Motor Disorders

Third Edition

Motor Disorders

Third Edition

Edited by

David S. Younger, M.D.

Clinical Associate Professor
Department of Neurology
New York University School of Medicine;
Attending Physician
Section of Neurology
Department of Medicine
Lenox Hill Hospital
New York, New York

Foreword by
Michael J. Aminoff, M.D.
Professor and Executive Vice Chair, Neurology
Past Editor, *Muscle & Nerve*
University of California, San Francisco
San Francisco, California

Marketed and distributed exclusively by the American Association of Neuromuscular and Electrodiagnostic Medicine-AANEM

Published by:

David S. Younger, MD, PC
david.younger@nyumc.org

ISBN: 978 0 615 70565-1

Design and composition by Dorie McClelland, springbookdesign.com.

Cover engraving from *Dictionnaire, Universal, D'Histoire Naturelle, Atlas*, by Charles D'Orbigny, Chez Les Èditeurs, L. Houssiaux Et C, Paris, 1861

Index by S.A. Fifer, sa.fifer.graffito@runbox.com.

Printed in Canada by Friesens.

Library of Congress Cataloging-in-Publication Data available upon request.

Care has been taken to confirm the accuracy of the information presented and to describe generally accepted practices. However, the authors, editors, and publisher are not responsible for errors or omissions or for any consequences from application of the information in this book and make no warranty, expressed or implied, with respect to the currency, completeness, or accuracy of the contents of the publication. Application of this information in a particular situation remains the professional responsibility of the practitioner. The authors, editors, and publisher have exerted every effort to ensure that drug selection and dosage set forth in this text are in accordance with current recommendations and practice at the time of publication. However, in view of ongoing research, changes in government regulations, and the constant flow of information relating to drug therapy and drug reactions, the reader is urged to check the package insert for each drug for any change in indications and dosage and for added warnings and precautions. This is particularly important when the recommended agent is a new or infrequently employed drug. Some drugs and medical devices presented in this publication have Food and Drug Administration (FDA) clearance for limited use in restricted research settings. It is the responsibility of health care providers to ascertain the FDA status of each drug or device planned for use in their clinical practice.

10 9 8 7 6 5 4 3 2 1

DEDICATION

I have had the good fortune to work alongside the contributors, all experts in their field, and exceptional in their dedication and willingness to collaborate on this edition. I am also privileged to have a supportive family, my spouse Holly and sons Adam and Seth, who allowed me the time to pursue this book.

Contents

III. SPINAL CORD DISEASES

IV. THE NEURONAL DEGENERATIONS

V. NEUROREHABILITATION

Contributing Authors

Pasquale Accardo, MD
Chief, Division of Developmental Pediatrics
Department of Pediatrics
Virginia Commonwealth University School of Medicine
Richmond, Virginia

Jung H. Ahn, MD
Medical Director, Neurological Rehabilitation
Department of Rehabilitation Medicine
New York University School of Medicine
New York University Langone Medical Center
New York, New York

Steven M. Albert, PhD
Department of Behavioral and Community Health Services
Graduate School of Public Health
University of Pittsburgh
Pittsburgh, Pennsylvania

Anthony A. Amato, MD
Vice-Chairman
Department of Neurology
Brigham and Women's Hospital
Harvard Medical School
Boston, Massachusetts

Stanley H. Appel, MD
Director, Methodist Neurological Institute
Director, MDA-ALS Research and Clinical Center
Chair, Department of Neurology
Methodist Neurological Institute
Weill Medical College of Cornell University
Houston, Texas

John R. Bach, MD
Vice-Chair, Departments of Physical Medicine and
Rehabilitation
Department of Physical Medicine and Rehabilitation
New Jersey Medical School
Newark, New Jersey

Richard J. Barohn, MD
Gertrude and Dewey Ziegler Chairman
Department of Neurology
Kansas University School of Medicine
Kansas City, Kansas

Jacqueline A. Bello, MD
Director, Division of Neuroradiology
Montefiore Medical Center
Department of Radiology
Albert Einstein College of Medicine
Bronx, New York

Andrew Blitzer, MD, DDS
New York Center for Voice and Swallowing Disorders
Head and Neck Surgical Group
St. Luke's/Roosevelt Hospital Center
New York, New York

Thomas H. Brannagan III, MD
Director, Peripheral Neuropathy Center
Neurological Institute
College of Physicians and Surgeons
Columbia University
New York New York

Mitchell F. Brin, MD
Senior Vice President, Development
Head, Therapeutic Area for Botox® and Neurology
Allergan Incorporated
Irvine, California

Mark B. Bromberg, MD, PhD
Professor of Neurology
Director, Neuromuscular Fellowship Program
Department of Neurology
University of Utah School of Medicine
Salt Lake City, Utah

Robert H. Brown Jr., MD, PhD
Professor and Chair
Department of Neurology
Director, Day Neuromuscular Research Laboratory
University of Massachusetts Medical School
Worcester, Massachusetts

Pedro Ciarlini, MD
Department of Pathology
Division of Neuropathology
Brigham and Women's Hospital
Harvard Medical School
Boston, Massachusetts

Marinos C. Dalakas, MD
Professor
Clinical Neuroscience
Neuromuscular Disease
Imperial College
London, United Kingdom;
Neuroimmunology Unit
University of Athens Medical School
Athens, Greece

Josep O. Dalmau, MD, PhD
IDIBAPS and Service of Neurology
Hospital Clinic
University of Barcelona
Barcelona, Spain

Mazen M. Dimachkie, MD
Director, Electromyography Laboratory and Neuromuscular
Diseases
Department of Neurology
University of Kansas Medical Center
Kansas City, Kansas

Salvatore DiMauro, MD
Lucy G. Moses Professor of Neurology
Director Emeritus, H. Houston Merritt Clinical Research
Center for Muscular Dystrophy and
Related Diseases
Associate Chair, Laboratory Research and Training
Department of Neurology
Neurological Institute
College of Physicians and Surgeons,
Columbia University
New York, New York

Michal E. Eisenberg, MD
Departments of Neurology and Rehabilitation
Hospital for Joint Diseases
New York University School of Medicine
New York, New York

Mark A. Ferrante, MD
Professor, Department of Neurology
Director, EMG Laboratory
University of Tennessee Health Science Center
Memphis, Tennessee

Joel Gutiérrez, MD, PhD
Research Director, Cuban Institute of Neurology
Cuba Institute of Neurology
Havana, Cuba

Steven J. Frucht, MD
Professor
Director, Movement Disorders
Department of Neurology
Robert and John M. Bendheim Parkinson and Movement
Disorders Center
Mount Sinai Medical Center
New York, New York

Umberto De Girolami, MD
Professor and Chief
Division of Neuropathology
Department of Pathology
Brigham and Women's Hospital
Harvard Medical School
Boston, Massachusetts

Tamara S. Greene, MD
General Neurologist
Neurology Specialists of Decatur
Decatur, GA

Robert C. Griggs, MD
Professor of Neurology
University of Rochester School of Medicine and Dentistry
Strong Memorial Hospital
Rochester, New York

Ehsan Hadi, MD
Division of Movement Disorders
Department of Neurology
Loma Linda University Medical Center
Loma Linda, California

Christina Hadzitheodoro, BA
Columbia School of General Studies
New York, New York

Asao Hirano, MD
The Harry M. Zimmerman Professor of Neuropathology
Department of Pathology
Albert Einstein College of Medicine
Montefiore Medical Center
Bronx, New York

Michio Hirano, MD
Professor of Neurology
Associate Director, Adult Muscular Dystrophy Association
Neuromuscular Clinic
Neurological Institute
College of Physicians and Surgeons
Columbia University
New York, New York

Laura Herbelin, BS
Department of Neurology
Neuromuscular Section
University of Kansas Medical Center
Kansas City, Kansas

Christopher W. Hess, MD
Movement Disorders Group and Clinical Motor Physiology
Laboratory
Department of Neurology
Columbia University
New York, New York

Paul P. Huang, MD
Chief of Neurosurgery
Bellevue Hospital
Site Director, New York Downtown Hospital
Department of Neurology and Neurosurgery
New York University School of Medicine
New York, New York

Brian Sun-Hoon Im, MD
Instructor
Department of Rehabilitation Medicine
New York University School of Medicine
New York, New York

Samay Jain, MD
Department of Neurology
Movement Disorders Division
University of Pittsburgh Medical Center
Pittsburgh, Pennsylvania

Burk Jubelt, MD
Professor of Neurology
State University of New York
Upstate Medical University College of Medicine
University Hospital
Syracuse, New York

Christian Krarup, MD, DMSc
Department of Clinical Neurophysiology
Copenhagen University
Rigshospitale
Copenhagen, Denmark

Hirofumi Kusaka, MD
Professor and Chair
Department of Neurology
Kansai Medical University
Kansai Medical University Hospital
Moriguchishi, Osaka, Japan

Norman Latov MD, PhD
Professor
Department of Neurology
Weill Cornell Medical College
New York, New York

Heather A. Lau, MD
Division of Neurogenetics
Department of Neurology
New York University School of Medicine
New York University Langone Medical Center
New York, New York

Yvonne W. Lui, MD
Section Chief, Neuroradiology
Department of Radiology
New York University School of Medicine
New York University Langone Medical Center
New York, New York

Thornton B. Alexander Mason II, MD, PhD
Department of Pediatrics and Neurology
Sleep Center
Perelman School of Medicine
University of Pennsylvania
Philadelphia, Pennsylvania

Nisha Mehta, MD
Department of Radiology
Division of Neuroradiology
New York University School of Medicine
New York University Langone Medical Center
New York, New York

Suraj A. Muley, MD
Director, Neuromuscular Institute
Barrow Neurological Institute
University of Arizona
Phoenix, Arizona

Jacob A. Neufeld, MD, MSPH
Medical Director, Pediatric Rehabilitation
Department of Children's Pediatric Rehabilitation
Children's Hospital and Research Center
Oakland, California

Mile Nikolic, PhD
Department of Clinical Neurophysiology
University of Copenhagen/Panum
Rigshospitalet
Copenhagen, Denmark

Gareth J. Parry, MD
Professor Emeritus, University of Minnesota Medical School
Department of Neurology
University of Minnesota Medical School
Minneapolis, Minnesota

Gregory M. Pastores, MD
Chief, Division of Neurogenetics
Department of Neurology
New York University School of Medicine
New York University Langone Medical Center
New York, New York

Paloma Gonzalez-Perez, MD
Day Neuromuscular Research Laboratory
University of Massachusetts Medical School
Worcester, Massachusetts

James M. Powers, MD
Professor of Pathology and Neurology
Department of Pathology and Laboratory Medicine
University of Rochester School of Medicine and Dentistry
Rochester, New York

Seth L. Pullman, MD
Professor
Department of Neurology
Director, Clinical Motor Physiology Laboratory
Neurological Institute
College of Physicians and Surgeons
Columbia University
New York, New York

Eytan Raz, MD
Department of Radiology
Division of Neuroradiology

New York University School of Medicine
New York University Langone Medical Center
New York, New York

John-Ross Rizzo, MD
Department of Rehabilitation Medicine
New York University School of Medicine
New York University Langone Medical Center
New York, New York

Ana-Marie Rojas, MD
Department of Rehabilitation Medicine
New York University School of Medicine
New York University Langone Medical Center
New York, New York

Gustavo C. Roman, MD
Department of Medicine
University of Texas Health Science Center
Audi L. Murphy Memorial Veterans Hospital
San Antonio, Texas

Michael Rose, MD
Consultant and Honorary Senior Lecturer in Neurology
Department of Neurology
King's College Hospital
London SE5 8AZ, United Kingdom

Myrna R. Rosenfeld, MD, PhD
IDIBAPS and Service of Neurology
Hospital Clinic
University of Barcelona
Barcelona, Spain

Barry Rodstein, MD, MPH
Chief, Physical Medicine and Rehabilitation Division
Medicine Department
Bay State Health
East Longmeadow, Massachusetts
Tufts University Medical School
Springfield, Massachusetts

Saud A. Sadiq, MD
Director, Multiple Sclerosis Research Center of New York
Multiple Sclerosis Research Center of New York
Albert Einstein College of Medicine of Yeshiva University
New York, New York

Keivan Shifteh, MD
Chief, Head and Neck Radiology
Division of Neuroradiology
Montefiore Medical Center
Albert Einstein College of Medicine
Bronx, New York

Laura E. Simionescu, MD
State University of New York

Upstate Medical University College of Medicine
University Hospital
Syracuse, New York

Stefano Simonetti, MD
Clinica Dermatologica
Azienda Ospedaliera di Perugia
Ospedale Santa Maria della Misericordia
Perugia, Italy

Ericka P. Simpson, MD
Director, ALS Clinical Research Division
Director, Neurology Residency Program
Co-Director, MDA-ALS Research and Clinical Center
Department of Neurology
Methodist Neurological Institute
Weill Cornell Medical College of Cornell University
Houston, Texas

Anuradha Singh, MD
Director, Bellevue Epilepsy Center
Bellevue Hospital Center
Department of Neurology
New York University School of Medicine
New York University Langone Medical Center
New York, New York

James W. Stark, MD
International Multiple Sclerosis Management Practice
New York, New York

Celia F. Stewart, PhD
Department of Communicative Sciences and Disorders
New York University School of Culture, Education and Human Development
New York, New York

David M. Swope, MD
Clinical Director, Movement Disorders
Director, Neurology Clinical Research Center
Loma Linda University Medical Center
Loma Linda, California

Jilda N. Vargus-Adams, MD, MSc
Division of Pediatric Rehabilitation
Department of Pediatrics and Physical Medicine and Rehabilitation
University of Cincinnati College of Medicine
Cincinnati Children's Hospital Medical Center
Cincinnati, Ohio

Jennifer Werely, MD
Department of Neurology
New York University School of Medicine
New York University Langone Medical Center
New York, New York

David S. Younger, MD
Clinical Associate Professor of Neurology
New York University School of Medicine
New York University Langone Medical Center
Attending Physician
Department of Medicine
Section of Neurology
Lenox Hill Hospital
New York, New York

Douglas W. Zochodne
Department of Clinical Neurosciences
Hotchkiss Brain Institute
University of Calgary
Calgary, Alberta, Canada

Preface to the Third Edition

Motor Disorders is twenty years old. The essence of the first edition was published in 1993 in the *Seminars in Neurology* as a two-part collection of articles, entitled "The differential diagnosis of progressive flaccid weakness," followed a month later by, "The differential diagnosis of progressive spastic paraparesis." Molded in content by Michael Brooke's monograph, *A Clinician's Guide to Neuromuscular Disorders*, the book entitled, *Motor Disorders* was organized instead into five sections with the goal of presenting concise, scholarly articles in the principal areas of motor disease. The second edition, which was expanded in depth and topic list, had the imprints of the emerging advances in neuromuscular and neurodegenerative molecular diagnosis, gene therapy, and neuro-rehabilitation. The book was welcomed by many colleagues, neurology residents, and medical students, although like the preceding editions, it had narrowly focused content. The original authors were gathered once again, along with new contributors, to produce the third edition of *Motor Disorders* with an even more challenging list of chapters. A return to the larger, more readable font of the first edition was accomplished by stringent editing and sorting through outdated reference citations.

I am pleased to convey my appreciation to Spring Book Design for their diligent page, figure, and table layouts, and indexing; and to a cadre of research assistants who assisted in typing, checking reference citations, and formatting manuscripts. It is hoped that this edition of *Motor Disorders*, like the ones before it, will benefit a generation of clinical professionals, well-versed in genetics, neurophysiology, and basic science and caring for patients, the suffering and resiliency of whom never ceases to inspire me.

Foreword

It is a privilege to introduce this book to its intended readership. Earlier editions have already received wide recognition and are deservedly familiar to many clinicians. In 1993, David Younger was the editor of two issues of Seminars in Neurology that focused on motor disorders, and he subsequently expanded these into the first edition of this book, published in 1999. A second, edition appeared in 2005. This new—third—edition cements and enhances the reputation gained by those earlier editions. The book continues to provide a detailed and practical account of motor disorders that will appeal to specialists as well as to general physicians and trainees while, at the same time, providing a convenient but thorough summary of advances in the field. The intent of the book is to bring together the entire spectrum of motor disorders and thereby aid in the evaluation, diagnosis, and distinction of these various disorders. In fact, it does far more than that, providing an account of any disorder with motor manifestations, and doing so through the perspective of many different subspecialties in order to provide a truly comprehensive but concise account of the subject matter.

Motor disorders are commonly seen in clinical practice, but their treatment is often limited and their management in many instances is unsatisfactory. Dramatic advances have occurred in the neurosciences since the last edition of this book was published, especially in genetics, immunology, neurophysiology, imaging, and pharmacology. These advances should have helped clinicians by suggesting new approaches to diagnosis and to patient care. In fact, they have not had as big an impact as might have been expected, in part because it is so difficult for practitioners to keep abreast of new developments in the field and appraise the accumulating literature and also because of the increasing tendency for subspecialization among physicians. The new edition of this book provides updates both of technological advances and of the fundamental basis of motor disorders, and translates these into clinical practice. It will therefore serve as a valuable resource for those wanting to learn more about these disorders and keep up with recent advances.

The editor, David S. Younger, is an associate professor of neurology at the New York University School of Medicine and an attending physician at its affiliated acute-care teaching hospital in Manhattan. He is a well-respected clinician, teacher, and clinical investigator who has authored studies on different aspects of neurological function, focusing mainly on the peripheral nervous system and neuromuscular function. His breadth of knowledge, as reflected by the fact that he authored or coauthored 33 of the chapters in this book, has made him a particularly skilled editor of the present volume. He has done an excellent job of determining the breadth and scope of the volume, ensuring a consistently high standard for all the chapters, and editing and melding them into a single comprehensive account. I congratulate him on his achievement. The individual authors—many of whom are internationally recognized experts—have critically appraised the latest developments in their field while also providing a thorough clinical account of various motor disorders.

The book has expanded since the last edition and now contains 71 chapters written by 70 authors and divided into five sections. Twelve of the chapters are new, and the remaining chapters have all been updated. The first section consists of 15 chapters dealing with various general topics such as correlative neuroanatomy, neuroimaging, the neurophysiology of motor control and the use of neurophysiological techniques for various diagnostic purposes, neuromuscular pathology, genetics, vestibular and laryngeal disorders. vasculitis, and various research aspects. This is followed by a large section on nerve and muscle diseases, another section on spinal cord diseases, a section on neuronal degenerations, and a final section on neurorehabilitation. The chapters are generally written clearly in an easy, flowing style, and are well illustrated, often supplemented by diagrams and tables. Many of the illustrations are in color. The book is attractively produced, has an easy-to read format, and contains bibliographies that are impressively up to date.

This new edition of *Motor Disorders* will become widely accepted as a standard work of reference. I welcome its publication, recommend it with enthusiasm, and congratulate Dr. Younger for producing such an outstanding volume.

Michael J. Aminoff, MD, DSc, FRCP

PART I

General Considerations

CHAPTER 1

Correlative Neuroanatomy

David S. Younger

Human motor function requires the coordinated function of the major components of the central nervous system (CNS), namely the spinal cord, medulla oblongata, pons, midbrain, cerebellum, diencephalon, and cerebral hemispheres. Injury to any of these structures due to stroke, tumor, infection, genetic defects, and other causes can lead to disturbances in speech, limb and truncal strength, coordination, balance, and body homeostasis. This chapter considers the development, normal structure, and correlative neuroanatomy of the CNS and its constituent elements. Aspects of this topic can be found in several classical (1–3) and current (4) sources.

EMBRYOLOGY

The spinal cord develops from the wall of the neural tube composed of a single layer of columnar ectodermal cells that divide rapidly from the central canal along three layers, from internal to external, including ependymal, mantle, and marginal. The ependymal layer is converted into the ependyma that lines the central canal with processes that pass outward to the periphery. The mantle portion develops into the future gray columns with differentiation from interconnected spongioblasts into syncytia of neuroglial cells. Germinal cells develop into neuroblasts and nerve cells defined by their shape and location in the grey substance. The marginal layer, devoid of nuclei, forms the supporting substance of white matter tracts. The sulcus limitans, which extends from the lateral wall of the neural tube to the midbrain, delimits the dorsal and ventral lamina with afferent fibers that synapse on cells derived from the former, and efferent connections arising from cells of the latter. The efferent fibers include somatic nerves that innervate striated muscles and autonomic or visceral nerves that originate from the upper part of the basal lamina to innervate smooth muscle, blood vessels, and glandular elements. Anterior spinal nerve roots derive from axons of neuroblasts in the ventral mantle layer while posterior roots develop from spinal ganglia cells that differentiate from neural crest. Spongioblast ganglia cells migrate with developing neurons along spinal nerves, becoming Schwann cell sheaths along the peripheral nerve axon processes to be later separated from each other by myelin. The posterior and anterior nerve roots join beyond the spinal ganglia to form spinal nerves which then divide into anterior, posterior, and visceral rami. The later rami transit sympathetic ganglia and parasympathetic nerve trunks to distribute to cervical, thoracic, abdominal, and pelvic viscera.

The brain develops from an expanded part of the anterior wall of the neural tube. Three flexures divide the developing brain into the forebrain or future cerebral hemisphere, midbrain or future mesencephalon, and hindbrain or future pons and medulla while the lateral wall of the developing brain, like that of the notochord or developing spinal cord below, is divided by sulcus limitans into dorsal and ventral lamina. The oculomotor nucleus is the most rostal group of somatic cells innervating striated muscles, as the hypothalamus is the most rostral end of autonomic cells. The cavity of the hindbrain develops into the fourth ventricle with the appearance of the cephalic flexure. The cerebellum appears from a thickening of the roof of the hindbrain, and the pons as a thickening of its floor and lateral wall, while thickening of the floor and lateral walls forms the medulla oblongata with the roof under the developing cerebellum. The development of the medulla and pons follows that of the spinal cord with dorsal and ventral lamina divided by the sulcus limitans, and the differentiation of ependymal, mantle and marginal cell layers. Fibers from ganglia of the neural crest are directed into the dorsal lamina as neuroblasts accumulate in the mantle layer while areas of the ventral lamina correspond to columns of future brainstem motor nuclei.

The cerebellum derives from areas of ectodermal thickening along the cephalic border of the fourth ventricle known as the rhombic lip, and attaches to the medulla, pons, and midbrain respectively, via three paired cerebellar peduncles, inferior, middle, and superior, that connect the cerebellum with the spinal cord, brain stem, and higher levels of the neuraxis. A series of five deep fissures developmentally, structurally, and functionally divide the cerebellum into its principal lobes and lobules. The posterolateral fissure separates the flocculonodular lobe, the phylogenetically oldest part, or archicerebellum, closely related to the vestibular system, from the body of the cerebellum, which in turn divides into anterior and posterior lobes by the second and deepest fissure to appear, the primary fissure. The anterior lobe, or paleocerebellum, lies rostral to the primary fissure and is most concerned with the regulation of extensor muscle tone. The cerebellar hemispheres, or neocerebellum, the largest and phylogenetically newest portion, contained between the primary and posterolateral fissures, is functionally divided into three sagittal zones of cortex, vermal, paravermal, and lateral, that relate to four masses of deep nuclei, from medial to lateral, namely fastigal, emboliform and globos, and dentate nuclei for the coordination of skilled voluntary movements.

The midbrain exists for a short time as a thin-walled cavity interposed between the forebrain in front, and the hind-brain behind, until the cerebral acqueduct is formed while its basal lamina increases in thickness to form the cerebral peduncles. Neuroblasts grouped in relation to the sides and floor of the cerebral acqueduct form the oculomotor and trochlear nuclei and nerves. The dorsal lamina forms the quadrigeminal plate that later develops into the inferior and superior tectum.

The forebrain shows the same constituents as the spinal cord and medulla, with separation into ventral and dorsal lamina. Before closure of the cranial neural tube, the two lateral diverticula corresponding to the optic vesicles appear with peripheral stalks and give rise to the retina and optic nerves. The anterior portion of the dorsal lamina of the cerebral hemispheres rapidly expands into large pouches, the cavities of which form rudiments of the lateral ventricles that communicate via the interventicular foramen while the lamina terminalis persists as a rudiment of the median forebrain wall that stretches from the interventricular foramen to the recess at the base of the optic stalk. The anterior portion of the forebrain, or telencephalon, becomes separated from the posterior portion, or diencephalons, while the

cavity of the latter develops into the third ventricle. Paired thalami develop from the dorsal lamina of the diencephalon and are subsequently hidden when the cerebral hemispheres grow backward over them. Eminences of the ventral lamina give rise to the paired lateral geniculate bodies, pineal body and posterior commissure. The ventral part of the wall of the diencephalon develops into the mammillary bodies and tuber cinereum of the hypothalamus, optic vesicles and chiasm. The adenohypophysis arises from a diverticulum of the ectodermal lining while the roof plate remains thin and invaginates to form the choroid plexus. The walls of the telencephalic cavities thicken to form the cerebral hemispheres, each differentiating into rhinencephalon, corpus striatum, and neopallium. The rhinencephalon forms the olfactory tract and bulb, anterior perforated substance, septum pellucidum, subcallosal, supracollosal, dentate gyris, fornix, hippocampus and uncus, which become continuous posteriorly with the anterior end of the temporal lobe. The primitive corpus striatum grows backward and downward to form the temporal lobe, caudate, putamen, and globus pallidus. The neopallium forms the remaining portions of the cerebral hemispheres, including the major commissures termed corpus callosum, fornix, and anterior commissure, which arise from the lamina terminalis and the septum pellucidum. The outer surface of the hemispheres develops major fissures, including the choroidal, hippocampal, calcarine, central sulcus, and Syvian fissure as well as the frontal, parietal, and temporal operculum that covers the insula. Neuroblasts from the ependymal and mantle layers migrate into the deep part of the outer marginal layer and develop into cells of the cerebral cortex, emerging as outgrowths of cells or corpora striata and thalami and, later, the fibers of the cortex into the underlying white matter substance in the course of myelination that begins about the time of birth and continues until puberty.

SPINAL CORD

The spinal cord can be considered as a series of superimposed segments, each relating to a specific peripheral myotome and dermatome through the attachment of paired spinal nerves that become oriented progressively more obliquely and downward from their initial adjacent position in embryogenesis as a consequence of the relative inequality in growth rates of the spinal cord and the vertebral column. Two enlargements, one cervical and the other lumbar, correspond to the nerves that innervate the arms and legs. Two fissures, one anterior and another posterior, divide the spinal cord into two symmetrical parts joined in the middle by anterior and posterior white matter commissures. The internal structure of the spinal cord reveals symmetrical anterior, lateral, and posterior columns of gray

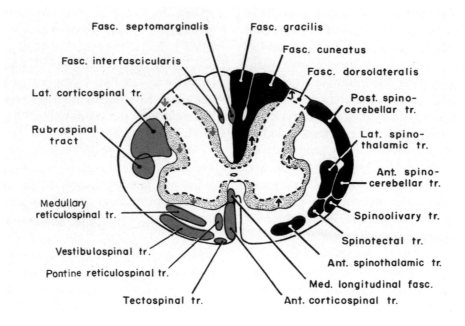

FIG. 1. Tracts of the spinal cord. Ascending tracts are shown in black and descending are shown in grey color. Reproduced from reference 3, with permission.

substance, the quantity of which varies on transverse section with the spinal level, namely small in the thoracic level and increased in the cervical and lumbar enlargements, joined in the middle around the central canal. The anterior columns contain somatic motor neurons separated from the cord surface by bundles of intramedullary nerve root fibers yet to emerge. The lateral gray column identified mainly in upper cervical, thoracic, and mid-sacral levels, corresponds to preganglionic cells of the autonomic nervous system. The posterior column corresponds to the central processes of corresponding dorsal roots separated from the cord surface by a thin layer of white matter termed the *tract of Lissauer*. Incoming fibers of the posterior column give rise to long fibers that divide in a T-shaped fashion, with some remaining in a single segment, others ascending or descending to adjoining segments, or traversing longer distances before synapsing at a distance.

Longitudinal fiber tracts of the spinal cord are broadly grouped into three bundles or fasciculi including anterior, lateral, and posterior (Figure 1), best appreciated in Weigert myelin stained preparations after lesion of the cell body of origin (Figure 2). Three fiber tracts of importance to motor function in the anterior fasciculus include the direct and indirect vestibulospinal fasciculi that derive from ipsilateral vestibular nuclei that descends to spinal levels for the modification of equilibratory and antigravity reflexes, and the medial longitudinal fasciculus (MLF) that interconnects the cervical cord, vestibular complex, and oculomotor nuclei for visual fixation. Four descending fiber tracts located in

the lateral fasciculus with additional motor importance include the lateral corticospinal, rubrospinal, reticulospinal and olivospinal tracts. The lateral corticospinal tract, also known as the final common pathway of voluntary motor function, extends throughout the entire length of the spinal cord interconnecting large pyramidal cells of motor cortex with concentric layers of anterior horn cells (AHC)

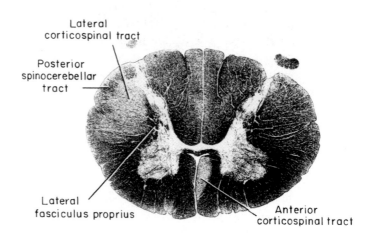

FIG. 2. Transverse section through the cervical enlargement of an individual with a medullary pyramid tract lesion. There is degeneration and demyelination of the crossed left lateral corticospinal tract and uncrossed anterior corticospinal tract after Weigert myelin staining. Reproduced from reference 3, with permission.

with those corresponding to the arm located most medially next to those to the trunk, and those to the legs more peripherally. The uncrossed rubrospinal, and crossed lateral reticulospinal tracts, both of questionable motor significance in humans, arise from the midbrain tegmentum and terminate upon AHC. The olivospinal tract arises from the inferior olivary nucleus and descends to cervical levels. Four fiber tracts ascend in the lateral fasciculus, including the dorsal and ventral spinocerebellar tracts, both relatively phylogenetically old and of questionable function and derived from lumbar levels, enters the cerebellum passing respectively through the inferior and superior peduncles. Two other tracts, the spinotectal and lateral spinothalamic tracts, derived from dorsal column cells, cross at spinal levels and, respectively, ascend to the midbrain and ventral nucleus of the thalamus. Two posterior fasciculi, cuneatus and gracilis, located medial to the posterior median septum, convey discriminatory joint position, vibration, and skin touch sensation derived from the central processes of ipsilateral posterior nerve roots that synapse in the posterior column, and separate from each other in cervical and upper thoracic levels to ascend to second order nuclei of the same name in the medulla.

The arterial organization of the spinal cord presents a simple intramedullary network associated with a highly variable complex extramedullary one. A single anterior spinal artery that extends downward along the ventral aspect of the cord ensures supply of the anterior two-thirds of the cord, while two posterior spinal arteries irrigate the dorsal three-fourths of the posterior columns. A perimedullary anastomotic system gives off a few branches to the periphery of the cord. An extramedually network is assured by cervicothoracic, middle thoracic, and thoracolumbar territories. The rostral territory, which extends from C1 to T4, is comprised of radicular arteries stemming from collaterals of the vertebral and subclavian arteries contributing to the anterior spinal artery, and dorsal radicular branches of the aorta contribute to the posterior spinal artery. A middle territory is supplied by anterior and posterior spinal arteries. A caudal territory is supplied from the single lumbar artery of Adamkiewicz.

The clinical symptomatology and classification of spinal cord injury depends upon the level of the lesion, the extent of damage in the transverse and longitudinal planes, whether the onset is sudden or gradual, and the nature of the insult. Acute spinal cord ischemia syndrome (ASCIS) (5–10) develops at any age, but frequently affects individuals in the fifth to seventh decades with infarction typically of the middle zone that is the most poorly vascularized in the territory of the anterior and posterior spinal arteries due to dependence of more or less single vessels. Atherosclerosis, arterial thombosis of feeding vessels or the aorta, dissection, aneurysm, cholesterol emboli, vasculitis, embolism, surgery, catheterization

procedures, sustained arterial hypotension, and spondylotic vertebral spurs that compress spinal arteries, and impaired blood supply to the cord contribute to the etiopathogenesis of ASCIS. Onset may be bilateral or unilateral due to radicular artery disease followed by central and transverse infarcts due to extensive spinal cord hypoperfusion and arteriopathy. The short-term outcome of ASCIS is favorable in up to two-thirds of patients.

The most serious spinal cord insult is *traumatic severance* of one or more segments, depending upon the type and extent of injury, leading to disorganization of the anatomical compartments at the level of injury, including incoming and outgoing anterior and posterior roots, descending and ascending long fiber tracts between peripheral end organs and supraspinal centers, and eventual replacement by dense fibrous scar tissue. Spinal cord *injury in continuity* is defined by the preservation of the outer shell of the cord, including meningeal coverings with disruption of the segmental anatomical organization and replacement by glial or fibrous tissue as in the case following crash injuries of the spine, transverse myelitis, or a vascular ischemic episode. *Physiological interruption* of the spinal cord results in a temporary loss of conductivity without permanent damage or alteration of the anatomical arrangement of the involved spinal cord segments as in concussion, manipulation of a dislocated vertebra, and inadvertent damage during a neurosurgical procedure. Regardless of the proximate cause, *acute complete spinal cord* injury in the transverse plane generally results in loss of voluntary movements of the skeletal muscles at and below the level of the lesion, which in thoracic and lumbar segments results in selective leg weakness or paraplegia, while involvement of cervical regions leads to quadriplegia. Whereas a lesion of descending corticospinal tract fibers classically results in upper motor neuron (UMN) signs of contralateral paralysis, hyperreflexia, Hoffman and Babinski signs, and ankle clonus, injury to AHC neurons and their peripherally running axons leads to lower motor neuron (LMN) signs of weakness, wasting, and fasciculation. Acute spinal cord injury incurs another pattern of motor and additional sensory signs. The muscles innervated by affected segmental levels in spinal cord injury leads to flaccid paralysis, of the LMN type, with loss of reflex activity, tone, and eventual atrophy unless some AHC escape destruction, whereas below the level of the lesion paralysis is first flaccid then spastic. Sensory disturbances in the immediate early, and later stages of complete transverse spinal cord lesions lead to acute interruption of superficial and deep sensibility, including touch, pressure, pain, temperature, position, and vibration as a result of loss of afferent conduction through the posterior columns, anterior and lateral spinothalamic tracts, and ventral and dorsal spinocerebellar tracts. The area of loss of pain perception is, as a rule, larger than that of touch sensitivity due to the overlapping nature of the latter, often with a border of hyperpathia above the lesion leading to band-like tightness, burning pain, and an unpleasant sensation with minor pressure or tactile encounter, termed *allodynia*. There can be unpleasant phantom limb sensations or mistaken perceptions such as the position of a limb in extension instead of flexion, and unpleasant burning pain in a paralyzed limb. Involvement of a particular spinal segment leads to clinically recognizable syndromes. For example, a traumatic lesion of C5 spinal cord segment due to fracture, dislocation, or compression along the respective vertebrae produces neck pain that intensifies with movement of the head and neck, combined with paresthesia along the respective cervical dermatome. There may be respiratory embarrassment due to diaphragm paralysis associated with spastic tetraplegia, focal sensory, and motor loss in the C5 dermatome and myotomes leading to LMN biceps, deltoids, biceps, brachialis, brachioradialis, and supinator weakness, with partial denervation in levator scapulae, rhomboids, supraspinatus, and infraspinatus due to contributing C4 root innervation, and overt sparing of the trapezoid and sternocleidomastoid due to their higher level of innervation. With time, diaphragmatic function resumes as a result of phrenic nerve reinnervation.

Lower spinal cord injury, particularly of the conus, leads to bladder, bowel, and sexual disturbances, loss of postural control due to impairment in sensation around the hips with progressive loss of the upright posture as the level of injury is higher in the cord. Bladder retention results from flaccid destrusor muscle paralysis with loss of volitional and reflex bladder function. However, the bladder wall is not completely atonic due to autonomous intramural innervation and inherent elasticity of the wall. When the resistance of the external urethral sphincter exceeds intravesicular pressure there can be partial bladder emptying due to overflow incontinence. In later stages of spinal injury and recovery, two types of bladder function occur, *automatic* and *autonomous*, depending upon whether the spinal lesion occurs respectively, above or at the level of the thoracolumbar junction affecting the bladder center in the lumbosacral segment of the cord. An automatic bladder displays a heightened detrusor reflex response to bladder distension whereas the autonomous bladder is often incapable of provoking appropriate emptying bladder-wall contractions. Long-term reconditioning of bladder function depends upon developing reflex micturition at regular intervals to avoid incontinence. Analogous disturbances in bowel function as a result of spinal cord injury leads to paralyzed peristalsis with impaired bowel sounds, fecal retention, and impaction due to loss of the integrity of the spinal center in the lumbosacral cord of motor and sensory impulses that govern the coordinated action of defecation in the first stage of cord or cauda equine lesions followed by the development

of autonomic reflex activity or autonomous defecation, and intestinal reconditioning. Sexual function, like bladder and bowel function, also depends upon the coordinated motor action. In the initial phase of spinal injury there is loss of erection and ejaculation in the male, and loss of orgasm during intercourse following penile penetration in the female. In the later stage of complete spinal injury, there is an automatic erection reflex to tactile stimulation and reflex contraction of the muscles of ejaculation potentially strong enough to elicit contraction of the seminal vesicles, prostate gland, and passage of seminal fluid through the urethra. It is possible for a paraplegic woman to become impregnated and deliver a normal baby, although the final stages of labor in such cases may be greatly diminished.

Incomplete lesions of the spinal cord demonstrate greater variation depending upon the etiology, level of the lesion, and the degree of damage to neural elements that may be either diffuse or circumscribed, affecting distinct portions of the cord resulting in dissociated syndromes. Segmental LMN paralysis combined with spasticity, dissociated analgesia, and temperature sensory loss occurs with combined lesions of the anterior horn, corticospinal, and anterolateral spinothalamic tracts as a result of fracture dislocation of the spine, anterior spinal artery occlusion, and epidural spinal cord compression by tumor. Spastic ataxia occurs with combined lesions of the posterior columns and lateral corticospinal tract as a result of posterior spinal artery insufficiency, traumatic and compressive lesions of the spinal cord, as well as subacute combined degeneration associated with B12 deficiency, and type 1 spinocerebellar degeneration, also known as Friedrich ataxia. The central syndrome of syringomyelia presents with dissociated touch, analgesia, and temperature sensation in a cape-like distribution, weakness and wasting of small hand muscles, and tendon reflex loss due to expansion of the cavity in the transverse plane, and sensory disturbance in the face or over the greater part of the body and legs with expansion in either direction of the vertical plane, due to disruption of crossing posterior root and spinothalamic fibers. Hemisection of the spinal cord (11) presents with ipsilateral LMN paralysis and band-like analgesia and temperature sensory loss and hypo- or anhidrosis at the level of the lesion. The upper extent of contralateral pain and temperature sensory loss is situated a few segments below the level of the lesion due to involvement of spinothalamic fibers that enter the cord but do not cross for a few segments.

MEDULLA

The medulla extends from the spinal cord to the lower end of the pons. Four cranial nerves emerge from the medulla, including the hypoglossal, accessory, vagus, and glossopharyngeal. The internal structure changes rapidly above the

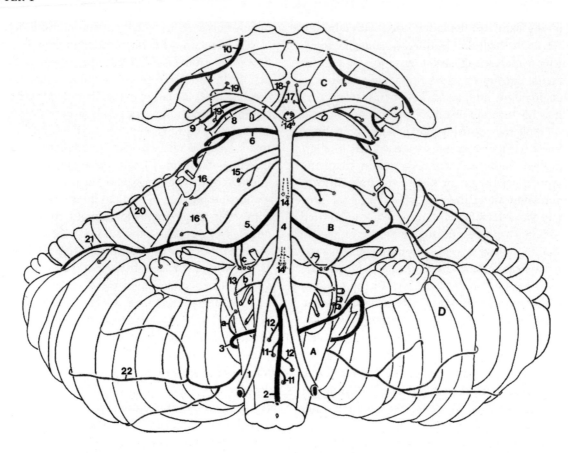

1. Vertebral artery
2. Anterior spinal artery
3. Posterior inferior cerebellar artery
4. Basilar artery
5. Anterior inferior cerebellar artery
6. Superior cerebellar artery
7. Posterior cerebral artery
8. Collicular artery
9. Posteromedial choroidal artery
10. Anterior choroidal artery
11. Anteromedial group of medullary arteries
12. Anterolateral group of medullary arteries
13. Lateral group of medullary arteries
    (a. inferior rami arising from the posterior inferior cerebellar artery; b. middle rami arising from the vertebral artery; c. superior rami arising from the anterior inferior cerebellar artery)

14. Anteromedial group of pontine arteries penetrating the basilar sulcus (14′ arteries penetrating the foramen coecum; 14″ arteries penetrating the interpeduncular fossa, inferior rami of the interpeduncular fossa)
15. Anterolateral group of pontine arteries
16. Lateral group of pontine arteries
17. Anteromedial group of mesencephalic arteries (middle rami of the interpeduncular fossa)
18. Anterolateral group of mesencephalic arteries (superior rami of the interpeduncular fossa)
19. Lateral group of mesencephalic arteries
20. Branches of the superior cerebellar artery
21. Branches of the anterior inferior cerebellar artery
22. Branches of the posterior inferior cerebellar artery

FIG. 3. Anterior view of the general arrangement of the brainstem and cerebellar arteries. Medulla **(A)**, Pons **(B)**, Midbrain **(C)**, and Cerebellum **(D)**. Reproduced from, Tatu L, Vuiller F. Moulin T. Anatomy of the circulation of the brain and spinal cord. *Handb of Clin Neurol 2009*; 92:247–281, with permission.

spinal cord. The corticospinal tracts decussate, producing changes in their position from lateral to ventral. The fasciculi cuneatus and gracilis end in relay nuclei from which internal arcuate fibers sweep ventrally and decussate to lie in the medial lemnisci of either side. The inferior olivary nuclei on either side of the midline give rise to olivocerebellar fibers that decussate in the raphe and enter the inferior cerebellar peduncle. The ventral spinothalamic tract joins the lateral tract of the same name, and the dorsal spinocerebellar tract leaves the medulla to enter the inferior cerebellar penducle. With spreading apart of the embryonic neural tube, the hypoglossus nucleus situates near the midline, adjacent to the nucleus ambiguous and motor nucleus of the glossopharyngeal, to innervate laryngeal, pharyngeal, and masticatory muscles. The cranial portion of the accessory nerve that innervates muscles of the larynx, and the motor nucleus of the vagus nerve that gives rise to preganglionic parasympathetic fibers to innervate smooth muscles

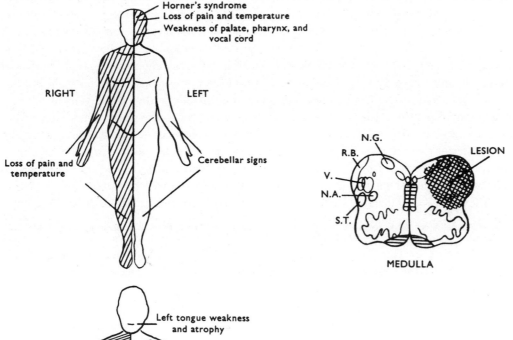

FIG. 4. Lateral medullary syndrome. Infarcted area of the left dorsolateral medulla produces signs demonstrated on the left side of the figure. NG: nucleus gracilis; RB: inferior cerebellar peduncle; V: descending root and tract of the trigeminal nucleus; NA: nucleus ambiguous; ST: lateral spinothalamic tract. Reproduced from reference 2, with permission.

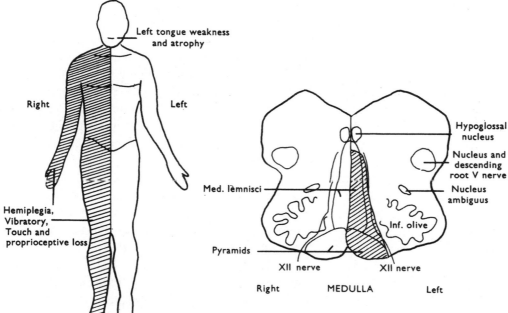

FIG. 5. Medial medullary syndrome. Infarcted area of the left medial medulla produces signs demonstrated in the left side of the figure. Reproduced from reference 2, with permission.

and the heart, are all located dorsolaterally. The trigeminal nucleus is surrounded by the spinal trigeminal tract and the nucleus of the solitary tract, which lies ventrolaterally to the dorsal motor nucleus of the vagus and receives visceral afferent fibers for taste from the facial and glossopharyngeal nerve. The sensory nucleus of the vagus nerve, like the solitary tract, receives visceral afferent fibers from vagus and glossopharyngeal nerves. The cochlear and vestibular nuclei lay posterolaterally giving rise, respectively, to the lateral lemniscus tract and central vestibular connections concerned with hearing and equilibrium. The vascular supply of the medulla can be divided into anteromedial, anterolateral, lateral, and posterior territories (12). Anteromedial and anterolateral vessels arise from the vertebral artery, and anterior spinal artery rami supply the medial

medulla. The lateral vessels arise from the vertebral artery, posterior inferior cerebellar (PICA), anterior inferior cerebellar (AICA), and basilar arteries and supply the lateral medulla. The posterior vasculature of the lower medulla arises from the posterior spinal artery, while upper medulla vasculature derives from the PICA. The vascular supply of the brainstem and cerebellum is shown in Figure 3.

For practical purposes there are two medullary syndromes, a medial and lateral, that is most often due to vascular occlusion or embolism resulting in infarction however, other disease processes, including primary and metastatic tumor, hemorrhage, and infection can lead to medullary brainstem injury. The lateral medullary syndrome (Figure 4) (13) results from occlusion of the vertebral artery or PICA. Clinical manifestations include ipsilateral Horner syndrome of ipsilateral ptosis, meiosis, endophthalmos, and loss of facial sweating; ipsilateral limb ataxia, facial pain, temperate and light touch sensory loss, dysarthria, dysphagia, dysphonia, contralateral sensory loss and vertigo, resulting respectively, from interruption of sympathetic fibers, spinocerebellar tract, descending trigeminal tract, nucleus ambiguous, crossed spinothalamic tract, and vestibular nucleus or its connections. The less often encountered medial medullary syndrome (14) presents with ipsilateral lingual weakness and atrophy, and contralateral spastic hemiplegia and posterior column sensory loss due to involvement of the hypoglossus nucleus and exiting fibers (Figure 5) and yet decussated ipsilateral medial lemnicus and corticospinal tracts, while pain and temperature sensation are unaffected. Bilateral median medullary infarction that presents with tetraplegia, bilateral lingual weakness and wasting, and posterior column sensory loss, is less often encountered due to bilateral origin of the anterior spinal artery.

PONS

The pons is separated from the medulla by a furrow in which the abducens, facial, and vestibulocochlear nerves appear. The ventral pons contains transverse corticobulbar fiber bundles that course laterally to enter the middle cerebellar peduncle, while three groups of longitudinal fasciculi enter the pons through the cerebral peduncles. Corticopinal tract fibers enter the middle third of the cerebral peduncle and continue caudally as the pyramidal tract. Aberrant corticobulbar fibers enter the pons through the medial margin of the peduncle and turn dorsally, ending upon cranial motor nuclei. Frontopontine and parietotemporopontine fiber bundles, situated in the lateral one-third of the cerebral peduncle, terminate on pontine nuclei and cross to the opposite side to ascend through the middle cerebellar peduncle to the cerebellar cortex, ending as mossy fibers. Three motor nuclei reside in the pons, including the nucleus of the abducens nerve, which is situated close to the floor of the ventricle, the nucleus of the facial nerve, which lies in the ventrolateral column of motor nuclei and sends its roots through the substance of the pons in proximity to the abducens, and the nucleus of the trigeminal nerve, which is the most rostral of the ventrolateral motor pontine nuclei that forms the motor root of the trigeminal nerve. There are six sensory nuclei in the pons, including the main sensory nucleus of the trigeminal nerve situated lateral to the motor nucleus that receives ascending trigeminal afferent fibers, and the nucleus of the descending trigeminal tract, which sends ascending fibers across the midline to the thalamus, subserving the same function for the head as the posterior columns and spinothalamic fibers do for the body. The superior, medial, lateral, and inferior vestibular nuclei are situated in the lateral floor of the fourth ventricle, while

the dorsal and ventral cochlear nuclei reside on the dorsolateral surface of the inferior cerebellar peducle. Vestibular fibers pass caudally into the direct vestibulospinal tract and connect with secondary vestibular centers. Crossing acoustic fibers from cochlear nuclei enter the trapezoid body and ascend in the lateral lemniscus rostrally to relay in the inferior colliculus and more rostrally in the medial geniculate body. The arterial vascular supply to the pons includes anteromedial and anterolateral groups of vessels that arise from the basilar artery, a lateral group that arises from the AICA and basilar termed *lateral pontine arteries*, and a posterior group that arises from the superior cerebellar artery.

Modern appreciation of brainstem vascular syndromes was initially fostered by recognition of basilar artery occlusion (15), vascularization of brainstem penetrating basilar branch occlusions (16–18), and the consequences of vertebral stenosis in the neck (19), leading to expected territories of possible infarction (Figure 6). A ventrocaudal pontine syndrome (20), now known to be most commonly caused by occlusion of circumferential branches of the basilar artery, presents with strabismus, diplopia, and lateral abduction palsy of the ipsilateral eye due to interruption of abducens fibers and nucleus of the facial nerve, contralateral hemiparesis due to interruption of corticospinal tract fibers, and contralateral decrease in temperature and pain sensation due to lesion in the lateral spinothalamic tract. Middle and rostal ventral pontine lesions lead to contralateral hemiparesis, and bilateral lesions lead to paraparesis due to interruption of basis pontine fibers. The addition of ipsilateral conjugate gaze paralysis, cerebellar incoordination, ipsilateral facial and crossed sensory loss of the limb and trunk resulting respectively, from disruption of supranuclear abducens, inferior cerebellar peduncle, spinal trigeminal root, and medial lemniscal tract projections describes the ventral tegmental syndrome (21) due to occlusion of circumferential branches of the basilar artery. A rostal tegmental pontine syndrome (22) gives rise to paralysis of ilpsilateral conjugate gaze, contralateral pain, temperature, and touch sensory loss, ipsilateral cerebellar incoordination, and rubral tremor owing to disruption, respectively, of supranuclear oculomotor pathways, spinothalamic and medial lemniscal tracts, and superior cerebellar peduncle fibers. A middle tegmental pontine syndrome, most often due to occlusion of short circumferential and paramedian perforating branches of the basilar artery gives rise to ipsilateral facial pain and temperature anesthesia, cerebellar incoordination, and masticatory muscle paralysis, with contralateral hemibody pain, temperature, and touch sensory anesthesia respectively, due to disruption of the sensory nucleus of the trigeminal nerve, spinothalamic tract, superior cerebellar peduncle, motor nucleus of the trigeminal nerve, and medial lemniscus. A caudal pontine tegmentum syndrome (23) caused by occlusion of short circumferential

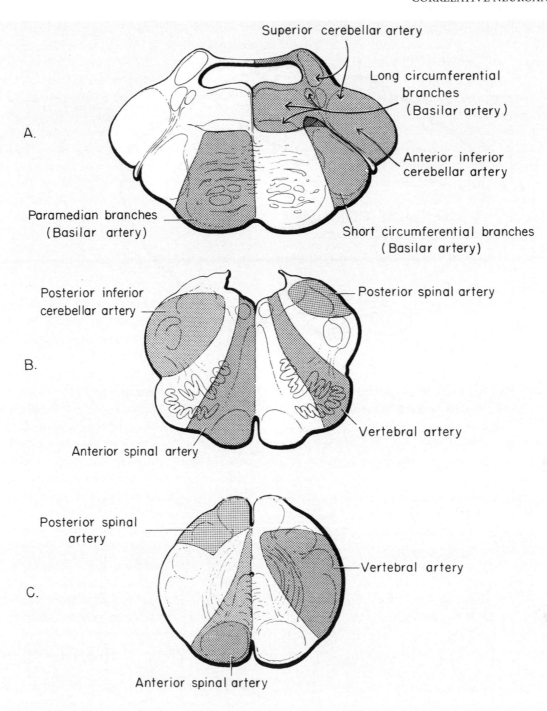

FIG. 6. Diagram of the arterial supply of the medulla and pons. **(A)** Pons, **(B)** Medulla, **(C)** upper cervicomedullary level. Reproduced from reference 3, with permission.

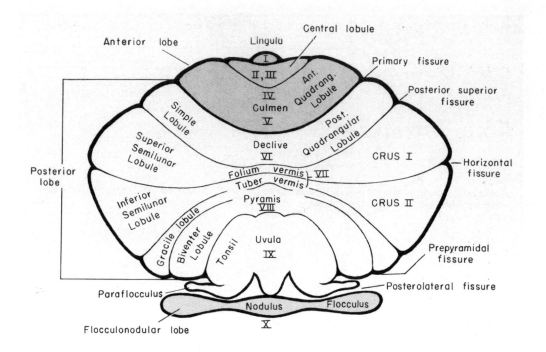

FIG. 7. Schematic diagram of the fissures and lobules of the cerebellum. Reproduced from reference 3, with permission.

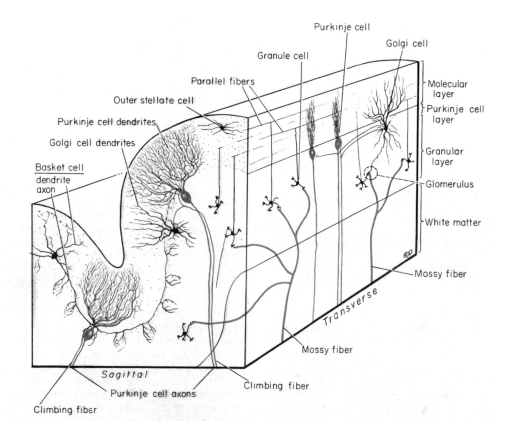

FIG. 8. Schematic diagram of a cerebellar folium in sagittal and transverse planes showing cellular layers and fiber arrangements. Reproduced from reference 3, with permission.

branches of the basilar artery or AICA disrupts supranuclear and nuclear abducens and facial fibers, spinothalamic tract, medial lemniscus, spinal trigeminal root, and inferior cerebellar peduncle tracts, leading to ipsilateral paralysis of conjugate gaze toward the side of the lesion, abducens and facial paralysis, ipsilateral cerebellar incoordination, contralateral hemiparesis, and touch, pain, and temperature sensory loss. Midpontine basilar syndromes are most often due to occlusion of short circumferential and paramedian perforating basilar branches that disrupt trigeminal nerve, pontine nuclei, and corticospinal tract projections leading to ipsilateral paralysis of mastication, decrease in facial sensory modalities, ipsilateral ataxia, and contralateral hemiparesis. Large unilateral basilar pontine infarction lead to pure motor hemiparesis involving the face, arm, and leg, and UMN signs of the opposite limbs, suggesting extension to the opposite side, while topographically smaller ischemic lesions placed in median, dorsomedian, and paramedian locations lead to clumsy hand-dysarthria, dysmetria-dysarthria, and facial paresis-dysarthria syndrome. Lateral pontine lesions (24) give rise to ipsilateral cerebellar incoordination and facial anesthesia, contralateral hemiparesis, pain and temperature anesthesia owing respectively, to disruption of the middle cerebellar peduncle, root of the trigeminal nerve, spinothalamic and trigeminal tracts.

CEREBELLUM

The fully developed cerebellum is divided into the three phylogenetic portions, archicerebellum in the floculonodular lobe, paleocerebellum rostral to the primary fissure, and neocerebellum between the primary and posterolateral fissures extending to the midline (Figure 7). Three well-defined layers, molecular, Purkinje, and granular, and cell types are found in each grey-white folia (Figure 8). An outer molecular layer comprises small external stellate cells and inner basket cells, dendritic arborizations of Golgi and Purkinje cells, and parallel oriented axons of granule cells that form synaptic connections with Purkinje cell dendrites that have a cell body at the junction of the molecular and nuclear layer below. Granule cells give rise to dendrites that end in glomeruli, and unmyelinated fibers that ascend vertically to the molecular cell layer above, coursing parallel to the long axis of a folium, resembling telegraph wires that make synaptic contact with the spiny processes of Purkinje cells. The dentrites of Golgi type II cells found in the upper granular layer extend throughout all layers of the cortex in contact with parallel fibers of the molecular layer, and in glomeruli of the granular layer. Impulses conveyed to dendrites in the molecular layer by parallel fibers result in excitation of a narrow band of Purkinje cells in the longitudinal axis of the folia, flanked on either side by Purkinje cells inhibited

by excited basket, Golgi, and stellate cells. Axons of Purkinje cells and their collaterals that represent the efferent cerebellar cortical pathways make synaptic contact with Golgi cells in the granular cell layer below to release the inhibitory neurotransmitter γ-amino-butyric acid (GABA), which in turn inhibits granule cells, the disinhibition of which allows further excitation of Purkinje cells. Projections from sensorimotor cortex end somatotopically upon longitudinally oriented pontine nuclei that crosses in the middle cerebellar peduncle and terminate as mossy fibers, while the inferior cerebellar peduncle consists of ipsilateral afferent and efferent fibers that relay primary and secondary vestibulocerebellar projections reciprocally from the floculonodular lobule and fastigal nuclei as climbing fibers. All parts of the cerebellar cortex project upon the deep cerebellar nuclei forming three sagittal organized zones of longitudinally oriented strips of cortex to which Purkinje cells project, including a medial or vermal zone to the fastigal nucleus, a paravermal zone to paired emboliform and globose nuclei, and a lateral or hemispheric zone to paired dentate nuclei. Although Purkinje cells exert inhibitory influences upon deep cerebellar nuclei, these neurons maintain high-frequency excitatory discharge, implying that unless spontaneously active, they must receive excitatory inputs from extracerebellar sources sufficient to overcome the tonic inhibitory output from the cerebellar cortex. The superior cerebellar peduncle is the largest efferent bundle formed by fibers arising from deep cerebellar nuclei that projects to the contralateral red nucleus, and from there is relayed to localized areas of ventrolateral and posterolateral thalamic nuclei and motor cortex. Impulses from dentate nuclei influence motor cell activity in the cerebral cortex while the latter exerts influence upon lower spinal levels. Cerebellar mechanisms assure the smooth and orderly sequence of agonist and antagonist muscle contraction that characterizes skilled voluntary movement and the maintenance of equilibrium and posture through the processing of afferent stretch receptor input from spinocerebellar and cuneocerebellar tracts.

Cerebellar arterial supply depends upon three long arteries, PICA, AICA, and superior cerebellar artery (SCA) (25). The PICA typically originates from the vertebral artery and gives off medial and lateral branches to the inferior vermis and the inferior and posterior surfaces of the cerebellar hemispheres. The AICA usually arises from the bottom third of the basilar artery and rarely, the posterior cerebral artery (PCA), and supplies the anterior surface of cerebellar lobules, floculus, and middle cerebellar peduncle, and gives rise to the internal auditory artery. The AICA supplies the middle cerebellar peduncle and the lower part of the pontine tegmentum. The SCA arises from the top of the basilar artery and divides into medial and lateral branches to supply the superior half of the cerebellar hemispheres and vermis, as well as the dentate nuclei; however, these two branches sometimes arise independently from the basilar artery. Long cerebellar arteries give rise to pial vessels, although few in number, at the cerebellar surface to form vascular lamina without anastomosis. Short, middle, and long intracortical vessels contribute to the three vascular layers within the cerebellar cortex, superficial, middle, and deep layers with the first situated within the molecular layer, the middle within the Purkinje cell layer, and the deep within the granular layer. Arteries parallel to the cerebellar surface, so-called parallel arteries, are in close relation to the Purkinje cells and their likely nutritional source (26).

Cerebellar disorders can be generally recognized by the presence of inaccurate and incoordinated limb movements, action tremor, oculomotor and speech disturbances, broad-based ataxic gait, pendulous reflexes, and subtle cognitive and behavioral changes. The pattern of connections within folia with uncrossed or crossed and recrossed circuitry explains the ipsilateral nature of most deficits. Despite the uniform cytoarchitecture, cerebellar circuitry produces characteristic disturbances attributed to one of the three forementioned sagittal zones (27). A midline cerebellar syndrome arises from cerebellar tumors such as a medulloblastoma leading to disequilibrium, often without limb ataxia due to disruption of vestibulocerebellar connections. The head may be rotated to the opposite side of the lesion with spontaneous nystagmus and a fast component toward the side of the lesion that worsens with gazing in that direction. Neocerebellar lesions that occur with stroke, tumor, and multiple sclerosis (MS) typically involve one hemisphere and its projections to the ipsilateral dentate nucleus. This results in ipsilateral hypotonia, action tremor, and loss of check during forceful contractions due to lack of engagement of antagonist muscles, and imbalance of stance and gait accompanied by a tendency to fall to the side of the lesion due to defective control of the affected leg, with loss of associated movements such as swinging of the arms. Decomposition of movements leads to dysmetria in finger-to-nose and heel-to-knee tests of accurary, and dysdiadichokinesis manifested as abnormal rapid alternating and successive movements. There can be disturbances in speech articulation, respiration, and phonation that convey an explosive, hesitant, and slow scanning quality.

Ischemic stroke in the territories of the PICA, AICA, and SCA territories leads to other expected syndromes (28–30). Those in the PICA are most often related to occlusion of the intracranial part of the vertebral artery due to cardiogenic or artery-to-artery embolism that affects both the brainstem and cerebellum. A medial pattern of PICA infarction involves the dorsal base and ventral apex of the cerebellum and the dorsolateral medulla leading to one of three syndromes, one with pseudolabyrinthine signs with or without concomitant dysmetria, ataxia, and lateropulsion, a partial or complete laterally medullary syndrome, and one that is clinically silent. A lateral PICA territory infarct that involves the anterolateral caudal cerebellar hemisphere is most often due to atherosclerosis of the vertebral artery and presents with unsteadiness, gait ataxia, dysdiadochokinesia, and ipsilateral body sway; rarely, there may be acute isolated vertigo. An AICA territory infarct results from atherosclerotic occlusion of the caudal basilar artery and presents with ipsilateral trigeminal sensory loss, facial palsy, hearing loss, Horner syndrome, limb dysmetria, contralateral pain and temperature sensory loss. An infarct in the territory of the SCA, generally caused by cardioembolism, may be seen in association with basilar artery occlusion, and presents with ipsilateral dysmetria, Horner syndrome, contralateral abducens nerve palsy, contralateral pain and temperature sensory loss. An SCA territory infarct presents with headache, gait ataxia, and vomiting. Eye movement disturbances are often encountered in cerebellar infarcts, including multidirectional nystagmus, upbeat nystagmus in primary gaze, and contrapulsion of saccades in SCA territory infarcts, and horizontal nystagmus, contralateral rebound nystagmus, and visual tilt illusions in PICA territory infarcts.

MIDBRAIN

The midbrain is divided into three parts, the tectum or corpora quadrigemina, the tegmentum that continues rostrally from the pons, and the crus cerebri or cerebral peduncles of descending corticofugal fibers. In the transition from lower brainstem levels, the fourth ventricle is replaced by the cerebral aqueduct. The superior medullary velum is replaced by the corpora quadrigemina, which is arranged in superior and inferior pairs. The superior brachium continues into the lateral geniculate body that carries fibers from the optic tract and the occipital cortex to the superior colliculus. The inferior brachia carry fibers from the lateral lemnisci and inferior colliculi to the medial geniculate bodies. The cerebral peduncles, located on the lower surface separated by the interpeduncular fossa just below the substantia nigra, have two major components, a cell rich compact, and reticular zone. The ventral surface of each peduncle is crossed from medial to lateral by the superior cerebellar and posterior cerebral arteries. Each peduncle consists of longitudinally oriented efferent fibers classically grouped into three areas from medial to lateral, fronto-pontine, corticospinal, and temporo-pontine fibers. Seven white matter tracts pass through the midbrain, including the lateral lemniscus tract that passes through the midbrain to terminate in the inferior colliculi; the spinotectal tract that terminates in the superior colliculi; the tectospinal tract that arises from the superior colliculi and projects to the oculomotor nucleus and MLF to coordinate horizontal eye movements; and the medial lemniscus, which together with the trigeminal lemniscus from the trigeminal main sensory nucleus and the ventral and lateral spinothalamic tracts, all continue to the ventral tier thalamic relay nuclei. The rubrospinal tract arises from the red nucleus and decussates in the ventral tegmentum of the midbrain to the spinal cord.

Five nuclei are situated in the midbrain, namely the oculomotor and trochlear that occupy dorsal and midline positions and innervate eye muscles; the Edinger-Westphal nucleus that gives rise to uncrossed pre-ganglionic parasympathetic fibers that emerges with somatic root fibers of the oculomotor nerve and projects to the ciliary ganglion and along post-ganglionic fibers to the pupilloconstrictor muscle; the nucleus of the mesencephalic root of the trigeminal nerve that subserves proprioceptive function for muscles of mastication; and the red nucleus that receives contralateral projections from the superior cerebellar peduncles, globus pallidus, and frontal lobe of the cortex and projects ipsilaterally to the corpora quadrigemini and ventral lateral (VL) nuclei of the thalamus. The paired inferior colliculi relay projections to the medial geniculate body, which in turn project upon the auditory cortex. Cells of the inferior colliculus encode sound localization tonotopically with spatiotemporal discharge patterns. The superior colliculi differ in organization that more closely resembles cerebral cortex with four layers, zonale, outer gray, superficial white, and stratum middle and deep gray and white. It receives projections from the retina via the optic tract, the cerebral cortex, inferior colliculus, and spinal cord. Superficial layers receive most of the input from the retina and visual cortex for the detection of movement in the visual field, with deeper layers arriving from other sources. Crossed retinotectal fibers leave the optic tract rostral to the lateral geniculate to project to the superior colliculus from homonymous retinal portions of each eye. Corticotectal fibers from frontal, temporal, parietal, and occipital cortex enter the stratum opticum and pass into superficial and middle gray layers. Brainstem afferents arise from the inferior colliculus and auditory relay nuclei, and those from spinal projections arise from nucleus cuneatus, lateral cervical, and spinal trigeminal nucleus.

The MLF is a central component of the visual motor system that interconnects oculomotor and abducens nuclei with other components of the brain. Efferent tectothalamic fibers arising from superficial superior collicular layers project ipsilaterally to the dorsal and ventral lateral geniculate body, pretectum, and pulvinar nucleus, the latter of which, in turn, projects to Brodmann areas 18 and 19 of visual cortex. In animals, unilateral lesions of the superior colliculus results in contralateral visual field neglect, loss of spatial discrimination, and impaired tracking behavior. Stimulation of the superior colliculus, by contrast leads to contralateral conjugate deviation of the eyes, suggesting a specialized function in head and eye movements to localize and follow visual stimuli. The neural pathways for ocular movements is augmented by the MLF which conducts axons from the pontine center for lateral conjugated eye movements to the homolateral abducens and through decussation to the contralateral oculomotor to innervate the medial rectus. Supranuclear control of voluntary eye movements includes projections from the frontal cortex and occipital related to visual fixation that descend via the internal capsule and decussate caudal to the oculomotor nucleus to synapse in the region of the contralateral abducns nucleus. Vestibular connections to the MLF contribute to vestibular nystagmus with slow and rapid components due to the presence of two distinct kinds of vestibular elements, phasic or canal, and tonus elements in the brainstem that are connected peripherally to the canal organs and centrally to the eye muscles that evoke nystagmus in relation to canal stimulation. A unilateral lesion of either vestibular element evokes spontaneous nystagmus due to the unopposed action of the opposite side, leading to directional change. One last important nuclear group is the substantial nigra, which also presents two divisions, a pars compacta region that possesses high concentrations of dopamine and is the principal source of striatal dopamine, while the enzyme glutamic acid decarboxylase (GAD), utilized in the synthesis of GABA, and serotonin (5-HT) are found in high concentration in the pars reticulata. Afferent substantia nigra fibers arise from the caudate and putamen, both segments of the globus pallidus, the pedunculopontine, and dorsal nucleus of the raphe, while efferent connections arise principally from pars compacta project to all portions of the caudate and putamen, forming a closed feedback loop. Nigrothalamic fibers arising from pars reticulata project to the ventral anterior, ventral lateral, and dorsomedial thalamic nuclei, and contribute to pallidothalamic projections, which collectively constitute the major output system of the corpus striatum.

Eye movement disturbances typically occur in association with midbrain lesions. Three midbrain syndromes, including upper, middle and lower, can be differentiated clinically (31). Upper midbrain injury leads to conjugate vertical gaze palsy, with isolated up-, down-gaze and combined disturbances, slow smooth pursuit, torsional nystagmus, pseudoabducens palsy, convergence-retraction nystagmus, disconjugate vertical gaze palsy, skew deviation, ocular tilt reactions, and see-saw nystagmus. Middle midbrain injury that interrupts nuclear and fascicular oculomotor nerve fibers in a middle paramedian midbrain infarct, typically leads to nuclear oculomotor nerve palsy, whereas lateral midbrain infarction spares the oculomotor nucleus. Internuclear ophthalmoplegia (INO) is a clue to the presence of a midbrain lesion with an anterior and posterior syndrome. The former is characterized by impaired convergence associated with paralysis of the medial rectus muscle on horizontal conjugate gaze toward the side of the lesion, while the posterior type leads to paralysis of the medial

16 / CHAPTER 1

rectus in conjugate horizontal gaze sparing convergence. Both produce monocular nystagmus of the abducting eye with a localization of the posterior type near the abducens level, and anterior type more rostral. The commonest causes of INO are MS and brainstem lacunar strokes.

Clinical syndromes of the midbrain present with alternating hemiplegia due to unilateral damage of nuclei and adjacent descending fiber tracts, disturbances of consciousness due to pathological involvmenent of the mesencephalic reticular formation, and decerebrate rigidity due to damage of structures subserving the regulation of motor tone. The entity of mesencephalic stroke was described in 1853 (32), followed soon after by descriptions of alternating hemiplegic syndromes (33–35). The lower red nucleus syndrome described by Benedikt (33) consists of ipsilateral paralysis of the oculomotor nerve, contralateral decrease in touch, position, and vibration sensation, contralateral rigidity, chorea and athetosis, respectively, due to interruption of ipsilateral ocular motor nerve fibers, medial lemniscus, substantia nigra, and red nucleus due to unilateral infarction in the territory of the interpeduncular branches of the basilar and PCA. Probably the best known alternating hemiplegic syndrome of the cerebral peduncle, described by Weber (34), (Figure 9) consists of ipsilateral oculomotor paresis, contralateral hemiparesis with supranuclear involvement of the facial and hypoglossal nerves, contralateral ataxia and rigidity, respectively, due to infarction and interruption of ipsilateral oculomotor, corticospinal, corticopontine fibers, and substantia nigra fibers, in the territory of interpeduncular branches of the PCA and posterior choroidal artery. A third syndrome described by Claude (35) consists of ipsilateral oculomotor paresis, contralateral asynergia, ataxia, dysmetria, dysdiadochokinesis due to interruption of oculomotor nerve fibers and cerebellothalamic pathways due to infarction and interruption in the territory of paramedian branches of the

basilar artery. Presumptive evidence of a mass lesion in the ventral interpedicular area is suggested by the combination of cranial nerve palsies and corticospinal tract involvement, with ensuing paralysis of the arms and legs. The syndrome of single- or double-sided ataxia and extraoccular nerve palsies due to expanding tumors of the quadrigeminal region, wherein cerebellar involvement is ascribed to pressure on the vermis or brachia conjunctiva without involvement of the red nucleus (36). The syndrome of contralateral ataxia and choreiform hyperkinesias without paresis of the oculomotor nerve is most often due to a pathological process located in the anterior part of the red nucleus and the area ventral to it (37). A syndrome of upward gaze, convergence paralysis, and papillary areflexia is caused by pretectal compression by a pinealoma or craniopharyngioma (38). The Sylvian aqueduct syndrome, most often ascribed due to a vascular lesion of the periaqueductal grey matter, includes impaired vertical gaze, retraction nystagmus, papillary abnormalities, convergence and vertical nystagmus, convergence spasm, and extraocular palsies. Decerebrate rigidity leading to sustained rigidity of antigravity muscles of the trunk and lower limbs denotes damage to the mesencephalic pontine junction in cases of severe head trauma, brainstem compression by infratentorial tumors, and transtentorial herniation.

DIENCEPHALON

The diencephalon is classified into five components, each with its own afferent and efferent connections and nuclear groups. The first is the thalamus that is further topographically divided into numerous nuclei with respect to the internal medullary lamina, a sheet-like packet of nerve fibers that course rostral to caudal along the length of the thalamus (Figure 10). The second is the metathalamus

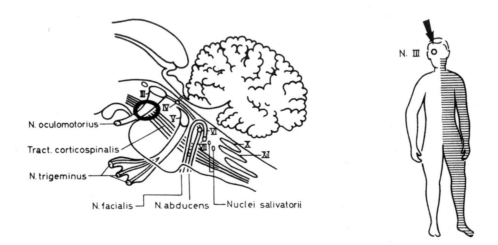

FIG. 9. Weber syndrome. Striped bars indicate motor deficiency. Reproduced from reference 2, with permission.

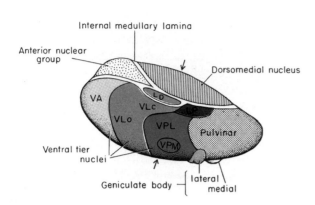

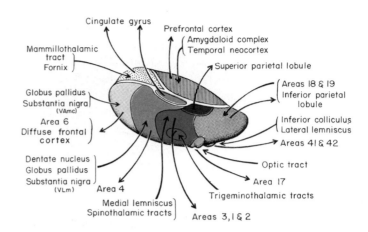

FIG. 10. Schematic diagram of the major thalamic nuclei. Reproduced from reference 3, with permission.

FIG. 11. Schematic diagram of the principal afferent and efferent thalamic projections. Reproduced from reference 3, with permission.

that comprises the medial and lateral geniculate bodies. The third is the epithalamus that includes the trigonum habenula, pineal body, and posterior commissure. The fourth is the subthalamus that separates it by fibers of the internal capsule. The last component is the hypothalamus that includes the rostral, middle, and lateral preoptic region, each with specialized function.

The afferent and efferent projections of the thalamic nuclei shown in Figure 11 converge into four peduncles. An anterior or frontal peduncle connects the frontal lobe with medial and anterior thalamic nuclei subserving connections with the hypothalamus, and indirectly with the hippocampus via the mammillary nuclei, fornix, and cingulate gyrus and entorhinal cortex subserving visceral and emotional function. A superior or centroparietal peduncle connects portions of the frontal and parietal lobes with ventral tier nuclei carrying general sensory impulses from the face and body terminating in the postcentral gyrus. A posterior or occipital peduncle connects the occipital and posterior parietal convolutions with the caudal thalamus, including the optic radiation from the lateral geniculate body to calcarine cortex concerning visual information. An inferior or temporal peduncle transmits auditory radiations from the medial geniculate body to the transverse gyrus of Heschel concerning auditory information. Descending cortical fibers pass through the white matter region of the hemispheres and converge toward the brainstem in the corona radiata and enter a compact fiber area termed the *internal capsule*, shown schematically in Figure 12. The internal capsule is bordered medially by the thalamus and caudate and laterally by the lentiform nuclei. In the horizontal plane the anterior limb of the internal capsule lies between the lentiform and caudate nuclei and contains anterior thalamic radiations and prefrontal corticopontine fibers. The genu contains corticobulbar and corticoreticular fibers. The

posterior limb contains corticospinal, frontopontine, superior thalamic radiations, and a smaller contingent of corticotectal, corticorubral, and corticoreticular fibers tracts. Corticospinal tract fibers are somatotopically arranged in the compact region of the posterior half of the posterior limb with those destined for cervical, thoracic, and lumbosacral segments arranged in rostrocaudal sequence. The retrolenticular portion of the posterior limb contains

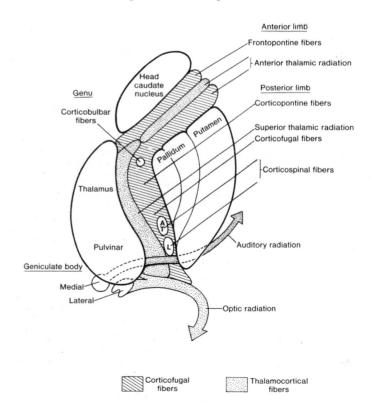

FIG. 12. Schematic diagram of the right internal capsule shown in horizontal section. Reproduced from reference 3, with permission.

posterior thalamic optic radiations while a sublenticular portion contains inferior thalamic and auditory radiations.

Rostral anterior nuclei receive projections from the fornix and mammillary nuclei via the mammillothalamic tracts, and reciprocally project to the cingulum and cingulate gyrus though the anterior limb of the internal capsule. The dorsomedial (DM) nucleus occupies the area between the internal medullary lamina and periventricular gray matter and relays projections from the amygdaloid complex, rostral frontal, and orbitofrontal cortex back to the entire frontal cortex concerned with the integration of consciousness and feeling tones as evidenced by the degeneration of dorsomedial cells after prefrontal lobotomy. The centromedian (CM), parafascicular, and rostral intralaminar nuclei are positioned along the internal medullary lamina and receive ascending projections from the brainstem reticular formation via the central tegmental tract, and the frontral lobe, as well as pallidofugal fibers from the thalamic fasciculus on the way to VA and ventral lateral (VL) thalamic nuclei, which are relayed in turn to sensory and motor cortex. The lateral nuclear mass consists of lateral dorsal, lateral posterior, and pulvinar nuclei arranged in rostrocaudal sequence, and are mainly concerned with integrative functions, especially those concerned with contralateral visual hemifield projections to occipital and striate cortex. A ventral nuclear mass is divided into four nuclei, VA, VL, ventral posterolateral (VPL) and ventral posteromedial (VPM). Afferent connections of the ventral anterior nucleus arise from the globus pallidus, substantia nigra, diffuse cortical areas, and intralaminar nuclei, and are relayed to frontal cortex. The VL receives crossed dentatorubrothalamic and pallidofugal fibers via the thalamic fasciculus, and projections from the substantia nigra and precenral cortex that relayed to areas 4 and 6 of the precental motor cortex important in motor control. The VPL nucleus relays projections from the medial lemniscus and spinothalamic tract to areas 3, 2, and 1 of postcentral sensory cortex. The VPM nucleus receives visceral and somatic afferent projections from the head, face and intraoral structures along crossed projections from the spinal and principal sensory trigeminal nuclei, which ascends in association with the medial lemniscus, trigeminal lemniscus, and lateral spinothalamic tract respectively, for pain, temperature, and discriminative sensation; and ipsilateral gustatory fibers from the nucleus solitarius in the central tegmental tract. A posterior thalamic nuclear complex that receives spinothalamic fibers is concerned with perception of pain and noxious stimuli, and projects to retroinsular cortex.

Bilateral medial geniculate bodies lying under the pulvinar, and lateral geniculate bodies located on the lateral part of the posterior end of the thalamus, which comprise the metathalamus, respectively relay auditory and visual projections via designated brachia of the inferior and superior colliculi, and terminate in areas 41 and 42 of the superior temporal gyrus, whereas other fibers sweep around through the retrolenticular portion of the internal capsule to reach area 17 of the occipital cortex surrounding the calcarine fissure. Each half of the contralateral binocular field is represented in all layers of the lateral geniculate bodies, with crossed and uncrossed fibers ending in different layers such that any small area can be shown to correspond to a column of cells extending radially through all six nuclear layers parallel to the lines of projection. The lamination of the medial geniculate body is similar to that of the lateral geniculate body except that the cellular laminae are not separated by bands of myelinated fibers. The cortical projection of the medial geniculate body to the superior temporal convolution, via the geniculotemporal auditory radiation, is presumed to have tonotopic localization in which high tones are located medially and low tones are represented laterally and anteriorly. The habenula nucleus of the epithalmus is part of a reflex olfactory pathway along with the stria medullaris, medial forebrain bundle, and fornix. The pineal body lies in a depression between the superior colliculi and splenium of the corpus callosum, and is a rudiment photosensitive organ.

The subthalamus or diencephalic tegmentum, separates the thalamus from the internal capsule, and lies in proximity to the tegmental Field of Forel, a rostral continuation of reticular nuclei, from which dentato-, rubro- and reticulothalamic connections continue forward toward the thalamic fasciculus of Forel. Two well-formed pallidothalamic fiber tracts originate in medial globus pallidus termed the *ansa lenticularis* and *lenticular fasciculus* or Field H2 of Forel, and merge in Forel field H to enter the thalamic fasciculus and terminate in the ventral tier thalamic nuclei joined by ascending fibers from contralateral deep cerebelllar nuclei that project in a non-overlapping manner to areas 4 and 6 of premotor cortex. Neurons of the subthalamic nucleus are separated from the lateral thalamic nucleus by the zona incerta.

The hypothalamus is the part of the diencephalon concerned with visceral, autonomic, and neuroendocrine functions. It is comprised of a periventricular region under the ependyma of the third ventricle, a middle region that is divided into a rostral supraoptic and paraventricular and tuberal infundibula portions, a caudal mammillary area, and lateral preoptic area. The third ventricle is formed above by the choroid plexus that invaginates its roof, anteriorly by the lamina terminalis, posteriorly by the pineal body, posterior commissure and cerebral acqueduct, and laterally by the thalamus. The columns of the fornix curve in front of the interventricular foramen beneath the corpus callosum. Two neurosecretory nuclei, supraoptic and paraventricular are located in the rostral hypothalamus and release vasopressin or antidiuretic hormone (ADH) important in regulation of water metabolism, and oxytocin important in childbirth. Both hormones are stored in the posterior lobe of the pituitary whereupon electrical stimulation of the cell bodies results in the generation of a conducted action potential along the axon processes to trigger the release of hormone packaged as dense granules within membranous vesicles bound to carrier proteins known as neurophysins at nerve endings in the neurohypophysis. The action of ADH is to retain water from kidney tubules and counterbalance increases in osmolality in the blood. The effect of oxytocin is to initiate uterine muscle contraction and secretion of myoepithelia of mammary gland alveoli with pregnancy and childbirth. While there is evidence that the supraoptic nucleus is related mainly to vasopressin, and paraventricular nucleus to oxytocin, in fact both hormones are found in each nucleus, but cells associated with each hormone show regional separation. An infundibular portion of the hypothalamus, located behind the anterior hypothalamic area and the mammillary bodies, is believed to be the origin of efferent hypothalamic connections that descend through the lateral brainstem tegmentum into the anterolateral columns of the spinal cord. Tuberal nuclei in the infundibular region, particularly the arcuate nucleus, project upon capillary loops near the sinusoids of the hypophysial portal system, wherein secretory granules can be demonstrated at their nerve endings. Fibers of the tuberoinfundibular tract convey releasing hormones, which are transported via the hypophysial portal vessels to the anterior lobe of the pituitary where they modulate the synthesis and secretion of adenohypophysial hormones including growth hormone (GH) for the growth of bone; thyroid stimulating hormone (TSH) for thyroidal function; adrenocorticotrophic hormone (ACTH) for the adrenal gland function, including secretion of corticosteroids; the gonadotrophic hormones, follicle stimulating hormone (FSH) and luteinizing hormone (LH), important in normal sexual function; and prolactin which is important in lactation. Paired mammillary nuclei, divided into medial and lateral portions that receive connections from the medial forebrain bundle, thalamus, and inferior mammillary peduncle arising in the mesencephalic tegmentum, and give rise to a descending mamillo-tegemental tract (the bundle of Vicq d'Azyr) to the anterior thalamic nuclei.

Afferent connections of the hypothalamus arise from the medial forebrain bundle, pre- and post-commisural fibers from the fornix, stria terminalis of the amygdaloid complex, tractus solitarius, dorsal tegmental bundle, and retina. The median forebrain bundle arises from olfactory areas, including the periamygdaloid region and septal nuclei, and passes through the preoptic and hypothalamic regions to the anterior perforated substance. Hippocampo-hypothalamic fibers that originate from the hippocampal formation form the fornix, precommisural fibers of which are distributed to septal nuclei, the lateral preoptic region, and the dorsal hypothalamic area. Posterior commissural fibers project to the hypothalamus and terminate in the medial mammallary nucleus. Amygadalo-hypothalamic fibers found in the stria terminalis from the amygdaloid complex distribute to the preoptic, anterior, ventromedial and arcuate hypothalamic nuclei. Ascending serotonergic fibers arising mainly from nuclei of the brainstem raphe also ascend in the median forebrain bundle to the lateral hypothalamus. General visceral afferents from the nucleus solitarius project upon preoptic nuclei, while special visceral afferent fibers of the nucleus solitarius project to posterior lateral regions of the hypothalamus. Ascending noradrenergic fibers originating in the locus ceruleus ascend in the dorsal tegmental bundle and distributes to dorsomedial, supraoptic, and paraventricular hypothalamic nuclei. Retinohypothalamic projections arise from retinal ganglionic cells and project to the suprachiasmatic nuclei. The principal efferent connections of the hypothalamus include the medial forebrain that projects rostrally from the lateral hypothalamus to the medial septal nuclei and hippocampal formation via fimbria of the fornix, and caudally from the medial and periventricular hypothalamus to midbrain, tectal gray matter, and spinal levels along the dorsal longitudinal fasciculus, and others that descend from mammillary nuclei in the mammillo-thalamic and mammilo-tegmental tracts to the lower brainstem.

Clinical syndromes arising from lesions in the thalamus should be considered in the context of its highly specialized function and blood supply. The thalamus functions as a neuronal subsystem for the high fidelity transmission of information with the capacity to synchronize and desynchronize its input store and modify signals for output to other areas of the neuraxis, especially higher cortical areas. Subspecialized nuclei of the ventral tier, for example, process the intensity and localization of discriminative sensation, and point-to-point auditory and visual information, respectively, via projections from the ascending medial lemniscus tracts to the VPL nucleus and along fiber projections from the medial and lateral geniculate bodies, whereas motor processes are influenced by deep cerebellar and globus pallidus projections to VL and VA nuclei and motor cortex. By contrast, associational nuclei have reciprocal connections with other diencephalic nuclei and association cortex for the intergration of complex behaviors.

The blood supply of the thalamus, shown in Figure 13, is derived from the basilar, paired posterior cerebral, and posterior communicating arteries (PComA) from which smaller branches arise, including thalamoperforator and medial posterochoroidal arteries that supply the middle, anterior, posterior and intralaminar nuclei; thalogeniculate and lateral posterior choroidal vessels that subserve lateral geniculate and ventral tier nuclei; and tuberothalamic arteries that arise from posterior communicating vessel that supply the anterior thalamus. Lenticulostriate

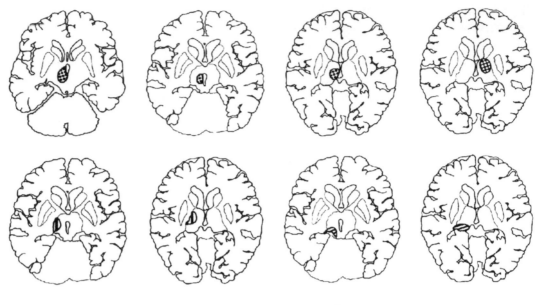

■■■ Posterior thalamo-subthalamic paramedian arteries *thalamo-perforate*

■■■ Anterior thalamo-subthalamic paramedian arteries *tuberothalamic or polar*

▥▥ Infero-lateral arteries *thalamo-geniculate*

▨ Posterior choroidal arteries

(A)

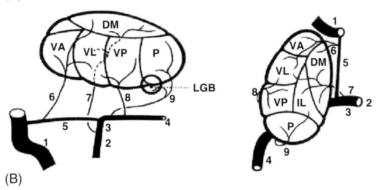

(B)

FIG. 13. Arterial supply of the thalamus. 1: Internal carotid artery, 2: basilar artery, 3: posterior cerebral artery (P1), 4: posterior cerebral artery, 5: posterior communicating artery, 6: tuberothalamic or polar, 7: thalamoperforate or paramedian, 8: thalamogeniculate or inferolateral, 9: posterior choroidal. Abbreviations: LGB: lateral geniculate body, DM: dorsomedial nucleus, VA: ventral anterior nucleus, VP: ventral posterior nucleus, P: pulvinar, IL: intralaminar nuclei. Reproduced from, De Freitas GR, De H Christoph D, Bogousslavsky J. Topographical classification of ischemic stroke. *Handb Clin Neurol* 2009; 93:425–452, with permission.

branches of the middle cerebral artery (MCA) supply the head and body of the caudate, anterior limb, genu and anterior portion of the posterior limb of the internal capsule, putamen, and lateral globus pallidus (Figure 14). Unilateral infarction in the territory of thalamoperforator vessels produces disturbances of arousal, memory, language, and visual deficits due to involvement of cortical relay and intralaminar nuclei. Infarction in the inferolateral thalamus affecting ventral tier nuclei, due to selective involvement of thalamogeniculate vessels, leads to a syndrome characterized by contralateral sensory loss, asterognoisis, hemiataxia, neurogenic pain, transitory hemiparesis, choreic and athetotic movements. Lesions that disrupt the thalamocortical and corticofugal fibers tract in the internal capsule that result from thrombosis and hemorrhage along the anterior choroidal, striate, and capsular branches of the MCA, produce widespread disturbances owing to the compact nature of the fiber tracts.

Clinical syndromes of the hypothalamus typically alter autonomic and neuroendocrine function. Parasympathetic function appears to reside in anterior, medial, supraoptic and preoptic hypothalamic areas and the ventricular portion of the tuber cinereum, stimulation of which leads to increased vagal and sacral responses characterized by reduced heart rate, peripheral vasodilatation, and increased tonus and motility of the intestine. Sympathetic function, however, appears to reside in the lateral and posterior hypothalamus, stimulation of which leads to pupillary dilatation, piloerection, cardioacceleration, increased blood pressure, rate and amplitude of respiration, and inhibition of the gut and bladder. Central syndromes of dysautonomia occur in Parkinson disease (PD), multisystem atrophy (MSA), progressive supranuclear palsy (PSP), Machado-Joseph disease, and senile dementia of the Alzheimer type (SDAT) (39). A lesion of the supraoptic nucleus leads to diabetes insipidus characterized by polyuria due to inhibition of ADH. Tumors and other pathological processes of the hypothalamus and hypophysis lead to abnormal sexual development and endocrinopathies of various types due to hyper- or hypo-end-organ secretion, often in association with elevated prolactin levels, ballooning of the sella turcica, compression of optic chiasm, optic tract fibers, and headache.

BASAL GANGLIA

Broadly defined, the caudate, putamen, and globus pallidus, together with the substantia nigra, subthalamic, and red nucleus, comprise the extrapyramidal motor system. Its connections with the amygdaloid complex, dentate nucleus, inferior olives, and portions of the frontal lobe of the cerebral cortex contribute additional important connections to extrapyramidal function. The caudate and putamen, which together form the corpus striatum, have an embryological derivation from neostriatum along the striatal ridge of the telencephalic vesicle. Afferent connections to the caudate and putamen arise from ipsilateral excitatory corticostriate fibers from virtually all regions of the neocortex that have glutamate as their neurotransmitter, as well as amygdaloid, intralaminar, and medial thalamic nuclei, pars compacta of the substantia nigra, and serotonergic projections arising from dorsal raphe nuclei along the median forebrain bundle to the striatum. Efferent projections include striopallidal and strionigral fibers that pass ventrally through the internal capsule to the globus pallidus, while strionigral projections from the putamen pass medially to the globus pallidus. Striopallidal fibers are considered to have mainly GABA as their neurotransmitter, and the globus pallidus is itself rich in glutamic acid decarboxylase (GAD), the enzyme that synthesizes GABA. High concentrations of dopamine are located in terminal varicosities of strionigral fibers. Major afferents to the globus pallidus arise from the striatum and subthalamic nucleus, but not cerebral cortex, thalamus, or substantia nigra. Pallidofugal fibers can be found in the ansa lenticularis, lenticular fasciculus, and pallidotegmental fibers, which all arise from the medial pallidal segment and pallidosubthalamic fibers that arise from the lateral pallidal segment. The pallidofugal fibers area is arranged rostal to caudal with the ansa lenticularis most rostral, the lenticular fasciculus intermediate, and pallidosubthalamic fibers most caudal. The substantia nigra is a large nucleus mass that lies dorsal to the crus cerebri and is divided into a pars compacta and reticulata that contains high concentrations of GAD. It receives afferent projections from the striatum, globus pallidus, subthalamic nucleus, dorsal nucleus of the raphe, and pedunculopontine nucleus, and projects dopaminergic fibers back to the striatum and dorsal nucleus of the raphe, with other nondopaminergic efferents via nigrothalamic, nigrotectal, and nigrotegmental tracts.

The blood supply to the striatum is provided mainly by lenticulostriate arteries that are terminal vessels without anastomosis (Figure 14). They supply the putamen and pallidum, the upper part of the anterior limb and genu of the internal capsule, and the anterior part of the posterior limb, head, and body of the caudate nucleus. The rostromedial parts of the head of the caudate nucleus is supplied by the medial striate artery of Heubner while the tail of the caudate and the caudal part of the caudate nucleus and the caudal part of the putamen receive branches of the anterior choroidal artery. The lateral segment of the globus pallidus is supplied by branches of both lateral striate and anterior choroidal arteries. The lateral part of the medial pallidal segment receives branches from the anterior choroidal artery, and the medial most pallidum is supplied by branches of the posterior communicating artery (PoComA). Lacunar

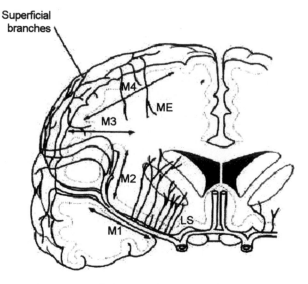

Superficial
branches

FIG. 14. Segments of the middle cerebral artery. See text. Abbreviations: LS: lenticulostriate arteries, ME: medullary arteries. Reproduced from, De Freitas GR, De H Christoph D,Bogousslavsky J. Topographical classification of ischemic stroke. *Handb Clin Neurol* 2009; 93:425–452, with permission.

infarcts involving the basal ganglia and internal capsule result from occlusion or severe stenosis of one of the penetrating arteries and manifest principally as pure motor hemiplegia. Pure motor hemiplegia involving the face, arm, and leg was noted in 2 of 5 pathologically studied patients, unaccompanied by sensory signs, visual field defect, aphasia, or apractognosia, in association with putamino-capsulo-caudate lesions extending variably from the putamen to the body of the caudate, across the posterior limb of the internal capsule in the territory of lenticulostriate branches (40). Later studies of serial sections of the involved basal ganglia in capsular infarcts leading to similar pure motor hemiplegia or hemiparesis involving the face, arm, and leg implicated penetrating arteries, traced throughout their length, and obstructive vascular lesions were found in 9 histopathological preparations (41), including 2 that revealed atheromatous plaque with a superimposed thrombus, 4 that showed atheromatous plaque associated with severe stenosis including 1 with lipohyalinosis, and 3 with patent vessels suggesting embolism (in 2) or an uncertain mechanism of infarction. It is of interest that capsular infarction of the basal ganglia was not associated with other motor phenomena, including hyperkinetic movements. Tremor at rest is most commonly in PD due to loss of dopamine rich cells of the pars compacta of the substantia nigra. Athetotic movement is slow and writhing, often seen in association with lesions of the globus pallidus, whereas, pathological processes involving the caudate nucleus, such as Huntington disease (HD), are associated with chorea that present

as brisk, graceful, involuntary movements due to low concentration of GABA. Ballism is violent, flinging movements that result from discrete lesions in the subthalamic nucleus or its connections. Such movements represent positive or release phenomena implying that the causative lesion removes control of regulating influences.

CEREBRAL HEMISPHERES

The cerebral hemispheres are the largest portion of the brain, divided from front to back by the longitudinal cerebral fissure, and in the middle by the corpus callosum, fornix, and septum pellucidum. The surfaces of the hemispheres have visible gyri and sulci, and fissures that divide the hemispheres into frontal, parietal, temporal, and occipital lobes. The Brodmann map is a useful system for designating cortical areas that are cytoarchitecturally and functionally different (Figure 15). The frontal lobes are situated anterior to the precentral gyrus and divided into three regions: the primary motor area or precentral gyrus (area 4), premotor (area 6 and part of 8), and prefrontal regions (area 10, 45, 46). Three sulci, precentral, superior, and inferior, divide the frontal lobe into four gyri, anterior central, superior, middle, and inferior frontal. The frontal operculum denotes a small region of cortex that covers the insula, and is comprised of three parts, namely pars orbitalis (area 47), triangularis (area 45), and opercularis (area 44), that relates to spontaneous and articulate speech. The corticospinal tracts, which convey impulses for highly skilled volitional movements to lower motor neurons, arises largely from giant pyramidal cells in motor, adjacent premotor cortex, and supplemental motor area located in the mesial frontal lobe above the cingulate gyrus. Frontal cortical eye fields, responsible for conjugate deviation of the eyes to the opposite side, correspond to area 8 along the caudal part of the middle frontal gyrus extending to the inferior frontal gyrus. Crossing anterior corpus colossal fibers link the dominant frontal lobe with the contralateral side, assuring skilled movements of the opposite hand. The parietal lobes are separated respectively, from the frontal, occipital, and temporal lobes by the central sulcus, parieto-occipital fissure, and posterior ramus of the lateral fissure. An intraparietal sulcus found along the lateral surface of the lobe delimits a superior and inferior parietal lobule, the latter of which is divided into supramarginal (area 40) and angular gyri (area 39). The parietal lobe is concerned with sensation and localization of body position and objects in space. However, even more specialized function of spontaneous repetition is located in the supramarginal gyrus, as are writing, calculation, finger recognition, and right-left awareness in the angular gyrus. The temporal lobe is bound by the Sylvian fissure above and laterally, by the hippocampal fissure

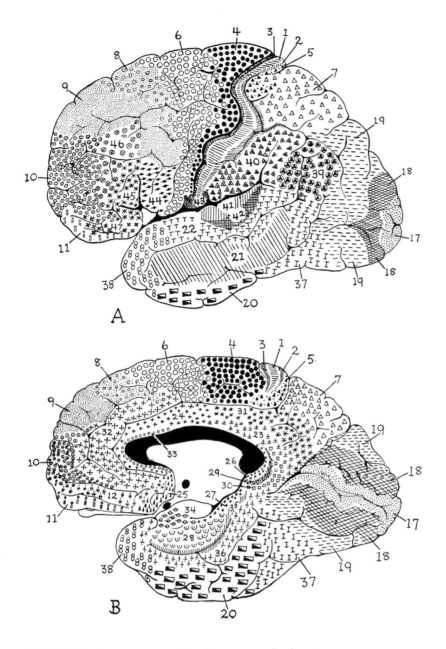

FIG. 15. Brodmann areas of the human cerebral cortex. Reproduced from reference 3, with permission.

and peristriate (area 19) association cortex for visuointegrative function. The dominant occipital lobe is connected to the other side by crossing fibers of the splenium of the corpus callosum for the processing of higher cortical functions relating to reading, color, movement, shapes, and face discrimination.

Archipallium is the oldest cortical derivative that includes the hippocampal formation, dentate, fascicular and supracallosal gyri. The hippocampal formation develops from the medial embryonic wall of the hemisphere along the hippocampal fissure that invaginates into the inferior horn of the ventricle becoming the hippocampus the lips of which give rise to the parahippocampal gyrus and dentate, covered by white matter termed the *alveus* or axons of hippocampal cells that converge to form the fimbria of the fornix. The septal region includes the subcallosal and paraterminal gyri, beneath which are located lateral and medial nuclei. The septal region receives afferent projections from the hippocampal formation via the fornix, and mamillary peduncles via the median forebrain bundle. Efferent septal fibers project to the habenular nucleus via the stria medullaris, as well as to the lateral hypothalamus and midbrain tegmentum via the median forebrain bundle, and the hippocampal formation via the fornix. Afferent fibers to the hippocampal formation arise mainly from the entorhinal area and distribute to the dentate gyrus and hippocampus, while others derive from the medial septal nuclei, which in turn are relayed to the entorhinal area via cingulate cortex and the cingulum. The hippocampal formation does not receive afferent input directly from the olfactory bulb or anterior olfactory nucleus. The limbic system contains neuronal connections that begin in the septal area and extend in a paramedian zone through the preoptic region and hypothalamus into the rostral mesencephalon, along with the interconnections of the fornix to the hippocampus, entorhinal cortex, cingulate gyrus, anterior nucleus of the thalamus, and mammillary bodies of the hypothalamus in a closed loop.

The term *rhinencephalon* refers to the olfactory brain and its components and projections, including those of the olfactory bulb, olfactory tract, olfactory tubercle and striae, anterior olfactory nucleus, amygdaloid complex, and prepyriform cortex. The central processes of bipolar cells, located in the olfactory epithelium, converge to form fascicles of the olfactory nerve that pass through foramina in

medially, and posteriorly by the occipital lobe and the inferior parietal lobule. It is divided by superior and middle sulci into three parallel gyri, superior, middle, and inferior. In the middle of the superior transverse temporal gyrus, deep into the lateral fissure, resides the auditory receptive area or Hesch gyrus (area 41), surrounded by auditory association cortex (area 42 and 22) subserving auditory integrative function. The occipital lobe presents three surfaces, lateral, medial, and tentorial. The lateral surface is divided into superior and inferior gyri by a lateral sulcus, and the medial surface is divided by the calcarine fissure dividing it into the cuneus and lingual gyri, surrounded by primary striate cortex (area 17), and adjacent parastriate (area 18) the cribiform plate of the ethmoid bone to the olfactory bulb where axon terminals synapse upon primary olfactory neurons. The efferent axons of the primary olfactory neurons enter the olfactory tract as secondary olfactory fibers and pass toward the anterior perforated substance where they divide into lateral and medial striae covered by gray substance respectively forming the lateral and medial olfactory gyri. The principal strial fibers pass toward the primary olfactory cortex, which includes the prepyriform cortex and periamygdaloid area, and project to area 28 of the entorhinal cortex, also known as the secondary olfactory area, and in turn to the hippocampal formation, as well as to the anterior insular area and frontal cortex via the uncinate fasciculus. However, no fibers from the olfactory tract or prepyriform cortex project to this hippocampal formation. The amygdaloid nuclear complex is situated in the dorsomedial portion of the temporal lobe covered by rudimentary cortex, and is continous with the uncus of the parahippocampal cortex. Olfactory afferent input to the amygdala arises from the lateral olfactory tract via the olfactory bulb and terminates in the basolateral nucleus. The most prominent efferent pathways from the amygdala travel in the stria terminalis to anterior and preoptic nuclei of the hypothalamus, septal region, and midline periventricular nuclei of the thalamus.

The neopallium displays neuroanatomical features of higher cortical organization through cellular lamination with six fundamental layers, and a columnar function organization, which as an elementary unit of the cortex, contains afferent, efferent, and interneuronal fiber systems necessary for the formation of complete cortical circuits. The columnar units are interconnected by short neuronal links through corticocortical and thalamic connections that permit the spread of horizontal cortical excitation and inhibition. Electrical stimulation of the primary motor cortex evokes discrete isolated contralateral movements via connections of the corticospinal tract and innervation of muscles concerned with specific movements, individual muscles, or a discrete body part such as flexion or extension of a single finger joint, twitching of the corner of the mouth, or protrusion of the tongue, depending upon the area of the motor homunculus that is stimulated. The premotor region that lies rostral to the motor area also contributes to the corticospinal tract. A supplementary motor area, which occupies the medial surface of the superior frontal gyrus rostral to area 4, appears to govern postures, complex patterned movement, and infrequent incoordinated movements. Movement, motor control, muscle tone, posture, and other motor activities are affected by inputs to motor cortical areas from subcortical centers, including crossed cerebellothalamic and uncrossed pallidothalamic fibers that project to ventral tier nuclei in a non-overlapping fashion, and in turn are relayed to areas

4 and 6. Ventral tier neurons show increased activity prior to any movement, suggesting that they play a role in its initiation. Corticoreticular, corticopontine, and corticothalamic fiber projections arise from diverse areas of the neocortex but the largest number arise from motor and premotor areas in the governance of movement. Corticoreticular fibers descend in association with corticospinal tract fibers to terminate upon circumscribed areas of the medulla and pons. Corticopontine fibers arising mainly from pyramidal cells in layer V, superficial to giant pyramidal cells from areas 4, 3, 1, 2, and 5, parts of the visual cortex, project somatotopically upon longitudinally oriented pontine nuclei, exerting excitatory action and conveying impulses from cerebral cortex to broad regions of the contralateral neocerebellum via mossy fibers. Cortical areas receiving projections from particular thalamic nuclei give rise to reciprocal corticothalamic projections passing back to the same nuclei, in addition to those from areas 4 and 6 of frontal and prefrontal cortex to dorsomedial nucleus, ventral tier, and intralaminar nuclei to affect further refinements in motor and sensory function.

The cortical branches of the cerebral hemispheres are derived from the internal carotid artery (ICA), which gives rise to the anterior cerebral artery (ACA) and MCA, and PCA formed by the bifurcation of the basilar artery. Each ICA arises from the ipsilateral common carotid artery, on the left arising from the left side of the aortic arch, and on the right, from the brachiocephalic artery. Each ICA takes its origin from the respective common carotid artery (CCA) at the carotid bifurcation, and is subdivided into seven segments as it ascends in the neck and intracranially, including the cervical (C1), petrous (C2), lacerum (C3), cavernous (C4), clinoid (C5), ophthalmic (C6), and communicating (C7) segments (Figure 16). The C1, or carotid bulb, enters the carotid canal of the skull in the petrous bone marking the C2 segment, becoming vertical and then horizontal, with a genu in between, before emerging under the petrolingual ligament as the C3 segment. The C4 segment, which courses through the cavernous sinus before emerging through the dura mater of its roof in the region of the clinoid as the C5 portion, and extending up to the origin of the (PComA) as the C6 segment. The main continuing branch of the ICA is the MCA, while the smaller ACA and the anterior communicating artery (AComA), PComA, and PCA respectively contribute the anterior, middle, and posterior portions of the circle of Willis connecting the vertebrobasilar and carotid systems. The ACA is divided into five segments, A1-5 (Figure 17). The A1 segment first gives rise to the recurrent artery of Heubner to supply the head of the caudate, anterior inferior internal capsue, anterior globus pallidus, putamen, and hypothalamus. The ACA continues as the A2 segment and pericallosal artery from which orbitofrontal and frontopolar arteries take their origin. The

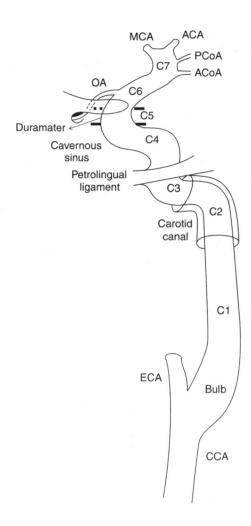

FIG. 16. Schematic representation lateral view, of the seven ICA segments. See text. Reproduced from, Kumral E, Topcuoglu MA, Onal MZ. *Handb Clin Neurol* 2009; 93:485–536, with permission.

callosomarginal artery continues above and beyond the corpus callosum to the central sulcus in the medial interhemispheric surface, giving rise to the anterior, middle, and posterior frontal arteries along its A3 segment. A paracentral artery arises from the A4 segment, as do superior and inferior parietal arteries from the A5 segment. The MCA arises as a stem, which gives rise to lenticulostriate arteries after which it bifurcates into a superior and inferior division and up to 12 cortical branches, originating from the MCA that supply the lateral surface of the frontal and parietal lobes, and superior temporal lobe (Figure 14). The orbitofrontal, prefrontal, precentral, Rolandic and anterior and posterior parietal arteries arise from the superior division in a territory while the angular, temporooccipital and temporopolar; anterior, posterior, and middle temporal arteries emerge from the inferior division. Four MCA segments are recognized according to anatomical landmarks, including

a horizontal sphenoidal M1 that contains the stem as it extends laterally in the Sylvian fisssue where the MCA subdivides into prebifurcation and postbifurcation portions, a vertical insular M2, horizontal opercular M3, and the M4 segment that provides the cortical branches that begin at the surface of the Sylvian fissure and extend over the cortical surface. The PCA arises from the basilar artery in the pontomesencephalic junction, courses around the midbrain and anastomoses with the PComA before dividing into cortical branches. Two segments, a precommunal or P1, which extends from the bifurcation to the origin of the PComA, and a postcomunal or P2, which continues into cortical branches. The P1 segment gives rise to interpeduncular arteries, thalamoperforate arteries, and medial posterior choroidal arteries that supply the median midbrain and thalamus. The P2 segment gives rise to thalamogeniculate branches and the lateral posterior choroidal artery that supplies the superficial portion of the pulvinar, lateral geniculate, and medial temporal lobe. The three terminal cortical branches include the posterior temporal, parieto-occipital, and calcarine arteries that respectively supply the inferomedial temporal lobe, medial occipital lobe, and visual areas.

Cerebral ischemia and infarction due to atherosclerotic stenosis and embolism can be localized to discrete areas of the cortex with some assurance, based upon knowledge of the underlying pathogenic mechanism. Whereas stenotic occlusive ICA lesions present with transient hemispheric ischemia, or transient monocular blindness, or amaurosis fugax, depending upon the degree of residual flow and collateral flow, the mechanism of artery-to-artery or distal embolic occlusion along different portions of the ACA and MCA stem and their cortical branches is more varied,

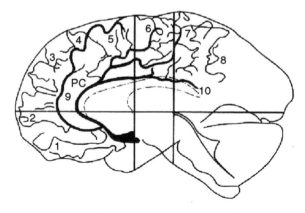

FIG. 17. Diagram of the main branches of the anterior cerebral artery on the medial surface of the brain. 1: orbitofrontal, 2: frontopolar, 3: anterior internal frontal, 4: middle internal frontal, 5: posterior internal frontal, 6: paracentral, 7: precuneal, 8: parieto-occipital, 9: callosomarginal, 10: posterior pericallosal, PC: pericallosal. Reproduced from, Kumral E, Topcuoglu MA, Onal MZ. *Handb Clin Neurol* 2009; 93:485–536, with permission.

and results in at least five stroke patterns, including hemispheric, subcortical, mixed, multiple small strokes, and watershed infarction, further recognizable by the neurological findings and associated neurobehavioral changes. In the most extreme case, there is deterioration of consciousness, contralateral homonymous hemianopia, hemiplegia, hemisensory disturbance, and gaze palsy.

Cerebral dominance and handedness are well recognized predictors of the localization of speech and language and other neurobehavioral processes, with 90% of the population, and nearly all right-handed individuals, left-hemisphere dominant. The dominant hemisphere is primarily concerned with the processing of speech and language functions while the nondominant hemisphere is concerned with spatial relations. The assertion that the central sulcus divides the cerebral cortex into an area of anterior motor and executive function, and a posterior area of sensory and receptive function, assumes that intracerebral and transcallosal neural pathways are interlinked. For example, dominant temporal areas for receptive comprehension of spoken and written language with motor areas of the hand, and muscles of speech, such that words can be repeated out loud or copied. The disturbance that follows damage to the frontal operculum or Broca area is commonly confused with Broca aphasia, named for Broca's original patient (42) who had an initial lesion of the inferior frontal region. However, both that patient and other similar patients are now known to have routinely sustained much larger areas of injury encompassing the operculum, insula, and adjacent cerebrum, often extending to the territory of the superior division of the MCA. Such patients exhibit protracted mutism, followed weeks to months later by spoken language that features hesitancies and agrammatism, and mildly disturbed language comprehension, the severity of which reflects the size of the lesion. Pathoanatomical studies show that the speech disturbance resulting from localized infarction of the Broca area also presents instead by mutism, but it is replaced by rapidly improving dyspraxia and effortful articulation, without significant disturbance in language function (43). The related entity of transcortical motor aphasia is characterized by grammatical capabilities in writing that is superior to speech, in which words can be repeated and copied without spontaneous communication. It is still not clear what factors mediate the varied presentation of individual patients and the recovery of language or speech.

Interruption of both parietal and temporal lobe function leads to discrete neurological syndromes that manifest alteration in cognitive and language function. Pathological involvement of the dominant parietal lobe along the angular gyrus (area 39) leads to finger agnosia, acalculia, right-sided disorientation, and agraphia (44), whereas isolated injury of non-dominant parietal lobe cortex leads instead to contralateral neglect, anosognosia, and constructional apraxia. Impaired spontaneous repetition is the main feature of conduction of aphasia word due to interruption of the supramarginal gyrus (area 40), associated with fluent output and frequent phonemic substitutions. Slight deafness that follows unilateral interruption of the primary auditory center is denser after bilateral injury. Auditory agnosia or cortical deafness, which precludes sound recognition and discrimination, is similar to pure word deafness characterized by the inability to comprehend words. Both occur in the presence of intact hearing for other types of sounds and intact written language comprehension due to interruption of bilateral auditory centers or unilateral dominant lobe injury.

Regions and pathways involved in the processing of visual stimuli occupy a large portion of the cerebral cortex with increasing segregation of information from the retina to the occipital cortex. The recognition of disturbances of color (achromatopsia), facial recognition (propagnosia), localization (simultanagnosia), manual localization (optic ataxia), gaze paresis (ocular apraxia), visual distortion (metamorphopsias), reading without writing difficulty (alexia without agraphia), and pure cortical blindness, that result from disturbances in and around the occipital cortex, emphasize the topographically distinct functions of cortical visual system processing.

Normal aging, dementia, and other disease processes impact upon memory. The histopathological and biochemical changes in aging include neuronal and neuropil loss, and sclerosis most evident in the hippocampus and temporal lobe. Alzheimer disease is characterized by extracellular plaques consisting of aggregates of the 42-amino acid amyloid-b (Ab) peptide and intracellular neurofibrillary tangles within neurons consisting of paired helical filaments of tau protein that hyperphosphorylate in the presence of aggregated amyloid Ab peptide. They emerge first in the hippocampal formation and later throughout the cerebral cortex. A characteristic amnesia occurs in the setting of Wernicke-Korsakoff syndrome due to thiamine deficiency and chronic alcoholism. Specific areas of the brain susceptible to injury include the hypothalamus, mammillary bodies, periaqueductal region of the midbrain, and superior cerebellar vermis that develop necrosis, gliosis, and vacuolation. Affected patients manifest the acute illness of Wernicke syndrome that includes nystagmus, ataxia, and confusion, followed later by Korsakoff syndrome of amnestic confabulation.

REFERENCES

1. Goss CM. *Gray's Anatomy of the Human Body. The Peripheral Nervous System.* Lea and Febiger: Philadelphia, 1956; 977–1023

2. Vinken PJ, Bruyn GW, eds. *Handb Clin Neurol.* North-Holland: Amsterdam, vol 2, 1978.

3. Carpenter MB and Sutin J. *Human Neuroanatomy.* 8th ed. Williams and Wilkins: Baltimore, 1983.

4. Kandel ER, Schwartz JH, Jessell TM. *Principles of Neural Science.* 4th ed. McGraw-Hill; New York, 2000.

5. Skvortsova VI, Bahar SZ. Spinal strokes. *Handb Clin Neurol* 2009; 93:683–702.

6. Younger DS, Kass RM. Vasculitis and the nervous system. *Neurol Clin* 1997; 15:737–758.

7. Bendixen B, Younger DS, Hair L, et al. Cholesterol emboli syndrome: a patient with peripheral neuropathy. *Neurology* 1992; 42:428–430.

8. Chesire WP, Santos CC, Massey EW, et al. Spinal cord infarction: etiology and outcome. *Neurology* 1996; 321–330.

9. Shibuya R, Yonenobu K, Yamamoto K, et al. Acute arm paresis with cervical spondylosis: three case reports. *Surg Neurol* 2005; 220–228.

10. Kumral E, Polat F, Gulluoglu H, et al. Spinal ischaemic stroke: clinical and radiological findings and short term outcome. *Eur J Neurol* 2011; 2:232–239.

11. C-É Brown-Séquard, De la transmission croisée des impressions sensitives par la moelle épinière. *Comptes rendus de la Société de biologie* 1851; 2:33–44.

12. Tatu L, Moulin T, Bogousslavsky J, et al. Arterial territories of the human brain: brainstem and cerebellum. *Neurology* 1996; 47:1125–1135.

13. Wallenberg A. Acute bulbar affection (Embolie der art. Cerebellar post inf Sinister). *Arch Psychiat Nervenkr* 1895; 27:505–540.

14. Dejerine J. *Semiologie des affections du systeme nerveux.* Paris: Masson et Cie, 1914.

15. Kubik CS, Adams RD. Occlusion of the basilar artery-a and pathological study. *Brain* 1946; 69:73–121.

16. Biemond A. Thrombosis of the basilar artery—the vascularization of the brain stem. *Brain* 1951; 74:300–317.

17. Lhermitte J, Trelles JO. L'arteriosclerose du tronc basilaire et ses consequences anatomo-cliniques. *Jb. Psychiat Neurol* 1934; 51:91–107.

18. Millikan CH, Siekert RG. Studies in cerebrovascular disease I. The syndrome of intermittent insufficiency of the basilar artery syndrome. *Proc Mayo Clin* 1955; 30:61–68.

19. Hutchinson EC, Yates PO. The cervical portion of the vertebral artery. A clinico-pathological study. *Brain* 1956; 79:319–331.

20. Millard M. Gaz hebd. *Bull Soc Anat Paris* 1856; 31:217–221.

21. Foville A. Note sur une paralysie peu connue de certains muscles de l'oeil et sa liason avec quelques points de l'anatomie et de la physiologie de la protuberance annulaire. *Bull Soc Anat Paris* 1858; 23:293–414.

22. Raymond F, Cestan R. Le syndrome protuberantiel superior. *Gaz Hop Paris* 1903; 76:829–834.

23. Grasset. Un type special de paralysie alterne motrice (type Foville): paralysie des members d'un cote, du facial total et de l'hemioculomoteur rotateur des yeux de l'autre. *Rev Neurol* 1900; 9:586–630.

24. Marie P, Foix C. Formes cliniques et diagnostic de l'hemiplegie cerebelleuse syphilique. *Sem med* 1913; 33:145–152.

25. Amarenco P, Hauw JJ. Anatomy of the cerebellar arteries. *Rev Neurol* 1989; 145:267–276.

26. Duvernoy H, Delon S, Vannson JL. The vascularization of the human cerebellar cortex. *Brain Res Bull* 1983; 11:419–480.

27. Grimaldi G, Manto M. Topography of cerebellar deficits in humans. *Cerebellum* 2011, Jan. 15 (Epub ahead of print).

28. Amarenco P. The spectrum of cerebellar infarctions. *Neurology* 1991; 41:973–979.

29. Amarenco P, Hauw JJ. Cerebellar infarction in the territory of the anterior and inferior cerebellar artery. A clinicopathological study of 20 cases. *Brain* 1990; 113:139–155.

30. Amarenco P, Hauw JJ. Cerebellar infarction in the territory of the superior cerebellar artery: a clinicopathological study of 33 cases. *Neurology* 1990; 1383–1390.

31. Moncayo J, Bogousslavsky J. Vertebro-basilar syndromes causing oculo-motor disorders. *Curr Opin Neurol* 2003; 16:45–50.

32. Marotte M. Observation de remollissement cerebral gauche, avec lesion du nerf oculaire commun. *Union Medicale* 1853; 7:407–408.

33. Benedikt M. Tremblement avec paralyzie croisée du moteur oculaire commun. *Bull med* 1889; 3:547–548.

34. Weber HD. A contribution to the pathology of the crura cerebri. *Tr Med chir* 1863; 46:121–139.

35. Claude H. *Soc Neurol* 1912; Febr 1 and June 27.

36. Nothnagel H. Topische diagnostic der Gehirnkrankheiten. 1879; A Hirschwald.

37. Foix C, Masson A. Le syndrome de l'artere cerebrale posterior. *Press med* 1923; 31:361.

38. Parinaud H. Paralysie des movements asssocies des yeux. *Arch Neurol* 1883; 5:145.

39. Chaudhuri KR, Hu M. Central autonomic dysfunction. *Handb Clin Neurol* 2000; 75, 161–202.

40. Fisher CM, Curry HB. Pure motor hemiplegia of vascular origin. *Arch Neurol* 1965; 13:30–44.

41. Fisher CM. Capsular infarcts. The underlying vascular lesions. *Arch Neurol* 36:65–73.

42. Broca P. Remarques sur le siege de la faculte du language articule, suivies d'une observation d'apheme. *Bull Soc Anat* 1861; 6:330–357.

43. Mohr JP, Pessin MS, Finkelstein S, Funkenstein HH, Duncan GW, Davis KR. Broca aphasia: pathologic and clinical. *Neurology* 1978; 28:311–324.

44. Gerstmann J. Syndrome of finger agnosia, disorientation for right and left, agraphia and acalculia. *Arch Neurol Psychiatry* 1940; 44:398–408.

CHAPTER 2

Brain Neuroimaging

Eytan Raz, Nisha Mehta, Yvonne W. Lui

Neuroimaging employing computer tomography (CT) and magnetic resonance imaging (MRI) and other neuroimaging techniques have an essential role in the diagnosis and management of motor disorders. This chapter provides an in-depth overview of brain imaging techniques, correlative neuroanatomy, and clinicopathological neuroradiological correlations of the spectrum of CNS motor disorders.

NEUROIMAGING TECHNIQUES

Computed Tomography

This technology employs variable x-ray attenuation of the different types of brain tissues to generate axial images (Figure 1), a process that takes a few moments, precluding the need for sedation, and user-friendly in non-cooperative patients, children, and trauma victims. It readily identifies calcium deposits and acute blood products important in clue to diagnosis of several conditions. Although widely available and low in cost, its limitations include relatively low soft tissue contrast resolution, radiation exposure, and artifacts arising from bone and metallic foreign objects. It is nonetheless the imaging modality of choice when MRI is contraindicated as for example in patients with implantable devices such as a pacemaker.

Conventional and Functional Magnetic Resonance Imaging

This technology, which harnesses the intrinsic magnetic properties of atomic nuclei arising from an odd number of body protons or neutrons, has an ever expanding range of clinical indications. Depending upon the type of tissue in which they reside, proton nuclei will release energy upon placement in a strong external magnetic field and subjected to radiofrequency waves that can be spatially localized and converted into gray-scale images for neuroradiographic interpretation. Several MRI sequences combined to elucidate normal brain structure as well as pathological changes (Figure 2). Clinical protocols that optimally image the brain in multiple planes include T_1, and T_2 weighted, fluid attenuated inversion recovery (FLAIR) and diffusion weighted imaging (DWI) sequences. The clinical question at hand and the intrinsic sensitivities of specific imaging technique dictate other possible sequences that should be employed. For example, T_2 gradient echo images sensitive to paramagnetic substances such as some hemoglobin degradation products and mineralization, and DWI, sensitive to acute ischemia, infectious processes including prion-related Creutzfeld-Jacob disease (CJD), and hypercellular tumors (1); and diffusion tensor imaging (DTI), a more sophisticated form of DWI, can demonstrate the axonal organization of the brain which would otherwise be unappreciated employing conventional MRI (Figure 3). The administration of intravenous gadolinium followed by the acquisition of T_1-weighted sequences assesses the integrity of the blood brain barrier (BBB).

Blood-oxygen level dependent (BOLD)-functional MRI (fMRI) measures the relative concentration of capillary oxygenated hemoglobin in excess of the increased oxygen tissue demand that results from neural activity and the increase in cerebral blood flow (CBF) and related hemodynamics. Motor paradigms using fMRI can be employed to localize hand and foot motor cortical areas of particular importance to neurosurgeons in preparing patients for particular procedures, and researchers investigating a variety of neurodegenerative motor disorders (Figure 4).

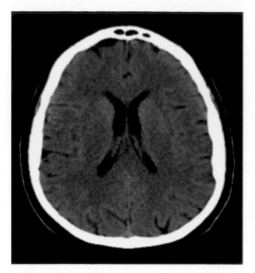

FIG. 1. Normal brain CT. Images are obtained at the level of the lateral ventricles demonstrates normal appearance of the brain.

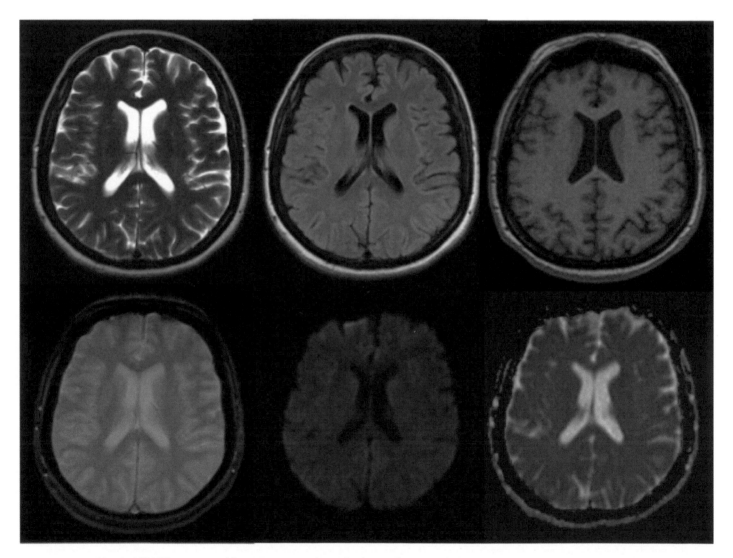

FIG. 2. Normal brain MRI. The protocol for MRI proceeding clockwise from top left includes T_2-, FLAIR, T_1-, T_2* gradient echo, diffusion and apparent diffusion coefficient (ADC) map images. The deep gray matter nuclei appear hypointense on T_1-weighted images and hyperintense on T_2-, FLAIR, and T_2*-weighted images compared to adjacent white matter.

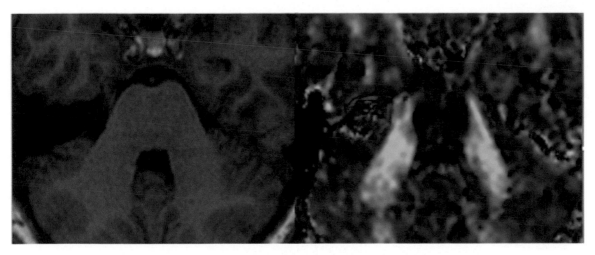

FIG. 3. Diffusion tensor imaging. Axial T₁-weighted images of the pons (left image) and color-coded orientation map (right image). The principal colors red, green, and blue represent fibers running left to right, anterior to posterior, and superior to inferior. The white matter, which appears homogeneous on the T₁-weighted images, is resolved into the complex architecture of separate bundles.

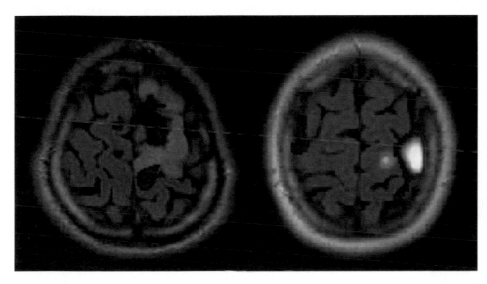

FIG. 4. Preoperative planning with fMRI. In the right image, the hand motor area is seen and activated laterally with respect to a glioblastoma multiforme. In the left image, the motor cortical area of the foot is located along the medial aspect of the precentral gyrus. Courtesy of Dr. Emmanuelle Tinelli, Sapienza University, Rome, Italy.

NEURORADIOLOGICAL CORRELATES OF MOTOR NEUROANATOMY

Most of the key anatomical structures involved in human motor function are well seen using neuroimaging. This section reviews salient motor radiographic CNS neuroanatomy.

Motor Pathways

The corticospinal tracts (CST) are the principal motor pathways of the brain that originates in each cerebral hemisphere from the fifth layer of mainly primary motor cortex, but also from premotor and supplementary motor areas. The central sulcus is an important landmark dividing the frontal lobe anteriorly from the parietal lobe posteriorly. While precise distinction between Brodmann areas is not possible with conventional neuroimaging, the central sulcus is readily identifiable. The motor cortex is organized spatially in such a manner that the area controlling the leg is medial and superior in the paracentral lobule, while the area that controls the arm lies inferiorly and laterally (2). The motor hand areas are recognized by an omega-shape on axial imaging located in the middle aspect of the precentral gyrus (Figure 5, 6). In certain instances the precision in neuroanatomical correlation can be so precise as to predict the neurological deficit with careful review of brain neuroimaging (3) (Figure 7). The CST is composed of the axons of upper motor neurons (UMN) that originate in the primary motor cortex and travel through the white matter of the centrum semiovale, coalescing in the corona radiate and continuing into the posterior limb of the internal capsule and cerebral peduncles of the midbrain (4). From there,

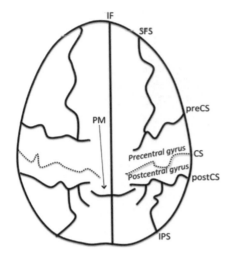

FIG. 5. The central sulcus. Abbreviations: superior frontal sulcus: SFS; precentral sulcus: preCS; central sulcus: CS; postcentral sulcus: postCS; pars marginalis: PM; interhemispheric fissure: IF; intraparietal sulcus: IPS. Courtesy of Dr. Marco Fiorelli, Sapienza University, Rome, Italy..

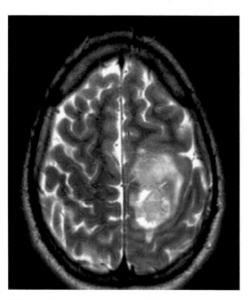

FIG. 6. Glioblastoma multiforme. Axial T_2-weighted image.

the tracts continue in the ventral aspect of the pons toward the medulla where most of the fibers decussate across the midline and continue caudally in the lateral funiculi of the spinal cord. Using DTI imaging and post-processing tractography, it is possible to isolate and depict the CST and other important neuroanatomical tracts (Figure 8).

Cranial Nerves

All but three of the 12 cranial nerves (CN) participate in motor function, including CN 3, 4, 5, 6, 7, 9, 10, 11, and 12 (Figure 9). Using high resolution heavily fluid sensitive sequences, it is possible to identify multiple portions of the CN.

Cerebral Deep Gray Matter and Cerebellum

The extrapyramidal system is a neural network involved in the coordination of movement, which is modulated by various brain structures, including the deep gray matter structures and the cerebellum, the evaluation of which is important in assessing motor function. The larger deep gray matter nuclei are readily identifiable on both CT and MRI (Figure 10). The gray matter is hyperdense on CT because of the higher density of cells compared to fatty axons present in white matter. Gray matter is hypointense on T_1-weighted MRI and hyperintense on T_2-weighted images compared with white matter. It is easy to distinguish the lenticular nucleus comprised of the globus pallidus medially and the putamen laterally, from the caudate nucleus, which is divided into a head that indents the frontal horn of the lateral ventricle, a body which constitutes the lateral wall of the lateral ventricles, and tail that follows the contour of the lateral ventricle. The thalami are ovoid structures oriented slightly obliquely facing the third ventricle in the median line. They are indirectly involved in motor control through connectivity with the cerebellum, pallidum, and reciprocal connections in motor and premotor cortex. The cerebello-thalamo-cortical tract coordinates motor synergies and postures. The substantia nigra, located in the midbrain, is divided into the pars reticulata and the pars compacta; the latter provides input to the basal ganglia supplying dopamine whereas the pars reticulata provides output to other brain structures. In normal subjects, components of the substantia nigra are discernible on MRI, depicted as hypointense areas in the posterior region of cerebral peduncle corresponding to the pars reticulata, whereas hyperintense areas between the pars reticulata and the red nucleus identify the pars compacta (5). The red nucleus is a rounded midbrain gray matter structure involved in motor coordination that is also readily identifiable on MRI in axial images of the brainstem (6). Each subthalamic nucleus is a small gray matter structure located ventrally to the thalamus, medial to the internal capsule, and dorsal to the substantia nigra,

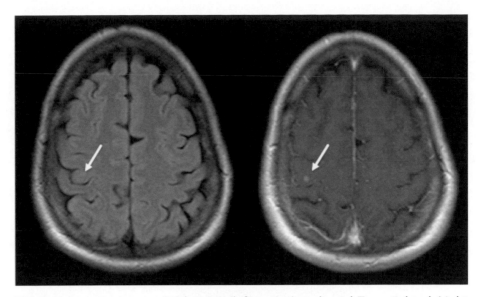

FIG. 7. Metastatic cancer. Axial FLAIR (left image) and axial T_1- weighted (right image) were obtained after the administration of intravenous contrast demonstrating a small focal lesion located in the right precentral gyrus.

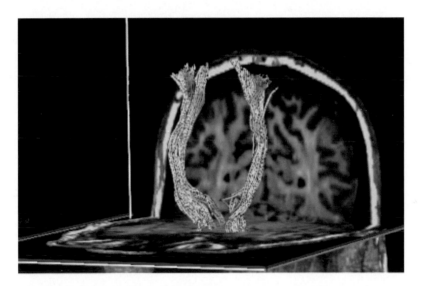

FIG. 8. Metastatic cancer. Axial FLAIR (left image) and axial T1- weighted (right image) were obtained in FIG. 8. Tractography of the bilateral corticospinal tracts superimposed on 3D T1-weighted images. Average fiber orientation is estimated from diffusion anisotropy at each pixel and a line is propagated from a pixel of interest following the fiber orientation with resultant bundles isolated and represented separately. After the administration of intravenous contrast demonstrating a small focal lesion located in the right precentralgyrus.

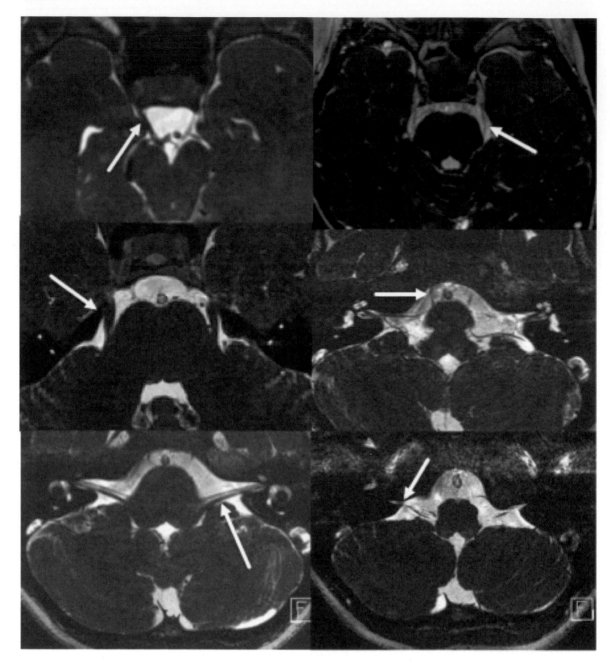

FIG. 9. Cranial nerves. High resolution fluid-sensitive 3D axial sequences proceeding clockwise from the upper left corner illustrating the normal appearance of the oculomotor, trochlear, trigeminal, abducens, facial, vestibulocochlear, and glossopharyngeal nerves.

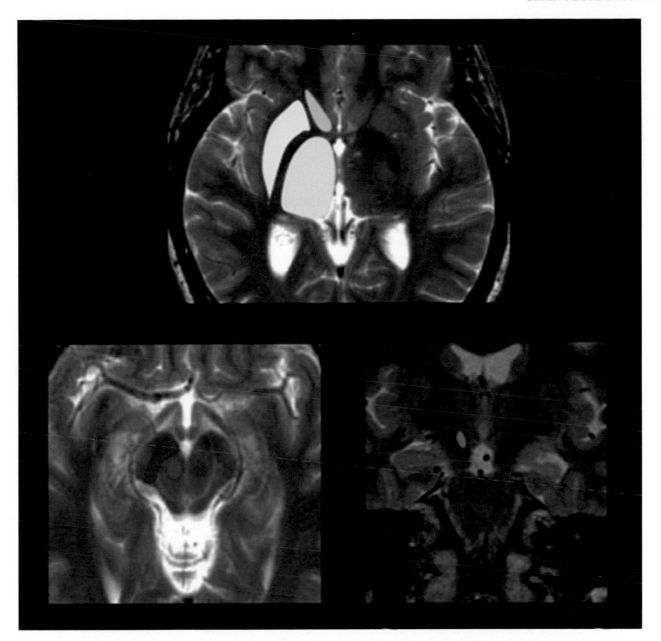

FIG. 10. Deep cerebral gray nuclei. The lenticular nucleus (colored yellow), the head of the caudate nucleus (colored green), the thalamus (colored light blue), substantia nigra (colored dark blue), red nucleus (colored red) and subthalamic nucleus (colored orange).

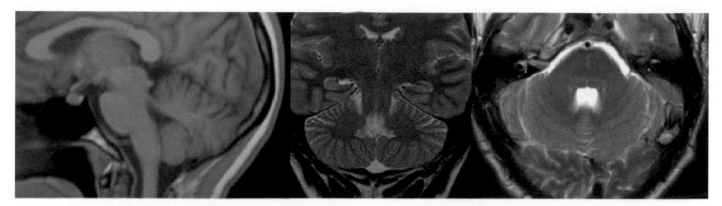

FIG. 11. The cerebellum. Proceeding top left to right, sagittal T_1-, and coronal T_2-weighted images demonstrate the cerebellum, middle cerebellar peduncles, folia, and vermis.

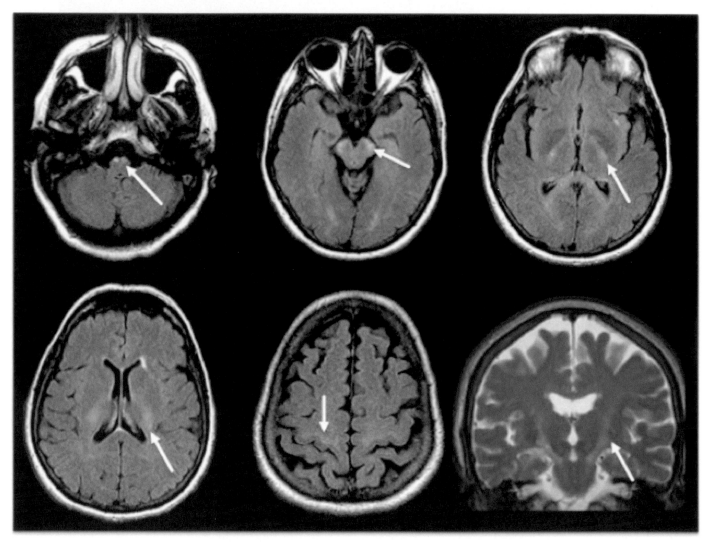

FIG. 12. Amyotrophic lateral sclerosis. Axial FLAIR coronal T_2-weighted MRI demonstrate abnormal hyperintensity of the corticospinal tracts at various cerebral and brainstem levels.

that is identifiable using high resolution coronal T_1 images (7). The cerebellum plays an important role in motor control. Located below the tentorium posterior to the brainstem, the two cerebellar hemispheres, tightly packed folia, midline vermis, and deep dentate nuclei are all readily identifiable on brain imaging. The cerebellum connects to the brain stem through the superior, middle, and inferior cerebellar peduncles (Figure 11) (8).

NEURODEGENERATIVE DISORDERS

Amyotrophic lateral sclerosis

This neurodegenerative disease of the motor neurons leads to the relentless progression of UMN and lower motor neuron (LMN) degeneration while sparing cognition. Pathologically, there is selective degeneration of motor neurons in the motor cortex, brainstem, and spine. The neuroimaging changes on MRI include characteristic hyperintense signals on T_2-weighted images in the CST extending from the motor cortex through the medulla due to diffuse bilateral Wallerian degeneration (Figure 12) (9). These findings are best seen on coronal images, which show the entirety of the CST on a single slice extending from the corona radiata to the brainstem (Figure 12) (10). Serial exams may show progressive sequential atrophy of the frontal, anterior temporal and parietal lobes (Figure 13). It is important to evaluating the CST for abnormal signals, keeping in mind that in normal individuals there can be reduced myelin staining along parietopontine tract fibers in the posterior portion of the posterior limb of the internal capsule compared to the remainder of the internal capsule, leading to abnormally appearing hyperintense signals on T_2-weighted and FLAIR images (11).

Huntington Disease

This neurodegenerative genetic disorder affects muscle coordination and cognitive function. Although symptoms can vary among affected individuals, the earliest manifestation is typically incoordinated body movements and unsteady gait, followed by progressive decline in cognitive abilities, and psychiatric disturbance leading to dementia. The pathological changes in Huntington disease (HD) affect the entire brain with disproportionate involvement of the caudate and putamen nuclei. The neuroimaging findings that occur late in the disease include the characteristic "box-car" appearance of the frontal horns of the lateral ventricles due to the atrophy of the caudate nuclei, with associated frontal lobe atrophy (Figure 14). Juvenile HD is associated with abnormal T_2-weighted signal intensity in the putamen and globus pallidus. The caudate nuclei can

be objectively assessed by measurement of the intercaudate distance, which is >2 centimeter (cm) HD compared to maximum of 1.2 cm in normal individuals; and the bicaudate ratio calculated by the intercaudate distance divided by the distance between the inner tables, that is usually >0.17 in HD compared to 0.12 in normal individuals (12). Chorea-acanthocytosis is another movement disorder that shows striatal shape alterations (13) with atrophy of the caudate and putamen nuclei on MRI (Figure 15).

Parkinson Disease

Affected individuals with Parkinson disease (PD) manifest initial symptoms of rigidity, tremor, bradykinesia and gait disturbance followed later by cognitive and behavioral disturbances, leading to dementia; other symptoms include sensory, sleep, and emotional problems. Although most patients with idiopathic onset are older than age 50, early onset is associated with genetic forms. The pathological basis is degeneration of dopaminergic neurons of the pars compacta of the substantia nigra. There is nonspecific atrophy on CT imaging, while MRI shows narrowing of the pars compacta with loss of the usual hyperintensity that progressively extends laterally to medially resulting in an ill-defined border between the pars compacta and red nucleus (Figure 16). Dopaminergic brain function measured by single photon emission tomography (SPECT) employing the radiotracers ioflupane (^{123}I) (DaTSCAN™) or iometopane (Dopascan™) and positron emission tomography (PET) employing fluorodeoxyglucose (^{18}F) shows reduced dopaminergic activity in the basal ganglia in PD. Advances in magnetic resonance volumetry, diffusion-weighted imaging, magnetization transfer imaging, and proton magnetic resonance spectroscopy (MRS) provide additional quantification of basal ganglia function in the differentiation of PD and atypical Parkinsonian disorders (APD) (14).

Multiple System Atrophy

Patients with multiple system atrophy (MSA) present in the sixth to seventh decade of life with movement, balance, and autonomic disturbances, although the hallmark of the disorder is an akinetic-rigid syndrome with slow initiation of movement, genitourinary disturbances and cerebellar ataxia. There are three recognized clinical subtypes termed: cerebellar (MSA-C), extrapyramidal (MSA-P), and autonomic (MSA-A). The pathological findings include loss of neurons and gliosis in the striatum, brainstem, and cerebellum. Neuroimaging differentiates MSA from PD by the demonstration of middle cerebellar peduncle and pontine atrophy and abnormal signal on MRI due to loss of transverse cerebellopontine fibers (15). The classical image of a hot-cross bun in MSA refers to the cruciform pontine hyperintensity seen in

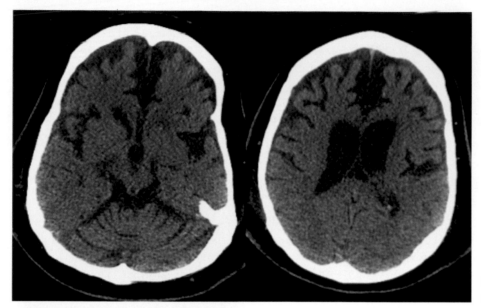

FIG. 13. Amyotrophic lateral sclerosis. CT shows selective frontal lobe atrophy.

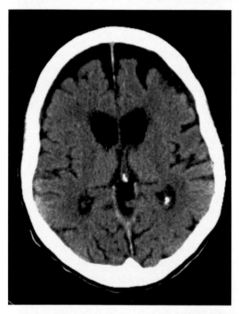

FIG. 14. Huntington disease. Axial CT image of the box-car appearance of the frontal horns of the lateral ventricles due to the atrophy of the caudate nuclei with associated frontal lobe atrophy.

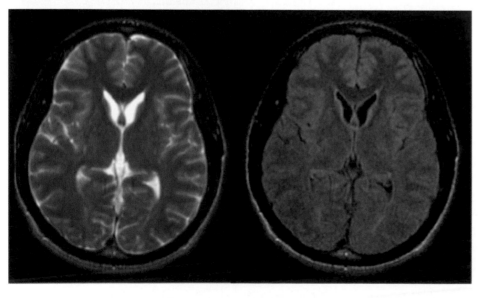

FIG. 15. Chorea acanthocytosis. Axial T$_2$-weighted (left image) and axial FLAIR (right image) show atrophy of the caudate nuclei and putamen.

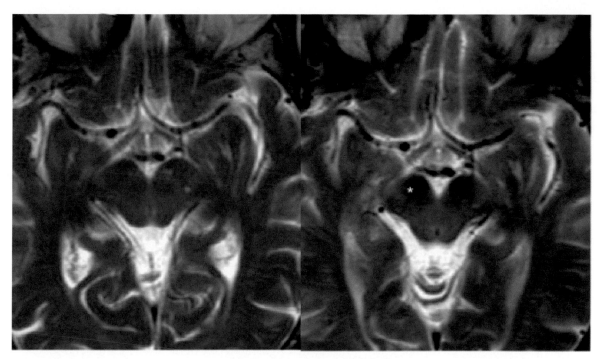

FIG. 16. Parkinson disease. Axial T_2-weighted (left image) demonstrates loss of distinction between the substantia nigra and the surrounding structures, with metallic deposit (*) associated with abnormal susceptibility-T_2-hypointense signal (right image) in the location of the substantia nigra associated with midbrain atrophy.

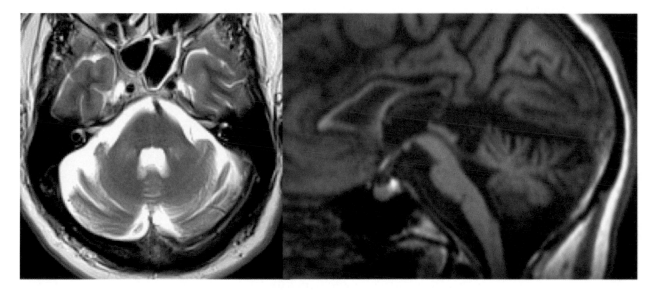

FIG. 17. Multiple system atrophy. Axial T2- (left image) and sagittal T1-weighted (right image) demonstrates cerebellar, middle cerebellar peduncles, and pontine atrophy, with T2 hyperintensity of the middle cerebellar peduncle and the hot-cross-bun sign visible on the axial image.

axial T_2-weighted MRI as a result of the loss of cerebellopontine fibers with sparing of CST and pontine tegmentum (Figure 17); atrophy of the putamen can also be seen. Although the hot cross bun sign is more common in MSA-C, similar to abnormal putamen signal intensity in MSA-P, neither have enough specificity to be used to reliably differentiate between the MSA subtypes (16).

Progressive Supranuclear Palsy

This atypical Parkinsonian disorder is associated with progressive axial rigidity, vertical gaze palsy, dysarthria, and dysphagia. Atypical patients can present with progressive apraxia of speech and nonfluent aphasia (17) and spastic paraparesis due to corticospinal tract degeneration (18); other reported patients have frontal lobe syndrome and subcortical dementia (19), corticobasal syndrome with increased cortical tau burden (20), or a Parkinsoniam syndrome initially difficult to differentiate from Parkinson disease (21). At least three pathogenic mutation in the 17q21.1 locus of the tau gene *MAPT* cause pathologically confirmed PSP phenotype, and variability in the MAPT gene is a major risk factor in the development of PSP. Neuropathological criteria for typical include a high density of neurofibrillary tangles and neuropil threads in the basal ganglia and brainstem with *tau*-positive astrocytes or their processes in involved areas, while atypical cases have an altered severity or distribution from this typical pattern (22). Conventional and advanced quantitative MR technologies improve the diagnostic accuracy of PSP. In addition to the expected finding of atrophy of the midbrain and the superior cerebellar peduncle, dilatation of the third ventricle and T_2-periacqueductal hyperintensities are often present. The average putaminal-apparent diffusion coefficient (putaminal-ADC$_{ave}$) ascertained on DWI, which is typically elevated in areas of the brain undergoing degeneration in DWI, was significantly increased in the PSP compared to patients with PD whose putaminal-ADC$_{ave}$ were similar to those of healthy subjects (23). A midbrain to pons area ratio <0.15; exaggerated concave lateral border of midbrain visible on axial MRI; and thinning of superior colliculus on sagittal MRI that contrasts with the normal convex shape, and is referred to as the penguin or hummingbird sign (Figure 18) (24, 25), add further accuracy to the neuroradiological diagnosis of PSP.

Corticobasal Degeneration

Corticobasal degeneration (CBD) is a sporadic neurodegenerative disorder of mid- to late-adult life characterized by basal ganglia dysfunction leading to asymmetrical Parkinsonism, rigidity, gait disturbances, and cortical dysfunction manifesting apraxia, aphasia, alien-limb phenomenon, and dementia often of the frontal lobe type. The term corticobasal syndrome (CBS) has been used interchangeably because the pathology of CBD is confirmed in about 50% of patients; moreover, these patients may be affected by other tauopathies such as Pick disease, PSP, Alzheimer or prion disease (18). While cortical atrophy, ballooned neurons, and degeneration of the substantia nigra have been emphasized, more recent neuropathological criteria for CBD include cortical and striatal tau-positive neuronal and glial lesions, especially astrocytic plaques and thread-like lesions in both white matter and gray matter, along with neuronal loss in focal cortical regions including the superior frontal superior parietal, and pre- and post-central gyri, and in the substantia nigra, differentiating CBD from other tauopathies (26). Notwithstanding, patients with pathologically confirmed CBD can have clinical presentations including progressive asymmetrical rigidity and apraxia, progressive aphasia, and frontal lobe dementia. Those with clinically diagnosed CBD demonstrate cortical atrophy, frequently asymmetric and mainly frontoparietal, putaminal hypointensity, and increased signal intensity in the motor cortex and subcortical white matter on T_2-weighted MRI, and have significantly increased putaminal-ADC$_{ave}$ on DWI that distinguishes them from PD but not from PSP (23).

Ataxia-Telangiectasia

Ataxia-telangiectasia (AT) is a multisystem autosomal recessive genetic disorder characterized by childhood-onset of cerebellar ataxia, oculocutaneous telangiectasia, recurrent bronchopulmonary infections, and varying states of immunodeficiency, with increased incidence of neoplasms. Neuroradiological evaluation by MRI shows vermian atrophy, inferior vermian hypoplasia, enlargement of the fourth ventricle and cisterna magna, best seen on sagittal T_1-weighted MRI, and cerebellar hemispheric atrophy on coronal T_1-weighted images (27).

Wilson Disease

Wilson disease (WD) is a disorder of copper metabolism that affects individuals of age 3 to 50 years due to abnormal deposition of copper in the brain and liver. The early neurologic sequelae include tremor, poor coordination, loss of fine motor control, micrographia, chorea, and choreoathetosis followed by a rigid dystonia syndrome of facial masking and gait disturbances. Other features include dysarthria, drooling, and swallowing difficulty, more common in older individuals. The neuropsychiatric manifestations include mood disturbance, depression, poor impulse control, changes in school performance, and deterioration of fine motor skills. Liver biopsy shows markedly increased copper content and cirrhosis. Brain MRI demonstrates atrophy and signal changes (28, 29), the former evident in T_1-weighted multiplanar images,

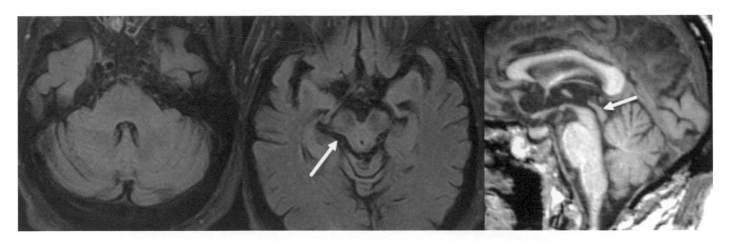

FIG. 18. Progressive supranuclear palsy. Axial FLAIR (left and middle images) and sagittal T$_1$-weighted (right side image) demonstrate marked midbrain atrophy with exaggerated concave lateral border (left arrows) and thinning of the superior colliculus (right arrow) in sagittal images. Courtesy of Drs. Patrizia Pantano and Cristina Piattella, Sapienza University, Rome, Italy.

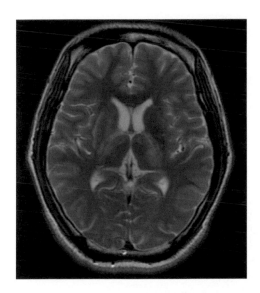

FIG. 19. Wilson disease. Axial T$_2$-weighted MRI demonstrates right outer putaminal and bilateral capsulo-thalamic hyperintensities (arrow).

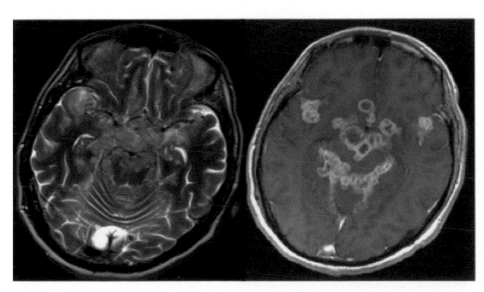

FIG. 20. Tuberculous cranial neuropathies. Axial T$_2$- (left image) and T$_1$-weighted (right image) after administration of intravenous contrast (right image) demonstrates ring-enhancing diffuse meningeal nodules in the suprasellar, ambient, middle cerebral artery, and superior cerebellar cisterns.

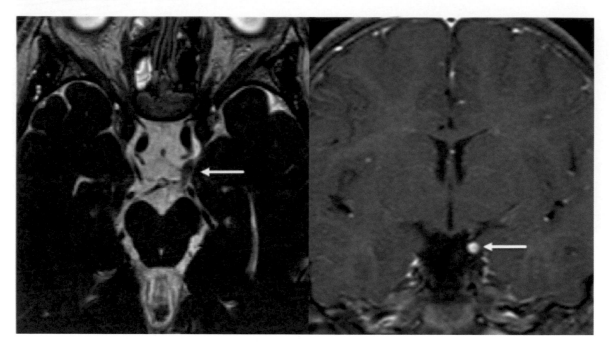

FIG. 21. Opthalmoplegic migraine. There is enlargement of the cisternal portion of the oculomotor nerve (left arrow) with enhancement (top arrow) after administration of intravenous contrast, associated with oculomotor palsy.

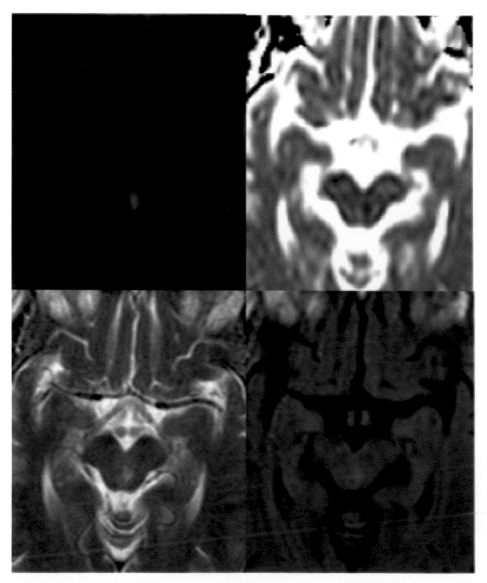

FIG. 22. Acute midbrain infarction in the region of the left oculomotor nerve. Proceeding clockwise from top left image, axial DWI, axial ADC map, axial T$_2$-weighted and FLAIR MRI show a punctate focus of acute infarction.

greatest in the cerebrum, followed by the brain stem and cerebellum; in a minority of patients, cerebellar and brainstem atrophy can be disproportionately severe compared to cerebral atrophy. Whereas the atrophy is often diffuse, the signal changes can be focal, multifocal, asymmetrical, or symmetrical in T_1-weighted and FLAIR axial sequences in the putamen, caudate, thalamus, globus pallidus, midbrain, and pons (Figure 19); abnormal brainstem hyperintensities in the midbrain lead to the face of giant panda sign. Proton and phosphorous MRS (*H MRS* and *P MRS*) have added further insight into the understanding of WD, wherein mean ratios of N-acetyl aspartate (NAA), a marker of neuronal integrity, and its ratio to choline (NAA/Cho) or creatinine (NAA/Cr) were both reduced in patients with WD compared to control indicating neuronal loss, or a biochemical correlate of a tissue-specific dysfunction even though the NAA/Cho and NAA/Cr ratios continue to decrease even after receiving copper reducing therapy (29).

Pantothenate Kinase-Associated Neurodegeneration

Neurodegeneration with brain iron accumulation is a genetic disorder caused by mutation in the PANK2 gene that encodes pantothenate kinase (PKAN) that leads to the clinical expression of dystonic postures, choreoathetosis, rigidity, dysarthria, tremor, and CST involvement leading to progressive spastic paraplegia. The classic form of PKAN presents in the first decade of life with rapidly progressing disease and loss of ambulation by 15 years. An atypical form has onset in the second decade with slower progression and maintenance of independent ambulation. An intermediate form has early onset and overall slow progression. The typical findings of neuroimaging include peripheral T2 hypointense signal changes due to iron deposition, and abnormal central hyperintense signals due to gliosis in the globus pallidus, creating the "eye of the tiger" sign.

Cranial Nerve Palsies

Cranial nerve palsies can be caused by inflammatory, vascular-ischemic mechanisms, direct-infectious and post-infectious autoimmune, neoplastic, genetic and systemic processes that are amenable to cranial neuroimaging. Evaluation of the muscles of the face, the neck and orbit is important to assess cranial nerve involvement. Infective leptomeningitis leads to multiple extra-axial cranial nerve palsies (Figure 20) whereas migraine headache prompts attention to a vascular-mediated cause (Figure 21). Unilateral ophthalmoparesis results from either intramedullary ischemic posterior midbrain infarction interrupting nuclear and exiting oculomotor nerve fibers (Figure 22) or extramedullary cavernous carotid aneurysmal compression (Figure 23); nerve sheath tumors lead to unilateral

cranial nerve paralysis in the territory of the cranial nerve within which they originate (Figure 24).

Congenital Muscular Dystrophy

This heterogeneous group of inherited disorders leads to fatal infantile hypotonia. Three types of congenital muscular dystrophy (CMD) are associated with major brain anomalies (30), further definable by brain neuroimaging, including Fukuyama CMD, Santavuori muscle-eye-brain (MEB) disease, and Walker-Warburg syndrome (WWS). Cobblestone cortex with cerebellar and brainstem hypoplasia, dysmorphic cerebellum, often accompanied by subcortical cerebellar cysts, and delayed myelination starting in the subcortical instead of the deep white matter occur in Fukuyama CMD. The brain malformations associated with WWS include ocular anomalies, cobblestone polymicrogyric brain tissue with ventriculomegaly, cephalocele, agenesis of corpus callosum, flat or Z-shaped brainstem with kinking of the pons, and vermian hypoplasia (Figure 25). The brain anomalies associated with Santavuori MEB disease are intermediate between Fukuyama and WWS. One extracranial imaging manifestations of CMD is fatty replacement of atrophic muscles.

MITOCHONDRIAL DISEASE

Mitochondrial disorders affect individuals of all ages, from infancy to adulthood lead to motor disorders lead to uncoupling of oxidative oxidative phosphorylation at various levels of the Krebs cycle and electron transport chain due to maternally inherited defects in mitochondrial DNA (mtDNA) or nuclear DNA (nDNA). Affected individuals present with diverse symptoms and signs of encephalomyopathy, manifested by lactic acidosis, hypotonia, myopathy, seizures, psychomotor delay, hearing loss, ataxia, spasticity, myoclonus, stroke-like episodes, and dystonia. Although neuroimaging employing MRI and MRS provides sensitive although often non-specific evidence of alterations in structure or function of deep and cortical gray matter and the state of global myelination, the distribution and specific pattern depend upon the specific disease phenotype. The finding of symmetrical or patchy hypointense signal changes on T_1-weighted brain images, and hyperintense signal changes T_2-, and FLAIR images in the deep gray matter conforming to the original shape of the nuclei are the commonest brain MRI findings in mitochondrial disease and should direct the further evaluation (31, 32).

Motor findings are encountered in Leigh syndrome and the syndromes of myoclonic epilepsy with ragged red fibers (MERRF) and mitochondrial encephalomyopathy with lactic acidosis and stroke-like episodes (MELAS). Leigh syndrome is an early onset progressive neurodegenerative

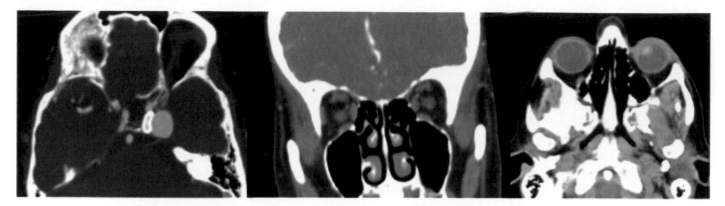

FIG. 23. Internal carotid artery aneurysm. Orbital CT imaging of the cavernous segment of the internal carotid artery shows an aneurysm with compression of the abducens nerve and atrophy of lateral rectus innervated muscle. The aneurysm has been treated with a flow-diverting stent.

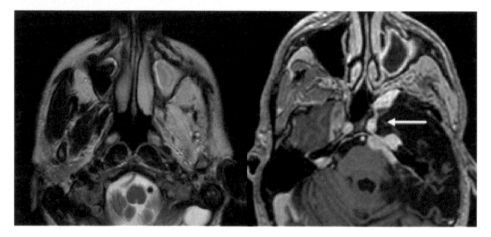

FIG. 24. Trigeminal schwannoma. Axial T_2-weighted (left image) shows unilateral hyperintensity of the external pterygoid, tensor veli palatini and masseter muscles. Postcontrast T_1-weighted (right image) demonstrate the trigeminal schwannoma located at the level of Meckel cave.

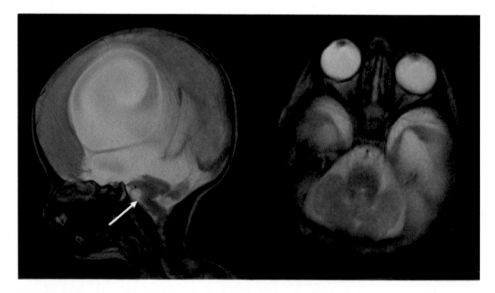

FIG. 25. Neonatal Walker-Warburg syndrome. Sagittal (left image) and axial T_2-weighted (right image) demonstrate ventriculomegaly, agenesis of corpus callosum, typical Z-shaped brainstem, kinking of the pons, and buphthalmos. (Courtesy of Dr. Sarah Milla, Pediatric Neuroradiology, NYU.)

disorder affecting oxidative phosphorylation. Although the neuropathological changes vary with the underlying gene defect, which may include focal bilateral lesions in the brainstem, thalamus, basal ganglia, cerebellum, and spinal cord associated with demyelination, gliosis, necrosis, spongiosis, and capillary proliferation, the associated clinical symptoms depend upon which areas of the CNS are involved. The latter include symptoms and signs of global developmental delay, feeding and swallowing difficulties, vomiting, spasticity, brainstem dysfunction, dystonia, abnormal eye movements, and multiorgan involvement. At least five separate mutations of different modes of inheritance mediated by X-linked (XL) recessive, autosomal recessive (AR), and mitochondrial maternal inheritance affecting complexes I, II, II, IV, and V of the respiratory chain have been described (33). Brain MRI demonstrates progressive bilateral areas of abnormal high signal intensity on T_2-weighted images in the basal ganglia and others typically in brainstem and periacqueductal gray matter (Figure 26).

The syndrome of MERRF presents with the primary features of myoclonus, seizures, cerebellar ataxia, and myopathy, however optic atrophy, sensorineural deafness, peripheral neuropathy, spasticity, and even dementia may be encountered. The underlying gene defect is an mtDNA mutation in the *tRNA* gene resulting in an A>G or T>C transition. Skeletal muscle biopsy shows RRF on Gomori trichrome muscle histochemistry. Neuroradiological findings include progressive atrophy of the cerebellum and cerebellar peduncles (Figure 27).

The syndrome of MELAS is also genetically heterogeneous with variable clinical phenotype. The disorder is associated with features of CNS involvement including seizures, hemiparesis, hemianopsia, cortical blindness, and episodic vomiting, caused by mutation in one of several pathogenic mitochondrial genes. In some patients with phenotypic MERRF/MELAS overlap, such that the relative amount of mutant mtDNA tRNA-lys in one point mutation gene correlated with the severity of the clinical presentation manifesting myoclonic epilepsy, sensorineural deafness, ataxia, and stroke-like episodes at presentation in a 3-generation kindred (34). The overlap of MERRF/MELAS was similarly manifested in a mother and daughter, the former of whom developed myoclonic jerks, generalized seizures and dementia 18 years before manifestation of later at age 37 years before development of blindness, stroke-like episodes, and bilateral occipital lobe atrophy on brain CT, consistent with MELAS. Her daughter who, at age 15, developed myoclonic seizures, generalized tonic-clonic seizures, paroxysmal hearing loss, ataxia, and elevated lactate levels in blood and CSF, cerebral atrophy and bilateral basal ganglia calcification on brain CT, and many RRF on muscle biopsy, remained MERRF (35). The pathophysiology of stroke in patients with MELAS is not well understood but there is

a postulated role for mitochondrial angiopathy, vascular dysfunction, and hyperemia mitochondrial-mediated cytopathic mechanisms resulting in energy failure and altered neuronal excitability (36). Measurement of a mitochondrial energy-generating system (MEGS) capacity, encompassing mitochondrial enzymatic oxidative phosphorylation reactions, which reflects overall mitochondrial function, correlates better in skeletal muscle tissue with mutation load than analysis of individual respiratory chain enzymatic activities of complex I, III, and IV (37).

Multiple Sclerosis

Multiple sclerosis is a chronic inflammatory–demyelinating CNS disorder affecting more than 400,000 persons in the United States and two million worldwide, of whom approximately 85% manifest a primary relapsing-remitting clinical disease. Unrecognized and, therefore, untreated, evolves along a secondary progressive course with steadily increasing disability; 20% of patients, the majority of whom have been treated, follow a relatively benign course (38, 39). The neuroradiological features of MS were recently reviewed (40). The prompt and accurate diagnosis of MS is based upon clinical recognition with MRI representing the most important objective diagnostic tool because of its unique sensitivity in fulfilling the two prerequisites of dissociation of the disease in time and space, showing abnormalities in up to 95% of patients with clinically definite MS (41). The typical lesions discerned on MRI are a reflection of the underlying pathology that includes focal demyelination, axonal injury, inflammation, gliosis, and remyelination, in a predominant periventricular and callososeptal location with a characteristic ovoid appearance and finger–like extensions into adjacent white matter. While hyper- and hypointense lesions noted on gadolinium-enhanced T_1 weighted sequences signify the counterparts of disease dissociation in time and space, they are not always seen simultaneously in a single examination of a new presentation, but together in an established patient (Figure 28) yield an accuracy of 80% in diagnosing clinically definite MS, exceeding that of prior investigators that emphasized the total number of lesions instead of their location and character (41, 42). The use of 3D fast FLAIR to obtain 1-mm sagittal sections through the brain reveal many periventricular and subcallosal lesions that might otherwise go undetected on conventional axial T_2-weighted sequences (43). Diffusion tensor imaging (DTI) is a valuable tool for investigating the variety of pathological features of T_2 visible lesions in which there may be variable degrees of tissue damage with more severely abnormal mean diffusivity equal to the magnitude of diffusion present in non-enhancing T1-hypointense lesions representing areas of irreversible tissue disruption, gliosis, and axonal loss; and consequent loss of the structural barrier to water diffusion (44). Investigators have described

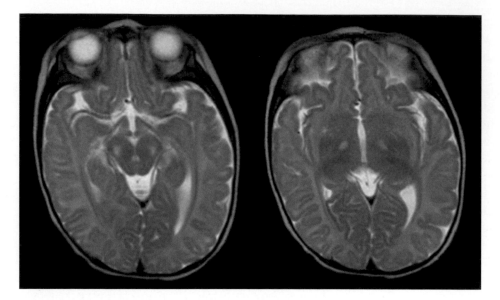

FIG. 26. Leigh disease. T$_2$-weighted (right image) of the basal ganglia; periaqueductal gray matter and midbrain (left image) show areas of abnormal high signal intensity.

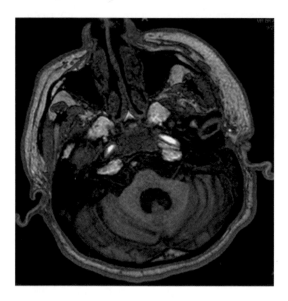

FIG. 27. The syndrome of mitochondrial encephalomyopathy with ragged-red fibers. Axial T$_1$-weighted MRI demonstrates marked atrophy of the cerebellar peduncles.

the application of DTI to detection of subtle or occult microscopic pathology in normal appearing white and gray matter (NAWM and NAGM) that show a steady and moderate increase of the apparent diffusion coefficient (ADC) which parallels the development of new contrast enhancing plaques, and tapers after cessation of enhancement suggesting that new lesions are preceded by progressive subtle tissue alterations beyond the resolution of conventional MRI (45). Global whole brain N-acetylaspartate (WBNAA) measurements employing ^1H MRS, a marker of neuronal integrity, parallels the course of axonal and neuronal damage in relapsing and remitting and benign forms of MS, the latter of which display up to 35% lower WBNAA levels than control subjects (46).

Ischemic Stroke

Acute stroke due to ischemic infarction (ACI) occurs when a cerebral artery is occluded and a core of brain tissue dies. However, surrounding the infarcted area is hypoperfused tissue at further risk of infarction termed the ischemic penumbra. Deep brain ischemia leads to a cascade of potentially reversible physiological changes, including the failure of Na$^+$/K$^+$ channels that results in cytotoxic edema with the net uptake of water in affected brain tissue and narrowing of the extracellular matrix due to reduction in Brownian molecular motion (47). It is precisely the goal of acute stroke management to accurately ascertain the site, size, age, and vascular territory of an ischemic lesion

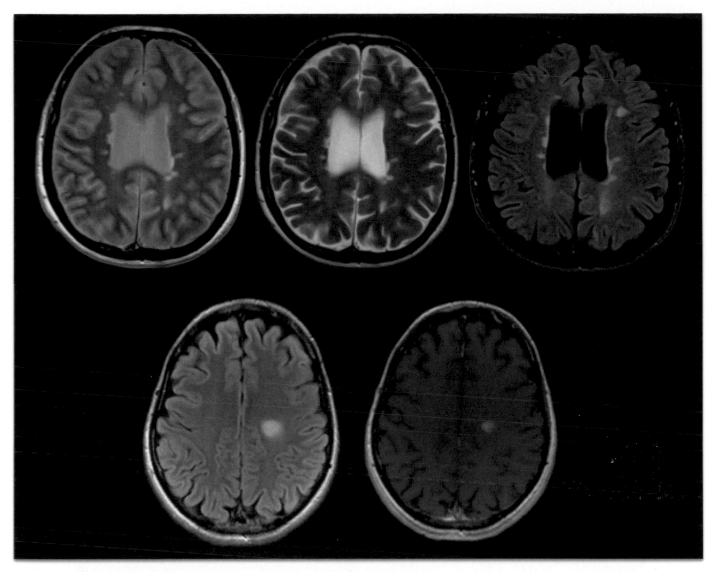

FIG. 28. Multiple sclerosis. Axial proton density, T$_2$-weighted and FLAIR (upper panel of images) demonstrate typical periventricular and subcortical white matter lesions with the major axis perpendicular to the lateral ventricles in a patient with long-standing disease. FLAIR and T$_1$-weighted (bottom images) demonstrate an enhancing demyelinating lesion in the centrum semiovale of another patient with a clinially isolated syndrome.

within hours of symptom onset by early brain neuroimaging, and to consider one of many treatment protocols, including intravenous recombinant tissue plasminogen activator (rtPA) and other measures to restore or improve perfusion, without which the infarcted core may continue to enlarge and progressively replace ischemic tissue in the penumbra (48). The categorization of subtypes of ischemic stroke, previously based primarily on risk factor profiles, clinical features of the stroke, and the findings on brain imaging employing CT and MRI, shifted in the direction of etiopathogenesis recognizing five essential types for the purposes of acute management in clinical trials, including large-artery atherosclerotic embolic and thrombotic (Figure 29), moderate and high-risk cardioembolic, small-vessel

occlusive lacunar (Figure 30), and those due to other (Figure 31) causes, and those undetermined or with negative or incomplete evaluations (49). Although non-contrast CT of the brain has been a criterion standard for evaluation of patients with suspected stroke, and to which all other brain imaging studies are compared, it is relatively insensitive in detecting acute and small cortical or subcortical infarctions especially in the posterior fossa. With the advent of rtPA treatment, there has been growing interest in using CT to identify subtle early signs of ischemic brain injury and arterial occlusion that might affect decisions about treatment beyond the tissue clock criteria based upon the most favorable outcome of the ischemic penumbra, which dictates that rtPA be administered within 3 hours of symptom onset for

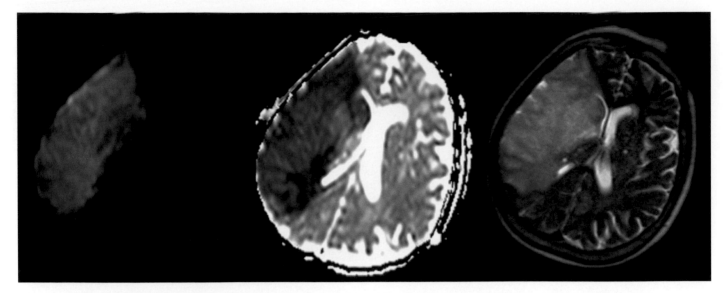

FIG. 29. Middle cerebral artery territory infarction. Proceeding left to right, diffusion weight imaging, ADC map, and T2-weighted MRI demonstrate massive ischemic infarction in the territory of the middle cerebral artery with diffusion restriction, reduced ADC signal, and right hemispheric mass effect.

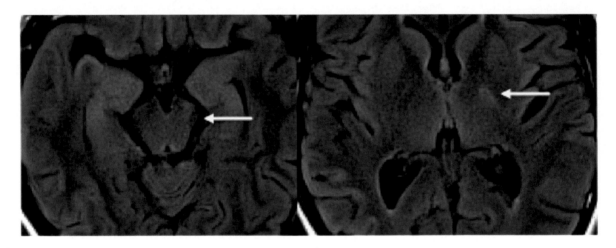

FIG. 30. Capsular lacunar motor infarction. Axial FLAIR MRI demonstrates a small internal capsule lacunar infarction (left image) and left cerebral peduncle (right image) atrophy consistent with Wallerian degeneration of the corticospinal tract.

the most favorable outcome, defined as complete or nearly complete neurological recovery 3 months after stroke onset (50). Recent advances in the use of perfusion-CT (PCT) employing whole-brain perfusion and dynamic perfusion that allow differentiation of reversible and irreversible ischemia and thus identification of the ischemic penumbra, and helical CT angiography (CTA) to rapidly and noninvasively evaluate vascular stenoses and occlusions, all have the advantage of rapid data acquisition and performance with conventional CT equipment available at most hospital centers, but the disadvantage of the need for iodine contrast and additional radiation exposure (51).

Although standard MRI sequences employing T1-, T_2-weighted, and proton density MRI are not superior to CT in the early detection of ischemic stroke or hematoma (52), DWI detects ischemic regions within minutes of symptoms as well as relatively small cortical and subcortical lesions including those of the brainstem and cerebellum, and valuable information about the vascular territory with a sensitivity and specificity that approaches 100% (51). The combination of perfusion-weighted imaging (PWI) that shows area of reduced cerebral perfusion with DWI to depict areas of irreversible injury, leads to mismatched areas, the PWI often being larger than DWI, representing

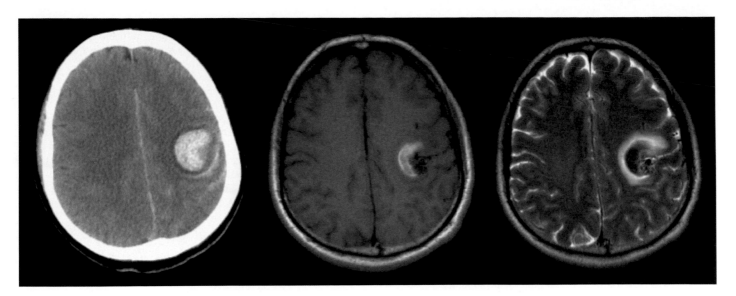

FIG. 31. Arteriovenous malformation. Proceeding left to right, CT shows a hemorrhagic cortical-subcortical lesion (left image) with hyperintense signal changes on T_1-weighted image and hypointense signal change on T_2-weighted images surrounding the AVM nidus.

the tissue at risk in the penumbra (52). Among 35 patients that underwent sequential neuroimaging for acute ischemic stroke that included DWI, PWI, T_2-weighted images, and MRA, 21 had a PWI/DWI mismatch and MRA evidence of vessel occlusion and T_2-weighted imaging indicative of

of infarction. They were subjected to rtPA within 3 hours of stroke onset and demonstrated significant recanalization and reduction in infarct size consistent with salvation of at-risk ischemic tissue (53).

REFERENCES

1. Schaefer PW, Grant PE, Gonzalez RG. Diffusion-weighted MR imaging of the brain. *Radiology* 2000; 217:331–345.
2. Lehéricy S, Duffau H, Cornu P, et al. Correspondence between functional magnetic resonance imaging somatotopy and individual brain anatomy of the central region: comparison with intraoperative stimulation in patients with brain tumors. *J Neurosurg* 2000; 92:589–598.
3. Hattingen E, Good C, Weidauer S, et al. Brain surface reformatted images for fast and easy localization of perirolandic lesions. *J Neurosurg* 2005; 102:302–310.
4. Jang SH. A review of corticospinal tract location at corona radiata and posterior limb of the internal capsule in human brain. NeuroRehabilitation 2009; 24:279–283; Lemon RN. Descending pathways in motor control. *Ann Rev Neurosci* 2008; 31:195–218.
5. Oikawa H, Sasaki M, Tamakawa Y, et al. The substantia nigra in Parkinson disease: proton density-weighted spin-echo and fast short inversion time inversion-recovery MR findings. *AJNR* 2002; 23:1747–1756.
6. Pu Y, Liu Y, Hou J, et al. Demonstration of the medullary lamellae of the human red nucleus with high-resolution gradient-echo MR imaging. *AJNR* 2000; 21:1243–1247.
7. Slavin KV, Thulborn KR, Wess C, et al. Direct visualization of the human subthalamic nucleus with 3T MR imaging. *AJNR* 2006; 27:80–84.
8. Schmahmann JD, Doyon J, McDonald D, et al. Three-dimensional MRI atlas of the human cerebellum in proportional stereotaxic space. *Neuroimage* 1999; 10:233–260.
9. Kalra S, Arnold D. Neuroimaging in amyotrophic lateral sclerosis. *Amyotrophic Lateral Sclerosis and Other Motor Neuron Disorders* 2003; 4:243–248.
10. Terao S, Sobue G, Yasuda T, et al. Magnetic resonance imaging of the corticospinal tracts in amyotrophic lateral sclerosis. *Journal of the Neurological Sciences* 1995; 133:66–72.
11. Mirowitz S, Sartor K, Gado M, et al. Focal signal-intensity variations in the posterior internal capsule: normal MR findings and distinction from pathologic findings. *Radiology* 1989; 172:535–539.
12. Aylward EH, Schwartz J, Machlin S, et al. Bicaudate ratio as a measure of caudate volume on MR images. *AJNR* 1991; 12:1217–1222.
13. Walterfang M, Looi JCL, Styner M, et al. Shape alterations in the striatum in chorea-acanthocytosis. *Psychiatry Res* 2011; 192:29–36.
14. Mahlknecht P, Hotter A, Hussl A, et al. Significance of MRI in diagnosis and differential diagnosis of Parkinson's disease. *Neurodegener Dis* 2010; 7:300–318.
15. Köllensperger M, Wenning GK. Assessing disease progression with MRI in atypical-parkinsonian disorders. *Mov Disord* 2009; 24 Suppl 2:S699–702.
16. Bhattacharya K, Saadia D, Eisenkraft B, et al. Brain magnetic

resonance imaging in multiple-system atrophy and Parkinson disease: a diagnostic algorithm. *Arch Neurol* 2002; 59:835–842.

17. Josephs KA, Boeve BF, Duffy JR, et al. Atypical progressive supranuclear palsy underlying progressive apraxia of speech and nonfluent aphasia. *Neurocase* 2005; 11:283–296.

18. Josephs KA, Katsus O, Beccano-Kelly DA, et al. Atypical progressive supranuclear palsy with corticospinal tract degeneration. *J Neuropathol Exp Neurol* 2006; 65:396–405.

19. Bigio EH, Brown DF, White CL 3rd. Progressive supranuclear palsy with dementia: cortical pathology. *J Neuropathol Exp Neurol* 1999; 58:359–364.

20. Tsubol Y, Josephs KA, Boeve BF, et al. Increased tau burden in the cortices of progressive supranuclear palsy presenting with corticobasal syndrome. *Mov Disord* 2005; 20:982–988.

21. Williams DR, de Silva R, Pavior DC, et al. Characteristics of two distinct clinical phenotypes in pathologically proven progressive supranuclear palsy: Richardson's syndrome and PSP-Parkinsonism. *Brain* 2005; 128:1247–1258.

22. Hauw J-J, Daniel SE, Dickson D, et al. Preliminary NINDS neuropathological criteria for Steel-Richardson-Olszewski syndrome (progressive supranuclear palsy). *Neurology* 1994; 44:2015–2019.

23. Rizzo G, Martinelli P, Manners D, et al. Diffusion-weighted brain imaging study of patients with clinical diagnosis of corticobasal degeneration, progressive supranuclear palsy and Parkinson's disease. *Brain* 2008; 131:2690–2700.

24. Quattrone A, Nicoletti G, Messina D, et al. MR imaging index for differentiation of progressive supranuclear palsy from Parkinson disease and the Parkinson variant of multiple system atrophy. *Radiology* 2008; 246:214–221.

25. Groschel K, Kastrup A, Litvan I, et al. Penguins and hummingbirds: midbrain atrophy in progressive supranuclear palsy. *Neurology* 2006; 66:949–950.

26. Dickson DW, Bergeron C, Chin SS, et al. Office of Rare Diseases neuropathological criteria for corticobasal degeneration. *J Neuropathol Exp Neurol* 2002; 61:935–946.

27. Farina L, Uggetti C, Ottolini A, et al. Ataxia-telangiectasia: MR and CT findings. *J Comput Asst Tomogr* 1994; 18:724–727.

28. Singh P, Ahluwalia A, Saggar K, et al. Wilson's disease: MRI features. *J Pediatr Neurosci* 2011; 6:27–28.

29. Sinha S, Taly AB, Ravishankar S, et al. Wilson's disease: 31P and 1H MR spectroscopy and clinical correlation. *Neuroradiology* 2010; 52:977–985.

30. Barkovich AJ. Neuroimaging manifestations and classification of congenital muscular dystrophies. *AJNR* 1998; 19:1389–1396.

31. Barkovich AJ, Good WV, Koch TK, et al. Mitochondrial disorders: analysis of their clinical and imaging characteristics. *AJNR* 1993; 14:1119–1137.

32. Saneto RP, Friedman SD, Shaw DWW. Neuroimaging of mitochondrial disease. *Mitochondrion* 2008; 8:396–413.

33. DiMauro S, Schon EA. Mitochondrial respiratory-chain diseases. *New Engl J Med* 2003; 348:2656–2668.

34. Zeviani M, Muntoni F, Savarese N, et al. A MERRF/MELAS overlap syndrome associated with a new point mutation in the mitochondrial DNA tRNA-lys gene. *Europ J Hum Genet* 1994; 1:80–87.

35. Nakamura M, Nakano S, Gato Y, et al. A novel point mutation in the mitochondrial tRNA (ser[UCN]) gene dectected in a family with MERRF/MELAS overlap syndrome. *Biochem Biophys Res Commun* 1995; 214:86–93.

36. Testai FD, Gorelick PB. Inherited metabolic disorders and stroke part 1: Fabry disease and mitochondrial myopathy, encephalopathy, lactic acidosis, and stroke-like episodes. *Arch Neurol* 2010; 67:19–24.

37. Janssen AJM, Schuelke M, Smeitink JAM. Muscle 3243A-G mutation load and capacity of the mitochondrial energy-generating system. *Ann Neurol* 2008; 63:473–481.

38. Weinshenker BG, Bass B, Rice GP, et al. The natural history of multiple sclerosis: a geographically based study. 1. Clinical course and disability. *Brain* 1989; 112:133–146.

39. Lublin FD, Reingold SC. Defining the clinical course of multiple sclerosis: results of an international survey. National Multiple Sclerosis Society (USA) Advisory Committee on Clinical Trials of New Agents in Multiple Sclerosis. *Neurology* 1996; 46:907–911.

40. Filippi M, Rocca MA. MR imaging of multiple sclerosis. *Radiology* 2011; 259:659–681.

41. Paty DW, Oger JJF, Kastrukoff LF, et al. MRI in the diagnosis of MS: a prospective study with comparison of clinical evaluation, evoked potentials, oligoclonal bands, and CT. *Neurology* 1988; 38:180–185.

42. Fazekas F, Offenbacher H, Fuchs S, et al. Criteria for an increased specificity of interpretation in elderly subjects with suspected multiple sclerosis. *Neurology* 1988; 38:1822–1825.

43. Hashemi RH, Bradley WG, Chen DY, et al. Suspected multiple sclerosis: MR imaging with a thin-section fast FLAIR pulse sequence. *Radiology* 1995; 196:505–510.

44. Inglese M, Bester M. Diffusion imaging in multiple sclerosis: research and clinical implications. *NMR Biomed* 2010; 23:865–872.

45. Werring DJ, Brassat D, Droogan AG, et al. The pathogenesis of lesions and normal-appearing white matter changes in multiple sclerosis: a serial diffusion MRI study. *Brain* 2000; 123:1667–1676.

46. Rigotti DJ, Gonen O, Grossman RI, et al. Global N-Acetyl-aspartate declines even in benign multiple sclerosis. *AJNR* 2011; 32:204–209.

47. Wintermark M, Fiebach J. Imaging of brain parenchyma in stroke. *Handb Clin Neurol* 2009; 94:1011–1019.

48. Wintermark M, Fiebach J. Imaging of brain parenchyma in stroke. *Handb Clin Neurol* 2009; 94:1011–1019.

49. Adams HP Jr, Bendixen BH, Kappelle LJ, et al. Classification of subtype or acute ischemic stroke. Definitions for use in a muticenter clinical trial. Toast. Trial of Org 10172 I Acute Stroke Treatment. *Stroke* 1993; 24:35–41.

50. The National Institute of Neurological Disorders and Stroke rt-PA Stroke Study Group. Tissue plasminogen activator for acute ischemic stroke. *N Engl J Med* 1995; 333:1581–1587.

51. Adams HP Jr, del Zoppo G, Alberts MJ, et al. Guidelines for the early management of adults with ischemic stroke. *Circulation* 2007; 115:e478–e534.

52. Mohr JP, Biller J, Hilal SK, et al. Magnetic resonance versus computed tomographic imaging in acute stroke. *Stroke* 1995; 26:807–812.

53. Jansen O, Schellinger P, Fiebach J, et al. Early recanalization in acute ischaemic stroke saves tissue at risk defined by MRI. *Lancet* 1999; 353:2036–2037.

CHAPTER 3

Spinal Cord Neuroimaging

Keivan Shifteh, Jacqueline A. Bello

Plain radiograph, also known as x-radiation or X-ray, computed tomography (CT), and myelography combined with X-ray and CT, often fail to demonstrate spinal cord lesions until gross expansion of the spinal cord or spinal canal occurs. Magnetic resonance imaging (MRI) produces images of the spinal cord with excellent anatomic detail. Its ability to noninvasively evaluate the spinal cord has revolutionized the diagnosis and treatment of spinal cord lesions. It is currently the imaging modality of choice for evaluating the spinal canal and its contents. The noninvasive and multiplanar capability of MRI makes it ideal for the detection, characterization, and determination of the extent of spinal cord lesions, including primary and metastatic tumors, inflammatory and infectious processes, vascular lesions, cystic lesions such as syringomyelia and hematomas, and congenital lesions associated with dysraphism. It is the preoperative imaging modality of choice to narrow differential diagnosis and guide surgical resection of lesions Although CT offers greater spatial resolution, MRI produces superior contrast resolution that facilitates characterization of spinal canal contents, including spinal cord parenchyma, cerebrospinal fluid (CSF), epidural fat that surrounds the thecal sac, vertebral venous structures, bone, and ligaments. Localization of a spinal lesion to the intramedullary, intradural extramedullary or extradural compartment employing MRI is the first step in establishment of a differential diagnosis.

A routine MRI examination of the spinal cord includes unenhanced sagittal and axial T_1-weighted spin-echo sequences utilizing short repetition time (TR), short echo time (TE) and T_2-weighted spin-echo sequences with long TR, and long echo time (TE). Sagittal short T1 inversion recovery (STIR) sequence are useful in detecting subtle intramedullary lesions, while gadolinium-enhanced sagittal

and axial T_1-weighted images should be performed for suspected tumors to better characterize them and delineate their extent. The normal anatomy of the spinal canal is easily discerned by MRI, revealing its oval shape and smooth contour, while the spinal cord, surrounded by CSF in the subarachnoid space yields intermediate signals on both T_1- and T_2-weighted images, and is separated from the epidural space by the dura (Figure 1).

This chapter illustrates the neuroradiologic imaging characteristics and clinical presentation of intramedullary neoplasms, including astrocytomas, ependymomas, hemangioblastomas, gangliogliomas, paragangliomas, dermoid tumors, intramedullary spinal cord metastasis (ISCM), and lymphoma, as well as non-neoplastic spinal cord lesions, among them multiple sclerosis (MS), transverse myelitis, syringomyelia, spinal cord infarction (SCI), and arteriovenous malformations (AVM). Neuroimaging of the spinal cord was recently reviewed (1).

NEOPLASMS OF THE SPINAL CORD

Spinal cord neoplasms account for 4% to 10% of central nervous system (CNS) tumors (2) as well as 20% of adult tumors and 35% of pediatric tumors (3). Most spinal cord tumors are malignant with 90% to 95% classified as gliomas, the majority of which are ependymomas and astrocytomas. Non-glial neoplasms, including hemangioblastomas, paragangliomas, metastases, lymphoma, and primitive neuroectodermal tumors (PNET) are less common. The majority of spinal cord neoplasms are low-grade lesions that enhance with contrast, and while the management and treatment of such tumors has progressed, the optimum standard of care

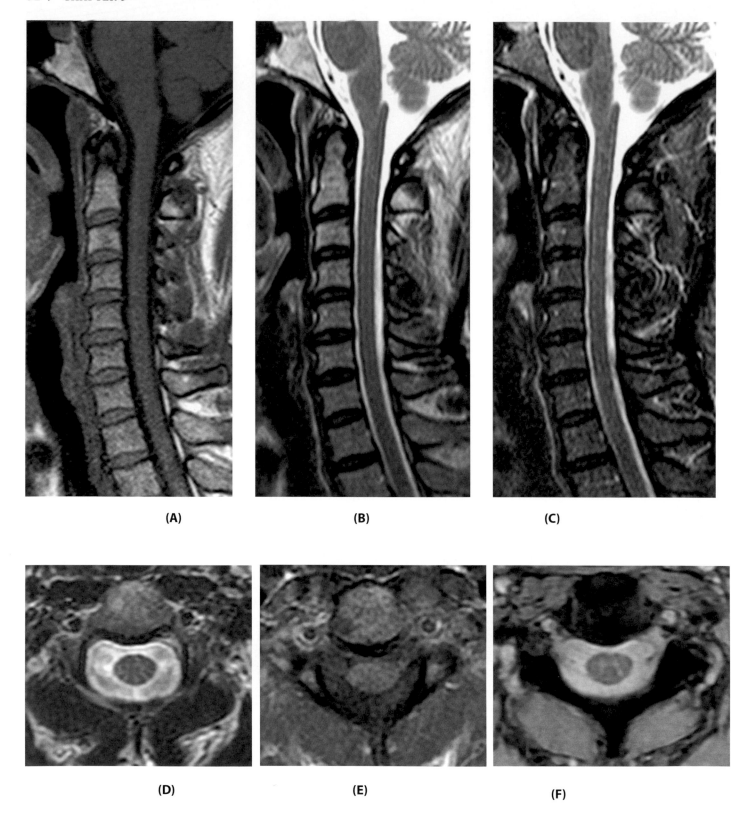

(A)　　　　　　　　**(B)**　　　　　　　　**(C)**

(D)　　　　　　　　**(E)**　　　　　　　　**(F)**

FIG. 1. (A–F). Normal anatomy. Sagittal T_1- and T_2-weighted STIR MRI, and axial T_1- and T_2-weighted images demonstrate normal anatomy of the cervical spine and cord.

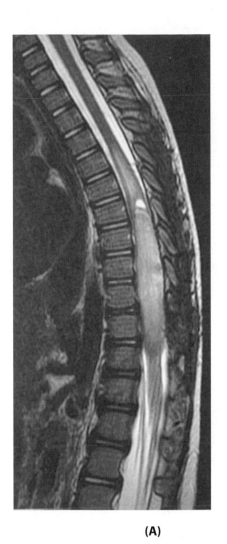
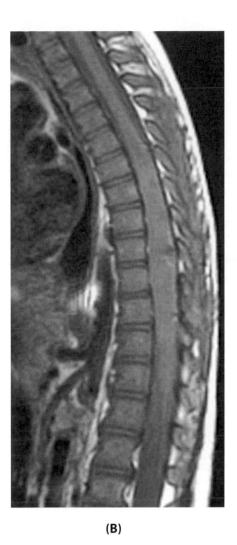
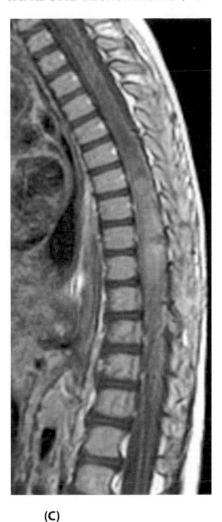

(A)   (B)   (C)

FIG. 2. (A–C). Astrocytoma. Sagittal T_2- and T_1-weighted pre- and post-contrast MRI demonstrate an infiltrate mass within the spinal cord with poorly-defined margins. The mass is hyperintense to the spinal cord signal on T_2-weighted images and isointense on T_1-weighted images with cord expansion and abnormal enhancement following administration of intravenous contrast.

remains unclear (4). Surgery is the mainstay of treatment and modern techniques have improved the extent of resection with completely excised tumors demonstrating the most favorable prognosis. The outcome of radiation therapy (RT) in the treatment of spinal cord gliomas is less certain than its brain counterpart; however, most authorities agree that it has a utility after biopsy or partial tumor resection to improve local control. Other mediating factors in the outcome of spinal cord gliomas include tumor pathology, patient age, extent of surgery, and adjunct treatment.

Three principles should be applied to the MRI evaluation of intramedullary spinal lesions, including the presence of expansion, enhancement, and concomitant cystic changes. The absence of expansion suggests a non-neoplastic process (5), while enhancement of a lesion, especially in two orthogonal planes after the intravenous administration of gadolinium contrast are important determinants of intramedullary spinal neoplasms (6-8) and essential in the planning of surgery. The absence of both spinal cord expansion and contrast enhancement does not exclude an intramedullary neoplasm. Both tumoral and non-tumoral cysts are associated with intramedullary spinal tumors, although non-tumoral cysts are typically located at the rostral or caudal pole of the solid tumor. Such cysts, which generally represent reactive dilatation of the central canal or hydromyelia do not enhance with contrast (9), while tumoral cysts, which may be part of the tumor, will demonstrate peripheral contrast enhancement.

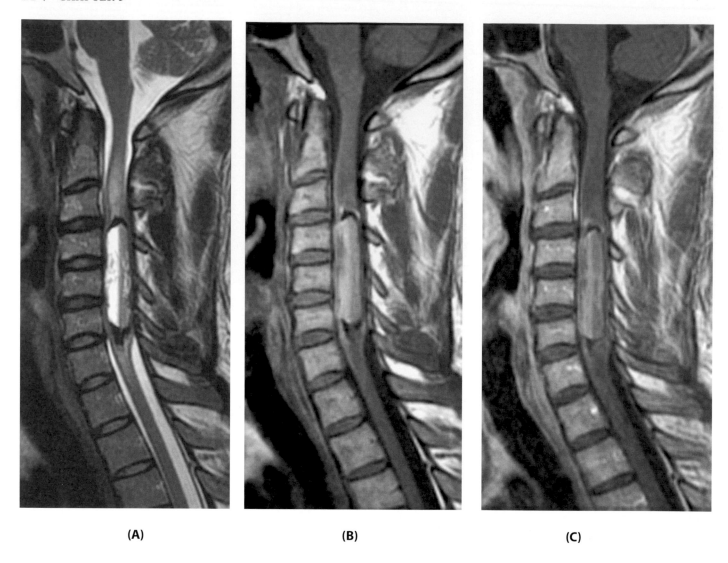

(A) **(B)** **(C)**

FIG. 3. (A–C). Ependymoma. Sagittal T_2- and T_1 pre- and post-contrast MRI demonstrate a well-defined mass with a fluid level expanding in the spinal cord. The rim of signal hypointensity noted on all sequences is due to hemosiderin deposition at the poles of the tumor, a classic finding for ependymoma.

Astrocytomas

Up to one-third of these tumors present in the spinal cord, and second in prevalence to ependymomas in adults, spinal astrocytomas are the most common pediatric intramedullary tumors. Unlike those of the brain, spinal cord astrocytomas are usually low-grade. They are a heterogeneous group of malignant neoplasms with varied clinical, radiographic, histological features, and prognosis. Morphologically, astrocytomas can be categorized into fibrillary and pilocytic subtypes with the former tending to undergo anaplasia and become progressively malignant. Grade I astrocytoma refers to the pilocytic type, a less aggressive tumor with better prognosis. Spinal cord pilocytic astrocytomas (PA), which account for 21% of pediatric intramedullary glial tumors (10), grow insidiously and evolve over months

to years often without neurologic deficit, occurring in order of frequency, in thoracic, cervical, and lumbar spinal segments. Fibrillary astrocytomas are further divided into well-differentiated astrocytoma (grade II), anaplastic astrocytoma (grade III), and glioblastoma (grade IV).

Neuroimaging reveals poorly defined margins in most tumors, with iso- to hypointense signals relative to the spinal cord on T_1-weighted images, and hyperintense signal intensities on T_2-weighted images (Figure 2), often in association with fusiform spinal cord expansion. Contrast enhancement of the tumor may be faint or prominent, and located in a central, peripheral, or diffuse distribution, however, non-enhancing spinal cord PA can also occur. The T_1 and T_2 signal intensity will vary depending upon the presence of secondary calcification and alterations in the structural complexity of cystic portions of tumor, the latter

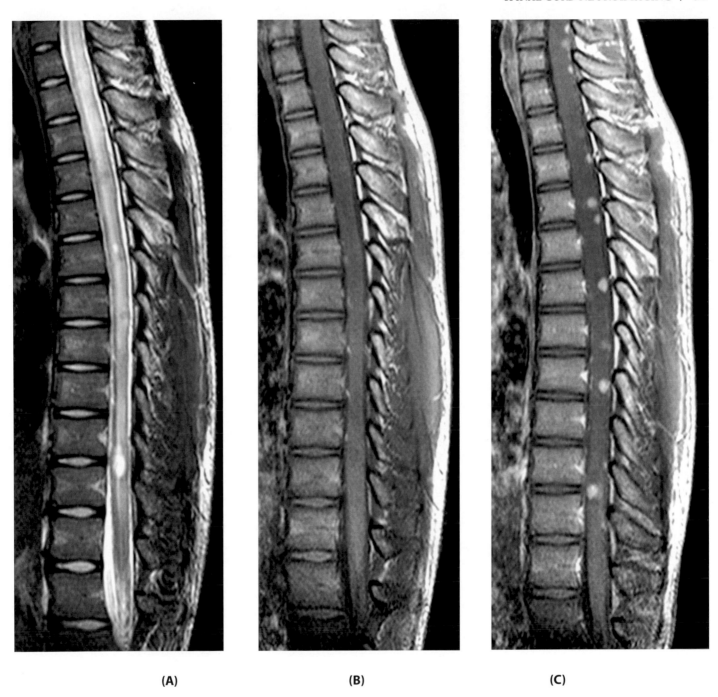

(A) (B) (C)

FIG. 4. (A–C). Hemangioblastoma. Sagittal T_2- and T_1-weighed pre- and post-contrast MRI demonstrate multiple nodular enhancing lesions throughout the spinal cord following the administration of intravenous contrast in this patient with Von Hippel-Lindau disease and hemangioblastomas. Extensive cord edema is seen on T_2-weighted images.

of which occurs in 25% to 38% of lesions. However, hemorrhage, necrosis, and hypervascularity are uncommon features. The length of spinal cord involvement is usually up to seven vertebral segments, and since astrocytomas arise from cord parenchyma and not from the central canal, they are located eccentrically within the posterior columns in more than one-half (57%) of patients; holocord astrocytomas, by

comparison, involve the entire cord. Although grade I and II astrocytomas may lack objective signs of neurologic dysfunction resulting in delayed detection, patients with grade III and IV lesions can present with rapidly progressive symptoms of shorter duration (11). Spinal cord astrocytomas typically produce local or radicular pain, paresthesia, and dysesthesia (12), compared to ependymomas, which usually present with dysesthesia (13). Motor dysfunction correlates with the level of the lesion, leading to prominent arm weakness and even torticollis in cervical lesions (12), and nearly always accompanies later stage cord lesions producing gait disturbances, spasticity, bowel and bladder incontinence (14); scoliosis may be an associated or incidental feature. Hydrocephalus, which indicates widespread leptomeningeal spread of the tumor, is more common in high-grade spinal astrocytomas than low-grade tumors (15), as well as 60% of preoperative intramedullary glioblastoma multiforme (16).

Ependymoma

Up to one-third of ependymomas present in the spinal cord and are the most common adult spinal glial tumor of the fourth and fifth decade, comprising 60% of primary spinal cord and filum terminale neoplasms (17). Unlike infiltrative astrocytomas, which typically undergo biopsy and partial resection, ependymomas are well circumscribed and easier to resect at surgery (18). Intramedullary ependymomas occur more often in women while myxopapillary ependymomas are encountered in younger men. Myxopapillary ependymomas are located in the conus and filum terminale, accounting for up to 90% of conus tumors overall (19), while intramedullary ependymomas are commonest in cervical and thoracic regions where they expand in the fusiform manner over three to four spinal segments; cystic formation is noted in up to 50% of tumors.

Patients with intraspinal ependymomas often present with mild symptoms without focal deficits, leading to a delay in neuroimaging and detection; subarachnoid hemorrhage is infrequently encountered. Two-thirds of patients complain of neck or back pain, and roughly one-half have a sensory deficit and motor weakness, with bowel or bladder dysfunction in about 15% of cases (13). The predominance of sensory symptoms noted in 85% of patients (13) is likely related to the central location of most tumors, although dominant motor symptoms are associated with very large tumors. Myxopapillary ependymoma presents with low back pain with or without radiculopathy, and variable leg weakness, and bladder and bowel dysfunction, depending upon the tumor extent and local compression (19).

Plain radiographic studies of patients with spinal ependymomas may show scoliosis, spinal canal widening, and scalloping of the vertebral bodies (20). However MRI typically reveals iso- or hypointense signals relative to spinal cord on T_1-weighted sequences, with signal hyperintensity on T_1-weighted images suggesting underlying hemorrhage, and T_2-weighted images demonstrating heterogeneous signal intensity. Intravenous administration of gadolinium typically shows well-defined margins and some degree of enhancement (21). A cap sign noted in 20% to 33%

of tumors presents as a rim of signal hypointensity on T_2-weighted images due to hemosiderin deposition at the poles of the tumor (Figure 3). Hemorrhage is common in ependymomas and other vascular tumors such as paragangliomas and hemangioblastomas (22), as was spinal cord edema noted in up to 60% of patients (23). Patients with myxopapillary ependymomas should undergo contrast-enhanced MRI of both the spine and brain even though solitary intramedullary lesions occur infrequently due to intracranial seeding.

Intraspinal ependymomas are believed to arise from ependymal cells of the central canal, conus, and filum terminale, and by direct CSF dissemination. Up to 76% of ependymomas occurred centrally in the spinal cord, consistent with a theoretical central ependymal cell origin, with singular, often polar, cysts reported in up to 84% of patients (24).

Given the slow growth and well-circumscribed nature of these tumors, early and wide surgical resection with or without post-operative RT in intramedullary ependymomas generally assures a favorable outcome that, despite long-term follow-up studies that might suggest otherwise, approaches five-year survival of 92% (25, 26). However, a less favorable prognosis can be seen in tumors that enlarge slowly in the cord with prominent motor imparting increased surgical risk (13).

Hemangioblastoma

These benign vascular tumors of the CNS are the most common primary posterior fossa neoplasm in adults but rarely present in the spinal cord. Hemangioblastomas account for approximately 1.6% to 5.8% of all spinal cord tumors and are associated with von Hippel Landau disease in up to one-third of patients (27), making MRI of the brain and spine an important recommended screening in patients with that family history. Up to one-third of patients have pain, sensory, or motor involvement, and as with other primary intramedullary spinal neoplasms, a long clinical course is generally the rule, with mean duration of symptom of up to 38 months. Up to one-third of patients have von Hippel Lindau syndrome with preceding retinal or cerebellar involvement. Rarely, these tumors may be a source of subarachnoid hemorrhage, hematomyelia, and polycythemia due to upregulation of erythropoietin (27).

Up to three-quarters of spinal hemangioblastomas are intramedullary, with solitary spinal lesions in 80% of patients, usually under age 40 years, presenting with impaired proprioception and multiple lesions characteristic of von Hippel Landau syndrome (Figure 4).

They appear as isointense signals on non-contrast enhanced T_1-weighted images, and hyperintense on

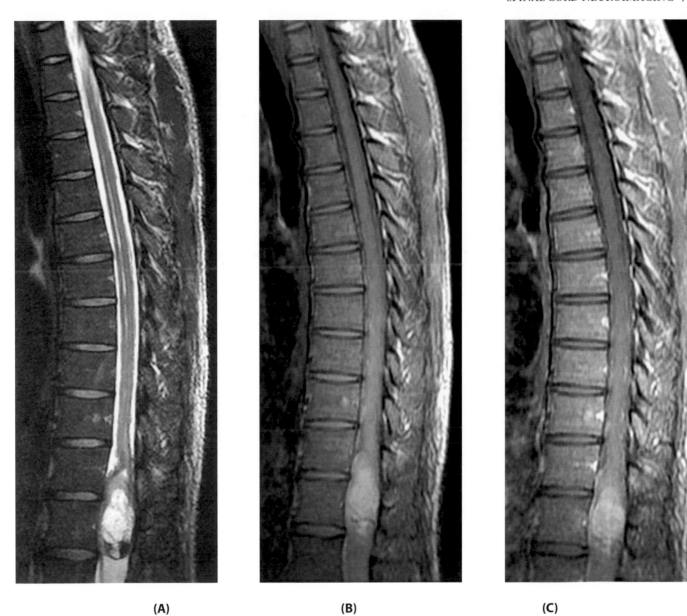

(A)   **(B)**   **(C)**

FIG. 5. (A–C). Ganglioglioma. Sagittal T_2- and T_1-weighted pre- and post-contrast MRI demonstrate a well-defined enhancing mass in the region of the conus. An area of hypointensity is noted within the lower pole of the mass on T_2-weighted images secondary to hemosiderin deposition. The mass is hyperintense on T_1-weighted images with mild enhancement following the administration of intravenous contrast.

T_2-weighted images, with characteristic signal voids due to flow within vascular structures, with variable diffuse spinal cord expansion and edema. Contrast-enhanced images show one or more intensely enhancing nodules within, or distinct from, the cyst wall. Some tumors will demonstrate a classic cystic mass with an enhancing mural nodule typical of cerebellar hemangioblastoma. Conventional spinal and magnetic resonance angiography (MRA) reveals a highly vascular mass with an intense prolonged tumor stain and prominent feeding arteries and draining veins.

Recognizing a well-defined mass of homogeneous signal intensity facilitates the differentiation of these lesions from spinal arteriovenous fistulae (SAF).

Intramedullary tumors can involve the intradural and extradural space, while extramedullary hemangioblastomas form attachments to the dorsal spinal cord pia and nerve roots (28). Hemangioblastomas result in spinal cord enlargement, and 55% are associated with cyst or syrinx (27). Complete removal of spinal hemangioblastomas alone (29), in association with von Hippel-Lindau syndrome

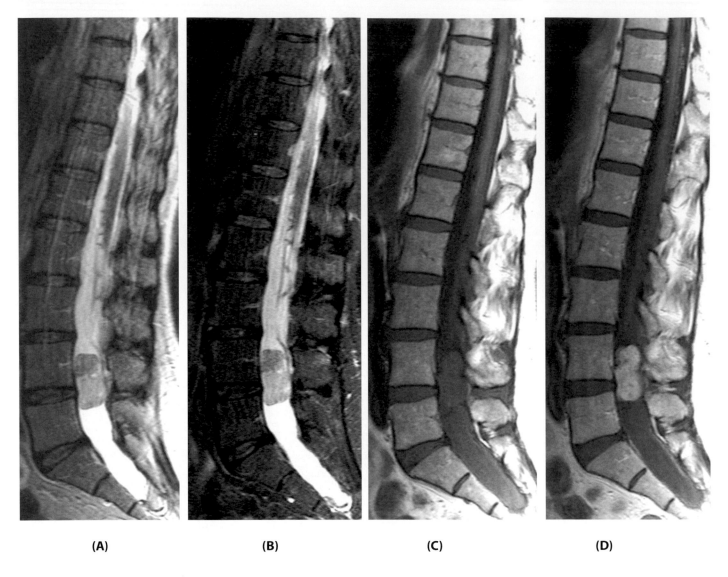

(A)   **(B)**   **(C)**   **(D)**

FIG. 6. (A–D). Paraganglioma. Sagittal T_2-weighted STIR, and T_1-weighted pre- and post-contrast MRI demonstrate a well-defined mass in the spinal canal at the L4-5 level. The mass demonstrates areas of hyperintensity on T_2-weighted images and is isointense to the conus signal on T_1-weighted images with abnormal enhancement following the administration of intravenous contrast. Prominent vessels are seen in the region of the conus extending to the lesion related to the hypervasculity of the lesions.

(30), and those complicated by intramedullary hemorrhage (31) have generally been accomplished with serious complications and low mortality, and complications in up to 7% of patients including residual neurological impairment or paraplegia (30) employing standard microsurgical operative techniques.

Gangliogliomas

These tumors, which are found throughout the CNS, constituting up to 6.25% of all primary CNS tumors and 1.1% of spinal tumors, although most often in the temporal lobes and supratentorial region of the brain, occur in patients of all ages, from 2.5 to 80 years, with a peak incidence in the first three decades of life without sex predominance (31). Affected patients most often present with back pain, limb weakness, and clinical signs of a progressive myelopathy with variable pain, motor and deficit, gait disturbance, and sphincter dysfunction (32), and a duration of symptoms that varies from months to up to five years (33)).

Neuroimaging employing MRI reveals hyperintense, isointense, hypointense, and heterogeneous signal changes on T_1-weighted images, and hyperintense signal changes on T_2-weighted images. The majority of spinal gangliogliomas enhance to some degree after contrast administration (33) (Figure 5), but up to 15% of tumor do not show typical enhancement. Surrounding edema is less common in spinal gangliogliomas than spinal ependymomas and astrocytomas (34), with more than eight spinal segments typically involved, resulting in lesion lengths twice those of astrocytoma and ependymoma. Osseous changes, which include remodeling and scoliosis and bone remodeling, occurs, respectively in 93% and 43% of patients, more commonly in gangliogliomas than in other spinal tumors (34).

These tumors, which are generally detected later in life due to characteristic slow growth with insidious progression of neurological deficit, can have eccentric location and contain tumor cysts (32). Their malignant potential is low, but such tumors can disseminate in the CNS. As a consequence of slow growth these tumors have an overall favorable prognosis with anticipated five-year and ten-year survivals, respectively, of 89% and 83%, and a recurrence rate of 27%, three to four times that of brain gangliogliomas (32).

Total surgical resection and close follow-up is the mainstay treatment with the extent of resection determining outcome; the role of chemotherapy is unclear, however tumor recurrence warranting a second resection should lead to consideration of adjuvant RT.

Paraganglioma

These tumors, which account for 0.3% of all neoplasms (35) arise from paraganglia cells closely associated with the autonomic nervous system with adrenal and extra-adrenal components; tumors arising from the first component are termed *pheochromocytomas,* and those originating from extra-adrenal sites are termed *paragangliomas*. Tumors of the carotid body and jugular foramen, respectively, termed *carotid body* and *glomus jugulare tumors*, account for 90% of paragangliomas.

Affected patients present with low back pain and sciatic pain, and as with other spinal neoplasms, with a prolonged duration of symptoms of four years. These tumors occur more commonly in men with a mean age of 46 years at presentation.

Paragangliomas of the spinal canal are usually found in the intradural and extramedullary compartment with an affinity for the cauda equina and filum terminale (36).

Neuroimaging employing MRI can reveal a well-circumscribed mass with isointense signals relative to the spinal cord on T_1-weighted images, and iso- to hyperintense signal changes on T_2-weighted images. Hemorrhage commonly occurs, demonstrating a low-signal-intensity rim, or cap sign on T_2-weighted images. Intense contrast enhancement of these highly vascular lesions is a constant finding. Serpentine structures along the surface and within the tumor nodule typically demonstrate signal void due to flow

(Figure 6). Catheter angiography of paragangliomas demonstrate intense early blushing that persists into the early venous and late arterial phases.

Complete surgical excision is the recommended therapy for paragangliomas, preceded by preoperative embolization in lesions greater than three centimeters (cm) in size. Since most paragangliomas are relatively radioresistant, RT is not recommended as primary therapy but may have a palliative role in those with unresectable tumors and residual post-operative lesions, and as a primary treatment modality in patients deemed not to be suitable candidates, or, who decline surgery (36).

Dermoid Tumors

These cysts, which account for 1.1% of all intraspinal tumors comprising fluid, soft tissue, calcium, and fat are benign congenital, slow-growing tumors that cause symptoms in adulthood (37) with slight male predominance. Arising from ectopic embryonic ectodermal rests within the spinal canal at the time of neural tube closure, 60% occur in an extramedullary location and 40% intramedullary. With only 21% of dermoid tumors spinal in location, one-half occur in the upper thoracic region, with a nearly equal remaining proportion in the cervical and lumbosacral regions. Dermoid tumors are associated with dysraphism and dorsal dermal sinus in 20% of lesions, and may be associated with other bony malformations and tethering of the spinal cord (38). Affected patients most often present with slowly progressive radiculopathy, myelopathy, and cauda equina syndrome.

Neuroimaging employing MRI typically demonstrates heterogeneous signal intensity changes due to varying amounts of soft tissue, fat, calcium, and hemorrhage. High signal changes from fat tissue seen on T_1-weighted images relate to the lipid component (Figure 7). Fat suppression MRI techniques confirm the diagnosis with enhancement of the soft tissue component after contrast administration. The differential diagnosis of the neuroimaging findings of a dermoid tumor includes teratoma and lipoma due to the high lipid content of the lesion.

Dermoid tumors may have two distinct portions, a lipid and a more solid or more fluid part. They can rupture, spreading content throughout the CSF spaces, leading to hydrocephalus, meningitis, and arachnoiditis. Rupture can occur spontaneously, with trauma, and after surgical manipulation. However, given the indolent benign nature of the majority of lesions, conservative management, especially of asymptomatic lesions, is usually recommended (39).

Metastasis

Up to 3% of spinal cord neoplasms are ISCM, with most discovered incidentally at postmortem examination (40). Nearly

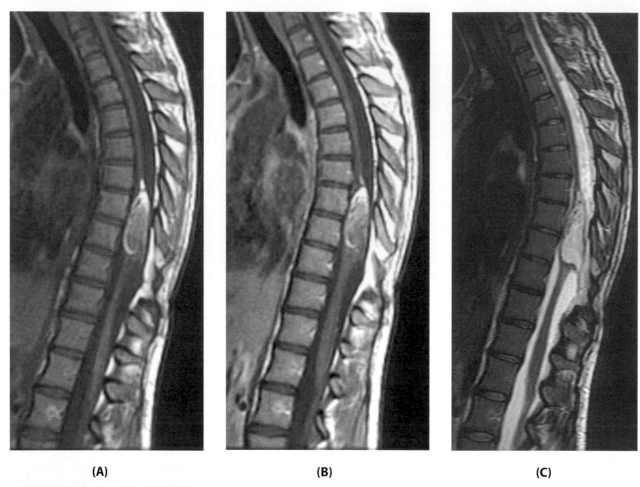

(A)

(B)

(C)

(D)

FIG. 7. (A–D). Dermoid. Sagittal T$_1$-weighted pre- and post-contrast; sagittal T$_2$-weighted and STIR MRI demonstrates a well-defined lesion within the spinal cord with areas of hyperintensity on T$_1$-weighted images representing fat that saturates the STIR sequence.

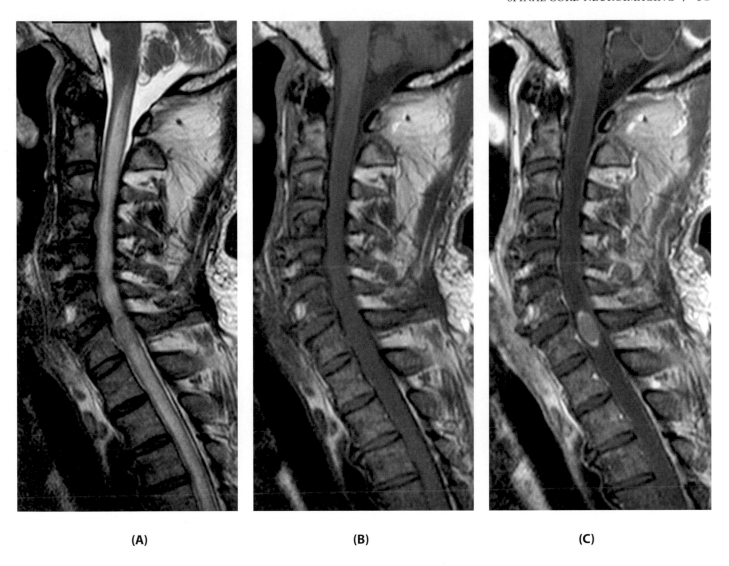

(A)   (B)   (C)

FIG. 8. (A–C). Metastases. Sagittal T_2- and T_1-weighted pre- and post-contrast MRI demonstrates a well-defined mass that is isointense to the spinal cord signal on T_2- and T_1-weighted images with abnormal enhancement following the administration of intravenous contrast. Extensive edema is present throughout the visualized portion of the spinal cord.

50% are from a primary lung cancer with other primary tumors of origin including breast, colorectal, melanoma, and lymphoma, however a primary source is unknown in 5% of affected patients (5). The arterial supply and Batson venous plexus are possible spreading routes (41).

Most affected patients with ISCM will complain of pain, paresthesia, weakness, and bowel and bladder dysfunction in 60%, and those with a rapidly deteriorating neurological condition, especially those with myelopathy, hemicord syndrome of Brown-Sequard syndrome, and elderly patients.

Neuroimaging employing MRI demonstrates the intramedullary lesion, with spinal cord expansion and associated edema disproportionate to the underlying solitary tumor that extends over several vertebral segments. The lesion demonstrates hypointense signal changes on T_1-weighted images,

hyperintense signal changes on T_2-weighted images with enhancement after contrast administration (Figure 8). These MRI findings are not specific for ISCM and may be seen in hemangioblastomas, MS, and acute disseminated encephalo-myelitis (ADEM), sarcoidosis, and transverse myelitis.

A clinicopathological study of 13 patients disclosed two distinct patterns of spinal cord involvement indicating spread of tumor to the cord by two different routes. In nine cases a deep ISCM unassociated with leptomeningeal carcinomatosis suggested hematogenous spread from a remote primary, while four cases with focal or multifocal direct extension of leptomeningeal metastatic tumor across the pia into the spinal cord parenchyma (40).

RT with corticosteroids is effective palliative therapy, however, when ISCM is the outcome of rapidly progressing

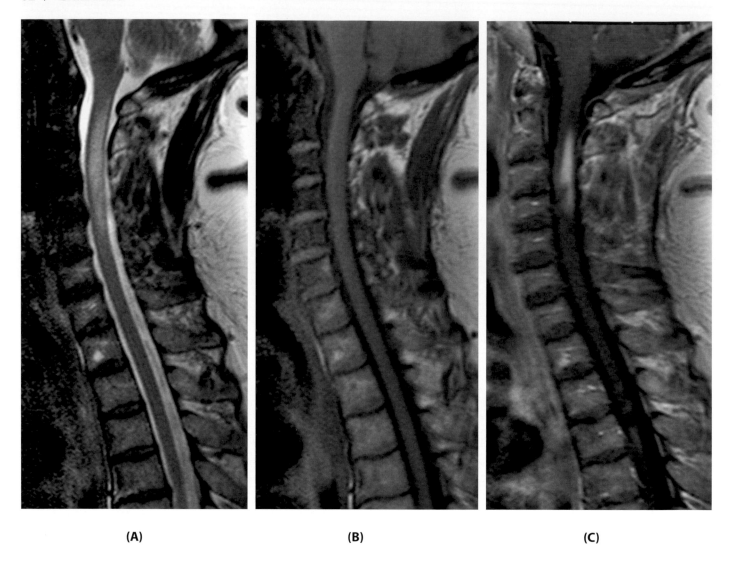

(A)　　　　　　　　　　(B)　　　　　　　　　　(C)

FIG. 9. (A–C). Lymphoma. Sagittal T_2- and T_1-weighted pre- and post-contrast MRI demonstrate edema within the spinal cord from C1 to C4. Abnormal enhancement following the administration of intravenous contrast is noted within the spinal cord.

systemic malignancy, the underlying cancer dictates an overall poor prognosis and short life expectancy (42). There are isolated reports of the successful removal of ISCM employing microsurgical resection (43, 44). By comparison, epidural spinal cord compression arising from metastatic breast, lung, and kidney tumors, with preferential involvement of the thoracic region, and a similar presentation of pain, motor, and sensory deficits similar to ISCM, has a relatively favorable prognosis with RT alone or in combination with decompressive laminectomy, with up to 75% of living patients remaining ambulatory at six months (45).

Lymphoma

Intramedullary spinal lymphoma can be a primary tumor or secondary to systemic lymphoma, which is estimated to occur, respectively, with a frequency of between one and three percent overall in the latter, often with leptomeningeal involvement at the time of diagnosis (46), and so infrequently as a manifestation of primary CNS lymphoma (PCNSL), that only 14 histologically verified patients have been reported (47). Although PCNSL is the most frequent primary brain tumor in patients with acquired immune deficiency syndrome (AIDS), only two patients had underlying immune disorders, and the clinical presentation of affected patients correlated with tumor site in the spinal cord that included sensory, motor, gait and bladder disturbances (47, 48), owing to a lesion in the cervical, thoracic, or cervicothoracic regions in 11 patients, and in the thoracolumbar, lumbar, or entire cord by regions, or the entire cord by MRI, in all so-studied (47). The findings of MRI in spinal PCNSL include isointense signal changes relative to spinal cord signal on T_1-weighted images and hyperintense signal changes on T_2-weighted images, with enhancement intensely after contrast administration (Figure 9) that may be focal, multicentric, irregular, or homogenous. While these findings, which are nonspecific for spinal PCSNL and include the possible diagnosis of glioma, metastatic tumor, and CNS inflammatory disease such as transverse myelitis, the latter of which is made more likely when the neuroradiological findings are combined with moderate non-malignant cell pleocytosis. The diagnosis of spinal PCNSL should be confirmed whenever possible by biopsy. High-dose methotrexate chemotherapy alone, or in combination with radiotherapy, substantially prolongs survival beyond 30 months (49); corticosteroids may have short-time benefit (50), suggesting the importance of early diagnosis and initiation of treatment.

NON-NEOPLASTIC LESIONS

Multiple Sclerosis

Multiple sclerosis is the most common CNS inflammatory disorder, affecting young adults in Western countries with pronounced inter-individual variability and unpredictable clinical course, from neurologically asymptomatic to severe sequela and disability (51). Brain MRI contributes to the diagnosis and management of MS including the monitoring of treatment response and prediction of disease progression (51), and is the most sensitive paraclinical test showing abnormalities in up to 95% of patients with clinically definite MS (52). Early criteria for the diagnosis of MS emphasized the total number of brain lesions (53); however, more recent appraisals emphasized the sort of lesion and where they were found (54). Of four possible MRI parameters, gadolinium-enhancement, infratentorial, juxtacortical, and periventricular lesions, which were investigated to build a regression model with a diagnostic accuracy of 80% for developing MS (54), only two emerged as most predictive, abnormal gadolinium-enhancement and juxtacortical lesions. The former suggests lesions involved in the phase of inflammation and active demyelination, while the latter, most evident on FLAIR sequences, relates to involved myelinated axons (54). Callosal and subcallosal lesions, long considered to be relevant to the neuroradiologic diagnosis of MS and probably undetected on conventional axial T_2-weighted sequences, are more readily visualized on 1-mm sagittal sections using 3D fast FLAIR sequences.

The concurrence of optic neuritis and spinal cord involvement without brain involvement per se, constitutes neuromyelitis optica (NMO). The clinical presentation of MS varies with the segment and extent of spinal cord involvement in the transverse and longitudinal planes. However, symptoms and signs of myelopathy are the most salient in those with spinal cord involvement alone or in association with lesions of the brain, manifesting hyperreflexia, clonus, and Babinski signs, long-tract sensory signs, cerebellar disturbances, and bladder, bowel and sexual dysfunction. Up to 85% of patients have a classical relapsing-remitting course defined by periods of new or worsening neurologic dysfunction followed by partial or complete clinical recovery. Spinal lesions occur most often in the cervical cord but are also common in thoracic cord and conus regions. Exclusive spinal cord involvement occurs in 2% to 10% of patients.

The initial clinical demyelinating event in the brain and spinal cord can be established with certainty by employing MRI, providing a baseline for comparison to subsequent clinical episodes. Neuroradiological studies employing spinal MRI in MS reveal eccentric peripherally located plaques that do not respect the boundary between white and gray matter. Such lesions typically involve the dorsolateral regions of the cord and occupy less than one-half the cross-sectional area of the spinal cord, with most lesions spanning fewer than two vertebral segments (Figure 10). The plaques appear as well- or ill-defined lesions of signal hyperintensity on T_2-weighted images, while larger active lesions may be associated with spinal cord expansion and edema. Chronic lesions will often result in focal cord atrophy. Acute and sub-acute demyelinating plaques will demonstrate enhancement for two to eight weeks after onset while chronic lesions fail to contrast enhance. Acute MS can mimic a spinal cord neoplasm, especially when there are peri-lesional cysts and hemorrhage, as well as acute disseminated encephalomyelitis (ADEM), infarction, and sarcoidosis, emphasizing the importance of correlating imaging with both clinical and other laboratory data.

Transverse Myelitis

Transverse myelitis is an inflammatory disturbance due to a variety of etiologies. It leads to severe acute or subacute motor or sensory symptoms, often with sphincter dysfunction, and associated intramedullary signal abnormality on spinal cord MRI. Transverse myelitis is classified as partial or complete according to the extent of the lesion in the transverse orientation of the spinal cord, and acute, subacute, or chronic depending on the clinical course. Like optic neuritis, acute partial transverse myelitis (APTM) is considered a clinically isolated syndrome (CIS) important in the clinical

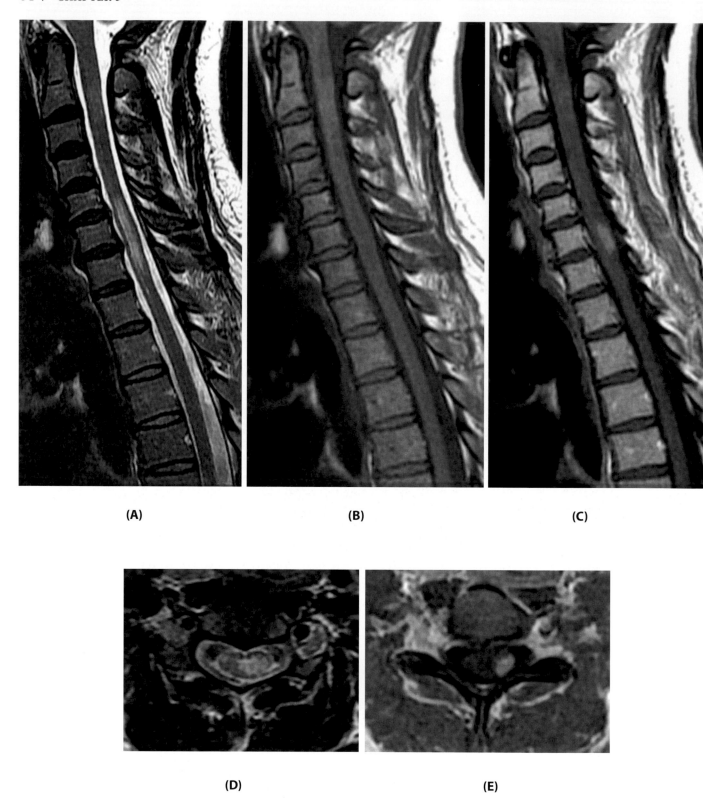

(A)   **(B)**   **(C)**

(D)   **(E)**

FIG. 10. (A–E). Multiple sclerosis. Sagittal T_2- and T_1-weighted pre- and post-contrast axial T_2- and T_1-weighted post-contrast MRI demonstrate edema within the spinal cord with focal abnormal enhancement after the administration of intravenous contrast at C6. Axial imaging depicts the abnormal enhancement as less than two-thirds of the cross-sectional area of the spinal cord, a classic finding for multiple sclerosis.

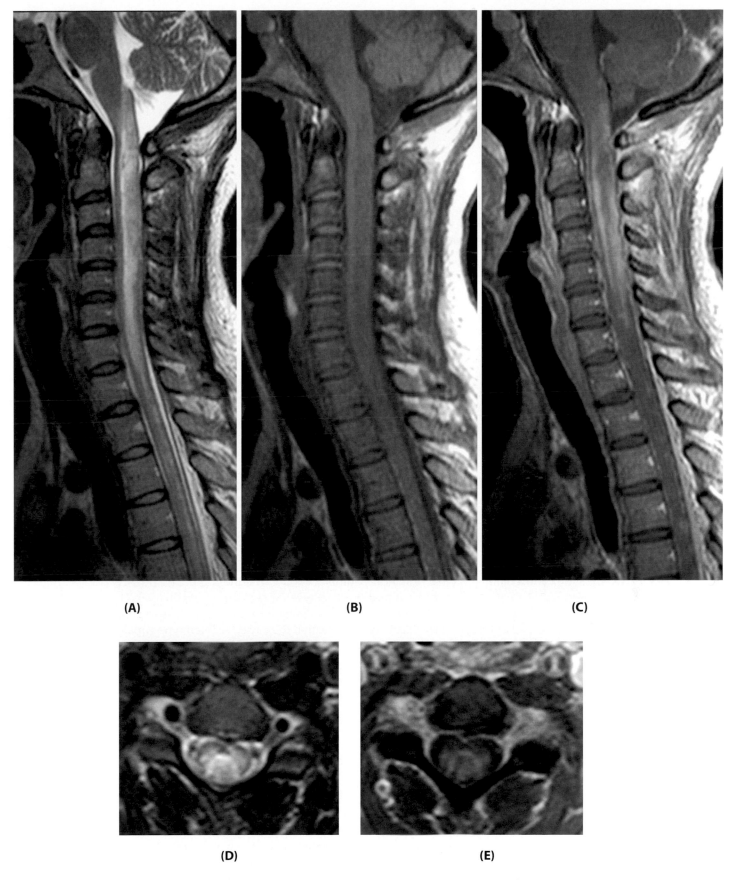

FIG. 11. (A–F). Transverse myelitis. Sagittal T_2- and T_1-weighted pre- and post-contrast axial T_2- and T_1-post-contrast MRI demonstrate an abnormal area of signal hyperintensity throughout the cervical spinal cord on T_2-weighted images with abnormal enhancement following the administration of intravenous contrast. Axial imaging depicts the abnormal enhancement as more than two-thirds of cross-sectional area of the spinal cord, a classic finding for transverse myelitis.

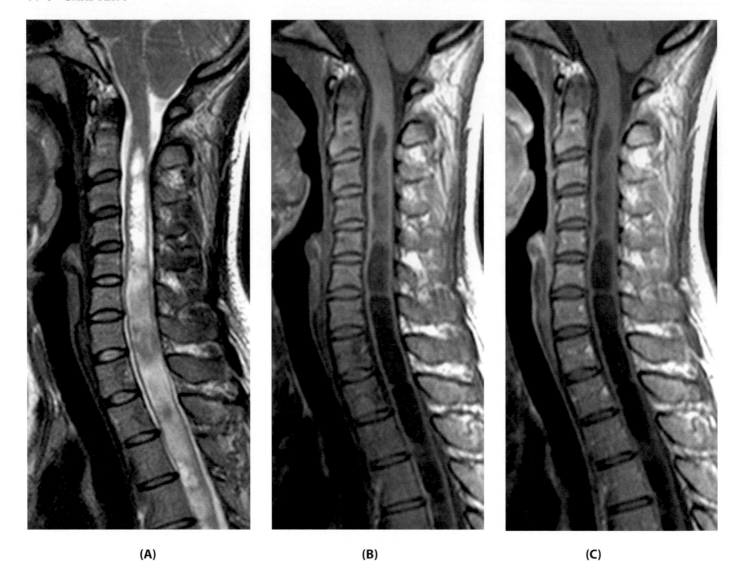

(A)   **(B)**   **(C)**

FIG. 12. (A–C). Syrinx and Chiari type I malformation. Sagittal T_2- and T_1-weighted pre- and post-contrast MRI demonstrate a large cystic cavity within the spinal cord which follows CSF signal intensity on T_2- and T_1-weighted images. There is no associated abnormal enhancement following administration of intravenous contrast. The spinal cord is expanded and CSF pulsation artifact is present within the cavity. A Chiari type 1 malformation is noted with tonsillar descent.

conversion to MS. The duration of symptoms in APTM lasts between 48 hours and three weeks with rapidly progressive neurological dysfunction (55); more severe and long-lasting symptoms and signs develop with complete transverse myelitis. Acute transverse myelitis is frequently associated with back pain, acute sensory and motor deficits, and tendon reflex changes. Sensory disturbances and weakness are, respectively, related to the interruption of ascending long tract fibers and descending corticospinal tracts, in addition to interruption of efferent motor fibers transversing the pericornual white matter before exiting the cord.

Neuroimaging employing MRI demonstrates abnormal intramedullary signal intensities that hypointense on T_1-weighted images, and hyperintense on T_2-weighted images. The spinal cord may be of normal caliber or mildly expanded. Following administration of gadolinium, the abnormal areas may demonstrate enhancement, in a pattern that suggests involvement of up to two-thirds of the spinal cord cross-sectional area, with most lesions spanning two or more longitudinal vertebral segments (Figure 11).

Long-term follow-up of patients with APTM showed that axial plane MRI with contrast injection was helpful in predicting the conversion to MS, especially when lesions occupied more than one vertebral level, occupied the posterolateral or lateral portion of the spinal cord, and showed gadolinium enhancement (55) in contrast to those with an undetermined relation to MS, in whom spinal MRI lesions were preferentially localized to only one vertebral segment, centrally located in the spinal cord, and often lacked gadolinium enhancement. The prognosis of transverse myelitis is variable, with recovery occurring over several weeks to months. Treatment with corticosteroids leads to full recovery in up to one-half of patients.

Syringomyelia

Syringomyelia is a CSF-filled cavity within the spinal cord that is eccentric to the central canal and lined by glial cells. It may be congenital or secondary to trauma, ischemia, or neoplasm. Hydromyelia refers to dilatation of the central canal, lined by ependymal cells and in direct communication with the fourth ventricle. Syringomyelia, which may be seen in association with Chiari I and II malformations, does not communicate with the fourth ventricle and is believed to be caused by increased pressure transmitted along the Virchow-Robin spaces, resulting in cystic cavity formation. The resolution of most MRI studies may not be sufficient to separate these entities, so these cavities are often grouped together and referred to as *syringohydromyelia* or *syrinx*. Clinical symptoms include back pain, radicular pain, headache, stiffness, weakness or pain in the extremities, spastic paraparesis, and loss of extreme temperature sensation, especially in the hands, with preservation of position sense, proprioception, and light touch. Patients may have an associated scoliosis. Spinal MRI demonstrates a cystic cavity within the spinal cord, which follows CSF signal intensity on all pulse sequences, without associated abnormal enhancement. The spinal cord may or may not be expanded and CSF pulsation artifact may be seen within the cavity (Figure 12).

Spinal Cord Infarction

Spinal cord infarction (SCI) is relatively rare, accounting for approximately 1% of strokes (56). The spinal cord is supplied by a single anterior spinal artery, two posterior spinal arteries, and the artery of Adamkiewicz, a branch of a lower left intercostal artery arising from the aorta. Spinal cord infarction results from any etiology that interrupts blood flow to the spinal cord, including aortic aneurysm rupture or repair, aortic dissection, spinal artery embolism, atherosclerotic disease, surgical cross-clamping, vasculitis,

coagulopathy, hypotension, and venous congestion. Anterior spinal artery occlusion may result in an anterior spinal cord syndrome manifesting paralysis, pain, and loss of temperature sensation, whereas occlusion of posterior spinal artery occlusion leads to the posterior column syndrome of impaired sensation of touch, position, and vibration. The clinical history is important in distinguishing SCI from similar appearing entities as, for example, the suddenness of the neurological deficit in SCI. Common locations for infarct are the thoracic and thoracolumbar cord, due to tenuous watershed blood supply.

Neuroradiological evaluation employing MRI demonstrates abnormal hyperintense signal intensity on T_2-weighted images within the central gray matter or the entire cross-sectional area of the spinal cord (Figure 13). The spinal cord may be of normal caliber or mildly expanded. Susceptibility artifacts from a heterogeneous magnetic environment limit the use of diffusion-weighted imaging for detection and early diagnosis of cord infarct (57) Acute SCI can be distinguished from neoplastic processes by enhancement after contrast injection in the latter, and demyelinating lesions which typically involve the dorsolateral regions of the cord and occupy less than one-half of the cross-sectional spinal cord area.

Spinal cord arteriovenous malformations

Arteriovenous malformations (AVM) occur throughout the spinal cord, but are commonly located in the thoracolumbar region. Intramedullary AVM are supplied by multiple arteries arising from both the anterior and posterior spinal arteries, and drained by the coronal venous plexuses, which are often enlarged and tortuous. Spinal cord AVM have no sex predilection and are commonly diagnosed in childhood and early adulthood (58). Clinical symptoms of progressive myelopathy with exacerbation and remission, and subarachnoid hemorrhage are attributed to venous congestion, hemorrhage, mass effect, and steal phenomena.

Neuroradiological evaluation of spinal cord AVM employing MRI reveals conglomerates of dilated vessels devoid of signal due to flow best demonstrated on T2-weighted sequences, whereas heterogeneous signal changes due to blood products are noted on T1-weighted images; contrast enhancement is variable. Serpiginous structures along the surface of the cord representing tortuous feeding arteries and distended draining veins may be appreciated (Figure 14). There may be apparent spinal cord edema with expansion of the cord. Selective spinal angiography can define the exact type of AVM to plan embolization and microsurgical treatment (59).

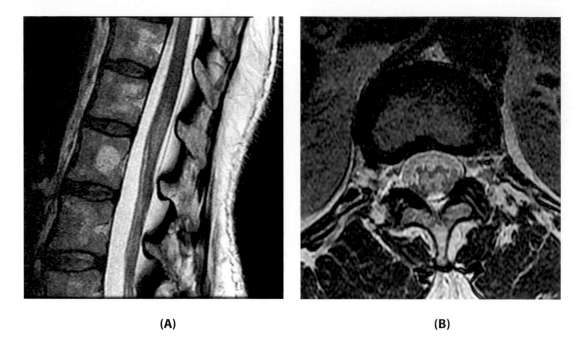

(A)   **(B)**

FIG. 13. (A–B). Infarction. Sagittal T$_2$- and axial T$_2$-weighted MRI demonstrate an abnormal area of signal hyperintensity within the conus due to infarction and edema involving the gray matter.

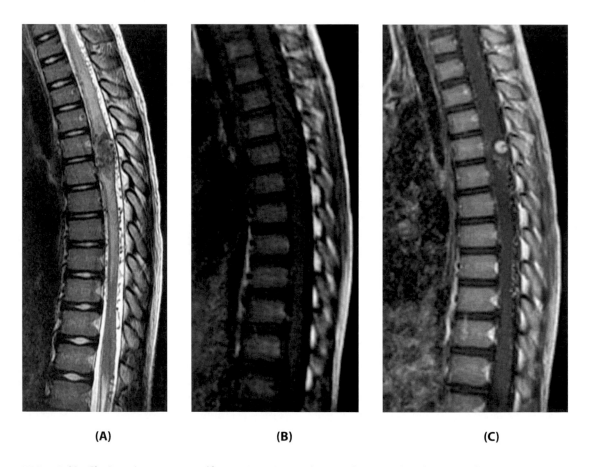

(A)   **(B)**   **(C)**

FIG. 14. (A–C). Arteriovenous malformation. Sagittal T$_2$- and T$_1$-weighted pre- and post-contrast MRI demonstrate serpiginous structures along the surface of the spinal cord representing tortuous feeding arteries and distended draining veins. Edema is present within the spinal cord with expansion of it.

REFERENCES

1. Do-Dai DD, Brooks MK, Goldkamp A, et al. *Curr Probl Diagn Radiol* 2010; 39:160–185.

2. Zorlu F, Ozyigit G, Gurkaynak M, et al. Postoperative radiotherapy results in primary spinal cord astrocytomas, *Radiother Oncol* 2005; 74:45–48.

3. Constantini S, Houten J, Miller D, et al. Intramedullary spinal cord tumors in children under the age of 3 years. *J Neurosurg* 1996; 85:1036–1043.

4. Kim MS, Chung CK, Choe G, et al., Intramedullary spinal cord astrocytoma in adults: Postoperative outcome. *J Neurooncol* 2001; 52:85–94.

5. Takemoto K, Matsumura Y, Hashimoto H, et al. MR imaging of intraspinal tumors: capability in histological differentiation and compartmentalization of extramedullary tumors. *Neuroradiology* 1988; 30:303–309.

6. Parizel PM, Balériaux D, Rodesch G, et al. Gd-DTPA enhanced MR imaging of spinal tumors. *AJR* 1989; 152:1087–1096.

7. Dillon WP, Norman D, Newton TH, Bolla K, Mark AS. Intradural spinal cord lesions: Gd-DTPA enhanced MR imaging. *Radiology* 1989; 170:229–237.

8. Bydder GM, Brown J, Niendorf HP, et al. Enhancement of cervical intraspinal tumors in MR imaging with intravenous gadolinium-DTPA. *J Comput Assist Tomogr* 1985; 9:847–851.

9. Epstein FJ, Farmer JP, Schneider SJ. Intraoperative ultrasonography: an important surgical adjunct for intramedullary tumors. *J Neurosurg* 1991; 74:729–733.

10. Rauhut F, Reinhardt F, Budach V, et al. Intramedullary pilocytic astrocytomas-a clinical and morphological study after combined surgical and photon or neutron therapy. *Neurosurg Rev* 12 (1989), pp. 309–313.

11. Epstein FJ, Farmer JP, Freed D. Adult intramedullary astrocytomas of the spinal cord. *J Neurosurg* 1992; 77:355–359.

12. Houten JK, Cooper PR. Spinal cord astrocytomas: presentation, management and outcome. *J Neurooncol* 2000; 47:219–224.

13. Epstein FJ, Farmer JP, Freed D. Adult intramedullary spinal cord ependymomas: the result of surgery in 38 patients. *J Neurosurg* 1993; 79:204–209.

14. Constantini S, Houten J, Miller D, et al. Intramedullary spinal cord tumors in children under the age of 3 years. *J Neurosurg* 1996; 85:1036–1043.

15. Cohen AR, Wisoff JH, Allen JC, et al. Malignant astrocytomas of the spinal cord. *J Neurosurg* 1989; 70:50–54.

16. Bell WO, Packer RJ, Seigel KR, et al. Leptomeningeal spread of intramedullary spinal cord tumors. *J Neurosurg* 1988; 69:295–300.

17. Sparaco M, Morelli L, Piscioli S. et al. Primary myxopapillary ependymoma of the cerebellopontine angle: report of a case. *Neurosurg Rev* 2009; 32:241–244.

18. Kahn J, Loeffler JS, Niemierko A, et al. Long-term outcomes of patients with spinal cord gliomas treated by modern conformal radiation techniques. *Int J Radiation Oncol Biol Phys* 2011; 81:232–238.

19. Moelleken SM, Seeger LL, Eckardt JJ, et al. Myxopapillary ependymoma with extensive sacral destruction: CT and MR findings, *J Comput Assist Tomogr* 1992; 16:164–166.

20. Ferrante L, Mastronardi L, Celli P, et al. Intramedullary spinal cord ependymomas: a study of 45 cases with long-term follow-up. *Acta Neurochir* 1992; 119:74–79.

21. Kahan H, Sklar EML, Post MJ, et al. MR characteristics of histopathologic subtypes of spinal ependymoma. *AJNR* 1996; 17:143–150.

22. Fine MJ, Kricheff II, Freed D, et al. Spinal cord ependymomas. MR imaging features. *Radiology* 1995; 197:655–658.

23. Brotchi J, Fischer G. Treatment. In: Fischer G, Brotchi J, eds. *Intramedullary spinal cord tumors*. Stuttgart, Germany: Thieme, 1996; 60–84.

24. Froment JC, Balériaux D, Turjman F, et al. Diagnosis: neuroradiology. In: Fischer G, Brotchi J, eds. *Intramedullary spinal cord tumors*. Stuttgart, Germany:Thieme, 1996; 33–52.

25. Gomez DR, . Missett BT, Wara WM, et al. High failure rate in spinal ependymomas with long-term follow-up. *Neuro-Oncology* 7:254–259.

26. Zaucha R, Sosinska-Mielcarek K, Zander I, et al. Spinal cord ependymoma: retrospective analysis of treatment outcomes of 14 patients. *Journal of Radiotherapy in Practice* 2004; 4:155–160.

27. Baker KB, Moran CJ, Wippold FJ II, et al. MR imaging of spinal hemangioblastoma. *AJR* 2000; 174:377–382.

28. Arbelaez A, Castillo M, Armao D. Hemangioblastoma of the filum terminale. *AJR* 1999; 173:857–858.

29. Yasargil MS, Antic J, Laciga R, et al. The microsurgical removal of intramedullary spinal hemangioblastomas. Report of twelve cases and a review of the literature. *Surg Neurol* 1976; 6:141–148.

30. Neumann HPH, Eggert HR, Weigel K, et al. Hemangioblastomas of the central nervous system. A 10-year study with special reference to von Hippel-Lindau syndrome. *J Neurosurg* 1989; 70:24–30.

31. Yu JS, Short MP, Schumacher J, et al. Intramedullary hemorrhage in spinal cord hemangioblastoma. *J Neurosurg* 1994; 81:937–940.

32. Hamburger C, Buttner A, Weis S. Ganglioglioma of the spinal cord: report of two rare cases and review of the literature. *Neurosurgery* 1997; 41:1410–1416.

33. Satyarthee GD, Mehta VS, Vaishya S, Ganglioglioma of the spinal cord: report of two cases and review of literature. *J Clin Neurosci* 2004; 11:199–203.

34. Patel U, Pinto RS, Miller DC, et al. MR of spinal cord ganglioglioma. *AJNR* 1998; 19:879–887.

35. Ojhaa BK, Sharmaa MC, Rastogia M, et al. Dumbbell-shaped paraganglioma of the cervical spine in a child. Pediatric *Neurosurgery* 2007; 43:60–64.

36. Moran CA, Rush W, Mena H. Primary spinal paragangliomas: a clinicopathological and immunohistochemical study of 30 cases. *Histopathology* 1997; 31:167–171.

37. Lunardi P, Missori P, Gagliardi FM, et al. Long-term results of the surgical treatment of spinal dermoid and epidermoid tumors. *Neurosurgery* 1989; 25:860–864.

38. Sharma NC, Chandra T, Sharma A, et al. Long-segment intramedullary spinal dermoid. *Indian J Radiol Imaging* 2009; 19:148–50.

39. Bailey IC. Dermoid tumors of the spinal cord. J Neurosurg 1970; 33:676–681.

40. Costigan DA, Winkelman MD. Intramedullary spinal cord metastasis: a clinicopathological study of 13 cases. *J Neurosurg* 1985; 62:227–233.

41. Edelson RN, Deck MD, Posner JB. Intramedullary spinal cord metastasis: clinical and radiographic findings in nine cases. *Neurology* 1972; 22:1222–1231.

42. Wu F-Z. Inramedullary spinal metastasis from breast cancer. *Arch Neurol* 2010; 67:360.

43. Findlay JM, Bernstein M, Vanderlinden RG, et al. Microsurgical resection of solitary intramedullary spinal cord metastases. *Neurosurg* 1987; 21:911–915.

44. Iplikcioglu AC, Hatiboglu MA, Ozek E, et al. Surgical removal of spinal mass lesions with open door laminoplasty. *Cen Eur Neurosurg* 2010; 71:213–218.

45. Gilbert RW, Kim J-H, Posner JB. Epidural spinal cord

compression from metastatic tumor: diagnosis and treatment. *Ann Neurol* 1978; 3:40–51.

46. Balmaceda C, Gaynor JJ, Sun M, et al. Leptomeningeal tumor in primary central nervous system lymphoma: recognition, significance, and implications. *Ann Neurol* 1995; 38: 202–209.

47. Pels H, Vogt I, Klockgether T, et al. Primary non-Hodgkin's lymphoma of the spinal cord. *Spine* 2000; 25: 2262–2264.

48. Schild SE, Wharen RE, Jr, Menke DM, et al. Primary lymphoma of the spinal cord. *Mayo Clin Proc* 1995; 70:256–260.

49. Abrey LE, Yahalom J, DeAngelis LM. Treatment for primary CNS lymphoma: the next step. *J Clin Oncol* 2000; 18:3144–3150.

50. Herrlinger U, Schabet M, Eichhorn M, et al. Prolonged corticosteroid-induced remission in primary central nervous system lymphoma: report of a case and review of the literature. *Eur Neurol* 1996; 36:241–24.

51. Noseworthy JH, Lucchinetti C, Rodriguez M, et al. Multiple sclerosis. *N Engl J Med* 2000; 343:938–52.

52. Paty DW, Oger JJF, Kastrukoff LF, et al. MRI in the diagnosis of MS: a prospective study with comparison of clinical evaluation, evoked potentials. oligoclonal bands, and CT. *Neurology* 1988; 38:180–185.

53. Fazekas F, Offenbacher H, Fuchs S, et al. Criteria for an increased specificity of MRI interpretation in elderly subjects with suspected multiple sclerosis *Neurology* 1988; 38:1822–1825.

54. Barkhof F, Filippi M, Miller DH, et al. Comparison of MRI criteria at first presentation to predict conversion to clinically definite multiple sclerosis. *Brain* 1997; 120:2059–2069.

55. Bourre B, Zephir H, Ongagna J-C, et al. Long term follow-up of acute partial transverse myelitis. *Arch Neurol* 2012; 69:357–362.

56. Sandson TA, Friedman JH. Spinal cord infarction: report of 8 cases and review of the literature. *Medicine* 1989; 68:282–92.

57. Loher TJ, Bassetti CL, Lövblad KO, et al. Diffusion-weighted MRI in acute spinal cord ischaemia. *Neuroradiology* 2003; 45:557–561.

58. Panciani PP, Fontanella M, Crobeddu E, et al. Spontaneous occlusion of a spinal arteriovenous malformation: is treatment always necessary? *Neurosurg Spine* 2010; 12:397–401.

59. Boström A, Krings T, Hans FJ, et al. Spinal glomus-type arteriovenous malformations: microsurgical treatment in 20 cases. *J Neurosurg Spine* 2009; 10:423–429.

CHAPTER 4

Neurophysiology of Clinical Motor Control

Christopher W. Hess, Seth L. Pullman

In this chapter we present an overview of clinically relevant issues in the physiology of motor control. Anatomic structures and pathways, pathophysiology, and clinical phenomenology are described within the context of motor control and behavior in a select number of representative movement disorders. This is an outline of the basic principles and current understanding of motor disorders. We specifically provide an overview of key anatomic pathways and review common movement disorders including hypokinetic movement disorders such as Parkinsonism, hyperkinetic syndromes such as dystonia, tremor, and myoclonus, and abnormalities of gait and posture.

ANATOMY OF KEY PATHWAYS INVOLVED IN MOTOR CONTROL

Voluntary motor control is a product of complex interactions between topographically and functionally diverse brain structures and pathways, including the motor and sensory cortex, basal ganglia, thalamus, cerebellum, brainstem, and spinal cord (Figure 1). Coordinated movement is achieved through the integration and modulation of cortical signals by these interconnected structures that are transmitted to the thousands of motor neurons and interneurons at the corresponding level of the spinal cord. The motor neuron and the muscle fibers that it innervates constitute the motor unit, which is the final common pathway and the smallest functional unit of the motor system. The motor unit and all its associated muscle fibers, tendons, bones, and joints work together to produce movement or isometric force.

The corticospinal tracts (CST) originate from the motor cortex in Brodmann's area 4, the premotor cortex in

Brodmann's area 6, and the parietal cortex in somatosensory areas 3, 1, and 2, at a ratio of 3:3:4, respectively. These glutaminergic fibers travel through the posterior internal capsule into the brainstem, forming the pyramids. They adopt a somatotopic arrangement in the spinal cord with ventromedial subdivisions projecting onto spinal motor neurons and interneurons to innervate axial and proximal muscles; dorsolateral subdivisions project onto the dorsolateral motor neuron and interneuron pools that innervate limb muscles. The CST fibers originating from primary somatosensory parietal cortex project primarily onto the dorsal horn of the spinal cord. Corticobulbar fibers originating in a similarly somatotopic pattern project to nuclei of the brainstem, dorsal columns, and pons, some of which then project to the cerebellum.

The basal ganglia are a group of subcortical nuclei in the telencephalon that are functionally composed of multiple, somewhat segregated circuits, each of which receives input from different areas of the cortex and is concerned with different aspects of cognition and behavior, including eye movements, motivation and reward, working memory, and executive functioning (Figure 2). Different sub-regions of the nuclei that make up the basal ganglia subserve these different functional loops. The caudate nuclei and putamen function together to form the striatum, and serve as the primary input nuclei to the basal ganglia, receiving glutaminergic excitatory input from primarily cortical and some thalamic regions, as well as neuromodulatory dopaminergic input from the substantia nigra pars compacta (SNc) and the ventral tegmental area (VTA). The major output nuclei of the basal ganglia are the internal segment of the globus pallidus (GPi) and the substantia nigra pars reticulata (SNr), which ultimately project back to the cortex, largely through

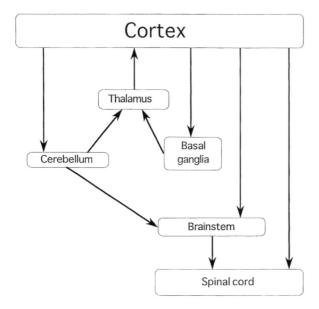

FIG. 1. Parallel projections of the cortex to multiple levels of the motor system, including two parallel reentrant systems (cortex-cerebellum-thalamus-cortex and cortex-basal ganglia-thalamus-cortex).

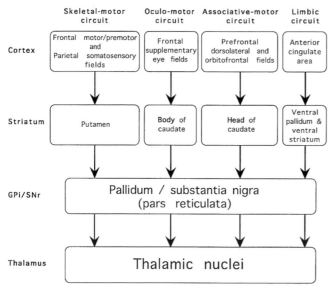

FIG. 2. Functional segregation of the basal ganglia. Somatotopy is maintained in the internal globus pallidus/substantia nigra pars reticulata (GPi/SNr) and in the thalamus; the latter projects back to the cortex.

projections to the ventrolateral (VL) and ventroanterior (VA) nuclei of the thalamus. In addition to these established basal ganglia nuclei, other structures such as the pedunculopontine nucleus (PPN), lateral habenula, and zona incerta (ZI) are being investigated as potential contributors to motor control processing in the basal ganglia (1).

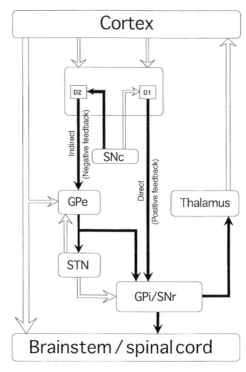

FIG. 3. Functional basal ganglia anatomy of movement disorders. The white arrows indicate glutaminergic excitatory effects. Cortically initiated activation of both pathways results in a net inhibition of the internal globus palidus/substantia nigra pars reticulata (GPi/SNr) through the direct pathway and a net facilitation of the GPi/SNr through the indirect pathway. The former results in increased movement (positive feedback to the cortex due to inhibition of inhibitory influences), and the latter results in decreased movement (negative feedback to the cortex). Substantia nigra pars compacta (SNc) stimulation, however, facilitates movements through its effect on both pathways, namely the activation of the direct (positive feedback) pathway and the inhibition of the indirect (negative feedback) pathway. Conversely, the decreased SNc influences, as occurs in Parkinson disease, and inhibits the generation of movement. GPe, external globus pallidus, STN, subthalamic nucleus.

The cerebellum plays an important role in the regulation and real-time adjustment of movement and the coordination of motor control and sensory information. It receives cortical input via pontine nuclei, and afferent somatic sensory information from the dorsal spinocerebellar and cuneocerebellar tracts. Feedback from spinal motor pathways travel directly to the cerebellum in the ventral and rostral spinocerebellar tracts, and indirectly through projections from the inferior olivary nucleus and reticular formation. These pathways convey information about ongoing movements and are processed in local synaptic relays that eventuate on cerebellar Purkinje cells, which project to the deep cerebellar nuclei and the vestibular nuclei. The output of the deep cerebellar nuclei is transmitted through the superior cerebellar peduncle to the VL thalamus and the red nucleus, and represents motor control information that has been scaled, focused, refined, and/or corrected in order to optimize motor control. In addition to its involvement in skeletal and eye muscle movement, the cerebellum also plays a role in balance, sensory perception, cognition, and affective functions (2); moreover, connections between the cerebellum and the basal ganglia are more direct than previously thought (3).

Descending pathways from the brainstem are the most primitive phylogenic motor pathways. Critical descending pathways in motor control include the ventromedial and dorsolateral pathway groups. The ventromedial pathway includes the reticulospinal tract originating from the reticular formation in the medulla and pons, the lateral and medial vestibulospinal tracts originating from the lateral and medial vestibular nuclei, and the tectospinal tract originating from the tectum and superior colliculi. The fibers of these pathways project bilaterally and widely over disparate segments of the spinal cord and synapse on motor neurons and interneurons, including long propriospinal neurons that control proximal and axial muscles. These tracts mediate gross postural adjustments, particularly in the reticulospinal tract, and head control and eye movement coordination mostly by the tectospinal tract. The reticulospinal pathways have been shown to be important in the generation of the startle response to sudden and intense acoustic stimuli (4). The ventromedial pathways receive multiple inputs from the interstitial nucleus of Cajal, the serotonergic raphe, and the noradrenergic locus ceruleus nuclei. Dorsolateral pathways include the rubrospinal and rubrobulbar fibers. The former originates from the magnocellular red nucleus and projects onto dorsolateral motor neurons and interneurons of a small number of spinal segments. These neurons innervate the muscle of the limbs in parallel to the dorsolateral division of the corticospinal tract. Similarly, the rubrobulbar fibers project to the facial nuclei, the sensory trigeminal nuclei, and the cuneate and gracile dorsal column nuclei.

The spinal cord has interconnected segmental circuits consisting of motor and sensory neurons and hundreds of thousands of interneurons at each level, all of which work together to mediate movement, sensation, and virtually all reflexes below the neck. Injections of spinal cord axons with anatomic tracers show that corticospinal neurons and spinal motor neurons have a connection pattern that is somatotopically both convergent and divergent; namely, a corticospinal neuron synapses on several motor neurons and an individual motor neuron receives projections from several corticospinal neurons (5). This arrangement ensures synchrony and balance between neighboring motor neurons that innervate muscle fibers of functionally related muscles.

CLINICAL DISORDERS OF MOTOR CONTROL—HYPOKINETIC SYNDROMES

Parkinson Disease and Related Syndromes

In 1957, Carlsson and coworkers (6) demonstrated that reserpine caused an akinetic-rigid Parkinsonian syndrome that could be reversed by dopamine. Three years later, Ehringer and Hornykiewicz (7) discovered that PD was a state of profound dopamine deficiency in the brain and later attributed it to degeneration of the SNc. Since then, a number of functional models of the basal ganglia in both normal and diseased states have been proposed to explain the influence of the basal ganglia on motor control. While to date no model of basal ganglia function is considered to be conclusive and without inconsistencies, these models continue to provide a useful framework from which to study and understand the role of the basal ganglia in motor functioning (8).

Early models of motor functioning in the basal ganglia emphasized the importance of two parallel motor circuits of basal ganglia processing; a "direct" pathway that promoted movement and an "indirect" pathway that suppressed it. In both pathways, dopaminergic modulation acts to enhance movement, but the net effect of each circuit and the direct effect of dopamine is based on their respective dopamine receptor type and the number of inhibitory connections within the circuits (Figure 3).

In the striatum, the predominant neuron is the medium spiny GABAergic neuron (MSN), which receives glutaminergic excitatory input from the cortex and thalamus and dopaminergic input from the SNc. Dopamine receptors are located along the dendritic spines and shafts of MSN, whereas corticostriatal glutaminergic synapses are located almost exclusively on the head of the dendritic spines, allowing for dopaminergic modulation of corticostriatal transmission (9). The direct pathway consists of inhibitory projections from striatal MSNs that contain substance-P and dynorphin and project directly to the GPi/SNr. This direct pathway loop from the cortex and back has two inhibitory synapses and is thus a net excitatory pathway that promotes movement. As direct pathway MSN neurons express D_1 receptors, dopamine has an excitatory modulatory effect on cortical input to MSNs and further promotes movement.

In the indirect pathway, striatal MSN that contain enkephalin have inhibitory projections directed to the GPe, which in turn has inhibitory projections to both the GPi/SNr and the STN. The STN has excitatory projections back to the GPe and directly to the GPi. There are three inhibitory synapses in this loop from and back to the cortex, and therefore its net effect is to inhibit movement. As indirect pathway MSN express D_2 receptors, dopamine has an inhibitory modulatory effect on cortical input to MSN in this pathway, promoting movement by inhibiting the pathway (10).

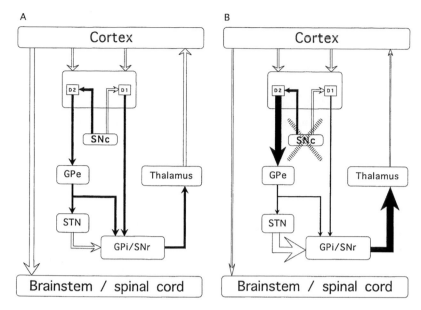

FIG. 4. Changes in basal ganglia circuitry in **(A)** the normal state compared with **(B)** Parkinson disease. GPe, exterior globus pallidus; GPi, interior globus apllidus; SNc, substantia nigra pars compacta; SNr, substantia nigra pars reticulata; STN, subthalamic nucleus.

Under normal conditions, the direct and the indirect pathways can be thought of as "balanced," ensuring normal motor control. Specific lesions in the basal ganglia that disrupt this balance could explain the development of a hyper- or hypokinetic state. The degeneration of SNc neurons which occurs in PD would result in excess indirect pathway activity and the subsequent hypokinetic state seen in PD and animal models (Figure 4) (11–13). That neuronal discharges in the STN and the GPi are increased compared with the GPe in 1-methyl-4-phenyl-1-1,2,3,6-tetrahydropyridine (MPTP) lesioned animals and PD patients (14) and clinical improvement is achieved after GPi (15–17) and STN DBS or lesions (18–20) lends credence to this model. However, a number of observations have demonstrated that this model is limited and incomplete; for instance, patients with GPi lesions generally do not become hyperkinetic, and GPe and motor thalamus lesions do not produce hypokinesia as would be expected by this simple model (21–23). Recent anatomically studies have shown that neurons of the direct and indirect pathways are not completely segregated (24), and single neurons have been shown to project to both the GPe and GPi (25, 26).

Subsequent models of basal ganglia functioning have expanded on this basic model, utilizing new observations and emphasizing different aspects of basal ganglia functioning. The anatomic model outlined above provided the frame for a theory of basal ganglia functioning in which the direct and indirect pathways play a role in the selection of specific movements and the suppression of unwanted movements though the scaling and focusing of movements in a center-surround model (27). This model would explain the hypokinesia seen in PD as excessive inhibitory focusing of movement through a proposed fast "hyperdirect" and the indirect pathways with inadequate motor activation in the direct pathway (28).

More recently, models have focused upon neural firing patterns of basal ganglia nuclei rather than absolute increases or decreases in firing rates. In both animal models and in patients with PD off medications, basal ganglia neurons in the parkinsonian state exhibit prominent alterations of their discharge patterns, with a greater tendency toward hyper-synchronous burst firing in multiple nuclei in the basal ganglia as demonstrated by local field potentials. In addition, neurons in the basal ganglia, thalamus, and cortex demonstrate abnormal oscillatory firing patterns, particularly in the beta band (10–30 Hz), but also in the alpha range and at frequencies closer to PD resting tremor (28, 29). Both levodopa administration and deep brain stimulation have been shown to suppress beta band oscillations, with correlation between the degree of improvement in bradykinesia and rigidity and the degree of reduced beta band synchronization and activity after levodopa administration (30). Thus abnormal oscillatory activity and forced synchronization might impair the ability of individual basal ganglia neurons to encode spatial and temporal aspects of motor function (30, 31). However, oscillatory activity in animal models develops relatively late, after clinical signs of parkinsonism, and systemic dopamine receptor antagonists do not produce substantial oscillations despite the presence of clinical parkinsonism, suggesting that while oscillations may be a component of advanced disease, they are not the primary cause of hypokinesia (22, 32, 33).

Given the beneficial effects of pallidal stimulation on both hypokinetic as in PD, and hyperkinetic movement patterns such as dystonia, the major motor symptoms of diseases ascribed to the basal ganglia might instead be due to interference of abnormal basal ganglia neurotransmission in normal cortical motor functioning. In this model, the basal ganglia do not play a role in movement generation or direct facilitation, but do so in a more subtle fashion in motor function. Deep brain stimulation could then be considered as interrupting abnormal transmission from dysfunctional basal ganglia to the cortex, with disconnection of basal ganglia contributions to motor control being less detrimental than allowing corrupted signals to reach the cortex (24, 28). This is supported by studies finding functional neuroimaging activation patterns in the motor cortices are normalized by deep brain stimulation (34). While current thinking is beginning to trend away from attributing a direct role in the generation and direct selection of movement to the basal ganglia, more research is clearly needed to delineate the specific contributions to motor processing by the basal ganglia.

In addition to idiopathic Parkinson disease, parkinsonism secondary to dysfunction of the basal ganglia and its connections can occur in Parkinson-plus syndromes, such as multiple system atrophy (MSA), progressive supranuclear palsy (PSP), corticobasal degeneration (CBD), as well in other neurodegerative disease and in secondary parkinsonism disorders. The various parkinsonian syndromes are discussed in more detail elsewhere in this volume.

CLINICAL DISORDERS OF MOTOR CONTROL—HYPERKINETIC SYNDROMES

Hyperkinetic movement disorders characterized by a relative excess of movement include dystonia, hemiballismus, chorea and athetosis, myoclonus, tremor, ataxia, tics, akathisia, and stereotypies, discussed further below.

Dystonia

Dystonia is characterized by sustained muscle contractions that cause twisting, repetitive movements, and abnormal postures due to co-contraction of agonist and antagonist muscles, often with a constant pattern of repeated muscle involvement (1). Agonist muscle activation is often prolonged and excessive, with overflow into both regional synergistic muscles and distant parts of the body. Co-contraction of antagonist muscles is often counter-productive to the intended movement. Dystonia can be task-specific, and often has a "geste antagoniste" or tactile or proprioceptive sensory trick that reduces symptoms. It can be classified by age of onset, distribution, or etiology, and whether primary or secondary (35).

Primary dystonias can be early- or late-onset, and have no underlying structural brain abnormalities. While the list of primary genetic dystonias continues to expand, the prototypical disease is primary torsion dystonia or Oppenheim dystonia (DYT 1), which is due to a deletion in the *TOR1A* gene encoding the TorsinA protein, which functions as a

molecular chaperone in the nuclear envelope and endoplasmic reticulum (36). Adult-onset focal dystonia is more common, and includes blepharospasm, spasmodic torticollis and focal task-specific dystonias (FTSD) such as writer's cramp (37). Musicians are especially prone to FTSD due in part to their intense training and years of performing complex repetitive movements. While FTSD has a frequency of 1:3,400 in the general population, it is 1:200 or higher among musicians (38, 39).

Secondary dystonias include dystonia-plus syndromes, psychogenic dystonias, and those that occur as part of or in association with other neurologic diseases, such as dystonia-plus syndromes, hereditary neurodegenerative dystonias, and dystonia associated with parkinsonism. Dystonia can occur at peak L-dopa doses in PD or paradoxically in patients during "off" periods, when they are most hypokinetic, such as in the morning (40).

The pathophysiology of dystonia is thought to involve a loss of motor inhibition at multiple levels of the neuraxis, reducing movement selectivity and allowing excessive activity clinically seen as motor overflow (41). Abnormalities in sensory processing, neuroplasticity, and somatotopic cortical organization have been demonstrated in animal models, (42) and imaging studies have demonstrated abnormal sensorimotor cortex size, reduced white matter fractional anisotropy in subgyral motor cortex, increased glucose metabolism in the cortex and basal ganglia, and altered basal ganglia dopamine receptor binding (43). Secondary dystonias have been shown to occur in association with lesions of multiple brain areas, including the basal ganglia, brainstem, and cerebellum (44).

FTSD may be caused by an exaggeration of normal mechanisms of brain plasticity. The postulated basis of task-driven changes in dystonia relates to the dynamic synapse concept of Hebb where neuronal connectivity is modulated by activation (45). Plastic reorganization of the cortex has been demonstrated by augmentation of the finger projection areas after repetitive tasks, or with practice (46). While this may improve performance, it also sets the stage for dystonia (46–48).

Hemiballismus, Chorea, and Athetosis

Hemiballismus refers to involuntary and irregular high amplitude, flinging movements secondary to contraction of the proximal limb and associated axial muscles (49). It is relatively rare and can develop acutely or subacutely, and can transition to less violent hemichorea as the patient recovers from the offending neurological insult (50). Structural lesions such as stroke, are the commonest cause of hemiballismus, but metabolic abnormalities such as nonketotic hyperglycemia can produce symptoms as well (51). Hemiballismus has traditionally been considered to be

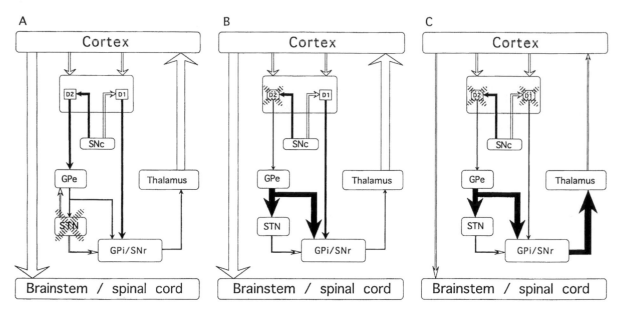

FIG. 5. Changes in basal ganglia circuitry in **(A)** hemiballism, **(B)** early, and **(C)** late Huntington disease. GPe, exterior globus pallidus; GPi, interior globus pallidus; SNc, substantia nigra pars compacta; SNr, substantia nigra pars reticulata; STN, subthalamic nucleus.

secondary to damage to the contralateral STN, which has been supported by animal models. However, lesions of the STN in patients with PD rarely have been reported to cause hemiballismus, and lesions of the GPi which according to traditional thinking should worsen hemiballismus, can actually be an effective treatment. In addition, more recent series describe lesions in the lentiform nucleus as more common causes of hemiballismus in stroke patients, with symptoms sometimes occurring due to isolated lesions of the contralateral cortex or thalamus (50, 52, 53).

Chorea is defined as rapid continual and unsustained involuntary movements that flow randomly and irregularly from one body part to another (1). It is a relatively common hyperkinetic movement disorder, due to its occurrence in a wide variety of genetic, metabolic, endocrinologic, pharmacologic, infectious, neoplastic, vascular, immunological, post-surgical, and structural brain disorders (54), including levodopa-induced dyskinesias. It is most useful to classify chorea based on these underlying causes, and accompanying neurologic symptoms and clinical history are often helpful in differential diagnosis.

The underlying pathophysiologic cause of chorea is thought to involve abnormal functioning of basal ganglia thalamocortical pathways, in which abnormal decreased inhibitory activity of the GPi upon the motor thalamus results in motor cortical disinhibition. This can occur secondary to excess direct pathway activity, as might occur in levodopa-induced dyskinesias, or abnormal indirect pathway activity, as occurs in Huntington disease (HD) secondary to degeneration of MSN neurons projecting to the lateral globus pallidus (55). Figure 5 illustrates the changes

that might occur in basal ganglia functioning in patients with hemiballismus and HD. In late stage HD, output of the direct pathway is also compromised, resulting in the motor incoordination, abnormal eye movements, and parkinsonism seen late in the disease.

Athetosis is a slow writhing form of chorea that can sometimes be mistaken for dystonia due to the transient sustained postures that can occur. It is most commonly encountered as part of cerebral palsy or perinatal birth injury, and can occur as part of a continuum with, or in conjunction with, choreic movements, termed choreoathetosis.

Tremor

Tremor is characterized by rhythmic oscillations of part of the body around one or more joints (56). It can occur at rest or action, with action tremors further divided into postural tremor and kinetic tremor, occurring during active voluntary movement. Kinetic tremor also can be isolated to task-specific activities. The underlying etiology of tremor can be considerable, and includes both normal physiologic and pathologic causes.

Physiologic tremor (PT) is generated and mediated both peripherally and centrally. The peripheral component of PT contributes irregular very low amplitude and variable oscillations, usually 8 to 12 Hz, depending on the physiologic characteristics of mass, stiffness, and other properties of the involved body part. The central component of PT, often referred to as the "central oscillator," also contributes weak 8- to 12-Hz oscillations and probably many higher frequency and low-amplitude oscillations. Exaggerated physiologic tremor (EPT) has the same peripheral and central components as PT, but there is greater participation of the stretch reflex and the 8- to 12-Hz central oscillator. Inertial loading will decrease the frequency of the mechanical-reflex component of PT in a manner analogous to adding weight to a traditional metronome.

The various pathologic tremors can be divided into those occurring with rest and with action. Causes of rest tremors include parkinsonism, long-standing essential tremor (ET), midbrain and thalamic lesions, and occasionally dystonia or tremorogenic medications. Action tremor can result from ET, dystonia, structural lesions of the cerebellum or its pathways, medications or toxins, and sometimes as a component of PD tremor. High frequency (>13 Hz) tremor commonly referred to as orthostatic tremor can occur with weight bearing and isometric contraction, most often presenting with complaints of inability to stand still due to subjective sensation of unsteadiness, pain, or shakiness.

The cause of pathologic tremors is specific to their underlying etiology, but most are thought to involve abnormal functioning in cerebellothalamocortical pathways. In essential tremor, for example, positron emission tomography (PET) and functional MRI (fMRI) have shown increased olivary metabolic function and increased regional blood flow in the cerebellum and associated structures. Magnetic resonance spectroscopy (MRS) and pathologic studies have also demonstrated abnormalities in the cerebellum (57). Pathologic tremors can have a peripheral cause, termed neuropathic tremor, secondary to central processing of distorted peripheral input due to concomitant neuropathic disease.

The differential diagnosis of tremor disorders is mostly clinical, with key aspects of the history and examination pointing toward specific etiologies. Hand tremor that is relatively symmetric and initially occurs only with posture or action and later progresses to include a horizontal head tremor typical of essential tremor, while a gradually progressive unilateral resting tremor can herald the onset of tremorous PD. A patient who complains of unsteadiness, thigh pain and inner shakiness upon standing that resolves with sitting or walking will be recognized as orthostatic tremor prior to confirmatory electrophysiologic testing. Careful neurologic examination is equally as important as a proper history. A postural tremor that occurs after a slightly delay in the outstretched hands is likely to be a re-emergent PD rest tremor, while failure to notice subtle abnormal posturing of the hand when writing could lead to a failure to correctly diagnose dystonic tremor.

Though multiple rating scales and physiologic techniques have been developed, there is currently no universally accepted method of rating or measuring tremor. Various rating scales have been developed and have been proven useful in clinical research (58, 59). A variety of computerized neurophysiologic techniques have also been developed that have been helpful in both the diagnosis of clinically complicated patients and the study of tremor mechanisms.

Among the various movement disorders, tremor is particularly amenable to quantitative mathematical analysis because movements are quasi-sinusoidal. Modern computers make data acquisition, processing, and analysis rapid and efficient. Several different techniques exist to objectively measure tremor. The most commonly used is the electronic detection of motion by accelerometry. Miniature accelerometers can be attached to the affected part of the body and do not interfere with voluntary or involuntary movements. Tremor frequency and amplitude are the most important and commonly evaluated characteristics. Sampling rates should be at least double the highest tremor frequency of interest for accurate frequency analysis, and low-pass filtering and other techniques can be used to further improve signal-to-noise ratios. Tremor displacement amplitudes can be determined accurately to less than 0.1 mm using accelerometric data.

Simultaneous surface electromyography (EMG) provides information about motor unit recruitment and synchronization with tremor activity and the relationship of the synergistic muscles. The EMG signal is often processed by rectification, integration, or smoothing to place its frequency profile into the tremor range. Combining accelerometry and surface EMG techniques, including EMG-to-movement and side-to-side frequency coherences, EMG topography, reflex responses, and tremor amplitude ratios during different clinical tasks contribute to the characterization and separation of the different tremor etiologies. Comparison of clinical tremor rating tasks and computerized tremor analysis reveal that in evaluating and grading tremor clinically, the gradations of amplitude severity perceived by clinicians is dictated by the Weber-Fechner laws of psychophysics such that the discernible size of amplitude change is proportional to the initial tremor amplitude, and perceived clinical change in amplitude is related logarithmically, the linearity of clinical scales (60).

Objective evaluation of tremor is also possible through computerized analysis of drawn Archimedean spirals, a task that has long been subjectively assessed by clinicians in evaluating tremor. Spirals drawn on a digitizing tablet can be analyzed with regard to time, position, and pen pressure, and can be mathematically "unraveled" and averaged together, allowing multiple tremor indices, such as frequency, direction, and amplitude to be captured and evaluated. In addition, other characteristics, such as drawing speed and acceleration, loop-to-loop width tightness and variation, and drawing pressure over time can be used to address questions of basic motor control research and to evaluate other movement disorders. Computerized spiral analysis has been demonstrated to correlate highly with the

UPDRS and to discern abnormalities in the clinically unaffected limb of patients early PD compared to controls (61), and have been used in epidemiologic studies of ET (62).

Combining the physiologic methods described above can help the clinician in cases of tremor in which the underlying cause is challenging. For example, the elderly patient presenting with longstanding bilateral hand tremor of low frequency and slightly worse on one side, in association with a nonspecifically slow gait could have ET or PD. Analysis of variables such as the shape of tremor waveforms, coherence and amplitude between limbs, consistency of tremor direction during spirals, movement acceleration and deceleration, and tightness of drawn spirals can help to differentiate the two diseases. Various other tremorous disorders can also be effectively evaluated and quantified with physiologic techniques (63–66).

Myoclonus

Myoclonus is defined as sudden, brief, "shock-like" movements caused by muscle contraction or inhibition in activity (67) that lead to quick body movements or limb jerks. EMG shows abrupt instantaneous increases or silent periods of muscle discharges (68). A remarkable number of different pathologic conditions result in similar-appearing jerks, yet no single biochemical or physiologic mechanism is common to all of them. Myoclonus occurs in more pathologic and normal physiologic conditions than any other movement disorder. It can be focal, multifocal, segmental, axial, or generalized; symmetric or asymmetric; periodic or aperiodic; present at rest or triggered by action; stimulus sensitive or independent.

An etiologic classification separates myoclonus into physiologic, essential, epileptic, and secondary causes. Physiologic myoclonus includes hypnic jerks and hiccups, and some exercise or anxiety induced movements. Essential myocloni include those hereditary or sporadic diseases in which myoclonus is the prominent or only clinical finding and it is not secondary to other causes other than genetic. Epileptic myoclonus occurs in the setting of epilepsy, and can occur in isolation or in combination with other types of seizure activity. The list of secondary causes of myoclonus is multitudinous; it can be seen in dementias, diseases of the basal ganglia and cerebellum, central nervous system infections, and toxic and metabolic insults, just to name a few.

Classification based on physiologic origin of myoclonus is also useful, though minor variations in how myoclonus is classified physiologically are often found (67, 69). Myoclonus of cortical origin is most common, includes most movements easily recognized as myoclonus. Cortical myoclonus analyzed by back-averaging EMG-EEG-derived information incorporates brief duration EMG discharges measuring <75

msec, high amplitude cortical somatosensory evoked potentials (SEP), and a preceding cortical discharge derived from motor cortex at intervals consistent with conduction along CST fiber pathways. Other forms of myoclonus include subcortical, brainstem, spinal cord, and peripheral, and are comprised of longer duration EMG bursts, sometimes with segmental muscle activity in axial or limb myotomes. Spinal myoclonus can be generated by discrete spinal lesions or more diffusely in the propriospinal interneurons (70).

Distinguishing myoclonus from other movement disorders can sometimes be difficult and requires specialized physiologic tests in addition to the clinical examination for accurate phenomenologic classification. In general, the rapid speed and short duration of movements or lapses in muscle tone, combined with the lack of patterned muscle activity (as seen in dystonia); the randomness or flowing quality seen in chorea; sustention after muscle stretch seen in clonus mechanisms; or sinusoidal and without discrete intervals between jerks help to properly identify myoclonus clinically. The physiologic investigation of myoclonus includes direct and intercorrelation of surface EMG signals, electroencephalographic measurement of cortical activity, and sensory evoked potential evaluation (71). Surface-EMG is useful in determining the rate of onset and burst durations of myoclonic jerks, patterns of antagonist actions, and the order of muscle activation up or down the brainstem or spinal cord. Although there are no specific burst durations, diagnostic of myoclonus, irregular EMG bursts with co-contracting antagonist activity lasting 10 to 50 msec in duration are characteristic of cortical myoclonus, whereas EMG bursts of up to 300 msec can be seen in brainstem and spinal segmental myoclonus.

STANCE, BALANCE, AND GAIT

Correct upright standing posture or stance involves maintaining the body center of mass (COM) vertically aligned over the feet, which serve as the base of support (BOS). The vertical line passing through the COM, known as the line of gravity, is approximately 3 to 8 cm anterior to the ankles (72). The movement that occurs as this line fluctuates during real-time corrections and adjustments to muscle activity and position is called postural sway (1). Maintenance of postural control requires continuous central nervous system processing, based on feedback provided by the special senses, mainly visual and vestibular, as well as information from muscles, joints, and cutaneous receptors. It can be separated into static postural control, in which COM can be variable but the BOS and supporting surface are fixed, and dynamic postural control, which begins when the BOS begins to vary as well, such as during the initiation of walking (73).

Walking is achieved through a repeating series of rhythmic leg and hip flexion and extension movements with concomitant hip and trunk stabilization in the supporting leg. This is achieved though the crucial integration of sensory and motor feedback information, allowing the maintenance balance and proper posture in an environment that can be constantly changing. The step cycle in locomotion is divided into the swing phase, when the foot is swinging forward as in stepping, and the support or stance phase, when the foot is planted with the leg moving backward. The rhythmic alternation between flexion and extension that occurs during walking is mediated by neural networks in the spinal cord, termed Central Pattern Generators (CPG), that receive sensory information from the limbs and project to higher central nervous system structures (74) (Figure 6). These spinal CPGs are responsible for the elementary locomotion that occurs in felines with spinal cord transections (75).

Above the spinal cord, imaging studies have demonstrated that a large number of structures, including primary sensory and motor cortices, supplementary motor area, frontal and parahippocampal cortex, basal ganglia, and the cerebellum, are all active during human locomotion (76). Specific locomotor regions are thought to exist in the pontomedullary reticular formation, mesencephalon, subthalamic nucleus, cerebellum, and the pedunculopontine nucleus (77, 78). Signals underlying fine control of locomotion are transmitted from higher brain structures through the corticospinal and rubrospinal pathways, while vestibulospinal, propriospinal, and reticulospinal pathways transmit information relating to initiation of gait and continued maintenance of postural control (79).

The capacity for normal gait is influenced by almost every aspect of cognitive function. Gait abnormalities can therefore be vastly more complicated than direct deficits in static postural control and recovery from perturbation or the initiation and maintenance of locomotion. Normal ambulation first requires the ability to *choose* the most appropriate route and navigate obstacles in real time and the capacity to *judge* the risk of falling in different situations, and secondarily, the facility to *execute* appropriate responses to these decisions, while integrating and multitasking concurrent physical and situational demands (80). Thus, a patient with early progressive supranuclear palsy whose balance and gait is only mildly impaired but impulsive, may fall more often than a patient with multiple system atrophy (MSA) with more prominent balance and gait impairments. On the opposite side of the spectrum, patients with a gait disorder who have suffered a serious fall can develop a fear of falling that is more crippling than their actual ambulatory deficit.

Although a detailed review is outside the scope of this chapter, gait disorders can be classified by level of dysfunction within the nervous system as low, middle, and high, or by the specific clinical syndromes that characterize them. For example, pain can produce the reduced stance phase in the effected limb seen in antalgic gait, and neuropathy

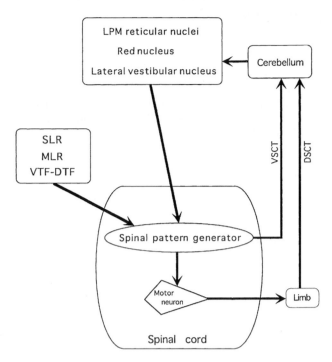

FIG. 6. Simplified connections between the "spinal pattern generator" and multiple supraspinal motor levels involved in gait and posture control. LPM, lateral pontomedullary (reticular nuclei); MLR, mesencephalic locomotor region; SLR, subthalamic locomotor region; VSCT, DSCT, ventral, dorsal spinocerebellar tracts; VTF-DTF, ventral, dorsal tegmental fields.

resulting in foot drop or sensory ataxia can produce the high stepping seen in neuropathic gait. A spastic limb can produce the circumducting, scissoring quality seen in spastic or hemiparetic gait, and cerebellar disorders can result in the wide-based staggering quality seen in ataxic gait.

Advances in computer processing, technology, and newer acquisition techniques that allow detailed quantitative and objective assessment of gait can be combined for more comprehensive analysis. Multichannel surface or fine-wire EMG can be recorded and transmitted wirelessly, allowing analysis of patterns of muscle activity, contraction patterns of agonist and antagonist muscle groups, and objective evidence of focal muscle dysfunction (81). Walkways with embedded, pressure-sensitive sensors allow measurement of step rate, length, and width, as well as the percentage time spent in the various phases of gait and the stride speed in cm/sec (82, 83). Passive multi-camera systems can be used in conjunction with infrared lights and reflective markers to capture kinematic data of walking in three dimensions (84). As technological advances continue, objective quantitative gait analysis will likely become more readily available and commonly used in clinical settings.

REFERENCES

1. Fahn S, Jankovic J, and Hallett M. *Principles and practice of movement disorders.* 2nd ed. New York: Elsevier, 2011.
2. Massaquoi SG. Physiology of clinical dysfunction of the cerebellum. *Handb Clin Neurol* 2012; 103:37–62.
3. Bostan AC, Strick PL. The cerebellum and basal ganglia are interconnected. *Neuropsychol Rev* 2010; 20:261–270.
4. Wu MF, Suzuki SS, Siegel JM. Anatomical distribution and response patterns of reticular neurons active in relation to acoustic startle. *Brain Research* 1988; 457:399–406.
5. Humphrey DR, Freund HJ. Motor control: concepts and issues: report of the Dahlem Workshop on Motor Control: Concepts and Issues. Dec 3–8, 1989; *Dahlem Workshop Reports* 1991.
6. Carlsson A, Lindqvist M, Magnusson T. 3, 4-Dihydroxyphenylalanine and 5-hydroxytryptophan as reserpine antagonists. *Nature* 1957; 180:1200.
7. Ehringer H, Hornykiewicz O. Distribution of noradrenaline and dopamine (3-hydroxytyramine) in the human brain and their behavior in diseases of the extrapyramidal system. *Klin Wochenschr* 1960; 38:1236–1239.
8. Gale JT, Amirnovin R, Williams ZM, et al. From symphony to cacophony: pathophysiology of the human basal ganglia in Parkinson disease. *Neurosci Biobehav Rev* 2008; 32:378–387.
9. Betarbet R, Turner R, Chockkan V, et al. Dopaminergic neurons intrinsic to the primate striatum. *J Neurosci* 1997; 17:6761–6768.
10. Shen W, Flajolet M, Greengard P, et al. Dichotomous dopaminergic control of striatal synaptic plasticity. *Science* 2008; 321:848–851.
11. DeLong MR, Coyle JT. Globus Pallidus lesions in the monkey produced by kainic acid: histologic and behavioral effects. *Appl Neurophysiol* 1979; 42: 95–97.
12. Kato M, Kimura M. Effects of reversible blockade of basal ganglia on a voluntary arm movement. *J Neurophysiol* 1992; 68:1516–1534.
13. Mink JW, Thach WT. Basal ganglia motor control. III. Pallidal ablation: normal reaction time, muscle cocontraction, and slow movement. *J Neurophysiol* 1991; 65:330–351.
14. Vitek JL, KY, Turner R. Neuronal activity in the internal (GPi) and external (GPe) segments of the globus pallidus (GP) of parkinsonian patients is similar to that in the MPTP-treated primate model of parkinsonism. *Soc Neurosci Abstr* 1993; 19:1584.
15. Dogali M, Fazzini E, Kolodny E, et al. Stereotactic ventral pallidotomy for Parkinson's disease. *Neurology* 1995; 45(4):753–761.
16. Laitinen LV, Bergenheim AT, Hariz MI. Leksell's posteroventral pallidotomy in the treatment of Parkinson's disease. *J Neurosurg* 1992; 76:53–61.
17. Sutton JP, Couldwell W, Lew MF, et al. Ventroposterior medial pallidotomy in patients with advanced Parkinson's disease. *Neurosurgery* 1995; 36:1112–1116; 1116–1117.
18. Ford B, Winfield L, Pullman SL, et al. Subthalamic nucleus stimulation in advanced Parkinson's disease: blinded assessments at one year follow up. *J Neurol Neurosurg Psychiatry* 2004; 75:1255–1259.
19. Kumar R, Lang AE, Rodriguez-Oroz MC, et al. Deep brain stimulation of the globus pallidus pars interna in advanced Parkinson's disease. *Neurology* 2000; 55 Suppl6:S34–39.
20. Stover NP, Okun MS, Evatt et al. Stimulation of the subthalamic nucleus in a patient with Parkinson disease and essential tremor. *Arch Neurol* 2005; 62:141–143.
21. Canavan, AG, Nixon, PD, Passingham, RE. Motor learning in monkeys (Macaca fascicularis) with lesions in motor thalamus. *Exp Brain Res* 1989; 77:113–126.
22. DeLong M, Wichmann T. Update on models of basal ganglia function and dysfunction. *Parkinsonism Relat Disord* 2009; 15 Suppl 3:S237–240.
23. Soares J, Kliem MA, Betarbet R, et al. Role of external pallidal segment in primate parkinsonism: comparison of the effects of 1-methyl-4-phenyl-1,2,3,6-tetrahydropyridine-induced parkinsonism and lesions of the external pallidal segment. *J Neurosci* 2004; 24:6417–6426.
24. Turner RS, Desmurget, M. Basal ganglia contributions to motor control: a vigorous tutor. *Curr Opin Neurobiol* 2010; 20:704–716.
25. Obeso JA, Marin C, Rodriguez-Oroz C, et al. The basal ganglia in Parkinson's disease: current concepts and unexplained observations. *Ann Neurol* 2008; 64 Suppl 2: S30–46.
26. Shepherd GM. *The synaptic organization of the brain.* 5th ed. New York: Oxford University Press, 2004.
27. Mink JW. The basal ganglia: focused selection and inhibition of competing motor programs. *Prog Neurobiol* 1996; 50:381–425.
28. Wichmann T, DeLong MR, Guridi, J, et al. Milestones in research on the pathophysiology of Parkinson's disease. *Movement Disorders* 2011; 26:1032–1041.
29. Nambu A. Seven problems on the basal ganglia. *Curr Opin Neurobiol* 2008; 18:595–604.
30. Brown P, Eusebio, A. Paradoxes of functional neurosurgery: clues from basal ganglia recordings. *Movement Disorders* 2008; 23:12–20; quiz 158.
31. Hammond C, Bergman H, Brown, P. Pathological synchronization in Parkinson's disease: networks, models and treatments. *Trends Neurosci* 2007; 30:357–364.
32. Leblois A, Meissner W, Bioulac B, et al. Late emergence of synchronized oscillatory activity in the pallidum during progressive Parkinsonism. *Eur J Neurosci* 2007; 26:1701–1713.
33. Mallet N, Pogosyan A, Sharott A, et al. Disrupted dopamine transmission and the emergence of exaggerated beta oscillations in subthalamic nucleus and cerebral cortex. *J Neurosci* 2008; 28:4795–4806.
34. Grafton ST, Turner RS, Desmurget M, et al. Normalizing motor-related brain activity: subthalamic nucleus stimulation in Parkinson disease. *Neurology* 2006; 66:1192–1199.
35. Geyer HL, Bressman SB. The diagnosis of dystonia. *Lancet Neurol* 2006; 5:780–790.
36. Ozelius LJ, Bressman SB. Genetic and clinical features of primary torsion dystonia. *Neurobiol Dis* 2011; 42:127–135.
37. Evatt ML, Freeman A, Factor S. Adult-onset dystonia. *Handb Clin Neurol* 2011;100: 481–511.
38. Nutt JG, Muenter MD, Melton, LJ, 3rd, et al. Epidemiology of dystonia in Rochester, Minnesota. *Adv Neurol* 1988; 50:361–365.
39. Schuele SU, Lederman RJ. Long-term outcome of focal dystonia in instrumental musicians. *Adv Neurol* 2004; 94:261–266.
40. Kidron D, Melamed E. Forms of dystonia in patients with Parkinson's disease. *Neurology* 1987; 37:1009–1011.
41. Hallett M. Neurophysiology of dystonia: The role of inhibition. *Neurobiol Dis* 2011; 42:177–184.
42. Cassidy A. Pathophysiology of idiopathic focal dystonia. *ACNR* 2010; 10:14–18.
43. Breakefield, XO, Blood, AJ, Li, Y, Hallett, M, Hanson, PI, and Standaert, DG. The pathophysiological basis of dystonias. *Nat Rev Neurosci* 2008; 9(3):222–234.
44. Standaert DG. Update on the pathology of dystonia. *Neurobiol Dis* 2011; 42:148–151.

45. Hebb DO. *The organization of behavior; a neuropsychological theory.* New York: Wiley, 1949.

46. Elbert T, Candia V, Altenmuller E, et al. Alteration of digital representations in somatosensory cortex in focal hand dystonia. *Neuroreport* 1998; 9:3571–3575.

47. Byl NN, Melnick M. The neural consequences of repetition: clinical implications of a learning hypothesis. *J Hand Ther* 1997; 10:160–174.

48. Tinazzi M, Priori A, Bertolasi L, et al. Abnormal central integration of a dual somatosensory input in dystonia. Evidence for sensory overflow. *Brain* 2000; 123:42–50.

49. Grandas F. Hemiballismus. *Handb Clin Neurol* 2011; 100:249-260.

50. Hawley JS, Weiner, WJ. Hemiballismus: Current concepts and review. *Parkinsonism and Related Disorders* 2012 Feb; 18(2):125-9. Epub 2011 Sep 17.

51. Shannon KM. Hemiballismus. *Curr Treat Options Neurol* 2005; 7:203–210.

52. Chung SJ, Im JH, Lee MC, et al. Hemichorea after stroke: clinical-radiological correlation. *J Neurol* 2004; 251:725–729.

53. Parees I, Hernandez-Vara J, Alvarez-Sabin, J. Post-stroke hemichorea: observation-based study of 15 cases. *Rev Neurol* 2010; 51:460–464.

54. Walker RH. Differential diagnosis of chorea. *Curr Neurol Neurosci Rep* 2011; 11:385–395.

55. Shoulson I, Young AB. Milestones in Huntington disease. *Movement Disorders* 2011; 26:1127–1133.

56. Elble RJ, Koller WC. *Tremor.* The Johns Hopkins series in contemporary medicine and public health. Baltimore: Johns Hopkins University Press, 1990.

57. Elble RJ, Deuschl G. An update on essential tremor. *Curr Neurol Neurosci Rep* 2009; 9:273–277.

58. Louis ED, Barnes L, Albert SM, et al. Correlates of functional disability in essential tremor. *Movement Disorders* 2001; 16;914–920.

59. Stacy MA, Elble RJ, Ondo WG, et al. Assessment of interrater and intrarater reliability of the Fahn-Tolosa-Marin Tremor Rating Scale in essential tremor. *Movement Disorders* 2007; 22:833–838.

60. Elble RJ, Pullman SL, Matsumoto JY, et al. Tremor amplitude is logarithmically related to 4- and 5-point tremor rating scales. *Brain* 2006; 129:2660–2666.

61. Saunders-Pullman, R, Derby C, Stanley K, et al. Validity of spiral analysis in early Parkinson's disease. *Movement Disorders* 2008; 23:531–537.

62. Cohen O, Pullman S, Jurewicz E, et al. Rest tremor in patients with essential tremor: prevalence, clinical correlates, and electrophysiologic characteristics. *Arch Neurol* 2003; 60:405–410.

63. Floyd AG, Yu QP, Piboolnurak P, et al. Kinematic analysis of motor dysfunction in Niemann-Pick type C. *Clinical Neurophysiology* 2007; 118:1010–1018.

64. Hsu AW, Piboolnurak PA, Floyd AG, et al. Spiral analysis in Niemann-Pick disease type C. *Movement Disorders* 2009; 24:1984–1990.

65. Pullman SL, Ford B, Elibol B, et al. Cutaneous electromyographic silent period findings in brachial dystonia. *Neurology* 1996; 46:503–508.

66. Pullman SL, Watts RL, Juncos JL, et al. Movement amplitude choice reaction time performance in Parkinson's disease may be independent of dopaminergic status. *J Neurol Neurosurg Psychiatry* 1990; 53:279–283.

67. Caviness JN, Truong, DD. Myoclonus. *Handb Clin Neurol* 2011; 100:399–420.

68. Shibasaki H. Neurophysiological classification of myoclonus. *Neurophysiologie Clinique/Clinical Neurophysiology* 2006; 36:267–269.

69. Chang VC, Frucht, SJ. Myoclonus. *Current Treatment Options in Neurology* 2008; 10:222–229.

70. Chokroverty S, Walters A, Zimmerman T, et al. Propriospinal myoclonus: a neurophysiologic analysis. *Neurology* 1992; 42:1591–1595.

71. Shibasaki H. AAEE minimonograph #30: Electrophysiologic studies of myoclonus. *Muscle Nerve* 1988; 11:899–907.

72. Elble RJ, Moody C, Leffler K, et al. The initiation of normal walking. *Movement Disorders* 1994; 9:139–146.

73. Granacher U, Muehlbauer T, Gollhofer A, et al. An intergenerational approach in the promotion of balance and strength for fall prevention—a mini-review. *Gerontology* 2011; 57:304–315.

74. Le Ray D, Juvin L, Ryczko D, et al. Supraspinal control of locomotion: the mesencephalic locomotor region. *Progress in Brain Research* 2011; 188:51–70.

75. Pearson KG. Generating the walking gait: role of sensory feedback. *Progress in Brain Research* 2004; 143:123–129.

76. Fukuyama H, Ouchi Y, Matsuzaki S, et al. Brain functional activity during gait in normal subjects: a SPECT study. *Neuroscience Letters* 1997; 228:183–186.

77. Jahn K, Deutschlander A, Stephan T, et al. Imaging human supraspinal locomotor centers in brainstem and cerebellum. *Neuroimage* 2008; 39:786–792.

78. Nutt JG, Horak FB, Bloem BR. Milestones in gait, balance, and falling. *Movement Disorders* 2011; 26:1166–1174.

79. Drew T, Prentice S, Schepens, B. Cortical and brainstem control of locomotion. *Progress in Brain Research* 2004; 143:251–261.

80. Snijders AH, van de Warrenburg BP, Giladi N, et al. Neurological gait disorders in elderly people: clinical approach and classification. *Lancet Neurol* 2007; 6:63–74.

81. Frigo C, Crenna, P. Multichannel SEMG in clinical gait analysis: a review and state-of-the-art. *Clinical Biomechanics* 2009; 24:236–245.

82. McDonough AL, Batavia M, Chen FC, et al. The validity and reliability of the GAITRite system's measurements: A preliminary evaluation. *Arch Phys Med Rehabil* 2001; 82:419–425.

83. Hollman JH, McDade EM, Petersen RC. Normative spatiotemporal gait parameters in older adults. *Gait and Posture* 2011; 34:111–118.

84. Nakao S, Komatsu K, Sakai W, et al. Gait and posture assessments of a patient treated with deep brain stimulation in dystonia using three-dimensional motion analysis systems. *J Med Invest* 2011; 58:264–272.

CHAPTER 5

Electrodiagnostic Studies in Motor Disorders

Mark A. Ferrante

The electrodiagnostic (EDX) examination, which is an extension of the clinical neurologic examination, provides important information about the peripheral nervous system (PNS), some of which cannot be obtained in any other manner. It includes nerve conduction studies (NCS), needle electromyography (EMG), and a variety of special studies including F waves, H responses, and repetitive motor nerve stimulation (RMS). Motor NCS (MNCS) and needle EMG assess the motor system from the lower motor neurons (LMN) in the brainstem and spinal cord to the muscle fibers they innervate. In addition, the needle examination also provides some information about upper motor neurons (UMN) in the central nervous system. Sensory NCS assess the sensory system from the sensory neurons located in the dorsal root ganglia (DRG) to the recording or stimulating site, whichever is more distal. This chapter reviews aspects of PNS anatomy, pathophysiology of electrodiagnosis, technical and diagnostic features of the EDX examination, and its correlation with specific motor unit disorders.

ANATOMIC CONSIDERATIONS

Cortical UMN give rise to corticospinal (CST) and corticobulbar tract fibers that synapse with the LMN located within the brainstem and spinal cord. The smallest element of skeletal muscle movement is the product of an individual motor unit, which consists of a single LMN, its axon, and all of the muscle fibers that it innervates across the intervening neuromuscular junctions (NMJ). Motor axons that exit from the same spinal cord segment fuse to form a single ventral root, which subsequently joins the fused sensory axons to form a mixed spinal nerve. The latter exits the intervertebral foramen and gives off a posterior branch, the posterior primary ramus, which is the source of paraspinal muscle innervation and sensation to the dorsal aspect of the neck and trunk. The remaining sensory and motor axons continue as the anterior primary ramus (APR), the latter of which intermingle to form the cervical, brachial, thoracic, and lumbosacral somatic plexuses. The fibers that supply muscle innervation and sensation to the ventral and lateral aspects of the trunk and all parts of the limbs are shown in Figure 1. Motor and sensory nerve fibers segregate into independent motor and sensory nerves and nerve branches.

The muscles innervated by the motor axons derived from LMN of the same spinal cord segment are referred to as a myotome, or muscle domain, of a particular spinal cord segment, whereas the cutaneous region innervated by sensory axons derived from the same spinal cord segment is termed a *dermatome*. The muscle domains of the more distally located PNS elements are readily deduced and are important for competent performance of the study and accurate localization of any identified abnormalities. The muscle domains of the cervical and lumbosacral roots and of the trunk and cord elements of the brachial plexus are shown in Tables 1–4; and those of the brachial plexus elements are shown in Table 5 (1). Illustrations of the dermatomes (Figures 2–5) and the sensory domains of the cutaneous nerves of the body are shown (Figures 6–9), as are the course and muscle innervation of the named median, ulnar, radial, femoral, tibial, and peroneal nerves (Figures 10–16).

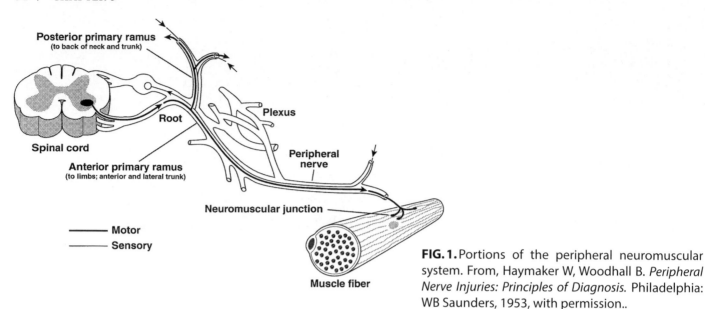

FIG. 1. Portions of the peripheral neuromuscular system. From, Haymaker W, Woodhall B. *Peripheral Nerve Injuries: Principles of Diagnosis.* Philadelphia: WB Saunders, 1953, with permission..

TABLE 1. Muscle domains of the cervical root elements

C-5:	Rhomboideus major and minor, **supraspinatus, infraspinatus, deltoid, biceps, brachioradialis**
C-6:	Supraspinatus, infraspinatus, **deltoid, biceps**, triceps, anconeus, **brachioradialis**, extensor carpi radialis, **pronator teres, flexor carpi radialis**
C-7:	**Triceps, anconeus**, extensor carpi radialis, extensor digitorum communis, extensor carpi ulnaris, **pronator teres, flexor carpi radialis**
C-8:	Extensor digitorum communis, extensor carpi ulnaris, extensor pollicis brevis, **extensor indicis proprius, flexor pollicis longus, pronator quadratus, abductor pollicis brevis,** flexor carpi ulnaris, **flexor digitorum profundus, abductor digiti minimi, adductor pollicis, first dorsal interosseous**
T-1:	Flexor pollicis longus, **pronator quadratus, abductor pollicis brevis,** flexor carpi ulnaris, **flexor digitorum profundus, abductor digiti minimi, adductor pollicis, first dorsal interosseous**

Our muscle preferences are shown. Paraspinal muscles belong to all root elements and therefore are not listed. Muscles shown in bold type are more likely to be involved with disease of the listed root element.

TABLE 2. Muscle domains of the lumbosacral root elements

L-2:	**Iliacus**
L-3:	**Iliacus, adductor longus, vastus lateralis, vastus medialis, rectus femoris**
L-4:	**Adductor longus, vastus lateralis, vastus medialis, rectus femoris, tibialis anterior,** extensor hallucis
L-5:	**Tensor fascia lata, gluteus medius,** gluteus maximus, **semimembranosus, semitendinosus, tibialis anterior, extensor hallucis, peroneus longus, extensor digitorum brevis, tibialis posterior, flexor digitorum longus,** gastrocnemius (lateral head)
S-1:	Tensor fascia lata, gluteus medius, **gluteus maximus, biceps femoris (short head), biceps femoris (long head), extensor digitorum brevis,** tibialis posterior, flexor digitorum longus, **gastrocnemius (lateral head), gastrocnemius (medial head), soleus, abductor hallucis, abductor digiti quinti pedis**
S-2:	Biceps femoris (short head), biceps femoris (long head), gastrocnemius (medial head), **soleus, abductor hallucis, abductor digiti quinti pedis**

Our muscle preferences are shown. Paraspinal muscles belong to all root elements and therefore are not listed. Muscles shown in bold type are more likely to be involved with disease of the listed root element.

TABLE 3. Muscle domains of the trunk elements

Upper trunk	Middle trunk	Lower trunk
Supraspinatus	Pronator teres	Flexor pollicis longus
Infraspinatus	Flexor carpi radialis	Abductor pollicis brevis
Biceps	Triceps	Extensor carpi ulnaris
Deltoid	Anconeus	Extensor digitorum communis
Teres minor	Extensor carpi radialis	Extensor pollicis brevis
Triceps	Extensor carpi ulnaris	Extensor indicis proprius
Pronator teres	Extensor digitorum communis	Flexor carpi ulnaris
Flexor carpi radialis	Extensor indicis proprius	Flexor digitorum profundus- 3,4
Brachioradialis		Abductor digiti minimi
Extensor carpi radialis		First dorsal interosseous

Our muscle preferences are shown. Paraspinal muscles belong to all root elements and therefore are not listed. Muscles shown in bold type are more likely to be involved with disease of the listed root element.

TABLE 4. Muscle domains of the cord elements

Upper cord	Middle cord	Lower cord
Biceps	Deltoid	Flexor pollicis longus
Pronator teres	Teres minor	Abductor pollicis brevis
Flexor carpi radialis	Triceps	Flexor carpi ulnaris
	Anconeus	Flexor digitorum profundus- 3,4
	Brachioradialis	Abductor digiti minimi
	Extensor pollicis brevis	First dorsal interosseous
	Extensor carpi radialis	
	Extensor indicis proprius	
	Extensor digitorum communis	
	Extensor carpi ulnaris	

TABLE 5. SNAP domains of the brachial plexus elements and incidence

Upper trunk: LABC (100%); Med-D1 (100%); radial (60%); Med-D2 (20%); Med-D3 (10%)
Middle trunk: Med-D2 (80%); Med-D3 (70%); radial (40%)
Lower trunk: Uln-D5 (100%); DUC (100%); MABC (100%); Med-D3 (20%)
Lateral cord: LABC (100%); Med-D1 (100%); Med-D2 (100%); Med-D3 (80%)
Posterior cord: radial (100%)
Medial cord: Uln-D5 (100%); DUC (100%); MABC (100%); Med-D3 (20%)

Values in parentheses indicate the approximate incidence of involvement for the various brachial plexus elements (8).
SNAP, sensory nerve action potential; LABC, lateral antebrachial cutaneous; Med-D1, median, recording first digit; Med-D2, median, recording second digit; Med-D3, median, recording third digit; Uln-D5, ulnar, recording fifth digit; DUC, dorsal ulnar cutaneous; MABC, medial antebrachial cutaneous.

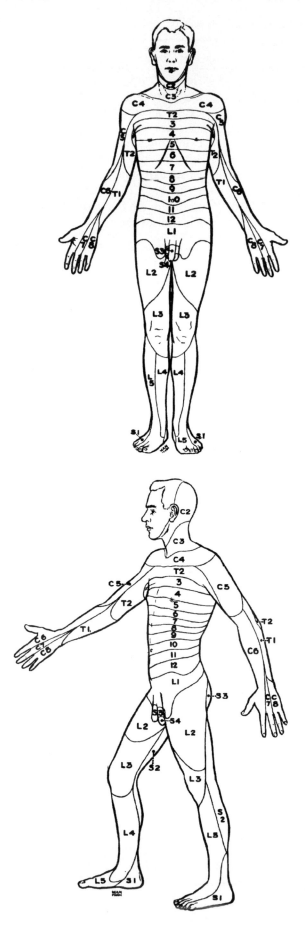

FIG. 2. Anterior view of the dermatomes of the body. The C-2 dermatome adjoins the cutaneous nerve distribution of the mandibular division of the fifth cranial nerve. The arrows indicate the lateral extensions of the T-3 dermatome. From, Haymaker W, Woodhall B. *Peripheral Nerve Injuries: Principles of Diagnosis.* Philadelphia: WB Saunders, 1953, with permission..

FIG. 3. Anterolateral view of the dermatomes of the body. From, Haymaker W, Woodhall B. *Peripheral Nerve Injuries: Principles of Diagnosis.* Philadelphia: WB Saunders, 1953, with permission..

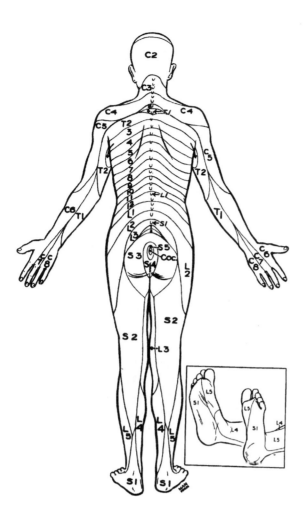

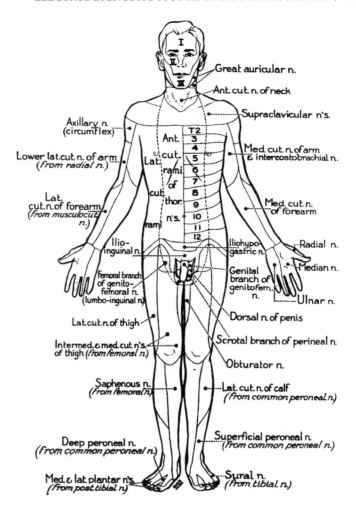

FIG. 4. Posterior view of the dermatomes of the body. Note the absence of a C-1 dermatome. The arrows in the region of the vertebral column identify the T-1, L-1, and S-1 vertebral processes, whereas those in the axillary regions indicate the lateral extent of the T-3 dermatome. The inset shows the dermatomes of the plantar aspects of the feet. From, Haymaker W, Woodhall B. *Peripheral Nerve Injuries: Principles of Diagnosis.* Philadelphia: WB Saunders, 1953, with permission.

FIG. 6. Anterior view of the cutaneous distributions of the peripheral nerves of the body. The intercostal nerves are indicated on the left side of the trunk by numbers, the cutaneous distributions of the branches of the anterior primary rami are shown on the right side of the trunk, and the asterisk just below the scrotum lies within the field of the posterior cutaneous nerve of the thigh. From, Haymaker W, Woodhall B. *Peripheral Nerve Injuries: Principles of Diagnosis.* Philadelphia: WB Saunders, 1953, with permission.

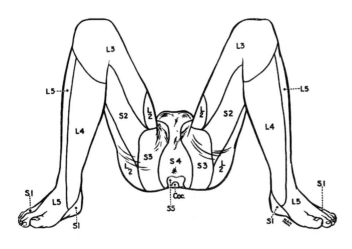

FIG. 5. The dermatomes of the perineum and lower extremities. From, Haymaker W, Woodhall B. *Peripheral Nerve Injuries: Principles of Diagnosis.* Philadelphia: WB Saunders, 1953, with permission.

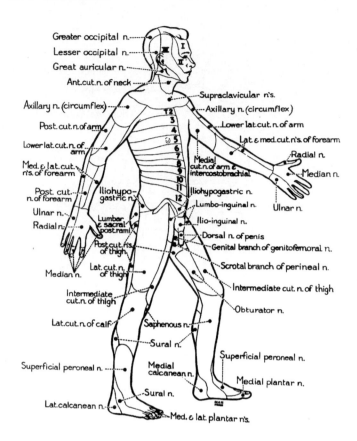

FIG. 7. Anterolateral view of the cutaneous distributions of the peripheral nerves of the body. The roman numerals indicate the ophthalmic (I), maxillary (II), and mandibular (III) divisions of the fifth cranial nerve. From, Haymaker W, Woodhall B. *Peripheral Nerve Injuries: Principles of Diagnosis.* Philadelphia: WB Saunders, 1953, with permission.

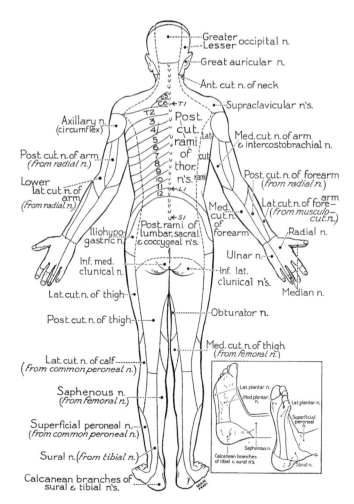

FIG. 8. Posterior view of the cutaneous distributions of the peripheral nerves of the body. The broken lines indicate the boundaries of the cutaneous supply of the posterior primary rami. From, Haymaker W, Woodhall B. *Peripheral Nerve Injuries: Principles of Diagnosis.* Philadelphia: WB Saunders, 1953, with permission.

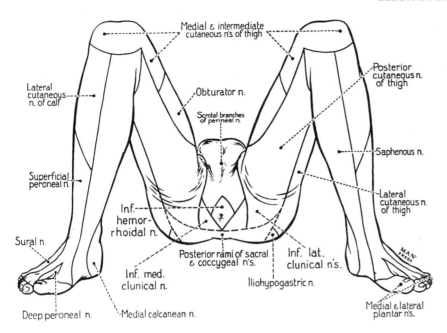

FIG. 9. The cutaneous distributions of the peripheral nerves of the perineum and lower extremities. From, Haymaker W, Woodhall B. *Peripheral Nerve Injuries: Principles of Diagnosis.* Philadelphia: WB Saunders, 1953, with permission.

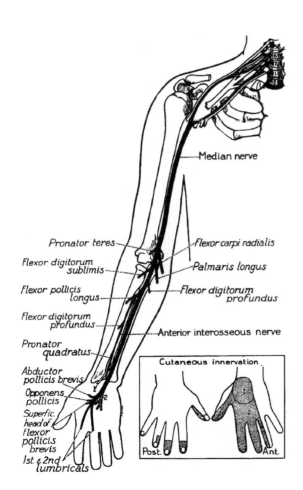

FIG. 10. The course and distribution of the median nerve and the muscles it supplies. The inset shows the cutaneous boundaries of the palmar cutaneous (1) and the palmar digital (2) nerve branches. From, Haymaker W, Woodhall B. *Peripheral Nerve Injuries: Principles of Diagnosis.* Philadelphia: WB Saunders, 1953, with permission.

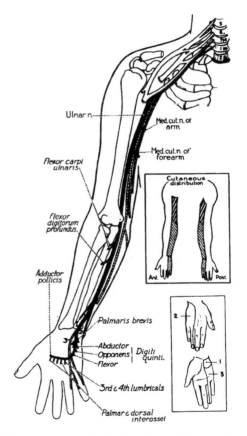

FIG. 11. The course and distribution of the medial cutaneous nerves of the arm and forearm and the ulnar nerve and the muscles supplied by the latter. The patterns of the three nerves are duplicated in the upper inset. The lower inset shows the cutaneous boundaries of the palmar (1), dorsal ulnar cutaneous (2), and superficial terminal (3) branches of the ulnar nerve. From, Haymaker W, Woodhall B. *Peripheral Nerve Injuries: Principles of Diagnosis.* Philadelphia: WB Saunders, 1953, with permission.

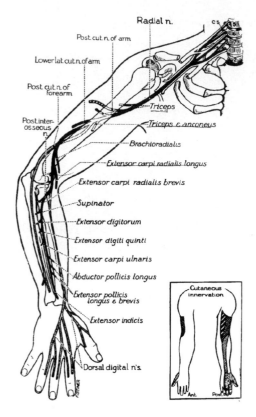

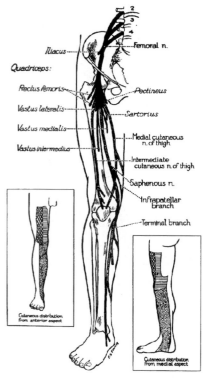

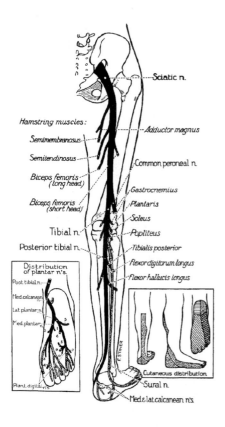

FIG. 12. The course and distribution of the radial nerve and the muscles it supplies. The patterns of the cutaneous nerves are duplicated in the inset. From, Haymaker W, Woodhall B. *Peripheral Nerve Injuries: Principles of Diagnosis.* Philadelphia: WB Saunders, 1953, with permission.

FIG. 13. The course and distribution of the femoral nerve and the muscles it supplies. The patterns of the cutaneous nerves are duplicated in the inset. The broken line indicates the boundaries between the infrapatellar and terminal branches of the saphenous nerve. From, Haymaker W, Woodhall B. *Peripheral Nerve Injuries: Principles of Diagnosis.* Philadelphia: WB Saunders, 1953, with permission.

FIG. 14. The course and distribution of the sciatic, tibial, posterior tibial, and plantar nerves and the muscles they supply. The patterns of the cutaneous nerves are duplicated in the inset. From, Haymaker W, Woodhall B. *Peripheral Nerve Injuries: Principles of Diagnosis.* Philadelphia: WB Saunders, 1953, with permission.

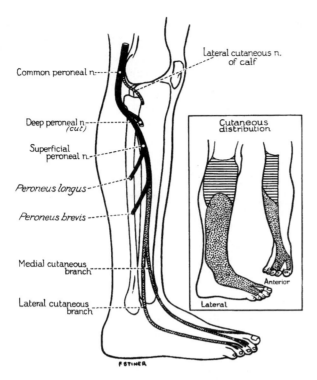

FIG. 15. The course and distribution of the superficial fibular nerve and the muscles it supplies. The patterns of the cutaneous nerves are duplicated in the inset. From, Haymaker W, Woodhall B. *Peripheral Nerve Injuries: Principles of Diagnosis.* Philadelphia: WB Saunders, 1953, with permission.

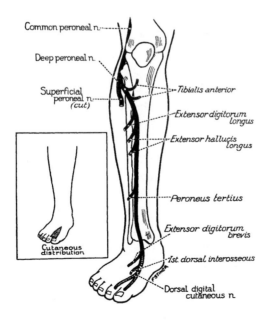

FIG. 16. The course and distribution of the deep fibular nerve and the muscles it supplies. Its cutaneous distribution is shown in the inset. From, Haymaker W, Woodhall B. *Peripheral Nerve Injuries: Principles of Diagnosis.* Philadelphia: WB Saunders, 1953, with permission.

NERVE CONDUCTION STUDIES

Standard NCS assess the large myelinated nerve fibers of named sensory, motor, and mixed nerves while thinly myelinated and unmyelinated fibers that transmit pain and temperature are unavailable for study. When a peripheral nerve is electrically depolarized by negative charge accumulation beneath the cathode of the stimulator, bidirectionally propagating nerve fiber action potentials are generated. Two electrodes positioned away from the stimulation site record the summation of these potentials, termed the *evoked response*. The electrode closest to the stimulation site is the active, or G1 electrode, and the more distant one is termed the reference, or G2 electrode. The electrical activity recorded by these two electrodes is amplified differentially and displayed on the oscilloscope screen. The actual performance of NCS is deceptively simple. With sensory or mixed NCS, the G1 and G2 electrodes are positioned over the nerve under study, whereas they are placed at the motor point of the muscle belly and along the tendon for G1 and G2 electrodes, respectively, when motor NCS are being performed. A ground electrode is affixed between the stimulating and recording sites to reduce shock artifact. The nerve is then stimulated, beginning with a low stimulus intensity that is progressively increased until a response is evoked. At this point, the stimulus intensity is continually increased until the size of the response ceases to increase. At this point, the stimulus is supramaximal and the response is maximal. Whenever NCS are performed, various components of the response are evaluated. These provide information concerning the conduction status of the nerve fibers being assessed, information that often is unobtainable from clinical examination and other laboratory studies.

Sensory Nerve Conduction Studies

The recorded sensory nerve action potential (SNAP) is the summation of many evoked sensory nerve fiber action potentials. These recordings are generally made with surface recording electrodes placed proximal or distal to the stimulating electrodes termed *orthodromic* or *antidromic techniques*, respectively. The antidromic technique is preferable because it produces higher SNAP amplitudes and less patient discomfort.

We measure the following waveform parameters of the nerve response: amplitude, duration, morphology, and peak latency. When a nerve conduction velocity (NCV) is desired, it is obtained by the calculation at two sites of stimulation to avoid the falsely slowed

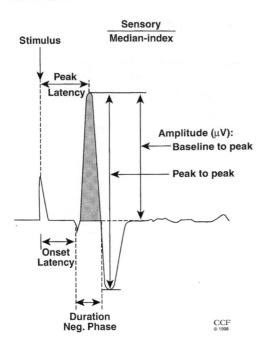

FIG. 17. The various components of the sensory nerve conduction response. From, Levin KH, Shields RW Jr, Wilbourn AJ. Electromyography/Electrodiagnosis. In: Isley MR, Krauss GL, Levin KH, et al., eds. *Electromyography/Electroencephalography.* Redmond, WA: SpaceLabs Medical, Inc., 1993, with permission.

values obtained with single point stimulation related to tissue transit and nerve fiber activation times. The response components for a sensory NCS are illustrated in Figure 17.

Since the waveform morphology can be biphasic or triphasic depending on the particular sensory NCS being performed, the amplitude of the SNAP, in microvolts (μv), can be defined in more than one manner. Triphasic responses are measured from the trough of the initial positive component to the peak of the subsequent negative component, and from the baseline to the peak of the initial negative component when the response is biphasic. The SNAP amplitude reflects the number of functioning axons, their relative conduction rates, and the distance between the stimulation and recording sites. A longer distance decreases the amplitude by increasing temporal dispersion among the individual sensory nerve fiber action potentials.

The amplitude is considered abnormal when it falls below control values or individual laboratory norms. When the amplitude value is 50% or less of the value of the contralateral homologous response, it is considered to be relatively abnormal. The duration in milliseconds (ms) is the time between the onset and termination of the first negative phase of the SNAP. The latency and NCV reflect the rate of conduction along the stimulated axons. One or both can be reported, depending on whether the distance between the stimulating and recording electrodes is predefined or

variable. However, due to the incorporated tissue transit and nerve fiber activation times, the calculated NCV value obtained with single-site stimulation will be an underestimate; consequently, it is possible for a recorded response with a normal peak latency to be associated with a slightly abnormal NCV. When the NCV is interpreted as abnormal, a falsely positive interpretation results.

A constant distance between the stimulating and recording electrodes, rather than a landmark, is employed for two reasons. First, it eliminates the need for a calculated NCV, thereby permitting the elapsed time or latency in ms to be directly compared without manipulation. Second, it removes the effects of temporal dispersion on the amplitude of the recorded responses when collected along nerve segments of varying length. The onset latency reflects the conduction rate along the fastest conducting fibers, whereas the peak latency corresponds to the average NCV of the conducting fibers. Although there are theoretical reasons why onset latencies are more sensitive, peak latencies are preferable because of the ease of identification and the lack of published studies indicating their greater diagnostic value. Although the NCV displayed in m/s can be calculated by dividing the distance between the stimulating and recording sites by the time required in ms for some portion of the SNAP to appear after the nerve is stimulated, the calculated value is falsely slowed. To avoid this inaccuracy, sensory NCV should be calculated using a two-point stimulation technique in which the sensory nerve is stimulated both proximally and distally, generating a proximal sensory response and a distal one. By dividing the surface distance in mm between the two stimulation sites by the latency difference in ms between the peak latencies of the two recorded responses, a NCV value is obtained. This approach can be helpful in the assessment of patients with a suspected polyneuropathy.

Sensory NCS are required to localize lesions involving the sensory system; for example, paraneoplastic sensory neuronopathy (PSN) due to circulating anti-Hu antibodies directed against DRG, CNS neurons, and tumor nuclei, and are more sensitive indicators than motor NCS in the detection of axon loss and focal demyelinating lesions and, not infrequently, the only NCS abnormality identified. For example, the peak latency value of the median SNAP in the carpal tunnel syndrome (CTS), a disorder that produces focal demyelination in its earliest stages, becomes abnormal before the distal motor latency value does. When the pathophysiology transitions from pure demyelination to mixed demyelination and axon loss, the SNAP amplitude value becomes reduced in isolation or to a greater degree than that of the motor response. Sensory NCS are the only component of the EDX study that assesses the PNS. A significant drawback of sensory NCS, however, is its greater vulnerability to physiologic, physical, and unrelated pathologic factors

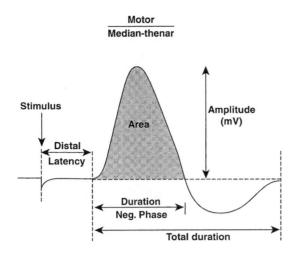

Motor
Median-thenar

FIG. 18. The various components of the motor nerve conduction response. From, Levin KH, Shields RW Jr, Wilbourn AJ. Electromyography/Electrodiagnosis. In: Isley MR, Krauss GL, Levin KH, et al., eds. *Electromyography/Electroencephalography*. Redmond, WA: SpaceLabs Medical, Inc., 1993, with permission.

reflected in the small size of the SNAP, rendering it vulnerable to obesity, edema, physiologic temporal dispersion, temperature, and trivial trauma. This explains why, even among normal individuals, they can be more technically challenging than motor NCS. Temperature is an important determinant of sensory NCS as cooling of the limb increases the SNAP amplitude and duration, prolongs its latency, and decreases the NCV. Whenever a prolonged latency and decreased CV and normal SNAP amplitude are encountered warming is probably the problem and may otherwise be wrongfully ascribed to demyelination. Individuals >60 years of age can normally have bilaterally non-elicited sural and superficial peroneal SNAP. Although many different sensory NCS are available, the frequency with which they are used varies among EMG laboratories.

It is advisable to routinely record the median (recording index finger), ulnar (recording fifth finger), radial (recording the thumb base), sural (recording lateral malleolus) and superficial fibular (recording dorsum of ankle), however other reliable nonstandard studies [e.g., the median (recording thumb and middle finger), the lateral and medial antebrachial cutaneous, and the dorsal ulnar cutaneous studies] also are useful, especially in the localization of axon loss brachial plexus lesions (1). Saphenous and lateral femoral cutaneous NCS are unreliable for routine clinical use, making study of the lumbar plexus challenging.

Motor Nerve Conduction Studies

Only orthostatic motor NCS are performed using the belly-tendon method wherein the recorded response represents the summation of the muscle fiber action potentials (AP) generated by the stimulated motor axons, each of which is termed a compound muscle action potential (CMAP). The innervation ratio or number of muscle fibers innervated per motor axon explains why motor responses measured in mv are so much larger than sensory responses measured in μv. This magnification effect significantly reduces CMAP vulnerability to physiologic, physical, and pathologic factors. Measured CMAP parameters include amplitude, duration, latency, CV, and waveform morphology. The CMAP morphology is biphasic because placement of the G1 electrode over the motor point of the muscle results in a CMAP response recorded at its inception. If the initial positive phase is absent, the CMAP amplitude is measured from baseline to peak. CMAP are more resistant to physiologic temporal dispersion permitting the distance between the stimulating and recording electrodes to be greater allowing assessment of longer nerve segments compared to sensory NCS, and rendering them adequate for the localization of focal demyelinating conduction block.

It is seldom necessary to stimulate proximal to the supraclavicular level along spinal motor root in the arm or proximal to the popliteal fossa level in the leg. When distances are kept constant between the stimulating and recording sites, latencies can be measured and directly compared to normative laboratory values. Distal latency is never used to calculate the motor nerve CV value, because in addition to the desired motor nerve conduction time, it also incorporates the tissue transit and nerve fiber activation times, NMJ transmission, and muscle fiber conduction times.

Accurate assessment of motor nerve conduction requires stimulation at two separate sites resulting in distal and proximal evoked responses, the latency values of which are employed to calculate the motor NCV. With other intervening factors equal, the difference between the proximal and distal latencies reflects the time required for the impulses to travel from the proximal stimulation site to the distal one. The motor NCV expressed in m/s between the two sites of stimulation is calculated by dividing the distance between the two sites in mm by the latency difference in ms (Figure 18).

The median, ulnar, peroneal, and posterior tibial motor responses, respectively recording from the abductor pollicis brevis (APB), abductor digiti minimi (ADM), extensor digitorum brevis (EDB), and abductor hallucis (AH) muscles, comprise the standard motor NCS, with other optional, limb and cranial motor nerves.

When the nerve under study can only be stimulated at one site as, for example, along the axillary nerve and recording from the deltoid muscle, or along the spinal accessory nerve and recording from the trapezius muscle, only distal motor response parameters are analyzed. Triphasic and biphasic mixed NCS are technically challenging, especially

In obese individuals, and aside from plantar and palmar mixed NCS, they offer little additional information over conventional NCS.

ELECTROPHYSIOLOGIC MANIFESTATIONS OF VARIOUS NERVE LESIONS

Nerve Conduction Studies

The pathologic responses to nerve injury are essentially limited to axon loss, focal demyelination, or some combination of the two. Axon disruption causes the distal stump of the involved axon to degenerate, termed *Wallerian degeneration,* rendering it incapable of conducting action potentials leading to axonal loss and conduction failure. Lesions that produce axon disruption and either LMN or DRG cell loss, are identifiable by a loss of the amplitude of the recorded response. Such changes are more noticeable in the sensory nerves, which are more sensitive to a given percentage of axon disruption than the corresponding CMAP amplitude.

A loss of approximately 50% of the axons of a mixed nerve leads to comparatively lower amplitudes in the SNAP responses compared to those of the CMAP, which appears to follow a more linear relationship. Whereas latency and CV measurements tend to be normal in partial axon loss lesions, indicating preservation of the fastest conducting fibers rather than the total number of conducting fibers, when the underlying disorder involves all or most of the fastest conducting fibers, latency and CV measurements may be mildly abnormal, and substantial slowing can be seen when a severe axon loss lesion is followed by successful regeneration reflecting the smaller diameter, higher impedance, thinner myelin sheaths, and increased capacitance of the regenerating nerve fibers.

The observed alterations with demyelinating lesions depend on its severity with such processes tending to affect the largest and fastest conducting fibers. Mild demyelinating lesions cause widening of the nodal gap and slowing of the rate of propagation of nerve fiber action potentials leading to prolongation of distal latencies and decreased CV with all of the propagating impulses reaching their target organ in a delayed manner. More pronounced demyelination is similar to axon disruption with propagating impulses blocked and unable to traverse the lesion site. As a result, the amplitude of the recorded response is decreased when the stimulus is applied proximal to the lesion. Thus, with both axon loss and demyelinating conduction block, the amplitude of the response is the most important parameter measured, with the degree of amplitude reduction dependent on the number of nerve fibers affected. Unlike axon loss processes in which the recorded response amplitudes are low or unobtainable, regardless of the site

TABLE 6. Electrodiagnostic abnormalities of the motor neuraxis

1. Upper motor neuron
   Normal sensory NCS
   Decreased spatial recruitment
   Decreased temporal recruitment
2. Intraspinal canal lesion
   Normal sensory NCS
   Abnormal motor NCS—uncommon
   Fibrillation potentials
   MUAP configuration changes
   Neurogenic MUAP recruitment
3. Postganglionic lesions
   Abnormal sensory NCS
   Abnormal motor NCS
   Fibrillation potentials
   Increased MUAP duration
   Neurogenic MUAP recruitment
4. Pure motor axon lesion
   Normal sensory NCS
   Abnormal motor NCS (+/-)
   Fibrillation potentials
   Increased MUAP duration
   Neurogenic MUAP recruitment
5. Terminal nerve branch(es)
   Disintegration of the motor unit
   Normal sensory NCS
   Abnormal motor NCS (+/-)
   Fibrillation potentials
   Decreased MUAP duration and amplitude
   Polyphasic potentials
   Early recruitment
6. NMJ disorders
   Disintegration of the motor unit
   As listed in no. 5
   Abnormal RSS
7. Muscle disorders
   Disintegration of the motor unit
   As listed in no. 5

None, some, or all of the above-listed EDX abnormalities may be observed, depending on the degree of severity of the underlying disorder.
EDX: electrodiagnostic; NCS: nerve conduction studies; MUAP: motor unit action potential; RSS, repetitive nerve stimulation studies.

of stimulation, with focal demyelinating conduction block lesions, the recorded response amplitude varies with the site of stimulation because the lesion does not affect conduction proximal or distal to the demyelinated region.

Conduction block may go undetected unless the stimulating and recording sites straddle the lesion; the exception to this is in early axonal disruption prior to the development of Wallerian degeneration. Four to seven days after Wallisian degeneration and axonal disruption, but before enervation has occurred, the pathophysiologic contributions to the lesion can be estimated by comparing the amplitude of the distal CMAP from the symptomatic side, with that from the asymptomatic side leading to an estimate of the contribution of axon disruption. The difference between the proximal and distal motor response amplitudes can be used to calculate the percentage of motor nerve fibers affected by the demyelinating conduction block. For example, when the CMAP amplitude is 5 mV with stimulation distal to the lesion, 2.5 mV upon stimulation proximal to the lesion, and 10 mV on the contralateral side, then 50% of the nerve fibers are affected by axon loss, 25% by demyelinating conduction block, and 25% conduct normally.

When a focal demyelinating conduction block lesion is suspected, further evaluation utilizing more proximal stimulation sites, such as at the elbow, spiral groove, axilla, and supraclavicular fossa can be undertaken. Once identified, further localization can be determined using stimulation applied at progressively more distal sites until the proximally identified amplitude reduction normalizes, the so-called inching technique.

The clinical correlation of the motor axonal pathophysiology is that clinical weakness occurs when propagating nerve fiber action potentials fail to reach their my fiber target, an outcome that occurs only with axon loss–induced conduction failure or demyelinating conduction block, but would not be expected to occur with lesions producing solely demyelinating conduction slowing. However, regarding the sensory axons, fixed sensory deficits would be expected with dropout of propagating SNAP, a condition that requires either axon loss–induced conduction failure or demyelinating conduction block. Regardless of the type of nerve fiber lesion, demyelinating conduction slowing has little clinical accompaniment more so an electrodiagnostic phenomenon (Table 6).

Needle Examination

This is the most sensitive test for detecting motor axon loss lesions and the only portion of the EMG examination capable of identifying disorders involving the UMN system and, for practical purposes, the muscle fibers themselves. Both concentric and monopole needle electrodes are used. The former are hollow and contain a thin, centrally located metal wire that is surrounded by an insulating resin. The tip of the wire is exposed distally and functions as the G1 electrode, whereas the intramuscular portion of the cannula functions as the G2 electrode. Monopole needles are composed of a metal shaft that is coated with Teflon, except at its tip, which functions as the G1 recording electrode. It is used

in conjunction with a separate surface electrode that functions as the G2 recording electrode. The electrical activity recorded by the G1 and G2 leads of the needle electrode passes through a differential amplifier and the voltage difference between them is displayed on an oscilloscope. The sound characteristics of the recorded responses are fed into an audio system. The standard needle examination includes a sampling of distal, middle, and proximal limb muscles of different root, plexus, and nerve origins, and paraspinal muscles; some of the more commonly studied muscles of several upper extremity muscle domains are displayed in Tables 1–4. When a myopathy is suspected, this approach is modified (2). The three phases of the needle examination include needle insertion, rest, and activation.

Insertion Phase

This phase includes the initial needle insertion through the skin and into the muscle, followed by small advances. Insertional activity is derived from needle-induced mechanical excitation of muscle fibers and follows each advancement, typically lasting less than one-third of a second. Several advancements are made in one direction, at which point the needle is brought back to the skin surface without exiting and advanced in a different direction. This is repeated until the muscle is thoroughly studied. When fat or connective tissue replaces muscle, the insertional activity decreases and ultimately disappears when the muscle tissue is completely replaced. Increased insertional activity is present when various types of electrical potentials follow the needle advancements such as snap-crackle-pop, or abnormal such as brief trains of positive sharp waves, although neither represent increase in the insertional activity produced by needle advancement (3).

Rest Phase

The rest phase is the period of time between needle advancements, when the needle is held motionless in a relaxed muscle. Both normal and abnormal spontaneous activity may be observed during this phase. End-plate noise, a type of normal spontaneous activity, occurs when the needle electrode records activity from a nearby end-plate region, a location typically painful for the patient. End-plate noise consists of two distinct types of electrical activity, miniature end-plate potentials (MEPP) and end-plate spikes.

Miniature EPP are irregular, short duration, low amplitude, monophasic, negative waveforms that produce a sound reminiscent of seashell noise. They reflect the spontaneous release of individual quanta of acetylcholine (ACh). End-plate spikes are irregular, biphasic waveforms with an initial negative phase. They are longer in duration and higher amplitude than MEPP, and sound like sputtering fat in a frying pan. During the rest phase, several types of abnormal spontaneous activity may be observed.

Fibrillation potentials are regularly firing potentials that result from spontaneous repetitive activation of muscle fibers that have been denervated for three or more weeks. They fire with metronomic regularity at 1 to 15 Hz and are the most common type of abnormal spontaneous activity encountered. They are the sine qua non of motor axon loss and have two morphologies, a biphasic spike form and a positive sharp wave (PSW) form, with both morphologies representing the same electrical activity but different relationship to the needle electrode and muscle fiber membrane.

A myofiber unable to generate spontaneous fibrillation potentials may be abnormal enough to generate brief trains of insertional PSW when injured and mechanically depolarized by the advancing needle tip. In this setting, the term insertional positive wave is applied. This form of electrical activity typically precedes the appearance of fibrillation potentials by about one week. It is important to differentiate insertional positive waves from the PSW form of fibrillation potentials because the former indicates recent denervation in the past three weeks.

Fibrillation potentials must also be differentiated from end-plate spikes. Compared with end-plate spikes, the initial phases of fibrillation potentials are positive. Following muscle fiber denervation, ion channel changes develop that produce 0.5- to 15-Hz autonomous muscle fiber depolarization. Although these potentials are best characterized by their metronomic regularity, irregularity may be noted in the acute setting. The high innervation ratio of most limb muscles accounts for the extreme sensitivity of the needle examination for the detection of motor axon loss. With disruption of just a single motor axon, fibrillation potentials develop in all of the muscle fibers of that motor unit, a degree of severity not discernible by motor NCS or clinical examination. Fibrillation potentials are commonly seen in primary muscle disorders, such as polymyositis, whenever a portion of the muscle fiber is separated from its end-plate due to segmental myonecrosis. Myopathic fibrillation potentials are identical to neurogenic ones but, unlike the latter, may fire at very slow rates. Although fibrillation potentials themselves are nonspecific, their distribution has a strong localizing role, and their size and density yields information on disease duration and severity, respectively. Large amplitude fibrillation potentials are observed in the acute setting and their density is proportional to the severity of motor axon disruption. They persist until reinnervation occurs or degeneration of the muscle fibers is complete.

Fasciculation potentials fire irregularly and have the configuration of motor unit action potentials (MUAP). They represent the spontaneous activation of individual motor units or of portions of motor units. They signify irritability rather than denervation. Their firing frequency varies from a few per minute to one per second. Their significance is determined by the company they keep. They are of little importance in isolation except in the clinical syndrome of benign fasciculation, but are quite important when accompanied by fibrillation potentials or prolonged duration MUAP, as in motor neuron disease.

Complex repetitive discharges (CRD) derive from the near-synchronous firing of multiple muscle fibers, with one fiber ephaptically pacing the others. They typically have a bizarre appearance, usually continuously disrupt the baseline, and have an abrupt onset and cessation. Although the amplitude, duration, configuration, and frequency vary among different CRD trains, these aspects are essentially constant for an individual one. These nonspecific discharges observed in both neuropathic and myopathic disorders are a sign of chronicity, typically indicating that the lesion is of at least six months duration.

Myotonic discharges are action potentials of single muscle fibers that also occur in trains. Like fibrillation potentials, there are two distinct morphologies, a spike form and a PSW appearance. Their firing frequency and amplitude continuously change, producing a characteristic pitch variation that has been likened to a diving airplane. These potentials, which typically reflect muscle membrane disorders, occur with clinical myotonia, including myotonic dystrophy, myotonia congenita, and paramyotonia congenita, or without myotonia as in polymyositis, acid maltase deficiency, hypothyroidism, hyperkalemic periodic paralysis, diazocholesterols and monocarboxylate drugs.

Grouped repetitive discharges are the repeated firing of groups of several potentials that display a simple waveform. The time period between individual potentials within the group is termed the *intrapotential interval*, whereas the time period separating each group of potentials is termed the *interpotential interval*; the latter is usually silent, unlike the case with complex repetitive discharges. The number of potentials composing a group and their firing frequency can vary. When two or more grouped repetitive discharges fire concurrently and typically asynchronously since they are independent, the term *myokymia* is applied. Facial myokymia is commonly seen in association with multiple sclerosis and pontine glioma, whereas limb myokymia occurs in radiation-induced plexopathy and multifocal motor neuropathy (MMN), and generalized myokymia in chronic inflammatory demyelinating polyradiculoneuropathy (CIDP) and gold intoxication (4).

Cramp potentials, like fasciculation activity, are abnormal MUAP. Two characteristic features of cramp potentials are their rapid firing rate and synchronicity. Normally, motor unit recruitment proceeds in single motor unit increments, from the smaller motor units to the larger ones. Although single MUAP are readily analyzed at the lower levels of MUAP recruitment, higher levels impede the recognition of individual MUAP. With a cramp potential, the involved MUAP are recruited synchronously and each one fires at frequencies well above the typical 40 Hz maximum. This feature likely accounts for the associated pain and likely reflects cramp-induced ischemia. Cramp potentials have a strong association with fasciculation activity. Among patients with abundant fasciculation, cramping is a frequent complaint. Conversely, among patients with frequent cramping, fasciculation are commonly observed. Cramp potentials can be benign or associated with a serious disorder, such as motor neuron disease. Cramp-like fasciculation potentials reflect irritability.

Activation Phase

During this phase, the patient voluntarily contracts the muscle under study, with the needle electrode held stationary while the recruitment, firing pattern, and morphology of the evoked MUAP are examined. Individual muscle fiber action potentials of a particular motor unit do not contribute equally to the observed MUAP since those nearest to the recording electrode provide a significant contribution to the MUAP amplitude and its rise time, although all of the muscle fiber action potentials contribute to its duration. They fire almost regularly with gentle contraction at a basal rate of 5 to 10 Hz and demonstrate a stable waveform morphology. With increasing contractile force, more MUAP appear on the oscilloscope screen, a phenomenon termed *spatial recruitment*, and those recruited increase the firing rate, a feature termed *temporal recruitment*. Together, they assure smooth increments in muscle contraction force. Individual MUAP become unrecognizable with increasing recruitment until a full interference pattern is present.

Recruitment is abnormal when it is reduced or neurogenic, and early and myopathic. Reduced recruitment refers to decreased spatial recruitment, a reflection of motor unit dropout. The latter occurs with disorders that impede action potential propagation from the LMN to the muscle fibers belonging to that motor unit, such as LMN and motor axon disorders that result in Wallerian degeneration with axon loss conduction failure, and in demyelinating disorders resulting in conduction block.

An advanced stage of MUAP dropout results in a discrete interference pattern. Normally, individual MUAP cannot be discerned at the upper end of their normal firing range because as spatial recruitment increases it becomes impossible to detect individual MUAP. However, with impaired spatial recruitment, MUAP of the functioning motor units are detectable and, for that reason, are distinguishable at the upper end of their firing range. This pattern is referred to as neurogenic recruitment as it demonstrates both a reduced number of MUAP and rapid firing rate. Although poor effort can occur in malingering, conversion disorder,

pain, and UMN disorders, wherein the numbers of MUAP are decreased, they do not produce a rapid firing rate. Both spatial and temporal recruitment are normal in lesions that produce demyelinating conduction slowing because they do not produce motor unit dropout and, consequently, do not impede the generation of muscle force.

Early recruitment exists when spatial recruitment is excessive for the degree of force generated. It occurs in disorders that produce disintegration of the motor unit as, for example, lesions that affect the terminal axon branches, NMJ, and myofibers. Since the number of muscle fibers per activated LMN is decreased, the amount of force generated by a given motor unit is reduced. More motor units are required to produce a given amount of contractile force. For this reason, motor unit recruitment proceeds at a faster than expected rate and, consequently, a full interference pattern is associated with a submaximal effort.

An abnormal recruitment pattern is observed with UMN lesions wherein both spatial and temporal recruitment are decreased and the interference pattern is incomplete. This MUAP firing pattern occurs with incomplete effort, and unlike the faster firing frequency observed with neurogenic recruitment, active MUAP fire at their basal rate.

The morphology of an observed MUAP can be described in terms of its external and internal configuration. The external configuration refers to the duration and amplitude of the potential. Whereas UMN lesions are positioned proximal to the LMN with an unchanged motor unit territory, fiber density, duration and amplitude of the MUAP, LMN lesions lead to axonal disruption produces denervation throughout the motor unit, and incomplete nerve lesions leads to collateral sprouting by unaffected motor axons that reinnervates some of the denervated myofibers. The latter process, which is associated with an increased innervation ratio, expansion of myofiber territory, and density, imparts an increase in the CMAP duration and amplitude as seen in static and remote poliomyelitis and other slowly progressive disorders in which there is both myofiber reinnervation that keeps pace with denervation and associated chronic neurogenic MUAP changes. When motor unit dropout follows demyelinating conduction block, MUAP configuration is unaffected since the motor axons remain in continuity and muscle fiber denervation is absent.

The motor unit territory and muscle fiber density are decreased in disorders that produce disintegration of the motor unit with shortening of the MUAP duration and lowering of MUAP amplitude, a process that is reminiscent of myopathy, but so noted in other disorders characterized by disintegration of the motor unit. The internal configuration of an MUAP instead refers to its phases and area under the curve between any two baseline crossings, and its turns or directional changes not crossing the baseline. Whereas UMN lesions do not result in changes in MUAP configuration, those involving the LMN and motor axon loss typically increase the number of MUAP phases and turns through collateral sprouting.

Demyelinating conduction block of motor axons leads to motor unit dropout, but the internal configurations of the remaining MUAP are unaffected. When demyelinating conduction block affects individual terminal nerve branches, disintegration of the motor unit occurs, and with significant degrees of muscle fiber loss, the number of turns and phases increase.

Polyphasic MUAP, defined as those with more than four phases, constitute up to 10% of the MUAP of any normal muscle. While chronic neurogenic MUAP appear polyphasic, the more apparent abnormality is the increase in MUAP duration. The primary diagnostic value of polyphasic MUAP is in the recognition of disorders that cause disintegration of the motor unit such as myopathy, and in the identification of early proximal-distal reinnervation that presents initially with reduced myofiber regeneration per motor axon and MUAP similar to those of motor unit disintegration, slow conduction rates along recently regenerated terminal axons, and a MUP duration that is markedly prolonged with satellite potentials.

Timing of the Electrodiagnostic Examination

At the onset of focal axon loss and demyelinating conduction block, there is an impedance of impulse transmission across the lesion site, with normal distal SNAP and CMAP, and low amplitude or absent responses proximal to the site of the lesion. Needle EMG reveals a neurogenic recruitment pattern in a partial lesion, and absence of voluntary MUAP in muscles innervated by the affected motor nerve fibers in complete lesions. The lesions that disrupt motor axons results in a drop-out of individual MUAP that contribute to the CMAP, which follows a temporal pattern of Wallerian degeneration, commencing by day three and reaching a nadir in presence of near- or complete absence of evoked CMAP at, above, or below the lesion. Demyelinating lesions manifesting conduction block lead to abnormal CMAP responses observed only after stimulation at or above the lesion with normal responses evoked distal to the lesion due to the lack of associated pathophysiologic effects. These two pathophysiologic processes may not be easily separable in the first five to seven days following the onset of clinical weakness, however a similar pattern of Wallerian degeneration follows sensory axon disruption, with abnormalities appearing slightly later as manifested by decay in the SNAP amplitude around day six and reaching a nadir by day 11. At that time, needle examination remains unchanged, however between days 15 to 20, denervated myofibers produce trains of PSW in response to needle insertion and advancement, persisting for up to one week, and then replaced by fibrillation potentials.

Lesions producing significant demyelinating conduction block can disrupt motor axons and not uncommonly lead to the appearance of large number of fibrillation potentials, especially in the setting of severe or acute presentations. For this reason, it is never wise to estimate the severity of the lesion based on the number of observed fibrillation potentials, rather the severity should be based upon the degree of amplitude decrement in the evoked CMAP.

Denervated muscle fibers can become reinnervated or progress to complete degeneration. Two factors enhance reinnervation, one fast and the other slow. The faster one is by collateral sprouting wherein normal unaffected motor axons generate branches that grow peripherally, adopting denervated myofibers. Collateral sprouting proceeds in intact motor axons of an incomplete lesion, with a success that is inversely proportional to the completeness of the lesion. The second mechanism of reinnervation is through regrowth from the proximal axon stump, a process that proceeds slowly at a rate of about one inch per month. Proximal-to-distal regeneration occurs best when the distance between the site of the lesion and the denervated muscles is short, however affected muscles that are separated by more than 20 to 24 inches from the lesion site experience ineffective reinnervation by the mechanism of regrowth, and can only be reinnervated by collateral sprouting.

Special Studies

H Responses

H responses are elicited by stimulating the tibial nerve in the popliteal fossa, with the cathode oriented proximally and recording from the gastrocnemius-soleus complex. Low stimulus intensities activate large Ia sensory fibers because of their lower activation threshold compared to motor fibers. The evoked action potentials reach the S-1 segment of the spinal cord and activate LMN at that segment. The latter generate action potentials that propagate distally to produce the H-wave response at the recording site. As the stimulus intensity is increased the H-wave amplitude also increases but with eventual activation of motor nerve fibers bidirectional propagating motor nerve fiber action potentials are generated, the proximally propagating ones of which collide with Ia sensory fibers, negating some of the action potentials contributing to the H-response leading to disappearance of the response. H responses are particularly useful in the detection of generalized sensory polyneuropathy and S-1 radiculopathy, and like other sensory and motor responses, the amplitude and not latency is the more sensitive measurement. They are consistently elicited from the gastrocnemius-soleus muscle complex but decrease with aging and, in fact, can be absent bilaterally in those older than age 60 years and in others with S-1 radiculopathy, and following lumbar laminectomy.

F Waves

F waves are elicited by the supramaximal stimulation of a motor nerve leads to bidirectional propagating action potentials with those traveling distally producing the M-wave, and others traveling proximally reaching the spinal cord LMN. Depending upon the state of excitation of the latter, backfiring can occur in 5 to 10% of LMN, resulting in centrifugally propagating motor nerve fiber action potentials, which in turn, are recorded distally as F-waves. Unlike H responses, they can be elicited from any motor nerve, and are theoretically useful in the detection of proximal nerve lesions, especially in the setting of demyelinating lesions, and in the early detection of Guillain Barré syndrome (GBS).

Repetitive Nerve Stimulation

Repetitive nerve stimulation (RNS) is performed in patients with suspected NMJ disorders wherein safety factors for NMJ transmission is compromised despite the overabundance of ACh release from axon terminals, ample number of postsynaptic receptors, and narrowness of the cleft separating the presynaptic and postsynaptic membranes, all of which generally ensure muscle fiber depolarization and generation of a muscle fiber action potential. Disorders that impede NMJ transmission can be identified by RNS first at low stimulation rates of 2 to 3 Hz such as the post-synaptic disorder of acquired autoimmune myasthenia gravis (MG) compared to incremental responses at rates of 40 Hz or more, that indicate a presynaptic NMJ disorder such as Lambert-Eaton myasthenic syndrome (LEMS). The stimulation and recording techniques are identical to those of individual motor NCS except successive trains of motor responses are collected and the amplitude or area compared to baseline to detect abnormal decremental changes, followed by an exercise period of 30 to 120 seconds that initially corrects the decrement, but successive trains at minute intervals leads to more profound decrement due to post-activation exhaustion of quanta of ACh at the synaptic cleft.

ELECTRODIAGNOSTIC FEATURES OF NEUROMUSCULAR DISORDERS

Incomplete Voluntary Effort

The combination of weak muscles that yield normal CMAP amplitudes and a needle EMG examination that reveals reduced MUAP recruitment is generally due to functional disorders causing incomplete voluntary effort or an underlying UMN disorder. Pain can limit effortful muscle contraction that remains normal up to the point at which the patient stops muscle activation, and hysterical conversion disorders and malingering can lead to variations in the MUAP. The electrodiagnostic features of clinical give-away weakness and alternating agonist-antagonist contraction patterns is associated with the sudden disappearance of MUAP activation and poorly synchronized MUAPs firing in bursts.

Upper Motor Neuron Disorders

Sensory and motor NCS, late responses, and the insertion and rest phases of the needle examination are normal in UMN disorders. However, because they can lead to impaired spatial and temporal MUAP recruitment, the activation phase of the needle examination during maximal effort can show a reduced number of MUAP that fire at the lower end or below the normal range, depending upon the threshold of the individual motor units that generate the MUAP (5). Regardless of the degree of coaxing, affected patients cannot recruit more MUAP or increase their firing rate. Since the muscle fiber density and territory of the motor units remain unaltered, the observed MUAP configurations are normal. Occasional patients with severe UMN lesions may have MUAP after stimulus-induced involuntary response, such as stroking the sole of the foot while recording from the tibialis anterior muscle, that exceeds that observed with voluntary activation. A possible hint to a UMN disorder can be a tremulous, poorly synchronized MUAP firing pattern.

Spinal Canal and Spinal Cord Disorders

The intraspinal canal contains the spinal cord with the anterior horn cells (AHC) and their exiting motor axons, the primary ventral rootlets and centrally directed preganglionic sensory axons. Intrinsic spinal cord disorders affect the CST and AHC, intraparenchymal portions of peripherally directed motor axons, preganglionic sensory axons, or a combination thereof. Electrodiagnostic studies do not recognize the segment of preganglionic or postganglionic sensory axon, or DRG and may have normal sensory NCS and H responses that assess the S-1 preganglionic sensory fiber. Anterior horn cell injury results in Wallerian degeneration of the affected motor axons that leads to muscle fiber denervation throughout the territories of the respective motor units, especially those that do not produce MUAP, with associated normal SNAP, and normal, low amplitude, or absent CMAP responses, with insertional PSW that appear from day 15 to day 20 after injury, and are later replaced by fibrillation potentials that appear from day 21 to 35 and persist until the muscle fiber is either reinnervated or degenerates.

Fasciculation potentials are a common finding in AHC disorders, particularly amyotrophic lateral sclerosis (ALS). Since spatial recruitment is impaired due to a dropout of whole motor units, the activation phase of the needle EMG shows a decreased number of firing MUAP at a faster than normal rate. Collateral sprouting from unaffected motor axons increases the muscle fiber territory and density of the rein-nervated motor units; consequently, the remaining MUAP become increased in duration and possibly amplitude. Rein-nervation may fail to keep pace with denervation, leading to absent or delayed H- and M-wave response amplitudes, and normal minimal F-wave latency and impersistence.

Acute poliomyelitis, now infrequent in developed countries due to widespread vaccination, leads to asymmetric distribution and absence of chronic MUAP changes, while remote poliomyelitis has already present myofiber rein-nervation. The evoked CMAP are normal due to collateral sprouting, and needle EMG shows altered firing rate and external configuration of MUAP coupled with sparse spontaneous activity comprised of a small number of very low amplitude fibrillation potentials, or absence of spontaneous activity. Abnormal needle examination features may be observed in seemingly unaffected muscles, however like those involved, the myofiber territories and densities of the surviving motor units are significantly increased.

There are five distinguishing electrodiagnostic features of ALS including asymmetry, abnormality of routine motor NCS, widespread fasciculation with less-affected muscles showing them even more and the more affected muscles revealing more fibrillation potentials and MUAP loss, and in contrast to poliomyelitis, a rate of denervation that far exceeds the capacity for reinnervation, leading to more prominent PSW and fibrillations than MUAP configurational changes, and combined UMN and LMN firing patterns. Similar to other motor neuron disorders, needle EMG abnormalities should be established in muscles of three limbs, including those of bulbar and thoracic paraspinal segments, not innvervated by the same nerve or root segment.

In the spectrum of spinal muscular atrophy (SMA), both Werdnig-Hoffman (SMA1) and Wohlfart-Kugelberg-Welander disease (SMA3) shows predominantly proximal symmetric abnormalities and occasional fasciculation with differing degrees of chronic MUAP changes. However SMA1 demonstrates widespread, rapid involvement of brainstem and the somatic LMN, with denervation out-pacing reinnervation, and needle abnormalities resembling ALS, while SMA3 has slower progression of reinnervation.

Kennedy disease or bulbospinal neuronopathy, is an X-linked recessive disorder distinguished by involvement of sensory and motor neurons (6-8) with electrodiagnostic features non-uniform low amplitude or non-elicited SNAP and less frequently low amplitude CMAP, which together suggest sensory neuropathy or neuronopathy. Needle examination reveals sparse fibrillation potentials and pronounced chronic neurogenic MUAP changes consistent with slow progression. Although the distribution of the electrical abnormalities is generalized, they may be more pronounced or restricted to the area at onset.

Primary Root Disorders

Disorders of the spinal roots or radiculopathy, are the commonest reasons for referral to an EMG laboratory. There are four important reasons to consider electrodiagnostc studies in the setting of presumed radiculopathy. First, it will localize the process and correctly identify the predominant pathophysiology. Second, unlike neuroimaging studies, which show false-positive or incidental findings, electrodiagnostic analysis rarely reveals false positive findings when performed by experienced electrodiagnosticians. Third, serial electrical assessment can be used to follow the course of the radiculopathic process. Finally, when the clinical diagnosis is in doubt, electrodiagnostic studies will redirects the evaluation toward the more appropriate diagnosis.

The dorsal and ventral roots consist, respectively, of sensory and motor axons, and with the exception of the S-1 preganglionic sensory fibers assessed by the H-response, the sensory root axons are preganglionic and unavailable for study by conventional sensory NCS, which instead assesses the DRG and the postganglionic sensory axons. Accordingly, sensory NCS are typically unaffected by intraspinal canal disorders and radiculopathy, which is unfortunate because isolated sensory root involvement is the most frequent clinical type of radiculopathy (9). The results of motor NCS are variable depending on the particular root and number of roots affected, as well as the underlying pathophysiology, severity of the lesion, and timing of the study. Significant CMAP amplitude reduction is infrequent, even in muscles of an affected myotome, because most lesions affect a minority of motor axons in a root, a feature that facilitates collateral sprouting and CMAP normalization.

Most muscles are innervated by more than one root, which facilitates reinnervation via collateral sprouting. Basic motor NCS address the C-8, T-1, L-5, and S-1 roots, whereas non-routine motor NCS are required to assess the other roots such as the phrenic CMAP for the C3 to C5 roots. The distribution of radicular disorders influences the likelihood of identifying motor NCS abnormalities as, for example, when the cause is demyelinating conduction block, which may not be recognized by routine motor NCS and hence go undetected by needle examination due to its lower sensitive to this pathophysiology.

Axonal loss related to axonal disruption, which is the more common pathophysiology associated with a radiculopathy, is readily discerned on needle examination. Needle EMG is abnormal in the acute phase from three weeks to two months after the onset of the lesion, before collateral sprouting occurs. Based on the innervation ratio of most of the studied skeletal muscles, hundreds of muscle fibers are denervated for each involved motor axon during this time period, and the insertion and rest phases of the needle examination show positive sharp waves and fibrillation potentials.

It is uncommon for a muscle to be so severely denervated by a monoradiculopathy so as to produce abnormal MUAP firing patterns. Once collateral sprouting occurs, chronic neurogenic MUAP changes become apparent. Acute radiculopathy is classically diagnosed by the finding of fibrillation potentials in a myotomal limb distribution with paraspinal muscle involvement. The H-response amplitude, more than the latency, is a sensitive marker of S-1 radiculopathy, whereas F-wave responses are usually normal. Nonetheless, the presence of myotomal fibrillation potentials and chronic neurogenic MUAP changes is usually consistent with either chronic, ongoing active radiculopathy or a recent active root lesion superimposed upon a long-standing pre-existing one. The increased frequency of active denervation in distal muscles is related to the nature of the reinnervation process, which proceeds earlier in proximal than distal muscles. The sensitivity of the electrodiagnostic study increases with involvement of multiple contiguous roots as in the cauda equina syndrome due to substantively more apparent muscle denervation, which presents more abundant fibrillation activity, as well as low amplitude or non-elicited CMAP, and a neurogenic MUAP recruitment pattern. Well-defined radiculopathies are often associated with normal electrodiagnostic findings due to involvement of sensory fibers alone or roots that cannot be adequately assessed, such as the L-2 root. Often, the study is performed before fibrillation potentials have had time to develop or after the spontaneous activity has disappeared due to concomitant reinnervation.

Plexus Disorders

Electrodiagnostic studies are helpful in the diagnosis of plexopathies (10). They reveal motor abnormalities and fibrillation potentials indicative of axon loss in mild lesions and decreased CMAP amplitudes and MUAP loss with more severe ones. Involvement of sensory NCS as manifested by SNAP amplitude reduction out of proportion to the degree of axon loss, and the absence of paraspinal denervation distinguish plexopathy from radiculopathy.

The cervical plexus, which is comprised of the APR of the C-1 through C-4 roots that lie in the lateral neck, is the most difficult of the plexuses to assess in the EMG laboratory. The phrenic nerve represents an exception because phrenic nerve conduction and needle examination of the diaphragm can be performed and may be of assistance in identifying the nature and site of respiratory insufficiency (11). The brachial plexus, extending from the lower cervical vertebrae to the axilla and suspended along with the neck and shoulder, is the most frequently injured somatic plexus.

Anatomically, the brachial plexus is composed of five APR, three trunks, six divisions, three cords, and several named derived nerves. The C-5 through T-1 APR combine to form the three trunks of the brachial plexus in the following manner: the C-5 and C-6 roots combine to form the upper trunk, the C-8 and T-1 roots join to form the lower trunk, and the C-7 root continues as the middle trunk. Each trunk in turn divides into anterior and a posterior divisions that individually separate and unite to form the posterior, lateral cord, and medial cords. The five named nerves of the brachial plexus, median, ulnar, radial, musculocutaneous, and axillary, enter the arm, while the suprascapular, dorsal scapular, and long thoracic nerves take their origin more proximally. The divisions of the brachial plexus are situated behind the clavicle, which permit its disorders to be grouped as supraclavicular and infraclavicular, a system that has both diagnostic and prognostic utility. Disorders affecting the supraclavicular portion are most often due to severe traction, are often confused with radiculopathy, and carry a poor prognosis, whereas infraclavicular lesions, also traumatic in origin, are more frequently mistaken for mononeuropathy multiplex, and associated with a more favorable outcome.

The supraclavicular plexus can be subdivided into upper, middle plexus, and lower plexus components, each of which has its own sensory and muscle domains and, thus, its own unique electrodiagnostic manifestations (12). Since most brachial plexus lesions cause some degree of axon loss–induced conduction failure and because the SNAP and muscle domains of each brachial plexus element are known, the investigation of axon loss brachial plexopathy is usually straightforward (13). Disorders that produce demyelinating conduction block along plexus fibers distal to the mid-trunk level can be identified by comparing the CMAP amplitude of the response obtained with supraclavicular fossa stimulation with the one obtained upon distal stimulation. A clue to the presence of proximal demyelinating conduction block is the combination of a relatively normal CMAP recorded from a muscle with significant reduction in MUAP recruitment on needle examination.

The appropriate electrodiagnostic for plexopathy depends upon the presumptive diagnosis and the findings as the study unfolds. However, the median SNAP is of little usefulness in the presence of CTS, similarly F-waves are generally unhelpful, and certain patterns of abnormality can assist in the localization and etiology of brachial plexopathy as, for example, true neurogenic thoracic outlet syndrome (14).

Lumbar and sacral plexopathies are encountered far less frequently and their location renders them less vulnerable to trauma. The limited number of sensory and motor NCS available for assessment makes them more difficult to evaluate. Femoral motor and sensory NCS that assess motor and sensory axons derived from the L-2 through L-4 spinal cord segments that traverse the lumbar plexus may be useful in the diagnosis of lumbar plexopathy, particularly when a postganglionic sensory response can be determined (15). Fibrillation potentials in femoral- and obturator-innervated muscles justify a tentative diagnosis of a lumbar plexopathy when the lumbar paraspinal muscles are spared. Needle examination can differentiate lumbar plexopathy from peripheral nerve lesions.

Whereas a lumbar plexus lesion involving the L-3 and L-4 motor axons in clinically suspected femoral mononeuropathy can be excluded when needle abnormalities are found in obturator-innervated muscles, a moderate to severe axon loss sacral plexopathy can be diagnosed with involvement of peripheral L-5 and S-1 sensory fibers. However, sacral plexopathy, which occurs most often among the elderly, among whom lower extremity SNAP often are absent bilaterally, unilateral abnormalities may be indicative of a postganglionic lesion regardless of age. One difficulty with the diagnosis of sacral plexopathy is the tendency for the underlying disorder to be bilateral; accordingly, side-to-side SNAP amplitude comparisons are of limited value. Routine motor NCS, which assess the L-5 to S-2 nerve fibers, do not differentiate between the overlap of sensory and motor axonal contribution to sciatic nerve and sacral plexus disorders, however needle EMG abnormalities in the glutei and tensor fascia lata muscles support a sacral plexus etiology; H-response abnormalities, which appear when S-1 sensory or motor fibers are affected, are of little value in discriminating between a sciatic nerve and plexus lesion.

Peripheral Nerve Disorders

These disorders can be subdivided clinically into focal mononeuropathy, mononeuropathy multiplex, and generalized polyneuropathy, and pathologically, as due to demyelination, axon loss, or both. Peripheral neuropathy produces variable electrical findings depending on the rapidity of onset, underlying pathophysiology, distribution, severity, acuteness of duration, and sensory or motor fibers involved. Electrodiagnostic studies detect demyelinating conduction slowing, demyelinating conduction block, axon loss–induced conduction failure, or some combination thereof, and contribute to an understanding of the pathophysiology and severity of an acquired mononeuropathy. Serial examination of the latter is of particular importance in decisions as to conservative or surgical management, based upon following the reinnervation of the lesion.

The underlying pathophysiology of CTS and ulnar entrapment at the elbow are usually the result of demyelinating conduction slowing, whereas neoplasm-induced neuropathy is usually a consequence of axon loss-induced conduction failure. Both types of pathophysiology can occur in a given mononeuropathy and it is possible to estimate the relative percentages of each pathophysiology for prognostic purposes as, for example, in recording both from the abductor digiti minimi (ADM) and first dorsal interosseus (FDI) along the ulnar nerve (16).

The pathophysiology of sudden mononeuropathy is either demyelinating conduction block, axon loss-induced conduction failure, or a combination thereof, examples of which include common fibular neuropathies at the fibular

TABLE 7. Characteristic pathophysiology of various mononeuropathies

Disorder	Pathology/pathophysiology
Long thoracic neuropathy	Axon loss/CF
Suprascapular neuropathy	Axon loss/CF
Axillary neuropathy	Axon loss/CF
Radial neuropathy—spiral groove	Axon loss/CF and demyelination/CB
Posterior interosseous neuropathy	Axon loss/CF
Ulnar neuropathy	
Across the elbow	Axon loss/CF and demyelination/CB, CS
At the wrist	Axon loss (demyelination)/CF (CB)
Anterior interosseous neuropathy	Axon loss/CF
Carpal tunnel syndrome	Demyelination/CSa
Femoral neuropathy	Axon loss (demyelination)/CF (CB)
Sciatic neuropathy	Axon loss/CF
Fibular neuropathy—fibular head	Axon loss/CF and demyelination/CB
Tarsal tunnel syndrome	Axon loss (demyelination)/CF (CS)

The pathologies and pathophysiologies shown in parentheses occur less frequently.
aAxon loss and CF appear later in the course of carpal tunnel syndrome.
CF, conduction failure; CB, conduction block; CS, conduction slowing.

head, radial neuropathy at the spiral groove, and selected ulnar neuropathy at the elbow, the first two of which characteristically present, respectively, with foot and wrist drop, indicating loss of excitability of the subserving myofibers. Inasmuch as demyelinating processes due to abrupt trauma typically resolve after a 6- to 8-week period, a result of axon loss obtain afterward, excludes a demyelinating pathophysiology with the exception of tourniquet paralysis, which may show prolonged conduction block lasting up to 10 months. However, some examples of demyelinating conduction block lesions can last longer, including those resulting from continuation of the traumatic phenomenon as, for example, elbow leaning sustaining ulnar neuropathy at the elbow, and leg crossing perpetuating a common a fibular lesion at the fibular head; persistent demyelinating conduction block along axons exposed can persist indefinitely in non-traumatic radiation-induced brachial plexopathy and multifocal motor neuropathy.

It is possible to separate the contribution of demyelinating conduction block and resultant clinical weakness with likely anticipated early recovery from sustained axon loss pathophysiology. This is accomplished by comparisons of the distal CMAP amplitude recorded from the affected side, the contralateral distal homologous response, and ipsilateral proximal response wherein the difference between the two distal CMAP amplitudes reflects the percentage of the lesion related to axon loss, while the difference between the proximal and distal CMAP amplitudes on the symptomatic side reflects the percentage of demyelinating conduction block. The most frequently encountered mononeuropathies are shown in Table 7.

Acquired polyneuropathies are due to either demyelination or axonal loss, whereas many, but not all, genetic neuropathies are demyelinating, with the exception of Charcot-Marie-Tooth (CMT) neuropathy type II and porphyria, which are hereditary disorders axon loss-associated. Chronic sensorimotor axon loss polyneuropathy has a typical electrodiagnostic and temporal progression that parallels the clinical course. The pathologic process starts distally with a stocking distribution that evolves to a stocking-glove pattern. In its mildest form and excluding isolated sensory involvement, initial findings are noted distally in intrinsic foot muscles on needle EMG examination in the form of fibrillation potentials. The sural, superficial fibular, plantar nerves, and H responses which are more sensitive to axon loss are involved first, followed later by motor nerve involvement such that needle EMG findings appear in the foreleg in association with already diminishing H-wave and SNAP amplitudes in the leg, even before sensory responses are affected in the arms. Sustained denervation of intrinsic foot muscles leads to diminished motor NCS responses, MUAP dropout, and features of axon loss on needle EMG examination. When H responses and lower extremity

SNAP responses are non-elicited, the SNAP amplitudes in the upper extremities have begun to diminish. Later, diminished motor NCS responses appear with distal changes more pronounced than proximal, followed by modest slowing of motor NCV due to loss of the fastest conducting fibers. The definition of distal symmetrical polyneuropathy for research purposes, and the evaluation thereof, has been extensively reviewed (17, 18).

The most prominent NCS parameter of the inherited demyelinating polyneuropathy CMT type I is conduction slowing characterized by prolonged sensory and motor peak latencies, with sensory NCS more abnormal and often non-elicited in the legs and of decreased amplitude, increased duration, and peak latency prolongation in the arms, compared to motor parameters. Since there is uniformly affliction along the length of the nerves, the synchrony of impulse conduction along individual nerve fibers is preserved and, consequently, the morphology of the recorded motor waveforms, including their amplitudes, are less distorted than those observed with acquired demyelinating polyneuropathy. When present, dispersion of the motor response typically occurs distally.

The degree of slowing in CMT may be of diagnostic importance in suggesting the abnormal inherited defect as, for example, in patients with peripheral myelin protein (PMP) gene duplications that typically manifest median motor NCV at or <30 meters per second (m/sec), whereas males with connexin 32 gene mutations demonstrate motor NCV at or >30 m/sec, as compared to children with myelin protein zero (MPZ) gene mutations with motor NCV typically <15 m/sec (19). Despite the predominant demyelinating pathophysiology, a mild amount of fibrillation activity is often noted in needle EMG of the distal leg muscles, along with prominent chronic neurogenic MUAP changes.

Acute and chronic acquired demyelinating polyradiculoneuropathies display various combinations of low amplitude or non-elicited motor and sensory responses, prolonged duration and distal latencies of elicited CMAP and SNAP, decreased CV, demyelinating conduction block, and a degree of axon loss. Non-uniform slowing and reduced synchrony result in an increase in the negative phase duration and a reduction in the CMAP amplitude. Disproportionate involvement of proximal, middle, or distal segments of the peripheral nerves leads to variable challenges in assessing conduction block, especially when present above the popliteal fossa in the leg.

Proximal conduction block should be considered in setting of a neurogenic MUAP recruitment pattern in the activation phase of the needle examination with normal or near-normal CMAP. Distal demyelination and conduction block of terminal nerve branches may be confused with a myopathy when there is selective drop out of fibers with secondary disintegration of the motor unit with early recruitment of short duration and low amplitude MUP. An axonal loss pathophysiology is, instead, suggested by distally diminished wrist and ankle CMAP amplitudes combined with proximal CMAP amplitudes. The SNAP abnormalities and the degree of demyelinating conduction slowing tend to be more pronounced in CIDP than GBS.

Electrodiagnostic criteria have been proposed for differentiating primary demyelinating from primarily axonal processes (20). However, mixed demyelinating and axonal polyneuropathies show features of both axon loss and demyelination, an example of which is diabetes mellitus, which can manifest both pathophysiology, alone or in association with superimposed median or ulnar entrapment. Polyneuropathies variably involve sensory, motor, and autonomic axons, however some affect only one type of fiber. Pure sensory polyneuropathy can be divided into acquired and hereditary forms, with less pronounced clinical severity in acquired forms, and more pronounced distal and uniform involvement in the genetic types. The electrical abnormalities noted in the hereditary forms are usually most pronounced in the lower extremities and uniform along the affected axons, whereas those associated with the acquired forms may not show lower extremity predominance and a non-uniform nature.

Neuromuscular Junction Disorders

These can be divided into presynaptic and postsynaptic types, classic examples of which are LEMS and MG, respectively. The latter is an autoimmune disorder that results from postsynaptic ACh receptor destruction, simplification of the postsynaptic membrane, and widening of the synaptic cleft, lowering the safety factor of NMJ transmission and producing or predisposing the patient to NMJ transmission failure. Clinical weakness has a proximal predominance with frequent ocular and bulbar involvement. Fatigability is the clinical hallmark of the disorder, and sustained effort and exercise enhance the electrical abnormalities in MG, however a single stimulation does not induce fatigue, and CMAP, late responses, and needle EMG examination are generally all normal, unless moment-to-moment amplitude variation of single-firing MUAPs is specifically sought during the activation phase of the needle examination or unless the disorder has advanced enough to cause disintegration of the motor unit, in which case myopathic-appearing MUAP may be observed. The electrodiagnostic maneuver of choice to demonstrate the defect in MG is low-frequency RNS at 2–3 Hz, which induces a reduction in the size of immediately releasable ACh, thereby diminishing the number of ACh-containing vesicles released with each subsequent stimulus.

In normal individuals, the safety factor for NMJ transmission ensures maximum CMAP responses with each stimulation and a uniform appearance of evoked CMAP to a train of stimuli. However, in MG 2 to 3-Hz RNS leads to progressively smaller MUAP, which in turn produces progressively smaller CMAP and the so-called decremental response. This physiologic explanation explains the less than complete activation of all myofibers composing the motor unit. Sustained effort or exercise further reduces the safety factor for NMJ transmission, worsening the degree of CMAP decrement. In mild generalized MG, basic NCS are normal, however slow RNS performed at two or more sites is usually diagnostic when chosen from one proximal site such as the spinal accessory nerve and upper trapezius, facial nerve, and orbicularis oculi or oris, and a distal system among them, the median nerve and APB or ulnar nerve and ADM. Cold temperature can normalize defective NMJ transmission and the abnormal decremental response induced by slow RNS. When uninformative, single-fiber EMG should be performed because of its higher yield.

The presynaptic membrane is the site of disease in the autoimmune disorder LEMS due to antibodies that bind to calcium channels producing presynaptic membrane disorganization and a decrease in the number of active zone particles. Depolarization, which normally increases the intracellular calcium concentration of the nerve terminal and facilitates the release of ACh-containing vesicles, instead releases less vesicles in LEMS with each nerve fiber depolarization. This decrease is substantial and severely lessens the number of muscle fiber action potentials generated by nerve fiber activation. Since the NMJ disorders have no effect on the sensory NCS, the latter are normal as in MG. However, unlike the latter, routinely recorded CMAP amplitudes are typically less than 10% of normal; needle EMG also shows moment-to-moment amplitude variation and MUAP with a pseuomyopathic appearance. Although slow RNS may lead to further decreases of the amount of ACh released with repetitive stimulation and CMAP decrement, fast RNS at 40 to 50-Hz increases the intracellular calcium concentration of the nerve branch terminal, and significantly increases the amount of ACh released with a resultant increase in the CMAP size, the so-called incremental response. Since fast RNS is painful and a similar outcome can be expected b voluntary exercise, those with an initially low CMAP amplitude instead undergo 10 seconds of exercise and single motor unit stimulation, which if it leads to a 100% or more increment, is followed by fast RNS to confirm the presynaptic pathophysiology.

Myopathic Disorders

Myopathy refers to a heterogeneous group of muscle disorders. The varied electrical manifestations associated with myopathy reflect differences in underlying physiology, pathology, stage of disease, and the effect of treatment. Electrodiagnostic studies are generally normal in myopathy, although the CMAP amplitudes may be significantly reduced when the recorded muscles are severely affected. All of the electrodiagnostic features of a myopathic process are nonspecific and can be seen with both terminal peripheral nerve and NMJ disorders. Nonetheless, when present in certain patterns and combinations, the likelihood of a myopathy increases. Several modifications of the electrodiagnostic study are required whenever a myopathy is suspected. Given that a generalized process is suspected, an arm and leg should be assessed, including a peroneal and median motor, and sural and median sensory NCS. As myopathic processes have a proximal predominance, the needle examination should include a greater number of proximal muscles, including paraspinal and limb girdle muscles. When inclusion body myopathy (IBM) is suspected, muscles of the flexor compartment of the forearm, such as the flexor pollicis longus and pronator teres, and the anterior thigh, such as the quadriceps, are added. Since muscle involvement may be patchy, a more thorough assessment of each muscle, often including two or more separate needle electrode insertion sites, is necessary. Sensory NCS are always normal, and motor NCS are typically abnormal when the myopathy is severe or when non-routine studies of the musculocutaneous nerve and biceps, and fibular nerve and tibialis anterior muscle are studied.

The most frequent electrodiagnostic abnormalities are fibrillation potentials, myopathic MUAP, and early motor unit recruitment. Fibrillation potentials are the commonest form of spontaneous activity observed in myopathies and indicate muscle fiber denervation. In the setting of a myopathy, they imply muscle fiber transection or splitting in such

a manner as to separate the fibrillating muscle fiber segment from the segment containing the end-plate. They also occur in polymyositis (PM) and dermatomyositis (DM)), rapidly progressive dystrophies, toxic myopathies, infectious myopathies, rhabdomyolysis, acid maltase deficiency, and myotubular myopathy. As myopathic MUAP and early recruitment reflect motor unit disintegration, they are not specific for a myopathy, and myotonic potentials and complex repetitive discharges may also be observed.

Despite its diagnostic limitations, the electrical examination has several potential uses among patients with suspected myopathic disorders. First, depending on the findings, the disorder can be assignable to a particular category; for example, based on the presence of prominent fibrillation potentials or myotonic discharges. This usually permits the list of possibilities to be substantially shortened. Second, the electrical studies can be useful in identifying a muscle suitable for biopsy. Ideally, it should be involved, but not end stage, and obtained on the side contralateral to the muscle examined to avoid needle-induced inflammatory and structural changes. Third, it can be used to serially assess the disease and to assist in management decisions, such as when a patient with PM develops increased weakness during steroid treatment and it is unclear whether the increase in weakness represents an exacerbation of PM or emerging corticosteroid myopathy. The former shows fibrillation potentials on needle examination, whereas the latter does not. Fourth, muscles not clinically amenable to evaluation can be assessed. Fifth, the electrodiagnostic study can reorient the evaluation, especially when a myopathic process proves to be an incorrect assumption.

REFERENCES

1. Ferrante MA, Wilbourn AJ. The utility of various sensory nerve conduction responses in assessing brachial plexopathies. *Muscle Nerve* 1995; 18:879–889.
2. Wilbourn AJ. The electrodiagnostic examination with myopathies. *J Clin Neurophysiol* 1993; 10:132–148.
3. Wilbourn AJ. An unreported, distinctive type of increased insertional activity. Muscle Nerve 1982; 5:S101 S105.
4. Mitsumoto H, Wilbourn AJ, Subramony SH. Generalized myokymia and gold therapy. *Arch Neurol* 1982; 39:449–450.
5. Frontera WR, Grimby L, Larsson L. Firing rate of the lower motoneuron and contractile properties of its muscle fibers after upper motoneuron lesion in man. *Muscle Nerve* 1997; 20:938–947.
6. Kennedy WR, Alter M, Sung JH. Progressive proximal spinal and bulbar muscular atrophy of late onset: a sex-linked trait. *Neurology* 1968; 18:671–680.
7. Harding AE, Thomas PK, Baraitser M, et al. X-linked recessive bulbospinal neuronopathy: a report of 10 cases. *J Neurol Neurosurg Psychiatry* 1982; 45:1012–1019.
8. Ferrante MA, Wilbourn AJ. The characteristic electrodiagnostic features of Kennedy's disease. *Muscle Nerve* 1997; 20:323–329.
9. Wilbourn AJ, Aminoff MJ. AAEE Minimonograph #32. The electrodiagnostic examination in patients with radiculopathies. *Muscle Nerve* 1998; 21:1612–1631.
10. Ko K, Shung DH, Kang MJ, et al. Clinical, electrophysiological findings in adult patients with non-traumatic plexopathies. *Ann Rehabil Med* 2011; 35:807–815.
11. Bolton CF. AAEM minimonograph #40: Clinical neurophysiology of the respiratory system. *Muscle Nerve* 1993; 16:809–818.
12. Ferrante MA. Brachial plexopathies: Classification, causes, and consequences. *Muscle Nerve* 2004; 30:547–568.
13. Ferrante MA, Wilbourn AJ. The utility of various sensory nerve conduction responses in assessing brachial plexopathies. *Muscle Nerve* 1995; 18:879–889.
14. Ferrante MA. The Thoracic outlet syndromes. *Muscle Nerve* 2012; 45:780–795.
15. Oh SJ, Hatanaka Y, Ohira M, et al. Clinical utility of sensory nerve conduction of medial femoral cutaneous nerve. *Muscle Nerve* 2012; 45:195–199.
16. Friedrich JM, Robinson LR. Prognostic indicators from electrodiagnostic studies for ulnar neuropathy at the elbow. *Muscle Nerve* 2011; 43:596–600.
17. England JD, Gronseth GS, Franklin G, et al. Distal symmetrical polyneuropathy: a definition for clinical research. Report of the Amerian Academy of Neurology, the American Association of Electrodiagnostic Medicine, and the American

Academy of Physical Medicine and Rehabilitation. *Neurology* 2005; 64:199–207.

18. England JD, Gronseth GS, Franklin G. et al. Practice parameter: evaluation of distal symmetric polyneuropathy: role of laboratory and genetic testing (an evidence based review). Report of the American Academy of Neurology, American Association of Neuromuscular and Electrodiagnostic Medicine, and American Academy of Physical Medicine and Rehabilitation. *Neurology* 2009; 72:185–192.

19. Deymeer F, Matur Z, Poyraz M, et al. Nerve conduction studies in Charcot-Marie-Tooth disease in a cohort from Turkey. *Muscle Nerve* 2011; 43:657–664.

20. Bromberg MB. Review of the evolution of electrodiagnostic criteria for chronic inflammatory demyelinating polyradiculoneuropathy. *Muscle Nerve* 2011; 43:780–794.

CHAPTER **6**

Electrophysiology of the Motor Unit

Stefano Simonetti, Miki Nikolic, Christian Krarup

The motor unit (MU) is the smallest functional unit of skeletal muscle, and its electrophysiologic characteristics are central in the diagnosis of neuromuscular disorders associated with partial denervation and myopathy. Since the introduction of electromyography (EMG), it has been apparent that the interpretation of the electrical activity of muscle is influenced by both technical and biologic factors and that the variability of the individual muscle requires quantitation for proper evaluation. With the introduction of computer technology, this quantitative evaluation has become less time consuming; however, the methods themselves influence the results of the interpretation (1). This chapter reviews the different methodologies of MU action potential (MUAP) analysis, parameters of EMG interpretation, and principal pathophysiological alterations.

DEFINITION OF THE MOTOR UNIT

The MU was defined as the motoneurone, its axon, and innervated myofibers (2). Multilead electrode studies reveal that the MU territory is approximately circular or elliptical with a diameter, for example, in the brachial biceps muscle of 15 mm with space for 15 to 30 MU (3, 4). The myofibers of a MU from one MU placed within 300 μm of a myofiber of the same motor unit is only 50%. Single-fiber recording shows that about 1.5 myofibers belong to the same motor unit indicating that the pickup area comprises about 6 MU, with a larger concentration of myofibers at the center of the M than along its periphery. Myofibers have different physiological, biochemical, and mechanical properties, as are the composition, size, and number of MU in individual muscles. This is of importance because involvement of MU

in a given disease may be influenced by the individual properties. The recruitment of MU during the development of force is not random such that it is possible to examine the characteristics of individual unit with weak force.

Classification of Motor Units

All muscle fibers in the individual motor unit have a similar histochemical profile. There are three main groups of MU according to physiological, mechanical, biochemical, and histochemical criteria (Table 1) that comprise a continuum (5, 6) with fast-twitch comparatively larger, greater twitch tension, lower twitch:tetanus ratio, and greater force potentiated by repetitive stimulation, faster motor axonal conduction velocity, larger motor neuron diameter, and lower input resistance (7). The innervation ratio, defined as the number of myofibers innervated by a single α-motor neuron, varies in individual muscles from 5 to 20 fibers in the extraocular eye muscle to more than 2,000 in the gastrocnemius. The innervation ratio, the main determinant of the force each MU can produce, and the force per unit area, are similar among different fiber myotypes. The innervation ratio is subject to influence by both biologic factors and pathologic lesions, with increasing age-associated with a reduction in motor neuron number and an increase in the innervation ratio due to collateral sprouting, further influenced by pathologic processes that cause axonal or neuronal degeneration. Collateral sprouting has a marked influence on the physiologic parameters of the MU and is of major importance as a compensatory mechanism that delays or reduces the degree of weakness.

Table 1
Classification of MU

Motor unit type	Myofiber type		
	Mitochondrial enzymes	Muscle fiber ATPase activity (pH 9.4)	Physiological classification and oxidative metabolism
Slow fatigue, resistant	Type C (strong mitochondrial staining)	Type 1 (weak activity)	Slow-twitch, oxidative
Fast fatigue, resistant	Type B (intermediate mitochondrial staining)	Type 2a (strong activity)	Fast-twitch, oxidative glycolytic
Fast fatigue, susceptible	Type A (weak mitochondrial staining)	Type 2b (strong activity)	Fast-twitch, glycolytic

Gradation of Force

Muscle increases force output by recruitment of additional MU and the modulation of the discharge frequency of different MU, as well as, potentiation, fatigue, and change in stiffness related to prior activity. At low levels of force additional MU are recruited before changes in firing rate. An increase in force is associated with recruitment to about 80% of the maximum force, whereas 20% derive from an increase in discharge frequency. Additional MU may be recruited at a force level of 50%, and the remaining force level is determined by rate coding that ensures more precise gradation. With reflex movement and during gradual increasing force production, the sequence of recruitment of motor units follows the size principle wherein small, low-force, slow-twitch, fatigue-resistant motor units are recruited at low levels of force, whereas the largest fatigable MU are recruited at maximal levels. During rapidly increasing force and ballistic movement, MU may be recruited independent of size. The input–output relationship of the motor neuron is under additional suprasegmental control such that the order of recruitment may be changed according to the specific task. The order of recruitment can vary with altered afferent input and with disease states and injury. The rise times of MU action potentials (MUAP) in fast twitch muscle is faster than in slow contracting muscle without appreciable differences in shape, amplitude, and duration. With steady isometric contraction, MU that are active at the beginning of the contraction and remain so, with a time-dependent replacement of active MU by others believed to delay fatigue. Human muscle fires at 2 to 3 Hz during slow ramp contraction and with slight effort reach a stable regular firing rate of 5 to 7 Hz. At maximum effort, discharge frequencies vary somewhat in different muscles but rarely increase above 30 to 40 Hz, however at brisk brief contractions, discharge rates of 150 Hz can be recorded. The firing rates of MU with different recruitment thresholds suggest that at moderate force, the low-threshold MU have higher maximal firing rates than high-threshold ones which instead seem to have higher and phasic discharge rates at higher forces.

Motor Unit Number

The number of functioning MU in a given muscle is of considerable interest both in distinguishing neurogenic from myopathic processes as the cause of weakness, and in following MU loss in neurogenic disorders. Considerable efforts have been made in developing methods of MU number estimation (MUNE) by recording single MUAP evoked by electrical stimulation and during voluntary contraction (8–10). Such methods include manual incremental stimulation, computer-assisted incremental stimulation, multiple-point threshold stimulation, analysis of F waves, spike-triggered averaging (STA) of MUAP, and statistical methods (11). A basic common principle is the determination of the size of the AP of a representative MU divided into the size of the maximal compound muscle response which is considered to be the algebraic sum of MU responses. A number of assumptions are made to determine the representative quantal MU response, whether obtained as the force of the MU or the MUAP. These assumptions pertain to activation of individual α-motor axons at low levels of stimulation and may be influenced by fluctuating activation of several axons with similar thresholds or alternation. To reduce alternation the nerve may be stimulated at several points along its length by multiple point stimulation and the very first all-or-nothing response is used to measure the MUAP. However, the stimulation at different sites along the length of the nerve does not take into consideration branching of the α-motor axon that increases distally and may take place at considerable distance from the nerve. Analysis of F waves to extract MUAP information reduces alternation, although the firing of α-motoneurones may be influenced by the increased excitability in central nervous system (CNS) disorders with corticospinal tract (CST) degeneration as occurs in amyotrophic lateral sclerosis (ALS); a supposed single unit response may be the result of a simultaneous activation of a number of MU. Little is known about the activated MU type and there could be a bias either toward larger or smaller MU. This method, while time-consuming, is inapplicable to many conditions characterized by denervation.

Alternation due to overlapping axon thresholds has been used statistically in the Poisson distribution of discrete events. The average size of MUAP at different levels of stimulation can be assessed from the variance of a series of 30 measurements. Estimates of MU size at each intensity are averaged to produce single motor unit potential amplitude which can be divided into the maximal CMAP response to obtain the MUNE. The questionable assumptions are that the probability of individual motor units firing to a specific stimulus is distributed according to the Poisson distribution of discrete events and thus, that MU of similar threshold should have the same size. The sampled MU should be representative of those in the recording area and the probability of response to each successive stimulus should not be affected by the response to the prior stimulus and remain unchanged during the evaluation period. Concerning the last assumption, the instability of single MU responding to a constant stimulus leading to an underestimation of MUNE could present a problem in cases with significant axon loss and reinnervation. The algorithm and statistical method for MUNE disregards MU of very small and very large sizes, and estimates MU from a wider response range than other techniques. Rather than using electrical stimulation of single motor axons, MUNE may be carried out during voluntary contractions. The individual MUAP are recorded with a concentric needle, and using spike-triggered averaging, the surface recordings of associated MUAP are then recorded. This method avoids the possibility of alternation and extends the applicability of MUNE to proximal muscles, but at slight effort, small motor units may be preferentially recruited and the number of motor units therefore overestimated. Contamination from a different MU or fasciculation potentials are possible and the method is time-consuming, available only in limited EMG units with the need for patient cooperation. To improve upon these limitations, decomposition-enhanced spike-triggered averaging extracts multiple MUAP trains from a given contraction through a series of a signal processing and pattern recognition algorithms, rapidly analyzing MUAP at higher degrees of effort (12). However, in all methods of MUNE, the MU response, whether it is a MUAP or a mechanical twitch response, must remain stable during repeated stimulations and arithmetically adds to yield the maximal compound response. Despite the potential sources of error, MUNE obtained by different methods in the same muscles yield comparable results in both the number and size of MUAP. Repeated measures show stable results over time in normal subjects whereas the number decreases in those with ALS (13). Direct anatomic assessment of MU counts are comparable with physiologic measures. In factoring counts of large myelinated fibers of a motor nerve to assess the number of α-motor axons, it should be recognized that sensory fibers can comprise up to 60% of the total number of large myelinated fibers with a diameter >6 to 7 μm.

MUAP PARAMETERS

Needle EMG examination by a concentric needle electrode referenced to the cannula or a monopolar electrode insulated with Teflon and referenced to a surface electrode at a frequency setting of 2 to 10k Hz, leads to recording areas of 0.07 mm² and 0.17 mm² respectively. Published control values have generally been obtained using concentric needle electrodes (14). The EMG examination, which is divided into three parts, includes first inspection of activity at rest for diverse forms of spontaneous activity resulting from denervation such as fibrillation potentials and positive sharp wave (PSW), fasciculation, myotonia, complex repetitive discharges (CRD), miniature end-plate potentials (MEPP), and end-plate spikes. Next, recording during low levels of voluntary effort to obtain individual MUAP is followed by recording during maximal voluntary effort to evaluate the interference pattern.

The MUAP is a compound signal reflecting the summation and cancellation of phases of the AP from individual muscle fibers in the MU. With intracellular recordings, the AP is a monophasic waveform of about 100 mV, whereas the extracellular potential is a volume-conducted derivative of the rate of membrane depolarization. The MUAP represents the spatial and temporal summation of these bi- and triphasic spikes, wherein the negative spike in the normal muscle is obtained from 2 to 3 fibers within 0.5 to 1 mm of the electrode. The contribution of activity from fibers at a slightly longer distance to the spike is negligible because of the steep spatial decay of the high-frequency spike. In contrast, the slow initial and terminal positive phases represent activity from fibers at greater distances because the decay of these slow components is much smaller. The amplitude of the spike is determined by the proximity of the closest active fibers. The amplitude, shape, and duration of the MUAP reflect the architecture of the MU. Recorded outside the end-plate region, the MUAP typically has three phases, including an initial positive phase, a negative spike, and a terminal positive phase. A negative afterpotential is sometimes recorded and is enhanced when the lower limiting amplifier frequency is set above 2 Hz. At the end-plate region, the MUAP is biphasic in shape with a sharp negative onset. In some instances, the MUAP may be split up into more phases, reflecting a greater asynchrony of discharges. In normal humans, the number of polyphasic MUAP, with 5 or more phases comprise an average of 3% of normal control subject MUAP. When 20 to 25 MUAP are recorded, less than 12% of the total number of are polyphasic. In the deltoid and facial muscles, less than 25% are polyphasic, and similarly, less than 20% in the vastus lateralis and the anterior tibial muscles. A MUAP may contain a late spike separate from the main spike. These so-called satellite potentials represent action potentials of a single or a few fibers temporally dispersed from the main bulk of the fibers in the motor unit and occur in disease states and contribute up to 3% of MUAP of healthy muscle. A stationary far-field positive potential is sometimes recorded during the positive terminal phase of the MUAP, with monopolar needle electrode, represents extinction of the action potential at the myotendinous transition (15). There are three MUAP parameters are of clinical importance including duration, peak-to-peak amplitude, and the number of phases (Figure 1).

MUAP Duration

The duration of the MUAP, which reflects the temporal dispersion of activity of fibers constituting the MU, is primarily due to the spatial distribution of end-plates measuring 20 to 30 mm along myofibers with a conduction velocity of 3 to 5 m/sec, as well as the number of muscle fibers present in a

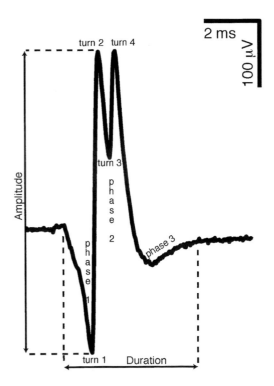

FIG. 1. MUAP from normal muscle recorded with concentric needle electrode. The measured parameters and the different components are indicated.

semicircle 2.5 mm from the active recording surface and the diameter of muscle fibers in the MU. The MUAP is measured from its first deflection from the baseline to the return of the terminal positive phase (Figure 1). The duration measured on film recordings is highly dependent on amplifier settings. Normal laboratory values obtained at a gain of100 μV/cm showed a measured duration that was shorter at lower gain settings and longer at higher gains. Modern digitalized equipment reveals a deviation and return to baseline determined by amplitude and slope criteria (16). The duration of individual normal MUAP vary by a factor of 3- to 5-fold, ranging from 5 to 15 msec, for example, in the brachial biceps with variability mainly due to the differences in myofiber content of MU. It is necessary to record 20 to 30 MUAP at different sites in the muscle to obtain a representative sample. The duration of simple MUAP, is defined by the presence of four or fewer phases, whereas polyphasic MUAP are averaged separately and together, and the results compared with age-matched control subjects. The normal range is defined as the normal mean ± 20%. The MUAP duration is the most important parameter to distinguish myopathic disorders with a loss of muscle fibers from chronic neurogenic disorders, with an increased number of muscle fibers due to collateral sprouting (17).

MUAP Amplitude

MUAP amplitude is measured peak-to-peak from the most positive to the sequentially most negative peak, however phase cancellation reduces the MUAP amplitude to less than the sum of individual fiber potentials, or even that of a single myofiber potential, depending upon the proximity within about a 0.5 mm diameter of the closest 2 to 15 myofibers of the MU, and is proportional to the number and density of fibers in the MU. The large effect of distance between active fibers and the recording surface can lead to variations in MUAP amplitude, as well as the type of electrode employed, with larger amplitudes using monopolar electrodes. It is important to identify the crisp sound of discharging MUAP indicating optimal placement to active MU. Manipulation of the electrode should be avoided to avert recording larger amplitude MUAP, with most laboratories requiring MUAP amplitudes >100% of normal control values to be clearly abnormal. It is generally recommended to accept MUAP with a rise time of no more than 0.5 msec, as measured from the maximum positive to the maximum negative peak, recognizing that it may vary with the number of myofibers that summate to generate the MUAP, increasing in chronic partial denervation with reinnervation, and decreasing in myopathy due to myofiber loss. In practice, MUAP with slow rise times and amplitudes of less than 50 μV should be excluded. The rise time is inversely related to the amplitude of the MUAP but, if less than 2 msec, has little influence on the duration of the

MUAP that is determined by the slow initial and terminal phases of the MUAP (18).

MUAP Shape

MUAP can be simple or polyphasic, the latter demonstrating long or short duration in myopathy depending on the degree of muscle fiber regeneration. It is important to separately calculate the amplitude and duration of simple and polyphasic MUAP, and to collect more MUAP than necessary in case additional ones are needed (19). Voltage reversals of the MUAP that do not result in baseline crossings are termed *turns* if they have an amplitude of more than 100 μV. There is variability in the shape of successive MUAP discharges, or *jiggle* (20) not due to electrode displacement that is more pronounced in myasthenia gravis (MG) and in early collateral sprouting with immature axonal sprouts.

MUAP Firing Rates

The firing rates of MUAP are not usually considered in routine EMG studies. Deafferentiation reduces the firing rate, emphasizing the impact of proprioceptors. Increased firing rates can occur in neuropathy and various CNS disorders.

Biological and Physical Factors

Age

MUAP duration increases from age 20 to 80 years and varies in different muscles (21), and appears to be influenced by collateral sprouting that leads to MU remodeling that starts in the third decade due to progressive anterior horn cell (AHC) loss (22). The increase in MUAP duration at ages less than 20 years is probably due to growth. Single-fiber EMG (SFEMG) show an increase in fiber density with age >60 years (23) that may be partly due to a reduction in muscle mass and fiber diameter (24). The increase in fiber density leads to an increase in the amplitude of initial and terminal phases, with a longer duration of the MUAP without change in the overall MUAP amplitude as a result of aging.

Temperature

There is a reduction in muscle fiber and axon conduction velocity with low temperature and an increase in MUAP duration with a reduction in intramuscular temperature. The mean MUAP duration increases by 6% per °C between 30 and 36°C, and by 9% per °C from 22 to 30°C. At normal intramuscular temperatures, the MUAP does not change enough to cause errors in diagnosis, however at temperatures less than 32°C, considerable errors can occur. MUAP polyphasia increases from about 3% at 37°C to 25% at 29°C.

The amplitude of the MUAP can increase or decrease at low temperatures due to variable phase cancellations. The MUAP duration is prolonged at low temperature with unchanged amplitudes and turns (25).

Special Electrodes

Since concentric electrodes may record a somewhat distorted MUAP depending upon its location within the MU (26), there has been interest in developing other types to examine the architectural features of the MUAP. Multilead electrodes contain up to 14 recording areas placed 1 mm apart, each with a surface corresponding to that of a concentric needle to determine the spatial distribution of individual spikes, delineating the shape and territory of the MU. Normal MU are circular in shape with a larger concentration of myofiber at the center than at the periphery (4) in agreement with earlier histochemical findings (27). In myopathy, the size of the MU is decreased but increased in neurogenic lesions (28, 29). In accordance with the presumption that larger MU can result from increased fiber density resulting in spike activity seen at a longer distance, multilead SFEMG showed that the density of fibers within the MU was increased in neurogenic lesions without a change in the corresponding territory (30).

Scanning EMG

A concentric needle is pulled through the MU and the corresponding MUAP is recorded at 50-μm intervals and averaged by means of a trigger-potential obtained from an SFEMG needle placed within the same MU (31). Spatial profiles show that a single major negative peak is present in one-half of control patients with some showing up to four peaks. The scans of patients with myopathy show increased fractionation of the MU with a larger number of spikes, whereas the number of silent areas with an activity of less than 50 μV is decreased in neurogenic lesions due to MU reinnervation. The relatively normal scan length supports the view of newly incorporated muscle fibers originating within the original MU territory and that collateral branches do not cross fascicular borders. In most cases, this technique will not distinguish between neurogenic lesions and myopathy possibly, because of the contribution of regeneration in the latter (32).

Macro EMG

The MUAP recorded with a concentric needle is a relatively poor indicator of the total MU activity. Recording with an electrode with a surface area 15 mm in length improves the evaluation of the size of the MU by sampling a larger portion of it, triggered by a potential recorded through a SFEMG lead incorporated in the same electrode, and averaged to reduce the contribution of activity from other MU.

The area and amplitude of the MUAP are correlated with the number and size of muscle fibers in the entire MU (33), whereas the duration is difficult to accurately measure. A variant of this method (34) combines a macro- and concentric needle electrode. The amplitude of the macro MUAP increases with age due to reinnervation after motor neuron loss; such changes can be found in progressive neurogenic lesions. The size of the MUAP decreases in ALS and postpolio syndrome indicating loss of large MU (35, 36). Mean MUAP amplitude is normal or slightly reduced in myopathy due to increased density of MU myofibers (37).

EMG Surface Recording

Surface recordings employing elaborate electrode arrays and spike triggering may be useful to assess end-plate distribution, muscle tendon transition, MU depth, firing rate, and MUAP propagation along myofibers.

Bipolar Needle Electrodes

Two concentric leads are placed together in the cannula and the electrical activity is recorded between them (38). The pickup area, which is restricted and thus unsuitable for MUAP evaluation, is used to exclude volume-conducted electrical activity from a distance.

ANALYSIS OF MOTOR UNIT ACTIVITY

MUAP in Disease

Sampling of a representative number of MU is necessary because of the large variability in innervation ratio, durations, and amplitudes of MUAP in individual muscles. Since reliance on the visual impression of MUAP characteristics is inaccurate (Figure 2), a mean MUAP duration or amplitude >95% confidence limit is suggested to establish abnormality. Mild disease and heterogeneous affection of the muscle by myositis and monoradicular disease can lead to outlier abnormal mean duration and amplitude values (39). It is important to obtain signals uncontaminated by activity from adjacent MU. MUAPs are recorded by the use of a trigger circuit at low efforts and a delay that allows the whole MUAP to be included on the oscilloscope to measure total duration and amplitude and to ensure that the signal is derived from a single MU, undisturbed by activity from other MU. The template method has the inherent bias toward higher amplitude MUAP, making it important to ensure that all MUAP at the needle position are included in the analysis. It is usually possible to record 2 to 3 MUAP at each site at low effort. A sampling should include recordings from 3 to 4 needle positions with at least 0.5 cm between each of 3 to 4 recording sites to ensure that the sampling is distributed over the entire muscle without overlap of individual MU. Even though modern integrated EMG machines allow the recording, storing, and analysis of MUAP to proceed faster and easier, the bias of the sampling may be such that only triggered MUAP are captured with exclusion of smaller MUAP. The reliability of MUAP analysis depends on the expertise of the examiner. For this reason it is necessary to keep hard copies or computer data files of all recordings to ensure that the MUAP amplitude and duration means and standard deviations (SD) are obtained from different and undisturbed MU. The calculated parameters of simple and polyphasic MUAP should be expressed separately when the degree of polyphasia is increased.

Automatic EMG Analysis

Automated EMG analysis systems (AEAS) permit the analysis of individual MUAP firing patterns (FP) during different degrees of voluntary effort. Systems aimed at constructing the FP for each recorded MU are termed decomposition systems and require user interaction in some decision making. In all such systems, MUAP identification is a multistep task that begins with recording, amplification, filtering, and sampling of the EMG signal; segmentation of the signal into time intervals that contain EMG activity whether single MUAP or superimposed MUAP; clustering of signals into MUAP according to certain fulfilled criteria; followed in some systems by resolution of superimposed MUAP; and display of identified MUAP, with parametric measurements and, in some, presentation of partial or complete firing patterns.

Originally designed to resemble as closely as possible the manual system developed by Buchthal and colleagues (40), the template system designed by Andreassen (41) assigns sequential signals to templates according to whether the power of the signal differs by less than 12% from that of the template with MUAP assigned when four matching potentials are accepted.

A multi-MUP analysis system (42) analyzes a 4.8-second signal and the parametric measurements of the potential MUAP shape to assign potentials to matching classes, and the resolved MUAP are averaged for measurements of parameters, however only a partial firing pattern is produced.

In the automatic decomposition (AD) EMG system developed by McGill and Dorfman (43), a 10-second signal is initially high-pass filtered using a first- or a second-order differentiating filter to enhance spikes with a fast rise time. The spikes are detected according to a preset threshold and subsequently transformed to a frequency domain and classified using template matching. The identified MUAP are averaged for measurements. Superimposed MUAP are not resolved, however only a partial firing pattern is used to confirm MUAP assignment.

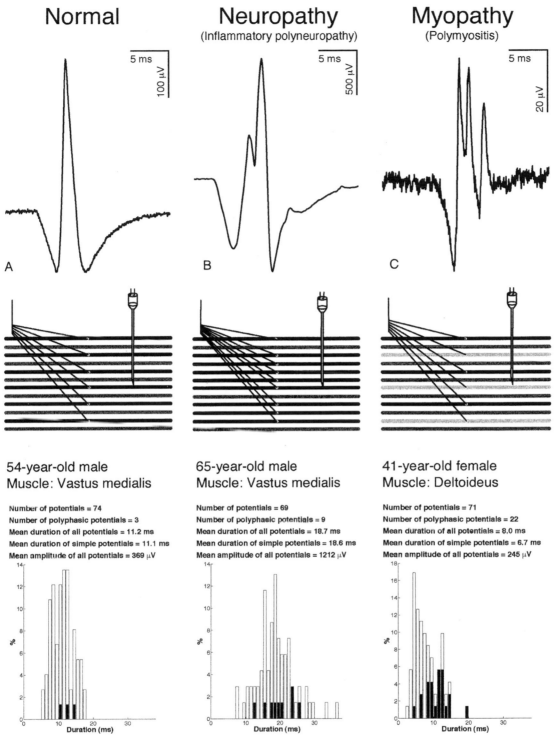

Normal

Neuropathy
(Inflammatory polyneuropathy)

Myopathy
(Polymyositis)

5 ms
100 µV

5 ms
500 µV

5 ms
20 µV

A

B

C

54-year-old male
Muscle: Vastus medialis

Number of potentials = 74
Number of polyphasic potentials = 3
Mean duration of all potentials = 11.2 ms
Mean duration of simple potentials = 11.1 ms
Mean amplitude of all potentials = 369 µV

65-year-old male
Muscle: Vastus medialis

Number of potentials = 69
Number of polyphasic potentials = 9
Mean duration of all potentials = 18.7 ms
Mean duration of simple potentials = 18.6 ms
Mean amplitude of all potentials = 1212 µV

41-year-old female
Muscle: Deltoideus

Number of potentials = 71
Number of polyphasic potentials = 22
Mean duration of all potentials = 8.0 ms
Mean duration of simple potentials = 6.7 ms
Mean amplitude of all potentials = 245 µV

FIG. 2. MUAP recorded with concentric needle electrodes. MUAP were extracted using the EMG-PAD system. **(A)** Normal subject; **(B)** patient with polyneuropathy; **(C)** patient with myopathy. The topmost traces are examples of MUAP from each muscle. The middle drawing is a schematic interpretation of distribution of muscle fibers. Black bars (A to C) indicate muscle fibers from the active MU; dark gray bars **(A to C)** indicate muscle fibers from a non-active motor unit; light gray bars **(C)** indicate degenerated myofibers belonging to the active MU. The lowermost histogram shows the distribution of durations of MUAP in the muscles. The white bars indicate simple potentials and the black bars indicate polyphasic potentials (4% in **A**, 13% in B, 31% in **C**). Mean parametric values are indicated above the histograms. In **B**, the duration of the MUAP was 51% prolonged and the amplitude was 427% increased; whereas in **C**, the duration of simple potentials was shortened by 41%, as were all potentials shortened by 29% with normal amplitude.

The system developed by Haas and Meyer (44) has a selectable degree of decomposition such that a fast extraction of the MUAP parameters for a routine clinical examination or a more time-consuming complete decomposition for research can be chosen.

Another EMG decomposition system called EMGTools extracts the constituent MUAP and FP for quantitative analysis from the EMG signal recorded at slight effort for clinical evaluation (45). Samples of electrical activity are obtained by a concentric needle electrode at a frequency of 23.5 kHz, first separating the EMG signal into segments containing MUAP activity, clustered by a minimum spanning tree method. This leads to a partition consisting of cluster-containing isolated MUAP and clusters composed of superimposed MUAP. The number of segments in a cluster is used to detect potentials from one MU. From each of these clusters, a template is selected. The clusters containing superimposed MUAP are analyzed by a recursive algorithm. The cross-correlation between superimposed MUAP and a template are computed, and time shifts with high correlation are detected. The template is subtracted for each of these time shifts, and a subsequent pass through the algorithm processes the residual segments. The output of the decomposition algorithm include MUAP parameters, MUAP plots, and FP.

Instead of decomposing EMG signals at weak effort, the decomposition system developed by LeFever and De Luca (46) separates the EMG signal into constituent MUAP trains at high contractile force, and the recording is carried out using a quadripolar needle electrode that allows each MU to be defined by three different MUAP, giving a unique description of the MUAP at high contractile force when the EMG signal consists of discharges from many MUAP.

Turns-Amplitude Analysis

In this analysis, the number of turns, defined as a change in voltage of 100 μV that may arise as a peak in a MUAP or interaction between MUAP in the interference pattern, and the mean amplitude difference between turns are measured within a fixed duration epoch (47). The number of turns reflects the number of active MU, proportion of polyphasic MUAP, and firing rate. The mean amplitude increases with increased force output and with the amplitudes of recruited MUAP. The number of turns at a force equal to 30% of the maximal voluntary force discriminates between myopathy, neurogenic lesions, and controls, wherein the number of turns increases in those with myopathy, as does the mean amplitude between turns in patients with neurogenic lesions. An increase in the ratio of turns/mean amplitude is also a sensitive indicator of myopathy, whereas a reduced ratio is associated with neurogenic disorders. The number of small intervals between turns is increased in myopathy, and decreased in neurogenic disorders. A turns-amplitude

analysis of the interference pattern at 30% of maximal effort has a diagnostic yield similar to the analysis of MUAP at low effort and is not further improved by analysis at forces greater than 30% of maximum (48). In an effort to reduce the cooperation required of the patient, the turns-amplitude analysis can be modified to obtain measurements independent of measured force, including measurements of the number of turns as a function of the mean amplitude at 3 to 5 force levels from minimum to maximum. A scatter plot which forms a cloud with myopathy and neurogenic lesions deviates in opposite directions (49). A peak ratio method uses the ratio of turns-to-mean amplitude as a function of increasing force (50, 51). Patients with myopathy have a higher peak ratio and an increased number of intervals <1.5 msec, whereas those with neurogenic lesions deviate in the opposite directions. The interference pattern can be studied by power spectral analysis in patients with neuromuscular disorders leading to a shift toward lower frequencies.

PATHOPHYSIOLOGIC CHANGES OF THE MUAP

The primary aim of the EMG examination is to determine whether weakness is due to myopathy or to neurogenic lesion. Appropriately chosen proximal and distal weak muscles are examined at rest for spontaneous muscle fiber activity at rest. In control and affected muscle, the end-plate zone shows miniature EPP and spontaneous muscle fiber discharges with a sharp negative onset. Outside the end-plate zone, propagated action potentials are rarely recorded in normal muscle. In myopathy, fibrillation activity is found when there is muscle fiber necrosis associated with myositis and some types of muscular dystrophy, rarely in mitochondrial myopathy and thyrotoxicosis, whereas denervation activity indicative of failure of reinnervation is seen in neurogenic disorders, which may endure for some time after the injury has occurred as in poliomyelitis. Fibrillation potentials, PSW activity, and CRD arise from groups of myofibers in both myopathic and neurogenic lesions. Fasciculation potentials, recognized as irregular discharges of groups of muscle fibers that can occur in normal muscle and in those with myositis and neurogenic lesions, have longer discharge intervals. Analysis of the MUAP at weak effort has a central position in the EMG examination because the duration, amplitude, and shape of the MUAP recorded with a concentric or a monopolar needle electrode reflects the architecture of the motor unit. The basic pathophysiological changes in myopathy are conduction failure and degeneration of myofibers in the individual MU that reflects the stage of the disease and compensatory regenerative mechanisms. At early stages of the disorder, muscle contraction may be affected at the level of excitation-contraction coupling leading to mild or unspecific MUAP changes. The incidence of polyphasic potentials is increased in those with myopathy for at least 2 reasons. First, myofibers may be lost leading to reduced summated MUAP amplitude and duration (Figure 2). Second, regeneration of muscle fibers from satellite cells is associated with polyphasic potentials due to increased dispersion caused by a reduced conduction velocity along the regenerated muscle fibers and collateral nerve sprouts. The incidence of polyphasic potentials is related to the duration of the MUAP and to the number of regenerating basophilic fibers at muscle biopsy. At an early stage of myopathy, the incidence of long duration polyphasic potentials is increased, whereas they decrease with advancing severity (52). The presence of long polyphasic potentials can lead to the erroneous conclusion of a neurogenic disorder. To avoid this error, measurement of the duration of simple MUAP is performed separately (Figure 2). Chronic partial denervation leads to enlarged MU due to reinnervation by collateral sprouting. Reinnervation due to axonal regeneration leads to polyphasic short duration nascent MU, however in such cases the mean MUAP duration of 20 to 30 MUAPs is usually prolonged with low amplitudes of the severely polyphasic MUAP. Chronic neuropathy is associated with MUAP of increased duration, amplitude, and polyphasia (Figure 2), the latter of which arise from dispersion of slowly conducting reinnervated and atrophic myofibers and axonal sprouts. Early reinnervation along immature sprouts leads to pronounced variability or jiggle, with intermittent dropout of segments of the MUAP. In long-standing neurogenic lesions, such as remote poliomyelitis are associated with a high incidence of polyphasic potentials which may be near normal due to maturing collateral sprouts. The postpolio syndrome is associated with an extended sprout tree that can show regressive changes with degeneration of sprouts, however, there can also be motor neuron degeneration leaving motor units with a smaller innervation ratio. Those with ALS manifest enlarged simple and polyphasic MUAP due to long-standing reinnervation and coupled-discharges of more than one motor unit. Quantitative EMG confirms widespread lower motor neuron involvement in patients with early ALS including clinically non-involved regions suggesting that maintenance of force is due to compensatory reinnervation in early disease and that this capacity may decline at later stages (53).

It is often helpful to supplement the study with turns-amplitude analysis of the interference pattern in those where MUAP analysis findings are uninformative. This aspect of muscle function allows examination at higher degrees of muscle force than the weak effort required to study individual MUAP. Evaluation of the interference pattern at maximal voluntary effort is an integral part of the EMG examination and gives a semiquantitative measure of the presence of MU loss. Normal cooperative individuals produce a maximal voluntary contraction associated with a full recruitment pattern wherein individual MUAP cannot be distinguished, and the measured amplitude of the envelope curve of the interference pattern is in the range of 2 to 4 mV (54). However in myopathy, the interference pattern, which is generally full and of lower amplitude than normal, starts abruptly at lower levels of effort than in controls, and in severe myopathy associated with extensive muscle fiber loss, may be reduced and show less pronounced summation than in normal muscle. In neurogenic lesions, the recruitment pattern is reduced in moderate cases with loss of MU and discrete in severe patients wherein individual MUAP stand out from the otherwise flat baseline between successive discharges. In chronic motor neuron disorders with reinnervation due to collateral sprouting, the amplitude of the reduced or discrete interference pattern increases, reaching values of 8 to 10 mV.

REFERENCES

1. Nikolic M, Krarup C. Challenges in computerized MUAP analysis. *Suppl Clin Neurophysiol* 2009; 60:233–246.
2. Liddell EGT, Sherrington CS. Recruitment and some other factor on reflex inhibition. *Proc R Soc Lond* 1925; B97:488–518; Sherrington CS. Recruitment and some other factors on reflex inhibition. *Proc Roy Soc Lond* 1925; B97:488–518.
3. Buchthal F, Guld C, Rosenfalck P. Volume conduction of the spike of the motor unit potential investigated with a new type of multielectrode. *Acta Physiol Scand* 1957; 38:331–354.
4. Buchthal F, Guld C, Rosenfalck P. Multielectrode study of the territory of a motor unit. *Acta Physiol Scand* 1957; 39:83–104.
5. Buchthal F, Schmalbruch H. Motor unit of mammalian muscle. *Physiol Rev* 1980; 60:90–142.
6. Close RI. Dynamic properties of mammalian skeletal muscles. *Physiol Rev* 1972; 52:129–197.
7. Krarup C. Evoked responses in normal and diseased muscle with particular reference to twitch potentiation. *Acta Neurol Scand* 1983; 68:269–315.
8. Sica R, McComas A. Review of MUNE over 30 years. In: Bromberg MB, ed. Motor unit number estimation (MUNE) *Clin Neurophysiol* (Suppl 55). Amsterdam: Elsevier, 2003; 3–13.
9. Daube JR. MUNE by statistical analysis. In: Bromberg MB, ed. Motor unit number estimation (MUNE) *Clin Neurophysiol* (Suppl 55). Amsterdam: Elsevier, 2003; 51–71.
10. Bromberg MB. Spike triggered averaging MUNE technique. In: Bromberg MB, ed. Motor unit number estimation (MUNE) *Clin Neurophysiol* (Suppl 55), Amsterdam: Elsevier, 2003:99–107.
11. Lomen-Hoerth C, Slawnych MP. Statistical motor unit number estimation. From theory to practice. *Muscle Nerve* 2003; 28:263–272.
12. Boe SG, Stashuk DW, Doherty TJ. Motor unit number estimation by decomposition-enhanced spike-triggered averaging: control data, test-retest reliability, and contractile level effects. *Muscle Nerve* 2004; 29:693–699.
13. Shefner JM, Cudkowicz ME, Zhang H, et al. The use of statistical MUNE in a multicenter clinical trial. *Muscle Nerve* 2004; 30:463–469.

14. Rosenfalck P, Rosenfalck A. *Electromyography—sensory and motor conduction. Findings in normal subjects.* Copenhagen: Laboratory of Clinical Neurophysiology, Rigshospitalet, 1975; 1–49.

15. Gydikov A, Kosarov D. Extraterritorial potential field of impulses from separate motor units in human muscles. *Electromyogr Clin Neurophysiol* 1972; 12:283–305.

16. Stålberg E, Andreassen S, Falck B, et al. Quantitative analysis of individual motor unit potentials: a proposition for standardized terminology and criteria for measurement. *J Clin Neurophysiol* 1986; 3:313–348.

17. Buchthal F. Electromyography in the evaluation of muscle disease. *Neurol Clin* 1985; 3:573–598.

18. Barkhaus PE, Nandedkar SD. On the selection of concentric needle electromyogram motor unit action potentials: is the rise time criterion too restrictive? *Muscle Nerve* 1996; 19:1554–1560.

19. Trojaborg W. Quantitative electromyography in polymyositis: a reappraisal. *Muscle Nerve* 1990; 13:964–971.

20. Stålberg EV, Sonoo M. Assessment of variability in the shape of the motor unit action potential, the "jiggle," at consecutive discharges. *Muscle Nerve* 1994; 17:1135–1144.

21. Bischoff C, Machetanz J, Conrad B. Is there an age-dependent continuous increase in the duration of the motor unit action potential? *Electroencephalogr Clin Neurophysiol* 1991; 81:304–311.

22. Tomlinson BE, Irving D. The numbers of limb motor neurons in the human lumbosacral cord throughout life. *J Neurol Sci* 1977; 34:213–219.

23. Stålberg E, Thiele B. Motor unit fibre density in the extensor digitorum communis muscle. Single fibre electromyographic study in normal subjects at different ages. *J Neurol Neurosurg Psychiatry* 1975; 38:874–880.

24. Roos MR, Rice CL, Vandervoort AA. Age-related changes in motor unit function. *Muscle Nerve* 1997; 20:679–690.

25. Bertram MF, Nishida T, Minieka MM, et al. Effects of temperature on motor unit action potentials during isometric contraction. *Muscle Nerve* 1995; 18:1443–1446.

26. Buchthal F, Erminio F, Rosenfalck P. Motor unit territory in different human muscles. *Acta Physiol Scand* 1959; 45:72–87.

27. Edström L, Kugelberg E. Histochemical composition, distribution of fibres and fatiguability of single motor units. Anterior tibial muscle of the rat. *J Neurol Neurosurg Psychiatry* 1968; 31:424–433.

28. Buchthal F, Rosenfalck P, Erminio F. Motor unit territory and fiber density in myopathies. *Neurology* 1960; 10:398–408.

29. Erminio F, Buchthal F, Rosenfalck P. Motor unit territory and muscle fiber concentration in paresis due to peripheral nerve injury and anterior horn cell involvement. *Neurology* 1959; 9:657–671.

30. Stalberg E, Schwartz MS, Thiele B, et al. The normal motor unit in man. A single fiber EMG multielectrode investigation. *J Neurol Sci* 1976; 27:291–301.

31. Stålberg E, Antoni L. Electrophysiological cross section of the motor unit. *J Neurol Neurosurg Psychiatry* 1980; 43:469–474.

32. Stålberg E, Dioszeghy P. Scanning EMG in normal muscle and in neuromuscular disorders. *Electroencephalogr Clin Neurophysiol* 1991; 81:403–416.

33. Stålberg E. Macro EMG, a new recording technique. *J Neurol Neurosurg Psychiatry* 1980; 43:475–482.

34. Jabre JF. Concentric macro electromyography. *Muscle Nerve* 1991; 14:820–825.

35. Grimby G, Stålberg E, Sandberg A, et al. An 8-year longitudinal study of muscle strength, muscle fiber size, and dynamic electromyogram in individuals with late polio. *Muscle Nerve* 1998; 21:1428–1437.

36. Sandberg A, Stålberg E. Changes in macro electromyography over time in patients with a history of polio: a comparison of 2 muscles. *Arch Phys Med Rehabil* 2004; 85:1174–1182.

37. Hilton-Brown P, Stålberg E. Motor unit size in muscular dystrophy, a macro EMG and scanning EMG study. *J Neurol Neurosurg Psychiatry* 1983; 46:996–1005.

38. Buchthal F, Guld C, Rosenfalck P. Action potential parameters in normal human muscle and their dependence on physical variables. *Acta Physiol Scand* 1954; 32:200–218.

39. Stålberg E, Bischoff C, Falck B. Outliers, a way to detect abnormality in quantitative EMG. *Muscle Nerve* 1994; 17:392–399.

40. Buchthal F. *An introduction to electromyography.* København, Stockholm, Oslo: Scandinavian University Books, 1957; 7–43.

41. Andreassen S. Methods for computer-aided measurement of motor unit parameters. Ellington RJ, Murray NMF, Halliday AM, eds. *The London symposia* (EEG Suppl 39). New York: Elsevier, 1987; 13–20.

42. Stålberg E, Falck B, Sonoo M, et al. Multi-MUP EMG analysis-a two year experience in daily clinical work. *Electroencephalogr Clin Neurophysiol* 1995; 97:145–154.

43. McGill KC, Cummins KL, Dorfman LJ. Automatic decomposition of the clinical electromyogram. *IEEE Trans Biomed Eng* 1985; 32:470–477.

44. Haas WF, Meyer M. An automatic EMG decomposition system for routine clinical examinations and clinical research. ARTMUP- automatic recognition and tracking of motor unit potentials. In: Desmedt JE, ed. *Computer-aided electromyography and expert systems.* Amsterdam: Elsevier Science Publishers B.V. (Biomedical Division), 1989; 67–81.

45. Nikolic M, Krarup C. EMGTools, an adaptive and versatile tool for detailed EMG analysis. *IEEE Trans Biomed Eng* 2011; 58:2707–2718.

46. LeFever RS, De Luca CJ. A procedure for decomposing the myoelectric signal into its constituent action potentials - Part I: Technique, theory, and implementation. *IEEE Trans Biomed Eng* 1982; 29:149–157.

47. Willison RG. Analysis of electrical activity in healthy and dystrophic muscle in man. *J Neurol Neurosurg Psychiatry* 1964; 27:386–394.

48. Fuglsang-Frederiksen A, Lo MM, Dahl K. Integrated electrical activity and number of zero crossings during a gradual increase in muscle force in patients with neuromuscular diseases. *Electroencephalogr Clin Neurophysiol* 1984; 58:211–219.

49. Stålberg E, Chu J, Bril V, Nandedkar S, et al. Automatic analysis of the EMG interference pattern. *Electroencephalogr Clin Neurophysiol* 1983; 56:672–681.

50. Liguori R, Dahl K, Fuglsang-Frederiksen A. Turns-amplitude analysis of the electromyographic recruitment pattern disregarding force measurement. I. Method and reference values in healthy subjects. *Muscle Nerve* 1992; 15:1314–1318.

51. Liguori R, Dahl K, Fuglsang-Frederiksen A, et al. Turns-amplitude analysis of the electromyographic recruitment pattern disregarding force measurement. II. Findings in patients with neuromuscular disorders. *Muscle Nerve* 1992; 15:1319–1324.

52. Buchthal F. Electrophysiological signs of myopathy as related with muscle biopsy. *Acta Neurol* (Napoli) 1977; 32:1–29.

53. Krarup C. Lower motor neuron involvements examined by quantitative electromyography in amyotrophic lateral sclerosis. *Clin Neurophysiol* 2011; 122:414–422.

54. Buchthal F, Kamieniecka Z. The diagnostic yield of quantified electromyography and quantified muscle biopsy in neuromuscular disorders. *Muscle Nerve* 1982; 5:265–280.

CHAPTER 7

Autonomic Electrophysiological Assessment

Joel Gutiérrez

The autonomic nervous system (ANS) regulates multiple reflex actions. Most of the tests employed to evaluate the ANS provide an overview of the functional state of these reflex arcs. The ideal test should be simple to perform, noninvasive, reproducible, sensitive, specific, safe and appropriate for longitudinal studies. The availability of computer-based techniques has facilitated functional assessment of the ANS (1, 2). However, the information provided by autonomic testing is only useful when the indication is derived from proper prior analysis of the clinical history and physical examination of the patient, allowing for a hypothesis that can be tested. Properly performed and interpreted, ANS testing can be used to confirm the presence of an ANS disturbance and the involved functional pathways, as well as the extent, intensity, and site of injury. There are standard sources of autonomic neurophysiological investigation and ANS disturbances (3, 4).

HISTORICAL BACKGROUND

In the second century, Galen described the paravertebral chains and their central and peripheral extensions as "tubes driving the animal spirit" to achieve "sympathy" or connection between the different parts of the body. The notion of a single functional unit persisted until the 16th century when the intercostal or sympathetic nerves were regarded as an independent anatomical entity. The term *intercostal nerve* was replaced by *great sympathetic nerve*, recognizing its role in cardiac autonomic innervation. Experimental dissection of the vagus nerve followed speculation of its role in cardiovagal innervation and heart rate (HR) modulation. Soon after recognition of the vegetative nervous system, which

encompassed the enteric plexuses of Meissner and Auerbach, vascular sympathetic tone was described. Langley, a physiologist in the late 19th century, is credited with use of the term ANS and recognition of the sympathetic and parasympathetic subdivisions, each with its distinctive anatomical and functional features.

ANATOMY AND PHYSIOLOGY

The ANS consists of a set of afferent pathways, a central nervous system (CNS) integrating complex in the brain and spinal cord, and two distinct efferent limbs, sympathetic and parasympathetic, each with preganglionic and postganglionic neurons. The parasympathetic division is topographically more restricted than the sympathetic division. The bodies of the preganglionic parasympathetic neurons are located in the brainstem nuclei of cranial nerve 3, 7, 9, and 10, and in the 2nd, 3rd and 4th sacral segments of the spinal cord. Preganglionic fibers originate in the Edinger-Westphal, upper and lower salivatory, ambiguous, and dorsal motor nuclei. Long, predominantly cholinergic parasympathetic preganglionic fibers travel relatively considerable distances to the sphenopalatine, submandibular and otic cranial nerve ganglia located in the vicinity of the effector organs, which in turn originate short, predominantly cholinergic parasympathetic postganglionic fibers, which innervate the effector organs. Vagal preganglionic fibers innervate all thoracic viscera and digestive tract up to the splenic flexure of the colon. The vagus and glossopharyngeal nerves contain afferent fibers that convey information to the CNS as to changes in blood pressure (BP) and HR essential in the integration of the baroreflex. Sacral segments provide parasympathetic innervation to the pelvic organs and the segments of the colon not innervated by the vagus nerves.

The sympathetic nervous system consists of preganglionic sympathetic neurons located in the intermediolateral horn of the thoracic and lumbar spinal segments that elaborate short nerves that innervate postganglionic neurons located in the prevertebral, paravertebral, and previsceral sympathetic ganglia, from whence long postganglionic axons innervate effector organs. Postganglionic axons are generally thin and unmyelinated, measuring <5 microns (μ), innervate smooth muscles of blood vessels, heart, endocrine glands and parenchymatous organs. Autonomic neurons of the spinal cord are innervated by the ventromedial and ventrolateral regions of the medulla oblongata, median raphe nucleus, and paraventricular nuclei of the hypothalamus. Central efferent fibers follow a pattern of

topographical innervation similar to a ladder, triggering a massive response, owing to the high degree of divergence of their circuits, or local responses limited to a limb or body region, as may be appropriate. Multiple neurotransmitters are involved in the integration of these responses including the monoamines epinephrine, norepinephrine, and serotonin; the neuropeptides substance P, vasopressin, oxytocin, and glutamate; the amino acids glutamate, GABA, and glycine; however, adrenalin is the predominant neurotransmitter at postganglionic synapses. Several neurotransmitters can coexist in a single autonomic neuron.

Postganglionic axons originating in thoracic and lumbosacral ganglia travel long distances to innervate the abdominal viscera and blood vessels of the legs, at times measuring >50 centimeters in length. Considering that such axons can attain a diameter of approximately 1.2 μ, the volume of these axons may reach about 565,000 μm³, in contrast to the volume of

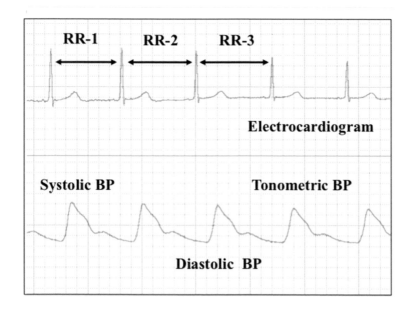

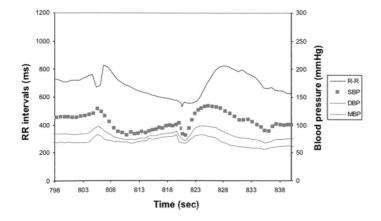

FIG. 1. Top panel: Electrocardiogram and beat by beat blood pressure recordings. Bottom panel: Curves of RR intervals variability and blood pressure (systolic, mean and diastolic) vs. time while the subject performs a Valsalva maneuver to activate autonomic cardiovascular reflexes.

the soma of these neurons of only 14,000 μm^3. These morphological characteristics, together with its constant activity, make sympathetic fibers especially vulnerable to injury.

Although parasympathetic and sympathetic effects have been traditionally regarded as antagonistic, it is now apparent that the interrelationship in more complex and context sensitive. For example, the specific effects of the autonomic innervation of a particular organ does not depend only on the type of autonomic organ receptor present, but the level of pre-activation at the time of neurotransmitter stimulation. Activation of the sympathetic nervous system evokes a diffuse response preparing the body for situations requiring high metabolic demand and physical activity, such as those of pupillary and bronchial dilation, increased HR and BP, decreased gastrointestinal motility, vasoconstriction, and increased glycogenolysis, but selectively activation can also occur. Whereas the parasympathetic nervous system regulates more restricted functions associated with resting activity, activation of this division promotes stages of energy conservation expressed as decreases in HR and BP, pupillary constriction and increased bronchial and gastrointestinal activity.

The baroreflex is the most important cardiovascular reflex for the control of rapid BP oscillation (5). It is triggered by activation of stretch receptors located in the carotid sinus and the aortic arch, and afferent fibers that convey information along the glossopharyngeal and vagus nerves to the solitary tract nucleus of the brainstem. Multiple connections related to the central autonomic network depart from the solitary tract nucleus to other areas of the CNS related to HR and BP control. These connections are the functional and anatomical bases of the short-term regulation of BP. The ANS acts upon three elements to maintain satisfactory control of BP, including the heart, venous return, and systemic vascular resistance. Efferent arms of the ANS that communicate with these components are the sympathetic and parasympathetic innervation of the heart and the sympathetic innervation of the smooth muscle of peripheral blood vessels, such that activation of arterial baroreceptors excites the sympathetic vasomotor and inhibit the cardiovagal control centers of the brainstem. For example, a decrement in BP reduces the activity of vascular stretch receptors, thereby decreasing vagal excitation and sympathetic inhibition, resulting in reduced cardiovagal activity and increased sympathetic output to blood vessels, translated as tachycardia and vasoconstriction. This combination of cardiac and vascular adjustments ultimately restores BP to its original level, with a reverse process occurring in situations that instead increase BP. These fine-tuning changes occur very quickly with a time profile such that cardiovagal activity that changes HR occur in the first to second beat after changes in BP, whereas sympathetic influences on HR and arterial vasomotor tone takes several seconds to reach a clinical expression. These features should

be taken into account in the design, implementation, and interpretation of functional tests for the clinical examination of the ANS.

TESTS OF AUTONOMIC FUNCTION

Although most tests are easy to perform, their interpretation is difficult due to the multiplicity of factors that can affect the responses and the complexity of the pathways and reflexes involved. Consequently, in clinical practice it is more reliable to perform a battery of ANS tests than a single test, the results of which will be complementary to each other, increasing clinically reliability. Particular attention should be given to the influence of factors that may increase or decrease the sensitivity of the tests, as for example, subjects who demonstrate completely normal vasoconstriction when tested under controlled laboratory conditions despite faulty vasoconstriction that leads to orthostatic hypotension under specific circumstances, such as strenuous exercise, emotionally stressful situations, and a hot environment.

It is advisable to perform the tests simulating factors that ordinarily trigger autonomic failure. Individual laboratories should have their own reference values corrected for the potential confounding among them, such as age, body mass index, laboratory conditions, and the characteristics of the recording protocols, such as the method of analysis, posture, test duration, order of application, levels of hydration, concurrent medication, prior consumption of caffeinated beverages, degree of physical activity, and emotional state.

Autonomic lesions can be underestimated both in the clinical and research setting due to their subclinical course, as well as the mistaken attribution to a primary disturbance of the affected organ such as tachycardia erroneously attributed to heart failure instead of deficient cardiovagal control, and the relative insensitivity of vascular sympathetic testing. The ANS, which regulates a wide range of biological functions, is amenable to standardized study of cardiovascular and sweat-reflexes testing, with beat-to-beat HR variation (HRV), commonly employed to explore cardiovagal regulation, while variations in BP are used to assess the influence on sympathetic vasomotor sympathetic tone. Maneuvers that assess the integrity of cardiovascular reflexes can be performed simply by manual evaluation of the radial pulse and blood pressure taken with an ordinary sphygmomanometer, while more sophisticated and sensitive evaluation of these functions is required to record and mathematically analyze the HRV and beat-to-beat BP variations.

The 1996 Task Force report of the American Academy of Neurology evaluated the safety, reproducibility, ease of performance, and sensitivity of available ANS tests (6). Those most useful to evaluate parasympathetic function included HRV during deep breathing with calculation of an expiratory and inspiratory ratio (I/E), Valsalva maneuver (VM) with calculation of the Valsalva ratio; HRV at rest and with active standing with calculation of the 30:15 ratio of the maximum RR interval at 30 divided by the minimal interval at 15 seconds; while the recommendation for sympathetic function testing included BP response to the VM, during muscle contraction and active standing, and sudomotor test of sympathetic skin response (SSR) and quantitative sudomotor axon reflex test (QSART).

Heart Rate Variability

The autonomic regulation of HR depends upon the interactions between cardiovagal innervation, β-adrenergic sympathetic innervation, and the influence of circulating hormones. In physiologic conditions, the HR fluctuates according to the metabolic needs of the organism with a variation that is most evident during physical exertion and states of high emotional stress; however HRV is a permanent phenomenon in normal subjects. The quantification of these variations is one of the most widely used tests to explore the ANS. Under physiological conditions, HR increases during inspiration and decreases during respiration termed *respiratory sinus arrhythmia* (RSA). Atropine and surgical destruction of the vagus nerves eliminates or reduces the RSA, suggesting that cardiovagal innervation is essential to its generation. The reflex arc of the RSA includes vagal afferent fibers from alveolar and thoracic aorta stretch receptors, carotid baroreceptors, dorsal motor ambiguous and vagus cranial nerve nuclei, and vagal efferent fibers to the heart (5). The analysis of HRV requires the recording of an electrocardiogram (EKG) rhythm strip from lead II with clearly identifiable R waves. The intervals between consecutive R waves are manually or automatically measured producing a series of values of successive RR intervals. Most programs for the analysis of HRV plot RR intervals against time in their sequence of appearance (Figure 1). Visual inspection of HRV curves gives an overview of the variability of RR intervals duration during the measured time period but that can be followed by different types of mathematical methods, including analyses in time or spectral domains. Such studies, termed *RR variability* or *RR intervalometry,* are recorded at rest and with activating maneuvers, including deep breathing at six cycles per second, VM, and active standing (7).

HRV with Deep Breathing

Patients are instructed to inhale and exhale deeply at a frequency of six cycles per minute (0.16 Hz), with each cycle lasting 10 seconds, comprised of five inspirations and expirations, a frequency that generates the most intense variations in the HRV. Some laboratories use visual signals on a monitor to guide the patient. It is advisable to record lead II of the resting ECG for 60 seconds before and after the maneuver. The commonest errors include completion of the breathing in less than 5 seconds and an inadequate respiratory effort. The commonest quantification of the change in HRV induced by deep breathing is the E/I ratio calculated by dividing the maximum and minimum RR intervals obtained during the deep breathing maneuver (Figure 2), and measurement of the average of three maximal and minimal values obtained in three respiratory cycles, discarding the first cycle. Alternatively, the difference in the ratio of the longest and shortest intervals of three cycles with maximal variation can be computed, wherein a result greater than 15 beats per minute (bpm) can be considered normal and 10 bpm abnormal. Deep breathing responses are highly dependent upon patient age and the intensity of the respiratory cycles. Alteration of HRV to deep breathing is considered a sensitive marker of impaired cardiovagal parasympathetic innervation with both afferent and efferent branches of this reflex mediated by the vagus nerves (8). Given its simplicity of implementation and high sensitivity, it is widely employed in research investigations of parasympathetic ANS function, especially in prediction of the progression of diabetic autonomic neuropathy, wherein a prospective study of 373 insulin-dependent diabetic children without clinical manifestations of autonomic neuropathy determined that one-third had changes in HRV to deep breathing over a seven-year period (9). The sensitivity of deep breathing ratio, which exceeds other tests of parasympathetic function, led to the assertion that incorporation of HRV to VM and active standing did not lead to additional benefit in discerning parasympathetic ANS dysfunction (10).

Valsalva maneuver

The complex hemodynamic and autonomic changes induced by a VM depend on multiple interactions between blood pressure, venous return, and the baroreflex, making the calculated VR sensitive to dysfunction of both the sympathetic and parasympathetic ANS divisions. Subjects are instructed to blow vigorously into a mouthpiece or mask applied over the mouth, sustaining a pressure of 40 mm Hg for 15 seconds while quantifying the expiratory force with a digital or aneroid manometer attached to the mask through a cannula. Subjects are encouraged to watch the pressure gauge to monitor the intensity of the respiratory excursion, which continues throughout the period of strain, emanating from the lungs and not the mouth alone and, guided by the examiner inform the patient when to start and end the strain. The recording should commence 60 seconds before and up to 60 seconds after the performance of the strain phase, and is repeated several times until at least two trials yield reproducible waveforms. Repeated maneuvers should be separated by intervals of three minutes to avoid overlapping the effects of adjacent strains. The VR, defined as the longest RR interval following completion of the maneuver, divided by the shorter RR interval recorded during the strain phase (Figure 3), is sufficient to evaluate the parasympathetic division, while cardiovagal innervation is more complex, since the resultant HR changes are secondary to systemic alterations BP. Whereas both deep breathing and VR ratios explore HRV induced by cardiovagal innervation, these indices have a different physiological basis,

with the E/I ration dependent solely upon afferent and efferent nerve fibers that course through the vagus nerves (11). In order to make a proper interpretation of the cardiovascular changes induced by a VM, it is necessary to evaluate both HR and BP reflective of primary cardiovagal and α-adrenergic vascular impairment (12). The increased VR in patients with peripheral neuropathy results from concomitant impairment of vascular α-adrenergic and spares cardiac β-adrenergic autonomic innervation (11).

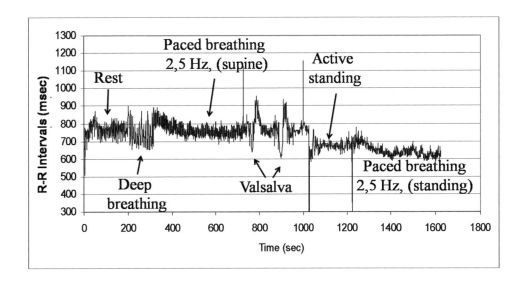

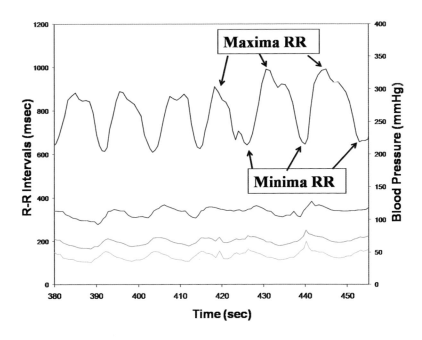

FIG. 2. Top panel: Effects of activating maneuvers on heart rate variability. Bottom panel: Calculation of deep breathing ratio. RR intervals are recorded while the subject is breathing at a frequency of six cycles per minute (five seconds inspiration and five seconds expiration). The maxima and minima of the three widest respiratory cycles (arrows) are visually identified in the RR intervals curve. The deep breathing ratio is derived by dividing the RR maximum by the RR minimum for each cycle and averaging their results.

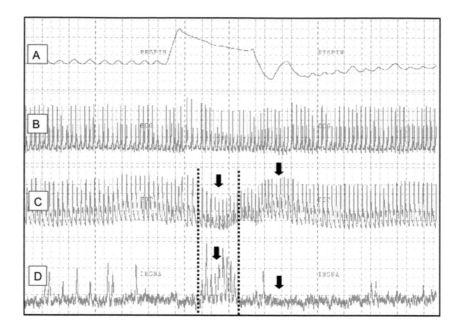

FIG. 3. Correlation between beat-to-beat blood pressure and muscle sympathetic nerve activity during a Valsalva maneuver. **(A)** Monitoring the duration and intensity of the respiratory effort. **(B)** Electrocardiogram. **(C)** Tonometric recordings of beat-to-beat blood pressure. **(D)** Microneurographic recordings of muscle nerve sympathetic activity from a peripheral nerve. Note that sympathetic nerve activity increases in response to blood pressure reduction in phase II and decreases following blood pressure recovery in phases IIB and IV (arrows).

Heart Rate Variability with Active Standing

The HR changes that occur during the first 30 seconds of active standing depend mainly upon cardiovagal regulation mediated by parasympathetic inhibition of the baroreflex with beat-to-beat recording showing an HR peak beginning between 3 and 12 seconds after standing, reaching a maximum value at 15 seconds, followed by a decrease in HR, which starts at 20 seconds and reaches a maximum value at 30 seconds. The ratio of the maximum RR interval at 30 seconds divided by the minimum interval at 15 seconds, termed *the 30:15 ratio,* is a reliable indicator of cardiovagal function and cardiac autonomic neuropathy. Patients are instructed to actively stand up, being careful not to detach any recording electrodes or generate movement artifact. The determination of the 30:15 ratio requires recording of the initial 30- to 40-second period of active standing; however, the test is usually extended for a longer time of 5, 15, or 30 minutes to explore long-term HR and BP responses generated by the postural change. As with the VM, the correct interpretation of HR changes induced by active standing requires the simultaneous recording of EKG and beat-to-beat BP. The Valsalva and 30:15 ratios, which are

less sensitive markers of cardiovagal dysfunction than the deep breathing ratio, depend instead upon complex central and peripheral interactions, rendering them less sensitive to mild autonomic abnormalities (13). All these ratios are reproducible in healthy subjects but show a clear decline with age, as does the HRV, which is sensitive to the presence of ectopic beats, technical artifacts, cardiac arrhythmias, inadequate identification of R waves, and wrong quantification of RR intervals. The reliability of these indicators is severely limited in patients with HR >100 bpm.

Heart Rate Variability at Rest

The HRV at rest can be quantified in the time and spectral, or frequency domains, the former in a given period of time, one minute, five minutes, or 24 hours, with a coefficient of variability, defined as the count of the number or percentage of intervals that exceed certain duration, as the commonest employed indicator thereof, followed by the standard deviation of RR intervals, and the square of the differences between consecutive RR intervals (6). Spectral domain analysis, which quantifies the frequency and intensity of periodic changes of HRV in a period of time, shows that rapid HRV oscillations depend upon the influence of breathing patterns and cardiac activity mediated by the parasympathetic system while slow changes in HRV are related, BP under control of both parasympathetic and sympathetic influences. The ratio of low-frequency (LF) and high-frequency (HF) bands (LF/HF) are useful indicators of the balance between the parasympathetic and sympathetic divisions (14). A promising application is the potential of estimating the relative contribution of the two ANS divisions in the control of HR more effectively than other methods of analysis (15). The spectral power of the HF band, which has traditionally been accepted as a reliable indicator of cardiovagal activity, is superior to that of the LF band that depends instead upon the combination of sympathetic, parasympathetic, and mixed cardiac influences. The study of the balance between parasympathetic and sympathetic influences on the cardiovascular system is important because it has been extensively demonstrated that subjects with absolute or relative predominance of sympathetic activity are more likely to suffer myocardial infarction, cardiac arrhythmias, hypertension, sudden death, gout, obesity, and premature aging than those with more balanced ANS function (16).

Beat-to-Beat Blood Pressure and Vascular Sympathetic Control

The autonomic innervation of blood vessels and skin is mainly under the control of the sympathetic nervous system. The ANS is essential for the short-term regulation of BP, including the fast compensation of transient changes that occur a few seconds after postural, hemodynamic, and emotional changes. Given the extended length of the sympathetic fibers throughout peripheral nerve trunks, it is likely that in the course of some neurological diseases, as for example, length-dependent neuropathy, peripheral sympathetic fibers are commonly injured earlier or more severely than parasympathetic fibers, the paths of which are usually much shorter (17, 18). The recording of beat-to-beat BP changes is essential for evaluating the sympathetic control of peripheral blood vessels. Early investigations employing catheters inserted inside peripheral arteries provided accurate data but were invasive and painful, and if continued in this manner, such analyses would have remained in research. Fortunately, non-invasive devices are available to record beat-to-beat BP for clinical use, and depending upon the transducer used, are of two types, photoelectric-cell-based sensors (Finometer, Finapres, Nexfin™) and those that monitor the mechanical deformation of the arterial wall with a tonometric transducer (COLIN) laboratories (19–21). These transducers transform beat-to-beat BP oscillations into a curve as a function of time in which systolic peaks and diastolic valleys of each cardiac cycle amenable to identification and measurement (Figure 3) (22).

Valsalva maneuver

The VM is considered the best method to explore the functional state of peripheral vascular innervation (23). The VM is comprised of four distinctive phases (Figure 4). Phase I is associated with an increase in BP due to the mechanical compression of the thoracic great vessels associated with transient bradycardia lasting one to two seconds. Phase IIA is associated with a progressive decrease in BP, lasting five to seven seconds, induced by reduced venous return and lowered cardiac output that follows compression of the great thoracic veins and baroreflex-mediated tachycardia that fails to reverse the fall in BP. Phase IIB is associated with progressive recovery of BP, which lasts five to seven seconds, that results from the combined activation of the vascular α-adrenergic vasomotor- and cardiovagal-mediated tachycardia, initiated in phase IIA. Phase III is the mirror image of phase I wherein the brief drop in BP caused by mechanical decompression of thoracic great vessels leads to progressive tachycardia. During phase IV the release of mechanical thoracic compression abruptly increases venous return and cardiac output, which in association with ongoing vasoconstriction, overshoots BP well above baseline values, reaching a maximum in five seconds followed by a decline toward normal levels. The HR curve reveals a reflex bradycardia that reaches maximum in a few seconds after BP maximum and then falls to normal levels.

Whereas BP recovery in phase II relies more upon increased vascular resistance mediated by α-adrenergic fibers than increased HR mediated by cardiovagal parasympathetic inhibition (24), BP recovery during phase IV is a consequence of the combined effects of vascular α-adrenergic, cardiac β-adrenergic, and cardiovagal functions. Mild α-adrenergic sympathetic disturbances yield delayed or impaired BP recovery during phase II with preserved phase IV. The differences between the physiological mechanisms underlying phases II and IV is shown by the administration of selective parasympathetic and sympathetic blocking medications. The administration of the α-adrenergic antagonist phentolamine produces a decrease in BP during phase II and an increase in BP during IV in normal subjects, while the β-adrenergic antagonist decreases the physiological increase in BP in phase IV without affecting BP in phase II, indicating that BP and HR changes in phase II are more dependent on α-adrenergic innervations, while those of phase IV are more reliant on β-adrenergic cardiac innervation. In general, a greater importance is attached to marked changes or absence of phase IV, and the reduction of BP recovery in phase IIA or its absence in phase IIB (25). The magnitude of quantifiable BP changes referenced to pre-maneuver baseline values, expressed as a percentage of the decrement of BP, reached during phase IIA is a quantitative and standardized way of comparing to normal reference values. Such quantification

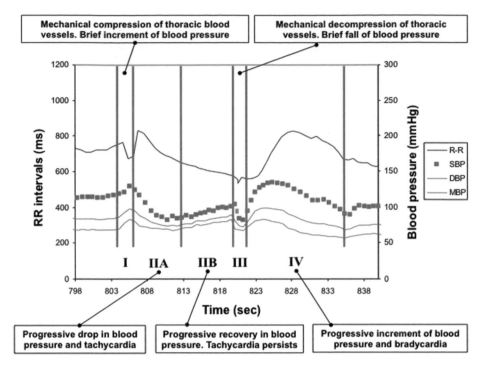

FIG. 4. Curves of RR interval duration (top tracing) and beat-to-beat systolic blood pressure (lower tracing) vs. time, recorded in a healthy subject while performing a standardized Valsalva maneuver. The heart rate and blood pressure changes associated with this maneuver are typically subdivided into four phases, I to IV. Phases I and III are mainly due to mechanical compression of the large thoracic blood vessels.

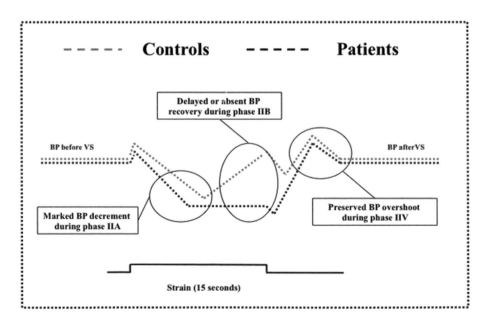

FIG. 5. Abnormalities in blood pressure changes during the Valsalva maneuver in patients with autonomic disorders in the course of peripheral neuropathy. Blood pressure drop during phase IIA is deeper and more prolonged in patients with polyneuropathy than in normal controls. These patients also have a poor recovery of blood pressure in phase IIB (remains below baseline values). However, both groups have a similar blood pressure recovery in phase IV.

may be more useful in detecting α-adrenergic abnormalities, such as those associated with peripheral neuropathy, than other markers of the sympathetic ANS (26). The BP changes that occur during the VM have been studied in patients with diabetic, alcoholic, demyelinating and nutritional neuropathies, and in those with neurally mediated syncope and orthostatic hypotension, in the early stages of which there may be delayed or ineffective recovery of BP during phase II, with other phases remaining normal (Figure 5).

Active and Passive Standing

The sympathetic control of vascular tone is essential for maintaining BP during standing, and the changes therein provide valuable information of the integrity of the baroreflex and other autonomic reflexes (5). Standing and gravitational stress evokes an immediate displacement of 500 to 1000 milliliters of blood to the lower part of the body, reducing BP and activating the baroreflex, with resultant adjustments in vascular tone and HR. After several seconds the slight drop in BP generates a vagal inhibitory response and reflex tachycardia that reaches a peak at 15 seconds, which in association with progressive vasoconstriction, is followed by recovery in BP and reflex bradycardia that reaches a maximum at 30 seconds. Over the ensuing one to two minutes, the BP remains steady in most subjects due to combined sympathetic and cardiovagal adjustments. Most of the ANS changes related to standing occur within the first five minutes while the long-term control of BP includes hormonal changes that influence vascular tone and fluid displacement. While initial active standing in normal subjects leads to a slight decrease in BP and increase in HR of less than 30 bpm, in those with orthostatic hypotension, BP is severely reduced in the first few seconds and minutes after active standing, accompanied by a reciprocal increase in HR. The criteria that define postural hypotension vary between laboratories, but a symptomatic drop in systolic BP >30 mm Hg is abnormal; however, a severe drop in BP should lead to consideration of poor vascular sympathetic tone. A drop in BP may be associated with either tachycardia or bradycardia, depending upon the primary underlying cause of the hypotension.

Patients with chronic orthostatic hypotension experience persistent and pronounced tachycardia, a situation encountered in postural tachycardia syndrome (POTS). Whereas normal subjects undergoing passive tilting of 60 degrees to 90 degrees can develop a slight transient drop in systolic, diastolic, and mean BP that recovers in one minute, and HR that increases from 10 to 20 bpm, those with significant adrenergic impairment have inadequate compensatory vasoconstriction leading to postural hypotension and a progressive fall in BP even during passive standing. The sensitivity of the tilt-table test for confirming neutrally-mediated syncope varies from 40% to 60% with up to 50% of patients with a compatible clinical history demonstrating completely normal tilt-table results. Accordingly, those with suspected neurally-mediated syncope that manifest normal HR and BP responses to passive standing should be studied for at least 30 to 45 minutes to increase the sensitivity of the study (5).

SUDOMOTOR REFLEXES

The regulation of body temperature is an important function of the ANS, and the control of sweating is essential for thermal homeostasis. Central and peripheral sudomotor sympathetic function is assessed by recording the responses of sweat glands to various types of stimuli. Such studies are especially useful in the early detection of small fiber neuropathy lesions (27).

Thermoregulatory Sweat Test

This test involves the application of a substance on the region of the body under examination, capable of changing color when body temperature is raised after placement in a room with elevated temperature, or following exposure to a heating lamp to stimulate sweating in regions of the body under investigation. The most commonly employed substances are starch iodide and corn starch with calcium carbonate, which change to a darker color upon contact with sweating than areas with absent or decreased sweating demonstrating topographic patterns of sudomotor disturbances. However, these studies are unable to differentiate central from peripheral autonomic disorders, or those due to preganglionic or postganglionic sympathetic sudomotor disturbances (28).

Sweat Imprinting

In this test, silicone mold or other easily imprintable substances are applied over the body in the regions of postganglionic sympathetic-innervated sweat glands and are activated by iontophoretically applied pilocarpine, leading to the accumulation of droplets of dermal sweat that becomes trapped in the mold, the volume of which can be ascertained (29). The association of severe reduction in sweating with normal response to iontophoresis is consistent with a preganglionic or central autonomic injury.

Sympathetic Skin Response

The sympathetic skin response (SSR) is a late electrical response of hairless skin characterized by a long reflex arc that involves central and peripheral ANS components, the former of which include synaptic connections from the posterior hypothalamus to the brainstem reticular formation

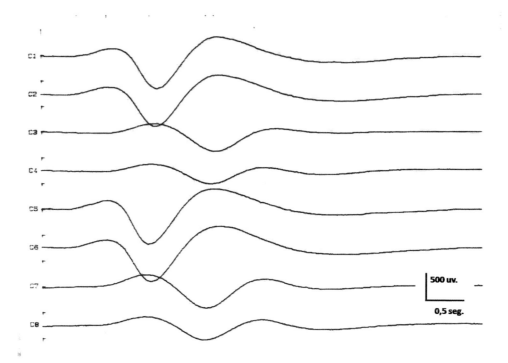

FIG. 6. Sympathetic skin responses recorded in the four limbs. C1 and C5: Right palms; C2 and C6: Left palms; C3 and C7: Right plants; C4 and C8: Left plants; The onset latencies were approximately 1.5 seconds in the upper limbs and 2 seconds in the lower limbs (delay: 1 second).

and spinal cord, and the latter of which include pre-and postganglionic sympathetic sudomotor fibers and the sweat glands. Under physiological conditions of normal room temperature, the skin of the soles and palms is usually 10 to 25 millivolts more negative than that of other body regions, with spontaneous electrical oscillation. The SSR is generated in the deeper layers of the glabrous skin, due to the reflex activation of sweat glands, stimulated by acetylcholine-secreting sudomotor sympathetic efferent fibers. The final morphology of the electrical responses recorded in the skin surface depends on the interaction between sweat glands and the surrounding skin tissue. Latency, amplitude, and morphology of the SSR are highly variable in the same subject during a given experimental session (30).

Central efferent fibers related to the SSR originate in the hypothalamus and travel caudally and ipsilaterally through the lateral columns of the spinal cord, synapsing upon preganglionic sympathetic neurons of the intermediate horn of the spinal cord. Preganglionic sympathetic fibers innervating the arms exit the spinal cord at the T4 to T7 spinal cord levels, while those innervating the legs depart from T10 to T12 segments. Postganglionic sympathetic fibers give rise to sympathetic sudomotor fibers that innervate sweat glands of the hands and feet.

These recordings are influenced by emotional, auditory, and light stimuli, and in order to avoid the interference of these external factors, they should be performed in a quiet, sound proof, and temperature-controlled room. Active electrodes are placed on hairless skin of the palms and soles and referenced to electrodes located on the hairy skin of the dorsum of the hands and feet. Electrophysiological activity is collected simultaneously from the arms and legs for 5 to 10 seconds after the stimulus. (Figure 6). Square pulses of electrical current lasting 0.2 ms, with an intensity of 10 to 30 mA, 2- to 3-fold the sensory threshold, are delivered to the subject at irregular intervals of 30 to 60 seconds, with varying intensity, to any sensory nerve; however, the supraorbital, median, sural, and posterior tibial are routinely used. If stimulation of a particular nerve is not effective to generate responses, others can be tried to avoid the effect of focal lesions of the afferent reflex. Electrical stimuli that fail to evoke responses can be switched to auditory, emotional, or light stimulation, as well as brisk and deep inspiration to induce SSR. With an average conduction velocity of 1 to 2 m/s, conduction through type C postganglionic fibers and sweat-gland activation account for more than 95% of the SSR latency. The total amplitude of the SSR depends on the interaction of two components, the activation of the sweat gland itself, and the influence of the surrounding skin tissue. Given its intrinsic vulnerability to emotional factors, the amplitude of the SSR shows 35% to 45% variability, decreasing with age with up to one-half of normal subjects age 60 years or older demonstrating no recordable SSR. Accordingly, as a result of the expected physiological variability, some consider the SSR abnormal only when absent (30).

One advantage of the SSR is that it can be recorded with simple technology available in most clinical neurophysiology laboratories. The SSR has been used extensively in the study of diabetic, acute demyelinating, nutritional, and toxic peripheral neuropathies, and in CNS disorders including Parkinson disease (PD), multiple system atrophy (MSA), multiple sclerosis (MS) and stroke. It is severely decreased or absent in patients with severe autonomic neuropathy; however, responses may remain within normal limits in up to 50% of patients of varying degrees of diabetic, uremic, amyloid, and alcoholic peripheral neuropathy, even in the presence of clinical dysautonomia. The responses have no predictable clinical-electrophysiological correlation (31), and for uncertain reasons, absence of SSR should not be considered a unique result of sympathetic skin denervation because other factors can affect local skin conductance, including trophic and callous skin changes. The diagnostic sensitivity of the SSR is higher in patients with PD, MSA, pure autonomic failure (PAF), and traumatic spinal cord injury than in patients with peripheral neuropathy.

Tetraplegic patients with spinal cord injuries above the T_3 segment demonstrate absent SSR in the arms and legs (32).

An important factor in the interpretation of SSR is whether the causative lesion affects pre- or postganglionic fibers. The most useful test to demonstrate injury to postganglionic sudomotor sympathetic fibers is the quantitative sudomotor axonal reflex test (QSART), which is performed by iontophoretically introducing pilocarpine into the dermis to directly stimulate the sweat glands. Action potentials of activated glands travel antidromically to the nearest axonal branching point where they are propagated to the other sweat glands innervated by the same postganglionic fiber, from which an electrical response can be recorded and quantified. Therefore, the functional integrity of the postganglionic axons is essential for the onset of normal QSART responses (2). Concomitantly, absent SSR and normal QSART responses suggest abnormality along preganglionic sudomotor fibers or of the CNS, a pattern which can be observed in those with MS, spinal cord injury, and stroke. Whereas abnormality of SSR and QSART testing show a high correlation, the QSART is more sensitive than the SSR. The QSART can be evaluated also in proximal portions of the arms and legs to prove the existence of a length-dependent pattern. In the interpretation of the QSART, it should be noted that a normal QSART does not exclude the existence of central or preganglionic disorders, because this test does not assess these levels of the sudomotor pathways.

REFERENCES

1. Hilz MJ, Dutsch M. Quantitative studies of autonomic function. *Muscle Nerve* 2006; 33:6–20.
2. Low PA. Testing the autonomic nervous system. *Semin Neurol* 2003; 23:407–421.
3. Appenzeller O, Oribe E. Testing autonomic reflexes. In: *The autonomic nervous system.* 5th ed, New York: Elsevier, 1997.
4. Low PA, Polinsky R, Kaufmann H, Freeman R, Eds. *Autonomic function and dysfunction.* Part A. Baltimore: Williams and Wilkins, 1998.
5. Wieling W, Shepherd JT. Initial and delayed circulatory responses to orthostatic stress in normal humans and in subjects with orthostatic intolerance. *Int Angiol* 1992; 11:69–82.
6. Assessment: Clinical autonomic testing report of the Therapeutics and Technology Assessment Subcommittee of the American Academy of Neurology. *Neurology* 1996; 46:873–880.
7. Ewing DJ, Campbell IW, Clarke BF. Heart rate changes in diabetes mellitus. *Lancet* 1981; 1:183–186.
8. Low PA. Autonomic nervous system function. *J Clin Neurophysiol* 1993; 10:14–27.
9. Stella P, Ellis D, Maser RE, Orchard TJ. Cardiovascular autonomic neuropathy (expiration and inspiration ratio) in type 1 diabetes. Incidence and predictors. *J Diabetes Complications* 2000; 14:1–6.
10. May O, Arildsen H. Assessing cardiovascular autonomic neuropathy in diabetes mellitus: How many tests to use? *J Diabetes Complications* 2000; 14:7–12.
11. Opfer-Gehrking TL, Low PA. Impaired respiratory sinus arrhythmia with paradoxically normal Valsalva ratio indicates combined cardiovagal and peripheral adrenergic failure. *Clin Auton Res* 1993; 3:169–173.
12. Benarroch EE, Opfer-Gehrking TL, Low PA. Use of the photoplethysmographic technique to analyze the Valsalva maneuver in normal man. *Muscle Nerve* 1991; 14:1165–1172.
13. Ewing DJ, Martyn CN, Young RJ, Clarke BF. The value of cardiovascular autonomic function tests: 10 years' experience in diabetes. *Diabetes Care* 1985; 8:491–498.
14. Niskanen J, Tarvainen MP, Ranta-aho PO, et al. Software for advanced HRV analysis. *Computer Methods and Programs in Biomedicine* 2004; 76:73–81.
15. Task Force of the ESC and NASPE. Heart rate variability. Standards of measurement, physiological interpretation, and clinical use. *Circulation* 1996; 93:1043–1108.
16. Sica DA. The importance of the sympathetic nervous system and systolic hypertension in patients with hypertension: benefits in treating patients with increased cardiovascular risk. *Blood Press Monit* 2000; 5(Suppl 2):S19–S25.
17. Gutiérrez JV, García H, Sánchez J, et al. The topographic diagnosis of the sympathetic nervous system lesions in Cuban epidemic neuropathy. The value of the sympathetic skin response. *Rev Cubana Med Trop* 1998; 50:245–248.
18. Low VA, Sandroni P, Fealey RD, et al. Detection of small-fiber neuropathy by sudomotor testing. *Muscle Nerve* 2006; 34:57–61.
19. Schutte AE, Huisman HW, Van Rooyen JM, et al. Sensitivity

of the Finometer device in detecting acute and medium-term changes in cardiovascular function. *Blood Press Monit* 2003; 8:195–201.

20. Maestri R, Pinna GD, Robbi E, et al. Noninvasive measurement of blood pressure variability: accuracy of the Finometer monitor and comparison with the Finapres device. *Physiol Meas* 2005; 26:1125–1136.

21. Zion AS, Bartels MN, Wecht JM, et al. Evaluation of blood pressure and baroreflex sensitivity by radial artery tonometry versus finger arteriolar photoplethysmography. *Am J Hypertens* 2003; 16:371–374.

22. Langewouters GJ, Settels JJ, Roelandt R, et al. Why use Finapres or Portapres rather than intra-arterial or intermittent non-invasive techniques of blood pressure measurement? *J Med Eng Technol* 1998; 22:37–43.

23. Denq JC, O'Brien PC, Low PA. Normative data on phases of the Valsalva maneuver. *J Clin Neurophysiol* 1998; 15:535–540.

24. Sandroni P, Benarroch EE, Low PA. Pharmacological dissection of components of the Valsalva maneuver in adrenergic failure. *J Appl Physiol* 1991; 71:1563–1567.

25. Ferrer MT, Kennedy WR, Sahinen F. Baroreflexes in patients with diabetes mellitus. *Neurology* 1991; 41:1462–1466.

26. Gutiérrez J, Molina L, Mustelier R, et al. Autonomic reflexes in hereditary sensorimotor neuropathy type I. *Muscle Nerve* 2002; 28:S56.

27. Low VA, Sandroni P, Fealey RD, Low PA. Detection of small-fiber neuropathy by sudomotor testing. *Muscle Nerve* 2006; 34:57–61.

28. Fealey, RD, Low, PA, Thomas, JE. Thermoregulatory sweating abnormalities in diabetes mellitus. *Mayo Clin Proc* 1989; 64:617–628.

29. Kennedy, WR, Navaro X. Sympathetic sudomotor function in diabetes neuropathy. *Arch Neurol* 1989; 1182–1186.

30. Shahani, BT, Halperin, JJ, Boulu, et al. Sympathetic skin response: a method of assessing unmyelinated axon dysfunction in peripheral neuropathies. *J Neurol Neursurg Psychiatry* 1984; 47: 536–542.

31. Gutiérrez JV, García H, Sánchez J, Ortega L. [The topographic diagnosis of the sympathetic nervous system lesions in Cuban epidemic neuropathy. The value of the sympathetic skin response]. *Rev Cubana Med Trop* 1998; 50(Suppl):245–248.

32. Arunodaya, GR, Taly, AB. Sympathetic skin response: a decade later. *J Neurol Sci* 1995; 129:81–89.

CHAPTER **8**

Muscle and Nerve Biopsy Pathology

Umberto De Girolami, Pedro Ciarlini, Anthony A. Amato, David S. Younger

This chapter reviews muscle and nerve biopsy, including the indications for their performance, the light and electron microscopic (EM) findings of normal skeletal muscle and of peripheral nerve, and the general reactions to injury seen in disease of skeletal muscle and of peripheral nerve. The scope is not all inclusive; rather, the aim is to stress fundamental principles and illustrate them with key figures. The past several decades have witnessed enormous advances in the understanding of muscle disease and the underlying basis of myalgia (1), fostered by classic detailed studies of normal (2, 3) and abnormal skeletal muscle tissue obtained by open biopsy in a variety of neuromuscular disorders employing light microscopic (4, 5) and ultrastructural analysis (6), as well as detailed investigations of tissue obtained at postmortem examination (7). These advances have been detailed in several dedicated clinical neuromuscular (8–12) and neuropathology (13) texts to which advanced students of this topic may be directed.

Modern peripheral nerve disease, which has been influenced by strides in the understanding of normal morphology across all ages (14), and the abnormal histopathologic changes in response to injury (15–19), remains an invaluable diagnostic tool (20–22). The procedure, which has typically been under closer scrutiny than muscle biopsy for a variety of reasons, not the least of which is the perceived association with untoward side effects, notwithstanding the anticipated irreversible loss of sensory function accompanied with the removal of a significant piece of nerve tissue to properly perform the requisite histological studies (23–25), is often preceded by less invasive analysis of intraepidermal and dermal nerve fiber studies (26–28).

MUSCLE BIOPSY

Before undertaking a muscle biopsy and/or nerve biopsy, patients should undergo thorough neurological and medical evaluation inclusive of the examination of other potentially affected family members. Laboratory assessment generally includes assessment of the serum creatine kinase (CK) assay, detailed nerve conduction, and concentric needle electromyography, and sometimes magnetic resonance imaging to guide the choice of a muscle that is clinically and electrophysiologically affected, but not overly damaged, to avoid sampling of tissue at the end stage of disease. The surgical procedure should be performed by a neurologist or surgeon experienced in the performance of biopsy surgery, at centers with a neuropathologist knowledgeable in the processing and interpretation of neuromuscular disorders. The quadriceps, deltoid, biceps brachii, or triceps (at some institutions) muscles are preferred sites of biopsy for disorders that have a clinical presentation characterized by proximal weakness; the extensor digitorum longus, tibialis anterior, or gastrocnemius muscles are sampled in patients where the clinical presentation indicates a distal myopathy. Communication including the primary physician or neurologist who requested the biopsy and will be following the patient, the individual who actually performs the biopsy, and the neuropathologist is absolutely essential to ensure that the correct muscle is biopsied. However, in our experience, there are formidable technical obstacles that preclude the utmost quality of the resulting tissue sections.

TISSUE PROCESSING

Three sets of procedures for the preparation of sections needing microscopic examination are ordinarily processed.

Paraffin Sections

Paraffin-embedded sections oriented for cross- and longitudinal sections are extremely useful to assess the extent of disease in the difference connective tissue compartment, including inflammatory reaction involving the muscle and supporting connective tissues; these are also useful to determine vessel abnormalities and infiltration by tumor or abnormal deposits.

Frozen Sections and Histochemistry

Cryostat sections of snap-frozen muscle in the cross-sectional plane and, in some centers, the longitudinal plane as well, are also used routinely. The frozen sections are stained with standard hematoxylin and eosin (H&E) and with the modified Gomori trichrome stain as the initial survey sections. Secondly, a battery of enzyme histochemical reactions is run. The adenosine triphosphatase (ATP) reactions at acid pH 4.3 and 4.6, and alkaline pH 9.4, are used to evaluate the proportion of type 1 and type 2 fibers and subtypes, as well as their shape, size and distribution. Specific histochemical reactions are performed to assess lipid content using Oil Red O and Sudan Black stains, while glycogen content is assessed by reactions with the Periodic acid-Schiff (PAS) stains, with and without diastase; in muscle fibers, as well as mitochondrial and oxidative enzyme activities employing nicotinamide adenine dinucleotide-tetrazolium (NADH-TR), succinate dehydrogenase (SDH), cytochrome-c-oxidase (COX) reactions. Frozen sections can be used for the immunohistochemical localization of membrane-associated proteins using a standard panel that includes dystrophin, as well as dystroglycan, sarcoglycan, and merosin reactivity.

Immunoperoxidase studies using the large number of commercially available antibodies can be performed on paraffin sections, and sometimes frozen sections as well. For example, the panoply of monoclonal antibodies used in hematopathology can be used to identify lymphocyte subsets or membranolytic complement activity.

Plastic Sections and Electron Microscopy

The third procedure is plastic embedding for light-microscopic examination of one micron semi-thin sections and ultrastructural study of ultrathin sections mounted on copper grids. These are particularly useful to identify abnormalities in the integrity of the myofibrillar contractile apparatus, organelles, and abnormal accumulations of proteins, lipids, or glycogen.

Morphometric analysis

Morphometric analysis is performed only in specialized centers possessing the required equipment and expertise to evaluate the tissue. The techniques are intended to demonstrate statistically important differences in the size, shape, and distribution of fiber types using the battery of histochemical stains described above. They can be especially useful in evaluating muscle biopsies of children, where even the well-trained observer may have difficulty with fine discrimination of relative proportions of affected fibers. Age-matched control comparisons can be extremely valuable. Morphometric analysis of cross-sections of muscle may be carried out either after photography or directly by image analysis.

Biochemical studies

Finally, the definitive identification of specific mitochondrial electron-transport abnormalities, genetically determined disorders of membrane-associated proteins, or metabolic derangements requires that frozen tissue be sent out to specialized centers that can perform the required biochemical or molecular/genetic analysis.

NORMAL ANATOMY

Aspects of normal muscle anatomy are shown in Plate I, Figures 1–6. Much information can be gained from a detailed examination of the overall architecture of muscle biopsy tissue. In cross-section, the muscle fibers are polygonally-shaped, with little intervening space between them and are fairly uniform in size. Neuromuscular spindles are recognized as bag-like structures (about 50–100 μm in diameter) containing rounded intrafusal fibers and bounded by a connective tissue capsule. The nuclei of muscle fibers are ordinarily located next to the subsarcolemma, although even in specimens without any apparent neuromuscular disease, as many as three to five percent of fibers may have more centrally located or "internalized" nuclei.

Muscle fibers are embedded in multiple connective tissue compartments. Individual muscle fibers are surrounded by the endomysium, which normally is a thin, delicate network of strands between the fibers and also contains the capillaries. Individual muscle fascicles are enclosed in the perimysium, comprised of concentric strands of connective tissue enclosing the fascicle. Muscle fascicles are separated from each other by the epimysium, which contains adipose tissue, the arterial and venous supply to the fascicle, and peripheral nerves. The fascia and tendons are contiguous to the epimysium.

An important neurophysiological construct in the understanding and interpretation of muscle biopsy findings is the

Plate I. Normal Muscle

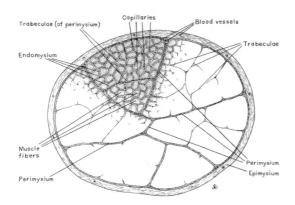

FIG. 1. Diagram illustrating cross section of skeletal muscle with its different connective tissue compartments. Reproduced with permission from SG Silverberg's *Principles and Practice of Surgical Pathology,* Churchill Livingston: New York, 1990.

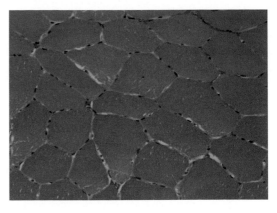

FIG. 2. H&E stained cryostat cross section of adult skeletal muscle. Note the polygonal shape of the myofibers.

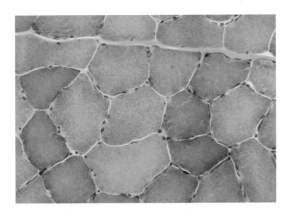

FIG. 3. Modified Gomori trichrome stain of snap-frozen skeletal muscle illustrating the inconspicuous endomysial connective tissue in normal skeletal muscle (*=perimysium).

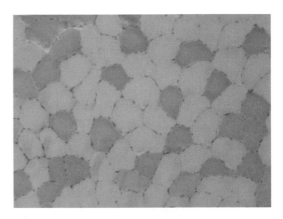

FIG. 4. ATPase reaction at pH 4.2 (snap-frozen skeletal muscle). The dark staining fibers are type 1. Note the almost random arrangement of the different fiber types.

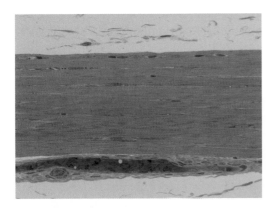

FIG. 5. Toluidine blue semi-thin plastic-embedded section (1 μm) showing a longitudinal view of the skeletal muscle, with good demonstration of cross-striations.

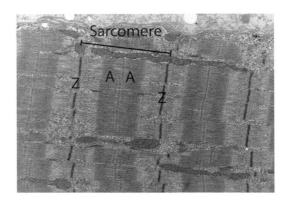

FIG. 6. Electron microgram illustrating the normal ultrastructure of the sarcomere (Z=Z lines, A=anisotropic bands with thick myosin filaments).

concept of the motor unit that refers to a single motor neuron and its motor axon, responsible for the innervation of a population of myocytes. The motor neuron, furthermore, is responsible for determining the histochemical type of the muscle innervated, be they Type-1 or -2 fibers. Normally, in human beings, the muscle fibers belonging to a given motor unit are not adjacent, but are spatially dispersed in a muscle fascicle over a distance of several millimeters. On histochemical reactions that type the fibers, the muscle appears as a mosaic checkerboard of the two fiber types. In the adult, the number of type 1, 2A, and 2B fibers are roughly comparable in the muscles that are usually studied in a proportion of type 1:30 to 40%, type 2A:20 to 30%, type 2B:40 to 50%, and type 2C 1 to 2%. The percentages of each fiber type varies with the particular muscle studied, but also according to sex, age, and physical state, making it necessary to evaluate the results in comparison to normative data of closely matched controls. Also, the number of fibers within each motor unit is proportional to the refinement of movement, so the ratio is low in the lumbrical or extraocular muscles and high in the gluteus and limb-girdle muscles.

The appearance of normal muscle just described applies to adults; in infants and very young children, the muscle fibers are rounded and only take on a polygonal cross-sectional shape later in development, from age three to six years. Furthermore, as the mean fiber diameter is a function of age, analysis of muscle biopsies in infants and children requires comparison to normal values for age. Nevertheless, variability of fiber diameter is not a function of age, i.e., excessive variation in fiber diameter is abnormal even in infants. There may be normally increased variability in fiber size and shape near tendinous insertions, sites that should be avoided in biopsy, and certain muscles such as the extraocular muscles, diaphragm, and paraspinal muscles.

BASIC REACTIONS OF SKELETAL MUSCLE TO INJURY

The features of muscle pathology are shown in Plate II, Figures 1–11. However, before considering the spectrum of pathologic change in muscle fibers, it is important to recognize that histologic artifacts frequently occur, first and foremost of which are those due to improper tissue freezing that present as small, rounded, empty, evenly distributed spaces within the muscle fiber in association with intracellular microcrystal ice formation. Tissue fixed in formalin destined for paraffin-embedding and not appropriately stretched with a muscle biopsy clamp or other device, can become distorted during fixation and is rarely properly oriented. Paraffin sections, under these circumstances, commonly show contraction artifacts that preclude fine morphological analysis of muscle fibers. There are many

artifacts encountered in the preparation of sections for electron microscopy. These are invariable due to preparation artefact, related to delayed fixation and improper processing of tissue.

Two broad diagnostic categories of muscle disease are recognizable on muscle biopsy, namely neurogenic and myopathic muscle diseases. These major subdivisions denote fundamental differences in the pathogenesis of the muscle injury. Neurogenic atrophy is prototypical of diseases characterized by interruption of any aspect of the innervation of the fiber be it due to anterior horn cell in the spinal cord or brainstem, motor root, peripheral nerve, intramuscular nerve twig, or neuromuscular junction abnormalities. Pathologic examination of the muscle alone ordinarily cannot determine the precise locus; correlative clinical and neurophysiologic data are critical requisites to be integrated for the interpretation of the clinical issue. Myopathy, on the other hand, is the result of a process whereby the primarily insult involves a pathologic process affecting constituents of the muscle fiber itself, resulting in structural abnormalities and potential destruction of the cell. The parameters listed below should be considered in the histopathological differentiation of these two categories of muscle disease.

Variations in Muscle Fiber Size and Shape

The first parameters evaluated are the uniformity of muscle fiber size or diameter, and shape. Fibers should be relatively uniform in size, although the mean diameter increases up to the age of 15 years. If a considerable population of small or larger fibers is present, the condition is termed excessive variation in fiber size. So-called small angulated fibers, that is, smaller than normal fibers, having a roughly triangular shape, are never a normal feature. Hyper-contracted fibers are characterized by a distinctly round cross-sectional appearance in a background of somewhat smaller polygonal fibers and moderate hyperchromasia. They can occur in biopsies with no other evidence of neuromuscular disease, and are particularly frequent in muscular dystrophies.

Atrophy and Hypertrophy

Hypertrophy consists of increases in size of the muscle fibers, often associated with loss of their usual polygonal outline. Physiological hypertrophy of type-2 fibers is reportedly seen in athletes, but definitive data on the biopsy appearance of muscle changes in response to training is lacking. In pathological skeletal muscle, hypertrophied fibers are a compensatory change, and are often accompanied by structural changes such as internalized nuclei and split fibers.

Atrophic fibers may be rounded in myopathic processes, or angulated as a result of fiber splitting found in type 2 fiber atrophy, and in neurogenic processes in adults. In the end

Plate II. Muscle pathology

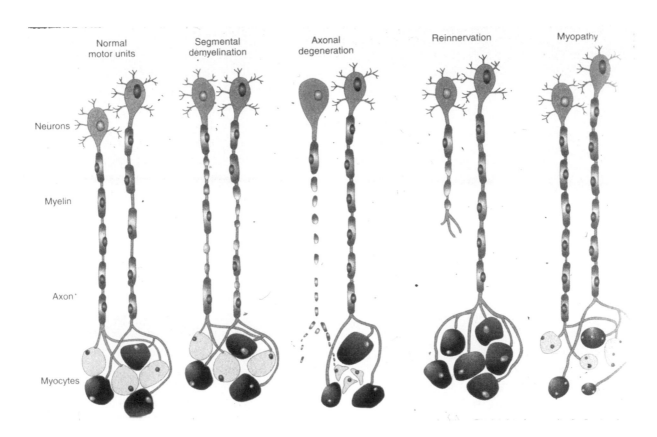

FIG. 1. Diagram illustrating overall pathological processes occurring predominantly in the peripheral nerve (left side), including reinnervation, as well as skeletal muscle proper (far right). Adapted with permission from: Anthony DS, Frosch MP, De Girolami U. *Peripheral Nerve and Skeletal Muscle.* In, Kumar V, Abbas AK, Fausto N, Aster JC, eds. Robbins and Cotran Pathological Basis of Disease, 8th ed., Philadelphia: Saunders Elsevier, 2010.

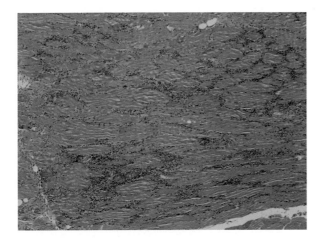

FIG. 2. Endomysial inflammatory infiltrate in a patient with inflammatory myopathy (H&E). Compare with Plate I, Figure 2.

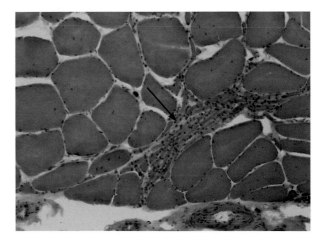

FIG. 3. Representative section of denervation atrophy (group atrophy, arrow), (H&E).

Plate II. Muscle pathology

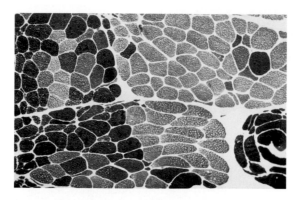

FIG. 4. ATPase at pH 4.2 illustrating fiber-type grouping (chronic denervation/reinnervation; notice also the presence of many small angulated fibers) compare with normal random distribution, Plate I, Figure 4.

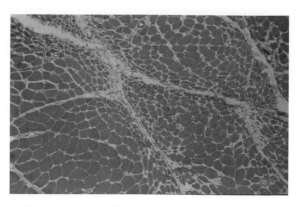

FIG. 5. Marked perifascicular atrophy in a patient with dermatomyositis (H&E).

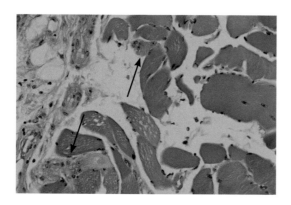

FIG. 6. Regenerating (basophilic) fibers (arrows) (H&E). Note the reactive nuclear characteristics with open chromatin and prominent nucleoli.

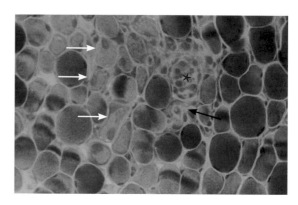

FIG. 7. Degenerating fibers (black arrow), some undergoing myophagocytosis (*), and regenerating fibers (white arrows, note large reactive nuclei) in a patient with dystrophinopathy. Note the increase in endomysial connective tissue (modified Gomori trichrome stain; compare with Plate 1, Figure 3).

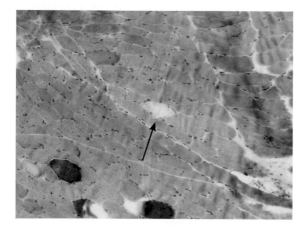

FIG. 8. Necrotic fiber in a patient with toxic myopathy (arrow); note the pale staining of the sarcoplasm.

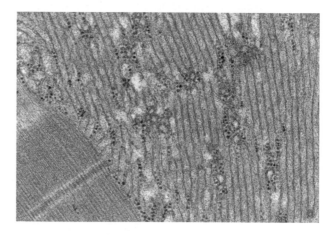

FIG. 9. Electron micrograph showing tubular aggregates adjacent to the sarcomere.

Plate II. Muscle pathology

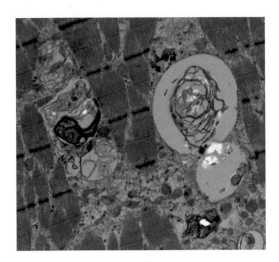

FIG. 10. Electron micrograph showing vacuoles of different stages with whorled figures in a patient with familial hypokalemic periodic paralysis.

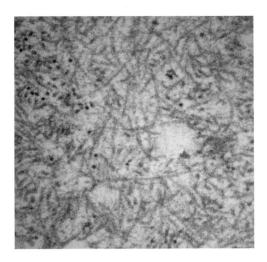

FIG. 11. Electron micrograph of sarcoplasmic tubular inclusions in a patient with inclusion body myositis.

stages of atrophy, the atrophic fibers form nuclear bags or clusters of sarcolemmal nuclei within shrunken muscle cells largely devoid of myofibrillar material. In the late stage of a severe myopathic or neurogenic process, the muscle can be severely damaged and is referred to as end stage. It is largely replaced by fibroadipose connective tissue with few remaining atrophic fibers and it is often impossible to infer the etiologic basis of the initial insult. It is important to determine the distribution of the atrophic fibers; they may occur randomly or be grouped together in clusters. Fascicular or group atrophy, a hallmark of denervation, consists of aggregates of atrophic fibers that occupy part of a fascicle. This process differs from the perifascicular atrophy seen in dermatomyositis in which atrophic fibers line the edges of the fascicles, and the transition to atrophy is gradual. Randomly scattered atrophic fibers are less characteristic of a specific pathologic process; when they involve both fiber types, they may represent early stages of denervation.

Atrophy may select a particular fiber type, wherein type 1 atrophy is usually seen in adults with myotonic dystrophy and also in some childhood congenital myopathies, perhaps due to developmental arrest. Type 2 atrophy is very frequent and mainly involves type 2B fibers, so noted in a variety of conditions, including immobilization, chronic debilitating disorders, and steroid treatment.

Abnormal Predominance or Deficiency of Myofiber Type

The prevalence of type 1 and type 2 or, more precisely, type 2A and 2B, is dependent on the specific muscle biopsied. For the most frequently biopsied sites, the deltoid, quadriceps, biceps, and gastrocnemius muscle, an abnormal predominance of fiber type is recognized when the proportion of fibers exceeds 55% type 1 or 80% type 2 fibers. Type 1 fiber predominance can be seen in congenital myopathies. Type 2 fiber predominance is found in amyotrophic lateral sclerosis. Cases of central hypotonia often show aberrations of fiber type proportions in the absence of overt denervation. Type 2B deficiency, sometimes total, and/or the presence of type 2C fibers may be seen in certain myopathic processes.

The mechanisms underlying the assignment of a fiber type are not well understood. It has been stated that fiber type is determined by the innervating motor neuron; however, embryologic studies also suggest that myofibers generated at different times in development have an autonomous, genetically regulated program to develop into specific fiber types.

Structural Anomalies of Muscle Fibers

Nuclear Anomalies

Central displacement of the nuclei or internalized nuclei is considered abnormal when present in over three to five percent of the fibers. The biologic basis of this phenomenon is not clear; however it is a marker of fibers which have regenerated or are in the process of regeneration. Relatively unremarkable-appearing nuclei may be internalized in hypertrophic fibers, possibly representing a preliminary stage in the process of fiber splitting. In certain diseases, notably myotonic dystrophy, on longitudinal sections of muscle, nuclei can be seen to aggregate closer together and line up in chains; these are referred to as *nuclear chains*. Intranuclear inclusions may be seen in certain disorders, including inclusion body myositis, and oculopharyngeal muscular dystrophy.

Split Fibers

This anomaly is especially seen in hypertrophic fibers. In cross-section, splitting presents as a fissure originating from the surface of a muscle fiber. This fissure may be branched or contain a capillary. It may become more ill-defined in the center of the fiber or extend to another edge of the fiber. Multiple splits may lead to grouping of angulated muscle fibers of the same histochemical type, a phenomenon sometimes termed *myopathic grouping*. The mechanism of splitting is not settled. Its significance is doubtful at myotendinous junctions.

Fiber Necrosis

Fiber necrosis or *degeneration* are interchangeabe terms for the hallmark of dystrophic, inflammatory, and toxic myopathic processes. Conversely, the presence of many necrotic fibers should cast doubt on a diagnosis of a neurogenic process, although it may be seen in the late stages of neurogenic atrophy. In H&E-stained preparations, necrotic fibers show a homogenization and glassy appearance of the cytoplasm and poor staining. In longitudinal sections, there is pallor and loss of cross striations. There is also loss of staining with PAS and NADH-TR stained sections. Over time, fibers become vacuolated and eventually are invaded by inflammatory cells extending across the basement membrane. Later, admixtures of macrophages, T-lymphocytes, predominantly CD8+, and regenerating myoblasts arising from neighboring muscle fibers may be seen within the muscle tube. This stage ends with the migration of inflammatory cells toward the adjacent blood vessels. In some conditions, muscle fiber necrosis is segmental and this phenomenon is best seen in longitudinal sections. Invasion of inflammatory cells into a seemingly histologically intact non-necrotic fiber is said to be characteristic of polymyositis.

Basophilic Fibers

These fibers correspond to regenerating muscle fibers, rich in ribonucleic acids (RNA). On H&E preparations the fibers have a basophilic cytoplasm, express neural cell adhesion molecule, may be either weakly striated or nonstriated, and possess vesicular nuclei with prominent nucleoli. Regeneration may result in complete restitution of the muscle fiber or leave sequelae such as variation in the shape and size of fibers. Regenerative lesions are either scattered randomly or occur in small clusters.

Target Fibers

These may be detected in standard preparations, but are particularly well seen with NADH-TR. True target fibers are particularly, but not exclusively, seen in type 1 fibers. They are composed of three concentric zones, including a central pale zone, which lacks oxidative enzyme activity; a dark, annular intermediate zone, which is rich in oxidative enzymes, and a normal peripheral zone. They are often found in denervation. A targetoid fiber is one in which the intermediate zone is absent, and is considerably less specific.

Moth-Eaten Fibers

These are recognized in oxidative enzyme preparations. They present as ill-defined zones of enzyme loss, resulting in a disorganized aspect of the intermyofibrillary network. They are not specific and are seen in a wide range of conditions, including inflammatory myopathies, malignant hyperpyrexia, or denervation.

Ring Fibers

Striated annulets, ringbinden or ring fibers, are formed by myofibrils that are normal in structure, but abnormally arranged to be perpendicular to the muscle fiber axis as seen on cross-section. Lateral sarcoplasmic masses present as delicately granulated nonstriated clear areas that are filled with oxidative enzymes and are situated between the sarcolemmal membrane and a central myofibrillary zone of normal appearance. These two abnormalities may be seen in myotonic dystrophy and other dystrophies and myotonic disorders.

Vacuoles

Clear spaces within the muscle cell, of variable size and location, are seen with H&E and other stains, and have variable pathological significance best determined after a battery of special stains, and sometimes only after electron microscopic study. They occur in a variety of disorders: non-lysosomal storage diseases such relating to glycogen in McArdle disease, and lipids in carnitine deficiency; lysosomal storage diseases recognized by the acid phosphatase reaction and by identification of the stored material as, for example, glycogen in Pompe disease and autofluorescent lipofuscin pigment in ceroid lipofuscinosis. Autophagic vacuoles with lysosomal hyperactivity, revealed by the acid phosphatase reaction, occur in chloroquine myopathy, whereas the rimmed vacuoles of inclusion body myositis (IBM) are comprised of an outer granular and basophilic border is granular on H&E that stains reddish with the modified Gomori trichrome stain; EM reveals membranous debris and intermediate filaments. Vacuoles may be produced by dilatation of the internal membrane systems as occurs in periodic paralysis; whereas those due to dilatation of the T transverse tubular system, and seen amid healthy regions of the sarcoplasm next to recent zones of segmental necrosis, with accumulation of sarcotubular material identified by ultrastructural analysis, occurs in sarcotubular myopathy. Finally, other vacuoles can result from the disappearance of myofibrils as, for example, in dermatomyositis, or have a reticulated honeycomb appearance typical of critical illness myopathy.

Ragged Red Fibers

These subsarcolemmal and/or intermyofibrillary aggregates are the hallmark of mitochondrial myopathy. They appear reddish with modified Gomori trichrome stain, hence the name, and bluish with H&E. These aggregates, which are essentially formed by abnormal mitochondria, are filled with oxidative enzymes and, therefore, stain strongly with the NADH-TR and SDH reactions. Ultrastructurally, they are associated with accumulation of glycogen and, especially, of lipids. Although strongly indicative of mitochondrial myopathy when found before the age of 60 years, scattered ragged red fibers may also be found in muscle tissue of elderly individuals in non-mitochondrial disorders. Conversely, their absence does not exclude the diagnosis of a mitochondrial cytopathy.

Tubular Aggregates

Presenting as well-limited zones that are usually subsarcolemmal and stain blue with hematoxylin-eosin and red with Gomori trichrome, tubular aggregates affect mainly type 2 fibers. They are strongly positive with NADH-TR, but are SDH-negative. By electron microscopy, their appearance is that of aggregates of tubules arranged in an organ-pipe pattern. These structures are not specific, but are often encountered in dyskalemic paralysis and represent the chief histological skeletal muscle anomaly seen in the myalgia/cramps syndrome associated with tubular aggregate myopathy.

Interstitial Changes

Some of the changes seen in the interstitial tissue may have diagnostic significance and establish the etiology of the process with certainty, e.g., sarcoidosis and polyarteritis nodosa, and amyloidosis. Increased endomysial connective tissue or "endomysial fibrosis" is less specific, but suggests muscular dystrophy. In end stage muscle of whatever cause, there is infiltration and replacement of muscle by adipose tissue. Discrete inflammatory cellular infiltrates may be seen in a variety of conditions: to some extent in muscular dystrophies such as dystrophinopathies and dysferlinopathies; and more floridly in inflammatory myopathies, such as dermatomyositis, polymyositis, and inclusion body myositis. The topography and also the cellular composition of the inflammatory infiltrates are important clues to establish an etiologic basis.

NERVE BIOPSY

Peripheral neuropathy is believed to be one of the most common disorders encountered in neurologic practice. However, with advances in clinical electrophysiology and molecular diagnostics, the clinical indications to perform a nerve biopsy in patients with peripheral neuropathy have decreased in comparison to those for a muscle biopsy. Also, the reasons for this change in medical practice are that, for the most part, experience has shown that the structural abnormalities seen in various types of neuropathy are not specific for any one disease process. Furthermore, even if almost invariably the nerve chosen for biopsy is a sensory nerve, there has always been the concern that a nerve biopsy is an invasive procedure usually associated with a permanent sensory deficit and, not uncommonly, neuralgia. In spite of these considerations, many cases of peripheral neuropathy remain unexplained and nerve biopsy has been used to attempt to better understand the disease process. Important indications for a nerve biopsy in adults include the evaluation of a patient where there is a strong clinical suspicion of vasculitis or amyloid polyneuropathy based on the neurological examination and laboratory studies. Ordinarily, the diagnosis chronic inflammatory demyelinating polyneuropathy (CIDP) does not require biopsy confirmation, unless there are atypical presentations. Directed nerve biopsy is sometimes performed in cases of asymmetric poly/mononeuropathy with focal signal changes on neuroimaging, searching for inflammation as in focal CIDP, sarcoidosis, perineuritis, and tumor infiltrates in neurolymphomatosis and leukemia, or peripheral nerve tumors. In parts of the world where leprosy is endemic, nerve biopsy, in conjunction with skin biopsy, is used to diagnose leprosy. Molecular studies performed in commercial laboratories are now used for the diagnosis of certain hereditary neuropathies such as Charcot-Marie-Tooth (CMT) disease, but nerve biopsy can be useful in trying to understand cases where these studies are inconclusive. In patients suspected of having polyglucosan body (PGB) neuropathy characterized by polyradiculoneuropathy, spasticity, and incontinence often associated with central nervous system (CNS) abnormalities, nerve biopsy can be diagnostic.

In general, nerve biopsy should only be performed in laboratories where there is technical and professional expertise in the performance and interpretation of paraffin embedded sections of nerve and appropriate staining techniques, frozen section histology, plastic embedding, and preparation of semi-thin sections (STS) and EM. In children, analysis of nerve biopsies is also greatly aided by the use of morphometric methods. As indicated above for muscle biopsies, careful coordination of efforts between the clinical team and the laboratory is required for the proper analysis of nerve biopsies.

A peripheral nerve biopsy is taken from a purely sensory nerve that is affected clinically and by nerve conduction studies. The sural nerve is the most common nerve chosen for biopsy and is mostly sensory in the majority of patients. We recommend biopsying the sural nerve in the mid-shin, approximately one-third to one-fourth of the distance from ankle to knee, approximately where the nerve is stimulated on nerve conduction studies. Patients should be informed that complications of nerve biopsy may cause a permanent loss of sensation on the lateral aspect of the ankle and foot as well as pain that may last for several months after the procedure. We suggest a superficial fibular nerve biopsy when vasculitic neuropathy is suspected and there is involvement of the fibular nerve, because the underlying peroneus brevis muscle can also be biopsied through the same incision site, thereby increasing the diagnostic yield. The superficial radial nerve can be biopsied if only the hand is involved, but as this leads to permanent numbness of the dorsum of the hand, we usually do not do this. In cases where the process involves only the proximal nerves, a fascicular nerve biopsy of a lesion in the root, plexus, or proximal nerve may be required. Obviously, in neoplastic disease, the affected nerve is excised, be it sensory, motor, or both.

Biopsy and Tissue Processing

Nerve biopsies should only be performed in institutions that are particularly equipped to process the tissue and have the expertise to interpret the results. The neuropathology laboratory should be alerted prior to the biopsy to allow preparation for the special handling that is required. Care should be taken by the neurologist or surgeon performing the biopsy to handle the nerve as little as possible during dissection and to avoid infiltration by local anesthetic. A resection of a segment of nerve 3- to 5cm in length is recommended. In order to prevent coiling of the specimen immediately after removal, it can be gently stretched over a tongue depressor or other suitable device. The nerve biopsy specimen is then allocated so as to be able to perform five types of studies.

Paraffin-Embedded Sections

The proximal and distal segments of the nerve are usually the ones used for paraffin embedding. These are fixed in 10% buffered formalin processed for cross and longitudinal sections. Paraffin sections are especially useful to evaluate the connective tissue components of nerves, including epineurium, perineurium, and endoneurium; blood vessels, and any abnormal deposits such as amyloid with Congo red immunofluorescence. The standard stains used on paraffin sections include H&E, elastic tissue stains, Masson trichrome, silver impregnation for axons, and stains for myelin. The sections can also be processed with stains that will demonstrate microorganisms such as methenamine silver stains for fungi, Gram stains for bacteria, and those for mycobacteria. Various markers can be employed to identify different types of inflammatory cells, including T- and B-lymphocytes, and macrophages. Immunoperoxidase studies with armamentarium of commercially available antibodies can be applied to the sections for demonstration of neurofilament proteins, myelin, and others.

Plastic-Embedded Sections

The middle third of the nerve tissue specimen is fixed in 2.5% buffered glutaraldehyde and embedded in plastic after fixation and staining with osmium tetroxide. Plastic embedded 1μm STS, cut in the transverse and longitudinal plain and stained with toluidine blue is the best method to examine the fine structural details of both myelinated and unmyelinated fibers and their distribution. The use of STS also allows for quantitative assessment of axonal density, myelin thickness, and subcellular structures that cannot easily be visualized with routine histology. Plastic embedding of the tissue is also the only technique that allows for ultrastructural evaluation. In a few specialized laboratories around the world, immuno-EM is performed to identify specific proteins or other substances at the ultrastructural level.

Quantitative analysis is typically done on STS or EM sections. Morphometric analysis is time-consuming and requires a substantial investment in equipment. From a clinical point of view, it is often not necessary, and is usually reserved for research purposes or in approach to very specific differential diagnosis. A well-trained observer can reliably assess the density of myelinated fibers, an estimate of the degree of loss of large or small fibers, and the presence and the severity of demyelinating and/or axonal lesions, without the expense of quantitative assessment. Morphometric analysis of cross-sections of the nerve may be carried out either after photography or directly by image analysis.

Teased Fiber Analysis

In order to perform teased fiber analysis, after aldehyde fixation and osmication and softening in glycerin, single myelinated fibers measuring 1 cm long are separated from each other and from their surrounding connective tissues utilizing fine needles under direct visualization with a dissecting microscope. Light microscopic examination of the teased fibers demonstrates the relative positions of nodes of Ranvier, the length of internodes, integrity and caliber of the axons, and thickness of the overlying myelin, and thus can be helpful in discriminating primary axonopathies from primary demyelinating neuropathies. The technique also allows for the demonstration of abnormalities in the thickness of the myelin as, for example, tomacula, or evidence of disintegration of the myelin/axon. Since the preparation of individual teased nerve fibers is very time-consuming, the technique is often reserved for evaluation in specific problematic cases.

Frozen Tissue for Immunofluorescence and Biochemical Studies

Part of the tissue is frozen in isopentane cooled by liquid nitrogen or directly on the cryostat with appropriate embedding medium, and transverse sections are cut on the cryostat. Direct immunofluorescence studies on frozen sections can be carried out using specific antibodies to identify abnormal deposits of immunoglobulins in endoneurium or in myelinated fibers. The last bit of tissue is quickly frozen in isopentane cooled by liquid nitrogen and stored in the ultra-low freezer for potential biochemical or genetic studies.

Skin Biopsy Analysis of Dermal-Intraepidermal Nerve Twigs

Over the past ten years or so, several specialized centers around the world have developed techniques to evaluate small sensory nerve fibers within the skin, which have been found particularly useful in following patients with small fiber sensory and/or autonomic neuropathies. Fixed or unfixed skin punch biopsies are cut and processed for immunoperoxidase studies with the antibody PGP9.5. An assessment is then made as to the deviation from normal in the density and extent of simplification of the arborization of the nerve twigs with the epidermis and in the dermis and skin adnexal structures.

NORMAL ANATOMY

Features of normal peripheral nerve anatomy are shown in Plate III, Figures 1–7. Individual nerve fibers of normal peripheral are embedded and packets in connective tissue compartments. Within each fascicle myelinated and unmyelinated nerves and their supporting cells are surrounded by delicate connective tissue strands containing blood vessels, termed the *endoneurium*. Nerve fascicles are bounded by the perineurium, a complex structure with important physiologic barrier functions consisting of multiple overlapping concentric layers of specialized connective tissue cells called *perineurial cells*. The epineurium is the fibroadipose connective tissue which surrounds the fascicules of nerve and contains the blood vessels supplying the nerve.

Schwann and Remak Cells, and Myelin Sheaths

The organization of a myelinated peripheral nerve fiber is such that the axon emanating form the cell body of the neuron is surrounded by a myelin sheath. The myelin sheath is interrupted at regular intervals along its length. The space between two adjacent myelinated segments is the node of Ranvier. The myelinated segment of nerve between one node of Ranvier and the next is referred to as an *internode*. Normally, the length of an internode is fairly constant along the axon and is proportional to the diameter of the axon. Individual myelin internodes extend from just beyond the neuronal cell body to just before the axon terminal.

Schwann cells are the supporting cells of individual myelin internodes. They appear in abundance within the endoneurial compartment, identifiable as cells with a pale nucleus and evenly-dispersed chromatin. A Schwann cell can be distinguished with certainty from endoneurial fibroblasts on EM because it is surrounded by basement membrane. In longitudinal sections of nerve, elongated Schwann-cell nuclei are normally roughly equidistant from the two adjacent nodes of Ranvier, positioned roughly toward the middle of the internode. In mature nerves, the cytoplasm, between the inner lamella of the myelin sheath and the axon, and between the outermost myelin lamella and the cell membrane, is sparse. EM examination demonstrates that Schwann-cell cytoplasm contains endoplasmic reticulum, a Golgi apparatus, mitochondria, sometimes a centriole, and complex multilamellar lipid membranous granules termed π *granules* or *granules of Reich*.

The myelin sheath is made up of regularly arranged concentric lamellae with a 12- to 17-nm periodicity, forming major dense lines separated by electron-lucent zones in which one or two inter-period lines can be observed. Discontinuity in the compaction of the lamellae is seen at the Schmidt-Lanterman incisures. Here, invaginations of Schwann cell cytoplasm penetrate openings of the major dense lines.

The specialized Schwann cell that supports unmyelinated fibers and does not form myelin is known as the *Remak cells*. In a given cross-section, a single Remak cell can surround and support multiple unmyelinated axons, and in the absence of nodes, they are evenly distributed along the length of the fiber.

Axons

The ratio of unmyelinated nerve fibers to myelinated nerve fibers in the sural nerve is approximately 4 to 1. The normal diameter of myelinated fibers ranges from 2 to 12 μm in a bimodal distribution with peaks at 3 to 6 μm and 9 to 12 μm.

Plate III: Normal nerve

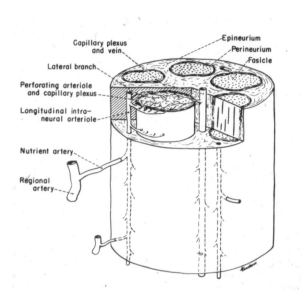

FIG. 1. Diagram illustrating the general organization of a peripheral nerve.

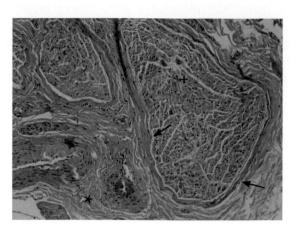

FIG. 2. H&E stained cross-section of a peripheral nerve showing the epineurium (*), perineurium (arrows) and endoneurium (+).

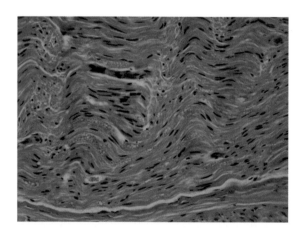

FIG. 3. H&E stained longitudinal section of a peripheral nerve with a characteristic wavy profile seen in paraffin-embedded sections. The majority of the nuclei seen are from Schwann cells.

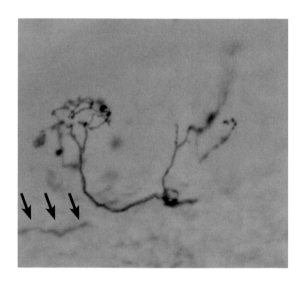

FIG. 4. Skin biopsy stained with PGP9.5 showing epidermal arborization of small fibers. Arrows indicate transition between dermis (inferior) and epidermis (superior).

Plate III: Normal nerve

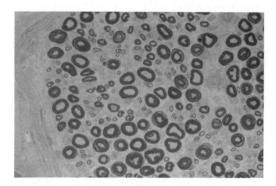

FIG. 5. Semi-thin transverse section of plastic-embedded sural nerve showing the normal distribution of axons of different sizes with appropriate thickness of myelin in relation to axon diameter (toluidine blue).

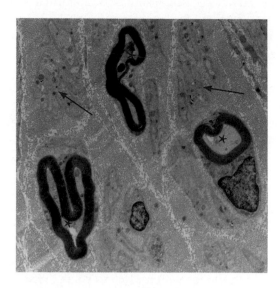

FIG. 6. Electron micrograph showing myelinated (*) and unmyelinated (arrows) fibers.

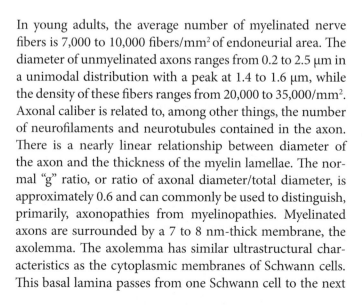

FIG. 7. Teased nerve fiber preparation showing two normal myelinated fibers at a node of Ranvier (arrows).

In young adults, the average number of myelinated nerve fibers is 7,000 to 10,000 fibers/mm² of endoneurial area. The diameter of unmyelinated axons ranges from 0.2 to 2.5 μm in a unimodal distribution with a peak at 1.4 to 1.6 μm, while the density of these fibers ranges from 20,000 to 35,000/mm². Axonal caliber is related to, among other things, the number of neurofilaments and neurotubules contained in the axon. There is a nearly linear relationship between diameter of the axon and the thickness of the myelin lamellae. The normal "g" ratio, or ratio of axonal diameter/total diameter, is approximately 0.6 and can commonly be used to distinguish, primarily, axonopathies from myelinopathies. Myelinated axons are surrounded by a 7 to 8 nm-thick membrane, the axolemma. The axolemma has similar ultrastructural characteristics as the cytoplasmic membranes of Schwann cells. This basal lamina passes from one Schwann cell to the next

without interruption at the nodes of Ranvier. The cytoplasm within the axons, the axoplasm, contains longitudinally oriented mitochondria, smooth endoplasmic reticulum, multivesicular bodies, neurofilaments, and microtubules. Neurofilaments have a mean diameter of 10 nm, whereas microtubules contain a central lumen and have an external diameter of approximately 25 nm.

BASIC REACTIONS OF PERIPHERAL NERVE TO INJURY

The abnormalities found in peripheral nerves in various disease states can be categorized into one of three groups: 1) Disorders that primarily affect axons, 2) Those that primarily affect myelin, and 3) Others that involve the connective tissues elements, including blood vessels such as peripheral nerve vasculitis, infiltrative disorders, including infection, neoplasms and abnormal deposits such as amyloid; and combinations thereof. Diverse aspects of peripheral nerve biopsy pathology and injury are illustrated in Plate IV, Figures 1–8.

Primary Axonal Degeneration

Primary axonal degeneration occurs as a result of acute injury that disrupts the continuity of the nerve as might happen in traumatic or surgical severance of the nerve, or crush, or following a neoplastic, vascular, metabolic, or infectious process that focally or diffusely destroys the nerve. Following such acute damage, the cellular events that occur in the distal part of the nerve from the site of injury are referred to as Wallerian degeneration. These consist of gradual disintegration of all components of the nerve, beginning with the formation myelin ovoids called digestion chambers, which are axonal fragments surrounded by myelin breakdown products. In time, there is a macrophage response, and the end stage of the process is fibrous replacement of the distal portion of the nerve. On STS and EM, one sees disruption of the myelin sheath and clustering, and swelling of organelles within axons.

Whether or not there is successful regeneration of nerve down the severed stump depends on the relative integrity of the tissue at the site of the gap. If extensive scar formation develops at the site of injury, the proximal stump will attempt to regenerate. As the nerves regenerate, Schwann cells proliferate within the tube formed by the original Schwann cell basal lamina. Two to five regenerating axonal sprouts emerge from the proximal stump of the sectioned nerve axons and grow slowly at a rate of 1 mm per day. This process results in the morphologic appearance of clusters of small, thinly-myelinated groupings of regenerating fibers.

One of the most common forms of subacute or chronic axonal degeneration is referred to as dying-back neuropathy or progressive distal axonopathy characterized by length-dependent degeneration beginning at the most distal portions of axons. The clinical correlate is involvement of the feet before the hands.

In the chronic or late stages of axonal degeneration, the principal morphologic features include a reduction in the number of myelinated axons and an increase in endoneurial connective tissue without much evidence of the active axonal degeneration seen in the acute process. Occasional disintegrating fibers and macrophage activity may be seen. Degeneration and attempted regeneration may be seen in a given specimen. Axonal regeneration is characterized by the sprouting of thinly myelinated axonal extensions that form clusters of small, closely-packed fibers and is best appreciated on STS viewed in cross-section and EM.

Teased nerve fiber preparations may also demonstrate the different stages of degeneration and regeneration where fragmentation and dissolution of the fiber may be seen at various stages of disintegration.

Axonal degeneration can be seen in neuronopathies or ganglionopathies, processes wherein the primary abnormality is thought to be in the cell body of the neuron. Since the irreversible process occurs in the cell body, regeneration is impossible and the projecting axon degenerates, beginning at the most distal portions of the axon. In the case of destruction of an anterior horn cell neuron, the degeneration begins at the periphery or the most distal portions of the cell, or toward the CNS, in a neuron located in the dorsal root ganglion in which the projections might be in the dorsal columns. The histological appearance on light and electron microscopy is comparable to what was described above for dying back axonal degeneration, except for the lack of regenerating axonal sprouts.

The process known as axonal atrophy is characterized by a reduction in the cross-sectional diameter of the fiber with retention of its circular outline. Axonal atrophy predominantly affects the large diameter fibers. Expansion of the axonal diameter, sometimes segmental, occurs in certain hereditary neuropathies such as hereditary giant axonal neuropathy; and in toxic neuropathies such as hexane neuropathy, wherein axonal swelling results from focal or multifocal accumulation of neurofilaments and other organelles. Intra-axonal inclusions, including PGB, corpora amylacea, and Lafora bodies can be seen in certain polyneuropathies, such as PGB disease.

Primary Demyelination

Primary demyelinating disorders of peripheral nerve are, by definition, those conditions where the site of injury is directed to the myelin sheath or the sustaining Schwann cells. The principal morphologic manifestation of primary demyelination is segmental damage to myelin internodes in arbitrary sequence, while preserving others, with preservation of the axon at the site of myelin injury. Experimental animal studies have shown that demyelination begins at the node of Ranvier and proceeds with unwrapping and disintegration of the myelin. Subsequently, Schwann cells and macrophages phagocytize broken down myelin. When demyelination involves only very short stretches of nerve fiber measuring <15 mm, the affected internode may be remyelinated by the surviving Schwann cell. Longer stretches of demyelination call upon proliferation of Schwann cells in order to re-myelinate the segments. Segmental demyelination can be demonstrated well in tease fiber preparations. In STS and EM in cross-sections reveal "naked" axons, i.e., individual axons of a caliber that would normally be myelinated which are

Plate IV. Nerve pathology

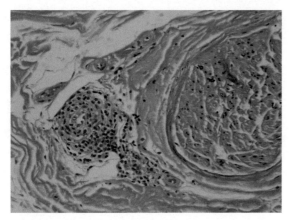

FIG. 1. Vasculitis affecting a blood vessel in the epineurium (H&E).

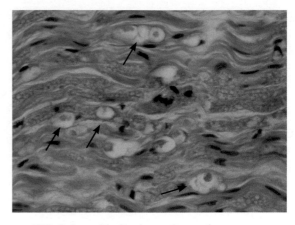

FIG. 2. Longitudinal section of a nerve showing acute axonal degeneration with multiple axonal injury (arrows) (H&E).

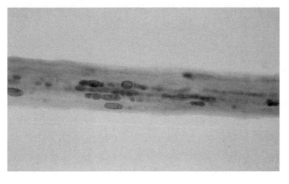

FIG. 3. Teased nerve fiber preparation showing axonal degeneration with myelin breakdown products (compare with Plate III, Figure 7).

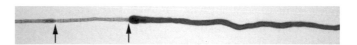

FIG. 4. Teased nerve fiber preparation showing segmental demyelination (between arrows).

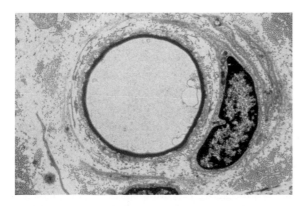

FIG. 5. Electron micrograph showing thinly myelinated large axon.

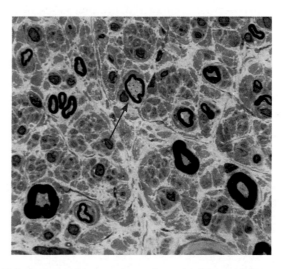

FIG. 6. Semi-thin section of nerve showing loss of large myelinated axons. Note the disproportionately thin myelin sheath of the large axon indicated by the arrow.

Plate IV. Nerve pathology

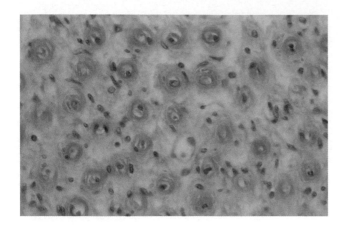

FIG. 7. Cross-section of peripheral nerve illustrating onion bulb formation (H&E).

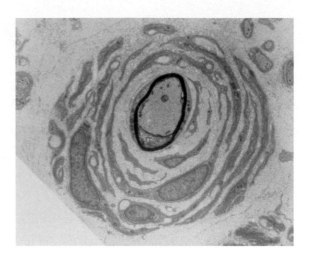

FIG. 8. Electron micrograph of an onion bulb formed by concenaround a thinly myelinated axon.

denuded of myelin. As the process of regeneration of the demyelinated segment proceeds, tease fiber preparations demonstrate shorter than normal internodes with relatively thin myelin sheaths. On STS and EM, myelinated nerve fibers have a disproportionately thin myelin sheath compared to the axon diameter.

In some hereditary neuropathies, the thickness of the myelin sheath may be segmentally greater than normal or hypermyelinated and ultrastructurally, there appears to be an excess of myelin lamellae relative to the diameter of the axon with redundant, abnormally folded loops of myelin. Tomacula are sausage-like expansions along the length of the fiber that can be demonstrated with teased fiber preparations. Tomacula are characteristic of hereditary neuropathy with predisposition for pressure palsies, but can be seen in autosomal recessive hereditary neuropathies such as CMT1 and CMT4.

With repeated episodes of segmental demyelination and remyelination, Schwann cells proliferate along with their basement membranes and align concentrically around a thinly myelinated or demyelinated axon, which is otherwise intact. This process is referred to as "onion bulb" formation and is best appreciated on semi-thin sections and electron microscopy.

Other Myelin Lesions

In certain polyneuropathies there is incomplete compaction of the outermost myelin lamellae at the ultrastructural level. Widening of myelin lamellae may stem from abnormalities

and genetically determined mutations of certain proteins in compact myelin, such as myelin protein zero (P_0). This phenomenon may also be observed in neuropathies due to IgM monoclonal gammopathy with antibodies directed against myelin-associated glycoprotein (MAG). In some forms of toxic neuropathy, due to chloroquine, hydroxychloroquine, and amiodarone exposure, abnormal vacuoles with myeloid debris, curvilinear, or dense lamellar inclusions are evident within Schwann cells.

PROCESSES AFFECTING SUPPORTING STRUCTURES

Evaluation of peripheral nerve also requires analysis of the connective tissue supporting structures. Endoneurial connective tissue proliferation is seen in peripheral neuropathies of long-standing, irrespective of etiology or basic pathologic process. Endoneurial blood vessels may be abnormally thick in certain metabolic diseases, such as diabetes. The perineurium may be the site of degenerative changes, also in diabetes. The epineurium is well assessed in plastic-embedded sections and may be the site of infiltration by neoplasm; inflammatory, infectious and autoimmune-mediated inflammation, including vasculitis alone or associated with abnormal deposits such as amyloid that affect the endoneurial compartment. Deposition of complement and membrane attack complex on vessel walls may be seen using immunohistochemistry stains in certain forms of vasculitis.

REFERENCES

1. Filosto M, Tonin P, Vatterni G, et al. The role of muscle biopsy in investigating isolated muscle pain. *Neurology* 2007; 68:181–186.

2. Brooke MH, Engel WK. The histographic analysis of human muscle biopsies with regard to fiber types. 1. Adult male and female. *Neurology* 1969; 19:221–233.

3. Brooke MH, Engel WK. The histographic analysis of human muscle biopsies with regard to fiber types. 2. Diseases of the upper and lower motor neuron. *Neurology* 1969; 19:378–393.

4. Brooke MH, Engel WK. The histographic analysis of human muscle biopsies with regard to fiber types. 3. Myotonias, myasthenia gravis, and hypokalemic periodic paralysis. *Neurology* 1969; 19:469–477.

5. Brooke MH, Engel WK. The histographic analysis of human muscle biopsies with regard to fiber types. 4. Children's biopsies. *Neurology* 1969; 19:591–605.

6. Engel AG, Banker BQ. Ultrastructural changes in diseased muscle. In, Engel AG, Franzini-Armstrong C, eds., *Myology*, 3rd ed. New York: McGraw-Hill, 2004.

7. Johnson MA, Polgar J, Leightman D, et al. Data on the distribution of fiber types in thirty-six human muscles. An autopsy study. *J Neurol Sci* 1973; 18:111–129.

8. Dubowitz V, Sewry CA. The biopsy: normal and disease muscle. In Dubowitz V, Sewry CA, eds, *Muscle biopsy—A practical approach.* 3rd ed. Philadelphia: Saunders Elsevier, 2007.

9. De Girolami U, Frosch M, Amato AA. Biopsy of nerve and muscle. In, Samuels M, Feske S, eds. *Office Practice of Neurology*, 2nd ed., Philadelphia: Harcourt Health Sciences, 2003.

10. Anthony DS, De Girolami U, Shapiro F. Muscle biopsy. In, Jones HR, De Vivo DC, Darras BT, eds. *Neuromuscular diseases of infancy, childhood and adolescence. A clinician's approach.* New York: Butterworth Heinemann, 2003.

11. Engel AG, The muscle biopsy. In Engel AG, Franzini-Armstrong C, eds., *Myology*, 3rd ed. New York: McGraw-Hill, 2004.

12. Dumitru D, Amato AA. Introduction to myopathies and muscle tissue's reaction to injury. In, Dumitru D, Amato AA, Swartz MJ, eds. *Electrodiagnostic Medicine,* 2nd ed., Philadelphia: Hanley and Belfus, 2002.

13. Banker BQ, Engel AG. Basic reactions of muscle. In, Engel AG, Franzini-Armstrong C, eds. *Myology*, 3rd ed. New York: McGraw-Hill, 2004.

14. Ferreire G, Denef J-F, Rodriguez J, et al. Morphomeric studies of normal sural nerves in children. *Muscle Nerve* 1985; 8:697–704.

15. Asbury A, Johnson PC. *Pathology of peripheral nerve.* Philadelphia: Saunders, 1978.

16. Amato AA, Russell J. *Neuromuscular disease.* New York: McGraw-Hill, 2008.

17. Dyck PJ, Dyck PJB, Engelstad J. Pathologic alternations of nerves. In, Dyck PJ, Thomas PK, eds. *Peripheral Neuropathy*, 4th ed. Philadelphia: WB Saunders, 2005.

18. Richardson EP Jr., De Girolami U. *Pathology of the peripheral nerve.* Philadelphia: WB Saunders, 1995.

19. Sroeder JM. *Pathology of peripheral nerves. An atlas of structural and molecular pathological changes.* Berlin: Springer, 2001.

20. Midroni G, Bilbao JM. *Biopsy diagnosis of peripheral neuropathy.* Boston: Butterworth-Heinemann, 1995.

21. Schweikert K, Fuhr P, Probst A, et al. Contribution of nerve biopsy to unclassified neuropathy. *Eur Neurol* 2007; 57:86–90.

22. Lacomis D. Clinical utility of peripheral nerve biopsy. *Curr Neurol Neurosci Rep* 2005; 5:41–47.

23. Weiss J, Brandner S, Lammens M, et al. Processing of nerve biopsies: a practical guide for neuropathologists. *Clin Neuropathol* 2012; 31:7–23.

24. Hilton DA, Jacob J, Househam L, et al. Complications following sural and superficial peroneal nerve biopsies. *J Neurol Neurosurg Psychiatry* 2007; 78:1271–1272.

25. Ruth A, Schulmeyer FJ, Roesch M, et al. Diagnostic and therapeutic value due to suspected diagnosis, long term complications, and indication for sural nerve biopsy. *Clin Neurol Neurosurg* 2005; 107:214 217.

26. Herman DN, Griffin JW, Hauser P, et al. Intraepidermal nerve fiber density, sural nerve morphometry and electrodiagnosis in peripheral neuropathies. *Neurology* 1999; 53:1634–1640.

27. Sommer C, Lauria G. Skin biopsy in the management of peripheral neuropathy. *Lancet Neurol* 2007; 6:632–642.

28. Lauria G, Hsieh ST, Johansson O, et al. EFNS/PNS Guideline on the use of skin biopsy in the diagnosis of small fiber neuropathy. Report of a joint task force of the European Federation of Neurological Societies and the Peripheral Nerve Society. *J Peripher Nerv Syst* 2010; 15:295–301.

CHAPTER 9

Cytopathology and Ultrastructure of CNS Motor Diseases

Hirofumi Kusaka, David S. Younger, Asao Hirano

The past decade has witnessed extraordinary advances in our understanding of central nervous system (CNS) motor diseases. In no other disorder is this as evident as in motor neuron diseases (MND) and the prototypical disorder, amyotrophic lateral sclerosis (ALS). The application of cytolopathological and ultrastructural methodologies have enhanced our understanding of ALS and related motor neuron diseases (MND). MND, in the singular tense, stands for the prototypic clinicopathologic disorder, ALS, due to upper motor neuron (UMN) and lower neuron (LMN) dysfunction, and primary lateral sclerosis (PLS) and progressive spinal muscular atrophy (SMA) and their related disorders are, respectively, due to selective UMN and LMN dysfunction. The disease-related genes in genetic and sporadic forms of ALS are shown in Table 1.

CLASSICAL SPORADIC ALS

With more than 90% of cases of sporadic occurrence, the prototypical neuropathologic findings of ALS include selective loss of large neurons in the anterior horns and large nerve fibers in the lateral funiculi of the spinal cord, and atrophic dark neurons, especially ones laden with lipofuscin pigment, and chromatolytic neurons (Figure 1A) (1). A few normal-looking neurons (Figure 1B) and their processes appear atrophic is tissue sections, and chromatolytic cytoplasm contains bundles of neurofilaments mixed with lipofuscin and rough endoplasmic reticulum. Alterations are present in the Golgi apparatus (2, 3) when stained with an MG-160 antibody. The Bunina body is the best-known cytoplasmic inclusion in ALS (4). It appears as eosinophilic small masses in hematoxyline and eosin (H&E) and

tissue sections immunostained by rabbit anti-cystatin-C serum (Figure 1C). It is immunopositive for transferrin and peripherin and negative for ubiquitin (5, 6), and is composed of electron-dense amorphous materials and variously-sized vacuoles without a limiting membrane (Figure 1D) that contain cytoplasmic elements and neurofilaments. A second, round hyaline inclusion (RI) has halos and cores indistinguishable from the Lewy body-like hyaline inclusions (LBHI) found in familial ALS (FALS) (7). The RI may instead lack halos and have small cores with vacuolar parts, irregular margins, and attached filamentous materials. It reacts with anti-ubiquitin, anti-TDP 43, and anti-optineurin antibodies (Figure 1E, F), and stains weakly with anti-phosphorylated neurofilament antibodies. Bundles of 15- to 20-nm-thick filaments and 10-nm neurofilaments intermingle in various proportions, forming round collections without a limiting membrane (Figure 1G). A third, the skein-like inclusion (SLI), has a filamentous structure clearly recognizable by anti-ubiquitin antibody staining, that varies from a single filament or coarse meshwork of filaments (Figure 1H, 1I) to a dense collection of filaments indistinguishable from RI (8). This inclusion consists of bundles of thick filaments with a diameter of 15- to 20-nm and hollow space in its center. Electron-dense granules are located in a distribution similar to RI filaments. The accumulation of neurofilaments characteristic of sporadic ALS consists of argyrophilic round structures or spheroids, with a diameter greater than 20 micrometers (Figure 1B), derived from the accumulation of phosphorylated neurofilaments found in the proximal portion of LMN axons; bundles of LMN neurofilaments correspond to chromatolytic cytoplasmic changes.

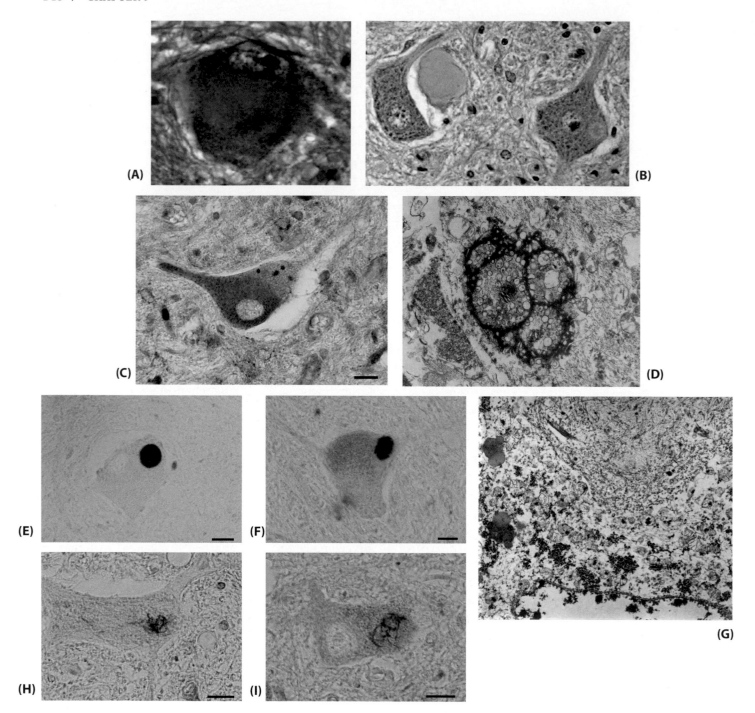

FIG. 1. Lumbar AHC in Sporadic Classical ALS. A chromatolytic but relatively atrophic neuron is occasionally seen in the lower motor neuron nuclei **(A)**. The remaining neurons are also atrophic (wide black arrow) and sometimes contain a round hyaline inclusion (thin black arrow) **(B)**. A large spheroid, which is presumed to have arisen from a proximal segment of the axon, is also seen (B; white broad arrow). Anti-cystatin C antibody clearly depicts Bunina bodies **(C)**. Ultrastructurally, the Bunina body is composed of electron-dense amorphous material studded with many vacuoles and tubules, making a conspicuous structure as a whole **(D)**. Round hyaline inclusions are immunopositive for ubiquitin and TDP-43 **(E),** as well as optineurin **(F)**. Ultrastructurally, round inclusions are a collection of crisscrossing filaments of 15 to 25 nm in diameter and of various lengths, without a limiting membrane (arrows). The filaments are coated with electron-dense granules. The nucleus is seen at the bottom of the figure **(G)**. Skein-like inclusions are distinctly depicted by anti-ubiquitin antibody as well as anti-TDP-43 and anti-optineurin antibodies **(H & I)**. A and B: H&E stain; C: Anti-cystatin C antibody stain; E and H: Anti-TDP-43 antibody stain; F and I: Anti-optineurin anbibody; Bar = 10 μm

TDP PROTEINOPATHY IN SPORADIC AND FALS

The *TARDBP* gene encodes the 43 kDa TAR DNA-binding protein, pathogenic mutations at the 1p36.22 locus which were detected in some patients that developed fronto-temporal lobe degeneration (FTLD), fronto-temporal dementia (FTD) and TDP43-positive inclusions (FTLD-TDP), with or without signs of MND (9, 10), and later in others with sporadic or FALS (11-13). TDP-43 is the major protein of ubiquitinated inclusions in ALS-TDP or ALS10 (Table), the neuropathology of which is characterized by abnormal cytoplasmic accumulation of TDP-43 in neurons and glia of the brainstem motor nuclei, spinal cord anterior horns, and associated white matter tracts. Neuronal cytoplasmic inclusions in motor neurons vary from small granules and filamentous skeins (Figure 1H, I) to round hyaline inclusions that are positive for ubiquitin (Figure 1E, F). Cells that contain cytoplasmic TDP-43 aggregates appear to have lost normal nuclear-associated immunoreactivity (ir), with large neurons of the primary motor cortex affected in the same way. Although Bunina bodies are negative for TDP-43, such aggregates may prove to be an important diagnostic feature in sporadic ALS and a minority of FALS with *TARDBP* gene mutations.

Although progression of both LMN and UMN disease is an essential pathological feature of ALS, there is accumulating evidence that the neurodegenerative process may be present in non-motor systems, associated with various so-called negative features, including eye movement, sensory, bowel and bladder, and cognitive disturbances. Among a cohort of sporadic ALS patients in which disease duration exceeded 10 years, particularly among those exposed to chronic artificial respiratory support (14), there was widespread occurrence of TDP-43 cystatin C-ir neuronal (NCI) and glial cytoplasmic inclusions (GCI), not only in motor neuron systems, but in other portions of the brain, including the globus pallidus, thalamus, inferior olivary nucleus, brain reticular formation, amygdala, frontal and temporal cortices, and the hippocampus. The demonstration of ubiquinated (UI) skein-like or round inclusions in hippocampal dentate granule cells (UDG) differentiated a type-2 distribution of TDP-43-ir NCI that was highly predictive of dementia.

A subset of patients PLS and concomitant FTLD (15-17) demonstrated aggregates of LMN TDP-43 protein without other apparent pathology, as did those with PSMA (18), implying a relation to TDP-43 proteinopathy.

It is estimated that 15% of patients with FTLD develop ALS, whereas about 50% of patients with ALS develop various degrees of cognitive impairment. Such patients may be considered to have TDP-43 proteinopathy since TDP-43 is found in clinically affected patients with FTLD, with or without frank dementia (19). The associated neuropathological features include frontal and temporal lobe atrophy, sponginess of cortical layer II, and ubiquitinated round neuronal inclusions in the cerebral cortex, including the hippocampus with TDP-43.

TABLE 1. Disease-related genes in familial and sporadic ALS

Type	Onset	Mode of Inheritance	Locus	Gene	Encoded Protein	Presence of Sporadic Patients
ALS1	adult	AD	21q22.1	SOD1	Cu/Zn superoside dismutase	+
ALS2	juvenile	AR	2q33-35	ALS2	alsin	
ALS3	adult	AD	18q21			
ALS4	juvenile	AD	9q34	SETX	senataxin	
ALS5	juvenile	AR	15q15-21	SPG11	spatacsin	
ALS6	adult	AD	16p11.2	FUS	fused in sarcoma	+
ALS7	adult	AD	20p13			
ALS8	adult	AD	20q13.33	VAPB	VAMP-associated protein B	
ALS9	adult	AD	14q11	ANG	angiogenin	+
ALS10	adult	AD	1q36	TARDBP	TAR DNA-binding protein	+
ALS11	adult	AD	6q21	FIG4	PI(3,5) P(2)5-phosphatase	+
ALS12	adult	AR/AD	10p15-p14	OPTN	optineurin	+
	adult	AD	12q24	DAO	D-amino acid oxidase	
ALS+FTD1	adult	AD	9q21-22			
ALS+FTD2	juvenile	AD	9p13.2-21.3			

AD: autosomal dominant
AR: autosomal recessive

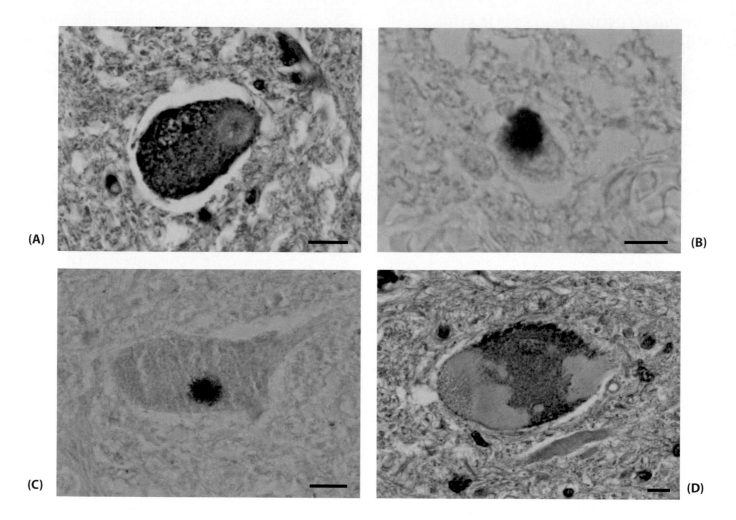

Fig. 2. Familial ALS with SOD-1 mutations. A patient with *SOD-1* mutation (A4V), and Lewy body-like hyaline inclusions that have a core and halo **(A)**. Lewy body-like hyaline inclusions are immunopositive for SOD-1 **(B)** and ubiquitin **(C)**. A patient with a different *SOD-1* mutation (I113T) that shows an inclusion containing a conglomerate of neurofilaments in a large neuron in a lumbar anterior horn **(D)**. A and D: H&E. stain; B: Anti-SOD-1 antibody stain; C: Anti-ubiquitin antibody stain; Bar = 10 μm

FALS WITH POSTERIOR COLUMN INVOLVEMENT

Hirano and colleagues (20) reported patients with predominantly LMN dysfunction beginning in the legs that was fatal within a year. At postmortem examination there was posterior and spinocerebellar tract involvement, neuronal cell loss in Clarke nucleus, with minimal corticospinal tract (CST) degeneration. The remaining large anterior horn cells (AHC) contained LBHI (Figure 2A), and large swollen rod-like axons were filled with parallel bundles of neurofilaments, without Bunina bodies or spheroids (21); an A4V mutation of the superoxide dismutase-1 (*SOD*-1) gene was confirmed (22). Since the discovery of a mutation in the *SOD1* gene on chromosome 21 (23), more than 140 pathogenic mutations have been reported, accounting for about 15 to 20% of FALS, and 1 to 3% of affected sporadic ALS patients. Several causative genes and chromosomal loci have been elucidated with most of the *SOD1*-related FALS patients demonstrating autosomal dominant (AD) inheritance. The neuropathological features of FALS or ALS1 are distinguished by degeneration in the middle root zone of the posterior column, in Clarke nucleus, and along ascending spinocerebellar tracts, with neuronal LBHI and astrocytic hyaline inclusions (HI), and absence of Bunina bodies and spheroids (24). Neuronal LBHI are eosinophilic structures with homogeneous core and pale halo, while astrocytic HI appear as a homogenous round mass when stained with H&E (Figure 2A). Ultrastructurally, both inclusions are composed of 15-25-nm-thick filaments studded with granular materials, and immunoreact with SOD-1 antibody, ubiquitin and phosphorylated neurofilaments, but not with TDP-43 (Figure 2B, 2C). However, patients with a C111Y *SOD1* gene mutation showed many LBHI that were immunopositive for both SOD1 and TDP-43 (25). In patients with 1113T *SOD1* mutation (26), neurofilamentous conglomerate inclusions (NFCI) (Figure 2D) are considered characteristic in the absence of LBHI, however both NFCI and LBHI are found in one patient with 1113T *SOD1* mutations (27). Therefore, further studies are needed as for genotype-phenotype correlations.

JUVENILE ALS AND BASOPHILIC INCLUSION BODY DISEASE

Juvenile ALS (ALSJ) is indistinguishable from sporadic ALS except for onset before age 25 years, associated negative features such as eye movement and sphincter disturbances, and variable course. Since early clinical and pathological descriptions of the disorder (28, 29), the cause has been ascribed to several genes and chromosomal loci, among them autosomal recessive inherited (AR) homozygous mutations at the 2q33.1 locus of the *ALS2* gene encoding alsin in ALS2, and

AD inherited heterozygous mutations at the 9q34.13 locus of *SETX* gene encoding sentaxin in ALS4. Postmortem spinal cord tissue in two patients with ALS4 showed atrophic spinal cords with marked loss of AHC and degeneration of CST, as well as neurons of dorsal root ganglia (DRG) and posterior columns, with axonal spheroids in the spinal gray matter, dorsal root entry zones, and peripheral nerves (30). Neuronal intracytoplasmic inclusions were noted in a sporadic ALSJ patient (31) and basophilic inclusions (BI) (32) were noted in the motor system, and in extra-motor areas of another patient. Similar intraneuronal BI were noted in UMN and LMN of two sporadic adult ALS patients (33, 34). These non-argyrophilic inclusions stain positive for cystatin-C; faintly with H&E and anti-ubiquitin antibodies, and react distinctively with Nissl stain (Figure 3A). Ultrastructurally, they consist of interlacing thick filaments 15- to 25-nm in diameter, decorated with ribosome-like granules, without a limiting membrane (Figure 3B), mRNA-related protein, T-cell intracellular antigen 1 (TIA-1), and stress related granules have been implicated in the formation of BI (Figures 3C-F) (35). Considering the widespread occurrence of BI with an emphasis on the motor neuron system and several atypical clinical features, we adopted the term basophilic inclusion body disease (BIBD) for the atypical MND in adulthood (36). Others have described BI in adult-onset sporadic disease (37), in association with FTD (38), and classic and generalized variants of Pick disease (39), in which inclusions occurred, not only in AHC, but in cerebral cortex and subcortical structures.

FTLD-FUS

Analogous to the identification of mutations in the *TARDBP* gene as the cause of most patients with FTLD and SOD1-negative ALS, pathologic mutations in the gene encoding the fused in sarcoma (FUS) protein as the cause of FALS or ALS6 (Table) (40, 41). FUS, originally discovered as a component of fusion oncogenes in human cancers, belongs to the family of multifunctional DNA/RNA-binding proteins, with a structure analogous to TDP-43. This nucleoprotein, which continuously shuttles between the nucleus and the cytoplasm, has been implicated, like TDP-43, in numerous cellular processes, including cell proliferation, DNA repair, transcription regulation, and RNA and microRNA processing. Although most FTLD were characterized by cellular inclusion bodies composed of either tau (FTLD-tau) or TDP-43 (FTLD-TDP), up to 15% of patients remained, including a number of uncommon FTLD subtypes in which the pathological protein was unknown (42). The recognized clinical, genetic, and pathological overlap between ALS and FTD, and the high degree of functional homology between FUS and TDP-43, prompted additional investigations that revealed that inclusions of several of the tau/

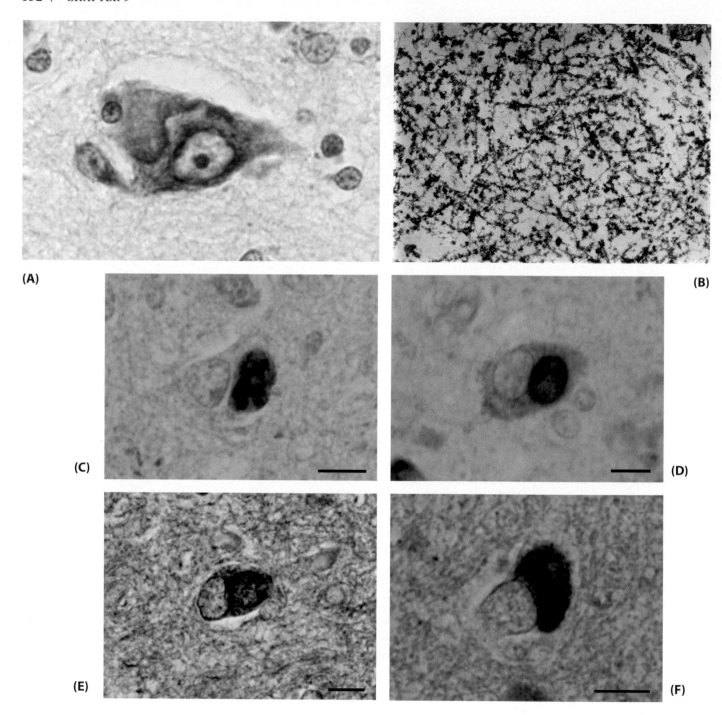

(A)

(B)

(C)

(D)

(E)

(F)

Fig. 3. Basophilic inclusions. A large, irregularly-shaped cytoplasmic structure with a distinct baso-philic rim without a clear halo or core is seen in a Betz cell **(A)**. Ultrastructurally, the basophilic inclusion in neurons in the lumbar anterior horn is composed of randomly arranged thick filaments of vari-ous lengths. The filaments are studded with ribosome-like granules **(B)**. Immunohistochemically, the basophilic inclusions are distinctly immuno-positive for p62 **(C)**. Messenger RNA-related proteins such as polyadenylate-binding protein 1 **(D)**. They are immunoreactive with antibodies against an effector for stress granule formation, T-cell intracellular antigen 1 **(E)**. They are immunoreactive with antibodies against FUS **(F)**. C–F: A neuron in the occipital cortex. A: Nissel stain; C: Anti-p62 antibody stain; D: Anti-polyadenylate-binding protein 1 antibody stain; E: Anti-T cell intracellular antigen1 antibody stain; F: Anti-FUS antibody stain. Bar = 10 μm

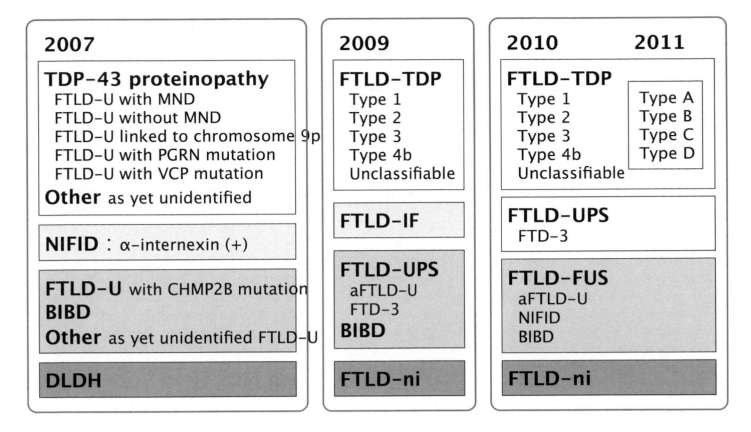

FIG. 4. Classifications of Tau-Negative FTLD.
Abbreviations: aFTLD-U: atypical frontotemporal lobar degeneration with ubiquitinated inclusions; BIBD: basophilic inclusion body disease; DLDH: dementia lacking distinctive histologic feature; FTD-3: frontotemporal dementia linked to chromosome 3; FTLD: frontotemporal lobar degeneration; FTLD-ni: frontotemporal lobar degeneration with no inclusions; FTLD-U: frontotemporal lobar degeneration with ubiquitin-positive, tau negative inclusions; IF: intermediate filament; MND: motor neuron disease; NIFID: neuronal intermediate filament inclusion disease; PGRN: progranulin gene; UPS: ubiquitin proteosome system; VCP: valosin-containing protein gene.

TDP-43-negative FTLD were FUS-ir positive (43–45). One such group was those with TDP-43-negative FTLD and ubiquinated inclusions (FTLD-U) (42), originally referred to as aFTLD-U (46, 47). Recognizing that ubiquitin-positive inclusions were FUS-ir, and their shared FUS accumulation was the most prominent molecular pathology, it was recommended that both FUS-ir cases and those with characteristic neuronal cytoplasmic inclusions of BIBD, and others with neuronal intermediate filament inclusion disease (NIFID) (45), be grouped together under the designation FTLD-FUS (42). Together with ALS patients and *FUS* mutations, they also comprise the category termed *FUS* proteinopathy or *FUSopathy* (43). Patients with ALS and FUS mutations comprise heterogeneous neuropathologies that correlate with disease severity and the specific mutations (48). Among sporadic and familial ALS-FUS patients with both juvenile and adult-onset, and four different *FUS* mutations so studied, the two distinct patterns included

frequent BI and round FUS-ir NCI as the feature of early-onset cases, including two with the p.P525L mutations, and tangle-like NCI and numerous FUS-ir GCI among those with the p.R521C mutations. Related explanations for the etiopathogenesis of motor neuron degeneration include derangement and impairments in nuclear transport (49) and ALS/FTLD-U-linked RNA metabolism, with disruption of autophagic processes causing further aggregation of toxic stress granules (50–52).

OPTINEURIN AND ALS

Homogyzous or heterozygous mutation at the 10p13 locus of optineurin gene (OPTN), originally reported as the causative gene for primary open-angle glaucoma-1E, has since been considered the causative gene in a subset of FALS patients (ALS12) (Table) (53) that included a cohort of Japanese individuals from two families of consanguineous marriages, thought to be unrelated but who shared a haplotype for a 0.9-Mb region containing the *OPTN* gene, including three patients homozygous, and four others heterozygous, respectively, for null or missense gene mutations, suggestive of AD inheritance with incomplete penetrance. The age at onset of ALS, which varied in clinical phenotype, was from 30 to 60 years, with prolonged and relatively slow disease progression before respiratory failure and supervened.

Neuropathological findings were available for a 66-year-old woman heterozygous for the E478G missense mutation and a disease course lasting about 10 years, featuring both upper and lower motor dysfunction, as well as mood and personality changes, and her two sisters who developed similar motor neuron signs (54). They showed slight frontotemporal lobe atrophy, and in addition to upper and motor neuron degeneration, the remaining lower motor neurons showed TDP-43 positive skein-like neuronal cytoplasmic inclusions, as well as glial inclusions that were immunonegative for optineurin, without Bunina bodies or RI. Whereas eosinophilic cytoplasmic regions of AHC showed intense immunoreactivity for optineurin, optineurin-positive inclusions with distinct margins were not discernible. Therefore, this case showed cytopathological features of both TDP-43 and optineurin abnormalities, suggesting a close link to TDP-43 proteinopathy. Optineurin was detected in RI (Figure 1F) and SLI (Figure 1I) in patients with sporadic classical ALS with TDP-43 pathology, in LBHI of familial ALS with *SOD-1* mutations (53), and in BI of sporadic BIBD patients (55). Subsequent investigations showed optineurin pathology in Alzheimer, Huntington, and Creutzfeldt-Jakob disease (56), and absence of immunohistochemically detectable optineurin in LBHI in ALS-SOD1 (57), as well as a relatively low incidence of optineurin abnormality in ALS, suggesting a minor pathogenic role for optineurin in ALS (58, 59). Despite the occurrence of novel mutations of the *OPTN* gene among Danish and Italian families with sporadic and FALS (60, 61), dysfunction of this gene seems to be a rare cause of ALS with or without FTLD (62, 63).

INFLUENCE OF FTLD ON ALS CLASSIFICATION

The classification of tau-nagative FTLD is shown in Figure 4. FTLD is the second to third commonest cause of degenerative dementia after Alzheimer disease and dementia with Lewy bodies (64). The neuropathological freatures of FTLD are associated with the clinical entities of frontotemporal dementia (FTD), semantic dementia (SD), and progressive non-fluent aphasia (PFNA). The findings are heterogeneous, with the common feature of relatively selective degeneration of the frontal and temporal lobes (65). Recent advances in the biochemical composition and molecular defect of the associated intracellular protein inclusions prompted a protein-based nomenclature for FTLD, wherein major subdivisions reflected the protein abnormality presumed to be pathogenic or most characteristic of the individual condition, substituting FTLD-tau for tau-positive FTLD, which include PiD, corticobasal degeneration (CBD), progressive supranuclear palsy (PSP), agryrophilic grain disease (AGD), multiple system tauopathy with dementia (MSTD) subtypes; and FTLD-TDP and FTLP-UPS, respectively, for TDP-43-positive and TDP-43-negative FTLD; and FTLD-IF for NIFID (65). One year later, additional nomenclature (42) suggested instead FTLD-FUS for FTLD-IF with other nomenclature remaining essentially the same (65).

Analogously, as TDP-43 was identified as a major constituent of ubiquinated inclusions in a subset of FTLD-U as well as in sporadic ALS, suggesting a link between FTLD and ALS (66, 67), the accumulation of TDP-43 was confirmed in familial FTLD with progranulin mutations (68, 69) and in FTLD with MND due to valosin-containing protein (*VCP*) gene mutations (70). They are collectively called TDP-43 proteinopathies (71). The discovery of a *FUS* gene mutation in a subset of familial ALS (ALS6) (72, 73) led to the confirmation of FUS protein as a major constituent of inclusions in aFTLD-U, BIBD and NIFID. This was followed by identification of TDP-43 in both FTLD and ALS, ascertaining a close link between ALS and dementia with most ALS patients exhibiting type B pathology, and others type A (Figure 4) (74), TDP-43 is not the only causative protein in ALS associated with dementia. Patients with *MAPT* (FTDP-17), progranulin (*PGRN*), valosin-containing protein (*VCP*), charged multi-vesicular protein 2B (*CHMP2B*), *DCTN1*, *ANG*, *DJ1*, and *SOD1* mutations, as well as patients with NIFID, BIBD, and FTLD-no inclusions (FTLD-ni), also known to show a clinical picture of ALS associated with FTD or dementia.

Both FTLD and ALS, which comprise heterogeneous groups of diseases, have an inherent propensity toward multi-system involvement and variability in clinical phenotype ranging from autonomic, pyramidal, and extrapyramidal, to cognitive involvement, even in those with the same protein abnormality. Analogous to the nosology of FTLD, sporadic and FALS can be considered in the context of the associated protein constituent, ALS-TDP, ALS-SOD1, ALS-FUS, and ALS-OPTN. Further detailed neuropathological studies based on molecular pathology are needed to explore the essential pathogenesis of ALS.

REFERENCES

1. Hirano A, Donnenfeld H, Sasaki S, Nakano I. Fine structural observations of neurofilamentous changes in amyotrophic lateral sclerosis. *J Neuropathol Exp Neurol* 1984; 43:461–470.

2. Gonatas NK, Stieber A, Mourelatos Z, et al. Fragmentation of the Golgi apparatus of motor neurons in amyotrophic lateral sclerosis. *Am J Pathol* 1992; 140:731–737.

3. Matsumoto S, Kusaka H, Ito H, Imai T. Golgi apparatus and intraneuronal inclusions of anterior horn cells in amyotrophic lateral sclerosis: an immunohistochemical study. *Acta Neuropathol* 1996; 91:603–607.

4. Rowland LP. T.L. Bunina, Asao Hirano, and the post mortem cellular diagnosis of amyotrophic lateral sclerosis. *Amyotroph Lateral Scler* 2009; 10:74–78.

5. Mizuno Y, Amati M, Takatama M, et al. Transferrin localizes in Bunina bodies in amyotrophic lateral sclerosis. *Acta Neuropathol* 2006; 112:597–603.

6. Mizuno Y, Fujita Y, Takatama M, et al. Peripherin partially localizes in Bunin bodies in amyotrophic lateral sclerosis. *J Neurol Sci* 2011; 302:14–18.

7. Kato T, Katagiri T, Hirano A, et al. Lewy body-like hyaline inclusions in sporadic motor neuron disease are ubiquitinated. *Acta Neuropathol* 1989; 77:391–396.

8. Sasaki S, Maruyama S. Ultrastructural study of skein- inclusions in anterior horn neurons of patients with motor neuron disease. *Neurosci Lett* 1992; 147:121–124.

9. Neumann M, Sampathu DM, Kwong LK, et al. Ubiquitinated TDP-43 in frontotemporal lobar degeneration and amyotrophic lateral sclerosis. *Science* 2006; 314:130–133.

10. Arai T, Hasegawa M, Akiyama H, et al. TDP-43 is a component of ubiquitin-positive tau-negative inclusions in frontotemporal lobar degeneration and amyotrophic lateral sclerosis. *Biochem Biophys Res Commun* 2006; 351:602 611.

11. Sreedharan J, Blair IP, Tripathi VB, et al. TDP-43 mutations in familial and sporadic amyotrophic lateral sclerosis. *Science* 2008; 319:1668–1672.

12. Yokoseki A, Shiga A, Tan CF, et al. TDP-43 mutation in familial amyotrophic lateral sclerosis. *Ann Neurol* 2008; 63:538–542.

13. Kabashi E, Valdmanis PN, Dion P, et al. TARDBP mutations in individuals with sporadic and familial amyotrophic lateral sclerosis. *Nat Genet* 2008; 40:572–574.

14. Nishihira Y, Tan CF, Onodera O, et al. Sporadic amyotrophic lateral sclerosis: two pathological patterns shown by analysis of distribution of TDP-43-immunoreactive neuronal and glial cytoplasmic inclusions. *Acta Neuropathol* 2008; 116:169–82.

15. Konagaya M, Sakai M, Matsuoka Y, Konagaya Y, Hashizume Y. Upper motor neuron predominant degeneration with frontal and temporal lobe atrophy. *Acta Neuropathol* 1998; 96:532–536.

16. Nishii M, Ito H, Kinoshita Y, et al. An autopsy report of a patient with motor neuron disease manifesting long-term clinical course. *Neuropathology* 2009; 29:203–205.

17. Kwong LK, Neumann M, Sampathu DM, et al. TDP-43 proteinopathy: the neuropathology underlying major forms of sporadic and familial frontotemporal lobar degeneration and motor neuron disease. *Acta Neuropathol* 2007; 114:63–70.

18. Geser F, Stein B, Partain M, et al. Motor neuron disease clinically limited to the lower motor neuron is a diffuse TDP-43 proteinopathy. *Acta Neuropathol* 2011; 121:509–517.

19. Dickson DW, Josephs KA, Amador-Ortiz C. TDP-43 in differential diagnosis of motor neuron disorders. *Acta Neuropathol* 2007; 114: 71–79.

20. Hirano A, Kurland LT, Sayre GP. Familial amyotrophic lateral sclerosis. A subgroup characterized by posterior and spinocerebellar tract involvement and hyaline inclusions in the anterior horn cells. *Arch Neurol* 1967;16:232–243.

21. Hirano A, Nakano I, Kurland LT, et al. Fine structural study of neurofibrillary changes in a family with amyotrophic lateral sclerosis. *J Neuropathol Exp Neurology* 1984; 43:461–470.

22. Shibata N, Hirano A, Kobayashi M, et al. Intense superoxide dismutase-1 immunoreactivity in intracytoplasmic hyaline inclusions of familial amyotrophic lateral sclerosis with posterior column involvement. *J Neuropathol Exp Neurol* 1996; 55:481–490.

23. Siddique T, Figlewicz DA, Pericak-Vance MA, et al. Linkage of a gene causing familial amyotrophic lateral sclerosis to chromosome 21 and evidence of genetic locus heterogeneity. *N Engl J Med* 1991; 324:1381–1384.

24. Kato S. Amyotrophic lateral sclerosis models and human neuropathology: similarities and differences. Acta Neuropathol 2008;115:97–114.

25. Sumi H, Kato S, Mochimaru Y, et al. Nuclear TAR DNA binding protein 43 expression in spinal cord neurons correlates with the clinical course in amyotrophic lateral sclerosis. *J Neuropathol Exp Neurol* 2009; 68:37–47.

26. Locate G, Balkh RH, Al-Lose MT, et al. Familial ALS with extreme phenotypic variability due to the I113T SOD1 mutation. *Amyotroph Lateral Scler* 2010; 11:232–236.

27. Nakamura S, Ito H, Asayama S, et al. A case of familial amyotrophic lateral sclerosis with I113T SOD1 mutation. *Neuropathology* 2010; 30:449–451.

28. van Bogaert L. La sclerose laterale amyotrophique et la paralysie bulbaire progressive chez l'enfant. *Rev Neurol* 1925; 1:180–192.

29. Wohlfart G, Swank RL. Pathology of amyotrophic lateral sclerosis. Fiber analysis of the ventral roots and pyramidal tracts of the spinal cord. *Arch Neurol Psych* 1941; 46:783–799.

30. Chance PF, Rabin BA, Ryan SG, et al. Linkage of the gene for an autosomal dominant form of juvenile amyotrophic lateral sclerosis to chromosome 9q34. *Am J Hum Genet* 1990; 62:633–640.

31. Oda M, Akagawa N, Tabuchi Y, Tanabe H. A sporadic juvenile case of the amyotrophic lateral sclerosis with neuronal intracytoplasmic inclusions. *Acta Neuropathol* 1978; 44:211–216.

32. Matsumoto S, Kusaka H, Murakami N, et al. Basophilic inclusions in sporadic juvenile amyotrophic lateral sclerosis: an immunocytochemical and ultrastructural study. *Acta Neuropathol* 1992; 83:579–583.

33. Kusaka H, Matsumoto S, Imai T. An adult-onset case of sporadic motor neuron disease with basophilic inclusions. *Acta Neuropathol* 1990; 80:660–665.

34. Kusaka H, Matsumoto S, Imai T. Adult-onset motor neuron disease with basophilic intraneuronal inclusion bodies. *Clin Neuropathol* 1993; 12:215–218.

35. Fujita K, Ito H, Nakano S, et al. Immunohistochemical identification of messenger RNA-related proteins in basophilic inclusions of adult-onset atypical motor neuron disease. *Acta Neuropathol* 2008; 116:439–445.

36. Kusaka H, Matsumoto S, Okamoto K, et al. Basophilic inclusion body disease presenting as an atypical motor neuron disease in adulthood. *J Neuropathol Exp Neurol* 1992; 51:322.

37. Sasaki S, Toi S, Shirata A, et al. Immunohistochemical and ultrastructural study of basophilic inclusions in adult-onset motor neuron disease. *Acta Neuropathol* 2001; 102:200–206.

38. Ishihara K, Araki S, Ihori N, et al. An autopsy case of frontotemporal dementia with severe dysarthria and motor neuron disease showing numerous basophilic inclusions. *Neuropathology* 2006; 26:447–454.

39. Munoz-Garcia D, Ludwin SK. Classic and generalized variants

of Pick's disease: A clinicopathological, ultrastructural, and immunocytochemical comparative study. *Ann Neurol* 1984; 16:467–480.

40. Kwiatkowski TJ Jr, Bosco DA, Leclerc AL, et al. Mutations in the FUS/TLS gene on chromosome 16 cause familial amyotrophic lateral sclerosis. *Science* 2009; 323:1205–1208.

41. Vance C, Rogelj B, Hortobágyi T, et al. Mutations in FUS, an RNA processing protein, cause familial amyotrophic lateral sclerosis type 6. *Science* 2009; 323:1208–1211.

42. Mackenzie IRA, Neumann M, Bigio EH, et al. Nomenclature and nosology for neuropathologic subtypes of frontotemporal lobe degeneration: an update. *Acta Neuropathol* 2010; 119:1–4.

43. Munoz DG, Neumann M, Kusaka H, et al. FUS pathology in basophilic inclusion body disease. *Acta Neuropathol* 2009; 118: 617–627.

44. Neumann M, Rademakers R, Roeber S, et al. Frontotemporal lobar degeneration with FUS pathology. *Brain* 132:2922–2931.

45. Neumann M, Roeber S, Kretzschmar HA, et al. Abundant FUS pathology in neuronal intermediate filament inclusion disease. *Acta Neuropathol* 2009; 118:605–616.

46. Mackenzie IRA, Foti D, Woulfe J, et al. Atypical frontotemporal lobar degeneration with ubiquitin-positive, TDP-43-negative neuronal inclusions. *Brain* 131:1282–1293.

47. Roeber S, Mackenzie IRA, Kretzschmar HA, et al. TDP-43-negative FTLD-U is a significant new clinicopathological subtype of FTLD. *Acta Neuropathol* 2008; 116:147–157.

48. Mackenzie IR, Ansorge O, Strong M, et al. Pathological heterogeneity in amyotrophic lateral sclerosis with FUS mutations: two distinct patterns correlating with disease severity and mutation. *Acta Neuropathol* 2011; 122:87–98.

49. Ito D, Seki M, Tsunoda Y, et al. Nuclear transport impairment of amyotrophic lateral sclerosis-linked mutations in FUS/TLS. *Ann Neurol* 2011; 69:152–162.

50. Ito D, Suzuki N. Conjoint pathologic cascades mediated by ALS/FTLD-U linked RNA-binding proteins TDP-43 and FUS. *Neurology* 2011; 77:1636–1643.

51. Gitler AD, Shorter J. RNA-binding proteins with prion-like domains in ALS and FTLD-U. *Prion* 2011; 5(3). Epub ahead of print.

52. Sun Z, Diaz Z, Fang X, et al. Molecular determinants and genetic modifiers of aggregation and toxicity for the ALS disease protein FUS/TLS. *PLoS Biol* 2011; 9:e1000614.

53. Maruyama H, Morino H, Ito H, et al. Mutations of optineurin in amyotrophic lateral sclerosis. *Nature* 2010; 465:23–226.

54. Ito H, Nakamura M, Komure O, et al. Clinicopathologic study on an ALS family with a heterozygous E478G optineurin mutation. *Acta Neuropathol* 2011; 122:223–229.

55. Ito H, Fujita K, Nakamura M, et al. Optineurin is co-localized with FUS in basophilic inclusions of ALS with FUS mutation and in basophilic inclusion body disease. *Acta Neuropathol* 2011; 121:555–557.

56. Osawa T, Mizuno Y, Fujita Y, et al. Optineurin in neurodegenerative disease. *Neuropathology* 2011 Feb 1; Epub ahead of print.

57. Deng HS, Bigio EH, Zhai H, et al. Differential involvement of optineurin in amyotrophic lateral sclerosis with or without SOD1 mutaions. *Ann Neurol* 2011; 68:1057–1061.

58. Hortobágyi T, Troakes C, Nishimura AL, et al. Optineurin inclusions occur in a minority of TDP-43 positive ALS and FTLD-TDP cases and are rarely observed in other neurodegenerative disorders. *Acta Neuropathol* 2011; 121:519–527.

59. Solski JA, Williams KL, Yang S, et al. Mutation analysis of the optineurin gene in familial amyotrophic lateral sclerosis. *Neurobiol Aging* 2011 Oct 17; Epub ahead of print.

60. Tümer Z, Bertelsen B, Gredal O, et al. A novel heterozygous nonsense mutation of the OPTN gene segregating in a Danish family with ALS. *Neurobiol Aging* 2011, Aug 25; Epub ahead of print.

61. Del Bo R, Tiloca C, Pensato V, et al. Neurodegenerative disease: Novel optineurin mutations in patients with familial and sporadic amyotrophic lateral sclerosis. *J Neurol Neurosurg Psychiatry* 2011; 82; 1239–1243

62. Suhihara K, Maruyama H, Kamada M, et al. Screening for OPTN mutations in amyotrophic lateral sclerosis in a mainly Caucasian population. *Neurobiol Aging* 2011; 32:1923.e9–1923.e10.

63. Fecto F, Siddique T. Making connections: Pathology and genetic link of amyotrophic lateral sclerosis with frontotemporal lobe dementia. *J Mol Neurosci* 2011; 45:663–675.

64. Mackenzie IR, Rademakers R, Neumann M. TDP-43 and FUS in amyotrophic lateral sclerosis and frontotemporal dementia. *Lancet Neurol* 2010; 9:995–1007.

65. Mackenzie IRA, Neumann M, Bigio EH, et al. Nomenclature for neuropathologic subtypes of frontotemporal lobar degeneration: consensus recommendations. *Acta Neuropathol* 2009; 117:15–18.

66. Neumann M, Sampathu DM, Kwong LK, et al. Ubiquitinated TDP-43 in frontotemporal lobar degeneration and amyotrophic lateral sclerosis. *Science* 2006; 314:130–133.

67. Arai T, Hasegawa M, Akiyama H, et al. TDP-43 is a component of ubiquitin-positive tau-negative inclusions in frontotemporal lobar degeneration and amyotrophic lateral sclerosis. *Biochem Biophys Res Commun* 2006; 351:602–611.

68. Cruts M, Gijselinck I, van der Zee J, et al. Null mutations in progranulin cause ubiquitin-positive frontotemporal dementia linked to chromosome 17q21. *Nature* 2006; 442:920–924.

69. Baker M, Mackenzie IR, Pickering-Brown SM, et al. Mutations in progranulin cause tau-negative frontotemporal dementia linked to chromosome 17. *Nature* 2006; 442:916–919.

70. Neumann M, Mackenzie IR, Cairns NJ, et al. TDP-43 in the ubiquitin pathology of frontotemporal dementia with VCP gene mutations. *J Neuropathol Exp Neurol* 2007; 66:152–157.

71. Kwong LK, Neumann M, Sampathu DM, Lee VM, Trojanowski JQ. TDP-43 proteinopathy: the neuropathology underlying major forms of sporadic and familial frontotemporal lobar degeneration and motor neuron disease. *Acta Neuropathol* 2007; 114:63–70.

72. Kwiatkowski TJ Jr, Bosco DA, Leclerc AL, et al. Mutations in the FUS/TLS gene on chromosome 16 cause familial amyotrophic lateral sclerosis. *Science* 2009; 323:1205–1208.

73. Vance C, Rogelj B, Hortobágyi T, et al. Mutations in FUS, an RNA processing protein, cause familial amyotrophic lateral sclerosis type 6. *Science* 2009; 323:1208–1211.

74. Mackenzie IR, Neumann M, Baborie A, et al. A harmonized classification system for FTLD-TDP pathology. *Acta Neuro Pathol* 2011; 122:111–113.

CHAPTER 10

Neurogenetic Evaluation of Motor Disorders

Gregory M. Pastores, Heather A. Lau

Advances in the field of genetics and related specialties have enabled the discovery of the molecular basis of a range of inherited neurological disorders (1). Although in most instances these findings have not resulted in curative treatment, there have been varied applications. In medical practice, characterization of genetic etiology yields several benefits. The rapid diagnostic confirmation on a patient with a suspected neurogenetic problem, performed on blood or other tissue samples to extract DNA, obviates the need for serial investigations, such as a muscle biopsy in the diagnosis of Duchenne muscular dystrophy (DMD). Pre-symptomatic, prenatal diagnosis, and when appropriate, early intervention employing directed treatment are available options (e.g., employing enzyme replacement therapy (ERT) can be immensely beneficial in the potentially fatal childhood disorder of Pompe disease). Moreover, counseling of patients regarding prognosis and management can deter medical errors such as therapy that may be instituted for presumed multiple sclerosis (MS) in a patient with an inherited leukodystrophy. Such benefits may extend to family members in terms of carrier detection and at-risk counseling (2). The current chapter will focus on general principles relevant to neurogenetic disorders.

GENERAL CONCEPTS

A range of defects can arise in particular genes that can lead to disease. These include nucleotide substitutions that result in a missense or nonsense mutation that encodes part of a gene sequence (exon) that can generate a transcript (mRNA) that is prematurely degraded and lost via non-sense mediated decay, or a nonfunctional protein product that is significantly truncated and missing key components (3). In instances where the mutation results in the genera-tion of a misfolded protein, a quality control system within the endoplasmic reticulum (ER) may mark the protein for ultimate degradation via the ubiquitin-proteasome (UPS) pathway (4). A gene sequence can also be subject to com-plete or partial deletion, or its sequence altered by a recom-bination event or the use of a cryptic splice site during transcription, which leads to the generation of a dysfunc-tional protein.

Occasionally, mutations in a particular gene may lead to the suppression of other genes as a consequence of epi-genetic changes such as DNA methylation (5). In such cases, a closed chromatin configuration results in the loss of accessibility to transcription factors, effectively silencing the gene's expression. This process was implicated in Rett syndrome due to mutations in the methyl-CpG-binding protein-2 (*MECP2*) gene (6). X-chromosome inactivation or lyonization is a normal epigenetic mechanism, wherein one X chromosome in females is silenced to equalize gene expression or dosage between XY males and XX females (7). Skewed X-inactivation is one explanation for symp-tomatic female carriers of an X-linked trait, wherein the X chromosome bearing the mutation is predominantly active.

A gene defect can result in a gain of toxic function or a novel property for the resulting gene product, which then causes a disruption in a particular cellular/biochemical path-way. Infrequently, the defect may not be an alteration of the gene sequence but a consequence of changes in its expression pattern, as seen with facioscapulohumeral muscular dystro-phy (FSHD). Through linkage analysis, FSHD was mapped to chromosome 4q35, although the causal gene defect has not been identified (8). It is now recognized that normal individuals have >10 *D4Z4* repeats and normally methylated chromatin, with *DUX4* expression turned off. In both FSHD1 and FSHD2, relaxation of chromatin structure allows *DUX4* expression leading to the production of toxic *DUX4* protein products. One confounding factor relates to the observation that *DUX4* expression occurs if there is a permissive genetic background containing a polyadenylation signal (Poly A). Further studies are required to establish the link between genetic changes and clinical FSHD expression.

IMPACT OF MODE OF INHERITANCE

Two alterations may explain development of disease in autosomal dominant (AD) disorders when only one of the 2 alleles is mutated. A mutation can lead to a dominant negative effect when the defective gene product effectively abrogates the function of the normal gene product or its interacting partner. For instance, patients with LGMD2A and calpain 3 (*CAPN3*) gene defect can harbor mutations at D705G and R448H associated with retained proteolytic activity but nevertheless cause muscular dystrophy, attributed to reduction in CAPN3's ability to bind to titin, resulting in myofiber structural instability, shown *in vitro* (9).

An AD mutation can likewise lead to a reduction of the gene product to a level below a threshold necessary for maintenance of normal function, termed *haplo-insufficiency state*, such as may be seen with acute intermittent porphyria, wherein reduction of the relevant enzyme activity to one-half normal level is not adequate to prevent development of symptoms (10). This contrasts with many autosomal recessive (AR) inherited enzyme deficiency disorders such as Tay-Sachs disease trait, wherein carriers who have one defective allele are unaffected because of sufficient residual enzyme activity from the corresponding normal allele.

FACTORS INFLUENCING PHENOTYPIC EXPRESSION

Abolition of gene product function is usually associated with a more severe form of the disease, often characterized by early symptom onset and rapid progression (11). In some instances, the gene is altered but the product is not completely lost and there may even be residual function leading to an attenuated form of the disease with a later age of onset and more insidious course.

Although once thought that characterization of the genotype would assist in accurate prediction of the phenotype, more often there was lack of perfect concordance. Such observations suggested the influence of other factors in ultimate disease expression. These so-called modifiers may be other genes or gene products that interact with the primary

defect or environmental aspects such as diet and concurrent medications. Severe neurotoxicity occurs in patients with Charcot-Marie-Tooth (CMT) disease who are prescribed vincristine for acute lymphoblastic leukemia (12). Similarly, in the mitochondrial disorder Leber hereditary optic neuropathy (LHON), there may be large variability in clinical expression that can be modulated by several factors including downregulation of another gene, optic atrophy (*OPA1*), environmental factors such as smoking, and anatomic elements such as predisposition of the optic nerve head to axonal loss (13). *OPA1* is a dynamin-like mitochondrial GTPase in which mutations of the encoding gene lead to an AD form of optic atrophy (14).

IDENTIFYING CAUSAL GENE DEFECTS

High-throughput sequence capture methods and next-generation sequencing technologies are proving to be productive means for identifying causal gene defects, particularly in sporadic and rare disorders not amenable to linkage type study analyses (15). Exome sequencing, or targeting exome capture, has enabled the discovery of the genetic basis of a number of rare Mendelian disorders such as Kabuki, Miller, and Fowler syndromes (16, 17). Such strategies will eventually enhance the ability to make a rapid diagnosis in clinical settings, provide therapy if available, and enable appropriate counseling regarding prognosis and reproductive implications. It is anticipated that technological advances will reduce the cost of the testing of panels of relevant genes in those with a suspected inherited neurologic disorders.

NEUROPATHOLOGIC CONSIDERATIONS

The way in which a gene defect ultimately leads to disease is poorly understood in many inherited neurologic motor disorders. Although the gene defect may reside in every nucleated cell of an affected individual, among patients with different neurologic disorders there clearly are specific populations of cells within the central nervous system (CNS) and peripheral nervous system (PNS) that are selectively vulnerable, as for example, upper motor neuron (UMN) and lower motor neurons (LMN), genetic disturbances of which result in inherited forms of amyotrophic lateral sclerosis (ALS) (18), or equivalent disturbances of dopaminergic neuronal function that lead to Parkinson disease (PD) (19).

The basis of disease-specific patterns of clinical expression is the subject of intense scrutiny, and remains to be elucidated. In certain instances, the pattern of involvement or disease manifestation can be clearly correlated with the corresponding configuration of gene expression as, for example, in the SCA28 form of inherited ataxia, wherein mutation in the ATPase family gene 3-like 2 (*AFG3L2*) gene, which is selectively expressed in cerebellar Purkinje neurons and involved in the maintenance of the mitochondrial proteome (20). In other instances, the relevant tissue-specific pattern of gene expression may be related more to the profile of its interacting partners, as may be the case in myotonic dystrophy types 1 (DM1) and 2 (DM2), wherein transcribed CTG repeats in the 3-prime-untranslated region of the dystrophia myotonica protein kinase (*DMPK*) gene are expressed in tissues affected by DM1, while intronic CCTG expansion in the *MBNL* gene occur in DM2, which elaborates a protein that functions as a target-specific regulator of pre-mRNA splicing (21). In these instances, mutant proteins become neurotoxic to specific cell subtypes due to highly selective protein-protein interactions driven by the unique properties of the pathogenic protein.

One disease producing genetic mechanism involves errors of RNA processing leads to alternative splicing and transcript editing. In the normal situation, these processes are a means of generating various products from a single gene, illustrating why the number of genes in humans is far less than had been anticipated, given the wide diversity of protein products. RNA processing involves multiple different players, and several genes. This is illustrated by the contribution of the transcriptional repressor TARDBP gene, which encodes the TAR DNA-binding protein (TDP43), and the fused in sarcoma (FUS) gene that encodes the regulatory transcription nucleoprotein; the cognate protein products are involved in RNA-processing pathways implicated in inherited ALS (22, 23). Other examples include defects in a particular gene that encodes proteins called snRNP, critical factors in the assembly of the survival of motor neurons gene 1 (*SMN1),* mutations of which cause spinal muscular atrophy (SMA (24). Splicing errors may also explain variability in clinical manifestations when the same gene is involved, such as occurs in disruption of the open reading frame of the *dystrophin* gene, resulting in the classic DMD phenotype; whereas preservation of the reading frame leads instead to the milder Becker phenotype (25).

Discovery of the gene defects can lead to the elucidation of novel mechanisms of disease. For example, mutations in the *ABHD12* gene encoding abhydrolase domain containing 12, the cause of AR polyneuropathy, hearing loss, ataxia, retinitis pigmentosa, and cataract (abbreviated as PHARC) (26) due to an enzymatic defect of 2-arachidonoyl glycerol (2-AG) hydrolysis, involved in the metabolism of an endogenous transmitter acting on cannabinoid receptors. Dysregulation of the endocannabinoid system has not been previously implicated in ataxia or any other neurodegenerative disorders. This discovery and others may ultimately enable development of rational therapies based on understanding of disease processes.

The elucidation of disease mechanisms is, in turn,

shedding new light on poorly understood physiology, illustrated by the recent characterization of defects in selonoprotein N (*SEPN1*), a cause of congenital muscular dystrophy (CMD) (27). Studies indicate SEPN1is involved in the regulation of ryanodine receptors and cellular redox homeostasis, as well as the regulation of satellite cell function. Pathogenic mutations have been identified in the gene encoding selenocysteine insertion sequence-binding protein 2 (*SECISBP2* or *SBP2*), which mediates the generation of selenoproteins. Affected individuals with *SBP2* mutations have axial muscular dystrophy with features similar to the myopathy caused by mutations in *SEPN1*, and shared molecular pathways may explain the commonalities in clinical presentations (28).

As shown above, investigation of putative disease mechanisms may reveal convergent disease pathways that explain overlapping clinical manifestations. Several studies suggest the function of RNA-processing proteins is affected by their sequestration by trinucleotide repeat expanded mRNA (29). As there is extensive coupling between RNA processing events, it is likely that multiple physiologic pathways are disrupted. Adult-onset of symptoms could reflect the protracted time it takes to breach a pathologic threshold in post-mitotic cells within muscle and brain, with somatic expansion of the repeats over an individual's lifespan. Another basis for diseases with shared features can be disruption of a particular signaling pathway as may be seen in NeuroCardioFacioCutaneous (NCFC), Noonan, CFC, and Costello syndrome, wherein distinct causal gene defects lead to abnormalities of RAS-MAP kinase signaling and similar manifestations (30).

A common feature of several neurological diseases is the presence of abnormal protein aggregates, which can be in the form of extracellular and intracellular protein deposits that develop respectively, from amyloid β-protein as in senile plaques in Alzheimer disease (AD), or α-synuclein in Parkinson disease (PD) (31). Although the relationship between deposits and neuronal loss is not fully understood, there is agreement that these observations are surrogate markers of specific neurodegenerative disorders.

In several disorders, including those associated with motor neuron disease (MND), spastic paraplegia, and peripheral neuropathy, gene defects that encode proteins that have a role in both anterograde and retrograde axonal transport have been identified (32). Similarly, genetic disorders associated with leukodystrophy are causally related to genes that encode proteins with roles in the generation and maintenance of myelin (33).

Neuronal loss and dysfunction related to genetic defects are likely mediated by one or more pathologic mechanisms, including excitotoxicity and oxidative stress. Misfolded proteins within the endoplasmic reticulum (ER) may overwhelm ER-associated degradation (ERAD), resulting in activation of ER-stress responses, and triggering a vicious cycle that ultimately leads to cell death or dysfunction (34).

Special considerations apply to mitochondrial disorders related to the distinctive role of these organelles in cellular metabolism and the presence of separate mitochondrial DNA (mtDNA), as each cell may contain several mitochondria, each with a different burden of mutation (35). Cells in the brain and muscle with an increased demand for aerobic metabolism can be compromised by mtDNA mutation-impairing ATP generation. Those with exclusively mutant mtDNA termed *homoplasmy*, may demonstrate a more severe phenotype, in contrast to those with a mixed population of mutant and normal mtDNA termed *heteroplasmy*. For instance, a high load of the mtDNA T8993G mutation leads to fatal childhood maternally inherited Leigh syndrome (MILS), whereas a lower mutant threshold causes the syndrome of neuropathy, ataxia and retinitis pigmentosa (NARP) (36). Recent investigations have shown that the mtDNA background may also play an important role in modulating the biochemical defects and clinical outcome in NARP/MILS (37).

CLINICAL IMPLICATIONS

Several lessons have been learned from characterization of gene defects associated with different neurogenetic disorders. These have led to recognition of various phenomena, which are important to understand so test results can be placed in their proper context.

Genetic heterogeneity, which refers to the manifestation of a single phenotype despite different mutated genes, describes a diverse group of genetic neurological disorders. The equivalent phenotypes of limb girdle muscular dystrophy type 1 (LGMD1) and type 3 (LGMD2A) derive, respectively, from mutation in the myotillin (*MYOT*) gene, which leads to a defective structural protein important in stabilizing and anchoring thin filaments to the Z-disc during myofibrillogenesis, while calpain-3 (*CAPN3*) encodes a different muscle-specific calcium-activated neutral protease that plays a role in disassembling sarcomeric proteins (38). When testing for a limited number of genes, a negative result may not exclude the clinical diagnosis under consideration. As new gene defects are described on a regular basis, it is generally worthwhile to re-examine a patient without an etiologic diagnosis, if several years have passed since testing was last performed.

Variable expressivity refers to the different patterns of clinical manifestations that occur with the same mutation, suggesting the influence of other factors and modifiers that interact with the gene defect to cause the disease. This observation implies patients with the same clinical diagnosis and gene defect can have a different disease course.

The presence of disease modifiers and how they exert their influence is an area of limited knowledge. There is immense interest in unraveling this phenomenon as it may provide insights into biochemical or cellular pathways that may be modifiable pharmacologically to delay disease onset or slow its progression.

Penetrance refers to the likelihood of manifesting a dominantly inherited disease phenotype such that when low, not every carrier of the gene defect will necessarily develop the disease, as in mutations of the torsin (*TOR*) gene and the leucine-rich repeat kinase 2 (*LRRK2*) gene associated with increased risk respectively, of developing torsion dystonia and PD (39, 40). All relatives of an affected individual may be a carrier of the same gene defect and should undergo appropriate genetic counseling, as they can still pass on a genetic trait to their descendant even when asymptomatic. Thus, no assumptions about carrier status should be made based on the presence or absence of symptoms in a relative of an affected person.

Anticipation, which refers to the increasing severity of an AD-inherited disorder in subsequent generations, occurs in inherited ataxia caused by dynamic mutations comprised of multiple iterations of tri-, tetra-, or penta-nucleotide repeats, in contrast to nucleotide substitutions that involves, instead, single base defects or point mutations (41).

Imprinting is an epigenetic process that leads to parent-specific expression of certain genes, as may occur in two distinct neurodevelopmental disorders, Prader Willi (PWS) and Angelman syndrome (AS). *De novo* paternal deletions of the imprinted *NDN*, and *SNRPN* genes, and possibly other genes within the chromosome region 15q11-q13, lead to PWS, manifested by diminished fetal activity, obesity, muscular hypotonia, mental retardation, short stature, hypogonadotropic hypogonadism, small hands and feet. *De novo* maternal deletions involving the same chromosome region and involving the gene encoding the ubiquitin-protein ligase E3A gene (*UBE3A*) lead to AS, associated with mental retardation, and movement, balance and behavioral disturbances, with severe limitations in speech (42). Imbalanced chromosome translocations leading to inherited small interstitial deletions or mutations in the *UBE3A* gene can be transmitted from an asymptomatic parent, without detection by prenatal testing.

Germline or *gonadal mosacism* refers to the occurrence of affected siblings in whom the mutation has not been established in a parent (43). Such may be the case in unsuspected families with an affected DMD boy in whom the gene defect may reside in the gamete of seemingly unaffected carrier parent as the mutation is not found in parental DNA obtained from blood or other tested tissues specimens. This infrequent event, an important confounder, raised in the counseling of families, can help in educating them about concerns related to future reproductive risks and available options.

Founder effects, a phenomenon of shared identity by common descent, which explains the increased frequency of certain conditions within a particular group of disorders such as hereditary inclusion body myopathy (IBM) among Ashkenazi Jews due to glucosamine (UDP-N-acetyl)-2-epimerase (*GNE*) mutations, with a carrier frequency of 1 in 20 susceptible individuals (44). The AR progressive fatal infantile neurodegenerative disorder Tay Sachs disease (TSD), is caused by mutation in the alpha subunit of the hexosaminidase (*HEXA*) gene among Ashkenazi Jews, the causality of which has been associated with a limited number of mutations. Screening programs can be introduced that offer a high detection rate within the community. Indeed, among the ultra-Orthodox Jews, screening prior to marriage introductions has led to the reduction in the incidence of TSD without the need for pregnancy terminations, as matches or marriages between carriers are discouraged.

CLUES TO GENETIC DIAGNOSIS

Initial clues to the diagnosis of a genetic disorder may be derived from careful clinical and laboratory analysis of the affected patient by a trained geneticist. Currently, readily available random genetic testing that employ disease-based panels are cost ineffective and run the risk of engendering spurious results such as incidental sequence alternations or changes whose significance is uncertain. Evolving techniques employed in genetic diagnosis are anticipated to bring the costs of testing down significantly.

Clues to the cause of myopathic disorders with an LGMD phenotype commences with a family pedigree to elucidate the pattern of inheritance, supplemented by electrodiagnostic studies and direct histological examination of muscle tissue (as indicated). The presence of dystrophic muscle pathology should prompt the performance of specific immunostaining and western blot analysis for evidence of a corresponding sarcoglycanopathy, calveolinopathy, calpainopathy, dysferlinopathy, or α-dystroglycanopathy (45). The demonstration of complete or partial protein deficiency can then be pursued by molecular analysis of the suspected gene mutation.

Clues to the cause of an inherited peripheral neuropathy may similarly be obtained by rigorous evaluation employing electrodiagnostic studies and histopathological examination of an affected cutaneous nerve, prompting appropriately selective molecular testing of the relevant suspected gene involved (46). The cutaneous nerve tissue findings of giant axonal swellings filled with densely packed bundles of neurofilaments and segregation of other axoplasmic organelles should suggest giant axonal neuropathy (GAN) due to AR mutations at the 16q23.2 locus of the *GAN* gene encoding gigaxonin (47). Similar giant axons containing

disorganized neurofilaments are noted in patients with AD CMT2E caused by mutation at the 8p21.2 locus of the *NEFL* gene (48). Focally folded myelin sheaths are seen in cutaneous nerve biopsy of patients with AR CMT4B due to mutation at the 11q21 locus of the *MTMR2* gene (49), while distinctive Schwann cell proliferation with multiple small onion bulbs occur in AR CMT4C due to homozygous or compound mutation at the 5q32 locus of the *SH3TC2* gene (50). Two allelic forms of CMT, AD type 2A2 and HMSN6, due to heterozygous mutation at the 1p36.22 locus of the *MFN2* gene, respectively, show loss of large myelinated fibers but no myelin abnormalities (51) or a mixed axonal pattern of axonal and demyelinating neuropathy with small onion bulbs (52).

ASSIGNMENT OF A GENE DEFECT

The demonstration of a gene sequence alteration does not automatically assign the cause of a disease to a specific genetic defect. Instead, the process of assigning a gene defect proceeds through a series of well-defined steps. First, the suggestion of causality requires functional correlation, such as elaboration of the mutant protein or demonstration of a loss of function as in absent or diminished enzyme activity. Second, assignment of a given genetic defect requires proof of a given pattern of segregation and inheritance, such that the mutation is detectable in affected relatives but absent in unaffected family members. Third, identification of the mutation in other patient cohorts, but not in the general population of otherwise healthy people, suggests even stronger causality. A fourth step involves detailed molecular analyses *in silico* of the gene sequence change employing certain computerized programs directing attention to the corresponding amino acid sequence, and the potential consequences of a change in protein structure. A next step involves identification and clarification of the gene defect, especially with regard to origin by carrier parents, transmission within a family, or the presence of a *de novo* gene mutation.

The identification of the causal basis of many genetic diseases, which in several instances may be polygenic, has enabled classification of those as well as others with often shared phenotypes. For example, a conceptual framework based upon the role or function of the defective gene product has impacted on the approach toward understanding of diverse forms of congenital muscular dystrophy (CMD). The CMD phenotype results from pathogenic mutation in more than one gene encoding a defective structural protein or enzyme (53). Structural proteins implicated in CMD include those localized to the sarcolemma, as well as others to the nuclear and basement membranes.

The elucidation of genetic mechanisms has also derived from experimental murine models of a given disease employing recombinant genetic techniques. Such studies can provide valuable information on the natural history of the disorder and the identification of cellular events prior to the onset of symptoms. On the other hand, the presence of murine models that do not exactly mimic the human situation, even when the same gene (ortholog) is involved, has promoted a shift in interest in the use of patient-derived samples, pluripotent stem cells and cells subjected to cellular reprogramming strategies in the investigation of disease pathophysiology (54). Such methodologies may also prove useful in screening of potential therapies.

The delineation of disease pathogenesis can lead to rational or directed therapies aimed at correcting the root problem instead of relieving symptoms. For many genetic disorders, management is little more than supportive; however, potential therapeutic options directed at genetic, molecular, and biochemical pathways are being intensively scrutinized. Such strategies have been envisioned in disorders characterized by abnormal protein folding in which ER quality control processes instead divert the newly synthesized protein toward premature degradation. These situations have prompted consideration of pharmacologic chaperones to rescue mutant proteins so their maturation and delivery to their appropriate subcellular localizations can be completed (55). The increase in residual protein function in these cases may be sufficient to ameliorate disease phenotype. Disorders in which the gene defect results in the introduction of a premature stop codon might be effectively managed by compounds such as ataluren (PTC124) that allow readthrough (56). The prospects for gene therapy remain promising with ERT already available in several lysosomal disorders, including glycogen storage disease type II (Pompe) caused by α–glucosidase deficiency (57, 58). So far, somatic gene therapy trials involving the transplant of transduced myoblasts have failed to demonstrate efficacy (59).

SUMMARY

The pace of gene discovery has accelerated, from initial linkage-based studies requiring DNA samples from multiple families of several affected individuals, to candidate gene positional cloning, microarray methods, exome sequencing and next-generation sequence analysis. These advances have significantly reduced cost, and offer a promise of a rapid, cost-effective approach to facilitate the diagnosis of inherited neurologic motor disorders. Genetic studies have led to increased understanding of atypical patterns of inheritance and insights into disease mechanisms that may ultimately lead to disease-modifying therapies (60–62).

REFERENCES

1. Zoghbi HY, Warren ST. Neurogenetics: advancing the "next-generation" of brain research. *Neuron* 2010; 68:165–173.
2. Bird TD. Approaches to the patient with neurogenetic disease. *Clin Lab Med* 2010; 30:785–793.
3. Nicholson P, Mühlemann O. Cutting the nonsense: the degradation of PTC-containing mRNAs. *Biochem Soc Trans* 2010; 38:1615–1620.
4. Mehnert M, Sommer T, Jarosch E. ERAD ubiquitin ligases: multifunctional tools for protein quality control and waste disposal in the endoplasmic reticulum. *Bioessays* 2010; 32:905–913.
5. Sultan FA, Day JJ. Epigenetic mechanisms in memory and synaptic function. *Epigenomics* 2011; 3:157–181.
6. Guy J, Cheval H, Selfridge J, et al. The role of MeCP2 in the brain. *Ann Rev Cell Dev Biol* 2011; 27:631–652.
7. Wutz A. Gene silencing in X-chromosome inactivation: advances in understanding facultative heterochromatin formation. *Nat Rev Genet* 2011; 12:542–553.
8. Statland JM, Tawil R. Facioscapulohumeral muscular dystrophy: molecular pathological advances and future directions. *Curr Opin Neurol* 2011; 24:423–428.
9. Ermolova N, Kudryashova E, Difranco M, et al. Pathogenicity of some limb girdle muscular dystrophy mutations can result from reduced anchorage to myofibrils and altered stability of calpain 3. *Hum Mol Genet* 2011; 20:3331–3345.
10. Lin CS, Lee MJ, Park SB, et al. Purple pigments: the pathophysiology of acute porphyric neuropathy. *Clin Neurophysiol* 2011; 122:2336–2344.
11. Gieselmann V. What can cell biology tell us about heterogeneity in lysosomal storage diseases? *Acta Paediatr Suppl* 2005; 94:80–86.
12. Nishikawa T, Kawakami K, Kumamoto T, et al. Severe neurotoxicities in a case of Charcot-Marie-Tooth disease type 2 caused by vincristine for acute lymphoblastic leukemia. *J Pediatr Hematol Oncol* 2008; 30:519–521.
13. Tońska K, Kodroń A, Bartnik E. Genotype-phenotype correlations in Leber hereditary optic neuropathy. *Biochim Biophys Acta* 2010; 1797:1119–1123.
14. Landes T, Leroy I, Bertholet A, et al. OPA1 (dys) functions. *Semin Cell Dev Biol* 2010; 21:593–598.
15. Moorhouse MJ, Sharma HS. Recent advances in i-Gene tools and analysis: microarrays, next generation sequencing and mass spectrometry. *Indian J Biochem Biophys* 2011; 48:215–225.
16. Bamshad MJ, Ng SB, Bigham AW, et al. Exome sequencing as a tool for Mendelian disease gene discovery. *Nat Rev Genet* 2011; 12:745–755.
17. Ku CS, Naidoo N, Pawitan Y. Revisiting Mendelian disorders through exome sequencing. *Hum Genet* 2011; 129:351–370.
18. Ferraiuolo L, Kirby J, Grierson AJ, et al. Molecular pathways of motor neuron injury in amyotrophic lateral sclerosis. *Nat Rev Neurol* 2011; 7:616–630.
19. Crosiers D, Theuns J, Cras P, et al. Parkinson disease: insights in clinical, genetic and pathological features of monogenic disease subtypes. *J Chem Neuroanat* 2011; 42:131–141.
20. Mariotti C, Bella DD, Di Donato S, et al. Spinocerebellar ataxia type 28. *Handb Clin Neurol* 2012; 103:575–579.

21. Sicot G, Gourdon G, Gomes-Pereira M. Myotonic dystrophy, when simple repeats reveal complex pathogenic entities: new findings and future challenges. *Hum Mol Genet* 2011; 20:R116–R123.

22. Kolb SJ, Sutton S, Schoenberg DR. RNA processing defects associated with diseases of the motor neuron. *Muscle Nerve* 2010; 41:5–17.

23. Joyce PI, Fratta P, Fisher EM, et al. SOD1 and TDP-43 animal models of amyotrophic lateral sclerosis: recent advances in understanding disease toward the development of clinical treatments. *Mamm Genome* 2011; 22:420–448.

24. Coady TH, Lorson CL. SMN in spinal muscular atrophy and snRNP biogenesis. *Wiley Interdiscip Rev RNA* 2011; 2:546–564.

25. Morrison LA. Dystrophinopathies. *Handb Clin Neurol* 2011; 101:11–39.

26. Fiskerstrand T, H'mida-Ben Brahim D, Johansson S, et al. Mutations in ABHD12 cause the neurodegenerative disease PHARC: An inborn error of endocannabinoid metabolism. *Am J Hum Genet* 2010; 87:410–417.

27. Cagliani R, Fruguglietti ME, Berardinelli A, et al. New molecular findings in congenital myopathies due to selenoprotein N gene mutations. *J Neurol Sci* 2011; 300:107–113.

28. Schoenmakers E, Agostini M, Mitchell C, et al. Mutations in the selenocysteine insertion sequence-binding protein 2 gene lead to a multisystem selenoprotein deficiency disorder in humans. *J Clin Invest* 2010; 120:4220–4235.

29. Krzyzosiak WJ, Sobczak K, Wojciechowska M, et al. Triplet repeat RNA structure and its role as pathogenic agent and therapeutic target. *Nucleic Acids Res* 2012; 40:11–26.

30. Wright EM, Kerr B. RAS-MAPK pathway disorders: important causes of congenital heart disease, feeding difficulties, developmental delay and short stature. *Arch Dis Child* 2010; 95:724–730.

31. Lee SJ, Lim HS, Masliah E, et al. Protein aggregate spreading in neurodegenerative diseases: Problems and perspectives. *Neurosci Res* 2011; 70:339–348.

32. Blackstone C, O'Kane CJ, Reid E. Hereditary spastic paraplegias: membrane traffic and the motor pathway. *Nat Rev Neurosci* 2011; 12:31-42.

33. Boespflug-Tanguy O, Labauge P, Fogli A, et al. Genes involved in leukodystrophies: a glance at glial functions. *Curr Neurol Neurosci Rep* 2008; 8:217–229.

34. Kimata Y, Kohno K. Endoplasmic reticulum stress-sensing mechanisms in yeast and mammalian cells. *Curr Opin Cell Biol* 2011; 23:135–142.

35. Lax NZ, Turnbull DM, Reeve AK. Mitochondrial mutations: newly discovered players in neuronal degeneration. *Neuroscientist* 2011; 17:645–658.

36. D'Aurelio M, Vives-Bauza C, Davidson MM, et al. Mitochondrial DNA background modifies the bioenergetics of NARP/MILS ATP6 mutant cells. *Hum Mol Genet* 2010; 19:374–386.

37. D'Aurelio M, Vives-Bauza C, Davidson MM, et al. Mitochondrial DNA background modifies the bioenergetics of NARP/MILS ATP6 mutant cells. *Hum Mol Genet* 2010; 19:374–386.

38. Broglio L, Tentorio M, Cotelli MS, et al. Limb-girdle muscular dystrophy-associated protein diseases. *Neurologist* 2010; 16:340–352.

39. Ozelius LJ, Bressman SB. Genetic and clinical features of primary torsion dystonia. *Neurobiol Dis* 2011; 42:127–135.

40. Drolet RE, Sanders JM, Kern JT. Leucine-rich repeat kinase 2 (LRRK2) cellular biology: a review of recent advances in identifying physiological substrates and cellular functions. *J Neurogenet* 2011; 25:140–151.

41. Matos CA, de Macedo-Ribeiro S, Carvalho AL. Polyglutamine diseases: the special case of ataxin-3 and Machado-Joseph disease. *Prog Neurobiol* 2011; 95:26–48.

42. Piedrahita JA. The role of imprinted genes in fetal growth abnormalities. *Birth Defects Res A Clin Mol Teratol* 2011; 91:682–692.

43. Delhanty JD. Inherited aneuploidy: germline mosaicism. *Cytogenet Genome Res* 2011; 133:136–140.

44. Zlotogora J. Multiple mutations responsible for frequent genetic diseases in isolated populations. *Eur J Hum Genet* 2007; 15:272–278.

45. Bushby K. Diagnosis and management of the limb girdle muscular dystrophies. *Pract Neurol* 2009; 9:314–323.

46. Wilmshurst JM, Ouvrier R. Hereditary peripheral neuropathies of childhood: A brief overview for clinicians. *Neuromuscul Disord* 2011; 21:763–775.

47. Tazir M, Nouioua S, Magy L, et al. Phenotypic variability in giant axonal neuropathy. *Neuromuscul Disord* 2009; 19:270–274.

48. Fabrizi GM, Cavallaro T, Angiari C, et al. Giant axonal and neurofilament accumulation in Charcot-Marie-Tooth disease type 2E. *Neurology* 2004; 62:1429–1431.

49. Quattrone A, Gambardella A, Bono F, et al. Autosomal recessive hereditary moor and sensory neuropathy with focally folded myelin sheaths: clinical, electrophysiologic, and genetic aspects of a large family. *Neurology* 1996; 46:1318–1324.

50. Kessali M, Zemmouri R, Guilbot A, et al. Clinical, electrophysiologic, neuropathologic, and genetic study of two large Algerian families with an autosomal recessive demyelinating form of Charcot-Marie-Tooth disease. *Neurology* 1997; 48.867–873.

51. Muglia M, Zappia M, Timmerman V, et al. Clinical and genetic study of a large Charcot-Marie-Tooth type 2A family from southern Italy. *Neurology* 2001; 56:100–103.

52. Ippel EF, Wittebol-Post D, Jennikens FGI, et al. Genetic heterogeneity of hereditary motor and sensory neuropathy type VI. *Child Neurol* 1995; 10:459–463.

53. Sparks SE, Escolar DM. Congenital muscular dystrophies. *Handb Clin Neurol* 2011; 101:47–79.

54. Chang KH, Bonig H, Papayannopoulou T. Generation and characterization of erythroid cells from human embryonic stem cells and induced pluripotent stem cells; an overview. *Stem Cells Int* 2011; Article ID 791604.

55. Valenzano KJ, Khanna R, Powe AC, Boyd et al. Identification and characterization of pharmacological chaperones to correct enzyme deficiencies in lysosomal storage disorders. *Assay Drug Dev Technol* 2011; 9:213–235.

56. Rowe SM, Clancy JP. Pharmaceuticals targeting nonsense mutations in genetic diseases: progress in development. *BioDrugs* 2009; 23:165–174.

57. Bowers WJ, Breakefield XO, Sena-Esteves M. Genetic therapy for the nervous system. *Hum Mol Genet* 2011; 20:R28–R41.

58. Beck M. Therapy for lysosomal storage disorders. *IUBMB Life* 2010; 62:33–40.

59. Shadrach JL, Wagers AJ. Stem cells for skeletal muscle repair. *Philos Trans R Soc Lond B Biol Sci* 2011; 366:2297–2306.

60. Gropman AL, Adams DR. Atypical patterns of inheritance. *Semin Pediatr Neurol* 2007; 14:34–45.

61. Hammond SM, Wood MJ. Genetic therapies for RNA missplicing diseases. *Trends Genet* 2011; 27:196–205.

62. Wilton SD, Fletcher S. RNA splicing manipulation: strategies to modify gene expression for a variety of therapeutic outcomes. *Curr Gene Ther* 2011; 11:259–275.

CHAPTER 11

Neurologic Hereditary Metabolic Diseases of Infancy and Childhood

David S. Younger

Neurologic hereditary metabolic disease (NHMD) can lead to motor disturbances that become clinically evident from the neonatal period through early and late infancy to childhood, each with a purported biochemical, molecular or cytogenetic defect, and unique genetic inheritance pattern. An appreciation of these disorders is essential to a clear understanding of the natural history, prognosis, and therapeutic decisions, including genetic counseling for prenatal diagnosis and carrier detection, and in the selection of potentially effective treatments to preserve neurological function and forestall deterioration. Even though each of the NHMD is exceedingly rare, the group as a whole is not, with an estimated prevalence of 1:5,000 (1).

CLASSIFICATION

The vast number of NHMD can be categorized into one of three possible etiopathogenic disturbances causing: 1) Storage of large molecule metabolism such as glycolipids and glycoproteins as occurs in lysosomal, leukodystrophy, and peroxisomal storage disorders affecting multiple visceral organs and the nervous system over time; 2) Altered small molecule metabolism as, for example, amino acids as in amino acid and organic acidurias, and urea cycle disorders that lead to early acute toxicity; 3) Glycolytic, fatty acid, and mitochondrial metabolic disturbances with deficient energy production resulting in slowly progressive and static motor disturbances and intermittent crises. Another method of classification is by age at onset from neonatal to early and late infancy or childhood. The genetic basis of the NHMD includes autosomal recessive (AR), dominant (AD), X-linked (XL), and mitochondrial DNA (mtDNA) inheritance.

MOTOR ASSESSMENT

The neurological evaluation of motor function and motor behavior in infancy and early childhood can be challenging. Systemically addressed, it can provide helpful information in the diagnosis of a NHMD, and in identifying patients likely to benefit from early intervention (2). The available methods to assess and objectify motor function from birth to six years vary widely and differ in validity and reliability. They include modifications of the standard pediatric neurological examination, which generally incorporates aspects of cognition, cranial nerve function, skeletal muscle tone, strength, coordination, posture, and reflexes (3, 4); condensed neurological assessments with standardized scoring (5–12); instruments that focus on observations of milestones and specific aspects of motor behavior (13, 14); and others that focus on assessment of the quality of motor behavior, including postural adjustments (15–17). The most accurate assessment is achieved through a combination of the neurological examination, achieved milestones, and assessment of the quality of motor behavior.

OVERVIEW OF NHMD IN DIFFERENT STAGES OF CHILDHOOD

Clues to the presence of a NHMD in the neonatal period may occur in a low Apgar score at birth, and impaired alertness resulting in lethargy, stupor, or coma. In addition, pupillary changes, impaired visual acuity, and oculomotor function leading to altered visual fixation and tracking. There may be abnormal postures and automatisms of the trunk and limbs, impairment of the Moro response, and abnormal supporting, placing, stepping reactions, palmar grasping, and tonic neck reflexes. Reduced sucking and swallowing mechanisms and seizures may occur, the latter presenting clinically with momentary apnea, tonic turning, posturing, eye and limb jerks, flexor and extensor spasms.

Electroencephalography (EEG) may show more severely disorganized background rhythms, multifocal and periodic bursts of epileptiform sharp waves, and intervening depressions that correspond to clinical flexor spasms as noted in hypsarrythmia. Associated findings suggestive of an NHMD include disturbance of the respiration, a peculiar odor of the urine, cardiomyopathy, organomegaly, and polycystic kidneys; dysmorphic facial features, micro- and macrocephaly, skeletal changes, disturbed skin and hair, and ocular abnormalities such as cataracts, corneal opacities, and retinal degeneration. Concomitant hypoglycemia, metabolic acidosis, and ketosis are features suggestive of the aminoacidopathy and organic acidopathy, defects in biotin metabolism, and disturbances in carbohydrate metabolism. Marked hyperammonemia and respiratory alkalosis occur in urea cycle disorders.

Lactic acidosis in blood and cerebrospinal fluid (CSF) are clues of an underlying mitochondrial disorder affecting pyruvate and respiratory chain reactions, while hypoglycemia and ketone bodies are seen in disorders of mitochondrial fatty acid oxidation. Elevated saturated very long-chain fatty acids (VLCFA) suggest multisystem peroxisomal disease belonging to one of two groups, one with virtual absence of peroxisomes and peroxisomal function, and a second with single enzyme deficiencies of β-oxidation.

Suspicion of an early infantile NHMD in the first year of life arises in infants with neurological regression, delayed or arrested development, and lack of visual interest in the surroundings, as well as poor head control, inability to roll over, sit unsupported, or productively use the hands due to poor motor control.

Predictive ocular abnormalities present in this age group include cataracts, corneal opacities, macular cherry red spot, macular degeneration, optic atrophy, chorioretinal degeneration, nystagmus, and supranuclear gaze palsies. Other important neurological phenomena include concomitant rigidity, hypotonia, peripheral neuropathy, extrapyramidal features including chorea, athetosis, dystonia, or ataxia, and abnormal respiratory movements. There may be non-neurological abnormalities such as vomiting, feeding disturbance; spleno-, cardio-, and hepatomegaly, dysmorphic facial features, skeletal changes, short stature, skin and hair features, renal tubular dysfunction, and abnormal bone marrow cell inclusions.

Early infantile NHMD can be divided into those that present with relentless progression or intermittent remission. In the first category are lysosomal storage disorders, sialidoses, glycogenoses, infantile leukodystrophies, and selective enzymopathies associated with cutaneous signs and frequent seizures as may be seen in oculocerebral syndrome of Lowe, inborn errors of aminobutyric acid, amino and organic acids, and disturbed glycosylation. The remitting disorders can be divided into those with disturbed pyruvate metabolism and mitochondrial fatty acid oxidation culminating in episodic nonketotic hypoglycemia, and inherited disorders of amino and organic acid metabolism leading to intermittent ketoacidosis including maple syrup urine disease (MSUD), and late onset urea cycle.

A late infantile NHMD presents in the second year of life with three suggestive patterns. One is progressive loss of motor function, such as children who have achieved independent locomotion, then develop increasing difficulty in doing so, due to motor regression or superimposed pyramidal, extrapyramidal, cerebellar, and peripheral nerve involvement, alone or in combination.

Disorders of onset of walking and limb coordination include metachromatic leukodystrophy (MLD), neuroaxonal dystrophy, ataxia telangietasia (AT), late infantile Neimann Pick disease, GM1 and GM2 gangliosidoses, Krabbe disease, Gaucher disease type III, and late infantile Leigh disease.

A second pattern of an NHMD is the occurrence of intermittent attacks of acute neurological dysfunction with irritability, lethargy, confusion, seizures, ataxia, and coma, suggestive of amino acid and organic acidopathy, and mitochondrial disease.

A third presentation of NHMD is intellectual impairment with intellectual and behavior disturbances leading to mental retardation, auditory and visual impairment, often in association with distinctive facial features and skeletal changes, as may be seen in the mucopolysaccharidoses (MPS), mucolipidoses (ML), and disorders of glycoproteinoses.

Childhood and adolescent NHMD present, in addition, with action myoclonus, extrapyramidal features, diffuse cerebrospinal involvement, behavioral and cognitive changes, and isolated stroke disorders. Action myoclonus is associated with progressive myoclonic epilepsies and present with polymyoclonus, seizures, and ataxia. Late childhood extrapyramidal involvement due to involvement of the basal ganglia leads to rigidity, involuntary movements, tremor, muscle spasm, and abnormal postures. The findings of juvenile Parkinson disease (PD) include rigidity, tremor, and akinesia; whereas chorea typifies juvenile Huntington (HD), Wilson (WD), and chorea acanthocytosis (ChAc). The forceful postures of dystonia occur in primary torsion and focal hereditary dystonia, whereas secondary dystonias may result from pallidal iron deposition as in Hallevorden Spatz disease.

Diffuse cerebrospinal involvement is characteristic of lysosomal, peroxisomal, and mitochondrial disorders that resemble those of infancy. Personality, behavioral, and mental regression, accompanied by psychiatric outbreaks and progressive dementia, occurs in HD, adrenoleukodystrophy (ALD), WD, HD, juvenile neuronal ceroid lipofuscinosis (NCL), MLD, GM2 gangliosidosis, Leigh syndrome, Lafora disease, amino and organic acidopathy, and Lesch-Nyan disease. Isolated strokes occur in disturbed homocystine metabolism and Fabry disease.

SPECIFIC CONDITIONS

Urea Cycle Disorders

The inborn amino acid and organic acid disorders have been reviewed (18–20). The overall incidence of urea cycle disorders is 1:30,000 live births. Deficiency of a cofactor producing enzyme, N-acetylglutamate synthetase (NAGS), and five catalytic enzymes, carbamoylphosphate synthetase-1 (CPS I), ornithine transcarbamylase (OTC), arginosuccinic acid synthetase (ASS) and arginosuccinate lyase (ASL), and arginase-1 (ARG1) are at fault in the urea cycle disorders that disturb the conversion of ammonia to urea in the Krebs cycle. Neonates affected by a urea cycle disorder generally present with poor feeding and acute episodes of vomiting, under-activity, irritability, bulging of the fontanelles, and progressive lethargy due to hyperammonemia and cerebral edema after protein consumption.

Arginase deficiency progresses into childhood with growth and intellectual failure, hyperactivity, and progressive spastic paraplegia. Almost all of the urea cycle disorders manifest AR inheritance with the exception of XL-OTC deficiency. The gene defects have been assigned to mutations at the 17q21.31 locus of the NAGS gene encoding NAGS; the 2q34 locus of the CPS1 gene encoding CPS; the Xp11.4 locus of the OTC gene encoding OTC; the 9q34.11 locus of the ASS1gene encoding ASS; the 7q11.21 locus of the ASL gene that encodes ASL; and the 6q23.2 locus of the ARG1 gene encoding ARG1 (Table 1).

Once a presumptive or conclusive diagnosis of a urea cycle disorder is established, treatment should be tailored to the specific biochemical defect. The acute care is directed toward returning blood ammonia and glutamine levels to normal to prevent irreversible neurological injury and death. Effective therapy starts with dialysis in emergent situations and dietary modification, installing high calorie, low protein diet supplements with essential amino acids, adding intravenous citrulline in cases of CPS, OTC, and AS, and intravenous arginine in ASS and ASL deficiency. Parenteral sodium benzoate, sodium phenylacetate, and phenylbutyrate can facilitate the excretion of excessive nitrogen by acting as an ammonia scavenger. Liver transplantation is the most effective means of preventing hyperammonemic crises in selected patients but has substantial risk related to rejection and immunosuppressant medication toxicity.

Prenatal diagnosis is possible by analysis of DNA extracted from fetal cells by amniocentesis at 15 to 18 weeks gestation and chorionic villus sampling (CVS) at 10 to 12 weeks gestation, if the disease causing alleles of a family member with urea cycle disorder are known. In families in which the mutation cannot be detected by molecular genetic analysis, linkage analysis is an option. Preimplantation genetic diagnosis may be available in selected disease-causing mutations.

Amino Acid and Organic Acid Disorders

Three disorders, hyperornithinemia-hyperammonemia-homocitrullinuria (HHH), nonketotic hyperglycinemia (NKH), and MSUD result from AR inborn errors amino acid metabolism. Affected neonates typically develop rapidly evolving vomiting, lethargy, stupor, coma, and even respiratory failure following the introduction of protein feeding. Brain computed tomography (CT) and magnetic resonance imaging (MRI) show variable cerebral edema and developmental defects, especially in the corpus callosum, whereas EEG exhibits hypsarrythmia and infantile spasms with sustained illness. The underlying defect in HHH is a mutation at the 13q14.11 locus of the SCL25A15 gene that encodes mitochondrial ornithine transporter (Table 1). The underlying defect in NKH is a mutation at the 9p24.1 locus of the GLDC gene that encodes P protein (Table 1). Maple syrup urine disease results from a mutation at the 19q13.2 locus of the E1 subunit of the BCKDHA gene that encodes α–keto acid dehydrogenase (Table 1).

Four other AR inherited disorders lead to significant illness in the neonatal period, sulfite oxidase deficiency, isovaleric and proprionic acidemia, and methylmalonic aciduria (MMA). In its classic severe form, sulfite oxidase deficiency manifests shortly after birth with feeding difficulty, hypomotility, hypotonia, potentially fatal neonatal seizures, metabolic crises, and eventual death at an early age. It results from a disease-causing mutation at the 12q13.2 locus of the SUOX gene that encodes sulfite oxidase (Table 1). Isovaleric acidemia presents shortly after birth with vomiting, lethargy, hypotonia, tremor, myoclonic jerks, seizures, and hypothermia. Clues to the diagnosis include acidosis without ketosis, and distinctive sweating feet or cheesy odors in the urine and sweat that permeate the infant's room, combined with elevated urinary isovaleryl glycine. The underlying genetic defect is caused by a mutation at the 15q15.1 locus of the IVD gene that encodes isovaleryl-CoA dehydrogenase (Table 1). Treatment of both is focused on management of ketoacidosis and hyperammonemia.

Propionic and MMA present shortly after birth with crises of metabolic acidosis after protein feeding, accompanied by anorexia, vomiting, lethargy, hyperventilation, and seizures. Glycine levels are elevated in the serum and urine,

TABLE 1. The Genetic Basis of NHMD of Infancy and Childhood

Disease	Enzyme Deficiency	Gene; OMIM[1]
Urea Cycle Disorders[AR]		
N-acetylglutamate synthetase deficiency	N-acetylglutamate synthetase	NAGS; 237310
Carbamoylphosphate synthetase-1 deficiency	Carbamoyl-phosphate synthetase	CPS1; 608307
Ornithine transcarbamylase deficiency[XL]	Ornithine transcarbamylase	OTC; 311250
Arginosuccinic acid synthetase deficiency	Arginosuccinate synthetase	ASS1; 215700
Arginosuccinate lyase deficiency	Arginosuccinate lyase	ASL; 207900
Arginase deficiency	Arginase-1	ARG1; 207800
Amino Acid and Organic Acid Disorders[AR]		
Hyperonithineemia-hyperammonemia-homocitrullinuria	Mitochondrial ornithine transporter	SLC25A15; 238970
Nonketotic hyperglycinemia	P-protein	GLDC; 605899
Maple syrup urine disease	α-Keto acid dehydrogenase	BCKDHA; 248600
Sulfite oxidase deficiency	Sulfite oxidase	SUOX; 606887
Isovaleric acidemia	Isovaleryl-CoA dehydrogenase	IVD; 243500
Propionic acidemia	Propiony-CoA carboxyclase	PCCA/B; 606054
Methylmalonic aciduria	Methylmalonyl-CoA mutase	MUT; 251000
Mitochondrial Deficiency Disorders[AR]		
Disturbances of pyruvate metabolism and respiratory chain defects		
Pyruvate dehydrogenase deficiency[XL]	Pyruvate decarboxylase	PDHA1; 300502
Pyruvate carboxylase deficiency	Pyruvate carboxylase	PC; 608786
NADH-ubiquinone oxidoreductase Fe-S protein 4 deficiency	NADH-ubiquinone oxidoreductase	NDUFS4; 602694
Fatal infantile cardioencephalomyopathy	Cytochrome c oxidase	SCO2; 604377
Progressive external ophthalmoplegia[AD/R; mtDNA]	DNA polymerase	POLG; 157640
Kearns-Sayre syndrome[mtDNA]		tRNA; 530000
MELAS[mtDNA]		MTTL1 (3243A-G); 540000
Leigh syndrome[AR, XL, mtDNA]	Cytochrome c oxidase	SURF1; 185620
Mitochondrial DNA depletion syndrome 1 (MNGIE type)	Thymidine phosphorylase	TYMP; 603041
Disturbances of fatty acid oxidation		
Primary systemic carnitine deficiency	Carnitine transporter OCTN2	SLC22A5; 212140
Lethal neonatal carnitine palmityoltransferase II deficiency	Carnitine palmitoyltransferase II	CPT2; 608836
Carnitine-acylcarnitine translocase deficiency	Carnitine-acylcarnitine translocase	SLC25A20; 212138
Acyl-CoA dehydrogenase, very long-chain deficiency	VLCAD	ACADVL; 201475
Acyl-CoA dehydrogenase, short-chain deficiency	SCAD	ACADS; 201470
Acyl-CoA dehydrogenase, medium-chain deficiency	MCAD	ACADM; 201450
3-hydroxyacyl-CoA dehydrogenase deficiency	SCHAD	HADHSC; 231530
Long-chain 3-hydroxyacyl-CoA dehydrogenase	LCHAD	HADHA; 609016
Trifunctional protein deficiency	Mitochondrial trifunctional protein	HADHA/B; 609015
Peroxisomal Biogenesis Disorders[AR]		
Zellweger syndrome	Peroxin	PEX1; 214100
Neonatal adrenoleukodystrophy	Peroxin	PEX1; 202370
Infantine Refsum disease	Peroxin	PEX1; 266510
Glycogenoses and Fructose Disorders[AR]		
Fructose-1,6-bisphosphatase deficiency	Fructose-1, 6-biphosphatase	FBP1; 229700
Fructose intolerance	Aldolase B	ALDOB; 229600
Glycogen storage disease La	Glucose-6-phosphatase	G6PC; 232200
Glycogen storage disease II (Pompe)	Acid alpha-1,4-glucosidase	GAA; 232300

Disease	Enzyme Deficiency	Gene; OMIM[1]
Lysosomal Disorders[AR]		
Neurolipidoses		
Tay-Sachs disease	Alpha subunit of HexA	HEXA; 272800
Sandhoff	Beta subunit of HexA	HEXB; 268800
GM2-gangliosidosis, AB Variant	GM2 activator	GM2A; 272750
GM1-gangliosidosis, type I	Beta-galactosidase-1	GLB1; 230500
Neimann-Pick, type A	Sphingomyelinase	SMPD1; 257200
Neimann-Pick type B	Sphingomyelinase	SMPD1; 607616
Gaucher disease, type II	Acid beta-glucosidase	GBA; 230900
Gaucher disease, type III	Acid-beta-glucosidase	GBA; 231000
Farbers lipogranulomatosis	Ceramidase	ASAH1; 228000
Mucopolysaccharidoses (MPS)		
MPSIH (Hurler)	Alpha-L-iduronidase	IDUA; 607014
MPSI-HS (Hurler-Scheie)	Alpha-L-iduronidase	IDUA; 607015
MPSI-S (Scheie)	Alpha-L-iduronidase	IDUA; 607016
MPSII (Hunter) [XL]	Iduronate 2-sulfatase	IDS; 309900
MPSIIIA (Sanfilippo A)	N-sulfoglucoasmine sulfohydrolase	SGSH; 252900
MPSIIIB (Sanfilippo B)	N-alpha-acetylglucosaminidase	NAGLU; 252920
MPSIIIC (Sanfilippo C)	Acetyl-CoA:a-glucosaminide N-acetyltransferase	HGSNAT; 252930
MPSIII D (Sanfilippo D)	N-acetylglucosamine-6-sulfatase	GNS; 252940
MPSIVA (Morquio A)	Galactosamine-6-sulfate sulfatase	GALNS; 253000
MPSIVB (Morquio B)	Beta-galactosidase	GLB1; 253010
Mucolipidoses (ML)		
MLI	Neuraminidase	NEU1; 256550
MLII	GLcNAc-phosphotransferase	GNPTAB; 252500
MLIII	GLcNAc-phosphotransferase	GNPTAB; 252600
MLIV	Mucolipin-1	MCOLN1; 252650
Neuronal ceroid lipofucsinoses		
Infantile	Palmitoyl-protein thioesterase 1	PPT1; 256730
Late infantile	Tripeptidyl-peptidase 1	TPP1; 204500
Juvenile	Battenin	CLN3; 204200
Glycoproteinoses		
Mannosidosis, Alpha B	Alpha-mannosidase	MAN2B1; 248500
Mannosidosis, Beta A	Beta-mannosidosis	MANBA; 248510
Fucosidosis	Alpha-L-fucosidase	FUCA1; 230000
Galactosialidosis	Cathespin A	CTSA; 256540
Aspartylglucosammonuria	Glycosylasparaginase	AGA; 208400
Leukodystrophies		
Krabbe disease	Galactocerebrosidase	GALC; 245200
Metachromatic leukodystrophy	Arylsulfatase A	ARSA; 250100
Multiple sulfatase deficiency	Multiple sulfatases	SUMF1; 272200
Pelizaeus-Merzbacher disease[XL]	Proteolipid protein-1	PLP1; 312080
Adrenoleukodystrophy[XL]	Adrenoleukodystrophy protein	ABCD1; 300100
Canavan disease	Aspartoacylase	ASPA; 271900
Alexander disease[AD]	Glial fibrillary acidic protein	GFAP; 203450
Hereditary Extrapyramldal Disorders[AR]		
Wilson disease	Ceruloplasmin	ATP7B; 277900
Huntington disease[AD]	Huntingtin	HTT; 143100
Juvenile Parkinson disease	Parkin	PARK2; 600116
Choreoacanthocytosis	Chorein	VPS13A; 200150
Lesch-Nyhan syndrome[XL]	HPRT	HPRT1; 300322

Disease	Enzyme Deficiency	Gene; OMIM[1]
Torsion dystonia[AD]	Torsin-A	DYT1; 128100
Dopa-responsive dystonia[AD]	GTP cyclohydrolase I	GCH1; 128230
Myoclonic dystonia[AD]	ε-sarcoglycan	SGCE; 159900
Dystonia-Parkinsonism[AD]	N, K-ATPase	ATP1A3; 128235
Hallevorden-Spatz disease	Pantothenate kinase 2	PANK2; 234200
Hereditary Spastic Paraplegia[XL]		
MASA syndrome (SPG1)	Neural cell adhesion molecule L1	L1CAM; 303350
Spastic paraplegia 2 (SPG2)	Myelin proteolipid protein	PLP1; 312920
Allan-Herndon-Dudley syndrome	Monocarboxylate transporter-8	SLC16A21; 300523
MAST syndrome (SPG21)	33-kD acidic-cluster protein	SPG21; 248900
Progressive Ataxias[AR]		
Spinocerebellar ataxia-27[AD]	Fibroblast growth factor-14	FGF14; 609307
Mitochondrial DNA depletion syndrome 7 (IOSCA)	Twinke/twinky proteins	C10orf2; 271245
Friedreich ataxia 1	Frataxin	FXN; 229300
Disorders Associated with Seizures[AR]		
Biotinidase deficiency	Biotinidase	BTD; 253260
Menkes disease[XL]	ATPase alpha polypeptide	ATP7A; 309400
Mitochondrial DNA depletion syndrome 4A (Alpers)	Mitchondrial DNA polymerase γ	POLG; 2037000
GLUT1 deficiency syndrome	GLUT1 transporter	SLCA1; 606777
Myoclonic epilepsy of Unverricht and Lundborg	Cystatin B	CSTB; 254800
Myoclonic epilepsy 2A (Lafora)	Laforin	EPM2A; 254780
Myoclonic epilepsy 2B	Malin	NHLRC1; 254780
MERRF[mtDNA]		MTTK; 545000
Familial Polyneuropathies[AD]		
Classic Refsum disease[AR]	Phytanoyl-CoA hydrolase/peroxin-7	PHYH/PEX7; 266500
Transthyretin amyloidosis	Transthyretin	TTR; 105210
Fabry disease[XL]	α-galactosidase A	GLA; 301500
Charcot-Marie-Tooth (CMT) Disease		
CMT1A	Peripheral myelin protein 22	PMP22; 118220
CMT1B	Myelin P0 protein	MPZ; 118200
CMT1C	LPS-induced TNF-alpha factor	LITAF; 601098
CMT1D	Early growth response protein 2	ERG2; 607678
CMT2A2	Mitofusin-2	MFN2; 609260
CMT2B	GTPase late endosomal protein	RAB7; 600882
CMT2D	Glycyl tRNA synthetase	GARS; 601472
CMT2E	Light polypeptide neurofilament protein	NEFL; 607684
CMT2F	Heat-shock 27-kD protein-1	HSPB1; 606595
CMT4A[AR]	Ganglioside-induced differentiation-Associated protein 1	GDAP1; 214400
CMT4F[AR]	Periaxin	PRX; 145900
CMTX1[XL]	Gap junction beta-1 protein	GJB1; 302800
HNPP	Peripheral myelin protein 22	PMP22; 162500
Hereditary Sensory and Autonomic Neuropathy (HSAN)		
HSAN IA	Serine palmitoyltransferase 1	SPTLC1; 162400
HSAN II[AR]	Serine/threonine-protein kinase WNK1	WNK1; 201300
HSAN IIB[AR]	Protein FAM13	FAM134B; 613115
HSAN III[AR]	Elongator complex protein 1	IKBKAP; 223900
HSAN IV[AR]	Neurotrophic tyrosine kinase-1 receptor	NTRK1; 256800
HSAN V[AR]	Nerve growth factor-β	NGFB; 608654

[1]OMIM: Online Mendelian Inheritance in Man (http://www.ncbi.nim.nih.gov/omim/).

accompanied by neutropenia. The underlying genetic defect in proprionic acidemia is a mutation at the 3q22.3 locus of the *PCCB* gene encoding propiony-CoA carboxylase, while mutation at the 6p12.3 locus in the *MUT* gene in MMA encodes methylmalonyl-CoA mutase (Table 1). While similar in principle, therapy depends upon the biochemical defect, the location of the metabolic block, and the effect of the resulting toxic compounds. Parenteral administration of sodium bicarbonate, glucose, and adequate fluids corrects acidosis, hypoglycemia, and hypovolemia. Later, metabolic formulas deficient in the particular precursor amino acid for each disorder, with adequate calories supplied as carbohydrates and fat, can be given orally, or as total parenteral nutrition during gastrointestinal illness or surgery. Adjunctive compounds such as thiamine, hydroxocobalamin, and non-absorbed antibiotics can be given respectively in MSUD, MMA, and propionate acidemia to reduce the levels of toxic metabolites.

Combined liver-kidney transplantation in selected patients with MMA can lead to a marked reduction in serum and urine methylmalonic acid levels, as well as a cessation of metabolic decompensations (21), but carries the risk of rejection and toxicity from immunosuppressant medications.

Prenatal testing is available by amniocentesis in isovaleric, propionic acidemia, and MMA, and via fetal cell analysis by CVS in MSUD. Preimplantation genetic diagnosis may also be available for families in which the disease-causing mutations have already been identified.

Mitochondrial Deficiency Disorders

There are several excellent reviews of inborn mitochondrial defects (22–24). Mitochondrial disorders present with disturbances in pyruvate, respiratory chain metabolism, and fatty acid oxidation due to mutations of nuclear and mtDNA, the former leading to AR, AD, and XL inheritance patterns, and the latter to maternal inheritance.

The incidence of infantile mitochondrial myopathy is estimated to be 1:51,000, while mitochondrial encephalomyopathies in preschool children less than six years of age is 1:11,000.

Two disorders of pyruvate metabolism include XL inherited pyruvate dehydrogenase (PDH) complex and AR pyruvate carboxylase (PC) enzyme deficiency. Both have variable clinical expression with severe neonatal or early infantile onset to relatively benign late infantile and childhood forms, with the most severely afflicted manifesting low birth weight, weak suck, hypotonia, lethargy, dysmorphic features often progressing to fatal respiratory distress, and cerebral deficits on neurological bedside examination and neuroimaging.

Pyruvate dehydrogenase deficiency results from mutations at the Xp22.12 locus of the *PDHA1* gene that encodes the α subunit of pyruvate decarboxylase (Table 1), the first of three enzymes in the PDH complex, while the β subunit of the E1 enzyme is encoded by the PDHB gene on chromosome 3p.

Pyrvuate carboxylase deficiency results from a mutation at the 11q13.2 locus of the *PC* gene that encodes the enzyme pyruvate decarboxylase (Table 1). Two respiratory chain defects arise from mutations in the nuclear genome leading to deficiency of NADH-ubiquinone oxidoreductase Fe-S protein 4 and cytochrome-c oxidase (COX), both of which present with rapidly progressive lactic acidosis, hypotonia, seizures, coma, and respiratory failure. NADH-ubiquinone oxidoreductase Fe-S protein 4 is the first multisubunit enzyme complex of the mitochondrial respiratory chain and plays a vital role in cellular ATP production, removing electrons from NADA and passing them by a series of protein-coupled redox centers to the electron acceptor ubiquinone. The deficiency disorder is due to a mutation at the 5q11.2 locus in the *NDUFS4* gene that encodes NADH-ubiquinone oxidoreductase (Table 1).

Unlike PC deficiency, those affected by PDH deficiency present with normal lactate to pyruvate ratio in the plasma and the cerebrospinal fluid (CSF) lactate levels are higher than those in the blood, giving rise to the term *cerebral lactic acidosis*. Enzyme activity assays in serum, immunoblot and sequence analysis of the respective genes make the diagnosis of these two disorders. Treatment focuses on providing alternative energy sources, hydration, and correction of metabolic acidosis during acute decompensation. Thiamine and lipoic acid, which can optimize PDHC activity may be useful in PC deficiency to reduce plasma and urine pyruvate and lactate concentrations through alternative routes of pyruvate metabolism. Carrier dectection is available for at-risk family members.

Two predictable phenotypes associated with mtDNA deletions include progressive external ophthalmoplegia (PEO) and Kearns-Sayre syndrome (KSS). The syndrome of PEO consists of ptosis, ophthalmoplegia, and variable proximal limb weakness. The multisystemic disorder KSS is defined by the obligatory triad of onset before age 20 years, pigmentary retinopathy, PEO, and one of the following: cardiac conduction block, CSF protein content >100 mg/dL, and cerebellar ataxia. Other frequent but not invariable findings include short stature, hearing loss, dementia, diabetes mellitus, hypoparathyroidism, and growth hormone deficiency. A few individuals with PEO have other manifestations of KSS but do not fulfill all the clinical criteria.

The diagnosis of an mtDNA deletion syndrome relies upon the presence of characteristic clinical findings, and in KSS, the presence of ragged red fiber (RRF) in muscle biopsy tissue with the modified Gomori trichrome stain, hyperactive fibers with succinate dehydrogenase (SDH) stain, decreased staining for COX, and activity of respiratory chain complexes containing mtDNA-encoded subunits in muscle extracts. Autosomal dominant PEO with mtDNA deletions-1 (PEO1) is caused by a mutation at the 15q26.1 locus of the *POLG* gene (Table 1), as well as in multiple mtDNA genes. Although more than 150 different mtDNA deletions occur with KSS, one 4977 bp known as m.8470_13446del4977 is the most frequently encountered. However, for all mtDNA mutations, clinical expressivity depends upon the tissue distribution, relative abundance of mutant mtDNA, and the threshold effect or vulnerability of the organ affected. Treatment of the manifestations in KSS includes consideration of a cardiac pacemaker, hearing aid or cochlear implant, and administration of coenzyme Q10 and L-carnitine in both PEO and KSS. Prenatal diagnosis of mtDNA mutation, while theoretically possible, is problematic.

Mitochondrial encephalomyopathy with lactic acidosis and seizures (MELAS) is a genetically heterogeneous disorder with onset between age 2 to 10 years, generalized tonic clonic seizures, episodic recurrent headache, anorexia, and vomiting in association with mitochondrial myopathy, serum and CSF lactic acidosis, elevated CSF protein, and areas of T2-signal abnormality on brain MRI in the posterior cerebrum not confined to the distribution of major arteries; early psychomotor development is always normal. The most frequent mutations in MELAS are at m.3243A>G in the tRNA gene MT-TL1 encoding tRNA leucine 1 in up to 80% of patients (Table 1), and in the MT-ND5 gene encoding NADH-ubiquinone oxidoreductase subunit 5, and other mtDNA tRNA genes in the remaining cases. Mutations can be present in all tissues, including blood in typical MELAS. Targeted mutation analysis is clinically available for the most common MT-ND5 mutation. No specific treatment exists for MELAS, however, coenzyme Q10 and L-carnitine may be of some benefit.

Leigh syndrome of subacute relapsing encephalopathy presents in infancy with psychomotor regression or delay and manifestations of disease in the brain stem and basal ganglia. It is uncommonly due to an mtDNA deletion, and more often due to a mutation at the 9q34.2 locus of SURF1 gene associated with COX deficiency (Table 1).

One other disorder, mitochondrial neurogastrointestinal encephalomyopathy, (MNGIE) or mitochondrial DNA depletion syndrome type-1, has AR onset in the first to fifth decade with ptosis, PEO, gastrointestinal dysmotility presenting with nausea, reflux, cachexia or pseudo-obstruction, and peripheral demyelinating neuropathy (25). Brain MRI shows leukoencephalopathy with relative sparing of the corpus callosum. The diagnosis of MNGIE is supported by RRF and complex IV COX defects in muscle biopsy tissue, mtDNA depletion relative to nuclear DNA, an increase in plasma thymidine concentrations, and decrease in thymidine phosphorylase activity in leukocytes. The disorder is caused by a homozygous or compound heterozygous mutation at the 22q13.33 locus of the TYMP gene that encodes thymidine phosphorylase (Table 1).

Fatty acids are an important source of energy, and mitochondrial fatty acid oxidation (FAO) is the principal pathway for oxidation of FA. Peroxisomes play an indispensable role in FAO by catalyzing b-oxidation of a range of FA, and FA derivatives not handled by mitochondria. The mitochondrial b-oxidation system is required for the degradation of FA derived from different sources, including diet, de novo synthesis, release from adipose tissue, and from different intracellular sources including the peroxisome and lysosome. Fatty acids are rapidly activated to corresponding CoA esters by one of a variety of acyl-CoA synthetases and traverse the mitochondrial inner membrane by the carnitine shuttle. Once inside, the acyl-CoA esters can be b-oxidized and fully degraded to CO_2 and H_2O. Patients with suspected mitochondrial b-oxidation defects present with distinctive clinical findings and a characteristic acylcarnitine profile according to the individual underlying b-oxidation defect.

The mitochondrial carnitine cycle requires the concerted action of three distinct proteins, carnitine palmitoyltransferase I (CPT I), the mitochondrial carnitine/acylcarnitine carrier (CACT), and carnitine palmitoyltransferase II (CPT II), all three of which are membrane bound with the noticeable difference that CPTI and CACT, but not CPT II, are integrally membrane bound. Carnitine palmitoyltransferase II is loosely associated with the inner face of the mitochondrial inner membrane, and CACT is required for the transport of acylcarnitine into the mitochondria in exchange for free carnitine. The cycle is completed by CPT II that reconverts the acylcarnitine back to corresponding acyl-CoA, which is then a substrate for the b-oxidation system.

Three related deficiency disorders, primary carnitine, CPT II, and CACT deficiency have distinctive childhood disturbances. Primary carnitine deficiency presents with acute episodes of lethargy, somnolence, hypoglycemia, hepatomegaly, cardiomegaly, and hypoketotic hypoglycemia. Carnitine levels are less than 5% of normal in plasma, muscle, and liver. The disorder is caused by mutation at the 5q31.1 locus of the SLC22A5 gene encoding the sodium ion-dependent carnitine transporter protein OCTN2 (Table 1). The consequence is impairment of skeletal and heart muscle FAO, and renal wasting of carnitine with low serum levels and impaired ketogenesis.

Prolonged treatment with oral carnitine results in increased muscle strength, improved cardiomyopathy, and repletion of carnitine levels in plasma, muscle, and liver. In the related disorder muscle carnitine deficiency, lipid storage myopathy occurs with low muscle carnitine but normal liver and serum carnitine levels.

Lethal neonatal forms of CPT II and CACT deficiency occur days after birth or in the first year of life, characterized by lethargy, hypotonia, liver failure, cardiac abnormalities, hypoketotic hypoglycemia, seizures, and eventual coma, with elevation of serum and urine C12-C18 acylcarnitines. Differentiation of the two disorders relies upon molecular testing for targeted mutation analysis of the most common disease-causing mutations, respectively at the 1p32.3 locus of the CPT2 gene that encodes CPT II, and at the 3p21.31 of the SCLC25A20 gene that encodes CACT (Table 1).

An infantile form of CPT II deficiency leads to severe multisystem disease, while the myopathic form presents in infancy to adulthood with exercise-induced myalgia and weakness, and recurrent episodes of myogloubinura. Treatment includes dietary modification to reduce long-chain dietary fat, increase the calories as carbohydrates, and providing carnitine to convert toxic long-chain acyl-CoA, and substituting medium-chain triglycerides. Prenatal diagnosis is available for families at known risk for an affected pregnancy by DNA extracted from cultured aminiocytes and chorionic villi.

The β–oxidation process involves the concerted action of multiple mitochondrial enzymes, including a series of substrate and chain-length specific acyl-CoA dehydrogenases, 3-hydroxyacyl-CoA dehydrogenases, and 3-ketoacyl-CoA thiolases to catalyze the cyclic release of acetyl-CoA units, and electron transfer flavoprotein (ETF) enzymes. The latter of which is not directly involved in FA β-oxidation, plays an essential role in transferring electrons coming from acyl-CoA dehydrogenases to the respiratory chain at the level of coenzyme Q. The oxidation of long-straight-chain acyl-CoA involves the sequential action of very long- (VLCAD, C14-C20 fatty acyl-CoA), medium- (MCAD; C6-C10 fatty acyl-CoA), and short-chain (SCAD; C4-C6 fatty acyl-CoA) acyl-CoA dehydrogenases, synthesized in the cytosol as precursor proteins and transported in their mature form to the mitochondria, either bound to the inner mitochondrial membrane as VLCAD where it accepts long-chain acyl-CoA as substrate, or in the mitochondrial matrix by SCAD and MCAD. Each enzyme shares approximately 40% amino acid identity or similarity within the catalytic domain.

In humans, LCAD does not play a significant role in FAO. As one of the first enzymes in the FAO spiral, the enzyme VLCAD controls a critical point in the supply of electrons to the respiratory chain and the pathway to production of ketones so critical in the transition from fetal to neonatal survival. Very long-chain acyl-CoA dehydrogenase (ACADVL) deficiency is associated with three phenotypes, severe early onset cardiac and multiorgan failure in early infancy with hypotonia, hypoketotic hypoglycemia, and cardiac disturbance; a childhood form with hypoketotic hypoglycemia and hepatomegaly without cardiomyopathy; and a late-onset form of episodic rhabdomyolysis and exercise intolerance without hypoglycemia.

Diagnosis in clinically suspected individuals is confirmed by acylcarnitine analysis by tandem mass spectroscopy, with elevated levels of C14:1, and deranged β-oxidation in cultured fibroblasts showing accumulation of excess tetradecanoyl C14 carnitine.

Very long-chain acyl-CoA dehydrogenase deficiency is caused by homozygous or compound heterozygous mutation at the 1713.1 locus of the ACADVL gene encoding VLCAD (Table 1). Diet modification that is low in fat and supplemented with calories through medium-chain triglycerides can reverse cardiac dysfunction and prevent cognitive impairment. Carrier and prenatal diagnosis are available.

Affected infants with SCAD deficiency may be well at the time of diagnosis through the intervention of newborn screening programs, or present with variable failure to thrive, hypotonia, seizures, feeding difficulty, ketotic hypoglycemia, and developmental delay.

Diagnosis is established by the presence of excess serum butyrylcarnitine (C4). The disorder is caused by mutation at the 12q24.31 locus in the ACADS gene encoding SCAD (Table 1). Deficiency of MCAD presents with intolerance to prolonged fasting, recurrent episodes of hypoglycemic coma with C6-C14 dicarboxylic aciduria, impaired ketogenesis, and low plasma and tissue carnitine levels that may be severe and even fatal. The disorder is caused by a mutation at the 1p31.1 locus of the ACADM gene encoding MCAD (Table 1).

Mitochondria contain short- and long-chain 3-hydroxyacyl-CoA dehydrogenase (SCHAD, LCHAD) as part of mitochondrial trifunctional protein (MTP), both of which are required for the oxidation of long-straight-chain acyl-CoA. Affected infants with 3-hydroxyacyl-CoA dehydrogenase deficiency can present with sudden death syndrome (SIDS) proceeded by hypotonia, hypoglycemia, hepatic steatosis, and hypoketotic dicarboxylic aciduria, while older adolescents may present variably with juvenile recurrent myoglobulinura, hypoketotic hypoglycemic encephalopathy, and cardiomyopathy.

The cause of SCHAD is a mutation at the 4q25 locus of the HADHSC gene encoding SCHAD (Table 1). Long-chain 3-hydroxyacyl-CoA dehydrogenase (LCHAD) deficiency is also associated with SIDS, feeding problems, impaired consciousness, early-onset cardiomyopathy, hypoglycemia, neuropathy, and pigmentary retinopathy due to a disease causing mutation at the 2p23.3 locus of the HADHA gene encoding LCHAD (Table 1). Mitochondrial trifunctional protein (MTP) enzyme catalyzes LCHAD, long-chain enoyl-CoA hydratase, and long-chain thiolase activity in mitochondrial β-oxidation; deficiency thereof is characterized by decreased activity of all three enzymes. Classic MTP deficiency is classified into three phenotypes, including, neonatal onset of severe lethal condition resulting in SIDS, infantile onset of a Reye-like syndrome, and late-onset myopathy, neuropathy, and rhabdomyolysis. These disorders are due to mutation at the 2p23.3 locus of the α- or β-subunits, respectively, of the *HADHA* and *HADHB* genes encoding MTP (Table 1).

Peroxisomal Biogenesis Disorders

There are several excellent reviews of peroxisomal bio-genesis disorders (PBG) (26–28). These multisystemic AR inherited disorders manifest prominent neurological features due to disturbances in peroxisomal function. Three such disorders, Zellweger syndrome (ZS), neonatal ALD (NALD), and infantile Refsum disease (IRD) form the spectrum of PBD or the Zellweger syndrome spectrum (ZSS), with an estimated incidence of 1:100,000, with ZS the most severe, and IRD the least severe.

Patients with ZS present with profound neonatal hypotonia, craniofacial dysmorphism, and inability to feed, seizures, and frequently die during the first year of life without psychomotor development. Neonatal ALD presents with hypotonia, facial dysmorphism, seizures, absent psychomotor development, retinopathy, deafness, and survival into adolescence. Patients with IRD present with mental retardation, dysmorphic features, hepatomegaly, sensorineural deafness, retinal pigmentary degeneration, anosmia, and survival into late childhood, adolescence, and adulthood.

Biochemical testing of saturated plasma VLCFA by gas chromatography and mass spectroscopy is the first step in the evaluation of suspected patients with a PBD with elevation of C26:0 and C26:1 and increased ratios of C24:C22 and C26:C22 most consistent with a peroxisomal biochemical defect. However, the degree of VLCFA plasma elevation may vary, with a small percentage of patients demonstrating modest elevations; and two types of peroxisomal mosaicism can lead to issues in interpreting biochemical results. Plasma VLCFA concentration may be increased while fibroblast VLCFA content is normal in Type 1 mosaicism, or there may be disparity in matrix proteins imported in peroxisomes in adjacent cells of tissues of the same individual (Type 2).

Neuroimaging shows hypomyelination, cortical gray abnormalities, and germinolytic cysts highly best seen on diffusion-weighted and tensor MR sequences. Absence of peroxisomes in cultured fibroblasts or liver tissue supports the diagnosis of a PBD later confirmed by molecular genetic testing for a disease-causing mutation in one of the 12 peroxin *PEX* genes that encode peroxins, the proteins required for normal peroxisome assembly. A mutation at the 7q21.2 locus in the *PEX1* gene is the most common (Table 1), seen in up to 68% of all affected individuals. Treatment is symptomatic and aimed at supplying adequate calories, hearing aids for sensorineural deafness, removal of symptomatic cataracts, supporting liver function, bile acid therapy to prevent stone formation, and early intervention for

seizures. Prenatal diagnosis is available through biochemical and molecular genetic testing of fetal cells obtained at amniocentesis or CVS.

Disorders of Carbohydrate Metabolism

There have been several recent reviews of this subject (29–31). There are two glycogen storage disease (GSD), each with a unique phenotype and age at onset. The incidence of GSD varies from 1:100,000 (GSD I) to 1:14,000 (GSD II). Type II Type I (Pompe) presents at age three to four months with a doll-like face of fat cheeks, thin extremities, short stature, and protuberant abdomen, and episodes of neonatal hypoglycemia, lactic acidosis, early infantile hypoglycemic seizures, and hepatomegaly. The diagnosis is established in clinically suspected patients with abnormal glucose, lactate, uric acid, triglycerides, and lipid levels.

The disorder is due to a mutation in the 17q21.31 locus of the *G6PC* gene encoding glucose-6-phosphatase (Table 1). Treatment is aimed at preventing normal glucose levels and hypoglycemia, frequent daytime feeding, nighttime intragastric continuous glucose infusion, and ultimately a diet high in complex carbohydrates. Prenatal diagnosis is available in instances of family-specific mutations from fetal cells obtained by amniocentesis and CVS, and for carrier detection in potentially affected sibs.

Type II GSD (Pompe) presents with early infantile hypotonia, weakness, macroglossia, and visceromegaly, without hypoglycemia or ketosis. There are juvenile and adult forms in which skeletal muscle involvement dominates the clinical picture. Affected adults usually present with skeletal muscle weakness and cramps and may have respiratory failure. Serum CK levels are a reliable marker for the skeletal muscle disease. The diagnosis is confirmed by biochemical assays showing absent or decreased enzyme activity in peripheral blood cells, skin fibroblasts, or muscle biopsy. The diagnosis is suspected by examination of muscle biopsies and confirmed by cultured fibroblasts for the deficient enzyme that is absent in infantile onset forms and markedly decreased in late-onset cases. The disorder results from a disease-causing mutation at the 17q25.3 locus of the *GAA* gene that encodes α-1,4-glucosidase, also known as acid maltase (Table 1).

Enzyme replacement therapy should be initiated as soon as the diagnosis of Pompe disease is established with alglucosidase in infantile and late-onset Pompe disease, which when compared to untreated cohorts leads to improved acquisition of motor skills, reduced need for ventilatory assistance, and overall improved survival (32). Experimental gene therapy, gel-mediated delivery of recombinant Adeno-associated virus (rAAV)1/2 vectors, significantly augmented ventilatory function at initial and late phases of disease in an experimental model of Pompe disease (33).

Two AR inborn errors of fructose metabolism affect newborns in the first week of life with an estimated incidence of 1:20,000 to 1:30,000 births: fructose-1,6-biphosphatase deficiency, and fructose-1, 6-biphosphate aldolase B enzyme deficiency. Fructose-1,6-biphosphate enzyme deficiency is associated with neonatal lactic acidemia, ketosis, and hypoglycemia due to impaired gluconeogenesis and a disease-causing mutation at the 9q22.32 locus of the *FBP1* gene encoding fructose-6-biphosphatase-1 (Table 1). Infants with fructose 1, 6-biphosphate aldolase B enzyme deficiency, or hereditary fructose intolerance develop profound near-fatal hypoglycemia, vomiting, and seizures, beginning after the first protein-fed meal, followed by hypotonia, hyperventilation, irritability, lethargy, and coma, due to disease-causing mutation at the 9q31.1 locus of the *ALDOB* gene encoding aldolase B (Table 1).

The diagnosis is established by demonstration of the deficient enzyme in liver and jejunal biopsy. Acute episodes are treated with intravenous infusion of glucose and sodium bicarbonate; otherwise, avoidance of fasting. Children with hereditary fructose intolerance should have restriction of dietary fructose.

Lysosomal Storage Disorders

There are several excellent recent reviews of the lysosomal storage disorders (LSD) (34–37). They generally display AR inheritance and result from the accumulation of non-degraded substances present in membrane bound intracellular bodies termed *lysosomes*. The incidence of LSD as a group is estimated to be 1:7700. They are classified according to the nature of the stored lysosomal substance: neurolipidoses, MPS, ML, NCL, glycoproteinoses, and glycogenoses.

The neuronopathic lysosomal disorders have provided valuable lessons into the strategy of gene therapy (38) that employs one of three approaches: injection of the deficient enzyme directly into the nervous system via recombinant vector coupled either with rAAV (39) encoded LSD specific peptide motifs into loop IV of the AAV2 capsid followed by peripheral injection of epitope-modified AAV (40), or by *ex vivo* gene transfer into hematopoietic or multipotent neural cell lines employing a retroviral vector (41).

Three infantile neurolipidoses, all GM$_2$ gangliosidoses, manifest AR inheritance and result in storage of G_{M2} ganglioside from defects in the lysosomal enzymes hexosaminidase A (HexA) in Tay-Sachs disease (TSD), hexosaminidase B (HexB) in Sandhoff disease, and the G_{M2} activator protein in AB variant. Tay-Sachs disease is 100 times more common in Ashkenazi Jews than in non-Jewish infants and has a carrier frequency of 1:31 in North American Jews compared to 1:300 in Sephardic Jews and non-Jews. It is a progressive neurodegenerative disorder, which in the classic acute infantile form, is characterized by progressive developmental retardation, loss of motor skills, a cherry red spot on fundoscopy caused by a grey white area of lipid-laden retinal ganglion cells that encircle the fovea centralis encircles, and startle response to sound, beginning at age three to six months. This is followed by seizures, blindness, spasticity, and death by four years. A subacute juvenile form begins with ataxia and incoordination between age two to ten years, with cognitive, motor skill, visual decline, and progressively fatal decerebrate rigidity by the second decade. Enzymatic studies on leukocytes reveal absence of HexA activity.

Infants with Sandhoff disease are further distinguished by hepatosplenomegaly and skeletal deformities. Urinary N-acetylglucosamine containing oligosaccharides are found in the urine along with foam cells in the bone marrow, with absent HexA and HexB enzyme activity in leukocyte and cultured fibroblasts. The basic enzyme defect of absent component A of total hemoxaminidase was first shown by Okada and O'Brien (42).

Tay-Sachs is due to a disease-causing mutation at the 15q23 locus of the α subunit of the HEXA gene that encodes the α subunit of HexA (Table 1). Individuals with infantile TSD have two null alleles without HexA enzyme activity, whereas those with juvenile-onset are usually compound heterozygotes for a null allele and one that results in residual low HexA activity.

Children with Sandhoff disease harbor a disease-causing mutation at the 5q13.3 locus of the β subunit of HEXB gene encoding the β subunit of HexB involved in the lysosomal breakdown of G_{M2} gangliosides (Table 1). The AB variant of G_{M2} activator deficiency, with a similar clinical phenotype, results from the absent intralysosomal activator necessary for hydrolysis of G_{M2} gangligoside by HexA that leads to the accumulation of G_{M2} gangliosides and related lysosomal glycolipids mainly of neuronal cells. It is caused by mutation at the 5q33.1 locus of the GM2A gene (Table 1).

Treatment of HexA deficiency is supportive. Although early experiments of intravenous enzyme-replacement therapy (ERT) were unsuccessful due to its large molecular weight, neuronal-corrective gene therapy via intracerebroventricular replacement of modified human β-hexosaminidase B is in experimental stages (43, 44). Genetic counseling of TSD is important for Ashkenazi Jews identifying specific HEXA mutations for carrier detection, preimplantation genetic diagnosis, and prenatal testing of fetal cells obtained by amniocentesis and CVS.

Three other neurolipidoses, all sphingolipidoses with prominent neurovisceral involvement, include G_{M1} gangliosidosis type I, NPD, Gaucher disease (GD), and Farber disease occur with an estimated frequency of 1:57,000 (Gaucher) to 1:250,000 (NPD).

Landing and colleagues (45) gave the first description of G_{M1} gangliosidosis type 1. It presents in early infancy with rapid psychomotor deterioration beginning within 6 months of birth with associated generalized CNS involvement, hepatosplenomegaly, facial dysmorphia, macular cherry red spot, skeletal dysplasia, facial dysmorphisms, and early death. There is complete absence of acid β-galactosidase activity in leukocytes and cultured fibroblasts. Vacuolated lymphocytes are noted in peripheral blood and bone marrow smears, and galactose-containing oligosaccharides and keratan sulfate are excreted in urine.

GM1-gangliosidois is caused by a mutation at the 3p22.3 locus in the GLB1 gene that encodes β−galactosidase (Table 1). A type II late infancy or juvenile onset form shows generalized CNS involvement, psychomotor deterioration, seizures, skeletal involvement, and survival into childhood, with absent hepatosplenomegaly and cherry red spot.

Niemann-Pick disease is divided into types A, B and C (NPA, NPB, and NPC). Type A is characterized by infantile hepatomegaly and typical macular cherry red spot, followed several months later by psychomotor regression and delayed development manifesting impaired swallowing, an acousticomotor startle response, hypotonia, seizures, rigidity, and opisthotonus. Sphingomyelin accumulates in all tissues, including the brain and autonomic ganglia that pathologically shows intralysosomal lipid inclusions. Type B, which is also due to deficient sphingomyelinase, leads to visceral accumulation of sphingomyelin, sparing the CNS. Diagnosis of both types rests upon the demonstration of reduced sphingomyelinase activity in peripheral leukocytes, fibroblasts, and visceral organ tissues, and the demonstration of a pathogenic mutation in the 11p15.4 locus of the SMPD1 gene (Table 1).

Juvenile Niemann-Pick disease (NPC) occurs in late infancy, manifesting progressive encephalopathy, loss of motor skills, and visceromegaly. Diagnosis rests upon the finding of vacuolated storage cells terms foam cells, and others containing blue granules referred to as sea-blue histiocytes in bone marrow smears. The disorder is not caused by a deficiency in sphingomyelinase, but instead by a disturbance of cholesterol, processing that leads to neurovisceral lysosomal and endosomal accumulation of unesterified cholesterol with the majority of affected patients manifesting a mutation at the 18q11.2 locus of the NPC1 gene in NPC type C1 (NPC1), and at the 14q24.3 locus of NPC2 in NPC2 that respectively encode a membrane protein localized to endosomes, and a lysosomal protein with cholesterol-binding properties (Table 1). There is yet no specific recommended treatment, however, substrate reduction therapy (SRT) employing miglustat crosses the blood brain barrier and led to improved supranuclear palsy and swallowing disturbances in a randomized controlled trial of patients with NPC (46), but not in an open label study of patients with G_{M2} gangliosidosis, despite reduction of lysosomal inclusions in peripheral white blood cells

(WBC) (47). An inflammatory component was postulated in G_{M1} and G_{M2} gangliosidoses, prompting consideration of the possible beneficial effects of anti-inflammatory therapy. The latter prompted a clinical investigation of non-steroidal anti-inflammatory drugs in mouse models of GM2 gangliosidosis and NPC that subsequently demonstrated improvement in motor function and survival when administered alone or in combination with other therapeutic approaches such as SRT with miglusatat (48).

Gaucher disease encompasses a spectrum of clinical phenotypes with types 2 and 3 characterized by primary neurological disease, and type 1 primarily bone, hepatic, lung, and hematologic involvement. Those with onset before age two years with limited psychomotor development and a rapidly deteriorating course, and with death by age four years, are classified as type 2 acute neuronopathic GD. Those with onset before age two and a more slowly progressive course, often survive to the fourth decade and are categorized as type 3 subacute neuronopathic GD. Although individuals with type 1 non-neuropathic GD lack primary CNS involvement, secondary neurological sequelae may develop as a result of bone disease, including osteopenia, vertebral compression, spinal cord and nerve root impingement, and cerebral embolism after long bone fracture. Types 2 and 3 manifest bulbar, oculomotor, cognitive disturbances (type 2), oculomotor apraxia, seizures, and progressive myoclonic epilepsy (type 3).

The diagnosis is suggested by assay of glucosylceramidase in leukocytes or other nucleated cells and cultured fibroblasts, and the identification of disease-causing mutations at the 1q22 locus of the GBA gene that encodes β-glucosidase (Table 1). Bone marrow and other body tissues show characteristic Gaucher cells composed of mononuclear phagocytic cells engorged by intracellular glucosylceramide. There is no specific treatment for GD, however ERT utilizing taliglucerase alfa (49), SRT employing the inhibitor of glucosylceramide synthetase eliglustat tartrate (50), chaperone-mediated ERT employing small molecules that are active-site inhibitors and at low doses promote refolding and correct trafficking of mutated and wild type proteins, including iminisugar isofagomine (51, 52), and gene therapy involving the introduction of GBA into hematopoietic stem cells (53) have all shown promise.

Infants with Farber disease present with joint swelling, deformity, subcutaneous nodules, malnutrition, dysphonia, and progressive mental deterioration due to granulomatous deposition. The diagnosis is confirmed by the demonstration of reduced activity of acid ceramidase in cultured leukocytes and skin fibroblasts, and the demonstration of a disease-causing mutation at the 8p22 locus of the ASAH1 gene encoding ceramidase (Table 1).

The MPS are a group of NHMD caused by a lack of specific lysosomal enzymes involved in the degradation of glycosaminoglycans (GAG), which results in a wide range of phenotypic syndromes. Four types of MPS, I to IV, have progressive multisystem neurological involvement. MPS type I presents with Hurler as the most severe, Hurler-Scheie as intermediate, and Scheie the least severe. However, there are no biochemical or molecular genetic differences, and the clinical findings overlap.

The MPSI Hurler phenotype is characterized by normal initial bone and psychomotor development that yields to coarsening of facial features caused by storage of GAG, namely heparan and dermatan sulphate in soft tissues of the eye, orofacial area, facial and skeletal bone dysostosis, growth retardation, thickening of the alae nasi, lips, ear, tongue, oropharynx, calvarium, and heart, and other viscera by age one to two years, with incipient hearing loss and increased pressure hydrocephalus that further compromises intellectual abilities.

Testing for MPS includes assay for urinary GAG, demonstration of deficient activity of α-L-iduronidase, a glycosidase that removes non-reducing terminal alpha-L-iduronide residues during lysosomal degredation of the GAG heparan sulphate and dermatan sulphate, and molecular genetic testing for a mutation at the 4p16.3 locus of the *IDUA* gene encoding α-L-iduronidase (Table 1).

The attenuated MPSI Hurler-Scheie or Scheie syndrome is characterized by onset between ages 3 and 10 years of more pronounced skeletal, joint, eye, hearing, cardiac, liver and spleen storage symptoms, and less intellectual impairment or risk of communicating hydrocephalus; however, progressive compressive cervical myelopathy may occur as a result of thickening of the dura.

The disorder is caused by mutation at the 4p16.3 locus of the *IDUA* gene that encodes α-L-idronidase (Table 1). In general, the severe MPSI phenotype is correlated with a severe *IDUA* allele and resultant paucity of enzyme activity, whether in a homozygous or compound heterozygous state, in contrast to attenuated MPSI phenotype which is usually associated with one severe allele and a second that permits some residual enzyme activity. Male infants with XL MPSII (Hunter) have normal developmental milestones but develop coarsening of facial features, macrocephaly, macroglossia, hydrocephalus, joint and skeletal contracture, sensorineural hearing loss, intellectual decline, carpal tunnel syndrome, compressive cervical myelopathy, hepatosplenomegaly, and cardiovascular involvement.

The diagnosis of MPSII is established by urine assay for GAG, demonstration of deficient iduronate 2-sulfatase enzyme activity, and molecular genetic testing for mutations at the Xq28 locus of the *IDS* gene that encodes iduronate 2-sulfatase (Table 1). MPSIII includes four Sanfilippo types, A through D, all AR, due to the deficiency of a different enzyme: heparan N-sulfatase (type A); α-N-acetyl-glucosaminidase (type B); acetyl CoA: α-glucosaminide

acetyltransferase (type C); and N-acetylglucosamine 6-sulfatase (type D). There is a common phenotype of normal or retarded early psychomotor development, followed by intellectual arrest, speech delay, and behavioral disturbances that become manifest by age two years. Signs of motor impairment become evident by the end of the first decade of life as walking becomes unsteady, hands clumsy, and ambulation ceases. There are mild skeletal and somatic disturbances, visceromegaly, thickened calvarium, stunted growth, and overall shortened life span. Sensorineural hearing loss develops as a result of recurrent ear infections and ossicle deformities. Spinal cord compression and nerve root impingement develops as a result of MPS storage, meningeal membrane thickening, and C1-2 vertebral subluxation.

The MPSIIIA phenotype is the most common, severe, and rapidly progressive due to mutations at the 17q25.3 locus of the *SGSH* gene that encodes N-sulfoglucosamine sulfohydrolase (Table 1). Experimental brain tissue of MPSIIIA mice show increased autophagosomes resulting from impaired autophagosome-lysosome fusion, decreased ability to degrade aggregation-prone proteins, accumulation of ubiquitin-positive inclusions, and increased numbers of dysfunctional mitochondria consistent with the block in lysosomal autophagy (54). Those with MPSIIIB demonstrate homozygous or compound heterozygous mutation at the 17q21.2 locus of the *NAGLU* encoding N-α-acetylglucosaminidase (Table 1). Patients with MPSIIIC harbor mutation at the 8p11.21 locus of the *HGSNAT* gene encoding heparan acetyl-CoA:α-glucosaminide N-acetyltransferase (Table 1).

Those with MPSIIID reveal mutations at the 12q14.3 locus of the *GNS* gene encoding N-acetylglucosamine-6-sulfatase (Table 1).

All MPSIII types show decreased residual or absent enzyme activity in plasma, yet only heparan sulfate is excreted in the urine. MPS IV (Morquio) types A and B are characterized by intracellular accumulation of keratin sulfate and chondroitin-6-sulfate.

The disorder is caused by mutation at the 16q24.3 locus in the *GALNS* gene encoding galactosamine-6-sulfate sulfatase (Table 1). Prenatal diagnosis of MPS is possible by amniocentesis and CVS. Without effective therapy, the lifespan of children with MPS is shortened as a result of cardiac and respiratory failure with death in infancy in MPS I, by age 10 in MPS II, and in teens to adulthood in severe forms of MPS III and IV.

The available modes of ERT include L-iduronidase for MPS I and idursalfase for MPS II (55). Gene therapy entails the peripheral injection of epitope-modified AAV for brain endothelial targeting expressing β-glucuronidase, which in MPS mice reconstituted the deficiency enzyme activity throughout the brain, reduced the levels of lysosomal storage product, and improved disease phenotype (40). Substrate reduction therapy using flavonoids, such as daidzein and kaempferol, has been used in MPS III. Hematopoietic stem cell transplantation (HSCT) modified the neuropsychological development of Hurler disease when performed early in the course of the disease (56).

The four types of ML (I to IV) are AR inherited and resemble MPS with storage instead of lipids and polysaccharides. The disorder was first termed "lipomucopolysaccharidosis" by Spranger et al. (57) and later ML I (58) by the same author in a description of a 12-year-old patient with mental retardation, hypotonia, ataxia, myoclonus, seizures, coarse facies, short trunk, barrel chest, spinal deformity, sensorineural hearing loss, and cherry red spot.

The cause of MLI is a mutation at the 6p21.33 locus of the NEU1 gene that encodes the lysosomal enzyme α-neuraminidase (Table 1). Mucolipidosis II (I cell) presents at birth with hypotonia, mental retardation, claw hand deformity, carpal tunnel syndrome, and the ophthalmic triad of corneal clouding, retinopathy, and hyperopic astigmatism, as well as coarse facial features, thick tight skin, gingival hyperplasia, and congenital hip dislocation.

The diagnosis of MLII is suggested by excessive urinary secretion of oligosaccharides and normal urinary excretion of GAG, including acid MPS, to exclude Hurler MPS I, with near complete inactivity of N-acetylglucosamine-1-phosphotransferase. The disorder results from homozygous or compound heterozygous mutation at the 12q23.2 locus of the GNTPAB gene encoding N-acetylglucosamine-1-phosphotransferase (Table 1).

Mucolipidosis Type III (Pseudo-Hurler) generally presents by age 3 years with developmental delay, short stature, joint pain, stiffness, coarsening of facial features, dysostosis multiplex, osteoporosis, and mild organomegaly. Biochemical testing shows excessive urinary excretion of oligosaccharides, normal urinary excretion of GAG, and deficiency of the enzyme N-acetylglucosamine-1-phosphotransferance in enzymatic assay. The cause of the disorder is a mutation at the 12q23.2 locus of the GNPTAB gene encoding the α subunit of GLcNAc-phophotransferase (Table 1), and is phenotypically less severe than the allelic disorder MLII. ML type IV presents predominantly in Ashkenazi Jews, with corneal clouding from birth or early infancy followed by psychomotor retardation that is apparent by the end of the first year of life. The disease results from a mutation at the 19p13.2 locus of the MCOLN1 gene that encodes mucolipin-1 (Table 1) that is required for efficient transport and delivery of material from late endosomes and autophagosomes to lysosomes. Prenatal testing, preimplantation genetic diagnosis, and carrier detection counseling is available in families with known disease-causing mutations. Treatment is supportive, however bone marrow transplantation (BMT) is available for MLII.

The NCL are degenerative storage disorders with common clinical and pathological features due to abnormal lysosomal storage of autofluorescent ceroid and lipofuscin in the CNS and visceral organs (59). The NCL disorders can be categorized by individual distinguishing phenotypic and genotypic features, and the specific enzyme deficiency. The mode of inheritance is AR with the exception of adult onset which may be AR or AD. Three deficient lysosomal enzymes have been identified in WBC, fibroblasts, and chorionic villi.

Infantile NCL (INCL; CLN1) (Santavuori-Haltia) presents with arrest and regression of psychomotor abilities in the first year of life leading to incoordination, hypotonia, and myoclonus that interrupts standing, gait, and acquired motor abilities, followed by progressive spastic paraparesis, seizures, and visual failure by the second year of life. There is progressive isoelectric flattening of the EEG commensurate with the eventual vegetative state of later childhood. Affected children fail to thrive, develop microcephaly and the disease is lethal by age 10.

Children with late infantile NCL (LINCL; CLN2) (Jansky-Bielschowsky) instead present with seizures, myoclonus, slowing of developmental milestones, progressive ataxia, spasticity, and blindness.

Diagnosis of both infantile and late-infantile NCL is aided by the finding of macular degeneration and optic atrophy, slow photic stimulation driven occipital spikes, and leukoencephalopathy in brain neuroimaging. Children with late infantile NCL survive into late adolescence.

Those with juvenile NCL (JNCL; CLN3) (Batten; Spielmeyer-Vogt) present with visual loss, epilepsy, motor and intellectual deterioration, and survival into the late teenage period. Testing strategy in NCL includes initial screening of deficient enzyme activity suggested by the clinical subtype INCL, LINCL, or JNCL and if informative, proceeding to molecular genetic testing for targeted mutation and sequencing of the gene associated with each phenotype. Supportive evidence of NCL may be obtained by finding one of several types of peripheral blood inclusions, including translucent lymphocyte vacuoles, azurophilic neutrophil hypergranulations, vacuolated lymphocytes, and intralysosomal inclusions on ultrastructural study of biopsied skin, sweat gland, muscle, and myenteric plexus tissue that demonstrate intralysosomal accumulations of curvilinear bodies, fingerprint-like deposits, and other lamellar inclusions.

Infantile NCL is due to a mutation at the 1p34.2 locus of PPT1 (CLN1) encoding palmitoyl-protein thioesterase, whereas LINCL results from a mutation at the 11p15.4 locus of TPP1 (CLN2) encoding tripeptidyl-peptidase, and JNCL (CLN3) results from a mutation at the 16p11.2 locus of CLN3 gene encoding battenin (Table 1).

Human and animal forms of the disorders are divided into two categories based on the material accumulated in lysosomes, however the relation between the genetic defects associated with the major NCL forms, the accumulation of storage material, and CNS tissue damage or dysfunction is still not well understood. Although individuals with NCL manifest lysosomal storage in many tissues and organs, severe degeneration and cell loss mainly affects neurons.

The NCL proteins may be most critical for the metabolism of neurons and it is uncertain whether the storage is caused by the properties of NCL proteins or the metabolic factors present in neurons. There is no effective treatment, however a phase I study of the safety of LINCL, using direct injection of AAV2 containing the CLN2 vector that encoded the deficient enzyme TTP-1 into each hemisphere, in 10 affected children showed a trend toward less decline in clinical and brain MRI indices when compared to historical controls (60).

Phosphocysteamine, a known lysosomotrophic drug that mediates the depletion of lysosomal ceroids, prevents their re-accumulation, and inhibits apoptosis, was used in the treatment of individuals with mutations in CLN1 (61). A unified rating scale has been developed to measure the rate of decline in physical and functional capability domains applicable to clinical trials (62).

Four glycopoteinoses, α- and β-mannosidosis, fucosidosis, galactosialidosis, and aspartylglucosaminuria, present with inborn defects of lysosomal glycoprotein degradation and AR inheritance. Infants with α- and β-mannosidosis present in the first year of life to early childhood, with progressive psychomotor retardation, hepatosplenomegaly, coarse facial features, dysostosis multiplex, recurrent infection, deafness, lenticular and corneal opacities. The diseases result from pathogenic mutations respectively at the 19p13.2 locus of the *MA2B1* encoding α-mannosidase, and the 4q24 locus of the *MANBA* gene encoding β-mannosidase (Table 1).

Fucosidosis occurs in two forms: type I, characterized by rapid psychomotor regression and severe neurological deterioration beginning at six months of age, with death by the first decade; and type II with milder psychomotor retardation and neurological signs. Affected children demonstrate spastic quadriplegia and decerebrate posturing, in addition to salivary gland enlargement and angiokeratoma. The disorder is caused by mutations at the 1p36.11 locus of the *FUCA1* gene encoding α-L-fucosidase (Table 1).

Galactosialidosis presents with clinical manifestations typical of a lysosomal disorder, including coarse facies, cherry red spots, vertebral changes, foam cells in the bone marrow, and vacuolated lymphocytes. Three phenotypic subtypes are recognized. An early infantile form is associated with fetal hydrops, edema, ascites, visceromegaly, skeletal dysplasia, and early death. A late infantile type is characterized by hepatosplenomegaly, growth retardation, cardiac involvement, and rare occurrence of neurologic signs. A non-lethal juvenile form manifests myoclonus, ataxia, angiokeratoma, and mental retardation, without visceromegaly.

The disorder results from disease-causing mutations at 20q13.12 locus of the *CTSA* gene encoding cathepsin A (Table 1) with resultant combined deficiency of β-galactosidase and neuraminidase secondary to a defect in the protective protein/cathepsin A.

Children with aspartylglycosaminuria present in the first year of life with recurrent infection, diarrhea, mental retardation, behavioral disturbances, coarse facial features, lenticular opacities, skeletal dysplasia, and mitral valve insufficiency. The disorder results from disease-causing mutations at the 4q34.3 locus of the *AGA* gene that encodes aspratylglycoaminase (Table 1). Experimental BMT has been suggested for fucosidosis, α-mannosidosis, and aspartylglycosaminuria.

INFANTILE LEUKODYSTROPHIES

There are seven infantile leukodystrophies due to failure of myelin synthesis or pathological demyelination, with or without concomitant peripheral nerve demyelination. They included three AR storage disorders, two of them sphingomyelinoses, Krabbe disease and MLD, and the other, multiple sulfatase deficiency (MSD), intermediate between them; two XL disorders, Pelizaeus-Merzbacher (PMD), which is due to deficiency in proteolipid protein (PLP), and the other, juvenile adrenoleukodystrophy (ALD), a peroxisomal disorder; and two others, Canavan disease (CD) and Alexander disease, respectively AR and AD in inheritance, associated with primary disturbances of oligodendrocytes and astrocytes or Rosenthal fibers.

Infantile Krabbe disease (globoid cell leukodystophy), with an incidence of 1:100,000 live births, typically manifests three stages, beginning with arrest of motor and mental development, irritability, hypersensitivity to auditory, tactile, or visual stimuli; muscle hypertonicity, and seizures. At this time, the CSF protein content may be elevated and peripheral neuropathy may already by evident.

The second stage is characterized by motor and mental deterioration and marked spasticity with optic atrophy.

The third stage manifests blindness, decerebrate paralysis and lack of contact with surroundings followed by death by two years of age. Approximately 10% to 15% of children present with late-onset disease, typically beginning in early (six months to three years) or late childhood (three to eight years) with normal early infancy until symptoms of weakness, visual loss, and intellectual deterioration supervene, followed by progressive paraparesis and peripheral neuropathy and blindness in up to one-half of patients. Late-infantile MLD instead presents with early development and walking until 30 months, followed by progressive gait difficulty and falls due to progressive flaccid paraparesis and hypotonia from predominant peripheral neuropathy or spastic paraparesis from underlying corticospinal tract degeneration, or a combination of the two.

Late-onset juvenile onset, which may develop at any age beyond three years, and an adult form arbitrarily demarcated from the former at age 16 years, manifest slower progression and in the latter, psychiatric symptomatology often leading to the erroneous diagnosis of schizophrenia at onset. The diagnosis of a leukodystrophy is suggested by symmetric abnormal white matter hyperintensities on T_2-weighted MRI sequences with sparing of subcortical U-fibers and cerebellar white matter in MLD.

A mechanism of cytotoxic mediated oligodendrocyte breakdown of previously formed myelin is postulated in Krabbe disease, and an inborn error of myelin composition of myelin is proposed in MLD. The EEG, which may be normal in the initial stages of either disease, gradually regresses. Electrodiagnostic studies show uniform slowing of nerve velocities consistent with a genetic etiopathogenesis. Krabbe disease results from mutation at the 14q31.3 locus of the *GALC* gene encoding galactocerebroside (GALC), whereas MLD results from mutation at the 22q13.33 locus of the *ARSA* gene encoding arylsulfatase A (Table 1).

Carrier testing by measurement of GALC enzyme activity in Krabbe disease is not reliable because of the wide range of enzymatic activities in carriers and non-carriers, but molecular genetic testing can be used for carrier detection in at-risk families and to identify presymptomatic infants who will benefit from HSCT to ameliorate neurological outcome (63, 64). Carrier detection via ARSA enzymatic activity in MLD does not discriminate between MLD and ARSA pseudodeficiency with activities up to 20% of normal without MLD.

Severe neonatal MSD resembles infantile MLD with progressive loss of motor and mental abilities and skeletal changes. There are attenuated late-infantile and juvenile-onset forms with slower progression and an overall prevalence of 1:40,000 to 1:160,000 in different populations with an even high prevalence in consanguineous populations. The disorder is caused by homozygous and compound heterozygous mutation at the 3p26.1 locus of the sulfatase-modifying factor-1 (*SUMF1*) gene encoding arylsulfatase A (ARSA) (Table 1). Although there is no effective treatment for the CNS manifestations of this disease, which is usually fatal in childhood, HSCT performed early in the stages of juvenile MLD stabilizes cognitive ability and improved neuroimaging and nerve conduction studies (NCS) (65).

The *PLP1* gene-related XL disorders of the CNS include a range of phenotypes from PMD to spastic paraplegia 2 (SPG2). In the U.S., the prevalence of PMD is 1:200,000 to 1:500,000. Severe neonatal PMD presents with pendular nystagmus, pharyngeal weakness, stridor, hypotonia, and stridor, followed by cognitive impairment, severe spasticity, ataxia, limited verbal expression, and aspiration. Affected children die during infancy and childhood. Male children with classic PMD present with nystagmus, hypotonia,

titubation, ataxia, and spastic quadriparesis, beginning in the first five years of life, with impaired cognitive abilities and ambulation, if present, requiring assistive devices. Life expectancy is not severely shortened.

Since the bulk of myelination occurs during the fist two years of life, T2 weighted MRI may not show definitive abnormalities until age 1 or 2 years. Visual, auditory, and somatosensory evoked potentials show normal to near-normal peripheral latencies but severely prolonged or absent central latencies. The disorder is due to mutation at the Xq22.2 locus of *PLP1* encoding proteolipid protein-1 (Table 1). Prenatal testing is available for carrier women with known family PLP1 mutations after first determining the sex by DNA analysis of fetal cells at amniocentesis or CVS, and if male, analyzing them further for known disease-causing mutations, although the phenotype may not be accurately predicted since phenotypes of varying severity may coexist in the same kindred and sib ship.

The XL peroxisomal disorder ALD affects the nervous system and adrenal cortex, leading to progressive CNS demyelination and adrenal insufficiency with an estimated prevalence of 1:20,000 to 1:50,000. The commonest cerebral childhood form has an onset between four and eight years of age with slowed mentation, psychological disturbance, dysarthria, attention deficit, parietal lobe disorder, progressive hemianopia, blindness, hearing loss, hemiplegia, seizures, and dementia. Brain neuroimaging shows contrast enhancing parieto-occipital demyelination.

The related disorder, adrenomyeloneuropathy (AMN) presents with slowly progressive spastic paraparesis and peripheral neuropathy. Saturated VLCFA are abnormal in 99% of males with ALD with increased concentration in the plasma and in cultured skin fibroblasts, with accumulation in the brain and adrenal cortex. Testing at-risk women for carrier status is a two step process beginning with measurement of plasma VLCFA followed by molecular genetic testing since 20% of women carriers will have normal plasma levels. The disorder results from mutation at the Xq28 locus of the *ABCD1* gene that encodes the adrenoleukodystrophy protein ALDP (Table 1), a member of the ATP-binding cassette protein transporter family. Dietary treatment with restriction of VLCFA, combined with oral 4:1 mixture of glyceryl trioleate ad glyceryl trierucate, lowers plasma VLCFA levels.

Canavan disease presents in late infancy after initial normal early birth and development, with macrocephaly followed by optic atrophy, poor visual tracking, disturbed head control, and developmental delay leading to inability to sit, stand, walk, or talk. Affected infants interact socially, laugh, smile, reach for objects, and raise their head in the prone position, but with increasing age hypotonia is replaced by spasticity, sleep disturbance, seizures, and feeding difficulties necessitating nasogastric or gastrostomy feeding. A milder juvenile form is characterized by normal or mildly delayed motor and speech development requiring interventional therapy.

The diagnosis of CD relies on the demonstration of excessive urinary excretion of N-acetylaspartic acid (NAA), white matter disease on brain neuroimaging, and elevated levels of NAA in blood, CSF, and skin fibroblast culture. Molecular genetic testing demonstrates mutation at the 17p13.2 locus of the ASPA gene encoding aspartoacylase (Table 1), which hydolyzes NAA into aspartic acid and acetate; the absence thereof leads to abnormal toxic concentration of NAA in oligodendrocytes causing demyelination and other signs of the disorder. Most reported cases of CD are of Ashkenazi Jewish origin with a carrier frequency of 1:40 for the most common mutations. Biochemical genetic testing is available for couples in whom one partner is a known carrier and the other is of unknown status, by measurement of NAA in amniotic fluid using liquid chromatography tandem mass spectroscopy (66).

Associated neuropathologic changes include spongy degeneration with astocytic swelling and normal neurons. There is no known effective treatment. *In vivo* gene transfer, well-tolerated in two human subjects, did not alter the clinical course compared to untreated subjects (67). Oral lithium citrate for two months led to improvement in alertness and social interactions without gross motor functional changes, and an overall drop in NAA in the basal ganglia on proton magnetic resonance imaging and mild improvement in frontal white matter myelination in T1MR in six other children (68). As a consequence of the potentially high carrier rate in individuals of Ashkenazi Jewish ancestry, and the availability of genetic counseling and prenatal diagnosis, screening programs have been initiated for the commonest ASPA mutations located at p.Glu285Ala, p.Tyr231Z, and p.Ala305Glu.

Alexander disease is a very rare disorder of cortical white matter with neonatal, infantile, and juvenile forms. The disorder first described by Alexander (69) included megalencephaly in infancy accompanied by progressive spasticity and dementia with features similar to those of CD. Affected neonates present with severe motor and intellectual disturbance, intractable seizures, papilledema, megalencephaly, hydrocephalus, bulging fontanelles, and increased intracranial pressure in association with aqueduct stenosis, with death in the first two years of life. Brain neuroimaging shows contrast enhanced extensive white matter changes with elevated signal intensity on T2-weighted sequences in the ventricular lining, periventricular rim, frontal white matter, optic chiasm, fornix, basal ganglia, thalamus, dentate nuclear, and brainstem. Onset in infancy presents with progressive psychomotor retardation with loss of developmental milestones, megalencephaly hydrocephalus, seizures, spasticity, ataxia, and survival up to early teenage years. A juvenile form presents,

instead, with gradual loss of intellectual function, seizures, megalencephaly, bulbar or pseudobulbar signs, swallowing, breathing difficulty, ataxia, and spasticity. The CSF protein content is elevated with increased levels of αβ-crystallin and heat shock protein HSP 27, and increased levels of glial fibrillary acidic protein (GFAP). Electroencephalography demonstrates frontal slowing.

Prior to the availability of molecular genetic testing in Alexander disease, the diagnosis relied upon immunohistochemical staining for the presence of intra-astrocytic aggregates of GFAP, vimentin, αβ-crystallin, and HSP-27 present in Rosenthal fibers in brain biopsy and postmortem brain tissue. Rosenthal fibers are not unique to Alexander disease but occur in a preponderant fashion in Alexander disease as well in other systemic illnesses.

The disorder is due to mutation at the 17q21.31 locus of the GFAP gene (Table 1). The infantile and juvenile forms of Alexander disease are caused by de novo mutation. Parents of molecularly confirmed cases typically do not have clinical features or identifiable GFAP mutations. The pathogenesis of the disease is not well understood. The GFAP mutants may harbor a defective protein that alters the oligomerization or solubility of the protein synthesized from the normal allele, inhibit proteasomal activity in astrocytes, or disturb the normal interaction between astrocytes and oligodendrocytes resulting in hypomyelination or demyelination (70). There is no specific therapy for Alexander disease.

HEREDITARY EXTRAPYRAMIDAL DISORDERS

Five disorders should be considered in a child with extrapyramidal neurological disease, including WD, juvenile HD and PD (JPD), ChAc, and Lesch-Nyhan syndrome (LNS) with diverse inheritance including AR (WD, JPD, ChAc), AD (HD), and XL (LNS) patterns.

Wilson disease was first described as progressive lenticular degeneration associated with cirrhosis of the liver (71). It is a disorder of copper metabolism that affects individuals of age 3 to 50 years with a prevalence of 1:30,000, leading to abnormal deposition of copper in the brain and liver even before hepatic, neurologic, hematologic, or psychiatric disturbances supervene (72). The neurologic sequelae can be divided into an early onset predominant movement disorder comprised of tremor, poor coordination, loss of fine motor control, micrographia, chorea, and choreoathetosis; and later onset rigid dystonia syndrome with mask-like facies, rigidity, and gait disturbances. Concomitant pseudobulbar involvement includes dysathria, drooling, and swallowing difficulty and is more often seen in older individuals. The neuropsychiatric manifestations of mood disturbance, depression, poor impulse control, changes in school performance, and deterioration of fine motor skills is seen in those with more advanced liver involvement. Kayser-Fleicher rings are noted on slit-lamp eye examination by the time neurological signs, hepatosplenomegaly, and cirrhosis occurs, and results from copper deposition in Descemet membrane of the cornea, one of the highest areas of copper storage body wide. Although not specific for WD, they are seen in patients with copper accumulation secondary to cholestatic liver disease and autoimmune hepatitis.

The diagnosis of WD is supported by reduced levels of serum ceruloplasmin, total serum copper, and elevation of nonceruloplasmin-bound copper. Liver biopsy shows markedly increased copper content and cirrhosis. Brain MRI demonstrates abnormal T_1 and hyperintense T_2 weighted signals in the caudate nucleus, while positron emission tomography (PET) shows reduced glucose consumption in the striatum, cerebellum, thalamus, and cortex. Molecular genetic testing reveals homozygous or compound heterozygote mutations at the 13q14.3 locus of the *ATP7B* gene (Table 1). Gene mutations that completely prevent function of the gene produce a more severe phenotype than certain types of missense mutations, with the most severe ones resulting in onset of symptoms before age 12. Low ceruloplasmin activity that normally transfers copper to copper-containing enzymes such as COX, which is markedly reduced in homozygotes, is less so in heterozygotes with the mutated gene who generally do not develop clinically evident WD. The goal of the therapy is to initiate copper chelation therapy employing D-penicillamine or triethylene tetramine dihydrochloride. Orthotopic liver transplantation is reserved for those who fail to respond or cannot tolerate medical therapy. Genetic counseling is available for parents and offspring of a proband, both of whom are obligate carriers, and in sibs who have a 25% chance of being affected, 50% chance of being an asymptomatic carrier, and 25% chance of being unaffected or a carrier.

Juvenile HD (73), defined as onset before age 20 years, comprises less than 10% of all HD cases and is usually transmitted from an affected father than mother with high penetrance, anticipation, and mutation during spermatogenesis. The prevalence of HD is 3 to 7:100,000 in individuals of western European descent. Affected children present with clumsiness, gait difficulty, rigidity, chorea, or choreoathetosis, dysarthria, myoclonus, and psychiatric disturbance after a period of normal psychomotor development, culminating in dementia. The commonest signs at onset among 29 French juvenile HD patients included cognitive and psychiatric disturbances in two-thirds, with motor signs at a mean of six years later; the remaining one-third presented with myoclonic head tremor, chorea, and progressive cerebellar signs (74). Brain neuroimaging shows atrophy of the caudate nucleus and putamen, while FDG-PET imaging shows hypometabolism in the caudate nucleus with selective neural cell loss, and 50% reduced binding at serotonin and muscarinic cholinergic receptors.

The diagnosis of HD rests on a positive family history, characteristic clinical findings, and detection of an expansion of 37 or more CAG trinucleotide repeats at the 4p16.3 locus of the *HTT* gene encoding huntingtin (Table 1), while normal individuals show a range of 9 to 36 CAG repeats. The risk of inheriting an *HTT* allele with CAG size of 35 is 10%.

Pharmacologic therapy of HD is limited to symptomatic treatment of chorea, hypokinesia, rigidity, myoclonic hyperkinesia, and psychiatric disturbances, including depression, psychosis, and aggression. However, experimental strategies have focused on inhibition of apoptosis, excitotoxicity, huntingtin aggregation and proteolysis, inflammation, oxidative damage, modulation of transglutamase activity, mitochondrial function, and transcriptional activity (75). A longitudinal study of persons at risk for HD was formed to study future therapeutic trials of HD (76).

The Parkin type of JPD is defined by onset before age 40 years and differs clinically and pathologically from classic late-onset PD. Although the exact prevalence is not known, it appears to be similar in all populations. Bradykinesia, tremor, and bradykinesia are common presenting signs, along with distal leg dystonia, hyperreflexia, abnormal behavior, and psychiatric manifestations.

The disease is slowly progressive over decades with atypical features, including peripheral neuropathy, autonomic dysfunction, and cerebellar ataxia. A cohort of Japanese PDJ patients (77) demonstrated onset of gait disturbance beginning at age 10 years with slow progression to assisted walking due to ataxia and frozen gait associated with tremor, diurnal fluctuation, and improvement after a nap or night's sleep that dissipated with age.

Laboratory evaluation shows diminished sensory nerve action potential (SNAP) amplitudes on NCS, and marked reduction in fluorodopa (FDOPA) uptake in caudate and putamen compared to the nigrostriatal pattern of idiopathic PD. Neuropathologic examination demonstrates neuronal loss, gliosis, and occasional neurofibrillary tangles in the medial and ventrolateral substantia nigra, and locus ceruleus with Lewy body inclusions.

Juvenile PD is caused by mutation at the 6q26 locus of the *PARK2* gene encoding parkin (Table 1) that ubiquitinates α synuclein and is involved in ubiquitin-mediated proteolytic pathways, which when defective in PDJ, leads to an accelerated loss of nigral neurons. Two simple heterozygous *PARK2* mutation carriers developed clinical symptoms of PDJ, suggesting that heterozygosity was a risk factor for disease expression, while heterozygous copy number variations in the PARK2 gene was noted in a similar percentage of controls, suggesting no increased risk (78, 79).

Management focuses upon an assessment of the severity and presence of atypical signs using the Unified Parkinson Disease Rating Scale (UPDRS) (80). PDJ responds well to levodopa and other dopaminergic agents, but there appears to be earlier occurrence of severe levodopa-induced dyskinesia, and a more favorable response to anticholinergic than dopaminergic medication than class PD. (81). Subthalamic deep brain stimulation, with its inherent benefits and side effects, may be considered. Carrier detection using molecular genetic analysis is available once the mutation has been identified in the proband. The offspring of an individual with PDJ are obligate heterozygotes.

Familial ChAc is a rare disorder with 500 to 1000 known cases, characterized by progressive neurodegeneration, red-cell acanthocytes, and onset from 8 to 62 years. It was described with at least two other syndromes as neuroacanthocytosis (82, 83). Neurological impairment includes chorea, involuntary orofaciolingual and pharyngeal dyskinesia, dysarthria, dysphagia, dystonic spasms, akinesia, cognitive impairment, psychiatric features and organic personality disorder in over one-half, and seizures in a third of patients.

Laboratory studies show acanthocytosis on peripheral blood smear and variably elevated serum creatine kinase (CK). Brain neuroimaging shows nonspecific cerebral, and, less often, caudate atrophy. Postmortem examination in one patient later showed extensive neuronal loss and gliosis affecting the striatum, pallidum, and substantia nigra. The disorder is caused by mutation at the 9q21.2 in the *VPS13A* gene encoding chorein (Table 1). Obligate heterozygotes do not show acanthocytosis. There is no specific treatment.

Lesch-Nyhan syndrome (LNS) presents with mental retardation, spastic cerebral palsy, choreoathetosis, uric acid urinary stones, self-mutilation of the fingers and lips, and XL inheritance. In 1965, Nyhan and colleagues (84) noted a 200-fold increase in the conversion of C(14)-labeled glycine to uric acid; two years later, excessive purine synthesis in LNS was attributed to deficiency of the enzyme hypoxanthine guanine phosphoribosyltransferase (HPRT) (85). It is now known that LNS is caused by a mutation at the Xq26.2-q26.3 locus of the HPRT1 gene encoding HPRT (Table 1), with a prevalence of 1:380,000. There is variable disease severity in patients with LNS, with an inverse relationship between HPRT enzyme activity, measured in intact cells, and clinical severity (86) and phenotypic variability across and among generations. The latter was apparent in one family of five individuals with a common mutation, including a child with classic LNS, delayed development, spasticity, dystonia and self-injurious behavior; and two each with either an intermediate phenotype of mild cognitive impairment, learning disability, dystonia, and increased uric acid without self-injurious behavior, and mild spasticity, gout, and normal intelligence. These observations suggested that each individual had a different expression of the mutant and wild type transcript and that those with the same genotype might not necessarily display an identical phenotype (87).

A 3-generation family carrying the same missense mutation showed similar phenotypic variability as follows. The proband presented at about age one year with increased uric acid levels followed by delayed development. A cousin was diagnosed with LNS at age 26 months with mild generalized hypotonia, delayed motor development, focal dystonia of the legs, developmental impairment, and speech delay. The proband's grandfather was more severely affected with borderline cognitive function, severe dyslexia, spasticity, and flexion contractures leading to motor impairment that was attributed to childhood cerebral palsy (86).

Patients with classic LNS demonstrate deficient enzyme activity in cultured fibroblasts, while those with partial HPRT deficiency designated LNS variants have reduced but not deficient HPRT enzyme activity.

Others with an intermediate form are indistinguishable from LNS with normal or near-normal intelligence and no self-injurious behavior.

The origin of self-injurious behavior in LNS has been postulated to be related to primary HPRT and secondary dopamine deficiency. Support of this hypothesis derives from several lines of evidence. Postmortem examination in three patients with LNS showed a marked reduction in dopamine content in the caudate and putamen (88). Patiens experimentally depleted of dopamine displayed self-injurious behavior similar to LNS (89). HPRT-deficient mutant mice showed a reduction in tyrosine hydroxylase and reduced numbers of striatal dopamine transporters (90). Brain PET imaging employing a dopamine analog in patients with LNS showed abnormally few dopaminergic nerve terminals and cell bodies (91). Experimental mouse neuroblastoma cell lines demonstrated that HPRT-deficiency regulates early developmental programming of dopamine neurons, findings that were seen in HPRT deficient human neuroblastoma cell lines (92). Genetic screening for LNS can be performed in fetal cells obtained by amniocentesis and CVS.

Dystonia is characterized by involuntary sustained muscle contractions affecting one or more sites of the body causing twitching, repetitive movements, and abnormal postures (93). They range from athetosis to rapid, shock-like myoclonic jerks, are sometimes rhythmic, and may be accompanied by tremor. Over time, dystonia occurs with less specific movements, eventually at rest, and causes sustained abnormal postures. The earlier the age at onset, the most likely it is to generalize and have a more severe course. The prevalence of dystonia ranges from 1:10,000 to 1:200.

The heritable dystonic syndromes are classified as primary dystonia, dystonia-plus, heredodegenerative, and paroxysmal dyskinesia syndromes. Non-heritable dystonia is usually secondary to another insult, most commonly drug-induced (tardive dystonia) by antipsychotic medication, L-dopa and phenothiazine antiemetic medication.

Childhood-onset dystonia syndromes occurs in the primary dystonia syndrome (DYT1) also known as dystonia musculorum deformans and idiopathic torsion dystonia (ITD). Four other dystonia-plus syndromes include dopa-responsive dystonia (DYT5), myoclonus-dystonia (DYT11), rapid-onset dystonia-parkinsonism (DYT12); pantothenate kinase-associated neurodegeneration (PKAN) or neurodegeneration with brain iron accumulation 1 (NBIA1) respectively, with AD (DYT1, DYT5, DYT 11, and DYT12) or AR inheritance (PKAN).

Children with DYT1 present in childhood or adolescence with involuntary postures of the limbs, trunk, or neck, with early onset cases the most severe, and generalization within three years. The disease is caused by a three-base pair GAG deletion at the 9q34 locus of the *DYT1* gene encoding torsin A (Table 1), an ATP-binding protein that appears to have a chaperone role in vesicle fusion, membrane trafficking, protein folding, and cytoskeletal dynamics.

Conventional brain MRI is normal in carriers of the *DYT1* gene mutation, however diffusion tensor MRI with fractional anisotropy showed microstructural white matter changes indicative of altered connectivity in the sensorimotor cortex (94). Brain PET shows reduced caudate and putamen D2 receptor availability in carriers compared to controls (95). Anticholinergic medication has been effective in some patients.

Dopa responsive dystonia (DRD, DYT5), or Segawa syndrome, presents insidiously between ages one and nine years, with dystonic postures or movement of one limb and involvement of all limbs within five years of onset. Nygard and colleagues (96) noted an extrapyramidal disorder characterized by childhood onset of leg and axial dystonia followed by Parkinsonism and a long-lasting response to levodopa (97).

The disorder is caused by mutation at the 14q22.2 locus of the *GCH1* gene encoding GTP cyclohydrolase I (Table 1) that is involved in the conversion of GTP to tetrahydrobiopterin, the cofactor for tyrosine hydroxylase, and the rate-limiting enzyme for dopamine synthesis. Disturbed dopamine synthetic capacity and reduced arborization of striatal dopamine terminals appear to be the underlying pathophysiology in DRD despite preservation of nigrostriatal dopaminergic neurons (98). An AR form of this disorder is caused by a mutation in the tyrosine hydroxylase gene. Oral phenylalanine identifies both symptomatic and asymptomatic carriers of the *GCH1* gene.

Myoclonic dystonia (DYT11) leads to proximal myoclonic jerking often associated with dystonia, usually torticollis, or writer cramp with onset in the first or second decade of life. Symptoms often respond to alcohol and clonazepam therapy, and the disorder generally pursues a benign course, however many patients have psychiatric abnormalities including obsessive-compulsive disorder (99).

This disorder is caused by a mutation at the 7q21.3 locus of the *SGCE* gene encoding ε-sarcoglycan (Table 1). Severe and refractory patients respond to deep brain stimulation of the internal pallidum (100). The syndrome of dystonia-parkinsonism (DYT12) was described in a large Indiana family characterized by unusually rapid evolution of acute or intermittent dystonia and Parkinsonism with onset during childhood or adolescence, and slow progression (101). The main dystonic features include dystonia of the face, arms, and legs, Parkinsonism, dysarthria, mutism, dysphagia, and drooling in association with broad-based gait, bradykinesia, and hypomimic face.

Brain MRI is generally normal, however early brain PET shows striatal hypermetabolism followed by decreased metabolic activity in later scans (102). The disorder is caused by heterozygous mutation at the 19q13.2 locus of the *ATP1A3* gene encoding the a-3 subunit of N, K-ATPase (Table 1). There is a moderate or absent response to dopamine agonists. Pantothenate kinase-associated neurodegeneration is characterized by progressive iron accumulation in the basal ganglia and other regions of the brain.

First described by Hallervorden and coworker (103) and later retracted after recognition of Hallervorden's active involvement in the euthanasia program in Germany during World War II, the disorder termed PKAN includes dystonic postures, choreoathetosis, rigidity, dysarthria, tremor, and coticospinal tract involvement leading to progressive spastic paraplegia. The classic form of PKAN presents in the first decade of life with rapidly progressing disease and loss of ambulation by 15 years. An atypical form has onset in the second decade with slower progression and maintenance of independent ambulation. An intermediate form has early onset and overall slow progression.

Brain MRI shows pronounced bilateral hypointensity of the globus pallidus because of iron accumulation and a central high-signal area of necrosis, the tiger eye sign.

The disorder is caused by mutation at the 20p13 locus of the *PANK2* gene that encodes pantothenate kinase 2 (Table 1). There is no known effective treatment, however some patients have been treated with tried iron chelation, dopaminergic and anticholinergic agents.

HEREDITARY SPASTIC PARAPLEGIA

Hereditary spastic paraplegia (HSP) is characterized by insidiously progressive leg weakness and spasticity. It is classified as "uncomplicated" or "pure" (pHSP) if neurologic impairment is limited to progressive lower-extremity spastic weakness, hypertonic urinary bladder disturbance, and mild diminution of vibration and joint position sensation; and "complicated" ("complex") (cHSP) when accompanied by systemic involvement or other neurologic features such as seizures, dementia, amyotrophy, extrapyramidal disturbance, or peripheral neuropathy (104). The disorders are transmitted by AD, AR, and XL recessive modes of inheritance.

There are presently 32 HSP loci and 11 HSP-related genes. Four well-documented genotypes occur in children, all cHSP phenotypes with an estimated prevalence of 1:100,000. Two are XL congenital, including spastic paraplegia-1 (SPG1) (105), and Allan-Herndon-Dudley syndrome (AHDS) (106), and two arise in childhood, 1 AR (SPG21) (107), and XL (SPG2) (108).

The acronym MASA was originally suggested by Bianchine and Lewis (109) to describe a Mexican-American kindred of three generations of SPG1 characterized by mental retardation, aphasia, shuffling gait, and adducted thumbs, in addition to small body size, microcephaly, exaggerated lumbar lordosis and hyperactive leg reflexes, distinguishing it from XL aqueductal stenosis by the absence of congenital hydrocephalus, which was absent in their patients. The disorder is due to mutation at the Xq28 locus of the *L1CAM* gene encoding the L1 cell adhesion molecule L1CAM (Table 1).

The occurrence of hydrocephalus, MASA, SPG1, and agenesis of the corpus callosum in other families with *L1CAM* mutation prompted the acronym CRASH for corpus callosum hypoplasia, mental retardation, adducted thumbs, spastic paraplegia, and hydrocephalus (110). X-linked aqueductal stenosis or hydrocephalus is now known to be an allelic disorder. An animal model of CRASH targeting the L1CAM gene in mice results in smaller than wild-type animals with weak incoordinated hind legs, with diminished size of the descending corticospinal tracts and enlarged ventricles (111). Allan and colleagues (112) described kindred of males affected by severe mental retardation spanning six generations, hypotonia at birth, and later development of impaired motor function with few ever walking, and most with generalized muscular atrophy, joint contraction, and hyporeflexia. Further study of this family revealed, in addition, dysarthria, ataxia, athetosis, spastic paraplegia, hyperreflexia, clonus, and Babinski signs more consistent with cHSP. The disorder is due to mutation at the Xq13.2 locus of the *SLC16A2* gene encoding monocarboxylate transporter-8 (Table 1).

In 1967 Cross and coworkers (113) described recessively inherited presenile dementia with onset in late teens or twenties and slowly progressive spastic paraparesis and basal ganglia involvement in an Amish kindred. Further analysis of the kindred by Simpson and coworkers (114) showed subtle childhood onset of slowly progressive cHSP with cerebellar and extrapyramidal signs, thin corpus callosum and white matter abnormalities on brain neuroimaging. The disorder is due to a mutation at the 15q22.31 locus of the *ACP33* gene encoding 33-kD acidic-cluster protein (Table 1).

Johnston and McKusick (115) reported a sex-linked recessive form of pure spastic paraplegia with later development of nystagmus, dysarthria, sensory disturbance, mental retardation, and variable optic atrophy, followed by muscle wasting, joint contracture, cerebellar signs, and crutches or wheelchair assistance in early adult life. Later postmortem examination in one of the members showed degeneration of corticospinal and spinocerebellar tracts. The disorder is due to a mutation at the Xq22.2 locus of the *PLP1* gene encoding myelin proteolipid protein (Table 1). There is no specific medication for HSP apart from physical and occupational therapy, and drugs to reduce spasticity and clonus. Prenatal diagnosis is available for some forms of HSP by analysis of DNA extracted from fetal cells at amniocentesis or CVS.

HEREDITARY ATAXIA

The hereditary ataxias are characterized by slowly progressive gait incoordination gait often associated with poor coordination of hands, speech, eye movements, and cerebellar atrophy. The hereditary ataxias can be categorized by mode of inheritance into AD, AR, XL, and mitochondrial, with a prevalence of the AD disorders of 3:100,000. Most of the AD cerebellar ataxias (ADCA) are numerically designated as spinocerebellar ataxia (SCA1 to36). Although nearly all have an average onset in the 3rd to 4th decade of life, some (SCA 13, 27, EA1, EA2) have onset in childhood. SCA13 presents with slowly progressive early childhood gait and limb ataxia, titubation, hypotonia, dysarthria, nystagmus, mental retardation, motor developmental delay, and corticospinal tract signs (116). Brain MRI shows moderate cerebellar and pontine atrophy. The disorder is due to a heterozygous mutation at 19q13.333 locus in the voltage-gated potassium channel, Shaw-related subfamily, member-3 gene *KCNC3* (Table 1) (117).

SCA27 presents with late childhood ataxia and tremor of the arms, orofacial dyskinesia, nystagmus, dysarthria, and psychomotor delay. Brain MRI shows cerebellar atrophy. The disorder is due to mutation at the 13q33.1 locus in the *FGF14* gene encoding fibroblast growth factor-14 (Table 1) (118). Two episodic ataxias, EA1 and EA2, present with spells of incoordination, imbalance, and variably progressive ataxia (119). EA1 is caused by mutation at the 12p13.32 locus of the potassium channel gene *KCNA1*, while EA2 results from a mutation at the 19p13.2 locus of the calcium ion channel gene *CACNA1A* (Table 1).

Two hereditary ataxias, infantile-onset spinocerebellar ataxia (IOSCA) and Friedrich ataxia (FRDA), manifest AR inheritance. The syndrome of IOSCA, which refers to the syndromes of opthalmoplegia, hypoacusis, ataxia, hypotonia, and athetosis (OHAHA) (120) and originally was regarded as a form of spinocerebellar ataxia (121) is now classified as an mtDNA depletion syndrome (122) based on the finding of mtDNA in the brain and liver of affected children. It is due to homozygous or compound heterozygous mutation at the 10q24.31 locus of the nuclear-encoded *C10ORF2* gene encoding the twinkle and twinky proteins (Table 1) (123).

Friedrich ataxia is characterized by progressive gait and limb ataxia, dysarthria, dorsal column sensory loss, limb weakness, absent reflexes, and Babinski signs in the first or second decade of life before the end of puberty (124). Other variable features include visual defects, scoliosis, pes cavus, and cardiomyopathy. It is one of the most common forms of AR ataxia, occurring in 1:50,000 individuals. It is caused by a GAA trinucleotide repeat expansion at the 9q21.11 locus of intron 1 of the *FXN* gene encoding frataxin (Table 1). Normal individuals have 5 to 30 GAA repeat expansions, while affected individuals have from 70 to 1,000 GAA triplets (125).

Molecular genetic evaluation is available for SCA 13, SCA27, EA1 and 2, IOSCA and FRDA, and many other ADCA but should be individualized whenever possible. It is virtually the only means of diagnosis in an individual with ataxia and no family history.

DISORDERS ASSOCIATED WITH SEIZURES

Three groups of hereditary metabolic disorders are recognized under this category. The first category consists of early infancy disorders presenting with cutaneous signs and seizures, among them biotinidase deficiency and Menkes disease. The second group includes infants with constant severe seizures, including Alpers or Alpers-Huttenlocher syndrome (AHS), and glucose transporter protein (GLUT1) deficiency. Others occur in older children and young adults characterized by progressive myoclonic epilepsy, notably Unverricht-Lundborg and Lafora disease (LD) (respectively designated EPM1 and EMP2A), and myoclonic epilepsy with RRF (MERRF). The inheritance patterns include AR (biotinidase deficiency, Alpers, GLUT1 deficiency, EPM1 and 2A), XL (Menkes), and mtDNA (MERRF).

Deficiency of biotinidase, the enzyme that cleaves biotin from biocytin, presents in early infancy with severe myoclonic seizures, skin rash, developmental delay, hypotonia, ataxia, and episodes of metabolic acidosis (126). Organic aciduria and biotinidase deficiency in serum, leukocytes, and cultured skin fibroblasts make the diagnosis certain.

The disorder is due to a mutation at the 3p25.1 locus of the *BTD* gene encoding biotinidase (Table 1). Newborn screening for biotinidase deficiency identifies children with profound (less than 10% of mean normal) and partial deficiency (10% to 30%). Treatment of children with severe enzyme inactivity show pronounced rapid clinical and biochemical improvement except for residual neurological damage, while those with partial untreated deficiency often do not exhibit symptoms unless they are stressed by prolonged infection. On the basis of newborn screening, the incidence of biotinidase deficiency is 18.4 cases per million live births. Turkish children homozygous for null mutations in *BTD* manifest hearing loss whereas those without hearing loss are homozygous for missense mutations leading instead to residual enzyme activity. Prompt treatment of those with the homozygous null mutations prevents later hearing loss (127).

Menkes described a sex-linked recessive disorder affecting male infants characterized by early growth retardation, peculiar hair, and focal cerebral and cerebellar degeneration. Severe neurological impairment began one to two months after birth and progressed rapidly to decerebration (128). The hair was stubby, white, and showed microscopic twisting, with varying diameter across the length of the shaft and fractures at regular intervals. The term *kinky hair disease* proved a useful designation in alerting pediatricians to possible new cases, which occur in 1 per 298,000 live births (129). Later evidence of the defect in copper metabolism and copper deficiency due to involvement of at least five defective cuproenzymes explained several, but not all, of the aspects of the disorder, including tyrosinase for depigmentation of hair and skin pallor, lysyl oxidase for frayed and split arterial intima due to a defect in elastin and collagen cross-linking, monoamine oxidase for kinky hair, COX for hypothermia, and ascorbate oxidase for skeletal deformities (130). A clearer understanding of the molecular pathogenesis and cytopathology soon followed (131).

The disorder is due to mutation at the Xq21.1 locus of the *ATP7A* gene encoding the Menkes protein (MNK) Cu (2+)-transporting ATPase, α-polypeptide (Table 1). The MNK protein, which is normally localized to the transGolgi network, rapidly relocates to the plasma membrane upon exposure to excessive copper where it then functions in copper efflux, removing copper from the cytoplasm by transporting it into vesicles through which it cycles. Carrier status for Menkes disease is suggested by examination of multiple hairs at scattered scalp sites for pili torti. First trimester prenatal diagnosis can be performed using a specific DNA probe (132). There is no effective treatment and empiric daily injections of copper restore serum levels but not those of the brain.

Alpers-Huttenlocher syndrome, or mtDNA depletion syndrome 4Λ, was initially described in a four-month-old child with intractable seizures (133). Sandbank and coworkers (134), and later Harding (135), extended the neurologic, electrophysiologic, and histopathological features among other patients that included the clinical triad of psychomotor retardation, intractable epilepsy, and liver failure, with neuropathological evidence of cerebral cortical degeneration, neuronal loss, astroglial proliferation, and abnormal electron dense mitochondrial inclusions. De Vries (136), Wiltshire (137), and Kurt and colleagues (138) described other children with progressive epileptic encephalopathy and liver involvement and molecular genetic defects in the *POLG* gene.

The estimated frequency of AHS is 1:100,000. Brain neuroimaging reveals cerebral atrophy and low density lesions in the medial occipital lobes. The cause of Alpers syndrome is due to homozygous or compound heterozygous mutation at the 15q26.1 locus of the *POLG* gene encoding mtDNA polymerase γ (Table 1). The *POLG*-related disorders comprise a continuum of overlapping phenotypes that exemplify the diversity that can result from mutations in a given gene. Biochemical deficiencies in pyruvate metabolism, NADH oxidation, and global reduction in the respiratory chain complexes I, II/III, and IV activity, and mtDNA polymerase γ activity have all been described.

Alpers-Huttenlocher syndrome affects 1:51,000 people. It is generally believed that the cellular mtDNA content reflects not only upon the genotype, but on the eventual phenotype, with biallelic *POLG* mutations developing the most severe clinical phenotype, early onset before age 1 year, hepatic involvement, and death before age 2 to 3 years.

Originally thought to be distinct entities, *POLG*-related disorders include in addition to AHS, childhood myocerebrohepatopathy spectrum (MCHS) of myopathy or hypotonia with developmental delay or encephalopathy and liver dysfunction; myoclonic epilepsy, myopathy, and sensory ataxia (MEMSA), formerly termed SCA with epilepsy; ataxia neuropathy spectrum (ANS), including disorders previously termed mitochondrial recessive ataxia syndrome (MIRAS) and sensory ataxia, neuropathy, dysarthria, and ophthalmoplegia (SANDO); AR and AD PEO (139, 140).

Glucose transporter deficiency syndrome-1 was first recognized by DeVivo among two infants with hypoglycorrhachia, seizures, developmental delay, and diminished transport of hexose into isolated red blood cells (RBC), and attributed to a defect in glucose transport across the blood-brain barrier (141). A decade later, Wang (142) described heterozygous mutations of *GLUT1*. Seizure types varied, including tonic clonic, myoclonic, atypical absence, and atonic, often in association with staring spells, apneic episodes, episodic eye movements, and motor disability in the first few months of life, aggravated by a carbohydrate load and rapidly responsive to ketogenic diet, not anticonvulsants (143, 144). Other intermittent phenomena include ataxia, myoclonic jerks, dystonic postures, confusion, lethargy, sleep disturbance, and headache while other described patients displayed global developmental delay, moderate mental retardation, dysarthria, and spasticity.

Laboratory criteria for the disorder include hypoglycorrhachia, low CSF to blood glucose ratio, low to normal CSF lactate, and reduced erythrocyte glucose uptake and decreased GLUT1 immunoreactivity in erythrocyte membranes.

The disorder is due to mutation at the 1p34.2 locus of the *SLC2A1* gene encoding the GLUT1 transporter. GLUT1 deficiency syndrome type 2 is an allelic disorder with a less severe phenotype. There are no firm estimates of the incidence or prevalence of GLUT1 deficiency. The persistent decrease in glucose in the developing brain is the uniform finding in both disorders, which Pascula and coworkers (145) classified as infantile neuroglycopenia. Hypothesizing glucose serves a dual capacity in the developing brain, acting both as a fuel and signaling molecule.

Myoclonus presents as asymmetrical asynchronous involuntary muscle jerks in various parts of the body, increased by voluntary movement and proprioceptive stimuli. It is associated with a propensity for seizures, ataxia, and dementia. Unverricht (146) and Lundborg (147) reported a type of progressive myoclonic epilepsy that occurred at around age 10 and progressed to incapacity with only mild mental deterioration. Histologic studies of the brain showed degenerative changes without inclusions.

Lundborg's report was one of the earliest examples of AR inheritance and the first statistical analysis testing the recessive hypothesis in humans. Eldridge (148) referred to the disorder as a Baltic type of myoclonic epilepsy and noted stimulus- and photo-sensitive myoclonus, with worsening upon awakening, and synchronous spike wave discharges on EEG. Although phenytoin was associated with progressive motor and intellectual deterioration, valproic acid led to marked improvement.

Patients with EPM1 present with adolescent-onset myoclonic epilepsy, absence of drop attack seizures typically upon awakening, polymyoclonus, progressive cerebellar ataxia, and spasticity. Symptoms typically worsen in the first six years after onset, stabilize and improve in early adulthood with little or no cognitive decline and variable survival, differentiating it from myoclonic epilepsy with Lafora bodies in which intelligence was affected and the disease invariably fatal. The incidence of the disorder in Finland is about 1:20,000 with far fewer cases in the rest of the world.

The disorder is caused by a mutation at the 21q22.3 locus of the *CSTB* gene encoding cystatin B (Table 1), leading to disturbance in the cysteine protease cystatin B associated with widespread neuronal degeneration that predominates in the cerebellar cortex, basal ganglia, dentate nuclei, brainstem, and spinal cord. There is no effective treatment. Lafora disease presents in childhood with seizures, myoclonus, mental deterioration, and dementia. Brain neuroimaging shows cerebellar atrophy.

Lafora bodies (LD), composed of PAS positive, abnormally branched, glycogen molecules or polyglucosans, are found in biopsies of skin sweat glands, liver, muscle, and neurons. Although LD occurs worldwide, the exact incidence and prevalence are not yet known.

Lafora disease results from mutation at the 6q24.3 locus of the *EPM2A* gene that encodes the dual-specificity protein phosphatase laforin, or a mutation at the 6p22.3 locus of the *NHLRC1* gene encoding malin (Table 1), a protein ubiquitin ligase that interacts with laforin and localizes with the latter in the endoplasmic reticulum. Together, the two genes regulate critical processes involved in the pathogenesis of LD (149).

Fukuhara and colleagues (150) reported the syndrome of MERFF, a mitochondrial encephalomyopathy that included childhood myoclonus, generalized seizures, mental deterioration, intention tremor, ataxia, weakness, atrophy, foot deformity, acidosis with elevated blood lactate, and pyruvate. Short stature, ataxia, and sensorineural hearing loss were recognized later. A specific mutation in mtDNA was first demonstrated by Shoffner and colleagues (151), leading to multiple deficiencies in enzyme complexes of the respiratory chain, most prominently in complex I of COX, consistent with a defect in translation of all mtDNA-encoded genes. The genetic basis of MERRF most commonly results from an A-to-G mutation at nucleotide 8344 of *tRNA* gene of mtDNA (152).

FAMILIAL POLYNEUROPATHIES

Infantile and childhood familial polyneuropathies are clinically and genetically heterogeneous. Peripheral nervous system (PNS) disturbances may predominate and precede signs of more widespread CNS and systemic involvement, as in Refusm disease, transthyretin (TTR) amyloidosis, and Fabry disease, or the singular clinical manifestation as in the Charcot Marie Tooth (CMT) disorders, with AR (Resfum), AD (TTR), and XL (Fabry) inheritance or a combination thereof (CMT).

Adult Refsum disease is distinguished clinically from infantile Refsum disease that belongs to the group of PBD disorders with a different phenotype and genetic basis. Presentations late in the first decade of life with anosmia, visual loss due to pigmentary retinal degeneration, gait disturbance due to peripheral sensory neuropathy, sensory neural hearing loss leading to deafness, cerebellar ataxia, ichthyosis, cardiac conduction abnormalities, cardiomyopathy, and skeletal malformations (153).

The four cardinal features described by Refsum (154) of retinitis pigmentosa, neuropathy, ataxia, and raised CSF protein concentration are rarely seen in a single individual. Patients were found to have accumulation of phytanic acid, an unusual branch-chain fatty acid in tissues and body fluids, as a result of disturbed α-oxidation of phytanic acid and deficient activity of phytanoly-CoA hydroxylase due to

mutation at 10p13 locus of the *PHYH* gene in Refsum disease-1 (Table 1) (155). Decreased phytanic acid oxidation was later observed in human cells. The disorder is due to a mutation at the 6q23.3 locus of the *PEX7* gene encoding peroxin-7 (Table 1), the receptor for peroxisomal-targeting signal type 2 (PTS2) (156).

Treatment is based upon dietary restriction of phytanic intake which helps resolve icthyosis, along with plasmapheresis or lipid apheresis for acute arrhythmias and severe neuropathy. A high calorie diet prevents mobilization of phytanic acid into the plasma.

Amyloidosis is a systemic disorder characterized by extracellular deposition of TTR, composed of insoluble amyloid protein fibrils in peripheral nerves, eye, heart, and kidney (157, 158) leading to peripheral neuropathy, carpal tunnel syndrome, autonomic insufficiency, cardiomyopathy, and gastrointestinal features, and occasionally associated with vitreous opacities and renal insufficiency. Before the emergence of molecular genetics the familial amyloid polyneuropathies were initially classified by phenotypic features and ethnicity (159). Formally termed *familial amyloid polyneuropathy* (FAP), TTR-familial amyloid neuropathy type I presents in Portuguese, Swedish, and Japanese cohorts with childhood onset of distal sensory neuropathy in the legs followed by motor neuropathy and eventual foot drop and upper limb involvement, autonomic dysfunction, cardiomyopathy, vitreous opacities, nephropathy, neurogenic ulcers, and arthropathy.

TTR-familial amyloid neuropathy type II presents in Indiana/Swiss or Maryland/German cohorts with carpal tunnel syndrome; sensorimotor and autonomic neuropathy with visceral organ involvement, and cardiomyopathy and nephropathy in the advanced stages of the disease. Sural nerve biopsy tissue stains positive with Congo red immunofluorescence for amyloid protein, and antithyretin antibodies for TTR protein.

This form of hereditary amyloidosis is caused by mutation at the 18q12.1 locus of the *TTR* gene encoding TTR (Table 1). The vast majority of individuals with familial TTR amyloidosis are heterozygous for a *TTR* mutation, however homozygotes present with incomplete penetrance, earlier onset, more severe clinical course and widespread amyloid deposition (160).

In addition to hereditary amyloidosis, there are two other forms of systemic amyloidosis, immunoglobulin (AL) amyloidosis, or primary amyloidosis associated with monoclonal paraproteinemic light chains as the amyloid fibrils, and reactive (AA) amyloidosis, or secondary amyloidosis that occurs in association with chronic inflammatory disorders with fibrils derived from amyloid A protein that circulates as an acute phase reactant.

Like other amyloid proteins, the pathogenic potential of the TTR protein lies in the extensive β sheet structure, which upon pathogenic mutation disrupts the stability of the TTR molecule, dissociating it into proamyloidogenic monomers (161). One non-TTR neuropathic disease, Finnish FAP type IV, presents with corneal lattice dystrophy, cranial neuropathy, bulbar signs, skin changes, peripheral neuropathy, and renal failure due to mutation at the 9q33.2 locus of the GSN gene encoding gelsolin (162).

Familial amyloid polyneuropathy type III is a non-neuropathic visceral type associated with mutation in APOA1. Patients younger than 60 years of age with polyneuropathy of the legs or autonomic neuropathy alone, and no significant cardiac or renal involvement, should be considered for orthotopic liver transplantation, which removes the main production site of the amyloidogenic protein and results in rapid disappearance of the variant TTR protein from the serum halting progression of peripheral and autonomic neuropath (163). Treatment in all types is supportive.

Fabry disease is a systemic disorder that manifests painful acroparesthesia occurring as episodic crises of burning pain in the distal extremities in childhood and early adolescence signalling onset of the disease, first described as purpura papulosa haemorrhagica Hebrae (164), and vascular lesions at other sites thought to result from lipid deposition. Later investigators (165) identified corneal opacities termed *cornea verticillata* in individuals of either gender, allowing heterozygous carrier females to be identified. Other features include neuropathic pain, cerebral small vessel vasculopathy, sensorineural deafness, widespread autonomic dysfunction, renal failure, and cardiovascular disease, the latter two of which curtail life expectancy, depending upon the aggressiveness of management.

The incidence of Fabry disease varies from 1:55,000 male births to 1:4,600 individuals based upon newborn screening studies (166). The disease should be considered in the differential diagnosis of older boys and young men with cryptogenic neuropathic pain (167) and unexplained stroke (168), especially of the posterior circulation wherein a combination of abnormalities of the vessel wall, blood components, and abnormal hemodynamics occurs, leading to a 20-fold increased risk of ischemic stroke and transient ischemic attacks compared to the general population (169). Female carriers are often asymptomatic or minimally symptomatic. The disorder results from mutations at the Xq22.1 locus of the GLA gene encoding α-galactosidase A (α-Gal A) (Table 1), which is deficient in plasma, leukocytes, and cultured skin fibroblasts, and leads to increased levels of globotriaosylceramide and related glycosphingolipids and found in the plasma, urinary sediment, and cellular lysosomes of blood vessels, nerve, tissues, and organs throughout the body.

Neuropathological examination reveals deposition of storage products in central and autonomic neurons, along peripheral axons of the intermediolateral spinal gray, and in dorsal column and visceral brainstem nuclei. Two recombinant or gene-activated human α-Gal-A ERT, algalsidase-β and algalsidase-α, have been evaluated in clinical trials to prevent the primary manifestations of Fabry disease, but only the former has been approved by the FDA for use in the U.S. A double-blind randomized placebo-controlled phase III clinical trial of agalsidase-β demonstrated clearance of GL-3 from endothelial cells of the kidney, heart, and skin, with absence of microvascular endothelial deposits of GL-3 as compared to the placebo group, who experienced none of the beneficial effects (170). The risk of major clinical events including death, myocardial infarction, stroke, end- stage renal disease, and a 33% increase in serum creatinine concentration was reduced by 54% by agalsidase in a phase IV double-blind placebo-controlled trial (171). Demonstration of decreased α-Gal A enzyme activity is diagnostic of the carrier state, however some carriers will have activities in the normal range, making it unreliable for routine detection. Those at risk should undergo ophthalmologic examination for the characteristic whorl-like corneal opacities by slit-lamp microscopy or molecular genetic testing if the GLA family is known. Prenatal testing by measurement of α-Gal-A enzyme activity can be performed in fetal cells obtained by amniocentesis or by CVS.

The classification of CMT hereditary neuropathy has not been an easy task since the original description by Charcot and Marie (172) and Tooth (173). The phenotypic, genotypic subtypes, and molecular genetic testing strategies of CMT neuropathy, the commonest inherited neuromuscular disorder affecting 1: 2500, has been the subject of several recent reviews (174). They result from mutations in over 30 causative genes expressed in Schwann cells and neurons responsible for the diversity of clinical phenotypes with AD, AR, and XL inheritance. There are six recognized AD CMT1 genes and associated chromosomal loci that lead to clinically indistinguishable subtypes due to mutation or sequence changes separately at the 17p12 locus of the PMP gene in CMT1A and CMT1E; the 1q22.3 locus of MPZ in CMT1B; the 16p13.13 locus in LITAF in CMT1C; the 10q21.3 locus of EGR2 in CMT1D; and the 8p21.2 locus of NEFL in CMT1F (Table 1).

Affected children with a classic CMT1 phenotype present in the first or second decade with a delay in the onset of walking before or after 15 months, depending upon the clinical severity and degree of uniform motor nervous conduction velocity (NCV) slowing, which is typically between 15 and 25 m/s, in association with palpably hypertrophic nerves, pes cavus foot deformity, and bilateral extensor foot weakness. The clinical progression is typically slow, with fewer than 5% of patients becoming wheelchair dependent.

There are 15 chromosomal loci of AD CMT2 (CMT2A1 and 2; 2B, B1, B2, 2C-L and N) that correspond to mutation at the 1p36.22 locus of the KIF1B and MFN2 genes in CMT2A1 and 2; the 3q21.3 locus of the RAB7A gene in

CMT2B; the 1q22 locus of the *LMNA* gene in CMTB1, the 19q13.33 locus of *MED25* in CMT2B2; the *TRPV4* gene of CMT2C; the 7p14.3 locus of the *GARS* gene in CMT2D; the 8p21.2 locus of the *NEFL* gene of CMT2E; the 7q11.23 locus of *HSPB1* in CMT2F; the *GDAP1* gene in CMT2H and K; the 12q24.23 locus of *HSPB8* in CMTL; and the 16q22.1 locus of *AARS* in CMT2N (Table 1).

Patients affected with CMT2 present with pes cavus foot deformity, axonal peripheral neuropathy characterized by less disabling distal muscle weakness, wasting, less prominent sensory loss, normal or near-normal motor NCV, non-hypertrophic nerves, and less prominent foot drop than those with CMT1. There are four recognized chromosomal loci of AD intermediate CMT (CMTDI) that include linkage to chromosome 10q24.1-q25.1 in CMTDIA; the 19p13.2 locus of *DNM2* in CMTDIB; the 1p35.1 locus of *YARS* in CMTDIC; and the 1q23.3 locus of *MPZ* in CMTDID (Table 1). Patients affected with CMTDI, manifest a relatively typical CMT phenotype with clinical and pathological evidence of both abnormal myelin and axonopathy, and motor NCV that overlap with those of CMT1 and CMT2. There are nine chromosomal loci of AR CMT4 and eight CMT4 subtypes (CMT4A, B1, B2, C-F, H, J) that specifically correspond to mutation at the 8q13-q21.1 locus of the *GDAP1* gene in CMT4A; at the 11q22 locus of *MTMR2* in CMT4B1; at the 11p15 locus of *SBF2* in CMT4B2; the 5q32 locus of *SH3TC2* in CMT4C; the 8q24.3 locus of *NRDG1* in CMT4D; the 10q21.1-q22.1 locus of the *ERG2* in CMT4E; the 19q13.1-q13.2 locus of *PRX* in CMT4F; the 12p11.2-q13.1 locus of *FGD4* in CMT4H; and the 6q21 locus of *FIG4* in CMT4J (Table 1).

Originally described as hypertrophic polyneuropathy by Dejerine-Sottas (175), the clinical features in affected infants and children born to unaffected parents manifest pes cavus, ataxia, pes cavus, kyphoscoliosis, distal sensory and motor deficits, and muscular atrophy predominating in the legs, progressing in a length-dependent patter, with palpably hypertrophic nerves, Argyll-Robertson pupils, very slow motor NCV, elevated CSF protein, and onion bulb formation (176).

Finally, five chromosomal loci of XL CMT (CMTX1-5) respectively localize to the Xq13.1 locus of *GJB1* and Xp22.2, Xq26, Xq24-q26.1, and the Xq22-q24 locus of the *PRPS1* gene (Table 1). X-linked dominant CMT type 1, the most common form of CMTX, presents in male children from infancy to early childhood with delayed motor development, sensorineural hearing loss, tremor, pathologic fractures, and transient CNS disturbances. Axon loss, as reflected in low amplitude compound muscle action potentials, is present in all patients, and carrier females show abnormal neurologic or neurophysiologic features of a lesser degree (177).

The growing number of genes attests to the complexity of pathways and purported mechanisms that contribute to CMT etiopathogenesis, making genetic testing ever more important in understanding the pathogenetic mechanisms. The latter include disturbances in transcriptional regulation, protein turnover, protein synthesis, stress responses, apoptosis, Schwann cell-axonal interactions, axonal transport, and mitochondrial dysfunction.

A related PMP22 genetic disorder termed *hereditary neuropathy with liability to pressure palsies* (HNPP) presents in the second or third decade of life with painless episodes of recurrent sensory and motor demyelinating neuropathy attributed to one or more nerves, and AD inheritance. The most commonly affected nerves are the peroneal at the fibular head leading to foot drop, the ulnar nerve at the elbow simulating a tardy ulnar palsy, the median nerve at the wrist resembling carpal tunnel syndrome, the radial nerve resembling a wrist drop, and brachial plexopathy presenting as brachial neuritis.

Occasional patients present with progressive mononeuropathy, CMT- or chronic inflammatory demyelinating disease-like progression, progressive muscular atrophy, CNS white matter lesions, and scapuloperoneal syndrome. Nerve conduction studies show demyelinating mononeuropathy with superimposed conduction block as the basis of weakness, with varying degrees of axonal loss reflective of the clinical severity and duration, typically without active denervation on needle electromyography (EMG). Sural nerve biopsy shows sausage-like elongations called tomaculi. The disorder results from point and frame-shift mutations at the 17p12 locus of the *PMP22* gene (Table 1).

Genetic testing in CMT and related disorders should be considered for the accurate diagnosis and classification recognizing however, that not every patient may wish to undergo such analysis due to personal convictions or limited financial resources. Two large analyses, one evidence literature based, and the other retrospective of a single institutional cohort, together suggested that genetic testing in CMT should be guided by the clinical phenotype, inheritance pattern, and electrodiagnostic features employing multi-tier algorithms for the likeliest involved genes and corresponding CMT subtypes (178, 179).

Genetic screening starts with studies for duplication or deletion mutation in *PMP22* for CMT1A and HNPP in classic phenotypes, positive family history, and slow upper-extremity motor NCV, typically 15 to 35 m/sec, as well as *GJB1* for CMTX in the absence of male-to-male transmission. If this is uninformative or there is male-to-male transmission, the second tier of genetic testing includes *MPZ* mutation studies for an unusual presentation of CMT1B, followed by a third-tier study, *LITAF* and *EGR2* mutations in CMT1C and CMT1D, *GDAP1*, and *PRX* in CMT4A and CMT4F, and the other uncommon CMT4 subtypes.

Whereas severely slow-motor NCV, typically less than 15 m/sec, were characteristic of CMT1A or CMT1B, a delayed age at onset of walking at or before 15 months was not encountered with *MPZ* mutation instead of the predicted duplication in *PMP22* (180).

Patients with a classic CMT phenotype, positive family history, and intermediate motor MCV, typically 35 to 45 m/sec, should be studied first for mutations in *GJB1* for CMT1X in the absence of male-to-male transmission, and *MPZ* for CMT1b in the presence of male-to-male inheritance, followed by testing for AR and CMTDI forms, depending upon the inheritance pattern. If axonal CMT is suggested instead by severe onset in infancy and childhood of a classical phenotype with normal or unobtainable motor NCV, such patients should undergo genetic studies for CMT2A and *GJB1* for CMT1X, or *MPZ* for CMT1B for later onset patients unless there is evidence of male-to-male inheritance, in which case only CMT1B would be warranted. If the foregoing is uninformative, it is appropriate to include genetic studies for AR CMT, including *RAB7* for CMT2B; *GARS* for DMT2D; *NEFL* for CMT2E; and *HSPB1* mutation for CMT2F.

Although there is no effective therapy, several scientific approaches have been considered. Treatment with prednisone or intravenous immune globulin produced variable levels of improvement in patients with CMT1 with sudden deterioration and inflammation in nerve biopsy tissue (181). Therapy with ascorbic acid in a mouse model and antiprogesterone therapy with onapristone in a transgenic rat model of CMT1A both showed improvement (182, 183), whereas ascorbic acid did not benefit patients so studied (184).

Supportive measures include bracing with ankle-foot orthotic, protective pads at the elbows and knees, avoidance of positions that predispose to focal compression, such as crossing of legs and sustained repetitive movements of the wrists and elbows, rapid weight loss, and avoidance of neurotoxic medications (185).

FAMILIAL DYSAUTONOMIAS

Hereditary sensory and autonomic neuropathies (HSAN) affect peripheral sensory and autonomic neurons with variable motor involvement (186). Dyck and Ohta classified HSAN into four subtypes HSAN1 to four based upon mode of inheritance, symptoms at onset, clinical course, and pathology of neurons or axons affected (187). There has been increasing appreciation of the genetic, clinical neurophysiology, biochemical, and autonomic features of this group of disorders (188). They are uncommon disorders with AD (HSAN1) and AR (HSANII) inheritance, and an overall incidence of 30:100,000.

Hicks described HSAN1A in an English family with perforating ulcers of the feet, shooting pains, and deafness, with an age range at onset of 15 to 36 years (189). Other clinical features known to occur include pupillary abnormalities, neuropathic pain, diminished sensation and sweating, gangrene, osteomyelitis, and variable distal motor involvement often eventuating in wheelchair dependency.

Electrodiagnostic studies remain normal until later in the disease. Cutaneous sensory nerve biopsy tissue is consistent with axonal degeneration, although small myelinated fibers are more affected than large ones, presumably as a result of slow axonal degeneration. Neuropathological finding include marked changes in posterior columns, posterior roots, and dorsal root ganglia (DRG) with a predilection for distal lumbosacral dermatomes.

The disorder is caused by heterozygous mutation at the 9q22.31 locus of the *SPTLC1* gene encoding serine palmitoyltransferase 1 (Table 1). The related disorder HSAN1B presents with sensory axonal neuropathy, cough, gastroesophageal reflux, and impaired laryngeal sensation and a cytogenetic location at 3p24-p22.

First described as neurogenic acro-osteolysis (190) and hereditary sensory neuropathy with a similarly to Morvan disease (191), children with HSAN2A and 2B present in infancy or early childhood with hypotonia and prominent autonomic involvement, including acral ahidrosis, gustatory sweating, tonic pupils, oromotor incoordination, constipation from gastrointestinal dysmotility, urinary incontinence from bladder dysfunction, intermittent fever, and apnea. There is marked loss of limb and truncal sensation leading to painless trophic ulcers and undetected fractures of the hands and feet. Children with HSAN2B, in addition, have mild motor neuropathy of the legs.

Sensory NCS reveal absent or reduced SNAP amplitudes with relatively preserved or reduced motor NCV, and needle EMG shows minimal fibrillation and neurogenic motor recruitment (186). Cutaneous sensory nerve biopsy tissue shows pronounced loss of small myelinated fibers, segmental demyelination, remyelination, and decreased unmyelinated fibers consistent with an axonal process.

The disorders are due to a mutation at the 12p13.33 locus of the *WNK1* gene encoding serine/threonine-protein kinase WNK1 in HSAN2A, and at the 5p15.1 locus of the *FAM134B* gene encoding protein FAM123B in HSAN2B (Table 1).

Riley and coworkers (192) described HSAN3 among five Jewish patients with defective lacrimation, episodic hypertension, hyperhidrosis, cyclic vomiting, and skin blotching. Later investigators noted lack of an axon flare after intradermal histamine (193), absence of lingual fungiform papillae (194), and Ashkenazi Jewish descent.

Affected children develop infantile hypotonia, developmental motor delay, swallowing difficulty, gastrointestinal dysfunction, cyclic vomiting episodes, blood pressure fluctuation, hypohydrosis, absent overflow tears with crying (alacrima), vasomotor instability, indifference to pain and temperature, impaired taste, neuropathic joint deformity, scoliosis, and emotional instability with intact intelligence.

Cutaneous sensory nerve biopsy tissue shows a decreased number of nonmyelinated axons and small-diameter myelinated axons, differentiating it from other sensory neuropathies. Neuropathological evaluation shows progressively reduced size and number of DRG and dorsal column myelinated axons, with decreased numbers of sympathetic preganglionic neurons in the intermediolateral columns and sympathetic ganglia and corresponding peripheral nerve terminals innervating blood vessels. The disorder is caused by mutation at the 9q31.3 locus in the *IKBKAP* gene encoding elongator complex protein 1 (Table 1).

Swanson and colleagues (195) described two brothers with congenital insensitivity to pain and anhidrosis, defective temperature sensation, and normal appearing sweat glands on skin biopsy. Postmortem examination showed absence of small primary sensory ganglia and neurons, with degeneration of roots and Lissauer's tracts (196).

Children with HSAN4 develop profound autonomic and sensory deficits, while hypotonia and delayed motor milestones that occur in infancy and childhood normalize with age. Anhidrosis predisposes to fever, while insensitivity to superficial and deep pain leads to corneal ulceration, while oral self-mutilation and fingertip biting contributes to inadvertent bone fractures and joint trauma. There may be learning disturbances, cognitive impairments, hyperactivity, and emotional liability.

Electrodiagnostic studies are usually normal. Skin biopsy shows lack of eccrine sweat gland and skin innervation. Quantitative sudomotor axon reflex and sympathetic skin response testing are abnormal. Cutaneous sensory nerve biopsy tissue shows decreased numbers of unmyelinated and small myelinated fibers. Neuropathological studies demonstrate atrophy and near complete absence of first-order afferent system components, including DRG neurons and their peripheral axons, Lissauer and brainstem

trigeminal nerve spinal tracts of the spinal cord, and brainstem commensurate with deficient pain and temperature sensation. The disorder is caused by mutation at the 1q23.1 locus of the NTRK1 gene encoding neurotrophic tyrosine kinase-1 receptor (Table 1).

Low (197), and later Dyck (198), described children with a congenital sensory neuropathy characterized by loss of pain and temperature sensation (199), insensitivity to pain, and self-mutilation of the lips, tongue, and fingers with mild autonomic involvement (200). Children with HSAN5 typically present in early infancy with congenital insensitivity to deep pain and decreased sweating. There is selective loss of pain and thermal sensation affecting the extremities leading to painless injuries, and mild autonomic involvement suggested by skin blotching, anhidrosis or hypohydrosis, and episodes of increased body temperature.

Electrodiagnostic studies are typically normal. Cutaneous sensory nerve biopsy tissue shows selective reduction in small myelinated fibers with normal population of unmyelinated fibers.

HSAN type V is due to mutation at the 1p13.2 locus of the NGFB gene (Table 1), however one novel missense homozygous mutation showed genetic linkage to the NTRK1 gene in an AR fashion with homozygosity in markers across the NTRK1 region (201).

Treatment of HSAN is supportive with careful maintenance of adequate nutrition and hydration to counteract orthostatic hypotension, avoidance of aspiration due to gastroesophageal reflux and vomiting, and attention to possible hypertension, cardiac arrhythmia, and foot ulcers.

This chapter is dedicated to Edwin H. Kolodny, MD, Bernard A. and Charlotte Marden Professor and former Chair of the Department of Neurology, New York University School of Medicine, whose devoted career in the elucidation and treatment of NHMD inspired me to write this review.

REFERENCES

1. Kolodny, EH, Fattal-Valevski A. Degenerative disorders. In, BL Maria, ed. *Current Management in Child Neurology*, 3rd ed. BC Decker, 265–276.
2. Heineman KR, Hadders-Algra M. Evaluation of neuromotor function in infancy-A systematic review of available methods. *J Dev Behav Pediatr* 2008; 29:315–323.
3. De Groot I, Hopkins B, Touwen BC. A method to assess the development of muscle power in preterms after term age. *Neuropediatrics* 1992; 23:172–179.
4. Haataja K, Mercuri E, Regev R, et al. Optimality score for the neurological examination of the infant at 12 and 18 months of age. *J Pediatr* 1999; 135:153–161.
5. Caputi AJ, Accardo PH, Vining EP et al. Primitive reflex profile. A pilot study. *Phys Ther* 1978; 58:1061–1065.
6. Ellison PH, Horn IL, Browning CA. Construction of an infant neurological international battery (Infanib) for the assessment of neurological integrity in infancy. *Phys Ther* 1985; 65:1326–1331.
7. Bayley N. *Manual for the Bayley scales of infant development.* 2nd ed. San Antonio: The Psychological Corp, 1995.
8. Bayley N. *Baley scales of infant and toddler development.* 3rd ed. San Antonio: Harcourt Assessment Inc., 2006.
9. Falio MR, Fewell RR. *Peabody Development Motor Scales: Examiner's Manual.* 2nd ed. Texas: Pro-Ed, 2000.
10. Chandler LS, Andrews MS, Swanson MW. *Movement assessment of infants (MAI).* Rolling Bay: Infant Movement Research, 1980.
11. Gorga D, Stern F. *The neuromotor behavioral inventory.* New York: NY Hospital-Cornell Medical Center, 1979.
12. Miller LJ, Roid GH. *The TIME toddler and infant motor evaluation, a statistical assessment.* San Antonio: Therapy Skill Builders, 1994.

13. Piper MC, Darrah J. *Motor assessment of the developing infant.* Philadelphia: Saunders, 1994.

14. Persson K, Stromberg B. Structural observation of motor performance (SOMP-I) applied to neonatally healthy full term infants at the ages of 0–10 months. *Early Hum Dev* 1995; 40:127–143.

15. Campbell SK, Kolobe TH, Osten ET, et al. Construct validity of the test of infant motor performance. *Phys Ther* 1995; 75:585–596.

16. Einspieler C, Prechtl HFR, Bos AF, et al. Prechtl's method on the qualitative assessment of general movements in preterm, term, and young infants. *Clinics in Developmental Medicine*, No. 167, London: Mac Keith Press, 2004.

17. Hadders-Algra M. General movements: a window for early identification of children at risk for developmental disorders. *J Pediatr* 2004; 145:512–518.

18. Knerr I, Weinhold N, Vockley J, et al. Advances and challenges in the treatment of branched-chain amino/keto acid metabolic defects. *J Inherit Metab Dis* 2011 Feb 3. PubMed ID 21290185

19. Lanpher BC, Gropman A, Chapman KA, et al. Urea cycle disorders overview. In: GeneReviews at GeneTest: Medical Genetics Information Resource (database online). Copyright, University of Washington, Seattle. 1993–2011. Available at http://www.genetests.org. Accessed 1/16/12

20. Seashore MR. The organic acidemias: an overview. In: GeneReviews at GeneTest: Medical Genetics Information Resource (database online). Copyright, University of Washington, Seattle. 1993–2011.Available at http://www.genetests.org. Accessed 1/16/12.

21. Mc Guire PJ, Lim-Melia E, Diaz GA, et al. Combined liver-kidney transplant for the management of methylmalonic aciduria: a case report and review of the literature. *Mol Genet Metab* 2008; 93:22–29.

22. DiMauro S. Pathogenesis and treatment of mitochondrial myopathies: recent advances. *Acta Myol* 2010; 29:333–338

23. DiMauro S, Garcone C. Metabolic disorders of fetal life: glycogenoses and mitochondrial defects of the mitochondrial respiratory chain. *Semin Fetal Neonatal Med* 2011; 16:181–189

24. DiMauro S, Hirano M. Pathogenesis and treatment of mitochondrial disorders. *Adv Exp Med Biol* 2009; 652:139–170.

25. Nishino I, Spinazzola A, Papdimitriou A, et al. Mitochondrial neurogastrointestinal encephalopathy: an autosomal recessive disorder due to thymidine phosphorylase mutatons. *Ann Neurol* 2000; 47:792–800.

26. Steinberg SJ, Dodt G, Raymond GV et al. Peroxisome biogenesis disorders. *Biochim Biophys Acta* 2006; 1763:1733–1748.

27. Shimozawa N, Nagase T, Takemoto Y, et al. Molecular and neurologic findings of peroxisome biogenesis disorders. *J Child Neurol* 2005; 20:326–329.

28. Ebberink MS, Mooijer PA, Gootjes, et al. Genetic classification and mutational spectrum of more than 600 patients with a Zellweger syndrome spectrum disorder. *Hum Mutat* 2011; 32:59–69.

29. Mayatepek E, Hoffmann B, Meissner T. Inborn errors of carbohydrate metabolism. *Best Pract Res Clin Gastroeterol* 2010; 24:607–618.

30. Bouteldja N, Timson DJ. The biochemical basis of hereditary fructose intolerance. *J Inherit Metab Dis* 2010; 33:105–112.

31. DiMauro S, Garcone C. Metabolic disorders of fetal life: glycogenoses and mitochondrial defects of the mitochondrial respiratory chain. *Semin Fetal Neonatal Med* 2011; 16:181–189.

32. Kishnani PS, Corzo D, Leslie ND, et al. Early treatment with alglucosidase alpha prolongs long-term survival of infants with Pompe disease. *Pediatr Res* 2009; 66:329–335.

33. Mah CS, Falk DJ, Germain SA, Kelley JS, et al. Gel-mediated delivery of AAV1 vectors corrects ventilatory function in Pompe mice with established disease. *Mol Ther* 2010; 18:502–510.

34. Schultz ML, Tecedor L, Chang M, et al. Clarifying lysosomal storage diseases. *Trends Neurosci* 2011; 34:401–410.

35. Filocamo M, Morrone A. Lysosomal storage disorders: molecular basis and laboratory testing. *Hum Genomics* 2011; 5:156–169.

36. Jardim LB, Villanueva MM, de Souza CF, et al. Clinical aspects of neuropathic lysosomal storage disorders. *J Inherit Metabol Dis* 2010; 33:315–329.

37. Bellettato CM, Scarpa M. Pathophysiology of neuropathic lysosomal storage disorders. *J Inherit Metab Dis* 2010; 33:347–362.

38. Schiffmann R. Therapeutic approaches for neuronopathic lysosomal storage disorders. *J Inherit Metab Dis* 2010; 33:373–379.

39. Cearley CN, Wolfe JH. A single injection of an adeno-associated virus vector into nuclei with divergent connections results in widespread vector distribution in the brain and global correction of a neurogenetic disease. *J Neurosci* 2007; 27:9928–9940.

40. Chen YH, Chang M, Davidson BL. Molecular signatures of disease brain endothelia provide new sites for CNS-directed enzyme therapy. *Nat Med* 2009; 15:1215–1218.

41. Biffi A, De Palma M, Quattrinti A, et al. Correction of metachromatic leukodystrophy in the mouse model by transplantation of genetically modified hematopoietic stem cells. *J Clin Invest* 2004; 113:1118–1129.

42. Okada, S., O'Brien, J. S. Tay-Sachs disease: generalized absence of a beta-D-N-acetylhexosaminidase component. *Science* 1969; 165: 698–700.

43. Matsuoka K, Tamura T, Tsuji D, et al. Therapeutic potential of intracerebroventricular replacement of modified human β-hexosaminidase B for GM2 gangliosidosis. *Mol Ther* 2011; 19:1017–24.

44. Tsuji D, Akeboshi H, Matsuoka K, et al. Highly phosphomannosylated enzyme replacement therapy for GM2 gangliosidosis. *Ann Neurol* 2011; 69:691–701.

45. Landing BH, Silverman FN, Craig JM, et al. Familial neurvisceral lipidosis. An analysis of eight cases of a syndrome previously reported as "Hurler-variant," "pseudo-Hurler disease" and "Tay-Sachs disease with visceral involvement." *Am J Dis Child* 1964; 108:503–522.

46. Patterson MC, Vecchio D, Prady H, et al. Miglustat for treatment of Niemann-Pick C disease: a randomized controlled study. *Lancet Neurol* 2007; 6:765–772.

47. Maegawa GH, Banwell BL, Blaser S, et al. Substrate reduction therapy in juvenile GM2 gangliosidosis. *Mol Genet Metab* 2009; 98:215–224.

48. Smith D, Wallom KL, Williams IM, et al. Beneficial effects of anti-inflammatory therapy in a mouse model of Niemann-Pick disease type C1. *Neurobiol Dis* 2009; 36:242–251.

49. Zimran A, Loveday K, Fratazzi C, et al. A pharmacokinetic analysis of a novel enzyme replacement therapy with Gene-Activated human glucocerebrosidase (GA-GCB) in patients with type 1 Gaucher disease. *Blood Cells Mol Dis* 2007; 39:115–118.

50. Lukina E, Watman N, Arreguin EA, et al. mprovement in hematological, visceral, and skeletal manifestations of Gaucher disease type 1 with oral eliglustat tartrate (Genz-112638) treatment: 2-year results of a phase 2 study. *Blood* 2010; 116:4095–4098.

51. Khanna R, Benjamin ER, Pellegrino L, et al. The pharmacological chaperone isofagomine increases the activity of the Gaucher disease L44P mutant form of beta-glucosidase. *FEBS J* 2010; 277:1618–1638.

52. Steet R, Chung S, Lee WS, et al. Selective action of the iminosugar isofagomine, a pharmacological chaperone for mutant forms of acid-beta-glucosidase. *Biochem Pharmacol* 2007; 73:1376–1383.

53. Enquist IB, Nilsson E, Ooka A, et al. Effective cell and gene therapy in a murine model of Gaucher disease. *Proc Natl Acad Sci USA* 2006; 103:13819–24.

54. Settembre C, Fraldi A, Jahreiss L, et al. A block of autophagy in lysosomal storage disorders. *Hum Molec Genet* 2008; 17: 119–129.

55. Wraith JE. Enzyme replacement therapy for the management of the mucopolysaccharidoses. *Int J Clin Pharmacol Ther* 2009; 47(Suppl 1):S63–S65.

56. Peters C, Shapiro EG, Krivit W. Neuropsychological development in children with Hurler syndrome following hematopoietic stem cell transplantation. *Pediatr Transplant* 1998; 2:250–253.

57. Spranger JW, Wiedemann HR, Tolksdorf M, et al. Lipomucopolysaccharidose: eine neue Speicherkrankheit. *Z. Kinderheilk* 1968; 103:285–306.

58. Spranger JW, Gehler J, Cantz M. Mucolipidosis I-a sialidosis. *Am J Med Genet* 1977; 1:21–29.

59. Goebel HH, Wisniewski KE. Current state of clinical and morphological features in human NCL. *Brain Pathol* 2004; 14:61–69.

60. Worgall S, Sondhi D, Hackett NR, et al. Treatment of late infantile neuronal ceroid lipofuscinosis by CNS administration of a serotype 2 adneo-associated virus expressing CLN2 cDNA. *Hum Gene Ther* 2008; 19:463–474

61. Zhang Z, Butler JD, Levin SW, Wisniewski KE, et al. Lysosomal ceroid depletion by drugs: therapeutic implications for a hereditary neurodegenerative disease of childhood. *Nat Med* 2001; 7:478–484.

62. Kwon JM Adam H, Rothberg PG, et al. Quantifying physical decline in juvenile neuronal ceroid lipofuscinosis (Batten disease). *Neurology* 2011; 77:1801–1807).

63. Escolar ML, Poe MD, Provenzale JM, et al. Transplantation of umbilical-cord blood in babies with infantile Krabbe's disease. *N Engl J Med* 352:2069–2081.

64. Prasad VK, Kurtzberg J. Emerging trends in transplantation of inherited metabolic diseases. *Bone Marrow Transplant* 2008; 41:99–100.

65. Pierson TM, Bonnemann CG, Finkel RS, et al. Umbilical cord blood transplantation for juvenile metachromatic leukodystrophy. *Ann Neurol* 2008; 64:583–587.

66. Al-Dirbashi OY, Jurdi W, Imtiaz F, et al. Reliable prenatal diagnosis of Canavan disease by measuring N-acetylaspartate in amniotic fluid using liquid chromatography tandem mass spectroscopy. P*renat Diagn* 2009; 29:477–480.

67. Leone P, Janson CG, Bilaniuk L, et al. Aspartoacylase gene transfer to the mammalian central nervous system with therapeutic implications for Canavan disease. *Ann Neurol* 2000; 48:27–38.

68. Assadi M, Janson C, Wang DJ, et al. Lithium citrate reduces excessive intra-cerebral N-acetyl aspratate in Canavan disease. *Eur J Paediatr Neurol* 2010; 14:354–359.

69. Alexander WS. Progressive fibrinoid degeneration of fibrillary astrocytes associated with mental retardation in a hydrocephalic infant. *Brain* 1949; 72:373–381.

70. Messing A, Goldman JE, Johnson AB, Brenner M. Alexander disease: new insights from genetics. *J Neuropathol Exp Neurol* 2001; 60:563–573.

71. Wilson SAK. Progressive lenticular degeneration: a familial nervous system disease associated with cirrhosis of the liver. *Brain* 1912; 34:295–507.

72. Ala A, Schilsky ML. Wilson disease: pathophysiology, diagnosis, treatment, and screening. *Clin Liver Dis* 2004; 8:787–805.

73. Ribai P, Nguyen K, Hahn-Barma V, et al. Psychiatric and cognitive difficulties as indicators of juvenile Huntington disease onset in 29 patients. *Arch Neurol* 2007; 64:813–819.

74. Ribai P, Nguyen K, Hahn-Barma V, et al. Psychiatric and cognitive difficulties as indicators of juvenile Huntington disease onset in 29 patients. *Arch Neurol* 2007; 64:813–819.

75. Bonelli RM, Hofmann P. A systematic review of the treatment studies in Huntington's disease since 1990. *Expert Opin Pharmacother* 2007; 8:141–153.

76. Huntington Study Group PHAROS Investigators. The PHAROS (Prospective Huntington At Risk Observational Study) cohort enrolled. *Arch Neurol* 2006; 63:991–996.

77. Takahashi H, Ohama E, Suzuki S, et al. Familial juvenile parkinsonism: clinical and pathological study in a family. *Neurology* 1994; 44:437–441.

78. Hoenicka J, Vidal L, Morales B, et al. Molecular findings in familial Parkinson disease in Spain. *Arch Neurol* 2002; 59:966–970.

79. Kay DM, Stevens CF, Hamza TH, et al. A comprehensive analysis of deletions, multiplications, and copy number variations in PARK2. *Neurology* 2010; 75:1189–1194.

80. Fahn S, Elton R, Members of the UPDRS Development Committee. In: Fahn S, Marsden CD, Calne DB, Goldstein M. eds. *Recent Developments in Parkinson's Disease*, vol 2. Florham Park, NJ. Macmillan Health Care Information 1987; 153–163, 293–304.

81. Mitsui T, Kawai H, Sakoda S, et al. Hereditary parkinsonism with multiple system degeneration: beneficial effect of anticholinergics, but not of levodopa. *J Neurol Sci* 1994; 125:153–157.

82. Hardie RJ. Acanthocytosis and neurological impairment: a review. *Q J Med* 1989; 71:291–306.

83. Brin MF. Acanthocytosis. In: Goetz CG, Tanner CM, Aminoff MJ, eds. In: *Handbook of Neurology* 1993; 19:271–299.

84. Nyhan WL, Olivier W J, Lesch M. A familial disorder of uric acid metabolism and central nervous system function. *J Pediat* 1965; 67:257–263.

85. Seegmiller JE, Rosenbloom FM, Kelley WN. Enzyme defect associated with a sex-linked human neurological disorder and excessive purine synthesis. *Science* 1967; 155:1682–1684.

86. Sarafoglou K, Grosse-Redlinger K, Boys, et al. Lesch-Nyhan variant syndrome: variable presentation in 3 affected family members. *Arch Neurol* 2010; 67:761–764.

87. Hladnik U, Nyhan W L, Bertelli M. Variable expression of HPRT deficiency in 5 members of a family with the same mutation. *Arch Neurol* 2008; 65:1240–1243.

88. Lloyd KG, Hornykiewicz O, Davidson, et al. Biochemical evidence of dysfunction of brain neurotransmitters in the Lesch-Nyhan syndrome. *New Eng J Med* 1981; 305:1106–1111.

89. Breese GR, Criswell HE, Duncan GE, et al. A dopamine deficiency model of Lesch-Nyhan disease: the neonatal-6-OHDA-lesioned rat. *Brain Res Bull* 1990; 25:447–484.

90. Jinnah HA, Wojcik BE, Hunt M, et al. Dopamine deficiency in a genetic mouse model of Lesch-Nyhan disease. *J Neurosci* 1994; 14:1164–1174.

91. Ernst M, Zametkin AJ, Matochik JA, et al, Presynaptic dopaminergic deficits in Lesch-Nyhan disease. *New Eng J Med* 1996; 334:1568–1572.

92. Ceballos-Picot I, Mockel L, Potier MC, et al. Hypoxanthine-guanine phosphoribosyl transferase regulates early developmental programming of dopamine neurons: implications for Lesch-Nyhan disease pathogenesis. *Hum Molec Genet* 2009; 18:2317–2327.

93. Fahn S, Marsden CD, Calne DB. Classification and investigation of dystonia. In: Marsden CD, Fahn S, eds. *Movement disorders 2*. London: Butterworth, 1987; 332–358.

94. Carbon M, Kingsley, PB, Su S, et al. Microstructural white matter changes in carriers of the DYT1 gene mutation. *Ann Neurol* 2004; 56:283–286.

95. Carbon M, Niethammer M, Peng S, et al. Abnormal striatal and thalamic dopamine neurotransmission: genotype-related features of dystonia. *Neurology* 2009; 72:2097–2103.

96. Nygaard TG, Duvoisin RC. Hereditary dystonia-parkinsonism syndrome of juvenile onset. *Neurology* 1986; 36:1424–1428.

97. Nygaard TG, Marsden CD, Fahn S. Dopa-responsive dystonia: long-term treatment response and prognosis. *Neurology* 1991; 41:174–181.

98. Segawa M, Nomura Y, Nishiyama N. Autosomal dominant guanosine triphosphate cyclohydrolase I deficiency (Segawa disease). *Ann Neurol* 2003; 54:S32–S45.

99. Schule B, Kock N, Svetel M, et al. Genetic heterogeneity in ten families with myoclonus-dystonia. *J Neurol Neurosurg Psychiatry* 2004; 75:1181–1185.

100. Azoulay-Zyss J, Roze E, Welter ML, et al. Bilateral deep brain stimulation of the pallidum for myoclonus-dystonia due to epsilon-sarcoglycan mutations: a pilot study. *Arch Neurol* 2011; 68:94–98.

101. Dobyns WB, Ozelius LJ, Kramer PL, et al. Rapid-onset dystonia-parkinsonism. *Neurology* 1993; 43: 2596–2602.

102. Anselm IA, Sweadner KJ, Gollamudi S, et al. Rapid-onset dystonia-parkinsonism in a child with a novel ATP1A3 gene mutation. *Neurology* 2009; 73:400–401.

103. Hallervorden J, Spatz H. Eigenartige Erkrankung im extrapyramidalen System mit besonderer Beteiligung des Globus pallidus und der Substantia nigra.: Ein Beitrag zu den Beziehungen zwischen diesen beiden Zentren. *Z Ges Neurol Psychiat* 1922; 79:254–302.

104. Bot ST, van de Warrenburg, BPC, Kremer HPH, et al. Child neurology: hereditary spastic paraplegia in children. *Neurology* 2010; 75(19):e75–79.

105. Bianchine JW, Lewis RC, Jr. The MASA syndrome: a new heritable mental retardation syndrome. *Clin Genet* 1974; 5:298–306.

106. Schwartz CE, May MM, Carpenter NJ, et al. Allan-Herdon-Dudley syndrome and the monocarboxylate transporter 8 (MCT8) gene. *Am J Hum Genet* 2005; 77:41–53.

107. Simpson MA, Cross H, Proukakis C, et al. Maspardin is mutated in Mast syndrome, a complicated form of hereditary spastic paraplegia associated with dementia. *Am J Hum Genet* 2003; 73:1147–1156.

108. Inoue K. PLP1-related inherited dysmyelinating disorders: Pelizaeus-Merzbacher disease and spastic paraplegia type 2. *Neurogenetics* 2005; 6:1–16.

109. Bianchine JW, Lewis RC, Jr. The MASA syndrome: a new heritable mental retardation syndrome. *Clin Genet* 1974; 5:298–306.

110. Fransen E, Lemmon V, Van Camp et al. CRASH syndrome: clinical spectrum of corpus callosum hypoplasia, retardation, adducted thumbs, spastic paraparesis and hydrocephalus due to mutations in one single gene, L1. *Europ J Hum Genet* 1995; 3:273–284.

111. Dahme M, Bartsch U, Martini R, et al. Disruption of the mouse L1 gene leads to malformations of the nervous system in mice. *Nature Genet* 1997; 17:346–349.

112. Allan W, Herndon CN, Dudley FC. Some examples of the inheritance of mental deficiency: apparently sex-linked idocy and microcephaly. *Am J Ment Defic* 1944; 48:325–334.

113. Cross HE, McKusick VA. The mast syndrome. A recessively inherited form of presenile dementia with motor disturbances. *Arch Neurol* 1967; 16:1–13.

114. Simpson MA, Cross H, Proukakis C, et al. Maspardin in mutated in Mast syndrome, a complicated form of hereditary spastic paraplegia associated with dementia. *Am J Hum Genet* 2003; 73:1147–1156.

115. Johnston AW, McKusick VA. A sex-linked recessive form of spastic paraplegia. *Am J Hum Genet* 1962; 14:83–94.

116. Herman-Bert A, Stevanin G, Netter JC. Rascol O, et al. Mapping of spincerebellar ataxia 13 to chromosome 19q13.3-q13.4 in a family with autosomal dominant cerebellar ataxia and mental retardation. *Am J Hum Genet* 2000; 67:229–235.

117. Waters MF, Minassian NA, Stevanin G, et al. Mutations in voltage-gated potassium channel KCNC3 cause degenerative and developmental nervous system phenotypes. *Nature Genet* 2006; 38:447–451.

118. Misceo D, Fannemel,M, Baroy T, et al. **SCA27** caused by a chromosome translocation: further delineation of the phenotype, *Neurogenetics* 2009; 10:371–374.

119. Jen JC, Graves TD, Hess EJ, et al. CINCH Investigators. Primary episodic ataxias: diagnosis, pathogenesis and treatment. *Brain* 2007; 130:2484–2493.

120. Kallio AK, Jauhiainen TA. A new syndrome of opthalmoplegia, hypoacusis, ataxia, hypotonia, and athetosis [OHAHA]. *Adv Audiol* 1985; 3:84–90.

121. Koskinen T, Santavuori P, Sainio K, et al. Infantile onset spinocerebellar ataxia with sensory neuropathy: a new inherited disease. *J Neurol Sci* 1994; 121:50–56.

122. Hakonen AH, Goffart S, Marjavaara S, et al. Infantile-onset spinocerebellar ataxia and mitochondrial recessive ataxia syndrome are associated with neuronal complex I defect and mtDNA depletion. *Hum Molec Genet* 2008; 17:3822–3835.

123. Nikali K, Suomalainen A, Saharinen J, et al. Infantile onset spinocerebellar ataxia is caused by recessive mutations in mitochondrial proteins twinkle and twinky. *Hum Molec Genet* 2005; 14:2981–2990.

124. Delatycki MB, Williamson R, Forrest SM. Friedreich ataxia: an overview. *J Med Genet* 2000; 37:1–8.

125. Al-Mahdawi S, Pinto RM, Varshney D, et al. GAA repeat expansion mutation mouse models of Friedreich ataxia exhibit oxidative stress leading to progressive neuronal and cardiac pathology. *Genomics* 2006; 88:580–590.

126. Wolf B, Heard GS, Weissbecker KA, et al. Biotinidase deficiency: initial clinical features and rapid diagnosis. *Ann Neurol* 1985; 18:614–617.

127. Sivri HSK, Genc GA, Tokatli A, et al. Hearing loss in biotinidase deficiency: genotype-phenotype correlation. *J Pediat* 2007; 150:439–442.

128. Menkes JH, Alter M, Steigleder GK, et al. A sex-linked recessive disorder with retardation in growth, peculiar hair and focal cerebral and cerebellar degeneration. *Pediatrics* 1962; 29:764–779.

129. Menkes JH. Kinky hair disease. *Pediatrics* 1972; 50:181–182.

130. Menkes JH. Kinky hair disease: twenty five years later. *Brain Dev* 1988; 10:77–79.

131. De Bie P, Muller P, Wijmenga C, Klomp L, et al. Molecular pathogenesis of Wilson and Menkes disease: correlation of mutations with molecular defects and disease phenotypes. *J Med Genet* 2007; 44:673–688.

132. Turner Z, Tonnesen T, Bohmann J, et al. First trimester prenatal diagnosis of Menkes disease by DNA analysis. *J Med Genet* 1994; 31:615–617.

133. Alpers BJ. Diffuse progressive degeneration of gray matter of cerebrum. *Arch Neurol Psychiat* 1931; 25:469–505.

134. Sandbank U, Lerman P. Progressive cerebral poliodystrophy-Alpers'

disease: disorganized giant neuronal mitochondria on electron microscopy. *J Neurol Neurosurg Psychiat* 1972; 35:749–755.

135. Harding BN. Progressive neuronal degeneration of childhood with liver disease (Alpers-Huttenlocher syndrome): a personal view. *J Child Neurol* 1990; 5:273–287.

136. De Vries MC, Rodenburg RJ, Morava E, et al. Multiple oxidative phosphorylation deficiencies in severe childhood multi-system disorders due to polymerase gamma (POLG1) mutations. *Europ J Pediat* 2007; 166:229–234.

137. Wiltshire E, Davidson G, DiMauro S, et al. Juvenile Alpers disease. *Arch Neurol* 2008; 65:121–124.

138. Kurt B, Jaeken J, Van Hove J, et al. A novel POLG gene mutation in 4 children with Alpers-like hepatocerebral syndromes. *Arch Neurol* 2010; 67:239–244.

139. Ashley N, O'Rourke A, Smith C, et al. Depletion of mitochondrial DNA in fibroblast cultures from patients with POLG1 mutations is a consequence of catalytic mutations. *Hum Molec Genet* 2008; 17:2496–2506.

140. Milone M, Massie R. Polymerase gamma 1 mutations: clinical correlations. *Neurologist* 2010; 16:84–91.

141. DeVivo DC, Trifiletti RR, Jacobson RI, et al. Defective glucose transport across the blood-brain barrier as a cause of persistent hypoglycorrhachia, seizures, and developmental delay. *N Engl J Med* 1991; 325:703–709.

142. Wang D, Kranz-Ebie P, DeVivo DC. Mutations analysis of GLUT1 (SLC2A1) in Glut-1 deficiency syndrome. *Hum Mutat* 2000; 16:224–231.

143. Wang D, Pascual JM, Yang H, et al. Glut-1 deficiency syndrome: clinical, genetic, and therapeutic aspects. *Ann Neurol* 2005; 57:111–118.

144. Brockmann K, Wang D, Korenke CG et al. Autosomal dominant Glut-1 deficiency and familial epilepsy. *Ann Neurol* 2001; 50:476–485.

145. Pascual JM, Wang D, Hinton V, et al. Brain glucose supply and the syndrome of infantile neuroglycopenia. *Arch Neurol* 2007; 64:507–513.

146. Unverricht H. Ueber familiaere myoclonie. *Dtsch Z Nervenheilk* 1895; 7:32–67.

147. Lundborg HB. Erbgang der progressive myoklonusepilepsie [Myoklonie-epilepsie, Unverricht's familiaere myoklonie]. *Z Ges Neurol Psychiat* 1912; 9:353–358.

148. Eldridge R, Iivanainen M, Stern R, et al. "Baltic" myclonus epilepsy: hereditary disorder of childhood made worse by phenytoin. *Lancet* 1983; 322:838–842.

149. Singh S, Ganesh S. Lafora progressive myoclonus epilepsy: a meta-analysis of reported mutations in the first decade following the discovery of the EPM2A and NHLRC1 genes. *Hum Mutat* 2009; 30:715–723.

150. Fukuhara N, Tokiguchi S, Shirakawa K, et al. Myoclonus epilepsy associated with ragged-red fibers (mitochondrial abnormalities): disease entity or a syndrome? Light- and electron-microscopic studies of two cases and a review of the literature. *J Neurol Sci* 1980; 47:117–133.

151. Shoffner JM, Lott MT, Lezza AMS, et al. Myolconic epilepsy and ragged-red fiber disease (MERRF) is associated with a new mitochondrial DNA tRNA-lys mutation. *Cell* 1990; 61:931–937.

152. Shoffner JM, Lott MT, Lezza, AMS et al. Myoclonic epilepsy and ragged-red fiber disease (MERRF) is associated with a mitochondrial DNA tRNA-lys mutation. *Cell* 1990; 61:931–937.

153. Skjeldal OH, Stokke O, Refsum S, et al. Clinical and biochemical heterogeneity in conditions with phytanic acid accumulation. *J Neurol Sci* 1987; 77:87–96.

154. Refsum S. Heredopathica atactica polyneuritiformis: a familial syndrome not hitherto described. *Acta Psychiatr Scand* Suppl. 1946; 38:1–303.

155. Jansen GA, Wanders RJA, Watkins PA, et al. Phytanoly-coenzyme A hydroxylase deficiency-the enzyme defect in Refsum's disease (Letter). *N Eng J Med* 1997; 337:133–134.

156. Mihalik SJ, Morrell JC, Kim D, et al. Identification of PAHX, a Refsum disease gene. *Nature Genet* 1997; 17:185–189.

157. Hund E, Linke RP, Willig MD, Grau A. Transthyretin-associated neuropathic amyloidosis: pathogenesis and treatment. *Neurology* 2001; 56:431–435.

158. Ando Y, Nakamura M, Araki S. Transthyretin-related familial amyloidotic polyneuropathy. *Arch Neurol* 2005; 62:1057–1062.

159. Hund E, Linke RP, Willig MD, et al. Transthyretin-associated neuropathic amyloidosis: pathogenesis and treatment. *Neurology* 2001; 56:431–435.

160. Tojo K, Sekijima Y, Machida K, et al. Amyloidogenic transthyretin Val30Met homozygote showing unusually early-onset familial amyloid polyneuropathy. *Muscle Nerve* 2008; 37:796–803.

161. Sekijima Y, Wiseman RL, Matteson J, Hammarstrom P, et al. The biological and chemical basis for tissue-selective amyloid disease. *Cell* 2005; 121:73–85.

162. Meretoja J. Genetic aspects of familial amyloidosis with corneal lattice dystrophy and cranial neuropathy. *Clin Genet* 1973; 4:173–185.

163. Adams D, Samuel D, Goulon-Goeau C, et al. The course and prognostic factors of familial amyloid polyneuropathy after liver transplantation. *Brain* 2000; 123:1495–1504.

164. Fabry J. Ein beitrag zur kenntnis der purpura haemorrhagica nodularis [Purpura pupulosa hemorrhagica Hebrae]. *Arch Derm Syph* 1898; 43:187–200.

165. Franceschetti AT, Philippart M, Franceschetti A. A study of Fabry's disease. I. Clinical examination of a family with cornea verticillata. *Dermatologica* 1969; 138:209–221.

166. Spada M, Pagliardini S, Yasuda M, et al. High incidence of later-onset Fabry disease revealed by newborn screening. *Am J Hum Genet* 2006; 79:31–40.

167. MacDermot KD, Holmes A, Miners AH. Aderson-Fabry disease: clinical manifestations and impact of disease in a cohort of 98 hemizygous males. *J Med Genet* 2001; 38:750–760.

168. Rolfs A, Bottcher T, Zschiesche M, et al. Prevalence of Fabry disease in patients with cryptogenic stroke: a prospective study. *Lancet* 366; 1794–1796.

169. Schiffmann R. Fabry disease. *Pharm Ther* 2009; 122:65–77.

170. Thurberg BL, Rennke H, Colvin RB, et al. Globotriaosylceramide accumulation in the Fabry kidney is cleared from multiple cell types after enzyme replacement therapy. *Kidney Int* 2002; 62:1933–1946.

171. Banikazemi M, Bultas J, Waldek S, et al. Agalsidase-beta therapy for advanced Fabry disease: a randomized trial. *Ann Intern Med* 2007; 146:77–86.

172. Charcot JM, Marie P. Sur une forme particuliere d'atrophie musculaire progressive, souvent familiale, debutant par les pieds et les jambs et atteignant plus tard les mains. *Rev Med* 1886; 6:97–138.

173. Tooth HH. *The peroneal type of progressive muscular atrophy*. London: HK Lewis; 186.

174. Patzko A, Shy ME. Update on Charcot-Marie-Tooth disease. *Curr Neurol Neurosci Rep* 2011; 11:78–88.

175. Dejerine J, Sottas J. Sur la nevrite interstitielle, hypertrophique et progressive de l'enfance. *C R Soc Biol* 1893; 45:63–96.

176. Plante-Bordeneuve V, Said G. Dejerine-Sottas disease and hereditary demyelinating polyneuropathy of infancy. *Muscle Nerve* 2002; 26:608–621.

177. Yiu EM, Geevasinga N, Nicholson GA, et al. A retrospective review of X-linked Charcot-Marie-Tooth disease in childhood. *Neurology* 2011; 76:461–466.

178. England JD, Gronseth GS, Franklin G, et al. Practice parameter:

evaluation of distal symmetric polyneuropathy: role of laboratory and genetic testing (an evidence-based review). *Neurology* 2009; 72:185–192.

179. Saporta ASD, Sottile SL, Miller LJ, et al. Charcot-Marie-Tooth disease subtypes and genetic testing strategies. *Ann Neurol* 2011; 69:22–33.

180. Saporta ASD, Sottile SL, Miller LJ, et al. Charcot-Marie-Tooth disease subtypes and genetic testing strategies. *Ann Neurol* 2011; 69:22–33.

181. Ginsberg L, Malik O, Kenton AR, et al. Coexistent hereditary and inflammatory neuropathy. *Brain* 2004; 127:193–202.

182. Passage E, Norreel JC, Noack-Fraissignes P, et al. Ascorbic acid treatment corrects the phenotype of a mouse of Charcot-Marie-Tooth disease. *Nat Med* 2004; 10:396–401.

183. Meyer zu Horste G, Prukop T, Liebetanz D, et al. Antiprogesterone therapy uncouples axonal loss from demyelination in a transgenic rat model of CMT1A neuropathy. *Ann Neurol* 2007; 61:61–72.

184. Micallef J, Attarian S, Dubourg O, et al. Effect of ascorbic acid in patients with Charcot-Marie-Tooth disease type 1A; a multicenter, randomized, double-blind, placebo-controlled trial. *Lancet Neurol* 2009; 8:1103–1110.

185. Weimer LH, Podwall D. Medication-induced exacerbation of neuropathy in Charcot Marie Tooth disease. *J Neurol Sci* 2006; 242:47–54.

186. Dyck PJ. Neuronal atrophy and degeneration predominantly affecting peripheral sensory and autonomic neurons. In: *Peripheral neuropathy*. PJ Dyck, JW Griffin, PA Low. WB Saunders: Philadelphia, 1993; 1065–1093.

187. Dyck PJ, Ohta M. Neuronal atrophy and degeneration predominantly affecting peripheral sensory neurons. In: *Peripheral neuropathy*. PJ Dyck, PK Thomas, EH Lambert, eds. Philadelphia: WB Saunders, 1975.

188. Hilz MJ. Assessment and evaluation of hereditary sensory and autonomic neuropathies with autonomic and neurophysiological examinations. *Clin Auton Res* 2002; 12(Suppl 1):I33–I43.

189. Hicks EP. Hereditary perforating ulcer of the foot. *Lancet* 1922; 199:319–321.

190. Giaccai L. Familial and sporadic neurogenic acro-osteolysis. *Acta Radiol* 1952; 38:17–29.

191. Heller IH, Robb P. Hereditary sensory neuropathy. *Neurology* 1955; 5:15–29.

192. Riley CM, Day RL, Greeley DM, et al. Central autonomic dysfunction with defective lacrimation: report of five cases. *Pediatrics* 1949; 3:468–478.

193. Smith AA, Dancis J. Response to intradermal histamine in familial dysautonomia: a diagnostic test. *J Pediat* 1963; 63:889–894.

194. Smith AA, Farbman A, Candis J. Absence of taste-bud papillae in familial dysautonomia. *Science* 1965; 147:1040–1041.

195. Swanson AG. Congenital insensitivity to pain with anhidrosis: a unique syndrome in two male siblings. *Arch Neurol* 1963; 8:299–306.

196. Swanson AG, Buchan GC, Alvord ED Jr. Anatomic changes in congenital insensitivity to pain: absence of small primary sensory neurons in ganglia, roots and Lissauer's tract. *Arch Neurol* 1965; 12:12–18.

197. Low PA, Burke WJ, McLeod JG. Congenital sensory neuropathy with selective loss of small myelinated fibers. *Ann Neurol* 1978; 3:179–182.

198. Dyck PJ, Mellinger JF, Reagan TJ, et al. Not "indifference to pain" but varieties of hereditary sensory and autonomic neuropathy. *Brain* 1983; 106:373–390.

199. Low PA, Burke WJ, McLeod JG. Congenital sensory neuropathy with selective loss of small myelinated fibers. *Ann Neurol* 1978; 3:179–182.

200. Dyck PJ, Mellinger JF, Reagan TJ, et al. Not "indifference to pain" but varieties of hereditary sensory and autonomic neuropathy. *Brain* 1983; 106:373–390.

201. Houlden H, King RHM, Hashemi-Nejad, et al. A novel TRK Λ (NTRK1) mutation associated with hereditary sensory and autonomic neuropathy type IV. *Ann Neurol* 2001; 49:521–525.

CHAPTER 12

Vertigo and Vestibular Disorders

David S. Younger

Labyrinthine function is important in the composition of coordinated movement and body equilibrium. Further, proper balance and posture require continuous information about the position and motion of all body parts, including the head and eyes. The head and eyes must be able to function independently of one another, allowing for visual fixation on a moving target, even when the head is in motion. In addition, the position and movement of the eyes must be compensated on non-visual cues. These varied tasks are fulfilled by the vestibular system, so-named for its position in the vestibule of the inner ear.

The term *vertigo* means a turning sensation, sense of movement, either in the individual or in external space that involves a defect, true or perceived, in the equilibrium of the body. Almost all affected patients report slight or more interference with consciousness of the body often chosing terms of giddiness and dizziness to describe the sensation. Vertigo also conveys involuntary movement, whether perceived or apparent, of external space and objects.

Inner ear disease is the commonest cause of vertigo with resultant dizziness, incoordination, imbalance, and disequilibrium. Vertigo and its associated findings can also result from peripheral lesions of vestibular neurons and their peripheral axons, as well as intraaxial lesions of the brainstem, cerebellum, and cerebrum. When I teach labyrinthine disorders and vertigo to medical students, I tell them that intact vestibular function enabled early Americans to ride horseback in pursuit of moving animal prey, with bow and arrow in hand, poised for engagement with exquisite hand and eye coordination. While survival today rarely involves such extraordinary motor tasks, patients with vertigo will tell you that it is a very incapacitating state.

This chapter reviews the terminology, clinical presentation, differential diagnosis, laboratory evaluation, etiopathogenesis, and treatment of disorders associated with labyrinthine disorders, dizziness, and vertigo. The prior edition of this chaper did not discuss postconcussive disorders in the cause of vertigo and dizziness, which has been added to this chapter, emphasizing its clinical importance.

VESTIBULAR LABYRINTH

The inner ear or labyrinth is composed of bony and membranous portions found in the petrous part of the temporal bone (Figure 1). The membranous labyrinth consists of fine membranes of a simple epithelium, which becomes more complex in certain regions, that differentiates into sensory receptor cells sensitive to accelerated movement and altered positions of the head. The vestibular portion of the membranous labyrinth consists of the otolith organs, the utricle, saccule, and the semicircular ducts. The two otolith organs lie in the midportion of the inner ear vestibule, while the semicircular canals are placed in the bony semicircular canals separated by thin connective sheaths.

The arterial and venous circulation to the labyrinth and eighth nerve is derived from the basilar artery (Figure 2); therefore, as might be anticipated, dizziness and vertigo can be cardinal signs of basilar artery occlusion. The internal auditory artery supplies the peripheral apparatus of the auditory and vestibular systems, arising from the anterior inferior cerebellar artery in 83% of individuals, and directly from the basilar artery in 17%. After supplying the eighth nerve, the internal auditory artery continues as a small vessel of approximately 200 microns in diameter, giving rise to three branches that supply the membranous

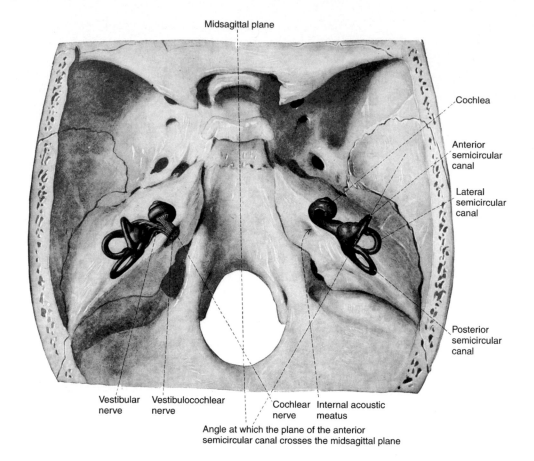

Midsagittal plane

Cochlea

Anterior semicircular canal

Lateral semicircular canal

Posterior semicircular canal

Vestibular nerve

Vestibulocochlear nerve

Cochlear nerve

Internal acoustic meatus

Angle at which the plane of the anterior semicircular canal crosses the midsagittal plane

(A)

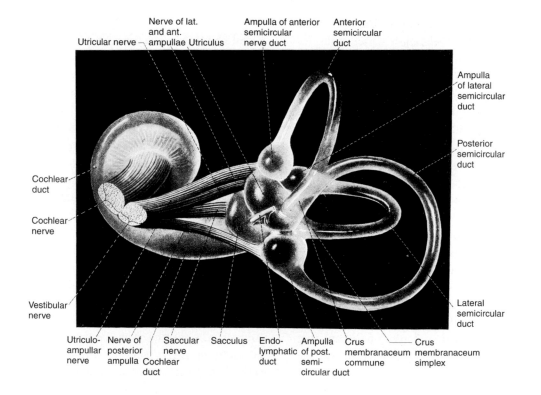

Nerve of lat. and ant. ampullae

Utriculus

Utricular nerve

Ampulla of anterior semicircular nerve duct

Anterior semicircular duct

Ampulla of lateral semicircular duct

Posterior semicircular duct

Cochlear duct

Cochlear nerve

Vestibular nerve

Lateral semicircular duct

Utriculo-ampullar nerve

Nerve of posterior ampulla

Cochlear duct

Saccular nerve

Sacculus

Endo-lymphatic duct

Ampulla of post. semi-circular duct

Crus membranaceum commune

Crus membranaceum simplex

(B)

FIG. 1. Anatomic depiction of the bony **(A)** and membranous **(B)** labyrinth. From, Clemente CD. *Anatomy. A regional atlas of the human body.* Philadelphia, Lea & Febiger 1975, figures 592, 593, with permission.

labyrinth. First, the anterior vestibular artery, which nourishes the superior part of the saccule, macula of the utricle, and cristae ampullares of the horizontal and superior vertical ducts. Second, the vestibulocochlear artery, which supplies the macula and the greater part of the saccule and then divides into two branches, one that runs to the body and inferior part of the utricle, and the crista ampullares of the posterior vertical duct, and the other to the basal turn of the cochlea. Third, the cochlear artery, which supplies the spiral arteries to the upper cochlear turns, anastomosing with twigs of the artery to the basal turn from the vestibulocochlear branch. Microscopically, the labyrinth has an abundance of capillaries. The venous circulation is comprised of the anterior and posterior vestibular veins, which drain into the vestibular aqueduct.

The bony labyrinth is filled with perilymphatic fluid, which resembles cerebrospinal fluid in its higher concentration of sodium ions, whereas the membranous labyrinth contains endolymphatic fluid that differs in a higher concentration of potassium ions, more similar to that of intracellular fluid. The maintenance of the ionic balance between the two appears to be essential for proper vestibular functioning. The fluid spaces of the bony labyrinth are in communication with the subarachnoid space via the cochlear aqueduct, also with an active maintenance of fluid pressure balances.

VESTIBULAR SENSORY END ORGAN

Just before its termination in the utricle, each semicircular duct dilates in the area of the ampulla, wherein the epithelium thickens in the ampullary crest containing specialized mechanoreceptors termed *vestibular hair cells*, innervated by peripheral processes of bipolar sensory neurons in the ampullary nerve. The hair cell receptor is an exquisitely sensitive mechanoelectric transducer that is directionally sensitive to bending of the hairs or kinocilium. The ampullary crest is covered by a gelatinous mass called the cupula. Rotation of the head causes fluid in the semicircular ducts to displace the hair cells of the crest, which alters the level of activity of the nerve fibers innervating them. Paired ducts on either side of the head work together. For example, movement of the head to the left causes endolymph to move to the right as a result of inertia. This moves stereocilia in the left duct in the direction of their axis of polarity, exciting the afferent fibers to increase their firing rate. Since the majority of vestibular neurons are spontaneously active, the excitatory event is likened more to an upregulation of activity rather than a simple turning on or off. Afferent fibers innervating the hair cells discharge spontaneously at a frequency of 100 spikes per second. With bending of them in one direction there is an increase in the rate of discharge, which decreases when they

bend in the other direction. Hair cells in the macula of the utricle and saccule are also arranged in an orderly pattern. The hair cells of the utricle are located in a specialized epithelium like that of the ampullary crest. Their cilia project into the otolith membrane, an overlying gelatinous matrix studded with otolith. Their kinocilium do not face in a single direction, with the result that the utricle can respond to tilt or to linear acceleration in any one of several directions.

VESTIBULAR NEURAL PATHWAYS

The cell bodies of the afferent fibers of the vestibular system reside in the ganglion of Scarpa, adjacent to the internal auditory meatus. The superior division innervates the macula of the utricle, the anterior portion of the macula of the saccule, and ampulla of the horizontal and anterior semicircular ducts. The inferior division innervates the posterior part of the macula of the saccule and the ampulla of the posterior duct. Centrally directed axons of Scarpa ganglionic cells join with those of the spiral ganglia of the cochlea in the vestibulocochlear or eighth cranial nerve. The vestibular nerve takes an oblique course dorsally and medially on a level with the caudal pole of the abducens nucleus, passing medial to the restiform body and lateral to the descending root of the fifth nerve, while the cochlear fibers rest dorsally and medially at the caudal border of the pons ventral to the restiform body. The vestibular nerve then divides into ascending and descending roots, forming a flat band that lies parallel and dorsal to the descending root of the fifth nerve and abuts laterally upon the masses of the various vestibular nuclei. The latter are divided by sharp constriction opposite the incoming vestibular nerve at the level of the lateral recess of the fourth ventricle. The cells that lie rostral to the constriction related to the ascending root of the vestibular nerve constitute the superior vestibular nucleus. Those that lie caudal to the constriction and are related to the descending root of the vestibular nerve constitute the medial vestibular nucleus. The lateral nucleus of Deiters, with its large cells, occupies a prominent part of the region of the constriction, traversing it and the associated vestibular roots from side to side.

The roots of the vestibular nerve with the vestibular nuclei extend rostrally to the level of the motor nucleus of the fifth cranial nerve, and caudally to well below the level of entry of the eighth nerve as far as the caudal extremity of the twelfth nucleus. Associated with the descending vestibular root are many nerve cells that constitute its descending nucleus. In contrast to the vestibular nerve, the cochlear nerve also separates into two groups, one passing to the dorsal cochlear nucleus on the lateral aspect of the restiform body, and the other passing in a ventromedial direction to the ventral cochlear nucleus. It envelopes the vestibular nerve in its course, joins the trapezoid body and superior olivary nucleus that lie ventral to the facial nucleus, without descending fibers or nuclei, or cochlear elements caudal to the dorsal cochlear nucleus. Most of the neurons arising from the cochlear nuclei cross the midline to the opposite trapezoid body and superior olivary nucleus, thereafter passing cranially in the lateral lemniscus.

The vestibular nuclear complex is thus comprised of the lateral vestibular nucleus of Deiters, superior vestibular nucleus, the medial vestibular nucleus, and the inferior descending vestibular nucleus. They occupy a large portion of the medulla beneath the floor of the fourth ventricle. Each nuclear group has a distinctive architecture and set of connections in the central nervous system (CNS), notably with the oculomotor nuclei, cerebellum, reticular formation, and spinal cord. Collectively, their projections and interconnections allow for the smooth coordination and execution of spinal locomotion, postural motor adjustments, and oculomotor reflexes, including visual fixation and pursuit, which compensates for linear and angular accelerative movements of the head and body in space.

The ventral portion of the lateral vestibular nucleus receives primary vestibular input from the macula of the utricle and the semicircular ducts, and contributes to vestibulo-ocular pathways, whereas the dorsal portion receives input from the cerebellum and the spinal cord. Cells of the dorsal portion project to the spinal cord in the lateral vestibulospinal tract where they facilitate the effect on both α and γ motor neurons that innervate muscle of the limbs, the tonic effect of which is to excite extensor muscles of the legs and inhibit flexor muscles to enable upright posture. Some neurons also respond selectively to tilting of the head the magnitude of their discharge, which increases with further angles of tilt. One portion of the lateral vestibular nucleus receives direct inhibitory input from Purkinje cells of the cerebellar vermis, electrical stimulation of which experimentally reduces decerebrate rigidity resulting from transaction of the brainstem above the level of the vestibular nuclei.

Fibers from the medial and superior vestibular nucleus receive input from the ampullae of the semicircular ducts. The former gives rise to the medial vestibulospinal tract, which terminates in the cervical cord upon motor neurons innervating the neck muscles, with participation in the reflexive control of neck movement, especially in coordination with eye movements. Both the medial and superior vestibular nuclei participate largely in the vestibulo-ocular reflex, sending their axons into the medial longitudinal fasciculus that runs beneath the midline of the fourth ventricle. Tilting of the head to one side reflexively rotates the eyes in the opposite direction, helping to maintain visual fixation. The voluntary control of eye movements is independent of vestibular input and resides mainly in the cerebral cortex in the frontal eye fields. The inferior vestibular nucleus receives primary vestibular and cerebellar input from the semicircular ducts, utricle, and saccule, and from the vermis of the cerebellum to integrate and relay information to higher levels in the brainstem as well as the projection of efferent fibers to ipsilateral vestibulospinal tract and vestibulo reticular pathways.

VESTIBULAR MECHANISMS OF MOVEMENT AND POSTURE

The spinal cord and brainstem are functionally organized into distinct medial and lateral motor systems innervating the neck and back. Within the lateral group of motor neurons, the most medial motor innervates proximal muscles while those more lateral innervate distal limb and axial muscles. Ventrally located motor neurons innervate extensor muscles, while dorsally placed ones innervate flexor muscle groups. The brainstem modulates the motor neurons and interneurons through four systems: First, medial pathways that terminate in the ventromedial part of the spinal gray matter, influencing motor neurons that innervate axial and proximal muscles. Second, lateral pathways that terminate in dorsolateral portions influencing distal limb muscles. Third, an aminergic pathway of axons to the entire spinal cord located in the ceruleospinal system of the pontomedullary reticular formation that descends to lateral columns. Fourth, the aminergic raphe-spinal serotonergic pathway that descends to both lateral and ventral columns. The medial pathway has a greater significance for the vestibular system since it incorporates the medial and lateral vestibulospinal and reticulospinal tracts, and the tectospinal tract. These pathways descend in the ipsilateral ventral column of the spinal cord and terminate on interneurons of the intermediate zone and some ventral motor neurons, influencing axial musculature. The reticulospinal tracts collectively have excitatory and inhibitory effects on interneurons and motor neurons important in the maintenance of posture, integrating information from vestibular and cerebellar nuclei. Corticoreticulospinal pathways originating from pre-motor cortex synapse with reticulospinal neurons and descend to spinal levels in the corticoreticulospinal tract, important in suppression of spinal reflexes. Tectospinal pathways that originate in the superior colliculus have an important role in the coordination of eye and head movements, including some under partial control by the cortex via the cortico-tectospinal tract.

The lateral pathways involved in motor control include the rubrospinal tract, which originates in the red nucleus of the midbrain and descends through the medulla to dorsolateral portions of the spinal cord, influencing distal limb muscles, and the corticospinal tract (CST), the largest descending tract from primary motor cortex located in the precentral gyrus of the frontal lobe, electrical stimulation of which evokes movements of different contralateral limb muscle groups. The lateral and ventral tracts terminate in approximately the same region as the lateral and medial descending brainstem systems, upon motor nuclei of the lateral portion of the ventral horn and upon interneurons of the intermediate zone. Corticobulbar fibers terminate mainly upon contralateral trigeminal, hypoglossal, and upon bilateral facial motor nuclei of the brainstem to control muscle of the head and face. The fact of several levels of control on motor neurons contributes to the recovery of function that can occur after lesions of one or another component, with younger patients typically recovering more muscle strength and function than older individuals, as a result of the transfer of function from one parallel system, including the corticospinal tract, to another, as well as the sprouting of other axons into synaptic areas vacated by degenerating axons.

Postural stability in standing and walking depends upon the receipt of sensory input from three types of receptors: muscle proprioceptors that sense change in length and tension, vestibular receptors that sense sway through head motion, and visual receptors that detect movement of the visual field. Whereas postural responses elicited by muscle proprioceptors have a relatively short latency triggered at 70 to 100 ms, vestibular and visual responses are almost twice as slow. However only vestibular, not visual or proprioceptive information, allow the CNS to distinguish whether the head and external environment are in motion. Diverse mechanisms align our head and body with respect to gravity and contribute to postural stability. They include vestibular reflexes evoked by changes in the position of the head, and neck reflexes triggered by tilting, bending, or turning of the neck. Both produce coordinated effects on limb muscle groups. Movement of the head also evokes a vestibular ocular reflex (VOR) that stabilizes visual images on the retina.

Other vestibular reflexes contribute to the maintenance of a vertical head position with respect to gravity, including the vestibulocolic and vestibulospinal reflexes, evoked by sensory input from otolith organs that inform the brain about the direction of gravity and the acceleration produced during head movement in the horizontal and sagittal planes. The vestibulocolic reflex counteracts head movements to keep it stable, as for example, when the head tilts forward without bending of the neck. The vestibulospinal reflex contracts limb muscles during a fall wherein tilting of the head forward produces extension of the arms and flexion of the legs, a combination of movements that reduces the impact of a fall. Whereas neck and vestibular reflexes are synergistic in the neck, they appear antagonistic in the limbs. In contrast to simpler reflexes, vestibular and neck reflexes can produce complex patterns of facilitation and inhibition of motor neurons innervating widely distributed muscle groups.

Vestibular neurons that project to the spinal cord via the two vestibulospinal tracts influence spinal circuits due to interconnections with the pontine and medullary reticular formation, which in turn projects to the spinal cord via two reticulospinal tracts, influencing axial muscle control of the neck and back. Specifically, input from the semicircular ducts and otolith organs project axons from the medial and inferior vestibular nuclei to cervical and thoracic muscle segments in the medial vestibulospinal tract where they terminate on medial motor neurons leading to inhibitory action on contralateral neck and back motor neurons. Input to motor neurons of the arms from otolith organs mediated by neurons in the lateral vestibular nucleus, which project ipsilaterally to all segment of the spinal cord in the lateral vestibulospinal tract, act to facilitate extensor motor neurons and inhibit flexor motor neurons of both the arms and legs.

NYSTAGMUS

The semicircular ducts of the vestibular labyrinth signal how fast the head rotates in response to head movement. The oculomotor system responds by moving the eyes at a velocity equal and opposite to the direction of head movement velocity to stabilize visual fixation of the external world on the retina. The compensatory slow phase of the eyes toward the edge of the orbit, averted by a rapid reversal of the direction across the center of gaze, is called the *fast phase* of nystagmus. The combination of the slow and fast phase results in a rhythmic oscillatory pattern termed *vestibular or spontaneous nystagmus*, or *nod* in Greek, because like head nodding, the slow phase of head dropping is counteracted by a fast phase as it snaps back to the erect position. Nystagmus has a saw-tooth character with the directionality defined by the rapid recovery or fast phase. Spontaneous vestibular nystagmus is defined as first degree to the right when present only on right lateral gaze, and absent in the straight-ahead position or on left lateral gaze. Second-degree nystagmus to the right is present on straight-ahead gaze and more marked on right lateral gaze. Third-degree nystagmus to the right is present on left lateral gaze, more brisk in the straight-ahead position, and brisk on right lateral gaze. Recognizing that the eyes remain still when the head is stationary because of the balanced tonic discharge of all six semicircular ducts, nystagmus can be regarded as a marker of disease, assisting in the localization of the lesion to the labyrinth and CNS vestibular connections. Nystagmus, which occurs with rotation of the subject or the periphery in the light, ceasing in the dark, is termed *rotatory nystagmus*. It exhibits the same alteration of slow and fast components of vestibular nystagmus, and shares a common mechanism in vestibular nuclei and their brainstem connections.

The neuroanatomical connections subserving horizontal VOR are located in the brainstem (Figure 3). As conceived, medial vestibular excitatory axons synapse

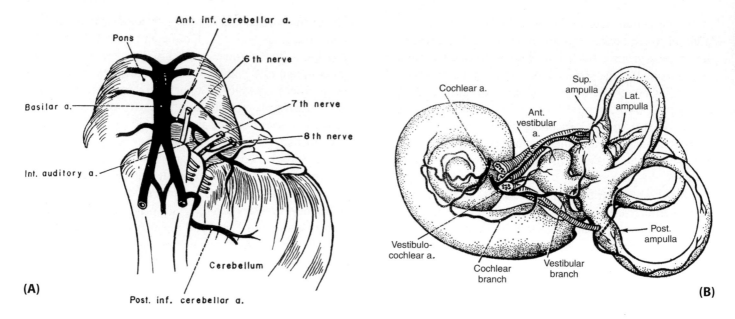

FIG. 2. Origin of the internal auditory artery from the inferior cerebellar artery **(A)**. Blood supply to the membranous labyrinth **(B)**. From, Fisher CM. Vertigo in cerebrovascular disease. *Arch Otolaryngol* 1967; 85:531, with permission.

with and excite motor axons of the left abducens nucleus and left lateral rectus muscle contralateral to the direction of rotation, and interneurons whose axons ascend in the ipsilateral medial longitudinal fasciculus (MLF) to excite right medial rectus neurons. Medial vestibular inhibitory axons synapse with and inhibit motor axons of the right lateral rectus and left medial rectus in the direction of rotation. The supranuclear pathways of optokinetic nystagmus (OKN) are shown in Figure 4. Nerve fibers from each optic tract pass to the ipsilateral external geniculate body and backwards, to the occipital cortex, while others pass directly to the superior colliculus and thence to eye muscle nuclei to subserve slow deviation of the eyes and the slow component of OKN. Cerebral pathways are the second supranuclear component of OKN, with the cortex of each side, or rather a particular region of it, although not an essential part of the primary reflex, exerting a reinforcing effect. The areas of the cortex that have been implicated by experimental lesion studies in the reinforcement of OKN include the supramarginal and angular gyri. The optokinetic system responds well to slow visual motion induced by slow head movement excited by a stripped rotating drum, which rotates between 72 to 360 degrees per second, with a variable angle of axis of rotation, and a continuously variable, instantaneous speed, and reversal switches, allowing for the investigation of nystagmus in all possible directions and planes.

CALORIC TESTING

The peripheral mechanism of caloric stimulation can be explained on the basis of convection currents in the endolymph of the external semicircular ducts. The main type of abnormality of OKN, directional preponderance of induced nystagmus, historically followed unilateral labyrinthine destruction by suppurative infective processes, so noted to be a striking preponderance of post-rotational nystagmus toward the unaffected ear, in accordance with the convention of the direction of nystagmus in terms of its fast component. Early appreciation of caloric testing considered nystagmus qualitatively as an all-or-none phenomenon indicative of vestibular function following strong stimulation with ice water, and a negative response accepted as a paralyzed labyrinth.

Modern appreciation of caloric testing commenced with standardization of the caloric method in which caloric testing in a series of patients observed before and after labyrinthectomy for unilateral Meniere disease noted development of two distinct abnormalities of induced nystagmus following the operation. First, as expected, there was abolition of the responses of the affected ear. Secondly, there was striking accentuation of the nystagmus toward the unaffected ear evoked by the hot stimulus. In other words, there was directional preponderance of caloric nystagmus toward the unaffected ear. As with

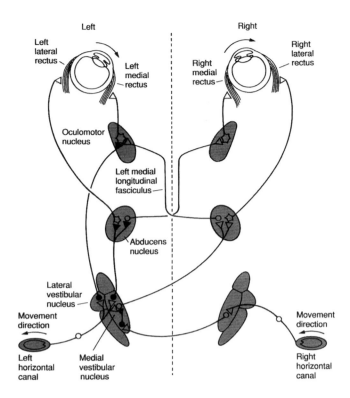

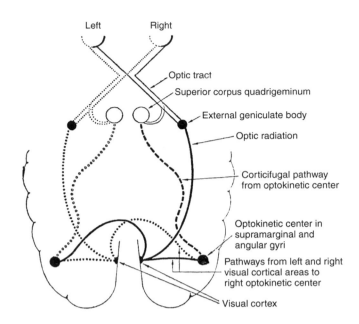

FIG. 3. Brainstem pathways for the horizontal VOR that subserve rotatory nystagmus. From, Kandel ER, Schwartz JH, Jessel TM. *Principles of Neural Science.* 3rd ed., New York, Elsevier, 1991, pg. 670, with permission.

FIG. 4. Cerebral mechanism of optokinetic nystagmus From, Dix MR. Modern tests of vestibular function, with special reference to their value in clinical practice. *Brit Med J* 1969; 3:318, with permission.

post-rotational nystagmus, this directional preponderance showed a marked diminution with time.

Later investigators refined the methodology, providing ease and comfort for the patient, improved accuracy and reproducibility, and revealing the features of directional preponderance. The features of directional preponderance and canal paresis were discerned not only in partial unilateral lesions of the labyrinth, tumors and lesions of the eighth nerve, Meniere disease, but also in unilateral lesions of the vestibular nuclei brought about, for example, by an occlusive lesion of the posterior inferior cerebellar artery, and cortical lesions, such as those in the posterior temporal lobe toward which the directional preponderance is directed.

As classically described at the bedside (Figure 5), the subject's head position brings the external canal into the vertical plane, in which its sensitivity is maximal. Although modern techniques employ cold and warm air, tap water at temperatures of 30 degrees and 44 degrees centigrade were initially used to bring about equal and opposite cupular deflections when instilled in the external canal for 40 seconds, the effects of which were measured in terms of the time interval between the application of the stimulus and the end of the nystagmus response, with the observations carried out in the

eyes straight-ahead position of gaze, and thus of the so-called second-degree nystagmus type. The method of recording caloric nystagmus in normal subjects is shown schematically in Figure 6. Continuous lines represent time of three minutes divided into intervals of 10 seconds, and dotted lines representing response durations. The recorded reactions are numbered 1 to 4 from above. Reactions of 1 and 4 consist of nystagmus with a rapid component to the right, whereas those of 2 and 3 are nystagmus to the left. Four important deviations, left and right canal paresis and directional preponderance are shown in Figure 7. With lesions of the eighth nerve and labyrinth, canal paresis was often associated with directional preponderance, to the opposite side, presumably due to a loss of tonic impulses originating in the utricle of the otolith. Directional preponderance was found to be a valuable sign of lesions of the vestibular areas in the brainstem wherein the direction was away from the side of the lesion, and toward the cerebral hemispheric lesion.

The Nylen-Barany test for positional vertigo is performed by seating the patient on the edge of the examining table and abruptly having him lie down with the head hanging 45 degrees backward and turned 45 degrees to one side with observation for the development of vertigo and

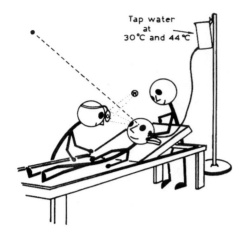

FIG. 5. Caloric test procedure. From, Cawthorne T, Dix MR, Hallpike CS, et al. The investigation of vestibular function. *Brit Med Bull* 1956; 12:132, with permission.

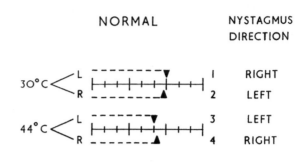

FIG. 6. Normal caloric nystagmus recording. From, Carmichael EA, Dix MR, Hallpike CS. Observations upon the neurological mechanism of directional preponderance of caloric nystagmus resulting from vascular lesions of the brainstem. *Brain* 1965; 88:56, with permission.

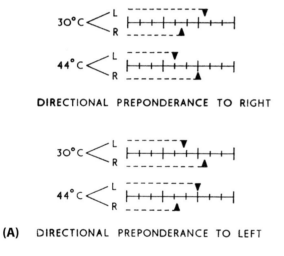

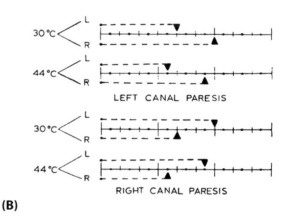

FIG. 7. Directional preponderance **(A)** and canal paresis **(B).** From, Cawthorne ST, Dix MR, Hood JD, Harrison MS. Vestibular syndromes and vertigo. Differential diagnosis between central and peripheral involvement. *Handb Clin Neurol* 1969; 2:374, with permission.

nystagmus and the time of onset, duration, and direction of the quick phase of nystagmus; it is then repeated with the head turned to the opposite side. The evoked nystagmus, which occurs after a latent period of several seconds, exhibits both horizontal and rotatory components directed toward the ear placed undermost in the test position, and adapts rapidly. Benign peripheral positional nystagmus implicates a unilateral otolith lesion. An alternative explanation for this type of nystagmus is the presence of neoplasm of the posterior fossa.

Whereas the optokinetic system involuntary stabilizes the eyes in space with head movement, smooth voluntary pursuit moves the eyes in space to keep a single target on the fovea by taking into account the speed of the moving target. Drugs, fatigue, alcohol, and distraction can all degrade the quality of smooth pursuit.

The rapid eye movements that occur when a subject looks at a target that suddenly moves away from the fovea, resulting in maintenance of the position for another 200 ms or so, moving quickly to bring it back onto the fovea, is called a *saccade*. It resembles the quick phase of nystagmus, but unlike smooth pursuit that requires a visual stimulus, saccades can also occur in response to sound, tactile stimuli, memories, location in space, and verbal commands. Like the VOR, the saccadic reflex adapts to changes in muscle function, such as when there is weakness of one of the extraocular muscles.

Dissociated nystagmus is a term that has been used to describe rhythmic oscillations that are different in the two eyes. At one extreme, the nystagmus may be present in one eye alone, termed *monocular nystagmus* or *spasmus nutans*. In other circumstances, the eyes may demonstrate vertical, horizontal, rotatory, or simultaneously different or similar direction but simply greater in one eye than in the other. Included in the category of dissociated nystagmus are asymmetrical nystagmus associated with aberrant regeneration of the third nerve, wherein one eye may move vertically while the other eye moves horizontally; nystagmus with amblyopia, as seen in vertical oscillations with unilateral blindness of infancy; see-saw nystagmus, such as in those with parachiasmal lesions, wherein movement of one eye has a different direction from that of the other eye; convergence or divergence nystagmus, in which there are simultaneous abductive movements of the eyes; and dissociated nystagmus accompanying lesions of the posterior fossa. Cogan (1) reported 14 patients with dissociated nystagmus, including among them, eight patients with brainstem and cerebellum lesions of neoplastic, demyelinative, degenerative, or vascular etiopathogenesis. Horizontal, vertical, and rotatory features of nystagmus were noted, with the eye on the side of the lesion of greater oscillation. With lateralized lesions, the homolateral eye was ordinarily the one with the greater oscillation. A slight reduction in acuity was noted that was attributed to the nystagmus.

Internuclear ophthalmoplegia is a distinct clinical and pathological entity associated with lesions of the medial longitudinal fasciculus, the symptoms of which include deficient adduction of one or both eyes on horizontal gaze, jerk nystagmus of the abducting eye, and vertical nystagmus usually evoked by upward gaze (2). Adduction on attempted convergence may or may not be preserved. The internuclear ophthalmoplegia was initially divided into an anterior and posterior variety according to whether adduction or abduction was involved, assuming that impulses from the pontine center for conjugate gaze to the medial rectus nuclei traversed the anterior portion of the medial longitudinal fasciculus, while that to the lateral rectus traversed the posterior portion. There is a bilateral form of internuclear ophthalmoplegia in which adduction of both eyes was impaired, and a unilateral form in which adduction of one eye was profoundly limited while adduction of the other eye was normal. Subclinical internuclear ophthalmoplegia was proposed for patients without relevant ocular symptoms who show a lag in

movement of the adducting eye on conjugate gaze to either side but no limitation in its end position. On being instructed to look to the right or left, the patient with subclinical internuclear ophthalmoplegia shows a normal saccade of the abducting eye but a distinct lag or sliding in of the adducting eye. The abducting eye usually develops nystagmus at the extreme of conjugate gaze but the nystagmus with subclinical internuclear ophthalmoplegia is not as constant as with the full-blown syndrome.

Downbeat nystagmus characteristically has a fast component downward and it is usually but not always, most marked when the gaze is directed downward. Whereas upbeat nystagmus is a common symptom of lesions in the posterior fossa or in several types of drug intoxication, downbeat nystagmus is relatively infrequent. Cogan (3) described the clinical features of 27 patients with downbeat nystagmus. Surprisingly labyrinthine involvement, as evidenced by vertigo, was noted in only two patients, a 55-year-old man with vertical nystagmus on downward gaze and unsteadiness of gait and vertigo after cervical injury and a 31-year-old woman with a posterior fourth ventricle ependymoma who developed conjugate gaze palsy and downbeat nystagmus as the presenting ocular signs along with vertigo, headache, and tinnitus. Other associated proximate etiologies unassociated with labyrinthine involvement included sphenoid meningioma, demyelinating disease, alcoholic cerebellar atrophy, platybasia, syphilis, diabetes, Arnold Chiari malformation, arachnoid adhesions, and pontine ischemia.

HISTORY AND NEUROLOGICAL EXAMINATION

An accurate description of the subjective experience of vertigo should be obtained in the patient's own words. Once the type of complaint has been ascertained, two determinations should be made. The first, to identify related neurological, otological, cardiac, psychiatric, gastrointestinal, visual, and other systemic symptoms, and the second is to determine whether the patient's symptoms bear any relation to position and motion, specifically upon changing position and maintaining a particular posture. Finally, the intermittency or constancy of symptoms should be noted, with particular attention paid to the continuous, intermittent, or paroxysmal nature of the symptoms. Information on the overall course of the illness, medications tried, and precipitating events should be recorded. Careful questioning is the first step in the differentiation of vertigo from dizziness. Dizziness implies something other than true vertigo, with the hallucination of motion that patients sense themselves or suspect of their surroundings, the nearest approximation of which may be lightheadedness, unsteadiness, or faintness. The association of symptoms with head motion, eyes closed, neck position, nausea, vomiting, sweating, and especially tinnitus, hearing loss, sensation of wooziness or other subtle disturbances of consciousness during paroxysms, may be present. Vertigo resulting from CNS lesions, in comparison to those with peripheral labyrinthine and eighth-nerve lesions, tends to be of longer duration, less severe, inconstant, or likely to precipitate with head turning and postures, and is more often associated with a disturbance of consciousness, although rarely associated with tinnitus and deafness.

The likeliest peripheral nervous system (PNS) and CNS causes of vertigo should be contemplated in the differential diagnosis. The principal causes of peripheral vertigo to be considered include intrinsic disorders of the ear such as otitis, mastoiditis, local trauma, labyrinthine disturbances including Meniere disease, benign positional vertigo, vestibular neuronitis, ototoxic drugs, otosclerosis, and cerebellopontine angle tumors, further separable by detailed neurological examination and laboratory evaluation. The main causes of CNS vertigo include brainstem and cerebellar ischemia, infarction, tumor, demyelinating disease, head trauma, meningitis, migraines, epilepsy, and psychogenic disease, also further separable by detailed evaluation.

The neurological examination should include assessment of mental status, cranial nerve, motor function, sensory function, and coordination, including the Romberg's test with the head in three position; careful assessment of stance and walking, including tandem gait, and past-pointing; and assessment of tendon reflexes according to standard practice. Although adequate evaluation of hearing depends mainly upon the results of formal audiologic testing, gross evaluation for hearing thresholds and asymmetries between the sides can be performed by noting the distance spoken and whispered voice is heard from either ear with the opposite one blocked. Hearing tests with a 512-cycle tuning fork may give useful information regarding the nature and type of hearing loss, whether conductive or sensorineural. It is also the most effective instrument in the Weber's test that is performed by placing the vibrating tuning fork about three inches from the patient's ear with the blades of the fork perpendicular to the ear, while establishing the level of air conduction by comparing side to side as to its equality and threshold. The tuning fork is then placed on the mid forehead and the patient is asked whether the tone is appreciated in the better hearing ear, which confirms the suspicion of sensorineural hearing loss, or in the poorer hearing ear, more compatible with conductive hearing loss.

The Rinne test incorporates placement first of the vibrating tuning fork with the shaft firmly opposed to the mastoid process, and then about three inches from the side of the ear to ascertain which sound is louder. Conductive hearing loss disturbances yield better bone conduction than air, whereas sensorineural hearing loss is suggested by louder air conduction than bone sound transmission.

In the setting of dizziness, the physical examination should also include a notation of heart rate, cardiac rhythm, palpation of carotid pulses, and auscultation of great vessel bruits. Blood pressure determinations should be performed lying and standing immediately and after three minutes, with forced expiration at 40 mm Hg for fifteen seconds as a Valsalva maneuver; carotid sinus stimulation for ten seconds; observation with turning of the head, sitting and standing, with eyes open and closed, and while walking, followed by hyperventilation for three minutes. Neuro-ophthalmic examination should comprise routine tests of visual and ocular motor function, as well as special studies of vestibulo-ocular and pursuit movement.

LABORATORY EVALUATION

The battery of laboratory studies should be appropriate to the patient's complaints, contemplating the likeliest diagnosis. It may be possible to arrive at the correct localization of the cause of vertigo or dizziness with little or no laboratory studies, especially in a young patient or in a patient with a previously diagnosed labyrinthine or CNS illness associated with vertigo. However, advanced age, superimposed systemic illnesses, and other factors may confound the clinical presentation of vertigo, and make it necessary to broaden the spectrum of diagnostic possibilities, leading to a more detailed evaluation. Serum chemistries, complete blood count, erythrocyte sedimentation rate, thyroid function tests, hepatitis B and C tests, *Borrelia burgdorferi* serology, quantitative immunoglobulins, immunofixation electrophoresis, Lyme serology, B12 measurement, C-reactive measurement protein, antibodies to SSA and SSB in Sjögren syndrome; antinuclear antibody and antibodies to double-stranded DNA in lupus erythematosus; antinuclear cytoplasmic antibodies; antibodies to thyroglobulin; microsomes, ribonuclear protein, and Sm antigens; 3- to 5-hour glucose tolerance testing, and HgA1c for diabetes mellitus are all relatively inexpensive, informative, and can provide the necessary clues to treatable disturbances.

A standard 12-lead electrocardiogram with rhythm strip should be performed, and if warranted, tilt-table testing and 24-hour Holter monitoring for rhythm disturbances in patients with palpitations, frank dizziness, or presumed orthostatic intolerance. Magnetic resonance imaging (MRI) of the brain and internal auditory canals, blink reflex electrophysiology, and brainstem auditory evoked responses (BAER) should be performed promptly if there is suspicion of a static or evolving CNS process, preceded by audiological studies employing binaural loudness balancing, simultaneous binaural median-plane localization, and other tests of hearing for filtered, masked, and binaural speech.

Electronystagmography (ENG) has been the cornerstone

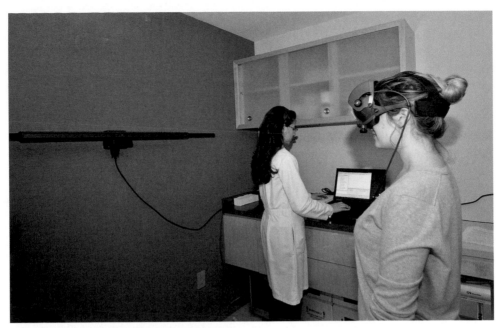

FIG. 9. Computerized algorithm driven videonystagmography (VNG). The patient wears video goggles, fixates on an infrared target while the examiner operates a laptop computer in a darkened room. Caloric testing is performed in the usual manner.

of vestibular diagnosis, employing electrodes applied around the patient's eyes to record eye movements in response to numerous test maneuvers using the evoked corneoretinal potential. However, traditional ENG has been supplanted by newer techniques of measuring eye movement, termed *videonystagmography* (VNG), using video goggles and automated infrared signals and cameras to preserve a film clip of the actual testing, which can be accomplished in the light and dark (Figure 9). Ocular motility is assessed using a sequence of maneuvers, including evoked gaze, saccades, and tracking movements; optokinetic, positional and spontaneous nystagmus in response to bithermal caloric testing; and the Nylen Barany maneuver. Although the analysis has generally been carried out by very experienced assessors, automatic systems have computer algorithms that have been taught to locate and quantify maximum responses. Among 100 patients analyzed by conventional ENG ad newer VNG systems by either an experienced assessor or computer algorithm to compare the outcome of testing, there were few meaningful differences, however assessment of complex VNG were believed to be best analyzed by experienced assessors (4). The diagnostic evaluation of patients with the primary complaint of dizziness, while challenging, ultimately reveals that up to one-third of patients will have a peripheral vestibular disorder, including benign positional vertigo, single or recurrent acute episodes of peripheral vestibulopathy, Meniere disease, chronic labyrinthine imbalance, a cerebellopontine angle tumors, and other categorized vestibular disorders.

SPECIFIC DISORDERS ASSOCIATED WITH VERTIGO

Meniere Disease

Although first attributed to severe vertigo (5), this diagnosis was soon applied to all forms of labyrinthine vertigo, both slight and severe. Affected patients present with acute and recurrent peripheral vestibulopathy accompanied by hearing loss and tinnitus, often with a characteristic cochlear deficit on audiologic testing. Pathological features include gross dilatation of the endolymph system, which affects the scala media of the cochlea and the saccule, and degenerative change in the organ of Corti and stria vascularis with the formation of hydrops labyrinthi. Tests of cochlear function are of greatest clinical value because 100% of patients demonstrate loudness recruitment, with impaired speech discrimination; and abnormal caloric responses in the majority of patients.

Benign Positional Vertigo

Benign postural or positional vertigo or positional nystagmus, as first described, encompassed two distinct conditions, a peripheral labyrinthine disorder and a second vaguely attributed to a CNS lesion. The first type gained later acceptance as a disturbance of the otolith organ. Later clinicopathologic correlations associated positional nystagmus with intracranial tumors of the posterior fossa, so-called position-changing type, due to the change in direction when the position of the head was reversed. The position-changing type was separated from direction-fixed nystagmus, in which certain positions of the head produced nystagmus, the direction of which remained constant despite changes in head position. Of 127 patients with positional nystagmus described by Cawthorne (6), 10% had a CNS cause, most often mid-line cerebellar lesion, and 90% were due to static peripheral labyrinthine lesions. Positional nystagmus arises from an abnormal and paroxysmal response to the positional stimulation to the disorganized but not defunct utricular sensory cells. Spontaneous nystagmus and vertigo erupts with a latency of a few seconds following assumption of the provocative posture and adapts after a minute or so, fatiguing with repetition of the maneuver. A malignant variety occurs with space-occupying, demyelinating, and other lesions of the posterior fossa, often with immediate onset of nystagmus, with little or no adaptation, fatigue of nystagmus, or subjective vertigo.

Vestibular Neuronitis

This disorder was first diagnosed in patients with bouts of spontaneous vertigo lasting for hours and days, with variable residual peripheral labyrinthine or nerve paresis. Affected patients have no complaints of deafness or tinnitus, and assessment of cochlear function is normal. Although spontaneous and positional nystagmus are absent, ataxia of stance and gait are often present, and caloric testing reveals moderate to complete canal paresis without response; however, certain cases exhibit directional preponderance, and others a combination of directional preponderance and canal paresis. Among 100 patients of vestibular neuronitis described by Dix (7), 47 manifested bilateral caloric dysfunction, and 53 showed unilateral abnormalities. The disorder pursues a benign course and recovery of each acute attack is the rule.

Perilabyrinthtis

Perilabyrinthitis classically presents with severe disturbance of equilibrium, usually after mastoid surgery, with a remnant of hearing in the affected ear, evidence of vestibular function in the shape of an active fistula sign, and brisk responses to caloric stimulation. Specifically, labyrinthectomy or opening into the perilymph space with removal of the membranous external canal, with total loss of vestibular and cochlear function; and labyrinthotomy and opening of the perilymph space for the relief of deafness, both presented with potentially disabling vertigo (8).

Cerebrovascular Disease

Labyrinthine and cerebrovascular disorders are both frequent and at times coexist, making the interpretation of cause and effect especially challenging in a given patient. In 1967, C.M. Fisher (9) reviewed a personal series of strokes involving named cerebral and brainstem vessels in association with dizziness, embracing all vestibular symptomatology, whether or not there was a rotational component. Four of ten patients with sudden deafness, with or without other brainstem signs studied at postmortem examination, had vascular occlusion of the internal auditory artery or anterior inferior cerebellar artery on the affected side. Dizziness occurred in nine of ten patients, and was an unaccompanied first sign in three patients. Whereas labyrinthine disorders were customarily attributed at times to occlusion of small vestibular arteries, occlusion of the anterior inferior cerebellar and internal auditory artery seemed more likely to be the cause of sudden deafness.

Of 112 patients with basilar occlusion, 77% had dizziness associated with a rotatory feeling, a percentage that was similar for autopsied cases. A review of 50 patients in which there was strong evidence of a labyrinthine etiopathogenesis, rotation was noted in 90%. Dizziness was unaccompanied by deafness, tinnitus, or other localizing neurological symptoms or signs of stroke in one quarter of those with basilar stroke, and was usually in the form of a prodromal transient ischemic attack. In half of the patients, dizziness lasting hours or days was one of two or more initial symptoms that preceded further neurological phenomena, allowing separation from a labyrinthine etiopathogenesis. Coarse nystagmus, excessive imbalance, Horner syndrome, and vertical nystagmus are suggestive of basilar artery ischemia. The most common accompaniments of dizziness as an initial sign of basilar ischemia were, in the order of frequency, diplopia usually due to skew deviation, produced by paralysis of secondary vestibular fibers running to the medial longitudinal fasciculi affecting eye muscles asymmetrically and dysconjugately, followed by dysarthria, weakness, headache, numbness of the face or limbs, gait ataxia, cerebellar limb ataxia, and visual impairment. Silversides (10) noted that in typical basilar artery thrombosis, there was a frequent history of acute vertigo, weakness, nausea and vomiting, before development of coma. Among 65 patients suspected of basilar insufficiency (11) vertigo was the initial symptom of basilar artery thrombosis in 32 patients, and in later attacks in another five patients. Of 54 patients with vertebrobasilar insufficiency (12), 77% had vertigo. Basilar artery thrombosis with infarction of the brainstem is shown in Figure 10.

Based on clinicoanatomical localization, medullary lesions in vestibular nuclei above the level of the eighth nerve are those most likely associated with deafness, with clinical involvement of the nuclei and intramedullary fibers of the sixth and seventh cranial nerves, and the trigeminal complex subserving sensation over the entire ipsilateral half of the face, with resultant abducens and facial paresis, and widespread disturbance of trigeminal sensory function. Lesions

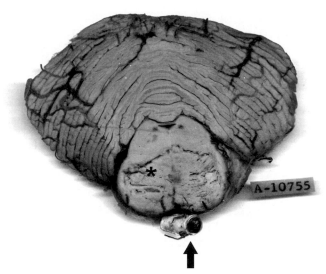

FIG. 10. Pontine infarction: basilar thrombosis in a gross specimen. Note the thrombus in the basilar artery (arrow), and the large ventral pontine infarction (*).

at the level of the eighth nerve resulted in deficits explained by involvement of the spintothalamic tract, restiform body, descending nucleus and tract of the fifth nerve, and nucleus ambiguous, resulting in hyperalgesia of the contralateral body and ipsilateral trigeminal nerve, with ipsilateral limb incoordination, and paralysis of the ipsilateral vocal cord and soft tissue palate. More caudally placed lesions led to involvement of the cuneate nucleus with sensory changes in the ipsilateral upper limbs. Such are the clinical neurologic manifestations of lateral medullary infarction (13). Although originally ascribed to occlusion of the posterior inferior cerebellar artery, occlusion of a vertebral artery and not of the posterior inferior cerebellar artery was more often the cause leading to a wedge-shaped infarct of the lateral medulla that included the inferior portion of the vestibular nucleus. Of 36 patients with lateral medullary infarction in the series by Fisher (9), only two had pathologically-proven occlusion of the posterior inferior cerebellar artery. Vertigo and nystagmus were seen in 51% and 61%, respectively, in the series reported by Sacco and colleagues (14); in 50% and 69% of patients, respectively, in the series by Fisher and colleagues (15); in 71% and 57% of patients studied by Peterman and Siekert (16); and in 100% and 50%, respectively, in the patients reported by Merritt and Finland (17). Among 43 patients with lateral medullary infarction reported by Norrving and Cronqvist (18), nystagmus was noted in 100% of patients. Kim and colleagues (19) studied 33 patients with lateral medullary infarction and found an overall incidence of vertigo and dizziness of 91%. Analysis of the magnetic resonance imaging (MRI) findings in a rostrocaudal manner revealed that 10 of 12 patients with lesions of the upper medulla or upper and middle medulla had vertigo and dizziness, and one patient had nystagmus on forward gaze, compared with vertigo and dizziness in all 13 patients with lesions in the lower medulla or lower and middle medulla, with six demonstrating nystagmus. Of eight additional patients with middle medullary lesions, seven had vertigo and dizziness. Nystagmus, vertigo and dizziness appeared to be more severe in those with caudal medullary lesions.

Nystagmus in lateral medullary syndrome is attributed to involvement of vestibular nuclei and their connections to the cerebellum, which begin at the caudal part of the medial and inferior vestibular nuclei. Among four patients reported by Ross and coworkers (20) with lateral medullary infarction, MRI demonstrated coexisting cerebellar infarction in three patients, similar to the study of Kim and colleagues (19) in which MRI of 33 such patients showed cerebellar infarcts in cases so studied. The vestibulocerebellar pathways run through the juxtarestiform body, a part of the inferior cerebellar peduncle, and in the posterolateral medulla, areas that tend to be spared in those with upper medullary lesions. Six of eight patients so studied in the series of Kim and colleagues (19) with lateral medullary infarction did not show nystagmus.

Carmichael and colleagues (21) summarized the vestibular findings in eight patients with unilateral lesions of the lateral medulla due to arterial occlusion. Those with lesions of the vestibular nuclei exhibited evidence of directional preponderance of caloric nystagmus to the side opposite to the lesion. Directional preponderance was attributed to damage to caudal vestibular nuclei. Such areas were thought to include utricular tonus elements and interpreted in terms of unilateral utricule lesions, the primary effect of which was to bring about a deviation toward the side of the lesion of the resting position of gaze.

Although lateral medullary infarction has been regarded overall as a benign condition, the outcome has not been uniformly favorable. Death from repeated brainstem ischemia culminating in cerebellar infarction, aspiration, cardiovascular and respiratory abnormalities, clot propagation, embolization, and involvement of the opposite vertebral artery occurred in 11% of patients during the acute phase of the stroke, with a recurring stroke rate of 1.9% per year afterward. Five of the patients had vertebrobasilar transient ischemic attacks 11 to 45 months after lateral medullary infarctions, symptoms included vertigo, diplopia, and numbness in the ipsilateral face and contralateral body (22).

Among 21 patients with pure motor hemiparesis due to pontine or capsular infarction studied by Nighoghossian and colleagues (23), transient gait ataxia and vertigo was noted in 57% of patients with pure motor hemiparesis, but in none with capsular infarcts, suggesting a relation of vertigo to brainstem vestibulocerebellar fibers. Of 26 patients with progressive unilateral pontine infarcts studied by Kunz and colleagues (24), a single patient had a history of vertebrobasilar transient ischemic attack with facial paresis, unsteady gait, and dizziness a month before the onset of acute pontine infarction, which in keeping with the neuroanatomic localization would probably have resulted in part from disturbance of corticopontocerebellar fibers, not the vestibular nuclei or its immediate connections. Bogousslavsky and colleagues (25) reported 22 patients with stroke and infarction of the upper, middle, and lower midbrain, respectively, in the territories of the posterior choroidal and posterior cerebral, superior cerebellar, and basilar artery, and paramedian basilar and short circumferential arteries, none of whom presented with vertigo or nystagmus, in keeping with the neuroanatomical localization and sparing of central vestibular connections.

Cerebellar Lesions

Over the decades, the existence of nystagmus in cerebellar lesions has been controversial. Early investigators admitted that lesions limited to the cerebellum produced a transient nystagmus, particularly if it affected deep cerebellar nuclei (26). However, there were few clinical studies on the influence of head position upon the appearance of spontaneous nystagmus. Experimental neuroanatomical studies (27, 28) linked cerebellar interconnections directly to the oculomotor neurons, the parapontine reticular formation horizontal gaze center, and the vestibular nuclei. Short latency potentials appear in the cerebellum when the eyes move, and stimulation of vermian and paravermian cerebellar regions produce saccadic and pursuit eye movements, while the flocculonodular lobe produce nystagmus and inhibit a post-rotatory and post-caloric nystagmus. Involvement of the vestibular or archicerebellum results from damage variably to the flocculonodular lobe, lingual, uvula, and parafloccular regions, whereas affected primates manifest disequilibrium consisting of oscillation of the head and neck, falling, titubation, gait ataxia, and nystagmus, the reverse of which followed unilateral labyrinthectomy.

The expected clinical symptoms and signs of vestibulocerebellar involvement in man include spontaneous nystagmus, which differs from labyrinthine disorders in the quick component toward the side of the lesion, similar to that of unilateral nodular lesions, and deviation of the eyes toward the side opposite the lesion, which is brought out more by fixation and is slower and more irregular in its excursion than true labyrinthine nystagmus. Cerebellar nystagmus is usually horizontal but may be vertical. Compensation is readily seen, and small superficial lesions demonstrate little nystagmus. Gait disturbance in vestibulocerebellar disease is characterized by unsteadiness in spite of the absence of frank limb ataxia, which is more commonly seen with corticopontocerebellar involvement. Rotation of head position is the other salient sign of cerebellar disease. Whereas a labyrinthine and vestibular nerve lesion leads to rotation

of the head with the occiput toward the side of the lesion, a lesion of the vestibulocerebellum, in particular unilateral flocculonodular lobe, leads to rotation of the head with the occiput to the opposite side.

Nonetheless, controversy persists as to whether the vestibular signs that result from cerebellar lesions in man are due to the cerebellum itself, or its connections with brainstem. Baloh and colleagues (29) conducted vestibulo-ocular tests in 15 patients with pure cerebellar, cerebellar and brainstem disease, and Friedreich ataxia (FA) to evaluate ocular signs thereof. Twelve patients had one or more types of spontaneous nystagmus, including eight with gaze nystagmus, three rebound, two positional, and one vestibular type. The latter instance might have suggested a possible second lesion in the peripheral labyrinth or brainstem. Caloric and rotatory-induced nystagmus was hyperactive in the pure cerebellar group and diminished in FA, while those with cerebellar and brainstem involvement had mixed responses. All patients demonstrated fixation instability and impaired smooth pursuit, with dysmetria of voluntary saccades, flutter, and rebound saccades. In addition, 60% of the patients had significant slowing of induced saccades. Hood and colleagues (30) studied 25 patients with rebound nystagmus and found a consistent pattern of bilateral or unilateral rebound nystagmus with neurological evidence of cerebellar involvement, markedly enhanced caloric responses, gait ataxia, a complaint of feeling unsteady rather than true vertigo, and deranged optokinetic responses.

Tumors

Acoustic neurofibromata are the best-known and commonest tumors of the cerebellopontine angle in the internal auditory meatus. Two stages of affliction have been recognized, an otological and neurological. The first is associated with slow and progressive destruction of cochlear and vestibular nerve fibers, with unilateral deafness, compensated vestibular dysfunction, and slight unsteadiness of gait and vertigo. The second stage is associated with expansion of the tumor from the internal auditory meatus, leading to brainstem compression. The diagnosis should be suspected in patients with headache, vertigo, dizziness, and hearing loss. Large tumors that compress the cerebellum and pons lead to impairment of the ipsilateral corneal reflex, peripheral facial nerve weakness, cerebellar incoordination, past pointing, and tandem imbalance. Magnetic resonance imaging of the cerebellopontine angle and mastoid demonstrates lesions of all sizes, including those which, when diagnosed early, can be successfully treated (Figure 11). Tests of cochlear function demonstrate abnormal pure tone audiometry. The vestibular assessment of unilateral acoustic neurofibromata was studied in detail by Dix and Hallpike (31). Spontaneous first-degree nystagmus was more forceful toward the contralateral

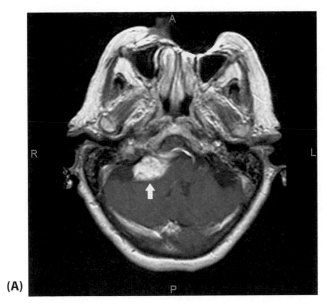

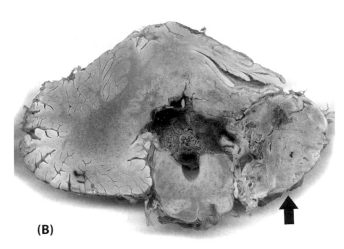

FIG. 11. Acoustic neurinoma. **(A)** Magnetic resonance imaging demonstrating acoustic neuroma of the cerebellopontine angle, and **(B)** a comparable gross anatomic specimen. The arrows demonstrate the tumor.

direction of gaze. Nystagmographic examination showed the nystagmus to be of a central or deviation maintenance type without alteration by positional changes. Optokinetic nystagmus elicited brisk responses to the contralateral side, with suppression of ipsilateral responses. Caloric testing showed directional preponderance to the contralateral side. In accordance with Alexander's law, the straight-ahead position of the eyes employed for caloric testing facilitated nystagmus to the contralateral side.

Brainstem auditory evoked responses in patients with eighth nerve tumors demonstrate prolongation of the I-III wave interpeak latency consistent with the proximal location of the tumor in the region of the proximal eighth nerve in close apposition to its synaptic connection with brainstem nuclei. Glomus jugulare tumors and sarcomas of the cerebellopontine angle, also recognized by multiple cranial nerve palsies, can be associated with vertigo. Congenital or primary cholesteatoma, recognized by slow progression of facial palsy and petrous bone erosion, accompanied by loss of cochlear and vestibular function, may be mistaken for a cerebellopontine angle tumor (32). Leukemia and other lymphoproliferative disorders likewise precipitated deafness and vertigo (33).

Tumors arising in the brainstem are an important cause of CNS vertigo. They occur more commonly in children than in adults, often with insidious onset of neurological symptoms and signs, with late occurrence, if at all, of increased intracranial pressure (ICP). For instance, among autopsy-verified case series, brainstem gliomas accounted for 12% of intracranial tumors reported both by Bailey and colleagues (34) and Walker and Hopple (35); 6% of tumors reported by Barnett and Hyland (36); and 5% of patients described by Smith and Fincher (37). Among 606 children with tumors observed at the Mayo Clinic in a 40-year period, by Keith and colleagues (38), 281 tumors were infratentorial, of which 30% each were astrocytoma or medulloblastoma, 12% ependymoma, 7% glioblastoma multiforme, and 21% other types. Among 48 brainstem tumors described by Bray and colleagues (39) one-half of patients presented with squint, headache, speech disturbance, and vomiting followed by personality change, swallowing difficulty, and lethargy. Corticospinal tract signs, hemiparesis, ataxia, Babinski signs, and involvement of multiple cranial nerve nuclei most commonly the seventh, ninth, tenth, sensory and fifth. Horizontal nystagmus was seen in over half the patients, and vertical nystagmus in 29%. A critical finding was gaze paralysis present in almost one half of patients at some time and the most important localizing lesion. Upgaze paralysis, a cardinal sign of upper midbrain compression, was noted in five patients. Among 90 verified tumors reported by Barnett and Hyland (40) involving the brainstem, glioma accounted for 40% of cases, ependymoma 23%, and pinealoma 9%, followed by papiloma, angioma, teratoma, hemangioendothelioma, and melanoma in the remaining patients. Initial symptomatology could be categorized into two main groups, those due to obstructive hydrocephalus, which usually accounted for ventricular tumors and a lesser proportion of brainstem and pineal tumors, and involvement of cranial nerve nuclei and long tracts, seen in two-thirds of those with primary brainstem tumors. In the latter, nystagmus was observed in one-quarter of patients, and cerebellar signs were usually present as a late manifestation in one-half and, infrequently, as the initial symptomatology. Bucy (41) noted nystagmus as a common finding with gliomas of the pons present in up to 38% of patients. Among 100 intracranial tumors in children (42), 63% were located in the posterior fossa, 52% were medulloblastoma or astrocytoma. Headache, vomiting, visual disturbance, staggering gait, and vomiting were the commonest initial symptoms. Dizziness and deafness were rare initial symptoms, seen in one patient each. Cawthorne and Hinchcliffe (43) described positional nystagmus of the central type among six patients with subtentorial metastatic lesions, emphasizing its potential localizing value in the CNS, particularly in vestibular centers of the cerebellum.

Unilateral cerebral lesions, especially of the temporal lobe, supramarginal, and angular gyrus can lead to vestibular disturbances with alteration in caloric and OKN testing. Carmichael and colleagues (44) studied the CNS localization of directional preponderance to the side of the lesion of caloric and OKN among patients with supratentorial lesions, stemming from widespread abnormality of one hemisphere to localized lesions, including gliomas, trigeminal angiomatosis, aneurysm, stroke, and meningiomas, that were either evident upon clinical grounds or later demonstrated at operation and at postmortem examination. Directional preponderance stemming from either caloric or OKN was absent in all subjects with lesions limited to the frontal lobe, the upper half of the parietal lobe, or the anterior half of the temporal lobe. Directional preponderance of caloric nystagmus to the side of the cerebral lesion without directional preponderance of optokinetic nystagmus was a constant finding in subjects with lesions of the posterior halves of the temporal lobes. Directional preponderance of both caloric nystagmus and optokinetic nystagmus was also a constant finding in subjects with lesions involving the supramarginal and angular gyri upon the same side. Surgical interference in the region of the supramarginal and angular gyrus in several of those subjects resulted in increase in directional preponderance of optokinetic nystagmus.

Heredodegenerative Disorders

Wadia (45) described 30 members of nine families with autosomal dominant spinocerebellar degeneration, with pronounced cerebellar ataxia and other signs, including chorea, facial weakness, and slow but full eye movement abnormalities. Spoendlin (46) studied two patients with FA, in whom histopathologically examined temporal bones showed selective degeneration of the primary cochlear neurons and, to a lesser degree, vestibular neurons and branches of the nerves, with little change in end organs at postmortem examination. These findings were correlated with the caloric inexcitability on both sides with complete loss of the ampullar nerve

fibers, with presumably remaining function of the maculae, although the latter function was not formally tested.

Craniovertebral Disease

The association of nystagmus with craniovertebral anomalies is well recognized. Thrush and Foster (47) studied 100 patients with communicating syringomyelia, of which 23% had nystagmus, without discernible pattern in the nystagmus or involvement of cranial nerves, limbs, or degree of descent of the cerebellar tonsils. Saez and colleagues (48) studied 60 patients with Arnold Chiari malformation treated with suboccipital decompression, in whom nystagmus was found in 43%, that was either of the downbeating vertical, horizontal, or rotatory types. Cogan and Barrows (49) noted horizontal and vertical nystagmus of the jerk type in all nine anatomically-proven patients with platybasia and Arnold Chiari malformation; three patients, in addition, had skew deviation and three had unexplained horizontal diplopia. The authors contended that the diagnosis of platybasia and Arnold Chiari malformation should be suspected when the foregoing ocular signs arise insidiously during adolescence, along with other evidence of brainstem and cerebellar involvement, especially when accompanied by neck pain, and provoked by sneezing and coughing. Spillane and colleagues (50) studied 24 patients with congential abnormalities of the foramen magnum causing disability, among them basilar impression, occipitalization of the atlas, chronic atlantoaxial dislocation, fusion of cervical vertebrae, and cerebellar ectopia, associated with nystagmus on lateral gaze in 63%, nine of whom were rotatory or oblique type with sustained vertical nystagmus, usually of a high amplitude, often slow type, with occasional oscillopsia, and six with spontaneous second-degree nystagmus of a very coarse nature. In all, nine had nystagmus movements when looking down, and four had vertical nystagmus looking up. Vertigo can be the presenting symptom of Paget disease of the skull, with involvement of the eighth nerves and labyrinthine capsules. Otosclerosis and other disorders involve the bony labyrinthine and capsule with resultant vertigo and unilateral conductive and mixed sensorineural deafness, and at times, a family history of otosclerosis.

Newborn children with torsion of the neck demonstrate horizontal ocular movements often interrupted by nystagmus beats; however, as long as the torsion of the neck is maintained the eyes retain a compensatory position. After optic fixation has been abolished, torsion of the neck in adults also leads to compensatory ocular movements with nystagmus, but the sustained compensatory ocular positions of newborns are rarely observed. Neck torsion nystagmus has been observed in patients with disorders that abolished vestibular reactions on angular acceleration. Local anaesthesia of paravertebral tissues of the neck causes a marked reduction in the number of nystagmus beats during torsion. Nystagmus has also been observed during small rotatory movements of the pelvic girdle with respect to the thorax (51). The contribution of injury to dorsal sensory nerve afferent input in the development of vertigo and nystagmus has been described (52). One posterior sympathetic cervical syndrome was comprised of rotatory vertigo with a tendency to fall and past point toward the side of procaine injections into deep cervical tissues lateral to the vertebral column, in association with bilateral tinnitus and ipsilateral Horner syndrome that persisted for up to an hour. Other patients with unilateral brachial neuritis, complaining of vertigo on assuming particular positions, had nystagmus directed toward the side of the diseased plexus. Unilateral section of the second and third cervical dorsal roots in two patients with severe torticollis led to position nystagmus that was directed toward the side of the operation. One patient who underwent transaction of the third and fourth cervical sensory roots for the removal of multiple neurinomas had severe bouts of vertigo induced by position change after recovery from anesthesia, and for days afterward showed positional nystagmus after rotation of the head with respect to the trunk and on turning the entire body along the longitudinal axis.

Multiple Sclerosis

Dam and colleagues (53) studied 82 patients with multiple sclerosis (MS) through a battery of clinical vestibular testing. Spontaneous nystagmus, positional nystagmus, and pathological differential caloric tests were noted in 60% of patients. Pathological horizontal OKN occurred in 57% of patients that was bilateral or bilateral and vertical, the latter of which suggested diffuse mesencephalic brainstem and bilateral hemispheric involvement combined with brainstem and cerebellar lesions, such as is seen in patients with widespread dissemination. In some patients, defective OKN was caused by a nuclear or internuclear ophthalmoplegia (INO), in whom a dissociated optokinetic nystagmus was found. Solinger and coworkers (54) evaluated eye movement abnormalities in 16 patients with multiple sclerosis with little or no clinically apparent eye movement disorder. Up to 25% had vestibular nystagmus with eyes closed, and one patient had typical rebound nystagmus. Aanta and colleagues (55) found either spontaneous or positional nystagmus in 60% of patients studied in the early stages of their disease. With caloric testing, unilateral hypoexcitability was noted in 18 patients and directional preponderance in 14 patients. Dam and coworkers (56) reported a similar incidence of vestibular abnormalities among 82 patients with MS, with impaired OKN in 44% of patients.

Bilateral internuclear ophthalmoplegia is the most common oculomotor manifestation of MS; conversely, it is one of the most common ways MS manifests due to predilection of the disease for the medial longitudinal fasciculus (MLF). The INO of MS may be complete, in which case neither eye adducts beyond the midline on attempted horizontal gaze, or it may be complete on one side and incomplete on the other; rarely is it strictly unilateral and then only for a short time during its evolution. The posterior variety is characteristically associated with paralysis of conjugate gaze to one or both sides. Bilateral INO occurs in brainstem disorders other than MS affecting the medial longitudinal fasciculus, including medulloblastoma and infiltrative gliomas of the brainstem, occlusive brainstem vascular disease, Arnold-Chiari malformation, and syphilis (57).

Infectious-Inflammatory Disorders

Apart from acute labyrinthitis, there are three other infective viral syndromes with vestibular involvement, including geniculate herpes zoster oticus (HZO) (58) and two uveoencephalitic disorders described by Vogt-Koyanagi and Harada (59). Syphilis and other granulomatous disorders can present with chronic aseptic meningitis located at the cerebellopontine angle causing vertigo and hydrocephalus, as can nonsyphilitic interstitial keratitis or Cogan syndrome, which presents with vertigo, deafness, tinnitus, leukocytosis, and eosinophilia, and association with polyarteritis nodosa (60).

The symptoms or signs of increased intracranial pressure in the setting of otitis media and chronic mastoiditis should also raise the possibility of otitic hydrocephalus first described in 1890 by Taylor (61), who commented: *It is important to remember what has now been verified in numerous cases, that in mastoid suppuration there is often double optic neuritis, with an entire absence of meningitis or of abscess, as proved by post-mortem examination, and by recovery after simple trephining the mastoid cells.*

Two clinical presentations were recognized, one type in the setting of otitis media and mastoiditis, often without other evident complications and relieved by draining of the CSF, the clinical presentation of which suggested tumor or abscess of the temporal lobe more than meningitis, with progressive headache, drowsiness, and papilledema. At operation, there is little evidence of osteitis, the roof of the atrium is intact, and the dura mater is under pressure. Postmortem examination showed congestion of the choroid plexus and edema of ependymal and subependymal tissues. The underlying process was ascribed to an excess of CSF in the subarachnoid space and ventricles that typically showed normal cell count and protein content. An alternative clinical syndrome was hydrocephalus, including a brief phase of headache and drowsiness with subsequent development of hemiparesis, seizure, papilledema, and increased intracranial pressure. Ventricular drainage is often necessary to alleviate the symptoms based on the assumption that the hydrocephalus is obstructive and a result of adhesions obliterating the effluent

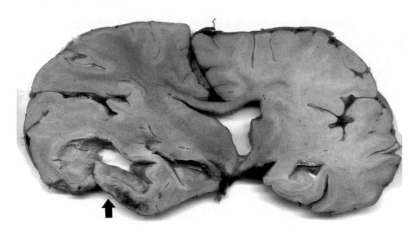

FIG. 12. Temporal lobe abscess shown at the arrow tip with suppurative otitis, mastoiditis, and hydrocephalus.

channels. Symonds (62) noted the occurrence of lateral sinus thrombosis in three patients with otitic hydrocephalus. However, against the hypothesis that it was causative was that if so, hydrocephalus would be a more frequent instead of a rare accompaniment of venous thrombosis.

There is a spectrum from benign otitic hydrocephalus to potentially fatal temporal lobe abscess (Figure 12), with the latter so suggested by toxic general appearance, papilledema, and focal neurologic signs, which can occur at any age accompanied by CSF under moderate pressure, cellular pleocytosis, and increased protein content, the differential diagnosis of which includes encephalitis, aneurysm, tuberculous and purulent pachymeningitis, leptomeningitis, arachnoiditis, and suppurative pyogenic abscess of the petrous pyramid.

Migraine

Bickerstaff (63) described 34 patients with basilar migraine, the majority of whom were adolescent girls. Premonitory symptoms of bilateral loss or disturbance of vision, vertigo, ataxia, dysarthria, tinnitus, tingling and numbness of the hands, feet, and around the lips and on the sides of the tongue, lasting less than an hour, were followed by severe throbbing occipital headache and vomiting, which although infrequent, were often related to menstruation. Eviatar (64) reviewed the results of vestibular testing in basilar artery migraine among 20 children, 16 of whom had abnormalities of bithermal caloric testing. Labyrinthine preponderance was found in one child with labyrinthine concussion and in six with symptoms suggesting ischemia of the territory supported by the basilar artery and the occipital branches of the posterior cerebral arteries. Directional preponderance was found in four children, with symptoms suggesting ischemia of the posterior temporal branches of the posterior cerebral arteries. Five children had both labyrinthine and directional preponderance. Normal ENG findings were present in four children and correlated with milder illness. Head trauma was the triggering factor for migraine in five children. Five children developed complex partial seizures and had evidence of directional preponderance (two children) and combined labyrinthine and directional preponderance (two children). The presence of abnormalities of ENG testing in children with basilar artery migraine correlated with the severity of the disease. Directional preponderance or labyrinthine and directional preponderance was more frequently correlated with ischemia in the posterior temporal branches of the posterior cerebral arteries and suggested a higher risk of developing vertiginous seizures when ischemic was prolonged. So-called reflex epilepsy differs in that the latter can often be precipitated by caloric stimulation.

Syncope and Vasovagal Syndrome

Both syncope and vasovagal syndrome due to different etiopathogenic mechanisms resulting in transient, decreased systemic blood pressure and resultant cerebral perfusion, can both be accompanied by rotational sensations.

Postconcussive Disturbances

While traumatic brain injury (TBI) can lead to prolonged vestibular involvement due to the direct effects of injury to the bony labyrinth and its contents, mild TBI (MTBI) that follows seemingly less significant head injury can be the cause of equally disabling vestibular complaints, even when there is little on bedside examination or office encounter to substantiate their presence weeks or months later. Two generally accepted definitions of concussion injury have been proposed. One is the entity termed *postconcussion syndrome* (PCS) as proposed by the International Classification of Diseases or ICD-10 (65); the other is so-called *postconcussion disorder* (PCD) proposed by the *American Psychiatric Association Diagnostic and*

Statistical Manual (DSM-IV-TR) (66), with considerable overlap but significant differences, particularly in time parameters, reliance on neuropsychological assessment, and the reliance on cognitive, physical and emotional residuals of concussive injury. According to the ICD-10 definition, PCS is diagnosed if symptoms persist one or more months after injury, while PCD is recognized by DSM-IV-TR after three or more months. While neuropsychological tests are often more reliable than subjective patient reports in quantifying cognitive impairment, ICD-10 and the DSM-IV-TR provide different guidelines, with the former allowing diagnosis of PCS on patient's subjective complaints without further documentation, and the DSM-IV-TR requiring documentation of cognitive deficits by neuropsychological testing. Both ICD-10 and DSM-IV-TR include similar symptoms under the categories of physical, cognitive and emotional impairment. The ICD-10 require three or more symptoms in those three categories to dagnose PCS, including difficulty with concentration, performing mental tasks, and memory (cognitive impairment) headache, dizziness, fatigue, irritability, and insomnia (physical impairment) and reduced tolerance to stress, emotional excitement, and alcohol consumption (emotional impairment). However the DSM-IV-TR includes vertigo, not mentioned by ICD-10, and requires, in addition, significant social or occupational impairments. The obvious solution would be to arrive at a present single definition for postconcussive deficits since a similar consensus was reached for the diagnosis of MTBI by the American Congress of Rehabilitation Medicine (67) and the WHO Collaborating Center Task Force on MTBI (68). The debate between brain-based and psychologically-based explanations for post-concussive injury has produced a flaw dichotomy with cognitive deficits, at times ascribed to psychogenic phenomena and others ascribed to brain damage, ignoring premorbid and comorbid factors. Some investigators have proposed a classification employing PCD with neuropathological features with objective evidence of brain injury by neuroimaging or neuropsychological testing; and others with a predominance of neurocognitive or psychopathology sparing objective brain injury, or mixed features (69).

Psychosomatic Disturbances

Psychosomatic disturbances occur in up to 30% of patients in a general medical practice, particularly in the setting of psychological stress and serious life events (70, 71) so-called, post-traumatic stress disorder (PTSD). It contains weightings for life events indicating their degree of stress that might be imposed, which cumulatively summed, can achieve etiological significance as a cause of illness such as vertigo and dizziness (72). Psychological reactions to physical illness were conceptualized in terms of psychological trauma, crisis, change in body, self-esteem, and stress, all of which can have important implications for patients with symptoms of labyrinthine disease, the symptoms of which can significantly impact upon body image and consciousness, and intensify psychological stressors.

Hallpike and colleagues (73) reviewed abnormalities of the caloric test results in diverse mental disorders and noted instead exaggerated activity of the caloric response. Drachman and Hart (74) carried out detailed evaluation of dizziness including neuro-otological studies that identified 23% of patients with hyperventilation syndrome, second only in frequency to peripheral vestibular disorders as the proposed etiopathogenesis of dizziness. The patients with hyperventilation syndrome generally equated the symptoms of hyperventilation with dizziness, imbalance, giddiness, and mental fuzziness. Two of 15 with a history of positional vertigo manifested positional nystagmus and vertigo with performance of the Nylen-Barany maneuver after hyperventilation. Nine patients or 9% were deemed to have psychogenic dizziness after detailed neuro-otological studies, including four patients deemed to be neurotic due to anxiety, depression, and hysteria. The patients with anxiety admitted to panic, fright, feeling of remoteness, and perspiration. Those with symptoms of depression admitted to difficulty in concentrating, with loss of energy, interest, appetite, and inordinate fatigue. The Minnesota Multiphasic Personality Inventory (MMPI) scores showed abnormal elevation of scores in the neurotic triad of depression, hysteria, and hypochondriasis. Four patients were psychotic, including two with chronic schizophrenia previously requiring institutionalization, and one with a probable diagnosis of schizophrenia. In the psychotic patients, the symptoms of dizziness did not conform to a recognizable pattern. A remaining patient had astasia-abasia imbalance and gait disturbance. Health care professionals should be aware of the literature on the social and psychological factors that contribute to bodily complaints, which may be useful in dealing with patients susceptible to psychogenic complaints including vertigo. Recognizing that anxiety, emotional stress, disturbances of self-esteem, and neurotic and hypochondriacal tendencies can all heighten the experience of somatic symptoms including vertigo. Mechanic (75) recommended that credible instructions be provided to patients with somatic symptoms in a sympathetic and supportive manner to avert attributional errors and new reasons for anxiety rather than giving blanket reassurances of health.

Medications

A variety of drugs can cause vertigo, among them, the narcotic analgesic meperidine; the anticonvulsants diphenhydantoin, ethosuximide, and primidone; the anti-hypertensive agent clonidine; the anti-inflammatory drugs aspirin and indomethacin; birth control medication; the parasympatholytic medication dicyclomine; the antibiotic medications gentamicin, griseofulvin, isoniazid, kanamy-cin, nalidixic acid, minocycline, polymyxin, streptomycin, sulfonamides, tobromycin, trimethoprim; the antiprotozoal and antihelminthic agents hydrochloroquine; the diuretics acetazolamide and furosemide; and the psychotropic medi-cations benzodiazepine, meprobamate, phenothiazine, and tricyclic antidepressants.

TREATMENT

There is no common treatment of vestibular disorders (76). The treatment of vestibular disorders should be tailored to the individual patient. While vestibular suppressant medica-tions are generally effective in both peripheral and central vestibular disorders, they provide only symptomatic relief of vertigo and nausea without altering the disease process. Anti-histamine, phenothiazine, butyrophenone, benzodiazeprine, and clonazepam can all be given orally with the expectation of symptom improvement for several hours, while the anti-cholinergic scopolamine can be given by transderm patch lasting up to 72 hours. Antiepileptic medications have been given with success for vestibular or reflex epilepsy and dis-abling paroxysmal vertigo. Beta-receptor blocker medica-tions can be given for basilar migraine, vestibular migraine, and benign recurrent vertigo. Betahistine is administered for Meniere disease. A trial of antibiotics can be given for pos-sible co-existing infections of the ear and temporal bone.

Corticosteroids have a role in vestibular neuronitis and auto-immune inner ear disease. Baclofen has been given with success in downbeat and upbeat nystagmus. Acetazolamine has been given in familial periodic vertigo. Vestibular nerve section is considered to be the most effective surgical treat-ment for control of intractable symptoms of vertigo second-ary to labyrinthine and eighth nerve function; however, the complications include CSF, meningitis, and intracranial fluid collections (77). There are retrosigmoid, translabyrinthine, retrolabyrinthine, and middle fossa surgical approaches. Among 36 patients who underwent vestibular nerve section for vestibular dysfunction owing to an anterior inferior cer-ebellar artery vascular loop, Meniere disease, head trauma, labyrinthine fistula, syphilitic labyrinthitis, or unknown causes thereof, 75% were improved and 25% were unchanged at 51 months follow-up (78). The most commonly practiced vestibular exercises are Cawthorne-Cooksey exercises, that incorporate eye and head movements in bed, sitting, stand-ing, and moving about a room to habituate abnormal ves-tibular responses.

Vestibular rehabilitation incorporating eye, head, and body exercises was superior to no therapy in a primary care setting among patients with disabling vertigo and dizziness (79). A double-blind placebo-controlled randomized trial of vestibular rehabilitation found that it was most helpful in providing locomotor stability (80). Post-traumatic ver-tigo, which occurs after blunt trauma to the head, neck, and craniocervical area without fractures, can lead to disabling vertigo that can be treated with a high success rate incor-porating medications, rehabilitation, and surgical therapy when there is rupture of the round window membrane, endolymphatic hydrops, and canalolisthiasis.

REFERENCES

1. Cogan DG. Dissociated nystagmus with lesions in the poste-rior fossa. *Arch Ophthal* 2002; 120:361–368.
2. Cogan DG. Internuclear ophthalmoplegia, typical and atypi-cal. *Arch Ophthal* 1970; 84:583–589.
3. Cogan DG. Down-beat nystagmus. *Arch Ophthal* 1968; 80:757–768.
4. Mallinson AI, Longridge NS, Pace-Asciak P, et al. Measuring caloric response: comparison of different analysis techniques. *J Vestib Res* 2010; 20:419–426.
5. Gowers WR. *A Manual of diseases of the nervous system.* Vol. II. Diseases of the brain and cranial nerves, general and functions diseases of the nervous system. Hafner Publishing, Darien, 1970; 782.
6. Cawthorne T. Positional nystagmus. *Ann Oto Rhinol Laryngol* 1954; 63:481–490.
7. Dix MR, Hallpike CS. The pathology, symptomatology and diagnosis of certain common disorders of the vestibular sys-tem. *Proc Royal Soc Med* 1952; 45:341–362.
8. Cawthorne T. Vestibular injuries. *Proc Royal Soc Med* 1946; 39:270-273.
9. Fisher CM. Vertigo in cerebrovascular disease. *Arch Otolaryng* 1967; 85:85-529-534.
10. Silversides JL. Basilar artery stenosis and thrombosis. *Proc Roy Soc Med* 1954; 47:290–293.
11. Williams D, Wilson GT. Major and minor syndromes of basilar insufficiency. *Brain* 1962; 85:741–773.
12. Bradshaw P, McQuaid P. The syndrome of vertebra-basilar insufficiency. *QJM* 1963; 32:279–296.
13. Wallenberg A. Acute bulbar affection (Embolie der art cerebel-lar post inf sinister). *Arch Psychiat Nervenkr* 1895; 27:505–540.
14. Sacco RL, Freddo L, Bello JA, et al. Wallenberg's lateral

medullary syndrome. Clinical-magnetic resonance imaging correlations. *Arch Neurol* 1993; 50:609–614.

15. Fisher CM, Karnes W, Kubik C. Lateral medullary infarction: the pattern of vascular occlusion. *J Neuropathol Exp Neurol* 1961; 20:103–113.

16. Peterman AF, Siekert RG. The lateral medullary (Wallenberg) syndrome: clinical features and prognosis. *Med Clin North Am* 1960; 44:887–895.

17. Merritt H, Finland M. Vascular lesions of the hind-brain (lateral medullary syndrome). *Brain* 1930; 53:290–305.

18. Norrving B, Cronqvist S. Lateral medullary infarction: prognosis in an unselected series. *Neurology* 1991; 41:244–248.

19. Kim JS, Lee JH, Suh DC, et al. Spectrum of lateral medullary syndrome. Correlation between clinical findings and magnetic resonance imaging in 33 subjects. *Stroke* 1994; 25:1405–1410.

20. Ross MA, Biller J, Adams HP Jr., et al. Magnetic resonance imaging in Wallenberg's lateral medullary syndrome. *Stroke* 1986; 17:542–545.

21. Carmichael EA, Dix MR, Hallpike CS. Observations upon the neurological mechanism of directional preponderance of caloric nystagmus resulting from vascular lesions of the brainstem. *Brain: a journal of neurology.* 1965; 88:51–74.

22. Norrving B, Cronqvist S. Lateral medullary infarction: prognosis in an unselected series. *Neurology* 1991; 41:244–248.

23. Nightoghossian N, Ryvlin P, Trouillas P, et al. Pontine versus capsular pure motor hemiparesis. *Neurology* 1993; 43:2197–2201.

24. Kunz S, Griese H, Busse O. Etiology and long-term prognosis of unilateral paramedian pontine infarction with progressive symptoms. *Eur Neurol* 2003; 50:136–140.

25. Bogousslavsky J, Maeder P, Regli F, et al. Pure midbrain infarction: clinical syndromes, MRI and etiologic patterns. *Neurology* 1994; 44:2032–2040.

26. Holmes G. The symptoms of acute cerebellar injuries. *Brain* 1917; 40:461–535.

27. Carpenter MB, Strominger NL. Cerebello-oculomotor fibers in the rhesus monkey. *J Comp Neurol* 1964; 123:211–229.

28. Carpenter MB. Lesions of the fastigal nuclei in the rhesus monkey. *Am J Anat* 1959; 104:1–34.

29. Baloh RW, Konrad HR, Honrubia V. Vestibulo-ocular function in patients with cerebellar atrophy. *Neurology* 1975; 25:160–168.

30. Hood JD, Kayan A, Leech J. Rebound nystagmus. *Brain* 1973; 96:507–526.

31. Dix MR, Hallpike CS. Observations on the clinical features and neurological mechanism of spontaneous nystagmus resulting from unilateral acoustic neurofibromata. *Acta Oto-Larygn* 1966; 61:1–22.

32. Cawthorne TE. Congenital cholesteatoma. *Arch Otolaryn* 1963; 78:248–252.

33. Hallpike CS, Spencer Harrison M. Clinical and pathological observations on a case of leukemia with deafness and vertigo. *J Laryng* 1950; 64:427–430.

34. Bailey P, Buchanan DN, Bucy P. *Intracranial tumors in infancy and childhood.* Chicago: University Chicago Press, 1939.

35. Walker AE, Hopple TL. *Brain tumors in children. J Pediat* 1949; 35:671.

36. Barnett HJ, Hyland HH. Tumours involving the brain-stem. A study of 90 cases arising in the brain-stem, fourth ventricle, and pineal tissue. *Quart J Med* 1952; 83:265–284.

37. Smith WA, Fincher EF. Intracranial tumors in children. *South M J* 1942; 35:547.

38. Keith HM, Craig WM, Kernohan JW. Brain tumors in children. *Pediatrics* 1949; 3:839–843.

39. Bray PF, Carter S, Taveras JM. Brainstem tumors in children. *Neurology* 8:1–7.

40. Barnett HJ, Hyland HH. Tumours involving the brain-stem. A study of 90 cases arising in the brain-stem, fourth ventricle, and pineal tissue. *Quart J Med* 1952; 83:265–284.

41. Bucy P. Round table discussion of tumors in children. *J Pediat* 1947; 30:716738.

42. Smith WA, Fincher EF. Intracranial tumors in children. *South M J* 1942; 35:547.

43. Cawthorne T, Hinchcliffe R. Positional nystagmus of the central type as evidence of subtentorial metastases. *Brain* 1961; 84:415–426.

44. Carmichael EA, Dix MR, Hallpike CS. Lesions of the cerebral hemispheres and their effects upon optokinetic and caloric nystagmus. *Brain* 77:345–372.

45. Wadia NH, Swami RK. A new form of heredo-familial spino-cerebellar degeneration with slow eye movements (nine families). *Brain* 1971; 94:359–374.

46. Spoendlin H. Optic and cochleovestibular degenerations in hereditary ataxias. *Brain* 1974; 97:41–48.

47. Thrush DC, Foster JB. An analysis of nystagmus in 100 consecutive patients with communicating syringomyelia. *J Neurol Sci* 1973; 20:381–386.

48. Saez RJ, Burton MO, Tanagihara T. Experience with Arnold-Chiari malformation, 1960 to 1970. *J Neurosurg* 1976; 45:416–422.

49. Cogan DG, Barrows LJ. Platybasia and the Arnold Chiari malformation. *Arch Ophthal* 1954; 52:13–29.

50. Spillane JD, Pallis C, Jones AM. Developmental abnormalities in the region of the foramen magnum. *Brain* 1957; 80:11–48.

51. Biemond A, De Jong JMBV. On cervical nystagmus and related disorders. *Brain* 1969; 92:437–458.

52. Biemond A, De Jong JMBV. On cervical nystagmus and related disorders. *Brain* 1969; 92:437–458.

53. Dam M, Johnsen NJ, Thomsen J, et al. Vestibular aberrations in multiple sclerosis. *Acta Neurol Scandinav* 1975; 52:407–416.

54. Solingen LD, Baloh RW, Myers L, et al. Subclinical eye movement disorders in patients with multiple sclerosis. *Neurology* 1977; 27:614–619.

55. Aanta E, Riekkinen PJ, Frey HJ. Electronystagmographic findings in multiple sclerosis. *Acta Otolaryngol* 1973; 75:1–5.

56. Dam M, Johnsen NJ, Thomsen J, et al. Vestibular aberrations in multiple sclerosis. *Acta Neurol Scand* 1975; 52:407–416.

57. Cogan DG. Internuclear ophthalmoplegia, typical and typical. *Arch Ophthal* 1970; 84:583–589.

58. Adams RD, Denny-Brown D, Fitzgerald PJ. Pathological features of herpes zoster: note on geniculate herpes. *Arch Neurol Psychiatry* 1944; 51:216–231.

59. Cooper A. Harada's disease and Vogt-Koyanagi syndrome: uveo-encephalitis. *Arch Ophthal* 1951; 45:367–376.

60. Oliner L, Taubenhaus M, Shapira TM, et al. Non-syphilitic interstitial keratitis and bilateral deafness (Cogan's syndrome) associated with essential polyangiitis (polyarteritis nodosa): review of syndrome with consideration of possible pathogenic mechanism. *N Engl J Med* 1953; 248:1001–1008.

61. Taylor F. *The practice of medicine.* London, J & A Churchill. 1890, 262.

62. Symonds CP. Otitic hydrocephalus: a report of three cases. *Brit Med J* 1932; 1:53–54.

63. Bickerstaff ER. Basilar artery migraine. *Lancet* 1961; 1:15–17.

64. Eviatar L. Vestibular testing in basilar artery migraine. *Ann Neurol* 1981; 9:126–130.

65. World Health Organization (WHO), *International Statistical Classification of Diseases and Related Health Problems*, 10th ed. World Health Organization: Geneva, Switzerland; 1992.

66. American Psychiatric Association Diagnostic Statistical Manual of Mental Disorders (DSM-IV-TR). 4th ed, text review. Washington DC, 2000.

67. Mild Traumatic Brain Injury Committee, ACORM, Head Injury Interdisciplinary Special Interest Group. Definition of mild traumatic brain injury. *J Head Trauma Rehab* 1993; 8:86–87.

68. Carroll L, Cassidy J, Holm L, et al. Methodological issues and research recommendations for mild traumatic brain injury: The WHO Collaborating Centre Task Force of Mild Traumatic Brain Injury. *J Rehab Med* 2004; 43:113–125.

69. Ruff RM. Mild traumatic brain injury and neural recovery: rethinking the debate. *NeuroRehabilitation* 2011; 28:167–180.

70. Spaulding WB. The psychosomatic approach in the practice of medicine. *International J Psychiatry in Medicine* 1975; 6:169–181.

71. Horowitz MJ, Kaltreider N, Alvarez W. Signs and symptoms of posttraumatic stress disorder. *Arch Gen Psychiatry* 1980; 37:85–92.

72. Holmes TH, Rahe RH. The social readjustment rating scale. *J Psychosomatic Research* 1967; 11:213–218.

73. Hallpike CS, Harrison MS, Slater E. Abnormalities of the caloric test results in certain varieties of mental disorder. *Acta Otol Laryngol* 1951; 39:151–159.

74. Drachman DA, Hart CW. An approach to the dizzy patient. *Neurology* 1972; 22:323–334.

75. Mechanic D. Social psychological factors affecting the presentation of bodily complaints. *N Engl J Med* 1972; 286:1132–1139.

76. Brandt T. Management of vestibular disorders. *J Neurol* 2000; 247:491–499.

77. Fucci MJ, Sataloff RT, Myers DL. Vestibular nerve section. *Am J Otolaryngol* 1994; 15:18–189.

78. Fucci MJ, Sataloff RT, Myers DL. Vestibular nerve section. *Am J Otolaryngol* 1994; 15:18–189.

79. Yardley L, Beech S, Zander L, et al. A randomized controlled trial of exercise therapy for dizziness and vertigo in primary care. *Brit J Gen Pract* 1998; 48:1136–1140.

80. Krebs DE, Gill-Body KM, Parker SW, et al. Vestibular rehabilitation: useful but not universally so. *Otolaryngol Head neck Surg* 2003; 128:240–250.

CHAPTER 13

Laryngeal Motor Disorders

David S. Younger

The cardinal functions of the larynx include phonation and breathing, as well as airway protection. Laryngeal paralysis results when some or all of the intrinsic laryngeal muscles fail to contract, causing decreased or absent motion and abnormal positions of the vocal cords. Weakness of laryngeal muscles and paralysis of the vocal cords is encountered in myopathic, neuromuscular junction, peripheral nerve disorders, motor neuron diseases, and stroke. Laryngeal nerve injury results from nerve compression, trauma, tumor metastasis, local tumor extension, and connective tissue disorders. Bulbar amyotrophic lateral sclerosis (ALS), poliomyelitis and postpolio syndrome, syringomyelia, and brainstem encephalitis all result in laryngeal dysfunction. The chapter is an introduction to the etiopathogenesis and clinical syndromes associated with central nervous system (CNS) and peripheral nervous system (PNS) disorders of the larynx. Aspects of this topic were recently reviewed (1).

LARYNGEAL ANATOMY

The laryngeal cartilages and vocal ligaments are shown in Figures 1A and B. The vocal ligature consists of elastic tissue attached anteriorly to thyroid cartilage and posteriorly to the vocal process of the arytenoid cartilage. It is surrounded by mucous membranes, which along with the vocalis muscle, forms the vocal fold. Laryngeal sound waves are produced by oscillations of the vocal folds initiated by puffs of air. The conus elasticus is a membrane consisting principally of yellow elastic fibers that interconnect the thyroid, cricoid, and arytenoid cartilages. It underlies the mucous membrane below the vocal folds and is overlaid to some extent by the cricothyroid muscle on the exterior of the larynx.

The larynbeal musculature is shown in Figures 2 A and B. The cricothyroid muscle consists of straight and oblique heads, with the former more vertical and inserting into the lower border of the lamina of the thyroid cartilage, while the oblique head is more horizontal and inserting onto the inferior horn of the thyroid cartilage. The cricothyroid muscle tilts the anterior part of the cricoid cartilage superiorly, and in doing so, the arytenoi cartilages, which are attached to the cricod, are pulled dorsally. In addition, the thyroid cartilage is pulled forward and downward. These actions increase the distance between the arytenoid and the thyroid cartilages, thereby increasing the tension of and elongating the vocal folds. The arytenoid muscle consists of a transverse portion which spans the zone between the two arytenoid cartilages horizontally, and an oblique portion that consists of two muscular fascicles that cross one another. Each of the two fascicles of the oblique portion extend from the base of one arytenoid cartilage to the apex of the other cartilage. The oblique arytenoid fibers that continue to the epiglottis along the aryepiglotic fold constitutes the aryepiglottis muscle. Transverse arytenoid muscle approximates the arytenoid cartilage and therefore closes the posterior part of the rima glottis. The oblique arytenoid and aryepiglottic muscles close the inlet to the larynx by pulling the aryepiglottic folds together and approximating the arytenid cartilages and the epidglottis. The posterior cricoarytenoids are the only abductors of the vocal cords while the lateral cricoarytenoids acting as antagonists, adduct the vocal folds. The posterior muscle abducts by pulling the base of the arytenoid cartilages medially and posteriorly, while the lateral muscle adducts by pulling these same cartilages anteriorly and laterally. The thyroarytenoid muscles are a thin sheet radiating from the thyroid cartilage principally backward

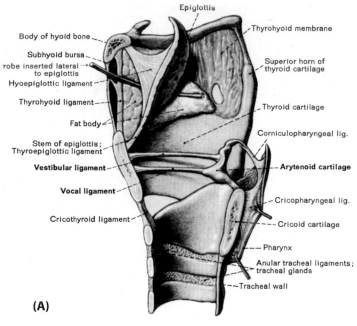

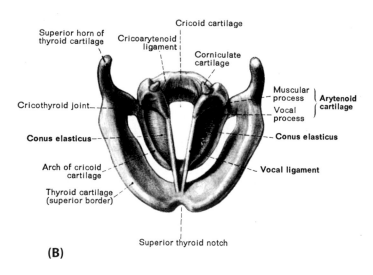

FIG. 1. Laryngeal cartilages and vocal ligaments, seen in the right half of the larynx **(A)** and from above **(B)** From reference 114, with permission.

toward the arytenoid cartilage. Its upper fibers continue to the epiglottis and, joining the aryepiglottic fibers, become the thyroepiglottic muscle. The thyroarytenoid muscles draw the arytenoid cartilages toward the thyroid cartilage and thus shorten, or relax, the vocal folds.

The positions of the rima glottides during various vocal maneuvers are shown in Figures 3 A–D, respectively, during forced inspiration, normal respiration, whispering, and phonation. During forced inspiration, the muscular processes of the arytenoid cartilages are fully abducted while the vocal processes of the cartilages are laterally rotated and retracted by the posterior cricoarytenoids, wheras during phonation and the emission of shrill tones, the vocal folds are approximated and the vocal ligaments tensed, resulting in a narrowing of the rima glottidis to a thin slit.

Motor innervation of the intrinsic laryngeal muscles originates in the nucleus ambiguus of the brainstem and in corresponding visceral efferent fibers of the vagus nerve, the principal branches of which include the superior and inferior laryngeal, or recurrent nerve. The course of the trunk of the vagus nerve in the neck and anterior mediastinum makes it particularly susceptible to surgical and traumatic injury, as well as compression by mass lesions. The nerve descends in the sheath common to the internal carotid artery and internal jugular vein in the neck. The left nerve is displaced ventrally onto the anterior surface of the esophagus. The inferior laryngeal or recurrent nerve ascends in the mediastinum on the right, posteriorly under the right subclavian artery, and, on the left, under the aortic arch. The recurrent laryngeal nerve is the principal motor nerve of the larynx and supplies all laryngeal muscles except the cricothyroid, which is supplied by the external branch of the superior laryngeal nerve. Additionally, the recurrent nerve provides sensory innervation to the mucous membrane of the larynx below the level of the vocal folds.

LARYNGEAL FUNCTION

The larynx closes during swallowing, preventing epitracheal aspiration of secretions or food. Aberrant exaggerated reflex activity, which is observed in laryngospasm, can be precipitated by endotracheal intubation, presence of a foreign body, or manipulation of the larynx during surgery. During normal breathing, the glottic opening widens by active abduction of the vocal cords during inspiration. Cough and clearing of the airway is produced by tight glottic closure, increasing subglottic pressure, sudden glottic release, and a burst of airflow clearing the airway. Speech results from the combined action of the larynx, tongue, and palate. Sound is generated by isotonic tension and vibration of the vocal cords. The shape and positioning of the

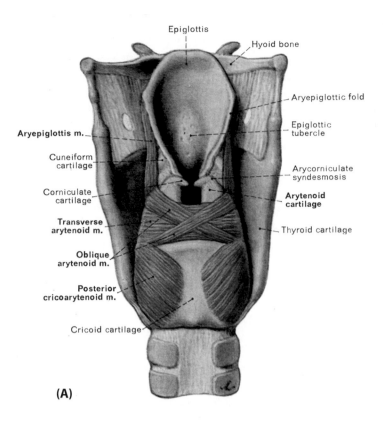

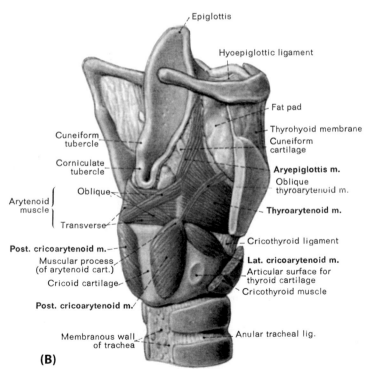

FIG. 2. Laryngeal musculature viewed from the ventrolateral **(A)** and dorsal **(B)** angles. From reference 114, with permission.

vocal cords during normal speech result from the combined action of the cricothyroid and thyroarytenoid muscles, which are involved in fine tuning of the voice, thereby affecting pitch and volume.

NEUROLOGICAL EXAMINATION

Clues to the cause of laryngeal weakness can be ascertained by a careful history that should include recent neck or mediastinal surgery, local trauma, tracheostomy, recent stroke, or transient ischemic attack. The neurological examination includes assessment of language, cranial nerve function, muscle strength, cerebellar function, sensation, and tendon reflexes.

Direct examination of the larynx should assure normal sensation and reflex responses. In particular, the clinician should observe the pattern of breathing, the quality and character of phonation, and the active swallowing of liquids and solids. Examination of the neck is necessary for detection of adenopathy, thyroid masses, and assessment of the mobility of the laryngeal framework. Sudden interruption of the sensory supply to the larynx may cause difficulty with swallowing and aspiration. This is usually due to a lesion of the internal ramus of the superior laryngeal nerve. The syndrome may result from surgical trauma, such as radical neck dissection, or operations on the supraglottic portion of the larynx. If the cricothyroid muscle is affected, or if signs implicate other cranial nerves or medullary pathways, the lesion is proximal to the bifurcation of the superior laryngeal nerve. When paralysis of the larynx is unilateral, symptoms are minimal and compensation is rapid. Absence of reflex response to palpation of the larynx may be an indication of sensory paralysis, but may also be seen in psychogenic disorders.

Laryngeal electromyography (EMG) and direct laryngoscopic examination are essential in the evaluation of laryngeal paralysis. Laryngeal EMG can assist in the differentiation of mechanical fixation from true weakness and paralysis. Direct laryngoscopic evaluation is essential in the identification of normal anatomy, vocal cord weakness, paralysis, and associated mass lesions such as laryngeal cancer.

DIAGNOSIS

Laryngeal or vocal cord paralysis may be classified by either the site of the lesion, whether supranuclear, bulbar, peripheral nerve, or muscular; and by the nature of the disorder, including inflammatory, neoplastic, traumatic, postsurgical, and idiopathic causes. The causative lesions of bilateral vocal cord paralysis are similar to those that cause unilateral

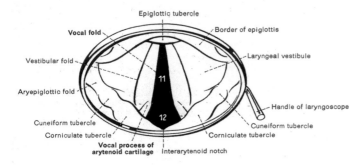

(A)

(B)

(C)

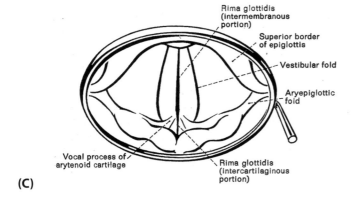

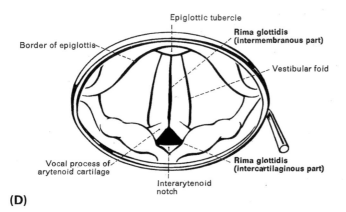

(D)

FIG. 3. The appearance of the rima glottides during forced or deep inspiration **(A)**, normal respiration **(B)**, whispering **(C)** and phonation or shrill tones **(D)**. From reference 114, with permission.

lesions. The clinical consequences of bilateral paralysis usually depend on the position of the cords; in general, the prognosis is more serious in cases of sudden onset. Bilateral paralysis after surgical injury may demand urgent relief by tracheostomy, but compression by tumor or aneurysm may cause only exertional dyspnea and stridor. In general, the nearer the cords to the midline, the greater the risk for respiratory insufficiency and more normal the voice. Conversely, the more the cords separate from the midline, the better the laryngeal airway, but the voice is weaker. Isolated paralysis of the superior laryngeal nerve is less common because it has a short course. Respiration is usually unaffected, but the voice may have a lower pitch and tire easily. Combined paralysis of the superior and recurrent laryngeal nerve may be caused by separate lesions in the respective nerves or an isolated vagal nerve lesion. Combined paralysis can also result from lesions in the upper part of the neck or in the region of the jugular foramen. In bilateral cases however, the lesion is usually in the medulla and, hence, other cranial nerves are often affected. In unilateral cases, the voice is hoarse, weak, and easily fatigued. Respiration is not affected and the glottic reflex is preserved by the bilateral sensory innervation. In bilateral cases, however, the voice is almost nonexistent, with a monotonous tone and lack of pitch change. Expectoration of secretions is difficult and stridor may be present. Aspiration is common.

Complete evaluation includes indirect laryngoscopy, neurologic examination, and complete serum blood tests for diabetes and thyroid disease. Chest radiograph and chest computed tomography (CT) and magnetic resonance imaging (MRI) should be performed in patients with left-sided paralysis to identify causative lesions before they enlarge enough to be palpable. Skull x-ray, head CT, and MRI evaluate the jugular foramen for masses and bony erosions. Endoscopy should include visualization of nasopharynx as well as passaage for air and food.

LARYNGEAL DISTURBANCES DUE TO CNS DISORDERS

Sporadic and Familial Amyotrophic Lateral Sclerosis

Motor neuron disease (MND) comprises a group of disorders characterized by progressive lower motor neuron (LMN) signs including weakness, wasting, and fasciculation, often with superimposed upper motor neuron (UMN) signs, including hyperreflexia, Hoffman, Babinski signs, and clonus, the combination of which makes the diagnosis of ALS inescapable. Paralysis of the abductor muscles of the vocal cords is noted in familial autosomal dominant (FALS-AD) and sporadic ALS (2). X-linked spinal bulbar atrophy, or Kennedy syndrome, presents with slowly progressive

LMN disease in adult men in association with gynecomastia and testicular atrophy; affected patients manifest laryngeal involvement. The molecular defect is an expansion of a CAG repeat in the first exon of the androgen receptor gene, which expands a polyglutamine tract within the receptor. One affected patient with X-linked spinal bulbar atrophy developed bilateral abductor vocal cord paralysis (3). Direct laryngoscopy showed a complete paralysis of both vocal cords in the paramedian position. It is generally agreed that vocal cord paralysis, when found in affected patients, can shorten their life expectancy. Childhood spinal muscular atrophy (SMA) presents with significant bulbar involvement and vocal cord paralysis (4–7). Children with SMA type 1 or Werdnig-Hoffmann disease, present at birth or in the first few months of life with hypotonia and lower motor neuron signs in the limbs and oropharynx, leading to death by two years of age from laryngeal paralysis, aspiration, and respiratory failure. Those with type 2 SMA achieve normal milestones up to about eight months of age, including sitting without support in spite of hypotonia, but fail to walk normally and can display variable oropharyngeal involvement. Affected children can survive into the third or fourth decade. Individuals with SMA type 3, or Wohlfart-Kugelberg-Welander syndrome, have their onset at any time after 18 months, typically in late childhood and adolescence as a proximal neurogenic muscular atrophy that may be confused with limb girdle muscular dystrophy. There may be an elevated serum creatine kinase (CK). Such patients present with a waddling gait, lumbar lordosis, genu recurvatum, and protuberant abdomen, or may appear thin like a stick man. Wirth (8) summarized the molecular genetic basis for SMA. Whereas up to 98% of causative deletions in autosomal recessive (AR) SMA are due to mutation at the 5q13.2 locus of the survival motor neuron (SMN) gene, the protein product of which is known to interact with RNA binding proteins, deletions in the neuronal apoptosis inhibitory protein (NAIP) are observed in patients affected by an acute form of SMA. Distal hereditary motor neuronopathy type VII is an AD disorder characterized by distal muscular atrophy and vocal cord paralysis, linkage of which was established to chromosome 2q14 in a large Welsh pedigree (9). The management of the oropharyngeal, laryngeal, and respiratory symptoms in the various syndromes of MND includes airway protection and voice, which may be improved with local therapy of the vocal cords, cricopharyngeal muscle myotomy, tracheostomy, feeding gastrostomy, parasympatholytic drugs, and, if necessary, laryngeal diversion, the primary disadvantage of which is the complete loss of phonation (10).

Acute poliomyelitis, now a rare cause of acute LMN paralysis in industrialized countries, is due to poliovirus infection of spinal anterior horn cells and other motor neurons. A minor illness occurs one to three days before onset of paralysis, with gastrointestinal complaints of nausea and vomiting, abdominal cramps, pain, diarrhea, and the systemic manifestations of sore throat, fever, malaise, and headache. The major illness includes all forms of CNS disease caused by the poliovirus, including aseptic meningitis or non-paralytic polio, polioencephalitis, bulbar polio, and paralytic poliomyelitis, that follows the minor illness by three to four days. Such patients can present with stiff neck, back pain, photophobia, headache, tremulousness, obtundation, agitation, myalgia, cramps, fasciculation, and radicular pain, Bulbar poliomyelitis, which occurs in 10 to 15 percent of paralytic patients, involves the seventh, ninth, and tenth cranial nerves and the medullary reticular formation, resulting in facial weakness, difficulty swallowing, and phonation, as well as variable nd respiratory difficulty, ataxic breathing, lethargy, obtundation, hypotension, hypertension, and arrhythmias. One reported patient with spinobulbar poliomyelitis had residual dysfunction of the ninth and tenth cranial nerves producing bilateral vocal cord paralysis and recurrent aspiration (11). Critical glottic stenosis developed 28 years after the initial episode of poliomyelitis, which appeared to be related to fibrosis of the intrinsic laryngeal muscles and ankylosis of the right cricoarytenoid joint. Accordingly, significant upper airway obstruction may develop as a late complication in those with stable neurological deficits and chronic immobility of the vocal cords.

Of the approximately 250,000 survivors of the polio epidemics, up to 25% experience progressive muscle weakness termed post-polio syndrome (PPS). In the order of decreasing occurrence, there may be symptoms of weakness, fatigue, arthralgia, myalgia, muscle atrophy, cold intolerance, respiratory insufficiency, and dysphagia. Nine patients with PPS were evaluated for swallowing complaints with comprehensive history, physical examination, acoustical voice analysis, and laryngeal video stroboscopic endoscopy, including three with laryngeal EMG (12) that revealed some degree of phonatory and laryngeal deficit, and in those with prominent dysphagia, vocal cord paralysis. Bilateral vocal cord paralysis was noted in one affected patient with bulbar and spinal involvement beginning at age 13, resulting in left facial, vocal cord, and hemidiaphragm paralysis that was treated by mechanical ventilation (13). Thirty-five years later, inspiratory and expiratory stridor was noted, leading to respiratory failure and tracheostomy. Laryngoscopic examination revealed bilateral vocal cord paralysis with near-midline fixation of the cords and pooling of secretions. The syndrome was attributed to progressive bulbar motor neuron weakness. Three patients with prior polio infection who presented with new complaints, including slowly progressive dyspnea, dysphagia, and hoarseness, were evaluated by video stroboscope and EMG that showed vocal cord abductor and adductor weakness, recurrent posterior glottic web in one patient, and laryngeal muscle denervation and reinnervation in two others (14). One patient benefited from tracheostomy, one from vocal cord medialization, and one from resection of interarytenoid scarring. Three additional patients with laryngeal changes in post-polio syndrome presented with dysphonia, vocal weakness, and fatigue. All three manifested abnormalities on video stroboscopic and laryngeal EMG.

Syringomyelia

Laryngeal weakness with vocal cord paralysis occurs in syringomyelia (15–17). In one patient (18) there was progressive loss of the pharyngeal reflexes with pooling of secretions in the upper esophagus and lower pharynx, requiring endotracheal intubation and feeding jejunostomy. At cervical laminectomy, the cavity was drained and repaired with improvement of pharyngeal reflexes, but there was aspiration two days after cervical laminectomy. Presumably, the syrinx extended into the brainstem to affect neurons of the nucleus ambiguus that normally control pharyngeal, laryngeal, and esophageal muscles. A 35-year-old patient who complained of noisy breathing for 15 years and had been treated for chronic asthma, developed acute breathing difficulty and was found to have stridor and bilateral abductor vocal fold palsy (19). A syrinx was found with associated type 1 Chiari malformation. Three other patients with communicating syringomyelia had acute presentations, including one with paraplegia, a second with acute respiratory distress secondary to bilateral vocal cord paralysis, and a third with symptoms of brainstem ischemia (20). Each had a communicating spinal cord syrinx associated with a posterior fossa and foramen magnum region anomaly, including a large posterior fossa arachnoid cyst in one, and Chiari malformations in the other two. Syringobulbia was found to be the cause of laryngeal stridor in an 11-year-old child who had chronic symptoms since birth, and suddenly died after development of respiratory obstruction due to vocal cord paralysis (21). Postmortem examination showed extensive bilateral syringobulbia with the greatest involvement in the nucleus ambiguous. Other brainstem tracts and nuclei were partially affected.

Arnold Chiari Complex

The classification of Chiari malformations, now termed Chiari complex (22), is based upon the relative position of the cerebellum and brainstem in relation to the foramen magnum and the upper cervical canal (23).

Types I and II are degrees of a similar abnormality in which a conical deformity of the posterior midline cerebellum and the elongated brainstem lies at or below the foramen magnum. Type 1 is divided into a classic and myelencephalalic form; symptomatic patients are treated with occipito-cervical surgical decompression. One MRI classification designated Chiari malformation in association with syringomyelia as type A, and those with evidence of frank herniation of the cerebellar tonsils below the foramen magnum alone as type B (24). Those with Chiari type II present with progressive hydrocephalus and typicallly require insertion of a cerebrospinal fluid (CSF) shunt. Chiari type III is associated with an occipito-cervical cephalocele and severe CNS malformations. Chiari type IV designates patients with myelomeningocele and severe cerebellar hypoplasia, the most common of which is probably the Dandy-Walker malformation, in which a defect in the inferior vermis is congruent with a ventricuocele of the enlarged fourth ventricle.

Affected infants and children can present symptomatic laryngeal and respiratory symptoms. The Arnold-Chiari malformation, in association with myelomeningocele, was considered the cause of progressive choking, apnea, and aspiration of 42 infants (25). Shunts were already in place and were thought to be functioning normally; however, at posterior fossa craniotomy, all had compression of the upper spinal cord. Mortality was highest (71%) in infants with rapidly progressive, irreversible symptoms. The Arnold-Chiari malformation and shunted myelomeningocele presented with adductor vocal cord paralysis and loss of laryngeal sensation for 10 months (26). Bilateral abductor vocal cord paralysis due to Arnold Chiari formation should be suspected in neonates and infants that present with high-pitched inspiratory stridor and airway compromise (27). Unilateral vocal cord paralysis suspected in an infant or child with hoarse voice, low-pitched cry, and breathy cry or voice should be evaluated with direct laryngoscopy with flexible fiberoptic nasopharyngolaryngoscope and photodocumentation using a videocassette recorder. Chiari malformation was suspected in a previously heatlthy 13-year-old boy without myelodysplasia who had mild scoliosis and complaints of nasal congestion, noisy nighttime breathing and difficulty sleeping (28). Flattening of the inspiratory loop on the flow-volume curve was found on pulmonary function testing, suggesting a variable extrathoracic obstruction due to a laryngeal lesion. Bilateral abductor vocal cord paralysis and sleep apnea developed precipitously following general anesthesia. Chiari malformations were discerned among six children by T1- and T2-weighted MRI with syndromes of failure to thrive, velopharyngeal incompetence, gastroesophageal reflux, or vagal hypertonia, leading to laryngeal obstruction due to vocal cord paralysis, paradoxical vocal cord motion, or laryngomalacia (29) and treated symptomatically before dccompressive surgery, which led to full functional recovery in five children. Linder and Lindholm (30) evaluated children born with a Chiari II malformation during their first 18 months; four of the 22 children studied by flexible fiberscopes had disturbed breathing; among those, two suffered from central apneic attacks as well as bilateral vocal fold motion impairment, one from apeneic spells only, and one from bilateral vocal fold motion impairment. All four had dysphagia with aspiration and respiratory symtpoms within the first three to six months of life. One infant with severe symptoms expired at age three months. The vocal fold paralysis, apeneic spells, and swallowing difficulties of another infant resolved following neurosurgical intervention.

Affected adults likewise present with symptomatic vocal cord paralysis due to type I Chiari malformations (31). Similarly, stridor and bilateral abductor vocal fold palsy was noted as well in a 35-year-old man with complaints of noisy breathing for 15 years, previously treated for chronic asthma (19); subsequent evaluation revealed syringomyelia with a Chiari type I malformation. Choi and coworkers (32) studied airway abnormalities in 16 patients with type I and 8 patients with type II Chiari malformation. Vocal cord impairment was noted in three patients with type II Chiari, including one each with unilateral paralysis, bilateral paresis, and paralysis, but in none of those with type I disease. Tracheostomy was necessary in three, all Chiari type II. Central sleep apnea was noted in five of six patients, and tracheostomy was needed in three patients, all with type II malformations, but in none of those with type I disease.

Stroke

Laryngeal dysfunction occurs with infarct of the brain, especially of the medulla. Venketasubramanian and colleagues (33) noted an overall frequency of 20.4% of vocal cord paresis with first-ever acute ischemic stroke among 54 patients, of whom 65 percent were lacunar, 22% cortical or subcortical, 9% lateral medullary, and 4% other brainstem infarcts. Vocal cord paresis was a constant feature of those with brainstem infarcts, but in only 11% of cortical and subcortical infarcts, and in 16% of those with lacunar infarcts. The vocal cord paresis was ipsilateral to the brainstem lesion in 80%, and contralateral to the lesion in all of those with cortical, subcortical, and lacunar infarcts.

Laryngeal hemiplegia caused by infarction of the medulla was recognized by Avellis in 1891 and named in his honor (34). Properly defined, affected patients manifest ipsilateral palatolaryngeal paresis and contralateral hemiparesis with or without hemihypoesthesia. One affected 72-year-old man with left supranuclear hypoglossal nerve palsy and right Avellis syndrome due to a medullary infarction was associated with a small lesion on brain MRI in the reticular formation medial to the nucleus ambiguous (35). Walther and Alevisopoulos (36) described a 65-year-old man with dysphagia and aspiration, associated with Horner syndrome, paralysis of the soft palate, and one vocal cord qualifying for Avellis' syndrome of palatolaryngeal hemiplegia.

Brain MRI demonstrated contrast enhancement in the dorsal upper medulla in the area of the IX and X nerve nuclei. He was clinically improved without residual neurological deficits three weeks later.

In 1985, Wallenberg (37) described a syndrome of the lateral medulla supplied by the posterior inferior cerebellar artery (PICA), which was later confirmed as postmortem examination and reported six years later (38). As summarized by Pearce (39), Wallenberg's patient presented with an attack of vertigo without loss of consciousness, and at the same time developed pain and hyperesthesia on the left side of the face and body, hypoesthesia of the right half of the face, and loss of pain and temperature sensitivity in the right limbs and right half of the torso, with retention of touch sensation. There was, in addition, paralysis of the left recurrent laryngeal nerve and paresis of the left hypoglossal muscle, with impaired swallowing, impaired sensation of the mucosa of the mouth, throat, and palate, and disturbed motility of the soft palate, which on the first day was bilateral, and later left-sided. The lateral medullary syndrome principally results from atherothrombotic short segment distal vertebral artery, long segment vertebral artery lesions sparing or involving the proximal portion of the vertebral artery with concomitant occlusion of the PICA, followed by artery dissection, isolated atherothrombotic PICA disease, moyamoya disease, and cardiogenic embolism (40, 41). Sacco and colleagues (42) collected retrospective data from a large reported series of Wallenberg's syndrome. Brain MRI abnormalities are evident in more than 90 percent of patients and varied in size. The prognosis for the majority of patients was good, with a large measure of functional independence.

It may be difficult for the examiner to recognize whether laryngeal muscle paresis or paralysis results from an UMN or LMN lesion, especially when the findings of Wallenberg syndrome are incomplete. Palmer and colleagues (43) assessed the utility of laryngeal EMG to discern the relative contribution of upper and lower motor neuron disease, including those with Wallenberg syndrome. Needle abnormalities at rest were significantly associated with lower motor neuron disease, whereas the pattern of motor unit action potential recruitment was a sensitive indicator of an upper motor neuron etiopathogenesis.

Dysphonia and soft palate dysfunction increase the accuracy of detecting aspiration after ischemic stroke in the medulla (44). Dysfunction of pharyngeal and laryngeal branches of the IX and X cranial nerve and ipsilateral vocal cord after brainstem infarct leads to swallowing difficulty and aspiration, revealed on modified barium swallow as sluggish pharyngeal peristalsis and absent swallowing reflex, treatment of which typically includes a multidisciplinary approach that includes percutaneous esophageal gastrostomy tube and intensive dysphagia rehabilitation (45).

Extrapyramidal Disorders

Abductor vocal fold palsy presents in the Shy-Drager syndrome with snoring and sleep apnea (46). Blumin and Berke (47) noted a frequency of 7% of patients with the diagnosis of multiple system atrophy (MSA) from among those with systemic neurodegenerative diseases presenting to a laryngologist for workup of dysphonia and later found to have bilateral vocal fold paresis. Isozaki and colleagues (48) found that vocal cord paralysis in hereditary cerebellar ataxia of the spinocerebellar ataxia (SCA) types 1 and 3 contrasted with that of MSA, with a more frequent occurrence of MSA than SCA 1 or 3, of 82% versus 29% and 16% respectively. All of the intrinsic laryngeal muscles, including the cricothyroid, interarytenoid, and posterior cricoarytenoid muscles, showed neurogenic atrophy in an autopsied patient with SCA1 and in four with SCA3.

LARYNGEAL DISTURBANCES DUE TO PNS DISORDERS

Lesions At or Proximal to the Nodose Ganglion

In general, lesions at or proximal to the nodose ganglion lead to involvement of the ipsilateral one-half of the larynx, with often involvement of other cranial nerves, whereas more distal lesions lead to selective neuropathic and muscular branch involvement. Disorders of the posterior cranial fossa, including meningioma, meningitis, or trauma, may affect several cranial nerves, including the vagus nerve. If the lesion is near the jugular foramen, the ninth, tenth, and eleventh nerves are affected. The twelfth nerve is not involved because it lies above the hypoglossal canal. Symptoms and signs include dysphagia, dysphonia, nasal regurgitation, torticollis, and an inability to raise the ipsilateral arm above shoulder level. This syndrome is most often caused by lymphadenopathy of the jugular foramen; other causes include thrombophlebitis and basilar skull fractures. Tapia syndrome includes ipsilateral paralysis of the tongue and vocal cord. The soft palate and cricothyroid muscles may be involved. The usual cause is a neoplasm in the lateral pharyngeal space where the hypoglossal nerve crosses the vagus nerve and internal carotid artery. General clues to the presence of laryngeal paralysis, in association with paralysis of the ninth to twelfth cranial nerves, is always an indication for careful investigation of the upper neck, base of the skull, and posterior pharyngeal fossa, as well as examination of the middle ear and nasopharynx with CT and MRI. Jugular bulb diverticula and tumors can be associated with lower cranial nerve palsies, including layrngeal dysfunction.

Hereditary Neuropathy

An inherited basis for laryngeal dysfunction should be considered when the family pedigree reveals a possible genetic basis for concomitant PNS disorders. Barbieri and colleagues (49) studied two brothers with AR late-onset cerebellar ataxia and severe dysphonia. Brain MRI showed vermian and hemipheric cerebellar atrophoy. Laryngofiberoscopy revealed laryngeal abductor paralysis. Neurophysiological studies showed a pure motor neuropathy. Laryngeal EMG is essential in the clinical categorization of the diverse forms of hereditary demyelinating and axonal neuropathy of the Charcot-Marie-Tooth (CMT) type before molecular genetic analysis for the causative gene mutation (50). Acute vocal cord paralysis was reported in hereditary neuropathy with liability to pressure palsies (51), a subtype of CMT disease, due to a mutation at the 17p chromosome. One reported family with CMT2C manifested autosomal dominant (AD) vocal cord paralysis during the first two decades of life due to recurrent laryngeal nerve palsy, in association with symptomatic chronic axonal polyneuropathy, abducens nerve palsy, and diaphragm weakness, and distinguished from types IIA in which axonal polyneuropathy was restricted to the limbs, and IIB, which is of early onset and associated with foot ulceration. Bilateral adductor vocal cord paralysis presenting with features of laryngeal incompetence is a rare form of congenital bilateral vocal cord paralysis, as an isolated disturbance or associated with Robinow syndrome and 22q chromosome deletion (52). Bilateral vocal cord paralysis was the presenting feature of a 9-year-old girl with Williams syndrome, a disorder manifested by growth deficiency, learning impairment, and typical facies, (53). Azevedo and colleagues (54) noted the occurrence of dysphonia, laryngeal paralysis, dysphagia among a review of 21 patients with Portuguese hereditary amyloid neuropathy.

Autoimmune Disorders

Laryngeal paresis may be the presenting feature of diverse acute and chronic autoimmune neuropathies, including acute inflammatory demyelinating polyradiculoneuritis, or Guillain Barré syndrome (GBS) (55), and chronic motor axonal neuropathy (56), with associated dyspnea, dysphonia, respiratory failure, and bilateral vocal cord paralysis responsive to immunomodulating therapy with intravenous gammaglobulin (IVIg) and plasma exchange (PE). One patient with idiopathic brachial plexopathy (57) presented with laryngeal paresis.

Systemic Illness

A systemic cause of presenting laryngeal dysfunction should be sought in patients with persistent constitutional complaints, as well as in chronic illness, debilitation, or a preexistent systemic condition. Dysphonia was the first clinical manifestation of a patient with granulomatous vasculitis of the Churg-Strauss syndrome (CSS), subsequently found to have paresis of the right vocal fold and reduction in adduction, together with incomplete glottic closure on video-laryngostroboscopy (58). Other patients with systemic necrotizing arteritis of the polyarteritis nodosa (PAN) type have been described (59). Laryngeal paralysis of the cricoarytenoid joint due to gouty arthritis with associated denervation atrophy of the posterior cricoarytenoid and arytenoideus msucles was reported by Gacek and colleagues (60).

Other causes of bilatarel vocal cord paralysis include diabetes mellitus (61), B12 deficiency (62), sarcoidosis (63), porphyria (64), mediastinal light chain (AL) amyloidosis (65), complete lung collapse and consolidation in cystic fibrosis (66), relapsing polychondritis (67), and lupus (68).

Infection

Bacteria infections can lead to life-threatening paraglottic laryngeal abscess, laryngeal dysfunction, and vocal cord paralysis (69). An infectious basis for bilateral vocal cord paralysis was noted in a patient with multifocal neuropathy and tick-borne relapsing fever (70), and others with recurrent laryngeal nerve paralysis associated with subclinical Lyme neuroborreliosis (LNB) (71) and clinically active LNB (72) prompting parenteral antibiotics, the latter of whom (72) evidenced intrathecal production of specific antibodies. Recurrent laryngeal nerve palsy was noted in association with intrathoracic mycobacteria (73), as was unilateral vocal cord paralysis homolateral to laryngeal mucosal varicella zoster virus (VZV) lesions localized to the larynx, covering the vestibule, arytenoid, false cord, and true vocal cord, but not extending to the hypopharynx or oropharynx (74). Other patients had bilateral vocal cord paralysis in association with herpes simplex virus (HSV) (75) and retroviral infection (76).

Cancer

A patient with known systemic cancer who develops hoarseness may be harboring compression of the recurrent laryngeal nerve by hilar adenopathy, direct tumor spread, a history of neurotoxic chemotherapy or mediastinal radiation, or infection. Immunosuppressed patients are at high risk for pharyngeal infection, especially of the lateral retropharyngeal space, as was the case of one patient with unilateral vocal cord paralysis associated with lymphoma and *Nocaridia farcinica* laryngeal abscess (77). Bronchogenic carcinoma with mediastinal metastases is a frequent cause of left recurrent nerve paralysis and

an indication of unresectability. Post-operative recurrent laryngeal nerve paralysis followed trans-hiatal resection for esophageal carcinoma (78). One patient with laryngeal mycosis fungoides, reported by Kuhn and colleagues (79), presented with vocal cord paresis progressing to paralysis. Another patient with prostatic carcinoma and metastasis to the larynx presented with vocal cord paralysis(80). Non-malignant thyroid swelling can cause recurrent laryngeal nerve paralysis. The neurologic complications of carcinoid tumor also include recurrent laryngeal nerve paralysis. Vocal cord paralysis occurred in 12 of 150 or 8% of breast cancer patients treated with postoperative therapy after radical mastectomy (81). Eleven of the 12 vocal cord paralyses were left-sided, and symptoms did not appear until two to 25 years after irradiation. Both mediastinal fibrosis and late radiation injury were proposed as explanations for the observed vocal cord paralysis. Vincristine-induced bilateral recurrent laryngeal nerve paralysis is a rare, but potentially life-threatening, complication and should be suspected when stridor is present. Vocal cord paralysis was the cause of stridor and dysphagia in a five-month-old infant with acute lymphoblastic leukemia after administration of four weekly doses of vincristine during induction therapy (82). Superior mediastinal syndrome due to a large unresectable cervico-mediastinal neuroblastoma had Horner syndrome, phrenic nerve palsy, and ipsilateral recurrent laryngeal nerve palsy (83). The child required prolonged mechanical ventilation but responded to chemotherapy and was free of tumor and completely recovered.

Cardiovascular Disease

Pediatric patients with congenital cardiac disease are predisposed to laryngeal anomalies owing to frequent intubation, prolonged ventilatory support, and recurrent laryngeal nerve injury leading to true vocal cord paralysis after repair surgery of the aortic arch (84). Non-surgical vocal cord paralysis occurs in association with thoracic aortic aneurysm, as did an equal number who underwent artificial vessel replacement (85). Pulmonary arterial stenting with occlusion of the arterial duct led to entrapment of the left recurrent laryngeal nerve between the coil used to close the arterial duct and the stent placed in the left pulmonary artery (86). Aortic aneurysm and atherosclerotic plaque are a rare cause of left vocal cord paralysis (87). Syphilitic aortic aneurysm, left auricular hypertrophy, atrial dilatation due to mitral stenosis, and cardiomegaly are all associated with lesions of the recurrent nerve. A 40-year-old man developed right vocal cord paralysis in association with dissection of the extracranial internal carotid artery with paresis of the right side of the soft palate (88).

Intoxications

Vocal cord paralysis can follow inadvertent injections and indirect exposure to medications and environmental toxins. Peritonsillar bupivicaine was administered preoperatively for an otherwise uneventful tonsillectomy to a five-year-old girl (89). She developed stridor and respirator distress following extubation and bilateral vocal cord paralysis was seen on laryngoscopy. One patient who underwent I^{131} therapy for a solitary toxic thyroid nodule experienced vocal cord paralysis, and was examined because of hoarseness one week after treatment; indirect laryngoscopy at the time confirmed right vocal cord paralysis (90). A 76-year-old man developed vocal cord paralysis due to lymph node involvement by silicosis identified by video-mediastinoscopy, which revealed granulomatous and fibrous recurrent lymph nodes encasing the left recurrent laryngeal nerve; the nerve was dissected and released from scar tissue, and followed by total recovery of his voice 15 weeks later (91). Organophosphate poisoning that lead to laryngeal paralysis was reported in a patient, leading to a difficult extubation due to bilateral vocal fold palsy that slowly recovered over time (92). Although collagen injections of the vocal fold rarely result in complications, Anderson and Sataloff (93) reported two patients in whom injected collagen formed firm submucosal deposits that interrupted the normal mucosal wave and produced significant dysphonia. Other complications included local abscess formation at the injection sites, hypersensitivity reactions, and induction of collagen vascular disease.

Trauma

Unilateral recurrent laryngeal neuropraxia followed placement of a laryngeal mask airway (94). Laryngeal examination revealed unilateral vocal cord paralysis. Recurrent bronchial cysts led to recurrent laryngeal nerve palsy in another patient (95). Of 521 patients undergoing total lobectomy and thyroidectomies, 37 or 7 experienced recurrent laryngeal nerve palsies, of whom 35 experienced complete recovery (96).

Operations for thyroid cancer, Graves' disease, and recurrent goiter demonstrated significantly higher recurrent laryngeal nerve palsy. Invasion of the recurrent laryngeal nerve was identified in 19% of patients with thyroid cancer. Total lobectomy with routine recurrent laryngeal nerve identification was recommended as a basic procedure in thyroid operations. Bilateral vocal cord paralysis was reported in a patient admitted with exacerbation of achalasia who developed acute respiratory distress from bilateral immobile vocal cords in whom imaging studies revealed impressive dilation of the cervical esophagus causing compression of both recurrent laryngeal nerves (97).

Recurrent laryngeal nerve injury was reported in association with central venous catheterization in a 29-year-old woman with aplastic anemia admitted for bone marrow transplantation (98); two other reported patients developed right vocal fold paralysis following right venous catheterization (99).

Tracheal tear, which requires fast and proper treatment, was reported in a 55-year-old man who struck his neck causing blunt trauma with cervical bruising, neck emphysema, and dyspnea (100). An end-to-end anastomosis of the trachea, as well as tracheostomy, was performed, and because of fracture of the larynx, an end laryngeal stent was employed to stabilize the lumen. Due to injury to both laryngeal nerves, the patient suffered dysphagia, whispered speech, and dyspnea on minimal exertion as long-term sequela. Tracheal diverticulum may similarly present with recurrent laryngeal nerve paralysis (101). Delayed onset of vocal cord paralysis occurred two weeks after exploration of a left vagus nerve stimulator in a child with intractable complex partial and generalized seizures (102). Unilateral vocal cord paralysis similarly developed after nasogastric tube insertion (103).

Any process involving either the vagus nerve, its recurrent laryngeal branch, or the external branch of the superior laryngeal nerve may cause paralysis of the vocal fold. One reported patient with degenerative disease of the cervical spine resulting in compression of the recurrent laryngeal nerve led to unilateral vocal cord paralysis (104). At least 80% of vocal fold paralyses occur after acute cervical diskectomy and fusion, and recover within 12 months of the procedure (105).

Vocal cord paralysis secondary to impacted esophageal foreign bodies was reported in two young children with respiratory symptoms, one of whom developed aphonia, and the other with stridor (106). Among 35 patients with blunt trauma injury from a motor vehicle accident or penetrating injury from a stab wound, 86% experienced acute external laryngeal injury leading to unilateral and bilateral vocal cord paralysis (107). Another reported patient who sustained blunt trauma to the neck sustained fracture of the thyroid cartilage and a retropharyngeal hematoma as an explanation for vocal cord paralysis (108). Self-injection injuries of the neck by intravenous drug users who lose peripheral venous access can lead to vocal cord paralysis and fragment foreign bodies (109). Pneumothorax is another proximate cause of vocal cord paralysis in patients with chronic obstructive pulmonary disease (110).

Neuromuscular Junction Disorders

Myasthenia gravis, an acquired autoimmune disorder of the neuromuscular junction (NMJ), is characterized by fluctuating ocular or oropharyngeal weakness, often with limb weakness. Weakness improves after administration of cholinergic drugs. Abnormal neuromuscular transmission is indicated by a decremental response of evoked motor responses after repetitive 3-per-sec nerve stimulation. Circulating antibodies to the acetylcholine receptor (AChR) are detected in up to 80% of affected patients. Severe oropharyngeal and laryngeal weakness and ineffective cough predisposes patients to aspiration, and overt aspiration likewise can precipitate crisis (111), defined as the need for mechanical ventilatory support. Evaluation by injection of edrophonium, repetitive nerve stimulation, AChR antibody titers, and CT of the chest for thymoma and glandular enlargement, should be performed in all cases to confirm the diagnosis of myasthenia gravis and provide basic data for further evaluation and management.

Acute botulism and the Lambert-Easton myasthenic syndrome (LEMS) are NMJ disorders characterized instead by presynaptic neuromuscular blockade. Both present with severe weakness of cranial muscles and the heightened risk of laryngeal weakness and aspiration. In suspected cases of botulism intoxication, laboratory confirmation includes detection of toxin in serum, stool, or in the contaminated food. Patients with LEMS are statistically predisposed to occult cancer of the lung, particularly when circulating N ad P/Q antibodies to voltage gated calcium channels are present. Electrophysiologic studies for abnormal increment help to establish the diagnosis, particularly if serologic and toxicology confirmation cannot be obtained.

Myopathic Disorders

If muscles of the oropharynx and larynx are involved, there is a risk of aspiration. Polymyositis is an acquired myopathy characterized by acute or subacute weakness evolving in weeks or months. There is usually histologic evidence of muscle inflammation. Dermatomyositis is defined by a characteristic rash in addition to proximal limb weakness. In one series of patients with confirmed pathology, oropharyngeal weakness with dysphagia was severe in 13 of 21 who had clinical evidence of overt aspiration and respiratory complications (112). Nine had rapidly progressive and unremitting symptoms, lasting a few months to one year before they died of respiratory complications. Six had histologic and clinical findings of dermatomyositis, two had polymyositis with either lupus or carcinoma of the lung; only one patient had "uncomplicated" polymyositis. Advances in therapy of respiratory failure have improved prognosis for survival. So-called myopathic pharyngoparalysis and layrngoparalysis was reported in three affected patients who presented with dysphagia, phonatory difficulty, abnormal EMG, and elevated CK; all were treated with corticosteroids with favorable benefit (113).

The muscular dystrophies are characterized by inherited, progressive weakness with variable age at onset, distribution, and disability. In infantile myotonic muscular dystrophy, severe oropharyngo laryngeal weakness may complicate feeding and lead to aspiration. In adult-onset cases, there is usually evidence of myotonia with facial, oropharyngeal, and limb weakness. Severe oropharyngeal weakness occurs late in the disease. Patients with oculopharyngeal muscular dystrophy and myotonic muscular dystrophy type 1 (DM1) can present with laryngeal stridor and vocal cord paralysis prompting video stroboscope and laryngeal EMG, and appropriate measures to safeguard the tracheobronchial system and prevent aspiration.

The metabolic myopathies, defined by known biochemical defects, can present with severe generalized weakness, infantile hypotonia, and feeding and respiratory difficulties. These include acid maltase deficiency, brancher enzyme deficiency, and cytochrome c-oxidase (COX) deficiency. Episodic muscular weakness, severe enough on rare occasions to cause complete paralysis, occurs in periodic paralysis due to primary excessive fluctuations of total body potassium. It can be precipitated by exogenous factors, including diet, cold, medication, and intercurrent infection.

REFERENCES

1. Younger DS. Neuromuscular disorders of the larynx. In: Blitzer A, Brin MF, Eds. *Neurologic disorders of the larynx,* 2nd ed. Thieme 2009; 216–226.
2. Raverdy P, Richer-Bigo A. Slowly progressive motor neuron disease associated with paralysis of the abductor muscles of the vocal cords. *Rev Neurol* 1990; 146:445–447.
3. Tomiyasu K, Saito T, Nukazawa T, et al. A case of X-linked bulbospinal muscular atrophy with bilateral abductor vocal cord paralysis. *Rinsho Shinkeigaku* 1996; 36:683–686.
4. Young ID, Harper PS. Hereditary distal spinal muscular atrophy with vocal cord paralysis. *J Neurol Neurosurg Psychiatry* 1980; 43:413–418.
5. Boltshauser E, Lang W, Spillmann T, et al. Hereditary distal muscular atrophy with vocal cord paralysis and sensorineural hearing loss: a dominant form of spinal muscular atrophy? *J Med Genet* 1989; 26:105–108.
6. Lapena JF Jr., Berkowitz RG. Neuromuscular disorders presenting as congenital bilateral vocal cord paralysis. *Ann Otol Rhinol Laryngol* 2001; 110:952–955.
7. Roulet E, Deonna T. Vocal cord paralysis as a presenting sign of acute spinal muscular atrophy SMA type 1. *Arch Dis Child* 1992; 67:352.
8. Wirth B. An update of the mutation spectrum of the survival motor neuron gene (SMN1) in autosomal recessive spinal muscular atrophy (SMA). *Hum Mutat* 2000; 15:228–237.
9. McEntagart M, Norton N, Williams H, et al. Localization of the gene for distal hereditary motor neuronopathy VII

(dHMN–VII) to chromosome 2q14. *Am J Hum Genet* 2001; 68:1270–1276.

10. Carter GT, Johnson ER, Bonekat HW, et al. Laryngeal diversion in the treatment of intractable aspiration in motor neuron disease. *Arch Phys Med Rehabil* 1992; 73:680–682.

11. Nugent KM. Vocal cord paresis and glottic stenosis: a late complication of poliomyelitis. *South Med J* 1987; 80:1594–1595.

12. Driscoll BP, Gracco C, Coelho C, et al. Laryngeal function in postpolio patients. *Laryngoscope* 1995; 105:35–41.

13. Cannon S, Ritter FN. Vocal cord paralysis in postpoliomyelitis syndrome. *Laryngoscope* 1987; 97:981–983.

14. Robinson LR, Hillel AD, Waugh PF. New laryngeal muscle weakness in post-polio syndrome. *Laryngoscope* 1998; 108:732–734.

15. Willis WH, Weaver DF. Syringomyelia with bilateral vocal cord paralysis. Report of a case. *Arch Otolaryngol* 1968; 87:468–470.

16. Lopez Gaston JI, Errea JM. Syringomyelobulbia and bilateral paralysis of vocal cords. *Neurologia* 1990; 5:298–299.

17. Holinger LD, Holinger PC, Holinger PH. Etiology of bilateral abductor vocal cord paralysis: a review of 389 cases. *Ann Otol Rhinol Laryngol* 1976; 85:428–436.

18. Bleck TP, Shannon KM. Disordered swallowing due to syrinx: correction by shunting. *Neurology* 1984; 34:1497–1498.

19. Abraham-Igwe C, Ahmad I, O'Connell J, et al. Syringomyelia and bilateral vocal fold palsy. *J Laryngol Otol* 2002; 116:633–636.

20. Zager EL, Ojemann RG, Poletti CE. Acute presentations of syringomyelia. Report of three cases. *J Neurosurg* 1990; 72:133–138.

21. Alcala H, Dodson WE. Syringobulbia as a cause of laryngeal stridor in childhood. *Neurology* 1975; 25:875–878.

22. Cama A, Tortori-Donati P, Piatelli GL, et al. Chiari complex in children-neuroradiological diagnosis, neurosurgical treatment and proposal of a new classification (312 cases). *Eur J Pediatr Surg* 1995; 5:35–38.

23. Caviness VS. The Chiari malformations of the posterior fossa and their relation to hydrocephalus. *Dev Med Child Neurol* 1976; 18:103–116.

24. Amer TA, El-Shman OM. Chiari malformation type 1: a new MRI classification. *Magn Reson Imaging* 1997; 15:397–403.

25. Park TS, Hoffman HJ, Hendrick EB, et al. Experience with surgical decompression of the Arnold-Chiari malformation in young infants with myelomeningocele. *Neurosurgery* 1983; 13:147–152.

26. Birns JW. An unusual form of laryngeal paralysis associated with Arnold-Chiari malformation. *Ann Otol Rhinol Laryngol* 1984; 93:447–451.

27. Grundfast KM, Harley E. Vocal cord paralysis. *Otolaryngol Clin North Am* 1989; 22:569–597.

28. Ruff ME, Oakes WJ, Fisher SR et al. Sleep apnea and vocal cord paralysis secondary to type 1 Chiari malformation. *Pediatrics* 1987; 80:231–234.

29. Portier F, Marianowski R, Morisseau-Durand MP, et al. Respiratory obstruction as a sign of brainstem dysfunction in infants with Chiari malformations. *Int J Pediatr Otorhinolaryngol* 2001; 57:195–202.

30. Linder A, Lindholm CE. Laryngologic management of infants with Chiari II syndrome. *Int J Pediatr Otorhinolaryngol* 1997; 39:187–197.

31. Blevins NH, Deschler DG, Kingdom TT, et al. Chiari-I malformation presenting as vocal cord paralysis in the adult. *Otolaryngol Head Neck Surg* 1997; 117:S191–S194.

32. Choi SS, Tran LP, Zalzal GH. Airway abnormalities in patients with Arnold Chiari malformation. *Otolaryngol Head Neck Surg* 1999; 121:720–724.

33. Venketasubramanian N, Seshadri R, Chee N. Vocal cord paresis in acute ischemic stroke. *Cerebrovasc Dis* 1999; 9:157–162.

34. Krasnianski M, Neudecker S, Schluter A, et al. Avellis' syndrome in brainstem infarctions. *Fortschr Neurol Psychiatr* 2003; 71:650–653.

35. Nakaso K, Awaki E, Isoe K. A case of supranuclear hypoglossal nerve palsy with Avellis' syndrome due to a medullary infarction. *Rinsho Shinkeigaku* 1996; 36:692–695.

36. Walther EK, Alevisopoulos G. "Palatolaryngeal hemiplegia" in transient brain ischemia-a contribution to neurogenic dysphagia. *Laryngorhinootologie* 1992; 71:588–591.

37. Wallenberg A. Akute bulbaraffektion (Embolie der arteria cerebelli post inf sinistra). *Archives fur Psychiatry* 1895; 27:504–540.

38. Wallenberg A. Anatomischer befund in einen als acute bulbaraffection (Embolie der art. Cerebellar post. Sinister) beshriebenen falle. *Arch Psych Nervenkrankh* 1901; 34:923–959.

39. Pearce JM. Wallenberg's syndrome. *J Neurol Neurosurg Psychiatry* 2000; 68:570.

40. Kim JS, Lee HJ, Choi CG. Patterns of lateral medullary infarction: vascular lesion-magnetic resonance imaging correlation of 34 cases. *Stroke* 1998; 29:645–652.

41. Wilkins RH, Brody IA. Wallenberg's syndrome. *Arch Neurol* 1970; 22:379–382.

42. Sacco RL, Freddo L, Bello JA, et al. Wallenberg's lateral medullary syndrome: clinical-magnetic resonance imaging correlations. *Arch Neurol* 1993; 50:609–614.

43. Palmer JB, Holloway AM, Tanaka E. Detecting lower motor neuron dysfunction of the pharynx and larynx with electromyography. *Arch Phys Med Rehabil* 1991; 72:214–218.

44. Kim H, Chung CS, Lee KH, et al. Aspiration subsequent to a pure medullary infarction: lesion sites, clinical variables and outcome. *Arch Neurol* 2000; 57:478–483.

45. Saltzman LS, Rosenberg CH, Wolf RH. Brainstem infarct with pharyngeal dysmotility and paralyzed vocal cord: management with a multidisciplinary approach. *Arch Phys Med Rehabil* 1993; 74:214–216.

46. Brown LK. Abductor vocal fold palsy in the Shy-Drager syndrome presenting with snoring and sleep apnea. *J Laryngol Otol* 1997; 111:689–690.

47. Blumin JH, Berke GS. Bilateral vocal fold paresis and multiple system atrophy. *Arch Otolaryngol Head Neck Surg* 2002; 128:1404–1407.

48. Isozaki E, Naito R, Kanda T, et al. Different mechanism of vocal cord paralysis between spinocerebellar ataxia (SCA1 and SCA3) and multiple system atrophy. *J Neurol Sci* 2002; 197:37–43.

49. Barbieri F, Pellecchia MT, Esposito E, et al. Adult-onset familial laryngeal abductor paralysis, cerebellar ataxia, and pure motor neuropathy. *Neurology* 2001; 56:1412–1414.

50. Dray TG, Robinson LR, Hillel AD. Laryngeal electromyographic findings in Charcot-Marie-Tooth disease type II. *Arch Neurol* 1999; 56:863–865.

51. Ohkoshi N, Kohno Y, Hayashi A, et al. Acute vocal cord paralysis in hereditary neuropathy with liability to pressure palsies. *Neurology* 2001; 56:1415.

52. Berkowitz RG. Congenital bilateral adductor vocal cord paralysis. *Ann Otol Rhinol Laryngol* 2003; 112:764–767.

53. Stewart FJ, Dalzell M, McReid M, et al. Bilateral vocal cord paralysis in Williams syndrome. *Clin Genet* 1993; 44:164–165.

54. Azevedo EM, Scaff M, Canelas HM, et al. Type 1 primary neuropathic amyloidosis (Andrade, Portuguese). *Arq Neuropsiquiatr* 1975; 33:105–118.

55. Yoskovitch A, Enepekides DJ, Hier MP. Guillain-Barré syndrome presenting as bilateral vocal cord paralysis. *Otolaryngol Head Neck Surg* 2000; 122:269–270.

56. Marchant H, Supiot F, Choufani G, et al. Bilateral vocal fold palsy caused by chronic motor axonal neuropathy. *J Laryngol Otol* 2003; 117:414–416.

57. Hyde GP, Postma GN, Caress JB. Laryngeal paresis as a

presenting feature of idiopathic brachial plexopathy. *Otolaryngol Head Neck Surg* 2001; 124:575–576.

58. Mazzantini M, Fattori B, Matteucci F, et al. Neuro-laryngeal involvement in Churg-Strauss syndrome. *Eur Arch Otorhinolaryngol* 1998; 255:302–306.

59. Fujiki N, Nakamura H, Nonomura M, et al. Bilateral vocal fold paralysis caused by polyarteritis nodosa. *Am J Otolaryngol* 1999; 20:412–414.

60. Gacek RR, Gacek MR, Montgomery WW. Evidence for laryngeal paralysis in cricoarytenoid joint arthritis. *Laryngoscope* 1999; 109:279–283.

61. Sommer DD, Freeman JL. Bilateral vocal cord paralysis associated with diabetes mellitus: case reports. *J Otolaryngol* 1994; 23:169–171.

62. Ahn TB, Cho JW, Jeon BS. Unusual neurological presentations of vitamin B(12) deficiency. *Eur J Neurol* 2004; 11:339–341.

63. Witt RI. Sarcoidosis presenting as bilateral vocal fold paralysis. *J Voice* 2003; 17:265–268.

64. Ratnavalli E, Veerendrakumar M, Christopher R, et al. Vocal cord palsy in porphyric neuropathy. *J Assoc Physicians India* 1999; 47:344–345.

65. Conaghan P, Chung D, Vaughan R. Recurrent laryngeal nerve palsy associated with mediastinal amyloidosis. *Thorax* 2000; 55:436–437.

66. Thompson RD, Empey DW, Bailey CM. Left recurrent nerve paralysis associated with complete lung collapse with consolidation in an adult with cystic fibrosis. *Respir Med* 1996; 90:567–569.

67. Hussain SS. Relapsing polychondritis presenting with stridor from bilateral vocal cord palsy. *J Laryngol Oto* 1991; 105:961–963.

68. Hari CK, Raza SA, Clayton MI. Hydralazine-induced lupus and vocal fold paralysis. *J Laryngol Otol* 1998; 112:875–877.

69. Fernandez PA, Fernandez-Nogueras JF, Moreno LJA. Paraglottic laryngeal abscesses. *Acta Otolaryngolol Esp* 2002; 53:435–438.

70. Olchovsky D, Pines A, Sadeh M, et al. Multifocal neuropathy and vocal cord paralysis in relapsing fever. *Eur Neurol* 1982; 21:340–342.

71. Karosi T, Racz T, Szekanecz E, et al. Recurrent laryngeal nerve paralysis due to subclinical Lyme borreliosis. *J Laryngol Otol* 2010; 124:336–338.

72. Martzolff L, Bouhala M, Dukic R, et al. [Recurrent nerve palsy due to Lyme disease: report of two cases]. *Rev Med Interne* 2010; 31:229–231.

73. Yew WW, Chau CH, Lee J, et al. Hoarseness due to recurrent laryngeal nerve palsy from intrathoracic mycobacteriosis. *Int J Tuberc Lung Dis* 2001; 5:1074–1075.

74. Nishizaki K, Onoda K, Akagi H, et al. Laryngeal zoster with unilateral laryngeal paralysis. *J Otorhinolaryngol Relat Spec* 1997; 59:235–237.

75. Pou A, Carrau RL. Bilateral abductor vocal cord paralysis in association with herpes simplex infection: a case report. *Am J Otolaryngol* 1995; 16:216–219.

76. Noda K, Isozaki E, Miyamoto K, et al. HTLV-1 associated myelopathy with bilateral abductor vocal cord paralysis-case report. *Rinsho Shinkeigaku* 1992; 32:324–326.

77. Cohen E, Blickstein D, Inbar E, et al. Unilateral vocal cord paralysis as a result of a Nocardia farcinica laryngeal abscess. *Eur J Clin Microbiol Infect Dis* 2000; 19:224–227.

78. Gockel I, Kneist W, Keilmann A, et al. Recurrent laryngeal nerve paralysis (RLNP) following esophagectomy for carcinoma. *Eur J Surg Oncol* 2005; 31:277–281.

79. Kuhn JJ, Wenig BM, Clark DA. Mycosis fungoides of the larynx. Report of two cases and review of the literature. *Arch Otolaryngol Head Neck Surg* 1992; 118:853–858.

80. Park YW, Park MH. Vocal cord paralysis from prostatic carcinoma metastasizing to the larynx. *Head Neck* 1993; 15:455–458.

81. Johansson S, Lofroth PO, Denekamp J. Left sided vocal cord paralysis: a newly recognized late complication of mediastinal irradiation. *Radiother Oncol* 2001; 58:287–294.

82. Anghelescu DL, De Armendi AJ, Thompson JW, et al. Vincristine-induced vocal cord paralysis in an infant. *Paediatr Anaesth* 2002; 12:168–170.

83. Kapoor V, Lodha R, Agarwala S. Superior mediastinal syndrome with Rowland-Payne syndrome: an unusual presentation of cervico-mediastinal neuroblastoma. *Pediatr Blood Cancer* 2005; 44:280–282.

84. Khariwala SS, Lee WT, Koltai PJ. Laryngotracheal consequences of pediatric cardiac surgery. *Arch Otolaryngol Head Neck Surg* 2005; 131:336–339.

85. Ishii K, Adachi H, Tsubaki K, et al. Evaluation of recurrent nerve paralysis due to thoracic aortic aneurysm and aneurysm repair. *Laryngoscope* 2004; 114:2176–2181.

86. Assaqqat M, Siblini G, Fadley FA. Hoarseness after pulmonary arterial stenting and occlusion of the arterial duct. *Cardiol Young* 2003; 13:302–304.

87. Gupta KB, Tendon S, Yadav RK. Left vocal cord paralysis and aortic arch aneurysm: an unusual presentation. *Indian J Med Sci* 2002; 56:443–444.

88. Nusbaum AO, Som PM, Dubois P, et al. Isolated vagal nerve palsy associated with a dissection of the extracranial internal carotid artery. *AJNR Am J Neuroradiol* 1998; 19:1845–1847.

89. Weksler N, Nash M, Rozentsveig V, et al. Vocal cord paralysis as a consequence of peritonsillar infiltration with bupivicaine. *Acta Anaesthesiol Scand* 2001; 45:1042–1044.

90. Coover LR. Permanent iatrogenic vocal cord paralysis after I-131 therapy: a case report and literature review. *Clin Nucl Med* 2000; 25:508–510.

91. Lardinois D, Gugger M, Balmer MC, et al. Left recurrent laryngeal nerve palsy associated with silicosis. *Eur Respir J* 1999; 14:720–722.

92. Indudharan R, Win MN, Noor AR. Laryngeal paralysis in organophosphorous poisoning. *J Laryngol Oto* 1998; 112:81–82.

93. Anderson TD, Sataloff RT. Complications of collagen injection of the vocal fold: report of several unusual cases and review of the literature. *J Voice* 2004; 18:392–397.

94. Kawauchi Y, Nakazawa K, Ishibashi S, et al. Unilateral recurrent laryngeal nerve neuropraxia following placement of a ProSeal laryngeal mask airway in a patient with CREST syndrome. *Acta Anaesthesiol Scand* 2005; 49:576–578.

95. Rice DC, Putnam JB Jr. Recurrent bronchogenic cyst causing recurrent laryngeal nerve palsy. *Eur J Cardiothorac Surg* 2002; 21:561–563.

96. Chiang FY, Wang LF, Huang YF, et al. Recurrent laryngeal nerve palsy after thyroidectomy with routine identification of the recurrent laryngeal nerve. *Surgery* 2005; 137:342–347.

97. Chegar BE, Emko P. Bilateral vocal cord paralysis secondary to esophageal compression. *Am J Otolaryngol* 2004; 25:361–363.

98. Salman M, Potter M, Ethel M, et al. Recurrent laryngeal nerve injury: a complication of central venous catheterization-a case report. *Angiology* 2004; 55:345–346.

99. Martin-Hirsch DP, Newbegin CJ. Right vocal fold paralysis as a result of central venous catheterization. *J Laryngol Otol* 1995; 109:1107–1108.

100. Sobiegalla M, von Hintzenstern U, Weidenbecher M Jr, et al. Tracheal rupture—a rare and dramatic emergency. *Anaesthesiol Reanim* 2003; 28:79–81.

101. Caversaccio MD, Becker M, Zbaren P. Tracheal diverticulum presenting with recurrent laryngeal nerve paralysis. *Ann Otol Rhinol Laryngol* 1998; 362–364.

102. Vassilyadi M, Strawsburg RH. Delayed onset of vocal cord paralysis after explanation of a vagus nerve stimulator in a child. *Childs Nerv Syst* 2003; 19:261–263.

103. To EW, Tsang WM, Pang PC, et al. Nasogastric-tube-induced unilateral vocal cord palsy. *Anaesthesia* 2001; 56:695–696.

104. Yoskovitch A, Kantor S. Cervical osteophytes presenting as unilateral vocal fold paralysis and dysphagia. *J Laryngol Otol* 2001; 115:422–424.

105. Morpeth JF, Williams MF. Vocal fold paralysis after anterior cervical diskectomy and fusion. *Laryngoscope* 2000; 110:43–46.

106. Virgilis D, Weinberger JM, Fisher D, et al. Vocal cord paralysis secondary to impacted esophageal foreign bodies in young children. *Pediatrics* 2001; 107:E101.

107. Sittitrai P, Ponprasert V. Acute external laryngeal injury. *J Med Assoc Thai* 2000; 83:1410–1414.

108. Levine RJ, Sanders AB, LaMear WR. Bilateral vocal cord paralysis following blunt trauma to the neck. *Ann Emerg Med* 1995; 25:253–255.

109. Kay DJ, Mirza N. Diagnosis and management of complications of self-injection injuries of the neck. *Ear Nose Throat J* 1996; 75:670–676.

110. Lazaro MT, Gonzalez-Anglada MI, Uson J, et al. Vocal cord paralysis due to pneumothorax in a patient with COPD. *Chest* 1994; 105:1297–1298.

111. Cohen M, Younger DS. Aspects of the natural history of myasthenia gravis: crisis and death. *Ann NY Acad Sci* 1981; 377:670–677.

112. Walton J, Adams R. *Polymyositis.* Edinburgh, Livingstone; 1958:38–74

113. Liu Z, Gu C, Hua W. The clinical characters of myopathic pharyngoparalysis and laryngoparalysis with three case reports. *Lin Chuang Er Bi Yan Hou K Za Zhi* 1999; 13:246–247.

114. Clemente CD. *Anatomy. A regional atlas of the human body.* Lea & Febiger, Philadelphia, 1975.

CHAPTER 14

Adult and Childhood Vasculitis of the Nervous System

David S. Younger

Vasculitis results in a variety of clinical neurological manifestations and Neuropathological changes in the central and peripheral nervous system (CNS and PNS). Unrecognized and therefore untreated, vasculitis leads to ischemia and injury of the involved tissues. Remarkable progress has been achieved in the pathogenesis, diagnosis and treatment of vasculitis of the CNS, making it an important topic for clinicians and researchers alike.

CLASSIFICATION AND NOSOLOGY

Vasculitis is defined as inflammation of blood vessel walls for at least some time during the course of the disease and affects arteries and veins of varying caliber. Two Chapel Hill Consensus Conferences (CHCC), one in 1994 (1), and the other in 2012 (2), provided consensus on nosology and definitions for the commonest forms of vasculitis. The revised CHCC nomenclature serves as a guide for the categorization of diverse forms of vasculitis based upon the vessels involved, and provides a scheme for the neurological aspects thereof (Table 1). Large vessel vasculitis (LVV) including giant cell arteritis (GCA) and Takayasu arteritis (TAK) affects the aorta, its major branches and analogous veins. Medium vessel vasculitis (MVV) inclusive of polyarteritis nodosa (PAN) and Kawasaki disease (KD) involves main visceral arteries and veins and initial branches. The category of small vessel vasculitis (SVV) recognizes involvement of intraparenchymal arteries, arterioles, capillaries, veins and venules, with a disease mechanism related to anti-neutrophil cytoplasmic antibody (ANCA) and immune complexes. The category of ANCA-associated vasculitis (AAV) includes granulomatosis with polyangiitis

(GPA) (Wegener granulomatosis [WG] type), eosinophilic granulomatosis with polyangiitis (EGPA) [Churg-Strauss syndrome [CSS]), and microscopic polyangiitis (MPA) (microscopic polyarteritis), while vasculitic disorders associated with immune complexes includes IgA vasculitis (IgAV) (Henoch-Schönlein purpura [HSP]), cryoglobulinemic vasculitis (CV), and hypocomplementemia urticarial vasculitis (HUV) associated with C1q antibodies. Vasculitis without a predominant vessel size and caliber, respectively from small to large, involving arteries, veins and capillaries, comprises the category of variable vessel vasculitis (VVV), characteristic of Behçet disease (BD) and Cogan syndrome (CS). The category of vasculitis associated with systemic disease includes vasculitis associated with rheumatoid arthritis (RA) and systemic lupus erythematosus (SLE) and other connective tissue disorders, wherein the vasculitic process is secondary to or associated with the underlying systemic disorder. There is a category of vasculitis associated with a probable specific etiology, such as substance abuse and infection designated by the specific vasculitic disorder with a prefix to denote the causative agent. The category of single-organ vasculitis (SOV) involves arteries or veins of any size in a single organ without features to indicate that it is a limited expression of a systemic vasculitis characterized by primary CNS vasculitis, nonsystemic peripheral nerve vasculitis (PNV), and isolated aortitis.

Recognizing that certain forms of vasculitis are more common in childhood and that some vasculitides display different disease courses compared to adult forms (3), the Pediatric Rheumatology European Society (PRES) and the European League against Rheumatism (EULAR) proposed specific classification criteria for the commonest childhood vasculitis syndrome (4) based upon vessel size, similar to

Table 1.
Childhood and Adult Vasculitides
with Nervous System Involvement

Large Vessel Vasculitis
  Giant cell arteritis
  Takayasu arteritis
  Idiopathic aortitis (IgG4)

Medium Vessel Vasculitis
  Polyarteritis nodosa
  Kawasaki disease

Small Vessel Vasculitis
  ANCA-Associated Vasculitis
    Microscopic polyangiitis
    Granulomatosis with polyangiitis (Wegener)
    Eosinophilic granulomatosis with polyangiitis
    (Churg-Strauss)

Immune-Complex Vasculitis
  Cryoglobulinemic vasculitis
  IgA vasculitis (Henoch-Schönlein)
  Hypocomplementemic urticarial vasculitis (C1q
  Vasculitis)

Variable Vessel Vasculitis
  Behçet Disease
  Cogan Syndrome

Primary CNS Vasculitis

Vasculitis Associated with Collagen Vascular Disease
  Systemic Lupus Erythematosus
  Rheumatoid Arthritis

Vasculitis Due to Substance Abuse
  Amphetamines
  Cocaine
  Opioids

Vasculitis and Infection
  Bacteria
  Viruses
  Neurosyphilis
  Mycoses
  Parasites
  HIV/AIDS

the CHCC nomenclature (2). In 2008, the EULAR, PRES, and the Pediatric Rheumatology International Trials Organization (PRINTO) reported their methodology and overall clinical, laboratory and radiographic characteristics for several childhood systemic vasculitides (5) followed by a final validated classification (6).

HISTORICAL OVERVIEW

The early history of vasculitis is debatable, but one fact is clear, the earliest patients with vasculitis appeared to have had neurologic involvement. According to Lamb (6), Kussmaul and Maier provided the first complete gross and microscopic description of a patient with leg pains, cramps, and tenderness so prominent that trichinosis was considered in an article entitled, "A hitherto undescribed peculiar disease of the arteries which is accompanied by Bright's disease and a rapidly progressive general paralysis of the muscles." At postmortem examination there was widespread arteritis that resembled syphilitic periarteritis. The disorder was named periarteritis for the inflammation around blood vessels. In 1908, Langcope (7) described the first American patient with periarteritis, a 35-year-old man with constitutional symptoms and subacute leg pains. Postmortem examination showed widespread necrotizing arteritis and nodules along small and medium sized vessels of the heart, liver, kidney, pancreas, testicles, brain, nerves and skeletal muscles, sparing the lungs and spleen. The histological lesions consisted of mononuclear cell infiltration, necrosis of internal and external elastic lamina of the media, fibrin deposition, aneurismal dilatation, perivascular inflammation of the adventitia, and intimal proliferation resulting in narrowing of arterial lumina.

Kernohan and Woltman (8) summarized the clinical and neuropathologic aspects of adult PAN, and Krahulik and colleagues (9) reported the postmortem neurologic findings of fulminant childhood PAN (cPAN). The dominant neurological picture of both adult and cPAN was a peripheral neuritis that occurred in one-half of patients early in the illness with a predilection for the legs. At postmortem examination, all had arteritic lesions along nutrient arteries of the peripheral nerves, and three-quarters had lesions in arteriae nervorum. The combination of acute and chronic lesions correlated with known exacerbations. Involvement of the CNS was estimated to occur in 8% of cases evident by clinically apparent brain infarcts resulting from occlusion of cerebral vessels which was often insidious in its progression. In PAN, as in the other systemic necrotizing arteritis, the vasculitic lesion proceeded in a characteristic manner (Figure 1) commencing with invasion of the intima, media and adventitia by polymorphonuclear cells, plasma cells, eosinophils, and lymphocytes, leading to swelling of the

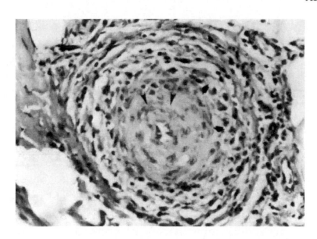

FIG. 1. This small muscular artery from muscle is from a patient with polyarteritis nodosa. In the third, or proliferative, phase illustrated here, chronic inflammatory cells replace the neutrophils of the second phase; there is evidence of necrosis of the media (arrows), early intimal proliferation (arrowheads), and fibrosis. The lumen is almost completely occluded. Ultimately, in the healing phase, this process is replaced by dense, organized connective tissue (stain, hematoxylin and eosin; original magnification, ×250).

media, and fibrinoid necrosis that clustered around the vasa vasorum, with fragmentation of the internal elastic lamina. There was focal deposition of perivascular connective tissue, vascular necrosis, and denuding of the endothelium, followed by vascular thrombosis, ischemia, aneurysm formation, rupture and hemorrhage. Healed lesions coexisted with active lesions. Harry Lee Parker conceptualized nerve and muscle biopsy in a discussion of the paper by Kernohan and Woltman (8) commenting, "It occurs to me that in any case in which polyarteritis nodosa may be suspected, it is advisable to take a biopsy from a peripheral nerve, muscle or artery." There are no published series confirming the correlation of the extent of systemic necrotizing arteritis that may be predicted by the singular finding of vasculitis in a cutaneous nerve biopsy specimen. Only one series (10) reported neither systemic nor isolated PNV was found at postmortem after diagnostic cutaneous nerve biopsy evidencing necrotizing vasculitis in life. A variant of PAN was recognized in very young children with mucocutaneous lymph node syndrome (11, 12). Although early publications used the term infantile PAN (13, 14), KD is the preferred term to describe this childhood syndrome with worldwide occurrence, affecting children of all ages and races. Both PAN and KD are prototypical examples of MVV.

Contemporaneously, SVV syndromes were recognized and differentiated from PAN. First described by Wohlwill in 1923 (15), Davson and colleagues (16) and Wainwright and Davson (17), described MPA among 34 patients that differed from PAN due to selective involvement of small microscopic arteries, arterioles, capillaries and venules including glomerular and pulmonary alveolar capillaries. Fever, arthralgia, purpura, hemoptysis, pulmonary hemorrhage, abdominal pain, and gastrointestinal bleeding likewise preceded the explosive phase of systemic necrotizing vasculitis that affected the kidney and lungs, with rapidly progressive glomerulonephritis and pulmonary capillaritis. Two of five deaths were attributed to CNS involvement by vasculitis during periods of disease respectively at four and eight months, however that could not be confirmed since postmortem examinations were not performed. The disorder was later reclassified by the CHCC (1, 2) as a necrotizing SVV with little or no immune-complex deposition that primarily affected the kidney and lungs. Medium-sized arteries might be involved even though the disease was predominantly considered to affect small-sized arteries, arterioles, capillaries and venules of the two organs most affected, with variable systemic necrotizing vasculitis.

The first patient with EGPA was probably Case 1 of Lamb (18) reported in 1914 under the heading of PAN. That patient, a 26-year-old man with two years of worsening asthma, developed fever, palpable purpura, nodular skin lesions, hemoptysis, vomiting, urinary difficulty and granular urinary casts. He died one month later and postmortem examination showed necrotizing arteritis of small arteries, with dense collections of extravascular eosinophils and tissue eosinophilia in the heart, stomach, and kidney. Decades later, Churg and Strauss (19) described the clinical and postmortem findings of thirteen patients with asthma, fever, and hypereosinophilia, accompanied by eosinophilic exudation, fibrinoid change, and granulomatous proliferation. That constituted the so-called allergic granuloma found within vessels walls and in extravascular connective tissue of major organ systems, leading to cardiac, pulmonary, gastrointestinal, skin, PNS and CNS manifestations. In 1977, Chumbley and coworkers (20) described thirty asthmatic patients from the Mayo Clinic over the period 1950 to 1974 with necrotizing vasculitis of small arteries and veins with extravascular granulomas and infiltration of vessels and perivascular tissue with eosinophilia. The lungs, peripheral nerves, and skin were most frequently involved, and renal failure was encountered in only one patient. Corticosteroids seemed to confer long-term survival. In 1984, Lanham and colleagues (21) emphasized that the combination of necrotizing vasculitis, tissue infiltration by eosinophils and extravascular granulomas suggested by Churg and Strauss (19), occurred contemporaneously in only a minority of patients. Moreover, such histological findings could be encountered as well in other granulomatous, vasculitic and eosinophilic disorders in the absence of clinical asthma, allergic rhinitis, sinusitis, pulmonary infiltrates, and cardiac involvement pathognomonic of EGPA. The authors described a phasic pattern of EGPA in which allergic disease preceded systemic vasculitis and eosinophilic tissue infiltrates that

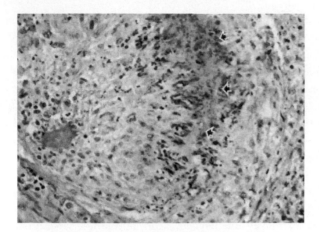

FIG. 2. Granulomatosis with polyangiitis. This small muscular artery is nearly completely destroyed. A large confluent area of fibrinoid degradation (arrows) is surrounded by neutrophils, palisading histiocytes, lymphocytes, plasma cells, and some giant cells (stain, hematoxylin and eosin; original magnification, ×250).

might occur in the absence of peripheral blood eosinophilia. Pulmonary infiltrates, upper respiratory tract and gastrointestinal disease often preceded the vasculitic component of the syndrome leading to cardiac, cutaneous, nervous system, renal, bone, and muscle involvement. In 1990, the American College of Rheumatology (ACR) (22) developed criteria for the classification of EGPA that included ascertainment of four or more of the following: asthma, eosinophilia of >10%, mononeuropathy or polyneuropathy, non-fixed pulmonary infiltrates on chest radiograph, paranasal sinus abnormality, and extravascular eosinophils on tissue biopsy that included an artery, arteriole or venule. These criteria were inadequate in differentiating the various clinicopathological expressions of SVV such that a patient with asthma and paranasal sinusitis could fit the designation of EGPA. The 1994 CHCC (1) characterized EGPA as an eosinophil-rich and granulomatous inflammatory process that involved the respiratory tract, with necrotizing vasculitis that affected small to medium-sized vessels such as capillaries, venules, arterioles and arteries, with associated asthma and eosinophilia.

In 1954, Godman and Churg (23) described the syndrome of GPA that included granuloma in the nasopharynx, sinuses and lower respiratory tract with focal segmental glomerulonephritis and disseminated small vessel vasculitis (Figure 2). Nervous system involvement in GPA was found in up to one-half of patients according to Drachman (24) who also described a patient with one month of headache that awakened him from sleep followed by rhinitis, nasal obstruction, epistaxis, mononeuropathy multiplex, confusion and hypertension. Active arteritis and necrotizing granulomata were found in the brain, not in

peripheral nerves. Two decades later, Fauci and colleagues (25) and Hoffman and colleagues (26) at the National Institutes of Health (NIH) respectively reported a prospective series of eighty-five patients with GPA, and a retrospective assessment of 180 patients followed for 6 months to 24 years, describing nervous system involvement in up to 23% of patients. There was a preponderance of mononeuritis multiplex with CNS abnormalities in 8 to 10% of patients. CNS involvement included stroke, cranial nerve abnormalities, and diabetes insipidus. Fauci and colleagues (25) established the efficacy of cyclophosphamide and prednisone in achieving complete remissions in 93% of patients as well as the tendency of patients to relapse and accrue additive mortality from both disease and treatment, however alternative immunosuppressant regimens were not equally effective (26). In a landmark article, Godman and Churg (27) concluded that MPA, EGRA and GPA were related to one another yet distinct from PAN. This astute conclusion was based mainly on pathological features was later substantiated by their common association with ANCA, but not so for PAN (28).

There ensued a renaissance in the understanding of primary systemic vasculitis with convincing clinical evidence to support an important role for ANCA in the development of AAV. Early observations of ANCA were provided by van der Woude and colleagues in 1985 (29), Falk and Jennette (30) and Goldschmeding and colleagues (31) in 1988, followed by progress in the differentiation of these subtypes and understanding of the eponymous manifestations (32). Proteinase 3 (PR3) is a serine protease found in the azurophilic granules of neutrophils and peroxidase-positive lysosomes of monocytes. Myeloperoxidase (MPO) which constitutes about 5% of the total protein content of the neutrophilic cell is localized to the same cellular compartment as PR3. However PR3 in contrast to MPO is also found on the plasma membrane of resting neutrophils and monocytes in many patients. Autoantibodies directed against PR3 and MPO are directed against multiple epitopes. Although sera from different patients may recognize different epitopes, all ANCA recognized restricted epitopes of PR3 involving its catalytic site (33). An AAV classification appears to better recognize ANCA disease and predict prognosis than any other existing clinical classification systems (34). However as with other autoimmune disorders, the etiology and pathogenesis appeared multifactorial, involving the interplay of initiating and predisposing environment and genetic factors. Important contributing factors to the mediation of vascular and extravascular inflammation included a loss of regulatory T- and B-cell function, acute neutrophilic cell injury with release of ANCA-antigens, cytokine priming of neutrophilic cells, subsequent complement activation by Fc and Fab2 engagement, and enhancement of complement dependent cytotoxicity with release of ANCA-antigens into the microenvironment (35–37). The ANCA lesion typical of GPA includes both vasculitic and granulomatous features in lung, with focal segmental glomerulonephritis typified pathologically by lysis of glomerular tufts, basement membrane disruption, accumulation of fibrinoid material, thrombosis of glomerular capillary loops, acute tubular necrosis, and scant deposition of immunoglobulin (Ig) and complement. There are genetic distinctions between MPO and GPA suggested by the strong association of PR3-ANCA disease with antigenic specificity of HLA-DP and the genes encoding α1-antitrypsin (SERPINA1) and PR3 (PRTN3), and HLA-DQ for MPO-ANCA (38). An immunofluorescence technique (IFT) has been standard method for routine determination of ANCA in vasculitis using ethanol-fixed human neutrophils as substrate. Two main immunofluorescence patterns are distinguished, a cytoplasmic (c-ANCA) and perinuclear (p-ANCA). The 1999 "International consensus statement on testing and reporting ANCA" (39) required laboratories to screen for ANCA by IFT and to confirm the specificity of fluorescent sera by enzyme-linked immunoassay (ELISA) for PR3 and MPO-ANCA. However, conventional ELISA using PR3 immobilized to the surface of the ELISA plate shows great variation in performance and often lacks sensitivity. Capture ELISA is superior in overall diagnostic performance to direct ELISA (40), but the sensitivity of capture ELISA may be reduced by the capturing antibodies hiding relevant epitopes. High sensitivity PR3 (hsPR3)-ANCA ELISA, which immobilizes PR3 via a bridging molecule to the plastic plate and preserves nearly all epitopes for the binding of ANCA, was superior to direct and capture techniques in GPA (41).

Hypersensitivity vasculitis leading to cutaneous vasculitis was conceptualized as an immunologic response to antigenic material associated with clinically evident purpura, and small vessel inflammation affecting arterioles, capillaries, and post-capillary venules. Between 1948 and 1952, Zeek (42, 43) separated the hypersensitivity vasculitides from allergic granulomatous angiitis, rheumatic arteritis, PAN, and GCA. Hemorrhage into the skin or palpable purpura was noted in virtually all patients resulting from extravasation of erythrocytes, pronounced endothelial swelling, polymorphonuclear and later mononuclear cell infiltration, followed by fibrosis, necrosis, fibrinoid deposits and visible polymorphonuclear debris termed leukocytoclasia (Figure 3). Zeek (44) likened hypersensitivity vasculitis to the anaphylactoid Arthus reaction produced by the experimental injection of horse serum into rabbits (45). Osler (46) first appreciated the relation of purpuric attacks to cerebral manifestations in the report of a patient with transient hemiparesis, and three others with potentially fatal cerebral hemorrhages. Gairdner (47) described HSP among twelve patients with anaphylactoid purpura including one child who developed rash, colic, melanotic stools, intussusception, and

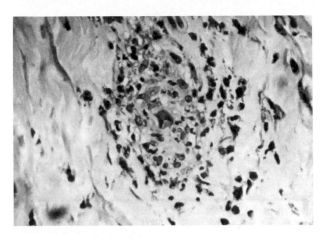

FIG. 3. This arteriole from muscle is from a patient with leukocytoclastic vasculitis. The entire vessel and perivascular tissue is infiltrated with polymorphonuclear leukocytes and some chronic inflammatory cells with necrosis and nuclear debris. The vascular lumen is nearly obliterated (stain, hematoxylin and eosin; original magnification, ×400).

hematuria followed by a typical exanthema and convulsion. She died three months later and postmortem examination showed scattered cortical hemorrhages associated with cerebral necrotizing arteriolitis. Levitt and Burbank (48) described the clinicopathological findings in two previously non-allergic patients with recurrent fatal attacks of HSP after injection of penicillin and ingestion of strawberries respectively that included glomerulonephritis alone or with systemic arteriolitis. The finding of IgA deposits in cutaneous blood vessel walls and in glomerular mesangial biopsies of patients with HSP and IgA nephropathy (IgAN) (49, 50) was circumstantially convincing enough to substitute the term IgAV for HSP.

Wintrobue and Buell (51) described cryoglobulinemia in a patient with progressive frontal headache, facial pain, Raynaud symptoms, recurrent nosebleeds, exertional dyspnea, palpitation, and changes in the eye grounds due to central vein thromboses. Postmortem examination showed infiltrating myeloma of the humerus and lumbar vertebra, and splenic enlargement. A unique plasma protein was detected that spontaneously precipitated with cold temperature and solubilized at high temperature differed from Bence-Jones proteinuria of other myeloma patients. Lerner and Watson (52) noted the association with purpura, and later Lerner and Watson (53) described its occurrence in 10% of pathological sera. Gorevic and colleagues (54) described mixed CV in forty patients, the clinical features of which included palpable purpura in all patients, polyarthralgia in three-quarters, and kidney involvement in slightly more than one-half, and deposits of IgG, IgM, and complement, or renal arteritis in a third of patients.

Recurrent attacks of erythematous, urticarial, and hemorrhagic skin lesions that lasted 24 hours at a time, associated with recurrent attacks of fever, joint swelling, abdominal distress, and depressed serum complement indicative of HUV were described by McDuffie and colleagues in 1973 (55), however small amounts of cryoglobulin were present at one time or another in the serum of each patient. When tested by immunodiffusion against purified preparations of rheumatoid factor (RF) and human C1q, two patients consistently produced bands against the former, and two others reacted strongly with purified C1q. Skin biopsies showed leukocytoclasia characteristic of necrotizing vasculitis in one patient; anaphylactoid purpura in two others, and mild nonspecific perivascular infiltration another. Immunofluorescence of skin specimens performed in three patients showed fixation of Ig in the patient with necrotizing vasculitis, while in two others with a pathological picture of anaphylactoid purpura or nonspecific dermal infiltrate, immunofluorescence was negative. Renal biopsy in two patients showed mild to moderate glomerulonephritis indistinguishable for those seen in other forms of chronic membranoproliferative glomerulonephritis. HUV differed from SLE due to more urticarial and purpuric skin lesions, and relatively mild renal or absent other visceral involvement. Moreover, serum speckled antinuclear and anti-DNA antibodies, and basement membrane Ig deposits were absent in those with HUV, also atypical for SLE. An etiopathogenesis related to chronic vascular inflammation resulting from deposits of immune complexes in small vessel walls seemed likely. Zeiss and colleagues (56) characterized C1q IgG precipitins from HUV sera that precipitated C1q in agarose gel among four additional patients. Wisnieski and Naff (57) showed C1q binding activity in IgG from HUV sera which suggested a relation to LE, but that view was later amended.

The historical account of the category of LVV spanned more than a century with notable advances in the past several years. Hutchinson provided the first clinical description of temporal arteritis (58), followed by a pathological description by Horton (59) more than fifty years after the description and designation of polymyalgia rheumatic (PMR) by Bruce (60) and Barber (61). Temporal arteritis was named for the site of granulomatous giant cell inflammation and vessel involvement (62). Those with biopsy-proven temporal arteritis and associated blindness due to vasculitic involvement of ophthalmic and posterior ciliary vessels were classified as cranial arteritis (63). The occasional finding of giant cell lesions along the aorta, its branches, and in other medium- and large-sized arteries at autopsy in other patients warranted the additional diagnosis of generalized GCA (64). The pathological heterogeneity of temporal arteritis was further demonstrated by the finding of intracranial lesions in eight patients who also qualified for the diagnosis of granulomatous angiitis of the nervous system (GANS) (65–70). PNS involvement in GCA was exceedingly uncommon (71). The earliest lesions of GCA (Figure 4) consisted of vacuolization of smooth muscle cells of the media, with enlargement of mitochondria, infiltration of lymphocytes, plasma cells, and histiocytes. With progression, there was extension of inflammation into the intima and adventitia leading to segmental fragmentation and necrosis of the elastic lamina, granuloma formation, and proliferation of connective tissue along the vessel wall. This eventuated in vascular thrombosis, intimal proliferation and fibrosis. One other LVV was described in the Japanese literature as

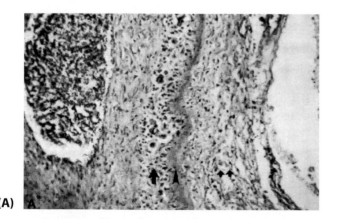

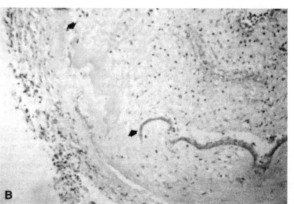

(A)

(B)

FIG. 4. Giant cell arteritis. A. In an early lesion of a large muscular artery, necrosis, inflammation, and giant cell formation (single arrow) can be seen immediately adjacent to the internal elastic lamina (arrowhead), which is undergoing degenerative changes, and there is some intimal proliferation (double arrows) (stain, hematoxylin and eosin; original magnification, ×100). B. This more advanced lesion has complete segmental destruction of the internal elastic lamina and virtually the entire media (arrows). Marked intimal proliferation has nearly occluded the lumen, and few inflammatory cells remain (stain, hematoxylin and eosin; original magnification, ×50).

unusual changes of the central vessels of the retina in the absence of peripheral arterial pulses in a woman (72). So-called pulseless disease (73), occlusive thromboaortopathy (74) or TAK disease (75), manifested constitutional complaints of malaise, fever, stiffness of the shoulders, nausea, vomiting, night sweats, anorexia, weight loss, and irregularity of menstrual periods weeks to months before the local signs of vasculitis were recognized in up to two-thirds of patients. It is the commonest large vessel vasculitis among Asian women.

One other form of inflammatory aortic disease or aortitis was coming to light in the surgical literature with equally broad and far-reaching implications for concepts of autoimmunity. In 1972, Walker and colleagues (76) noted that 10% of 217 patients presenting with abdominal aneurysms at Manchester Royal Infirmary between 1958 and 1969 for resection showed excessive thickening of aneurysm walls and perianeurysmal adhesions at operation. Subsequent histological examination of the walls of the aneurysms showed extensive active chronic inflammatory changes including plasma-cell infiltration. The clinical features of patients with inflammatory aneurysms differed from those with atherosclerotic disease due to generally younger age by a decade, lower incidence of rupture, lack of limb claudication, presence of peripheral pulses, less likelihood of unusual presenting features, elevated erythrocyte sedimentation rate (ESR), and absence of calcification on preoperative abdominal radiographs. In 1985, Pennell and coworkers (77) reported inflammatory aortic or iliac aneurysms in 4.5% of 2,816 patients undergoing repair for abdominal aortic aneurysm from 1955 to 1985. Ultrasound and CT imaging suggested the diagnosis respectively in 13.5% and 50% of patients, the former showing a sonolucent halo with clear definition of the aortic wall posterior to the thickened anterior and lateral aortic walls. In 2000, Rojo-Leyva and colleagues (78) noted idiopathic aortitis in 43% of 1,204 aortic specimens gathered over a period of 20 years. In 96% of the patients with idiopathic aortitis and aneurysm formation, aortitis was present only in the thoracic aorta. In 2001, Hamano and colleagues (79) noted a high concentrations of IgG4 associated with sclerosing pancreatitis characterized by obstructive jaundice, infrequent attacks of abdominal pain, irregular narrowing of the pancreatic duct, sonolucent swelling of the parenchyma, lymphoplasmacytic infiltration, fibrosis, and a favorable response to corticosteroid treatment. One year later, Hamano and coworkers (80) noted the association of sclerosing pancreatitis with raised concentrations of IgG4 among those with concomitant hydronephrosis that caused ureteral masses later diagnosed as retroperitoneal fibrosis (RPF). Histologic examination of ureteral and pancreatic tissues revealed abundant tissue infiltration by IgG4-bearing plasma cells. In the same year, 2008, three important observations were made. First, Sakata

and colleagues (81) concluded that inflammatory abdominal aortic aneurysm (IAAA) was related to IgG4 sclerosing disease. Second, Kasashima and colleagues (82) concluded that IAAA was an IgG-related disease (IgG4-RD) together with RPF. Third, Ito and colleagues (83) described a patient with IAAA, hydronephrosis caused by RPF, and high levels of IgG4 in whom treatment with corticosteroids led to clinical improvement and reduction in IgG4 levels. Histological inspection of the aortic wall specimen showed lymphocytoplasmacytic infiltration. Immunohistochemical analysis of the tissue showed IgG4-positive plasma cells. The findings suggested that IAAA had an etiopathogenesis similar to autoimmune pancreatitis and that some cases of IAAA and RPF might be aortic and periaortic lesions of IgG4-RD. One year later, in 2009, Khosroshahi and colleagues (84) described thoracic aortitis due to IgG4-RD with marked elevation of the serum IgG4 levels and progression to autoimmune pancreatitis; and Stone and coworkers (85) described IgG4-related thoracic aortitis with a media-predominant pattern of aortic wall infiltration and marked elevation of serum IgG4 levels, unequivocally linking IgG4-RD with thoracic lymphoplasmacytic aortitis.

Two forms of VVV, BD and CD, were recognized with very different clinical presentations and systemic involvement. Adamantiades (86) recognized the disorder of relapsing aphthous ulcers of the mouth, eye and genitalia, the clinicopathological details of which were described in later detail by Behçet (87, 88) in two Turkish patients. Nervous system involvement of a 28-year-old Yemenite with relapsing oral, genital and oral eruptions over four years, was accompanied by severe headache, memory loss, dizziness, lethargy, fatal seizures and coma. Postmortem examination showed perivascular inflammatory cell infiltration of the meninges, brain, and central retinal artery and optic nerve with necrotic cerebral lesions. Encephomyelopathy was detailed at postmortem examination in two Australian patients with BD (89) who presented with hemiparesis, while the other patient presented with pseudobulbar affect, vertical gaze palsy, nystagmus, and spastic paraplegias. Postmortem examination showed widespread lesions in cortical and brainstem white matter and hypothalamus, corresponding to small blood vessels including arterioles and veins that showed perivascular mononuclear cell infiltration. The first well-documented American patient with nervous system involvement of BD was described by Wolf and coworkers (90) in a 22-year-old woman with a five-year history of recurrent oral and genital ulceration, and a two-year course of progressive visual loss, headache, hemiparesis, ataxia, tremor, dysarthria, cranial nerve palsy, cerebellar and corticospinal tract disease, and mental deterioration, that responded to prednisone therapy.

Mogan and Baumgartner (91) described a 26-year-old man with recurrent pain, spasm and redness of the left eye with photophobia, excessive tearing, and marked conjuncti-val injection, followed by severe attack of dizziness, tinnitus, vertigo, nausea, vomiting, ringing in the ears, profuse per-spiration, and deafness. A diagnosis of recurrent interstitial keratitis and explosive Menière disease was made. In retro-spect he was probably the first reported patient with CS of nonsyphilitic interstitial keratitis (IK) (91). Vestibuloaudi-tory symptoms were later described by Cogan (92). Haynes and colleagues (93) set forth diagnostic criteria for typi-cal CS. In a review of 30 patients seen at the National Eye Institute of the NIH by Cogan (92, 94, 95), symptoms of IK developed abruptly and gradually resolved, associated with photophobia, lacrimation, and eye pain which might be uni-lateral or bilateral. Such symptoms tended to recur periodi-cally for years before becoming quiescent. Vestibuloauditory dysfunction was manifested by sudden onset of Menière-like attacks of nausea, vomiting, tinnitus, vertigo, and frequently progressive hearing loss that characteristically occurred before or after the onset of IK. However within one to six months of the onset of eye symptoms, auditory symptoms progressed to deafness over a period of one to three months, certainly no longer than two years. Cody and Williams (96) provided a description of atypical CS if another significant inflammatory eye lesion in addition to, or instead of IK such as scleritis, episcleritis, retinal artery occlusion, choroiditis, retinal hemorrhage, papilledema, exophthalmos, or tendon-itis. Haynes and colleagues (93) defined acute CS as the pres-ence of acute eye disease within two weeks of hearing loss, while inactive CS was applied to patients without active eye disease or vestibuloauditory dysfunction of greater than two weeks prior to study. With fewer than 100 reported children and young adults, the majority of reported patients with typ-ical CS have appeared as single case reports or patient series (93, 97–99, 100), without pathological confirmation (92, 94, 100, 101) or evidence of systemic vasculitis in a biopsy or at postmortem examination (95, 96, 102, 103). In contrast to Mogan and Baumgartner (91) and Cogan (92, 94), headache and other CNS manifestation do occur. Norton and Cogan (95) described a patient with atypical acute CS in whom headache preceded detection of superior central retinal artery branch occlusion and orbital edema.

The histopathologic appearance of vasculitis of the periph-eral nerve is similar regardless of whether the process is primary or secondary to underlying systemic vasculitis. His-torically, detailed neurovascular anatomy arose from the careful dissection of amputated limbs following injection of India ink to opacify peripheral nerve vessels in World War II veterans (104, 105). Such studies indicated that proximal stretches of each of the major nerves were supplied both by a single arterial vessel, such as in the axilla-to-elbow and knee-to-elbow segments located peripherally in the nerve trunk, and abundantly along their distal course by a suc-cession of microvessel which by their repeated division

and anastomosis, outlined an unbroken vascular net that assured continuous vascular supply. As there was no evi-dence for the presence of watershed zones of poor vascu-lar supply along major nerves of the arm or leg, ischemic paralysis of a limb should rarely if ever occur in the absence of widespread arteritis, abrupt occlusion of large named vessels, or focal nerve compression. A quarter-century later, Dyck and coworkers (106) ascribed ischemic centro-fascicular nerve fiber degeneration of named upper arm and thigh nerves in a patient with necrotizing angiopathic neuropathy due to poor vascular perfusion along presumed watershed zones of the upper arm and thigh regions. How-ever the clinical details of the patient were not given, the centrofascicular fiber loss was only pronounced in the legs, and extraneural blood vessels of the arms were not studied. Two decades later, Moore and Fauci (107) ascribed pro-gressive weakness and sensory loss in the arms and sub-sequently in the legs distally from the knees in Patient 8 with extensive mononeuritis multiplex due to infarction of specific peripheral nerves, culminating in ambulation with leg braces and good use of the hands. However, that patient was not studied pathologically. Vasculitis of the peripheral nerves leads to specific alterations in the arteriae nervo-rum with a caliber of 100 micrometers (μm) located in the epineurial compartment, as well as in peripheral nerve fas-cicles ensheathed by perineurium and endoneurium. The key elements of pathologically definite nonsystemic vascu-litic neuropathy, generally regarded as a form of SOV, are intramural inflammation accompanied by pathological evi-dence of vascular wall damage without evidence of systemic involvement (108).

Diverse syndromes of adult and childhood primary CNS vasculitis with very different clinical presentation,

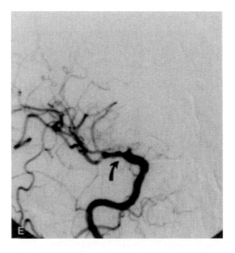

FIG. 5. Radiographic features of cerebral vasculitis. Ectasia and beading in the M1 segment and lack of flow in the A1 segment of the right anterior cerebral artery (arrow).

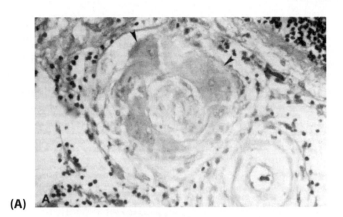
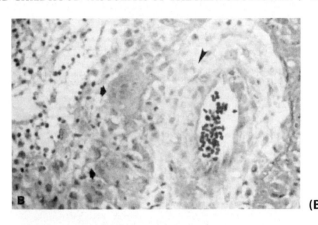

(A)   **(B)**

FIG. 6. Central nervous system vasculitis. A. The media and adventitia of this small leptomeningeal artery have been almost completely replaced by multinucleated giant cells (arrowheads). There is intimal proliferation with obliteration of the vascular lumen, and a dense, perivascular, mononuclear inflammatory infiltrate can be seen (stain, hematoxylin and eosin; original magnification, ×250). B. A somewhat larger leptomeningeal vessel shows necrosis of the media and internal elastic lamina with multinucleated giant cell formation (arrows), intimal proliferation (arrowhead), and lymphocytic infiltration of the adventitia and neighboring meninges (stain, hematoxylin and eosin; original magnification, ×250).

histopathology, and prognosis were described. Primary CNS vasculitis was first described by Harbitz in 1922 (109) in one patient with worsening headaches, mental change, and ataxia culminating in stupor, spastic paraparesis, coma and death in two years. A second patient presented with hallucination and confusion progressing to gait difficulty, stupor, coma and death in nine months. At postmortem examination both had granulomatous vasculitis of the meninges comprised of lymphocytes, multinucleate giant cells and epithelioid cells with vessel necrosis and extension into the brain along involved veins and arteries of varying caliber. Over the ensuing quarter century, additional patients were reported under the rubric of allergic angiitis and granulomatosis (110), giant cell arteritis (111), and sarcoidosis (112). Cravioto and Fegin (113) delineated the clinicopathologic syndrome of non-infectious granulomatous angiitis, and for two more decades, rare affected patients were identified in life, but there was no effective treatment. The identification of angiographic beading and a sausage-like appearance of cerebral vessels at sites of presumed arteritis (Figure 5) were first noted by Hinck and coworkers (114) in GCA, and later by Cupps and Fauci (115) in other patients with so-called, isolated angiitis of the CNS (IACNS). The angiographic features of presumed vasculitis along with the judged efficacy of a combination immunosuppressive regimen of oral cyclophosphamide and alternate day prednisone, including three patients with IACNS defined angiographically, and another with biopsy-proven GANS of the filum terminale, led to prospective diagnostic and therapeutic recommendations (116). At that time, investigators at the NIH regarded IACNS and GANS as equivalent entities with the former term emphasizing the restricted nature of the vasculitis

and the latter the granulomatous histology. Giant cells and epithelioid cells, usually found at autopsy in GANS (Figure 6), were an inconsistent finding in a meningeal and brain biopsy, and therefore considered unnecessary for antemortem diagnosis. In the same year of 1988, Calabrese and Mallek (117) proposed criteria for the diagnosis of primary angiitis of the central nervous system vasculitis (PACNS), while Younger and colleagues (118) contemporaneously described the limits of granulomatous angiitis of the brain (GAB) and nervous system (GANS) (119). The past quarter century has witnessed an expansion in the present understanding of primary CNS vasculitis in children and adults

Vasculitis due to drug abuse captured the interest of successive generations of investigators. The earliest reports of misuse of amphetamine sulfate occurred in 1937 when it was used by students to avoid sleep during examination periods (120). This was followed by reports of death by those who ingested the drug repeatedly as a stimulant for the same purpose (121) in a suicide attempt that resulted in a fatal intracerebral hemorrhage (122), or accidentally, when dexamphetamine and phenelzine were fatally ingested together decades later (123). During the Second World War, amphetamine and methamphetamine were used clinically and illicitly but their abuse soared in San Francisco after 1962 wherein it was illegally produced and distributed (124). By 2009, the United Nations Office on Drugs and Crime estimated that 16 to 51 million persons between the ages of 15 and 64 years consumed amphetamine drugs, with more than half using methamphetamine (125), exceeding the combined consumption of all other drugs of abuse except cannabis (126). Illicit amphetamine drugs are available in powder, capsule, tablet, and parenteral forms that

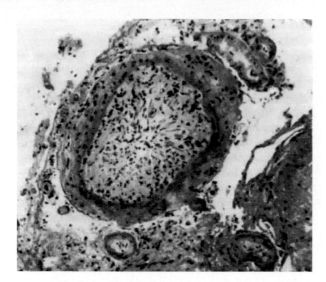

FIG. 7. Cerebral vasculopathy in a case of intracerebral hemorrhage associated with the use of phenylpropanolamine as an aid to weight loss. The profound intimal hyperplasia all but obliterates the vascular lumen. Polymorphonuclear leukocytes are in all three vascular layers but particularly the intima. The media are remarkably well preserved compared with cases of polyarteritis nodosa and leukocytoclastic vasculitis (stain, hematoxylin and eosin; original magnification, ×100).

can be swallowed, snorted or taken intra-nasally, smoked or injected with highly variable purity and dosage equivalence. Histologically confirmed cerebral vasculitis (Figure 7) due to amphetamine, methamphetamine and related agents is exceedingly rare which is surprising given the number of substances that could cause this disorder if there was a true association.

CLINICAL PRESENTATION AND LABORATORY EVALUATION

The clinical presentation of a patient with vasculitis of the nervous system depends on three factors: distribution of the involved neural vessels, spectrum of extra-neurologic organ involvement, and the severity and rate of progression of the underlying vasculitic process. Patients with systemic vasculitis will have other involved tissues besides peripheral nerve, brain and spinal cord, including the skin, joints, kidneys, lungs, and gastrointestinal tract, although the dysfunction may be extremely mild or subclinical and detectable only after extensive laboratory evaluation (107). Constitutional symptoms such as fever, weight loss, anorexia, myalgia, arthralgia, and nonspecific fatigue and weakness occur in about 80% of patients, but careful general examination and laboratory investigation is mandatory

to look for systemic abnormalities that may suggest a more generalized process. Two exceptions are patients with isolated PNV and primary CNS vasculitis in which systemic organ involvement by definition is lacking. Since the ischemic process in PNS vasculitis does not have a predilection for motor or sensory fibers, both modalities are nearly always affected. Most patients complain of deep aching discomfort in the affected limb that later evolves into burning dysesthetic pain. There may be restricted involvement such as unilateral foot drop or intrinsic hand muscle weakness due to single nerve involvement. However, multifocal nerve involvement is more typical at the outset, with up to one-half of patients presenting with mononeuropathy multiplex and a quarter to a third of patients demonstrating overlapping bilateral involvement resulting in distal symmetrical and asymmetrical polyneuropathy due to extensive confluent ischemic involvement at many levels of multiple nerve trunks (127). The clinical manifestations of primary CNS vasculitis range from minor to severe life-threatening signs of ischemia, although specific symptoms and signs depend upon the associated underlying mechanism. Affected adults and children present with headache, cognitive impairment, mood impairment, seizures, and focal deficits. It generally evolves in a stepwise or insidious fashion with progressive deficits culminating in quadriparesis, lethargy, coma and death due to additional ischemic lesions.

The clinical manifestations of primary and secondary CNS vasculitis range from minor to severe life-threatening signs of ischemia, although specific symptoms and signs depend upon the associated underlying mechanism.

There is general agreement on four principles in the diagnosis of vasculitis, especially applicable to the nervous system:

First, vasculitis of the CNS and PNS is a potentially serious disorder with a propensity for permanent disability owing to tissue ischemia and infarction; recognition of the neurologic manifestations is important in developing a differential etiologic diagnosis.

Second, undiagnosed and untreated, the outcome of vasculitis is potentially fatal.

Third, a favorable response to an empiric course of immunosuppressive and immunomodulating therapy should never be considered a substitute for the absolute proof of the diagnosis of vasculitis.

Fourth, histolopathologic confirmation of vasculitis is essential for accurate diagnosis, such as by brain and meninges biopsy when there is CNS involvement, and analysis of nerve and muscle biopsy tissue when PNS involvement is postulated.

Serologically-specific serum studies should be obtained in all patients guided by the clinical presentation and postulated etiologic diagnosis to avoid excessive cost and spurious results.

Electrodiagnostic studies are useful in the initial investigation of systemic vasculitis because they can identify areas of asymptomatic involvement and sites for muscle and nerve biopsy and distinguish the various neuropathic syndromes associated with peripheral nerve and muscle involvement. A wide sampling of nerves and muscles should be examined, both distal and proximal, using standard recording and needle electrodes for the performance of nerve conduction studies (NCS) and needle electromyography (EMG), at skin temperatures of 34°C, with comparison to normative data. Most patients with peripheral nerve vasculitis show evidence of active axonopathy acutely in a mononeuritis multiplex pattern and over time in a distal symmetric or asymmetric pattern. Quantitative motor unit potential (MUP) analysis can delineate whether proximal wasting and weakness are caused by myopathic or neurogenic disease. In clinically suspected patients, open biopsy of a cutaneous sensory nerve is indispensable in the evaluation of primary and secondary PNV. Collectively, the observed primary pathologic process is generally an axonopathy with correlative findings on light microscopy employing cryostat- and paraffin-stained hematoxylin and eosin (H&E) sections, and later by plastic embedded, 1-mm, semithin sections and teased nerve fiber studies. Such studies show Wallerian degeneration due to nerve ischemia and vasculitis in addition to the presence of myelin ovoids, myelin debris, macrophage recruitment along the course of degenerated fibers, marked fascicular depletion of myelinated and unmyelinated nerve fibers, and endoneurial fibrosis. Immunocytochemical studies including lymphocyte cell marker analysis and complement immunofluorescence can be performed to identify pathogenic components of the cell-mediated and humoral immune system present in active or chronic vasculitis.

Cerebrospinal fluid (CSF) analysis, electroencephalography (EEG), and CNS neuroimaging studies are integral to the diagnostic evaluation of most CNS disorders including vasculitis. Properly performed, lumbar puncture carries minimal risk and provides potentially useful information regarding possible underlying vasculitis so suggested by pleocytosis in excess of 5 cells/mm3, protein elevation > 100 mg/dL, and evidence of intrathecal synthesis of immunoglobulin (Ig) and oligoclonal bands. Molecular genetic, immunoassay, and direct staining techniques to exclude spirochetal, fungal, mycobacterial and viral infections, as well as cytospin examination of CSF for possible malignant cells should be performed. There are no typical EEG findings in CNS vasculitis. Magnetic resonance imaging (MRI) is more sensitive than computed tomography (CT), but both methods lack specificity in histologically confirmed cases. The most common MRI findings are multiple bilateral cortical and deep white matter signal abnormalities and enhancement of the meninges after gadolinium. High-resolution 3-Tesla MRI and MR angiography (MRA), CT angiography (CTA) and functional imaging of the brain provide complementary information. The former is useful in the evaluation of medium and large vessel disease, but can miss fine vessel contours better seen on cut-film or digital subtraction angiography (DSA). The abnormal diffuse and focal perfusion patterns seen on single photon emission-CT (SPECT) do not always correlate with neurologic symptoms or distinguish vasculitic from nonvasculitic vasculopathy. The claims that cerebral angiography shows diagnostic features has been modified. Beading of vessels is found in only about a third of patients with histologically proven CNS vasculitis, as well as in CNS infection, atherosclerosis, cerebral embolism, and vasospasm of diverse cause. Multiple microaneurysms, often seen on visceral angiography in systemic vasculitis, are distinctly rare in CNS vessels.

Brain, spinal cord, and meningeal biopsy are the gold standard for the diagnosis of CNS vasculitis, but false-negatives occur because of focal lesions and sampling errors. Radiographic studies that guide the biopsy site toward areas of abnormality probably improve the sensitivity, but this has not been formally studied. The risk of serious morbidity related to biopsy is less than 2.0% at most centers, which is probably less than the cumulative risk of an empiric course of long-term immunosuppressive therapy. There are no certain guidelines as to when to proceed to brain and meningeal biopsy. However, it would certainly be warranted if there were no other explanation for the progressive syndrome of fever, headache, encephalopathy, and focal cerebral signs, in association with CSF pleocytosis and protein content elevation >100 mg/dL (118).

LARGE VESSEL VASCULITIS

Giant Cell Arteritis

Giant-cell arteritis is a chronic granulomatous vasculitis of large and medium-sized vessels that frequently affected the thoracic aorta and its branches. There are several excellent recent reviews (128–132). Kermani and colleagues (128) reported a population–based incident cohort of 204 patients with GCA seen between 1950 and 2004 at the Mayo Clinic noting a mean age of diagnosis of 76 years, and a female to male ratio of 1.5:1. It is the most common vasculitis in populations with predominantly Northern European ancestry, with an annual incidence of 15 to 33 cases per 100,000 age 50 years and older (133). Both GCA and PMR, a related disorder, are both probably polygenic disease in which multiple environmental and genetic factors influence susceptibility and severity (134).

Two-thirds of patients complain of headache that typically emanates along tender granulomatous lesions of inflamed extracranial vessels and is resistant to standard analgesic agents. There may be tender red cords along the temple with scalp tenderness or occipital and nuchal pain. About one-half of patients report dysesthesia of the scalp and jaw claudication. The ocular manifestations of GCA include visual loss of varying severity in more than 90% of patients, notably anterior ischemic optic neuropathy (81%), central retinal artery occlusion (14%), cilioretinal artery occlusion (21%), posterior ischemic optic neuropathy (6%), and ocular ischemia (1%), and amaurosis fugax (30%) (135). There may be oculomotor disturbances resulting from vasculitis of the extraocular muscles, and vertigo and hearing impairment resulting from acute auditory artery involvement. Cervical myelopathy can result from anterior spinal artery involvement. Stroke, transient ischemic attacks and amaurosis fugax can occur as a result of arteritic involvement along the proximal intracranial carotid artery and extracranial vertebral artery to the point of dural attachment. There may be confusion with PMR and inflammatory myopathy in elderly individuals due to concomitant arthralgia and myalgia along the torso, shoulders, proximal arms, hips, and proximal thighs. The ESR is typically elevated to 100 millimeters per hour (mm/hr) or more.

Temporal artery biopsy is the only sure way of establishing the diagnosis. However, false negative findings on the contemplated affected side may be due to inadvertent sampling of a vasculitic-free length of vessel. The non-invasive assessment of LVV includes performance of color-Doppler sonography (CDS), contrast-enhanced high-resolution MRI combined with MRA, and contrast-enhanced CT combined with CTA to visualize the vessel wall and the lumen of large vessels. The signs of early inflammation that include vessel wall thickening and mural inflammation, as well as the late complications of stenosis and aneurysms, can be ascertained. ^{18}F-Fluorodeoxyglucose (FDG) positron emission tomography (PET) detects increased FDG uptake by metabolically active cells, including inflammatory cells infiltrating the vessel wall in vasculitis, while DSA is a useful modality to demonstrate luminal changes. Moreover, such studies can assist the surgeon in centering on an involved segment of vessel (136). Performance of CDS is better suited to study superficial vessels such as the internal and external carotid artery and its branches, while MR and CT are best suited for deep vessels. When performed together, they can be used to monitor disease extent and severity through the demonstration of early vascular changes in wall thickness and mural inflammation, to which PET can be added to ascertain active inflammation in vessels affected by GCA and TAK. The risk factors for GCA-related ischemic events include visual loss, prior ischemic events, marked intimal hyperplasia on temporal artery biopsy, elevated inflammatory markers, older age at diagnosis, hypertension, ischemic heart disease, and absence of systemic manifestations (137).

The classic histologic picture of granulomatous vasculitis, which is observed in about one-half of affected patients, eventuates in infiltration of vessel cell by giant cells at the junction between the intima and media, leading to thrombosis, intimal hyperplasia, and fibrosis (134). Weyland and colleagues (138) described local dendritic cells that recruit and activate CD4 T-cells that in turn direct the activity of effector macrophages. In response to the immune attack, the blood vessel forms lumen-stenosing intima. Multiple cascades of excessive T-cell reactivity contribute to the autoimmune features of GCA with helper T-cell (Th) types Th1 and Th17 immunity responsible for the early phase and TH1 immunity promoting chronic-smoldering inflammation. Restuccia and colleagues (139) described two subsets of GCA among forty-five patients including isolated vasa vasorum vasculitis and SVV surrounding an uninflamed temporal artery. The temporal artery biopsy of six patients considered negative at initial examination were later found to show vasa vasorum vasculitis in four patients, and combined vasa vasorum and SVV in two others, four of whom satisfied the 1990 ACR criteria for the classification of GCA (140), with typical headache complaints in up to 50% of those so studied.

GCA was classified according to the 1990 ACR criteria (140) designed to discriminate between different types of vasculitides. The five discriminatory features that included age greater than 50 years at onset, new onset of localized headache, temporal artery tenderness or decreased temporal artery pulse, ESR >50 mm/hr, and biopsy of an artery showing necrotizing arteritis characterized by a predominance of mononuclear cells or a granulomatous process with multinucleated giant cells. Unrecognized and therefore untreated or inadequately treated, there is a high likelihood of large artery complication. Nuenninghoff and coworkers (133) reported incident cases of large-artery complications representing 27% of 168 patients in a GCA cohort at the Mayo Clinic between 1950 and 1999 that included aortic aneurysm or dissection in 18%, large artery stenosis in 13%, cervical artery stenosis in 9%; and subclavian, axillary or brachial artery stenosis in 4%. Aortic insufficiency murmur was predictive of later aortic aneurysm or dissection, while diminished pulse or blood pressure or claudication of an arm, transient ischemic attack or stroke, and diplopia at time of diagnosis were associated with large-artery stenosis. Cranial symptoms such as headache, scalp tenderness, and swollen or nodular arteries at the time of diagnosis, were negative associated with large-artery stenosis. Kermani and colleagues (128) reported that the incidence of aortic aneurysm and dissection increased 5 years after GCA diagnosis and was associated with increased mortality.

Since the early reports of a salutary effect of corticosteroids on GCA in 1950 (141), corticosteroids have remained the standard of care because of their ability to reduce disease-related morbidity, mortality, and symptoms that negatively impact on quality of life. However they are not curative, do not prevent relapses, and are associated with significant toxicity (142). Disease related morbidity in GCA which largely results from cranial ischemic events or LVV, leads to visual loss in up to 20% of patients. While there is no treatment to date that has been found to completely reverse blindness once it has occurred, there is strong evidence to suggest that once corticosteroids have been started the risk of visual loss is low (143). For this reason, corticosteroids should be started while the diagnostic evaluation is in progress and continued for up to one year before tapering to the lowest maintenance levels. Retrospective studies showed that patients who are also on aspirin have a lower risk of cranial ischemic complications (144, 145). Apart from corticosteroids, there is ongoing interest in the use of infliximab for maintenance of corticosteroid-induced remission (146), abatacept (CTLA4-Ig) and the interleukin (IL)-6 receptor antagonist tocilizumab

Takayasu Arteritis

Individuals younger than 50 year of age, particularly women of Asian descent with granulomatous arteritis affecting the aorta and its branches, are most susceptible to TAK (2). The reported mean annual incidence of TAK was .4 per million in a population-study in eastern Denmark between 1990 and 2009 (147). For comparison, the UK General Practice Research Database (UKGPRD) (148) ascertained an overall annual incidence of TAK of .8 per million and a mean prevalence of 4.7 per million; among those age less than 40 years, the annual incidence was .3 per million. According to Mishima (149) the disease in Asia, where it is far more prevalent accounting for 1 in 3,000 persons at postmortem, TAK is more common in women most of whom are in their second or third decades of life. Since 1985, a nation-wide survey and a multicenter clinical study have been conducted in Japan by the Research Committee on systemic vascular disorders within the Ministry of Health and Welfare demonstrating that approximately 10% of TAK patients are men and the number of affected patients is estimated to be around 3,000, with 100 new cases being ascertained each year. The Research Committee reported the distribution of vascular lesions in autopsy cases in 1992 that showed preferential involvement of the ascending aorta, aortic arch, and thoracic aorta in three-quarters of cases between 1958 and 1984.

According to the 1990 ACR criteria (150), a patient was considered to have TAK when three of six criteria were present including age at disease less than or equal to 40 years; claudication of one or more extremities while in use especially the arms; decreased brachial artery pulse of one or both sides; blood pressure difference of >10 mmHg between the arms; audible bruit with auscultation over one or both subclavian arteries or over the abdominal aorta; arteriographic narrowing or occlusion of the entire aorta, its primary branches, or large arteries in the proximal upper or lower extremities, not due to arteriosclerosis, fibromuscular dysplasia, or similar causes. Such changes were expected to be focal and segmental. Ascertainment of three or more of the criteria yielded a sensitivity of 90.5% and a specificity of 97.8%.

Nakao and coworkers (76) noted nonspecific systemic clinical manifestations at onset among eighty-four patients with TAK that included malaise, fever, stiffness of the shoulders, nausea, vomiting, night sweats, anorexia, weight loss, and irregularity of menstrual periods weeks to months before the local signs of vasculitis were recognized (76). Absent pulses in the neck and limbs are symptoms of claudication and syncope may occur with bending of the head backward due to vasculitic-related circulatory insufficiency along the aorta and branches to the brain, face and limbs (76, 151). Headache may be associated with carotid arterial inflammation (152) and increased propensity to migraine (152, 153). There may be ischemic presentations of amaurosis fugax, monocular blindness, subclavian steal and carotid sinus syndrome, typically associated with audible neck and limb bruits, and asymmetry of pulses, all resulting from granulomatous vasculitis of the ascending and descending aorta and its major branches (154); (150). Kerr and colleagues (152) described the neurological manifestations in 60 patients with TAK that included visual aberration in 48% of those with and 18% of those without vertebral artery involvement, and among 40% of those with and 12% of patients without common carotid lesions. Permanent monocular blindness was attributed to TAK lesions in one patient, and eight of ten patients with transient ischemic attacks or cerebrovascular accidents had carotid or vertebral artery disease that anatomically corresponded to the observed neurological deficits. Cardiac disease was observed in 40% of the patients, of whom 20% had aortic regurgitation resulting from a dilated aortic root with separation of valvular leaflets. Riehl and Brown (151) described a 43-year-old Japanese woman who underwent neurological evaluation in 1961 at a United States medical center for complaints of dizziness, transient visual loss, and hypotension was later found to have a thrill over the chest that was interpreted to be an aortic arch aneurysm that was surgically corrected but she subsequently died of heart failure. At postmortem examination there was evidence of thrombosis of the aortic arch graft with complete obstruction of the great vessels and distal aortic stenosis. There was a massive infarction of the left temporoparietal region, left half of the midbrain, brainstem and cerebellum associated with thrombotic obliteration of the proximal portion of the left middle cerebral and left posterior cerebral arteries, as well as the anterior third of the basilar artery. Microscopic examination revealed widespread granulomatous arteritis of large and middle-sized vessels including the cerebral vessels, aortic arch and its tributaries, and the proximal stump of the left common carotid, with sparing of smaller arteries and arterioles.

Although arterial biopsy is impractical given the restriction of lesions to the aorta and its branches, MRA and conventional angiography demonstrates vessel irregularities, stenosis, poststenotic dilatations, aneurysmal formation, occlusions, and increased collateralization. Although the mechanism and distribution of headache differs between patients with GCA and TAK, there are strong similarities and subtle differences in the distribution of arterial disease on cerebral arteriography that suggest that the two disorders may exist nonetheless on a spectrum within the same or a similar disease (131).

Ishikawa (75) reported the natural history of TAK among fifty-four Japanese patients from 1957 to 1975 classified as uncomplicated (Group I), mono-complicated (Group II) and multicomplicated (Group III). The 5-year survival rate after the established diagnosis in the fifty-four patients was 83%. The major factors related to death among the eight patients so studied included fatal cerebral and cardiac events each in three, and aortic reconstruction surgery or steroid withdrawal in another patient. Ohigashi and colleagues (155) ascertained an improved prognosis among 106 consecutive patients with TAK with onset before 1999 compared to those diagnosed after 2000 (4.2% versus 0%) that was attributed to reduction in the time from onset to diagnosis, replacement of digital subtraction angiography (79% versus 9%) with ultrasound (6% versus 34%), CTA (24% versus 77%), MRA (21% versus 57%), and ¹⁸F-FDG PET (0% versus 20%); less frequent complications of moderate or severe aortic regurgitation, increase in the use and maximal dose of corticosteroids (70% versus 97%); and the use of first and second-line immunosuppressant agents (7% versus 42%). Surgical treatment of TKA was similar in those with onset before 1999 to others diagnosed after 2000 (22.5% versus 22.8%).

MEDIUM VESSEL VASCULITIS

Polyarteritis Nodosa

Polyarteritis nodosa is the prototypical MVV. In a retrospective study of 348 patients registered in the French Vasculitis Study Group (FVSG), who satisfied the 1994 CHCC criteria for the diagnosis of PAN between 1963 and 2005 (1), the most frequent clinical findings in order of occurrence were general in type in 93%, neurologic in

79%, urologic or renal in 50%, and cutaneous involvement in 50% of patients. The general presenting features of PAN included fever, weight loss, myalgia, and arthralgia. Neurological involvement included peripheral neuropathy and mononeuritis multiplex respectively in 74% and 70%, and CNS involvement in 4.6% of patients. Urologic and renal involvement included hematuria, proteinuria, new-onset hypertension, orchitis and testicular tenderness. Cutaneous involvement included purpura, skin nodules, and livedo reticularis. Histological proof of PAN was ascertained in 70% by a positive finding in nerve, muscle or skin. Altogether, 129 patients underwent nerve biopsy including 108 with peripheral neuropathy and the remainder without peripheral neuropathy, of whom vasculitic lesions were noted respectively in 83% and 81% (156) compared to muscle biopsy which showed vasculitis respectively in 68% and 60%. Angiography showed renal and gastrointestinal microaneurysms or stenosis respectively in 66% and 57% of patients. Patients with hepatitis B virus (HBV)-related PAN had more frequent peripheral neuropathy, abdominal pain, cardiomyopathy, orchitis, and hypertension than those with non-HBV-related PAN, with respective five-year relapse-free survival rates of 59% and 67% in scheduled therapeutic regimens of glucocorticoids and cyclophosphamide depending upon involvement in clinical trials, and according to the standard of care at the time of diagnosis (157, 158). The predictors of a poor prognosis were age >65 years, hypertension, and gastrointestinal involvement, and cutaneous manifestations or non-HBV-related PAN with higher rates of relapse. Henegar and colleagues (159) identified three positive predictive parameters (hepatitis B virus antigen and DNA in serum, arteriographic anomalies, and mononeuropathy or polyneuropathy) and 5 negative predictive parameters (IFT detection of ANCA, asthma; ear, nose and throat signs; glomerulopathy; and cryoglobulinemia) that yielded a 70.6% sensitivity for control vasculitides and 92.3% specificity for all controls, outperforming the ACR 1990 criteria in all analytical situations.

PAN is a rare childhood vasculitis. The classification criteria for cPAN requires histological evidence of necrotizing vasculitis in medium-or small-sized arteries or angiographic abnormalities demonstrating aneurysm formation or vascular occlusions, as a mandatory criterion, plus two of five features among them myalgia, skin involvement, hypertension, neuropathy, or abnormal urinalysis or impaired renal function (6), with disease manifestations ranging from a benign cutaneous form with clinical, laboratory and molecular characteristics of Familial Mediterranean Fever (160, 161) to severe disseminated multisystemic disease. Ozen and colleagues (162) studied 110 children of mean age 9 years, from twenty-one pediatric centers worldwide diagnosed with cPAN dividing them into four groups including systemic PAN (57%), cutaneous PAN (30%), and classic PAN with hepatitis B surface antigen (HBsAg) (4.6%); with 8% instead manifesting ANCA so qualifying for MPA. Cutaneous cPAN was confined to the skin and musculoskeletal system. There are reported children with serological and microbiologic evidence of preceding streptococcal infection (163). Patients with HBsAg-associated PAN were diagnosed with renal angiograms. Antiviral treatment was administered in most cases. Those with MPA had pulmonary-renal disease together or separately. Patients classified with systemic PAN had multiple system involvement, with constitutional symptoms and elevated acute phase reactants, with only six of forty-seven so tested manifesting a positive ANCA (some p- and c-ANCA and others not specified) by IF, with no elevated MPO-ANCA enzyme-linked immunosorbent assay (ELISA) titers. Corticosteroids and cyclophosphamide were administered with an overall mortality of 1.1%.

Kawasaki Disease

This MVV disorder is rather common in childhood with the highest incidence in Japan where it exceeds 120 per 100,000, affecting 80% of children less than 5 years of age with a boy-to-girl ratio of 1.5 to 2 (164, 165). Headache is an associated symptom along with cough, abdominal pain, arthralgia, and seizures noted in up to one-quarter of untreated patients (166). Those with abdominal pain and headache are older by a decade or more than those without these symptoms (166). Migraine and Raynaud phenomenon which coexist in some patients with KD may be reflective of similar vascular lesions indicative of the late consequences of extracoronary endothelial cell dysfunction (167). Endothelial damage occurs in the acute stages of the disease in small and medium size arteries (168) with a predilection for coronary arteries leading to aneurysm and ectasia formation (2) that typically occurs one to four weeks after the onset of fever in up to 25% of untreated children (169) at a rate that is higher in infants than older children. Several HLA gene polymorphisms have been implicated in KD including HLA-E in Taiwanese children, HLA-B35, HLA-B75, and HLA-Cw09 alleles in Korean patients; and HLA-DRB1*11 and HLA-DRB1*09 alleles with coronary complications (170). The standard of care involves administration of intravenous immune globulin (IVIg) during the acute illness, initially at high doses with tapering to lower doses during convalescence, followed by aspirin. Children with IVIg-resistant disease have higher serum IL6 levels before and after treatment than responsive children. Pulse methylprednisolone, low-dose methotrexate, warfarin, and infliximab have shown no substantial benefit over IVIg (170).

ANCA-ASSOCIATED SMALL VESSEL VASCULITIS

Granulomatosis with Polyangiitis

This disorder is characterized by the clinicopathologic complex of necrotizing granulomatous vasculitis of the upper and lower respiratory tract, glomerulonephritis, and variable degrees of small vessel vasculitis. The characteristic histopathology is a necrotizing granulomatous vasculitis which may be found in lung and renal biopsy tissue although the latter is less common. Instead, a focal, segmental glomerulonephritis is often seen. Other inflammatory or vasculitic phenomenon can be encountered such as leukocytoclastic vasculitis in skin lesions, and acute and chronic inflammation in sinus, retro-orbital, and tracheal tissues. A limited form of GPA without glomerulonephritis was described (171) that is a long-term disease stage or phenotype accounting for about 5% of all patients characterized by destructive and space-consuming lesions associated with relapse rates of 46% and local damage (172). The 1990 ACR criteria for the classification of GPA (173) which preceded routine ANCA testing, included the presence of two or more criteria including, nasal or oral inflammation (painful or painless oral ulcers or purulent or bloody nasal discharge); abnormal chest radiograph (showing nodules, fixed infiltrates or cavities); urinary sediment (showing microhematuria >5 red blood cells per high-power field, or red cell casts in urinary sediment); and granulomatous inflammation on biopsy tissue (within the wall of an artery or in the perivascular or extravascular area of an artery or arteriole). A proposed classification tree substituted hemoptysis for granulomatous inflammation on a tissue biopsy if the latter was not available. Baseline serum samples for 180 participants in the WG Etanercept Trial Research Group (WGET) found that when IFT, direct and capture ELISA ANCA testing were performed at baseline, 166 (92%) were seropositive, including 96% with severe disease and 83% with limited disease. Holle and colleagues (174) who prospectively compared hsPR3-ANCA ELISA to the IFT noted an excellent performance of hsPR3-ANCA ELISA in identifying GPA and other AAV disorders associated with PR3-ANCA suggesting that the former be used as screening test.

Nishino and colleagues (175) described neurological involvement in 34% of patients with GPA at the Mayo Clinic that included peripheral neuropathy in the majority, followed by external ophthalmoplegia, cranial neuropathy, cerebrovascular events, seizures, and cerebritis. Of five patients with presumed clinical vasculitis, cerebral angiography was negative in two; and of twelve patients studied at postmortem examination, findings of vasculitis were detected in only two patients. De Groot and colleagues (176) performed a prospective analysis of the clinical, electrophysiologic, radiologic, and serologic data of 128 GPA patients over 19 months, respectively noting PNS, CNS, and cranial nerve involvement in 43%, 7% and 4.7% of patients. Symmetrical sensorimotor polyneuropathy was noted in 31 patients compared with mononeuritis multiplex in 25 patients. Suppiah and colleagues from the European Vasculitis Study Group (EUVAS) trials (177) ascertained an overall prevalence of chronic neuropathy at any time up to 5 years in 15%, and a frequency of PNV at baseline of 8% among 506 AAV patients with PNV, that was significantly associated with systemic, cutaneous, mucous membrane and otolaryngologic manifestations of vasculitis. However, there was no association of peripheral neuropathy with renal, chest, cardiovascular, or abdominal vasculitis or overall mortality. The spectrum of CNS involvement in the patients described by de Groot (176) included granulomatous infiltration of the frontobasal cortex arising from adjacent paranasal sinuses, cerebral vasculitis, vacuolar myelopathy, and meningeal granulomatosis. The cranial nerves involved included the optic nerve, oculomotor, trigeminal and facial nerves alone or simultaneously attributable to contiguous infiltration of paranasal sinus granuloma. Cyclophosphamide and corticosteroids have been the cornerstone of remission-induction therapy for severe AAV since 1983 (25). Among 197 ANCA-positive patients with GPA or MPA in nine centers participating in the Rituximab in ANCA-Associated Vasculitis-Immune Tolerance Network (RAVE-ITN) Research Group multicenter, randomized, double-blind, double-dummy, non-inferiority trial (178), rituximab 375 mg per square meter (m2) body-surface area (BSA) per week for 4 weeks and cyclophosphamide 2 mg per kilogram of body weight per day was associated with achievement of the primary end point of remission of disease without use of prednisone at six months in 67% of study patients compared to 42% of controls.

Granulomatosis with polyangiitis in childhood has recently been reviewed (179). The criteria for cGPA requires the presence of three of the following six criteria including, abnormal urinalysis, granulomatous inflammatory on tissue biopsy, nasal-sinus-oral inflammation; subglottic, tracheal or endobronchial stenosis; abnormal chest radiograph or CT, and positive ANCA staining (6). Cabral and colleagues of A Registry for Childhood Vasculitis: e-entry (ARChiVe) Investigators Network (180) reported improved sensitivity and specificity of the 2009 EULAR/PRINTO/PRES classification criteria compared to the 1990 ACR criteria (173). Treatment and efficacy and safety data continue to be largely derived from adult GPA studies, however as described in ARChiVe, pediatric patients in the United States and Canada are being offered pulse methylprednisolone for 3 to 5 days, followed by oral prednisone, and cyclophosphamide orally or in intravenous regimens, followed by maintenance therapy, most frequently with methotrexate (180).

Microscopic Polyangiitis

Watts and colleagues applied the 1990 ACR criteria (181) and CHCC definitions (1) for systemic vasculitis to an unselected cohort of 130 patients with systemic vasculitis in a single district hospital in the United Kingdom between 1988 and 1994, ascertaining an annual incidence of MPA of 3.6 per million (182) compared to 3.6 per million for PAN. Together, four European clinical studies (183–186), one ultrastructural analysis (187), a Korean MPA clinical cohort study (188), and a recent clinical review (189) reported a total of 279 MPA patients with detailed clinicopathologic findings. Among thirty-four MPA patients described by Savage and colleagues (184) the clinical symptoms and signs at presentation were constitutional (67%), arthralgia (65%), purpura (44%), hemoptysis in (32%), abdominal pain (32%), mouth ulcers (21%), sensory peripheral neuropathy (18%), and CNS (headache, seizures) (18%). The clinical manifestations among 85 patients studied by Guillevin and colleagues (186) were instead renal (79%), weight loss (73%), skin involvement (purpura, livedo, nodules, urticarial) (62%), mononeuritis multiplex neuropathy (57%), fever (55%), arthralgia (50%), myalgia (48%), vascular manifestations (hypertension, cardiac failure, pericarditis) 50%, lung involvement (alveolar hemorrhage, pneumonitis, pleurisies) (24%), and CNS involvement (12%). Ahn and colleagues (188) noted pANCA or anti-MPO antibody positivity in 69% of Korean MPA patients, compared to 74.5% of positive ANCA in European patients, of whom 87% had a pANCA staining pattern; antibodies to PR3 were present in 8% of patients compared to MPO in 61% of those so studied as determined by ELISA. Renal function was impaired in 17% of the patients described by Savage and colleagues (184) and in all by the time of tertiary referral, further noting focal segmental necrotizing glomerulonephritis in all renal biopsies and in six postmortem examinations. Serra and colleagues (183) identified forty-two patients that manifested segmental necrotizing glomerulitis histologically in renal tissue including thirty-six who had evidence of extrarenal vasculitis of small vessels; 28 (77%) of whom were further judged to have a clinical diagnosis of vasculitis. Diagnostic histology in eighty-one of eighty-five patients described by Guillevin and colleagues (186) was obtained from renal biopsy in thirty-six patients demonstrating a pauci-immune glomerulonephritis, and in fifty-one others based on diagnostic features of vasculitis in skin, muscle, or nerve tissue. D'Agati and colleagues (187) reported renal vasculitis in arterial and arteriolar vessels in 1 μm-thick tissue sections from among twenty-four renal biopsies so studied. Among forty-three patients described by Adu and coworkers (185) forty patients had renal tissue for analysis that showed segmental thrombosing and necrotizing glomerulonephritis by biopsy (35 patients), nephrectomy (2 patients), or at postmortem examination (3 patients). The majority (37 patients) of lesions were acute, with capillary thrombosis and extracapillary proliferation forming crescents, while three other renal biopsy tissues showed only healed lesions. Twelve patients (30%) had evidence of renal extraglomerular vasculitis, including seven with arteritis (six of whom had arteriolitis) and five patients with arteriolitis without arteritis.

The treatment of MPA does not differ from other AAV. Moreover, the majority of prospective treatment trials of GPA have included MPA patients making the results applicable to both (178) even though differences in clinical presentation and outcomes could conceivably influence therapeutic strategies. An analysis of four prospective trials of 278 patients comparing PAN, MPA and EGPA (190) observed excess deaths during follow-up of MPA patients, with survival probability trends adjusted to the Five-Factor Score (FFS) (191) and the Birmingham Vasculitis Activity Score (BVAS) (192) that suggested increased mortality in MPA patients compared to the other forms of vasculitis. Of 53 patients studied by Serra and colleagues (183) all ten oliguric and untreated patients died at presentation. Among the remaining forty-three patients treated with varying immunosuppressive regimens including corticosteroids, cyclophosphamide, and azathioprine in varying combination, 33 (77%) survived the acute stage of disease, thirty of whom comprised a long-term analysis that showed stable vasculitis in 12 (40%), smoldering disease in 16 (53%) patients, and recurrent vasculitis in 2 (7%) patients. Savage and colleagues (184) noted an overall survival rate of 65%, and an actuarial survival rate of 70% at one year, with 65% at five years following treatment with prednisolone, azathioprine, and cyclophosphamide or plasma exchange in varying combination. Of five late deaths, two were from unrelated causes and at postmortem examination there was no evidence of disease activity. Two deaths, one from subarachnoid hemorrhage at four months, and another from brainstem stroke at eight months, were believed to be due to vasculitis. Adu and colleagues (185) noted an overall morality of 37% among forty-three patients following treatment with varying oral and intravenous immunosuppressant regimens in the first year following diagnosis, and a general trend toward excess mortality among twenty-four intravenously-treated compared to seventeen patients orally treated with corticosteroids and cyclophosphamide due to sepsis. Guillevin and colleagues (186) noted a relapse rate of 34% following treatment with varying immunosuppressant regimens of corticosteroids and cyclophosphamide or azathioprine, with a mortality of 33% at follow-up for a mean duration of 70 months. According to multivariate analysis, proteinuria was the only factor associated with increased mortality and cytotoxic drugs were significantly associated with lower mortality. Ahn and colleagues (188)

noted a survival rate among fifty-five patients with MPA of 94% at one year and 89% at three years with combination corticosteroids and cyclophosphamide or azathioprine given respectively to 86% and 13% of patients.

Childhood MPA is very uncommon. The criteria for diagnosis includes three of the following features including, abnormal urinalysis, granulomatous inflammation on tissue biopsy, nasal sinus inflammation, subglottic, tracheal, or endobronchial stenosis; abnormal chest radiograph or CT scan, and PR3 ANCA or cANCA staining (6). Those with cMPA accounted for four of the first 32 children in the United States/Canadian ARChiVe registry (180). Treatment of cMPA does not significantly differ from that of adults.

Eosinophilic Granulomatosis with Polyangiitis

There are a few large modern series of EGPA defined by ANCA status (193, 194). Among 383 patients enrolled in the French Vasculitis Study Group (FVSG) Cohort (193) who satisfied the ACR criteria (22) or CHCC definition for EGPA (1), the mean age at presentation was 50 years without sex predominance. Clinical manifestations at presentation included asthma (91%), peripheral neuropathy (51%), weight loss (49%), ear, nose and throat signs (48%), non-erosive sinusitis and polyposis (41%), skin lesions (39%), purpuric rash (22%), lung infiltrates (38%), gastrointestinal involvement (23%), renal manifestations (22%), cardiomyopathy (16%), CNS (5%), and cranial nerve involvement (3%). A total of 108 (31%) patients tested positive for ANCA with significantly more frequent ear, nose and throat, peripheral nerve and renal involvement, but less frequent cardiac manifestations. Healy and colleagues (194) described ninety-three patients with leukotriene receptor antagonist (LTRA)-drug-induced EGPA registered in the Food and Drug Administration Adverse Event Reporting System, who met criteria for case selection of known ANCA status and conformity to the ACR definition (22), alternatively a history of asthma, eosinophilia, and consistent histology on biopsy tissue or the postmortem findings of EGPA. So defined, the clinical manifestations included asthma (100%), peripheral blood eosinophilia (94%), pulmonary infiltrates (64%), chronic sinusitis (63%), peripheral neuropathy (51%), fever and night sweats (45%), purpuric rash (43%), arthralgia (35%), myalgia (33%); and cardiac (28%), gastrointestinal (17%), renal (17%), liver (15%), and CNS involvement (13%). Among those with peripheral neuropathy, mononeuritis multiplex was most commonly observed, while CNS involvement included visual impairment, cerebrovascular accidents, mental stage changes, cerebellar impairment, hemorrhagic events, and ptosis in order of decreasing frequency. Amaurosis fugax, superior oblique palsy, ischemic optic neuropathy, and scattered areas of retinal infarction may be presenting neuro-ophthalmologic manifestations of EGPA (195). Moreover, among 38 (41%) ANCA-positive patients described by Healy and colleagues (194) 15 demonstrated a positive ELISA, all of which were positive for anti-MPO. The finding of ANCA-negativity was associated with a decreased proportion of peripheral neuropathy, and an increased proportion of cardiac, gastrointestinal, pulmonary involvement, and outcome of a life-threatening events or death when compared to anti-MPO-positive cases.

Clues to the clinicopathologic limits of this disorder may be ascertained by examination for two diagnostically essential lesions, necrotizing vasculitis and extravascular necrotizing granulomas, with eosinophilic infiltrates (196), considered essential to the diagnosis of EGPA by Churg and Strauss (19), Chumbley and colleagues (20) and the CHCC (1), but not so by the ACR (22) that did not include the criteria of necrotizing vasculitis (22). Healy and colleagues (194) compared the occurrence of eosinophilic granuloma and necrotizing vasculitis among 46 ANCA-negative (46 patients) and 11 anti-MPO positive patients noting granulomas present respectively in one-third of tissue biopsy specimens of the former compared with none of eleven of the latter (risk difference ([RD] 32; p value .05), however necrotizing vasculitis and extravascular eosinophils were statistically insignificant between the two groups by odds ratio ([OR] computation. Among ninety-one patients reported in the literature with EGPA in whom detailed results of cutaneous nerve histopathology was available at postmortem in one patient (19) and at biopsy in the remainder (195, 197–203). Necrotizing vasculitis, extravascular granulomas, and tissue eosinophilia were found together in four nerves (203). Necrotizing vasculitis was noted alone in thirty-three nerves (19, 197, 199, 200–202) and in association with tissue eosinophilia in eight nerves (195, 198, 203), with indefinite (200) or absent vasculitis (195, 197, 202, 203) in thirty-four nerves without granuloma or tissue eosinophilia, and normal histology in twelve others (202). Among thirty-two patients with EGPA, seventeen underwent cutaneous nerve biopsy evidencing necrotizing vasculitis in 15 (88%), tissue eosinophilia in 12 (70%), and extravascular granuloma in 2 (12%). Muscle biopsy in 16 other patients showed necrotizing vasculitis in 4 (25%), and tissue eosinophilia in 2 (13%), none of which evidenced extravascular granuloma. Cutaneous nerve biopsy was not mentioned in four other studies (20, 21, 204, 205). Nor was there mention of tissue eosinophilia or extravascular granuloma in comparison groups of fifty-eight cutaneous nerve tissue biopsies from patients with multisystemic disease without evidence of EGPA, and isolated necrotizing peripheral nerve vasculitis (127, 206)) or conversely evidence of necrotizing vasculitis and either tissue eosinophilia or extravascular granuloma among eight patients with peripheral neuropathy and

hypereosinophilic syndrome to suggest a relation to EGPA (207–209). As regards the histopathology of CNS tissue in EGPA, Churg and Strauss (19) noted involvement in eight of thirteen postmortem studied patients, and cited cause of death in three patients due to subarachnoid (one patient) or cerebral hemorrhage (two patients). The FVSG Cohort remission-induction treatment of EGPA included corticosteroids for all patients, and additionally immunosuppressant therapy in 56% that included cyclophosphamide, azathioprine, methotrexate and rituximab. Altogether, one-half of the ANCA-positive patients received immunosuppressants as part of induction-remission therapy, 70% of whom continued therapy during follow-up in a proportion similar to the ANCA-negative group. Vasculitis relapse occurred in one-quarter of patients, with a greater frequency for ANCA-positive status (35% versus 22.5%). Conversely, the five-year relapse-free survival was 68% in ANCA-negative patients compared to 58% in those ANCA-positive. Deaths occurred at a mean of 5 years after diagnosis, and were attributed to cardiac events, infection, cancer, active vasculitis, and respiratory events.

Small numbers of children have been included in large studies of EGPA sufficient to allow comparisons to adults. Among 133 vasculitic patients in the ARChiVe registry, only two were reported to be of the EGPA type (170). The association between leukotriene antagonists and EGPA has been described (194, 210), a relation that cannot be explained further by corticosteroid withdrawal or pre-existing EGPA. There is a correlation between the HLA-DRB4 locus and the risk of EGPA and subsequent vasculitis severity (211). Three polymorphisms of the IL-10.2 haplotype are associated with ANCA-negative EGPA status and not GPA (212). The treatment of cEGPA is not dissimilar from adults.

IMMUNE COMPLEX-ASSOCIATED SMALL VESSEL VASCULITIS

Cryoglobulinemic Vasculitis

The presence in the serum of one or more Ig that precipitates below core body temperatures and redissolve on rewarming is termed cryoglobulinemia (213). All cryoglobulins have rheumatoid activity consisting of IgM and polyclonal IgG, and one-third had monoclonal IgM kappa components. Brouet and coworkers (214) provided a modern classification of cryoglobulinemia among eighty-six patients that included type 1, composed of a single monoclonal Ig; and types II and III as mixed cryoglobulinemia, composed of different Ig, with a monoclonal component in type II, and polyclonal Ig in type III. Type 1 was associated only with malignant hematologic disorders, while types II and III were associated with connective tissue and malignant hematologic disorders, and infectious diseases. In the absence of well-defined disease the presence of mixed cryoglobulinemia was termed "essential." Agnello and colleagues (215) demonstrated a strong association with concomitant hepatitis C virus (HCV) infection and a high rate of false negative serological tests in type II cryoglobulinemia. The finding of HCV virions and HCV antigen-antibody complexes in cryoprecipitates, most commonly associated with the RF, suggested an important role for HCV in the pathogenesis of mixed cryoglobulinemia similar to elevated antibodies to HCV in the serum of affected patients (216). The extrahepatic manifestations of chronic HCV infection included mixed cryoglobulins (217) and systemic vasculitis (218).

Disease manifestations attributed to cryoglobulinemia were found in 206 of 443 (47%) of patients from one center (219). The commonest symptom was purpura noted at presentation in 24% and during disease evolution in 15 to 33%, skin biopsy of which showed leukocytoclastic vasculitis. Neurologic manifestations were noted in 47 (23%) of which peripheral neuropathy was noted in 35 (17%) and CNS involvement in 12 (6%). Infection was the main etiologic factor noted overall in 75% of 443 patients, of which antibodies to HCV and human immunodeficiency virus (HIV) were respectively noted in 75% and 19%, and HBsAg in 3%. Concomitant autoimmune disorder was noted in 24%, hematologic disease in 7%, and essential cryoglobulinemia in 11% of patients. Type I (monoclonal IgG and IgMκ or IgGλ) cryoglobulinemia was diagnosed by immunofixation of the cryoprecipitate in 34% of patients, type II (IgMκ and polyclonal IgG) in 55%, type III in 2%, and other mixed (IgG- or IgM κ or λ) in 8%.

The frequency of HCV-negative and HCV-positive peripheral neuropathy ranged from 44% in the former to 74% in the latter (218, 220). Systemic vasculitis occurs in an estimated 10 cases per million (220) in mixed cryoglobulinemia with or without HCV (221) with a preponderance in the latter. Among 242 patients with noninfectious mixed CV in the CryoVas survey between 1995 and 2010 (222), peripheral neuropathy was noted overall in 125 (52%), with the greater frequency among those with type II (56%) compared with type III CV (22%). The overall frequency of sensorimotor (31%) types exceeded that of pure sensory (21%) neuropathy, as did those with either form in type II CV (33% and 23%) versus type II (19% and 3% respectively).

The frequency of CNS involvement in HCV-negative and HCV-positive CV ranges from nil (221) to 7% (222), 9% (218, 220) and 13% (223), with higher values in association with HCV-positivity, and some indication that increased prevalence in recent years may be due to more accurate diagnosis. With an overall mortality of 8.7% (223), and a 33% fatality rate (224), the symptom set of CNS involvement appears to be important factor in prognosis.

An inflammatory mechanism of nervous system involvement in CV has been demonstrated in histopathologic studies of several patients with cryoglobulinemia with or without HCV infection. Abramsky and Slavin (225) described polyneuropathy, encephalopathy, and seizures with corticospinal tract signs in a patient with mixed IgG-IgM cryoglobulinemia. Postmortem findings in that patient showed vasculitis in muscles, acute and subacute proliferative and membranous glomerulonephritis and multiple thrombotic occlusions of small intracerebral blood vessels with adjacent foci of ischemia accompanied by marked demyelination, without cerebral vasculitis. Gorevic and colleagues (55) described three patients with mixed cryoglobulinemia and peripheral neuropathy who presented with bilateral foot drop (one patient) or severe paresthesia. Sural nerve biopsy in one of the two latter patients revealed epineurial vasculitis. The same author (55) described two other patients had fatal CNS involvement, one of whom was studied at postmortem evidencing vasculitis of small- and medium-sized vessels. Bolay and coworkers (226) described a patient with progressive encephalomyelitis with rigidity associated with HCV infection. Postmortem examination in that patient showed perivascular lymphocytic cuffing, infiltration and neuronal loss mainly affecting the brainstem and cervical spinal cord in which polymerase chain reaction (PCR) detected HCV genome in the brain. Petty and colleagues (227) described a patient with type II cryoglobulinemia, stroke and seizures, who was found to have HCV RNA by PCR of HCV RNA and early infarction in brain biopsy tissue without vasculitis. In other patients (228, 229), a mechanism related to the cryoprecipitate has been postulated. Marshall and Malone (228) described a patient with circulating cyroglobulins, retinal hemorrhage, and pathological fractures who lapsed into fatal coma. At postmortem examination the bone marrow was infiltrated by myeloma cells. Vessels from various organs, notably small vessels of the brain, showed thrombi formed by a peculiar hyaline acidophilic material histologically identical to larger casts formed in the heart and great vessels, which was presumed to have precipitated curing cooling of the body after death. Ince and colleagues (229) described a patient with cryoglobulinemia and relapsing ischemic encephaloenteropathy. Postmortem examination in that patient showed a right basal ganglia hemorrhage, with multifocal small vessel occlusions in the brain by amorphous bland protein plugs and abundant intravascular Russell bodies in arterioles and venules with relative sparing of capillaries, and without inflammation.

The treatment of HCV-related CV is reviewed in detail (230). One concern has been the potential adverse side-effects of immunosuppressant therapy employing corticosteroids and cytotoxic agents on chronic viral infection. Alternatively, anti-viral therapy was heralded as a means to control the underlying infection that was driving immune complex formation and resultant vasculitis (231). The mainstay of therapy for HCV has been interferon (INF) alpha which can precipitate or worsen other autoimmune diseases, among them thyroid, rheumatoid arthritis, Sjogren syndrome, sarcoidosis, systemic lupus erythematosus, and immune-mediated hemolysis (232). One such patient with HCV-related mild sensory neuropathy and sural nerve biopsy evidence of necrotizing vasculitis, who was treated with subcutaneous INF alpha three times weekly, developed mononeuropathy multiplex after only two weeks of therapy (233). Aggressive optimal therapy of HCV-related CV with PEGylated (PEG)-INF alpha to improve the pharmacologic properties, and ribavirin with a protease inhibitor in the instance of HCV genotype 1 infection, should be considered as induction therapy for CV and administered for forty-eight weeks for all HCV genotypes (220). An induction phase of immunosuppression such as rituximab plus antivirals is recommended in patients with more severe HCV-related CV exemplified by worsening renal function, mononeuritis multiplex, extensive skin disease including ulcers and distal necrosis (230). Terrier and colleagues (222) showed a greater therapeutic efficacy of rituximab and corticosteroids compared with corticosteroids alone and alkylating agents with corticosteroids in achieving complete clinical, renal, and immunologic responses and a prednisone dosage of <10 mg per day at six months. However, this regimen was associated with severe infections, particularly when high doses of corticosteroids were employed. Plasmapheresis combined with immunosuppression can be useful in fulminant HCV-related CV to engender an immediate effect but should be continued to avoid post-pheresis rebound worsening. Rituximab, fludarabine, and cyclophosphamide treatment was an effective treatment for refractory CV associated with lymphoma (234). One-year, 2-year, 5-year, and 10-year survival rates of 91%, 89%, 79% and 65% respectively, have been reported in patients with CV (220) with fatalities related to serious infection in one-half and vasculitic flares in one-fifth.

Cryoglobulinemia is rarely reported in the pediatric literature. One comparison cohort (235) showed a significantly higher prevalence of prolonged fever, arthralgia, arthritis, and cutaneous involvement in children compared to adults. There are no prospective controlled trials of treatment in children to assess relative efficacy of the various available agents.

IgA Vasculitis/HSP

IgA vasculitis/HSP is the commonest vasculitis in children, with an incidence of 10 (236) to 20.4 per 100,000 (237) between the ages of 3 and 10 years (238), in association with a variety of drug, infectious and environmental precipitants.

The 1990 ACR criteria (239) for the identification of HSP included, age less than or equal to 20 years at disease onset, palpable purpura, acute abdominal pain, and tissue biopsy showing granulocytes in the walls of small arteries or venules. The presence of any two or more of these criteria distinguished 85 patients who were diagnosed as having HSP by physicians who submitted cases based on vasculitis criteria compared to 722 patients diagnosed with other forms of vasculitis, arriving at sensitivity of 87.1% and specificity of 87.7%. The addition of gastrointestinal bleeding in a classification tree format respectively increased sensitivity to 89.4% and specificity to 88.1%. The EULAR/PRINTO/PRES classification criteria (6) which recognizes the contribution of IgA deposits, differed in the mandatory finding of purpura with predominance in the legs, and the presence of one of the four including, diffuse abdominal pain, arthralgia or arthritis; a biopsy showing predominant IgA deposits, and renal involvement including proteinuria and hematuria. Derived from the analysis of 827 patients in the database, the calculated sensitivity, specificity for the clinical and laboratory findings in between the consensus panel and specific definition were respectively 100% and 87%.

Peru and colleagues (240) studied 254 children with IgAV/HSP between 2003 and 2006 with a distribution of skin, joint, gastrointestinal and renal manifestations respectively of 100%, 66%, 56% and 30%; nervous system manifestations were not mentioned. The clinical manifestations are protean (239) commencing with fever and palpable purpura, although early lesions can be urticarial (241). Arthralgia and abdominal pain precede, accompany or follow the rash. Melena is common as are signs of peritonitis. Proteinuria and hematuria are of variably severity and renal pathology may be of a mild glomerulitis to necrotizing or proliferative glomerulonephritis. Ozen and coworkers (6) noted palpable purpura, commonly in crops with lower limb predominance in 89% of patients, arthritis or arthralgia in 78%, diffuse abdominal pain in 60%, proteinuria and hematuria combined in 33%; and IgA deposition in 10% of children. According to Saulsbury (242), neurological complications are infrequently encountered including obtundation, seizures, aphasia, paresis, cortical blindness, chorea, ataxia, cranial neuropathy, peripheral neuropathy, and Guillain-Barré syndrome. Lewis and Philpott (243) described CNS complications in three children, two of whom developed xanthochromic CSF in association with severe headache, seizures, subarachnoid or intracerebral hemorrhage. Postmortem examination in one patient showed preglomerular arteriolitis. A third child had seizure and hypertension. Belman and coworkers (244) described CNS manifestations in two children, one of whom presented with status seizures, generalized headache, abdominal pain, left hemiparesis, hemianopia, and right gaze preference before cutaneous, renal and joint involvement;

a second patient presented with complex partial seizures with secondary generalization and postictal hemiparesis seven days after classic signs of IgAV/HSP. A third patient presented with PSN manifestation of brachial plexopathy and transient leg weakness during the course of IgAV/HSP. A review of the literature, inclusive of their patients, totally 79 patients, identified generalized seizures in 71%; mental status changes including behavior and depressed levels of consciousness in 71%; focal CNS deficits associated with aphasia, hemiparesis, paraparesis, quadriparesis, cortical blindness, chorea or ataxia in 33%, and headache in 9% of cases. Peripheral nervous involvement including mononeuropathy and polyneuropathy was noted in 13% of patients.

IgAV/HSP and IgAN share a number of clinical and immunologic features. Hinge region O-linked glycans of IgA1 are deficient in galactose (Gal) and sialic acid in IgAN (245–247) and IgAV/HSP children with nephritis (248, 249). IgA1 molecules deficient in sialic acid or Gal tend to aggregate and form macromolecular complexes (250). Hinge regions that interact with IgG antiglycan antibodies form IgA-IgG complexes, and underglycosylation of IgA1 hinge lead to a propensity for glomerular deposits (251). Patients with IgAV/HSP and IgAN have circulating abnormally glycosylated IgA1 and possibly glycan-specific IgG antibodies that form IgA1-IgG anti-IgA1 immune complexes (252). IgG antibodies directed against the abnormal glycosylation putatively bind to the IgA1 molecules in glomerular mesangium localizing in vessel walls causing inflammation (2). Soluble IgA and IgG aggregates catabolized by cultured rat mesangial cells induce the production of tumor necrosis factor (TNF)-alpha and IL-6 chemo-attractant cytokines (253). Murine and human mesangial cells possess a specific receptor for IgA1 that recognize hinge regions carbohydrates (254). Binding is increased with desialylation of the IgA1 molecule. There are two candidate receptors, an asialoglycoprotein (ASGPR) and Fc alpha (FcaR [CD89]). Pathogenic soluble receptor-IgA complexes in CD89 deficient transgenic mice spontaneously develop IgAN (255). Aberrant glycosylation of IgA in IgAV as suggested in IgAN with resultant polymerization and enhanced FcaR binding, may be the stimulus for FcaR shedding with subsequent deposition of the FcaR-IgA complexes in glomerular mesangium (242).

The treatment of IgAV/HSP remains empiric and largely supportive, with conflicting conclusions in retrospective and uncontrolled case series of immune suppression in severe HSP nephritis (170). Extrarenal manifestations can be managed by symptomatic treatment. A meta-analysis of 15 studies based on a comprehensive review of the literature in the Medline database from 1956 to 2007, and Cochrane Controlled Trials Registry among fifteen studies and over 1300 patients (256) found that early treatment conferred a protective effect on developing persistent renal disease (OR .43) and the likelihood of surgical intervention for abdominal pain (OR .75), as well as a statistically significant positive effect on shortening the duration of abdominal symptoms (OR.5.42).

Hypocomplementemic Urticarial Vasculitis (Anti-C1q Vasculitis)

Hypocomplementemic urticarial vasculitis is characterized by urticaria, migratory arthralgia, and persistent or intermittent hypocomplementemia. Affected patients develop urticarial, bullous, and purpuric skin lesions, sometimes severe angioneurotic edema and life-threatening laryngeal edema, accompanied by arthralgia and arthritis, conjunctivitis, episcleritis, uveitis, mild renal disease including glomerulonephritis, obstructive pulmonary disease, pericarditis, abdominal pain, and splenomegaly. Urticarial lesions affect capillary and postcapillary venues. Histopathologic examination of the persistent urticarial lesion (257) shows perivascular neutrophilic or less commonly lymphocytic infiltration, fibrinoid necrosis, leukocytoclastic vasculitis, with injury to the endothelial cells of the postcapillary venules, and erythrocyte extravasation. Direct immunofluorescence study of hemolytic uremic vasculitic syndrome HUV lesions shows immune complex and complement deposition in a granular pattern in and around blood vessels of the upper dermis, with Ig deposition, including IgG that binds to C1q where it activates complement (258). Besides complement cascade activation, C1q has been found to have other biological functions including a modulating effect on cellular functions within the adaptive immune response. Moreover, anti-C1q antibodies may have a direct pathogenic role in complement-mediated autoimmune disease including SLE and HUV (259). However it is not clear whether all anti-C1q autoantibodies have equivalent C1q-bindng specificity or clinical consequences (260). For example, anti-C1q antibody in SLE patients do not bind to reduced C1q but about 60% of HUV anti-C1q preparations do bind, a process that appears to be governed by the tertiary structure of the intact C1q collagen-like domain and recognition of specific epitopes by HUV preciptins on reduced and denatured C1q. C1q autoantibodies are also found in association with mixed cryoglobulinemia (261), monoclonal IgM gammopathy (262), fluoxetine ingestion (263), malignant disorders (264), and other connective tissue diseases apart from SLE (265). The 2012 Revised CHCC (2) considered replacing HUV with anti-C1q vasculitis, however consensus could only be reached to introduce this term in parenthesis.

Peripheral nervous system manifestations of HUV include peripheral neuropathy and cranial nerve palsies. Central nervous system involvement includes seizures, peudotumor cerebri, aseptic meningitis, and transverse myelitis (257, 266).

Antihistamines are the drug of choice with cutaneous lesions to control itching, but they may be insufficient in controlling the formation of immune complexes when given late in the inflammatory cascade. There is yet a consensus on the most effective therapeutic regimen. Plasmapheresis and IVIg are alternative modalities for immunosuppressant medications to control refractory skin lesions and in cases with renal involvement.

VARIABLE VESSEL VASCULITIS

Behçet Disease

This disorder is characterized by relapsing aphthous ulcers of the mouth, eye and genitalia (88). The most widely used diagnostic criteria of BD were formulated by the International Study Group (ISG) (267) that included recurrent oral ulcerations plus any two of genital ulceration, typical defined eye lesions, typical skin lesions, or positive pathergy. Recurrent oral ulcerations were categorized as minor aphthous, major aphthous, and herpetiform ulcerations that recurred at least three times in a 12-month period. Recurrent genital ulcerations were defined as aphthous ulceration and scarring. Eye lesions were defined as anterior uveitis, posterior uveitis or cells in the vitreous on slit lamp examination; and retinal vasculitis. Compatible skin lesions included erythema nodosum, pseudofolliculitis, papulopustular lesions, and aceneiform nodules in post-adolescent patients not receiving corticosteroids. A positive pathergy test of cutaneous hypersensitivity was defined as positive when a sterile pustule developed after twenty-four to forty-eight hours at the site of a needle prick to the skin (268). Although the usual onset of BD is in the third or fourth decade of life, pediatric onset patients have been described (269). Two population-based studies, both fulfilling ISG criteria (267) studied prevalence data for BD, including one from France (270) and another from the United States (271). The overall prevalence in France was 7.1 per 100,000, with immigrants of North African and Asian ancestry manifesting significantly higher prevalence rates of BD than those of European ancestry (17.5 per 100,000 compared with 2.4 per 100,000), comparable with those of North Africa and Asia. These suggested that BD risk was not related to age at immigration but a primarily hereditary basis. The point prevalence of BD in the United States was 5.2 per 100,000.

Genetic studies that focused on molecules related to innate immune responses (272) identified an association with endothelial nitric oxide eNOS gene located on chromosome 7q35-36, a variant of which causes deficient NOS and contributes to the pathogenesis of endothelial abnormalities, and increases thrombotic tendency in BD. Dhifallah and colleagues (273) identified a polymorphism of eNOS that was associated with BD susceptibility as well as skin lesions. Park and coworkers (274) identified single nucleotide polymorphisms of the promoter and exons regions in the cytotoxic T-lymphocyte antigen 4 (CTLA4) gene that predisposed to BD related to the immunological abnormalities and disease expression associated with BD. Kim and colleagues (275) noted that genital ulceration, eye involvement, and neurological BD (NBD) were associated with mannose-binding lectin 2 (MBL2) polymorphisms and production of high levels of MBL or functional MBL. Fei and colleagues (276) conducted a genome-wide study identifying a genetic association between BD and a single nucleotide polymorphisms (SNP) in KIAA1529, the BD-risk allele (rs2061634) that led to a substitution of serine to cysteine at amino acid position 995 in the KIAA1529 protein.

Uluduz and colleagues (277) studied two large Istanbul BD cohorts totaling 728 patients, ascertaining and comparing pediatric-onset (26 patients) and adult adult-onset (702 patients)-NBD. The mean age of pediatric-onset of BD and NBD onset were respectively 13 and 13.5 years; compared to adult-onset BD and NBD of 26 and 32 years. The commonest initial neurological symptom in the pediatric-onset patients was headache in 92% followed by seizures in 11.5%, compared to adult-onset BD that manifested corticospinal tract signs in 59% followed by headache in 58% and dysarthria in 23%. Significant differences in neurological involvement consisted of a higher frequency of cerebral venous sinus thrombosis (CVST) so noted in 88.5% of children and 17% of adults whereas parenchymal involvement was noted in 74.8% of adults compared to 11.6% of children. None of the children had associated cortical venous infarcts. Oral ulcers were noted in 100% of both groups, and there were no significant statistical differences in the occurrence of skin lesion, uveitis, or arthralgia, however genital ulcers were less common in children compared to adults (54% compared to 84%).

Headache may be due to migraine, tension-type headache, uveitis, or the direct consequence of NBD. A case-control study of headache in BD reported by Haghighi and colleagues (278) found that 65% of patients suffered from chronic headache due to migraine with aura in 1.7%, migraine without aura in 25%, tension headache in 24%, NBD in 8%, uveitis 3% and the remainder due to other factors. Frontal and occipital headache and deep-seated pain around the eyes were presenting symptoms in several patients with imminent florid involvement later studied at postmortem examination (89, 279–281), or as a clue to silent neurological involvement in other cohorts so studied (282). Cognitive impairment involving mainly memory functions occurs in BD without overt NBD, so noted in 46% of BD patients compared to none in control subjects, with high disease activity and prednisone dosage independently associated with cognitive impairment (283).

Siva and Saip (284) classified neurological involvement into two major primary types, one due to vascular-inflammatory mechanisms with focal or multifocal parenchymal involvement, presenting most often as a subacute brainstem syndrome, and another with few symptoms and more favorable prognosis, due to isolated cerebral venous sinus thrombosis and intracranial hypertension. A secondary form results instead from CNS involvement such as cerebral emboli from cardiac disease, intracranial hypertension from superior vena cava syndrome, and neurotoxicity of specific mediations employed in treatment. Mortality among neurologically-complicated clinicopathologically-confirmed cases (90) was 41%, with 59% occurring within one year of onset of neurological involvement. Among non-fatal cases, residual neurological signs are not uncommon. The neuropathological findings in BD in brain biopsies and postmortem examination have been remarkably consistent among patients over the past several decades evidencing perivascular cuffing of small meningovascular and parenchymal arteries and veins (89, 90, 279, 281, 285), rarely medium-sized arteries displaying fibrinoid degeneration and recanalization, and examples of venous thrombosis (280) generally with frank necrotizing vasculitis. The inflammatory cell infiltrates were generally comprised of lymphocytes, both T-, and B-cell, macrophages, rarely plasma cells and eosinophils, with reactive astrocytosis and microscopic gliosis in neighboring cerebral, cerebellar and brainstem white matter. Matsumoto and colleagues (286) noted large vessel lesions in seven of eight patients age 31 to 56 years with BD, including saccular aneurysms of the sinus of Valsalva or aortic arch, thoracic and abdominal aorta, pulmonary, femoral, and iliac arteries, and thrombotic occlusions in the pulmonary vein and superior and inferior vena. Aortitis was noted histologically in six of the eight patients that was active in one, scarred in six, and intermixed in another. Active aortitis was characterized by intense infiltration of inflammatory cells in the media and adventitia more frequently than in the interim with occasional giant cell formation. The scar stage was characterized by fibrous thickening of the intima and adventitia with condensation of the elastic lamina and proliferation of vasa vasorum with slight perivascular lymphocytic and plasma cell infiltrates. The patients with large venous occlusions had thrombophlebitis with luminal obstruction by organized thrombi.

CVST in BD presents with subacute or chronic onset of symptoms of isolated intracranial hypertension accompanied by headache, blurred vision, and diplopia (287) compared to those without BD in whom the onset is typically acute and associated with headache, hemiparesis, aphasia, and seizure. Venous infarcts occur in up to 63% of those with CVST of other causes, and in only 6% of patients with BD. The rarity of venous infarcts, long delay to diagnosis and clinical signs of isolated intracranial hypertension is more typical of BD-related CVST in which prothrombosis is presumed to commence as an endothelial dysfunction that takes longer to develop. Although anticoagulation would not be recommended for BD-related CVST, it might be considered in association with arterial occlusions; with both venous and arterial occlusive episodes warranting prompt consideration of corticosteroids alone or in association with another immunosuppressant agent.

Cogan Syndrome

Gluth (98) reviewed a cohort of CS seen at the Mayo Clinic between 1940 and 2002. The commonest symptoms at presentation were sudden hearing loss (50%), balance disturbance (40%), ocular irritation (32%), photophobia (23%), tinnitus (13%), and blurred vision (10%). Systemic symptoms noted alone at presentation included headache (40%), arthralgia (35%), fever (27%), myalgia (23%), abdominal pain (22%), rash (12%), peripheral neuropathy (10%), hematuria (7%), meningismis (5%), encephalitis (5%), and cerebral infarction. Otolaryngologic symptoms noted in the course of the disease included hearing loss (100%), vertigo or dizziness (90%), tinnitus (80%), ataxia (53%), oscillopsia (25%); similarly those related to inflammatory eye involvement included interstitial keratitis (77%), iritis or uveitis (37%), scleritis or episcleritis (23%), and conjunctivitis (10%). Laboratory evidence of elevated ANCA antibodies was detected in 10% of patients, both in a perinuclear pattern.

There is ample literature to attest to the variable caliber of vessels affected by the underlying vasculitic process. Pathologically-proven necrotizing vasculitis in association with CS was confirmed at postmortem examination alone in three patients (288–290), by examination of subcutaneous nodular tissue and amputated limbs in life, and later at postmortem examination in another patient (291); and by examination of biopsy tissue alone in ten living patients (288, 289, 292, 294–297). Crawford (288) observed three patients with systemic necrotizing vasculitis, both whom had headache at onset of CS. Postmortem examination in the first patient (Case 1) with frontal headaches and IK prior to onset of vestibuloauditory symptoms showed necrotizing arteritis involving small arteries and arterioles of the brain, gastrointestinal tract, and kidneys, in addition to cerebral edema and petechial hemorrhages. Eisenstein and Taubenhaus (289) reported a second postmortem description of CS and systemic vasculitis without preceding headache, in association with terminal heart failure (Case 1), in which fibrinoid necrosis of an affected aortic valve extended to the endocardium and intimal surface of the aorta. There was marked intimal thickening and fibrosis of several small intramural branches of the coronary arteries combined with dense perivascular infiltration by lymphocytes and polymorphonuclear cells. Fisher and Hellstrom (291) described a third patient with CS and systemic vasculitis, also without obvious headache, in whom initial biopsy of a subcutaneous nodule showed marked infiltration by polymorphonuclear cells throughout all coats and into the surrounding tissue of a large vein and artery, as well as in smaller arteries by a severe lymphocytic infiltrate. The amputated extremities of the same patient showed intense inflammatory cell infiltration and necrosis of the media of the distal tibial and smaller muscular arteries, with focal fibrous intimal thickening and rarely organized thrombi reminiscent of thromboangiitis obliterans or Buerger disease. Postmortem examination of the eyes and ears demonstrated IK, degeneration of the vestibular and spiral ganglia, edema of the cochlea and semicircular canals, and inflammation of the ligamentous spirale, without vascular changes. Vasculitic lesions noted in the amputated extremities were seen in some viscera. Cogan and Dickerson (290) described a patient with CS and fatal aortitis, also without preceding headache, noting severe thickening of small arteries of the aortic wall with reduplication of the elastica, and destruction of smooth and elastic tissue of the media, and infiltration of the intima and media by polymorphonuclear and mononuclear inflammatory cells. Vollerstein and coworkers (298) noted generalized aortic dilatation of the aorta at postmortem examination in one patient without mention of necrotizing vasculitis. An analysis of vessels other than the aorta in five patients, two had vasculitis in biopsy tissue of small muscular femoral arteries at the time of femoral arterial thrombosis; one patient had chronic venous inflammation at the site of thrombosis of the right arm, one had intimal fibrosis suggestive of resolved vasculitis, and one had a normal temporal artery biopsy. Darougar and colleagues (299) described a child with CS, antibodies to *Chlamydia psitaci*, and sudden cardiac arrest in whom postmortem examination showed destructive atrial and coronary artery, and aortic lesions in association with lymphocytic inflammation of the intima, without frank vasculitis:

Lunardi and colleagues (300) used pooled IgG immunoglobulin from eight patients with CS to screen a random peptide library to identify possible autoantibodies in CS. One isolated immunodominant peptide which showed similarly with the autoantigens SSA/Ro and reovirus III major core protein lambda1, and the peptide sequence of tyrosine phosphatase-1 (DEP-1/CD148), expressed on the sensory epithelia of the inner ear and on endothelial cells. IgG antibodies against the peptide purified from patient sera recognized DEP-1/CD148 protein, bound human cochlea, and inhibited proliferation of cells expressing DEP-1/CD148. The same antibodies bound *connexin*, gene mutations of which led to congenital inner-ear deafness, that induced the feature of CD in mice.

Most patients with CS (58%) treated with corticosteroids experience a favorable response in both vestibuloauditory and ophthalmologic manifestations, with the remainder demonstrating only ophthalmologic (23%) or vestibuloauditory improvement (19%) alone (98). Other therapies included methotrexate (23%), cyclophosphamide (10%), azathioprine (5%), entanercept (3%), hydroxchloroquine (2%), and IVIg (2%). Surgical cochlear implantation led to objective and subjective benefits with improved hearing recognition in 92% of patients (98).

Early recognition of the diagnosis of childhood CS is important in instituting corticosteroid therapy to preserve hearing, especially when hearing loss is a later occurrence. Such was the case in a 4-year-old girl with IK and ataxia who developed profound hearing loss over the ensuing two months when the diagnosis of CS was established and oral corticosteroid treatment commenced (301). A combination of oral and intravenous corticosteroids may be considered in children who partly but not fully improve. Chaudhuri and colleagues (302) described a 7-year-old boy who was promptly diagnosed after concomitant headache, IK and sensorineural hearing loss occurred leading to commencement of prednisone 1 mg per kilogram per day and prednisolone acetate ophthalmic 1% solution, leading to resolution of IK. The addition of pulse intravenous methylprednisolone 30 mg per kilogram per day for five doses in conjunction with a one-month course of prednisone however led to marked improvement in hearing loss.

Chronic auditory and ophthalmologic childhood disease may occur before recognition of CS similarly warranting aggressive management. Orsoni and colleagues (303) described two children with chronic ocular inflammation and hearing loss prompting consideration of CS. A 6-year-old boy had recurrent bilateral keratoconjunctivitis followed at age 13 by sudden hearing loss, headache, asthenia, and recurrent arthralgia leading to the diagnosis of CS. A 3-year-old boy had chronic bilateral uveitis from age 6 months, followed by sudden hearing loss at age 5 years accompanied by headaches and arthralgia prompting consideration of CS. Both children were treated with combination (non-corticosteroid) immunosuppressant for six months leading to resolution first of headache and arthralgia in the first two months in both children, followed by improvement in ocular inflammation and auditory symptoms.in the first child, but not in the other.

SINGLE ORGAN VASCULITIS

Primary Central Nervous System Vasculitis

Adult (116) and childhood isolated CNS angiitis (304), primary angiitis of the CNS (117), adult (305) and childhood primary CNS vasculitis (PCNSV) (306), GAB and GANS, are equivalent terms for a prototypical primary vasculitic disorder restricted to the CNS of diverse cause and clinico-pathologic expression. As originally defined, the diagnosis of PACNS (117), like IACNS (116) relied upon either classic angiographic or histopathologic features of angiitis within the CNS in the absence of systemic vasculitis or another cause for the observed findings. The typical patient with PACNS presented with headache of gradual onset often accompanied by the signs and symptoms of dementia, while only later developing focal neurological symptoms and signs. The clinical course might be rapidly progressive over days to weeks, or at times insidiously over many months with seemingly prolonged periods of stabilization. By comparison those with GAB (118) presented with headache, mental change, and elevated CSF protein content with or without pleocytosis. Hemiparesis, quadriparesis, and lethargy were associated with a poor prognosis and mandated the need for combined meningeal and brain biopsy to establish the diagnosis with certainty. Granulomatous giant cell and epithelioid cell infiltration in the walls of arteries of various caliber, from named cerebral vessels to small arteries and veins, was noted at postmortem examination. Salvarani and colleagues (305) diagnosed primary PCNSV in thirty-one patients by histopathology and seventy patients by angiography, in whom eighteen had a granulomatous inflammatory pattern, eight had a lymphocytic pattern, and five had an acute necrotizing pattern. Headache was the commonest symptoms so noted overall in 63% of patients, followed by abnormal cognition, hemiparesis and persistent neurological deficit. A granulomatous pattern of inflammation was seen most often in those with altered cognition and at an older age. Nor were there significant differences in survival when patients were stratified by treatment (prednisone alone versus prednisone and cyclophosphamide) or method of diagnosis (angiography or biopsy). Four manifestations at presentation were associated with increased mortality rate including focal neurological deficit, cognitive impairment, cerebral infarction, and large cerebral vessel involvement. Hajj-Ali and Calabrese (307) separated GANS from PACNS and the reversible cerebral vasoconstriction syndrome, so suggested by sudden, severe thunderclap-like headache with or without associated neurological deficits, and reversible angiographic findings not due to true vasculitis.

The past decade has revealed insights into childhood PACNS (cPACNS) (308), one of the many childhood inflammatory brain diseases that affect small and large vessels, as well as, anti-N-methyl D-asparatate receptor (NMDR) encephalitis, anti-neuronal antibody mediated diseases, and secondary CNS vasculitis in association with infection and rheumatic disease (309). Angiographically-negative small-vessel cPACNS (SVcPACNS) (306) leads to persistent headache, cognitive decline, mood disorder, focal seizures and abnormal brain neuroimaging in children. Among thirteen such children in whom detailed brain biopsy findings were available (310) the inflammatory cell infiltrate located in intramural arterioles, capillaries, or venules in eleven patients so studied, consisted predominantly of a mixture of lymphocytes and macrophages, with occasional plasma cells, polymorphonuclear cells, and eosinophils. Granulomatous inflammation and multinucleated giant cells were characteristically absent. Affected blood vessels were found in leptomeninges, cortex, and subcortical white matter in seven of nine specimens. The remaining two patients without definable vasculitis exhibited nonspecific perivascular lymphocytic inflammation. A similar pathology was noted in the distribution of large named cerebral vessels and single stenosis on cerebral angiography in a child with focal seizures and large arterial ischemic lesions (304).

Sound treatment begins with an accurate diagnosis and the exclusion of disorders that mimic primary CNS vasculitis. Unrecognized and therefore untreated, the prognosis is generally dismal. Cerebral angiography, high-resolution MRA and CTA, all provide complementary information however a small vessel vasculitis may escape detection, making it necessary to contemplate combined brain and meningeal biopsy for tissue confirmation. Treatment with corticosteroids offers the best assurance of arrest of progressive arteritis and forestalls cerebral damage, with added benefit in refractory patients with the addition of a second immunosuppressant such as azathioprine. One retrospective analysis (119) found that cyclophosphamide conferred little benefit over azathioprine in patients with GAB so treated and in fact, increased the risk for potentially fatal side effects.

Isolated Aortitis (IgG4)

Isolated noninfectious aortitis comprises disorders characterized by chronic inflammation within the aortic wall (311). The Japanese investigators of the Ministry of Health, Labor and Welfare Japan G4 team (312) concurred on the terminology IgG4-RD, a term that was similarly approved by members of a 2012 International Symposium on IgG4-Related Disease held in Boston, Massachusetts (313). The most recent CHCC nomenclature (2) regards isolated aortitis as an SOV with limited expression of IgG4-RD. In a twelve year nationwide Danish population-based study (314), aortic aneurysms and dissections were the most common indication for surgery so noted in 76% of patients. The prevalence of aortitis among 1,210 resected thoracic aorta samples was 6.1%, with nearly three-quarters being idiopathic and one-quarter associated with disease known to cause aortitis. Only 14% were linked to GCA and none to TAK. Among thirty-six patients reported by Rojo-Leyva and colleagues (78) with aortitis not related to prior systemic disease in which disease was restricted to the thoracic aortic aneurysmal segment, the mean age was 65 years (range 36 to 79 years). Only one patient of the thirty-six had systemic symptoms concurrent with aortic dissection. Eleven patients were treated with corticosteroid therapy in varying dosages, and none developed new aneurysms, while six of twenty-five not so treated developed additional aneurysms. In forty-seven of the fifty-two patients inflammation was part of the histopathologic features found within an aneurysm, and in 96% of those, disease was identified within the thoracic aorta while others occurred in the abdomen. The HLA DRB1*0405 and DQB1*0401 serotypes increased susceptibility to IgG4-RD in Japanese populations.

Large thoracic vessel FDG-uptake, useful in detecting inflammatory changes in affected patients similar to GCA (136) may have a role in the preoperative evaluation of aortic aneurysm to identity those with an underlying inflammatory autoimmune basis due to IgG4-RD. A review of sixty-four patients with mostly idiopathic aortitis undergoing ascending aortic aneurysm resection found additional vascular imaging abnormalities in 72% of patients (315), while another study (316) described manifestations of systemic arterial disease in two-thirds of forty-five patients with noninfectious aortitis, one-half of whom had idiopathic aortitis. Therefore it is plausible that a proportion of aortitis patients might have vasculitis affecting other vessels in addition to the aorta, although in some arterial disease might be due to atherosclerosis and hypertension (317).

Neurological involvement may be a clue to the diagnosis when there are ischemic cranial symptoms. Headache, so noted in 14% of patients with aortitis with concomitant GCA or TAK (317) may be a clue to infectious aortitis when it occurs in association with fever and other constitutional symptoms, or in association with another systemic inflammatory disorder (318).

The histopathologic analysis of biopsy specimens has been the cornerstone of the diagnosis of IgG4-RD. A 2012 consensus statement on the pathology of IgG4-RD by Deshpande and colleagues (319) proposed a terminology scheme for the diagnosis of IgG4-RD based upon the morphological appearance and tissue IgG4+ plasma cell counts in biopsy tissue. Three histopathologoical features associated with IgG4-RD included a dense lymphoplasmacytic infiltrate, fibrosis arranged at least focally in a storiform pattern, and obliterative phlebitis in morphological specimens. The majority of cells were T-cell with scattered B-cells, and an essential component of plasma cells with occasional eosinophils and macrophages. The storiform-type pattern of fibrosis resembled the spokes of a cart wheel with spindle cells radiating from a center, buried within the lymphoplasmacytic infiltrates. Some

needle biopsies may be deficient in the storiform pattern of fibrosis. Venous channels obliterated by the lymphoplasmacytic infiltrate require elastin stains for identification. While the presence of arteritis occasionally noted in some patients does not exclude the diagnosis of IgG4-RD, and necrotizing arteritis is not a feature of IgG4-RD, nonnecrotizing lymphocytoplasmic vascular infiltrates may occur. IgG4- immunostaining is the other essential aspect of the diagnostic evaluation of biopsy tissue in IgG4-RD. The finding of dense infiltrates of IgG4+ plasma cells that number >50 per high power field are highly specific for the diagnosis. The IgG4-to-IgG ratio was a more powerful tool than IgG4+ plasma cell counts, incorporating an IgG4+/IgG plasma cell ratio of >40% as a comprehensive cut-off in any organ. IgG4+ cells can be counted using a printed photograph of the microscopic field at a 40X lens, or counted directly under the microscope preferably in areas of intense IgG4 hot spots to be more representative. Most laboratories use a mouse monoclonal antibody again human IgG4 clones designed to bind to the Fc portion of the IgG4 molecule. After a thorough analysis, the histopathology can be rated highly suggestive, probable or insufficient to diagnose IgG4-RD.

The pathobiology of the IgG4 antibody is being understood (320). It represents less than 5% of the total IgG in healthy individuals but levels are tightly regulated. The unique biology has been reviewed by Nirula and colleagues (321). It has a unique structural and functional property that undergoes half antibody exchange in vivo resulting in recombined antibodies composed of two different binding specificities. Their production is driven in part by Th2 cytokines that mediate allergic reactions and IgE production. It does not activate complement pathways and has reduced effector function relative to other IgG subtypes. Yet it remains unclear as to whether IgG4 directly mediates the disease process or reflects a protective response induced by anti-inflammatory cytokines, making it simply a valuable biological marker of IgG4-RD.

A Japanese consensus management guideline (322) suggested the initiation of oral prednisolone for induction of remission at a dose of 0.6 mg per kilogram per day for 2 to 4 weeks, with tapering by 5 mg every one to two weeks based on clinical manifestations, biochemical blood tests, and repeated imaging, to a maintenance dose of 2.5 to 5 mg per day for up to 3 months. Re-administration of corticosteroids is advised for treating relapses. Treatment with azathioprine, mycophenolate mofetil and methotrexate can be used as corticosteroid sparing agents or as remission-maintenance drugs after corticosteroidinduced remissions. Patients with recurrent or refractory disease and B-cell depletion may be considered for rituximab (320).

Non-Systemic Peripheral Nerve Vasculitis

Vasculitic neuropathy is a heterogeneous disorder that presents in the setting of systemic vasculitis, but in some patients, necrotizing vasculitis may remain clinically and pathologically restricted to the PNS, affecting peripheral nerve and muscle tissue, analogous to primary CNS vasculitis, which is recognized by the revised 2012 CHCC (2) as a SOV and not just a limited expression of one of the systemic vasculitides. The Peripheral Nerve Society (108) established guidelines for the classification, diagnosis, investigation, and immunosuppressant treatment of isolated PNV so-called non-systemic vasculitic neuropathy (NSVN). Pathologically-definite vasculitic neuropathy was defined as meeting the pathological criteria for an active or chronic lesion respectively demonstrating cellular invasion of the walls of blood vessels and one or more signs of active or chronic lesions respectively showing signs of acute vascular damage (fibrinoid necrosis, endothelial loss/disruption, internal lamina loss/fragmentation, smooth muscle media loss/fragmentation/separation, acute thrombosis, vascular/perivascular hemorrhage or leukocytoclasia) or chronic vascular damage with repair (intimal hyperplasia, fibrosis of media, adventitial/periadventitial fibrosis or chronic thrombosis chronic thrombosis with recanalization), without evidence of another primary disease process that could mimic vasculitis pathologically such as lymphoma, lymphomatoid granulomatosis or amyloidosis. Probable vasculitic neuropathy included pathologically predominant axonal changes and perivascular inflammation accompanied by signs of active or chronic vascular damage or perivascular or vascular inflammation plus one of the many possible pathological predictors of vasculitis (vascular deposition of complement, IgM, or fibrinogen by direct immunofluorescence; hemosiderin deposits; asymmetric/multifocal nerve fiber loss or degeneration; prominent active axonal degeneration; myofiber necrosis, regeneration, or infarcts in concomitant peroneus muscle biopsy tissue [not explained by underlying myopathy]). Accordingly, NSVN was recognized by satisfaction of either pathologically definite or probable vasculitic neuropathy; without symptoms, signs, or laboratory evidence of involvement of other organs (demonstrable by laboratory evidence of PR3-, MPO-ANA, mixed cyroglobulins, SSA, SSB, Sm, RNP, Scl-70, centromere, dsDNA, CCP serology; ESR >100 mm per hour, tissue biopsy evidencing vasculitis in another organ other than muscle; serologic, PCR or culture evidence of a specific infection associate with vasculitis), and absence of predisposing vasculitic conditions or factors other than diabetes (connective tissue diseases, sarcoidosis, inflammatory bowel disease, active malignancy, HUV, cutaneous PAN, or drugs likely to cause vasculitis). Inflammation of microvessels less than 40 to 70 μm in diameter without vascular damage, so-called microvasculitis, was considered nonspecific, without a definite relation to necrotizing vasculitis.

There have only been a few postmortem studied patients with presumed NSVN. Kernohan and Woltman (8) reported a 54-year-old man with five years of progressive generalized painful peripheral neuropathy that was so severe before death that he was partially paralyzed, and unable to speak or swallow. Postmortem examination showed PAN limited to the nerve trunks of the arms and legs. The brain, cranial nerves, and spinal cord were normal except for early acute changes without evidence of vasculitis. Examination of all other organs failed to reveal a single vascular lesion, except one small artery in the capsule of the prostate gland. Torvik and Berntzen (323) described a 76-year-old woman with diffuse fever, pain, and central scotoma of the eye that improved with corticosteroids. A biopsy of the temporal artery and pectoralis muscle disclosed necrotizing arteries of small arteries and arterioles of the pectoral muscle, and in small adventitial vessels of the temporal artery without frank temporal arteritis. Postmortem examination showed no signs of vasculitis from any visceral organ as well as the CNS, only evidence of healed or slightly active vasculitis in numerous small arteries and arterioles of muscle and nerve tissue measuring 50 to 200 μ in diameter. Younger and colleagues (10) reported a 59-year-old diabetic patient with lumbosacral radiculoplexus neuropathy in whom sural nerve biopsy demonstrated non-necrotizing vasculitis with vessel wall inflammation and reactive luminal connective tissue suggesting recanalization of a thrombus. An adjacent nerve fascicle showed marked focal loss of myelinated nerve fibers. He was treated with intravenous corticosteroids and cyclophosphamide but died several weeks later. Postmortem examination showed no evidence of vasculitis in any visceral organ or in tissue blocks from the femoral, sciatic or extradural lumbar plexus. However there was perivascular epineurial and adjacent endoneurial vascular inflammation.

Kissel and colleagues (127) reported that 4.5% of 350 consecutive nerve biopsies performed at a single institution evidenced peripheral neuropathy secondary to necrotizing angiopathy. Six patients manifested a distal symmetrical sensorimotor polyneuropathy, while ten had a mononeuritis multiplex presentation, eight of whom had overlapping involvement of peripheral nerves that obscured the picture of mononeuritis. In three-quarters (12 patients), a specific underlying collagen vascular disease was not diagnosed despite extensive clinical, radiologic, and serological evaluation. Said and colleagues (206) studied 100 patients with necrotizing arteritis in muscle or nerve biopsy tissue that occurred in the context of a connective tissue disorder in fifty-five patients and in association with a disorder unrelated to connective tissue pathology in thirteen others. The commonest complaints at presentation in this cohort were specific cutaneous manifestation of vasculitis, including livedo, cutaneous necrosis, and nodules in one-third. Thirty-two patients had neuropathy only and necrotizing arteritis, the most common complaints of which were spontaneous pain of neurogenic or muscle origin (48%). More recently, Collins and colleagues (324) described forty-eight patients with NSVN, 85% of whom had extensive, overlapping involvement of multiple nerves. Fibular nerve and peroneus muscle tissue biopsy was 58% diagnostically sensitive compared to 47% for sural nerve biopsy for the diagnosis of vasculitis. Combination therapy with corticosteroids and cytotoxic agents was more effective than corticosteroids monotherapy for inducing remission and improving disability, with trends toward reduced relapses and chronic pain. Overall, 21% of patients died over the period of 63-month follow-up, five (10%) of whom were related to the disease or treatment, including two patients who succumbed to pulmonary emboli as a result of limited mobility of the legs or myocardial infarction in another; and two patients, one of whom had fatal sepsis and another metastatic bladder cancer as a consequence of cyclophosphamide toxicity.

Recommendations for the treatment of NSVN (108) include prednisone monotherapy unless there is rapidly progressive neuropathy consistent with the practice of small-to-medium vessel primary systemic vasculitis at the dose of 1 mg per kilogram per day, with tapering over one year to a low dose. Combination therapy employing cytotoxic drugs include cyclophosphamide, methotrexate, and azathioprine. Other agents such as IVIg may be effective as adjunctive therapy. Careful monitoring should be performed to observe desired therapeutic responses and to avoid potentially serious drug side effects.

VASCULITIS ASSOCIATED WITH COLLAGEN VASCULAR DISEASE

Systemic Lupus Erythematosus

The early concepts of the collagen-vascular disorders introduced by Klemperer (325, 326) stemmed from the appreciation of fibrinoid necrosis using collagen staining in patients with SLE. As collagen swells and fragments, it dissolves to form a homogeneous hyaline and granular periodic acid-Schiff (APS)-positive material. The latter fibrinoid material contained immunoglobulins, antigen–antibody complexes, complement, and fibrinogen. The organ-specific responses in the CNS of this fibrinoid material lead to recognizable clinical sequela due to vascular and parenchymal damage. Khamashta and colleagues (327) described the CNS manifestations of SLE that included those associated with focal ischemia such as transient ischemic attack, ischemic

infarction, and cerebral venous thrombosis; complications presenting as ocular ischemia including amaurosis fugax, retinal artery and vein thrombosis, cilioretinal artery occlusion, and choroidal infarction; and the sequelae of myelopathy, Guillain-Barré syndrome, migraine, chorea, and seizures. The ACR criteria for SLE (328) recognized only psychosis and seizures as attributes of CNS lupus. Borowoy and colleagues (329) noted a prevalence of neuropsychiatric lupus (NPSLE) of 6.4% in a cohort of 1,253 SLE patients defined by the ACR (330) compared to the reported estimates of NPSLE in 14 to 39% in children and adults. Headache was regarded as a non-specific minor NP manifestation of chronic disease, along with mild cognitive impairment and depression. According to Tomic-Lucic and colleagues (331) those with so-called late-onset SLE due to development of disease after age 50 years, had a frequency of NPSLE of 6.6% compared to 36.6% in early-onset disease along with a higher prevalence of comorbid conditions and higher Systemic Lupus International Collaborating Clinics/ACR damage index, despite less major organ involvement and more benign course. Once thought to be an important cause of CNS or cerebral lupus, true vasculitis was present in only 12% of postmortem examinations in the series of Johnson and colleagues (332); and in 26.7% of late-onset SLE patients compared to 16.6% of those with early-onset SLE. A comparison of the cumulative incidence of clinical manifestations in the two latter groups showed that seizures were more common in early-onset patients compared to later-onset patients (6.6% versus 0%), similarly for multiple cerebrovascular attacks (23.3% versus 3.3%), cranial and peripheral neuropathy (6.6% versus 3.3%). There was no mention of CNS vasculitis among 150 patients with SLE described by Estes and Christian (333). Neurological complications were noted in 30% of patients, which included focal deficits, seizures, dementia, stupor, and coma. Psychiatric involvement included organic affective, delusional and hallucinatory syndromes in 3.5% of 50 clinicopathologic cases of SLE, one-half of whom had CNS lesions compiled by Devinsky and colleagues (334). Feinglass and colleagues (335) noted neuropsychiatric manifestations at onset of SLE among 3% of 140 patients compared to 37% in the course of the illness; however headache was not specifically tabulated. Cerebral dysfunction in SLE can be caused by large vessel or small vessel involvement or both. In the series by Fienglass and colleagues (335), vasculitis was noted overall in 28% of patients, as well as in 46% of those with neuropsychiatric involvement compared to 17% of patients lacking neuropsychiatric involvement. Postmortem examination of the CNS in ten of nineteen fatalities showed two cases of multiple large and small infarcts, which in one of them, demonstrated inflammatory cell infiltrates in the walls of medium-sized vessels, and perivascular infiltrates around small arterioles. Although active CNS vasculitis was absent in the brain and spinal tissue of all fifty patients reported by Devinsky and colleagues (334), two had evidence of inactive healed CNS vasculitis so suggested by focal disruption of the elastic lamina and mild intimal proliferation of a single medium-sized artery, one of which had active systemic vasculitis of the PAN type, both of which evidenced Libman-Sacks endocarditis and embolic brain infarcts. Focal angiitis of the CNS with cyst-like formation around affected blood vessels was noted at postmortem in the patient described by Mintz and Fraga (336) with typical SLE rash, cutaneous vasculitis, and active neuropsychiatric involvement. Trevor and colleagues (337) summarized the literature of large named cerebral vessel occlusions from 1958 to 1965 noting one patient with an MCA stenosis progressing to occlusion and three others with angiographic ICA occlusions, adding three new patients and suggesting a relation of the occurrence to cerebral arteritis. Two women, one age 21 and the other age 42 years, presented with headache followed by focal neurological symptoms attributed respectively to lesions along the left middle cerebral artery (MCA) followed by right internal carotid artery (ICA) occlusions, and a right MCA stenosis progressing to occlusion in four months. A third patient had a left ICA occlusion without mention of headache. Johnson and colleagues (332) attributed the vasculitic nature of this process histopathologically to cerebral vasculitis mediated by acute inflammation and necrosis. Younger and colleagues (338) reported large named cerebral vessel occlusion attributed to circulating anticardiolipin antibodies in a young man in whom a vasculitis mechanism was not evoked.

A number of fluorescent antibody tests provide serological support of SLE. The antinuclear antibody (ANA) screen produces a homogenous pattern in the majority of patients, with antibodies to native double-stranded DNA (anti-dsDNA) and reactivity to the smith (Sm) and ribonucleoprotein (RNP) antigens, the combination of which constitutes the extractable nuclear antigen (ENA). Circulating IgG and IgM antibodies with an affinity for charged phospholipids, antiphospholipid antibodies (APA), some of which have procoagulant activity such as the lupus anticoagulant (LAC) and the generic anticardiolipin (aCL) antibody assay using cardiolipin as the antigen probe for APA are all important determinants of prothrombotic events, especially in the CNS wherein there is a propensity for occlusive microangiopathy.

Circulating SLE-related antibodies can impact on the CNS by affecting both vascular mechanisms and brain tissue directly (327). Immune complex mediated vasculitis probably affecting small vessels is thought to account for much of the damage in CNS lupus in spite of the paucity of cerebral vasculitis evident in the form of inflammatory infiltrates in vessel walls at postmortem examination.

In those with discrete vascular infarcts, there is a known association with the presence of circulating pathogenic antibodies which predisposes some individuals to a high risk of stroke due to both small and large vessel occlusion (338, 339). Lupus cerebritis and meningoencephalitis are two neurological disturbances that can be associated with preceding headache. So noted in up to 75% of patients with SLE depending upon criteria (340), an etiopathogenesis related to antibody-mediated neuronal dysfunction is likely given the lack of correlation of symptoms of NPSLE and CNS lesions at postmortem examination, together with the transient nature of the disturbance. Patients with SLE are predisposed to infectious episodes due to impaired B-cell function and humoral immunity, in addition to others receiving immunosuppressant medication rendered impaired in T-cell function and cell mediated immunity (340). The treatment of CNS Lupus should be guided by the tempo of the presenting neurological features, duration of disease activity, results of serological studies, comorbid disorders, and the presence of true vasculitis, with most patients offered corticosteroids and those with true vasculitis of the brain considered for combination or more aggressive immunosuppressant therapy. Despite less major organ involvement and decreased incidence of neurological complications overall, late-onset SLE has a poor prognosis because of the higher frequency of comorbid conditions, longer exposure to classical vascular risk factors and both the less likelihood of treatment with higher doses of corticosteroids and the concomitantly higher rate of complications to cyclophosphamide when administered (331).

Rheumatoid Arthritis

A joint working group from the ACR and the European League Against Rheumatism (EULAR) published the 2010 classification criteria for RA (341). Extra-articular RA (ExRA) occurrence is associated with increased comorbidity and mortality (342). Criteria for severe ExRA were proposed in 2004 (343). Active RA with high disease activity is associated with increased risk of severe ExRA manifestations. Major cutaneous vasculitis and vasculitis involving other organs, are two such ExRA occurrences (343). The diagnosis of RA vasculitis (RAV) has generally been ascertained according to the criteria of Scott and Bacon (344) so defined by the presence of one or more of the following: 1) mononeuritis multiplex; 2) peripheral gangrene; 3) biopsy evidence of acute necrotizing arteritis plus fever and weight loss; and 4) deep cutaneous ulcers or active ExRA disease if associated with typical digital infarcts or biopsy evidence of vasculitis. Watts and colleagues (345) reported an annual incidence of RAV of 11.6 per million inhabitants between 1988 and 1992 in the Norfolk area of the United Kingdom, and a rate of 3.6 per million between 1998 and 2002.

Myasoedova and coworkers (346) reported a retrospective population-based cohort study of 463 RA patients (mean age 55.6 years) followed for a mean of 6.3 years in Olmsted County, Minnesota, from 1995 to 2007, two-thirds of whom had rheumatoid factor (RF) positivity. The ten-year cumulative incidence of any ExRA manifestations (among them cutaneous and other organ vasculitis) was 50.1% and severe ExRA was 6.7%, similar to 147 patients who comprised the 1985 to 1994 cohort respectively of 46.2% and 9.7%. The ten-year cumulative incidence of vasculitis, but not other ExRA, was significantly lower in the 1995–2007 cohort (0.6%) compared to the 1985 to 1994 cohort (3.6%). The decrease in the cumulative ten-year incidence of RAV suggested that the pattern of occurrence of this ExRA manifestation might be changing in recent years. Notwithstanding, markers of RA severity including RA positivity, erosion and joint destructive changes (21% among those in the 1985 to 1994 cohort, compared to 29% in 1995 to 2007), use of methotrexate, other disease-modifying anti-rheumatic drugs, and use of systemic corticosteroids were significantly associated with ExRA development between 1995 and 2007. A near one-half difference in mortlity risk after the occurrence of severe ExRA in the 1995 to 2007 cohort compared with the 1985 to 1994 cohort (Hazard Ratio [HR] of 2.1 versus 0.6) was not statistically significant.

Vollerstein and colleagues (347) studied 52 patients with RAV at the Mayo Clinic between 1974 to 1981 who developed clinical vasculitis as demonstrated by classic ischemic skin lesions, mononeuritis multiplex, or a positive tissue biopsy in comparison to population controls. The median duration of RA was 10 years and the mean age of the cohort was 60 years. The initial manifestation of vasculitis was seen in skin (26 patients), nerve (20 patients) or both (3 patients), and mononeuritis multiplex presented in one (2 patients), two (9 patients), three (5 patients) or four nerves (4 patients). More than 90% of tissue biopsy specimens revealed vascular necrosis and inflammation. A diagnosis 80% of patients began therapy with aspirin and other non-steroidal anti-inflammatory drugs, however three-fourths continued or began corticosteroid therapy. Sixteen of the original 52 patients eventually received cytotoxic immunosuppressive therapy. Compared to the general population, those with RAV had decreased survival that was immediately evident and continued for six years. A previously reported incidence cohort (348), adjusted for referral bias, reported no difference in survival after the diagnosis of vasculitis between RAV and classic RA. The factors that predicted decreased survival of RAV in a univariate proportional-HR model included older age, failure to receive previous non-steroidal anti-inflammatory drugs, previous administration of cytotoxic immunosuppressive agents, a higher dose of corticosteroids at diagnosis, decision to continue or initiate corticosteroids, and abnormal urinary sediment.

Ouyang and coworkers (349) estimated CNS involvement in RA to be extremely uncommon, and other authors (350, 351) found CNS vasculitis to be decidedly rare. Puéchal and colleagues (352) found vasculitic involvement of vasa nervorum of both small- and medium-sized arteries indistinguishable from PAN in 64% of patients, with a mortality ranging from 28 to 44% according to the length of follow-up. Epineurial and perineurial vasculitis was observed with the same frequency among those with primary sensory neuropathy as others with predominant motor involvement, respectively 67% versus 64%. A greater extent of the neuropathy and motor involvement tended to predict decreased survival, however mononeuritis multiplex was not associated with a poorer five-year survival rate (57%) than was distal symmetrical sensory or sensorimotor neuropathy (55%). Scott and Bacon (344) reported that five patients (24%) died in the group receiving methylprednisolone and cyclophosphamide; postmortem examination in four of whom failed to demonstrate active vasculitis. By comparison, seven patients (29%) died receiving other treatments, of whom postmortem examination in one of two so studied showed active vasculitis.

Three forms of vasculitis classically occur in RA affecting all calibers of blood vessels from dermal postcapillary venules to the aorta, usually in association with circulating IgM and IgG rheumatoid factor as measured by the latex fixation test, decreased complement levels, and a positive ANA. The first form of vasculitis is a proliferative endarteritis of a few organs, notably the heart, skeletal muscle, and nerves characterized by inflammatory infiltration of all layers of small arteries and arterioles, with intimal proliferation, necrosis, and thrombosis. The second is fulminant vasculitis indistinguishable from PAN with less severe leukocytosis, myalgia, renal and gastrointestinal involvement, and bowel perforation. The third type takes the form of palpable purpura, arthritis, cryoglobulinemia, and low complement levels. The literature contains references to RAV with involvement of the CNS at postmortem examination in only nine patients.

Detailed postmortem findings evidencing CNS vasculitis have been reported in nine patients (349–351, 353–357). The neurological presentations included delirium, confusion, seizures, hemiparesis, Gerstman-like syndrome, blindness, and peripheral neuropathy. Postmortem examination showed widespread systemic vasculitis in three patients (353, 355, 356). Two patients demonstrated single major cerebral artery involvement including Case 1 described by Steiner and Gelbloom (351) with foci of fibrinoid deposition and early necrosis of muscle cells along the vertebral artery; and isolated necrotizing basilar arteritis in Case 3 of Klemper and coworkers (354). Case 2 of Steiner and colleagues (351) demonstrated arteritis of medium and small-sized vessels of the subarachnoid space extending to deep cerebral white matter.

The patient described by Pirani (353) was reported to have generalized PAN of the CNS. Patient 1 of Johnson and colleagues (356) was noted to have inflammatory lesions of the PAN type affecting meningeal arteries varying from acute necrotizing to subacute to partly healed ones. The patient described by Ouyang and colleagues (349) had isolated CNS vasculitis affecting the temporal lobes and brainstem with diffuse infiltrative thickening of the pia arachnoid, rheumatoid nodular formation, and inflammatory cell infiltration of leptomeningeal vessels and the immediately subjacent brain tissue including the midbrain, medulla, and upper cervical cord. The patient described by Ramos and Mandybur (350) displayed chronic perivasculitis, transmural chronic inflammatory cell infiltration with severe fibrinoid necrosis of the media of small leptomeningeal vessels and cortical arterioles. Case 3 of Sokoloff and Bunim (355) cited vasculitic brain lesions without further elaboration. Watson and coworkers (357) described a patient with necrotizing vasculitis affecting only the CNS present in both hemispheres, as well as, the pons and spinal cord.

Despite development of new and potent drugs for RA, there are no available evidence-based recommendations for treatment of systemic rheumatoid vasculitis (358). Complete remission of systemic rheumatoid vasculitis in nearly three-fourths treated with rituximab, with a significant decrease in daily prednisone dosage and an acceptable toxicity profile, made it a suitable therapeutic option to induce remission but maintenance therapy was necessary. Bartels and Bridges (359) recommended prednisone therapy to initially decrease systemic inflammation with a dose dependent upon the degree of systemic inflammation and level of organ system involvement. The presence of CNS involvement mandated intravenous corticosteroid therapy and consideration of cytotoxic or biologic agents, among them methotrexate, azathioprine, cyclophosphamide, anti-TNF agents and rituximab. Bartolucci and colleagues (360) reported the successful induction of a prompt symptomatic response in ten patients with systemic vasculitis not responsive to conventional treatment, including two with RA and associated vasculitis. Puechal and colleagues (361) demonstrated evidence of efficacy of adjunctive anti-TNF therapy and corticosteroids for treatment of active refractory systemic RAV with remission achieved in two-thirds of patients, and a significant decrease in prednisone dose, with a higher risk of infection in the most severely ill patients.

VASCULITIS DUE TO SUBSTANCE ABUSE

Amphetamines

Amphetamines are available in powder, capsule, tablet, and injectable fluid form, and can be swallowed, snorted or taken intra-nasally, smoked or injected with highly variable purity and dosage equivalence. Their potent systemic effects include elevation of blood pressure, pulse rate, and increased level of alertness, sometimes in association with insomnia, excitability, panic attacks, and aggressive behavior. Ecstacy refers to different hallucinogenic amphetamine derivatives that contain 3, 4-methylene-dioxymethamphetamine (MDMA) and 3, 4-methylenedioxyethylamphetamine (MDE) as the main components. Ecstacy alters brain serotonin concentrations, and postsynaptic 5-HT2 receptors play a role in the regulation of brain microvessel. The CNS toxic effects are mitigated through blockage of dopamine (DA) uptake and stimulation DA and norepinephrine (NE) release, as well as possible involvement upon serotonergic and endogenous opiate system. The neurotoxic effects of methamphetamine are believed to be mediated by multiple mechanisms including generation of free radicals, nitric oxide, excitotoxicity, mitochondrial dysfunction, apoptosis, and the induction of immediate early inflammatory genes and transcription factors. Methamphetamine is the most potent amphetamine and the most commonly abused. All forms of amphetamine administration increase the risk of stroke that may be ischemic, hemorrhagic and intraparenchymal (362) occurring with a frequency four times that of nonusers (363), surpassing the rate of hemorrhagic stroke caused by cocaine use with ORs respectively of 4.95 versus 2.33 (364). Amphetamines and methamphetamine are the second commonest cause of all strokes after cocaine, occurring largely in persons younger than 45 years.

Cintron and colleagues (365) described multi-organ arteritis including the CNS in a highly publicized report of fourteen Los Angeles multidrug abusers. The drug closest to a common denominator was methamphetamine used intravenously by all but two patients and exclusively by one. Acute vessel lesions of fibrinoid necrosis of the media and intima with infiltration by polymorphonuclear cells, eosinophils, lymphocytes and histiocytes, was followed by vascular elastic and vascular smooth muscle destruction resulting in lesions considered typical for PAN. Two patients one abbreviated D.G. and the other E.V., who injected methamphetamine via intravenous injection, had arterial lesions in cerebral, cerebellar, and brainstem pontine vessels however detailed histopathologic descriptions were not provided. Their report was followed by correspondence by Gocke and Christian (366) who contended that exposure to the Australia antigen of hepatitis B antigen was likely in their cohort (365) associated with circulating immune complexes and complement activation. The authors (367) responded that 30% of sera from drug abuse patients ultimately tested positive for the Australia antigen but those with antigen-positive sera who had used drugs others than methamphetamine had no evidence of angiitis when studied angiographically. Baden (368) wrote that he had not observed a causal relation between drug abuse and necrotizing arteritis at the Office of Chief Medical Examiner of New York City for the past one-half century among thousands of autopsied drug abusers, and that substantiation of necrotizing arteritis was presented in only four of the fourteen patients. Citron and Peters (367) responded that evidence of aneurysms noted in thirteen patients was in their opinion ample evidence of arteritis. Two decades later, cerebral vasculitis was demonstrated in a dubious report (369) of a three-week postpartum woman who took her first over-the-counter Dexatrim diet pill containing phenylpropanolamine in many months followed 90 minutes later by sudden headache, nausea vomiting. Brain CT showed subarachnoid blood with a frontal lobe hematoma and bilateral carotid angiography demonstrated diffuse segmental narrowing and dilatation of small, medium and large vessels and branches of the anterior and posterior circulation. Evacuation and histopathologic analysis of the hematoma showed necrotizing vasculitis of small arteries and veins with infiltration of polymorphonuclear leukocytes particularly prominent in the intima with fragmentation of the elastic lamina and areas of vessel occlusion. It was unclear whether the findings were related to primary or drug-related CNS vasculitis. Treatment with cyclophosphamide for 6 months was associated with almost complete resolution of cerebral angiographic abnormalities.

Amphetamine was not the definite agent of purported cerebral vasculitis in the patient described by Kessler and colleagues (370) with an acute intracerebral hemorrhage. Nor was amphetamine the causative agent in the patient reported by Bostwick (371) with ischemic stroke in two multi-drug abusers of heroin, cocaine, and amphetamine and beading of small tributaries of the middle cerebral artery (370). Neither was amphetamine the proven cause of vasculitis in occlusion of the right internal carotid artery (371). Postmortem examination in the first patient (370) showed occasional intramural mononuclear and polymorphonuclear cellular infiltration of small leptomeningeal arteries, while histopathology of the second patient (371) was not provided. Detailed histopathology was lacking in the patient described by Olsen (372) as "vasculitis and cerebritis" as the cause for subarachnoid hemorrhage in a drug abuser who injected methedrine and soon afterward lapsed into a fatal coma. Cerebral angiography that demonstrated typical features of vasculitis in conjunction with a skin biopsy that revealed granular deposits of IgM and C3 component around the lumina of small vessels of the upper dermis consistent with immune complex disease were the only supportive features of cerebral vasculitis in a patient who ingested methamphetamine and later developed headache, nausea and vomiting heralding subarachnoid hemorrhage, without other confirmatory histopathology (369). Corroborative histopathology was not sought in ten other often-cited patients (373–375). Moriya and Hashimoto (376), Shibata and coworkers (377), and Delaney and colleagues (378) each described patients with fatal intracranial hemorrhages following intravenous injection of amphetamine alone or after intranasal injection of methamphetamine. Postmortem examination in one patient (376) did not reveal vascular lesions, while that of the second patient (377) with evidence of necrosis of blood vessel walls along named cerebral arteries, failed to reveal cellular infiltration of vessel walls. Detailed gross and microscopic examination of the cerebral vessels in another patient (378) failed to show evidence of cerebral vasculitis. Moreover, there was no mention of vasculitic lesions at postmortem examination of the CNS among thirteen patients with purported vasculitis following fatal intravenous injection (379), oral ingestion of methamphetamine amphetamine sulfate or oral ingestion of combination dexamphetamine and phenelzine (380). There was no postmortem or brain biopsy studies to investigate the possibility of cerebral vasculitis among four other often-cited patients (381), one of whom was fatally self-injected with intravenous methamphetamine leading to cerebellar and brainstem hemorrhage, or in three other patients who survived ischemic infarction or lobar hemorrhage associated with inhaled or unknown modes of administered methamphetamine. Cerebral vasculitis was not mentioned in a recent series of thirty patients, one-third of whom carried the diagnosis of ischemic stroke, intracerebral hemorrhage, or subarachnoid hemorrhage (382). Nor were the postmortem findings of multiple large intracerebral vessels occlusions attributed to cerebral vasculitis in a patient with a fatal stroke, and attributed instead to accelerated atherosclerosis. Histopathology was not sought in two other fatal strokes or a patient with fatal subarachnoid hemorrhage (382).

Cocaine

Cocaine, which is derived from the leaves of the Erythroxylum coca plant found primarily in the eastern mountains of Peru, Ecuador, and Bolivia, is available for abuse as cocaine hydrochloride, a water-soluble white salt in crystal, granular, and white powder that can be sniffed and "snorted" intranasally or injected parenterally. The "free base" alkaloid form known as "crack" derives its name from the cracking sound that occurs after dissolution of the hydrochloride salt in water, heated, and mixed with ammonia with or without baking soda. This chemical reaction converts cocaine hydrochloride to a volatile form of the drug, almost pure cocaine. Street cocaine or the non-crack form is highly variable in purity, and often cut with various agents. The alkaloid free-based form, which is inhaled or smoked, is accompanied by higher blood concentrations and more pronounced euphoria. When smoked as free-base, it is absorbed into the pulmonary circulation and transmitted to the brain in <10 seconds. After appearance in the bloodstream, cocaine is rapidly hydrolyzed to benzoylecgonine which can be accurately tested in the urine. However levels may persist for up to 27 to 36 hours depending upon the route of administration and host cholinesterase activity. It is a highly potent CNS stimulant that rapidly crosses the blood-brain barrier due to its highly lipophilic properties. It is widely distributed through the brain with its major metabolites binding at receptors with varying affinities at presynaptic sites stimulating the release of dopamine from synaptic vesicles and blocking its reuptake. This results in enhanced dopaminergic neurotransmission, in addition to its local anesthetic properties. The underlying molecular neurobiology and genetics of the mu-1 and kappa opioid receptor systems which contributes to variability in drug addiction among susceptible individuals, is reviewed elsewhere (383, 384).

Ten histologically verified patients with cocaine-related vasculitis have been described (371, 385–391). In all but one patient (389) who had a long-standing cocaine habit with abuse sometime in the 6 months before onset of neurological symptoms immediately followed cocaine use that was intranasal in six patients, intravenous in two, smoked in one, and acquired via an unknown modality in another. Cerebral vasculitis was associated with cerebral hemorrhage in three patients and ischemia in seven, that typically began with abrupt onset of headache and focal hemiparesis so noted in six patients, and confusion or agitation and grand mal seizures that progressed to stupor, coma and death in three patients. The pathology of cerebral vasculitis was established by brain and meningeal biopsy in seven patients (385, 386, 388–391) at postmortem examination in two patients (371, 387), and by both in one patient (385). The underlying pathology of cerebral vasculitis was non-necrotizing with transmural mononuclear cell inflammation affecting small arteries and veins or the veins alone each in three patients, necrosis of small cerebral vessels associated with polymorphonuclear cell inflammation of small arteries and veins or large named vessels in two others, and perivascular cuffing of small arteries and veins in another. Among three patients so studied at postmortem examination, non-necrotizing small vessel vasculitis was noted in the brains of two patients without evidence of systemic involvement (385, 387), while necrotizing large vessel vasculitis was found in both the brain and systemic organs (371). Treatment consisting of corticosteroids was administered to seven patients, five of whom improved and two who died with refractory seizures despite anticonvulsant medication or as a consequence of infection, coma and decerebration.

Since the first reported patient with possible association of cocaine and ischemic stroke (392), both stroke and cerebral vasculitis have been described in the literature as features of cocaine drug abuse. One clinical series of twenty-eight patients (393) and another of fifteen patients (394) failed to identify vasculitis by cerebral angiography or in a patient studied at postmortem examination (393). Moreover, vasculitis was not suggested in a review of thirteen patients from nine published reports by the same authors (395) of cocaine-associated cerebrovascular complications. Other cases of presumed vasculitis suggested by intracranial arterial narrowing (396) in the absence of confirmed histopathology were contested as probably representing vasospasm following subarachnoid hemorrhage (397).

Heroin

The opioid drugs comprise a large number of agonists, antagonists and mixed agonist-antagonists. Also known as diacetylmorphine, heroin was first synthesized by the Bayer Company in 1889 as a less addictive morphine sulfate substitute, however it has since become cheaper and more readily available. Opioids or narcotic drugs have pharmacologic properties similar to those of morphine that include the derivatives morphine, hydrocodone, oxycodone, hydromorphone, codeine, fentanyl, meperidine, methadone, and opium. Whereas the source of opioids is the exudate of seed from the poppy plant, heroin is derived from acetylation of morphine. It is administered intravenously, intranasally and subcutaneously. A higher bioavailability of heroin is present after heating on foil for inhalation compared to smoking after heating. Intravenous injection leads to extreme euphoria that peaks at ten minutes followed by profound sedation and analgesia that lasts for up to one hour. Opiate overdose produces the triad of coma, respiratory depression and miosis. The medical complications of long-term heroin exposure includes endocarditis, pulmonary complications of embolism, pneumonia and granulomatosis or fibrosis; nephropathy, immunodepression, infection at the site of injection due to cellulitis, thrombophlebitis, and bacteremia and hepatitis due to needle sharing. It binds to endogenous opiate mu-1 receptors, which are responsible for most of the analgesic effects, and for the actions of the central nervous system and cardiovascular system leading to bradycardia, hypotension, and respiratory depression. Agonist actions at mu-2 receptors are responsible for respiratory depression, delayed gastrointestinal motility, miosis, and physical dependence. Agonist actions at kappa receptors lead to separate analgesia. Circulating serum morphine is transformed into morphine-3-glucuronide or morphine-6-glucuronide by the liver and the kidney. Most fatal and nonfatal overdoses occur when heroin is administered intravenously.

There are no convincing pathologically confirmed cases of heroin-induced cerebral vasculitis in the literature.

Moreover, among 134 victims of acute heroin intoxication for whom detailed neuropathologic studies were available, including eighteen patients who survived for periods of hours or days (398), none showed evidence of cerebral vasculitis, and only one showed a focus of lymphocytic perivascular inflammation. The brains of ten intravenous drug abusers who died from heroin overdoses, including one due to gunshot injury (399), likewise showed no evidence of cerebral vasculitis at postmortem examination, evidencing only a few perivascular mononuclear cells associated with pigment deposition.

Pathological confirmation was not obtained among four often-cited patients with heroin abuse and cerebral vasculitis studied after death by Brust and coworkers (392) and Adle-Biassette and colleagues (400). In three patients (392), cerebral vasculitis was considered possible after exclusion of bacterial or fungal endocarditis, focal ischemic during a period of shock after overdosage and hypoventilation, concomitant methamphetamine, drug allergy, and likely adulterants. One patient died in methadone detoxification and postmortem revealed a massive hemorrhage of the right basal ganglia however intracranial vessels were not examined. A second patient developed unconsciousness followed by seizures, global aphasia and right hemiparesis in association with multiple occlusions on cerebral angiography before expiring; however neuropathologic postmortem examination was not performed. A third patient who presented comatose with xanthochromic and bloody CSF and died, was found to have a left intracerebral hemorrhage with normal large vessels on postmortem examination however, the smaller cerebral vessels were not commented upon. Another often-cited pathological patient (400) in whom cerebral infarction and death followed the usual signs of recent heroin intake was found dead one morning with ischemic cardiac lesions of varying ages, cortical watershed infarcts and normal intracranial vessels at postmortem examination. Neither was confirmatory pathology sought among five often-cited surviving heroin abusers (401–405) who presented with focal strokes on neuroimaging after inhalation or intravenous injection evidencing likely cerebral vasculitis on cerebral angiography, one of whom admitted to intermittent lysergic acid diethylamide use (401). Citron and colleagues (365) did not identify those with heroin-related angiitis angiographically or histopathologically in their cohort of drug abuse related necrotizing angiitis.

VASCULITIS AND INFECTION

The category of infection-related vasculitides includes acute septic bacterial meningitis, CNS mycobacterial infection, spirochetal infection, viral agents notably varicella zoster virus (VZV), mycotic infections, parasitic agents, human T-lymphotropic virus infection and HIV/ AIDS. Recognition of an infection is important because prompt treatment may avert or lessen the severity of vasculitis. Many different pathogenic mechanisms have been proposed. Although blood vessels are relatively resistant to infection, certain pathogens can invade vessels and cause indirect damage through immune or toxic mechanisms. There may be cross-reacting antibodies, cellular immune responses with granuloma formation or immune complex deposition, and local activation of membranolytic complement. These immune responses may reflect a direct attack against blood vessel antigens or a cross-reactive attack mediated by molecular mimicry or an indirect bystander effect. Host immune responses to pathogens result in the production of factors with the potential for vascular damage. Examples of infection-triggered immunity include cryoglobulinemia associated with HCV and IgAV/ HSP evoked by streptococcal infection.

Acute Bacterial Meningitis

Purulent bacterial meningitis causes arteritis and thrombophlebitis of vessels due to infiltration of blood vessels as they traverse sites of exudation at the base of the brain and across foci of cerebritis, leading to vascular narrowing, cerebral ischemia, infarction, hemorrhage, abscess formation and true vasculitis. Adhesion of leukocytes to endothelial cells activates leukotrienes, complement, and platelet activating factors. Local cytokine activation leads to production of reactive oxygen species, arachidonic acid metabolites, excitatory amino acids, and proteolytic enzymes, which further damage vascular endothelia and surrounding tissue. Host and immune factors are equally important determinants of whether mycobacterial tubercles rupture in cisterns of the brain with a similar outcome of arteritis.

Syphilis

Meningovascular syphilis is the most common presentation of neurosyphilis, its pathologic features being those of an endarteritis with perivascular adventitial inflammation (406). Neurosyphilis, a form of tertiary syphilis, typically develops seven to ten years after an initial infection with inadequate treatment and tends to occur more frequently in patients with concurrently infected HIV/AIDS. It is the most common clinical manifestation of neurosyphilis comprising approximately 39 to 61% of all symptomatic cases of neurosyphilis (407). The resultant obliterative endarteritis affects blood vessels of the brain, spinal cord and leptomeninges precipitating substantial ischemic injury. Often referred to as Heubner arteritis, it involves medium-sized to large arteries with intimal inflammation and fibrosis. Classically a mononuclear specifically lymphoplasmacytic inflammation, a variant form termed Nissl-Alzheimer arteritis, characteristically affects small vessels and produces both adventitial and intimal thickening. Both types can lead to vascular thrombotic occlusions and cerebral infarction, with preferential involvement of the MCA. The search for the cause of stroke in young adults should include meningovacular syphilis as a potential etiology. A 35-year-old African American man without significant past medical history with meningovacular syphilis suffered fatal vertebrobasilar occlusion despite timely thrombolytic treatment and endovascular interventions. Postmortem examination revealed necrotizing vasculitis and extensive adventitial inflammation involving the basilar and vertebral arteries (408).

Varicella Zoster Virus

The VZV causes chickenpox in childhood and most children manifest only mild neurologic sequela. After it resolves, the virus becomes latent in neurons of cranial and spinal ganglia of nearly all individuals and reactivates in adult elderly and immunocompromised individuals to produce shingles. The resultant neurological syndromes generally include neuropathy, myelitis, stroke, and encephalitis (409, 410). Cerebral vasculitis may follow VZV ophthalmicus causing a spectrum of large-vessel vascular damage. Nagel and colleagues (411) reported with viral antigen without inflammation in media of late VZV vasculopathy, and thickening of the intima and inflammation of vasa vasorum in early VZV vasculopathy supporting a role of virus-induced inflammation in vessel wall remodeling. A characteristic syndrome of contralateral hemiplegia occurs in adults (412, 413) and rarely, in children (414). The syndrome of GAB was described in association with disseminated and non-ophthalmic VZV alone (118) and in association with lymphoma (415), with necrotizing arteritis and viral-like particles (416).

Fungal and Parasitic Infection

Four fungal species, *Aspergillus, Candida, Coccidiodes,* and *Mucormycetes* can lead to opportunistic infection in immunocompromised and severely disabled hosts and have the capacity to invade arteries of the CNS. Cysticercosis, the most common parasitic infection of the nervous system due to the tapeworm *Taenia solium,* leads to tissue cysts in the CNS within the subarachnoid space and basal cisterns, producing an arachnoiditis and small-vessel angiitis with resultant cerebral infarction.

HIV/AIDS

Early in the HIV/AIDs epidemic, it was clear that a significant proportion of infected persons were intravenous drug users. Their associated risk behavior exposed them to infection through sharing of contaminated needles thereby increasing the risk of spread of HIV and other blood-borne infections. The two postulated periods in the neurobiology of HIV when autoimmune disease manifestations can occur that appear to be significant for the development of cerebral vasculitis are shortly after seroconversion and before the spread of productive infection, and after initiation of highly active antiretroviral therapy (HAART) in association with the immune reconstitution inflammatory syndrome (IRIS) (417). The timing of early HIV invasion has been difficult to ascertain based on the presence of one or more well-recognized clinicopathological HIV/AIDS syndromes including HIV encephalitis, HIV-associated dementia and AIDS-dementia complex (418–420), all of which are indicative of symptomatic infection. HIV encephalitis is initially associated with myelin pallor and gliosis of the centrum semiovale found in more than 90% of brains from patients dying with AIDS (421). With increasing severity of symptomatic disease, multiple glial nodules with the multinucleated cells characteristic of HIV encephalitis occur throughout the white matter, basal ganglia, cerebral and cerebellar cortex, brainstem and spinal cord. HIV has been demonstrated in monocytes and multinucleated giant cells by electron microscopy, immunocytochemical techniques and in situ hybridization.

It has long been recognized that HIV antigens may be identified in CSF at or shortly after seroconversion and in asymptomatic HIV-positive subjects, including seropositive men with normal CD4+ cell counts, neuropsychological, neuroimaging and neurophysiological investigations. Histopathologic examination of the nervous system in presymptomatic individuals has virtually been confined to intravenous drug abusers since other risk groups have a very low mortality before development of AIDS. Six patients with non-necrotizing cerebral vasculitis were described in a postmortem series of presymptomatic HIV-seropositive drug abusers by Gray and colleagues (399). Seven other patients were described by Bell and colleagues (422) with lymphocytic infiltration of the walls of leptomeningeal and subarachnoid veins, without specific reference to cerebral vasculitis. Gray and colleagues (399) studied two cohorts of eleven patients, one HIV-seropositive and non-AIDS, and the other HIV-seronegative heroin abusers, ten patients in each of whom died from heroin overdose and another of a fatal gunshot wound. Neuropathological studies showed varying degrees of vascular inflammation including "true vasculitis" exemplified by dense vascular inflammation extending through the vessel wall, associated with leptomeningitis in six of the eleven HIV-seropositive AIDS-negative patients. However, there was neither mention of whether the inflammatory process involved both arteries and veins nor vessel caliber. Vascular inflammation was comparatively mild or absent and restricted to a few perivascular mononucleated cells associated with pigment deposition, without transmural vascular inflammation or meningitis in the HIV-seronegative cohort. HIV immunocytochemistry was negative in both cohorts and multinucleated giant cells, considered the hallmark of productive HIV infection in the brain and an essential neuropathologic feature of HIV encephalitis, were not seen. One year later, Bell and coworkers (422) described the neuropathologic findings of twenty-three intravenous drug users from the Edinburgh HIV Autopsy Cohort who died suddenly after seroconversion but while still in the presymptomatic stage of HIV infection. In comparison to ten HIV-negative intravenous drug users, twelve non-intravenous drug user controls, and nine patients with full-blown AIDS, who also died suddenly, seven of the presymptomatic HIV-positive patients showed infiltration of T-cell in the walls of veins in association with low-grade lymphocytic meningitis. Seven others demonstrated isolated lymphocytic meningitis, and one patient had focal perivascular lymphocytic cuffing and macrophage collections throughout the central white matter tissue of the brain and in basal ganglia. Neither conspicuous perivascular lymphocytic infiltration nor lymphocytic meningitis was noted in HIV-negative intravenous drug user controls, those with no drug association, or in those with full-blown AIDS. Neuropathological examination in presymptomatic HIV-seropositive patients failed to reveal characteristic lesions of HIV encephalitis and none of the subjects showed immunocytochemical evidence of p24 antigen in brain tissue. Nearly a decade later, Bell and colleagues (423) reiterated that in more than 50% of pre-AIDS cases so studied, the brain was characterized by a low-grade lymphocytic meningoencephalitis in which T-cell infiltration was present in leptomeninges and the perivascular compartment, with a very occasional HIV-p24 positive lymphocytes in the lymphocytic infiltrate, but not in brain parenchyma. Conversely, there was no clear evidence of vasculitis in intravenous drug users with HIV encephalitis in the Edinburgh HIV autopsy cohort (424).

The early CNS changes of HIV infection have been investigated among hemophiliacs examined after sudden death from intracranial hemorrhage and liver cirrhosis (425). Similar neuropathologic changes were sought in experimental animal models of simian immunodeficiency virus (SIV) syndrome (426) and feline immunodeficiency virus (FIV) infection (427) that included gliosis, occasional microglial nodules, perivascular mononuclear infiltrates, and occasional leptomeningeal meningitis, characteristically without multinucleated giant cells or evidence of HIV in the brain. HIV-infected cells were mainly perivascular and expressed macrophage markers in the SIV model suggesting transit of virus across the blood-brain barrier as the main source of entry into the CNS. Moreover, comparatively less pronounced vascular inflammation than that described in early HIV-infection associated with drug abuse suggested that intravenous drug abuse contributed to vascular inflammation.

The introduction of HAART has changed the incidence, course and prognosis of the neurological complications of HIV infection concomitant with almost undetectable viral load in plasma and a rise in circulating T-lymphocytes. One pathologically confirmed patient with cerebral vasculitis and IRIS was described by van der Ven and colleagues (428). An HIV-seropositive homosexual man developed dysarthria and dysphagia after HAART with worsening and appearance of limb paresis after discontinuation of the medication. Treatment with corticosteroids preceded recommencement of HAART but there was worsening with discontinuation of corticosteroids. Biopsy of a hyperintense fronto-pareital lesion on T2-weighted MRI showed small vessel lymphocytic vasculitis, with microglial activation in the surrounding parenchyma. A severe demyelinating leukoencephalopathy in association with intense perivascular infiltration by HIV-gp41 immunoreactive monocytes/ macrophages and lymphocytes was described by Langford and colleagues (429) in seven postmortem patients. All had IRIS after severe immunosuppression and treatment with HAART, and high not low levels of HIV replication were noted without consideration of cerebral vasculitis. Moveover, confirmatory neuropathology was not sought. Patel and coworkers (430) described a man with HIV-seropositive man who developed encephalitis 10 months after HAART in association with a lower thoracic dermatomal varicella zoster virus rash.

REFERENCES

1. Jennette JC, Falk RJ, Andrassay K, et al. Nomenclature of systemic vasculitides. Proposal of an international conference. *Arthritis Rheum* 1994; 37:187–192.

2. Jennette JC, Falk RJ, Bacon PA, et al. 2012 Revised International Chapel Hill Consensus Conference Nomenclature of Vasculitides. *Arthritis Rheum* 2013; 65:1–11.

3. Yildiz C, Ozen S. The specificities of pediatric vasculitis classification. *Presse Med* 2013; 42:546–550.

4. Ozen S, Ruperto N, Dillon MJ, et al. EULAR/PRES endorsed consensus criteria for the classification of childhood vasculitides. *Ann Rheum Dis* 2006; 65:936–941.

5. Ruperto N, Ozen S, Pistorio A, et al. EULAR/PINTO/PRES criteria for Henoch-Schönlein purpura, childhood polyarteritis nodosa, childhood Wegener granulomatosis and childhood Takayasu arteritis: Ankara 2008. Part I: Overall methodology and clinical characterization. *Ann Rheum Dis* 2010; 69:790–797.

6. Ozen S, Pistorio A, Iusan SM, et al. EULAR/PRINTO/PRES criteria for Henoch-Schönlein purpura, childhood polyarteritis nodosa, childhood Wegener granulomatosis and childhood Takayasu arteritis. Ankara 2008. Part II: Final Classification. *Ann Rheum Dis* 2010; 69:798–806.

7. Longcope WT. Periarteritis nodosa with report of a case with autopsy. *Bull Auyer Clin Lab*, Pennsylvania Hospital, 1908, volume 1.

8. Kernohan JW, Woltman HW. Periarteritis nodosa: a clinicopathologic study with special reference to the nervous system. *Arch Neurol* 1938; 39:655–686.

9. Krahulik L, Rosenthal M, Loughlin EH. Periarteritis nodosa (necrotizing panarteritis) in childhood with meningeal involvement. Report of a case with study of pathologic findings. *Am J Med Sci* 1935: 190:308–317.

10. Younger DS. Diabetic neuropathy: A clinical and neuropathological study of 107 patients. *Neurol Res Int* 2010, Article ID: 140379.

11. Kawasaki T. MLNS showing particular skin desquamation from the finger and toe in infants. *Allergy* 1967; 16:178–189.

12. Tanaka N, Naoe S, Kawasaki T. Pathological study on autopsy cases of mucocutaneous lymph node syndrome. *J Jap Red Cross Cent Hosp* 1971; 2:85–94.

13. Chamberlain JL, Perry LW. Infantile periarteritis nodosa with coronary and brachial aneurysms: a case diagnosed during life. *J Pediatrics* 1971; 78:1039–1040.

14. Landing BH, Larson EJ. Are infantile periarteritis nodosa with coronary artery involvement and fatal mucocutaneous lymph node syndrome the same? Comparison of 20 patients from North America with patients from Hawaii and Japan. *Pediatrics* 1977; 59:651–652.

15. Wohlwill F. Uber die mur mikroskopisch erkenbarre form der periarteritis nodosa. *Arch Pathol Anat* 1923; 246:377–411.

16. Davson J, Ball M, Platt R. The kidney in periarteritis nodosa. *QJM* 1948; 17:175–202.

17. Wainwright J, Davson J. The renal appearance in the microscopic form of periarteritis nodosa. *J Pathol Bact* 1950; 62:189–196.

18. Lamb AR. Periarteritis nodosa-a clinical and pathological review of the disease with a report of two cases. *Arch Intern Med* 1914; 14:481–516.

19. Churg J, Strauss L. Allergic granulomatosis, allergic angiitis, and periarteritis nodosa. *Am J Pathol* 1951; 27:277–301.

20. Chumbley LC, Harrison EG, DeRemee RA. Allergic granulomatosis and angiitis (Churg-Strauss syndrome). Report and analysis of 30 cases. *Mayo Clin Proc* 1977; 52:477–484.

21. Lanham JG, Elkon KB, Pussey CD, et al. Systemic vasculitis with asthma and eosinophilia: a clinical approach to the Churg-Strauss syndrome. *Medicine* 63:65–81.

22. Masi AT, Hunder GG, Lie JT, et al. The American College of Rheumatology 1990 criteria for the classification of Churg-Strauss syndrome (Allergic granulomatosis and angiitis). *Arthritis Rheum* 1990; 33:1094–1100.

23. Godman GC, Churg J. Wegener's granulomatosis: pathology and review of the literature. *Arch Pathol* 1954; 58:533–553.

24. Drachman DA. Neurological complications of Wegener's granulomatosis. *Arch Neurol* 1963; 8:45–55.

25. Fauci AS, Haynes BF, Katz P, et al. Wegener's granulomatosis: Prospective clinical and therapeutic experience with 85 patients over 21 years. *Ann Intern Med* 1983; 98:76–85.

26. Hoffman GS, Kerr GS, Leavitt RY, et al. Wegener granulomatosis: an analysis of 158 patients. *Ann Intern Med* 1992; 116:488–498.

27. Wegener's granulomatosis: Pathology and review of the literature. *Arch Pathol Lab Med* 1954; 58:533–553.

28. Guillevin L, Visser H, Noel LH, et al. Antineutrophil cytoplasm antibodies in systemic polyarteritis nodosa with and without hepatitis B virus infection and Churg-Strauss syndrome-62 patients. *J Rheumatol* 1993; 20:1345–1349.

29. van der Woude FJ, Rasmussen N, Lobatto S, et al. Autoantibodies against neutrophils and monocytes: tool for diagnosis and marker of disease activity in Wegener's granulomatosis. *Lancet* 1985; 1:425–429.

30. Falk RJ, Jennette JC. Anti-neutrophil cytoplasmic autoantibodies with specificity for myeloperoxidase in patients with systemic vasculitis and idiopathic necrotizing and crescentic glomerulonephritis. *N Engl J Med* 1988; 318:1651–1657.

31. Goldschmeding R, Cohen Tervaert JW, van der Schoot CE, et al. Autoantibodies against myeloid lysosomal enzymes: a novel class of autoantibodies associated with vasculitic syndrome [Abstract]. *Kidney Int* 1988; 34:558–559.

32. Gadola SD, Gross WL. The renaissance of granulomatous inflammation in AAV. *Nat Rev Rheumatol* 2012; 8:74–76.

33. Griffith ME, Coulthart A, Pemberton S, et al. Anti-neutrophil cytoplasmic antibodies (ANCA) from patients with systemic vasculitis recognize restricted epitopes of proteinase-3 involving the catalytic site. *Clin Exp Immunol* 2001; 123:170–177.

34. Lionaki S, Blyth ER, Hogan SL, et al. Classification of anti-neutrophil cytoplasmic autoantibody vasculitides: the role of anti-neutrophil cytoplasmic autoantibody specificity for myeloperoxidase or proteinase 3 in disease recognition and prognosis. *Arthritis Rheum* 2012; 64:3452–3462.

35. Savage CO, Gaskin G, Pusey CD, et al. Myeloperoxidase binds to vascular endothelial cells, is recognized by ANCA and can enhance complement dependent cytotoxicity. *Adv Exp Med Biol* 1993; 336:121–123.

36. Jennette JC, Falk RJ. Pathogenesis of ANCA-associated vasculitis: observations, theories, and speculations. *Presse Med* 2013; 42:493–498.

37. Free ME, Ciavatta DJ, Falk RJ. How antigens influence the disease: An immunologist point of view. *Presse Med* 2013; 42:577–579.

38. Lyons PA, Rayner TF, Trivedi S, et al. Genetically distinct subsets within ANCA-associated vasculitis. *N Engl J Med* 2012; 367:214–223.

39. Savige J, Gillis D, Benson E, et al. International consensus statement on testing and reporting of anti-neutrophil cytoplasmic antibodies (ANCA). *Am J Clin Pathol* 1999; 111:507–513.

40. Csernok E, Holle J, Hellmich B, et al. Evaluation of capture ELISA for detection of antineutrophil cytoplasmic antibodies against proteinase-3 in Wegener's granulomatosis:

first results from a multicenter study. *Rheumatology* 2004; 43:174–180.

41. Hellmich B, Csenok E, Fredenhagen G, et al. A novel high sensitivity ELISA for detection of antineutrophil cytoplasm antibodies against proteinase-3. *Clin Exp Rheumatol* 2007; 25 (Suppl 44):S1–S5.

42. Zeek PM, Smith CC, Weeter JC. Studies on periarteritis nodosa. III. The differentiation between the vascular lesions of periarteritis nodosa and of hypersensitivity. *Am J Pathol* 1948; 24:889–917.

43. Zeek PM. Periarteritis nodosa-a critical review. *Am J Clin Pathol* 1952; 22:777–790.

44. Zeek PM. Periarteritis nodosa and other forms of necrotizing angiitis. *N Engl J Med* 1953; 248:764–772.

45. Arthus M, Breton M. Lesions cutanées produites par les injections de sérum de cheval chez le lapin anaphylactisé par et pour ce sérum. *Compt Rend Soc de Biol* 1903; 55:1478–1480.

46. Osler W. The visceral lesions of purpura and allied conditions. *BMJ* 1914; 1:517–525.

47. Gairdner D. The Schönlein-Henoch syndrome (anaphylactoid purpura). *QJM* 1948; 17:95–122.

48. Levitt LM, Burbank B. Glomerulonephritis as a complication of the Schonlein-Henoch syndrome. *N Engl J Med* 1953; 248:530–536.

49. Faille-Kuyber EH, Kater L, Kooiker CJ, et al. IgA-deposits in cutaneous blood-vessel walls and mesangium in Henoch-Schonlein syndrome. *Lancet* 1973; 1:892–893.

50. Conley ME, Cooper MD, Michael AF. Selective deposition of immunoglobulin A1 in immunoglobulin A nephropathy, anaphylactoid purpura nephritis, and systemic lupus erythematosus. *J Clin Invest* 1980; 66:1432–1436.

51. Wintrobe MM, Buell MV. Hyperproteinemia associated with multiple myeloma. With report of a case in which an extraordinary hyperproteinemia was associated with thrombosis of the retinal veins and symptoms suggesting Raynauds disease. *Bull Johns Hopkins Hosp* 1933; 52:156–165.

52. Lerner AB, Watson CJ. Studies of cryoglobulins. I. Unusual purpura associated with the presence of a high concentration of cryoglobulin (cold precipitable serum globulin). *Am J Med Sci* 1947; 214:410–415.

53. Lerner AB, Watson CJ. Studies of cryoglobulins. II. The spontaneous precipitation of protein from serum at 5°C in various disease states. *Am J Med Sci* 1947; 214:416–421.

54. Gorevic PD, Kassab HJ, Levo Y, et al. Mixed cryoglobulinemia: clinical aspects and long-term follow-up of 40 patients. *Am J Med* 1980; 69:287–308.

55. McDuffie FC, Sams WM, Maldonado JE, et al. Hypocomplementemia with cutaneous vasculitis and arthritis. Possible immune complex syndrome. *Mayo Clin Proc* 1973; 48:340–348.

56. Zeiss CR, Burch FX, Marder RJ, et al. A hypocomplementemic vasculitic urticarial syndrome: Report of four new cases and definition of the disease. *Am J Med* 1980; 68:867–875.

57. Wisnieski JJ, Naff. Serum IgG antibodies to C1q in hypocomplementemic urticarial vasculitis syndrome. *Arthritis Rheum* 1989; 32:1119–1127.

58. Hutchinson J. On a peculiar form of thrombotic arteritis of the aged which is sometimes productive of gangrene. *Arch Surg* 1890; I:323–329.

59. Horton BT, Magath BT, Brown GE. Arteritis of temporal vessels: report of 7 cases. *Mayo Clin Proc* 1937; 12:548–553.

60. Bruce GM. Senile rheumatic gout. *BMJ* 1888; 2:811–813.

61. Barber HS. Myalgic syndrome with constitutional effects: polymyalgia rheumatic. *Ann Rheum Dis* 1957; 16:230–237.

62. Jennings GH. Arteritis of the temporal vessels. *Lancet* 1938; 1:424–428.

63. Bruce GM. Temporal arteritis as a cause of blindness: Review of the literature and report of a case. *Trans Am Ophthalmol Soc* 1949; 47:300–316.

64. Gilmour JR. Giant-cell chronic arteritis. *J Pathol Bacteriol* 1941; 53:263–277.

65. Jellinger K. Giant cell granulomatous angiitis of the central nervous system. *J Neurol* 1977; 215:175–190.

66. Kjeldsen M, Reske-Nielsen E. Pathological changes of the central nervous system in giant cell arteritis. *Acta Ophthalmol* 1968; 46:49–56.

67. McLean C, Gonzalez M, Dowling J. Systemic giant cell arteritis and cerebellar infarction. *Stroke* 1993; 24:899–902.

68. Morrison A, Abitol M. Granulomatous arteritis with myocardial infarction. *Ann Intern Med* 1955; 42:691–700.

69. Ritama V. Temporal arteritis. *Ann Med Exp Fenn* 1951; 40:63–87.

70. Save-Soderbergh J, Malmvall B, Anderson R, et al. Giant cell arteritis as a cause of death. *JAMA* 1986; 255:493–496.

71. Nesher G, Rosenberg P, Shorer Z, et al. Involvement of the peripheral nervous system in temporal arteritis-polymyalgia rheumatic. Report of 3 cases and review of the literature. *J Rheumatol* 1987; 14:358–360.

72. Takayasu M. Case with unusual changes of the central vessels in the retina [Japanese]. Acta Soc Ophthal Jap 1908; 12:554–555.

73. Shimizu K, Sano K. Pulseless disease [Japanese]. *Clin Surg* 1948; 3:377–342.

74. Ishikawa K. Natural history and classification of occlusive thromboaortopathy (Takayasu's disease). *Circulation* 1978; 57:27–35.

75. Nakao K, Ikeda M, Kimata S-I, et al. Takayasu's arteritis: clinical report of eighty-four cases and immunologic studies of seven cases. *Circulation* 1967; 35:1141–1155.

76. Walker DI, Bloor K, Williams G, et al. Inflammatory aneurysms of the abdominal aorta. *Brit J Surg* 1972; 59:609–614.

77. Pennell RC, Hollier LH, Lie JT, et al. Inflammatory abdominal aortic aneurysms: A thirty year review. *J Vasc Surg* 1985; 2:859–869.

78. Rojo-Leyva F, Ratliff NB, Cosgrove DM, et al. Study of 52 patients with idiopathic aortitis from a cohort of 1,204 surgical cases. *Arthritis Rheum* 2000; 43:901–907.

79. Hamamo H, Kawa S, Horiuchi A, et al. High serum IgG4 concentrations in patients with sclerosing pancreatitis. *N Engl J Med* 2001; 344:732–738.

80. Hamano H, Kawa S, Ochi Y, et al. Hydronephrosis associated with retroperitoneal fibrosis and sclerosing pancreatitis. *Lancet* 2002; 359:1403–1404.

81. Sakata N, Tashiro T, Uesugi N, et al. IgG4-positive plasma cells in inflammatory abdominal aortic aneurysm: The possibility of an aortic manifestation of IgG4-related sclerosing disease. *Am J Surg Path* 2008; 32:553–559.

82. Kasashima S, Zen Y, Kawashima A, et al. Inflammatory abdominal aortic aneurysm: Close relationship to IgG4-related periaortitis. *Am J Surg Path* 2008; 32:197–204.

83. Ito H, Kalzaki Y, Noda Y, et al. IgG4-related inflammatory abdominal aortic aneurysm associated with autoimmune pancreatitis. *Pathology International* 2008; 58:421–426.

84. Khosroshahi A, Stone JR, Pratt DS, et al. Painless jaundice with serial multiorgan dysfunction. *Lancet* 2009; 373:1494.

85. Stone JH, Khosroshahi A, Hilgenberg A, et al. IgG4-related systemic disease and lymphoplasmacytic aortitis. *Arthritis Rheum* 2009; 60:3139–3145.

86. Adamantiades B. Sur un cas d'iritis a hypopion recidivant. *Ann D'Ocul* 1931; 168:271–278.

87. Behçet H. Ueber rezidivierende, aphthöse, durch ein virus verursachte Geschwüre am Mund, am Auge und an den Genitalien. *Dermat Wchnschr* 1937; 105:1152–1157.

88. Behçet H, Matteson EL. On relapsing, aphthous ulcers of the mouth, eye and genitalia caused by a virus. 1937. *Clin Exp Rheumatol* 2010; 28(Suppl 60):S2–S5.

89. McMenemey WH, Lawrence BJ. Encephalomyelopathy in Behçet's disease. Report of necropsy findings in two cases. *Lancet* 1957; 2:353–358.

90. Wolf SM, Schotland DL, Phillips LL. Involvement of nervous system in Behçet's syndrome. *Arch Neurol* 1965; 12:315–325.

91. Mogan RF, Baumgarten CJ. Meniere's disease complicated by recurrent interstitial keratitis: Excellent results following cervical ganglionectomy. *West J Surg* 1934; 42:628.

92. Cogan DG. Syndrome of nonsyphilitic interstitial keratitis and vestibuloauditory symptoms. *Arch Ophthal* 1945; 33:144–149.

93. Haynes BF, Kaiser-Kupfer MI, Mason P, et al. Cogan's syndrome: Studies in thirteen patients, long-term follow-up, and a review of the literature. *Medicine* 1980; 59:426–441.

94. Cogan DG. Nonsyphilitic interstitial keratitis with vestibuloauditory symptoms. Report of four additional cases. *Arch Ophthalmol* 1949; 42:42–49.

95. Norton EWD, Cogan DG. Syndrome of nonsyphylitic interstitial keratitis and vestibuloauditory symptoms. A long-term follow-up. *Arch Ophthalmol* 1959; 61:695–697.

96. Cody DTR, Williams HL. Cogan's syndrome. *Laryngoscope* 1960; 70:447–478.

97. Bicknell JM, Holland JV. Neurologic manifestations of Cogan syndrome. *Neurology* 1976; 28:278–28.

98. Gluth MB, Baratz KH, Matteson EL, et al. Cogan syndrome: A retrospective review of 60 patients throughout a half century. *Mayo Clin Proc* 2006; 81:483–488.

99. Cody DTR, Williams HL. Cogan's syndrome. *Mayo Clin Proc* 1962; 37:372–375.

100. Pagnini I, Zannin ME, Vittadello F, et al. Clinical Features and outcome of Cogan syndrome. *J Pediatr* 2012; 160;303–307.

101. Vaiopoulos G, Sfikakis PP, Skoumas B, et al. Lack of response to corticosteroids and pulse cyclophosphamide therapy in Cogan's syndrome. *Clin Rheumatol* 1994; 13:110–112.

102. Quinn FB Jr, Falls HF. Cogan's syndrome. Case report and a review of etiologic concepts. *Trans Am Acad Ophthalmol Otolaryngol* 1958; 62:716–721.

103. Albrite Lt. Col. JP, Resnick DM. Cogan's syndrome. Case presentations. *Arch Otolaryngol* 1961; 74:501–506.

104. Sunderland S. Blood supply of the nerves of the upper limb in man. *Arch Neurol* 1945; 53:91–115.

105. Sunderland S. Blood supply of the sciatic nerve and its popliteal divisions in man. *Arch Neurol* 1945; 53:283–289.

106. Dyck PJ, Conn DL, Okazaki H. Necrotizing angiopathic neuropathy. Three-dimensional morphology of fiber degeneration related to sites of occluded vessels. *Mayo Clin Proc* 1972; 47:461–475.

107. Moore PM, Fauci AS. Neurologic manifestations of systemic vasculitis. A retrospective and prospective study of the clinicopathologic features and responses to therapy in 25 patients. *Am J Med* 1981; 71:517–524.

108. Collins MP, Dyck PJ, Gronseth GS, et al. Peripheral Nerve Society Guideline on the classification, diagnosis, investigation, and immunsuppressive therapy of non-systemic vasculitis neuropathy: executive summary. *J Peripher Nerv Syst* 2010; 15:176–184.

109. Harbitz F. Unknown forms of arteritis with special reference to their relation to syphilitic arteritis and periarteritis nodosa. *Am J Med Sci* 1922; 163:250–272.

110. Neuman W, Wolf A. Noninfectious granulomatous angiitis involving the central nervous system. *Trans Am Neurol Assoc* 1952; 77:114–117.

111. McCormack H, Neuberger K. Giant cell arteritis involving small meningeal and intracerebral vessels. *J Neuropathol Exp Neurol* 1958; 17:471–478.

112. Meyer J, Foley J, Campagna-Pinto D. Granulomatous angiitis of the meninges in sarcoidosis. *Arch Neurol* 1953; 69:587–600.

113. Cravioto H, Fegin I. Noninfectious granulomatous angiitis with a predilection for the nervous system. *Neurology* 1959; 9:599–607.

114. Hinck V, Carter C, Rippey C. Giant cell (cranial) arteritis. A case with angiographic abnormalities. *AJR* 1964; 92:769–775.

115. Cupps T, Fauci A. Central nervous system vasculitis. *Major Problems in Internal Medicine* 1981; 21:123–132.

116. Cupps TR, Moore PM, Fauci AS. Isolated angiitis of the central nervous system. Prospsective diagnostic and therapeutic experience. *Am J Med* 1983; 74:97–105.

117. Calabrese HL, Mallek JA. Primary angiitis of the central nervous system: report of 8 new cases, review of the literature, and proposal for diagnostic criteria. *Medicine* 1988; 67:20–39.

118. Younger DS, Hays AP, Brust JCM, et al. Granulomatous angiitis of the brain. An inflammatory reaction of diverse etiology. *Arch Neurol* 1988; 45:514–518.

119. Younger DS, Calabrese LH, Hays AP. Granulomatous angiitis of the nervous system. *Neurol Clin* 1997; 15:821–834.

120. Editorial: Benzedrine sulfate "pep pills." *JAMA* 1937; 108:1973–1974

121. Smith L. Collapse with death following the use of amphetamine sulfate. *JAMA* 1939; 113:1022–1023.

122. Gericke O. Suicide by ingestion of amphetamine sulfate. *JAMA* 1945;128:1098–1099.

123. Lloyd JT, Walker DR. Death after Combined Dexamphetamine and Phenelzine. *BMJ* 1965; 2:168–169.

124. Anglin MD, Burke C, Perrochet B, et al. History of the methamphetamine problem. *J Psychoactive Drugs* 2000; 32:137–141.

125. United Nations Office on Drugs and Crime. UNODC 2009 World Drug Report. Vienne, Austria: United Nations; 2009.

126. United Nations Office on Drugs and Crime. *World Drug Report 2000*. New York, NY: United Nations; 2000.

127. Kissel JT, Slivka AP, Warmolts JR, Mendell JR. The clinical spectrum of necrotizing angiopathy of the peripheral nervous system. *Ann Neurol* 1985; 18:251–257.

128. Kermani TA, Warrington KJ, Crowson CS, et al. Large-vessel involvement in giant cell arteritis: a population based cohort study of the incidence-trends and prognosis. *Ann Rheum Dis* 2012 Dec 19. [Epub ahead of print].

129. Salvarani C, Piptone N, Versari A, et al. Clinical features of polymyalgia rheumatic and giant cell arteritis. *Nat Rev Rheumatol* 2012; 8:509–521.

130. Weyand CM, Liao YJ, Goronzy JJ. The immunopathology of giant cell arteritis: Diagnostic and therapeutic implications. *J Neuro-Ophthalmol* 2012; 32:259–265.

131. Grayson PC, Maksimowicz-McKinnon K, Clark TM, et al. Distribution of arterial lesions in Takayasu's arteritis and giant cell arteritis. *Ann Rheum Dis* 2012; 71:1329–1334.

132. Maksimowicz-McKinnon K, Clark TM, Hoffman GS. Takayasu arteritis and giant cell arteritis. A spectrum within the same disease? *Medicine* 2009; 88:221–226.

133. Nuenninghoff DM, Hunder GG, Christianson TJH, et al. Incidence and predictors of large-artery complication (aortic aneurysm, aortic dissection, and/or large artery stenosis) in patients with giant cell arteritis. *Arthritis Rheum* 2003; 48:3522–3531.

134. Salvarani C, Cantini F, Boiardi L, et al. Polymyalgia rheumatic and giant cell arteritis. *N Engl J Med* 2002; 347:261–271.

135. Hayreh SS, Podhajsky PA, Zimmerman G. Ocular manifestations of giant cell arteritis. *Am J Ophthalmol* 1998; 125:509–520.

136. Blockmans D, Bley T, Schmidt W. Imaging for large-vessel vasculitis. *Curr Opin Rheumatol* 2009; 21:19–28.

137. Salvarani C. Assessment of vasculitis extent and severity. *Presse Med* 2013; 42:588–589.

138. Weyland CM, Liao J, Goronzy JJ. The immunopathology of giant cell arteritis: Diagnostic and therapeutic implications. *J Neuro-Ophthalmol* 2012; 32:259–265.

139. Restuccia G, Cavazza A, Boiardi L, et al. Small-vessel vasculitis surrounding an uninflamed temporal artery and isolated vasa vasorum vasculitis of the temporal artery. Two subsets of giant cell arteritis. *Arthritis Rheum* 2012; 64:549–556.

140. Hunder GG, Bloch DA, Michel BA, et al. The American College of Rheumatology 1990 criteria for the classification of giant cell arteritis. *Arthritis Rheum* 1990; 33:1122–1128.

141. Shick RM, Baggenstoss AH, Fuller BF, et al. Effects of cortisone and ACTH on periarteritis nodosa and cranial arteritis. *Mayo Clin Proc* 1950; 25:492–494.

142. Langford CA. Perspectives on the treatment of giant cell arteritis. *Presse Med* 2013; 42:609–612.

143. Aiello PD, Trautmann JC, McPhee TJ, et al. Visual prognosis in giant cell arteritis. *Ophthalmology* 1993; 100:550–555.

144. Lee MS, Smith SD, Galor, et al. Antiplatelet and anticoagulant therapy in patients with giant cell arteritis. *Arthritis Rheum* 2006; 54:3306–3309.

145. Nesher G, Berkun Y, Mates M, et al. Low-dose aspirin and prevention of cranial ischemic complications in giant cell arteritis. *Arthritis Rheum* 2004; 50:1332–1337.

146. Hoffman GS, Cid MC, Rendt-Zagar KE, et al. Infliximab for maintenance of glucocorticoid-induced remission of giant cell arteritis: a randomized trial. *Ann Intern Med* 2007; 146:621–630.

147. Dreyer L, Faurschou M, Baslund B. A population-based study of Takayasu's arteritis in eastern Denmark. *Clin Exp Rheumatol* 2011; 29:(Suppl 64):S40–42.

148. Watts R, Al-Taiar A, Mooney J, et al. The epidemiology of Takayasu arteritis in the UK. *Rheumatology* 2009; 48:1008–1011.

149. Mishima Y. Leriche Memorial Lecture at 24th World Congress 'Takayasu's arteritis in Asia'. *Cardiovascular Surg* 2001; 9:3–10.

150. Arend WP, Michel BA, Bloch DA, et al. The American College of Rheumatology 1990 criteria for the classification of Takayasu arteritis. *Arthritis Rheum* 1990; 33:1129–1134.

151. Riehl JL, Brown J. Takayasu's disease. *Arch Neurol* 1965; 12:92–97.

152. Kerr GS, Hallahan CW, Giordano J, et al. Takayasu arteritis. *Ann Intern Med* 1994; 120:919–929.

153. Grahm JR. Migraine: Clinical aspects. *Handb Clin Neurol* 1968; 5:45–58

154. Manno RL, Levine SM, Gelber AC. More than meets the eye. *Semin Arthritis Rheum* 2011; 40:324–329.

155. Ohigashi H, Haraguchi G, Konishi M, et al. Improved prognosis of Takayasu arteritis over the past decade. *Circ J* 2012; 76:1004–1011.

156. Pagnoux C, Seror R, Henegar C, et al. Clinical features and outcomes in 348 patients with polyarteritis nodosa. *Arthritis Rheum* 2010; 62:616–626.

157. Guillevin L, Cohen P, Mahr A, et al, and the French Vasculitis Study Group. Treatment of polyarteritis nodosa and microscopic polyangiitis with poor prognosis factors: a prospective trial comparing glucocorticoids and six or twelve cyclophosphamide pulses in sixty-five patients. *Arthritis Rheum* 2003; 49:93–100.

158. Guillevin L, Mahr A, Callard P, et al, for the French Vasculitis Study Group. Hepatitis B virus-associated polyarteritis nodosa: clinical characteristics, outcome, and impact of treatment in 115 patients. *Medicine* 2005; 84:313–322.

159. Henegar C, Pagnoux C, Puechal X, et al, for the French Vasculitis Study Group. A paradigm of diagnostic criteria for polyarteritis nodosa. *Arthritis Rheum* 2008; 58:1528–1538.

160. Tekin M, Yalcinkaya F, Turner N, et al. Clinical, laboratory and molecular characteristics of children with familial Mediterranean fever-associated vasculitis. *Acta Paediatr* 2000; 89:177–182.

161. Rogalski C, Sticherling M. Panarteritis cutanea benigna-an entity limited to the skin or cutaneous presentation of a systemic necrotizing vasculitis? Report of seven cases and review of the literature. *Int J Dermatol* 2007; 46:817–821.

162. Ozen S, Anton J, Arisoy N, et al. Juvenile polyarteritis: results of a multicenter survey of 110 children. *J Pediatr* 2004; 145:517–522

163. David J, Ansell BM, Woo P. Polyarteritis nodosa associated with streptococcus. *Arch Dis Child* 1993; 69:685–688.

164. Nakamura Y, Yashiro M, Uehara R, et al. Epidemiologic features of Kawasaki disease in Japan: results from the nationwide survey in 2005–2006. *J Epidemiol* 2008; 18:167–172.

165. Shulman ST, Rowley AH. Advances in Kawasaki disease. *Eur J Pediatr* 2004; 163:285–291.

166. Yun SH, Yang NR, Park SA. Associated symptoms of Kawasaki disease. *Korean Circ J* 2011; 41:394–398.

167. Constantinescu CS. Migraine and Raynaud phenomenon: possible late complications of Kawasaki disease. *Headache* 2002; 42:227–229.

168. Hirose S, Nagashima Y. Morphological observations on the vasculitis in the mucocutaneous lymph node syndrome. A skin biopsy study of 27 patients. *Eur J Pediatr* 1978; 129:17–27.

169. Khans A, Langford CA. Update on vasculitis. *J Allergy Clin Immunol* 2009; 123:1226–1236.

170. O'Neil KM. Progress in pediatric vasculitis. *Curr Opin Rheumatol* 2009; 21:538–546.

171. Carrington CB, Libow AA. Limited forms of angiitis and granulomatosis of Wegener's type. *Am J Med* 1966; 41:497–527.

172. Holle JU, Gross WL, Hull-Ulrich K, et al. Prospective long-term followup of patients with localized Wegener's granulomatosis: does it occur as persistent disease stage? *Ann Rheum Dis* 2010; 69:1934–1939.

173. Leavitt RY, Fauci AS, Bloch DA, et al. The American College of Rheumatology 1990 criteria for the classification of Wegener's granulomatosis. *Arthritis Rheum* 1990; 33:1101–1107.

174. Holle JU, Csernok E, Fredenhagen G, et al. Clinical evaluation of hsPR3-ANCA ELISA for detection of antineutrophil cytoplasmic antibodies directed against PR3. *Ann Rheum Dis* 2010; 69:468–469.

175. Nishino H, Rubino FA, DeRemee RA, et. Neurological involvement in Wegener's granulomatosis: An analysis of 324 consecutive patients at the Mayo Clinic. *Ann Neurol* 1993; 33:4–9.

176. de Groot K, Schmidt DK, Arlt AC, et al. Standardized neurologic evaluations of 128 patients with Wegener's granulomatosis. *Arch Neurol* 2001; 58:1215–1221.

177. Suppiah R, Hadden RDM, Batra R, et al. Peripheral neuropathy in ANCA-associated vasculitis: outcomes from the European Vasculitis Study Group Trials. *Rheumatology* 2011; 50:2214–2222.

178. Stone JH, Merkel PA, Spiera R, et al; for the RAVE-ITN Research Group. Rituximab versus cyclophosphamide for ANCA-associated vasculitis. *N Engl J Med* 2010; 363:221–232.

179. Twilt M, Benseler S, Cabral D. Granulomatosis with polyangiitis in childhood. *Curr Rheumatol Rep* 2012; 14:107–115.

180. Cabral DA, Uribe AG, Benseler S, et al, for the ARChiVe (A Registry for Childhood Vasculitis: e-entry) Investigators Network. Classification, presentation, and initial treatment of Wegener's granulomatosis in childhood. *Arthritis Rheum* 2009; 3413–3424.

181. Lightfoot RW Jr., Michel AB, Bloch DA, et al. The American College of Rheumatology 1990 criteria for the classification of polyarteritis nodosa. *Arthritis Rheum* 1990; 33:1088–1093.

182. Watts RA, Jolliffe VA, Carruthers DM, et al. Effect of classification on the incidence of polyarteritis nodosa and microscopic polyangiitis. *Arthritis Rheum* 1996; 39:1208–1212.

183. Serra A, Cameron JS, Turner DR, et al. Vasculitis affecting the kidney: presentation, histopathology and long-term outcome. *QJM* 1984; 201:181–207.

184. Savage COS, Winearls CG, Evans DJ, et al. Microscopic polyarteritis: presentation, pathology and prognosis. *QJM* 1985; 220:467–483.

185. Adu D, Howie AJ, Scott DGI, et al. Polyarteritis and the kidney. *QJM* 239:221–237.

186. Guillevin L, Durand-Gasselin B, Cevallos R, et al. Microscopic polyangiitis. Clinical and laboratory findings in eighty-five patients. *Arthritis Rheum* 1999; 42:421–430.

187. D'Agati V, Chander P, Nash M, et al. Idiopathic microscopic polyarteritis nodosa: ultrastructural observations on the renal vascular and glomerular lesions. *Am J Kidney Dis* 1986; 7:95–110.

188. Ahn JK, Hwang J-W, Lee J, et al. Clinical features and outcome of microscopic polyangiitis under a new consensus algorithm of ANCA-associated vasculitides in Korea. *Rheumatol Int* 2012; 32:2979–2986.

189. Villiger PM, Guillevin L. Microscopic polyangiitis: clinical presentation. *Autoimmunity Reviews* 2010; 9:812–819.

190. Gayraud M, Guillevin L, le Toumelin P, et al; and the French Vasculitis Study Group. Long-term followup of polyarteritis nodosa, microscopic polyangiitis, and Churg-Strauss syndrome. *Arthritis Rheum* 2001; 44:666–675.

191. Guillevin L, Lhote F, Gayraud M, et al. Prognostic factors in polyarteritis nodosa and Churg Strauss syndrome; a prospective study of 342 patients. *Medicine* 1996; 75:17–28.

192. Luqmani RA, Bacon PA, Moots RJ, et al. Birmingham Vasculitis Activity Score (BVAS) in systemic necrotizing vasculitis. *QJM* 1994; 87:671–678.

193. Comarmond C, Pagnoux C, Khellaf M, et al, for the French Vasculitis Study Group. Eosinophilic granulomatosis with polyangiitis (Churg-Strauss). *Arthritis Rheum* 2013; 65:270–281.

194. Healy B, Bibby S, Steele R, et al. Antineutrophilic cytoplasmic autoantibodies and myeloperoxidase autoantibodies in clinical expression of Churg-Strauss syndrome. *J Allergy Clin Immunol* 2013; 131:571–576.

195. Weinstein JM, Chui H, Lane S, et al. Churg-Strauss syndrome (Allergic granulomatous angiitis). Neuro-ophthalmologic manifestations. *Arch Ophthalmol* 1983; 101:1217–1220.

196. Lie JT and Members and Consultants of the American College of Rheumatology Subcommittee on Classification of Vasculitis. *Arthritis Rheum* 1990; 33:1074–1087.

197. Bouche P, Léger JM, Travers MA, et al. Peripheral neuropathy in systemic vasculitis: clinical and electrophysiologic study of 22 patients. *Neurology* 1986; 36:1598–1602.

198. Oh SJ, Herrera GA, Spalding DM. Eosinophilic vasculitis neuropathy in the Churg-Strauss syndrome. *Arthritis Rheum* 1986; 29:1173–1175.

199. Cavallaro T, Fenzi F, Lazzarino LG, et al. Peripheral neuropathy associated with allergic granulomatous angiitis (Churg-Strauss syndrome): clinical features and histological findings. *Ital J Neurol Sci* 1988; 9:595–598.

200. Hawke SHB, Davies L, Pamphlett R, et al. Vasculitic neuropathy. A clinical and pathological study. *Brain* 1991; 114:2175–2190.

201. Inoue A, Koh C-S, Tsukada N, et al. Allergic granulomatous angiitis and peripheral nerve lesion. *Intl Med* 1992; 31:989–993.

202. Guillevin L, Cohen P, Gayraud M, et al. Churg-Strauss syndrome. Clinical study and long-term follow-up of 96 patients. *Medicine* 1999; 78:26–37.

203. Hattori N, Ichimura M, Nagamatsu M, et al. Clinicopathological features of Churg-Strauss syndrome-associated neuropathy. *Brain* 1999; 122:427–439.

204. Abu-Shakra M, Smythe H, Lewtas J, et al. Outcome of polyarteritis nodosa and Churg-Strauss syndrome. An analysis of twenty-five patients. *Arthritis Rheum* 1994; 37:1798–1803.

205. Sehgal M, Swanson JW, DeRemee RA, et al. Neurologic manifestations of Churg-Strauss syndrome. *Mayo Clin Proc* 1995; 70:337–341.

206. Said G, Lacroix-Ciaudo C, Fujimura H, et al. The peripheral neuropathy of necrotizing arteritis: A clinicopathologic study. *Ann Neurol* 1988; 23:461–465.

207. Dorfman LJ, Ransom BR, Forno LS, et al. Neuropathy in the hypereosinophilic syndrome. *Muscle Nerve* 1983; 6:291–298.

208. Wichman A, Buchtal F, Pezeshkpour GH, et al. Peripheral neuropathy in hypereosinophilic syndrome. *Neurology* 1985; 35:1140–1145.

209. Monaco S, Lucci B, Laperchia N, et al. Polyneuropathy in hypereosinophilic syndrome. *Neurology* 1988; 38:494–496.

210. Bibby S, Healy B, Steele R, et al. Association between leukotriene receptor antagonist therapy and Churg-Strauss syndrome: an analysis of the FDA AERS database. *Thorax* 2010; 65:132–138.

211. Vaglio A, Martorana D, Maggiore U, et al. HLA-DRB4 as a genetic risk factor for Churg-Strauss syndrome. *Arthritis Rheum* 2007; 56:3159–3166.

212. Wieczorek S, Hellmich B, Arning L, et al. Functionally relevant variations of the interleukin-10 gene associated with antineutrophil cytoplasmic antibody-negative Churg-Strauss syndrome, but not with Wegener's granulomatosis. *Arthritis Rheum* 2008; 58:1839–1848.

213. Ferri C, Sebastiani M, Giuggioli D, et al. Mixed cryoglobulinemia: demographic, clinical, and serologic features and survival in 231 patients. *Sem Arthritis Rheum* 2004; 33:355–374.

214. Brouet JC, Clauvel JP, Danon F, et al. Biologic and clinical significance of cryoglobulins: a report of 86 cases. *Am J Med* 1974; 57:775–788.

215. Agnello V, Chung RT, Kaplan LM. A role for hepatitis C virus infection in type II cryoglobulinemia. *N Engl J Med* 1992; 327:1490–1495.

216. Ferri C, Greco F, Longombardo G, et al. Antibodies to hepatitis C virus in patients with mixed cryoglobulinemia. *Arthritis Rheum* 1991; 34:1606–1610.

217. Cacoub P, Poynard T, Ghillani P, et al. Extrahepatic manifestations of chronic hepatitis C. *Arthritis Rheum* 1999; 42:2204–2212.

218. Terrier B, Semoun O, Saadoun D, et al. Prognostic factors in patients with hepatitis C virus infection and systemic vasculitis. *Arthritis Rheum* 2011; 63:1748–1757.

219. Trejo L, Ramos-Casals M, Garcia-Carrasco M, et al. Cryoglobulinemia. Study of etiologic factors and clinical and immunologic features in 443 patients from a single center. *Medicine* 2001; 80:252–262.

220. Terrier B, Cacoub P. Cryoglobulinemia vasculitis: an update. *Curr Opin Rheumatol* 2013; 25:10–18.

221. Cacoub P, Costedoat-Chalumeau N, Lidova O, et al. Cryoglobulinemia vasculitis. *Curr Opin Rheumatol* 2002; 14:29–35.

222. Terrier B, Krastinova E, Marie I, et al. Management of noninfectious mixed cryoglobulinemia vasculitis: data from 242 cases included in the CryoVas survey. *Blood* 2012; 119:5996–6004.

223. Landau D-A, Scerra S, Sene D, et al. Causes and predictive factors of mortality in a cohort of patients with hepatitis C

virus-related cryoglobulinemic vasculitis treated with antiviral therapy. *J Rheumatol* 2010; 37:615–621.

224. Ramos-Cassals M, Robles A, Brito-Zeron P, et al. Life-threatening cryoglobulinemia: clinical and immunological characterization of 29 cases. *Semin Arthritis Rheum* 2006; 36:189–196.

225. Abramsky O, Slavin S. Neurologic manifestations in patients with mixed cryoglobulinemia. *Neurology* 1974; 24:245–249.

226. Bolay H, Söylemezoğlu F, Nurlu G, et al. PCR detected hepatitis C virus genome in the brain of a case with progressive encephalomyelitis with rigidity. *Clin Neurol Neurosurg* 1996; 98:305–308.

227. Petty GW, Duffy J, Huston J. Cerebral ischemia in patients with hepatitis C virus infection and mixed cryogloblinemia. *Mayo Clin Proc* 1996; 71:671–678.

228. Marshall RJ, Malone RGS. Cryoglobulinemia with cerebral purpura. *BMJ* 1954; 2:279–280.

229. Ince PG, Duffey P, Cochrane HR, et al. Relapsing ischemic encephaloenteropathy and cryoglobulinemia. *Neurology* 2000; 55:1579–1581.

230. Cacoub P, Ferrier B, Saadoun D. Hepatitis C virus mixed cryoglobulinemia vasculitis: Therapeutic options. *Presse Med* 2013; 42:523–527.

231. Sansonno D, Dammacco F. Hepatitis C virus, cryoglobulinemia, and vasculitis: immune complex relations. *Lancet Infect Dis* 2005; 5:227–236.

232. Conlon KC, Urba WJ, Smith JW, et al. Exacerbation of symptoms of autoimmune disease in patients receiving alpha interferon therapy. *Cancer* 1990; 65:2237–2242.

233. Boonyapisit K, Katirji B. Severe exacerbation of hepatitis C-associated vasculitic neuropathy following treatment with interferon alpha: a case report and literature review. *Muscle Nerve* 2002; 25:909–913.

234. Saadoun D, Pineton de Chambrun M, Hermine O, et al. Rituximab plus fludarabine and cyclophosphamide as a treatment for refractory mixed cryoglobulinemia associated with lymphoma. *Arthritis Care Res* 2013; 65:643–647.

235. Liou YT, Huang JL, Ou LS et al. Comparison of cryoglobulinemia in children and adults. *J Microbiol Immunol Infect* 2013; 46:59–64.

236. Saulsbury FT. Clinical update: Henoch-Schonlein purpura. *Lancet* 2007; 369:976–978.

237. Gardner-Medwin JM, Dolezalova P, Cummins C, et al. Incidence of Henöch-Schonlein purpura, Kawasaki disease, and rare vasculitides in children of different ethnic origins. *Lancet* 2002; 360:1197–1202.

238. Gedalia A. Henoch-Schönlein purpura. *Curr Rheumatol Rep* 2004; 6:195–202.

239. Mills JA, Michel BE, Bloch DA, et al. The American College of Rheumatology 1990 criteria for the classification of Henoch-Schönlein purpura. *Arthritis Rheum* 1990; 33:1114–1121.

240. Peru H, Soylemezoglu O, Bakkaloglu SA, et al. Henoch Schonlein purpura in childhood: clinical analysis of 254 cases over a 3-year period. *Clin Rheumatol* 2008; 27:1087–1092.

241. Allen DM, Diamond LK, Howell DA. Anaphylactoid purpura in children (Schonlein-Henoch syndrome). *Am J Dis Child* 1960; 99:833–854.

242. Saulsbury FT. Henoch-Schönlein purpura. *Curr Opin Rheumatol* 2001; 13:35–40.

243. Lewis IC, Philpott MG. Neurological complications in the Schönlein-Henoch syndrome. *Arch Dis Child* 1956; 31:369–370.

244. Belman AL, Leicher CR, Moshe SL, et al. Neurological manifestations of Schoenlein-Henoch purpura: Report of three cases and review of the literature. *Pediatrics* 1985; 75:687–692.

245. Suzuki H, Kiryluk K, Novak J, et al. The pathophysiology of IgA nephropathy. *J Am Soc Nephrol* 2011; 22:1795–1803.

246. Allen AC, Bailey EM, Barratt J, et al. Analysis of IgA1 O-glycans in IgA nephropathy by fluorophore-assisted carbohydrate electrophoresis. *J Am Soc Nephrol* 1999; 10:1763–1771.

247. Odani H, Kiki Y, Takahashi M, et al. Direct evidence for decreased sialylation and galactosylation of human serum IgA1 Fc O-glycosylated hinge peptides in IgA nephropathy by mass spectroscopy. *Biochem Biophys Res Comm* 2000; 271:268–274.

248. Saulsbury FT. Alternations in the O-linked glycans of IgA1 in children with Henoch-Schöenlein purpura. *J Rheumatol* 1997; 24:2246–2249.

249. Allen AC, Willis FR, Beattie TJ, et al. Abnormal IgA glycosylation in Henoch-Schoenlein purpura restricted to patients with clinical nephritis. *Nephrol Dial Transplant* 1998; 13:930–934.

250. Tomana M, Novak J, Julian BA, et al. Circulating immune complexes in IgA nephropathy consist of IgA1 with galactose-deficient hinge region and antiglycan antibodies. *J Clin Invest* 1999; 104:73–81.

251. Hiki Y, Kokubo T, Iwase H, et al. Underglycosylation of IgA1 hinge plays a certain role for its glomerular deposition in IgA nephropathy. *J Am Soc Nephrol* 1999; 10:760–769.

252. Suzuki H, Fan R, Zhang Z, et al. Aberrantly glycosylated IgA1 in IgA nephropathy patients is recognized by IgG antibodies with restricted heterogeneity. *J Clin Invest* 2009; 119:1668–1677.

253. Gomez-Guerrero C, Lopez-Armanda MJ, Gonzalez E, et al. Soluble IgA and IgG aggregates are catabolized by cultured rat mesangial cells and induce production of TNF-alpha and IL-6 and proliferation. *J Immunol* 1994; 153:5247–5255.

254. Gomez-Guerrero C, Gonzalez E, Egido J. Evidence for a specific IgA receptor in rat and human mesangial cells. *J Immunol* 1993; 151:7172–7178.

255. Launay P, Grossetete B, Arcos-Fajardo M, et al. Fcα receptor (CD89) mediates the development of immunoglobulin A (IgA) nephropathy (Berger's disease): evidence for pathogenic soluble receptor-IgA complexes in patients and CD89 transgenic mice. *J Exp Med* 2000; 191:1999–2000.

256. Weiss PF, Feinstein JA, Luan X, et al. Effects of corticosteroid on Henoch-Schonlein purpura: a systematic review. *Pediatrics* 2007; 120:1079–1087.

257. Buck A, Christensen J, McCarthy M. Hypocomplementemic urticarial vasculitis syndrome. *J Clin Aesthet Dermatol* 2012; 5:36–46.

258. Davis MDP, Daoud MS, Kirby B, et al. Clinicopathologic correlation of hypocomplementemic and normcomplementemic urticarial vasculitis. *J Am Acad Dermatol* 1998; 38:899–905.

259. Lienesch D, Sherman K, Metzger A, et al. Anti-C1q antibodies in patients with chronic hepatitis C infection. *Clin Exp Rheumatol* 2006; 24:183–185.

260. Jara L, Navarro C, Medina G, et al. Hypocomplementemic urticarial vasculitis syndrome. *Current Rheumatology Reports* 2009; 11:410–415.

261. Yasue T, Yasue A. Urticarial vasculitis with circulating immune complexes and mixed cryoglobulins: studies on pathogenesis. *J Dermatol* 1987; 14:597–603.

262. Borradori L, Rybojad M, Puissant A, et al. Urticarial vasculitis associated with a monoclonal IgM gammopathy. Schnitzler's syndrome. *Br J Dermatol* 1990; 123:113–118.

263. Roger D, Rolle F, Mausset J, et al. Urticarial vasculitis induced by fluoxetine [Letter]. *Dermatology* 1995; 191:164.

264. Sprossmann A, Muller RP. [Urticarial vasculitis syndrome in metastatic malignant testicular teratoma]. *Der Hautarzt* 1994; 45:871–874.

265. Asherson RA, D'Cruz D, Stephens CJ, et al. Urticarial vasculitis in a connective disease clinic: patterns, presentations, and treatment. *Semin Arthritis Rheum* 1991; 20:285–296.

266. Wisnieski JJ, Baer AN, Christensen J, et al. Hypocomplement-emic urticarial vasculitis syndrome. Clinical and serologic findings in 18 patients. *Medicine* 1995; 74:24–41.

267. International Study Group for Behçet's Disease. *Lancet* 1990; 335:1078–1080.

268. Sobel JD, Haim S, Shafrir A, et al. Cutaneous hyper-reactivity in Behçet disease. *Dermatologica* 1973; 146:350–356.

269. Özen S. Pediatric onset Behçet disease. *Curr Opin Rheumatol* 2010; 22:585–589.

270. Mahr A, Belarbi L, Wechsler B, et al. Population-based prevalence study of Behçet disease. Differences by ethnic origin and low variation by age at immigration. *Arthritis Rheum* 2008; 58:3951–3959.

271. Calamia KT, Wilson FC, Icen M, et al. Epidemiology and clinical characteristics of Behçet's disease in the US: a population-based study. *Arthritis Rheum* 2009; 61:600–604.

272. Dursun A, Durakbasi-Dursun HG, Dursun R, et al. Angiotensin-converting enzyme gene and endothelial nitric oxide synthase gene polymorphisms in Behçet disease with or without ocular involvement. *Inflamm Res* 2009; 58:401–405.

273. Dhifallah IB, Houman H, Khanfir M, et al. Endothelial nitric oxide synthase gene polymorphism is associated with Behcet's disease in Tunisian population. *Human Immunology* 2008; 69:661–665.

274. Park KS, Baek JA, Do JE, et al. CTLA4 gene polymorphisms and soluble CTLA4 protein in Behçet's disease. *Tissue Antigens* 2009 74:222–227.

275. Kim J, Im CH, Kang EH, et al. Mannose-binding lectin gene-2 polymorphisms and serum mannose-binding lectin levels in Behcet's disease. *Clin Exp Rheumatol* 2009; 27(Suppl 53):S13–S17.

276. Fei Y, Webb R, Cobb BL, et al. Identification of novel genetic susceptibility loci for Behçet's disease using a genome-wide association study. *Arthritis Research & Therapy* 2009; 11:R66 (doi:10.1186/ar2695.

277. Uluduz D, Kürtüncü M, Yapici et al. Clinical characteristics of pediatric-onset neuro-Behçet disease. *Neurology* 2011; 77:1900–1905.

278. Haghighi AB, Aflaki E, Ketabchi L. The prevalence and characteristics of different types of headache in patients with Behçet's disease, a case-control study. *Headache* 2008; 48:424–429.

279. Rubinstein LJ, Urich H. Meningo-encephalitis of Behçet's disease. Case report with pathological findings. *Brain* 1963; 86:151–160.

280. Kawakita H, Nishimura M, Satoh Y, et al. Neurological aspects of Behçet's disease. A case report and clinico-pathological review of the literature in Japan. *J Neurol Sci* 1967; 5:417–439.

281. Arai Y, Kohno S, Takahashi Y, et al. Autopsy case of neuro-Behçet's disease with multifocal neutrophilic perivascular inflammation. *Neuropathology* 2006; 26:579–585.

282. Koseoglu E, Yildirim A, Borlu M. Is headache in Behçet's disease related to silent neurologic involvement? *Clin Exp Rheumatol* 2011; 29 (Suppl 67):S32–S37.

283. Monastero R, Camarda C, Pipia C, et al. Cognitive impairment in Behçet's disease without overt neurological involvement. *J Neurol Sci* 2004; 220:99–104.

284. Siva A, Saip S. The spectrum of nervous system involvement in Behçet's syndrome and its differential diagnosis. *J Neurol* 2009; 256:513–529.

285. Hadfield MG, Aydin F, Lippman HR, et al. Neuro-Behçet's disease. *Clin Neuropathol* 1997; 16:55–60.

286. Matsumoto T, Uekusa T, Fukuda Y. Vasculo-Behçet's disease: a pathologic study of eight cases. *Hum Pathology* 1991; 22:45–51.

287. Yesilot N, Bahar S, Yilmazer S, et al. Cerebral venous thrombosis in Behçet's disease compared to those associated with other etiologies. *J Neurol* 2009; 256:1134–1142.

288. Crawford WJ. Cogan's syndrome associated with polyarteritis nodosa. A report of three cases. *Penn Med J* 1957; 60:835–838.

289. Eisenstein B, Taubenhaus M. Nonsyphilitic interstitial keratitis and bilateral deafness (Cogan's syndrome) associated with cardiovascular disease. *N Engl J Med* 1958; 258:1074–1079.

290. Cogan DG, Dickersin GR. Nonsyphilitic interstitial keratitis with vestibuloauditory symptoms. A case with fatal aortitis. *Arch Ophthal* 1964; 71:172–175.

291. Fisher ER, Hellstrom HR. Cogan's syndrome and systemic vascular disease. Analysis of pathological features with reference to its relationship to thromboangiitis obliterans (Buerger). *Arch Pathol* 1961; 72:572–592.

292. Oliner L, Taubenhaus M, Shapira TM, et al. Nonsyphilitic interstitial keratitis and bilateral deafness (Cogan's syndrome) associated with essential polyangiitis (periarteritis nodosa). A review of the syndrome with consideration of a possible pathogenic mechanism. *N Engl J Med* 1953; 248:1001–1008.

293. Leff TL. Cogan's syndrome: ocular pathology. *NY State J Med* 1967; 67:2249–2257.

294. Gelfand ML, Kantor T, Gorstein F. Cogan's syndrome with cardiovascular involvement: aortic insufficiency. *Bull NY Acad Med* 1972; 48:647–660.

295. Cheson BD, Bluming AZ, Alroy J. Cogan's syndrome: a systemic vasculitis. *Am J Med* 1976; 60:549–555.

296. Del Caprio J, Espinozea LR, Osterland SK. Cogan's syndrome in HLA Bw 17 [letter to the editor]. *N Engl J Med* 1976; 295:1262–1263.

297. Pinals RS. Cogan's syndrome with arthritis and aortic insufficiency. *J Rheumatol* 1978; 5:294–298.

298. Vollertsen RS, McDonald TJ, Younge BR, et al. Cogan's syndrome: 18 cases and a review of the literature. *Mayo Clin Proc* 1986; 61:344–361.

299. Darougar S, John AC, Viswalingam M, et al. Isolation of Chlamydia psittaci from a patient with interstitial keratitis and uveitis associated with otological and cardiovascular lesions. *Br J Ophthalmol* 1978; 62:709–714.

300. Lunardi C, Bason C, Leandri M, et al. Autoantibodies to inner ear and endothelial antigens in Cogan's syndrome. *Lancet* 2002; 360:915–921.

301. Podder S, Shepard RC. Cogan's syndrome: a rare systemic vasculitis. *Arch Dis Child* 1994; 71:163–164.

302. Chaudhuri K, Das RR, Chinnakkannan S. Reversible severe sensorineural hearing loss in a 7-year-old child. *Acta Paediatr* 2011; 100:322–323.

303. Orsoni JG, Zavota L, Vincenti V, et al. Cogan syndrome in children: early diagnosis and treatment is critical to prognosis. *Am J Ophthalmol* 2004; 137:757–758.

304. Lanthier S, Lortie A, Michaud J, et al. Isolated angiitis of the CNS in children. *Neurology* 2001; 56:837–842.

305. Salvarani C, Brown RD Jr., Calamia KT et al. Primary central nervous system vasculitis: analysis of 101 patients. *Ann Neurol* 2007; 62:442–451.

306. Benseler SM, deVeber G, Hawkins C, et al. Angiography-negative primary central nervous system vasculitis in children. *Arthritis Rheum* 2005; 52:2159–2167.

307. Hajj-Ali RA, Calabrese LH. Central nervous system vasculitis. *Curr Opin Rheumatol* 2009; 21:10–18.

308. Benseler SM. Central nervous system vasculitis in children. *Curr Rheum Rep* 2006; 8:442–449.

309. Twilt M, Sheikh S, Cellucci T, et al. Recognizing childhood inflammatory brain diseases in Canada [Abstract]. *Presse Med* 2013; 42:670.

310. Elbers J, Halliday W, Hawkins C, et al. Brain biopsy in children with primary small-vessel central nervous system vasculitis. *Ann Neurol* 2010; 68:602–610.

311. Stone JR. Aortitis, periaortitis, and retroperitoneal fibrosis, as manifestations of IgG4-related systemic disease. *Curr Opin Rheumatol* 2011; 23:88–94.

312. Umehara H, Okazaki K, Masaki Y, et al, and the Research Program for Intractable Disease by Ministry of Health, Labor and Welfare (MHLW) Japan G4 team. A novel clinical entity, igG4-related disease (IgG4RD): general concept and details. *Mod Rheumatol* 2012; 22:1–14.

313. Stone JH, Khosroshahi A, Deshpande V, et al. Recommendations for the nomenclature of IgG4-related disease and its individual organ system manifestations. *Arthritis Rheum* 2012; 64:3061–3067.

314. Schmidt I, Sunesen K, Kornum JB. Predictors for pathologically confirmed aortitis after resection of the ascending aorta: a 12-year Danish nationwide population-based cross sectional study. *Arthritis Res Ther* 2011; 13:R87.

315. Liang KP, Chowdhary VR, Michel CJ, et al. Noninfectious ascending aortitis: a case series of 64 patients. *J Rheumatol* 2009; 36:2290–2297.

316. Miller DV, Isotalo PA, Weyand CM, et al. Surgical pathology of noninfectious ascending aortitis: a study of 45 cases with emphasis on an isolated variant. *Am J Surg Pathol* 2006; 30:1150–1158.

317. Pipitone N, Salvarani C. Idiopathic aortitis: an underrecognized vasculitis. *Arthritis Research & Therapy* 2011; 13:119.

318. Gornik HL, Creager MA. Aortitis. *Circulation* 2008; 117:3039–3051.

319. Deshpande V, Zen Y, Chan JKC, et al. Consensus statement on the pathology of IgG4-related disease. *Modern Pathology* 2012; 25:1181–1192.

320. Stone JH, Zeri Y, Deshpande V. IgG-4 Related disease. *N Engl J Med* 2012; 366:539–551.

321. Nirula A, Glaser SM, Kalled SL, et al. What is IgG4? A review of the biology of a unique immunoglobulin subtype. *Curr Opin Rheumatol* 2011; 23:119–124.

322. Kamisawa T, Okazaki K, Kawa S, et al. Japanese consensus guidelines for management of autoimmune pancreatitis: III. Treatment and prognosis of AIP. *J Gastroenterol* 2010; 45:471–477.

323. Torvik A, Berntzen AE. Necrotizing vasculitis without visceral involvement. Postmortem examination of three cases with affection of skeletal muscles and peripheral nerves. *Acta Med Scand* 1968; 184:69–77.

324. Collins MP, Periquet MI, Mendell JR, et al. Nonsystemic vasculitis neuropathy. Insights from a clinical cohort. *Neurology* 2003; 61:623–630.

325. Klemperer P. Diseases of the collagen system. *Bull NY Acad Med* 1947; 23:581–588.

326. Klemperer P. The pathogenesis of lupus erythematosus and allied conditions. *Ann Intern Med* 1948; 28:1–11.

327. Khamashta MA, Cervers R, Hughes GRV. The central nervous system in systemic lupus erythematosus. *Rheumatol Int* 1991; 11:117–119.

328. Tan EM, Cohen AS, Fries JF, et al. The 1982 revised criteria for classification of systemic lupus erythematosus. *Arthritis Rheum* 1982; 25:1271–1277.

329. Borowoy AM, Pope JE, Silverman E, et al. Neuropsychiatric lupus: The prevalence and autoantibody associations depend on the definition: Results from the 100 Faces of Lupus Cohort. *Semin Arthritis Rheum* 2012; 42:179–185.

330. The American College of Rheumatology nomenclature and case definitions for neuropsychiatric lupus syndrome. *Arthritis Rheum* 1999; 42:599–608.

331. Tomic-Lucic A, Petrovic R, Radak-Perovic M, et al. Late-onset systemic lupus erythematosus: clinical features, course, and prognosis. *Clin Rheumatol* 2013, March 21 [Epub ahead of print].

332. Johnson RT, Richardswon EP. The neurological manifestations of systemic lupus erythematosus. *Medicine* 1968; 47:337–369.

333. Estes D, Christian CL. The natural history of systemic lupus erythematosus by prospective analysis. *Medicine* 1971; 50:85–95.

334. Devinsky O, Petito CK, Alonso DR. Clinical and Neuropathological findings in systemic lupus erythematosus: the role of vasculitis, heart emboli, and thrombotic thrombocytopenic purpura. *Ann Neurol* 1988; 23:380–384.

335. Feinglass EJ, Arnett FC, Dorsch CA, et al. Neuropsychiatric manifestations of systemic lupus erythematosus: Diagnosis, clinical spectrum, and relationship to other features of the disease. *Medicine* 1976; 55:323–339.

336. Mintz G, Fraga A. Arteritis in systemic lupus erythematosus. *Arch Intern Med* 1965; 116:55–66.

337. Trevor RP, Sondheimer FK, Fessel WJ, et al. Angiographic demonstration of major cerebral vessel occlusion in systemic lupus erythematosus. *Neuroradiology* 1972; 4:202–207.

338. Younger DS, Sacco R, Levine SR, et al. Major cerebral vessel occlusion in SLE due to circulating anticardiolipin antibodies. *Stroke* 1994; 25:912–914.

339. Levine SR, Welch KMA. The spectrum of neurologic disease associated with antiphospholipid antibodies. *Arch Neurol* 1987; 44:876–883.

340. McCaffrey LM, Petelin A, Cunha BA. Systemic lupus erythematosus (SLE) cerebritis versus Listeria monocytogenes meningoencephalitis in a patient with systemic lupus erythematosus on chronic corticosteroid therapy: The diagnostic importance of cerebrospinal fluid (CSF) of lactic acid levels. *Heart & Lung* 2012; 41:394–397.

341. Aletaha D, Neogi T, Silman AJ, et al. 2010 Rheumatoid arthritis classification criteria. An American College of Rheumatology/European League Against Rheumatism Collaborative Initiative. *Arthritis Rheum* 2010; 62:2569–2581.

342. Turesson C. Extra-articular rheumatoid arthritis. *Curr Opin Rheumatol* 2013; 25:360–366.

343. Turesson C, Jacobsson LT. Epidemiology of extra-articular manifestations in rheumatoid arthritis. *Scand J Rheumatol* 2004; 33:65–72.

344. Scott DG, Bacon PA. Intravenous cyclophosphamide plus methylprednisolone in treatment of systemic rheumatoid vasculitis. *Am J Med* 1984; 76:377–384.

345. Watts RA, Mooney J, Lane SE, et al. Rheumatoid vasculitis: becoming extinct? *Rheumatology* 2004; 2012; 43:920–923.

346. Myasoedova E, Crowson CS, Turesson C, et al. Incidence of extra-articular rheumatoid arthritis in Olmsted County Minnesota, in 1995–2007 versus 1985–1994: a population-based study. *J Rheumatology* 2011; 38:983–989.

347. Vollerstein RS, Conn DL, Ballard DJ, et al Rheumatoid vasculitis: survival and associated risk factors. *Medicine* 1986; 65:365–375

348. Rasker JJ, Cosh JA. Cause and age at death in a prospective study of 100 patients with rheumatoid arthritis. *Ann Rheum Dis* 2982; 40:115–120.

349. Ouyang R, Mitchell DM, Rozdilsky B. Central nervous system involvement in rheumatoid disease. *Neurology* 1967; 17:1099–1105.

350. Ramos M, Mandybur TI. Cerebral vasculitis in rheumatoid arthritis. *Arch Neurol* 1975; 32:271–275.

351. Steiner JW, Gelbloom AJ. Intracranial manifestations in two cases of systemic rheumatoid disease. *Arthritis Rheum* 1959; 2:537–545.

352. Puechal X, Said G, Hilliquin P, et al. Peripheral neuropathy with necrotizing vasculitis in rheumatoid arthritis. *Arthritis Rheum* 1995; 38:1618–1629.

353. Pirani CL, Bennett GA. Rheumatoid arthritis; a report of three cases progressing from childhood and emphasizing

certain systemic manifestations. *Bull Hosp Joint Dis* 1951; 12:335–367.

354. Kemper JW, Baggenstoss AH, Slocumb CH. The relationship of therapy with cortisone to the incidence of vascular lesions in rheumatoid arthritis. *Ann Intern Med* 1957; 46:831–851.

355. Sokoloff L, Bunim JJ. Vascular lesions in rheumatoid arthritis. *J Chronic Dis* 1957; 5:668–687.

356. Johnson RL, Smyth CJ, Holt GW, et al. Steroid therapy and vascular lesions in rheumatoid arthritis. *Arthritis Rheum* 1959; 2:224–249.

357. Watson P, Fekete J, Deck J. Central nervous system vasculitis inrheumatoid arthritis. *Can J Neurol Sci* 1977; 4:269–272.

358. Puéchal X, Gottenberg JE, Berthelot JM, et al. Rituximab therapy for systemic vasculitis associated with rheumatoid arthritis: Results from the Autoimmunity and Rituximab Registry. *Arthritis Care & Research* 2012; 64:331–339.

359. Bartels CM, Bridges AJ. Rheumatoid vasculitis: Vanishing menace or target for new treatments? *Curr Rheumatol Rep* 2010; 12:414–419.

360. Bartolucci P, Ramanoelina J, Cohen P, et al. Efficacy of the anti-TNF-α antibody infliximab against refractory systemic vasculitides: an open pilot stud on 10 patients. *Rheumatology* 2002; 41:1126–1132.

361. Puéchal X, Miceli-Richard C, Mejjad O, et al. Anti-tumor necrosis factor treatment in patients with refractory systemic vasculitis associated with rheumatoid arthritis. *Ann Rheum Dis* 2008; 67:880–884.

362. Fonseca AC, Ferro JM. Drug abuse and stroke. *Current Neurology and Neuroscience Reports* 2013; 13:325.

363. Petitti DS, S; Quesenberry, C; et al. Stroke and cocaine or amphetamine use. *Epidemiology* 1998; 9:596–600.

364. Westover AN, McBride S, Haley RW. Stroke in young adults who abuse amphetamines or cocaine: a population-based study of hospitalized patients. *Arch Gen Psychiatry* 2007; 64:495–502.

365. Citron BP, Halpern M, McCarron M, et al. Necrotizing angiitis associated with drug abuse. N Engl J Med 1970; 283:1003–1011.

366. Gocke DC, CI. Angiitis in drug abusers [Letter]. *N Engl J Med* 1971; 284:112.

367. Citron B, Peters R. Angiitis in drug abusers [Letter]. *N Engl J Med* 1971; 284:111–113.

368. Baden M. Angiitis in drug abusers [Letter]. *N Engl J Med* 1971; 284:111.

369. Glick R, Hoying J, Cerullo L, et al. Phenylpropanolamine: an over-the-counter drug causing central nervous system vasculitis and intracerebral hemorrhage. Case report and review. *Neurosurgery* 1987; 20:969–974.

370. Kessler JT, Jortner BS, Adapon BD. Cerebral vasculitis in a drug abuser. *J Clin Psychiatry* 1978; 39:559–564.

371. Bostwick DG. Amphetamine induced cerebral vasculitis. *Human Pathology* 1981;12:1031–1033.

372. Olsen ER. Intracranial hemorrhage and amphetamine usage. Review of the effects of amphetamines on the central nervous system. *Angiology* 1977; 28: 464–471.

373. Trugman J. Cerebral arteritis and oral methylamphenidate. *Lancet* 1988; 1:584–585.

374. Buxton N, McConachie NS. Amphetamine abuse and intracranial hemorrhage. *J Royal Coll Soc Med* 2000; 93:472–477.

375. Coroner's Report. Amphetamine overdose kills boy. *The Pharmaceutical Journal* 1976; 198:172.

376. Moriya FH, Y. A case of fatal hemorrhage in the cerebral ventricles following intravenous use of methamphetamine. *Forensic Science International* 2002;129:104–109.

377. Shibata S, Mori K, Sekine I, Suyama H. [An autopsy case of subarachnoid and intracerebral hemorrhage and necrotizing angiitis associated with methamphetamine abuse]. *Brain Nerve* 1988; 40:1089–1094

378. Delaney P, Estes M. Intracranial hemorrhage with amphetamine abuse. *Neurology* 1980; 30:1125–1128.

379. Hall CD, Blanton DE, Scatliff, JH; et al. Speed kills: fatality from the self-administration of methamphetamine intravenously. *South Med J* 1973; 66:650–652.

380. Byard RG, JR; Lokan, RJ. Amphetamine derivative fatalities in South Australia—Is "Ecstasy" the culprit? *Am J Forensic Med Pathol* 1998; 19: 261–265.

381. Perez JA, Jr., Arsura EL, Strategos S. Methamphetamine-related stroke: four cases. *J Emerg Med* 1999; 17:469–471.

382. Ho EL, Josephson SA, Lee HS, Smith WS. Cerebrovascular complications of methamphetamine abuse. *Neurocritical Care* 2009; 10:295–305.

383. Kreek MJ, Levran O, Reed B, et al. Opiate addiction and cocaine addiction: underlying molecular neurobiology and genetics. *J Clin Invest* 2012; 122:3387–393.

384. Kreek MJ, Bart G, Lilly C, al et. Pharmacogenetics and human molecular genetics of opiate and cocaine addictions and their treatments. *Pharmacol Rev* 2005; 57:1–26.

385. Krendel DA, Ditter SM, Frankel MR, et a. Biopsy-proven cerebral vasculitis associated with cocaine abuse. *Neurology* 1990; 40:1092–1094.

386. Fredericks RK, Lefkowitz DS, Challa VR, et al. Cerebral vasculitis associated with cocaine abuse. *Stroke* 1991; 22:1437–1439.

387. Morrow PL, McQuillen JB. Cerebral vasculitis associated with cocaine abuse. *J Forensic Sci* 1993;38:732–738.

388. Tapia JF, JM S. Case 27-1993-A 32- year-old man with the sudden onset of a right-sided headache and left hemiplegia and hemianesthesia. *N Engl J Med* 1993;329:117–124.

389. Merkel PA, Koroshetz WJ, Irizarry MC, et al. Cocaine-associated cerebral vasculitis. *Sem Arthritis Rheum* 1995; 25:172–183.

390. Martinez N, Diez-Tejedor E, Frank A. Vasospasm/thrombus in cerebral ischemia related to cocaine abuse [Letter]. *Stroke* 1996; 27:147 148.

391. Diez-Tejedor E, Frank A, Gutierrez M, et al. Encephalopathy and biopsy-proven cerebrovascular inflammatory changes in a cocaine abuser. *Eur J Neurol* 1998; 5:103–107.

392. Brust JC, Richter RW. Stroke associated with cocaine abuse? *NY State J Med* 1977; 77:1473–1475.

393. Levine SR, Brust JCM, Futrell N, et al. Cerebrovascular complications of the use of the "crack" form of alkaloidal cocaine. *N Engl J Med* 1990; 323:699–704.

394. Daras M, Tuchman AJ, Marks S. Central nervous system infarction related to cocaine abuse. *Stroke* 1991; 22:1320–1325.

395. Nolte KB, Gelman BB. Intracerebral hemorrhage associated with cocaine abuse. *Arch Pathol Lab Med* 1989; 113:812–813.

396. Kaye BR, Fainstat M. Cerebral vasculitis associated with cocaine abuse. *JAMA* 1987; 258:2104–2106.

397. Levine S, JCM B, Welch K. Cerebral vasculitis associated with cocaine abuse or subarachnoid hemorrhage? *JAMA* 1988; 259:1648–1649.

398. Oehmichen M, Meissner C, Reiter A, et al. Neuropathology in non-human immunodeficiency virus-infected drug addicts: hypoxic brain damage after chronic intravenous drug abuse. *Acta Neuropathologica* 1996; 91:642–646.

399. Gray F, Lescs MC, Keohane C, et al. Early brain changes in HIV infection: Neuropathological study of 11 HIV seropositive, non-AIDS cases. *J Neuropathol Exp Neurol* 1992; 51:177–185.

400. Adle-Biassette H, Marc B, Benhaiem-Sigaux N, et al. Cerebral infarctions in a drug addict inhaling heroin. *Archives D'Anatomie et de Cytologie Pathologiques* 1996; 44:12–17.

401. Lignelli GJ, WA B. Angiitis in drug abusers [Letter]. *N Engl J Med* 1971; 284:112–113.

402. Woods BT, Strewler GJ. Hemiparesis occurring six hours after intravenous heroin injection. *Neurology* 1972; 22:863–866.

403. Niehaus L, Meyer BU. Bilateral borderzone brain

infarctions in association with heroin abuse. *J Neurol Sci* 1998; 160:180–182.

404. Benoilid A, Collongues N, de Seze J, Blanc F. Heroin inhalation-induced unilateral complete hippocampal stroke. Neurocase 2012. doi: 10.1080/13554794.2012.667125.

405. Bartolomei F, Nicoli F, Swiader L, et al. [Ischemic cerebral vascular stroke after heroin sniffing. A new case]. *Presse Med* 1992; 21:983–986.

406. Kent ME, Romanelli F. Reexamining syphilis: an update on epidemiology, clinical manifestations, and management. *Ann Pharmacother* 2008; 42:226–236.

407. Burke JM, Schaberg DR. Neurosyphilis in the antibiotic era. *Neurology* 1985; 35:1368–1371.

408. Fend W, Caplan M, Matheus MG, et al. Meningovascular syphilis with fatal verebrobasilar occlusion. *Am J Med Sci* 2009; 338:169–171.

409. Amlie-Lefond C, Jubelt B. Neurologic manifestations of varicella zoster virus infections. Current Neurology *Neuroscience Reports* 2009; 9:430–434.

410. Kleinschmidt-DeMasters BK, Gilden DH. Varicella-zoster virus infections of the nervous system: clinical and pathologic correlates. *Arch Pathol Lab Med* 2001; 125:770–780.

411. Nagel MA, Traktinskiy I, Stenmark KR, et al. Varicella-zoster virus vasculopathy: immune characteristics of virus-infected arteries. *Neurology* 2013; 80:62–68.

412. Doyle P, Gibson G, Dooman C. Herpes zoster ophthalmicus with contralateral hemiplegia. Identification of cause. *Ann Neurol* 1983; 14:84–85.

413. Hilt D, Buchholz D, Krumholz A, et al. Herpes zoster ophthalmicus and delayed contralateral hemiparesis caused by cerebral angiitis: Diagnosis and management approaches. *Ann Neurol* 1983; 14:543–553.

414. Leis A, Butler IJ. Infantile herpes zoster ophthalmicus and acute hemiparesis following intrauterine chickenpox. *Neurology* 1987; 37:1537–1538.

415. Rosenblum W, Hadfield M. Granulomatous angiitis of the nervous system in causes of herpes zoster and lymphosarcoma. *Neurology* 1972; 22:348–354.

416. Reyes M, Fresco R, Chokroverty S, et al. Virus-like particles in granulomatous angiitis of the central nervous system. *Neurology* 1976; 26:797–799.

417. Nachega JB, Morroni C, Chaisson RE, Goliath R, Efron A, Ram M, et al. Impact of immune reconstitution inflammatory syndrome on antiretroviral therapy adherence. *Patient Preference and Adherence* 2012; 6:887–891.

418. Sharer LR, Kapila R. Neuropathologic observations in acquired immunodeficiency syndrome (AIDS). *Acta Neuropathologica* 1985; 66:188–198.

419. McArthur JC, Haughey N, Gartner S, et al. Human immunodeficiency virus-associated dementia: an evolving disease. *J Neurovirol* 2003; 9:205–221.

420. Price RW, Brew B, Sidtis J, et al. The brain in AIDS: central nervous system HIV-1 infection and AIDS dementia complex. *Science* 1988; 239:586–592.

421. Petito CK. Review of central nervous system pathology in human immunodeficiency virus infection. *Ann Neurol* 1988; 23(Suppl):S54–S7.

422. Bell JE, Busuttil A, Ironside JW, et al. Human immunodeficiency virus and the brain: investigation of virus load and neuropathologic changes in pre-AIDS subjects. *J Inf Dis* 1993; 168:818–824.

423. Bell JE, Arango JC, Anthony IC. Neurobiology of multiple insults: HIV-1-associated brain disorders in those who use illicit drugs. *J Neuroimmune Pharmacol* 2006; 1:182–191.

424. Connor MD, Lammie GA, Bell JE, et al. Cerebral infarction in adult AIDS patients: observations from the Edinburgh HIV Autopsy Cohort. *Stroke* 2000; 31:2117–2126.

425. Esiri MM, Scaravilli F, Millard PR, et al. Neuropathology of HIV infection in haemophiliacs: comparative necropsy study. *BMJ* 1989; 299:1312–1315.

426. Sharer LR, Michaels J, Murphey-Corb M, et al. Serial pathogenesis study of SIV brain infection. *J Med Primatol* 1991; 20:211–217.

427. Hurtrel M, Ganiere JP, Guelfi JF, et al. Comparison of early and late feline immunodeficiency virus encephalopathies. *AIDS* 1992; 6:399–406.

428. Van der Ven AJ, Van Oostenbrugge RJ, Kubat B, et al. Cerebral vasculitis after initiation antiretroviral therapy. *AIDS* 2002; 16:2362–2364.

429. Langford TD, Letendre SL, Marcotte TD, et al. Severe, demyelinating leukoencephalopathy in AIDS patients on antiretroviral therapy. *AIDS* 2002; 16:1019–1029.

430. Patel AK, Patel KK, Shah SD, et al. Immune reconstitution syndrome presenting with cerebral varicella zoster vasculitis in HIV-1-infected patient: a case report. *JIAPAC* 2006; 5:157–160.

CHAPTER **15**

Clinical Research Parameters in Neuromuscular Disease

Richard J. Barohn, Laura Herbelin, Mazen M. Dimachkie

Clinical research in neuromuscular disease has grown remarkably in the last several decades. At the simplest level, clinical research begins with simple case presentations describing unusual individual cases (1–7) that can be expanded to small and large case series (8–20), from which retrospective clinical data can be used to make statements about effectiveness of therapies used in the clinical setting (21, 22). Those can be followed by retrospective case reports, ideas for prospective series, and plans for future data collection. Such prospective series can be of the observational and interventional study types, in which the former is used to ascertain the natural history of a given disorder, while the latter involves an interventional drug or device. Interventional studies themselves may take the form of a simple case report (23) or lay the framework for a future large trial. (24). Observational research in neuromuscular disease involves direct participant contact and recording clinical measurements or reporting results from blood, muscle, nerve, skin, cerebrospinal fluid (CSF) samples, and neuroimaging procedures (25, 26), laying the groundwork for an in-depth analysis of one or more related parameters (27).

The availability of several large clinical databases such as the Medicare database, the Nationwide Inpatient Sample, and various electronic medical record systems (28–30) were used to address and answer important questions in myasthenia gravis (MG) comparisons of outcomes following therapeutic plasma exchange (PE) and intravenous immune globulin (IVIg) therapy, and utilization of hospital services and outcomes in others with amyotrophic lateral sclerosis (ALS). The types of clinical endpoints chosen for analysis can be as simple as survival or mortality (31), or a more complicated physiological measure such as quantitative muscle strength or vital capacity (VC). According to the Common Data Element (CDE) initiative of the National Institute of Neurological Disorders and Stroke (NINDS), the supplemental and exploratory data is essential to the development of common definitions, data-set capture, and recording, while promoting standards for clinical research in the neuromuscular community (www.commondataelements.ninds.nih.gov).

MOTOR NEURON DISEASES

Amyotrophic Lateral Sclerosis

Functional Rating Scale

The revised Amyotrophic Lateral Sclerosis Functional Rating Scale (ALSFRS-R), shown in Table 1, is the most widely used primary outcome measure in ALS clinical trials (32–42), demonstrating a reliable and reproducible correlation with quantitative strength testing (42, 43) without the necessity of specialized equipment and specialized training of clinical evaluators. The goal of a therapeutic research intervention in ALS is slowing the rate of decline of the ALSFRS by 15% to 30%, which is accepted to be approximately 1.0 unit per month in natural history trials. The ALSFRS-R, which scores 12 items on a scale of 0 to 4, takes about 10 minutes to perform in person or over the phone (44–46); nevertheless it has the disadvantage of insensitivity to small changes in neurologic function.

Table 1. Revised ALS Functional Rating Scale[1]

1. *Speech*
   4 Normal speech processes.
   3 Detectable speech disturbance.
   2 Intelligible with repeating.
   1 Speech combined with non-vocal communication.
   0 Loss of useful speech.

2. *Salivation*
   4 Normal.
   3 Slight but definite excess of saliva in mouth; may have nighttime drooling.
   2 Moderately excessive saliva; may have minimal drooling.
   1 Marked excess of saliva with some drooling.
   0 Marked drooling; requires constant tissue or handkerchief.

3. *Swallowing*
   4 Normal eating habits.
   3 Early eating problems—occasional choking.
   2 Dietary consistency changes.
   1 Needs supplemental tube feeding.
   0 NPO (exclusively parenteral or enteral feeding).

4. *Handwriting*
   4 Normal.
   3 Slow or sloppy: all words are legible.
   2 Not all words are legible.
   1 Able to grip pen but unable to write.
   0 Unable to grip pen.

5a. *Cutting food and handling utensils (patients without gastrostomy)*
   4 Normal.
   3 Somewhat slow and clumsy, but no help needed.
   2 Can cut most foods, although clumsy and slow; some help needed.
   1 Food must be cut by someone, but can still feed slowly.
   0 Needs to be fed.

5b. *Cutting food and handling utensils (alternate scale for patients with gastrostomy)*
   4 Normal.
   3 Clumsy but able to perform all manipulations independently.
   2 Some help needed with closures and fasteners.
   1 Provides minimal assistance to caregiver.
   0 Unable to perform any aspect of task.

6. *Dressing and hygiene*
   4 Normal function.
   3 Independent and complete self-care with effort or decreased efficiency.
   2 Intermittent assistance or substitute methods.
   1 Needs attendant for self-care.
   0 Total dependence.

7. *Turning in bed and adjusting bed clothes*
   4 Normal.
   3 Somewhat slow and clumsy, but no help needed.
   2 Can turn alone or adjust sheets, but with great difficulty.
   1 Can initiate, but not turn or adjust sheets alone.
   0 Helpless.

8. *Walking*
   4 Normal.
   3 Early ambulation difficulties.
   2 Walks with assistance.
   1 Non-ambulatory functional movement only.
   0 No purposeful leg movement.

9. *Climbing stairs*
   4 Normal.
   3 Slow.
   2 Mild unsteadiness or fatigue.
   1 Needs assistance.
   0 Cannot do.

10. *Dyspnea*
   4 None.
   3 Occurs when walking.
   2 Occurs with one or more of the following: eating, bathing, dressing (ADL).
   1 Occurs at rest, difficulty breathing when either sitting or lying.
   0 Significant difficulty, considering using mechanical respiratory support.

11. *Orthopnea*
   4 None.
   3 Some difficulty sleeping due to shortness of breath, does not routinely use >2 pillows.
   2 Needs extra pillows to sleep (>2).
   1 Can only sleep sitting up.
   0 Unable to sleep.

12. *Respiratory insufficiency*
   4 None.
   3 Intermittent use of BIPAP.
   2 Continuous use of BIPAP at night.
   1 Continuous use of BIPAP day and night.
   0 Invasive mechanical ventilation by intubation/ tracheostomy.

[1]Adapted from, Cedarbaum JM, Stambler N, Malta E, et al, and The BDNF ALS Study Group. The ALSFRS-R: a revised ALS functional rating scale that incorporates assessments of respiratory function. *J Neurol Sci* 1999; 169:13–21.

Strength Measures

Maximal Voluntary Isometric Contraction

Maximal voluntary isometric contraction (MVIC) testing is a standardized measure of the force of a muscular contraction by a transducer system that has been modified and adopted for ALS studies (47). Expressed as z-scores, and averaged to obtain a megascore (36–38, 48–52), it demonstrates a linear decline over time. An advantage of this modality is the greater sensitivity in detecting small changes in strength that might otherwise be missed in ordinal strength measures and function testing scales, while the disadvantages are the large size of the equipment, increased expense, and necessity of evaluator training. While hand-held dynamometry devices that measure strength in various muscle groups (31, 33, 34, 53–56) have good agreement with MVIC and ALSFR-S, there is need of the former to ascertain improvement in the slope of the deterioration curve in judging the success of any positive therapeutic intervention.

Manual Muscle Testing

Manual muscle testing (MMT) employing British Medical Research Council (MRC) scale of 0 to 5 is the commonest method of assessing strength in the clinical setting (32, 35, 49, 57–60), and correlates with MVICT in ALS patients. (61).

Respiratory Measurements

Respiratory insufficiency is the usual cause of death in patients with ALS and the decline in respiratory measures can be documented over the course of the illness. Although employed most often as secondary endpoint, forced VC is most commonly employed, with a decline that correlates other clinical trial endpoints (31, 32, 36–39, 53, 54, 62–68). Other measures include maximal inspiratory and expiratory positive pressures (PIM_{ax} and PEM_{ax}), and forced and slow vital capacity, which correlate with ALSFRS-R and MVIC (43).

Quality of Life Instruments

A number of generic quality of life instruments have been utilized in ALS studies, including a 36-item short-form (SF-36) (69–77), EuroQol (EQ)-5D (78–81), and the Sickness Impact Profile (SIP-19) (82–84); however, one Health Related Quality of Life (HRQOL) instrument, the McGill Quality of Life questionnaire (MQoL), consists of 16 items grouped into five subscales of questions comprising

Table 2. The ALS Specific Quality of Life Scale[1]
Single Item Global Impression

Please assess your overall quality of life over the past week (7 days).

Considering all parts of my life:
• physical,
• emotional,
• social,
• spiritual, and
• financial

Over the past week, the quality of my life has been:

Very bad									Excellent
01 2 3	4	5	6	7	8	9	10

[1]Adapted from, Felgoise S, Rodriguez J, Stephens H, et al. Validation of a shorter ALS-specific quality of life instrument: the ALSSQOL-R. *Amyotroph Lateral Scler* 2008; 9(Suppl):12–13.

physical and psychological well-being symptoms, and those of existential well-being and support (85, 86). Though this questionnaire does not correlate with measures of physical strength and function, it does with psychological, existential, and support subscores in the ALS population (87, 88). Viewing the Schedule for the Evaluation of Individual Quality of Life (SEIQoL), there is a correlation with physical strength, may function as well as ties to friends, hobbies, spiritual life/religion, and psychosocial or existential background (89). The ALS-specific quality of life (ALSSQoL) measure (90), composed of 46 items, scored on a 0 to 10 scale, incorporates the (HRQoL) and the McGill quality of life (MQoL) measures, the advantage of which is the focus on issues perceived to be meaningful for patients (Table 2). (91). One other ALS quality-of-life instrument is the ALS questionaireALSAQ-40 (92, 93).

Spinal Muscular Atrophy

Many of the scales used in ALS have been used in spinal muscular atrophy (SMA) (94, 95). The SMA functional rating scale (SMAFRS) was adapted from the ALSFRS to assess function in patients with SMA (94, 96). Patients or caregivers are asked to rate and compare their present function in eating, dressing of the upper and lower body, bathing, toileting and grooming, oral hygiene, turning in bed, and adjusting bed clothes, studied in childhood SMA (97)

In Pediatric SMA type I studies, other functional outcome measures have been shown to be reliable and are now routinely performed. Two of these procedures are the Test for Infant Motor Performance Screening Item (TIMPSI) (98–100) and the Children's Hospital of Philadelphia Infant Test of Neuromuscular Disorders (CHOP INTEND) (101).

The TIMPSI is a reliable and validated measure of postural and selective control of movements in infants less than five months of age. and the CHOP INTEND is a reliable, yet not validated, measure of SMA-1 motor skills.

Another method to measure gross motor maturation of infants from birth through the age of independent walking is the Alberta Infant Motor Scale (AIMS). This measurement gauges infant performance in their transition through four positions: supine, prone, sitting, and standing (102).

PERIPHERAL NEUROPATHY

Similar instruments have been validated for specific types of neuropathy, including distal symmetric diabetic polyneuropathy (DPN), Charcot-Marie-Tooth disease (CMT), acute inflammatory demyelinating polyneuropathy (AIDP), chronic inflammatory demyelinating polyradiculoneuropathy (CIDP), and multifocal motor neuropathy (MMN).

Diabetic Neuropathy

The Neuropathy Disability Score, later renamed the Neuropathy Impairment Score (NIS), which lists abnormal items in the neurologic examination, including cranial nerve, motor, sensory function, deep tendon reflexes (DTR), and estimating impairment severity, has been validated in clinical studies of acquired and genetic neuropathies including DPN, CIDP, and transthyretin (TTR)-related familial amyloid polyneuropathy (FAP) (103–105). An NIS of the lower limb (NIS-LL) derives from 14 bilateral items, including eight related to leg muscle power, scored 0 to 4 points in hip, knee, ankle and toes flexors and extensors; two in knee and ankle DTR scored 0 to 2 points, and four items pertaining to toe touch, pin perception, vibration, and position sensation, rated 0 to 2 points. There is a supplementary composite of seven neurophysioplogic parameters that provide minimal criteria for DPN, including detection of vibratory thresholds, fibular motor nerve conduction velocity (NCV), fibular distal motor latency, fibular compound muscle action potential (CMAP) amplitude, tibial distal motor latency, sural sensory nerve action potential (SNAP) amplitude, and changes in heart rate response to deep breathing (HRDB) (101), applied in the Nathan 1 trial of α-lipoic acid in DPN (102).

The Michigan Neuropathy Screening Instrument (103), a two-step approach based on self-reported history (Table 3), followed by examination of foot appearance, ulceration, ankle DTR, and foot sensation, is a valid screening tool (104), the composite values of which declined with worsening nerve conduction study (NCS) parameters in the placebo group of the natural history of diabetic neuropathy in the Zenarestat study (105).

The Total Neuropathy Score (TNS) (Table 4) (106), which comprised the combination of scored symptoms of sensation, motor and autonomic function, and signs of pinprick and vibratory perception, strength, and DTR, as well as instrument testing of quantitative vibratory sensory testing (QST) and sural and peroneal SNAP amplitudes, demonstrated excellent inter- and intra-rater reliability, cross-sectional validation, and correlations with all measures of DPN.

The Utah Early Neuropathy Score (UENS) (107), designed specifically to provide increased sensitivity to detect mild neuropathy and early diabetic small fiber neuropathy (SFN) and its progression by virtue of spreading sensory loss (Table 5), focused less on muscle weakness compared with the NIS-LL, correlated with changes in small-fiber neuropathy measures over a one-year follow-up. A variety of pain scales have been employed for painful DPN including the McGill pain questionnaire and its short form, visual analogue scale (VAS) 10-cm scale, and the Likert numeric pain rating scale. Secondary endpoint measures include physician and patient global impression of change, sleep interference, and quality-of-life questions.

In addition, measures of outcome in DPN included NCS and QST in the NIS-LL +7, and intraepidermal nerve-fiber density (IENFD) of a 3-mm punch biopsy specimen obtained 10 cm above the lateral malleolus or along the distal thigh, evaluated qualitatively and quantitatively by the cytoplasmic neuronal marker PGP 9.5 in the Fabry disease enzyme replacement therapy study (108). Secondary branching was excluded from quantification that, however, single IENF crossing the dermal–epidermal junction were counted with good intra- and inter-observer reliability. In idiopathic SFN (109) there is a high concordance rate between reduced foot IENF density and loss of pinprick sensitivity. Since quantification of IENF density assesses small fiber involvement better than sural nerve biopsy, it should be included as an end point in all prospective peripheral neuropathy trials. Patients with asymptomatic human immunodeficiency virus type I (HIV-1) infection with or without neurological signs, demonstrated lower IENF density and increased risk of progression to symptomatic HIV-associated distal sensory neuropathy six to twelve months later (110). The IENF density progressively declines with increased severity of clinical neuropathy (111). In a study of diet and exercise in those with impaired glucose tolerance and neuropathy, punch skin biopsy was the most sensitive measure of change in DPN over the course of a year, and increased IENF density at the proximal thigh correlated with decreased neuropathic pain intensity (112). The rate of IENF regeneration and subsequent quantitation after capsaicin chemical denervation was slower in asymptomatic subjects with DPN and HIV compared to healthy control subjects (113–115), consistent with the assumption

Table 3. Neuropathy Screening Instrument Questionnaire[1]

Part A: Please take a few minutes to answer the questions below about the feeling in your legs and feet. Check yes or no based on how you usually feel.

1. Are your legs and/or feet numb? Yes __ No __
2. Do you ever have any burning pain in your legs and/or feet? Yes __ No __
3. Are your feet too sensitive to touch? Yes __ No __
4. Do you get muscle cramps in your legs and/or feet? Yes __ No __
5. Do you ever have any prickling feelings in your legs or feet? Yes __ No __
6. Does it hurt when the bed covers touch your skin? Yes __ No __
7. When you get into the tub or shower, are you able to tell the hot water from the cold water? Yes __ No __
8. Have you ever had an open sore on your foot? Yes __ No __
9. Has your doctor ever told you that you have diabetic neuropathy? Yes __ No __
10. Do you feel weak all over most of the time? Yes __ No __
11. Are your symptoms worse at night? Yes __ No __
12. Do your legs hurt when you walk? Yes __ No __
13. Are you able to sense your feet when you walk? Yes __ No __
14. Is the skin on your feet so dry that it cracks open? Yes __ No __
15. Have you ever had an amputation? Yes __ No __

Part B: Physical Assessment

1. Appearance of feet:
   Right
   a. Normal 0 Yes 1
   b. If no, check all that apply:
      Deformities
      Dry skin, callus
      Infection
      Fissure
      Other: specify
   Left
   a. Normal 0 Yes 1
   b. If no, check all that apply:
      Deformities
      Dry skin, callus
      Infection
      Fissure
      Other: specify

2. Ulceration Right and Left
   Absent 0 or Present 1
   Ulceration Right and Left
   Absent 0 or Present 1

3. Ankle Reflexes Right and Left
   Present 0, Reinforcement 0.5, Absent 1
   Ankle Reflexes Right and Left
   Present 0, Reinforcement 0.5, Absent 1

4. Vibration at great toe
   Present 0, Decreased 0.5, Absent 1
   Vibration at great toe
   Present 0, Decreased 0.5, Absent 1

5. Monofilament
   Normal 0, Reduced 0.5 Absent 1
   Monofilament
   Normal 0, Reduced 0.5 Absent 1

[1]Adapted and modified from, Feldman EL, Stevens MJ, Thomas PK, et al. A practical two-step quantitative clinical and electrophysiological assessment for the diagnosis and staging of diabetic neuropathy. *Diabetes Care* 1994; 17:1281–1289.

Table 4. Total Neuropathy Score[1]

Parameter	Score				
	0	1	2	3	4
Sensory symptoms	None	Symptoms limited to fingers or toes	Symptoms extend to ankle or wrist	Symptoms extend to knee or elbow	Symptoms above knees or elbows, or functionally disabling
Motor symptoms	None	Slight difficulty	Moderate difficulty	Require help/ assistance	Paralysis
Autonomic symptoms	0	1	2	3	4 or 5
Pin sensibility	Normal	Reduced in fingers/ toes	Reduced up to wrist/ankle	Reduced up to elbow/knee	Reduced to above elbow/knee
Vibration sensibility	Normal	Reduced in fingers/ toes	Reduced up to wrist/ankle	Reduced up to elbow/knee	Reduced to above elbow/knee
Strength	Normal	Mild weakness	Moderate weakness	Severe weakness	Paralysis
Tendon reflexes	Normal	Ankle reflex reduced	Ankle reflex absent	Ankle reflex absent, others reduced	All reflexes absent
Vibration sensation (QST vibration)	Normal to 125% ULN	126 to 150% ULN	151 to 200% ULN	201 to 300% ULN	>300% ULN
Sural amplitude	Normal/reduced to <5% LLN	76 to 95% of LLN	51 to 75% of LLN	26 to 50% of LLN	0 to 25% of LLN
Peroneal amplitude	Normal/reduced to <5% LLN	76 to 95% of LLN	51 to 75% of LLN	26 to 50% of LLN	0 to 25% of LLN

QST = quantitative sensory test; ULN = upper limit of normal; LLN = lower limit of normal.

[1]Adapted from, Cornblath DR, Chaudhry V, Carter K, et al. Total neuropathy score: validation and reliability study. *Neurology* 1999; 53:1660–1664.

that serial IENFD measurement provides a clinically useful index of recovery to the salutary effects of neuropathy disease-modifying therapies.

Charcot-Marie-Tooth Disease

The Charcot-Marie-Tooth Neuropathy score (CMTNS), based on a modification of the TNS, placing more emphasis on motor function, contains nine assessments including three items of symptoms, four signs, and two neurophysiological parameters (Table 6). Sixty subjects so studied were divided into mild (CMTNS ≤10), moderate (CMTNS 11 to 20), and severe (CMTNS ≥21) categories, with >95% inter- and intra-investigator reliability across all measures of disability (116). Lack of standardization in the way the subjects were asked questions may have led to differences

in the interpretation of symptoms (117) and floor or ceiling effects, prompting design of the CMTNS2, which demonstrated favorable inter- and intra-rater reliability. Further longitudinal analyses are being carried out to ascertain whether CMTNS2 is more sensitive than CMTNS in detecting changes over time.

Immune-Mediated Neuropathy

Hughes and colleagues (118) employed a 7-point Guillain-Barré syndrome (GBS) disability scale ranging from 0 (normal) to 7 (dead) with 3 able to walk 5 meters with assistance. Employing this simple outcome measure in a clinical trial of plasma exchange (PE) (119, 120) and IVIg (121), with an improvement of one grade at four weeks, demonstrated respective efficacy in both treatment modalities. A

Table 5. The Utah Early Neuropathy Score[1]

Patient Name	
Study Number	
Visit	

The Utah Early Neuropathy Scale

Motor Examination   Left   Right

0   normal
2   weak

Great Toe Extension

Total both sides (out of 4)

Segments for pin sensation reporting

Left Leg   Right Leg

Pin Sensation: L   R

0   normal

1   for each segment with
     reduced sensation

2   for each segment with
     absent sensation

Total both sides (out of 24)

Allodynia/Hyperesthesia   L   R

0   normal

1   if present in toes or foot

Total both sides (out of 2)

Large Fiber Sensation   L   R

0   normal
1   diminished
2   absent

Great toe vibration

time   s   s

Great toe joint position

Total both sides (out of 8)

Deep Tendon Reflexes   L   R

0   normal
1   diminished
2   absent

Ankle

Total both sides (out of 4

Total Score (out of 42)

[1]Adapted from, Singleton JR, Bixby B, Russell JW, et al. The Utah Early Neuropathy Scale: a sensitive clinical scale for early sensory predominant neuropathy. *J Peripher Nerv Syst* 2008; 13:218–27.

Table 6. CMT Neuropathy Score[1]

Parameter	Score				
	0	1	2	3	4
Sensory symptoms	None	Limited to toes	Extend up to and may include ankle	Extend up to and may include knee	Extends above knees
Motor symptoms					
Legs	None	Trips, catches toes, slaps feet	AFO on at least 1 leg or ankle support	Cane, walker, ankle surgery	Wheelchair most of the time
Arms	None	Difficulty with buttons/zippers	Unable to do buttons or zippers but can write	Cannot write or use keyboard	Prosimal arms
Pin sensibility	Normal	Reduced in fingers/toes	Reduced up to and may include wrist/ankle	Reduced up to and may include elbow/knee	Reduced above elbow/knee
Vibration	Normal	Reduced at fingers/toes	Reduced at wrist/ankle	Reduced at elbow/knee	Redulced above elbow/knee
Strength					
Legs	Normal	4+, 4, or 4- on dorsiflexion	≤3 foot dorsiflexion	≤3 dorsiflexion and plantar flexion	Proximal weakness
Arms	Normal	4+, 4, or 4- on intrinsics or finger extensors	≤3 intrinsics or finger extensions	≤3 wrist extensors	Weak above elbow
Ulnar CMAP (Median)	>6 mV (>4 mV)	4.0-5.9 mV (2.8-3.9)	2.0-3.9 mV (1.2-2.7)	0.1-1.9 mV (0.1-1.1)	Absent (Absent)
Ulnar SNAP (Median)	>9 µV (>22 µV)	6.0-8.9 µV (14.0-21.9)	3.0-5.9 µV (7.0-13.9)	0.1-2.9 µV (0.1-6.9)	Absent (Absent)
Total (max. 36)					

AFO-ankle-foot orthosis; CMAP-compound muscle potential; SNAP-sensory nerve action potential

[1]Adapted from, Shy M, Blake J, Krajewski K, et al. Reliability and validity of the CMT neuropathy score as a measure of disability. *Neurology* 2005; 64:1209–1214.

CIDP study that compared IVIg and corticosteroids in the Inflammatory Neuropathy Cause and Treatment (INCAT) Group (122) introduced the INCAT Disability Scale (Table 7), comprised of ten disability items measuring composite motor function of the arms and legs, graded 0 to 5 in diminishing function, with 0 normal and 5 no movement. The INCAT group expanded the leg score in the inflammatory neuropathy Overall Disability Score Scale (ODSS) (123) that, instead, focused on upper and lower limb functions, consisting of an interview checklist, also scored 0 to 5 in the arms, and 0 to 7 in the legs, respectively, wherein 5 or 7 signified no purposeful movement and 0 was normal. To reduce a possible ceiling effect, the ODSS was modified to include climbing stairs and running, and was relabeled the Overall Neuropathy Limitations Scale (ONLS) (124). The INCAT Disability Scale was the primary outcome measure for later GBS, CIDP, and MMN trials (Table 7). The INCAT Disability Scale was employed in two other positive studies, one demonstrating efficacy (125) in a double-blind, placebo controlled trial of 10% caprylate/chromatography purified IVIg versus placebo administered every three weeks, and another that examined improvements and maintenance of health-related quality of life (126), ascertained by the SF-36 and the Rotterdam Handicap Scale. Other research trials in inflammatory demyelinating neuropathy have used MVIC testing using quantitative dynamometry, manual muscle strength testing, and an average muscle score (127).

Table 7. INCAT Disability Scale[1]

Arm disability

1 = Symptoms, in one or both arms, not affecting the ability to perform any of the following functions: doing all zips and buttons; washing or brushing hair; using a knife and fork together; and handling small coins
2 = Symptoms, in one arm or both arms, affecting but not preventing any of the above-mentioned functions
3 = Symptoms, in one arm or both arms, preventing one or two of the above-mentioned functions
4 = Symptoms, in one arm or both arms, preventing three or all of the functions listed, but some purposeful movements still possible
5 = Inability to use either arm for any purposeful movement

Leg disability

0 = Walking not affected
1 = Walking affected, but walks independently outdoors
2 = Usually uses unilateral support (stick, single crutch, one arm) to walk outdoors
3 = Usually uses bilateral support (sticks, crutches, frame, two arms) to walk outdoors
4 = Usually uses wheelchair to travel outdoors, but able to stand and walk a few steps with help
5 = Restricted to wheelchair, unable to stand and walk a few steps with help
Overall disability = Sum of arm and leg disability

[1]Adapted from, Hughes R, Bensa S, Willison H, et al. Randomized controlled trial of intravenous immunoglobulin versus oral prednisolone in chronic inflammatory demyelinating polyneuropathy. *Ann Neurol* 2001; 50:195-201.

MYASTHENIA GRAVIS

Quantitative MG Score

The quantitative MG score (QMG) (128) expanded and modified the scale developed by Bessinger and colleagues (129, 130) that consisted of eight items, each graded 0 to 3 with the score of 3 being the most severe. Tindall and colleagues (131, 132) expanded the scale to 13 items and used it as a primary efficacy measurement in two trials of the efficacy of cyclosporine, and Barohn and coworkers (133–135), in turn, replaced three subjective items in facial muscles, chewing and swallowing, rendering it more objective (Table 8), enabling it to reach the 95% confidence level in inter-rater reliability as a primary outcome measure, such that QMG scores did not differ by more than 2.63 units, translating to a required sample size of 17 patients in each treatment group, allowing the detection of a significant difference of power, 0.80. The QMG can be completed in 20 to 30 minutes. The only specialized equipment required are a spirometer and grip dynamometer. The first Myasthenia Gravis Foundation of America (MGFA) Task Force recommended the QMG be used in all prospective studies as therapy for MG (133). It has since been used in studies of mycophenolate mofetil, IVIg, and PE (136–140), employing post-intervention status definitions for clinical myasthenic remission, improvement, and worsening status (133).

Myasthenia Gravis Manual Muscle Testing

A disease-specific manual MMT can be performed at the bedside without specialized equipment (Table 9), addressing 30 muscle groups typically affected by MG including 6 cranial and 24 axial, measured on a scale of 0 to 4. The MG-MMT demonstrates good inter-rater reliability with a mean difference between scores of 1.3 +/- 1.8 points and correlates well with the QMG. However, there is a wide scatter of MG MMT values within general disease classifications, an issue also observed with QMG. Advantages of the MG MMT are that it can be easily performed by the physician as part of a routine clinical visit and requires no specialized equipment (141).

Myasthenia Muscle Score

The Myasthenia Muscle Score (MMS) sums nine independent functions that encompass cranial, neck, truncal, and limb strength with a total score that ranges from 0 to 100, and unlike those developed earlier, a highest score MMS indicates better strength and function (142, 143). Pulmonary function is not assessed in the MMS, but it is in the QMG.

Table 8. Quantitative MG Score[1]

TEST ITEMS WEAKNESS (SCORE)	NONE (0)	MILD (1)	MODERATE (2)	SEVERE (3)	Item Score (0,1,2 or 3)
1. Double vision on lateral gaze right or left (circle one), seconds	61	11–60	1–10	Spontaneous	
2. Ptosis (upward gaze), seconds	61	11–60	1–10	Spontaneous	
3. Facial Muscles	Normal lid closure	Complete weak, some resistance	Complete, without resistance	Incomplete	
4. Swallowing 4 oz./ 120 ml water	Normal	Minimal coughing or throat clearing	Severe coughing/ choking or nasal regurgitation	Cannot swallow (test not attempted)	
5. Speech following counting aloud from 1–50 (onset of dysarthria)	None at #50	Dysarthria at #30–49	Dysarthria at #10–29	Dysarthria at #9	
6. Right arm outstretched (90° sitting), seconds	240	90–239	10–89	0–9	
7. Left arm outstretched (90° sitting), seconds	240	90–239	10–89	0–9	
8. Vital Capacity (% predicted) mouthpiece or facemask (circle one; best of 3)	≥80%	65–79%	50–64%	<50%	
9. Right hand grip: (best of 2) male (KgW) female	≥45 ≥30	15–44 10–29	5–14 5–9	0–4 0–4	
10. Left hand grip: (best of 2) male (KgW) female	≥35 ≥25	15–34 10–24	5–14 5–9	0–4 0–4	
11. Head, lifted (45° supine), seconds	120	30–119	1–29	0	
12. Right leg outstretched (45° supine), seconds	100	31–99	1–30	0	
13. Left leg outstretched (45° supine), seconds	100	31–99	1–30	0	

TOTAL QMG SCORE (range 0–39) _____

[1]Adapted from, Barohn RJ, McIntire D, Herbelin L, et al. Reliability testing of the quantitative myasthenia gravis score. *Ann NY Acad Sci* 1998; 13; 841:769–772.

Table 9. Myasthenia Gravis Manual Muscle Test[1]

	Right	Left	Sum
Lid ptosis	___	___	___
Diplopia	___	___	___
Eye closure	___	___	___
Cheek puff	___	___	___
Tongue protrusion	___	___	___
Jaw closure	___	___	___
Neck flexion	___	___	___
Neck extension	___	___	___
Shoulder abduction (deltoid)	___	___	___
Elbow flexion (biceps)	___	___	___
Elbow extension (triceps)	___	___	___
Wrist extension	___	___	___
Grip	___	___	___
Hip flexion (iliopsoas)	___	___	___
Knee extension (quadriceps)	___	___	___
Knee flexion (hamstrings)	___	___	___
Ankle dorsiflexion	___	___	___
Ankle plantar flexion	___	___	___
Total score	___	___	___

Score each function as follows: 0, normal; 1, 25% weak/mild impairment; 2, 50% weak/moderate impairment; 3, 75% weak/severe impairment; 4, paralyzed/unable to do. In addition, record any condition other than MG causing weakness in any of these muscles.
[1]Adapted from, Sanders DB, Tucker-Lipscomb B, Massey JM. A simple manual muscle test for myasthenia gravis: validation and comparison with the QMG score. *Ann NY Acad Sci* 2003; 998:440-444.

MG Activities of Daily Living Profile

The MG Activity of Daily Living (ADL) Profile is a relatively simple eight-point questionnaire that focuses on common symptoms reported by MG patients (Table 10) and complements the QMG. Each item of the profile, graded 0 to 3, with the former normal and the latter most severe, correlates well with the QMG and has become a secondary efficacy measurement in various myasthenic clinical trials (144). It can be administered in less than ten minutes by unspecialized personnel; and it is worthy to note the MG-ADL is not a quality-of-life scale.

MG Composite Score

An MG composite score was developed that embodied the most useful features of the QMG, MGADL, and MG-MMT with the hope that this may be a more useful primary outcome measure in MG trials (145). A 3-point change in the scale, which meaningfully correlates with quality of life, the score has the advantages of items rigorously selected through a process that assessed performance during two randomized, controlled clinical trials involving more than 250 myasthenic patients that covers ten important functional domains most frequently affected by the disease, including bulbar and respiratory items. Moreover, the chosen items are appropriately weighted, and it is easy to administer, requiring less than five minutes to complete without the necessity of specialized equipment, and easy to interpret, taking less than ten seconds to calculate a total score. It is reliable, and demonstrates concurrent and longitudinal construct validity in the MG practice care setting. The second MGFA task force recommended the MG Composite in all prospective studies as therapy for MG (Table 11) (146).

Prednisone Dose as the Primary Endpoint

The dose of prednisone a patient was taking was the primary endpoint in a randomized, placebo-controlled trial of azathioprine in MG (147). Some investigators have returned to

Table 10. MG Activities of Daily Living Profile[1]

TEST ITEMS WEAKNESS (SCORE)	NONE (0)	MILD (1)	MODERATE (2)	SEVERE (3)	Item Score (0,1,2 or 3)
1. Talking	Normal	Intermittent slurring or nasal speech	Constant slurring or nasal, but can be understood	Difficult to understand speech	
2. Chewing	Normal	Fatigue with solid food	Fatigue with soft food	Gastric tube	
3. Swallowing	Normal	Rare episode of choking	Frequent choking necessitating changes in diet	Gastric tube	
4. Breathing	Normal	Shortness of breath with exertion	Shortness of breath at rest	Ventilator dependence	
5. Impairment of ability to brush teeth or comb hair	None	Extra effort, but no rest periods	Rest periods needed	Cannot do one of these functions	
6. Impairment of ability to arise from a chair	None	Mild, sometimes uses arms	Moderate, always uses arms	Severe, requires assistance	
7. Double vision	None	Occurs, but not daily	Daily, but not constant	Constant	
8. Eyelid droop	None	Occurs, but not daily	Daily, but not constant	Constant	

MG-ADL TOTAL SCORE (range 1–8) _____

[1]Adapted from, Wolfe GI, Herbelin L, Nations SP, et al. Myasthenia gravis activities of daily living profile. *Neurology* 1999; 52:1487–1489.

this as a primary endpoint and other quantitative scales as secondary endpoints. In an ongoing trial of methotrexate in MG, the prednisone area under the curve (AUC) was used as the primary endpoint with the goal of attaining the lowest prednisone AUC compared to placebo (148).

MG Quality of Life

Several MG-specific QOL scales have been developed, including the MG questionnaire (MGQ) and the 60-question MG-QOL 60 survey (77, 149, 150). A shorter version of 15 questions (MG-QOL15) correlated well with the larger scale, and was faster to perform. It is being utilized in most MG studies that are ongoing or being developed (150–152).

MYOPATHY

Manual Muscle Testing

A modified Medical Research Council grading system (153–159) expanded from the 0 to 5 scale to a 12-point system (Table 12) that, while simple to use, is ordinal and the differences between the various ranks are not equal. Best known for its use in the randomized blinded trial in Duchenne muscular dystrophy (DMD) (155–157, 159), the endpoint of MMT evidenced the favorable effect of prednisone in improving strength in affected boys so treated compared to placebo, similar to the salutary effect of deflazacort (160). Both MRC and MVICT have been employed in other myopathy trials with inconclusive or negative results, including the myostatin inhibitor trial for limb girdle muscular dystrophy (LGMD), facioscapulohumeral muscular dystrophy (FSH), Becker muscular dystrophy (BMD) (161), oxandrolone for DMD (158), inclusion body myositis (IBM) trials employing interferon-b (153, 154), rituximab in dermatomyositis-polymyositis (162), and etanercept for IBM (163). Other than the DMD, no other clinical trial in myopathy has evidenced improvement of strength or a slowing of the decline of strength over time employing MMT or MVIC as endpoint measures. Most prospective clinical trials employ a fixed or mobile hand-held device using MMT or MVIC methodology as endpoint measures.

Timed Functional Measurement

A timed six-minute walk was suggested as a primary outcome measure for a number of prospective myopathy clinical trials. Stemming from the cardiopulmonary experience (164), this methodology was later employed in a pivotal trial of a-glucosidase for Pompe disease, evidencing improvement in the six-minute walk of patients so treated compared to placebo (165). Since that time, other myopathy trials adopted the six-minute walk as a primary or secondary measure of muscle function, including a Phase 2b, dose-ranging study of ataluren (PTC124) in nonsense mutation of DMD/BMD (nmDBMD) (166). Other timed tests that assess muscle strength and function in myopathy studies include the timed get-up-and-go (167) and the 10-meter walk test (168). In DMD, timed Gower tests of the time to get up from chairs, and climb a standardized flight of stairs, have also been employed (160, 169). Several tests also assess motor skills in pediatric patients, including those that address turning sitting, standing, climbing stairs, jumping, hopping, walking, and running, some of which can be timed. Two such tests that instead assess motor skills are the North Star Ambulatory Assessment (NSAA) and the Gross Motor Functional Measurement (GMFM) battery. The North Star consists of 17 items and the GMFM consists of 88 items. There is a 66-item GMFM (170–172).

Pulmonary Function Testing

Pulmonary function testing (PFT) results were used as secondary outcome measures in the DMD prednisone (156) and Pompe α-glucosidase trial (173) in which forced vital capacity (FVC) showed a positive correlation with strength testing and a six-minute walk (173).

Quality of Life

The Individualized Neuromuscular Quality of Life questionnaire (INQoL) (174) is a neuromuscular disease-specific quality of life adult measure (174) comprised of 12 domains of daily activities, leisure, employment, relationship with partner, relationships with family, relationships with friends, general social interaction, and psychological impact on emotions, perception of the future, identity and self-image, independence, and coping strategies. For each domain patients are asked about the extent to which the neuromuscular disorder has an effect on a 5-point scale from "not at all" to "very much" effect, and the importance thereof. The INQoL questionnaire was used in trials of non-dystrophic myotonia employing mexiletine, and in dermatomyositis employing etanercept (23, 174–176). A pediatric neuromuscular disease-specific (PedsQol) instrument provides similar information with a fatigue module. A generic core module comprises 23 questions and a neuromuscular disease-specific module comprises an additional 25 questions (177–179).

Outcome Measures for Inflammatory Myopathy

Outcome measures for inflammatory myopathy parallel those used for genetic myopathy employing a combination of strength testing, PFT, and timed functional

Table 11. MG Composite Scale[1]

Ptosis, upward gaze (physician examination)	>45 seconds = 0	11 – 45 seconds = 1	1 – 10 seconds = 2	Immediate = 3
Double vision on lateral gaze, left or right (physician examination)	>45 seconds = 0	11 – 45 seconds = 1	1 – 10 seconds = 3	Immediate = 4
Eye closure (physician examination)	Normal = 0	Mild weakness (can be forced open with effort) = 0	Moderate weakness (can be forced open easily) = 1	Severe weakness (unable to keep eyes closed) = 2
Talking (patient history)	Normal = 0	Intermittent slurring or nasal speech = 2	Constant slurring or nasal but can be understood = 4	Difficult to understand speech = 6
Chewing (patient history)	Normal = 0	Fatigue with solid food = 2	Fatigue with soft food = 4	Gastric tube = 6
Swallowing (patient history)	Normal = 0	Rare episode of choking or trouble swallowing = 2	Frequent trouble swallowing e.g., necessitating changes in diet = 5	Gastric tube = 6
Breathing (thought to be caused by MG)	Normal = 0	Shortness of breath with exertion = 2	Shortness of breath at rest = 4	Ventilator dependence = 9
Neck flexion or extension (weakest) (physician examination)	Normal = 0	Mild weakness = 1	Moderate weakness (i.e., ~50% weak, +/- 15%) = 3	Severe weakness = 4
Shoulder abduction (physician examination)	Normal = 0	Mild weakness = 2	Moderate weakness (i.e., ~50% weak, +/- 15%) = 4	Severe weakness = 5
Hip flexion (physician examination)	Normal = 0	Mild weakness = 2	Moderate weakness (i.e., ~50% weak, +/- 15%) = 4	Severe weakness = 5

[1]Adapted from, Burns TM, Sanders DB, Conaway MR, et al. The MG Composite: a valid and reliable outcome measure for myasthenia gravis. *Neurology* 2010; 74:1434–1440.

Table 12. Manual Muscle Testing[1]

Grade	Modified Score	Description
5	5.0	Normal strength
5-	4.67	Uncertain muscle weakness
4+	4.33	Ability to resist against strong pressure throughout range of motion
4	4	Ability to resist against moderate pressure throughout range of motion
4-	3.67	Ability to resist against minimal pressure throughout range of motion
3+	3.33	Ability to move through full range of motion against gravity and to resist against minimal pressure through partial range of motion, the contraction breaks abruptly
3	3	Ability to move through full range of motion against gravity but unable to take any resistance
3-	2.67	Ability to move through partial range of motion against gravity
2	2.0	Ability to move through full range of motion with gravity eliminated
2-	1.67	Ability to move through partial range of motion only with gravity eliminated
1	1	A flicker of movement is seen or felt in the muscle
0	0	No contraction palpable

[1]Adapted from, The Muscle Study Group. A randomized, pilot trial of etanercept in dermatomyositis. *Ann Neurol* 2011; 70:427–436.

activities. A pilot study of etanercept in dermatomyositis (176) employed the average prednisone dose as a primary endpoint measurement. Such patients taking etanercept required less prednisone at the end of the study compared to patients receiving placebo suggesting that etanercept might have been beneficial.

Over the last decade, the Myositis Disease Activity Assessment Tool (MDAAT) (180) has been used to assess extramuscular disease activity and muscle function in dermatomyositis, polymyositis, and IBM. The Myositis Disease Activity Assessment Visual Analog Scale (VAS) (MYOACT) and the Myositis Intention to Treat Activity Index (MITAX) are, respectively, a series of physician assessments of disease activity in various organ systems using a Vasculitis Activity Index to assess the severity of activity, whereas the latter assesses specific manifestation in certain organ systems including constitutional, cutaneous, skeletal, gastrointestinal, pulmonary, cardiac, and muscle. The MYOACT consists of a 10-cm VAS for each organ system to score the overall severity of activity in a global extra muscular VAS. The MDAAT was an outcome measure in the rituximab trial of adult juvenile polymyositis and dermatomyositis (162), and as a secondary endpoint measurement in the etanercept for dermatomyositis pilot study (181). There are several core set measures (CSM), including patient or parent global VAS, physician global impression

VAS, a Health Assessment Questionnaire (HAQ) or Childhood HAQ disability index, elevation of muscle enzymes, a global extramuscular disease activity score based on composite assessment of disease activity on the constitutional, cutaneous, skeletal, gastrointestinal, pulmonary, and cardiac scales of the MDAAT. The definition of improvement was based on the International Myositis Assessment and Clinical Studies Group (IMACS) preliminary validated top-ranked response criterion of a ≥20% improvement in three of any six CSM, with no more than two worsening by ≥25%, but this could not include a worsening of strength on manual muscle testing (164). These IMACS outcome measures demonstrated excellent test–retest reliability in the etanercept trial (181).

The Inclusion Body Myositis Functional Rating Scale

The Inclusion Body Myositis Functional Rating Scale (IBM-FRS) is a 10-point disease-specific functional rating scale intended only for patients with IBM. It uses a 0 to 4 grading system with 4 being normal. The evaluator questions the patient about functional activities in the following areas: swallowing, handwriting, cutting food and handling utensils, fine motor tests, dressing, hygiene, turning in bed and adjusting covers, change in position from sitting to standing, walking, and climbing stairs (Table 13). The IBMFRS

Table 13. Inclusion Body Myositis Functional Rating Scale[1]

1. *Swallowing*
   4 Normal
   3 Early eating problems—occasional choking
   2 Dietary consistency changes
   1 Frequent choking
   0 Needs tube feeding

2. *Handwriting*
   4 Normal
   3 Slow or sloppy: all words are legible
   2 Not all words are legible
   1 Able to grip pen but unable to write
   0 Unable to grip pen

3. *Cutting food and handling utensils*
   4 Normal
   3 Somewhat slow and clumsy, but no help needed
   2 Can cut most foods, although clumsy and slow; some help needed
   1 Food must be cut by someone, but can still feed slowly
   0 Needs to be fed

4. *Fine motor tasks (opening doors, using keys & picking up small objects)*
   4 Independent
   3 Slow or clumsy in completing task
   2 Independent but requires modified techniques or assistive device
   1 Frequently requires assistance from caregiver
   0 Unable

5. *Dressing*
   4 Normal function
   3 Independent but with increased effort or decreased efficiency
   2 Independent but requires assistive devices or modified techniques (Velcro, snaps, shirts without buttons)
   1 Requires assistance from caregiver for some clothing items
   0 Total dependence

6. *Hygiene (bathing & toileting)*
   4 Normal
   3 Independent but with increased effort or decreased efficiency
   2 Independent but requires use of assistive devices (shower chair, raised toilet seat)
   1 Requires occasional assistance from caregiver
   0 Completely dependent

7. *Turning in bed and adjusting bed clothes*
   4 Normal
   3 Somewhat slow and clumsy, but no help needed
   2 Can turn alone or adjust sheets, but with great difficulty
   1 Can initiate, but not turn or adjust sheets alone.
   0 Unable or requires total assistance

8. *Sit to stand*
   4 Independent (without use of arms)
   3 Performs with substitute motions (leaning forward, rocking but without use of arms)
   2 Requires use of arms
   1 Requires assistance from a device or person
   0 Unable to stand

9. *Walking*
   4 Normal
   3 Slow or mild unsteadiness
   2 Intermittent use of an assistive device (AFO, cane, walker)
   1 Dependent on assistive device
   0 Wheelchair dependent

10. *Climbing stairs*
    4 Normal
    3 Slow with hesitation or increased effort; uses hand rail intermittently
    2 Dependent on hand rail
    1 Dependent on hand rail and additional support (cane or person)
    0 Cannot climb stairs

[1]Adapted from, Jackson CE, Barohn RJ, Gronseth G, et al, and The Muscle Study Group. Inclusion body myositis functional rating scale: A reliable and valid measure of disease severity. *Muscle Nerve* 2008; 37:473–476.

correlated with MMT and MVIC in two negative trials (103, 182, 183) employing Avonex for IBM and arimoclomol for IBM (unpublished data, clinicaltrials.gov NCT00769860).

Patient Report of Outcome Measures

A number of patient-based reported outcome measures are being developed for FSH and myotonic muscular dystrophy (DM1), however none has been used in a clinical trial thus far. We developed a patient-based report of outcome measures using an interactive voice response diary for patients with non-dystrophic myotonias involving hereditary sodium or chloride muscle defects, as a part of a natural history consortium of clinical investigation on neurologic channelopathies (CINCH) in North America and Europe. Patient Reported Outcome measures (PRO) are being used to characterize patient experiences of the disorder without the bias of interpretation by an interviewer. These measures can be collected in many formats from pen-and-paper questionnaire to interactive call-in responses and they can be used to establish outcomes as diverse as quality of life and symptom severity (184). The FDA has increasingly been encouraging industry to adapt PRO in public forums and it has published guidelines for the use of PRO measures by the industry. We developed an automated Interactive Voice Response diary (IVR) of real time in repeated patient-reported symptom frequency and severity in the natural history study. The patients called in by telephone and were prompted to answer a series of questions regarding stiffness, pain, fatigue, and weakness using the 1 to 9 keypad scale on the telephone with 1 being minimal and 9 being the worst-ever experience. We were able to demonstrate IVR to be a convenient technology that allowed patient reporting of repeated and real-time symptom frequency and severity. We then adapted an IVR system as an endpoint measure in the prospective randomized control trial of mexiletine for non-dystrophic myotonia completed in 2011 (23, 175, 185). The study, which involved 59 patients in a four-week cross-over trial, showed that mexiletine dramatically lowered patient-reported outcome measures of symptoms as reported by IVR, including stiffness (a primary outcome measure) as well as fatigue, weakness, and pain compared to those patients taking placebo.

REFERENCES

1. Barohn RJ, Kissel JT. Diabetic Muscle Infarction. *Muscle Nerve* 1992; 15:850–855.
2. Barohn RJ, McVey AL, DiMauro S. Adult acid maltase deficiency. *Muscle Nerve* 1993; 16:672–676.
3. Bazan C, Jackson C, Jinkins JR, et al. Gadolinium-enhanced MRI in a case of cytomegalovirus polyradiculopathy. *Neurology* 1991; 41:1522–1523.
4. Jackson CE, Barohn RJ. Improvement in the exercise test in periodic paralysis. *Muscle Nerve* 1992; 15:1069–1071.
5. Barohn RJ, Mendell JR, Brumback RA. Hyaline body myopathy. *Neuromuscul Disord* 1994; 4:257–262.
6. Jackson CE, Amato AA, Barohn RJ. Case of the month: Isolated vitamin E deficiency. *Muscle Nerve* 1996; 19:1161–1165.
7. Wolfe GI, Baker NS, Haller RG, Burns DK, Barohn RJ. McArdle's disease presenting with asymmetric, lateonset arm weakness. *Muscle Nerve* 2000; 23:641–645.
8. Barohn RJ, Miller RG, Griggs RC. Autosomal recessive distal dystrophy. *Neurology* 1991; 41:1365–1370.
9. Barohn RJ, Kissel JT, Warmolts JR, et al. Chronic inflammatory demyelinating polyradiculoneuropathy. Clinical characteristics, course and recommendations for diagnostic criteria. *Arch Neurol* 1989; 46:878–884.
10. Barohn RJ, Sahenk Z, Warmolts JR, et al. The Burns Garland syndrome ("Diabetic Amyotrophy"): Revisited 100 years later. *Arch Neurol* 1991; 48:1130–1135.
11. Barohn RJ, Jackson CE, Kagen-Hallet KS. Neonatal nemaline myopathy with abundant intranuclear rods. *Neuromuscul Disord* 1994; 4:513–520.
12. Sahenk Z, Barohn RJ, New P, et al. Taxol neuropathy: electrophysiologic and sural nerve biopsy study. *Arch Neurology* 1994; 51:726–729.
13. Amato AA, Gronseth GS, Callerame KJ, et al. Tomaculous neuropathy: a clinical and electrophysiologic study in patients with and without deletions in chromosome 17p11.2. *Muscle Nerve* 1996; 19:16–22.
14. Katz JS, Wolfe GI, Burns DK, et al. Isolated neck extensor myopathy: A common cause of dropped head syndrome. *Neurology* 1996; 46:917–921.
15. Katz JS, Wolfe GI, Bryan WW, et al. Electrophysiologic findings in multifocal motor neuropathy. *Neurology* 1997; 48:700–707.
16. Saperstein DS, Amato AA, Wolfe GI, et al. Multifocal acquired demyelinating sensory and motor neuropathy: The Lewis Sumner Syndrome. *Muscle Nerve* 1999; 22:560–566.
17. Van der Sluis RW, Wolfe GI, Nations SP, et al. Postradiation lower motor neuron syndrome. *J Clin Neuromuscul Dis* 2000; 2:10–17.
18. Katz JS, Wolfe GI, Andersson PB, et al. Brachial amyotrophic diplegia: A slowly progressive motor neuron disorder. *Neurology* 1999; 53:1071–1076.
19. Wolfe GI, Baker NS, Amato AA, et al. Chronic cryptogenic sensory polyneuropathies: clinical and laboratory characteristics. *Arch Neurol* 1999; 56:540547.
20. Amato AA, Barohn RJ, Jackson, CE, et al. Inclusion body myositis: treatment with intravenous immunoglobulin. *Neurology* 1994; 44:1516–1518.
21. Mittal M, Pasnoor M, Mummaneni RB, et al. Retrospective chart review of duloxetine and pregabalin in the treatment of painful neuropathy. *Int J Neurosci* 2011; 121:521–527.
22. Jackson CJ, Barohn RJ, Ptacek LJ. Paramyotonia congenita: improvement of the short exercise test with mexilitene therapy. *Muscle Nerve* 1994; 17:763–768.
23. Statland JM, Bundy BN, Wang Y, et al. and the Consortium for Clinical Investigation of Neurologic Channelopathies. Mexiletine for symptoms and signs of myotonia in non-dystrophic myotonia: A randomized controlled trial. *JAMA* 2012; 308 (13):1357–1365.
24. Barohn RJ, Levine EJ, Olson JO, et al. Gastric hypomotility in Duchenne's muscular dystrophy. *N Engl J Med* 1988; 319:15–18.

25. Barohn RJ, Gronseth GS, Amato AA, et al. Cerebrospinal fluid and nerve conduction abnormalities in HIV positive individuals. *J Neurol Sci* 1996; 136:81–85.

26. Olney RK. Clinical trials for polyneuropathy: the role of nerve conduction studies, quantitative sensory testing, and autonomic function testing. *J Clin Neurophysiol* 1998; 15:129–137.

27. Miller RG, Barohn RJ, Dubinsky R. Expanding the evidence base for therapeutics in myasthenia gravis. *Ann Neurol* 2010; 68:776–777.

28. Mandawat A, Kaminski HJ, Cutter G, et al. Comparative analysis of therapeutic options used for myasthenia gravis. *Ann Neurol* 2010; 68:797–805.

29. Dubinsky R, Chen J, Lai SM. Trends in hospital utilization and outcome for patients with ALS: analysis of a large US cohort. *Neurology* 2006; 67:777–780.

30. Bensimon G, Lacomblez L, Meininger V. A controlled trial of riluzole in amyotrophic lateral sclerosis. ALS/Riluzole Study Group. *N Engl J Med* 1994; 330:585–591.

31. Rosenfeld J, King RM, Jackson CE, et al. Creatine monohydrate in ALS: Effects on strength, fatigue, respiratory status and ALSFRS. *Amyotroph Lateral Scler* 2008; 9:266–272.

32. Gordon PH, Moore DH, Miller RG, et al, and the Western ALS Study Group. Efficacy of minocycline in patients with amyotrophic lateral sclerosis: a phase III randomized trial. *Lancet Neurol* 2007; 6:1045–1053.

33. Cudkowicz ME, Shefner JM, Simpson E, et al, and the Northeast ALS Consortium. Arimoclomol at dosages up to 300 mg/day is well tolerated and safe in amyotrophic lateral sclerosis. *Muscle Nerve* 2008; 38:837–844.

34. Cudkowicz ME, Shefner JM, Schoenfeld DA, et al. A randomized, placebo-controlled trial of topiramate in amyotrophic lateral sclerosis. *Neurology* 2003; 61:456–464.

35. BDNF Study Group. A controlled trial of recombinanat methionyl human BDNF in ALS: The BDNF Study Group (Phase III). *Neurology* 1999; 52:1427–1433.

36. Miller RG, Moore D, Young LA, et al, and the WALS Study Group. Placebo controlled trial of gabapentin in patients with amyotrophic lateral sclerosis. *Neurology* 1996; 47:1383–1388.

37. Miller RG, Moore II DH, Gelinas DF, et al. Phase III randomized trial of gabapentin in patients with amyotrophic lateral sclerosis. *Neurology* 2001; 56:843–848.

38. Kaufmann P, Thompson JLF, Levy G, et al. Phase II trial of CoQ10 for ALS finds insufficient evidence to justify phase III. *Ann Neurol* 2009; 66:235–244.

39. Miller RB, Moore DH, Forshew DA, et al. Phase II screening trial of lithium carbonate in ALS: examining a more efficient trial design. *Neurology* 2011; 77:973–979.

40. The ALS CNTF Treatment Study (ACTS) phase I–II Study Group. The amyotrophic lateral sclerosis functional rating scale. Assessment of activities of daily living in patients with amyotrophic lateral sclerosis. *Arch Neurol* 1996; 53:141–147.

41. Cedarbaum JM, Stambler N, Malta E, et al, and the BDNF ALS Study Group. The ALSFRS-R: A revised ALS functional rating scale that incorporates assessments of respiratory function. *J Neurol Sci* 1999; 169:13–21.

42. Miano B, Stoddard GJ, Davis S, et al. Inter-evaluator reliability of the ALS functional rating scale. *Amyotroph Lateral Scler* 2004; 5:235–239.

43. Gordon PH, Bheng B, Salachas F, et al. Progression in ALS is not linear but is curvilinear. *J Neurol* 2010; 257:1713–1717.

44. Kasarskis EJ, Dempsey-Hall L, Thompson MM, et al. Rating the severity of ALS by caregivers over the telephone using the ALSFRS-R. *Amyotroph Lateral Scler* 2005; 6:50–54.

45. Kaufmann P, Levy G, Montes J, Buchsbaum R, et. Al. Excellent inter-rater, intra-rater, and telephone-administered reliability of the ALSFRS-R in a multicenter clinical trial. *Amyotroph Lateral Scler* 2007; 8:42–46.

46. Atsuta N, Watanabe H, Ito M, et al. [Development of a telephone survey system for patients amyotrophic lateral sclerosis using the ALSFRS-R (Japanese version) and application of this system in a longitudinal multicenter study]. *Brain Nerve* 2001; 63:491–496.

47. Andres PL, Hedlund W, Finison L, et al. Quantitatvie motor assessment in amyotrophic lateral sclerosis. *Neurology* 1986; 36:937–941.

48. Ringel SP, Murphy JR, Alderson MK, et al. The natural history of amyotrophic lateral sclerosis. *Neurology* 1993; 43:1316–1322.

49. Great Lakes ALS Study Group. A comparison of muscle strength testing techniques in amyotrophic lateral sclerosis. *Neurology* 2203; 61:1503–1507.

50. Andres PL, Finison LJ, Conlon T. et al. Use of a composite scores (meagascores) to measure deficit in amyotrophic lateral sclerosis. *Neurology* 1988; 38:405–408.

51. Miller RG, Petajan JH, Bryan WW, et al. A placebo-controlled trial of recombinanat human ciliary neurotrophic (rhCNTF) factor in amyotrophic lateral sclerosis. *Ann Neurol* 1996; 39:256–260.

52. ALSCNTF Treatment Study Group. A double-blind placebo-controlled clinical trial of subcutaneous recombinant human ciliary neurotrophic factor (rhCNTF) in amyotrophic lateral sclerosis. *Neurology* 1996; 46:1244–1249.

53. Cudcowicz ME, Shefner JM, Schoenfeld DA, et al and the Northeast ALS Consortium. Trial of celecoxib in amyotrophic lateral sclerosis. *Ann Neurol* 2006; 60:22–31.

54. Miller RG, Bradley W, Cudkowicz M, et al, and the TCH346 Study Group. Phase II/III randomized trial of TCH346 in patients with ALS. *Neurology* 2007; 69:776–784.

55. Beck M, Giess R, Wurffel W, et al. Comparison of maximal voluntary isometric contraction and Drachman's hand-held dynamometry in evaluating patients with amyotrophic lateral sclerosis. *Muscle Nerve* 1999; 22:1265–1270.

56. Van der Ploeg R, Fidler V, Oosterhuis HJGH. Hand-held myometry: Reference values. *J of Neurol Neurosurg Psychiatry* 1991; 51:244–247.

57. Bensimon GB, Lacomblez L, Meninger V. A controlled trial of riluzole in amyotrophic lateral sclerosis. *New Engl J Med* 1994; 330:585–591.

58. Meninger V, Bensimon G, Bradley WR, et al. Efficacy and safety of xaliproden in amyotrophic lateral sclerosis: results of two phase III trials. *Amyotroph Lateral Scler* 2004 5:107–117.

59. O'Brien, Michael. *Aids to the Examination of the peripheral Nervous System* (5th ed). East Sussex England, Bailliere Tindall/WB Saunders, 2010.

60. Mendell J, Florence J. Manual muscle testing. *Muscle Nerve* 1990; 13:S16–S20.

61. Armon C, Ponraj E. Comparing composite scores based on maximal voluntary isometric contraction and on semi-quantitative manual motor testing in measuring limb strength in patients with ALS. *Neurology* 1996; 47:1589–1587.

62. Andres PL, Skerry LM, Munsat TL. Measurement of strength in neuromuscular disease. In: Munsat TL, ed. *Quantification of Neurologic Deficit*. Stoneham, MA: Butterworth, 1989: 87–100.

63. Stambler N, Charatan M, Cedarbaum J. Prognostic indicators of survival in ALS. *Neurology* 1998; 50:66–72.

64. Schiffman PL, Belsh JM. Pulmonary function at diagnosis of amyotrophic lateral sclerosis. Rate of deterioration. *Chest* 1993; 103:508–513.

65. Rosenfeld J, Blythe A, Johnson B, et al. Tidal volume may be a better index of respiratory function than forced vital capacity

in patients with motor neuron disease. In: 10th International Symposium on ALS/MND; Vancouver, Canada, 1999.

66. Kleopa KA, Sherman M, Neal B, et al. Bipap improves survival and rate of pulmonary function decline in patients with ALS [see comments]. *J Neurol Sci* 1999; 164:82–88.

67. ALS CNTF Treatment Study Group. A double-blind placebo-controlled clinical trial of subcutaneous recombinant human ciliary neurotrophic factor (rHCNTF) in amyotrophic lateral sclerosis. *Neurology* 1996; 46:1244–1249.

68. Fallat RJ, Jewitt B, Bass M, et al. Spirometry in amyotrophic lateral sclerosis. *Arch Neurol* 1979; 36:74–80.

69. Brazier JE, Harper R, Jones NM, et al. Validating the SF-36 health survey questionnaire: new outcome measure for primary care. *BMJ* 1992; 305:160–164.

70. Hayes V, Morris J, Wolfe C, et al. The SF-36 health survey questionnaire: is it suitable for use with older adults? *Age Ageing* 1995; 24:120–125.

71. Stucki G, Liang MH, Phillips C, et al. The Short Form-36 is preferable to the SIP as a generic health status measure in patients undergoing elective total hip arthroplasty. *Arthritis Care Res* 1995; 8:174–181.

72. Ware JE Jr, Sherbourne CD. The MOS 36-item Short-Form Health Survey (SF-36): I. Conceptual framework and item selection. *Med Care* 1992; 30:473–483.

73. Ware JE, Snow KK, Kosinski M, et al. *SF-36 Health Survey Manual and Interpretation Guide.* Boston: The Health Institute, New England Medical Center; 1993.

74. Ware JE, Kosinski M, Keller SD. *SF-36 Physical and Mental Health Summary Scales: A User's Manual.* Boston: The Health Institute, New England Medical Center; 1994.

75. Shields RK, Ruhland JL, Ross MA, et al. Analysis of health-related quality of life and muscle impairment in individuals with amyotrophic lateral sclerosis using the medical outcome survey and the Tufts Quantitative Neuromuscular Exam. *Arch Phys Med Rehabil* 1998; 79:855–862.

76. De Groot IJM, Post MWM, van Heuveln T, et al. Cross-sectional and longitudinal correlations between disease progression and different health-related quality of life domains in persons with amyotrophic lateral sclerosis. *Amyotroph Lateral Scler* 2007; 8:356–361.

77. Jenkinson C, Fitzpatrick R, Swash M, et al, and the ALS-HPS Steering Group. The ALS Health Profile Study: quality of life of amyotrophic lateral sclerosis patients and caregivers in Europe. *J Neurol* 2000; 247:835–840.

78. The EuroQoL Group. EuroQol-a new facility for the measurement of health related quality of life. *Health Policy* 1990; 16:199–208.

79. Kiebert GM, Green C, Murphy C, et al. Patients' health-related quality of life and utilities association with different stages of amyotrophic lateral sclerosis. *J Neurol Sci* 2001; 191:87–93.

80. Green C, Kiebert G, Murphy C, et al. Patients' health-related quality-of-life and health state values for motor neurone disease/amyotrophic lateral sclerosis. *Qual Life Res* 2003; 12:565–574.

81. Lopez-Bastida J, Perestelo-Perez L, et al. Social economic costs and health-related quality of life in patients with amyotrophic lateral sclerosis in Spain. *Amyotroph Lateral Scler* 2009; 10:237–243.

82. Bergner M, Bobbitt RA, Carter WB, et al. The Sickness Impact Profile: Development and final revision of a health status measure. *Med Care* 1981; 19:787–805.

83. McGuire D, Garrison L, Armon C, et al, and the SNJV/CNTF ALS Study Group. Relationship of the Tufts Quantitative Neuromuscular Exam (TQNE) and the Sickness Impact Profile in measuring progression of ALS. *Neurology* 1996; 46:1442–1444.

84. McGuire D, Garrison L, Armon C, et al. A brief quality-of-life measure for ALS clinical trials based on a subset of items from the sickness impact profile. The Syntex-Synergen ALS/CNTF Study Group. *J Neurol Sci* 1997; 152:S18–S22.

85. Cohen SR, Mount BM, Strobel MD, et al. The McGill quality of life questionnaire: a measure of quality of life appropriate for people with advanced disease. A preliminary study of validity and acceptability. *Palliat Med* 1995; 9:207–219.

86. Cohen SR, Mount BM, Bruera E. et al. Validity of the McGill Quality of Life Questionnaire in the palliative care setting: a multi-centre Canadian study demonstrating the importance of the existential domain. *Palliat Med* 1997; 11:3–20.

87. Gauthier A, Vignola A, Calvo A, et al. A longitudinal study on quality of life and depression in ALS patient-caregiver couples. *Neurology* 2007; 68:923–926.

88. Roach AR, Averill AJ, Segerstrom SC, et al. The dynamics of quality of life in ALS patients and caregivers. *Ann Behav Med* 2009; 37:197–206.

89. Felgoise SH, Steward JL, Bremer BA, et al. The SEIQol-DW for assessing quality of life in ALS: strengths and limitations. *Amyotroph Lateral Scler* 2009; 10:456–462.

90. Simmons Z, Bremer BA, Robbins RA, et al. Quality of life in ALS depends on factors other than strength and physical function. *Neurology* 2000; 55:388–392.

91. Felgoise S, Rodriguez J, Stephens H, et al. Validation of a shorter ALS-specific quality of life instrument: the ALSSQOL-R. *Amyotroph Lateral Scler* 2008; 9(Suppl):12–13.

92. Jenkinson C, Fitzpatrick R, Brennan C, et al. Evidence for the validity and reliability of the ALS Assessment Questionairre: The ALSAQ-40. *Amyotroph Lateral Scler* 1999; 1:33–40.

93. Jenkinson C, Levvy G, Fitzpatrick R, et al. The Amyotrophic Lateral Sclerosis Assessment Questionnaire (ALSAQ-40): Tests of data quality, score reliability and response rate in a survey of patients. *J Neurol Sci* 2000; 180:94–100.

94. Miller RG, Moore DH, Dronsky V, et al, and the SMA Study Group. A placebo-controlled trial of gabapentin in spinal muscular atrophy. *J Neurol Sci* 2001; 191:127–131.

95. Merlini L, et al. Motor function-muscle strength relationship in spinal muscular atrophy. *Muscle Nerve* 2004; 29:548–552.

96. Elsheikh B, Prior T, Zhang X, et al. An analysis of disease severity based on SMN2 copy number in adults with spinal muscular atrophy. *Muscle Nerve* 2009; 40:652–656.

97. Iannaccone ST, Hynan LS, Morton A, et al. The PedsQL in pediatric patients with spinal muscular atrophy: Feasibility, reliability, and validity of the Pediatric Quality of Life Inventory Generic Core Scales and Neuromuscular Module. *Neuromuscul Disord* 2009; 19:805–812.

98. Campbell, SK, Swanlund, A, et al. Validity of the TIMPSI for estimating concurrent performance on the test of infant motor performance. *Pediatr Phys Ther* 2008; 20:3–10.

99. Finkel RS, Hynan LS, et al. The test of infant motor performance: reliability in spinal muscular atrophy type 1. *Pediatr Phys Ther* 2008; 20:242–246.

100. Glanzman AM, Mazzone E, et al. The Children's Hospital of Philadelphia Infant Test of Neuromuscular Disorders (CHOP INTEND): test development and reliability. *Neuromuscul Disord* 2010; 20:155–161.

101. Morton JP, MacLaren DP, et al. Time course and differential responses of the major heath shock protein families in human skeletal muscle following acute nondamaging treadmill exercise. *J Appl Physiol* 2006; 101:176–182.

102. Piper MC, Pinnell LE, et al. Construction and validation of the Alberta Infant Motor Scale (AIMS). *Can J Public Health* 1992; 83(supll 2):S46–50.

103. Dyck PJ, Kratz KM, Lehman KA, et al. The Rochester Diabetic

Neuropathy Study: design, criteria for types of neuropathy, selection bias, and reproducibility of neuropathic tests. *Neurology* 1991; 41:799–807.

104. Bril V. NIS-LL: the primary measurement scale for clinical trial endpoints in diabetic peripheral neuropathy. *Eur Neurol* 1999; 41(Suppl):8–13.

105. Coelho T, Maia LF, Martins da Silva A, et al. Tafamidis for transthyretin familial amyloid polyneuropathy: A randomized, controlled trial. *Neurology* 2012; 79:785–792.

106. Dyck PJ, Davies JL, Litchy WJ, et al. Longitudinal assessment of diabetic polyneuropathy using a composite score in the Rochester Diabetic Neuropathy Study cohort. *Neurology* 1997; 49:229–239.

107. Ziegler D, Low PA, Litchy WJ, et al. Efficacy and safety of anti-oxidant treatment with α-lipoic acid over 4 years in diabetic polyneuropathy: the NATHAN 1 trial. *Diabetes Care* 2011; 34:2054–2060.

108. Feldman EL, Stevens MJ, Thomas PK, et al. A practical two-step quantitative clinical and electrophysiological assessment for the diagnosis and staging of diabetic neuropathy. *Diabetes Care* 1994; 17:1281–1289.

109. Moghtaderi A, Bakhshipour A, Rashidi H. Validation of Michigan neuropathy screening instrument for diabetic peripheral neuropathy. *Clin Neurol Neurosurg* 2006; 108:477–481.

110. Brown MJ et al. Natural progression of diabetic peripheral neuropathy in the Zenarestat study population. *Diabetes Care* 2004; 27:1153–1159.

111. Cornblath DR, Chaudhry V, Carter K, et al. Total neuropathy score: validation and reliability study. *Neurology* 1999; 53:1660–1664.

112. Singleton JR, Bixby B, Russell JW, et al. The Utah Early Neuropathy Scale: a sensitive clinical scale for early sensory predominant neuropathy. *J Peripher Nerv Syst* 2008; 13:218–227.

113. Schiffmann R, Hauer P, Freeman B, et al. Enzyme replacement therapy and intraepidermal innervation density in Fabry disease. *Muscle Nerve* 2006; 34:53–56.

114. Walk D, Wendelschafer-Crabb G, Davey C, et al. Concordance between epidermal nerve fiber density and sensory examination in patients with symptoms of idiopathic small fiber neuropathy. *J Neurol Sci* 2007; 255:23–26.

115. Herrmann DN, McDermott MP, Sowden JE, et al. Is skin biopsy a predictor of transition to symptomatic HIV neuropathy? A longitudinal study. *Neurology* 2006; 66:857–861.

116. Quattrini C, Jeziorska M, Boulton AJ, Malik RA. Reduced vascular endothelial growth factor expression and intra-epidermal nerve fiber loss in human diabetic neuropathy. *Diabetes Care* 2008; 31:140–145.

117. Smith AG, Russell J, Feldman EL, et al. Lifestyle intervention for pre-diabetic neuropathy. *Diabetes Care* 2006; 29:1294–1299.

118. Polydefkis M, Hauer P, Sheth S, et al. The time course of epidermal nerve fiber regeneration: studies in normal controls and in people with diabetes, with and without neuropathy. *Brain* 2004; 127:1606–1615.

119. Hahn K, Triolo A, Hauer P, et al. Impaired reinnervation in HIV infection following experimental denervation. *Neurology* 2007; 68:1251–1256.

120. Kluding PM, Pasnoor M, Singh R, et al. The effect of exercise on neuropathic symptoms, nerve function, and cutaneous innervation in people with diabetic peripheral neuropathy. *J Diabetes Complications* 2012; 26:424–429.

121. Shy M, Blake J, Krajewski K, et al. Reliability and validity of the CMT neuropathy score as a measure of disability. *Neurology* 2005; 64:1209–1214.

122. Murphy SM, Herrmann DN, McDermott MP, Reliability of the CMT neuropathy score (second version) in Charcot-Marie-Tooth disease. *J Peripher Nerv Syst* 2011; 16:191–198.

123. Hughes RA, Newsom-Davis JM, Perkin GD, et al. Controlled trial prednisolone in acute polyneuropathy. *Lancet* 1978; 2:750–753.

124. Guillain-Barré Syndrome Study Group. Plasmapheresis and acute Guillain-Barré syndrome. *Neurology* 1985; 35:1096–1104.

125. French Cooperative Group on Plasma Exchange in Guillain-Barré Syndrome: Role of replacement fluids. *Annals of Neurology* 1987; 22:753–761.

126. van der Meché FG, Schmitz PI, and the Dutch Guillain-Barré Study Group. A randomized trial comparing intravenous immune globulin and plasma exchange in Guillain-Barré syndrome. *N Engl J Med* 1992; 326:1123–1129.

127. Hughes R, Bensa S, Willison H, et al. Randomized controlled trial of intravenous immunoglobulin versus oral prednisolone in chronic inflammatory demyelinating polyneuropathy. *Ann Neurol* 2001; 50:195–201.

128. Merkies IS, Schmitz PI, van der Meché FG, et al. Inflammatory Neuropathy Cause and Treatment (INCAT) group. Clinimetric evaluation of a new overall disability scale in immune mediated polyneuropathies. *J Neurol Neurosurg Psychiatry* 2002; 72:596–601.

129. Graham RC, Hughes RA. A modified peripheral neuropathy scale: the Overall Neuropathy Limitations Scale. *J Neurol Neurosurg Psychiatry* 2006; 77:973–976.

130. Hughes RA, Donofrio P, Bril V, et al, and the ICE Study Group. Intravenous immune globulin (10% caprylate-chromatography purified) for the treatment of chronic inflammatory demyelinating polyradiculoneuropathy (ICE) study: A randomised placebo-controlled trial. *Lancet Neurol* 2008; 7:136–144.

131. Merkies ISJ, Bril V, Dalakas MC, et al. Health-related quality-of-life improvements in CIDP with immune globulin IV 10%. *Neurology* 2009; 72:1337–1344.

132. Mendell JR, Barohn RJ, Freimer ML, et al. Randomized controlled trial of IVIg in untreated chronic inflammatory demyelinating polyradiculoneuropathy. *Neurology* 2001; 56:445–449.

133. Barohn RJ. Standards of measurement in myasthenia gravis. *Ann N Y Acad Sci* 2003; 998:432–439.

134. Besinger UA, Toyka KV, Heininger K, et al. Long-term correlation of clinical course and acetylcholine receptor antibody in patients with myasthenia gravis. *Ann NY Acad Sci* 1981; 377:812–815.

135. Besinger UA, Toyka KV, Homberg M, et al. Myasthenia gravis: long-term correlation of binding and bungarotoxin blocking antibodies against acetylcholine receptors with changes in disease severity. *Neurology* 1983; 33:1316–1321.

136. Tindall RAS, Phillips JT, Rollins JA, et al. A clinical therapeutic trial of cyclosporine in myasthenia gravis. *Ann NY Acad Sci* 1993; 681:539–551.

137. Tindall RSA, Rollins JA, Phillips JT, et al. Preliminary results of a double-blind, randomized, placebo-controlled trial of cyclosporine in myasthenia gravis. *N Engl J Med* 1987; 316:719–724.

138. Jaretzski A III, Barohn RJ, Ernstoff RM, et al. Myasthenia gravis: recommendations for clinical research standards. *Ann Thorac Surg* 2000; 70:327–334.

139. Barohn RJ, McIntire D, Herbelin L, et al. Reliability testing of the quantitative myasthenia gravis score. *Ann NY Acad Sci* 1998; 841:769 772.

140. Barohn RJ. Video: how to administer the quantitative myasthenia test. Myasthenia Gravis Foundation of America, Inc., 1821 University Ave.W. Suite S256, St. Paul, MN 55104; 1996.

141. The Muscle Study Group. A trial of mycophenolate mofetil with prednisone as initial immunotherapy in myasthenia gravis. *Neurology* 2008; 71:394–399.

142. Wolfe GI, Barohn RJ, Sanders DB, McDermott MP, and The Muscle Study Group. Comparisons of outcome measures from a trial of mycophenolate mofetil in myasthenia gravis. *Muscle Nerve* 2008; 38:1429–1433.

143. Wolfe G, Barohn R, Foster B, et al. Randomized, controlled trial of intravenous immunoglobulin in myasthenia gravis. *Muscle Nerve* 2002; 26:549–552.

144. Zinman L, Ng E, Bril V. IV Immunoglobulin in patients with myasthenia gravis: a randomized controlled trial. *Neurology* 2007; 68:837–841.

145. Barth D, Nabavi Nouri M, Ng E, et al. Comparison of IVIg and PLEX in patients with myasthenia gravis. *Neurology* 2011; 76:2017–2023.

146. Sanders DB, Tucker-Lipscomb B, Massey JM. A Simple manual muscle test for myasthenia gravis: validation and comparison with the QMG score. *Ann NY Acad Sci* 2003; 998:440–444.

147. Gajdos P, Chevret S, Clair B, et al. Clinical trial of plasma exchange and high-dose intravenous immunoglobulin in myasthenia gravis. *Ann Neurol* 1997; 41:789–796.

148. Gaidos P, Simon N, de Rohan-Chabot P, et al. [Long-term effects of plasma exchange in myasthenia: results of a randomized study.] *Presse Med* 1983; 12:939–942.

149. Wolfe GI, Herbelin L, Nations SP, et al. Myasthenia gravis activities of daily living profile. *Neurology* 1999; 52:1487–1489.

150. Burns TM, Sanders DB, Conaway MR, et al. The MG Composite: a valid and reliable outcome measure for myasthenia gravis. *Neurology* 2010; 74:1434–1440.

151. Benatar M, Sanders DB, Burns TM, et al. Recommendations for myasthenia gravis clinical trials. *Muscle Nerve* 2012; 45:909–917.

152. Palace J, Newsom-Davis J, Lecky B. A randomized double-blind trial of prednisolone alone or with azathioprine in myasthenia gravis. *Neurology* 1998; 50:1778–1783.

153. Barohn RJ. Efficacy of methotrexate in myasthenia gravis. In. Clinicaltrials.gove [Internet]. Bethesda (MD): National Library of Medicine (US). [Accessed 2008 July 30].

154. Padua L, Evoli A, Aprile I, et al. Myasthenia gravis outcome measure: development and validation of a disease-specific self-administered questionnaire. *Neurol Sci* 2002; 23:59–68.

155. Burns TM, Graham CD, Rose MR, et al. Quality of life and measures of Quality of Life in patients with neuromuscular disorders. *Muscle Nerve* 2012; 46:9–25.

156. Burns TM, Conaway MR, Cutter GR, et al, and the Muscle Study Group. Less is more, or almost as much: a 15-item quality-of-life instrument for myasthenia gravis. *Muscle Nerve* 2008; 38:957–963.

157. Burns TM, Grouse CK, Wolfe GI, et al, and the MG Composite and MG-QOL15 Study Group. The MG-QOL15 for following the health-related quality of life of patients with myasthenia gravis. *Muscle Nerve* 2011; 43:14–18.

158. Muscle Study Group. Randomized pilot trial of betaINF1a (Avonex) in patients with inclusion body myositis. *Neurology* 2001; 57:1566–1570.

159. Muscle Study Group. Randomized pilot trial of high-dose betaINF-1a in patients with inclusion body myositis. *Neurology* 2004; 63:718–720.

160. Florence JM, Pandya S, King WM, et al. Clinical trials in Duchenne dystrophy: Standardization and reliability of evaluation procedures. *Phys Ther* 1984; 64:41–45.

161. Mendell JR, Moxley RT, Griggs RC, et al. Randomized, double-blind six-month trial of prednisone in Duchenne's muscular dystrophy. *N Engl J Med* 1989; 320:1592–1597.

162. Brooke MH, Griggs RC, Mendell JR, et al. Clinical trial in Duchenne dystrophy. I. Design of the protocol. *Muscle Nerve* 1981; 4:186–197.

163. Fenichel GM, Griggs RC, Kissel JT, et al. A randomized efficacy

164. Griggs RC, Moxley RT, Mendell JR et al. Duchenne dystrophy: Randomized controlled trial of prednisone (18 months) and azathioprine (12 months). *Neurology* 1993; 43:520–527.

and safety trial of oxandrolone in the treatment of Duchene dystrophy. *Neurology* 2001; 56:1075–1079.

165. Angelini C, Pegoraro E, Turella E, et al. Deflazacort in Duchenne dystrophy: study of long-term effect. *Muscle Nerve* 1994; 17:386–391.

166. Wagner KR, Fleckenstein JL, Amato AA, et al. A phase I/II trial of MYO-029 in adult subjects with muscular dystrophy. *Ann Neurol* 2008; 63:561–571.

167. Oddis CV, Reed AM, Aggarwal R. Rituximab in the treatment of refractory adult and juvenile dermatomyositis (DM) and adult polymyositis (PM)—the RIM study. *Arthritis Res* 2010; 62(Suppl 12):3844.

168. Barohn RJ, Herbelin L, Kissel JT, et al. Pilot trial of etanercept in the treatment of inclusion body myositis. *Neurology* 2006; 66(Suppl 1):S123–S124.

169. ATS Committee on Proficiency Standards for Clinical Pulmonary Function Laboratories. ATS Statement: guidelines for the six-minute walk test. *Am J Respir Crit Care Med* 2002; 166:111–117.

170. Van Der Ploeg AT, Clemens PR, Corzo D, et al. A randomized study of alglucosidase alfa in late-onset Pompe's disease. *New Engl J Med* 2010; 15:1396–1406.

171. Finkel R, Wong B, Bushby K, et al. Results of a Phase 2b, dose-ranging study of ataluren (PTC124) in nonsense mutation Duchenne/Becker muscular dystrophy (nmDBMD). *Neuromuscul Disord* 2010; 656–657.

172. Podsiadlo D, Richardson R. The timed "Up & Go": a test of basic functional mobility for frail elderly persons, *J Am Geriatr Soc* 1991; 39:142–148.

173. Wall JC, Bell C, Campbell S, et al. The Timed Get-up-and-Go test revisited: measurement of the component tasks. *J Rehabil Res Dev* 2000; 37:109–113.

174. Matias S, Nayak U, Isaacs B. Balance in elderly patient" The "Get Up and Go" Test. *Arch Phys Med Rehabil* 1986; 67:387–389.

175. Mazzone ES, Messina S, Vasco G, et al. Reliability of the North Star Ambulatory Assessment in a multicentric setting. *Neuromuscul Disord* 2009; 19:458–461.

176. Mayhew A, Cano S, Scott E, et al. Moving towards meaningful measurement: Rasch analysis of the North Star Ambulatory Assessment in Duchenne muscular dystrophy. *Dev Med Child Neurol* 2011; 53:535–542.

177. Russell DJ, Rosenbaum PL, Avery LM, et al. *Gross Motor Function Measure (GMFM-66 and GMFM-88) User's Manual.* London, United Kingdom: Mac Keith Press; 2002.

178. Kissel JT, McDermott MP, Natarajan R, et al, and the PSH-DY Group. Pilot trial of albuterol in facioscapulohumeral muscular dystrophy. *Neurology* 1998; 50:1402–1406.

179. Vincent K, Carr A, Walburn J, et al. Construction and validation of a quality of life questionnaire for neuromuscular disease (INQoL). *Neurology* 2007; 68:1051–1057.

180. Barohn RJ, Wang Y, Herbelin LL, et al, and the CINCH Study Group. Phase II therapeutice trial of mexiletine in non-dystrophic myotonia. *Neurology* 2011; 76(Suppl 4):A645.

181. The Muscle Study Group. A Randomized, Pilot Trial of Etanercept in Dermatomyositis. *Ann Neurol* 2011; 70:427–436.

182. Varni JW, Seid M, Knight TS, et al. The PedsQL 4.0 Generic Core Scales: sensitivity, responsiveness, and impact on clinical decision-making. *J Behav Med* 2002; 25:175–193.

183. Varni JW, Seid M, Kurtin PS. PedsQL 4.0: reliability and validity of the Pediatric Quality of Life Inventory version 4.0 generic core scales in healthy and patient populations. *Med Care* 2001; 39:800–812.

184. Varni JW, Seid M, Rode CA. The PedsQL: measurement model

for the pediatric quality of life inventory. *Med Care* 1999; 37:126–139.

185. Rider LG, Werth VP, Huber AM, et al. Measures of adult and juvenile dermatomyositis, polymyositis, and inclusion body myositis: Physician and Patient/Parent Global Activity, Manual Muscle Testing (MMT), Health Assessment Questionnaire (HAQ)/Childhood Health Assessment Questionnaire (C-HAQ), Childhood Myositis Assessment Scale (CMAS), Myositis Disease Activity Assessment Tool (MDAAT), Disease Activity Score (DAS), Short Form 36 (SF-36), Child Health Questionnaire (CHQ), physician global damage, Myositis Damage Index (MDI), Quantitative Muscle Testing (QMT), Myositis Functional Index-2 (FI-2), Myositis Activities Profile (MAP), Inclusion Body Myositis Functional Rating Scale (IBMFRS), Cutaneous Dermatomyositis Disease Area and Severity Index (CDASI), Cutaneous Assessment Tool (CAT), Dermatomyositis Skin Severity Index (DSSI), Skindex, and Dermatology Life Quality Index (DLQI). *Arthritis Care Res* 2011; 63(Suppl 11):S118–S157.

186. The Muscle Study Group. A randomized, pilot trial of etanercept in dermatomyositis. *Ann Neurol* 2011; 70:427–436.

187. Jackson CE, Barohn RJ, Gronseth G, et al. and The Muscle Study Group. Inclusion body myositis functional rating scale: A reliable and valid measure of disease severity. *Muscle Nerve* 2008; 37:473–476.

188. Barohn RJ. Arimoclomol in sporadic inclusion body myositis. In. Clinicaltrials.gov [Internet]. Bethesda (MD): National Library of Medicine (US). [Accessed 2008 Aug 8].

189. Chang CH. Patient-reported outcomes measurement and management with innovative methodologies and technologies. *Qual Life Res* 2007; 16 (Suppl 1):157–166.

190. Statland JM, Wang Y, Richesson R, et al. An interactive voice response diary for patients with non-dystrophic myotonia. *Muscle Nerve* 2011; 44:30–35.

PART II

Nerve and Muscle Diseases

CHAPTER 16

Isolated and Multiple Cranial Nerve Palsies

David S. Younger

In depth working knowledge of the correlative neuroanatomy of the cranial nerves is vital in neurological diagnosisand surgery, the essentials of which are the topic of this chapter. The reader is encouraged to refer to several excellent classical reviews (1–4).

Background

The twelve pairs of cranial nerves are individually named and designated by Roman numerals (CN I–XII), each with distinct functional components comprising diverse somatic, autonomic efferent, and afferent fiber types. They are attached to the base of the brain and transit the skull through foramina in the skull (Figures 1, 2). In the developing human embryo, they arise into two sets, one medial (oculomotor, trochlear, abducens, and hypoglossal nerves), and the other lateral (trigeminal, facial, glossopharyngeal, vagus, and accessory nerves) with motor constituents as outgrowths of neuroblast cells situated in the basal lamina of the mid and hindbrain, and sensory components derived from ganglionic rudiments of the neural crest (Figure 3).Their central processes grow inward, forming the roots of the nerves while the peripheral processes extend outward distributing their fiber connections.

ISOLATED CRANIAL NERVE PALSIES

Olfactory Nerve (CN I)

Bundles of unmyelinated nerve fibers subserving the sense of smell transmit information from olfactory cells that reside in both sides of the nasal cavity. They gather into bundles passing medially along the septum and laterally from the concha, ensheathed by dura, arachnoid, and pia of the brain, and pass through foramina of the cribiform plate before making synaptic connection with mitral cells in the olfactory bulb (Figure 4). Several hundred olfactory nerve fibers converge upon each mitral cell, giving rise to second order neurons that run in the olfactory tract thereby enhancing the sense of smell. Olfaction is tested at the bedside by asking the patient to smell substances such as coffee grounds. Anosmia or loss of smell, and paranosmia, an unpleasant sensation of smell, occur in up to 12% of cases of head injury and in other pathological conditions, resulting from lesions of one or both olfactory bulbs or tracts, with temporary or permanent loss of smell and recovery by three months in up to three-quarters of patients (5, 6).

Kennedy (7) described patients with unilateral atrophy of the olfactory and optic nerves combined with papilledema on the opposite side due to increased intracranial pressure. Other causes of unilateral anosmia include internal carotid artery aneurysm, orbital osteoma, suprasellar meningioma, and tumors of the sphenoid ridge and frontal lobes. Bilateral anosmia occurs with large pituitary lesions, hydrocephalus and chronic meningitis, Parkinson, Alzheimer disease, multiple sclerosis (MS), and B12 deficiency. Hyposmia or decreased olfaction occurs normally with aging. Paranosmia can present with olfactory hallucinations and epilepsy.

Optic Nerve (CN II)

This nerve (Figure 5) develops from a lateral tract of fibers along a diverticulum of the lateral aspect of the forebrain with supporting neuroglia and the prolongations of the three parts of the meninges of the brain. The peripheral

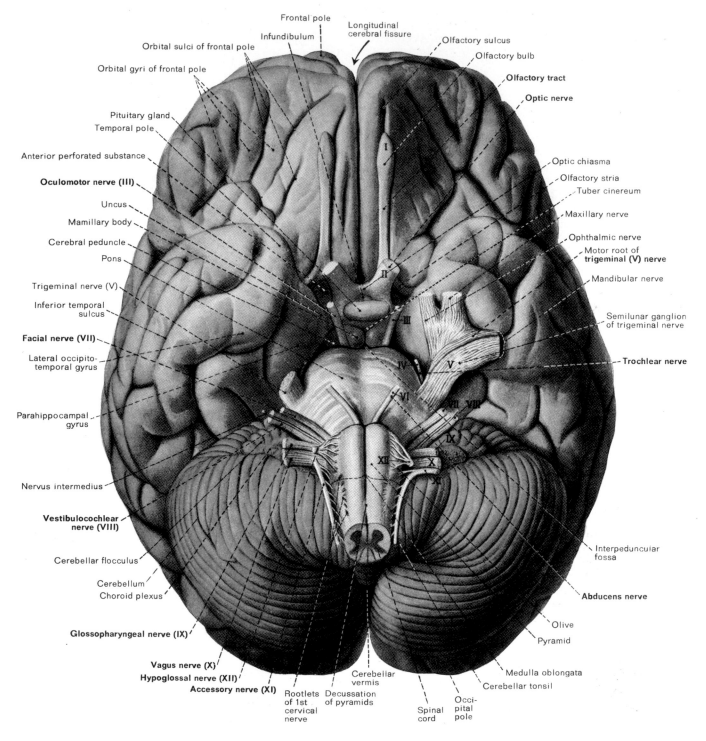

FIG. 1. Base of the brain showing cranial nerve roots.
Reproduced from reference 1, with permission.

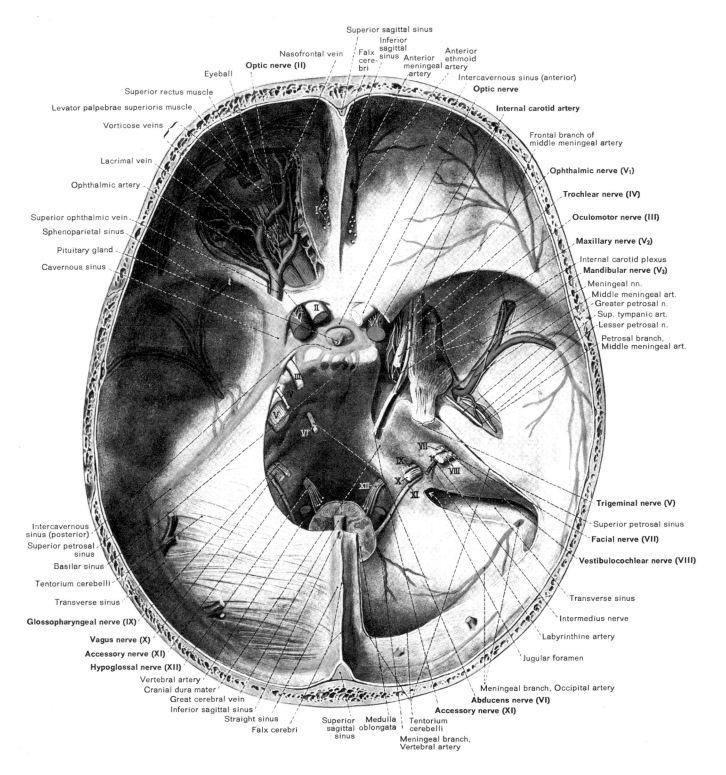

FIG. 2. Interior base of the skull showing the exit of cranial nerves.
Reproduced from reference 1, with permission.

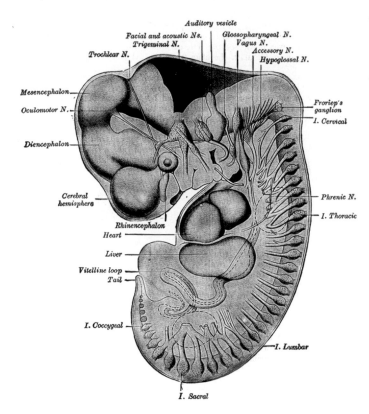

FIG. 3. Developing human embryo showing reconstruction of the brain, cranial and spinal nerves. Reproduced from reference 1, with permission.

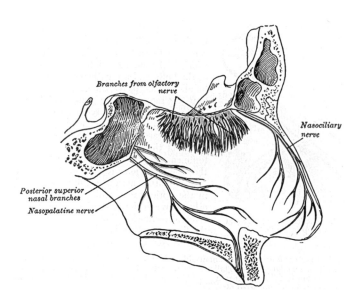

FIG. 4. Olfactory nerves along the septum of the nose. Reproduced from reference 1, with permission.

nerve axons of retinal ganglion cells comprising this nerve form four well-defined peripheral portions: (1) intraocular or bulbar; (2) intraorbital; (3) intraosseus or optic foramen, which traverses the optic canal; (4) and intracranial.

The short intraocular portion occupies the posterior scleral foramen where its fibers are unmyelinated. The intraorbital portion extends from the globe to the optic foramen wherein they myelinate supported by neuroglia and invested by pia, arachnoid, and dura, all of which become continuous with the lamina cribrosa allowing for unrestricted movement of the eyeball. The dura fuses with the sclera, periosteum, and annulus of Zinn, and the pia extends to the optic chiasm where it ensheaths the nerve fibers and provides capillary vascular support. As the nerve traverses the orbit it is surrounded in its anterior two-thirds by the nasociliary nerve, ophthalmic artery, superior ophthalmic vein, and the superior division of the oculomotor nerve.

As it leaves the globe it is then surrounded by posterior ciliary arteries, central retinal artery and vein, and nasociliary ophthalmic arteries. In the orbital apex, the optic nerve is surrounded superiorly by the superior rectus and levator of the lid, and trochlear and frontal nerves; inferiorly by the inferior division of the oculomotor nerve and the rectus inferior; medially by the rectus medialis; and laterally by the abducens nerve and rectus lateralis muscle. A short distance behind the bulb, the optic nerve is pierced by the central retinal artery and vein, and enters the orbital apex at right angles wherein it is subject to compression and papilledema. The optic nerve enters the optic canal through the optic foramen, located in the apex of the orbit, a short distance from the supraorbital margin. In the optic foramen portion, the nerve is bordered inferiorly by the ophthalmic artery just following its branch from the internal carotid; medially by a thin plate of bone separating it from the sphenoidal air cells; laterally by the inferior division of the oculomotor, nasociliary artery, abducens nerve, and ciliary ganglion; and superiorly by the three sheaths of dura, arachnoid, and pia that fuses to each other, which prevent it from being forced back and forth in the foramen.

Fibers of the intracranial optic nerve extend to the optic chiasm, resting on the anterior portion of the cavernous sinus and on the diaphragm sellae which overlies the pituitary gland. Each optic nerve is boarded superiorly by the frontal lobes, and laterally by the internal carotid artery, which attaches to the optic nerve by the ophthalmic artery. The optic fibers converge in the optic chiasm formed by their junction, which is most often situated over the diaphragm sellae, projecting backwards and bordered laterally by the cavernous sinuses. The chiasm is termed *prefixed* when it rests in the sulcus chiasmatic or over the diaphragm, and *postfixed* when it is over and behind the dorsum sella, the variations of which contribute to characteristic field defects

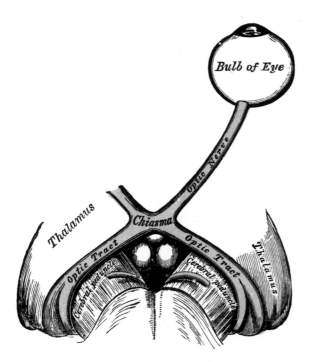

FIG. 5. Optic nerves and tracts. Reproduced from reference 1, with permission.

produced by tumors in this region. Visuotopically segregated nasal retinal fibers corresponding to temporal visual hemifields cross while temporal retinal fibers remain homolateral. Visual nerve fibers are destined for the lateral geniculate body while intermixed papillary axons diverge toward the pretectal nuclei of the midbrain, and other intermingled centrifugal efferent fibers that synapse with retinal amacrine and ganglionic cells and innervate retinal blood vessels.

The function of the optic nerve is tested by observing pupillary responsiveness, visual acuity, visual fields, and the appearance of the optic fundus. The papillary light response is mediated by afferent optic nerve fibers and efferent parasympathetic pupilloconstrictor nerve fibers. Anisocoria or inequality of the pupillary size is confirmed by the response of a bright light shown in either eye which should otherwise lead to a consensual and equal pupillary response. Accomodation is tested by asking the patient to focus on the examiner's finger, which is brought slowly inward. A swinging flashlight should not evoke a different papillary size but does so if there is a relative afferent papillary defect due to a lesion anterior to the optic chiasm. Visual acuity is tested at the bedside with a Snellen chart, near-vision cart or card, and by asking the patient to read, write, count fingers identify hand movements, and perceive light. Fundoscopic examination by ophthalmoscopy discerns the appearance of the optic disk, blood vessels, and retinal background. Visual field defects evoked by gross confrontation and perimetry offer valuable clues to the diagnosis of optic nerve lesions. Lesions along the optic nerve are clinically diverse, includ-

ing infectious and inflammatory disorders, compressive optic neuropathy from intracranial tumors, and vascular causes leading to anterior ischemic optic and radiation induced optic neuropathy. Patients presenting with bilateral anterior optic neuritis should be evaluated for papilledema, as well as Leber hereditary optic neuropathy, a mitochondrial disorder, especially in young men, that mimics optic neuritis and presents with unilateral central visual loss at the early stage before the fellow eye is involved.

The diagnosis of optic neuritis is suggested by the clinical tempo of visual loss, and confirmed by ophthalmologic examination. Central acuity is usually reduced, but 10% of patients have preserved central vision of at least 20/20. Patients who retain normal or near-normal acuity often have reduced color vision and contrast sensitivity out of proportion to central visual disturbance. The majority of affected patients have unilateral relative afferent pupillary defect. Central visual field loss and central scotoma account for 90% of the visual field defects, however others occur, including cecocentral, paracentral, arcuate, hemialtitudinal, and hemianopic types, as well as peripheral constriction and diffuse suppression. The optic disc is normal in up to two-thirds of patients with retrobulbar optic neuritis, and swollen in anterior optic neuritis or papillitis; hemorrhage at the disc margin occurs in less than 6% of patients.

The optic disc becomes pale weeks after the initial episode and transient reversible neurologic dysfunction can occur in response to exercise or exposure to heat, referred to as *Uhthoff symptom*. Pattern reversal visual evoked potentials (VEP), which record electrical activity along visual pathways from the optic nerves to the occipital cortex, show asymmetric inter-eye latency prolongation of the P100response consistent with a unilateral prechiasmatic lesion. Flash VEP can be used to confirm visual pathway integrity when the P100 is not seen with pattern VEP. Other disorders that cause a VEP disturbance include compressive lesions, congenital optic nerve anomalies, glaucoma, hereditary and toxic optic neuropathy, and papilledema. Magnetic resonance imaging (MRI) of the brain and optic nerves may reveal findings supporting optic neuritis alone or clinically silent ones instead suggestive of MS. Corticosteroids have long been the cornerstone of therapy for optic neuritis. The intravenous infusion of 250 mg of methylprednisolone every six hours for three days followed by 1 mg per kilogram of oral prednisone for 11 days was superior to oral prednisone or placebo for 14 days in the recovery of visual loss due to optic neuritis, preserves vision at six months, and lowers the rate of developing clinically definite MS for up to two years, and averts new MS attacks in clinically established patients (8–10).

Neuromyelitis optica (NMO) presents with acute transverse myelitis and bilateral optic or retrobulbar neuritis in association with NMO-IgG, a serum channelopathy auto-

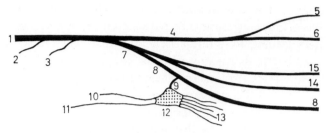

Diagram of third cranial nerve. 1, Trunk. 2, Communication with sympathetic. 3, Communication with ophthalmic nerve. 4, Superior ramus. 5, N. to levator palpebrae superioris. 6, N. to superior rectus. 7, Inferior ramus. 8, N. to inferior oblique. 9, Short (parasympathetic) root of ciliary ganglion. 10, Sympathetic root of ciliary ganglion. 11, Long (sensory) root of ciliary ganglion. 12, Ciliary ganglion. 13, Short ciliary nerves. 14, N. to inferior rectus. 15, N. to medial rectus.

FIG. 6. Schematic diagram of the oculomotor nerve. Reproduced from reference 4, with permission.

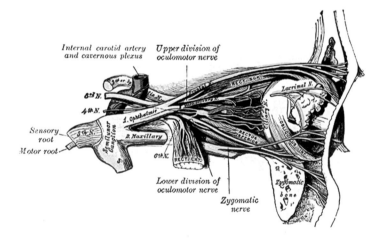

FIG. 7. Intraorbital oculomotor nerve. Reproduced from reference 1, with permission.

antibody that selectively binds to the aquaporin-4 water channel, a component of the dystroglycan protein complex located in astrocytic foot processes at the blood brain barrier (11). This disorder can be monophasic, relapsing, or progressive but tends to have a poorer prognosis and response to immunomodulation than straightforward MS.

Prechiasmal lesions involving one optic nerve lead to blindness or progressive central scotoma on the side of the lesion and a defect in the temporal field of the other eye, while those of the anterior angle of the chiasm originating in the third ventricle lead to isolated contralateral temporal field loss. Lesions of the body of the chiasm produced by intrasellar adenomas lead to bitemporal hemianopia as a resultof pressure from below. Pressure on the chiasmfrom above, characteristically due to a suprasellartumor or aneurysms of the anterior cerebral artery, result in lower bitemporal field defects, while mass lesions of the posterior angle of the chiasm originating in the interpeduncular space and hypothalamus produce selective field defects resulting from involvement of crossed nasal fibers from the opposite retina or uncrossed temporal fibers from the homolateral eye. Lesions lateral to the chiasm originating in the cavernous sinus, such as aneurysms of the internal carotid artery, affect uncrossed temporal and crossed nasal fibers from the opposite eye leading to contralateral homonymous hemianopia. Bilateral superior hemianopia occurs in developmental disorders that stretch or place pressure on the optic nerves, whereas bilateral inferior hemianopias typically follow intracranial hemorrhage.

Oculomotor Nerve (CN III)

Peripheral axons of the oculomotor nucleus exit the midbrain along the medial side of the cerebral peduncle and traverse the subarachnoid space in the interpeduncular cistern invested by pia where it passes between the superior cerebellar and posterior cerebral arteries near the termination of the basilar artery. The nerve pierces the dura between the anterior and posterior clinoid processes by passing between the free and attached borders of the cerebellar tentorium, and runs anteriorly embedded in the lateral wall of cavernous sinus superior to the trochlear, oculomotor, abducens, and ophthalmic branch of the trigeminal nerve in the cavernous sinus. It enters the superior orbital fissure between the two heads of the rectus lateralis muscles, separating into superior and inferior divisions (Figures 6, 7) where it joins a communication from the cavernous plexus carrying postganglionic sympathetic fibers from the superior cervical ganglion destined for long ciliary nerves to the pupillodilator muscle; and another communication from the ophthalmic division of the trigeminal nerve providing sensory innervation of the bulb and conjunctiva of the eye (Figure 8).

Fibers of the superior division carry sympathetic post-

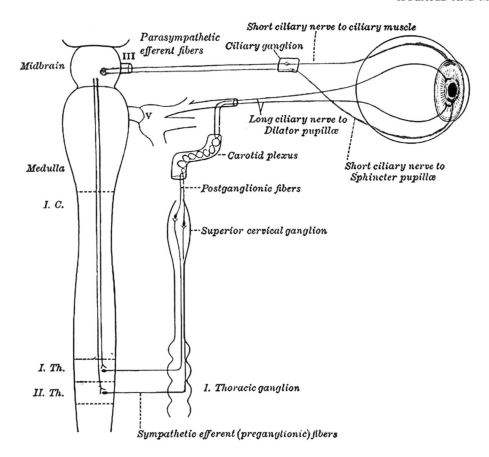

FIG. 8. Anatomical connections of the ciliary and superior cervical ganglion. Reproduced from reference 1, with permission.

ganglionic fibers from the cavernous plexus innervating the superior tarsus muscle to provide form and support of the eyelids. The inferior division has four branches including one each to the medial and inferior rectus, and inferior oblique muscles, and another to the root of the ciliary ganglion. In addition to providing efferent innervation to the medial and inferior recti and oblique muscles, fibers of the inferior division fibers carry preganglionic parasympathetic fibers to the ciliary root, the cell bodies of which originate in the Edinger-Westphal cell group of the oculomotor nucleus, which synapse in the ciliary ganglion and continue as postganglionic fibers along short ciliary nerves exiting the ganglion in two bundles. A superior and inferior bundle runs anteriorly with the ciliary arteries, one above and the other below the optic nerve, and pierces the sclera and pass to the inner surface of the ciliary body to innervate the ciliaris and pupillosphincter muscle.

Two communicating branches, formerly termed roots of the ciliary ganglion, include sensory fibers from nasociliary branches of the ophthalmic nerve that traverse short ciliary nerves on the way to the cornea, iris and ciliary body; another, via filaments from the cavernous plexus, contain postganglionic sympathetic fibers from the superior cervical ganglion that pass through the ciliary ganglion without

synapse to reach the pupillodilator muscle via long ciliary nerves, with those destined for innervation of blood vessels of the bulb transitting short ciliary branches.

Oculomotor function is examined by examining the position of the eyes in the six primary diagnostic directions of gaze noting positions in which the patient develops diplopia or pathological nystagmus (Figure 9), and observing the size of the pupil before and after direct light stimulation and accommodation, taking note of compensatory head positions. Complete oculomotor nerve palsy is recognized when the four extrinsic ocular muscles, medial, superior, inferior rectus, and inferior oblique and instrinsic eye muscles, including the superior levator palpebral, papillary sphincter, and ciliaris muscles governing papillary size, are involved by the pathological process. In addition, the eye is deflected outward and downward, with the upper eyelid almost completely covering the eyeball, and only slight upward movement from the frontal belly of the epicranius muscle with a fixed dilated pupil that is unreactive to light, accommodation, or lid closure. With intact sympathetic function, the pupil constricts to the installation of the meiotic cocaine. Partial oculomotor nerve palsy, which is more common, resembles initially recovering complete palsy. Abnormal movements include synkinesia, pupillary constriction on abduction, activation of the paralyzed medial or inferior rectus, and a pseudo-Von Graefe sign in which the upper lid descends slowly, not at all, or even retracts the eye upon looking down or toward the opposite side, following regeneration of a third nerve palsy.

Damage to the oculomotor nerve at its emergence from the midbrain produces the syndrome of oculomotor palsy and crossed hemiplegia due to concomitant lesion of the ipsilateral corticospinal tract (CST). The nerve is susceptible to compression near the cerebral peduncle where its fibers may be juxtaposed to mass lesions or aneurysms of the basilar, superior cerebellar, posterior cerebral, and posterior communicating arteries. The oculomotor nerve is also susceptible to injury along the superior orbital fissure where its superior division crosses the ophthalmic artery before giving off muscular branches to the superior rectus muscle, and along the clivus ridge by a subdural hematoma or local cerebritis. Concurrent involvement of the trigeminal, facial,

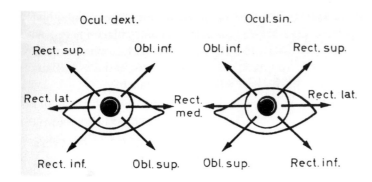

FIG. 9. The six diagnostic directions of gaze Reproduced from reference 1, with permission of the publisher.

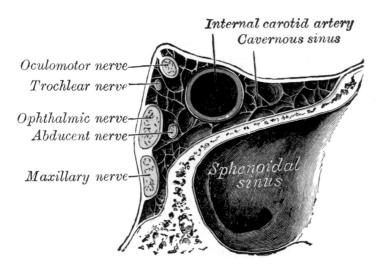

FIG. 10. Oblique section through the right cavernous sinus. Reproduced from reference 1, with permission.

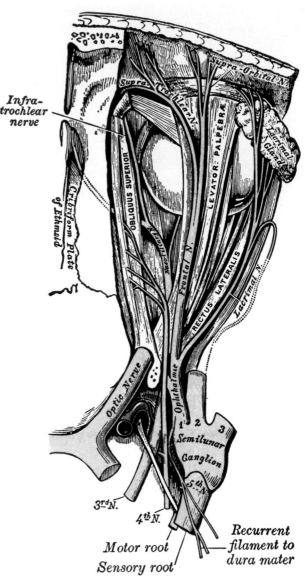

FIG. 11. Tochlear nerve and its branches in the orbit seen from above. Reproduced from reference 1, with permission.

and vestibulocochlear nerves suggests a proximal localization in the middle or anterior portion of the posterior cranial fossa, whereas associated trochlear, trigeminal, and abducens nerve involvement with incomplete oculomotor palsy infers a more distal localization such as the cavernous sinus or superior orbital fissure. The third cranial nerve is involved by infiltrative processes that penetrate the cranium through the foramen lacerum, leading to severe neuralgia due to involvement of the second division of the trigeminal nerve near the petrous ridge. Concomitant involvement of the oculomotor and facial nerve occurs in the sphenoidal sinus syndrome most often caused by meningiomas of the anterior cranial fossa. Ophthalmoplegia in the Miller Fisher syndrome, along with ataxia and areflexia, results from selective oculomotor nerve involvement.

Trochlear Nerve (CN IV)

This nerve exits the dorsal pons posterior to the inferior colliculus and winds forward around the midbrain, at first parallel to the posterior cerebral artery, then along the free edge of the cerebellar tentorium behind the posterior clinoid process where it pierces the dura lateral to the oculomotor nerve and takes its place in the lateral wall of the cavernous sinus (Figure 10). There it receives a sympathetic communication from the cavernous plexus and sensory fibers from the ophthalmic division of the trigeminal nerve and proceeds upward, crossing the oculomotor nerve to enter the orbit through the superior orbital fissure. It takes a position superior to the other nerves passing medially above the origin of the superior levator of the lid where it finally pierces the orbital surface of the superior oblique muscle (Figure 11). The trochlear nerve transmits somatic efferent fibers that innervate the superior oblique muscle, and conveys somatic afferent proprioceptive fibers to the mesencephalic nucleus of the trigeminal nerve.

The trochlear nerve is examined along with other oculomotor nerves by observing the excursions of the eyes in the six primary positions (Figure 9), noting any that evoke diplopia and a compensatory head position. Since the principal action of the superior oblique muscle is to depress the eye, an action that is most pronounced when placed on full adduction, full engagement of it can only be ascertained in down and inward gaze. Trochlear palsy leads to deflection of the eye upward and slightly inward. A compensatory head posture that consists of depression of the chin with tilting, and rotation of the head toward the normal eye, allows for more effective depressive action of the paretic muscle. Passive head tilting, often ineffective or hardly possible in true torticollis, is easily performed in children with functional torticollis in association with congenital trochear palsy. Its slender caliber makes the trochear nerve more vulnerable to injury in the course of meningitis than the oculomotor or abducens nerve, and more easily injured by minor head trauma.

Trigeminal Nerve (CN V)

This nerve with its two roots, and sensory much larger than the motor, provides cutaneous sensory innervation of the face, mucous membranes, and other internal cutaneous structures of the head, and motor innervation of masticatory muscles in its two roots through the three major divisions: ophthalmic, mandibular, and maxillary. The sensory root is comprised of central processes of the trigeminal or semilunar ganglion, and the motor root combines special visceral efferent fibers of mastication with reciprocal afferent proprioceptive innervation from sensory endings in those muscles to the mesencephalic nucleus. They pass anteriorly in the posterior cranial fossa under the tentorium to reach the trigeminal ganglion, which lies in a pocket of dura at the apex of the petrous portion of the temporal bone, lateral to the posterior cavernous sinus and the internal carotid artery at the foramen lacerum.

The greater superficial petrosal branch of the facial nerve and trigeminal motor root fibers pass under the ganglion, the latter exiting through the foramen ovale with the mandibular nerve. The trigeminal ganglion then divides into the ophthalmic, maxillary and mandibular divisions. The ophthalmic and maxillary nerves remain sensory in nature while sensory fibers of the maxillary are joined by extracranial motor root fibers.

Four small parasympathetic ganglia are associated with the trigeminal nerve complex, among them the ciliary ganglion with the ophthalmic, the sphenopalatine with the maxillary, and the otic, and submaxillary ganglia with the mandibular division (Figure 12). Altogether, the ophthalmic nerve innervates the skin and deep structures of the forehead and scalp from the upper eyelid to three-fifths of the vault of the skull and about 8 cm laterally from the midline; the root, tip and bridge of the nose; the eyeball, conjunctiva, cornea and iris; lacrimal glands and sac; mucous membrane of the frontal, sphenoidal, and ethmoidal sinuses; mucous membranes of the upper part of the nasal septum and lateral nasal cavity; and dura of the anterior cranial fossa, falx, and cerebellar tentorium (Figure 13). It departs from the trigeminal ganglia giving off a tentorial branch to the dura just prior to passing through the superior orbital fissure dividing into the lacrimal, frontal, and nasociliary nerves. The major branches of the ophthalmic nerve include the lacrimal, frontal, supratrochlear, supraorbital, nasociliary, long ciliary, infratrochlear, ethmoidal, and nasal nerves.

The lacrimal nerve enters the orbit through the superior orbital fissure where it runs along the border of the rectus lateralis. There it receives postganglionic parasympathetic fibers that pass from the cells of origin in the sphenopalatine ganglion through sphenopalatine nerves to the maxillary nerve and along the zygomatic and zygomaticotemporal nerves before being distributed with branches of the lacrimal nerve to innervate the lacrimal gland and adjacent conjunctiva. The frontal nerve enters the orbit through the superior orbital fissure where it divides into a small supratrochlear and larger supraorbital nerve. The supratrochlear nerve pierces the orbital fascia to innervate conjunctiva and skin of the medial upper lid, and after dividing into branches that pierce the corrugator and frontalis muscles, innervates the skin of the lower and mesial forehead. The supraorbital nerve leaves the orbit through the supraorbital notch and innervates the upper lid and continues to the forehead, dividing into medial and lateral branches beneath the frontalis muscle, the former of which pierces the muscle and innervates the scalp as posterior as the parietal bone, while the lateral branch pierces the galea aponeurotica and supplies the scalp to the lambda suture. One additional branch of the frontal nerve pieces the frontal bone to supply the mucous membranes of the frontal sinus. The nasociliary nerve enters the orbit along the medial wall of the cavity, passing through the ethomoid fissure as the anterior ethmoidal nerve and enters the cranial cavity just above the cribriform plate to the nasal cavity. There it branches into long ciliary nerves that accompany short ciliary nerves to distribute sensory afferents to the iris and cornea, and sympathetic fibers from the superior cervical ganglion to the pupillodilator muscle through communication between the cavernous sinus and ophthalmic nerve. The infratrochlear, anterior, and posterior ethmoidal and internal and external nasal

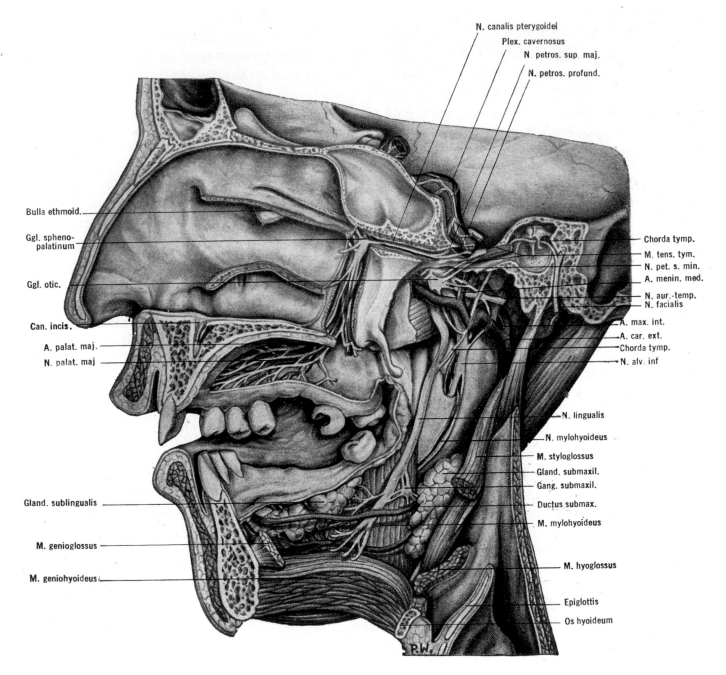

FIG. 12. Dissection showing the sphenopalatine, otic and submaxillary ganglia and associated structures. Reproduced from reference 1, with permission.

branches diverge from the nasociliary nerve and run anteriorly to the medial angle of the eye supplying sensation to the skin of the eyelids and side of the nose, conjunctiva, and lacrimal sac, as well as ethmoidal and frontal sinuses, anterior portion of the septum, and lateral wall of the nasal cavity, ala, and apex of the nose.

The maxillary nerve (Figure 14) supplies the skin and deep tissues of the upper lip, nose, cheek, and forehead contiguous with that supplied by the ophthalmic branch to the temporal ridge; mucous membranes of the maxil-

lary antrum, nasal fossa, and portions of the nasopharynx, hard and soft palate, upper gums, tonsils, pulp of the upper teeth, periosteum of the orbit, and dura of the middle cranial fossa. It passes horizontally first in the lateral wall of the cavernous sinus, then under the dura to the foramen rotundum, to cross the pterygopalatine fossa, entering the orbit through the inferior orbital fissure. There it becomes the infraorbital nerve and emerges into the face through the infraorbital foramen, dividing into branches for the skin of the face, nose, lower eyelid, and upper lip.

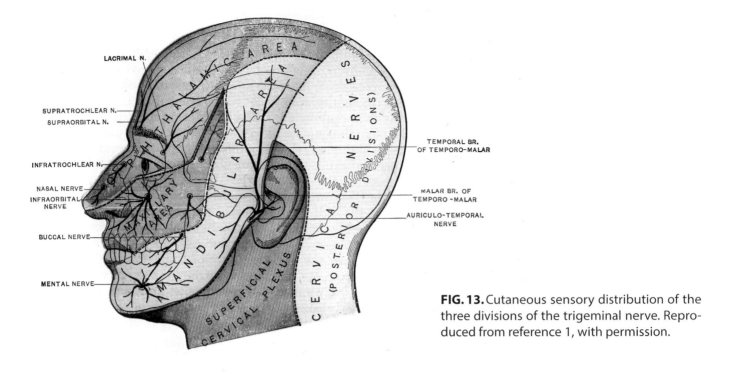

FIG. 13. Cutaneous sensory distribution of the three divisions of the trigeminal nerve. Reproduced from reference 1, with permission.

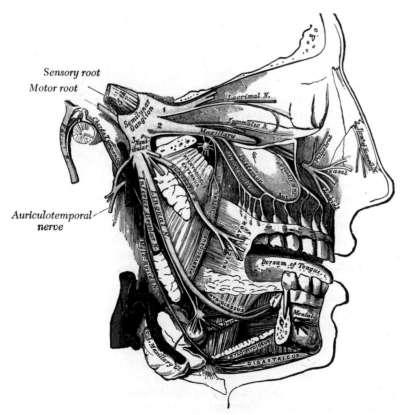

FIG. 14. The maxillary nerve and submaxillary ganglion. Reproduced from reference 1, with permission.

Those branches are divided into four groups, an intracranial nerve termed the middle meningeal nerve which accompanies the middle meningeal artery to supply the dura; three branches in the pterygopalatine fossa, namely the zygomatic nerve that sends a communicator, the zygomaticotemporal branch, to the lacrimal nerve through which postganglionic parasympathetic fibers from the sphenopalatine ganglion reach the lacrimal gland; and two others, the sphenopalatine and posterior superior alveolar branches. The sphenopalatine nerves serve as important communications between the sphenopalatine ganglion and the maxillary nerve providing transit for postganglionic parasympathetic secretomotor fibers to and from the ganglion back along the main maxillary nerve to the zygomatic nerve. Five additional branches, all sensory, termed orbital nerves, enter the orbit by the inferior orbital fissure and supply the periosteum and mucous membranes of the posterior ethmoidal and sphenoidal sinuses; and the greater and lesser palatine nerves that, respectively, pass through the pterygopalatine canal and emerge along the hard palate through the greater palatine foramen and supply the gums and mucous membranes of the hard palate, and adjacent soft palate, inferior nasal concha, middle and inferior meatuses; uvula, and tonsils (Figure 15).

Two other nerves, the posterior superior nasal branches and the pharyngeal nerves, enter the posterior nasal cavity and supply the lining of the posterior ethmoid sinuses and mucous membrane of the nasal portion of the pharynx posterior to the auditory tube. Two branches of the maxillary nerve originate in the infraorbital canal, the anterior and middle superior alveolar nerves, to innervate the premolar, incisor, and canine teeth, and the mucous membranes of the inferior meatus and nasal cavity floor communicating with nasal branches of the sphenopalatine nerves. Three maxillary nerve branches that originate in the face: the inferior palpebral branches, external nasal branches, and superior labra branches respectively, innervate the skin and conjunctiva of the lower lid, side of the nose and skin of the upper lip, mouth, and labial glands. Together with branches of the facial nerve, they form the infraorbital plexus.

The mandibular nerve is a mixed nerve with two large roots, one sensory and the other motor. The sensory fibers innervate skin and deeper structures of the temporal fossa, lower jaw, lower lip and chin; tympanic membrane, skin of the external auditory meatus, and upper half of the ear, and the mucous membranes of the mastoid air cells, floor of the mouth, lower gums, anterior two-thirds of the tongue, pulp of the lower teeth, temporomandibular joint, and dura of the posterior cranial fossa. Motor fibers innervate muscles of mastication, including the masseter, temporalis, and pterygoids as well as the mylohyoid and anterior belly of the digastric, tensor tympani, and veli palatine. The two roots that exit the middle cranial fossa through the foramen ovale

where it lies close to the otic ganglion unite outside the skull (Figure 16). The united main trunk gives off four branches, a meningeal branch to the dura, and nerves to the internal pterygoid, tensor veli palatine, and tensor tympani muscles, whereupon it divides into anterior and posterior divisions.

The anterior division receives a small sensory contribution and all of the remaining motor fibers innervate muscles of mastication and the skin and mucous membrane of the cheek. Buccal nerves innervate the masseter, temporalis, external pterygoid, and buccinator, skin overlying the cheek, mucous membrane of the mouth and neighboring gums. The posterior division of the mandibular nerve is mainly sensory with a small motor component that divides into three important branches: the auriculotemporal, lingual, and inferior alveolar nerves.

The auriculotemporal nerve arises close to the foramen spinosum and runs between the auricular and condyle of the mandible under the parotid gland to divide into superficial temporal branches. There are seven branches of the auriculotemporal nerve including a communicator from the facial nerve that carries sensory fibers that accompany the zygomatic, buccal, and mandibular branches of that nerve to supply the skin of those areas. A parotid branch and communicator from the otic ganglion carries postganglionic parasympathetic fibers from the glossopharyngeal nerve to supply secretomotor function to the parotid gland. Four sensory nerves including branches of the anterior auricular, external acoustis meatus nerves innervate the skin of the auricular and the external acoustis meatus. An articular branch innervates the temporomandibular joint, and superficial temporal branches that accompany the superficial temporal artery to the cranial vertex supply the skin of the temporal region.

The lingual nerve joins the chorda tympani nerve deep to the pterygoideus externus muscle and runs forward to the side of the tongue, passing between the hyoglossus muscle and submaxillary gland. The lingual nerve receives fibers from the chorda tympani that carry taste and preganglionic parasympathetic fibers to the submaxillary gland, as do short communicating nerves it receives from the submaxillary ganglion for distribution to the sublingual gland. Anterior terminal branches of the lingual nerve that innervate the anterior two-thirds of the tongue are communicated by the chorda tympani nerve, and subsequently innervate the mylohyoid muscle digastric muscles, canine and incisor teeth, and the skin of the chin. The inferior alveolar nerve accompanies the inferior alveolar artery in the mandibular canal and continues in the bone as far as the mental foramen where it divides into terminal branches.

Sensory trigeminal nerve function is assessed clinically by testing light touch and pinprick sensation along the three main divisions, V1 (forehead), V2 (cheek), and V3 (lower lip), and as well corneal reflexes in each eye via cotton appli-

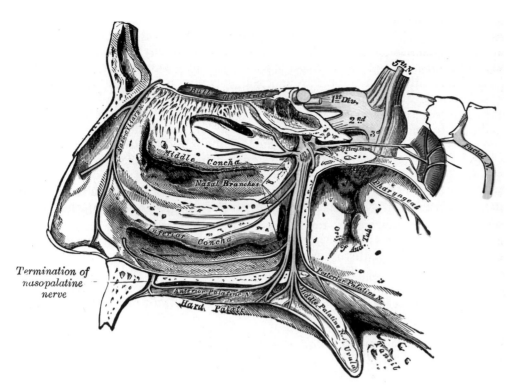

FIG. 15. The sphenopalatine ganglion and its branches. Reproduced from reference 1, with permission.

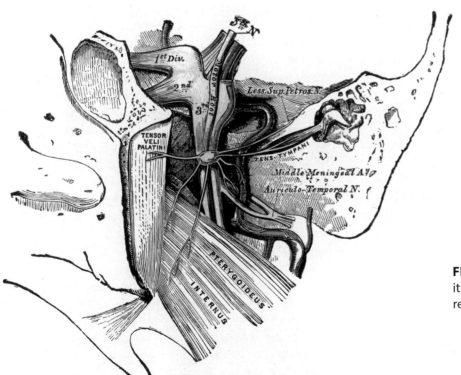

FIG. 16. The otic ganglion and its branches. Reproduced from reference 1, with permission.

cator. Motor function is ascertained by looking first for wasting of the temporal muscles and asking the patient to clench the jaw while palpating the masseter and temporalis muscles, trying to open the jaw against resistance and then trying to forcibly close it. The jaw jerk reflex is performed by asking the patient to let the mouth open loosely and percussing the chin against a resting finger, observing its movement.

Nuclear lesions of the trigeminal nerve present with muscle wasting detected as a flattening of the face above and below the zygoma. Lesions distal to the trigeminal ganglion tend to produce changes localized to the territory of one or two divisions while proximal lesions usually affect the whole or one side of the face. Lesions of the ganglion can produce variable patterns of distribution, but later the whole face tends to become affected. Pain, which is often severe, is a common accompaniment of lesions of the peripheral trigeminal nerve and ganglion caused by dental abscesses, caries, orbital tumor, or pseudotumor, tumors of the eye or jaw, sarcoid granulomas, cranial artery aneurysms, Wegener granulomatosis, vasculitis, cavernous sinus thrombosis, nasopharyngeal cancer, paranasal sinus infection, herpes zoster, neurofibromas and meningiomas, and metastases.

Frontal and maxillary bone fractures can injure the supraorbital and infraorbital nerves. Since autonomic connections to the salivary and lacrimal glands, pupils, and blood vessels travel with proximal branches of the trigeminal nerve, lesions in the nasociliary branch of the ophthalmic division can cause Horner syndrome (12). The latter consists of meiosis due to paralysis of the pupillodilator muscle, ptosis attributed to paralysis of the smooth muscle fibers of the lids, anhidrosis of the same side of the face due to a lesion of the nerve supply to the sweat glands, endopthalmos, as well as dryness of the nasal mucous membranes with lesions of the maxillary division.

Lesions of the sphenopalatine ganglion, zygomatic, and lacrimal nerves can suppress tearing in one eye. Salivary gland secretions are reduced by lesions situated in the lingual nerve after it has united with the chorda tympani nerve. Lesions of the trigeminal ganglion produce intense persistent or paroxysmal pain not localized to areas of one or more anatomical divisions but most often starts in the cheek and spreads over the face.

One particular infectious syndrome of the trigeminal ganglion, herpes zoster ophthalmicus (HZO), or shingles, is due to varicella zoster virus (VZV) infection localized to the ophthalmic division of the trigeminal nerve (13, 14). It is estimated that herpes zoster affects 20 to 30% of the population at some point in their lifetime and approximately 10 to 20% of these individuals will develop HZO. Moreover, it is estimated that approximately 50% of herpes zoster patients develop HZO without the use of suppressive antiviral therapy.

Herpes zoster ophthalmicus presents with vesicular rash over the forehead and eye; pain after the rash subsides, which is termed post-herpetic neuralgia. The complications of HZO include acute epithelial, stromal, and discoform keratitis, anterior uveitis, necrotizing retinitis, and cranial nerve palsies, the latter of which is most often due to vasculitis within the orbital apex or brainstem. Persistent vasculitis and neuritis can result in chronic ocular complications, especially post-herpetic neuralgia, which is seen in well over one-half of patients with HZO. Oral acyclovir, in conjuction with topical 3% acyclovir ointment, lubricants, and steroids for conjunctival, corneal, and uveal inflammation is recommended. The pain of post-herpetic neuralgia is treated with non-steroidal anti-inflammatory drugs and anti-epileptic agents. Varicella-zoster virus-specific cell mediated immunity, which keeps latent VZV in check, is boosted by periodic re-exposure, and is an important mechanism in preventing reactivation.

Vaccination of a lyophilized preparation of the Oka strain of live attenuated virus is suggested for at-risk patients, and has been shown to boost immunity against VZV in older patients. Disease processes that involve preganglionic trigeminal nerve roots tend to produce paresthesia, tingling, numbness, and sensory loss more than frank pain. Such involvement can be seen in transverse basal skull fractures, metastases, schwannoma, meningioma, chordoma, nasopharyngeal carcinoma, pituitary tumors, intracranial aneurysms, granulomatous and carcinomatous meningitis, sarcoidosis, and connective tissue disorders with concomitant involvement of the middle cranial fossa.

Although the entity of trigeminal neuralgia or tic doloreux was known for centuries, the first undisputed modern description of chronic paroxysmal trigeminal neuralgia or tic douloureux was that of Fothergill (15), who described onset in the fifth to sixth decade, primarily in women with excrutiating pain of sudden onset and brevity, precipitated by eating, talking, facial movements or light touches, and separated from toothache. It is now known that a family history increases its tendency for bilateral presentation, and although MS, hemifacial spasm, syringomyelia, and posterior fossa tumor can each be found in increased frequency, these are commonly accompanied by easily demonstrable focal signs. The initial pain is sometimes in a small area where it may remain; and, in others, it spreads to other areas and trigeminal divisions, with the mandibular and maxillary the commonest. Although by definition the disorder is paroxysmal, it is useful to differentiate between paroxysms or brief periods of pain, from runs or bouts of respectively either very brief or longer periods between paroxysms. Precipitating factors such as eating, talking and facial washing, and painful or not trigger areas, and relieving factors such as warmth, rubbing or stroking the painful area of skin, can remain consistent in the same patient. Treatment includes acupuncture, epileptic and non-epileptic drugs for non-emergency patients, and consideration of stereotactic radiosurgery, radiofrequency ablation, microvascular decompression, glycerol rhizotomy and cervicomedullary junction spinal cord stimulation for refractory cases (16–18). Other disorders to consider in the differential diagnosis of trigeminal neuralgia include glossopharyngeal neuralgia, temporomandibular disease, migraine, postherpetic neuralgia, dental pain, and atypical facial pain.

Abducens Nerve (CN VI)

This nerve that innervates the rectus lateralis muscle has its origin in the brainstem between the border of the pons and superior medulla. It exits the brainstem and pierces the dura along the dorsal sella of the sphenoid bone and runs through a notch below the posterior clinoid process where it traverses the cavernous sinus embedded in the lateral wall interposed between the oculomotor, trochlear, and ophthalmic nerves located above, the maxillary nerve below, and the internal carotid artery laterally, where it receives communicating sympathetic fibers from the carotid and cavernous sinus plexuses and the ophthalmic division of the trigeminal nerve (Figure 10). The nerve enters the orbit through the superior orbital fissure above the ophthalmic vein to pierce and enter the rectus lateralis muscle, which it innervates.

Abducens nerve palsy is ascertained by examining the position of the eyes in the six primary diagnostic directions of gaze, noting the position in which the patient develops diplopia, and taking note of compensatory head positions. Since the lateral rectus lateralis muscle abducts the eye, a newly affected patient will present with adduction of the affected eye and attempt to look in the direction of action of the paralyzed muscle to reduce diplopia. With long-standing palsy there can be a compensatory head posture due to contracture of bilateral medial recti serving as ipsilateral antagonist and contralateral synergist, as well the contralateral lateral rectus antagonist. Abducens palsy is encountered with intramedullary lesions, such as occlusion of a short circumferential basilar pontine branch in the Millard-Gubler syndrome of the ventrocaudal pontine tegmentum with abducens, and facial nerve palsy and contralateral CST involvement. A causal lesion along circumferential basilar branches, leads to the Foville syndrome of the dorsocaudal pontine tegmentum with ipsilateral trigeminal, abducens, facial nerve palsy, and contralateral sensory loss of the lower body due to involvement of the ipsilateral medial lemniscus. The addition of ipsilateral nystagmus and Horner syndrome occurs in a lower Foville syndrome due to occlusion of the posterior inferior cerebellar artery, and ipsilateral oculomotor palsy with an upper Foville syndrome. Extension of the disease process leads to a combination of Foville and Millard-Gubler syndromes with disturbance of hearing due to damage of cochlear fibers, while even more caudal extension of brainstem involvement leads to Gasperini syndrome of the dorsolateral caudal pontine tegmentum with ipsilateral trigeminal, abducens, facial paralysis, incomplete unilateral deafness, paralysis of conjugate eye movement, gaze deviation away from the lesion, and nystagmus with the quick phase toward the lesion. Damage to the abducens nucleus and ipsilateral pyramidal fibers before they decussate leads to Raymond syndrome of hemiplegia alternans of the caudal pons with ipsilateral abducens palsy and contralateral hemiplegia.

Facial Nerve (CN VII)

The two roots of this nerve, facial motor proper, and a second smaller sensory root, exit the inferior border of the ventral pons in a recess between the olivary complex and the inferior cerebellar peduncle and pass into the internal acoustic meatus. Accompanied by the vestibulocochlear nerve, they enter the petrous portion of the temporal bone, fusing together in the geniculate ganglion to enter the facial canal near the tympanic membrane and oval window. The nerve bends beside mastoid air cells to reach the stylomastoid foramen from which it exits into the substance of the parotid gland, crossing the external carotid artery, and dividing into superior temporofacial and inferior cervicofacial branches. The facial nerve gives off three sets of branches, one pair each along its anatomical course along the geniculate ganglion, facial canal, face, and neck (Figures 17, 18). Those from the geniculate ganglion include the greater superficial petrosal and deep petrosal nerves, the former of which runs on the anterior surface of the petrous portion of the temporal bone over cartilage of the auditory tube, crossing the internal carotid artery and uniting with the deep petrosal nerve to form the nerve of the Vidian nerve of the pterygoid canal that provides sensory innervation to the soft palate through the lesser palatine nerves.

The greater superficial petrosal nerve gives rise to a few filaments to the auditory tube and parasympathetic secretomotor innervation via the nervus intermedius and sphenopalatine ganglion to the lacrimal gland and other glands of the nasal cavity and palate, as well as postganglionic sympathetic innervation via the superior cervical ganglion, carotid plexus, and trigeminal branches to mucous membranes of the nasal cavity and palate. Two branches emanate from the facial canal: the motor branch to the stapedius muscle as the facial nerve proceeds downward past the tympanum, and the chorda tympani nerve branch just prior to emergence of the facial nerve from the stylomastoid foramen. The chorda tympani enters its own canal and emerges through an aperture between the tympanum and base of the pyramid, uniting with the lingual nerve in a groove joined by a communication from the otic ganglion

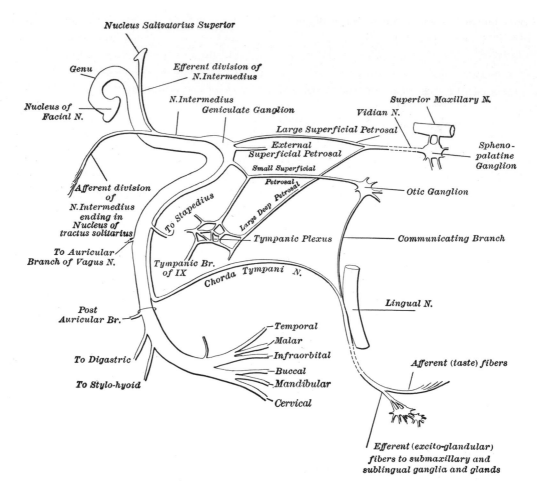

FIG. 17. The facial and intermedius nerve and their communications with other nerves. Reproduced from reference 1, with permission.

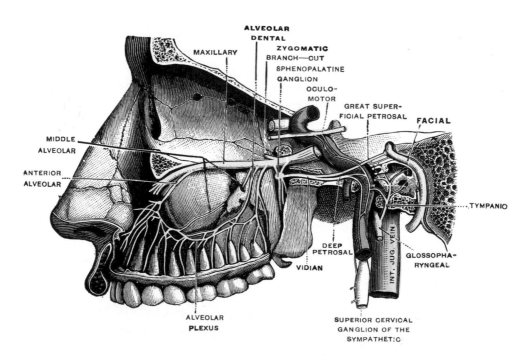

FIG. 18. The facial nerve and its connections. Reproduced from reference 1, with permission.

to transmit special sensory fibers for taste, and preganglionic parasympathetic secretomotor fibers from the nervus intermedius to the submaxillary, sublingual, lingual, and neighboring salivary glands.

In the face and neck, the facial nerve travels upwards in front of the mastoid process where it is joined by the auricular branch of the vagus nerve and muscular branches of the greater auricular and lesser occipital nerves, issuing fiber branches that innervate the digastric and stylohyoideus muscles, while temporal branches communicate with zygomaticotemporal branches of the maxillary nerve and auriculotemporal branches of the mandibular division of the trigeminal nerve. The temporal and auriculotemporal branches supply the frontalis and orbicularis oculi while others join supraorbital and lacrimal branches of the ophthalmic nerve. Zygomatic and buccal branches of the facial nerve are distributed across the face, respectively, in the region of the zygomatic arch to the lateral portion of the orbit to supply orbicularis oculi muscles; and below the orbit via an infraorbital plexus comprised of infraorbital branches of the maxillary division of the trigeminal nerve. Other branches innervate buccinator and orbicularis oris muscles of the mouth via communicating filaments of the mandibular branch of the trigeminal nerve, and muscles of the lower lip and chin traversing the side of the neck via trigeminal mandibular and cervical branches.

Clinical assessment of the facial nerve consists of inspection of the face for obvious paralysis suggested by visible drooping of the angle of the mouth and lower lid. The patient is observed attempting to raise the eyebrows, frown, wrinkle the forehead, scalp, and ears, wink, screw the eyes, move the nose, smile, whistle, snarl, purse the lips, pout, and dimple the chin. Dissociated unilateral voluntary weakness that improves with emotional stimuli is more characteristic of supranuclear facial palsy. Bilateral facial immobility due to Parkinson disease may be difficult to separate from bilateral infranuclear involvement. Intact taste on the anterior two-thirds of the tongue and lacrimation excludes a lesion proximal to the geniculate ganglion. Absence of hypersensitivity to sound and objective response of the stapedius reflex performed by comparing pure tones to either ear, excludes a significant lesion proximal to the origin of the nerve to the stapedius muscle. Peripheral facial nerve lesions can be grouped into seven clinically relevant anatomical localizations: 1) Posterior fossa; 2) Suprageniculate, between the internal auditory meatus and geniculate ganglion; 3) Transgeniculate involving the ganglion proper; 4) Suprastapedial, between the geniculate ganglion and branch to the stapedius muscle; 5) Infrastapedial, between the branch to the stapedius muscle and chorda tympani nerve; 6) Infrachordal, between the chorda tympani and stylomastoid foramen; and 7) Infraforaminal, distal to the stylomastoid foramen.

Facial paralysis associated with lesions of the posterior fossa resembles nuclear lesions that occur in compressive tumors of the cerebellopontine angle. Suprageniculate are typically unilateral, influenced by the position of the vestibulocochlear nerve upon the facial nerve and the scant connective tissue that makes it susceptible to compression by enlarging Schwannomas. Geniculate herpes zoster (HZO), described by Ramsey Hunt (19), is an example of a transgeniculate lesion. The Ramsey Hunt syndrome presents with malaise, fever, pain and, later, vesicles along the auricle and external auditory meatus with facial palsy, and vestibular and auditory symptoms including hyperacusis, hearing impairment, vertigo, ataxia, nystagmus, disturbances of salivation, lacrimation, taste, and varying involvement of neighboring cranial nerves.

Facial nerve contrast-enhanced MRI demonstrates linear enhancement of the nerve in its canal associated with perivasculitis of arteriae nervorum. Idiopathic or Bell palsy presents with suprastapedial, infrastapedial, or infrachordal facial nerve involvement. Suprastapedial localization leads to loss of taste in the anterior two-thirds of the tongue and impaired salivation without abnormal lacrimation or hyperacusis due to sparing of lacrimal, stapedius and chorda tympani nerves, whereas infrastapedial and infrachordal lesions, respectively, spare the stapedius and chorda tympani nerve branches leading to normal hearing and taste. Infraforaminal lesions due to trauma, tumors, and granulomatous disease of the parotid gland produce isolated facial palsy that includes the whole or part of the face.

Named in honor of Charles Bell who first described the syndrome in 1907 (20), Bell palsy presents with facial pain in and around the ear, cheek area, jaw, neck, or back of the head, typically in an individual of the second or third decade, without gender or seasonal preference. An affected patient demonstrates a wide-open affected eye due to loss of tone of the ipsilateral levator palpebrae muscle, flattened eyebrow, smooth forehead, droop of the lower eyelid slightly off the eyeball, obliteration of the nasolabial fold, and median pull of the tip of the nose toward the health side due to loss of muscle innervation. Lacrimation is more pronounced on the affected side due to paralysis of the orbicularis oculi muscle and the failure of tears to travel toward the inner can thus, as well as, paralysis of the lacrimal canal that ceases to take up the fluid. The tongue veers toward the healthy side due to the illusion created by hemiplegia of the mouth.

A striking feature is Bell phenomenon wherein the eyeball moves upwards and slightly outward when the patient forcibly shuts the weak eye. There may be inactive supraorbital (glabellar), blinking, glare (opticopalpebral), corneal, auriculopalpebral and cochleopalpebral (blinking with loud noise) reflexes. The disturbance of lacrimal secretion is caused by loss of functionality of the greater superficial petrosal nerve or geniculate ganglion, hyeraccusis due to paralysis of the nerve branch supplying the stapedius muscle, loss of taste along the anterior two-thirds of the tongue due to loss of innervation of the chorda tympani nerve, deviation of the chin toward the normal side when the mouth is opened, apparent deviation of the tongue, and slight semilateral paresis of the soft palate caused by loss of facial muscle innervation. Serial electrodiagnostic studies performed from onset through convalescence provides valuable information on lesion location, severity, pathophysiology and prognosis (21).

It is the propensity of the facial nerve to form a single bundle with dense thick connective tissue and near complete filling of the canal that probably renders it more susceptible and less tolerant of expansive lesions and focal inflammatory swelling leading to internal damage. In the first few days, electrically induced blink reflexes and assessment of peripheral facial nerve conduction studies provide information on the degree of demyelinating conduction block. After 10 days, the size of the compound muscle action potential (CMAP) reflects the relative functional loss of axons on the affected side, while after three weeks, needle electromyography can ascertain the presence and intensity of denervation.

If axonal damage predominates, regeneration and functional recovery proceed more slowly than if demyelination is the underlying injury. Convalescent studies may provide evidence of abnormal regeneration and changes in motor neuronal excitability characteristic of the postparalytic facial syndrome with muscle synkinesis, myokymia, involuntary muscle contractions, and hemifacial spasm. The latter consists of paroxysms of rapid irregular clonic twitching or phasic contraction starting around the eyes with eventual spread to ipsilateral facial muscles. A vascular mediated etiopathogenesis is considered likely in some cases by virtue of the improvement in hemifacial spasms after surgical intervention to empirically decompress the facial nerve at its root exit zone (22).

It is believed that extrinsic irritation of the facial nerve at the posterior fossa generates an antidromic bombardment of inputs to facial motor neurons. This leads to hyperexcitability and reflex firing due to kindling effects, often with demonstrable lateral spread of excitability between facial axons evident as reflex responses in the orbicularis oris to electrical stimuli applied over the supraorbital nerve when, in fact, the trigeminofacial reflex should instead be limited to the orbicularis oculi (23, 24).

The treatment of new-onset Bell palsy includes corticosteroids and antiviral agents, and occasionally surgical intervention with decompression of the facial canal depending upon the severity, stage of evolution, and electrodiagnostic findings (25, 26). The rationale for empiric corticosteroid administration is the salutary effect on demyelinating conduction block early in the course of the illness. While antivirals do not provide an additional objective benefit over corticosteroids alone in facial nerve recovery, nor should they be considered effective monotherapy for the disorder, one potential rationale for its adjuvant use with corticosteroids is to avert an outbreak of VZV rash, notably oticus, which would be further devastating to the facial nerve. Treatment with botulinum toxin markedly alleviates hemifacial spasm and the abnormal activity that occurs in patients with postparalytic facial syndrome (27).

The differential diagnosis of Bell palsy includes otitic facial paresis due to suppurative infection, petrous bone fracture, inner ear surgery, facial canal tumors, herpes zoster oticus, brainstem pathology affecting exiting peripheral facial nerve including infarction, hemorrhage, increased intracranial pressure, and resolving supranuclear lesions wherein superior facial muscles recover before those of the lower face.

Vestibulocochlear Nerve (CN VIII)

This nerve consists of two distinct sets of sensory nerve fibers organized into medial, vestibular, and lateral cochlear roots that, respectively, derive from bipolar cells in Scarpa and spiral ganglia. Peripheral processes of Scarpa ganglion located in the outer end of the internal auditory meatus and those of the spiral ganglion located along the inner edge of the osseous spiral lamina, send peripheral processes distally in the internal auditory meatus joined by the facial nerve, nervus intermedius of Wrisberg and the internal auditory artery and vein to the labyrinth. A superior branch innervates the utricle and ampulla of the superior and lateral semicircular canals, while an inferior branch innervates the saccule, and a posterior branch innervates the ampulla of the posterior semicircular canal that mediates balance and equilibrium; other branches innervate the organ of Corti concerned with hearing. Centrally, the vestibulocochlear nerve traverses the cerebellopontine angle where it enters the brainstem laterally at the junction of the pons and medulla.

Bedside tests of this nerve should be separated into those of hearing and vestibular function. Vestibular function is best understood by separating vestibular function into phasic or semicircular canal elements with central connections for the coordination of compensatory eye movements, chiefly in response to canal stimulation and tonic elements centered in the otolith organs of the utricle and saccule. Unilateral infranuclear vestibular nerve lesions interrupt this balance and are clinically manifested by nystagmus that is appreciated by examination of the eyes at rest, as well as in response to provocative testing.

Observation of the eyes should be made in a patient seated upright following the examiner's fingers, with fast excursions in both horizontal directions and in slow pursuit. Spontaneous nystagmus, defined by the direction of the quick component, is more evident, especially in peripheral vestibular lesions, when the direction of gaze is in the quick component, which in an excitatory lesion of the labyrinth emanates from the opposite affected ear. This explains why a patient suffering from an acute attack of labyrinthine vertigo lies curled on one side with the affected ear faced up and avoids looking in the direction of spontaneous nystagmus. Optokinetic nystagmus is evaluated by using a cloth strip with images that permit fixation or a rotating drum, whereas positional nystagmus can be evaluated by the Barany test maneuver with the patient resting comfortably on an examining table. Caloric testing is more complicated and requires a formal laboratory approach using oculonystagmography that ascertains the directionality of eye movements in response to positional changes and air stimulation in either ear, as a measure of the degree of canal paresis and directional preponderance.

Tests of cochlear nerve function are best carried out in a laboratory, however bedside examination in a quiet setting can also give clues to the cause of altered hearing. The patient should be asked to repeat spoken and whispered sounds, or listen to a ticking watch comparing the sound in the left and right ears. A 256 cps tuning fork applied to either mastoid and the external auditory meatus can estimate the degree of cochlear function and distinguish conductive from sensorineural hearing loss. The vibrating tuning fork should be applied to the mastoid process until the patient signals the end of the sound and then held near the external auditory meatus indicating better conductive function, such is a positive Rinne test. The Weber test is performed by placing the foot of the tuning fork on the forehead and asking the patient which ear seems to hear the vibrations best, wherein the side with a conductive hearing loss lateralizes vibrations to the affected ear, while those in the setting of sensorineural hearing loss lateralize to the unaffected side. Pure tone audiometry provides essential information regarding hearing thresholds, while brainstem auditory evoked responses (BAER) provide precise measurements of conduction time along peripheral and central auditory pathways. Together, they are complementary tools in the evaluation of childhood and adult disturbances due to acquired end organ cochlear diseases, compressive lesions of the proximal and distal vestibulocochlear nerve, brainstem nuclei and tracts subserving hearing.

Peripheral lesions of the vestibulocochlear nerve produce partial or complete deafness and vertigo. Combined deafness and vertigo most often results from drug intoxications; infections, notably meningitis; acoustic schwannomas; cerebellopontine angle tumors; Paget disease of the bone; head injury; and autoimmune insults. Attacks of severe vertigo that occur in Meniere disease due to endolymphatic distention, infectious illnesses that target Scarpa ganglia, and otosclerosis.

The syndrome of sudden sensorineural hearing loss is of particular importance (28). Individuals from childhood to late adulthood present with variably severe unilateral hearing loss associated with tinnitus and vestibular dysfunc-

tion that is typically unilateral but bilateral in about 5% of cases. The proximate mechanism of injury stems from peri- or postinfectious, vascular, and autoimmune mediated factors. Mumps, herpes viruses, cytomegalovirus, and influenza infections are found in about two-thirds of cases, however another well recognized cause is Lyme borreliosis in endemic areas.

The cochlea is supplied by an end artery and although vascular occlusion mediated by atherosclerosis, hypertension, vasospasm, hyperviscosity, and paradoxical embolism have been postulated as causes for sudden sensorineural hearing loss, there is little neuropathological evidence for its occurrence. Hypercholesterolemia, hypertension, and diabetes appear to be closely associated with sudden hearing loss in small case control studies, as are hypotension and migraine headaches in young adults, which could predispose an individual patient to reflex vasoconstriction and cochlear hypoxia. Susac syndrome presents with encephalopathy and hearing loss due to autoimmune endotheliopathy and branch artery occlusions of the retina, with involvement of the inner ear and cerebral microvasculature (29). Waldenstrom syndrome, multiple myeloma, systemic arteritis, Sjogren syndrome, relapsing polychondritis, Behcet disease, systemic lupus, ulcerative colitis, Crohn disease, Cogan syndrome, and those with serum antibodies directed against inner ear antigens appear to be at higher risk of developing autoimmune hearing loss.

A thorough serological and audiological evaluation should be performed and contrast-enhanced MRI of the brain and internal auditory canals should be performed to screen for acoustic neuroma, meningiomas, demyelinating lesions, thrombotic and hemorrhagic vascular events. Although prognosis is generally favorable with the majority of patients spontaneously improving by two weeks, there is a rationale for a trial of oral corticosteroids and intratympanic dexamethasone in oral non-responders, however efficacy has not been clearly established in either therapeutic modality.

Glossopharyngeal Nerve (CN IX)

Rootlets of this nerve emerge from the medulla in the groove between the olive and inferior peduncle adjacent to the vestibulocochlear, vagus, and accessory nerves, passing through the jugular foramen in a separate sheet of dura. Outside the skull the nerve runs anteriorly between the internal jugular vein, internal carotid artery, and styloid process, following the stylopharyngeus muscle and across its surface to the posterior border of the hyoglossus where it penetrates the palatine tonsil, base of the tongue, and adjacent glands. This portion of the nerve is comprised of superior and inferior ganglia, the lower one of which contains cells bodies of sensory nerve fibers that form connections with the vagus nerve via the auricular branch and the superior cervical sympathetic ganglion. Afterward the facial nerve divides into six terminal branches: tympanic, carotid sinus, pharyngeal, stylopharyngeus, tonsillar, and lingual nerves. The tympanic nerve fibers arise from the inferior ganglion and pass through the otic ganglion into a small bony opening in the petrous bone between the carotid canal and jugular fossa, continuing as the lesser superficial petrosal nerve with sensory branches distributed through the tympanic plexus to mucous membranes of the oval and round windows, tympanic membrane, auditory tube, and mastoid air cells. Preganglionic parasympathetic fibers originating in the root of the otic ganglion pass in the lesser superficial petrosal nerve synapsing in the otic ganglion, and transits via communication along the auriculotemporal branch of the trigeminal nerve to the parotid gland (Figure 19). The carotid nerve arises from the main glossopharyngeal trunk beyond its emergence in the jugular foramen and communicates with the nodose ganglion and pharyngeal branch of the vagus nerve where is continues along the anterior surface of the internal carotid artery to a dilated portion of the vessel termed the *carotid sinus* supplying afferent innervation to blood pressure baroreceptors. Glossopharyngeal pharyngeal branches join those of the vagus nerve and other sympathetic fibers to form the pharyngeal plexus that innervates the muscular coat of the pharynx. The stylopharyngeus branch supplies the muscle of the same name, whereas tonsillar branches innervate the soft palate, and those of the lingual branches innervate vallate papillae with afferent fibers for taste and sensory innervation of mucous membranes along the base of the tongue.

Glossopharyngeal nerve function is tested by ascertaining taste over the posterior third of he tongue, and appreciation of touch and pain sensitivity along the soft palate, tonsil, and posterior pharyngeal wall. Since the glossopharyngeal nerve supplies the afferent input for the palatal and pharyngeal reflexes, those should disappear in lesions of the glossopharyngeal nerve and its branches, as well as with damage of vagal efferents. The glossopharyngeal nerve can be damaged by vertebral artery lesions, tumors of the tongue and tonsil, and fractures of the styloid process.

First recognized by Weisenburg (30), glossopharyngeal neuralgia refers to pain along the glossopharyngeal nerve and its connections. It appears most often in young patients and in the older individuals, often without a history of prior illness. It presents with sudden and unexpected pain in the lower throat, along small cavities of the tonsil and base of the tongue, often radiating to the ears, external auditory meatus, lower jaw, and teeth. Patients observed during an attack may demonstrate contraction of the face and a characteristic cough in an effort to arrest the pain. Swallowing, yawning, sneezing, coughing, and extension of the tongue can precipitate attacks. Trigger zones, wherein anesthetic injection

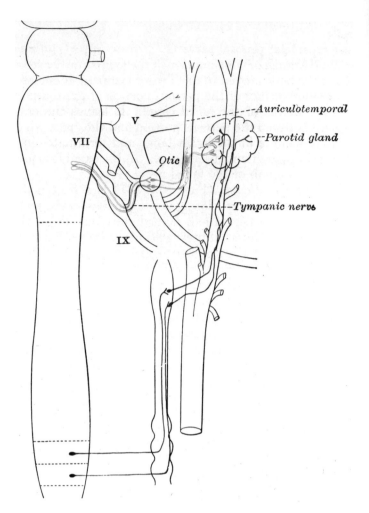

FIG. 19. The otic ganglion and its connections. Reproduced from reference 1, with permission.

can bring temporary cessation of the paroxysms, are important to document and coincide with areas of maximal pain, including the upper wall of the posterior pharynx, base of the tongue, and tonsillar cavities, pillars and base. Secondary forms of the neuralgia occur in rhinopharyngeal and laryngeal malignancies. Medication-resistant forms can be treated by cervical neurotomy at the root of nerve.

Vagus Nerve (CN X)

This nerve, the longest of the cranial nerves and with the most extensive innervation, originates from rootlets attached to the medulla between the olives and inferior cerebellar penduncle, passing through the jugular foramen accompanied by the accessory nerve, but separated from the glossopharyngeal nerve, forming two sensory ganglia, the superior jugular and nodose. Sensory nerve fiber input from the posterior fossa and ear join the nerve in the jugular foramen, traveling in the auricular nerve while the more inferior nodose ganglion emerges just after exit from the jugular foramen, receiving peripheral ramuses of the superior laryngeal nerve and other vagal branches to laryngeal, tracheal, bronchial, esophageal, and other thoracic and abdominal viscera. The motor fiber contribution from the cranial part of the accessory nerve occurs just distal to the nodose ganglion. Other nerve fiber communications contribute to the pharyngeal plexus and the superior laryngeal nerve. One branch provides motor innervation to the cricothyroid muscle and another conveys sensory impulses from the larynx as far down as the vocal cords. The vagal trunk passes vertically downward within the carotid sheath deep to, and beneath the internal jugular vein and internal and common carotid arteries (Figure 20), separating into right and left portions, each side giving a recurrent laryngeal nerve that innervates ipsilateral laryngeal muscles except for the cricothyroid.

The right vagus crosses the subclavian artery and continues along the side of the trachea to the lung where it spreads out in the pulmonary plexus below the diaphragm to the lesser curvature of the stomach, and divides into celiac and gastric branches. The left vagus enters the thorax between the left carotid and subclavian arteries, crossing the arch of the aorta to reach the pulmonary plexus and esophagus, and below the diaphgram to the anterior stomach, dividing into hepatic and gastric branches. Several branches of the vagus nerve exit at the jugular foramen, including a meningeal nerve to the dura of the posterior fossa and an auricular branch to the skin of the auricular and external auditory meatus. In the neck, pharyngeal branches are distributed to muscles and mucus membranes of the pharynx, soft palate, carotid body, and chemoreceptors sensitive to blood oxygen tension. A superior laryngeal nerve branch communicates with the superior cervical sympathetic ganglion and contributes to the pharyngeal plexus, and superior cardiac branches.

The recurrent laryngeal nerve arises more distally and runs upward in the neck to the larynx where it divides into cardiac, tracheal, esophageal, and laryngeal branches. In the thorax, the vagus nerve gives inferior cardiac branches that supply preganglionic parasympathetic efferent fibers that terminate along ganglion supplying heart muscle and the cardiac conduction system. Other thoracic branches include those to respective plexuses of bronchial, esophageal, gastric, hepatic, gall bladder, pylorus, duodenal, and celiac viscera.

The clinical examination of the vagus nerve commences with inspection of the soft palate duration phonation, and the application of a padded applicator to the surface of the uvula or soft palate, recognizing that the afferent limb of the palatal reflex runs in the glossopharyngeal nerve while the efferent limb transits the vagus. Unilateral vagal lesions lead to impaired soft palate elevation with deviation of the uvula toward the unaffected side. Absent palatal movement occurs in bilateral vagal lesions, afferent glossopharyngeal

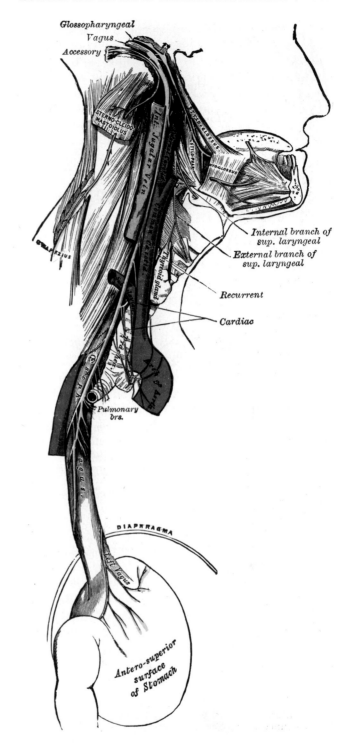

FIG. 20. Course and distribution of the glossopharyngeal, vagus, and accessory nerves. Reproduced from reference 1, with permission.

denervation, and in some normal individuals. Inspection during swallowing evidences drooping of the paralyzed side, nasal regurgitation, and lateral movement of one-half of the palatal and pharyngeal muscles. The voice is hoarse, weak, and tires easily with a breathy quality and ineffective cough. Direct laryngoscopy discerns the position of the vocal cords. Flexible endoscopic evaluation of swallowing with sensory testing (FEESST) assesses largyngophargeal discrimination thresholds by delivering air pulse stimuli to the mucosa innervated by the superior laryngeal nerve to elicit the laryngeal adductor reflex recognized as forceful adduction of the vocal folds. This procedure is complementary to videofluorscopic studies of swallowing in recognizing patients at risk for aspiration and pneumonia, including those with acquired unilateral fold immobility after partial laryngectomy, cardiac-related dysphagia following open heart surgery, stroke, progressive neuromuscular disorders, chronic cough and gastroesophageal reflux disease, and extraesophageal reflux with dysphagia (31–35).

Isolated lesions of the vagus nerve above the ganglia or the posterior fossa are rare and clinically insignificant unless bilateral. In the neck, vagal nerve lesions result from the complications of thyroidectomy or contiguous cancer involving the thyroid, pharynx, and upper esophagus. In the thorax, the left recurrent laryngeal nerve is prone to damage by contiguous carcinoma, compressive aortic aneurysm, sarcoidosis, toxic exposures, and polyneuritis. Intact superior laryngeal nerve function confers slight vocal cord movement on attempted phonation from contraction of the cricothyroid muscle. Total paralysis of laryngeal musculature results from lesions above the origin of the superior laryngeal nerve, and bilateral lesions of the vagal nerves at the inferior ganglion or above.

Vagus nerve stimulation has been used in the management of intractable childhood epilepsy, in those unsuitable for epilepsy surgery, and others with insufficient benefit from such a treatment (36). It reduces seizure frequency and has mild side effects. Effective stimulation in human subjects appears to be primarily mediated by afferent vagal fibers with synapses in the locus ceruleus, solitary tract, thalamus, and limb structures of the brainstem and cerebrum, mediated by the major inhibitory neurotransmitter gamma aminobutyric acid. Potential complications include infection, lead fracture, fluid collections around the stimulator, neck pain, and difficulty swallowing. Vagus nerve stimulation has been investigated in the management of advanced heart failure due to its presumed salutary effect of increasing parasympathetic tone on the production of nitric oxide and the reduction of the inflammatory process involved in heart failure, as well as in drug resistant daily chronic migraine headache with depression (37).

Accessory Nerve (CN XI)

This motor nerve consists of two parts, a cranial and a spinal portion. The cranial portion arises as roots from the medulla below the origin of the vagus nerve and runs laterally to jugular foramen where it interchanges and unites with the spinal portion. After passing through the foramen the cranial part joins the vagus nerve proximal to the nodose ganglion to which it distributes fibers along pharyngeal branches to the uvula, levator veli palatine, and pharyngeal constrictor muscle; and through superior and inferior laryngeal branches of the vagus nerve to muscles of the larynx and esophagus. The spinal accessory portion originates from motor cells in the upper fiber cervical segments of the spinal cord and emerges from it to pass through the foramen magnum and across the occipital bone to the jugular notch, penetrating the dura over the jugular bulb. It exchanges fibers with the cranial portion and passes posteriorly across the posterior triangle of the neck to the anterior border of the trapezius and sternocleidomastoid muscles which it innervates.

Examination of accessory nerve function begins with inspection and assessment of the strength of the trapezius and sternocleidomastoid muscles. The sternocleidomastoid muscle is tested by asking the patient to turn the chin against resistance, while the trapezius muscle is tested by asking the patient to shrug shoulders upward. Unilateral weakness of the sternocleidomastoid muscle leads to slight rotation of the head toward the affected side and lateral flexion of the head away from it. Trapezius muscle paralysis is associated with flattening of the line from the shoulder to the neck, scapular prominence when viewed frontward, and winging when viewed from the back due to its displacement downward and outwards, accentuated with passive abduction of the arm. Proximal lesions of the accessory nerve proximal to the sternocleidomastoid muscle involve both muscles, whereas a distal lesion leads to involvement of the trapezius muscle alone. Electrodiagnostic studies along the accessory nerve to the trapezius and sternocleidomastoid muscles are important in the evaluation of presumed accessory neuropathy due to neck trauma, radical neck dissection, oropharyneal and laryngeal cancer (38, 39).

Hypoglossal Nerve (CN XII)

The roots of this motor nerve to the tongue exit the medulla along its anterolateral surface between the pyramid and olives, piercing the dura opposite the hypoglossal canal in the occipital bone and emerging through the skull positioned under the internal carotid artery and internal jugular vein closely bound to the vagus nerve. It runs downward and becomes superficial near the angle of the mandible, loops around the occipital artery, and passes forward across the external carotid and lingual arteries below the tendon of the digastric and stylohyoid muscles between the mylohyoid and hyoglossus to the tip of the tongue. The hypoglossal nerve communicates with anterior primary divisions of the first and second cervical nerve that contain motor fibers for the supra-, and infrahyoid muscles, and sensory fibers

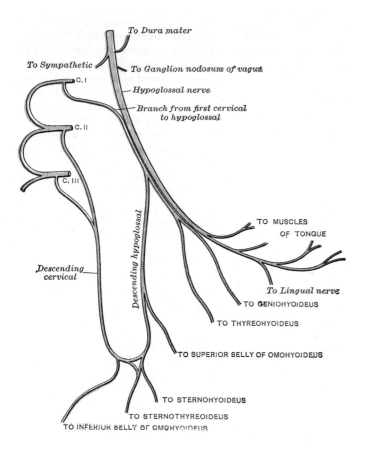

FIG. 21. The hypoglossal nerve. Reproduced from reference 1, with permission.

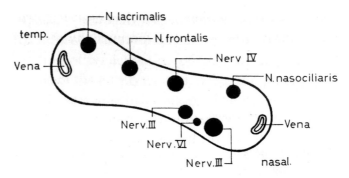

FIG. 22. The arrangement of nerves in the superior orbital fissure. Reproduced from reference 4, with permission.

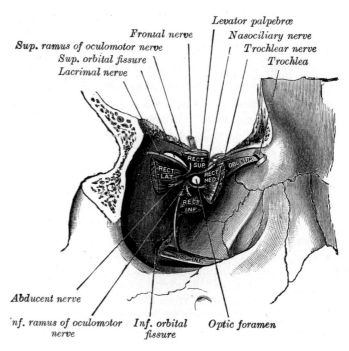

FIG. 23. Anatomic view of the superior orbital fissure and apex. Reproduced from reference 1, with permission.

from uppermost cervical dorsal root ganglia (Figure 21). A descending hypoglossal branch becomes the ansa hypoglossi that supplies the omohyoid, sternohyoid, and sternothyroid muscles. Other motor branches innervate the thyrohyoid, geniohyoid, styloglossus, hyoglossus, genioglossus and other intrinsic muscles of the tongue.

The examination of the hypoglossal nerve commences with inspection and examination of the tongue at rest, in forward and lateral protrusion, and forcible contraction against the inside cheek. Lesions of the hypoglossal nerve produce lingual weakness and wasting. True fibrillation or twitching is recognized as fine continuous irregular undulations through the mucous membrane of the tongue. Unilateral weakness of the tongue leads to deviation of the tip toward the paralyzed side with voluntary protrusion because of the unopposed action of the contralateral genioglossus muscle. Skull trauma, tumors, and vertebral aneurysms can cause hypoglossal nerve injury, as can a lesion of the neck in the vicinity of the carotid sheath, simultaneously injuring sympathetic fibers leading to ipsilateral tongue paralysis and Horner syndrome.

MULTIPLE CRANIAL NERVE PALSIES

Superior Orbital Fissure

First described by Rochon-Duvigneau (40), this syndrome includes paralysis of the oculomotor, trochlear, and abducens nerves resulting in total ophthalmoplegia with exophthalmos, fixed staring eyeball, dilated pupil, paralysis of accommodation and light reflex, ptosis, sensory loss of the ipsilateral cornea, forehead, and upper eyelid due to involvement of the ophthalmic branch of trigeminal nerve (Figures 22, 23). This becomes the orbital apex syndrome when the former is combined with impaired vision or total blindness due to concomitant involvement of the optic nerve in the optic canal (Figure 23). Such syndromes are usually associated with traumatic orbital or sphenoid skull fracture, hematoma, orbital infection, and neoplasms, including meningioma, cavernous angioma, optic nerve glioma, nasopharyngeal and bone tumors adjacent to the superior orbital fissure.

Cavernous Sinus Syndrome

First recognized by Foix (41), this is the syndrome of the lateral wall of the cavernous sinus (Figure 10) which gives passage to a number of elements from superior to inferior, the oculomotor, trochlear, ophthalmic and maxillary nerves, and the abducens nerve, which is suspended by connective tissue trabeculae within the venous sinus plexus. The maxillary nerve is related to the posterior portion of the sinus and soon diverges from the other nerves. The syndrome is essentially composed of unilateral ophthalmoplegia, starting with involvement of the abducens followed by ophthalmic and other branches of the trigeminal nerve, with unilateral exophthalmos and sympathetic paralysis.

Based upon the anteroposterior anatomy, three possible clinical presentations can be discerned. An anterior syndrome presents essentially the same as the superior orbital fissure syndrome with involvement of the optic nerve; a medial syndrome with involvement of extrinsic ocular muscles, ophthalmic and superior maxillary branches of the trigeminal nerve leads to complete ophthlamoplegia with sensory loss in the upper two branches of the trigeminal nerve. A posterior syndrome associated with trigeminal sensory and motor involvement and oculomotor paralysis is confined to the abducens nerve. The syndrome of the sphenopetrous fissure occurs in association with carotid artery aneurysm and paralysis of the abducens, with watering of the eyes indicative of involvement of the superior petrosal nerve, and progressive involvement of the trigeminal nerve involving the ophthalmic, superior and inferior maxillary nerves. Causes of the cavernous sinus syndrome include medially invasive craniopharyngioma, skull base invading nasopharyngeal tumors, saccular infraclinoid carotid artery aneurysms, traumatic carotid-cavernous fistula, cavernous sinus thrombophlebitis, and basal meningitis.

Gradenigo-Lannois Syndrome

Gradenigo (42) described the syndrome of acute otitis media, subacute ipsilateral pain in the eye and temporal region, and abducens nerve palsy in the preantibiotic era; other more common causes of this syndrome are tumors localized to the petrous apex, meningioma of the trigeminal cavity, sphenocavernous angle, neurinoma of the trigeminal nerve, and Gasserian ganglion tumor.

Paratrigeminal Syndrome

Raeder (43) described the association of a trigeminal nerve lesion and ipsilateral sympathetic involvement of the eye leading to frontal orbital pain along the ophthalmic nerve or its branches with meiosis, intact direct papillary light response, and absent pupillary dilatation upon installation of ophthalmic cocaine. The paratrigeminal area, the site of the causative lesions, is the area wedged between the trigeminal ganglion and vertical portion of the internal carotid artery as it passes up to the petrosal apex. The causative lesions include primary and metastatic tumors, aneurysm of the internal carotid artery, osteitis, and basilar meningitis.

Cerebellopontine Angle Syndrome

The cerebellopontine angle refers to the recess limited medially by the brainstem, anteriorly by the posterior wall of the petrous temporal bone, posteriorly by the middle cerebellar peduncle and the cerebellum, inferiorly by the cerebellar fossa of the occipital bone and the bundle of the glossopharyngeal, vagus, and accessory nerves, and superiorly by the tentorium cerebelli. The cerebellopontine cistern is traversed by the middle cerebellar and internal auditory branch of the vertebral artery, and the trigeminal, facial, and vestibulocochlear nerves. First described by Hennery and Koch (44), the cerebellopontine angle syndrome typically results from a compressive acoustic neuroma involving first the auditory, facial, and trigeminal nerves, then glossopharyngeal, vagus, and accessory nerves; and finally the brainstem, eventually blocking cerebrospinal fluid flow and causing intracranial hypertension. Cochlear signs include unilateral tinnitus, loss of auditory acuity, and eventual deafness, while vestibular involvement is suggested by vertigo with a sensation of rotation and horizontal rotatory nystagmus with the slow component directed to the affected side. Associated cranial nerve deficits depend upon the etiology of the cerebellopontine compression, with variable facial sensory loss and pain, hypoesthesia of the cornea, loss of the corneal reflex and of facial sensation along branches of the trigeminal nerve. Symptoms and signs of impending brainstem compression include cerebellar intention tremor, dysdiadochokinesis, hypotonia, strabismus due to abducens palsy, and involvement of the glossopharyngeal, vagal, and accessory nerves with palatal asymmetry, dysarthria, and dysphagia.

Acoustic neuromas are the most frequent tumors of the cerebellopontine angle, followed by meningioma, cerebellar hemangioma, glioma, cholesteatoma, and those of the fourth ventricle, including epidermoid cyst, tuberculoma, ependymoma, jugular glomus tumor, metastases, Hodgkin lymphoma, multiple myeloma, and non-neoplastic lesions such as basilar artery aneurysms and arachnoiditis.

Jugular Foramen Syndrome

Vernet (45) described the syndrome of glossopharygneal, vagus, and accessory nerve paralysis of the jugular foramen. Affected patients present with hoarseness, phonation, and swallowing difficulty with nasal regurgitation, and increased pharyngeal sections. Examination shows paralysis of the superior constrictor muscle of the pharynx manifested by distress at the end of swallowing and impairment of taste at the back of the tongue and hemianesthesia of the velum palatinum, pharynx, and larynx; and homolateral vocal cord, sternocleidomastoid, and trapezius muscle paralysis.

The causes of the jugular foramen syndrome include traumatic injury of the ear or neck; fracture of the petrous bone extending to the jugular foramen, nerve sheath tumors of the jugular foramen, metastases, chrondromas, acoustic neurinoma, invasive cancer of the pharynx and middle ear, and infectious processes due to arachnoiditis, osteitis, ear, nose, and throat abscess; and jugular vein phlebitis.

Once the glossopharygeal, vagus, and accessory nerves exit the jugular foramen they lie in the retrostyloid or posterior subparotid space limited anteriorly by the styloid process, posteriorly by the prevertebral aponeurosis, medially by the pharynx, and laterally by the sternocleidomastoid and diagastric muscles. The hypoglossal nerve exits the skull through its own canal and passes through the anterior condylar space, whereupon all of the aforementioned nerves are susceptible to base-of-the-brain lesions that produce a clinical presentation inseparable from the jugular foramen syndrome unless the hypoglossal nerve is involved, whereupon the disorder is termed the *anterior condyle syndrome.*

Selective paralysis of the accessory branch to the vagus nerve produces paralysis of one-half of the soft palate and one vocal cord termed *palatolaryngeal hemiplegia* manifested by a hoarse nasal voice. Involvement of both the accessory and spinal branch of the accessory nerve produces unilateral paralysis of the sternocleidomastoid and trapezius muscle in addition to paralysis of soft palate and one vocal cord, a variation of which leads to paralysis of the spinal part of the accessory nerve and the ipsilateral vocal cord without paralysis of the palate termed scapulolaryngeal hemiplegia.

A lesion anterior to the occipital condyle, situated in such a way that all the nerves passing through the jugular foramen and anterior condyle canal are affected, produces dysphonia; dysphagia; loss of taste along the posterior tongue; palatal, vocal cord, lingual, trapezius and sternocleidomastoid muscle paralysis. The possible causes of this syndrome include ear, skull base, parotid tumors, metastases, lymphoma, trauma, carotid artery aneurysms below the skull base, and jugular vein phlebitis. The syndrome of the subparotid space is caused by a parotid tumor that affects the four lower cranial and cervical sympathetic nerves leading to manifestations of the jugular foramen, anterior condyle, and Horner syndromes.

The syndrome of glossolaryngeal hemiplegia is manifested by ipsilateral lingual and vocal cord paralysis with variable involvement of the sternocleidomastoid and trapezius muscles and cervical sympathetic chain, and sparing the soft palate and pharynx. It is due to a causative lesion involving the glossopharyngeal and vagus nerve below the inferior ganglion that spares its pharyngeal branches, the most common causes of which are trauma and tumors of the skull base or parotid gland.

Unilateral paralysis of all 12 cranial nerves is caused by a tumor of the middle cranial fossa, rhinopharyngeal tumors that invade the skull base; ear, nose and throat tumors, and metastases of the base of the skull, as well as significant trauma and hematoma. Unilateral trigeminal neuralgia, oculomotor, trochlear and abducens ophthalmoplegia, and amaurosis due to involvement of the optic nerve proceeds with expansion, to involve the other cranial nerves in succession, known as *hemibase syndrome.*

REFERENCES

1. Goss CM. Gray's Anatomy of the Human Body. *The Peripheral Nervous System.* Lea and Febiger: Philadelphia, 1956; 977–1023
2. Taverner D. The localization of isolated cranial nerve lesions. *Handb Clin Neurol* 1978; 2:52–85.
3. Roger J, Bille J, Vigouroux RA. Multiple cranial nerve palsies. *Handb Clin Neurol.* 1978; 2:86–106.
4. Sachsenweger R. Clinical localisation of oculomotor disturbances. *Handb Clin Neurol* 1978; 2:286–357
5. Sumner D. Post-traumatic anosmia. *Brain* 1964; 87:107–120.
6. Haxel BR, Grant L, Mackay-Sim A. Olfactory dysfunction after head injury. *J Head Trauma Rehabil* 2008; 6:407–413.
7. Kennedy F. Retrobulbar neuritis as an exact diagnostic sign of certain tumors and abscesses in the frontal lobes. *Am J Med Sci* 1911; 142:355–368.
8. Beck RW, Cleary PA, Anderson MM, et al. A randomized, controlled trial of corticosteroids in the treatment of acute optic neuritis. *N Engl J Med* 1992; 326:581–588
9. Beck RW, Cleary PA, Trobe JD, et al. The effect of corticosteroids for acute optic neuritis on the subsequent development of multiple sclerosis. *N Engl J Med* 1993; 329:1764–1769.
10. Optic Neuritis Study Group. The five-year risk of multiple sclerosis after optic neuritis; experience of the Optic Neuritis Treatment Trial. *Neurology* 1997; 49:1404–1413.
11. Marignier R, Giraudon P, Vukusic S, et al. Anti-aquaporin-4 antibodies in Devic's neuromyelitis optica: therapeutic implications. *Ther Adv Neurol Disord* 2010; 3:311–321.
12. Horner F. Uber eine form von ptosis. *Klin Mbl.Augenheilk* 1869; 7:193-198.
13. Sanjay S, Huang P, Lavanya R. Herpes zoster ophthalmicus. *Curr Treat Options Neurol* 2011; 13:79–91.

14. Liesegang TJ. Herpes zoster ophthalmicus natural history, risk factors, clinical presentation, and morbidity. *Ophthalmology* 2008; 115:S3–12.

15. Fothergill J. Of a painful affection of the face. *Medical Observations and Enquiries* 1773; 5:129–142.

16. Yang M, Zhou M, He L, et al. Non-antiepileptic drugs for trigeminal neuralgia. *Cochrane Database Syst Rev* 2011; Jan 19:1CD004029.

17. Wiffen PJ, Derry S, Moore RA. Lamotrigine for acute and chronic pain. *Cochrane Database Syst Rev* 2011 Feb 16:2:CD006044.

18. Emril DR, Ho KY. Treatment of trigeminal neuralgia: role of radiofrequency ablation. *J Pain Res* 2010; 3:249–254.

19. Ramsey Hunt J. On herpetic inflammations of the geniculate ganglion. A new syndrome and its complications. *J Nerve Ment Dis* 1907; 34:73–96.

20. Bell Charles. On the nerves of the face, being a second paper on that subject. *Phil Trans* 1829; 111:317–330.

21. Valls-Sole J. Electrodiagnostic studies of the facial nerve in peripheral facial palsy and hemifacial spasm. *Muscle Nerve* 2007; 36:14–20.

22. Maroon JC. Hemifacial spasm. A vascular cause. *Arch Neurol* 1978; 35:481-483.

23. Nielsen VK. Pathophysiology of hemifacial spasm. 1. Ephaptic transmission and ectopic excitation. *Neurology* 1984; 34:418–426.

24. Nielson VK. Pathophysiology of hemifacial spasm. II. Lateral spread of the supraorbital nerve reflex. *Neurology* 1984; 34:427–431.

25. De Almeida JR, Khabori AI, Guyatt GH, et al. Combined corticosteroids and antiviral treatment for Bell palsy: a systematic review and meta-analysis. *JAMA* 2009; 302:985–993.

26. Gronseth GS, Paduga R. Evidence-based guideline update: steroids and antivirals for Bell palsy. Report of the Guideline Development Subcommittee of the American Academy of Neurology. *Neurology* 2012; 79:2209–2213.

27. Boroojerdi B, Ferbert A, Schwarz M, et al. Botulinum toxin treatment of synkinesia and hyperlacrimation after facial palsy. *J Neurol Neurosurg Psychiatry* 1998; 65:111–114.

28. Schreiber BE, Agrup C, Haskard DO, et al. Sudden sensorineural hearing loss. *Lancet* 2010; 375:1203–1211.

29. Saux A, Niango G, Charif M, et al. Susac's syndrome, a rare, potentially severe or lethal neurological disease. *J Neurol Sci* 2010; 297:71–73.

30. Weisenburg JM. Cerebello pontine tumor diagnosed for six years as tic doloreux. The symptoms of irritation of the ninth and twelfth cranial nerves. *JAMA* 1910; 59:1600–1604.

31. Schindler A, Ginocchio D, Peri A, et al. FEESST in the rehabilitation of dysphagia after partial laryngectomy. *Ann Otol Rhinol Laryngol* 2010; 119:71–76.

32. Tabaee A, Murry T, Axchommler A, et al. Flexible endoscopic evaluation of swallowing with sensory testing in patients with unilateral vocal fold immobility: incidence and pathophysiology of aspiration. *Laryngoscope* 2005; 115:565–569.

33. Doggett DL, Turkelson CM, Coates V. Recent developments in diagnosis and intervention for aspiration and dysphagia in stroke and other neuromuscular disorders. *Curr Atheroscler Rep* 2002; 4:311–318.

34. Phua SY, McGarvey LP, Ngu MC, et al. Patients with gastro-oesophageal reflux disease and cough have impaired larygopharyngeal mechanosensitivity. *Thorax* 2005; 60:488–491.

35. Aviv JE, Parides M, Fellowes J, et al. Endoscopic evaluation of swallowing as an alternative to 24-hour pH monitoring for diagnosis of extraesophageal reflux. *Ann Otol Rhinol Laryngol Suppl* 2000; 184:25–27.

36. Vonck K, De Herdt V, Boon P. Vagal nerve stimulation—a 15 year survey of an established treatment modality in epilepsy surgery. *Adv Tech Stand Neurosurg* 2009; 34:111–146.

37. Cecchini AP, Mea E, Tullo V, et al. Vagus nerve stimulation in drug-resistant daily chronic migraine with depression: preliminary data. *Neurol Sci* 2009; 30 (Suppl 1):S101–104.

38. Friedenberg SM, Zimprich T, Harper CM. The natural history of long thoracic and spinal accessory neuropathies. *Muscle Nerve* 2002; 25:535–539.

39. Sharkar K, Means KM. Accessory nerve conduction in neck dissection subjects. *Arch Phys Med Rehabil* 1990; 71:403–405.

40. Rochon-Duvigneaud. Quelques cas de paralysies de tous les nerfs orbitaires (ophtalmoplegie totale avec amaurose et anesthesia dans la domaine de o'ophtalmique) d'origine syphilique. *Arch Ophtal* 1896; 16:746–760.

41. Foix C. Syndrome de la paroi externe du sinus caverneux, ophtalmoplegie unilaterale a marche rapidement progressive. *Bull Soc Med Hop Paris* 1920; 44:1355–1361.

42. Gradenigo G. A special syndrome of endocranial otitic complications (paralyses of the motor oculi externus of otititc origin). *Ann Otol* 1904; 13:637.

43. Raeder JG. Paratrigeminal paralysis of ocular papillary sympathetic nerve. *Brain* 1924; 47:149.

44. Henneberg and Koch. Uber "central"neurofibromatose und die Geshwulste des Kleinhirnbrucken-winkels. *Arch Psychiat Nervenkr* 1902; 36:251–304.

45. Vernet M. Syndrome du trou dechire posterieur (paralysie des IX, X, XI). *Rev Neurol* 1918; 2:117–148.

CHAPTER 17

The Hypotonic Infant

Thornton B.A. Mason II, Darryl C. De Vivo

CLINICAL INSPECTION

Infantile hypotonia is suggested by the constellation of physical signs observed when a hypotonic or floppy infant is placed into a series of suspended postures. When placed supine with the arms lying flail to the side and the hips externally rotated in the frog-leg position gentle arm traction and elevation of the infant from the supine position causes the head to lag in retroflex at the neck (Figure 1). When supported in a seated position the hypotonic infant veers forward because of poor axial tone (Figure 2). With vertical suspension and the child held upright under the arms, the hypotonic infant will begin to slip through the examiner's hands. In prone position with the trunk supported, the affected infant slumps over the examiner's hand in an inverted U posture with the head and limbs limply hanging like a rag doll (Figure 3). When individual joints are passively moved by the examiner, there is decreased perceived resistance. The head of a hypotonic infant should be kept in midline during this evaluation of limb tone because turning it may inadvertently evoke a tonic neck reflex response promoting lateral tone asymmetry.

PATHOPHYSIOLOGY

Muscle tone is controlled in part by γ-motor neurons (MN) of the ventral horn of the spinal cord. Together with afferent muscle spindles and effector αMN, they form a feedback loop that adjusts resting muscle tone. When αMN and γMN are compromised, hypotonia and weakness can occur. Muscle tone is also regulated by upper motor neurons (UMN) and descending fibers of the corticospinal tracts

(CST), the final common pathway of voluntary movement. Experimental evidence supports the presence of areas of cortical inhibition, especially among them the supraorbital frontal lobe which, when stimulated, produces diffuse non-reciprocal inhibition of mono- and polysynaptic reflexes and muscle tone (1). The state of alertness is important when assessing tone since drowsiness may inadvertently be associated with decreased tone. Maturation of the central nervous system (CNS), in particular the CST, is also important since its development underlies normal passive muscle tone and postures at rest (2). A premature neonate has less tone than a full-term newborn because the CST do not fully myelinate until age two years. The status of the spinal cord MN is an important factor in primary CNS insults associated with central hypotonia in comparison to peripheral causes due to interruption of sequential connections of the peripheral processes of the αMN to skeletal muscle through the motor unit.

CAUSES OF INFANTILE HYPOTONIA

The differential diagnosis of infantile hypotonia is summarized in Table 1 along with age-appropriate investigations based on the specific clinical presentation. In general, it is helpful to separate conditions of the newborn period, defined as the first month of life, from those that occur later in the first year of life. While infantile spinal muscular atrophy (SMA) has onset in utero, the motor manifestations are usually delayed for two to three months after birth due to limited compensation of spinal cord MN. Severe hypotonia and weakness are accompanied by feeding difficulty, lingual fasciculation, and respiratory insufficiency. Skeletal muscle

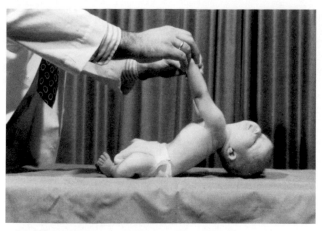

FIG. 1. Examination of the hypotonic infant. Gentle arm traction demonstrates a prominent head lag.

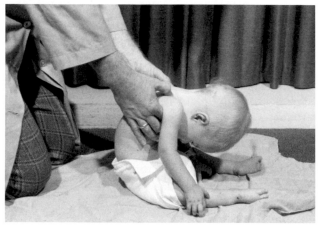

FIG. 2. In an upright seated position, there is decreased axial tone.

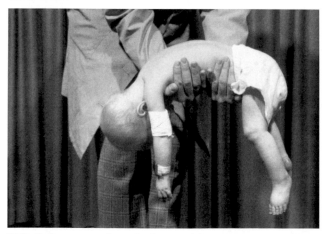

FIG. 3. Supported and elevated in a prone position, the floppy infant fails to right his head or to extend his extremities against gravity.

biopsy reveals hypertrophied fibers grouped among atrophic dying fibers. A family pedigree is indicative of autosomal recessive (AR) inheritance and mutation analysis confirms the diagnosis when it demonstrates a pathogenic mutation or deletion at the 5q13.2 locus in the telomeric copy of the *SMN* gene, known as *SMN1*; changes in the centromeric copy of SMN, termed *SMN2*, can favorably modify the phenotype. Death is nearly always caused by respiratory failure. Infants with congenital myotonic dystrophy or dystrophica mytonica 1 (DM1) also present at birth with severe weakness, often requiring ventilator and nutritional support for several weeks. Affected infants have prominent facial diplegia including tenting of the upper lip and a hatchet face when older. The family pedigree demonstrates autosomal dominant (AD) inheritance, and molecular genetic testing shows heterozygous trinucleotide CTG repeat expansion at the 19q13.32 locus of the dystrophia myotonica protein kinase gene, *DMPK*. After a prolonged stay in the nursery, affected infants may be well enough to go home but generally remain symptomatic. Neonatal myasthenia gravis (MG) affects newborn infants due to transplacental transfer of acetylcholine receptor (AChR) antibodies from a symptomatic mother. Clinical improvement of strength and muscle tone parallels clearance of maternally derived antibodies over several weeks. Radioimmunoassay of AChR antibodies in placental and newborn blood confirms the disorder. Small repeated doses of the acetyl-cholinesterase inhibitor neostigmine temporarily improves feeding.

Clues to the presence of CNS-related hypotonia may lie in the history of asphyxia at birth, demonstrated chromosomal abnormalities, discrete metabolic disturbances, and seizures. Concomitant abnormalities in electroencephalography (EEG) even in the absence of clinical seizures, support a central cause of hypotonia. Such patients will manifest normal or brisk deep tendon reflexes (DTR) often in association with Babinski signs and clonus, in comparison to those with absent DTR, without frank upper motor neuron (UMN) signs, in association with true limb weakness. The occurrence of asphyxia at birth is especially relevant when Apgar scores are low, there is documented resuscitation and respiratory support immediately after birth, and neurological examination shows signs of CNS involvement including decreased alertness and seizures. Over weeks to months, such infants may shows signs of spastic quadriparesis, while those remaining hypotonic for one or two years afterward may manifest a cerebellar syndrome with ataxia and incoordination (3). Fatally asphyxiated neonates evidence prominent ischemic necrosis of anterior spinal cord gray matter in a radially-oriented watershed distribution at postmortem examination due to hypoperfusion along the single anterior spinal artery and the paired dorsal spinal arteries (4, 5).

Table 1. Etiology of Infantile Hypotonia by Age at Onset
(Adapted from reference 48)

Disorders	PNS Disorders	CNS Disorders
Neonatal	Infantile SMA Congenital myopathies: multicore, nemaline, myotubular, fibertype disproportion CMD: Fukuyama, occidental, merosin deficient Metabolic myopathies: Pompe, mtDNA depletion, COX, glycogenosis type IV and V Subacute neuropathy: neonatal ADL	Perinatal brain injury: ischemic, hemorrhagic Chromosomal disorders Congenital hypothyroidism Genetic syndromes: PWS, Lowe, SLOS, ZS, FD In utero exposures and infection Failure to thrive syndromes Spinal cord injury or malformation: dysraphism, sacral agenesis, caudal regression
Age 1–6 months or Older	Infantile SMA Poliomyelitis Infantile botulism Acute periphral neuropathies: GBS, Diphtheria, tick-bite paralysis Connective tissue disorders: Ehlers-Danlos, Marfan Subacute and chronic neuropathy: MLD, Globoid cell, ALD, neuroaxonal dystrophy Congenital myasthenic syndromes	Biotinidase deficiency Metabolic cerebral degenerations Intoxication Spinal trauma Metabolic disorders: organic acidemia, RTA, Endocrine disorders: hypothyroidism Electrolyte disturbances: hypocalcium

Neurogenetic factors such as dysmorphic features may offer further clues to the etiology of infantile hypotonia and guide the investigation toward possible chromosomal disorders. Profound hypotonia at birth and in infancy are seen in isochromosome 12p mosaicism that underlies the Pallister mosaic aneuploidy syndrome, the clinical findings of which include coarse facies, prominent forehead, hypertelorism, sparse scalp hair, epicanthal folds, flat nasal bridge, and high-arched palate. Visualization by a Wood-lamp shows generalized pigmentary dysplasia (6). Terminal deletion of chromosome 2q is associated with infantile hypotonia, developmental delay, and craniofacial abnormalities including frontal bossing and micrognathia (7).

The inverted duplication 8p syndrome manifests hypotonia, feeding difficulty, and severe developmental delay, with associated dysmorphic features of posteriorly low-set and rotated ears, high-arched palate, forehead prominence, large mouth, and thin upper lip (8). The diagnosis of Gillespie syndrome is suggested by hypotonia in association with partial aniridia, fixed dilated pupils, mental retardation, and cerebellar involvement caused by a heterozygous mutation in the PAX6 gene on chromosome 11p13 (9). Trisomy 21 is associated with a large variety of phenotypes that vary in prevalence and expression,

including cardiac anomalies, Brushfield spots, and duodenal stenosis with neonatal hypotonia and mental retardation present in close to 100% of affected infants with Down syndrome (10). The Down syndrome chromosome region 1 (DCR1) is located on sub-band q22.2 of chromosome 21 and contains genes that result in specific trisomy 21 phenotypes, including hypotonia.

Two recently described genes in the DCR1 regions encode inwardly rectifying potassium (Kir) channels that are important regulators of resting membrane potential and cell excitability and also appear to regulate muscle tone (11). Hypothyroidism is a contributing cause of hypotonia, especially in Down syndrome wherein congenital onset presents with hypotonia in association with icterus, retardation of skeletal maturation and growth in length, abdominal distention, lingual hypertrophy, skin mottling, and macrocephaly (12). Infants with Down syndrome have a 35-fold or greater risk for primary hypothyroidism than infants in the general population. Accordingly, the American Academy of Pediatrics Committee on Genetics recommends thyroid screening tests at 4 to 6 months, 12 months, and annually in patients with Down syndrome because of the increased risk for acquired hypothyroidism (13).

Prader-Willi syndrome (PWS) is an AD disorder characterized by marked neonatal hypotonia, mental retardation, hyperphagia, and obesity after the first year of life but before age six years. The characteristic facial features include almond shaped eyes, narrow bifrontal diameter, small mouth with thin upper lip, and down-turned corners of the mouth. The affected hypogonadotrophic hypogonadal child manifests a micropenis, hypoplastic scrotum, and cryptorchidism (14, 15) as well as short stature and small hands and feet. The disorder results from deletion of the paternal copies of the imprinted *SNRPN* gene at the 15q11.2 locus; alternatively, there may be causative maternal uniparental disomy in which two different, apparently intact, maternal chromosomes are present, termed heterodisomy and absence of paternal genes as in otherwise typical PWS cytogenetics. A DNA methylation based test at the PW71 locus detects such pathogenic conditions (16). Conventional chromosome analysis, fluorescence in situ hybridization, and DNA polymorphism studies may distinguish the specific mutation in a given affected patient.

High-resolution chromosome analysis is not recommended for diagnosis of PWS because of the high rates of false-positive and false-negative results (16). Other genetic syndromes to consider in the setting of infantile hypotonia include Lowe oculocerebral syndrome (OCRL) due to X-linked mutation at the Xq25-q26 locus in the *OCRL1* gene with aminoaciduria, hydro-ophthalmia, cataracts, and mental retardation; and three other AR disorders: Smith-Lemli-Opitz syndrome (SLOS), characterized clinically by multiple congenital malformations and mental retardation due to mutation at the 11q13.4 locus in the *DHCR7* gene encoding sterol delta-7 reductase; the peroxisomal biogenesis disorder Zellweger syndrome (ZS) characterized clinically by craniofacial abnormalities and liver dysfunction due to mutation in one of several *PEX* genes; and Riley-Day syndrome of familial dysautonomia (FD), characterized clinically by profound autonomic dysfunction, labile blood pressure, hyperhidrosis, cyclic vomiting, skin blotching, and defective lacrimation with a corresponding mutation at the 9q31.3 locus of the *IKFKAP* gene.

Hereditary neurometabolic disorders (HNMD) should be considered in the differential diagnosis of infantile hypotonia because many such disorders can be accurately diagnosed and effectively treated. One such HNMD is biotinidase deficiency, which results in severe hypotonia, intractable seizures, and lactic acidosis (17, 18). It presents in infants age six months to one year of age, rarely several weeks after birth, with profound hypotonia, ataxia, visual and auditory impairment, developmental delay, alopecia, eczematous skin rash, and metabolic coma. Associated keto-lactic acidosis and organic acidemia is due to decreased activity of one of three biotin-dependent enzymes, pyruvate carboxylase, proprionyl CoA carboxylase, and β-methylcrotonyl CoA carboxylase. Serum biotinidase activity is assayed by quantitative calorimetric testing of blood-soaked filter paper samples as part of a newborn nursery screen. Undiagnosed and therefore untreated, it can be fatal, however the administration of 10 to 20 mg/day of biotin dramatically stops anticonvulsant-unresponsive seizures in a few days. Other features also resolve quickly, especially if biotin therapy is instituted promptly.

Marked hypotonia is also seen in rare pediatric disorders due to individual or combined deficiencies of the monoamine oxidase (MOA) neurotransmitters serotonin (SE), dopamine (DA), and norepinephrine (NE), due to deficiency of aromatic L-amino acid decarboxylase, succinic semialdehyde dehydrogenase deficiency, and tyrosine hydroxylase deficiency (19, 20). Diurnal fluctuation in axial hypotonia provides diagnostic support for tyrosine hydroxylase deficiency. In a recent review of patients with aromatic L-amino acid decarboxylase deficiency, the most common neonatal findings were hypotonia, feeding difficulties, and autonomic dysfunction, all affected children of which developed oculogyric crises in the first months of life (21). Reliable quantification of cerebrospinal fluid (CSF) biogenic amines establishes the diagnosis, and treatment options include the use of vitamin B6, dopamine agonists, and MAO inhibitors

Ehlers-Danlos syndrome is a heritable connective tissue disorder and an important cause of infant hypotonia. It is characterized by excessively stretchable, fragile, and easily bruised skin, and hyperextensible joints. The disease is transmitted with AD inheritance. The clinical phenotype of Marfan syndrome, another AD disorder, includes long thin extremities, ectopia lentis, and aortic aneurysm. The mucopolysaccharidoses (MPS) are rare lysosomal storage disorders of cartilage and bone due to accumulation of dermatan sulfate, heparan sulfate, and keratan sulfate. Affected children have variable skeletal system, eye, liver, spleen, and CNS disease. An MPS should be suspected when coarse facial features, corneal opacities, developmental delay, kyphosis, growth failure, and stiff joints occur. Urinalysis screening and skin fibroblast or lymphocyte testing are useful methods of laboratory diagnosis.

The pregnancy, birth, and family history can provide important clues to the cause of infant hypotonia. Parental consanguinity increases the likelihood of AR inherited disorders such as Pompe disease and congenital muscular dystrophy (CMD). An affected mother may be minimally symptomatic, and the diagnosis may emerge only after the birth of a severely affected child. Documented disturbance in the quality, timing of fetal movements its counts prompted further investigation of prenatal or neonatal onset of nemaline myopathy in a clinically suspected birth (22). Whereas infantile SMA may be accompanied by a decrease in brisk fetal movements during pregnancy due to the progressive loss of MN function, a paucity of movements throughout pregnancy should prompt consideration

TABLE 2. Laboratory Evaluation of Infantile Hypotonia

NCS	Peripheral neuropathies
	Brachial plexus injuries
Tetanic nerve stimulation	Botulism
	Neonatal MG
	Congenital myasthenic syndromes
EMG	Congenital myopathies
	Myotonic dystrophy
	SMA
	Metabolic myopathies
Skeletal muscle biopsy	Congenital myopathies
	Congenital muscular dystrophy
	Metabolic myopathies
Microbiology	Viral: Polio and other enteroviruses, Encephalitis
	Bacterial: Botulism, diphtheria; meningitis and sepsis
Serum antibody titers	Intrauterine infection: Toxoplasma, Rubella, CMV, Herpes
	Neonatal myasthenia gravis: AChR
Chromosomal studies	Down syndrome
	PWS
	Other dysmorphic syndromes
Serum chemistries	Endocrinopathies: calcium levels, thyroid homone levels
	Congenital myopathies, muscular dystrophy: serum CK
	Metabolic disorders: organic and amino acids, lactate, and pyruvate levels: ABG
	Neonatal ADL: saturated VLCFA
	Smith-Lemli-Opitz syndrome: choleserol
Cranial neuroimaging	Asphyxia
	Hemorrhage
	Dysgenetic syndromes, especially midline facial defects
	CMD (Fukuyama and merosin-negative)
	Leukodystrophies

of CMD or arthrogryposis. In utero toxin exposure may be revealed in the pregnancy history and herald dysmorphism and hypotonia, common examples of which include fetal exposure to alcohol, heroin, phenytoin, and trimethadione. Drugs administered to the mother during labor and delivery affect the newborn most dramatically at the time of birth with gradual improvement afterward. Recovery may be hastened by the administration of the opioid antagonist naloxone, or the benzodiazepine antagonist, flumazenil. Concomitant asphyxia, low Apgar scores and the need for delivery room resuscitation suggest prior sepsis or cerebral hemorrhage as the cause of central hypotonia. Appropriate cultures, acute and convalescent Toxoplasmosis, Rubella, Cytomegalovirus, and Herpes (TORCH) titers, cranial ultrasound imaging, and toxicology screens may point to a specific etiology of hypotonia.

The pattern of clinical involvement is also important. Asymmetrically decreased leg tone and weakness, along with fever, meningeal signs, CSF pleocytosis, and elevated protein content suggests poliomyelitis and other enteroviral infections. Viral cultures and polymerase chain reaction (PCR) may be helpful in identifying the responsible organism.

Cervical spine trauma and spinal cord injury can lead to sudden unexplained hypotonia and quadriparesis. Cranial nerve function remains intact. Electromyography (EMG) at the time of presentation may be normal and only later demonstrates denervation changes at affected spinal root segments. Immediate cervical spine immobilization with a hard collar is mandatory before imaging studies in clinically suspected cases. Skeletal survey may demonstrate other acute or healing fractures (23). Focal neonatal hypotonia may result from trauma as occurs with peripartum brachial plexus injury resulting in flaccidity of one arm, often in association with dystocia and fetal macrosomia. The upper brachial plexopathy, Erb-Duchenne paralysis may be associated with fracture of the clavicle or ipsilateral diaphragm paralysis, while infantile lower brachial plexopathy or Klumpke paralysis, is often accompanied by ipsilateral Horner syndrome. Inherited developmental anomalies may lead to neonatal hypotonia with selective involvement of the legs as may occur in spinal dysraphism, caudal regression syndrome, and sacral agenesis.

Guillain-Barré syndrome (GBS) is an important cause of acute ascending symmetric weakness, hypotonia, and areflexia of infancy (24). It leads to progressive proximal motor weakness of the legs, later followed by involvement of the arms, trunk, and face. Areflexia is common although trace reflexes of the biceps and knee jerk may be present. Elevation of the CSF protein content with few or no cells, termed *albuminocytologic dissociation*, should be documented over several weeks (25). Electrophysiological studies reveal reduced compound muscle action potential (CMAP) amplitudes to 50% of normal with prolongation of F-wave latencies even before the decrease in motor nerve conduction velocities (NCV), which are maximal by the third week of illness. Denervation potentials on needle EMG occur late in the course and are associated with a poor outcome (26). Treatment involves supportive care and careful monitoring of cardiac and respiratory status, and consideration of plasmapheresis and/or intravenous immunoglobulin (IVIg) therapy. Diphtheria, caused by *Corynebacterium diphtheria*, produces a generalized demyelinating polyneuropathy clinically similar to GBS. A protein exotoxin secreted by the organism inhibits myelin synthesis activates cytotoxic mechanisms. Treatment consists of anti-toxin administration and antimicrobial therapy. Tick paralysis is an acute illness similar to GBS that presents in the spring and summer months with hypotonia caused by tick attachment that leads to the secretion of neurotoxinladen saliva; prompt removal of the tick is rapidly curative (27). Subacute and chronic diffuse neuropathies that cause hypotonia include metachromatic leukodystrophy (MLD), globoid cell leukodystrophy or Krabbe disease, neonatal adrenoleukodystrophy (ALD), and infantile neuroaxonal dystrophy. Clues to their diagnosis may include a known family history, UMN signs, CSF protein elevation, and slow nerve NCV. Metachromatic leukodystrophy, globoid cell leukodystrophy, and adrenoleukodystrophy all demonstrate white matter abnormalities on cranial magnetic resonance imaging (MRI). In neonatal adrenoleukodystrophy, moderate to severe hypotonia hepatomegaly and retinitis pigmentosa are noted at birth or shortly thereafter. Increased plasma levels of very-long-chain fatty acids are found, often with raised phytanic acid and bile fluid trihydrocoprostanic acid levels, consistent with a deficiency of multiple peroxisomal enzymes (28). Infantile neuroaxonal dystrophy is an AR disease, with marked generalized hypotonia in late infancy. There is an overall regression of motor and language milestones, which may be accompanied by bilateral pyramidal signs, esotropia, and pendular nystagmus. Electroencephalography (EEG) demonstrates an admixture of high-amplitude 18- to 20-Hz beta activity. Cranial MRI, electrophysiology studies, and serum amino acid screens are generally all normal (29). The diagnosis can be ascertained on skin and conjunctival biopsy, where axonal spheroids are found in unmyelinated nerve fibers near

termination sites on skin appendages or dermal blood vessels. Electron microscopy (EM) reveals tuberomembranous and tuberocisternal profiles (29, 30). The accumulation of this material in the axon terminal suggests impaired axonal transport in infantile neuroaxonal dystrophy (30).

The causes of acute descending weakness may be due to a disorder of the neuromuscular junction. Weakness and hypotonia due to botulism develop in a previously healthy infant age two to six months, although cases have been described in the first two weeks of life (31, 32). The weakness is caused by ingestion of *Clostridium (C.) botulinum* spores which germinate in the infant gut and elaborate low levels of exotoxin. The toxin cleaves synaptobrevin, a membrane component of small synaptic vesicles, and impairs presynaptic axonal release of ACh, thereby producing weakness (33). Electrophysiological studies show decreased miniature end-plate potentials due to a decrease in quantal release of ACh upon nerve terminal depolarization (34). Clinical weakness typically begins with multiple cranial nerve palsies, leading to bilateral ptosis and dilated pupils with diminished light response. Poor feeding is due to decreased suck ability and pooling of secretions in the pharynx. The weakness descends to the trunk and limbs; bowel sounds are hypoactive, and constipation is common. Deterioration can be rapid and lead to progressive respiratory compromise requiring ventilator support (35). The most specific single electrophysiological test for botulism is an incremental response on repetitive motor nerve stimulation at 20 to 50 Hz. Concentric-needle EMG shows short-duration low-amplitude motor unit potentials (MUP) (34). Fecal material should be sent for culture of *C. botulinum* and for exotoxin identification. Environmental cultures, including soil and dirt samples from the home, honey, or other products that may have been fed to the infant, are sometimes positive, suggesting the specific source of infection. Most infant botulism in the United States is caused by group I organisms that elaborate toxin types A and B. Treatment of infantile botulism is supportive, but prompt treatment with Botulism Immune Globulin Intravenous (human) (BIG-IV) may reduce the length of hospital stay (31). Attention should be paid to avoiding any medications that might exacerbate the neuromuscular transmission deficit, in particular aminoglycoside antibiotics, which are sometimes initiated empirically at presentation for possible sepsis (32). Autonomic nervous system (ANS) dysfunction, especially with regard to cardiovascular responses, occurs in some infants with severe botulism and may persist beyond objective motor deficits (33). Full recovery is expected but may require several weeks to months. The congenital myasthenic syndromes are a heterogeneous group of rare conditions caused by a variety of genetic defects affecting neuromuscular transmission (36). Unlike neonatal and juvenile myasthenia gravis, they are not antibody mediated. Affected children manifest weakness and abnormal fatigability on exertion in the first two years of life and sometimes at birth. Neither plasma exchange nor immune suppression offer a demonstrable benefit, but some patients may respond favorably to cholinesterase inhibitors, quinidine, or 3, 4-diaminopyridine.

Primary muscle disease is an important cause of infantile hypotonia. The congenital myopathies are clinically and morphologically distinctive on skeletal muscle biopsy. They include multicore and central core disease, nemaline myopathy, myotubular or centronuclear myopathy, and congenital fiber type disproportion of small type I and large type II myofibers (37) each of which presents with true muscle weakness, feeding difficulty, decreased tendon reflexes, and respiratory failure, often in association with mental retardation, dysmorphic physical features, scoliosis, and congenital hip dislocation.

By comparison, CMD shows primary myopathic changes in a skeletal muscle biopsy without distinctive histochemical or ultrastructural features. Infants with CMD are symptomatic from birth or the first few months of life. They manifest hypotonia, delayed motor milestones, early and severe contractures, and joint deformity. Serum creatine kinase (CK) is up to 30 times normal in early disease stages and then decreases rapidly. The Fukuyama form of CMD caused by mutations in the gene encoding fukutin is characterized by severe mental retardation in all cases and seizures in about half. MRI reveals cerebral and cerebellar polymicrogyria reflecting a neuronal migration defect. Although affected children never walk, they may live into adulthood (38, 39). An occidental type of CMD occurs in infants from Western countries with clinical skeletal muscle involvement alone. A subset of both types has a specific absence of merosin, the α2 chain of laminin-2, by immunocytochemistry and immunoblot (40, 41). Fukuyama CMD shares a common disease mechanism of hypoglycosylation of α-dystroglycan with two other CMD, Walker-Warburg syndrome and muscle-eye-brain disease. The latter disorders due to mutations in the *POMT1* and *POMGnT* genes, respectively; further similarities include neuronal migration defects and ocular abnormalities (42).

Metabolic myopathies frequently cause myotonia and weakness. Pompe disease or glycogen storage disease (GSD) type II, is an AR metabolic myopathy due to deficiency of the enzyme acid maltase. Affected infants are normal at birth but soon develop generalized hypotonia, weakness, macroglossia, and hepatomegaly. Electrocardiogram abnormalities include giant QRS complexes, short PR interval, and ventricular hypertrophy. Echocardiography reveals concentric hypertrophic cardiomyopathy. Electromyography shows evidence of a generalized myopathy with occasional positive sharp wave activity, fibrillation potentials, bizarre repetitive discharges, and myotonic discharges in the absence of clinically detectable myotonia (43, 44). Muscle biopsy shows vacuolar myopathy that stains positively with the periodic acid-Schiff technique. Diastase digestion of fresh frozen tissue sections removes most vacuolar material, consistent with the presence of glycogen. EM shows glycogen sequestered into membrane-bound autophagic vacuoles (43, 44). Other metabolic myopathies that present with infantile hypotonia include the mitochondrial DNA depletion syndrome, cytochrome c oxidase (COX) deficiency, glycogenosis type IV or debrancher enzyme deficiency, and glycogenosis type V or myophosphorylase deficiency. Lactic acidosis is a frequent associated finding in mitochondrial DNA depletion syndrome and COX deficiency.

The possibility of an exogenous toxin should be considered in cases of acute and recurrent hypotonia. Although routine urine toxicology screens commonly detect drugs, one should remain alert to the continued possibility of a toxic substance when the initial screen is reported to be negative. In a report of Munchausen syndrome, chronic ipecac or emetine poisoning in infancy resulted in hypotonia, poor suck, and respiratory insufficiency (45). Carbamate and organophosphate poisoning results in meiosis, flaccid muscle tone; fasciculation; dyspnea; and stupor. Atropine sulfate in doses of 0.05 mg/kg repeated at regular intervals dramatically improves cholinergic crisis symptoms, including a depressed level of consciousness (46). Ingestion of ethylene glycol produces vomiting, irritability, acidosis, and hypotonia suggestive of a metabolic disorder. Organic acid analysis reveals glycolic acid and a positive anion gap, and urinalysis shows hematuria and calcium oxalate crystals (47).

Finally, after excluding all other etiologies, a benign condition may be the cause of infant hypotonia. Essential hypotonia is applied to otherwise healthy infants with unexplained hypotonia, normal strength and tendon reflexes, and normal physical characteristics. The presence of an older sibling with infantile hypotonia as an isolated finding and normal tone later in childhood is supportive.

ACKNOWLEDGMENT
Funding was provided by The Colleen Giblin Foundation.

REFERENCES

1. Sauerland EK, Knauss T, Nakamura Y, et al. Inhibition of monosynaptic and polysynaptic reflexes and muscle tone by electrical stimulation of the cerebral cortex. *Exp Neurol* 1967; 17:159–171.

2. Sarnat HB. Do the corticospinal and corticobulbar tracts mediate functions in the human newborn? *Can J Neurol Sci* 1989; 16:157–160.

3. Lesny IA. Follow-up study of hypotonic forms of cerebral palsy. *Brain Dev* 1979; 1:87–90.

4. Clancy RR, Sladky JY, Rorke LB. Hypoxic-ischemic spinal cord injury following perinatal asphyxia. *Ann Neurol* 1989; 25:185–189.

5. Rousseau S, Metral S, Lacroix C, et al. Anterior spinal artery syndrome mimicking infantile spinal muscular atrophy. *Am J Perinatol* 1993; 10:316–318.

6. Reynolds JF, Daniel A, Kelly TE. Isochromosome 12p mosaicism (Pallister mosaic aneuploidy or Pallister-Killian syndrome): report of 11 cases. *Am J Med Genet* 1987; 27:257–274.

7. Gorski JL, Cox BA, Kyine M, et al. Terminal deletion of the long arm of chromosome 2 in a mildly dysmorphic hypotonic infant with karyotype 46,XY,del(2)(q37). *Am J Med Genet* 1989; 32:350–352.

8. Feldman GL, Weiss L, Phelan MC, et al. Inverted duplication of 8p: ten new patients and review of the literature. *Am J Med Genet* 1993; 47:482–486.

9. Nelson J, Flaherty M, Grattan-Smith P. Gillespie syndrome: a report of two further cases. *Am J Med Genet* 1997; 71:134–138.

10. Kronenberg JR, Chen XN, Schipper R, et al. Down syndrome phenotypes: the consequences of chromosomal imbalance. *Proc Natl Acad Sci USA* 1994; 91:4997–5001.

11. Gosset P, Ghezala GA, Korn P, et al. A new inward rectifier potassium channel gene (KCNJ15) localized on chromosome 21 in the Down syndrome chromosome region 1 (DCR1). *Genomics* 1997; 44:237–241.

12. Virtanen M. Manifestations of congenital hypothyroidism during the 1st week of life. *Eur J Pediatr* 1988; 147:270–274.

13. Roberts HE, Moore CA, Fernhoff PM, et al. Population study of congenital hypothyroidism and associated birth defects, Atlanta, 1979–1992. *Am J Med Genet* 1997; 71:29–32.

14. Greenberg F, Elder FF, Ledbetter DH. Neonatal diagnosis of Prader-Willi syndrome and its implications. *Am J Med Genet* 1987; 28:845–856.

15. Holm VA, Cassidy SB, Butler MG, et al. Prader-Willi syndrome: consensus diagnostic criteria. *Pediatrics* 1993; 91:398–402.

16. Gillessen-Kaesbach G, Gross S, Kaya-Westerloh S, et al. DNA methylation based testing of 450 patients suspected of having Prader-Willi syndrome. *J Med Genet* 1995; 32:88–92.

17. Wolf B, Heard GS, Weissbecker KA, et al. Biotinidase deficiency: initial clinical features and rapid diagnosis. *Ann Neurol* 1985; 18:614–617.

18. Collins JE, Nicholson NS, Dalton N, et al. Biotinidase deficiency: early neurological presentation. *Dev Med Child Neurol* 1994; 36:268–270.

19. De Vivo DC, Johnston MV. Forward to supplement on pediatric neurotransmitter diseases. *Ann Neurol* 2003; 54 Suppl 6:S1–2.

20. Doummar D, Clot F, Vidailhet M, et al. Infantile hypokinetic-hypotonic syndrome due to two novel mutations of the tyrosine hydroxylase gene. *Mov Disord* 2009; 24: 943–945.

21. Pons, R, Ford B, Chiriboga CA, et al. Aromatic L-amino acid decarboxylase deficiency: clinical features, treatment, and prognosis. *Neurology* 2004; 62:1058–1065.

22. Kuwata T, Matsubara S, Ohkusa T, et al. Decreased fetal movement prompts investigation of prenatal/neonatal nemaline myopathy: the possible merit of fetal movement count. *J Obstet Gynaecol Res* 2011; 37:921–925.

23. Thomas NH, Robinson L, Evans A, et al. The floppy infant: a new manifestation of nonaccidental injury. *Pediatr Neurosurg* 1995; 23:188–191.

24. al-Qudah AA, Shahar E, Logan WJ, et al. Neonatal Guillain-Barré syndrome. *Pediatr Neurol* 1988; 4:255–256.

25. NINCDS ad hoc Guillain-Barré syndrome committee. Criteria for diagnosis of Guillain-Barré syndrome. *Ann Neurol* 1978; 3:565–566.

26. Cornblath DR. Electrophysiology in Guillain-Barré syndrome. *Ann Neurol* 1990; 27[Suppl]:S17–20.

27. Dworkin MS, Shoemaker PC, Anderson DE. Tick paralysis: 33 human cases in Washington State, 1946-1996. *Clin Infectious Dis* 1999; 19:1435–1439.

28. Aubourg P, Scotto J, Rocchiccioli F, et al. Neonatal adrenoleukodystrophy. *J Neurol Neurosurg Psychiatry* 1986; 49:77–86.

29. Ozmen M, Caliskan M, Goebel HH, et al. Infantile neuroaxonal dystrophy: diagnosis by skin biopsy. *Brain Dev* 1991; 13:256–259.

30. Kimura S. Terminal axon pathology in infantile neuroaxonal dystrophy. *Pediatr Neurol* 1991;7:116–120.

31. Infant botulism. New York City, 2001–2002. *MMWR Morb Mort Wkly Rep* 2003; 52:21–24.

32. Hurst DL, Marsh WW. Early severe infantile botulism. *J Pediatr* 1993;122:909–911.

33. Patural P, Goffaux P, Paricio C, et al. Infant botulism intoxication and autonomic nervous system dysfunction. *Anaerobe* 2009; 15:197–200.

34. Cornblath DR, Sladky JT, Sumner AJ. Clinical electrophysiology of infantile botulism. *Muscle Nerve* 1983; 6:448–452.

35. Smith GE, Hinde F, Westmoreland D, et al. Infantile botulism. *Arch Dis Child* 1989; 64:871–872.

36. Engel AG. Congenital myasthenic syndromes. *Handb Clin Neurol* 2008; 91:285–331.

37. Goebel HH. Congenital myopathies. *Acta Paediatr Jpn* 1991; 33:247–255.

38. Toda T, Segawa M, Nomura Y, et al. Localization of a gene for Fukuyama type congenital muscular dystrophy to chromosome 9q31-33. *Nat Genet* 1993; 5;283–286.

39. Kobayashi K, Nakahori Y, Miyake M, et al. An ancient retrotransposal insertion causes Fukuyama-type congenital muscular dystrophy. *Nature* 1998; 394:388–392.

40. Tome FMS, Evangelista T, Leclerc A, et al. Congenital muscular dystrophy with merosin deficiency. *CR Acad Sci III* 1994; 317:351–357.

41. Helbling-Leclerc A, Zhang X, Topaloglu H, et al. Mutations in the laminin a2-chain gene (LAMA2) cause merosin-deficient congenital muscular dystrophy. *Nat Genet* 1995; 11:216–218.

42. Vervoort VS, Holden KR, Ukadike KC, et al. POMGnT1 gene alterations in a family with neurological abnormalities. *Ann Neurol* 2004; 56:143–148.

43. Tsao CY, Boesel CP, Wright FS. A hypotonic infant with complete deficiencies of acid maltase and debrancher enzyme. *J Child Neurol* 1994; 9:90–91.

44. Van den Hout HMP, Hp W, van Diggelen OP, et al. The natural course of infantile Pompe's disease: 20 original cases compared with 133 cases from the literature. *Pediatrics* 2003; 112:332–340.

45. Berkner P, Kastner T, Skolnick L. Chronic ipecac poisoning in infancy: a case report. *Pediatrics* 1988; 82:384–386.

46. Sofer S, Tal A, Shahak E. Carbamate and organophosphate poisoning in early childhood. *Pediatr Emerg Care* 1989; 5:222–225.

47. Woolf AD, Wynshaw-Boris A, Rinaldo P, Levy HL. Intentional infantile ethylene glycol poisoning presenting as an inherited metabolic disorder. *J Pediatr* 1992; 120:421–424.

48. Mason TBS, De Vivo DC. The floppy infant syndrome. In: Rowland LP, ed. *Merritt's textbook of neurology*, 10th Ed. Baltimore: Williams & Wilkins, 2000.

CHAPTER 18

Inflammatory Myopathies

Donald S. Younger, Marinos C. Dalakas

Inflammatory myopathy (IM) comprises three major and distinct subsets including polymyositis (PM), dermatomyositis (DM), sporadic and hereditary inclusion body myositis (sIBM and hIBM); and the related disorder necrotizing autoimmune myopathy (NAM), which is considered in greater detail elsewhere (1–3). Although the presence of moderate to severe muscle weakness and endomysial inflammation are common features in all these conditions, respectively unique clinical, immunopathologic, and histologic criteria along with different prognosis and response to therapies characterize each subset. This chapter reviews the main clinical and histologic features of these diseases, their association with autoimmune conditions or viruses, and the underlying immunopathology. It also provides a practical approach to immunotherapeutic interventions.

CLINICAL DISORDERS

Polymyositis

Although first recorded by Wagner in 1863 (4), and named in the quarter century between 1954 and 1975, the distinctive clinical, electromyogaphic, serum muscle enzyme features, and histopathological aspects of PM and DM were described by Eaton (5), Walton and Adams (6), Rowland (7), Pearson and Rose (8), Rose and Walton (9), and Bohan and Peter (10), distinguishing it from progressive muscular dystrophy, and establishing the association with collagen vascular disorders.

The actual onset of PM cannot be easily determined. Unlike in DM, in which the rash secures early recognition, patients with PM do not have unique heralding clinical features. Affected patients present with subacute proximal muscle weakness and myalgia that develops subacutely, usually over weeks to months, and progresses steadily, without evidence of a rash, extraocular or facial muscle involvement, or history of similarly affected family member.

PM can be viewed as a syndrome of diverse etiology that occurs separately or in association with systemic autoimmune and systemic collagen vascular disorders, and certain parasitic, viral, retroviral, and bacterial infections. There may be a causal relation to concomitant toxic conditions and myotoxic drugs causing myopathic symptoms such as myalgia, often with transient or sustained elevation of serum creatine kinase (CK) levels that typically improves with discontinuation of the offending agent but does not lead to frank polymyositis.

Examples of drug-induced, typically non-IM, categorized under the rubric toxic myopathies (1, 11) include NAM and rhabdomyolysis due to statins, fibrates, ε-aminocaproic acid, and alcohol; mitochondrial myopathy resulting from exposure to zidovudine, elevudine, and statin medications; lysosomal and autophagic myopathy and neuromyopathy due to amiodarone and perihexiline; microtubular myopathy and neuromyopathy due to exposure to vincristine; emetine-induced myofibrilar myopathy, and acute quadriplegia myopathy.

With the exception of D-penicillamine, long-term, high-dose use of the antimalarial medications chloroquine and hydroxychloroquine, the anti-gout medication colchicine, interferon-α employed in the treatment of chronic active hepatitis, cyclosporine and tarolimus used to prevent solid organ transplant rejection, chronic administration of prednisone in doses greater than 20 mg daily, and long term use of the nucleoside analogue reverse transcriptase inhibitor

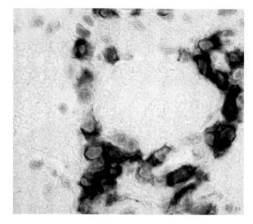

(A)

(B)

FIG. 1. Polymyositis. **(A)** A longitudinal section of muscle shows intense cellular infiltration within the fascicle. **(B)** Immunocytochemical staining reveals that the infiltrating cells invading the muscle fiber are mostly CD8+ T-cells.

zidovudine, such drugs typically elicit a toxic non-IM that differs histologically from PM and does not require immunosuppressive therapy. While statin medication can cause NAM and hyperCKemia, which are reversible upon cessation of the drug, they can also initiate an immune-mediated myopathy that persists after withdrawal of the drug and responds to immunosuppressant therapy. The proposed mechanism for this is induction by statins of endoplasmic reticulum (ER)-related stress response associated with up-regulation of main histocompatibility complex class 1 (MHC-1) expression and antigen presentation by myofibers (12).

Animal parasites such as the protozoa Toxoplasma, Trypanosoma, Cysticerci, and Trichinae instead produce a focal or diffuse IM known as parasitic PM, while suppurative or pyomyositis is caused by Saphylococcus, Streptococcus species, and other anaerobes are causes of pyomyositis; and *Borrelia (B.) burgdorferi* and Legionella pneumophila are infrequent causes of PM. Among viral agents, human immunodeficiency virus type 1 (HIV-1) and human T lymphotropic virus type 1 (HTLV-1) are retroviruses associated with polymyositis (13), while other viruses, such as enteroviruses and acute viral syndromes, cause severe myalgia and even transient elevation of serum CK levels that rarely if ever lead to frank polymyositis. However, PM can be seen in patients with systemic lupus erythematosus (SLE), Sjogren syndrome, and rheumatoid arthritis, whereas, IM associated with systemic sclerosis and mixed connective tissue disease when present, is more often associataed with DM. Nonetheless, PM occurs during the course of other systemic autoimmune disorders including Crohn disease, vasculitis, sarcoidosis, primary biliary sclerosis, adult Celiac disease, ankylosing spondylitis, Hashimoto thyroiditis, Lyme borrelosis, and acquired immune deficiency syndrome (AIDS).

Considering all of the possible pitfalls in the recognition and classification of PM, the diagnosis is bolstered by evaluation of serum muscle enzymes, electrodiagnostic studies, and confirmed by muscle biopsy. The most sensitive enzyme is the muscle CK level, which along with seemingly elevated liver transaminases and LDH that can misdirect the evaluation toward a cardiac or liver disease, parallels muscle disease activity, or remain normal in corticosteroid-treated patients and those with chronic PM. Needle electromyography (EMG) shows myopathic short-duration, low-amplitude, polyphasic voluntary motor unit potentials (MUP) that recruit rapidly with submaximal effort, associated with acute spontaneous activity at rest in the form of fibrillations, positive sharp waves, and complex repetitive discharges (CRD). Serological studies against nuclear and cytoplasmic antigens, which may be found in up to 20% of patients with inflammatory myopathy, are directed in the latter toward ribonucleoproteins involved in translation and protein synthesis. They include Jo-1 directed again the histidyl-transfer ribonucleic acid (RNA) synthetase anti-Jo-1, which accounts for 75% of synthetases, and the clinically most useful.

Muscle biopsy, which reveals immunocytochemical evidence of infiltrating CD8+ T-cells invading muscle fibers (Figure 1A, B), confirms the diagnosis in clinically compatible patients. Chahln and Engel (14) proposed criteria for PM similar to those suggested by van der Meulen and colleagues (15), including subacute, progressive limb muscle weakness with or without associated autoimmune disease or markers, compatible EMG findings, inflammatory endomysial exudate or invasion of non-necrotic muscle fibers by mononuclear cells, and perimysial or perivascular inflammation; and absence of clinical or pathological features of DM, necrotizing vasculitis, muscular dystrophy, or overlap syndromes, ascertaining PM in only 27 of 107 patients with inflammatory myopathy. With an estimated occurrence of PM, DM, and sIBM of 1 per 100,000 individuals, PM is the least common of the three disorders, and the most difficult to diagnose because other diagnoses need to be excluded. They include dysferlinopathy, facioscapulohumeral (FSH), and Becker muscular dystrophy (BMD), which are more common in younger patients but associated with variable endomysial inflammatory. Metabolic myopathy, endocrinopathy, mitochondrial myopathy, and other systemic illnesses including malabsorption, alcoholism, vasculitis, granulomatous disease, known treatment with potentially myotoxic agents, and necrotizing myopathy need to be excluded by clinical, electrodiagnostic and muscle biopsy studies.

Evidence suggests a T-cell-mediated and MHC-1 antigen-restricted process, a pervasive T-cell-mediated cytotoxic process directed against heretofore unidentified muscle antigens in PM, as suggested by the concomitant presence of CD8+ cells that, along with macrophages, initially surround healthy non-necrotic muscle fibers, eventually invading and destroying them, while adjacent myofibers and those remote from the areas of inflammation strongly express MHC-1 antigen absent from the sarcolemma of normal muscle fibers. The specificity of the T-cells has been examined by studying the gene rearrangement of T-cell receptors (TCR) of autoinvasive T-cells, with similar findings in both PM and IBM, indicating that those with the α-and β-TCR family are recruited to the muscle from the circulation (16).

Among the circulating T-cells, clonal expansion occurs only in cytotoxic CD8+ cells that express genes for perforin and infiltrate MHC-1-expressing muscle fibers (17). The process of antigen presentation and recognition by T-cells involves myofibers, autoinvasive CD8+ T-cells, and expression of costimulatory molecules B7-1, B7-2, BB1, CD40 or inducible costimulatory-ligand (ICOS-L) and the respective counter-receptors in the trimoleuclar complex. Cell-to-cell CD8+ T-cell interactions and signalng between infiltrating T-cells is facilitated by specific ligands and molecules recognized both on the surface of infiltrating T-cells and MHC-I-expressing myofibers. Upregulation of cytokines, chemokines, and metalloproteinases, including mRNA of interleukin (IL)-1, IL-2, tumor necrosis factor (TNF)-a and its receptor, interferon-gamma (INF-γ), T-cell growth factor-β, granulocyte-macrophage colony-stimulating factor, IL-6, and IL-10, some of which exert a direct cytotoxic effect on myofibers, while others are expressed in the endomysial inflammatory cells and in the neighboring extracellular matrix.

Adhesion of lymphocytes to muscle may be facilitated by metalloproteinases, a family of calcium-dependent zinc endopeptidases involved in the remodeling of the extracellular matrix, among them metalloproteinase-9 and metalloproteinase-2, which are upregulated in non-necrotic and MHC-1 expressing myofibers, and expressed on the autoinvasive CD8+ T-cells facilitating cell-to-cell contact with myofibers. The release of cytokines and chemokines, which upregulates the expression of vascular cell adhesion molecule-I and intracellular adhesion molecule-I in the endothelial cells, serve as ligands for the integrins, very late activation antigen (VLA)-4, and lymphocyte function associated antigen-1 expressed in T-cells that in turn, facilitate their exit through the blood vessel wall into the perimysial and endomysial spaces.

Anchored to cytoskeletal molecules in the nascent immunological synapse, the interaction of the TCR-MHC-1 complex with co-stimulatory molecules and their ligands commence the requisite process of antigen recognition while facilitating the attachment of T-cells to the muscle surface. Ensuing myofiber necrosis occurs as a result of released perforin granules by the autoinvasive T-cells, combined with the myotoxic effects of IFN-γ, IL-1, and TNF-α released by locally invasive macrophages.

Whereas myofiber death is mediated by necrosis and not apoptosis presumably as a result of the counterbalancing effect or protection of the anti-apoptotic molecules Bcl-2, human inhibitor of apoptosis-like protein (hILP), and Flice inhibitory protein (FLIP) that are upregulated in PM and IBM, up-regulated neural cell adhesion molecule (NCAM) on degenerating muscle fibers, enhances regeneration. A role for myeloid dendritic cells (mDC), potent antigen-presenting cells that can be found among the endomysial infiltrates of patients with PM, IBM, and DM (18) may be candidate cells for antigen presentation to surrounding T-cells, but their significance in inflammatory myopathies remains unknown.

Based on their immunoglobulin gene isotype, plasma cells, which appear to mature and expand in situ, implying an antigen-driven response (19), may reflect a peculiarity of the inflammatory response within the muscle microenvironment rather than a specific pathogenic response unique to PM. MHC-I upregulation may exert a stress effect to the endoplasmic reticulum (ER) of myofibers independent of T-cell-mediated cytotoxicity (20). The assembly and folding of MHC-I, which occurs in the ER and matures when bound to an antigenic peptide synthesized in the cytosol, is combined with a system of chaperone proteins, including calnexin, calreticulin, GRP94, GRP78, and ERP72 that form the MHC-loading complex, ensuring the proper maturation of MHC for antigen processing (21). If the MHC-class-I loading complex does not bind to suitable antigens, the heavy chain glycoprotein is misfolded and removed from the ER to the cytosol for degradation.

In PM and IBM, myofibers overloaded by MHC molecules and antigenic peptides sustain ER stress, similar to that observed in MHC-I transgenic mice, suggesting that overexpression of MHC-I alone may be sufficient to induce ER stress. This hypothesis is reasonable in explaining the continuous MHC-expression and chronic inflammation as seen in PM and IBM (21).

INCLUSION BODY MYOSITIS

First recognized as a distinct entity between 1967 and 1971, three independent groups identified distinct microtubular filamentous inclusions by electron microscopy (EM) in the muscle biopsies of affected patients with presumed PM (22–24). Sporadic IBM (sIBM) is the most frequently acquired myopathy in men over age 50 years and is no longer considered as rare as when first described, representing probably 16% to 28% of all inflammatory myopathies (25). With an estimated prevalence of 2.2 to 9.3 persons per million, depending upon case ascertainment, a mean age at onset generally of 56 years, and a mean delay between onset of symptoms and diagnosis of four years, sIBM is probably underdiagnosed. Involvement of distal muscles, especially foot extensors and deep finger flexors, which occurs in almost all patients, is a valuable clue to the early clinical detection. Some patients present with falls and buckling of the knees due to proximal leg weakness. Others present with weakness in the small muscles of the hands, especially finger flexors, and complain of inability to hold certain objects such as golf clubs, play the guitar, turn keys, or tie knots. The weakness and accompanying wasting is often asymmetric with selective involvement of the quadriceps, iliopsoas, deltoid, triceps, biceps, and most characteristically, flexor digitorum profundus finger muscles, with shared innervation by the median and ulnar nerves.

Dysphagia occurs in up to 60% of patients, especially late in the disease. A lower motor neuron (LMN) neurogenic disorder may be suspected when the serum CK is normal or if there are features of motor neuron involvement (26). Similarly, PM and muscular dystrophy should be considered when the CK is elevated more than 5- to 10-fold, especially if there is no response to a trial of corticosteroids aimed at PM. Sensory function may be normal or show distal age-related loss. Contrary to early suggestions, distal weakness is not on a neurogenic basis but is a feature of the distal myopathy as shown by macro electromyography EMG (27). In contrast to PM and DM, in which facial muscles are typically spared, mild facial muscle weakness occurs in 60% of patients with sIBM (28).

The diagnosis is confirmed by muscle biopsy that shows the characteristic histopathologic changes of rimmed vacuoles, small atrophic fibers, and characteristic cytoplasmic filamentous inclusions by EM in myonuclei (Figure 2A, B). Sporadic IBM can be associated with systemic autoimmune or connective tissue diseases in up to 20% of patients. The

progression is slow and steady with a degree of disability that is generally related to the duration of the disease. The IBM functional rating scale (IBMFRS) (29, 30) score from 10 graded categories, with a maximal score of 40 derived from aspects of swallowing, handwriting, cutting food and handling utensils, fine motor tasks, dressing, hygiene, turning in bed and adjusting covers, sit to stand, and walking and climbing functions, showed statistically significant correlations with composite maximal voluntary isometric contraction (MVIC) strength testing, the latter derived from elbow and knee flexor and extensor, and hand grip muscle evaluation; manual muscle testing (MMT), functional disability, and quality of life (QoL) measures (31).

The recognition that a four percent decline in predicted normal strength occurred in just a six-month period (32), and that the time from independent ambulation to walker use arose after 5.7 years of untreated disease, respectively among cohorts between the 6th to 8th decade (33), suggested that early diagnosis was important in arresting and slowing disease progression, particularly since short-term improvement or stabilization may be difficult to elicit with any given therapy (34).

Although the vast majority of IBM occurs sporadically, and is considered an IM due to both inflammatory and dysimmune causation, there is increasing interest in concurrent myodegenerative factors (35). Garlepp and colleagues (36) demonstrated characteristic rimmed vacuoles with immunohistochemical evidence of the β-amyloid fragment of the beta-amyloid precursor protein (β-APP or APP) and ubiquitin (UBB). Askanas and colleagues (37) noted vacuolar degeneration, congophilic inclusion, and clusters of colocalizing beta-amyloid and transthyretin (TTR) immunoreactivity in cultured skeletal muscle from a patient with sporadic IBM and cardiac amyloidosis and a mutation in the *TTR* gene, suggesting that the mutation may have predisposed to the development of IBM. Although nonspecific, a mean of 23% of sIBM tissue samples showed non-nuclear multiple curvilinear filamentous 43 kD Tar DNA binding-protein (TDP-43) immunoreactivity (38). A transgenic mouse model of IBM that showed signs of acute and chronic inflammation after administration of lipopolysaccharide (LPS), with exacerbation of motor decline compared to untreated mice, and increased levels of phosphorylated tau and β-amyloid (39). Treatment with a specific inhibitor of glycogen synthase kinase 3-β that reduces muscle phosphorylated-tau levels leads to motor improvement.

Baumbach and colleagues (40) reported hIBM among a family of Ashkenazi Jewish descent with autosomal dominant (AD) inheritance and mild early-, to mid-adult gait disturbances due to symmetric leg weakness that progressed over a decade or less to all limbs, with bulbar, respiratory, facial muscle, and cardiac involvement, and normal or mildly elevated CK levels. Muscle biopsy showed myopathic

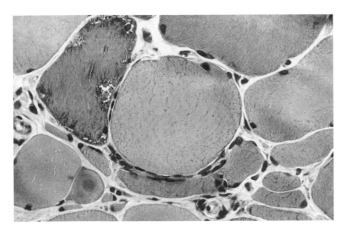

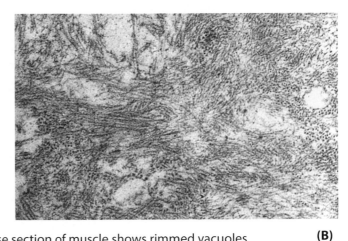

(A) **(B)**

FIG. 2. Inclusion body myositis. **(A)** A transverse section of muscle shows rimmed vacuoles and small atrophic fibers among big-size fibers. **(B)** Characteristic filamentous inclusion seen by electron microscopy in the cytoplasm within one vacuole of myonuclei.

features, rimmed vacuoles, and desmin present as abundant granulofilamentous deposits between individual myofibrils or adjacent to the sarcolemma. Autosomal dominant IBM type 1 (IBM1) is caused by heterozygous, homozygous, and compound heterozygous mutation at the 2q35 locus of the desmin (*DES*) gene (41). Among 159 patients with 40 different *DES* mutations described by van Spaendonck-Zwarts and colleagues (42), hIBM was shown in 54% and neurological signs were noted overall in 74%. A second hereditary form, IBM type 2 (IBM2), displayed autosomal recessive (AR) inheritance affecting individuals of Persian, Iranian, and Kurdish Jewish descent. The clinical picture originally described by Argov and Yarom (43) included progressive proximal and distal weakness of the arms and legs beginning after age 20, sparing the quadriceps muscles even in advanced stages, with gradual incapacitation within 10 to 20 years. Serum CK levels were normal or moderately elevated and nerve conduction studies (NCS) were normal. Muscle biopsy showed rimmed vacuolar myopathy wherein degenerating myofibers contained abnormal accumulations of β-amyloid protein. UDP-N-acetylglucosamine 2-epimerase/N-acetylmannosamine kinase (GNE) protein expression in subsequent tissue specimens showed immunoreactivity to NCAM, a fetal muscle antigen, expressed by many vaculolated fibers, with normal levels of GNE suggesting a usefulness of NCAM as a tissue marker of IBM2 and abnormal function of GNE (44, 45). Autosomal recessive IBM2 is caused by homozygous or compound heterozygous mutation at the 9p13.3 locus of the *GNE* gene (46), encoding GNE, the rate-limiting enzyme in the sialic acid biosynthetic pathway. Nonaka myopathy (47) is an allelic disorder with a similar phenotype as AR IBM2. Patients with AD IBM-3 (IBM3) were described by Darin and colleagues (48) in a multigenerational Swedish family with congenital joint contractures that normalized during childhood, external ophthalmoplegia, and non-progressive proximal weakness

and atrophy, most prominent in the pectoralis and quadriceps muscles starting from age 30 to 50 years. Muscle biopsy showed focal disorganization of myofilaments with dystrophic changes and rimmed vacuoles that contained cytoplasmic inclusions of 15- to 21-nm filaments. IBM3 is caused by mutations at the 17p13.1 locus of the myosin heavy chain 2 skeletal muscle adult (*MYH2*) gene (49, 50), encoding myosin heavy chain IIa. The frequent abnormality of type 2A fibers in the patients reported by Darin and colleagues (48) suggested that a mutation in the region of the *MYHC2A* gene encoding the major isoform of type 2A fibers was likely to result in dysfunctional myosin (50).

DERMATOMYOSITIS

This distinct childhood and adult clinical disorder is identified by a characteristic rash accompanying or, more often, preceding the muscle weakness. The skin manifestations include blue-purple discoloration on the upper eyelids or heliotrope rash with edema, a flat red rash on the face and upper trunk, and erythema of the knuckles with a raised violaceous scaly eruption or Gottron rash that later results in scaling of the skin. An erythematous rash also occurs on other body surfaces, including the knees, elbows, malleoli, neck, and anterior chest, often in a "V" sign, or on the back and shoulders, the so-called shawl sign; the latter can be exacerbated after exposure to the sun. In some patients the rash is pruritic, especially in the scalp, chest, and back. Dilated capillary loops at the base of the fingernails are characteristic of DM. The cuticles may be irregular, thickened, and distorted, and the lateral and palmar areas of the fingers may become rough and cracked, with irregular dirty horizontal lines, resembling mechanic's hands. The degree of weakness can be mild, moderate, or severe, leading to quadraparesis. At times, the muscle strength appears

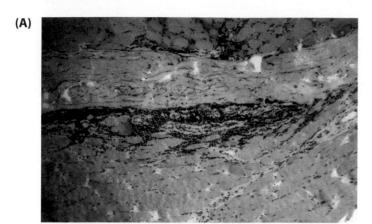

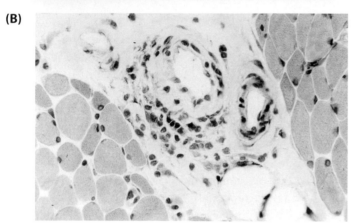

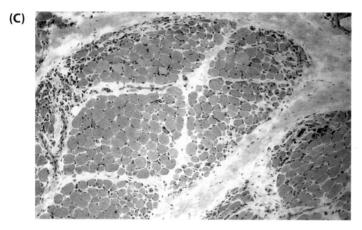

FIG. 3. Dermatomyositis. **(A)** A transverse section of muscle shows intense mononuclear cellular infiltration at the periphery of the fascicle that includes activated B cells and plasma cells. **(B)** Perivasculitis of an interfascicular vessel in mild disease. **(C)** Characteristic perifascicular atrophy in a transverse section of muscle.

normal, hence the term "dermatomyositis sine myositis," however in muscle biopsy in such cases shows significant cellular infiltration at the peripheral of a fascicle, perivasculitis of interfascicular vessels, and characteristic perifascicular atrophy (Figure 3A–C) similar to other more usual patients (51). In children, DM resembles the adult disease, except for more frequent extramuscular manifestations. A common early abnormality in children is misery, defined as an irritable child who feels uncomfortable, has a red flush on the face, is fatigued, does not feel well enough to socialize, and has a varying degree of proximal muscle weakness. A tiptoe gait due to flexion contracture of the ankles is also common. DM usually occurs alone or with systemic sclerosis and mixed connective tissue disease. Fasciitis and skin changes similar to those found in DM occur in patients with the eosinophilia-myalgia syndrome associated with the ingestion of contaminated L-tryptophan.

The etiopathogenesis of DM has been ascribed to local cell and humorally-mediated mechanisms involving endomysial CD4+, β-, and CD4+ T-cells, plasmacytoid DC (pDC) infiltration of muscle, and antibody and complement-mediated capillary injury of muscle (21, 52, 53). The perifascicular area, known to be a possible watershed region at the periphery of fascicules, appears to be targeted. Microarray studies assessing the pattern of gene expression shows it to be a region rich in local expression and upregulation of gene transcripts and proteins. Although the sequence of injurious mechanisms are not fully understood, an immune mediated microvasculopathy, commencing with C5b-9 membrane attack complex (MAC) complement activation and deposition along endothelial capillaries targeting endothelial cells with resultant ischemic myofiber damage (54–57), precedes other morphological muscle change. These include a reduction in the number of capillaries throughout the muscle, while lumina of remaining vessels dilate to compensate for the ischemic process associated with capillary tubuloreticular inclusions, focal myofiber atrophy at the periphery of fascicles, and deposits of complement and immunoglobulin. Many of the regenerating and degenerating perifascicular myofibers stain with antibodies against alkaline phosphatase desmin, and NCAM, and also stain with antibodies against a variety of molecules including transforming growth factor-(TGF)-b, and MHC-I, α/β-crystallin, cathepsins, amyloid precursor protein (APP), signal transducer and activator of transcription-1 (STAT-1), interferon-α/β, Mi-2 chromatin remodeling protein, Kallmann syndrome protein (KAL1), and myxovirus resistance A (MxA) protein, triggered by α/β-IF, and present within endothelial tubuloreticular inclusions.

Greenberg (58) proposed a revised model for the immunopathogenesis of DM based upon observations alone of the association of tissue pathology with interferon-α/β inducible proteins, and cited supporting evidence based upon several observations. First, tubuloreticular capillary inclusions develop *in vitro* with interferon exposure. Second, MxA is expressed ion in DM capillaries, and STAT-1 and MHC-I are induced in abnormal perifascicular myofibers by interferon-α/β. Third, perifascicular fibers are preferentially injured as a result of interferon-α/β production by locally concentrated perimysial perifascicular pDC, the latter leading to perifascicular atrophy through unidentified mechanisms. However, this model is unlikely for several reasons. It does not explain the reduced number of capillaries throughout the fascicle or in perifascicular regions, nor does it account for complement activation and MAC deposition on capillaries or the presence of other proteins expressed by perifascicular myofibers including NCAM, neonatal myosin heavy chain, Jo-1, cathepsin L, calpain, and α/β-crytallin, that have no known relationship to type 1 IF. Nor does the model of chronic overexpression of α/β interferon account for the salutary effects of intravenous immune globulin (IVIg) on the interception of complement-mediated MAC activation that leads to improvement in strength and amelioration of the muscle immunopathology (59, 60). Moreover, α/β-interferon inducible genes lack specificity or uniqueness for DM, as they are overexpressed in patients' blood not only in DM but also in PM (61). Furthermore, α/β-IF upregulation occurs in several connective tissue diseases including SLE and Sjögren syndrome.

NECROTIZING AUTOIMMUNE MYOPATHY

Necrotizing autoimmune myopathy (62) presents with clinical, electrophysiologic, serological aspects, and muscle biopsy features on that meet the major criteria of Bohan and Peter (10). Onset of symmetrical weakness progresses over weeks to months, although there may be acute severe weakness. Serum CK levels are elevated, often into the thoursand or more range. There are typical electromyographic features of acute myopathy including acute fibrillation activity (63), myopathic motor unit potential (MUP) that show a full recruitment pattern (64), and muscle-biopsy evidences myofiber necrosis, regeneration, basophilia, and prominent nucleoli, but without prominent inflammatory cell exudation. An autoimmune etiopathogenesis in some patients prompted investigators to classify NAM into idiopathic IM (65). In support of this is the finding of C5b-9 MAC expression in skeletal blood vessels in some affected patients (66) and the association with the myositis specific autoantibody (MSA) and the anti-synthetase antibody anti-PL12 (67, 68). One reported muscle tissue biopsy demonstrated scant cellular infiltrates comprised of rare T-lymphocytes and macrophages (68), similar to those of a minority of others, some of whom demonstrated upregulation of MHC class I and II

(2). There was a small, albeit insignificant, association with comorbid connective tissue disorders and malignancy in cohort studies (2). Some affected patients were purported to manifest a favorable response to immunosuppressant and immune modulatory therapy (2, 68), however they had rapidly progressing weakness and minimal response to corticosteroids that might otherwise have slowly improved untreated over time.

EXTRAMUSCULAR MANIFESTATIONS

In addition to the primary disturbance of skeletal muscles, there may be prominent extramuscular manifestations in patients with IM, including dysphagia, most prominent in IBM and DM, due to involvement of striated muscles of the oropharynx and distal esophagus; cardiac abnormalities consisting of atrioventricular conduction defects, tachyarrhythmia, low ejection fraction, and dilated cardiomyopathy alone or associated with hypertension or long-term steroid use; and respiratory involvement generally resulting from weakness of chest-cage muscles (69), drug-induced pneumonitis from methotrexate, and interstitial lung disease (ILD) (70). Interstitial lung disease (ILD) can precede inflammatory myopathy or accompany it as an associated feature in 5 to 40% of patients with PM and DM determined by roentgenography or by pulmonary function tests, most of whom have antiendothlial cell, primarily Jo-1 antibodies.

Such patients may be at at risk of increased fatality resulting from adult respiratory distress syndrome compared to those with PM without Jo-1 antibodies (71). The etiology and pathogenesis of ILD in PM and DM are unknown, however several factors have been implicated, including infectious agents, drug and chemical exposures, and immune mechanisms. Pulmonary capillaritis with varying degree of diffuse alveolar hemorrhage has also been described (72).

Subcutaneous calcification, sometimes extruding on the skin and causing ulceration and infection, is found in children and some adults with DM (73). Gastrointestinal ulceration, seen more often in children with DM, is due to vasculitis and infection. Joint contractures are seen, especially in children with DM. General systemic disturbances are seen, such as fever, malaise, weight loss, arthralgia, and Raynaud phenomenon, when the inflammatory myopathy is associated with a connective tissue disorder. Malignancy is also manifested with increased frequency in patients with biopsy-proven DM, modestly if at all in PM, but not in IBM associated with ovarian, pancreatic stomach, colorectal cancer, and non-Hodgkin lymphoma (74, 75). Two independent predictive factors for malignancy include older age at onset of inflammatory myopathy and male gender. It is the authors' practice to recommend a complete annual physical examination, with breast, pelvic, and rectal examinations, urinalysis, complete blood cell count, blood chemistry tests. and a chest x-ray film in all patients with IM because such tumors will usually be uncovered not by a radiological blind search, but by abnormal findings on their medical history, physical examination, and laboratory investigations.

DIAGNOSIS

The diagnosis of clinically suspected PM, DM, and sIBM is suggested by examination of serum CK levels and compatible findings on EMG, albeit definitively by muscle biopsy. Serum autoantibody studies, muscle imaging studies, and genetic analysis, can provide useful supportive information in some patients.

Serum Muscle Enzymes

The most sensitive serum enzyme is the CK, which in the presence of active disease can be elevated up to 50-fold or more, along with elevation in serum aspartate (SGOT), alanine aminotranferases (SGPT), lactate dehydrogenase (LDH), and aldolase levels. Although the CK parallels the disease activity, it can be normal in active DM and rarely, even in active PM. It is often normal in elderly patients in whom the body muscle mass may be reduced due to aging, and this may lead to a delay in recognition of the diagnosis (76). The serum CK level in sIBM rarely exceeds 1,000 U and is more often only several hundred units. The serum CK level may also be normal in patients with untreated, even active, childhood DM, and in those with PM and DM associated with a connective tissue disease, reflecting the concentration of the pathologic process in the intramuscular vessels and the perimysium.

Myositis-Specific Autoantibodies

Muscle-specific autoantibodies are directed against defined nuclear and cytoplasmic antigens found in patients with PM and DM (77, 78). The most commonly detected and best characterized autoantibody, called anti-Jo-1, is directed against histidyl-transfer RNA synthetase, and accounts for three quarters of all the anti-synthetases. It is diagnostically useful because up to 80% of patients with anti-Jo-1 antibodies have ILD. Seven other different synthetases described to date, anti-PL12 (alanine), anti-PL7 (threonine), anti-EJ (glycine), anti-OJ (isoleucine), anti-Zo (phenylalanine), anti-Ha (tyrosine), and anti-KS (asparagine), are detected overall in about 4% of patients with IM. Naked tRNA may be recognized by autoantibodies in one-third of anti-Jo-1, and in most anti-PL12 sera (79). Anti-SRP autoantibodies, recognized in a minority of patients, targets the co-translational translocation of secretory and membrane proteins to the membrane

of endoplasmic reticulum. Another MSA recognizes auto-antigenic forms of the Mi-2 antigen, a 220 kDa protein in a nuclear protein complex containing histone deacetylase and nucleosome remodeling activities (80).

Originally detected in up to 20% of myositis sera of patients with DM, increased Mi-2 expression was found preferentially in myofibers within fascicles affected by peri-fascicular atrophy, particularly in the centralized nuclei of small perifascicular myofibers expressing markers of regeneration, and in injured mouse muscle tissue where Mi-2 was upregulated during muscle regeneration in vivo (81). Anti-Mi2 autoantibodies were later found to be present in the sera of patients with PM and IBM using an enzyme linked immunoassay (ELISA) technique in which four overlapping fragments, NT, NM, CT, and M were used, whereas previous studies only employed the NM fragment thought to contain the major epitope region (82). Further analyses of autoantibody reactivity against different parts of the Mi-2B autoantigen (83) found no significant differences between patients with autoantibodies to different fragments, with the possible exception of an increased risk of cancer in those with reactivity to the N-terminal fragment.

Other serum autoantibodies associated with IM encountered in other disorders, with or without clinical signs of myositis, include those directed at PM/Scl and Mas, components of the U1 small nuclear RNP (snRNP), the cytoplasmic Ro RNP antigens Ro60/SSA, La/SSB, and Ro52. Finally, antibodies to antigens involved in protein synthesis, while specific for IM and characteristic of subsets of adult IM, are rare in pediatric IM. In juvenile DM, serological indicators of disease activity include neopterin, von Willebrand factor (vWF), vascular cell adhesion molecule-1 (VCAM-1), a-smooth muscle actin (SMA), TNF-α antigens, and type 1 interferon-regulated gene signature, with down regulation of MiR-126.

Electrodiagnostic Studies

The natural history of EMG abnormalities in IM is virtually unknown since most patients undergo some therapeutic intervention and serial EMG studies have not been performed. Several EMG indices include spontaneous activity at rest, recruitment with graded force and interference pattern at low force, MUP analysis, macro EMG, single fiber EMG (SFEMG), and muscle fiber conduction velocity (MFCV) measurements. Systematic investigation of these techniques suggests that detailed analysis by qualified electromyographers can lead to improved diagnosis, management, monitoring, and prognosis of IM.

Normal myofibers show no spontaneous electrical activity outside the motor endplate region located midway between the ends of the muscle, wherein miniature endplate potentials (MEPP) occur randomly due to spontaneous release of individual quanta of acetylcholine (ACh) and can be recorded easily with needle electrodes as monophasic negative waveforms <10uv and duration 1 to 3 ms. Acute denervation leads to downregulation of cholinetransferase, impaired neuromuscular transmission and increased sensitivity to ACh. These are accompanied by positive sharp wave and fibrillation potentials due to hyerexcitable spots along the muscle which trigger activity in neighboring myofibers and locked fibrillation or CRD when denervated groups of myofiber activate one another (84).

The amount of fibrillation is related to the disease activity (85). Within days, nerve sprouts emerge reaching denervated fibers, forming multiple contacts over several weeks leading to the incorporation of new fibers by surviving motor units. The typical finding of low amplitude and short duration unstable polyphasic MUP in primary myopathy, while interpreted as evidence of myofiber loss, is associated with other findings, including increasing fiber density (FD), increased jitter, and impulse-blocking, reflecting-impaired transmission, as well as normal macro EMG, which with regard to its large recording area from the entire motor unit, indicates a present regenerative process. Chronically, MUP amplitude and duration increase, assuming a stable neurogenic character. Reactivation of disease can be associated with recurrence of acute spontaneous activity, increased jitter and blocking in SFEMG, and unstable MUP.

The notion of a myopathic EMG, which was initially based upon qualitative visual analysis and acoustical impressions (86), was quantified using concentric needle EMG analysis of motor unit action potential (MUAP) features of amplitude, area, duration and complexity. Formally applied to IM, it showed a myopathic pattern of decreased mean MUP duration and area to amplitude ratio in 69% of studies among 37 patients at different points in the disease in the biceps brachii muscle that varied in clinical strength (87). Algorithms employing multi-MUAP analysis (MMA) aid in the extraction and analysis of 20 MUAP, the results of which were comparable to those obtained with an amplitude-triggered manual method, and when combined with interference pattern analysis (IPA), make MMA useful in documenting EMG abnormalities in IM (88).

Focused IPA of the EMG exceeded the sensitivity of detecting myopathy by amplitude-triggered manual quantitative MUP analysis by 14% (87, 89), showing an increase in the number of spike and amplitude of the envelope with increasing force measures from zero to maximal voluntary contraction (MVC). At weak effort or force, it was possible to identify individual MUP, whereas at higher efforts there was interference with summation and cancellation of MUAP components. The quantification of IPA, which is performed with automatic methods, expressed as the number of spikes per turn or number of turns per unit time, defined as the number of zero crossing of 100 μv per unit time, normally increases with force up to about 30% of MVC. The number of motor units and their firing rate, which influences the number of turns per second, is displayed as a power spectrum analysis, with displacement of the frequency pattern toward higher frequencies in patients with myopathy compared to normal individuals, due to the changes in individual MUP, resulting in an increase in the number of turns per second and a decrease in mean amplitude per turns. Whereas an increase in turns per second was attributed to increased firing rate, a study of myopathic motor unit firing rates at a force of 10% of maximum revealed no difference between patients with myopathy and normal controls (90). The impression of an increased firing rate in patients with myopathy is likely false, at least at a low force levels.

Although high-amplitude MUP, sometimes interpreted as a mixed neurogenic and myopathic pattern can sometimes be noted in IBM, they are usually of short-duration and likely generated from general or focal hypertrophy of myofibers close to a segment where the muscle fiber has split. A late-stage, more typical neurogenic pattern can be noted in IBM when there is concomitant neuropathy (91). The combination of normal or decreased macro-MUP with normal or borderline increased FD was seen in all patients with sIBM so studied by macro EMG (92), similar to other investigators (27).

The technique of MFCV, which employs a direct muscle-fiber stimulation and recording (93), yielded a prospective accuracy of 72% in the diagnosis of IM, compared to 60% for EMG alone, making it a potentially useful adjunctive electrodiagnostic examination.

Imaging Studies

Magnetic resonance imaging (MRI) is the method of choice for imaging muscle abnormalities (94, 95). Compared to computed tomography (CT) and ultrasound, it is quantitative, easily detects active inflammation, and it encompasses large fields. Although CT scanning is more sensitive in showing subcutaneous and fascial calcification in DM, MRI is useful in recognizing the selective pattern of muscle involvement in IBM, and in the recognition of active PM and DM. However, the diagnostic sensitivity of MRI has not been formally evaluated.

The classical method of quantification of inflammation by MRI is the calculation of T_1- and T_2-weighted relaxation times. Areas of inflammation within muscle tissue generally yield high values for T_1- and T_2-weighted images, whereas fat displays low T_1- and high T_2-values. Fat-suppressed STIR images improve the utility of T_2-weighted images, particularly in the case of PM and IBM wherein fat replacement and inflammation are prominent. Muscle MRI in active DM, PM and, to a lesser extent in IBM, shows multifocal or diffuse high-signal intensity of T_2-weighted STIR and non-fat saturated sequences. The STIR images can be evaluated quantitatively on the basis of the increased signal intensities in regions of inflammation.

Anticipated semi-automated computer analyses should be able to calculate a myositis index based upon histograms of signal intensities of STIR images, precluding observer bias. For the present, initially elevated T_1- and T_2-weighted values indicative of significant inflammation in a given patient can be followed by serial imaging to more normal values with effective therapy. MR elastography (MRE), which is a non-invasive technique that assesses the shear modulus or stiffness of muscle, was studied in nine subjects with active DM or PM, demonstrating a significant reduction in muscle stiffness compared to healthy controls during the relaxed condition (96). A commercial version of MRE available in Europe is known as the Fibroscan (Echosens, Paris). The cause of reduced stiffness, complex waveforms, and excessive fatigabilty, so noted, is conjectured to result from destruction of passive structures or elements such as intramuscular collagen. Temporary fatigue and alteration in the extracellular matrix in experimental rat skeletal muscle during progression of heart failure (97) could impact on the passive elements of human muscle tissue by disturbing the delicate balance or remodeling of muscle tissue by proteins, proteases, and protease inhibitors (96).

The finding of ILD, which frequently accompanies PM and DM, and confers a poorer prognosis, requires prompt diagnosis and aggressive management. An early diagnosis of ILD was ascertained by positive 18F-fluorodeoxyglucose (FDG) positron emission tomography (PET) CT scanning, prior to clinical onset of ILD and typical CT radiographic features in the lung of an adult Japanese woman with clinically amyopathic DM (CADM), normal CK levels, and elevated antibodies to the 140-kDa polypeptide, CADM-140, despite active myopathy on needle EMG, and abnormal high signal changes in the adductor magnus on axial and T_2-weighted MRI. However, CT scan of the lungs showed no sign of interstitial pneumonia (98).

Muscle Biopsy

Muscle biopsy has the potential to not only establish the histological diagnosis of DM, PM, and IBM, but also to exclude other morphologically distinct processes. Patients planning to undergo muscle biopsy should undergo thorough neurological and medical evaluation, inclusive of the examination of other potentially affected family members, and undergo detailed NCS and concentric needle EMG, not only to guide the choice of a muscle to one that is clinically and electrophysiologically affected, but also to avoid sampling one that is end-stage muscle tissue. The procedure should be performed by a neurologist or surgeon experienced in the performance of biopsy surgery at a center

with a dedicated neuromuscular neuropathologist. There should be communication between the treating neurologist, surgeon, and neuropathologist regarding the presumptive diagnosis to assure that the correct muscle is biopsied, distant from areas previously examined by needle EMG, and to assure that the correct tissue specimens are obtained for the needed histological studies. Both the vastus lateralis and biceps muscles are ideal for disorders accompanied by proximal weakness due to presumed IM.

Peripheral neuropathy, when present, is generally due to alternative causes in patients with DM and PM, whereas distal polyneuropathy should not be an unexpected finding on electrophysiological studies in patients with IBM, and should prompt consideration of biopsy of a distal cutaneous nerve and muscle, such as the medial gastrocnemius or tibialis anterior muscle. Twelve patients with sIBM or hIBM were described in whom the diagnosis of peripheral neuropathy was confirmed histologically by sural nerve biopsy with evidence of chronic axonopathy (99–101).

At least four specimens of muscle should be obtained caring to incise the muscle along natural longitudinal and cross-sectional epimysial tissue planes to optimize later histopathological sections, while minimizing tissue handling, blunt trauma, bleeding, and vascular compression. Separate pieces of muscle are placed in moist saline gauze, 10% formalin, and glutaraldehyde, and transported directly to the muscle laboratory for paraffin-embedded histology, snap-freezing, cryosections, EM, and a battery of tissue stains at varying pH. A complete analysis begins with the search for myopathic changes including myofiber necrosis, regeneration, and cellular infiltration, excluding fiber type grouping and other features of neurogenic disease. This is followed by tissue stains for glycolytic and oxidative myofiber metabolism, and other investigations employing monoclonal antibody probes that recognize lymphocyte subset subsets, macrophages, MHC and complement factors, as well as specimens for, collagen staining, and ultrastructural analysis.

Although the presence of inflammation is the histological hallmark, an exhaustive analysis is often necessary to differentiate the various types of IM, a process that often entails further sectioning of the tissue block when the expected morphologic features are lacking and the findings are ascribed to skip lesions or random sampling. PM is characterized by endomysial infiltrates of CD8+ T-cells, mostly within the fascicle, surrounding individually healthy myofibers that express MHC-1, resulting in phagocytosis and necrosis. Chronic disease results in increased connective tissue formation and reaction with alkaline phosphatase staining.

The histologic hallmarks of IBM include basophilic granular inclusions distributed around the edge of slit-like rimmed vacuoles, scattered angulated and round fibers that can occur in small groups, with eosinophilic cytoplasmic inclusions, and primary endomysial inflammation composed of CD8+ T-cells that invade myofibers in a pattern identical to, but often more severe than PM. Tiny deposits of Congo red and crystal violet-positive amyloid immunoreactive with β-amyloid protein, the type sequenced from the amyloid fibrils of blood vessels of patients with Alzheimer disease, is found in or adjacent to vacuoles in up to 80% of patients. Characteristic filamentous inclusions are seen by EM in the cytoplasm or in myonuclei prominently in the vicinity of the rimmed vacuoles. Although the demonstration of filaments by EM was at one time essential to the diagnosis of IBM, it is no longer necessary when all of the characteristic light microscopic features, including the amyloid deposits, are present. Furthermore, the filamentous inclusions are not specific for IBM but can be seen in other vacuolar myopathies. Cytoplasmic tubulofilaments, within vacuolated muscle fibers strongly immunoreact with tau, ubiquitin, chymotrypsin, and prion (102). Finally, abnormal mitochondria are seen as ragged red fibers (RRF) may be associated with mitochondrial DNA (mtDNA) deletions (103).

In DM, the endomysial inflammation is predominantly perivascular or in the interfascicular septae, around rather than within the muscle fascicles, with activation of B-cell, CD4+ T-cells, and plasma cells. Intramuscular blood vessels show endothelial hyperplasia with tubuloreticular profiles, fibrin thrombi and obliteration of capillaries, as well as degeneration, phagocytosis, and myofiber necrosis, often in groups, involving a portion of a muscle fascicle in a wedge-like shape or at the periphery of the fascicle due to microscopic infarction. The latter results in perifascicular atrophy characterized by two to ten layers of atrophic fibers at the periphery of the fascicles. Unlike PM and sIBM, which demonstrate uniform expression of MHC-1 along the surface of myofibers, it is evident only in the perifascicular area in DM. Extranodal lymphoid microstructures, indicative of a more severe course, were noted in inflamed muscle of new-onset juvenile DM, suggesting that lymphoneogenesis was a factor in the early disease process of that disorder (104).

Nonetheless, there are several possible pitfalls in the interpretation of muscle histology that can lead to misdiagnosis (105). The commonest one is an error in interpretation that fails to distinguish sIBM from PM, and PM from one of several inflammatory muscular dystrophies, including Duchenne muscular dystrophy, dysferlinopathy, calpainopathy, merosin deficiency, and sarcoglycanopathy that present with prominent endomysial inflammation. The latter disorders, unlike PM and sIBM, show myofiber necrosis due to macrophage invasion instead of cytotoxic lymphocytes, and even when present, lack the MHC-1/CD8+ T-cell complex typical of PM and sIBM. Diagnostic pathology may be absent due to skip lesions, necessitating further sectioning of the tissue block, or even a second biopsy, as may be the case when the typical findings of perifascicular

atrophy are present in an otherwise consistent case of DM lacking prominent inflammatory cell infiltrates, leading to a categorically non-specific result.

Up to 25% of patients were categorized by combined clinical and muscle biopsy tissue criteria as PM/IBM due to a biopsy diagnosis of PM with clinical features of IBM (14). In the same regard, one reported patient with severe progressive myopathy with clinical features of DM had muscle pathology instead typical of IBM, suggesting that the inflammatory process of the former triggered the pathological changes of the latter (106). Finally, failure to morphologically assess intramuscular blood vessels for endothelial hyperplasia, tubuloreticular inclusions, fibrin thrombi, capillary obliteration, or perform immunofluoroscence for the terminal components of complement activation, may preclude a certain diagnosis of DM.

TOWARD A UNIFIED PATHOGENESIS OF INFLAMMATORY MYOPATHY

Advances have been achieved in our understanding of the mechanisms underlying the development and persistence of IM. Genetic influences increase the risk of developing inflammatory myopathy regardless of age and ethnicity, however multiple genetic influences are probably involved in its etiopathogenesis. Human leukocyte antigen (HLA) genes encompass the strongest risk factor, however many non-HLA polymorphic foci also appear to influence the risk of inflammatory myopathy through encoded immunoglobulins, cytokines, and their receptors. HLA B8 and the MHC-1 allele first associated with childhood DM, was later found to be in linkage disequilibrium with HLA class II genes. HLA DRB1*0313 and the linked allele DQA1*0501 have the strongest association with subsets of inflammatory myopathy, both sporadic and familial, in Caucasian children and adults. Other class II alleles, such as DMA*0103 and DMB*0102, increase the risk of DM in Caucasian children. Some differences occur in ethnic minorities. For example, HLA DQA10501 but not DRB1*0301, increases the risk of adult inflammatory myopathy and juvenile DM in African-Americans, whereas, the HLA DQA1*0501 haplotype increases the risk of DM in Hispanic children but not adults. The non-HLA genetic factors of importance include polymorphic genes that encode immunoglobulin heavy chains, such as the Gm allotypes on chromosome 14 associated with immunoglobulin responses, one gene that encodes the IL-1 receptor antagonist located on chromosome 2 that increased the risk for DM in Caucasian children, and another that encodes the polymorphic site for the TNF-α promoter region that increased the risk of inflammatory myopathy in Caucasian children due to linkage with DRB1*0301.

Apart from the risk of disease susceptibility, genetic studies have shown an influence on disease progression and duration by the TNF-α-308 allele with the associated production of TNF-α that perpetuates the inflammatory response (107). The folding and transportation of MHC-1 through the ER is tightly regulated and critical, but overexpression leads to ER stress with critical significance to genetically and developmentally young myofibers and, by extension, those with juvenile DM (108). Gene expression profiling comparing transgenic expression of MHC-1 in experimental transgenic myositis mice associated with carly or late muscle development, respectively referred to as HT-L and HT-E, found a more severe and rapid disease in the young mice compared to adults, with alterations in multiple proteins relating to ER function, protein transport, Golgi function, the SNARE complex, or ubiquitination pathway, suggesting an attempt to clear the increase of the MCH-1 resident protein.

Host immunological factors independently contribute the greatest share of factors involved in the etiopathogenesis of IM. Observations of the co-culture of autologous myotubes and cytotoxic T-cells isolated from muscle in IM (109) suggested that myofibers not only participated in T-cell mediated recruitment, antigen presentation, and co-stimulation (110), but also contributed to the stimulation of autoreactive T-cells and secretion of pro-inflammatory cytokines, facilitating the recruitment of activated T-cells, contributing to self-sustained endomysial inflammation (111, 112). It is now known that the migration of activated leukocyte and T cell subsets of muscle tissue requires a coordinated sequence of cellular and molecular events mediated by CAM, cytokine, and chemokine molecules (113).

The functional roles for CAM, cytokines, and chemokines in the initiation of the inflammatory response has been explored in cultured human myoblast studies and in muscle tissue of patients with subsets of inflammatory myopathy, notably PM and DM. Muscles cells in inflammatory myopathy constitutively express various cell surface molecules such as CD54, CD106, MHC class I and II antigens, apoptosis related molecules, CD40, and other molecules (114).

INF-γ induces the constitutive expression of CD40 in human myoblasts and in other cell systems, including mononuclear cells and activated T-cells of the CD4+ and, to a lesser extent, CD8+ type. Cross-linked activated CD40 ligand expressing CD4+ T-cells interactive with CD40 on human myocytes play a role in augmenting inflammation via upregulation of CD54, CD106, CAM, and local cytokine production, notably IL-6, IL-8, and monocyte chemoattractant protein-1 (MCP-1). The constitutive expression of the pro-inflammatory cytokines IL-1α, IL-1β, IL-6, and TNF-α, and the chemokines IL-8, MCP-1, and regulated upon activation normal T-cell expressed and secreted (RANTES), further contribute to inflammatory cell recruitment from the bloodstream (115).

The relevance of increased chemokine expression has been demonstrated in muscle sections from affected patients (116). The chemokines MCP-1, macrophage inflammatory protein-(MIP)-1α and their transcripts were detected in muscle sections in infiltrating inflammatory cells and in neighboring extracellular matrix by immunohistochemistry and polymerase chain reaction (PCR).

The importance of pro-inflammatory cytokines by cultured normal muscle cells has also been studied in sIBM, which is also typified by inflammatory cell infiltration (117), however the site of sensitization and the mechanisms that trigger the inflammatory reaction are not well understood. Cultured muscle cells increased the constitutive production of IL-6 in response to local deposition of amyloid-b (Ab) protein in sporadic IBM, suggesting a pro-inflammatory effect of Ab in vacuolated fibers. Since IL-1β and TNF-α were produced by Ab-stimulated human monocytes, it is possible that one of the pathologic mechanisms leading to cytokine expression in IBM depends on Ab deposition, which activates myogenic cells to release Il-6 and mononuclear phagocytes to IL-1β and TNFα, that in turn enhances the production of IL-6 by muscle cells and the resulting proinflammatory events (118).

The association of PM and sIBM with viruses and the retroviruses, HIV-1 and HTLV-1 in humans and simian immunodeficiency virus (SIV), has been fundamental in understanding potential triggers of muscle immunity (112, 119, 120). A mechanism of molecular mimicry was proposed for coxsackievirus-associated IM because of structural homology between the Jo-1 and the genomic RNA of an animal picornavirus, the encephalomyocarditis virus, however PCR studies repeatedly failed to confirm the presence of such viruses in the muscle biopsies of patients so studied, rendering it unlikely, although not impossible, for them to be replicated in the muscles of patients with PM, DM, and IBM.

Retrovirus-associated PM in monkeys infected with SIV (121, 122) and in humans infected with HIV-1 and HTLV-I (13, 123) provide convincing evidence of an association with IM. HIV-1-associated-PM can be the first clinical indication of HIV infection or occur concurrent with the manifestations of acquired immune deficiency syndrome (AIDS) (13, 124). HIV-1 seroconversion can coincide with myoglobulinuria and acute myalgia, suggesting that myotropism for HIV-1 may be symptomatic early in the infection. In addition, HTLV-I causes PM, which may be the only manifestation of HTLV-1 infection, or in association with the myeloneuropathy tropical spastic paraparesis (TSP) (123, 124). IBM also occurs with HIV-1 and HTLV-I infection (125) and like PM, cellular inflammation is comprised of endomysial CD8+ T-cells, which with macrophages, invade and surround MHC-I–antigen-expressing non-necrotic muscle fibers. In PM, in situ hybridization, PCR, immunocytochemistry, and EM fail to detect retroviral antigens within the myofiber, however, retroviral antigens are found instead in occasional endomysial macrophages (125–127). A T-cell–mediated MHC-I–restricted cytotoxic process appears to be a common pathogenetic mechanism in both retroviral negative and retroviral-positive PM and IBM but, in the latter, viral-induced cytokines might have triggered the process by breaking tolerance.

The pathogenesis of sIBM is complex as the onset of myofiber damage is age-related and the disease is slowly and inexorably progressive with evidence of intramyofiber accumulation of conformationally modified proteins and multiprotein aggregates, several of which are congophilic and, therefore, generically termed amyloid, including APP, amyloid-beta protein (Ab42), antibodies to phosphorylated neurofilaments SMI-31, the transporter protein p62/SQSTMI, presenilin-1, apolipoprotein E, γ-tubulin, clusterin, α-synuclein, gelsolin, as well as the oxidative and cell stress-related proteins, APP, chymotrypsin, apolipoprotien E, and phosphorylated tau (128, 129). The abnormal accumulation of multiprotein aggregates has been attributed to increased transcription of several proteins, posttranslational modifications and misfolding, and inadequate protein disposal, collectively termed *abnormal myoproteostasis*, combined with, or provoked by, an aging intracellular milieu (130).

Whether these deposits are secondarily related to the chronicity of the disease or are generated de novo, contributing to disease pathogenesis, is unclear. Mitochondrial abnormalities, seen in up to 70% of sIBM patients and attributed to large-scale mtDNA deletions leading to cytochrome c oxidase (COX)-deficient myofibers impairing mitochondrial function, probably contribute to muscle weakness and wasting (131). They are associated with clonal expansion of mtDNA deletions and point mutations in segments of muscle fibers ranging from 75 um to more than 1,000 μ in length, the commonest of which is expansion of the common deletion, 4977 bp (131). The deletion breakpoints, which cluster in a few regions and are similar to those in human mtDNA, were not associated with mutations in the three nuclear genes *POLG1*, *ANT1*, and *C10orf2*, most often associated with multiple mtDNA deletions (131). The transfer of the *βAPP* gene on chromosome 21, using an adenovirus vector, which produces several alternatively spliced isoforms, the largest of which (APP-751 and APP-770) contain an insert of a Kunitz-type protease inhibitor (KP1) in their extracellular region, caused mitochondrial abnormalities in cultured normal human muscle, suggesting that *βAPP* may be responsible for mitochondrial and COX abnormalities in IBM muscle (132).

While the observation of abnormal tau immunoreactivity, accumulation of TDP-43, and mutations in the valosin-containing protein (*VCP*) gene, implicated in IBM, Paget disease, and frontotemporal dementia (IBMPFD) (133, 134), further supports a role for neurodegeneration, it is the interplay of neuroinflammation evidenced by a strong primary inflammatory response and overexpression of pro-inflammatory mediators, MHC-I antigen, and neurodegeneration, that distinguishes IBM (135).

The interrelation of inflammation and APP in sIBM is supported by the observation that IL-1 induces accumulation of β-amyloid in skeletal muscle (111, 135).

The inflammatory mediators IFN-γ and CXCL-9 correlate with protein and mRNA level of βAPP expression, and colocalize with β-amyloid proteins. The exposure of muscle cells to the pro-inflammatory cytokines IL-1β and IFN-γ leads to overexpression of APP with subsequent accumulation of β-amyloid, similar to induction of tau pathology induced by LPS-induced inflammation via glycogen synthase kinase-3-beta with accumulation of tau and β-amyloid (39).

The heat shock protein (HSP) molecule, αβ-crystallin, associated with cell stress and β-amyloid clearance and present in healthy-appearing IBM myofibers, stained doubly positive for APP and MHC-I antigen even before these myofibers showed β-amyloid deposits, other markers of vacuolar degeneration, or T-cell invasion(136, 137). Human myotubes exposed to IL-1β and INF-γ upregulated APP and αβ-crystallin with accumulationof β amyloid, suggesting that αβ-crystallin upregulation, along with other pro-inflammatory markers, are early events associated with cell stress-response that precedes accumulation of β-amyloid (137). The continuous stimulationof inflammatory factors in sIBM, may after a long period, induce a higher basal expression of APP and an increased sensitivity to de novo pro-inflammatory cytokines, triggering a self-perpetuating cycle (111, 112, 135, 138–140).

TREATMENT

The goal of therapy in inflammatory myopathy is to improve muscle strength and thereby improve overall function in activities of daily living. When strength improves, the serum CK also tends to fall, but the reverse is not always true because most immunosuppressive therapies can result in decrease of serum muscle enzymes without necessarily improving muscle strength. The orientation of treating the CK level instead of the muscle disease activity, best ascertained by serial muscle testing, functional measures of daily living, and electrodiagnostic studies, may still be so imprecise as to engender prolonged immunosuppressive drug therapy or erroneous assessment of drug efficacy. Although at present there is general reliance upon older medications such as the corticosteroids (CS) for initial therapy in IM, effective and target-oriented immunotherapy, focusing on immuno-pathogenic-specific mechanisms relevant to the particular subtype of IM, forms the basis for the rational use of available immune suppressants and modulators (62, 140–142).

Such therapy of DM focuses upon modulating or interrupting complement activation early in the disease, averting formation and deposition of the terminal components of complement on endomysial capillaries, and the later sequela of capillary destruction, perivascular inflammation, and perifascicular ischemia.

A similar target-oriented immunotherapy approach to PM and, to an extent, IBM, attempts to intercept clonally expanded CD8+ cytotoxic T-cells complexed with MHC-1, or to attenuate the epimysial infiltration associated with myofiber necrosis via the perforin pathway (21, 112, 143), However, the added features of neurodegeneration characterized by rimmed vacuoles and deposition of congophilic β-amyloid and other misfolded proteins in sIBM present challenges to effective therapy.

Current treatment options of IM, few of which have been studied in randomized, placebo-controlled trials sufficient to establish detailed algorithms, can be categorized into first-line therapy employing CS, second-line conventional agents, depending upon whether there is a documented response to CS, and third-line therapies employing new or emerging biological substances, especially in those who are unresponsive to conventional therapies.

First-Line Therapy

Corticosteroids

Prednisone exerts a beneficial effect by inhibiting recruitment and migration of lymphocytes to the areas of muscle inflammation while interfering with the production of lymphokines, including IL-1, which is secreted by activated macrophages-invading muscle fibers (144). CS-induced suppression of ICAM-1 may also be relevant to its action in IM since down-regulation of ICAM-1 prevents lymphocyte trafficking across the endothelial cell wall toward the muscle fibers. Other salutary effects can be attributed to the multiplicity of effects on the cell and humoral immune system, including inhibition of activated T- and B-cells, antigen-presenting cells (APC), and leukocytes at sites of inflammation, IFN-γ- induced MHC class II expression, macrophage differentiation, and complement interactions.

Since the effectiveness and relative safety of prednisone therapy will determine the future need for stronger immunosuppressive drugs, it is preferable to commence therapy with high doses, such as 80 to 100 mg per day and, after three to four weeks, gradually reduce the alternate off-day dose by 5 to 10 mg per week to 0, while watching for breakthrough of disease. With sustained improve-

ment, an attempt can be made to gradually taper the dose further by 5 to 10 mg every three to four weeks until the lowest possible dose that controls the disease is reached, after which the choice is made to add a steroid-sparing agent. However, if after tapering the alternate day dose to 0 there is no increase in muscle strength, then the patient should be deemed unresponsive and further reduction in dosage accelerated while empirically choosing from among appropriate second-line agents, based largely on the anticipated efficacy and safety ratio.

Patrick and Bohan (10) considered a responsiveness to CS as improved muscle strength, not just a lowering of serum muscle enzymes, whereas CS resistance was considered a lack of a clinical response after an empiric three to four month course of 60 mg of daily prednisone, after which consideration would be given to immunosuppressive medication, deeming that further therapy would not be expected to show beneficial results.

One series of 89 patients with PM (9), defined clinically and electrodiagnostically with compatible serum CK levels and muscle biopsy confirmation, ascertained a response rate leading to full or nearly full recovery among 29 of 62 (46%) surviving patients with PM after a course of 40 to 80 mg of daily prednisone that was reduced slowly over the course of months to a maintenance level of 5 to 15 mg and a reasonably stable symptom-free status. Overall mortality of 30% was adjusted to 16% after excluding 16 patients who died with malignant neoplasms. Alternate-day CS in neuromuscular diseases, first suggested by Engel and coworkers (145), spares the pituitary axis and reduces side effects of hypertension, fluid retention, glucose intolerance, cataracts, myopathy, avascular necrosis, osteoporosis, infection, gastric and duodenal ulcers, and psychosis.

There is some overlap in the choice of steroid-sparing agents for CS responders and non-responders, however CS-sparing agents employed in initial responders include azathioprine, methotrexate, and mycophenolate mofetil.

Azathioprine

The oral purine analog azathioprine, which metabolizes to the cytotoxic derivative 6-mercaptopurine, is an empirically useful long-term therapy for IM. It inhibits T-cell activation and T-cell-dependent antibody-mediated responses and is considered a safe alternative to prednisone. However, there are three drawbacks to its use. First, idiosyncratic side effects, most often gastrointestinal and flu-like, including pancreatitis and gastritis severe enough to warrant hospitalization, occur in approximately 10% of patients although rarely necessitate permanent withdrawal of the medication. Second, bone marrow suppression occurs in all patients, usually manifested by mild pancytopenia. Third, there is an expected long delay in the onset of the therapeutic effect of three months or more. Susceptibility to toxicity, which appears to be genetically dependent on inter-individual variations in thiopurine-S-methyl transferase (TPMT) enzyme activity, is based upon genetic polymorphisms of high-metabolizing versus low-metabolizing alleles (146). Taking all of these factors into account, most clinicians concur with the slow advancement of the dose over weeks, commencing with 50 mg/day and achieving maintenance levels of 2 to 3 mg/kg/day with careful monitoring of liver and bone marrow function indices.

Methotrexate

Methotrexate, an antagonist of folate metabolism that is administered orally or intravenously, was historically recommended as the immunosuppressant drug of choice in PM and DM because of an observed response rate greater than 75% without hepatic or other major toxicity (147). It has a faster mode of action than azathioprine, and while superiority of either agent as monotherapy has yet to be established, there was equivalent efficacy as adjunctive treatment when added to CS in a randomized, double-blind placebo-controlled trial (148). The starting dosage is 7.5 mg per week for three weeks, given 2.5 mg three times daily, gradually increasing it by 2.5 mg per week to a total of 20 to 25 mg. Pneumonitis is a side effect that can be difficult to distinguish from the ILD associated with Jo-1 antibodies. Other less common side effects include stomatitis, gastrointestinal symptoms, leukopenia, thrombocytopenia, and hepatotoxicity.

Mycophenolate Mofetil

Mycophenolate mofetil, a purine antimetabolite that has efficacy in the inhibition of solid organ transplant rejection medication, is a morpholinoethyl ester of mycophenolic acid that promptly inhibits new B- and T-cell production. With a profile similar to azathioprine, and a lag period of three to six months before the salutary effects of suppression of existing circulating lymphocytes are noted, it is typically employed after initial treatment with a first-line agent such as prednisone. It has a side effect profile like azathioprine and is well tolerated in daily divided doses of up to 3 grams per day. Myocphenolate mofetil at a dose of 1.5 grams daily was given to one patient with ankylosing spondylitis, ulcerative colitis, and severe refractory PM after other conventional treatment regimens, leading to considerable improvement of clinical and EMG findings within 6 months of commencement of therapy which allowed for tapering of CS (149).

Second-Line Therapy

Intravenous Immune Globulin

High-dose IVIG therapy is the most widely employed immunomodulating agent for autoimmune neurological disorders. Its beneficial effects in the treatment of IM is attributed to blocking of endomysial deposition of activated complement fragments, suppression of cytokines, especially ICAM-1, saturation of Fc receptors, and interference with the action of macrophages (59).

The first IVIg preparation, a 5% IgG concentration formulated in a 10% maltose and 0.1 molar glycine solution, was licensed in the United States in 1981 for combined immunodeficiency syndrome. It was prepared by the classic Cohn cold water alcohol fractionation processing of pooled plasma from at least 1000 normal donors and chemically modified by selective reduction with dithiothreitol, and alkylation with iodoacetamide.

Continuing research led to the development of a native 5% IVIg preparation in which the IgG molecule was chemically unmodified and stabilized in solution at pH 4.25 with 10% maltose added to provide isotonicity. A 10% IVIg solution using the same manufacturing method was licensed in 1992. Solvent detergent treatment, including partitioning steps, and incubation at low pH in the final container, has been effective in the removal and inactivation of enveloped viruses. A chromatographic purification process alleviates many labor-intensive and time-consuming intermediate steps, with a more closed manufacturing process to reduce risk of contamination, and provides a glycine-stabilized, purer final IVIg product that more closely reflects the IgG subclass distribution found in plasma.

The immunomodulating and anti-inflammatory actions of IVIg are provided by monthly doses of 2000 mg/kg per body weight, and given 400 mg per kg daily for up to five consecutive doses each month via slow drip with acetaminophen and diphenydramine pretreatment to prevent side effects, that include fever, chills, rash, erythema, flushing, headache, nausea, myalgia, arthralgia, abdominal cramps, and chest and back pain.

True anaphylactic reactions to IVIg can occur in recipients with documented prior allergies to immune globulins or antibodies, especially of the IgA type. Transient reversible renal insufficiency occurs in individuals with preexisting renal disease. Susceptible individuals can be identified by less- than-normal expected 24-hour creatinine clearance rates for age, and abnormal vascular perfusion on radionuclide scans. Aseptic meningitis rarely occurs several hours after treatment and resolves over several days with discontinuation of therapy.

One Class II study in DM, two Class I- studies, and one Class II study in sIBM (150) reported the findings of IVIg treatment. Dalakas and colleagues (60) studied efficacy of IVIg in refractory DM in a double-blind Class II crossover study of 15 adult patients showing improvement in five outcome measures after three months of treatment, including summed MRC scores of strength, neuromuscular symptom score, muscle cytoarchitecture, and muscle inflammation in repeat muscle biopsy specimens. Benefits were usually evident after the first month and clearly present after two months, but were generally short-lived and usually for not more than eight weeks. Repeated infusions at six to eight weekly intervals were generally necessary to maintain improvement.

Contemporaneously, Jann and coworkers (151) reported an uncontrolled study of the successful treatment of two patients with CS-resistant PM. Dalakas and colleagues (152) studied efficacy of IVIg in a double-blind study of 19 patients with sIBM, showing improvement in summed modified MRC score of strength, although insignificant compared to controls, was associated with significantly improved swallowing function in the treated group. Dalakas and colleagues (153) assessed the addition of high-dose prednisone to IVIg in sIBM showing a decline in the number of necrotic myofibers and endomysial inflammatory foci in the treated group, without significant clinical differences in summed or quantitative muscle strength testing three months after cessation of therapy compared to controls. Walter and coworkers (154) conducted a double-bind, placebo-controlled crossover study of the efficacy of IVIg in sIBM, showing significant improvement in the neuromuscular symptom score during the first six months of treatment, without other significant differences compared to controls.

Cyclophosphamide

Cyclophosphamide is an alkylating agent that can be given intravenously or orally at dosages of 2 to 2.5 mg/kg in 50-mg tablets three times daily. It has not been effective in

our experience (155) despite occasional promising results reported by others (156).

Rituximab

This monoclonal antibody against CD20+ B-cells causes prompt depletion of circulation B cells (157). Rituximab, administered 375 mg per m² weekly for four weeks, or two grams in divided biweekly doses of 1 gram each, is well-tolerated and possibly effective therapy for all types of IM (158), with few complications including that it can be easily managed with antihistamines and CS. Although infection is rare, progressive multifocal leukoencephalopathy can occur.

Tacrolimus

Formerly known as FK506, tacrolimus is structurally different from cyclosporine, although they share the ability to selectively inhibit transcription of cytokines, specifically IL-2. Although published experience is lacking, tacrolimus led to clinical improvement in one patient with refractory PM with ILD (159) and three others with sIBM as alternate therapy of cyclosporine-A, in combination with CS (160). An observation study of the effects of tacrolimus on thymic output in patients with refractory PM and DM (161) showed significantly attenuated T-cell receptor excision circle (TREC) content in cultured CD4+CD8+ cells from patients with normal total cell counts, indicating that tacrolimus therapy suppresses not only activated T-lymphocytes, but also some naïve T-cell subsets in IM.

Emerging Therapies

Involvement of activated complement, T- and B-cells, cytokines, adhesion and transmigration molecules in the pathogenesis of IM justifies off-label consideration of several new target-specific biological agents in selected patients, reviewed elsewhere (62, 146).

REFERENCES

1. Mastaglia FL, Needham M. Update on toxic myopathies. *Curr Neurol Neurosci Rep* 2012; 12:54–61.
2. Ellis E, Tan JA, Lester S, et al. Necrotizing myopathy: Clinico-serological associations. *Muscle Nerve* 2012; 189–194.
3. Dalakas MC. H. Autoimmune inflammatory myopathies. *Handb Clin Neurol* 2007; 86:273–301.
4. Wagner E. Fall Einer Seltnen Muskelkrankheit. *Arch Heilkd* 1863; 4:288.
5. Eaton LM. The perspective of neurology in regard to polymyositis. *Neurology* 1954; 4:245–263.
6. Walton JN, Adams RD. *Polymyositis.* Edinburgh: E&S. Livingston, 1958.
7. Rowland LP. Muscular dystrophies, polymyositis and other myopathies. *J Chronic Dis* 1958; 8:51–535.

8. Pearson CM, Rose AS. Myositis: The inflammatory disorders of muscle. *Res Publ Assoc Res Nerve Ment Dis* 1960; 38:422–478.
9. Rose AL, Walton JN. Polymyositis: A survey of 89 cases with particular reference to treatment and prognosis. *Brain* 1966; 89:747–768.
10. Bohan A, Peter JB. Polymyositis and dermatomyositis. *N Engl J Med* 1975; 344:344–347; 403–407.
11. Dalakas MC. Toxic and drug-induced myopathies. *J Neurol Neurosurg Psychiatry* 2009; 80:832–838.
12. Needham M, Fabian V, Knezivic W, et al. Progressive myopathy with up-regulation of MHC-1 associated with statin therapy. *Neuromuscl Disord* 2007; 17:194–200.
13. Dalakas MC, Pezeschkpour GH, Gravell M, et al. Polymyositis in patients with AIDS. *JAMA* 1986; 256:2381–2383.
14. Chahin N, Engel AG. Correlation of muscle biopsy, clinical

course, and outcome in PM and sporadic IBM. *Neurology* 2008; 70:418–424.

15. Van der Meulen MFG, Bronner IM, Hoogendijk JE, et al. Polymyositis: an overdiagnosed entity. *Neurology* 2003; 61:316–321.

16. O'Hanlon TP, Dalakas MC, Plotz PH, et al. Predominant TCR-alpha-beta-variable and joining gene expression by muscle-infiltrating lymphocytes in the idiopathic inflammatory myopathies. *J Immunol* 1994; 152:2569–2576.

17. Nishio J, Suzuki M, Miyasaka N, et al. Clonal biases of peripheral CD8 T cell repertoire directly reflect local inflammation in polymyositis. *J Immunol* 2001; 167:4051–4058.

18. Greenberg SA, Pinkus GS, Amato AA, et al. Myeloid dendritic cells in inclusion-body myositis and polymyositis. *Muscle Nerve* 2007; 35:17–23.

19. Bradshaw EM, Orihuela A, McArdel SL, et al. A local antigen-driven humoral response is present in the inflammatory myopathies. *J Immunol* 2007; 178:547–556.

20. Nagaraju K, Casciola-Rosen L, Lundberg I, et al. Activation of the endoplasmic reticulum stress response in autoimmune myositis: potential role in muscle fiber damage and dysfunction. *Arthritis Rheum* 2005; 52:1824–1835.

21. Dalakas MC. Mechanisms of disease: signaling pathways and immunobiology of inflammatory myopathies. *Nat Clin Pract Rheumatol* 2006; 2:219–227.

22. Chou SM. Myxovirus-like structures in a case of chronic polymyositis. *Science* 1967; 158:1453–1455.

23. Carpenter S, Karpati G, Wolff L. Virus-like filaments and phospholipid accumulation in skeletal muscle: study of a histochemically distinct chronic myopathy. *Neurology* 1970; 20:889–903.

24. Yunis EJ, Samaha FJ. Inclusion body myositis. *Lab Invest* 1971; 25:240–248.

25. Carpenter S, Karpati G, Heller I, et al. Inclusion body myositis: a distinct variety of idiopathic inflammatory myopathy. *Neurology* 1978; 28:8–17.

26. Dabby R, Lange DJ, Trojaborg W, et al. Inclusion body myositis mimicking motor neuron disease. *Arch Neurol* 58:1253–1256.

27. Luciano CA, Dalakas MC. A macro-EMG study in inclusion-body myositis: no evidence for a neurogenic component. *Neurology* 1997; 48:29–33.

28. Sekul EA, Dalakas MC. Inclusion body myositis: new concepts. *Semin Neurol* 1993; 13:256–263.

29. Barohn RJ, Herbelin BS, Kissel JT, et al. Pilot trial of etanercept in the treatment of inclusion body myositis. *Neurology* 2006; 66(Suppl 1):S123–S124.

30. Jackson CE, Barohn RJ, Gronseth G, et al, and the Muscle Study Group (MSG). Inclusion body myositis functional rating scale: a reliable and valid measure of disease severity. *Muscle Nerve* 2008; 37:473–476.

31. Sadjadi R, Rose MR, Muscle Study Group. What determines quality of life in inclusion body myositis? *J Neurol Neurosurg Psychiatry* 2010; 81:1164–1166.

32. Rose MR, McDermott MP, Thornton CA, et al. A prospective natural history study of inclusion body myositis: implications for clinical trials. *Neurology* 2001; 57:548–550.

33. Peng A, Koffman BM, Malley JD, et al. Disease progression in sporadic inclusion body myositis: observations in 78 patients. *Neurology* 2000; 55:296–298.

34. Griggs RC. The current status of treatment for inclusion-body myositis. *Neurology* 2006; 66(Suppl1):S30–S32.

35. Askanas V, Dalakas MC, Engel WK. Inclusion-body myositis. Clinical and pathologic aspects, and basic research potentially relevant to treatment. *Neurology* 2006; 66(Suppl 1):Si.

36. Garlepp MJ, Tabarias H, van Bockxmeer FM, et al. Apolipoprotein E epsilon-4 in inclusion body myositis. *Ann Neurol* 1995; 38:957–959.

37. Askanas V, Engel WK, McFerrin J, et al. Transthyretin val-122ile, accumulated A-beta, and inclusion-body myositis aspects in cultured muscle. *Neurology* 2003; 61:257–260.

38. Salajehheh M, Pinkus JL, Taylor JP, et al. Sarcoplasmic redistribution of nuclear TDP-43 in inclusion body myositis. *Muscle Nerve* 2009; 40:19–31.

39. Kitazawa M, Trinh DN, LaFerla FM. Inflammation induces tau pathology in inclusion body myositis model via glycogen synthase kinase-3-beta. *Ann Neurol* 2008; 64:15–24.

40. Baumbach LL, Neville HE, Ringel SP, et al. Familial inclusion body myositis: evidence for autosomal dominant inheritance (Abstract). *Am J Hum Genet* 1990; 47(Suppl):A48.

41. Goldfarb LG, Park K-Y, Cervenakova L, et al. Missense mutations in desmin associated with familial cardiac and skeletal myopathy. *Nature Genet* 1998; 19:402–403.

42. van Spaendonck-Zwarts KY, van Hesem L, Jongbloed JDH, et al. Desmin-related myopathy. *Clin Genet* 2011; 80:354–366.

43. Argov A, Yarom R. 'Rimmed vacuole myopathy' sparing the quadriceps: a unique disorder in Iranian Jews. *J Neurol Sci* 1984; 64:33–43.

44. Ricci E, Broccolini A, Gidaro T, et al. NCAM is hyposialyated in hereditary inclusion body myopathy due to GNE mutations. *Neurology* 2006; 66:755–758.

45. Krause S, Aleo A, Hinderlich S, et al. GNE protein expression and subcellular distribution are unaltered in HIBM. *Neurology* 2007; 69:655–659.

46. Eisenberg L, Avidan N, Potikha T, Hochner H, et al. The UDP-N-acetylglucosamine-2-epimerase/N-acetylmannosamine kinase gene is mutated in recessive hereditary inclusion body myopathy. *Nature Genet* 2001; 29:83–87.

47. Nonaka I, Sunohara N, Ishiura S, et al. Familial distal myopathy with rimmed vacuole and lamellar (myeloid) body formation. *J Neurol Sci* 1981; 51:141–155.

48. Darin N, Kyllerman M, Wahlstrom J, et al. Autosomal dominant myopathy with congenital joint contractures, opthalmoplegia, and rimmed vacuoles. *Ann Neurol* 1998; 44:242–248.

49. Martinsson T, Darin N, Kyllerman M, et al. Dominant hereditary inclusion-body myopathy gene (IBM3) maps to chromosome region 17p13.1. *Am J Hum Genet* 1999; 64:1420–1426.

50. Martinsson T, Oldfors A, Darin N, et al. Autosomal dominant myopathy: missense mutation (glu-706-to-lys) in the myosin heavy chain IIa gene. *Proc Nat Acad Sci* 2000; 97:14614–14619.

51. Otero C, Illa I, Dalakas MC. Is there dermatomyositis (DM) without myositis? *Neurology* 1992; 42(Suppl):388.

52. Dalakas MC, Hohfield R. Polymyositis and dermatomyositis. *Lancet* 2003; 362:971–982.

53. Greenberg SA, Pinkus JL, Pinkus GS, et al. Interferon-αβ-mediated innate immune mechanisms in dermatomyositis. *Ann Neurol* 2005; 57:664–678.

54. Kissel JT, Mendell JR, Rammohan KW. Microvascular deposition of complement membrane attack complex in dermatomyositis. *N Engl J Med* 1986; 314:329–334.

55. Kissel JT, Halterman RK, Rammohan KW, et al. The relationship of complement-mediated mirovasculopathy to the histologic features and clinical duration of disease in dermatomyositis. *Arch Neurol* 1991; 48:26–30.

56. de Visser M, Emslie-Smith AM, Engel AG. Early ultrastructural alterations in adult dermatomyositis, Capillary abnormalities precede other structural changes in muscle. *J Neurol Sci* 1989; 94:181–192.

57. Emslie-Smith AM, Engel AG. Microvascular changes in early and advanced dermatomyositis: a quantitative study. *Ann Neurol* 1990; 27:343–356.

58. Greenberg SA. Proposed immunologic models of the inflammatory myopathies and potential therapeutic implications. *Neurology* 2007; 69:2008–2009.

59. Basta M, Dalakas MC. High-dose intravenous immunoglobulin exerts its beneficial effect in patients with dermatomyositis by blocking endomysial deposition of activated complement fragments. *J Clin Invest* 1994; 94:1729–1735.

60. Dalakas MC, Illa I, Dambrosia JM, et al. A controlled trial of high-dose intravenous immunoglobulin infusions as treatment for dermatomyositis. *N Engl J Med* 1993; 329:1993–2000.

61. Walsh RJ, Kong SW, Yao Y, et al. Type I interferon-inducible gene expression in blood is present and reflects disease activity in dermatomyositis ad polymyositis. *Arthritis Rheum* 2007; 56:3784–3792.

62. Dalakas MC. Immunotherapy of inflammatory myopathies: practical approach and future prospects. *Curr Treat Options Neurol* 2011; 13:311–323.

63. Daube JR, Rubin DI. Needle electromyography. *Muscle Nerve* 2009; 39:244–270.

64. Gilchrist JM, Sachs GM. Electrodiagnostic studies in the management and prognosis of neuromuscular disorders. *Muscle Nerve* 2004; 29:165–190.

65. Amato AA, Barohn RJ. Evaluation and treatment of inflammatory myopathies. *J Neurol Neurosurg Psychiatry* 2009; 80:1060–1068.

66. Cong L, Pu C, Mao Y, et al. Role of C5b-9 expression in skeletal muscle blood vessels in necrotizing myopathy. *Nan Fang Yi Ke Da Xue Xue Bao*2012; 32:714–717.

67. Christopher-Suine L, Casciola-Rosen LA, Hong G, et al. A novel autoantibody recognizing 200-kd and 100-kd proteins is associated with an immune-mediated necrotizing myopathy. *Arthritis Rheum* 2010; 62:2757–2766.

68. Mehndiratta Pl Mehta S, Manjil SV, et al. Isolated necrotizing myopathy associated with ANTI-PL12 antibody. *Muscle Nerve* 2012; 46:282–286.

69. Selva-O'Callaghan, Sanchez-Sitjes L, Munoz-Gall X, et al. Respiratory failure due to muscle weakness in inflammatory myopathies: maintenance therapy with home mechanical ventilation. *Rheumatology* 2000; 39:914–914.

70. Hirakata M, Nagai S. Interstitial lung disease in polymyositis and dermatomyositis. *Curr Opin Rheumatol* 2000; 12:501–508.

71. Clawson K, Oddis CV. Adult respiratory distress syndrome in polymyositis patients with the anti-Jo-I antibody. *Arthritis Rheum* 1995; 38:1519–1523.

72. Schwarz MI, Sutarik JM, Nick JA, et al. Pulmonary capillaritis and diffuse alveolar hemorrhage: a primary manifestation of polymyositis. *Am J Respir Crit Care Med* 1995; 151:2037–2040.

73. Dalakas MC. Calcifications in dermatomyositis. *N Engl J Med* 1995; 333:978.

74. Buchbinder R, Forbes A, Hall SH, et al. Incidence of malignant disease in biopsy-proven inflammatory myopathy. *Ann Intern Med* 2001; 134:1087–1095.

75. Hill CL, Zhang Y, Sigurgeirsson B, et al. Frequency of specific cancer types in dermatomyositis and polymyositis: a population based study. *Lancet* 2001; 357:96–100.

76. Pautas E, Cherin P, Piette J-C, et al. Features of polymyositis and dermatomyositis in the elderly: a case-control study. *Clinical and Experimental Rheumatology* 2000; 18:241–244.

77. Garlepp MJ, Mastaglia FL. Autoantibodies in inflammatory myopathies. *Am J Med Sci* 2000; 319:227–233.

78. Mozaffar T, Pestronk A. Myopathy with anti-Jo-1 antibodies: pathology in perimysium and neighboring muscle fibers. *J Neurol Neurosurg Psychiatry* 2000; 68:472–478.

79. Brouwer R, Hengstman GJD, Vree Egberts W, et al. Autoantibody profiles in the sera of European patients with myositis. *Ann Rheum Dis* 2001; 60:116–123.

80. Zhang Y, LeRoy G, Seelig HP, et al. The dermatomyositis-specific autoantigen Mi-2 is a component of a complex containing histone deacetylase and nucleosome remodeling activities. *Cell* 1998; 95:279–289.

81. Mammen AL, Casciola-Rosen A, Hall JC, et al. Expression of the dermatomyositis autoantigen Mi-2 in regenerating muscle. *Arthritis Rheum* 2009; 60:3784–3793.

82. Hengstman GJD, Brouwer R, Vree Egberts WTM, et al. Clinical and serological characteristics of 125 Dutch myositis patients. Myositis specific autoantibodies aid in the differential diagnosis of the idiopathic myopathies. *J Neurol* 2002; 249:69–75.

83. Hengstman GJD, Vree Egberts WTM, Seelig HP, et al. Clinical characteristics of patients with myositis and autoantibodies to different fragments of the Mi-2B antigen. *Ann Rheum* 2006; 65:242–245.

84. Stalberg E. Invited review: Electrodiagnostic assessment and monitoring of motor unit changes in disease. *Muscle Nerve* 1991; 14:293–303.

85. Sandstedt P, Henriksson KG, Larsson L-E, et al. Quantitative electromyography in polymyositis and dermatomyositis: A long-term study. *Acta Neurol Scand* 1982; 65:110–121.

86. Pfeiffer G. The diagnostic power of motor unit potential analysis: an objective Bayseian approach. *Muscle Nerve* 1999; 22:584–591.

87. Barkhaus PE, Nandedkar SD, Sanders DB. Quantitative EMG in inflammatory myopathy. *Muscle Nerve* 1990; 13:247–253.

88. Nandekar SD, Barkhaus PE, Charles A. Multi-motor unit action potential analysis (MMA). *Muscle Nerve* 1995; 18:1155–1166.

89. Fuglsang-Frederiksen A. The utility of interference pattern analysis. *Muscle Nerve* 2000; 23:18–36.

90. Fuglsang-Frederiksen A, Smith T, Hogenhaven H. Motor unit firing intervals and other parameters of electrical activity in normal and pathological muscle. *J Neurol Sci* 1987; 78:51–62.

91. Stalberg E. Macro electromyography, an update. *Muscle Nerve* 2011; 44:292–302.

92. Barkhaus PE, Periquet MI, Nandedkar SD. Quantitative electophysiologic studies in sporadic inclusion body myositis. *Muscle Nerve* 1999; 22:480–487.

93. Blijham PJ, Hengstman JD, Ter Laak HJ, et al. Muscle-fiber conduction velocity and electromyography as diagnostic tools in patients with suspected inflammatory myopathy: a prospective study. *Muscle Nerve* 2004; 29:46–50.

94. Park JH, Olsen NJ. Utility of magnetic resonance imaging in the evaluation of patients with inflammatory myopathy. *Curr Rheumatol Rep* 2001; 3:334–345.

95. Mastaglia FL, Garlepp MJ, Phillips BA, et al. Inflammatory myopathies: clinical, diagnostic and therapeutic aspects. *Muscle Nerve* 2003; 27:407–425.

96. McCullough MB, Domire ZJ, Reed AM, et al. Evaluation of muscles affected by myositis using magnetic resonance elastrography. *Muscle Nerve* 2011; 43:585–590.

97. Rehn TA, Borge BA, Lunde PK et al. Temporary fatigue and altered extracellular matrix in skeletal muscle during progression of heart failure in rats. *Am J Physiol Regul Integr Comp Physiol* 2009; 297:R26–R33.

98. Sato S, Hirakata M, Kuwana M, et al. Autoantibodies to a 140-kd polypeptide, CADM-140, in Japanese patients with clinically amyopathic dermatomyositis. *Arthritis Rheum* 2005; 52:1571–1576.

99. Gengstman GJD, van Engelen BGM, et al. Familial inclusion body myositis with histologically confirmed sensorimotor neuropathy. *J Neurol* 2000; 415:882–884.

100. Amato AA, Gronseth GS, Jackson CE, et al. Inclusion body myositis: clinical and pathological boundaries. *Ann Neurol* 40:581–586.

101. Lindberg C, Oldfors A, Hedstrom A. Inclusion body myositis: peripheral nerve involvement. Combined morphological and

electrophysiological studies on peripheral nerves. *J Neurol Sci* 1989; 99:327–338.

102. Askanas V, Serdaroglu P, Engel WK, et al. Immunocytochemical localization of ubiquitin in inclusion body myositis allows its light-microscopic distinction from polymyositis. *Neurology* 1992; 42:460–461.

103. Santorelli FM, Sciacco M, Tanji K, et al. Multiple mitochondrial DNA deletions in sporadic inclusion body myositis: a study of 56 patients. *Ann Neurol* 1996; 39:789–795.

104. Lopez de Padilla C, Vallejo AB, Lacomis D, et al. Extranodal lymphoid microstructures in inflamed muscle and disease severity of new-onset juvenile dermatomyositis. *Arthritis Rheum* 2009; 1160–1172.

105. Dalakas MC. Review: An update on inflammatory and autoimmune myopathies. *Neuropathology and Applied Neurobiology* 2011; 37:226–242.

106. Layzer R, Lee HS, Iverson D, et al. Dermatomyositis with inclusion body myositis pathology. *Muscle Nerve* 2009; 40:469–471.

107. Pachman LM, Liotta-Davis MR, Hong DK, et al. TNF-alpha 308A allele in juvenile dermatomyositis. *Arthritis and Rheum* 2000; 43:2368–2377.

108. Li CK-C, Knopp P, Moncrieffe H, et al. Overexpression of MCH class I heavy chain protein in young skeletal muscle leads to severe myositis. Implications for juvenile myositis. *Am J Pathol* 2009; 175:1030–1040.

109. Hohlfeld R, Engel AG. Coculture with autologous myotubes of cytotoxic T cells isolated from muscle in inflammatory myopathies. *Ann Neurol* 1991; 29:498–507.

110. Wiendl H, Hohlfeld R, Kieseier BC. Immunobiology of muscle: advances in understanding an immunological microenvironment. *Trends Immunol* 2005; 26:373–380.

111. Schmidt J, Barthel K, Wrede A, et al. Interrelation of inflammation and APP in sIBM: IL-1 beta induces accumulation of beta-amyloid in skeletal muscle. *Brain* 2008; 131:1228–4050.

112. Dalakas MC Sporadic inclusion body myositis: diagnosis, pathogenesis and therapeutic strategies. *Nat Clin Prac Neurol* 2006:2:437–447.

113. Figarella-Branger D, Civatte M, Bartoli C, et al. Cytokines, chemokines, and cell adhesion molecules in inflammatory myopathies. *Muscle Nerve* 2003; 28:659–682.

114. Sugiura T, Kawaguchi Y, Harigai M, et al. Increased CD40 expression on muscle cells of polymyositis and dermatomyositis: role of CD40-CD40 ligand interaction in IL-6, IL-8, IL-15, and monocyte chemoattractant protein-1 production. *J Immunol* 2000; 164:6593–6600.

115. De Rossi M, Benison P, Baggy F, et al. Cytokines and chemokines are both expressed by human myoblasts: possible relevance for the immune pathogenesis of muscle inflammation. *International Immunology* 2000; 12:1329–1335.

116. Confalonieri P, Bernascni P, Megna P, et al. Increased expression of b-chemokines in muscle of patients with inflammatory myopathies. *J Neuropathol Exp Neurol* 2000; 59:164–169.

117. Baron P, Galimberti D, Meda L, et al. Production of IL-6 by human myoblasts stimulated with AB. Relevance in the pathogenesis of IBM. *Neurology* 2001; 57:1561–1565.

118. Meda L, Baron P, Prat E, et al. Proinflammatory profile of cytokine production by human monocytes and murine microglia stimulated with β-amyloid (25–35). *J Neuroimmunol* 1999; 93:45–52.

119. Leff RL, Love LA, Miller FW, et al. Viruses in the idiopathic inflammatory myopathies: absence of candidate viral genomes in muscle. *Lancet* 1992; 339:1192–1195.

120. Leon-Monzon M, Dalakas MC. Absence of persistent infection with enteroviruses in muscles of patients with inflammatory myopathies. *Ann Neurol* 1992; 32:219–222.

121. Dalakas MC, London WT, Gravell M, Sever JL. Polymyositis in an immunodeficiency disease in monkeys induced by a type D retrovirus. *Neurology* 1986; 36:569–572.

122. Dalakas MC, Gravell M, London WT, et al. Morphological changes of an inflammatory myopathy in rhesus monkeys with simian acquired immunodeficiency syndrome (SAIDS). *Proc Soc Exp Biol Med* 1987; 185:368–376.

123. Morgan O StC, Rodgers-Johnson P, Mora C, et al. HTLV-I and polymyositis in Jamaica. *Lancet* 1989; 2:1184–1187.

124. Dalakas MC, Pezeshkpour GH. Neuromuscular diseases associated with human immunodeficiency virus infection. *Ann Neurol* 1988; 23:S38–S48.

125. Cupler EJ, Leon-Monzon M, Miller J, et al. Inclusion body myositis in HIV-I and HTLV-I infected patients. *Brain* 1996; 6:1887–1893.

126. Illa I, Nath A, Dalakas MC. Immunocytochemical and virological characteristics of HIV-associated inflammatory myopathies: similarities with seronegative polymyositis. *Ann Neurol* 1991; 29:474–481.

127. Leon-Monzon M, Illa I, Dalakas MC. Polymyositis in patients infected with HTLV-I: the role of the virus in the cause of the disease. *Ann Neurol* 1994; 36:643–649.

128. Askanas V, Engel WK, Nogalska A. Inclusion body myositis: a degenerative muscle disease associated with intra-muscle fiber multi-protein aggregates, proteasome inhibition, endoplasmic reticulum stress and decreased lysosomal degradation. *Brain Pathol* 2009; 19:493–506.

129. Nogalska A, Terracciano C, D'Agostino C, et al. p62/SQSTM1 is overexpressed and prominently accumulated in inclusions of sporadic inclusion-body myositis muscle fibers, and can help differentiating it from polymyositis and dermatomyositis. *Acta Neuropathol* 2009; 118(3):407–13.

130. Askanas V, Engel WK, Nogalaska A. Pathogeneic considerations in sporadic inclusion-body myositis, a degenerative muscle disease associated with aging and abnormalities of myoproteostasis. *J Neuropathol Exp Neurol* 2012, July 16 (Epub ahead of print).

131. Oldfors A, Moslemi AR, Jonasson L, et al. Mitochondrial abnormalities in inclusion-body myositis. *Neurology* 2006; 66 (Suppl 1):S49–S55.

132. Askanas V, McFerrin J, Baque S, et al. Transfer of β-amyloid precursor protein gene using adenovirus vector causes mitochondrial abnormalities in cultured normal human muscle. *Proc Nat Aca Soc* (USA) 1996; 93:1314–1319.

133. Salajegheh M, Pinkus JL, Nazareno R, et al. Nature of "Tau" immunoreactivity in normal myonuclei and inclusion body myositis. *Muscle Nerve* 2009; 40:520–528.

134. Weihl CC, Temiz P, Miller SE, et al. TDP-43 accumulation in inclusion body myopathy muscle suggests a common pathogenic mechanism with frontotemporal dementia. *J Neurol Neurosurg Psychiatry* 2008; 79:1186–1189.

135. Dalakas MC. Interplay between inflammation and degeneration: using inclusion body myositis to study neuroinflammation. *Ann Neurol* 2008; 64:1–3.

136. Banwell BL, Engel AG. Alpha-β-crystallin immunolocalization yields new insights into inclusion body myositis. *Neurology* 2000; 54:1033–41.

137. Muth IE, Barthel K, Bähr M, et al. Proinflammatory cell stress in sporadic inclusion body myositis muscle: overexpression of alpha-β-crystallin is associated with amyloid precursor protein and accumulation of beta-amyloid. *J Neurol Neurosurg Psychiatry* 2009; 80:1344–1349.

138. Dalakas MC. Pathogenesis and therapies of immune-mediated myopathies. *Autoimmun Rev* 2012; 11:203–206.

139. Dalakas MC. Pathophysiology of inflammatory and autoimmune myopathies. *Presse Med* 2011; 40:e237–247.

140. Dalakas MC. Inflammatory muscle diseases: a critical review on pathogenesis and therapies. *Curr Opin Pharmacol* 2010; 10:346–352.

141. Dalakas MC. Advances in the treatment of myositis. *Nature Review Rheumatol* 2010; 6:129–137.

142. Dalakas MC. Therapeutic advances and future prospects in immune-mediated inflammatory myopathies. *Therapeutic Advances in Neurological Disorders* 2008; 1:157–166.

143. Wiendl H, Hohfield R, Kiessier BC. Immunology of muscle: advances in understanding an immunological environment. *Trends Immunol* 2005; 26:373–380.

144. Leon-Monzon M, Dalakas MC. Interleukin-1 (IL-1) is toxic to human muscle. *Neurology* 1994; 44:S132.

145. Engel WK, DeVivo DC, Warmolts JR, et al. High-single-dose alternate-day prednisone (HSAD-PRED) in neuromuscular diseases, II International Congress on Muscle Diseases; International Congress series No. 237, *Amsterdam:Excerpta Medica* 1971.

146. Dalakas MC. Immunotherapy of myositis: issues, concerns and future prospects. *Nat Rev Rheumatol* 2010; 6:129–37.

147. Metzger AL, Bohan A, Goldberg LS, et al. Polymyositis and dermatomyositis: combined methotrexate and corticosteroid therapy. *Ann Intern Med* 1974; 81:182–194.

148. Miller J, Walsh Y, Lecky BRF, et al. Randomised double blind trial of methotrexate and steroids compared with azathioprine and steroids in the treatment of idiopathic inflammatory myopathy. *J Neurol Sci* 2002; S53.

149. Schneider C, Gold R, Schafers M, et al. Mycophenolate mofetil in the therapy of polymyositis associated with a polyautoimmune syndrome. *Muscle Nerve* 2002; 25:286–288.

150. Patwa HS, Chaudhry V, Katzberg H, et al. Evidence-based guideline: Intravenous immunoglobulin in the treatment of neuromuscular disorders. Report of the Therapeutics and Technology Assessment Subcommittee of the American Academy of Neurology. *Neurology* 2012; 78:1009–1015.

151. Jann S, Beretta S, Moggio M, et al. High-dose intravenous human immunoglobulin in polymyositis resistant to treatment. *J Neurol Neurosurg Psychiatry* 1992; 55:60–64.

152. Dalakas MC, Sonies B, Dambrosia J, et al. Treatment of inclusion body myositis with IVIg: a double blind study. *Neurology* 1997; 48:712–716.

153. Dalakas MC, Koffman B, Fujii M, et al. A controlled study of intravenous immunoglobulin combined with prednisone in the treatment of IBM. *Neurology* 2001; 56:323–327.

154. Walter MC, Lochmuller H, Toepfer M, et al. High-dose immunogloubin therapy in sporadic inclusion body myositis: a double-blind, placebo-controlled study. *J Neurol* 2000; 247:22–28.

155. Cronin ME, Miller FW, Hicks JE, et al. The failure of intravenous cyclophosphamide therapy in refractory idiopathic inflammatory myopathy. *J Rheumatol* 1989; 16:1225–1228.

156. Bombardieri S, Hughes GRV, Neri R, et al. Cyclophosphamide in severe polymyositis. *Lancet* 1989; 1:1138–1139.

157. Dalakas MC. B cells as a therapeutic target in autoimmune neurological disorders. *Nat Clin Pract Neurol* 2008; 4:557–567.

158. Kosmidis ML, Dalakas MC. Practical considerations on the use of rituximab in autoimmune neurological disorders. *Ther Adv Neurol Disord* 2010; 3:93–105.

159. Oddis CV, Sciurba FC, Elmagd KA, et al. Tacrolimus in refractory polymyositis with interstitial lung disease. *Lancet* 1999; 353:1762–1763.

160. Quartuccio L, De Marchi G, Scott CA, et al. Treatment of inclusion body myositis with cyclosporine-A or tacrolimus: successful long-term management in patients with earlier active disease and concomitant autoimmune features. *Clin Exp Rheumatol* 2007; 25:246–251.

161. Kitsui T, Kuroda Y, Ueno S, et al. The effects of FK506 on refractory inflammatory myopathies. *Acta Neurol Belg* 2011; 111:188–194.

CHAPTER 19

Metabolic Myopathies

Michio Hirano, Salvatore DiMauro

Derived from the Greek meaning "conversion," metabolism has been used to denote all biochemical changes occurring in living organisms. Metabolism encompasses all cellular functions related to energy production. Thus, the term *metabolic myopathy* encompasses those clinical disorders in which muscle weakness or dysfunction result from defects in biochemical pathways of ATP production. Skeletal muscle is highly energy-dependent and, therefore, vulnerable to disorders of energy metabolism. This chapter reviews the clinical and biochemical features of the major metabolic myopathies. Readers are referred to more comprehensive reviews for further details (1–9).

Skeletal muscle uses three major sources of ATP: high-energy phosphate compounds such as phosphocreatine, glycogen, and fatty acids (10). The type and duration of muscle activity dictates the relative proportions of energy derived from these three energy sources. At rest, fatty acid oxidation accounts for the bulk of ATP production, whereas during the first several minutes of moderate exercise, high-energy phosphate compounds regenerate ATP from ADP. After five to ten minutes of exercise, glycogen becomes the major energy source, and after longer periods of exercise, fatty acids are the predominant sources of ATP. Both pyruvate, the end product of glycolysis, and fatty acids are transported into the mitochondrial matrix where they are processed to acetyl-CoA via the pyruvate dehydrogenase complex reaction and the sequential "turns" of beta-oxidation. Acetyl-CoA is metabolized through the Krebs cycle and oxidative phosphorylation to produce ATP. In the metabolic myopathies, the specifically affected energy-producing pathway determines the type of exercise that will provoke symptoms. For example, defects of glycolysis, such as myophosphorylase deficiency (McArdle disease), are evi-

dent after relatively short intervals of moderate to intense exercise, such as walking uphill or running at a rapid pace (11). By contrast, fatty acid metabolism disorders, such as carnitine palmitoyltransferase (CPT) II deficiency, are more likely to produce symptoms after prolonged exercising (12).

Although clinical manifestations of the metabolic myopathies are protean, three broad myopathic phenotypes can be discerned: fixed weakness that may be progressive; dynamic symptoms (e.g., recurrent acute muscle dysfunction such as stiffness, cramps, and transiently elevated creatine kinase [CK] with or without myoglobinuria); and both static and dynamic symptoms (13).

Individual metabolic myopathies are described below and grouped according to the metabolic pathway that is affected.

DEFECTS OF GLYCOGEN METABOLISM

During moderate- to high-intensity exercise, glycogen is the major source of stored energy for ATP production, primarily via aerobic glycolysis. However, intense exercise induces increased anaerobic glycogen catabolism that elevates serum lactate and extended strenuous exertion, especially in untrained subjects, causes fatigue, muscle burning and, under extreme duress, cramps and muscle breakdown with elevation of CK and myoglobinuria. In patients with defects of glycogen breakdown in muscle, impaired anaerobic and aerobic glycolysis causes exercise intolerance, muscle cramps, and myoglobinuria. In contrast, defects of glycogen synthesis in muscle generally cause static weakness. Of the 15 different glycogenoses that have been identified, 13 have associated neuromuscular syndromes (Table 1). The two

Table 1. Classification of myopathic glycogen storage diseases (GSD)

GSD type	Affected organs	Clinical manifestations	Defective Enzyme	Inheritance
0	Skeletal and heart muscle	Exercise intolerance and hypertrophic cardiomyopathy	Glycogen synthase 1	AR
	Skeletal and heart muscle	Myopathic weakness and hypertrophic cardiomyopathy	Glycogenin	AR
II. Infantile	Generalized	Cardiomegaly, weakness, hypotonia	Acid maltase	AR
	Skeletal muscle	Myopathy often simulating Duchenne muscular dystrophy	Acid maltase	AR
Childhood Adult	Skeletal muscle	Myopathy with early respiratory muscle weakness	Acid maltase	AR
III	Generalized	Hepatomegaly, fasting hypoglycemia, progressive weakness	Brancher	AR
IV	Generalized	Hepatosplenomegaly, liver cirrhosis, myopathy	Debrancher	AR
V	Skeletal muscle	Intolerance to intense exercise, cramps, myoglobinuria	Muscle phosphoryase	AR
VII	Skeletal muscle	Intolerance to intense exercise, cramps, myoglobinuria	Muscle phosphofructokinase	AR
VIII	Liver and skeletal muscle	Hepatomegaly, growth retardation, muscle hypotonia	Phosphorylase b kinase	AR
	Skeletal muscle	Exercise intolerance, myoglobinuria	Phosphorylase b kinase	AR
	Heart	Fatal infantile cardiomyopathy	Phosphorylase b kinase	AR
IX	Generalized	Hemolytic anemia, seizures, mental retardation, parkinsonism, intolerance to intense exercise, myoglobinuria	Phosphoglycerate kinase	AR
X	Skeletal muscle	Intolerance to intense exercise, cramps, myoglobinuria	Muscle phosphoglycerate mutase	AR
XI	Skeletal muscle	Intolerance to intense exercise, cramps, myoglobinuria	Muscle lactate dehydrogenase	XR
XII	Skeletal muscle	Intolerance to intense exercise, weakness, hemolytic anemia, fatigue, developmental delay, myoglobinuria	Aldolase A	AR
XIII	Skeletal muscle	Exercise intolerance, myoglobinuria	b-enolase	AR
XIV	Skeletal muscle	Exercise intolerance, cramps	Phosphoglucomutase 1	AR

non-myopathic glycogen storage diseases (GSD) are: type I due to glucose-6-phosphatase deficiency, which causes liver and kidney dysfunction, and type VI due to hepatic phosphorylase deficiency that affects the liver and erythrocytes. Types 0, II-V, VII, VIII, IX, and XI-XIV are inherited in an autosomal recessive (AR) pattern, whereas one form of GSD VIII and GSD X are inherited as X-linked traits. In this section, we describe the glycogenoses-causing myopathy.

GSD Types 0 and XV

Aglycogenoses due to deficiency of glycogen synthetase or glycogenin present with prominent cardiomyopathy along with myopathy, but rather than defects of glycogen catabo-

lism, these diseases are due to lack of glycogen synthesis, more succinctly described as aglycogenosis. The first is due to deficiency of glycogen synthetase in muscle, GSD type 0 (zero), indicating absence of glycogen in muscle. This rare condition has been described in only four patients from three families with AR mutations in the GSD1 gene encoding the muscle-specific isoform of glycogen synthetase. Three patients presented with juvenile-onset exercise intolerance. All had cardiomyopathy that was fatal in two and one had seizures. The fourth child without antecedent exercise intolerance, died suddenly while climbing stairs. The second aglycogenosis (GSD type XV) was identified in a 27-year-old man with myopathic weakness, cardiac arrhythmias, and depletion of glycogen in muscle due to compound heterozygous mutations in the GYG1 gene encoding glycogenin, the primer of glycogen synthesis that utilizes uridine diphosphate glucose (UDPG) to generate a short (~10 glucosyl units) glucose polymer, the nidus for new glycogen molecules.

GSD Type II: Acid Maltase Deficiency

Acid maltase deficiency (AMD) was first reported as idiopathic infantile hypertrophy of the heart (14). It is distinguished from other glycogenoses because the abnormal enzyme is lysosomal bound. Three clinical subtypes have been defined based on age-at-onset: infantile, childhood, and adult AMD forms (7). Infantile AMD, or Pompe disease, presents in the first six months of life with diffuse hypotonia and weakness, including respiratory muscles; however, muscle bulk can be increased and macroglossia is common. There is marked cardiomegaly and mild hepatomegaly. The disease is usually fatal within the first year, and death occurs invariably before age two years due to pulmonary and cardiac failure (15, 16). A milder infantile subtype has been described (17).

Childhood AMD typically presents with a delay in the onset of walking. The weakness of limb and axial muscles is slowly progressive, and in boys, the clinical picture, which often includes calf pseudohypertrophy, can resemble Duchenne muscular dystrophy. Respiratory muscle weakness typically causes death in the second or third decade.

Adult AMD is a slowly progressive myopathy beginning in the third or fourth decade without visceral organ involvement. Respiratory muscle weakness is out of proportion to the limb weakness and can be a clinical clue to the diagnosis. Serum CK is elevated in all forms of AMD. Electromyography (EMG) reveals small short-duration motor units with fibrillation, positive sharp waves, bizarre high-frequency discharges, and myotonic discharges. Muscle histology shows a vacuolar myopathy most prominent in the infantile form. The vacuoles are enlarged lysosomes engorged with periodic acid-Schiff (PAS)–positive diastase-digestible material and stains intensely for acid phosphatase. Electron microscopy confirms the presence of excess glycogen, both within lysosomes and free in the cytoplasm.

The molecular defect in the various forms of AMD resides in the gene that encodes acid alpha-1, 4-glucosidase (GAA), and over 200 pathogenic mutations have been identified (18). Whereas cytoplasmic glycogen is distributed uniformly in the other glycogen storage diseases, it is predominantly enclosed in lysosomal membranes in this form. Molecular genetic studies have revealed mutations in the lysosomal acid alpha-glucosidase gene. In infantile-onset Pompe disease, GAA activity is completely, or nearly completely, absent (<1% of normal activity in cultured fibroblasts), whereas in juvenile- or adult-onset patients,

residual GAA activity is higher (2–40% of normal activity in cultured fibroblasts) (19, 20).

The carrier frequency for AMD has been estimated at about 1 in 100, and based upon a calculated mutant gene frequency of 0.005, the expected number of affected births has been estimated to be 1 in 40,000 births (21). Carrier frequency calculations in Holland have estimated the overall frequency of AMD as 1 in 40,000 (1 in 138,000 for the infantile disorder and 1 in 57,000 for adult patients) (22). In Taiwan, the frequency of infantile-onset Pompe has been estimated to be higher ~1 in 35,000 (23).

In 2006, the U.S. Food and Drug Administration (FDA) and the European Medicines Agency (EMA) approved the use of recombinant human GAA (rhGAA) therapy in AMD, based largely on the results of a landmark paper of this enzyme replacement therapy (ERT) in 18 infants (24). In this study, rhGAA was infused intravenously at 20mg/kg (n=9) or 40 mg/kg (n=9) every other week for one year. Fifteen patients survived to age 18 months, whereas only 1 of 61 historical controls had lived to age 18 months. In a follow-up longer term open label study of 21 infants treated with rhGAA for 3–43 months (median 13 months), 71% (15/21) were alive, 44% (7/16) were ventilator-free, and 62% (13/21) attained new motor milestones indicating efficacy (25). However, virtually all of the patients (95%, 19/20) developed IgG antibodies to rhGAA because infants often have null mutations and no endogenous GAA protein (i.e., no cross-reactive immunological material [CRIM]). Anaphylactic reactions have been associated with rhGAA treatment. Not surprisingly, CRIM-negative status and high-sustained antibody titers have correlated with poor response to rhGAA (26). In contrast, in a cohort of 11 rhGAA-treated infantile-onset patients who survived to at least age five, all were CRIM-positive and showed sustained improvements in assessments of cardiac and motor functions but had residual muscle weakness, hearing loss, risk for arrhythmias, nasal speech, dysphagia, and osteopenia (27).

In comparison to infantile-onset Pompe disease, late-onset AMD has shown less dramatic response to rhGAA in the randomized placebo-controlled Late-Onset Treatment Study (LOTS)(28). After the 78-week treatment period, patients who received rhGAA showed significant, albeit mild, improvements in both primary outcomes: 6-minute walk test (+7.5% in rhGAA group vs. -1% in placebo arm, P-value 0.03) and vital capacity (+2.2% in rhGAA group vs. -4.2% in placebo arm, P-value 0.006). All of the patients developed anti-GAA antibodies by week 12 and 3/60 (5%) developed anaphylactic reactions. Based on this study and smaller open-label studies that suggested rhGAA efficacy, a consensus paper recommended that symptomatic late-onset patients be treated with rhGAA, ideally by a multidisciplinary team, and reevaluated after one year to assess whether ERT should be maintained (29).

GSD Type III: Debrancher Deficiency

The first reported patient with debrancher deficiency had a markedly enlarged liver, obesity, and small genitalia (30). Debrancher deficiency is clinically characterized by childhood-onset liver dysfunction with hepatomegaly, growth failure, fasting hypoglycemia, and occasionally hypoglycemic seizures (31). Symptoms resolve spontaneously at puberty, leading to more normal adult lives, although cirrhosis and hepatic failure may develop later (32). Myopathy presents in the third to fourth decade in 70% of patients and primarily affects distal leg and intrinsic hand muscles. The myopathy is slowly progressive and rarely incapacitating. Myoglobinuria occurred in one patient (33), and peripheral neuropathy and symptomatic cardiomyopathy were seen in others; however, laboratory evidence of myocardial ventricular hypertrophy is common. Serum CK is elevated in all patients with myopathy, and electrophysiological studies reveal myogenic changes but may also show decreased nerve conduction velocities.

Skeletal muscle biopsy shows severe vacuolar myopathy with PAS-positive vacuoles beneath the sarcolemma and between myofibrils. Ultrastructurally, they are mainly collections of free glycogen. Some glycogen-filled lysosomes are seen but are not as numerous as in AMD. Glycogen debrancher enzyme (GDE) is a 160-kDa polypeptide with both transferase and α-glucosidase catalytic functions. After muscle phosphorylase has shortened the peripheral chains of glycogen to about four glucosyl units, a partially digested polysaccharide is produced, called phosphorylase-limit-dextrin. The debrancher enzyme removes the residual oligosaccharide "twigs" through a two-step process catalyzed by 1, 4-1, 4-glucantransferase and amylo-1, 6-glucosidase (AGL) activities. The two activities are determined at separate catalytic sites on the polypeptide chain and can function independently of each other. Numerous mutations in the gene for debrancher enzyme have been identified. The overall incidence of glycogen debrancher deficiency in the United States is about 1 in 100,000 live births (34).

GSD Type IV: Brancher Deficiency

Glycogen branching enzyme (GBE) deficiency, or Andersen disease, presents predominantly as a severe, rapidly progressive disease of infancy clinically dominated by liver dysfunction. As recognized in a seminal paper published in 2004 (35), there are two main infantile presentations. The first is a perinatal disorder dubbed "fetal akinesia-deformation sequence" (FADS), characterized by multiple congenital contractures (arthrogryposis multiplex congenita), hydrops fetalis, pulmonary hypoplasia, craniofacial abnormalities, intrauterine growth retardation, abnormal amniotic fluid volume, and perinatal death. The second form, labeled "congenital" should probably be called "fatal infantile" because it presents at or soon after birth with hypotonia, muscle wasting, neuronal involvement, inconsistent cardiomyopathy, and early death. Of the eight patients reported by Bruno and colleagues (35) three had FADS, three had the congenital form, and two had childhood myopathy. Interestingly, there was a good correlation between molecular severity and clinical severity, which has been confirmed in several subsequent patients.

It is becoming increasingly clear that patients with congenital GBE deficiency present a clinical continuum from FADS to a rapidly fatal congenital multisystem disorder dominated by profound hypotonia, respiratory failure, and inconsistent cardiomyopathy (35–39). Detailed neuropathology in a few infants showed PG inclusions in neurons of the basal ganglia and thalamus, oculomotor and pontine nuclei, and periaqueductal neurons (36, 37, 39). In the medulla, PG deposits were found in the hypoglossal nucleus, the dorsal motor nucleus of the vagus, and the nucleus ambiguous. The motor neurons of the spinal cord are also severely affected (39), thus explaining how one of the patients we studied was initially diagnosed as spinal muscular atrophy type I until mutations in the *SMN1* gene were ruled out (38).

Patients may also present with juvenile onset myopathy. Three Turkish male siblings with chronic progressive myopathy were found to have a juvenile form of GBE deficiency with enzyme deficiency limited to muscle tissues with polyglucosan inclusions in myofibers, and otherwise normal enzyme activity in circulating erythrocytes and leukocytes of all three siblings and in the parents (40). A second patient with a juvenile myopathy, subclinical neuropathy, dilated cardiomyopathy, heart failure, dysmorphic features, had total branching enzyme deficiency in skeletal muscle and liver tissue (41).

In adults, GSD IV presents as adult polyglucosan body disease (PGBD), a neurological syndrome characterized by onset in the fifth to sixth decade of progressive upper and lower motor neuron dysfunction, sensory neuropathy, bladder and bowel incontinence and, in about 50% of the patients, dementia (42–44). Patients with liver involvement can have slight elevations of the serum CK. Electrophysiologic testing of adult polyglucosan body disease patients demonstrates axonal sensorimotor neuropathy. Cytometric studies reveal a neurogenic bladder. Basophilic intensely PAS-positive polysaccharide bodies partially resistant to diastase digestion are found in skin, liver, muscle, heart, nerve, and central nervous system (CNS) tissues. Ultrastructurally, the polysaccharide appears filamentous and finely granular.

Glycogen branching enzyme catalyzes the final step of glycogen synthesis by adding short glucosyl chains of about seven glucosyl units with α-1, 6-glucosidic bonds to linear peripheral chains of glycogen. The short glucosyl

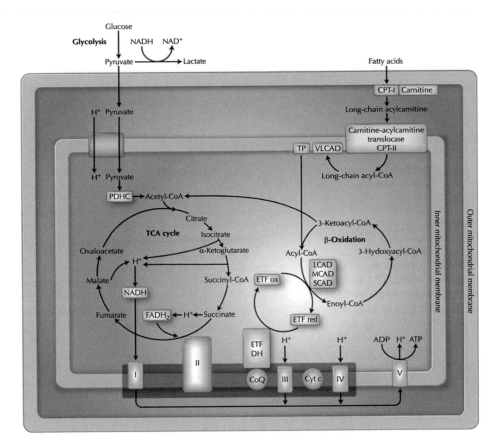

FIG. 1. Schematic representation of mitochondrial metabolism. Respiratory chain complexes or components encoded exclusively by the nuclear genome are light orange. Complexes containing some subunits encoded by the nuclear genome and others encoded by mitochondrial DNA are dark orange. CPT, carnitine palmitoyltransferase; PDHC, pyruvate dehydrogenase complex; CoA, coenzyme A; TCA, tricarboxylic acid; CoQ, coenzyme Q; Cyt c, cytochrome c. Modified from: reference 13, with permission.

twigs are elongated by glycogen synthetase. The diagnosis of homozygote and heterozygote GBE deficiency can often be made on the basis of branching enzyme activity in erythrocytes (45) or by GBE gene sequencing, which has revealed numerous mutations.

GSD Type V: Muscle Phosphorylase Deficiency

The patient of Dr. McArdle (11) was a 30-year-old man who experienced first myalgia and then weakness and stiffness with exercise of any muscle, including the masseter, which abated promptly with rest. Blood lactate did not increase after exercise, suggesting that the patient was unable to convert muscle glycogen into lactate. Schmid and coworkers (46, 47), and Mommaerts and colleagues (48) identified the cause of the disorder as a glycogenolytic defect in muscle due to the absence of myophosphorylase activity. Symptoms of fatigue, myalgia, and cramps generally occur during intense isometric exercise, such as lifting heavy weights, or during less-intense sustained dynamic exercise (49, 50).

A characteristic "second wind" phenomenon which occurs in individuals who slow down and rest briefly at the onset of symptoms allows for the resumption of exercise at the original pace. About one-half of patients experience acute muscle necrosis and myoglobinuria after exercise, while renal failure occurs in 4 to 25% (6, 51). About one-third develop fixed weakness, especially older patients.

Atypical clinical presentations include "tiredness" or poor stamina, progressive limb weakness in the sixth to seventh decade, severe generalized neonatal weakness with respiratory insufficiency and death in infancy, and delayed psychomotor development and mild proximal weakness. DiMauro and Hartlage (50) described an infant with severe McArdle disease who developed generalized rapidly progressive weakness at age 4 weeks and died at age 13 weeks of respiratory failure. Muscle biopsy showed complete absence of myophosphorylase activity and of the enzyme protein as indicated by immunodiffusion studies. Kost and Verity (52) described a patient with immobilizing cramps, stiffness, and myoedema that began at age 60. Abarbanel and colleagues (53) described a 59-year-old man with myophosphorylase deficiency who presented with long-standing painless and static weakness starting in childhood, in whom serum CK, EMG, and muscle biopsy were all consistent with a myopathic process in conjunction with accumulation of glycogen. Milstein and coworkers (54) described a premature infant of consanguineous parents with McArdle disease who demonstrated joint contractures and evidence of perinatal asphyxia.

Laboratory evaluation reveals elevation in the serum CK in greater than 90% of patients. Nerve conduction studies (NCS) are generally normal. EMG may be normal or show a myopathy. During spontaneous or exercise-induced contractures, the shortened muscles are electrically silent. Using 31P nuclear magnetic resonance (NMR) spectroscopy, Ross and colleagues (55) observed lack of cytoplasmic acidification during exercise with an excessive drop in the phosphocreatine: inorganic phosphate ratio. The forearm ischemic exercise test invariably causes muscle cramps and pain in patients with these glycolytic defects, however alternative protocols, including exercise without ischemia, show with equal accuracy in separating affected patients and healthy controls on the basis of post-exercise peak lactate-to-ammonia ratios. Two other tests use intermittent hand-grip contractions at 50% of maximal voluntary force or at 30% of maximal force (56).

Phosphorylase (α-1, 4-glucan orthophosphate glucosyl transferase) initiates glycogen breakdown by removing 1, 4-glucosyl residues phosphorylytically from the outer branches of glycogen and liberating glucose 1-phosphate (Figure 1). It is now known that muscle phosphorylase activity is decreased to less than 10% of normal due to a specific defect in the muscle isoform; liver and brain isoforms also have been identified. Muscle glycogen levels may be normal or elevated.

Molecular genetic studies have identified at least 129 mutations in the muscle phosphorylase gene (PYGM) (18, 57). The most common mutation in the United States, Spain, Italy, and the United Kingdom is a CGA(Arg) to TGA(stop) at codon 50 (p.R50X), which accounted for 43 to 77% of the mutant alleles, but is not encountered in Japanese patients (6, 51, 57–59).

Therapies to bypass the metabolic defect by oral administration of glucose and fructose have shown inconsistent results. Slonim and Goans (60) observed that a high-protein diet was associated with improvement in muscle endurance and strength. In a placebo-controlled crossover study of 12 McArdle patients, Vissing and Haller (61) noted that oral sucrose intake (75 grams) 30–40 minutes prior to exercise markedly improved exercise tolerance. They also reported that moderate aerobic exercise training improved exercise capacity via enhanced circulatory delivery and mitochondrial metabolism (62).

GSD Type VII: Phosphofructokinase Deficiency

Muscle phosphofructokinase (PFK) deficiency, or Tarui disease (63), is clinically indistinguishable from myophosphorylase deficiency, which is not surprising since both interfere with pyruvate production. The family originally reported by Tarui and colleagues (63) contained three affected children of consanguineous parents, a 20-year-old woman, and her 23- and 27-year-old siblings. All complained of easy fatigue with marked weakness, stiffness, and cramps in muscles subjected to vigorous and sustained exertion, relieved by rest and with no abnormalities thereupon at rest. Phosphofructokinase activity was absent in muscle tissue and one-half normal in erythrocytes. Layzer and colleagues (64, 65) noted that red cell PFK was composed of two immunologically related, but not identical, subunits, one of which was only present in muscle. Subsequent investigators noted patients with late-onset progressive myopathy associated with an abnormal muscle polysaccharide, elevated glucose-6-phosphate content, and activation of the chain-elongating enzyme glycogen synthase (66).

Laboratory studies generally reveal elevated serum CK, bilirubin, uric acid levels, and reticulocytosis. EMG shows myopathy with variable irritative features. In the United States, most patients have been of Ashkenazi Jewish origin. Muscle biopsy reveals accumulation of normal-appearing subsarcolemmal and intermyofibrillar glycogen and pockets of an abnormal polysaccharide that stains intensely with PAS but is resistant to diastase digestion. Ultrastructurally, this abnormal glycogen has a granular and filamentous appearance, similar to that in branching enzyme deficiency.

It is now recognized that PFK is a tetrameric enzyme. There are three subunits: M (muscle), L (liver), and P (platelet). Muscle contains exclusively the M isoform, whereas erythrocytes contain both the L and M subunits. PFK deficiency causes a block distal to glucose and fructose, which is, therefore, not improved by administration of these substrates. PFK-deficient patients depend on free fatty acids and ketones for ATP generation; therefore, exercise intolerance is worsened by high-carbohydrate meals that lower the blood levels of these compounds (67). The negative effect of glucose has been aptly described as an "out-of-wind" phenomenon (67).

At least 20 distinct mutations in the muscle phosphofructokinase subunit encoded by PFKM have been identified (6, 18). Treatment is problematic in myophosphorylase deficiency because glucose and fructose are not usable substrates.

GSD Type VIII: Phosphorylase-b-Kinase Deficiency

Phosphorylase-b-kinase (PHBK) deficiency is associated with five major phenotypes based on the mode of inheritance and tissue involvement: 1) liver disease, typically a benign condition of infancy or childhood with hepatomegaly, growth retardation, delayed motor development, fasting hypoglycemia, and usually inherited as an X-linked trait; 2) liver and muscle disease with a static myopathy inherited as an AR trait; 3) myopathy alone, inherited in an AR or X-linked recessive pattern; 4) severe hepatopathy with cirrhosis transmitted in an AR manner; and 5) fatal infantile cardiomyopathy, also inherited as an AR condition (6, 68–70). In patients with myopathy, the serum CK is variably increased (6). EMG reveals myogenic abnormalities. Muscle biopsy reveals subsarcolemmal glycogen predominantly in type IIb fibers. Ultrastructurally, the glycogen is free in the cytoplasm and appears normal.

PHBK is composed of the subunits α, β, γ, and δ that form an (αβγδ)4 complex. PHBK acts on two enzymes, glycogen synthetase and phosphorylase. Specifically, it converts phosphorylase from the less active β form to the more active α form while converting glycogen synthetase from the more active dephosphorylated state to a less active phosphorylated form. The γ-subunit is catalytic and is regulated by phosphorylation of the α- and β-subunits. Calcium sensitivity is conferred by the δ-subunit, which is tightly bound to calmodulin. *PHKA1*, the gene encoding the α-subunit of skeletal muscle phosphorylase kinase, resides in the X-chromosome while β-, γ-, and δ- subunits are autosomal.

The genes encoding the PBK subunits have been cloned, and the molecular defects are under investigation. Only about 15 patients with myopathic PhK deficiency have been reported, most of whom were men, suggesting X-linked inheritance. In agreement with this concept, all molecular defects identified thus far were in the *PHKA1* gene (71). A number of patients with myopathy due to mutations in muscle-specific PHKB deficiency have been reported. Two patients were heterozygous for single amino acid substitutions in *PHKB* that were of unclear significance (Q657K and Y770C) (72). In one man, myopathy and absent muscle PHK activity were caused by frameshift mutation in the gene encoding the a-subunit of *PHK* on chromosome Xq12-q13 (73).

Not surprisingly, patients with myopathic PHK deficiency clinically resemble individuals with a milder form of McArdle disease, which has been described as "McArdle light" (71). Formal cycle ergometry studies have confirmed the mild impairment of glycogenolysis; there was no change in lactate during dynamic submaximal exercise, and intravenous glucose infusion improved exercise tolerance, but to a lesser degree than in McArdle patients (74).

The molecular genetic cause of the fatal infantile cardiomyopathy with PHK deficiency has been elusive because there is no heart-specific PHK isoform, and mutations in the *PHK* subunit genes were excluded (72).

Type IX: Phosphoglycerate Kinase Deficiency

The clinical presentation of phosphoglycerate kinase (PGK) deficiency is highly variable (75, 76). DiMauro and colleagues (77) described recurrent myoglobinuria with PGK deficiency. Sugie and colleagues (78) demonstrated PGK deficiency in three unrelated mentally retarded men with myoglobinuria, of whom two had epilepsy and the other had hemolytic anemia. Neither organ-specific isozymes nor post-translational modifications appear to be responsible for the variable presentations since enzymes derived from different tissue in the same individual do not substantially differ in physical or biochemical characteristics. Rather, the variability appears to be the consequence of the unique biochemical properties of the individual PGK mutants. After DiMauro and coworkers (77) described X-linked PGK deficiency as the cause of myoglobinuria without hemolytic anemia, three new variants of PGK deficiency were reported, resulting in the definition of three clinical phenotypes: myopathic, hemolytic, and mixed (79).

Laboratory findings include a variably increased resting serum CK level and a normal EMG. Muscle biopsy generally shows nonspecific morphologic changes and mildly increased glycogen content. Muscle phosphoglycerate kinase activity is virtually undetectable in patients. Phosphoglycerate kinase deficiency is an X-linked recessive disorder due to a variety of *PGK* missense and splice site mutations (80, 81)

GSD Type X: Phosphoglycerate Mutase Deficiency

In 1981, DiMauro and colleagues (82) reported a 52-year-old man who became symptomatic in adolescence, but led a relatively normal life, including service in the army. Muscle phosphoglycerate mutase (PGAM) enzyme activity was 5 to 7% of normal. Other patients were reported by Bresolin, Kissel, Vita and coworkers (83–85). Recurrent cramps and myoglobinuria and exercise intolerance dominated the clinical presentation in affected patients. Muscle extracts from unaffected parents of the probands showed approximately 50% of normal PGAM enzymatic activity consistent with AR inheritance (83).

Muscle biopsies can be normal or show diffuse or patchy increase of glycogen; PGAM activity in muscle tissue is less than 10% of normal. The enzyme is a dimer composed of a muscle-specific (M) and a brain-specific (B) isoform. In patients with myopathy, mutations affect the M isoform. Cardiac muscle expresses both isoforms; hence, the BB isoform protects the heart from symptoms in PGAM-M deficiency.

Among five affected patient reported by Tsujino and coworkers (86), three were homozygous for a trp78-to-ter mutation, one was homozygous for an arg90-to-trp mutation, and a fifth was a compound heterozygote for trp78-to-ter and glu89-to-ala; four of the five patients were African American, and the other was Italian. Tsujino and coworkers (87) noted that two Caucasian patients, a brother and sister, were homozygous for a different missense mutation CGG (Arg)-to-TGG (Trp) at codon 90. Despite the small number of patients identified, the authors concluded that there is a common mutation in African Americans while there may be molecular heterogeneity in other ethnic groups. Hadji-georgiou and coworkers (88) noted a novel *PGAM*-M mutation in a Japanese family with partial PGAM deficiency: a G-to-A transition at nucleotide position 209, resulting in the substitution of a highly conserved glycine at codon 97 with aspartic acid (G97D). Two heterozygous family members for the G97D mutation presented with exercise intolerance and muscle cramps, indicating that heterozygous individuals can be symptomatic.

Treatment with dantrolene led to improvement in a patient with PGAM deficiency in whom tubular aggregates were noted in muscle in association with increased calcium adenosine triphosphatase and calcium content, leading to the suggestion that cramps in muscle PGAM-deficient patients can be caused by high calcium release from the sarcoplasmic reticulum relative to calcium uptake capacity (89).

GSD Type XI: Lactate Dehydrogenase Deficiency

Kanno and coworkers (90) described a family with deficiency of the M-subunit of lactate dehydrogenase type A (LDH-A). The proband was an 18-year-old man with exertional myoglobinuria and preamature fatigue. Forearm ischemic exercise test did not produce an increase in the blood lactate but marked increases in blood pyruvate and serum CK, with myoglobinuria. Kanno and coworkers (91) also reported this defect in glycogen metabolism in eight individuals from three Japanese families, two of which had first-cousin parents. Painful muscle stiffness and cramps afflicted one sibling from age nine, and a sister had complete absence of the M-subunit of LDH-A. LDH is a tetrameric enzyme comprised of LDH-A and LDH-B subunits. The M4 tetramer predominates in skeletal muscle. In LDH-deficient patients with myopathy, the low residual LDH activity in muscle, about 5% of normal, is due to the small amount of retained LDH-B tetramers. Although homozygosity for the lack of the LDH-A subunit leads to early postimplantation death in a mouse model (92), humans with complete absence of LDH-A survive. This is probably due to the fact that, in contrast to the mouse, LDH-B predominates in the human fetus.

Three affected women developed stiffness of the uterine muscle at the onset of delivery, necessitating cesarean section, whereas a few patients had a dermatologic disorder characterized by follicular papules and erythematous patches (93, 94).

A patient with a lack of LDH-A had a 20-bp deletion in exon 6 which resulted in a frameshift translation and premature termination (95). Absence of detectable protein was presumably due to rapid protein degradation. She complained of uterine stiffness during her pregnancy and in the early stages of delivery. The same mutation was identified in 18 other individuals from four affected families in Japan (95). Miyajima and colleagues (96) noted a similar gene defect among two affected adult sisters of consanguineous parents, who had muscle stiffness from early and late adolescence, and had similar complaints of dystocia.

Type XII: Aldolase A Deficiency

In 1996 (97), aldolase A deficiency was identified in a four-year-old boy with exercise intolerance, limb weakness, premature fatigue, developmental delay, hemolysis, and repeated bouts of rhabdomyolysis during febrile illnesses. The muscle biopsy did not reveal excess glycogen by histochemistry. However, it did show that aldolase activity level was 3.8% of normal by biochemical analysis. Sequencing of the aldolase A gene revealed a homozygous p.E206K mutation.

Aldolase A (ALDOA), or fructose-1,6-biphosphate aldolase is a glycolytic enzyme that catalyzes the reversible conversion of fructose-1,6-biphosphate to glyceraldehydes 3-phosphate and dihydroxyacetone phosphate. It is a tetrameric enzyme of identical 40,000 Da subunits. Vertebrates have three aldolase isozymes, aldolase A, B, and C, which are distinguishable by the electrophoretic and catalytic properties.

Forearm-Ischemic Exercise Test

The forearm-ischemic exercise test described in Table 2 is useful in corroborating the diagnosis of defects in the glycogenolytic or the glycolytic pathways that impair lactate production during exercise but frequently produce painful cramps in patients. Originally performed with ischemia (98); non-ischemic forearm exercise has been demonstrated to be effective and useful in diagnosing glycolytic disorders in adults without inducing cramps (56). The forearm ischemic exercise test can be difficult for children to perform; therefore, Bruno and colleagues (99) introduced a modified semi-ischemic protocol that requires blood pressure cuff inflation only to the mean arterial pressure. This modified test was used in children 7 to 16 years old and is most reliable in 11 to 16-year-old children. In normal adults, there is a 5- to 6 increase in blood lactate in the first three minutes after exercise, followed by a gradual decline to baseline level in later ones that does not generally occur in those with defects of the glycolytic pathway. In normal children, semi-ischemic forearm exercise elevated lactate by an average of 2.6-fold. Serum ammonia should rise 3- to 10-fold after exercise in both normal subjects and in patients with a glycogen metabolism defect. Patients with myophosphorylase deficiency generally show less than a

Table 2. Forearm Ischemic Test[1]

1. Explain the procedure to the patient.

2. Insert an indwelling sterile needle into the patient's antecubital vein. We prefer to use a 23-gauge butterfly needle. Collect blood for measurements of lactate, creatine kinase, and ammonia.

3. For children 11–16 years-old, place a sphygmomanometer cuff above the patient's elbow and inflate up to, but not above, the mean arterial blood pressure.

4. With constant encouragement, have the patient intermittently open and clench his or her fist (1 second maximum contraction and 1 second relaxation) for 1 min. The patient should squeeze a rolled-up sphygmomanometer cuff or handgrip dynamometer.

5. In children, after 1 min of exercise, the blood pressure cuff is deflated and the patient rests.

6. If the patient develops a cramp, tell the patient to stop exercising immediately and, in children, deflate the sphygmomanometer cuff to avoid excess muscle necrosis.

7. Blood samples, drawn at 1, 3, 6, and 10 min after exercise and placed on ice, are sent for lactate, ammonia, and creatine kinase measurements.

1. Adapted from references 56 and 99.

1.5-fold increase in venous lactate levels. If a patient develops muscle cramping during exercise, the test should be stopped immediately to reduce the risk of muscle necrosis. False-positive results arise because of suboptimal effort that may be suggested by the lack of rise in ammonia after ischemic exercise. If the patient's serum lactate level rises after exercise but the ammonia fails to rise significantly, then the diagnosis of myoadenylate deaminase (MAD) deficiency can be considered. While the forearm ischemic exercise test is helpful in supporting diagnoses of glycolytic disorders and MAD deficiency, confirmation by measurement of biochemical activities of enzymes, molecular genetic testing, or both is required.

DEFECTS OF LIPID METABOLISM

Lipids are the most important and efficient fuel source in the body. Fatty acids are vital during periods of fasting, particularly when liver glycogen stores are depleted a few hours after a meal. They serve three main functions: their partial oxidation in the liver produces ketones that are an important auxiliary fuel for almost all tissue, especially the brain; they provide a major energy source in cardiac and skeletal muscle, particularly during rest and during prolonged exercise; and ATP produced from fatty acid oxidation provides energy for gluconeogenesis and urea genesis. The normal fatty acid oxidation pathway is shown in Figure 2. Adipocytes liberate free fatty acids that are bound to serum albumin or incorporated into triglyceride-rich lipoproteins and transported to other tissues. Short 4-carbon- and medium 8-carbon-chain fatty acids freely cross the outer and inner mitochondrial membranes into the mitochondrial matrix where they are metabolized to CoA esters before beta-oxidation. By contrast, the mitochondrial membranes are impermeable to long-chain fatty acids (LCFA); therefore, at the outer mitochondrial and endoplasmic reticulum membranes, LCFA must first be converted to CoA-thioesters by long-chain acyl-CoA synthetase. To cross the inner mitochondrial membrane, the very-long-chain acyl-CoA (VLCA-CoA) and long-chain acyl-CoA (LCA-CoA) molecules are converted into acylcarnitine with release of free CoA by CPT I located on the inner side of the outer mitochondrial membrane. Carnitine acylcarnitine translocase transports very-long- and long-chain acylcarnitine across the inner mitochondrial membrane. Within the mitochondrial matrix, CPT II bound to the inner surface of the inner mitochondrial membrane exchanges CoA for carnitine to reform VLCA-CoA and LCA-CoA and liberate carnitine, which is shuttled back into the cytoplasm by the translocase.

VLCA-CoA, 14 to 24 carbon atoms in length, is processed by VLCA-CoA dehydrogenase, which is bound to the inner mitochondrial membrane and generates 2-trans-enoyl-CoA molecules. The VLCA-CoA molecules are processed by a trifunctional enzyme, which is also bound to the inner mitochondrial membrane and possesses three beta-oxidation enzymatic activities: long-chain enoyl-CoA hydratase, long-chain-l-3-hydroxyacyl-CoA dehydrogenase, and long-chain thiolase enzymes. This process shortens the acyl-CoA by two carbon molecules.

Acyl-CoAs of 4 to 18 carbons in length are oxidized by the beta-oxidation pathway in the mitochondrial matrix. Each cycle of the β-oxidation system shortens the acyl-CoA by two carbon fragments through four catalytic steps: acyl-CoA dehydrogenase, 2-enoyl-CoA hydratase, l-3-hydroxyacyl-CoA dehydrogenase, and 3-ketoacyl-CoA thiolase. The acetyl-CoA moiety produced at each turn of the β-oxidation spiral enters the Krebs cycle. There are three different mitochondrial matrix dehydrogenase enzymes, namely, short-chain acyl-CoA dehydrogenase, which acts on fatty acid of four to six carbon atoms; medium-chain acyl-CoA dehydrogenase (MCAD) for substrates of four to fourteen carbon atoms, and long-chain acyl-CoA dehydrogenase for substrates of 10 to 18 carbon atoms. Defects of fatty acid oxidation can occur at various points along the pathway from the transport of fatty acid into mitochondria to the beta-oxidation cycle as described below.

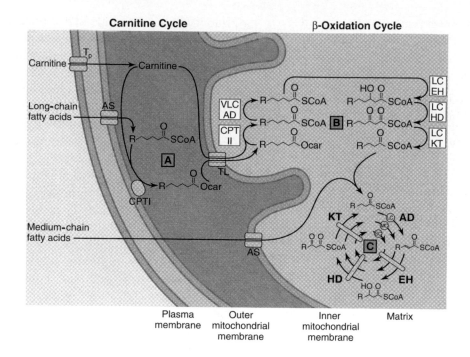

FIG. 2. Schematic representation of fatty acid oxidation. This metabolic pathway is divided into the carnitine cycle **(A)**, the inner mitochondrial membrane system **(B)**, and the mitochondrial matrix system **(C)**. The carnitine cycle includes the plasma membrane transporter, carnitine palmitoyltransferase I (CPT I). The reactions shown in B occur in the inner mitochondrial membrane. The carnitine-acylcarnitine translocase system and carnitine palmitoyltransferase II (CPT II). The inner mitochondrial membrane system includes the very-long-chain acyl-CoA dehydrogenase (VLCAD) and the trifunctional protein with three catalytically active sites. Long-chain acylcarnitines enter the mitochondrial matrix by the action of CPT II to yield long-chain acyl-CoAs. These thioesters undergo one or more cycles of chain shortening catalyzed by the membrane-bound system. Chain-shortened acyl-CoAs are degraded further by the matrix beta-oxidation system. Medium-chain fatty acids enter the mitochondrial matrix directly and are activated to the medium-chain acyl-CoAs before degradation by the matrix beta-oxidation system. Tp, carnitine transporter; TL, carnitine-acylcarnitine translocase; LC, long chain; EH, 2-enoyl-CoA hydratase; CoA, coenzyme A; VLC, very long chain; AD, acyl-CoA dehydrogenase; AS, arginosuccinate; HD, 3-hydroxyacyl-CoA dehydrogenase; CPT, carnitine palmitoyltransferase; KT, 3-ketoacyl-CoA thiolase; MC, medium chain; SC, short chain.

Carnitine Deficiency

L-Carnitine or 3-hydroxy-4-N-trimethylammoniobutanoate is a vital molecule for the transport of LCFA into mitochondria. Other physiologic functions of L-carnitine include buffering the acyl-CoA:CoASH ratio, scavenging potentially toxic acyl groups, and oxidizing branched-chain amino acids (100). About 75% of L-carnitine is derived from dietary sources, whereas the rest is synthesized in the liver and kidney; and 95% of the total body carnitine is stored in muscle.

Primary deficiency of L-carnitine is manifested in three phenotypic forms: dilated cardiomyopathy, myopathy, and hypoketotic hypoglycemia with recurrent encephalopathy. Patients frequently show overlapping phenotypes. The age at onset of symptoms ranges from one month to seven years

with a mean of two years (9). The cardiomyopathy is progressive and rapidly fatal unless treated with L-carnitine supplementation. The myopathic form of L-carnitine deficiency is the least common phenotype and is usually associated with cardiomyopathy, encephalopathy, or both. It presents with motor delay, hypotonia, and slowly progressive proximal limb weakness. Acute metabolic encephalopathy is associated with hypoketotic hypoglycemia in younger infants. The episodes are typically triggered by intercurrent illnesses and stress, which are often complicated by recurrent vomiting and decreased oral dietary intake. Persistent CNS signs develop due to severe hypoglycemic encephalopathy and cardiac or respiratory arrest.

Laboratory studies reveal low total and free serum carnitine concentrations, usually less than 10% of normal. The diagnosis can be confirmed by documenting decreased carnitine uptake in cultured skin fibroblasts. Mutations in the sodium-ion-dependent carnitine transporter gene have been identified as causes of primary carnitine deficiency (101, 102). Primary carnitine deficiency responds dramatically to oral L-carnitine therapy at daily divided doses of 100 to 200 mg/kg of body weight. Primary carnitine deficiency is important to identify because it is potentially treatable, whereas secondary deficiencies are more common and due to a variety of underlying metabolic defects. Causes of secondary carnitine deficiency include defects of β-oxidation; malnutrition; excessive carnitine loss, for example, in renal Fanconi syndrome; and valproic acid therapy that results in excessive carnitine excretion.

Carnitine Palmitoyltransferase Deficiency

Mitochondria contain two CPT enzymes, CPT I and II, both vital in the transport of LCFA into mitochondria. CPT I is located in the inner aspect of the outer mitochondrial membrane, whereas CPT II is bound to the inner aspects of the inner mitochondrial membrane (Figure 2). CPT I deficiency presents in infancy as attacks of potentially fatal, fasting-induced, hypoketotic hypoglycemia. The hypoglycemic episodes manifest as lethargy, coma, and seizures. They can lead to psychomotor developmental delay, hemiplegia, and generalized epilepsy. Myopathy is not a typical manifestation, and serum CK has been elevated in only two siblings (103); another patient had a lipid-storage myopathy (104). The diagnosis is confirmed by demonstrating decreased CPT I activity in cultured fibroblasts, leukocytes, or hepatocytes. CPT I activity is normal in skeletal muscle, which may be due to the existence of tissue-specific isoforms and accounts for the absence of clinical myopathy is probably due to tissue-specific isoforms. The first mutations in CPTI have been identified in patients with the hepatic form (105–107).

In contrast, CPT II deficiency has variable clinical manifestations. Three forms of CPT II deficiency have been described: infantile, late-infantile, and adult (108). The early infantile phenotype is rare: it presents at birth with severe hypoketotic hypoglycemia and generalized steatosis and can cause death in a few days. Multiple organ malformations are often present, including renal cystic dysplasia, nephromegaly, microgyria, neuronal heterotopia in the brain, and facial dysmorphism. The late-infantile hepatomuscular form is clinically similar to CPT I deficiency, with acute episodic fasting hypoglycemia and hypoketosis, lethargy, coma, and death. Seizures, hepatomegaly, cardiomegaly, arrhythmias, and pancreatitis have also been described (108). In both infantile forms, CPT II activity is less than 10% of normal.

The adult form of CPT II deficiency was first described in 1973 and is a common cause of exercise-induced myoglobinuria (12, 109). It typically presents in young adulthood with complaints of muscle pain and pigmenturia after prolonged exercise. Severe bouts of rhabdomyolysis with myoglobinuria can cause acute renal failure. Some infants have presented with acute muscle breakdown induced by fever. Adult patients may also have rhabdomyolysis precipitated by fever or other stress. CPT activity is less than 30% of normal. CPT II is a homotetrameric enzyme and the gene (CPT1) encoding the subunit has been characterized. Missense, frame-shift, and deletion mutations in CPT1 segregate with the clinical phenotypes. In the adult muscular form, the most common mutation is a c.439C>T transversion, which changes a highly conserved serine to leucine (p.S113L) (110, 111).

Carnitine-Acylcarnitine Translocase Deficiency

Patients with carnitine-acylcarnitine translocase deficiency are rare (108, 112). The first, described by Stanley and coworkers (112), was a young boy with stunted growth, recurrent vomiting, and coma from birth. At age 2.5 years, he had muscle weakness, cardiomyopathy, and fasting hypoglycemia. Hypoketosis, increased serum long-chain acylcarnitines, and normal CPT activity were later found. Carnitine-acylcarnitine translocase activity was less than 5% of normal control subjects.

β-OXIDATION DEFECTS

The breakdown of fatty acid in mitochondria requires two related systems: the inner mitochondrial membrane portion that metabolizes long-chain acyl-CoA and the mitochondrial matrix beta-oxidation spiral that acts on medium- and short-chain acyl-CoA (Figure 2).

β-Oxidation Defects of the Inner Mitochondrial Membrane System

Very-long-chain acyl-CoA dehydrogenase (VLCAD) deficiency presents in infancy with hypoketotic hypoglycemia, hepatic steatosis, cardiomyopathy, and elevated plasma levels of long-chain acylcarnitines (113). Metabolic acidosis, dicarboxylic aciduria, and increased serum CK with myoglobinuria have also been noted. Patients with recurrent myoglobinuria have the same clinical phenotype as those with CPT II deficiency. Immunoblot analyses for VLCAD have shown absence of the protein in fibroblasts from patients (5). The cDNA for the human VLCAD has been cloned, and a 105-base bp deletion in the gene has been identified in two unrelated infants (8, 108).

Patients with defects of trifunctional protein have isolated long-chain-L-3-hydroxyacyl-coA dehydrogenase (LCHAD) deficiency, whereas a small number of individuals have a combined defect of all three enzyme components. The clinical feature of LCHAD deficiency include onset in infancy, Reyes-like episodes, hypoketotic hypoglycemia with hepatic dysfunction, progressive myopathy, recurrent myoglobinuria, cardiomyopathy, and sudden infant death syndrome (9, 108). Jackson and coworkers (114) first reported the combined defect of the three trifunctional enzyme activities in an infant with recurrent limb weakness, hypotonia, and anorexia precipitated by intercurrent illnesses, who died at age 4.5 years during a severe metabolic crisis with an elevated serum CK, hyperammonemia, and lactic acidosis.

The treatment of patients with inner mitochondrial membrane defects of fatty acid metabolism is mainly dietary. Affected patients should avoid prolonged fasts and long-chain fatty acid ingestion. Intravenous glucose should be given during acute intercurrent illnesses (9, 108).

β-Oxidation Defects of the Mitochondrial Matrix System

The mitochondrial β-oxidation matrix spiral shortens the fatty acid backbone of acyl-CoA by two carbon fragments during each turn through the beta-oxidation spiral. The acetyl-CoA produced in this process is oxidized in the Krebs cycle. In addition, electron transfer flavoprotein (ETF) is reduced and provides reducing equivalents to the oxidative-phosphorylation pathway though the action of ETF CoQ oxidoreductase. Human diseases are caused by defects in several steps of this matrix system (Figure 2).

Defects of long-chain, medium-chain, and short-chain acyl-CoA dehydrogenases generally occur in infancy. Medium-chain acyl-CoA dehydrogenase (MCAD) is, along with CPT II deficiency, the most frequent defect of β-oxidation, with more than 200 identified patients and a disproportionately high incidence in Anglo-Saxon whites (115). MCAD typically begins in the first two years of life with fasting intolerance, nausea, vomiting, hypoketotic hypoglycemia, lethargy, and coma, however, clinical expression is variable and some patients are asymptomatic. MCAD activity in most tissues, including fibroblasts, lymphocytes, and liver, is low, generally 2% to 20% of normal. Early diagnosis and treatment can lead to a favorable outcome. Dietary therapy is aimed at avoidance of fasting and provision of adequate caloric intake. Most MCAD-deficient patients have a c.985A>G transition mutation, causing a lysine-to-glutamate substitution at amino acid 304 of the mature protein (p.K304E), which leads to impaired homotetrameric assembly and instability of the protein (116, 117). Long-chain acyl-CoA dehydrogenase deficiency is less common, and many reported patients instead have VLCAD deficiency. Short-chain acyl-CoA dehydrogenase deficiency has been documented in only a few patients with varying phenotypes, including one adult with progressive

myopathy and massive lipid storage in type I muscle fibers and in several infants with failure-to-thrive and nonketotic hypoglycemia who died in early childhood (118, 119).

Short-chain 3-hydroxyacyl-CoA dehydrogenase deficiency was identified in a nine-month-old child with episodes of hypoglycemia and Reyes-like encephalopathy (120). At age 16 years, she had an attack of hypoketotic hypoglycemia, acute myoglobinuria, and encephalopathy. She developed arrhythmia and died of a dilated cardiomyopathy. Deficiency of 2,4-dienoyl-CoA reductase was identified in muscle and liver of a dysmorphic infant with hypotonia who died at four months of age (121).

Multiple acyl-CoA dehydrogenase deficiency (MADD) or glutaric aciduria type II is a clinical syndrome characterized by metabolic acidosis, hypoketotic hypoglycemia, strong sweaty-feet odor, and early death. There are three distinct clinical presentations of MADD: a severe neonatal form with congenital abnormalities, a severe neonatal form without congenital abnormalities, and a mild later-onset form (9, 108). Pathology reveals fatty degeneration of kidney, liver, heart, and skeletal muscle. The biochemical abnormality is characterized by decreased activities of various acyl-CoA dehydrogenases with urinary excretion of large amounts of numerous organic acids. Three defects lead to MADD, namely ETF deficiency, ETF CoQ oxidoreductase deficiency, and riboflavin (B2)-responsive MAD.

Neutral Lipid Storage Myopathy

Neutral lipid storage diseases (NLSD) are AR disorders characterized by marked accumulation of lipid droplets in the cells of most tissues and circulating leukocytes. A key diagnostic feature common to both NLSDI and NLSDM is the appearance of large neutral lipid droplets in granulocytes (Jordans' anomaly) (122). Despite extensive accumulation of lipid droplets in all tissues, symptoms of NLSDM are limited to myopathy, sometimes with cardiomyopathy and hepatomegaly, without any involvement of the CNS or peripheral nervous system (PNS) (123). In 2007, Fischer and colleagues (124) identified compound heterozygous and homozygous mutations in PNPLA2, the gene encoding adipose triglyceride lipase (ATGL), causing NLSDM in three affected women from different families from The Netherlands, France, and Algeria. All three had myopathies and Jordans anomaly; two apparently had early onset with delays in walking. In addition, variable hepatomegaly was noted in two and one had cardiomyopathy. Reileich and colleagues (123) described six patients with NLSDM and PNPLA2 mutations with a recognizable phenotype of proximal limb weakness beginning in the late 20s and early 30s with early and prominent weakness of the shoulder girdle. Later in the disease, weakness was observed in finger extensors and foot flexors. CK was elevated more than five-fold above normal. One patient with a homozygous

PNPLA2 mutation presented with distal lipid storage myopathy (125), and an apparently healthy 18-year-old woman, serendipitously diagnosed with NLSDM (126), had unexplained high CK and muscle biopsy findings of massive lipid storage, indicating that lipid accumulation occurs over an extended period of time before muscle weakness developed.

Neutral Lipid Storage Myopathy with Ichthyosis

NLSD with icthyosis (NLSDI, also known as Chanarin-Dorfman syndrome) is clinically similar to NLSDM, but manifests prominent scaly skin lesions (ichthyosis) and earlier age-at-onset, usually before 20 years in most patients (126–131). Liver involvement with steatosis and hepatomegaly is common and may progress to cirrhosis. Other clinical features include steatorrhea, cataracts, and hearing loss. NLSDI is caused by mutations in *ABHD5*, which encodes CGI-58, an activator of ATGL (132).

DEFECTS OF MYOADENYLATE DEAMINASE

In 1978, myoadenylate deaminase (mAMPD) deficiency was first described in association with exercise-related myalgia and cramps (133). At present it is also detected in 1 to 3% of skeletal muscle biopsies in asymptomatic patients so studied (133). Fishbein (134) proposed two forms of mAMPD deficiency: primary or hereditary mAMPD deficiency characterized by myopathy, exercise intolerance, myalgia, and cramps with negligible or less than 1% of normal residual activity and lack of cross-reactive material in muscle; and secondary or acquired mAMPD deficiency, associated with other well-defined neuromuscular disorders, higher residual enzyme activity, and detectable cross-reactive material. In the forearm ischemic exercise test, affected patients show a normal elevation of venous lactate, but no rise in ammonia and inosine monophosphate, the products of the mAMPD reaction.

DEFECTS OF OXIDATIVE-PHOSPHORYLATION

General Considerations

Our understanding of the mitochondrial encephalomyopathies has advanced at an astoundingly rapid pace. Interested readers are referred to more in-depth reviews (135–139). In the 1960s, mitochondrial disease research focused on morphologic abnormalities of skeletal muscle, but many characteristic microscopic changes have since been noted in other tissues (140). Accordingly, in the mid-1960s, Shy and coworkers (141) described the typical ultrastructural alterations seen in mitochondrial myopathies, including an overabundance of ultrastructurally normal mitochondria or "pleoconial myopathy," enlarged mitochondria with disoriented cristae or "megaconial myopathy," and inclusions within mitochondria or so-called "paracrystalline" and "osmiophilic" inclusions. Engel and Cunningham (142) developed the modified Gomori trichrome stain that is still commonly used to identify fibers with subsarcolemmal accumulations of mitochondrial, referred to as "ragged red fibers (RRF)." Histochemical stains for mitochondrial enzymes are also used to identify excessive mitochondrial proliferation and to demonstrate specific enzyme defects. These stains include succinate dehydrogenase (SDH) and cytochrome-c-oxidase (COX).

In numerous, but certainly not all, mitochondrial diseases, RRF with ultrastructurally abnormal mitochondria are identified in skeletal muscle by the Gomori trichrome stain. SDH histochemistry reveals mitochondrial proliferation as darker than normal staining in subsarcolemmal regions of muscle fibers. However, the histologic abnormalities are neither specific nor sensitive enough to define all mitochondrial diseases. Morphologically abnormal muscle mitochondria have been detected in many conditions that are not primary oxidative-phosphorylation defects; for example, inflammatory myopathies (143, 144). Conversely, some conditions with defects of mitochondrial enzymes, mitochondrial (mt) DNA, or both, do not have morphologically abnormal mitochondria, including CPT II deficiency. Even in the group of mtDNA-related diseases, not all are characterized by RRF in muscle biopsy tissue. As a general rule, mutations in structural genes are not associated with ragged-red fibers; for example, Leber hereditary optic neuropathy (LHON) and neuropathy, ataxia, retinitis pigmentosa (NARP).

Assessing the respiratory chain enzyme activities or protein levels in tissues can be very informative. For example, biochemical defects of single respiratory chain enzymes have been identified in Leigh syndrome; however, mitochondrial respiratory chain disorders often do not conform to single enzyme defects. The measured enzyme activities may be normal or multiple enzymes can be affected. Therefore, a biochemical classification system can have limitations. Since the initial discoveries of the first mtDNA point mutation and large-scale deletions in 1988 (145–148), there has been an outburst of information relating to the underlying molecular genetic bases of these complex human diseases. Numerous mtDNA mutations have been identified, including duplications, depletions, multiple deletions, and more than 260 pathogenic point mutations (149–151).

One can gain a better understanding of mitochondrial disorders by considering the several unusual genetic characteristics of mitochondria. They are unique organelles because they possess their own genetic material, mtDNA, which is a small circular molecule of 16.5 kilobases (kb) (152). Each mtDNA encodes 22 transfer RNA, 13 polypeptides, and two ribosomal RNAs. The mtDNA-encoded polypeptides are functionally important because they are subunits of the respiratory chain. In addition, more than 1,000 mitochondrial proteins are encoded in the nuclear DNA (nDNA); thus, mitochondria are the products of two genomes. Defects in either genome can cause mitochondrial dysfunction.

Four important characteristics of mtDNA contribute to the expression of a given mt gene defect. The first is heteroplasmy. Each mitochondrion contains two to ten copies of mtDNA, and in turn, each cell contains multiple mitochondria. Therefore, there are thousands of copies of mtDNA in each cell. Mutations of mtDNA may be present in some mtDNA molecules (heteroplasmy) or in all molecules (homoplasmy). As a consequence of heteroplasmy, the proportion of a deleterious mtDNA mutation can vary widely. An individual that harbors a large proportion of mutant mtDNA will be more severely affected than one with a low percentage of the same mutation. Therefore, there is a spectrum of clinical severity among patients with a given mitochondrial mutation.

A second factor that can influence the expression of an mtDNA mutation in an individual is the tissue distribution of that mutation. In turn, variable tissue distribution broadens the clinical spectrum of pathogenic mtDNA mutations. The best example of tissue distribution affecting phenotype comes from large-scale mtDNA deletions. Infants with a high proportion of deleted mtDNA in blood can develop Pearson syndrome, characterized by sideroblastic anemia, often accompanied by exocrine pancreatic dysfunction (153). Presumably, these infants have a high proportion of deleted mtDNA in the bone marrow stem cells. Some children survive the anemia with blood transfusions and recover because the stem cells with a high proportion of deleted mtDNA are under a negative selection bias. Later in life, however, those same children can develop the multisystem mitochondrial disorder Kearns-Sayre syndrome (KSS), characterized by ophthalmoplegia, pigmentary retinopathy, onset before age 20, and cardiac conduction block (154, 155).

A third factor that determines the clinical manifestations of an mtDNA mutation is the tissue threshold effect. Cells with high metabolic activities are severely and adversely affected by mtDNA mutations; therefore, these disorders tend to disproportionately affect brain and muscle (encephalomyopathies).

A fourth unusual characteristic of mtDNA is maternal inheritance. During the formation of the zygote, the mtDNA is derived exclusively from the oocyte. Thus, mtDNA is transmitted vertically in a non-Mendelian fashion from the mother to both male and female progeny. This inheritance pattern is important to recognize in determining whether a family is likely to harbor an mtDNA mutation. A caveat to this principle is the fact that maternal relatives who have a lower percentage of an mtDNA muta-

tion may have fewer symptoms than the proband; thus, they may be oligosymptomatic or even asymptomatic. Therefore, in taking the family history, it is important to inquire about subtle symptoms and signs among maternally related family members that might be oligosymptomatic. Whereas Schwartz and Vissing (156) reported paternal inheritance of muscle mtDNA in a patient with exercise intolerance and an mtDNA mutation restricted to skeletal muscle, a subsequent analysis by Filosto and colleagues (157) failed to reveal paternal inheritance in ten sporadic patients with skeletal muscle-restricted mtDNA mutations, including five-point mutations in protein-coding genes, and five single mtDNA deletions.

These peculiar features of mitochondrial genetics contribute to the clinical complexity of human mitochondrial disorders. Variable heteroplasmy of mtDNA mutations produces an extensive range of disease severity, whereas tissue distribution and tissue threshold of mtDNA mutations explain the frequent but variable involvement of multiple organ systems. In addition to mtDNA mutations, nDNA defects can also cause mitochondrial dysfunction. In fact, nDNA encodes most electron transport chain components, and nDNA mutations have been demonstrated to cause defects in oxidative-phosphorylation and other metabolic pathways (139).

Mitochondrial Diseases due to mtDNA Mutations

Among the mitochondrial encephalomyopathy syndromes, three have been extensively characterized: KSS; mitochondrial encephalomyopathy, lactic acidosis, with stroke-like episodes (MELAS); and myoclonus epilepsy with RRF (MERRF) (154, 158, 159). In addition, numerous other clinical syndromes have been associated with oxidative-phosphorylation defects (136, 160, 161). Despite the complexity and the heterogeneity of mitochondrial disorders, there are several clinical themes common to all. First, they tend to affect children and young adults. Second, they are often multisystemic. Third, maternal inheritance is often pathognomonic of mtDNA point mutations, whereas patients with single large-scale rearrangements tend to be sporadic. Fourth, there is great variability of phenotypic expression in families with mtDNA point mutations.

Although the identification of mtDNA mutations has simplified diagnosis in most cases of mitochondrial encephalomyopathies, it has created new dilemmas. Genetic counseling of patients and their maternal relatives is difficult because heteroplasmy and variability of mutation tissue distribution make clinical outcome predictions tenuous. Similarly, prenatal diagnosis is also perilous. The molecular genetic information should be handled carefully because it can adversely affect medical insurability, employment opportunities, and the emotional status of patients.

Kearns-Sayre Syndrome

Kearns-Sayre syndrome is a multisystemic disorder defined by Rowland (157) by the obligatory triad of progressive external ophthalmoplegia (PEO), atypical salt and pepper retinopathy, and onset before age 20, with at least one of the following: cardiac conduction block, cerebellar ataxia, and cerebrospinal fluid (CSF) protein greater than 100 mg/dL. Other frequent but not invariable clinical manifestations include short stature, hearing loss, dementia, limb weakness, diabetes mellitus, hypoparathyroidism, and growth hormone deficiency (162). Pigmentary retinopathy affects low light vision more than visual acuity, hence patients complain of night-vision difficulties, and peripheral vision may be compromised by ptosis. Muscle involvement includes oropharyngeal dysfunction, and proximal more than distal limb weakness. Dysphagia results from incomplete opening of the upper esophageal sphincter, so-called cricopharyngeal achalasia (163). The heart block is of a conduction type, which can lead to complete heart block and the necessity of pacemaker insertion. Short stature results from growth hormone deficiency.

EMG and nerve conduction studies are generally consistent with myopathy, but neuropathy may coexist. Brain magnetic resonance imaging (MRI) may show leukoencephalopathy associated with cerebral and cerebellar atrophy, and basal ganglia lesions. Echocardiogram and electrocardiography (ECG) may show intrinsic heart disease and conduction block. Muscle biopsy typically shows RRF with the modified Gomori trichrome stain as well as COX-deficient myofibers. Biochemical studies of respiratory chain enzymes in muscle extracts usually show decreased activities of respiratory chain complexes containing mtDNA encoded subunits. The differential diagnosis of KSS and PEO should be differentiated from other disorders associated with ophthalmoplegia, including myasthenia gravis, oculopharyngeal muscular dystrophy, myotonic dystrophy, and autosomal dominant (AD) and AR PEO with multiple deletions of mtDNA.

Neuropathological changes include basal ganglia calcifications and spongy changes of the brain white matter. The mtDNA deletions are detectable in skeletal muscle, but rarely identified in blood so muscle biopsy is typically necessary to identify the molecular genetic defect.

Typically, KSS patients are sporadic because the mtDNA rearrangements seem to originate in oogenesis or early zygote formation. Long PCR analysis, which detects deletions throughout the mtDNA, has a high sensitivity and low specificity, and may be of limited use, especially in older individuals wherein mtDNA deletions may accumulate with age and lead to misdiagnosis. As a result, Southern blot is the preferred method of molecular diagnosis.

An ECG should be performed at regular intervals at least yearly to allow for the planning of pacemaker insertion. Diabetes can be treated with insulin administration. Hyperparathyroidism can be treated with surgery with later hormone replacement therapy. Patients at risk for pneumonia and aspiration can be studied with swallowing studies and dietary adjustment. Hearing aids and cochlear implants can assist hearing loss

Myoclonus Epilepsy and Ragged Red Fibers

MERRF is a multisystemic syndrome characterized by myoclonus, which is often the first symptom, followed by generalized epilepsy, ataxia, weakness, and dementia. Onset is usually in childhood after normal early development. Common findings also include hearing loss, short stature, optic atrophy, peripheral neuropathy, exercise intolerance, lipomas, lactic acidosis, and cardiomyopathy with Wolff-Parkinson-White (WPW) syndrome (159, 164). Most MERRF patients have a history of affected maternally related family members, although not all have the full syndrome. The diagnosis is based upon the presence of the following four elements: myoclonus, generalized epilepsy, ataxia, and RRF in the muscle biopsy.

As in KSS, diagnostic evaluation should include measurement of pyruvate and lactate in the blood and CSF, which are commonly elevated at rest and increase excessively after moderate activity. The CSF protein is typically elevated but rarely surpasses 100 mg/dl. The electroencephalogram shows generalized spike and wave discharges with background slowing, but focal epileptiform discharges can be seen. The ECG can show pre-excitation but heart block is not usually present. The EMG and NCS are consistent with myopathy but often shows co-existing axonal neuropathy. Brain MRI shows atrophy and basal ganglia calcification. Muscle biopsy typically shows RRF with the modified Gomori trichrome stain and fibers that fail to stain with COX. Biochemical studies of respiratory chain enzymes in muscle extracts usually show decreased activities of respiratory chain complexes containing mtDNA encoded subunits, especially COX.

In 1990, Shoffner and colleagues (165) identified an m.8344A>G mutation in the MT-TK gene was found in about 80% of MERRF patients tested (164). The m.8344A>G mutation can be associated with isolated myopathy resembling limb girdle muscular dystrophy, or with multiple lipomas of the neck and shoulder area, so-called Ekbom syndrome. Other clinical presentations of the mutation include spinocerebellar degeneration, and Leigh syndrome. At least five other mtDNA point mutations cause MERRF, including three additional MT-TK point mutations (m.8356T>C, m.8363G>A, and m.8361G>A) and two mutations in other tRNA genes (m.611G>A in MT-TF and m.15967G>A in MT-TP) (166–169). In families with a MERRF proband, oligosymptomatic and asymptomatic members harbor the same mtDNA mutation, but the phenotype is presumably attenuated by heteroplasmy and tissue distribution of the mtDNA mutation (170). Occasionally, patients present with MERRF-MELAS (171) or MERRF-KSS overlap syndromes (172, 173).

There is no clear correlation between the genotype and clinical phenotype for individual patients. Prenatal testing is possible by extraction of DNA from fetal cells obtained at amniocentesis and chorionic villus biopsy sampling; however, the specific mtDNA mutation in the mother must be identified before prenatal diagnosis is performed. In addition, as a result of mitotic segregation, the mtDNA mutational load in amniocytes and chorionic villi may not correspond with that of other fetal or adult tissues, nor is prediction of phenotype, age of onset, severity, or rate of progression possible.

Mitochondrial Encephalomyopathy, Lactic Acidosis, and Stroke-Like Episodes

This maternally inherited disorder has the defining clinical features of stroke-like episodes, typically before age 40, with encephalopathy manifested as seizures and dementia, and mitochondrial dysfunction with lactic acidosis and RRF in muscle tissue (158, 174). It is uncommon for more than one family member to have the full MELAS syndrome. In most pedigrees, there is only one MELAS patient with oligosymptomatic or asymptomatic relatives in the maternal lineage.

In typical cases, there is normal early psychomotor development with short stature is common. Onset of symptoms occurs frequently between the ages of two to ten years with seizures, recurrent headaches, anorexia, and vomiting. Exercise intolerance and proximal limb weakness can be an initial manifestation, followed by generalized epilepsy. Seizures can be associated with stroke-like episodes of transient hemiparesis, cortical blindness, altered mental consciousness, migraine headache, and residual cumulative motor impairment in adolescence and young adulthood. Other symptoms can include myoclonus, ataxia, episodic coma, optic atrophy, cardiomyopathy, pigmentary retinopathy, diabetes mellitus, hirsutism, gastrointestinal dysmotility, nephropathy, fever, drop attached, impaired gait, WPW syndrome of pre-excitation, cardiac conduction block, PEO, and sensorineural hearing loss. The typical range of death is from 10 to 35 years and is due to intercurrent infection and gastrointestinal obstruction; however, some individuals live into their sixth decade.

Laboratory testing should include determination of lactate and pyruvate in blood and CSF along with protein content, which rarely surpasses 100 mg/dl. During the stroke-like episodes, brain MRI typically shows lesions with increased FLAIR/T2 signals that do not conform to vascular territories, along with basal ganglia calcification. ECG may show cardiomyopathy, pre-excitation, and heart block. Electrodiagnostic studies show myopathy but neuropathy can coexist. Muscle biopsy demonstrates RRF with modified Gomori trichrome that also stain positively for COX, in contrast to other mtDNA-related disorders such as KSS and MERRF in which RRF do not react with COX histochemical stain. There may be an overabundance of mitochondria in smooth muscle and endothelial cells of intramuscular blood vessels, best revealed with SDH stain. Biochemical analysis of respiratory chain enzymes in muscle extracts shows multiple partial defects, especially involving complex I and IV. There are no clear correlations between genotype and clinical phenotype for individual patients.

There are at 30 causative mtDNA mutations (175), the commonest of which is the A-to-G transition at nucleotide 3243 in *MTTL1* encoding tRNALeu (UUR), first described by Goto and coworkers (177), and so-noted in about 80% of individuals with MELAS. Although the common MELAS mutation, m3243A>G, was identified more than 2 decades ago, the molecular consequences of the mutation are still incompletely understood. Muscle cells with the m.3243A>G mutation grown in tissue culture demonstrate respiratory deficiency (176). King and Attardi developed a cell line called rho-0 that replicates in the absence of mtDNA (177). The rho-0 cells can be fused with cytoplasts harboring mutant mtDNA forming cybrids. Cybrids with greater than 95% m.3243A>G mtDNA showed decreased rates of protein synthesis, lower levels of steady-state mitochondrial translational products, reduced oxygen consumption, and increased amounts of an unprocessed RNA fragment containing the mutant gene designated RNA-19 (178). Other investigators have demonstrated that high levels of the mutant tRNA decreased aminoacylation (covalent attachment of leucine to the tRNA), and were associated with hypomodification of the D-stem. These alterations may contribute to the decreased protein synthesis (179–182). An alternative theory, also based on cybrid work, is that the mutant tRNALeu (UUR) is less efficiently modified at the base corresponding to the wobble base of the codon, thereby leading to misreading of leucine codons as phenylalanine codons (183) due to lack of a post-transcriptional methyl-taurine modification of the anticodon wobble base (184). Cultured myoblasts from a patient with the m.3243A>G mutation revealed evidence of both amino acid misincorporation and moderate reduction of protein synthesis (185).

Treatments aimed at the primary biochemical defects in the mitochondrial encephalomyopathies consist mainly of symptomatic measures, the efficacy of which have been anecdotally observed. A trial of coenzyme Q10, 50 to 100 mg three times a day, and L-carnitine, 330 mg three times daily, may afford some benefit. Dichloroacetate inhibits pyruvate dehydrogenase specific kinase, thus activating pyruvate dehydrogenase complex and reducing lactate. Unfortunately, a double-blind randomized placebo-controlled trial of DCA showed no treatment benefit and the trial was terminated due to frequent peripheral nerve toxicity (186). L-arginine, a nitric oxide precursor, has been used to stimulate vasodilation in MELAS (187). In open-label studies, intravenous L-arginine administered shortly after the onset of a stroke-like episode seemed to improve outcomes while oral administration during interictal phases appeared to decrease the frequency and severity of stroke-like events (188, 189).

Mitochondrial Diseases Due to Nuclear DNA Mutations

Genomic Defects of the Mitochondrial Respiratory Chain and Oxidative-Phosphorylation

The first nDNA-causing mitochondrial respiratory chain defect was described 17 years ago in a pair of siblings with Leigh syndrome who were found to have compound heterozygous mutations in the flavoprotein subunit of complex II (190). Since then, additional mutations encoding subunits of all five respiratory chain/oxidative phosphorylation complexes have been identified in a growing number of patients mainly with Leigh syndrome (139). In addition to structural subunits, these multi-subunit enzyme complexes require assembly factors, when mutated, produce a defect of a mitochondrial respiratory chain/oxidative phosphorylation enzyme. In fact, the commonest causes of Leigh syndrome with complex IV deficiency are AR mutations in SURF1, which encode a protein required for COX biogenesis (191, 192).

Coenzyme Q10 (CoQ10) is a vital respiratory chain component that shuttles electrons from complexes I and II to complex III (193). Deficiency of CoQ10 is particularly noteworthy as it often responds to therapy, namely CoQ10 supplementation (194, 195). Clinical presentations of CoQ10 deficiency include: infantile-onset multisystemic diseases (predominantly encephalonephropathies); encephalomyopathies with the trial of brain involvement, myopathy with recurrent myoglobinuria, and RRF; cerebellar ataxia; nephropathy; and isolated myopathy. CoQ10 is synthesized within mitochondria. Primary CoQ10 deficiencies are due to mutations in one of the nuclear DNA genes required for CoQ10 biosynthesis whereas secondary forms are due to mutations in other genes. Primary CoQ10 deficiencies have been associated mainly with the infantile multisystemic diseases or predominant nephropathy due to mutations in PDSS1, PDSS2, COQ2, COQ6, and COQ9 (196–200). Mutations in ADCK3, which encodes a kinase that modulates CoQ10 synthesis, cause AR juvenile onset ataxia (201, 202). In a report of seven patients with the myopathic form of CoQ10 deficiency, mutations were identified in the ETFDH gene encoding electron-transferring flavoprotein dehydrogenase, also associated with glutaric aciduria type II (multiple acyl-CoA dehydrogenase deficiency [MADD]) (203). Patients with primary and secondary forms of CoQ10 deficiency (including individuals with ETFDH mutations) have improved with high CoQ10 doses (in children up to 10mg/kg/day and in adults up to 3,000mg daily).

Defects of Intergenomic Communication

The mitochondrial genome is dependent on nuclear DNA factors necessary for mtDNA replication, repair, transcription, and protein translation (204). A growing number of autosomal diseases have been associated with instability of mtDNA (e.g., depletion and multiple deletions) as well as mitochondrial protein synthesis defects that are collectively called defects of intergenomic communication. AD PEO with multiple deletions of mtDNA was the first of these disorders to be identified and, in most cases, is due to mutations in POLG encoding the catalytic subunit of mitochondrial DNA polymerase γ (151, 205). Mendelian forms of PEO or PEO-plus phenotypes with multiple mtDNA deletions have also been associated with mutations in the following genes: ANT1 (encoding the ADP/ATP translocator), PEO1 (DNA helicase), RRM2B (small subunit of p53-inducible ribonucleotide reductase), MPV17 (mitochondria protein of unknown function), and POLG2 (accessory subunit of polymerase γ) (206–211). MtDNA depletion syndrome was originally reported in infants with severe hepatopathy or myopathy (150). Both are usually fatal in early childhood, but a few patients with the myopathic form are alive in young adulthood. Myopathic mtDNA depletion is typically due to AR mutations in the mitochondrial thymidine kinase encoded by TK2 while the hepatocerebral form is often due to mutations in DGUOK encoding the mitochondrial deoxyguanosine kinase (212, 213). In addition, mutations in at least seven other genes (POLG, RRM2B, MPV17, PEO1, SUCLA2, SUCLG2, and TYMP) cause mtDNA depletion (214). Mitochondrial neurogastrointestinal encephalomyopathy (MNGIE) is an AR disorder that manifests PEO, gastrointestinal dysmotility, cachexia, peripheral neuropathy, and leukoencephalopathy (215). Muscle biopsies usually show neurogenic changes, RRF, depletion and multiple deletions of mtDNA. MNGIE is due to mutations in TYMP encoding thymidine phosphorylase, a cytosolic enzyme that is thought to contribute to the regulation of nucleotide pools in the mitochondria (216). Allogeneic hematopoetic stem cell transplantation (AHSCT including bone marrow transplant) has been demonstrated to improve the biochemical derangements and clinical manifestations in MNGIE, however transplant-related mortality has been high; therefore, further studies are necessary to assess this treatment (217, 218).

Defects of mtDNA translation typically manifest as severe infantile multisystemic disorders with encephalopathy as the predominant clinical feature (219), except in the juvenile-onset AR disorder, mitochondrial myopathy, lactic acidosis, and sideroblastic anemia (MLASA) caused by mutation in *PUS1* encoding pseudouridine synthetase 1, an enzyme that modifies cytosolic and mitochondrial transfer RNAs (220).

Defects of the Mitochondrial Lipid Milieu Composition

The inner mitochondrial membrane (IMM) contains phospholipids that are critical for the structure and integrity of the embedded respiratory chain proteins. Barth syndrome is a prototypical disorder of mitochondrial phospholipid metabolism with secondary respiratory chain defects (221). This X-linked recessive disorder is caused by mutations in *TAZ1*, encoding the monolyso-cardiolipin transacylase, which is required for cardiolipin remodeling (222). The disease is clinically characterized by mitochondrial cardiac and skeletal myopathy, cyclic neutropenia, and growth retardation with defects of respiratory chain enzyme activities.

A second disorder of the mitochondrial lipid milieu is an AR congenital myopathy with mental retardation and a protracted course (223). The cause is mutations in *CHKB*, encoding choline kinase beta, an enzyme required for the *de novo* synthesis of phosphatidyl choline and phosphatidylethanolamine (224). Muscle biopsies have shown strikingly enlarged mitochondria that were displaced to the periphery of the fibers.

The AR inherited disorder Sengers syndrome presents with congenital cataracts, hypertrophic cardiomyopathy, skeletal myopathy, exercise intolerance, and lactic acidosis, due to mutations in the *AGK* gene encoding acylglycerol kinase (225, 226). The *AGK* defect causes deficiency of phosphatidic acid and secondary decrease of ANT in the IMM.

Defects of Mitochondrial Dynamics

Mitochondria are not static organelles, but rather move, fuse, and divide in a dynamic fashion (227). A striking example of a defect of mitochondrial dynamics is mutations in *OPA1* that cause AD optic atrophy (DOA or Kjer disease) in isolation or in combination with sensorineural hearing loss, PEO, myopathy, ataxia, and axonal peripheral neuropathy (228, 229). Muscle biopsy tissue from patients with DOA-plus phenotypes show ragged-blue, COX-negative fibers, and multiple mtDNA deletions. OPA1 protein is required for fusion of the IMM; however, the causal link between *OPA1* defects and mtDNA instability has not been established.

Defects of Iron Metabolism

Mitochondrial respiratory chain enzymes contain redox active sites with metals (iron-sulfur clusters or copper). Defects of iron metabolism cause deficiencies of iron-sulfur containing enzymes such as aconitase and respiratory chain complexes I and II, which in turn cause mitochondrial diseases including Friedreich ataxia, neurodegeneration with brain iron accumulation (NBIA), and a rare AR myopathy clinically characterized by childhood-onset early fatigue, dyspnea, cardiomyopathy and tachycardia with mild exercise (230, 231). The disorder is static or slowly progressive, but patients may have life-threatening episodes of weakness, metabolic acidosis, and rhabdomyolysis. This disease has been observed in Sweden and Finland and is due to mutations in *ISCU*, which encodes the mitochondrial iron-sulfur cluster assembly protein, IscU (232–234).

Diagnostic Investigation of Mitochondrial Myopathies

Algorithms and criteria have been developed to diagnose mitochondrial encephalomyopathies, which are notoriously difficult to identify because of their clinical complexity and diversity (162, 235–237). Clues in the medical history that can suggest mitochondrial disease include: psychomotor retardation or regression, short stature, exercise intolerance, migraine headaches, sensorineural hearing loss, diabetes mellitus, atypical strokes, myoclonic epilepsy, or ptosis. Family history may reveal subtle suggestions of maternal inheritance when dealing with an mtDNA point mutation. For example, probands with MELAS often have relatives in the maternal lineage who may have migraine-like headaches or diabetes mellitus as the only manifestation of the same genetic defect.

Careful medical and neurologic examinations often reveal findings to the correct diagnosis. Affected patients are often short and thin. Multiple lipomatosis can be disfiguring in patients with MERRF or their maternal relatives (238). Dementia can be a prominent finding in KSS, MELAS, and MERRF (162). Cranial nerve functions may be impaired and affect particularly extraocular muscles, with ptosis and PEO, which are necessary to diagnose KSS but are sometimes seen in MELAS patients. Fundoscopy may reveal pigmentary retinopathy in KSS and, less commonly, in MELAS and MERRF. Optic atrophy is sometimes detected in MERRF patients. Peripheral neuropathy is more frequent in MERRF than in the other two syndromes. Sensorineural hearing loss is common in many mitochondrial encephalomyopathies.

The laboratory evaluation should include a complete blood count, with serum electrolytes, and calcium, phosphorous, liver function tests, blood urea nitrogen, creatine, CK, plasma venous and arterial lactate and pyruvate levels, amino acids, and carnitine profile. Urine should be obtained for amino acids, organic acids, and myoglobin. Plasma lactate and pyruvate are commonly elevated at rest in patients with mitochondrial encephalomyopathies and can increase dramatically after moderate exercise. The ECG may reveal pre-excitation in MELAS or MERRF and heart block in KSS or MELAS. Lumbar puncture may show elevation of the CSF protein content, especially in those with KSS, or reveal elevation of lactate and pyruvate levels, and amino acids. Electromyography and NCS are typically consistent with a myogenic process, although neurogenic changes may be detected in MERRF or MELAS. Brain computed tomography (CT) and MRI may reveal basal ganglia calcifications and atrophy. In patients with MELAS, atypical strokes do not conform to vascular territories but rather affect the cortex and adjacent white matter, particularly in the posterior cerebrum (239). ^{31}P-MRS will reveal potentially valuable information such as decreased high energy phosphate molecules (e.g., ATP and phosphocreatine) content.

Specialized evaluation for oxidative-phosphorylation defects has evolved from laboratory research and includes histologic studies performed directly on skeletal muscle, measurement of biochemical activities of mitochondrial respiratory chain enzymes, and molecular genetic analyses. With the application of next-generation sequencing to clinical diagnostic testing, screening of the whole mtDNA and panels of nuclear genes has become less expensive and is often used in routine clinical evaluations. Although already available for clinical use, whole exome sequencing is still expensive and has technical limitations, including incomplete coverage and paucity of information about the significance of the wide array of DNA variants. Nevertheless, as knowledge of the normal and abnormal genetic spectrum advances, whole exome and whole genome sequencing are likely to become part of routine clinical diagnostic testing for metabolic myopathies and other inherited disorders.

REFERENCES

1. DiMauro S, Garone C, Naini A. Metabolic myopathies. *Curr Rheumatol Rep* 2010; 12:386–393.
2. DiMauro S, Musumeci O. Metabolic Myopathies. In: Katirji B, Kaminski HJ, Preston DC, Ruff RL, Shapiro BE, eds. *Neuromuscular Disorders in Clinical Practice*. Boston: Butterworth Heinemann, 2002; 1128–1150.
3. Hirano M, Nishino I, DiMauro S. Mitochondrial Myopathies. In: Katirji B, Kaminski HJ, Preston DC, Ruff RL, Shapiro BE, eds. *Neuromuscular Disorders in Clinical Practice*. Boston: Butterworth Heinemann, 2002; 1151–1168.
4. Liang WC, Nishino I. Lipid storage myopathy. *Curr Neurol Neurosci Rep* 2011; 11:97–103.
5. DiMauro S, Bonilla E. Mitochondrial Encephalomyopathies. In: Engel AG, ed. *Myology*. New York: McGraw-Hill, 2004; 1623–1662.
6. DiMauro S, Hayes AP, Tsujino S. Nonlysosomal Glycogenoses. In: Engel AG, ed. *Myology*. New York: McGraw-Hill, 2004; 1535–1558.
7. Engel AG, Hirschhorn R, Huie ML. Acid maltase deficiency. In: Engel AG, ed. *Myology*. New York: McGraw-Hill, 2004; 1559–1586.
8. Di Donato S, Taroni F. Disorders of Lipid Metabolism. In: Engel AG, ed. *Myology*. New York: McGraw-Hill, 2004; 1587–1622.
9. De Vivo DC, Hirano M, DiMauro S. Mitochondrial disorders. In: Moser HW, ed. *Neurodystrophies and Neurolipidoses*. Amsterdam: Elsevier Science BV, 1997; 389–446.
10. Felig P, Wahren J. Fule homeostasis in exercise. *N Engl J Med* 1975; 293:1078–1084.
11. McArdle B. Myopathy due to a defect in muscle glycogen breakdown. *Clin Sci* 1951; 10:13–33.
12. DiMauro S, DiMauro-Melis PM. Muscle carnitine palmitoyltransferase deficiency and myoglobinuria. *Science* 1973; 182:929–931.
13. Berardo A, DiMauro S, Hirano M. A diagnostic algorithm for metabolic myopathies. *Curr Neurol Neurosci Rep* 2010; 10:118–126.
14. Pompe JC. Over Idiopatische Hypertrophie van het Hart. *Ned T Geneesk* 1932; 76:304–311.
15. van den Hout HM, Hop W, van Diggelen OP, et al. The natural course of infantile Pompe's disease: 20 original cases compared with 133 cases from the literature. *Pediatrics* 2003; 112:332–340.
16. Kishnani PS, Hwu WL, Mandel H, Nicolino M, Yong F, Corzo D. A retrospective, multinational, multicenter study on the natural history of infantile-onset Pompe disease. *J Pediatr* 2006; 148:671–676.
17. Slonim AE, Bulone L, Ritz S, Goldberg T, Chen A, Martiniuk F. Identification of two subtypes of infantile acid maltase deficiency. *J Pediatr* 2000; 137:283–285.
18. The Human Gene Mutation Database [online]. Available at: http://www.hgmd.org. Accessed August 24, 2012.
19. Hirschhorn R, Reuser AJ. Glycogen Storage Disease Type II: Acid α-Glucosidase (Acid Maltase) Deficiency. Scriver's Online Metabolic and Molecular Bases of Inherited Disease [serial online] 2006. Available at: http://dx.doi.org/10.1036/ommbid.135.
20. Kishnani PS, Steiner RD, Bali D, et al. Pompe disease diagnosis and management guideline. *Genet Med* 2006; 8:267–288.
21. Martiniuk F, Chen A, Mack A, et al. Carrier frequency for glycogen storage disease type II in New York and estimates of affected individuals born with the disease. *Am J Med Genet* 1998; 79:69–72.
22. Ausems MG, Verbiest J, Hermans MP, et al. Frequency of glycogen storage disease type II in The Netherlands: implications for diagnosis and genetic counselling. *Eur J Hum Genet* 1999; 7:713–716.
23. Chien YH, Chiang SC, Zhang XK, et al. Early detection of Pompe disease by newborn screening is feasible: results from the Taiwan screening program. *Pediatrics* 2008; 122:e39–45.
24. Kishnani PS, Nicolino M, Voit T, et al. Chinese hamster ovary cell-derived recombinant human acid alpha-glucosidase in infantile-onset Pompe disease. *J Pediatr* 2006; 149:89–97.
25. Nicolino M, Byrne B, Wraith JE, et al. Clinical outcomes after long-term treatment with alglucosidase alfa in infants

and children with advanced Pompe disease. *Genet Med* 2009; 11:210–219.

26. Kishnani PS, Goldenberg PC, DeArmey SL, et al. Cross-reactive immunologic material status affects treatment outcomes in Pompe disease infants. *Mol Genet Metab* 2010; 99:26–33.

27. Prater SN, Banugaria SG, Dearmey SM, et al. The emerging phenotype of long-term survivors with infantile Pompe disease. *Genet Med* 2012; 14:800–810.

28. van der Ploeg AT, Clemens PR, Corzo D, et al. A randomized study of alglucosidase alfa in late-onset Pompe's disease. *N Engl J Med* 2010; 362:1396–1406.

29. Cupler EJ, Berger KI, Leshner RT, et al. Consensus treatment recommendations for late-onset Pompe disease. *Muscle Nerve* 2012; 45:319–333.

30. Van Creveld S. Over een bijzondere stoornis in de koolhydraatstofwisseling in de kinderleeftijd. *Ned T Geneesk* 1928; 15:349–359.

31. Smit GPA, Fernandes J, Leonard JV, et al. The long-term outcome of patients with glycogen storage diseases. *J Inher Metab Dis* 1990; 13:411–418.

32. Fellows IW, Lowe JS, Ogilvie AL, Stevens A, Toghill PJ, Atkinson M. Type III glycogenosis presenting as liver disease in adults with atypical histological features. *J Clin Pathol* 1983; 36:431–434.

33. Brown BI. Debranching and branching enzyme deficiencies. In: Engel AG, Banker BQ, eds. *Myology*. New York: McGraw-Hill, 1986; 1653–1661.

34. Parvari R, Moses S, Shen J, Hershkovitz E, Lerner A, Chen YT. A single-base deletion in the 3'-coding region of glycogen-debranching enzyme is prevalent in glycogen storage disease type IIIA in a population of North African Jewish patients. *Eur J Hum Genet* 1997; 5:266–270.

35. Bruno C, van Diggelen OP, Cassandrini D, et al. Clinical and genetic heterogeneity of branching enzyme deficiency (glycogenosis type IV). *Neurology* 2004; 63:1053–1058.

36. Taratuto AL, Akman HO, Saccoliti M, et al. Branching enzyme deficiency/glycogenosis storage disease type IV presenting as a severe congenital hypotonia: muscle biopsy and autopsy findings, biochemical and molecular genetic studies. *Neuromuscul Disord* 2010; 20:783–790.

37. Konstantinidou AE, Anninos H, Gyftodimou Y, et al. Neonatal neuromuscular variant of glycogen storage disease type IV: histopathological findings leading to the diagnosis. *Histopathology* 2006; 48:878–880.

38. Tay SK, Akman HO, Chung WK, et al. Fatal infantile neuromuscular presentation of glycogen storage disease type IV. *Neuromuscul Disord* 2004; 14:253–260.

39. Herrick MK, Twiss JL, Vladutiu GD, et al. Concomitant branching enzyme and phosphorylase deficiencies. An unusual glycogenosis with extensive neuronal polyglucosan storage. *J Neuropathol Exp Neurol* 1994; 53:239–246.

40. Reusche E, Aksu F, Goebel HH, et al. A mild juvenile variant of type IV glycogenosis. *Brain Dev* 1992; 14:36–43.

41. Schroder JM, May R, Shin YS, et al. Juvenile hereditary polyglucosan body disease with complete branching enzyme deficiency (type IV glycogenosis). *Acta Neuropathol* 1993; 85:419–430.

42. Lossos A, Barash V, Soffer D, et al. Hereditary branching enzyme dysfunction in adult polyglucosan body disease: a possible metabolic cause in two patients. *Ann Neurol* 1991; 30:655–662.

43. Bruno C, Servidei S, Shanske S, et al. Glycogen branching enzyme deficiency in adult polyglucosan body disease. *Ann Neurol* 1993; 33:88–93.

44. Cafferty MS, Lovelace RE, Hays AP, et al. Polyglucosan body disease. *Muscle Nerve* 1991; 14:102–107.

45. Shin YS, Steiguber H, Klemm P, Endres W, et al. Branching enzyme in erythrocytes. Detection of type IV glycogenosis homozygotes and heterozygotes. *J Inherited Metab Dis* 1988; 2:252–254.

46. Schmid R, Hammaker L. Hereditary absence of muscle phosphorylase (McArdle's syndrome). *N Engl J Med* 1961; 264:223–225.

47. Schmid R, Mahler R. Chronic progressive myopathy with myoglobinuria: demonstration of a glycogenolytic defect in the muscle. *J Clin Invest* 1959; 38:2044–2058.

48. Mommaerts W, Illingworth B, Pearson CM, et al. A functional disorder of muscle associated with the absence of phosphorylase. *Proc Nat Acad Sci USA* 1959; 45:791–797.

49. DiMauro S, Hays AP, Tsujino S. Nonlysosomal glycogenoses. In: Engel AG, Franzini-Armstrong C, eds. *Myology*. 3rd ed. New York: McGraw-Hill, 2004; 1535–1558.

50. DiMauro S, Hartlage P. Fatal infantile form of muscle phosphorylase deficiency. *Neurology* 1978; 28:1124–1129.

51. Lucia A, Ruiz JR, Santalla A, et al. Genotypic and phenotypic features of McArdle disease: insights from the Spanish national registry. *J Neurol Neurosurg Psychiatry* 2012; 83:322–328.

52. Kost GJ, Verity MA. A new variant of late-onset myophosphorylase deficiency. *Muscle Nerve* 1980; 3:195–201.

53. Abarbanel JM, Potashnik R, Frisher S, Moses SW, Osimani A, Herishanu Y. Myophosphorylase deficiency: the course of an unusual congenital myopathy. *Neurology* 1987; 37:316–318.

54. Milstein JM, Herron TM, Haas JE. Fatal infantile muscle phosphorylase deficiency. *J Child Neurol* 1989; 4:186–188.

55. Ross BD, Radda GK, Gadian DG, et al. Examination of a case of suspected McArdle's syndrome by 31P nuclear magnetic resonance. *N Engl J Med* 1981; 304:1338–1342.

56. Kazemi-Esfarjani P, Skomorowska E, Jensen TD, et al. A nonischemic forearm exercise test for McArdle disease. *Ann Neurol* 2002; 52:153–159.

57. Tsujino S, Shanske S, DiMauro S. Molecular genetic heterogeneity of myophosphorylase deficiency (McArdle's disease). *N Engl J Med* 1993; 329:241–245.

58. Quinlivan R, Buckley J, James M, et al. McArdle disease: a clinical review. *J Neurol Neurosurg Psychiatry* 2010; 81:1182–1188.

59. Bruno C, Cassandrini D, Martinuzzi A, et al. McArdle disease: the mutation spectrum of PYGM in a large Italian cohort. *Hum Mutat* 2006; 27:718.

60. Slonim AE, Goans PJ. McArdle's syndrome: improvement with a high-protein diet. *N Engl J Med* 1985; 312:355–359.

61. Vissing J, Haller RG. The effect of oral sucrose on exercise tolerance in patients with McArdle's disease. *N Engl J Med* 2003; 349:2503–2509.

62. Haller RG, Wyrick P, Taivassalo T, et al. Aerobic conditioning: an effective therapy in McArdle's disease. *Ann Neurol* 2006; 59:922–928.

63. Tarui S, Okuno G, Ikua Y, et al. Phosphofructokinase deficiency in skeletal muscle. A new type of glycogenosis. *Biochem Biophys Res Comm* 1965; 19:517–523.

64. Layzer RB, Rowland LP, Bank WJ. Physical and kinetic properties of human phosphofructokinase from skeletal muscle and erythrocytes. *J Biol Chem* 1969; 244:3823–3831.

65. Layzer RB, Rowland LP, Ranney HM. Muscle phosphofructokinase deficiency. *Arch Neurol* 1967; 17:512–523.

66. Hays AP, Hallett M, Delfs J, et al. Muscle phosphofructokinase deficiency: abnormal polysaccharide in a case of late-onset myopathy. *Neurology* 1981; 31:1077–1086.

67. Haller RG, Lewis SF. Glucose-induced exertional fatigue in muscle phosphofructokinase deficiency. *N Engl J Med* 1991; 324:364–369.

68. Kilimann MW. Glycogen storage disease due to phosphorylase

kinase deficiency. In: Swallow DM, Edwards YH, eds. *Protein dysfunction in human genetic diseases.* Oxford: Bios Scientific Publishers, 1997; 57–75.

69. Mizuta K, Hashimoto E, Tsutou A, et al. A new type of glycogen storage disease caused by deficiency of cardiac phosphorylase kinase. *Biochem Biophys Res Comm* 1984; 119:582–587.

70. Servidei S, Metlay LA, Chodosh J, et al. Fatal infantile cardiopathy caused by phosphorylase b kinase deficiency. *J Pediatr* 1988; 113:82–85.

71. DiMauro S, Spiegel R. Progress and problems in muscle glycogenoses. *Acta Myol* 2011; 30:96–102.

72. Burwinkel B, Hu B, Schroers A, et al. Muscle glycogenosis with low phosphorylase kinase activity: mutations in PHKA1, PHKG1 or six other candidate genes explain only a minority of cases. *Eur J Hum Genet* 2003; 11:516–526.

73. Wuyts W, Reyniers E, Ceuterick C, et al. Myopathy and phosphorylase kinase deficiency caused by a mutation in the PHKA1 gene. *Am J Med Genet A* 2005; 133A:82–84.

74. Orngreen MC, Schelhaas HJ, Jeppesen TD, et al. Is muscle glycogenolysis impaired in X-linked phosphorylase b kinase deficiency? *Neurology* 2008; 70:1876–1882.

75. Tsujino S, Shanske S, DiMauro S. Molecular genetic heterogeneity of phosphoglycerate kinase (PGK) deficiency. *Muscle Nerve* 1995; 3:S45–49.

76. Spiegel R, Gomez EA, Akman HO, et al. Myopathic form of phosphoglycerate kinase (PGK) deficiency: a new case and pathogenic considerations. *Neuromuscul Disord* 2009; 19:207–211.

77. DiMauro S, Dalakas M, Miranda AF. Phosphoglycerate kinase deficiency: another cause of recurrent myoglobinuria. *Ann Neurol* 1983; 13:11–19.

78. Sugie H, Sugie Y, Tsurui S, Ito M. Phosphoglycerate kinase deficiency. *Neurology* 1994; 44:1364–1365.

79. Tonin P, Shanske S, Miranda AF, et al. Phosphoglycerate kinase deficiency: Biochemical and molecular genetic studies in a new myopathic variant (PGK Alberta). *Neurology* 1993; 43:387–391.

80. Sugie H, Sugie Y, Ito M, et al. A novel missense mutation (837T-->C) in the phosphoglycerate kinase gene of a patient with a myopathic form of phosphoglycerate kinase deficiency. *J Child Neurol* 1998; 13:95–97.

81. Fujii H, Kanno H, Hirono A, et al. A single amino acid substitution (157 Gly-Val) in a phosphoglycerate kinase variant (PGK Shizuoka) associated with chronic hemolysis and myoglobinuria. *Blood* 1992; 79:1582–1585.

82. DiMauro S, Miranda AF, Khan S, et al. Human muscle phosphoglycerate mutase deficiency: newly discovered metabolic myopathy. *Science* 1981; 212:1277–1279.

83. Bresolin N, Ro YI, Reyes M, et al. Muscle phosphoglycerate mutase (PGAM) deficiency: a second case. *Neurology* 1983; 33:1049–1053.

84. Kissel JT, Beam W, Bresolin N, et al. Physiologic assessment of phosphoglycerate mutase deficiency: incremental exercise test. *Neurology* 1985; 35:828–833.

85. Vita G, Toscano A, Bresolin N, et al. Muscle phosphoglycerate mutase (PGAM) deficiency in the first Caucasian patient. *Neurology* 1990; 40:297.

86. Tsujino S, Shanske S, Sakoda S, et al. The molecular genetic basis of muscle phosphoglycerate mutase (PGAM) deficiency. *Am J Hum Genet* 1993; 52:472–477.

87. Tsujino S, Shanske S, Sakoda S, et al. Molecular genetic studies in muscle phosphoglycerate mutase (PGAM-M) deficiency. *Muscle Nerve* 1995; 3:S50–53.

88. Hadjigeorgiou GM, Kawashima N, Bruno C, et al. Manifesting heterozygotes in a Japanese family with a novel mutation in the muscle-specific phosphoglycerate mutase (PGAM-M) gene. *Neuromuscul Disord* 1999; 9:399–402.

89. Vissing J, Schmalbruch H, Haller RG, et al. Muscle phosphoglycerate mutase deficiency with tubular aggregates: effect of dantrolene. *Ann Neurol* 1999; 46:274–277.

90. Kanno T, Sudo K, Takeuchi I, et al. Hereditary deficiency of lactate dehydrogenase M-subunit. *Clin Chim Acta* 1980; 108:267–276.

91. Kanno T, Sudo K, Maekawa M, et al. Lactate dehydrogenase M-subunit deficiency: a new type of hereditary exertional myopathy. *Clin Chim Acta* 1988; 173:89–98.

92. Merkle S, Favor J, Graw J, et al. Hereditary lactate dehydrogenase A-subunit deficiency as cause of early postimplantation death of homozygotes in Mus musculus. *Genetics* 1992; 131:413–421.

93. Yoshikuni K, Tagami H, Yamada M, et al. Erythematosquamous skin lesions in hereditary lactate dehydrogenase M-subunit deficiency. *Arch Dermatol* 1986; 122:1420–1424.

94. Takayasu S, Fujiwara S, Waki T. Hereditary lactate dehydrogenase M-subunit deficiency: lactate dehydrogenase activity in skin lesions and in hair follicles. *J Am Acad Dermatol* 1991; 24:339–342.

95. Maekawa M, Sudo K, Li S, et al. Analysis of genetic mutation in human lactate dehydrogenase-A (M) deficiency using DNA conformation polymorphism in combination with polyacrilamide gradient gel and silver staining. *Biochem Biophys Res Comm* 1991; 180:1083–1090.

96. Miyajima H, Takahashi Y, Suzuki M, et al. Molecular characterization of gene expression in human lactate dehydrogenase-A deficiency. *Neurology* 1993; 43:1414–1419.

97. Kreuder J, Borkhardt A, Repp R, et al. Brief report: inherited metabolic myopathy and hemolysis due to a mutation in aldolase A. *N Engl J Med* 1996; 334:1100–1104.

98. DiMauro S, Bresolin N. Phosphorylase deficiency. In: Engel AG, Banker BQ, eds. *Myology.* New York: McGraw-Hill, 1986: 1585–1601.

99. Bruno C, Bado M, Minetti C, et al. Forearm semi-ischemic exercise test in pediatric patients. *J Child Neurol* 1998; 13:288–290.

100. Hoppel C. The physiological role of carnitine. In: Ferrari R, DiMauro S, Sherwood G, eds. *L-carnitine and its role in medicine: from function to therapy.* London: Academic Press, 1992; 5–19.

101. Lamhonwah AM, Tein I. Carnitine uptake defect: frameshift mutations in the human plasmalemmal carnitine transporter gene. *Biochem Biophys Res Commun* 1998; 252:396–401.

102. Nezu J, Tamai I, Oku A, et al. Primary systemic carnitine deficiency is caused by mutations in a gene encoding sodium ion-dependent carnitine transporter. *Nat Genet* 1999; 21:91–94.

103. Haworth JC, Demaugre F, Booth FA, et al. Atypical features of the hepatic form of carnitine palmitoyltransferase deficiency in a Hutterite family. *J Pediatr* 1992; 121:553–557.

104. Bonnefont JP, Haas R, Wolff J, et al. Deficiency of carnitine palmitoyltransferase I. *J Child Neurol* 1989; 4:198–203.

105. IJlst L, Mandel H, Oostheim W, et al. Molecular basis of hepatic carnitine palmitoyltransferase I deficiency. *J Clin Invest* 1998; 102:527–531.

106. Gobin S, Bonnefont JP, Prip-Buus C, et al. Organization of the human liver carnitine palmitoyltransferase 1 gene (CPT1A) and identification of novel mutations in hypoketotic hypoglycaemia. *Hum Genet* 2002; 111:179–189.

107. Ogawa A, Yamamoto S, Kanazawa M, et al. Identification of two novel mutations of the carnitine/acylcarnitine translocase (CACT) gene in a patient with CACT deficiency. *J Hum Genet* 2000; 45:52–55.

108. Di Donato S, Taroni F. Disorders of lipid metabolism. In: Rosenberg RN, DiMauro S, Paulson H, Ptácek L, Nestler EJ, eds. *The Molecular and Genetic Basis of Neurologic and Psychiatric Disease.* Philadelphia: Lippincott, Williams & Wilkins, 2008; 610–623.

109. Tonin P, Rowland LP, Servidei S, et al. Metabolic causes of myoglobinuria. *Ann Neurol* 1990; 27:181–185.

110. Taroni F, Verderio E, Dworzak F, et al. Identification of a common mutation in the carnitine palmitoyltransferase II gene in familial recurrent myoglobinuria patients. *Nature Genet* 1993; 4:314–320.

111. Kaufmann P, el-Schahawi M, DiMauro S. Carnitine palmitoyltransferase II deficiency: diagnosis by molecular analysis of blood. *Mol Cell Biochem* 1997; 174:237–239.

112. Stanley CA, Hale DE, Berry GT, et al. Brief report: a deficiency of carnitine-acylcarnitine translocase in the inner mitochondrial membrane. *N Engl J Med* 1992; 327:19–23.

113. Bertrand C, Largilliere C, Zabot MT, et al. Very long chain acyl-CoA dehydrogenase deficiency: identification of a new inborn error of mitochondrial fatty acid oxidation in fibroblasts. *Biochim Biophys Acta* 1993; 1180:327–329.

114. Jackson S, Bartlett K, Land J, et al. Long-chain 3-hydroxyacyl-CoA dehydrogenase deficiency. *Pediatr Res* 1991; 29:406–411.

115. Roe CR, Ding J. Mitochondrial fatty acid oxidation disorders. Scriver's Online Metabolic and Molecular Bases of Inherited Disease [serial online] 2006. Available at: http://dx.doi.org/10.1036/ommbid.135.

116. Matsubara Y, Narisawa K, Miyabayashi S, et al. Identification of a common mutation in patients with medium-chain acyl-CoA dehydrogenase deficiency. *Biochem Biophys Res Commun* 1990; 171:498–505.

117. Yokota I, Saijo T, Vockley J, et al. Impaired tetramer assembly of variant medium-chain acyl-coenzyme A dehydrogenase with a glutamate or aspartate substitution for lysine 304 causing instability of the protein. *J Biol Chem* 1992; 267:26004–26010.

118. Turnbull DM, Bartlett K, Stevens DL, et al. Short-chain acyl-CoA dehydrogenase deficiency associated with a lipid-storage myopathy and secondary carnitine deficiency. *N Engl J Med* 1984; 311:1232–1236.

119. Amendt BA, Greene C, Sweetman L, et al. Short-chain acyl-coenzyme A dehydrogenase deficiency. Clinical and biochemical studies in two patients. *J Clin Invest* 1987; 79:1303–1309.

120. Tein I, De Vivo DC, Hale DE, et al. Short-chain L-3-hydroxy-acyl-CoA dehydrogenase deficiency in muscle: a new cause for recurrent myoglobinuria and encephalopathy. *Ann Neurol* 1991; 30:415–419.

121. Roe CR, Millington DS, Norwood DL, et al. 2,4-Dienoyl-coenzyme A reductase deficiency: a possible new disorder of fatty acid oxidation. *J Clin Invest* 1990; 85:1703–1707.

122. Jordans GH. The familial occurrence of fat containing vacuoles in the leukocytes diagnosed in two brothers suffering from dystrophia musculorum progressiva (ERB.). *Acta Med Scand* 1953; 145:419–423.

123. Reilich P, Horvath R, Krause S, et al. The phenotypic spectrum of neutral lipid storage myopathy due to mutations in the PNPLA2 gene. *J Neurol* 2011; 258:1987–1997.

124. Fischer J, Lefevre C, Morava E, et al. The gene encoding adipose triglyceride lipase (PNPLA2) is mutated in neutral lipid storage disease with myopathy. *Nat Genet* 2007; 39:28–30.

125. Ohkuma A, Nonaka I, Malicdan MC, et al. Distal lipid storage myopathy due to PNPLA2 mutation. *Neuromuscul Disord* 2008; 18:671–674.

126. Chanarin I, Patel A, Slavin G, et al. Neutral-lipid storage disease: a new disorder of lipid metabolism. *Br Med J* 1975; 1:553–555.

127. Dorfman ML, Hershko C, Eisenberg S, et al. Ichthyosiform dermatosis with systemic lipidosis. *Arch Dermatol* 1974; 110:261–266.

128. Miranda A, DiMauro S, Eastwood A, et al. Lipid storage myopathy, ichthyosis, and steatorrhea. *Muscle Nerve* 1979; 2:1–13.

129. Campagna F, Nanni L, Quagliarini F, et al. Novel mutations in the adipose triglyceride lipase gene causing neutral lipid storage disease with myopathy. *Biochem Biophys Res Commun* 2008; 377:843–846.

130. Cakir M, Bruno C, Cansu A, et al. Liver cirrhosis in an infant with Chanarin-Dorfman syndrome caused by a novel splice-site mutation in ABHD5. *Acta Paediatr* 2010; 99:1592–1594.

131. Bruno C, Bertini E, Di Rocco M, et al. Clinical and genetic characterization of Chanarin-Dorfman syndrome. *Biochem Biophys Res Commun* 2008; 369:1125–1128.

132. Lefevre C, Jobard F, Caux F, et al. Mutations in CGI-58, the gene encoding a new protein of the esterase/lipase/thioesterase subfamily, in Chanarin-Dorfman syndrome. *Am J Hum Genet* 2001; 69:1002–1012.

133. Fishbein WN, Armbrustmacher VW, Griffin JL. Myoadenylate deaminase deficiency: a new disease of muscle. *Science* 1978; 200:545–548.

134. Fishbein WN. Myoadenylate deaminase deficiency: inherited and acquired forms. *Biochem Med* 1985; 33:158–169.

135. DiMauro S, Schon EA. Mitochondrial respiratory-chain diseases. *N Engl J Med* 2003; 348:2656–2668.

136. DiMauro S, Schon EA. Mitochondrial disorders in the nervous system. *Annu Rev Neurosci* 2008; 31:91–123.

137. Schon EA, DiMauro S. Mitochondrial mutations: genotype to phenotype. *Novartis Found Symp* 2007; 287:214–225; discussion 226–233.

138. Schon EA, DiMauro S, Hirano M, et al. Therapeutic prospects for mitochondrial disease. *Trends Mol Med* 2010; 16:268–276.

139. Koopman WJ, Willems PH, Smeitink JA. Monogenic mitochondrial disorders. *N Engl J Med* 2012; 366:1132–1141.

140. Tanji K, Bonilla E. Optical imaging techniques (histochemical, immunohistochemical, and in situ hybridization staining methods) to visualize mitochondria. *Methods Cell Biol* 2007; 80:135–154.

141. Shy GM, Gonatas NK, Perez M. Childhood myopathies with abnormal mitochondria. I. Megaconial myopathy-pleoconial myopathy. *Brain* 1966; 89:133–158.

142. Engel WK, Cunningham CG. Rapid examination of muscle tissue: An improved trichrome stain method for fresh-frozen biopsy sections. *Neurology* 1963; 13:919–923.

143. Carpenter S, Karpati G, Eisen AA. A morphologic study of muscle in polymyositis: clues to pathogenesis of different types. In: *Amsterdam: Excerpta Medica* 1975; 374–379.

144. Carpenter S, Karpati G, Heller I, et al. Inclusion body myositis: a distinct variety of idiopathic inflammatory myopathy. *Neurology* 1978; 28:8–17.

145. Holt IJ, Harding AE, Morgan Hughes JA. Deletions of muscle mitochondrial DNA in patients with mitochondrial myopathies. *Nature* 1988; 331:717–719.

146. Lestienne P, Ponsot G. Kearns-Sayre syndrome with muscle mitochondrial DNA deletion. *Lancet* 1988; 1:885.

147. Wallace DC, Singh G, Lott MT, et al. Mitochondrial DNA mutation associated with Leber's hereditary optic neuropathy. *Science* 1988; 242:1427–1430.

148. Zeviani M, Moraes CT, DiMauro S, et al. Deletions of mitochondrial DNA in Kearns-Sayre syndrome. *Neurology* 1988; 38:1339–1346.

149. Schon EA, Przedborski S. Mitochondria: the next (neurode) generation. *Neuron* 2011; 70:1033–1053.

150. Moraes CT, Shanske S, Tritschler HJ, et al. MtDNA depletion with variable tissue expression: A novel genetic abnormality in mitochondrial diseases. *Am J Hum Genet* 1991; 48:492–501.

151. Zeviani M, Servidei S, Gellera C, et al. An autosomal dominant disorder with multiple deletions of mitochondrial DNA starting at the D-loop region. *Nature* 1989; 339:309–311.

152. Anderson S, Bankier AT, Barrel BG, et al. Sequence and organization of the human mitochondrial genome. *Nature* 1981; 290:457–465.

153. Rötig A, Colonna M, Bonnefont JP, et al. Mitochondrial DNA deletion in Pearson's marrow/pancreas syndrome. *Lancet* 1989; 1:902–903.

154. Kearns TP, Sayre GP. Retinitis pigmentosa, external ophthalmoplegia, and complete heart block. *Arch Ophthal* 1958; 60:280–289.

155. Rowland LP, Hays AP, DiMauro S, et al. Diverse clinical disorders associated with morphological abnormalities of mitochondria. In: Cerri C, Scarlato G, eds. *Mitochondrial Pathology in Muscle Diseases.* Padua: Piccin Editore, 1983; 141–158.

156. Schwartz M, Vissing J. Paternal inheritance of mitochondrial DNA. *N Engl J Med* 2002; 347:576–580.

157. Filosto M, Mancuso M, Vives-Bauza C, et al. Lack of paternal inheritance of muscle mitochondrial DNA in sporadic mitochondrial myopathies. *Ann Neurol* 2003; 54:524–526.

158. Pavlakis SG, Phillips PC, DiMauro S, et al. Mitochondrial myopathy, encephalopathy, lactic acidosis, and strokelike episodes: a distinctive clinical syndrome. *Ann Neurol* 1984; 16:481–488.

159. Fukuhara N, Tokiguchi S, Shirakawa K, et al. Myoclonus epilepsy associated with ragged-red fibres (mitochondrial abnormalities): disease entity or a syndrome? Light-and electron-microscopic studies of two cases and review of literature. *J Neurol Sci* 1980; 47:117–133.

160. DiMauro S, Hirano M, Schon EA. *Mitochondrial Medicine.* Oxon: Informa Healthcare, 2006.

161. DiMauro S, Schon EA, Hirano M, et al. Mitochondrial Encephalomyopathies: Diseases of Mitochondrial DNA. In: Rowland LP, Pedley TA, eds. *Merritt's Neurology,* 12th ed. Philadelphia: Wolters Kluwer, 2010; 679–685.

162. Hirano M, DiMauro S. Clinical features of mitochondrial myopathies and encephalomyopathies. In: Lane RJM, ed. *Handbook of Muscle Disease.* New York: Marcel Dekker Inc. USA, 1996; 479–504.

163. Kornblum C, Broicher R, Walther E, et al. Cricopharyngeal achalasia is a common cause of dysphagia in patients with mtDNA deletions. *Neurology* 2001; 56:1409–1412.

164. Silvestri G, Ciafaloni E, Santorelli F, et al. Clinical features associated with the A>G transition at nucleotide 8344 of mtDNA ("MERRF mutation"). *Neurology* 1993; 43:1200–1206.

165. Shoffner JM, Lott MT, Lezza AMS, et al. Myoclonic epilepsy and ragged-red fiber disease (MERRF) is associated with a mitochondrial DNA tRNALys mutation. *Cell* 1990; 61:931–937.

166. Silvestri G, Moraes CT, Shanske S, et al. A new mtDNA mutation in the tRNALys gene associated with myoclonic epilepsy and ragged-red fibers (MERRF). *Am J Hum Genet* 1992; 51:1213–1217.

167. Ozawa M, Nishino I, Horai S, et al. Myoclonus epilepsy associated with ragged-red fibers: a G-to-A mutation at nucleotide pair 8363 in mitochondrial tRNALys in two families. *Muscle Nerve* 1997; 20:271–278.

168. Rossmanith W, Raffelsberger T, Roka J, et al. The expanding mutational spectrum of MERRF substitution G8361A in the mitochondrial tRNALys gene. *Ann Neurol* 2003; 54:820–823.

169. Mancuso M, Filosto M, Mootha VK, et al. A novel mitochondrial tRNAPhe mutation causes MERRF syndrome. *Neurology* 2004; 62:2119–2121.

170. Silvestri G, Ciafaloni E, Santorelli FM, et al. Clinical features associated with the A-->G transition at nucleotide 8344 of mtDNA ("MERRF mutation"). *Neurology* 1993; 43:1200–1206.

171. Zeviani M, Muntoni F, Savarese N, et al. A MERRF/MELAS overlap syndrome with a new point mutation in the mitochondrial DNA tRNALys gene. *Eur J Hum Genet* 1993; 1:80–87.

172. Nishigaki Y, Tadesse S, Bonilla E, et al. A novel mitochondrial tRNALeu(UUR) mutation in a patient with features of MERRF and Kearns-Sayre syndrome. *Neuromuscul Disord* 2003; 13:334–340.

173. Emmanuele V, Silvers DS, Sotiriou E, et al. MERRF and Kearns-Sayre overlap syndrome due to the mitochondrial DNA m.3291T>C mutation. *Muscle Nerve* 2011; 44:448–451.

174. Hirano M, Pavlakis S. Mitochondrial myopathy, encephalopathy, lactic acidosis, and strokelike episodes (MELAS): current concepts. *J Child Neurol* 1994; 9:4–13.

175. Klopstock T, Hirano M. MELAS. In: Gilman S, ed. *Medlink Neurology.* San Diego: Medlink Corporation, 2012.

176. Kobayashi Y, Momoi MY, Tominaga K, et al. A point mutation in the mitochondrial tRNA(Leu)(UUR) gene in MELAS (mitochondrial myopathy, encephalopathy, lactic acidosis and stroke-like episodes). *Biochem Biophys Res Commun* 1990; 173:816–822.

177. King MP, Attardi G. Human cells lacking mtDNA: repopulation with exogenous mitochondria by complementation. *Science* 1989; 246:500–503.

178. King MP, Koga Y, Davidson M, et al. Defects in mitochondrial protein synthesis and respiratory chain activity segregate with the tRNALeu(UUR) mutation associated with mitochondrial myopathy, encephalopathy, lactic acidosis, and stroke-like episodes. *Mol Cell Biol* 1992; 12:480–490.

179. Chomyn A, Enriquez JA, Micol V, et al. The mitochondrial myopathy, encephalopathy, lactic acidosis, and stroke-like episode syndrome-associated human mitochondrial tRNALeu(UUR) mutation causes aminoacylation deficiency and concomitant reduced association of mRNA with ribosomes [In Process Citation]. *J Biol Chem* 2000, 275:19198 19209.

180. Helm M, Florentz C, Chomyn A, et al. Search for differences in post-transcriptional modification patterns of mitochondrial DNA-encoded wild-type and mutant human tRNALys and tRNALeu(UUR). *Nucleic Acids Res* 1999; 27:756–763.

181. Park H, Davidson E, King MP. The pathogenic A3243G mutation in human mitochondrial tRNALeu(UUR) decreases the efficiency of aminoacylation. *Biochemistry* 2003; 42:958–964.

182. Börner GV, Zeviani M, Tiranti V, et al. Decreased aminoacylation of mutant tRNAs in MELAS but not in MERRF patients. *Hum Mol Genet* 2000; 9:467–475.

183. Yasukawa T, Suzuki T, Ishii N, et al. Defect in modification at the anticodon wobble nucleotide of mitochondrial tRNA(Lys) with the MERRF encephalomyopathy pathogenic mutation. *FEBS Lett* 2000; 467:175–178.

184. Kirino Y, Yasukawa T, Ohta S, et al. Codon-specific translational defect caused by a wobble modification deficiency in mutant tRNA from a human mitochondrial disease. *Proc Natl Acad Sci USA* 2004; 101:15070–15075.

185. Sasarman F, Antonicka H, Shoubridge EA. The A3243G tRNALeu(UUR) MELAS mutation causes amino acid misincorporation and a combined respiratory chain assembly defect partially suppressed by overexpression of EFTu and EFG2. *Hum Mol Genet* 2008; 17:3697–3707.

186. Kaufmann P, Engelstad K, Wei Y, et al. Dichloroacetate causes toxic neuropathy in MELAS: a randomized, controlled clinical trial. *Neurology* 2006; 66:324–330.

187. Koga Y, Akita Y, Nishioka J, et al. MELAS and L-arginine therapy. Mitochondrion 2007; 7:133–139.

188. Koga Y, Akita Y, Nishioka J, et al. L-arginine improves the symptoms of strokelike episodes in MELAS. *Neurology* 2005; 64:710–712.

189. Koga Y, Ishibashi M, Ueki I, et al. Effects of L-arginine on the

acute phase of strokes in three patients with MELAS. *Neurology* 2002; 58:827–828.

190. Bourgeron T, Rustin P, Chretien D, et al. Mutation of a nuclear succinate dehydrogenase gene results in mitochondrial respiratory chain deficiency. *Nature Genet* 1995; 11:144–149.

191. Zhu Z, Yao J, Johns T, et al. SURF1, encoding a factor involved in the biogenesis of cytochrome c oxidase, is mutated in Leigh syndrome. *Nat Genet* 1998; 20:337–343.

192. Tiranti V, Hoertnagel K, Carrozzo R, et al. Mutations of SURF-1 in Leigh disease associated with cytochrome c oxidase deficiency. *Am J Hum Genet* 1998; 63:1609–1621.

193. Turunen M, Olsson J, Dallner G. Metabolism and function of coenzyme Q. *Biochim Biophys Acta* 2004; 1660:171–199.

194. Emmanuele V, Lopez LC, Berardo A, et al. Heterogeneity of Coenzyme Q10 Deficiency: Patient Study and Literature Review. *Arch Neurol* 2012; 69.

195. Quinzii C, Hirano M. Primary and secondary CoQ10 deficiencies in humans. *Biofactors* 2011; 37:361–365.

196. Heeringa SF, Chernin G, Chaki M, et al. COQ6 mutations in human patients produce nephrotic syndrome with sensorineural deafness. *J Clin Invest* 2011; 121:2013–2024.

197. Mollet J, Giurgea I, Schlemmer D, et al. Prenyldiphosphate synthase, subunit 1 (PDSS1) and OH-benzoate polyprenyltransferase (COQ2) mutations in ubiquinone deficiency and oxidative phosphorylation disorders. *J Clin Invest* 2007; 117:765–772.

198. Lopez LC, Schuelke M, Quinzii CM, et al. Leigh syndrome with nephropathy and CoQ10 deficiency due to decaprenyl diphosphate synthase subunit 2 (PDSS2) mutations. *Am J Hum Genet* 2006; 79:1125–1129.

199. Duncan AJ, Bitner-Glindzicz M, Meunier B, et al. A nonsense mutation in COQ9 causes autosomal-recessive neonatal-onset primary coenzyme Q10 deficiency: a potentially treatable form of mitochondrial disease. *Am J Hum Genet* 2009; 84:558–566.

200. Quinzii C, Naini A, Salviati L, et al. A Mutation in Para-Hydroxybenzoate-Polyprenyl Transferase (COQ2) Causes Primary Coenzyme Q10 Deficiency. *Am J Hum Genet* 2006; 78:345–349.

201. Mollet J, Delahodde A, Serre V, et al. CABC1 gene mutations cause ubiquinone deficiency with cerebellar ataxia and seizures. *Am J Hum Genet* 2008; 82:623–630.

202. Lagier-Tourenne C, Tazir M, Lopez LC, et al. ADCK3, an ancestral kinase, is mutated in a form of recessive ataxia associated with coenzyme Q10 deficiency. *Am J Hum Genet* 2008; 82:661–672.

203. Gempel K, Topaloglu H, Talim B, et al. The myopathic form of coenzyme Q10 deficiency is caused by mutations in the electron-transferring-flavoprotein dehydrogenase (ETFDH) gene. *Brain* 2007; 130:2037–2044.

204. Zeviani M, Carelli V. Disorders of nuclear-mitochondrial intergenomic signalling. In: Gilman S, ed. *Medlink Neurology.* San Diego: Medlink Corporation, 2012.

205. Van Goethem G, Dermaut B, Lofgren A, et al. Mutation of POLG is associated with progressive external ophthalmoplegia characterized by mtDNA deletions. *Nat Genet* 2001; 28:211–212.

206. Fratter C, Raman P, Alston CL, et al. RRM2B mutations are frequent in familial PEO with multiple mtDNA deletions. *Neurology* 2011; 76:2032–2034.

207. Kaukonen J, Juselius JK, Tiranti V, et al. Role of adenine nucleotide translocator 1 in mtDNA maintenance. *Science* 2000; 289:782–785.

208. Spelbrink JN, Li FY, Tiranti V, et al. Human mitochondrial DNA deletions associated with mutations in the gene encoding Twinkle, a phage T7 gene 4-like protein localized in mitochondria. *Nat Genet* 2001; 28:223–231.

209. Blakely EL, Butterworth A, Hadden RD, et al. MPV17 mutation causes neuropathy and leukoencephalopathy with multiple mtDNA deletions in muscle. *Neuromuscul Disord* 2012; 22:587–591.

210. Garone C, Rubio JC, Calvo S, et al. MPV17 mutations causing adult-onset multisystemic disorder with multiple mitochondrial DNA deletions. *Arch Neurol* 2012; in press.

211. Longley MJ, Clark S, Yu Wai Man C, et al. Mutant POLG2 disrupts DNA polymerase gamma subunits and causes progressive external ophthalmoplegia. *Am J Hum Genet* 2006; 78:1026–1034.

212. Mandel H, Szargel R, Labay V, et al. The deoxyguanosine kinase gene is mutated in individuals with depleted hepatocerebral mitochondrial DNA. *Nat Genet* 2001; 29:337–341.

213. Saada A, Shaag A, Mandel H, et al. Mutant mitochondrial thymidine kinase in mitochondrial DNA depletion myopathy. *Nat Genet* 2001; 29:342–344.

214. Suomalainen A, Isohanni P. Mitochondrial DNA depletion syndromes—many genes, common mechanisms. *Neuromuscul Disord* 2010; 20:429–437.

215. Garone C, Tadesse S, Hirano M. Clinical and genetic spectrum of mitochondrial neurogastrointestinal encephalomyopathy. *Brain* 2011; 134:3326–3332.

216. Nishino I, Spinazzola A, Hirano M. Thymidine phosphorylase gene mutations in MNGIE, a human mitochondrial disorder. *Science* 1999; 283:689–692.

217. Halter J, Schupbach WM, Casali C, et al. Allogeneic hematopoietic SCT as treatment option for patients with mitochondrial neurogastrointestinal encephalomyopathy (MNGIE): a consensus conference proposal for a standardized approach. *Bone Marrow Transplant* 2011; 46:330–337.

218. Hirano M, Marti R, Casali C, et al. Allogeneic stem cell transplantation corrects biochemical derangements in MNGIE. *Neurology* 2006; 67:1458–1460.

219. Chrzanowska-Lightowlers ZM, Horvath R, Lightowlers RN. 175th ENMC International Workshop: Mitochondrial protein synthesis in health and disease, 25–27th June 2010, Naarden, The Netherlands. *Neuromuscul Disord* 2011; 21:142–147.

220. Bykhovskaya Y, Casas K, Mengesha E, et al. Missense mutation in pseudouridine synthase 1 (PUS1) causes mitochondrial myopathy and sideroblastic anemia (MLASA). *Am J Hum Genet* 2004; 74:1303–1308.

221. Barth PG, Scholte HR, Berden JA, et al. An X-linked mitochondrial disease affecting cardiac muscle, skeletal muscle and neutrophil leucocytes. *J Neurol Sci* 1983; 62:327–355.

222. Bione S, D'Adamo P, Maestrini E, Gedeon AK, et al. A novel X-linked gene, G4.5. is responsible for Barth syndrome. *Nat Genet* 1996; 12:385–389.

223. Nishino I, Kobayashi O, Goto Y, et al. A new congenital muscular dystrophy with mitochondrial structural abnormalities. *Muscle Nerve* 1998; 21:40–47.

224. Mitsuhashi S, Ohkuma A, Talim B, et al. A congenital muscular dystrophy with mitochondrial structural abnormalities caused by defective de novo phosphatidylcholine biosynthesis. *Am J Hum Genet* 2011; 88:845–851.

225. Sengers RC, Stadhouders AM, Jaspar HH, et al. Cardiomyopathy and short stature associated with mitochondrial and/or lipid storage myopathy of skeletal muscle. *Neuropadiatrie* 1976; 7:196–208.

226. Mayr JA, Haack TB, Graf E, et al. Lack of the mitochondrial protein acylglycerol kinase causes Sengers syndrome. *Am J Hum Genet* 2012; 90:314–320.

227. Chan DC. Mitochondrial dynamics in disease. *N Engl J Med* 2007; 356:1707–1709.

228. Delettre C, Lenaers G, Griffoin JM, et al. Nuclear gene OPA1, encoding a mitochondrial dynamin-related protein, is mutated in dominant optic atrophy. *Nat Genet* 2000; 26:207–210.

229. Hudson G, Amati-Bonneau P, Blakely EL, et al. Mutation of OPA1 causes dominant optic atrophy with external ophthalmoplegia, ataxia, deafness and multiple mitochondrial DNA deletions: a novel disorder of mtDNA maintenance. *Brain* 2008; 131:329–337.

230. Sheftel A, Stehling O, Lill R. Iron-sulfur proteins in health and disease. *Trends Endocrinol Metab* 2010; 21:302–314.

231. Haller RG, Henriksson KG, Jorfeldt L, et al. Deficiency of skeletal muscle succinate dehydrogenase and aconitase. *J Clin Invest* 1991; 88:1197–1206.

232. Mochel F, Knight MA, Tong WH, et al. Splice mutation in the iron-sulfur cluster scaffold protein ISCU causes myopathy with exercise intolerance. *Am J Hum Genet* 2008; 82:652–660.

233. Olsson A, Lind L, Thornell LE, Holmberg M. Myopathy with lactic acidosis is linked to chromosome 12q23.3-24.11 and caused by an intron mutation in the ISCU gene resulting in a splicing defect. *Hum Mol Genet* 2008; 17:1666–1672.

234. Kollberg G, Tulinius M, Melberg A, et al. Clinical manifestation and a new ISCU mutation in iron-sulphur cluster deficiency myopathy. *Brain* 2009; 132:2170–2179.

235. DiMauro S, Tay S, Mancuso M. Mitochondrial encephalomyopathies: diagnostic approach. *Ann N Y Acad Sci* 2004; 1011:217–231.

236. Bernier FP, Boneh A, Dennett X, Chow CW, et al. Diagnostic criteria for respiratory chain disorders in adults and children. *Neurology* 2002; 59:1406–1411.

237. Morava E, van den Heuvel L, Hol F, et al. Mitochondrial disease criteria: diagnostic applications in children. *Neurology* 2006; 67:1823–1826.

238. Petty RK, Harding AE, Morgan Hughes JA. The clinical features of mitochondrial myopathy. *Brain* 1986; 109:915–938.

239. Hirano M, Ricci E, Koenigsberger MR, et al. MELAS: An original case and clinical criteria for diagnosis. *Neuromuscul Disord* 1992; 2:125–135.

CHAPTER 20

Childhood Muscular Dystrophies

David S. Younger

In the premolecular era, there were very few clues that different clinical and genetic forms of muscular dystrophy shared a common pathogenesis of membrane instability. Since the cloning of the gene for Duchenne muscular dystrophy (DMD) in late 1987 (1), our concepts have dramatically changed along with identification of novel skeletal muscle genes, including those encoding the extracellular matrix, sarcolemmal, cytoskeletal, cytosolic, and nuclear membrane proteins (2). A large number of genes encode components of the dystrophin-glycoprotein complex (DGC) (Figure 1), which links the intracellular cytoskeleton to the extracellular matrix, mutations of which lead to a loss of sarcolemma integrity and render myofiber susceptible to injury. Prototypical examples of muscular dystrophies include those associated with nuclear (Emery-Driefuss muscular dystrophy [EDMD], laminopathy), cytosolic (calpainopathy, dystroglycanopathy, Fukyama congenital muscular dystrophy (CMD) [FCMD]), cytoskeleton (dystrophinopathy, telethoninopathy), sarcolemma (calveolinoapthy, dysferlinopathy), extracellular matrix (dystroglycanopthy α-2 laminin and merosin CMD[LAMA2]), and the sarcoglycan-sarcospan complex (sarcoglycanopathies).

DYSTROPHIN-GLYCOPROTEIN COMPLEX

Dystrophin is a large protein molecule of molecular weight 427 kDa, localized to the cytoplasmic face of the skeletal muscle membrane in a subsarcolemmal location. The dystrophin domains include the amino terminus, the rod domain composed of 24-helical repeats, and a carboxy terminus (1). At the amino terminus, dystrophin is bound to the cytoskeletal protein f-actin. The carboxy terminus includes a binding site for the syntrophins, but more importantly its cysteine-rich region serves as a ligand to the dystroglycans. α/β-dystroglycan is encoded by a single gene on chromosome 3p21. Two proteins are proteolytically cleaved and undergo posttranslational modification. Whereas β–dystroglycan serves as the ligand for the cysteine-rich region of dystrophin, α-dystroglycan serves as the ligand for laminin-2 in the basal lamina. Thus, the dystroglycans establish a bridge across the membrane from the cytoskeleton and dystrophin to laminin-2 in the extracellular matrix.

The sarcoglycan subcomplex is an integral part of the DGC, composed of at least four transmembrane constituents: α-sarcoglycan (50 kDa, formerly called adhalin), β–sarcoglycan, -λ-sarcoglycan, and δ-sarcoglycan. Whereas laminins are ubiquitous integral constituents of the basal lamina of all tissues, the skeletal muscle form is designated laminin-2 and bears an integral relationship to the DGC as a separate component. Its heterotrimeric molecular structure is arranged in the shape of a cross with one heavy α-chain and one each β and λ chains. Originally called merosin, the laminin heavy chain of skeletal muscle and Schwann cells is designated laminin α2.

There is general agreement that the DGC confers stability to the muscle membrane. In DMD and the other muscular dystrophies, the serum CK elevation is usually seen at the time of birth and persists throughout life. Studies in DMD indicate that dystrophin deficiency disrupts the membrane localization for the dystroglycans and sarcoglycans. The same is true when the sarcoglycans are deficient, particularly α-sarcoglycan, where deficiency disrupts the integrity of localization for many components of the DGC. A strong argument favoring an integrated function

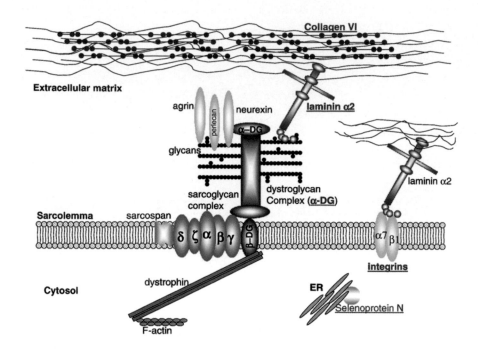

FIG. 1. Schematic representation of the dystrophin-glycoprotein complex. Adapted from reference 128, with permission.

of these proteins is the observed overlapping phenotypic aspects of DMD and Becker muscular distrophy (BMD), limb-girdle muscular distrophy (LGMD), and lamininopathy-related congenital muscular dystrophy (CMD) (3), such that tears along the DRG membrane from weakening of the sarcolemma could lead to excess calcium leakage into the muscle fiber, initiating a cascade of events culminating in myofiber necrosis and a muscular dystrophy phenotype.

DYSTROPHIN-ASSOCIATED MUSCULAR DYSTROPHY

Background

Dystrophin-associated muscular dystrophy ranges from severe DMD to milder BMD. DMD is the commonest X-linked recessive lethal disease with an incidence of approximately 1 in 3,500 newborns. Rowland and Layzer (4) provide an excellent historical review of the X-linked muscular dystrophies, in particular DMD. Edward Meryon (5) is credited with the first clearly recognizable description of the disease, later detailed by Duchenne (6) in the description of pseudohypertrophic and myosclerotic muscular paralysis.

Clinical Aspects

Clinical symptoms are unusual in the neonatal period; however, occasional patients, especially those with mental retardation, exhibit delayed motor milestones. In most instances, the disease is clinically apparent by age two to three years with relentless progression of weakness and wasting that more profoundly affects proximal leg muscles with ankle and hip contractures that ultimately limit function. Scoliosis is associated with wheelchair confinement that typically ensues about age 12.

Cardiac involvement is a consistent feature demonstrating fibrosis along the posterobasal portion of the left ventricular wall, with lesser involvement of the right ventricular septum, ventricle, and atrial myocardium, or conduction system. Congestive heart failure and cardiac arrhythmias occur in the later stages and during periods of stress from intercurrent infection. There is relative sparing of pulmonary function unless there is associated congestive heart failure. Smooth muscle gastrointestinal tract involvement may be overlooked, leading to chronic constipation, acute gastric dilatation and intestinal pseudo-obstruction with sudden vomiting, abdominal pain, and distention, and death if untreated. The average intelligence quotient may be one standard deviation below the mean; however, intellectual impairment, if present, does not progress. Most patients die of complications of respiratory insufficiency at about age 20.

The pattern of muscle wasting in BMD closely resembles that of DMD but the natural history permits distinction between the two disorders. Patients with BMD experience difficulties between ages 5 to 15 years, ambulate beyond age 15, and survive at least into the fourth to fifth decades, implying a clear distinction between the two disorders although there can be heterogeneity of clinical presentation and course of illness, emphasizing the continuous spectrum of dystrophin-associated muscular dystrophy ranging from very mild to severe involvement (7).

Laboratory Diagnosis

The laboratory diagnosis of boys affected by DMD is generally straightforward when progressive myopathic weakness with pseudohypertrophy of the calves is associated with a very high serum creatine kinase (CK) level along with confirmatory electromyography (EMG) and muscle biopsy. Elevation of the serum CK level was such a constant feature of DMD that it has become one of the essential criteria for presumptive diagnosis, although it occurs in other muscular dystrophies. In young patients it was usually 20- to 100-fold the upper limit of normal, while activities of other enzymes such as aldolase, lactate dehydrogenase (LDH), and glutamic oxaloacetic (SGOT) and pyruvic transaminases (SGPT), although increased, are usually less than 10-fold normal (8). Elevated in fetal blood obtained by placental puncture, the serum CK is characteristically very high at birth and continues to be so in the first few months of life (9), while in first decade and fluctuating during the transition from walking to wheelchair living thereafter dropping due to declining muscle mass (4). The abnormalities of CK and other enzymes in BMD are virtually identical to those of DMD patients. Electrophysiological studies served both as an aid to diagnosis as well as a method of understanding the pathophysiology of the disorder.

Although once widely used, conventional nerve EMG has been challenging in young children and in clinical practice it is usually abbreviated to examination of a few motor unit potentials (MUP) in the arms or legs. Fibrillation potentials were recorded at rest in at least one site in 28% (10) to 87% of patients (11), and attributed to segmental myofiber necrosis with isolation from nerve supply; an equal proportion of bizzare high frequency pseudomyotonic discharges were also noted (10, 11). Increased polyphasia, decreased MUP duration, and a myopathic pattern of excessive recruitment of MUP, with generally normal MUP amplitude, were recorded (10). However, when related to the stage of muscle involvement, polyphasia was more marked in early stages (10, 11) compared to fibrillation and mean MUP duration that were more commonly encountered in more advanced stages (11). The latter was attributed to loss or blocking of myofibers (12), making mean MUP dura-

tion, a cornerstone criterion of myopathy, potentially less useful in young children when the diagnosis of myopathy was most important (4). Among 39 patients with diverse forms of muscular dystrophy, including 12 patients with DMD (13). Single fiber EMG (SFEMG) and scanning EMG demonstrated normal volume conduction and cross section of motor unit length, with increased jitter and fiber density (FD). These findings were attributed to a localized increase in the number of muscle action generators with remodeling of the motor unit, myofiber loss, and reparative processes of fiber regeneration and reinnervation. The contribution of large fibers considered pathognomonic of DMD in muscle biopsy tissue were not typically seen in groups, and their contribution to the increased FD was attributed to myogenic mechanisms of splitting and branching of myofibers due to degenerative and regenerative phenomena, less so reinnervation with altered redistribution. The availability of automated EMG analysis systems, which permit extensive analysis with limited patient participation, has solved many of the logistical problems and redefined the utility of electrodiagnosis in myopathies such as DMD (14–17). Collectively they incorporate analysis of individual motor unit action potential (MUAP) firing patterns (FP) during different degrees of voluntary effort that proceeds in a multistep process beginning with recording, amplification, filtering, and sampling of the EMG signal. This is followed by segmentation of the signal into time intervals that contain EMG activity, whether single or superimposed MUAP with subsequent clustering of signals into MUAP according to certain fulfilled criteria, and displayed with parametric measurements. Automated turns analysis is performed as a function of the mean amplitude at three to five force levels from minimum to maximum, producing a scatter plot which forms a cloud with myopathy and neurogenic lesions, deviating in opposite directions. Among 188 patients with diverse neuromuscular disorders, including 21 with DMD in whom EMG and related clinical and muscle biopsy tissue were available for comparison, EMG was concordant with the diagnosis of myopathy in 87% of patients (18).

Muscle biopsy in patients with DMD classically shows increased numbers of internal nuclei, clusters of regenerating myofibers, scattered necrotic fibers, increased variation in fiber size with hypercontracted myofibers, and infiltration of fat and connective tissue and endomysial and perimysial fibrosis, the severity of which varies with the stage of the disease. Immunohistochemistry of frozen muscle sections using antibodies against dystrophin shows absent dystrophin staining in affected DMD patients, whereas unaffected individuals show normal dystrophin staining along the sarcolemma membrane, and immunoblot analysis of muscle extracts shows a severe defect of dystrophin with concentrations less than 3% of normal.

Molecular Basis of Dystrophinopathy

Approximately one-third of cases are the result of new mutations at the Xp21.2-p21.1 locus of the *DMD* gene encoding the 14-kb transcript, dystrophin. The gene spans more than 2,000 kilobases (kb) of genomic DNA and is composed of 79 exons, the enormity of which probably accounts for the high frequency of spontaneous mutations. Despite the large number of intragenic and flanking DNA polymorphisms, uncertainties may nonetheless remain in the prenatal diagnosis that is circumvented more by mapping more than use of restriction fragment length polymorphisms (RFLP). An algorithm for the molecular diagnosis of DMD or BMD begins with Western blot testing for dystrophin in males with clinically consistent features of CK, EMG and muscle biopsy, which if normal, proceeds to the study for other neuromuscular diseases (19). PCR testing and Southern blot analysis is performed to search for deletions and duplications in the *DMD* gene. Collectively, these procedures diagnose two-thirds of patients, and Southern blot permits prognostication of severity by distinguishing in-frame versus frameshift mutations in over 90% of samples. In the absence of deletion or duplications, one can proceed to RFLP-based linkage studies, which if informative, can be later used for carrier detection. Approximately 65% of DMD and BMD patients demonstrate large-scale deletions of several kilobases to greater than one million base pairs in the dystrophin gene, whereas duplications are found in approximately 5% of patients. The deletions are non-randomly distributed and occur primarily in the center, less frequently near the 58 end of the gene. Deletions disrupting the open reading frame result in the severe DMD phenotype, deletions that maintain the translational reading frame leading to production of a semi-functional truncated protein and the BMD phenotype. The reading frame rule explains the phenotypic differences observed in about 92% of affected patients with the exception of BMD patients that have out-of-frame deletions of exons 3 to 7. It has been proposed that an alternate splicing mechanism or new cryptic translational start sites account for the milder phenotype observed with deletion in exons 3 to 7 and the production of dystrophin (20). There are point mutations, small deletions, and duplications in the dystrophin gene in DMD patients (21, 22). Most of the point mutations result in dystrophin truncation consistent with the reading frame hypothesis; however, unlike deletion hot spots, the small mutations are private and randomly distributed throughout the gene. With the ability to perform direct DNA diagnostics in patients with deletion and duplications, the accuracy of carrier detection has significantly improved. Nevertheless, the carrier state of the mother of an isolated case should be interpreted cautiously from DNA testing. For example, when the mother has no detectable mutation of the dystrophin gene, the risk of carrier status still cannot be excluded because of the possibility of germline mosaicism (23). Mothers that do not harbor mutations of the dystrophin gene in peripheral blood leukocytes may still manifest mutations in a percentage of the oocytes. Such examples of germline mosaicism have important counseling implications. Sisters of Duchenne patients should be investigated independently of the outcome of DNA testing of the mother. Partial dystrophin deficiency was noted in monozygous twin carriers of the DMD gene, the manifesting carrier of which had a Turner genotype and likely uneven lionization, and the sister of whom had an affected child (24). A negative mutation result in the mother does not rule out a recurrence risk for future pregnancies, but the exact risk is unknown because there is no method to estimate the size of the mutant clone. The recurrence risk for the mother of a sporadic DMD case has been estimated to be as high as 14% (23). The Haldane rule (25), which predicted that one-third of cases of a genetic lethal X-linked recessive trait would be the consequence of a new mutation, suggested that the mutation rate for *DMD* might be higher in males (26). Tuffery-Giraud and colleagues (27) described a French database for mutations in the *DMD* gene, indicating that 24% of mutations were *de novo*. Among 624 index patients evaluated for *DMD* mutations (28), genomic rearrangements were noted in 38% of samples, deletions in 79%, including 31 with single-, and 157 with multi-exonic deletions, most of which fell between exons 8 to 13, and 45 and 52 of the gene. Duplications, detected in 18%, included 12 which involved single-, and 32 multiple exons; complex rearrangements were noted in 2.5% of samples. Among 106 DMD patients examined for variations in 29 genes (29), skeletal muscle mRNA profiling identified the G allele of rs28357094 in the promoter of the *SPP1* gene encoding osteopontin, which appeared to have a significant effect as a modifier of disease progression and response to corticosteroids.

In DMD, the absence of dystrophin leads to a drastic reduction in all components of the DGC that are normally synthesized but not properly assembled or integrated into the sarcolemma. Based on these observations, it is proposed that disruption of the DGC plays a key role in the cascade of events, leading to muscle cell necrosis. The absence of dystrophin causes a disruption of the linkage between the subsarcolemmal cytoskeleton and the extracellular matrix, leading to sarcolemmal instability, membrane tears, and muscle cell necrosis. Classical observations in the mdx transgenic mouse model of dystrophin deficiency showed the critical role of the cysteine-rich region (30–32) such that a dystrophin gene construct devoid of exons 64 to 70, responsible for transduction of the cysteine-rich domain, prevented localization of all components of the DGC. The observation of missense mutations that resulted in conformational changes of the molecular structure of dystrophin prevents proper assembly of the DGC (22). Other observations support a model whereby dystrophin deficiency, or small changes that alter the structural conformation of dystrophin, disrupt the DGC leading to membrane instability, predisposing the muscle to repeated insults, with calcium re-entry, myofiber breakdown, and a muscular dystrophy phenotype. Iwata and colleagues (33) demonstrated a muscular dystrophy phenotype in mdx mice by dominant-negative inhibition of transient receptor potential cation channel, subfamily V, member 2 (*Trpv2*), a principal candidate for Ca^{2+} entry pathways. Whereas dystrophin deficiency does not fully recapitulate the human disease in mdx mice, which shows milder skeletal muscle defects and potent regenerative myofiber capacity, mdx mice lacking the telomerase RNA component (TERC) develop severe progressive muscular dystrophy more consistent with the human phenotype associated with a decline in stem cell regenerative capacity that is ameliorated by transplantation of wild-type muscle stem cells in mdx/mTR mice (34). These findings are consistent with a model of stem cell exhaustion in maintaining the damage-repair cycle initiated by dystrophic deficiency. Increasing the expression of intramuscular heat-shock protein-72 (Hsp72) preserves muscle strength and ameliorates the dystrophic pathology in two mouse models of muscular dystrophy (35), as does treatment with BGP-15, a pharmacologic inducer of Hsp72 that protects against obesity-induced insulin resistance.

Treatment

The management of DMD is largely symptomatic, providing assistance to ambulation, prevention of scoliosis, and respiratory toilet. However, appropriate stretching of the heel cords, iliotibial bands, and hip flexors at a young age prevents contractures, and night splints may delay heel cord tightness. Segmental spinal stabilization corrects scoliosis. Patients with progressive curvatures measuring 35 to 45 degrees should be considered surgical candidates. A forced vital capacity of greater than 35% of predicted normal mean is recommended to prevent postoperative pneumonia. Anesthesia for patients with DMD should not include halogenated inhalational anesthetics or neuromuscular depolarizing agents such as succinylcholine because adverse reactions may occur that are similar, but not identical, to malignant hyperthermia (MH).

The Quality Standards Subcommittee of the American Academy of Neurology and the Practice Committee of the Child Neurology Society (36) identified several class I studies to guide treatment (37–43). In particular, prednisone and deflazacor led to improved muscle strength, pulmonary function, and functional ability in randomized, double-blind, controlled trials (38, 40) in as early as ten days,

reaching maximal improvement by three months. There was insufficient data comparing prednisone and deflazacort, an oxazolone analogue of prednisone, to determine if it has fewer side effects. It is available outside the US with an estimated dosage equivalency of 1:1.3 compared with prednisone, and administered at a dose of 0.9 mg/kg/day. Long-term studies indicate that a prednisone dose of 0.65 mg/kg/day can maintain improvement, but similar results cannot be achieved with alternate-day treatment (39). Prednisone should be offered at a dose of 0.75 mg/kg/day as treatment, maintaining that dose unless side effects require a decrease, whereupon the dose can be gradually tapered as low as 0.3 mg/kg/day, while maintaining significant improvement. Timed function tests, pulmonary function tests, and age at loss of independent ambulation are useful to assess benefits in research studies. An offer of treatment with prednisone should include a discussion of potential side effects, including weight gain, Cushingoid appearance, short stature, acne, and undesired hair growth, and gastrointestinal and behavioral side-effects. The salutary effects of prednisone in DMD, while not well understood, have been ascribed to alternation in mRNA levels of structural, signaling, and immune response genes, reduction in cytotoxic T-cells, lowering of calcium influx, increase in laminin expression and myogenic repair, retardation of muscle apoptosis and cell infiltrates, enhancement of dystrophin expression, improved neuromuscular transmission, attenuation of myofiber necrosis, and slowing in the rate of muscle fiber breakdown.

Gene therapy, which is not limited to replacement of defective genes, but also includes strategies using surrogate genes with alternative but effective means of improving cellular function or repairing mutations (44), has been limited to intramuscular injections of virus into a single muscle limited in scope in phase I trials with safety as the primary end point. In March 2006, six boys with frame-shift deletions of the dystrophin gene were enrolled in the first randomized, double-blind study (45) of adeno-associated virus (AAV) vector delivery of the *DMD* gene to one biopsy muscle while the other received saline or empty capsid, and concomitant testing of peripheral mononuclear cells in an interferon-g enzyme linked immunosorbent (ELISA) spot assay for reactivity to mini-dystrophin. Four of the patients were receiving standard corticosteroid therapy that was continued throughout the study. Intravenous methylprednisolone was administered prior to vector administration and repeated at one and two days to reduce local inflammation from intramuscular needle insertion. Muscle biopsy specimens were assessed on day 42 and 90 for dystrophin positive fibers recognized by double labeling with antibodies positive for N-terminal dystrophin. In all patients, vector DNA was detected in amounts ranging from 0.01 to 2.56 genome copies per diploid genome in the treated muscles but not in the untreated ones. Myofibers expressing mini-dystrophin protein were not detected in two biopsy specimens on day 90, but were on day 42. One patient had three or four dystrophin-positive fibers recognized by the N-terminal, as did another with one positive fiber that was negative for an antibody that detected the C-terminal, which is removed when dystrophin complementary DNA is miniaturized to accommodate the small insertion capacity of the AAV. The findings highlighted the future importance of experimental therapy designs to include monitors of self and nonself dystrophin epitopes to assure successful transgene delivery into DMD muscle.

LIMB GIRDLE MUSCULAR DYSTROPHY

Background

The term *limb-girdle muscular dystrophy* (LGMD) initially referred to a heterogeneous group of genetic disorders affecting predominantly shoulder and pelvic girdle musculature (46). With recognition of the diversity of inheritance patterns, and the clinical and genetic heterogeneity, that concept was transformed into classification nosology (47, 48), and complemented by a classification based upon the involved proteins and the underlying genetic defects (49). There are presently 24 different subtypes of LGMD (Table 1), of which eight display autosomal dominant (AD)-LGMD (AD-LGMD, LGMD1) inheritance, including LGMD1A to LGMD1H, in which a genetic basis has been established for myotilinopathy, laminopathy, and calveolinopathy; and 16 other subtypes that display autosomal recessive (AR)-LGMD (AR-LGMD, LGMD2) inheritance, including LGMD2A to LGMD2O, and Q), in which the genetic basis has been established for calpainopathy, dysferlinopathy; TRIM32; sarcoglycanopathy types γ-, α-, β-, and δ; and dystroglycanopathy due to fukutin (*FKTN*), fukutin-related protein (*FKRP*), 0-mannosyl transferase 1 (*POMT1*), protein-0-mannosyl transferase 2 (*POMT2*), and protein-0-mannose 1, 2-N-acetylglucosaminyltransferase 1 (*POMGnT1*) gene mutations. The historical achievements in the elucidation of the major AD and AR forms, respectively, LGMD1A, 1B, and 1C associated with deficiency of myotilin, lamin A/C, and calveolin 3; and LGMD2A, 2B, 2E, and 2F, associated with deficiency of calpain 3, dysferlin, β- and δ-arcoglycanopathy, recapitulate the achievements in molecular diagnosis of neuromuscular disease that remains unparalleled in its scope.

Myotilinopathy

First regarded as a late-onset muscular dystrophy (50), and later referred to as an adult-onset form of AD hereditary quadriceps myopathy (51), Gilchrist (52) and Speer and colleagues (53) demonstrated anticipation in subsequent generations, erroneously concluding a genetic basis due to expansion of an unstable trinucleotide repeat. That concept was later amended with elucidation of the sarcomeric protein myotilin (54). Reilich and colleagues (55) recently described an especially severe form of LGMD1A. The disorder, which is due to heterozygous mutation at the 5q31.2 locus of *MYOT*, is characterized clinically by adult-onset proximal muscle weakness, beginning in the hip girdle and later progressing to the shoulder girdle, with later distal weakness.

Laminopathy

First appreciated for AD weakness and association with cardiac disease in up to two-thirds of patients (56), the weakness in LGMD1B demonstrates two broad groups of patients (57) related to phenotypic clustering, one with childhood onset of predominant scapuloperoneal and facial weakness and a phenotype similar to EDMD and CMD due to toxic gain-of-function, and a second group with later adult onset of limb-girdle myopathy and cardiac disease attributed to loss of gene function secondary to haplo-insufficiency. Two unrelated adult-onset German patients had slow progression simulating proximal spinal muscular atrophy (58). The disorder is caused by mutation at the 1q22 locus of the *LMNA* gene encoding the nuclear envelope protein lamin A/C; EDMD and dilated cardiomyopathy type 1A are allelic disorders. In the same year, 1998, Minetti and colleagues (59) described a cohort with onset of AD weakness at about age five years, associated with calf hypertrophy, Gower sign, proximal weakness, up to 25-fold elevation in the CK level, nonspecific myopathic changes in biopsied muscle tissue, and two heterozygous mutations in the *CAV3* gene.

Calveolinopathy

In the same year, McNally and colleagues (60) determined the genomic organization of human caveolin 3, determining homozygosity for one *CAV3* mutation, and a heterozygous mutation in another affected patient, both of whom presented with weakness in the first decade of life. LGMD1C is caused by mutation at the 3p25 locus of the *CAV3* gene encoding caveolin 3. Missense mutation in the membrane-spanning region, and micro-deletion in the scaffolding domains of which, interfere with caveolin 3 oligomerization and disrupts caveolae formation at the muscle cell plasma membrane. A transgenic mouse model of LGMD1C demonstrates severe myopathy accompanied by caveolin-3 deficiency, suggesting a dominant effect of mutant caveolin 3 (61).

Calpainopathy

A premolecular analysis of muscular dystrophy (62) suggested that up to 59% of patients with the commonest fea-

Table 1.

Classification of Limb-Girdle Muscular Dystrophy

Disease Name[1]	Inheritance[2]	Gene[3]	Locus	Gene Product
LGMD1A	AD	*MYOT*	5q31.2	Myotilin
LGMD1B	AD (AR)	*LMNA*	1q22	Lamin A/C
LGMD1C	AD (AR)	*CAV3*	3p25	Calveolin 3
LGMD1D	AD	*LGMD1D*	7q36	--
LGMD1E	AD	*CMD1F*	6q23	--
LGMD1F	AD	*LGMD1F*	7q32.1-q32.2	--
LGMD1G	AD	*LGMD1G*	4q21.21	--
LGMD1H	AD	*LGMD1H*	3p25-p23	--
LGMD2A	AR	*CAPN3*	15q.15.1	Calpain 3
LGMD2B	AR	*DYSF*	2p13.2	Dysferlin
LGMD2C	AR	*SGCG*	13q12-q12	γ-Sarcoglycan
LGMD2D	AR	*SGCA*	17q21.33	α-Sarcoglycan
LGMD2E	AR	*SGCB*	4q12	β-Sarcoglycan
LGMD2F	AR	*SGCD*	5q33.3	δ-Sarcoglycan
LGMD2G	AR	*TCAP*	17q12	Telethonin (T-cap)
LGMD2H				
TRIM32 deficiency	AR	*TRIM32*	9q33.1	TRIM32
LGMD2I	AR	*FKRP*	19q13.3	Fukutin-related protein
LGMD2J	AR	*TTN*	2q31	Titin
LGMD2K	AR	*POMT1*	9q34.1	POMT1
LGMD2L	AR	*ANO5*	11p14.3	--
LGMD2M	AR	*FKTN*	9q31.2	Fukutin
LGMD2N	AR	*POMT2*	14q24.3	POMT2
LGMD2O	AR	*POMGNT1*	1p34.1	POMGNT1
LGMD2Q	AR	*PLEC*	8q24.3	--

[1]Classification of LGMD by the European Neuromusuclar Center (ENMC). From, Bushby KMD, Beckmann JS.
The 105th ENMC sponsored workshop: Pathogenesis in the non-sarcoglycan limb-girdle muscular dystrophies, Naarden, April 12–14, 2002, *Neuromuscul Disord* 2003; 13:80–90).

[2]AD: autosomal dominant; AR: autosomal recessive.

[3]HUGO Gene Nomenclature. From, Seal RL, Gordon SM, Lush MJ, et al. genenames.org: the HGND resources in 2011. *Nucleic Acids Res* 2011; 39(Database issue):D514-519.

tures of LGMD, namely asymmetric weakness and wasting of the pelvic and shoulder girdle muscles beginning in childhood, with spread to the legs over two decades, variable progression, severe gait disturbance, occasional contractures and facial involvement, could be ascribed to AR inheritance. Richard and colleagues (63) catalogued 15 nonsense, splice site, frameshift, or missense calpain mutations that cosegregated with LGMD2A in several families, six of whom had juvenile onset kindred from La Reunion Island, previously described by Fardeau and colleagues (64), explaining the paradox of multiple independent mutations rather than a single founder mutation by proposing a digenic inheritance model. Calpainopathy (65) is caused by homozygous or compound heterozygous mutation at the 15q15.1 locus of the CAPN3 gene encoding the proteolytic enzyme calpain 3.

Dysferlinopathy

Passos-Bueno and colleagues (66–68) characterized the genetic heterogeneity of LGMD2B, differentiating it from other AR types and confirming assignment to 2p. In a review of LGMD, Bushby (69), referred to the now-known allelic disorder Miyoshi myopathy and LGMD2B as dysferlinopathies. Patients with undetermined LGMD and Miyoshi myopathy phenotype with less than 20% dysferlin on skeletal muscle biopsy, as determined by Western blot analysis (70), correlated with pathogenic mutation in the DYSF gene. The disease is caused by mutation at the 2p13.2 locus of the DYSF gene encoding the skeletal muscle protein dysferlin. Miyoshi myopathy and distal myopathy with anterior tibial onset are allelic disorders.

Sarcoglycanopathy

Lim and colleagues (71) studied several Amish families with AR LGMD and identified a homozygous mutation in the SGCB gene with dramatic reduction in SGCB expression in the sarcolemma and concomitant loss of adhalin and SCGD, interpreted as disruption of a functional subcomplex within the DGC. Bonnemann and coworkers (72) identified novel mutations in the SGCB gene in several familial and sporadic childhood onset patients. Affected patients present with proximal symmetric weakness and atrophy of limb and trunk musculature, with average age at onset of seven years, and loss of walking between 12 and 38 years, with occasional calf hypertrophy and marked intrafamilial variability. Trabelsi and colleagues (73) identified biallelic mutations in more than two-thirds of patients with a clinical diagnosis of LGMD. The disorder is caused by mutation at the 4q12 locus of the SGCB gene encoding SGCB. Analogously, gypsies with mutations at the 13q12-q13 locus of the SGCG gene (74) encoding SGCG; at the

17q21 locus of the SGCA gene (75) encoding SGCA; and at the 5q33-q34 locus of the SGCD gene (76, 77) encoding SGCD in LGMD2F among severe Brazilian patients. Muscle biopsy in affected patients with LGMD2F showed lack of staining for SGCD as well as the other three components of the sarcoglycan complex SGCA, SGCB, and SGCG, with present but reduced quantity of dytrophin suggesting disruption of the entire complex. Affected patients studied by Duggan and colleagues (78) showed childhood onset of facial and proximal limb weakness with scapular winging, and frequent falls, with wheelchair dependence in the teens. The BIO14.6 hamster is a model for sarcoglycan-deficient LGMD due to deletion in the SGCD gene.

Epidemiology

Estimates of the prevalence for all forms of LGMD range from 1 in 14,500 to 1 in 123,000 (79, 80), while the carrier frequency of primary sarcoglycanopathy is estimated to be 1:150 to 1:211 (81, 82). There is also considerable reported geographic variation in the frequency of specific subtypes of LGMD. Among a cohort of Austrian LGMD patients, calpain 3 deficiency was present in 8%, dysferlinopathy in 5%, caveolin 3 and FKRP deficiency each in 3%; g-, b-sarcoglycanopathy, and lamin A/C deficiency each in 1%; while among those undiagnosed, 20% were dysferlin-defective and 58% were categorized as dysferlin-normal (83). By comparison, among 51% of 105 patients with LGMD in the Netherlands (84), DNA and protein analysis reached a molecular genetic diagnosis of calpainopathy, most frequently of the LGMD type, accounting for 21% of families, followed by sarcoglycanopathy in 16%, and LGMD21 associated with FKRP in 8%; however, no further subclassification could be made in the remaining 49%. Among a cohort of Italian LGMD patients, 26% had deficiency of calpain 3, 19% in dysferlin, 17% in one or more components of the sarcoglycans, 6% in FKRP, and 5% in caveolin 3; 27% of the remaining were undetermined.

Clinical Aspects

There are features common to all LGMD disorders (48). The age at onset varies within subtypes and between patients with the same mutation; however, onset in childhood and in teenage is usually encountered in deficiency of lamininopathy, calpainopathy, dystroglycanopathy, and sarcoglycanopathy. Whereas there is a specific tendency for proximal muscles to become weak and wasted (85), distal emphasis at onset or in the course of the disease can be seen in myotiliniopathy, laminopathy, calveoliopathy, and dysferlinopathy. Scapular involvement with prominent winging is a feature of calpainopathy and sarcoglycanopathy. Muscle hypertrophy is frequently encountered in calveolinopathy, sarcoglycanopathy, and FKRP; however, other muscles, including the tongue may be involved. Contractures are common in laminopathy including those with EDMD mutations and calpainopathy; scoliosis may be encountered in sarcoglycanopathy. Relative preservation of hip abductor muscles is seen in calpainopathy with severe involvement of posterior thigh muscles. Dysarthria is a feature of myotilinopathy, whereas rippling muscles and percussion-induced rapid muscle contractions are noted in calveoliniopathy.

Laboratory and Molecular Diagnosis

The serum CK is normal or elevated less than fivefold normal in AD-inherited myotilinopathy and laminopathy, and more than tenfold normal in those with calveolinopathy and others with AR inheritance. Nerve conduction studies exclude an alternative neuropathic basis, or may reveal concomitant neuropathy in those with laminiopathy. Needle EMG confirms the myopathic nature of the disorder, but generally do not offer additional specificity in refining the diagnostic subtype of LGMD. Similarly, quantitative EMG (QEMG) and muscle biopsy, while useful in detecting myopathic changes, failed to discriminate among patients with diverse forms of progressive muscular dystrophy, and showed poor concordance with muscle biopsy (18). Of ten patients so studied, nine showed myopathic electrophysiology in association with nonspecific muscle biopsy tissue abnormalities, in addition to marked myofiber atrophy in one-half of biopsies, and two showed group atrophy indicative of concomitant neurogenic impairment. Decomposition-based QEMG (DQEMG) employs a series of algorithms that decompose the needle-detected EMG signal into its constituent MUP trains (86), which revealed reduced mean MUP duration, MUP area, and area-to-amplitude ratio (AAR) among 15 patients with FSHD, LGMD, and BMD, more so among those more severely affected (87).

Whereas ultrasound detects muscular changes in children during initial screening, with a sensitivity of 25% for non-dystrophic processes and up to 100% in dystrophic myopathies (88–90), producing a brightly speckled pattern of increased echo in real-time from the muscle in patients with muscular dystrophy (91). It has the major advantage of being noninvasive, similar magnetic resonance imaging (MRI) that may add additional useful information regarding the pattern and severity of muscle involvement in patients with LGMD. Dystrophic changes such as fatty degeneration can be easily appreciated and sensitivity detected using T_1-, and T_2-weighted sequences; inflammatory changes such a muscle edema change can be depicted on T_2-weighted FLAIR (92) and STIR images (93) with applied rating scales (94–96). Atrophy is recognized radiographically by reduced muscle volume and hypertrophy by increased muscle volume, whereas pseudohypertrophy is apparent as fatty infiltration of muscle with increased volume. Although not yet established, contrast administration may be a valuable option for the assessment of connective tissue replacement. Quantitative MRI methodologies, including T_2 relaxation time measurements, muscle fat quantitation, magnetic resonance spectroscopy (MRS), and perfusion imaging techniques might be helpful in further analyzing pathological changes in striated muscle (97). The MRI approach to LGMD commences with ascertainment of patients with greater involvement of anterior than posterior compartment thigh muscles wherein gastrocnemius involvement typifies dystrophinopathy but is spared in sarcoglycanopathy. Posterior thigh compartment involvement exceeded that of the anterior compartment, in association with calf atrophy in dysferlinopathy, while focal or diffuse posterior leg muscle involvement sparing the anterior leg compartment, affecting soleus and medial gastroc muscles typified calpainopathy and *FKRP* mutation (92). Muscle MRI showed selective involvement of the glutei, adductor thigh, and hamstring muscles with severe involvement of posterior compartment of the legs in two patients with calpainopathy (93); with similar calf muscle changes in seven other patients, three of whom were ambulatory, regardless of severity (98). Muscle MRI revealed diffuse severe involvement of shoulder girdle muscles sparing quadriceps, Sartorius, and gracilis musculature with diffuse hyperintensity on STIR images in muscles with normal signal on T_1-weighted images in two patients with dysferlinopathy (93). A diamond on quadriceps sign on T_1-weighted MRI of the thighs indicative of a focal bulge-out of muscle fibers during forced contraction, was noted in eight patients with dysferlinopathy and in 13 patients with Miyoshi myopathy (MM), but not in those with sarcoglycanopathy (99). Imaging in several patients with α- and γ-sarcoglycanopathy (93) showed fatty atrophy of both shoulder girdle and pelvic girdle musculature, with focal hyperintensity in the triceps on STIR imaging, which was relatively spared on T_1-weighted images. Several patients so studied with *FKRP* mutations (93) were noted to have severe early involvement of the adductors, pectineus, obturator, and hamstring muscles on T_1-weighted imaging, with fatty degeneration and atrophy of the vasti, glutei, and tensor fascia latae, with sparing of the gracilis. Serratus, subscapularis, supra-, and infraspinati were affected earlier and more severely than other proximal muscles, while STIR imaging showed hyperintensity in muscles that were relatively spared on T_1-weighted imaging.

Cardiac involvement, most often a feature of myotilinopathy, laminiopathy, sarcoglycanopathy, and dystro glycanopathy, was associated with mild structural and functional cardiac abnormalities in nine patients with dysferlinopathy and seven patients with FKRP mutations, only one of whom had severe dilated cardiomyopathy, and otherwise normal left ventricular size and systolic function, with clinically inapparent cardiac disease on cardiac magnetic resonance (CMR) imaging (100).

Brain involvement is a frequent, but not constant, feature in patients with dystroglycanopathies, ranging hierarchically from isolated cerebellar cysts to more severe structural involvement affecting the brainstem and pons, including polymicrogyria and cobblestone lissencephalic changes indistinguishable from those found in muscle-eye-brain (MEB) disease and Walker-Warburg syndrome (WWS) due to mutations in genes encoding known or putative glycosyltransferase enzymes (101, 102). Brain MRI from 27 patients with mutations in *POMT1, POMT2, POMGnT1, FKTN* or *LARGE*, responsible for muscular dystrophy with abnormal glycosylation of dystroglycan (103), showed a spectrum of brain involvement. This ranged from normal or minimal ventricular dilatation in the patients with *FKTN* mutations to complete lissencephaly in those with WWS phenotype, pontine clefts in several patients with a MEB phenotype and in those with *POMGnT1, LARGE,* and *POMT2* mutations, and prominent cerebellar cysts in all of those with *POMGnT1,* but not *POMT1* and *POMT2* mutations. Brainstem and pontine abnormalities were common in patients with *POMT2, POMGnT1,* and *LARGE* mutations. Brain MRI, employed in ten patients with *FKRP* mutation as part of an extensive cognitive profile in patients with mild impairments in executive function and visuospatial planning (104) showed non-specific white matter abnormalities in four, moderate ventriculomegaly in two, mild enlargement of the subarachnoid spaces in three, and marked cerebellar atrophy in one patient, indicating that like *FKTN* mutations, abnormal glycosylation of α-dystrogycan in LGMD2I did not produce specific brain abnormalities seen on MRI.

Muscle biopsy probably yields the most useful information when undertaken at a center with expertise both in the performance of the biopsy and its interpretation. The muscle biopsied should be clinically and electrophysiologically affected, but not end-stage. Both the vastus lateralis and biceps brachii muscles are ideal for disorders accompanied by proximal weakness due to presumed muscular dystrophy. At least four specimens of muscle should be obtained caring to incise the muscle along natural longitudinal and cross-sectional epimysial tissue planes to optimize later histopathological sections, while minimizing tissue handling, blunt trauma, bleeding, and vascular compression. Separate pieces of muscle are placed in moist saline gauze, 10% formalin, and glutaraldehyde, and transported directly to the muscle laboratory for paraffin embed histology, snap-freezing, cryosections, electron microscopy (EM), and a battery of tissue stains at varying pH. A complete analysis begins with the search for myopathic changes, including myofiber necrosis, regeneration, and cellular infiltration, excluding fiber type grouping and

other features of neurogenic disease. This is followed by tissue stains for glycolytic and oxidative myofiber metabolism, and other investigations employing monoclonal antibody probes that recognize lymphocyte subsets, macrophages, main histocompatibility complex (MHC) and complement factors, immunofluorescence, collagen-staining studies, and ultrastructural analysis, and most importantly, muscle immunohistochemistry and quantitative analysis of proteins by Western blotting to distinguish primary and secondary immunohistochemical abnormalities.

More than a decade ago, the pathological and immunohistochemical evaluation of LGMD (105) recognized collections of inflammatory cells in up to a quarter of AR- and 10% of AD-LGMD subtypes respectively. Sarcoglycanopathy was discerned in about 25% of AR and sporadic patients, and the histological appearance of AR, AD, and sporadic LGMD were deemed to be essentially the same, with up to 80% of muscle biopsies demonstrating a predominantly dystrophic pattern, and 20% evidencing active myopathic features at the time of biopsy, 17% of which displayed associated neurogenic features (105). With further improvements in immunoanalytic methodology, it is possible to screen muscle tissue more effectively for primary and secondary changes. Whereas immunoblot protocols traditionally required the solubilization of a significant portion of a muscle biopsy specimen, improved methodologies for Western blot analysis such as termed single section Western blot (SSWB), requires only a single 8-µm biopsy cyrosection for simultaneous analysis of multiple disease candidates for a range of human muscular dystrophies, in particular LGMD subtypes (106), the spectrum of which is expanding as new gene loci are incorporated into the evaluative process. Whereas the primary changes in a muscle biopsy specimen showed decreased caveolin 3 labeling in a suspected patient with LGMD1C, regardless of the secondary loss of dysferlin, the converse may not be so in patients with LGMD2B attributed to dysferlinopathy in whom secondary calveolin 3 labeling as a result of the concomitant reduction in members of the DRC. The presence of inflammatory cells, more likely in LGMD2B than LGMD1C, may be a helpful finding. Rimmed vacuoles are an associated feature of myotilinopathy, telethoninopathy, and dystroglycanopathy. Molecular genetic testing of whole blood is commercially available for analysis of mutations in the *MYO, LMNA, CAV3, CAPN3, DYSF, SGCG, SGCAA, SGCB, SGCD,* and *FKRP* genes (107).

Treatment

There are no established drug treatments for LGMD; however, initial management should focus on aspects that improve quality of life and prolong survival through respiratory aids, weight control to prevent obesity, physical therapy to promote mobility and reduce contractures, mechanical assistive aids to maintain ambulation, orthopedic intervention to treat foot deformity and scoliosis, cardiologic care to treat cardiomyopathy; and genetic counseling for family planning, carrier detection and prenatal testing. Corticosteroids showed salutary benefit in patients with sarcoglycanopathy (108, 109) and *FKTN* gene mutations (110, 111). A trial of neutralizing antibody to myostatin (MYO-029) among different forms of LGMD2 showed adequate safety and tolerability but no improvement in measures of strength and function; however, the study was not powered to provide proof of efficacy (112). Gene therapy for LGMD has been investigated (113, 114) employing AAV as the vector for transgene expression of full length a-sarcoglycan (a-SG) cDNA, delivered by recombinant AAV (rAAV), with a muscle specific CK promoter (tMCK) to differentially regulate expression in skeletal muscle in conjunction with intravenous methylprednisolone at the same dose and time of administration to reduce local inflammation from intramuscular needle insertion as in a DMD trial (45). Mendell and colleagues (115, 116) showed persistent a-SG transgene expression for six months in two of three LGMD2D patients with concomitant expression of major histocompatibility complex (MHC) I expression, increase in muscle fiber size, and restoration of the full sarcoglycan complex. The patient who failed gene transfer demonstrated an early rise in neutralizing antibody titers and T-cell immunity to AAV, validated by enzyme-linked immunospot on the second day of gene injection, in clear distinction to other participants with satisfactory responses. Transplantation of genetically reprogrammed fibroblasts and myoblasts from LGMD2D patients to generate human-induced pluripotent stem cells (iPSC)-derived mesoangioblasts into a-SG-null immunodeficient mice generated muscle fibers that expressed a-SG, suggesting that transplantation of genetically corrected mesoangioblasts-like cells generated from iPSC from LGMD2D patients may be useful in the treatment in human subjects (117).

CONGENITAL MUSCULAR DYSTROPHY

The main CMD subtypes are classified by the mutated gene and protein products included among them, α-2 laminin and lamimin M chain (merosin) deficiency, the dystroglycanopathies, and LMNA-related CMD.

LAMA2

Laminin-2 is a heterotrimer composed of α-2, β-1, and γ-1 laminin subunits, and is the main laminin found in skeletal muscle. The *LAMA2* gene encodes the α-2 chain of laminin-2. Merosin, or laminin M chain (LAMM), is a basement membrane-associated protein found in striated muscle, peripheral nerve, and placenta, and is thought to contain the neurite-promoting site and the major cell binding sites in laminin (118). An antiserum against the synthetic peptide from the middle of the merosin cDNA sequence identified a 300-kDa polypeptide in placental extracts, indicating that the merosin polypeptide was similar in size to the laminin A chain. Vuolteenaho and colleagues (119) assigned human LAMM to chromosome 6q22-q23. Arahata and colleagues (120) found that merosin was reduced in myofibers of patients with Fukuyama CMD, suggesting that it played a role in the disorder. Complete LAMA2 deficiency is found in about one-half of patients with CMD associated with many loss-of-function mutations in neonatal-onset cases, and missense mutations in milder CMD with partial LAMA2 deficiency (121). Mutation positive patients with undetectable or greater reduced muscle expression of LAMA2 protein present with generalized hypotonia and severe weakness at birth and abnormal white matter signal changes on brain MRI (122).

Dystroglycanopathy

The dystroglycanopathies are a group of predominantly AR inherited muscular dystrophies that result from mutations in genes encoding known or putative glycosyltransferase enzymes, in which the hallmark is defective glycosylation of dystophin-associated glycoprotein1 (DAG1) leading to reduced expression of muscle glycosylated α-dystroglycan (103). Affected patients present structural changes in the brain and eyes included under the rubric Fukuyama CMD, MEB disease, and WWS. Mutations in six different genes, *POMT1*, *POMT2*, *POMGnT*, *FKTN*, *FKRP*, and *LARGE*, have been identified. Type A muscular dystropohy dystroglycanopathy (MDDG) is subtypes MDDGA1-7; as are type B into subtypes MDDGB1-6, respectively due to mutation at the 9q34.13 locus of POMT1 in MDDGA1 and B1; at 14q24.3 in *POMT2* in MDDGA2 and MDDGB2; at 1p34.1 locus of *POMGNT1* in MDDGA3 and B3; at 9q31.2 of *FKTN* in MDDGA4 and B4; at 19q13.32 locus of *FKRP* in MDDGA5 and MDDGB5; and at 22q12.3 of the *LARGE* gene in MDDGA6 and B6. Affected patients have frequent but inconstant brain involvement and abnormal cognitive development that ranges from normal, as in those described with the first *FKRP* mutations (123), to severe structural abnormalities including complete lissencephaly in those with WWS, to isolated cerebellar involvement and pontine cleft in those with MEB phenotype, all with associated learning difficulties, variable mental retardation, and early mortality. Three types of gross pathology include verrucous dysplasia, unlayered polymicrogyria, and agyric regions (124).

LMNA-Related CMD

Mercuri and colleagues (125) described a patient with inability to roll over at age five months, feeding difficulty, axial and limb weakness, foot deformity, and increased CK. Two additional patients with frank floppy or dropped head syndrome were later described (126) associated with mutations in *LMNA* and *SEPN1*. Other patients with severe early-onset weakness and decreased fetal movements *in utero*, absent motor development, severe hypotonia, diffuse limb and axial weakness, and foot deformities were characterized in association with 11 different *de novo* heterozygous *LMNA* mutations (127). The disorder is caused by heterozygous mutation at the 1q22 locus of the *LMNA* gene encoding lamin A/C; two allelic disorders, LGMD1B and EDMD2, have overlapping phenotypes.

The treatment for all forms of congenital muscular dystrophies is supportive. Anticonvulsant therapy is mandatory for those with seizures. Passive stretching to correct contractures, night splints, and serial plaster casts may be useful. Tenotomies may be necessary for some patients to facilitate standing and ambulation. Expression of laminin-α2 in dy^w and dy^{2J} mice, both partly deficient, causes some degree of rescue in the muscle phenotype with improved longevity and muscle morphology; transgenic expression of laminin-α1 is beneficial to the skeletal muscle and infertility phenotype of laminin-α2 deficient mice (128). Once thought to be simply disorders due to abnormalities and perturbation of the extracellular matrix, ongoing investigation into the pathogenesis of these disorders, including mechanisms of neuronal migration defects, and possible avenue of enzymatic modification of the glycosylation process of α-dystroglycan, may yet lead to novel future treatment options.

EMERY-DREIFUSS MUSCULAR DYSTROPHY

The term EDMD was suggested by Rowland (4) after the essential features were delineated by Emery and Dreifuss (129). The disease begins in infancy or early childhood at around age four or five, with pelvic girdle weakness, later involving the pectoral girdle muscles, with slow progression, cardiac involvement, contractures of the elbows, shortening of the Achilles tendons, mild pectus excavatum, and absence of pseuohypertrophic calves. Affected patients are typically very thin with normal facial musculature, restriction of neck flexion, contractures of the knees and manifested humeropcroneal distribution of weakness and wasting, with invariable toe-walking, absent reflexes, eventual distal leg weakness, and preservation of intellect and ambulation, the latter even until the sixth decade (129).

The serum CK is typically elevated two- to fourfold normal. Although originally studied patients (129) showed no evidence of denervation on gastrocnemius muscle biopsy, there were examples of myofiber necrosis, phagocytosis, and variation in myofiber size without fatty or connective tissue replacement. Electrodiagnostic studies usually show evidence of myopathy but quantitative EMG and SFEMG may demonstrate neurogenic aspects in increased mean MUP amplitude (130). Electrocardiographic features included varying degrees of atrial arrhythmia and bradycardia, which precede Wenckebach phenomenon, and complete atrioventricular heart block with syncope, potentially fatal ventricular arrhythmia, and sudden death. However, these is no strict correlation between the severity of the cardiac disease and the severity of limb weakness. One patient with EDMD studied at postmortem examination (131) met all five premolecular clinical criteria defined by the European Workshop on EDMD (132).

In 1994, Bione and colleagues (133) found a unique mutation that resulted in loss of all or part of the protein product, followed later by the amplication and sequencing of each of the six *EMD* exons (134). By the end of the twentieth century, there were a total of 26 causative mutations in the *EMD* gene, and the ubiquitous protein that immunostained only the nuclear membrane was found in skeletal, cardiac, and smooth muscles of patients with EDMD (135). From the first workshop of the MYO-CLUSTER project, European muscle envelope nucleopathies (EUROMEN) in 2000 (136) to the third meeting in 2002 (137), progress in the clinical and genetic spectrum of EDMD led to recognition of new insights into laminopathy and emerinopathy attributed to mutation in the *EMD* gene that corresponded to the X-linked form of EDMD, up to six phenotypes associated with mutation in the *LMNA* gene, and the cellular and cardiac consequences of these mutations. EDMD1 is caused by mutation at the xq28 locus of the *EMD* gene. Autosomal dominant EDMD2 is caused by heterozygous mutation at the 1q22 locus of the *LMNA* gene encoding lamin A/C. Two other forms, EDMD4 and EDMD5, both AD, are caused by heterozygous mutations, respectively, at the 6q25.1-q25.2 and the 14q23.2 loci of the *SYNE1* and *SYNE2* genes. Skin fibroblasts from EDMD patients with *SYNE1* and *SYNE2* mutations showed similar defects in nuclear morphology as those described in EDMD due to *LMNA* and *EMD* mutations (138). A loss of nesprin-1 and nesprin-2, respectively associated with *SYNE1* and *SYNE2*, plays an important role in the nesprin/emerin,/lamin complex, changes in stoichiometric binding which may be important in uncoupling the nucleoskeleton and cytoskeleton, contributing to the pathogenesis of EDMD.

REFERENCES

1. Koenig M, Hoffman EP, Bertelson EP, et al. Complete cloning of the Duchenne muscular dystrophy cDNA and preliminary genomic organization of the DMD gene in normal and affected individuals. *Cell* 1987; 50:509–517.

2. Cohn RD, Campbell KP. Molecular basis of muscular dystrophies. *Muscle Nerve* 2000; 23:1456–1471.

3. Mendell JR, Sahenk Z, Prior TW. The childhood muscular dystrophies: diseases sharing a common pathogenesis of membrane instability. *J Child Neurol* 1995; 10:150–159.

4. Rowland LP, Layzer RB. X-linked muscular dystrophies. *Handb Clin Neurol* 1979; 40:349–414.

5. Meryon E. ON the granular and fatty degeneration of the voluntary muscles. *Med Chir Trans* 1852; 35:73–85.

6. Duchenne GB. Recherches sur la paralysie musculaire pseudohypertrophicque, ou paralysie myosclerosique. *Arch Gen Med*, Series 6, 1868; 11:5–25.

7. Brooke MH, Fenichel GM, Griggs RC, et al. Duchenne muscular dystrophy: patterns of clinical progression and effects of supportive therapy. *Neurology* 1989; 39:475–481.

8. Munsat TL, Bahoh R, Pearson CM, et al. Serum enzyme alterations in neuromuscular disorders. *JAMA* 1973; 226:1536–1543.

9. Bradley WG, Hudgson P, Larson PF, et al. Structural changes in early stages of Duchenne muscular dystrophy. *J Neurol Neurosurg Psychiatry* 1972; 35:451–455.

10. Buchthal F. Electrophysiological signs of myopathy as related with muscle biopsy. *Acta Neurol* 1977; 32:1–29.

11. Desmedt JE, Borenstein S. Regeneration in Duchenne muscular dystrophy. Electromyographic evidence. *Arch Neurol* 1976; 33:642–650.

12. Buchtal F, Rosenblack P. Electrophysiological aspects of myopathy with particular reference to progressive muscular dystrophy. In: GH Bourne, N Golarz, eds. *Muscular dystrophy in animals and man.* Basel: Hafner, 1963; 193–262.

13. Hilton-Brown PER, Stålberg E. The motor unit in muscular dystrophy, a single fiber EMG and scanning EMG study. *J Neurol Neurosurg Psychiatry* 1983; 46:981–995.

14. Stålberg E, Falck B, Sonoo M, et al. Multi-MUP EMG analysis a two year experience in daily clinical work. *Electroencephalogr Clin Neurophysiol* 1995; 97:145–154.

15. McGill KC, Cummins KL, Dorfman LJ. Automatic decomposition of the clinical electromyogram. *IEEE Trans Biomed Eng* 1985; 32:470–477.

16. Nikolic M, Krarup C. EMGTools, an adaptive and versatile tool for detailed EMG analysis. *IEEE Trans Biomed Eng* 2011; 58:2707–2718.

17. Stålberg E, Chu J, Bril V, Nandedkar S, et al. Automatic analysis of the EMG interference pattern. *Electroencephalogr Clin Neurophysiol* 1983; 56:672–681.

18. Buchthal F, Kamieniecka Z. The diagnositic yield of quantified electromyography and quantified muscle biopsy in neuromuscular disorders. *Muscle Nerve* 1982; 5:265–280.

19. Beggs AH, Kunkel LM. Improved diagnosis of Duchenne/Becker muscular dystrophy. *J Clin Invest* 1990; 85:613–619.

20. Winnard AV, Mendell JR, Prior TW, et al. Frameshift deletions of exons 3–7 and revertant fibers in Duchenne muscular dystrophy: mechanisms of dystrophin production. *Am J Hum Genet* 1995; 56:158–166.

21. Prior TW. Perspectives and molecular diagnosis of Duchenne and Becker muscular dystrophies. Clin Lab Med 1995;15:927–941; Roberts RG, Gardner RJ, Bobrow M. Searching for the 1 in 2,400,000: a review of dystrophin gene point mutations. *Hum Mutat* 1994; 4:1–11.

22. Prior TW, Bartolo C, Pearl DK, et al. Spectrum of small mutations in the dystrophin coding region. *Am J Hum Genet* 1995; 57:22–33.

23. Prior TW, Papp AC, Snyder PJ, Mendell JR. Germline mosaicism in carriers of Duchenne muscular dystrophy. *Muscle Nerve* 1992; 15:960–963.

24. Bonilla E, Younger DS, Chang HW, et al. Partial dystrophin deficiency in monozygous twin carriers of the Duchenne dystrophy gene. *Neurology* 1990; 40:1267–1270.

25. Haldane JBS. The rate of spontaneous mutation of a human gene. *J Genet* 1935; 31:317–326.

26. Haldane JBS. Mutation in the X-linked recessive type of muscular dystrophy: a possible sex difference. *Ann Hum Genet* 1956; 20:344–347.

27. Tuffery-Giraud S, Beroud C, Leturca F, et al. Genotype-phenotype analysis in 2,405 patients with a dystrophinopathy using the UMD-DMD database: a model of nationwide knowledgebase. *Hum Mutat* 2009; 30:934–945.

28. Oshima J, Magner DB, Lee JA, et al. Regional genomic instability predisposes to complex dystrophin gene rearrangements. *Hum Genet* 2009; 126:411–423.

29. Pegoraro E, Hoffman EP, Piva L, et al. PP1 genotype is a determinant of disease severity in Duchenne muscular dystrophy. *Neurology* 2011; 76:219–226.

30. Rafael JA, Yoshihide S, Cole NM, et al. Prevention of dystrophic pathology in mdx mice by a truncated dystrophin isoform. *Hum Mol Genet* 1994; 3:1725–1733.

31. Rafael JA, Cox GA, Corrado K, et al. Forced expression of dystrophin deletion constructs reveals structure-function correlations. *J Cell Biol* 1996; 134:93–102.

32. Wells DJ, Wells KE, Asante G, et al. Expression of human full-length and minidystrophin in transgenic mdx mice: implications for gene therapy of Duchenne muscular dystrophy. *Hum Mol Genet* 1995; 4:1245–1250.

33. Iwata Y, Katanosaka Y, Arai Y, et al. Dominant-negative inhibition of Ca(2+) influx via TRPV2 ameliorates muscular dystrophy in animal models. *Hum Molec Genet* 2009; 18:824–834.

34. Sacco A, Mourkioti F Tran R, et al. Short telomeres and stem cell exhaustion model of Duchenne muscular dystrophy in nmdx/mTR mice. *Cell* 2010; 143:1059–1071.

35. Gehrig SM, van der Poel C, Sayer TA, et al. Hsp72 preserves muscle function and slows progression of severe muscular dystrophy. *Nature* 2012; 484:394–398.

36. Moxley RT III, Ashwal S, Pandya S, et al. Practice Parameter: Corticosteroid treatment of Duchenne dystrophy. Report of the Quality Standards Subcommittee of the American Academy of Neurology and the Practice Committee of the Child Neurology Society. *Neurology* 2005; 64:13–20.

37. Griggs RC, Moxley RT III, Mendell JR, et al. Duchenne dystrophy: randomized controlled trial of prednisone (18 months) and azathioprine (12 months). *Neurology* 1993; 43:520–527.

38. Mendell JR, Moxley RT III, Griggs RC, et al. Randomized, double-blind six-month trial of prednisone in Duchenne's muscular dystrophy. *N Engl J Med* 1989; 320:1592–1597.

39. Fenichel GM, Mendell JR, Moxley RT III, et al. A comparison of daily and alternate-day prednisone in the treatment of Duchenne dystrophy. *Arch Neurol* 1991; 48:575–579.

40. Griggs RC, Moxley RT III, Mendell JR, et al. Prednisone in Duchenne dystrophy. A randomized, controlled trial defining the time course and dose response. Clinical Investigation of Duchenne Dystrophy Group. *Arch Neurol* 1991; 48:383–388.

41. Rahman MM, Hannan MA, Mondol BA, et al. Prednisolone in Duchenne dystrophy. *Bangladesh Med Res Counc Bull* 2001; 27:38–42.

42. Backman E, Henriksson KG. Low-dose prednisolone treatment in Duchenne and Becker muscular dystrophy. *Neuromusc Disord* 1995; 5:233–241.

43. Fenichel GM, Florence JM, Pestronk A, et al. Long term benefit from prednisone therapy in Duchenne muscular dystrophy. *Neurology* 1991; 41:1874–1877.

44. Rodino-Klapac LR, Chicoine LG, Kaspar BK, et al. Gene therapy for Duchenne muscular dystrophy. Expectations and challenges. *Arch Neurol* 2007; 64:1236–1241.

45. Mendell JR, Campbell L, Rodino-Klapac I, et al. Dystrophin immunity in Duchenne's muscular dystrophy. *N Engl J Med* 2010; 363:1429–1437.

46. Walton JN, Nattrass FJ. On the classification, natural history and treatment of the myopathies. *Brain* 1954; 77:169–231.

47. Bushby KMD, Beckmann JS. The 105th ENMC sponsored workshop: pathogenesis in the non-sarcoglycan limb-girdle muscular dystrophies. Naarden, April 12–14, 2002. *Neuromusc Disord* 2003; 13:80–90.

48. Norwood F, de Visser M, Eymard B, et al. EFNS guidelines on diagnosis and management of limb girdle muscular dystrophies. *Eur J Neurol* 2007; 14:1305–1312.

49. Guglieri M, Straub V, Bushby K, et al. Limb-girdle muscular dystrophies. *Curr Opin Neurol* 2008; 21:576–584.

50. Bacon PA, Smith B. Familial muscular dystrophy of late onset. *J Neurol Neurosurg Psychiatry* 1971; 34:93–97.

51 Espir MLE, Matthews W. Hereditary quadriceps myopathy. *J Neurol Neurosurg Psychiatry* 1973; 36:1041–1045.

52. Gilchrist JM, Pericak-Vance, Silverman L, et al. Clinical and genetic investigation in autosomal dominant limb-girdle muscular dystrophy. *Neurology* 1988; 38:5–9.

53. Speer MC, Yamaoka LH, Gilchrist JH, et al. Confirmation of genetic heterogeneity in limb-girdle muscular dystrophy: linkage of an autosomal dominant form to chromosome 5qL. *Am J Hum Genet* 1992; 50:1211–1217.

54. Salmikangas P, Mykkanen OM, Gronholm M, et al. Myotilin, a novel sarcomeric protein with two Ig-like domain, is encoded by a candidate gene for limb-girdle muscular dystrophy. *Hum Molec Genet* 1999; 8:1329–1336.

55. Reilich P, Krause L, Schramm N, et al. A novel mutation in the myotilin gene (MYOT) causes a severe form of limb girdle muscular dystrophy 1A (LGMD1A). *J Neurol* 2011; 258:1437–1444.

56. van der Kooi AJ, Ledderhof TM, de Voogt WG, et al. A newly recognized autosomal dominant limb girdle muscular dystrophy with cardiac involvement. *Ann Neurol* 1996; 39:636–642.

57. Beneditti S, Menditto I, Degano M, et al. Phenotypic clustering of lamin A/C mutations in neuromuscular patients. *Neurology* 2007; 69:1285–1292.

58. Rudnik-Schoneborn S, Botzenhart E, Eggermann T, et al. Mutations in the LMNA gene can mimic autosomal dominant proximal spinal muscular atrophy. *Neurogenetics* 2007; 8:137–142.

59. Minetti C, Sotgia F, Bruno C, et al. Mutations in the caveolin-3 gene cause autosomal dominant limb-girdle muscular dystrophy. *Nat Genet* 1998; 18:365–368.

60. McNally EM, de Sa Moreira E, Duggan DJ, et al. Caveolin-3 in muscular dystrophy. *Hum Molec Genet* 1998; 7:871–877.

61. Sunada Y, Ohi H, Hase A, et al. Transgenic mice expressing mutant caveolin-3 show severe myopathy associated with increased nNOS activity. *Hum Molec Genet* 2001; 10:173–178.

62. Chung CS, Morton NE. Discrimination of genetic entities in muscular dystrophy. *Am J Hum Genet* 1959; 11:339–359.

63. Richard I, Broux O, Allamand V, et al. Mutations in the proteolytic enzyme calpain 3 causes limb-girdle muscular dystrophy type 2A. *Cell* 1995; 81:27–40.

64. Fardeau M, Hillaire D, Mignard C, et al. Juvenile limb-girdle muscular dystrophy: clinical, histopathological and genetic data from a small community living in the Reunion Island. *Brain* 1996; 119:295–308.

65. Richard I, Roudaut C, Saenz A, et al. Calpainopathy-a survey of mutations and polymorphisms. *Am J Hum Genet* 1999; 64:1524–1540.

66. Passos-Bueno MR, Richard I, Vainzof M, et al. Evidence of genetic heterogeneity in the autosomal recessive adult forms of limb-girdle muscular dystrophy following linkage analysis with 15q probes in Brazilian families. *J Med Genet* 1993; 30:385–387.

67. Passos-Bueno MR, Bashir R, Moreira ES, et al. Confirmation of the 2p locus for the mild autosomal recessive limb-girdle muscular dystrophy gene (LGMD2B) in three families allows refinement of the candidate region. *Genomics* 1995; 27:192–195.

68. Passos-Bueno MR, Vainzof M, Moreira ES, et al. Seven autosomal recessive limb-girdle muscular dystrophies in the Brazilian population: from LGMD2A to LGMD2G. *Am J Med Genet* 1999; 82:392–398.

69. Bushby KMD. The limb-girdle muscular dystrophies-multiple genes, multiple mechanisms. *Hum Molec Genet* 1999; 8:1875–1882.

70. Cacciottolo M, Numitone G, Aurino S, et al. Muscular dystrophy with marked dysferlin deficiency is consistently caused by primary dysferlin gene mutations. *Europ J Hum Genet* 2011; 19:974–980.

71. Lim LE, Duclos F, Broux O, et al. Beta-sarcoglycan: characterization and role in limb-girdle muscular dystrophy linked to 4q12. *Nature Genet* 1995; 11:257–265.

72. Bonnemann CG, Passos-Bueno MR, McNally EM et al. Genomic screening for beta-sarcoglycan gene mutations: missense mutations may cause severe limb-girdle muscular dystrophy type 2E (LGMD 2E). *Hum Mol Genet* 1996; 5:1953–1961.

73. Tabelsi M, Kavian N, Daoud F, et al. Revised spectrum of mutations in sarcoglycanopathies. *Europ J Hum Genet* 2008; 16:793–803.

74. Piccolo F, Jeanpierr M, Leturcq F, et al. A founder mutation in the gamma-sarcoglycan gene of gypsies possibly predating their migration out of India. *Hum Mol Genet* 1996; 5:2019–2022.

75. McNally EM, Yoshida M, Mizuno Y, et l. Human adhalin is alternatively spliced and the gene is located on chromosome 17q21. *Proc Natl Acad Sci USA* 1994; 91:9690–9694.

76. Nigro V, de Sa Moreira E, Piluso G, et al. Autosomal recessvie limb-girdle muscular dystrophy, LGMD2F, is caused by mutation in the delta-sarcoglycan gene. *Nat Genet* 1996; 14:195–198.

77. Passos-Bueno MR, Moreira ES, VAinzof M, et al. Linkage analysis in autosomal recessive limb-girdle muscular dystrophy (AR LGMD) maps a sixth form to 5q33-34 (LGMD2F) and indicates that there is at least one more subtype of AR LGMD. *Hum Mol Genet* 1996; 5:815–820.

78. Duggan DJ, Manchester D, Stears KP, et al. Mutations in the delta-sarcoglycan gene are a rare cause of autosomal recessive limb-girdle muscular dystrophy (LGMD2). *Neurogenetics* 1997; 1:49–58.

79. van der Kooi AJ, Barth PG, Busch HF, et al. The clinical spectrum of limb girdle muscular dystrophy. A survey in The Netherlands. *Brain* 1996; 119:1471–1480.

80. Urtasun M, Saenz A, Roudaut C, et al. Limb-girdle muscular dystrophy in Guipuzcoa (Basque Country, Spain). *Brain* 1998; 121:1735–1747.

81. Fanin M, Duggan DJ, Mostacciuolo ML, et al. Genetic epidemiology of muscular dystrophies resulting from sarcoglycan gene mutations. *J Med Genet* 1997; 34:973–977.

82. Hackman P, Juvonen V, Sarparanta J, et al. Enrichment of the R77C alpha-sarcoglycan gene mutation in Finnish LGMD2D patients. *Muscle Nerve* 2005; 31:199–204.

83. Lo HP, Cooper ST, Evesson FJ, et al. Limb-girdle muscular

dystrophy: Diagnostic evaluation, frequency and clues to pathogenesis. *Neuromusc Disord* 2008; 18:34–44.

84. van der Kooi AJ, Frankhuizen WS, Barth PG, et al. Limb-Girdle muscular dystrophy in the Netherlands. Gene defect identified in half the families. *Neurology* 2007; 68:2125–2128.

85. Bradley WG. The limb-girdle syndromes. *Handb Clin Neurol* 1979; 40:433–469.

86. Doherty TJ, Stashuk DW. Decomposition-based quantitative electromyography: methods and initial normative data in five muscles. Muscle Nerve 2003; 28:204–211.

87. Derry KL, Venance SL, Doherty TJ. Decomposition-based quantitative electromyography in the evaluation of muscular dystrophy severity. *Muscle Nerve* 2012; 45:507–513.

88. Pillen S, Arts IM, Zwarts MJ. Muscle ultrasound in neuromuscular disorders. *Muscle Nerve* 2008; 37:679–693.

89. Pillen S, Verrips A, van Alfen N, et al. Quantitative skeletal muscle ultrasound: diagnostic value I childhood neuromuscular disease. *Neuromusucul Disord* 2007; 17:509–516.

90. Pillen S, Morava E, van Keimpema M, et al. Skeletal muscle ultrasonography in children with dysfunction in the oxidative phosphorylation system. *Neuropediatrics* 2006; 37:142–147.

91. Heckmatt JZ, Dubowitz V. Real-time ultrasound imaging of muscles. *Muscle Nerve* 1988; 11:56–65.

92. Wattjes MP, Kley RA, Fischer D. Neuromuscular imaging in inherited muscle diseases. Eur Radiol 2010; 20:2447–2460.

93. Degardin A, Morillon D, Lacour A, et al. Morphologic imaging in muscular dystrophies and inflammatory myopathies. *Skeletal Radiol* 2010; 39:1219–1227.

94. Mercuri E, Talim B, Moghadaszadeh B, et al. Clinical and imaging findings in six cases of congenital muscular dystrophy with rigid spine syndrome linked to chromosome 1p (RSMD1). *Neuromuscul Disord* 2002; 12:631–638.

95. Fischer D, Kley RA, Strach K, et al. Distinct muscle imaging patterns in myofibrillar myopathies. *Neurology* 2008; 71:758–765.

96. Kornblum C, Lutterbey G, Bogdanow M, et al. Distinct neuromuscular phenotypes in myotonic dystrophy types 1 and 2. A whole body highfield MRI study. *J Neurol* 2006; 253:753–761.

97. Hsieh TJ, Wang CK, Hy C, et al. In vivo proton magnetic resonance spectroscopy for muscle metabolism in neuromuscular disorders. *J Pediatr* 2007; 151:319–321.

98. Mercuri E, Bushby K, Ricci E, et al. Muscle MRI findings in patients with limb girdle muscular dystrophy with calpain 3 deficiency (LGMD2A) and early contractures *Neuromuscul Disord* 2005; 15:164–171.

99. Pradhan S. Clinical and magnetic resonance imaging features of 'diamond on quadripceps'sign in dysferlinopathy. *Neurol India* 2009; 57:172–175.

100. Rosales XQ, Moser SJ, Tran T, et al. Cardiovasclar magnetic resonance imaging of cardiomyopathy in limb girdle muscular dystrophy 2B and 2I. *J Cardiovasc Magn Reson* 2011; 13:39.

101. Toda T, Chiyonobu T, Xiong H, et al. Fukutin and alpha-dystroglycanopathies. *Acta Myol* 2005; 24:60–63.

102. Muntoni F, Brockington M, Torelli S, et al. Defective glycosylation in congenital muscular dystrophies. *Curr Opin Neurol* 2004; 17:205–209.

103. Clement E, Mercuri E, Godfrey C, et al. Brain involvement in muscular dystrophies with defective dystroglycan glycosylation. *Ann Neurol* 2008; 64:573–582.

104. Palmieri A, Manara R, Bello L, et al. Cognitive profile and MRI findings in limb-girdle muscular dystrophy 2I. *J Neurol* 2011; 258:1312–1320.

105. van der Kooi AJ, Ginjaar HB, Busch HFM, et al. Limb girdle muscular dystrophy: a pathological and imunohistochemical reevaluation. *Muscle Nerve* 1998; 21:584–590.

106. Cooper ST, Lo HP, North KN. Single section Western blot. *Neurology* 2003; 61:93–97.

107. Pegoraro E, Hoffman EP. Limb-girdle muscular dystrophy overview. In, Pagon RA, Bird TD, Dolan CR, et al., editors. GeneReviews [Internet] Seattle (WA): University of Washington, Seattle, 1993–2012, Accessed 9/1/2012.

108. Angelini C, Fanin M, Menegazzo E, et al. Homozygous a-sarcoglycan mutation in two siblings: one asymptomatic and one steroid-responsive mild limb-girdle muscular dystrophy patients. *Muscle Nerve* 1998; 21:769–775.

109. Connolly AM, Pestronk A, Mehta S, et al. Primary a-sarcoglycan deficiency responsive to immunosuppression over three years. *Muscle Nerve* 1998; 21:1549–1553.

110. Godfrey C, Escolar D, Brockington M, et al. Fukutin gene mutations in steroid-responsive limb-girdle muscular dystrophy. *Ann Neurol* 2006; 60:603–610.

111. Darin N, Kroksmark AK, Ahlander AC, et al. Inflammatory and response to steroid treatment in limb-girdle muscular dystrophy 2I. *Eur J Paediatr Neurol* 2007; 11:353–357.

112. Wagner KR, Fleckenstein JL, Amato AA, et al. A phase I/II trial of MYO-029 in adult subjects with muscular dystrophy. *Ann Neurol* 2008; 63:561–571.

113. Daniele N, Richard I, Bartoli M. Ins and outs of therapy in limb girdle muscular dystrophies. *Int J Biochem Cell Biol* 2007; 39:1608–1624.

114. Mendell JR, Rodino-Klapac L, Sahenk Z, et al. Gene therapy for muscular dystrophy: Lessons learned and path forward. *Neurosci Lett* 2012, http://dx.doi.org/10.1016/j.neulet.2012.04.078.

115. Mendell JR, Rodino-Klapac LR, Rosales-Quintero XQ, et al. Limb-girdle muscular dystrophy type 2D gene therapy restores alpha-sarcoglycan and associated proteins. *Ann Neurol* 2009; 66:290–297.

116. Mendell JR, Rodino Klapac LR, Rosales XQ, et al. Sustained alpha-sarcoglycan gene expression after gene transfer in limb-girdle muscular dystrophy, type 2D. *Ann Neurol* 2010; 68:629–638.

117. Tedesco FS, Gerli MRM, Perani L, et al. Transplantation of genetically corrected human iPSC-dervied progenitors in mice with limb-girdle muscular dystrophy. *Sci Transl Med* 2012; 4:1–13.

118. Ehrig K, Leivo I, Argraves WS, et al. Merosin, a tissue-specific basement membrane protein, is a laminin-like protein. *Proc Natl Acad Sci USA* 1990; 87:3264–3268.

119. Vuolteenaho R, Nissinen M, Sainio K, et al. Human laminin M chain (merosin): complete primary structure, chromosomal assignment, and expression of the M and A chain in human fetal tissues. *J Cell Biol* 1994; 124:381–394.

120. Arahata K, Hayashi YK, Mizuno Y, et al. Dystrophin-associated glycoprotein and dystrophin co-localization at sarcolemma in Fukuyama congenital muscular dystrophy. *Lancet* 1993; 342:23–24.

121. Tezak Z, Prandini P, Marin M, et al. Clinical and molecular study in congenital muscular dystrophy with partial laminin alpha-2 (LAMA2) deficiency. *Hum Mutat* 2003; 21:103–111.

122. Di Blasi C, Piga D, Brioschi P, et al. LAMA2 gene analysis in congenital muscular dystrophy: new mutations, prenatal diagnosis, and founder effect. *Arch Neurol* 2005; 62:1582–1586.

123. Mercuri E, Brockington M, Straub V, et al. Phenotypic spectrum associated with mutations in the fukutin-related protein gene. *Ann Neurol* 2003; 53:537–542.

124. Takada K, Nakamura H, Tanaka J. Cortical dysplasia in congenital muscular dystrophy with central nervous system involvement (Fukuyama type). *J Neuropathol Exp Neurol* 1984; 43:395–407.

125. Mercuri E, Poppe M, Quinlivan R, et al. Extreme variability of phenotype in patients with an identical misssense mutation

in the lamin A/C gene: from congenital onset with severe phenotype to milder classic Emery-Dreifuss variant. *Arch Neurol* 2004; 61:690–694.

126. D'Amico A, Haliloglu G, Richard P, et al. Two patients with 'dropped head syndrome' due to mutations in LMNA or SEPN1 genes. *Neuromuscul Disord* 2005; 15:521–524.

127. Quijano-Roy S, Mbieleu B, Bonnemann CG, et al. De novo LMNA mutations cause a new form of congenital muscular dystrophy. *Ann Neurol* 2008; 64:177–186.

128. Lisi MT, Cohn RD. Congenital muscular dystrophies: new aspects of an expanding group of disorders. *Biochimica et Biophysica Acta* 2007; 1772:159–172.

129. Emery AEH, Dreifuss FE. Unusual type of bening X-linked muscular dystrophy. *J Neurol Neurosurg Psychiatry* 1966; 29:338–342.

130. Hopkins LC, Jackson JA, Elsas LJ. Emery-Dreifuss humeroperoneal muscular dystrophy: an X-linked myopathy with unusual contractures and bradycardia. *Ann Neurol* 1981; 10:230–237.

131. Thomas PK, Calne DB, Elliott CF. X-linked scapuloperoneal syndrome. *J Neurol Neurosurg Psychiatry* 1972; 35:208–215.

132. Yates JRW. European Workshop on Emery-Dreifuss Muscular Dystrophy. *Neuromuscul Disord* 1991; 1:393–396.

133. Bione S, Maestrini E, Rivella S, et al. Identification of a novel X-linked gene responsible for Emery-Dreifuss muscular dystrophy. *Nature Genet* 1994; 8:323–327.

134. Wulff, K, Parrish JE, Hermann FH, et al. Six novel mutations in the emerin gene causing X-linked Emery-Dreifuss muscular dystrophy. *Hum Mutat* 1997; 9:526–530.

135. Nagano A, Koga R, Ogawa M, et al. Emerin deficiency at the nuclear membrane in patients with Emery-Dreifuss muscular dystrophy. *Nature Genet* 1996; 12:254–259.

136. Bonne G, Capeua J, De Visser M, et al. 82nd ENMC international workshop, 5th international Emery-Dreifuss muscular dystrophy (EDMD) workshop, 1st Workshop of the MYO-CLUSTER project EUROMEN (European muscle envelope nucleopathies), 15–16 September 2000, Naarden, The Netherlands. *Neuromuscul Disord* 2002; 12:187–194.

137. Bonne G, Yaou RB, Beroud C, et al. 108th ENMC International Workshop, 3rd Workshop of the MYO-CLUSTER project: EUROMEN, 7th International Emery-Dreifuss Muscular Dystrophy (EDMD) Workshop, 13–15 September 2002, Naarden, The Netherlands. *Neuromuscul Disord* 2003; 13:508–515.

138. Zhang Q, Bethmann C, Worth NF, et al. Nesprin-1 and -2 are involved in the pathogenesis of Emery-Dreifuss muscular dystrophy and are critical for nuclear envelope integrity. *Hum Molec Genet* 2007; 16:2816–2833.

CHAPTER 21

Distal Myopathies

Mazen M. Dimachkie, Richard J. Barohn

OVERVIEW

Gowers (1) described distal myopathy in two patients with weakness confined to distal muscles. Over the next five years, Dejerine and Thomas (2) Campbell (3) and Spiller (4) reported other similar patients. Welander (5) established the existence of autosomal dominant (AD) distal myopathy in a large Scandanavian cohort, the impact of which was so influential that it was later referred to as Welander distal myopathy (WDM).

The distal myopathies are clinically and genetically heterogeneous. Affected kindred manifest weakness, primarily limited to foot and toe extensor muscles even in advanced stages of the disease, with variable mild proximal leg, distal arm, neck, and laryngeal muscle involvement in selected individuals.

Single mutations can lead to more than one clinical disorder, such as Myoshi myopathy (MM) and limb girdle muscular dystrophy (LGMD) type 2B, both caused by mutation at the 2p12-14 locus in the gene encoding dysferlin. There are six well described distal myopathy syndromes (Table 1). Myofibrillar myopathy and less common forms of distal myopathy are listed in Tables 2 and 3.

The approach to the patient with distal myopathy commences with consideration of the differential diagnosis of that pattern of weakness (6), facilitated by six key clinical questions (Table 4) and categorization into one of ten phenotypic patterns (Table 5) (7–14).

WELANDER DISTAL MYOPATHY: LATE-ADULT ONSET, TYPE 1

Welander (5) described AD distal myopathy among 249 patients in 72 Swedish families, and in 12 subsequent Finnish families with extensor hand and finger muscle involvement, later found to co-segregate, suggesting a founder effect (15, 16). Affected individuals develop symptoms in the mid-fifth decade and as late as age 77 years, but rarely before age 30. Proximal limb involvement rarely occurs in WDM with disease progression except in severe homozygous cases. Foot flexor muscles are initially affected in 40% of patients, and ankle dorsifexors in 25% of patients. Tendon reflexes remain present except for ankle and brachoradialis reflexes that are later lost with disease progression. Sensation is normal, although deficits may be found on quantitative temperature and vibration testing (17).

The serum creatine kinase (CK) level may be normal or slightly elevated (18, 19). Motor and sensory nerve conduction studies (NCS) are typically normal, and needle electromyography (EMG) shows occasional active spontaneous activity comprised of fibrillation potentials with myopathic motor unit potentials (MUP), although some authors (18–21) reported a mixed myopathic and neuropathic recruitment pattern. T_1 and T_2-weighted muscle magnetic resonance imaging (MRI) in 11 patients showed signal abnormalities in the distal anterior and posterior compartments of the legs, including the gastrocnemius, soleus, tibialis anterior (TA), extensor digitorum longus (EDL), and hamstrings (22). Muscle biopsy showed myopathic features, including variation in fiber size, increased connective tissue, fat deposition, central nuclei, and rimmed vacuoles in some (5, 18, 19, 23) but not all patients (21, 24, 25). Dis-

Table 1. Classification of Classic Distal Myopathy

Type	Inheritance Pattern	Gene Localization	Initial Weakness	CK Level	Muscle Biopsy Findings
Welander— late adult type 1	AD	2p13	Hands, fingers wrist extensors	NL Normal or mild increase	Myopathic; rimmed vacuoles in some cases
Udd— late adult type 2a	AD	2q31 *TTN*	Legs, anterior compartment	NL Normal or mild increase	Myopathic; rimmed vacuoles in some cases
Markesbery— Griggs late adult type 2b	AD	10q22.3-q23.2 *ZASP*	Legs, anterior compartment	NL Normal or mild increase	Vacuolar myopathy; myofibrillar features
Nonaka— early adult onset or sporadic	AR	9p13.3 *GNE*	Legs, anterior compartment	Mild to moderate increase, <5 x NL	Vacuolar myopathy type 1 (h IBM2)[1]
Miyoshi— adult type 2	AR or sporadic	2p13 *DYSF*	Legs, posterior compartment (LGMD 2B) β	10 to 150 -fold increased	Myopathic, usually no early vacuoles; "endstage" onset
Laing— early adult onset type 3	AD	14q11.2 *MYH7*	Legs, anterior compartment, in most	Increased <3x-fold increased	Moderate myopathic changes; no vacuoles

1. Autosomal recessive familial hereditary IBM2, also known as quadriceps sparing myopathy, has been genetically linked with the Nonaka distal myopathy (References 69, 72, 73).
2. LGMD type 2B has been genetically linked with Miyoshi distal myopathy (Reference 84).
Abbreviations: AD, autosomal dominant; AR, autosomal recessive; CK, creatine kinase; hIBM, hereditary inclusion body myopathy; LGMD, limb girdle muscular dystrophy; NL, normal.

organization and loss of myofibrils with accumulation of Z-disk material and 15- to 18-nm cytoplasmic and nuclear filaments have been noted in ultrastuctural and electron microscopic (EM) studies (18, 19, 23). Groups of small angular fibers can occur, suggestive of a neurogenic component (23). Sural nerve biopsy can demonstrate a moderate reduction in myelinated nerve fibers, without frank axonal degeneration, demyelination, or remyelination (23).

The clinical progression of WDM is generally so slow that affected patients continue to work without a reduction in life expectancy, while others homozygous for the causative genetic defect can have atypical relative rapid progression (5, 16).

TIBIAL MUSCULAR DYSTROPHY: LATE ONSET DISTAL MYOPATHY TYPE 2

Patients with AD late-onset distal tibial muscular atrophy (TMD) were described in English families by Sumner (26), in French-English and Finnish families by Markesbery (27), and others (28, 29). The recent identification of two distinct gene mutations in the titin and ZASP genes led to the elucidation of clinical subtypes.

UDD-Late Onset Distal Myopthy Type 2a

The estimated prevalence of AD TMD is 5 to 15 per 100,000 in Finland. Weakness typically begins in ankle dorsiflexor muscles after age 40. In non-Scandinavian patients, weakness involves finger and wrist extensor muscles over time (Figure 1) and proximal muscles. Whereas most Finnish patients progress slowly and rarely involve the arms or hands, (4), those of pedigrees from western Finland can

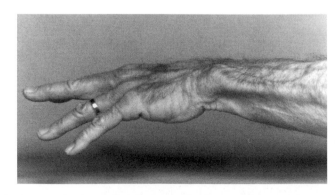

FIG. 1. Markesbery distal myopathy (late adult onset type 2). Note extensive forearm atrophy and weakness of finger extensors as patient attempts to raise fingers.

exhibit severe limb girdle syndrome (28–30). The serum CK is normal or slightly elevated, and EMG reveals active denervation and myopathic MUP. Muscle biopsy shows dystrophic tissue with single and multiple myofiber vacuoles. Magnetic resonance imaging in 22 patients so studied (22) showed fatty replacement of the TA muscle and EDL in eight patients, and in the hamstring and posterior leg compartment in 14 others. Tibial muscular dystrophy 2a is a titinopathy caused by mutations at the 2q31 locus of the *TTN* gene encoding the giant skeletal muscle protein titin (31). Mutation at Mex6 titin leads to abnormal titin-calpain-3 interaction (32). The Finnish mutation is due to a deletion and insertion of 11 consecutive base pairs changing four amino acid residues without interruption of the reading frame. Point mutation in Mex6 introduces a potentially harmful proline in the beta sheet structure, the exon of which corresponds to M-line titin in some cases, and in the calpain-3 binding site at the N2-A line in I-band titin. Protein studies in TMD shows secondary calpain-3 reduction in the homozygous state with apoptotic myonuclei.

Markesbery-Griggs-Late Onset Distal Myopthy Type 2b

TMD2b has been described among English, French, and Finnish families, with men marginally affected more than women. Similar to TMD2a, weakness begins in the anterior leg compartment after age 40. Hand weakness affects distal finger and wrist extensors and, late in the course, the proximal arms and legs. Progression is faster than in TMD2a, leading to more severe disability. The serum CK level is normal or mildly elevated and muscle biopsy demonstrates a vacuolar myopathy with myofibrillar features. One patient described by Markesbery (27) had cardiomyopathy with heart block and heart failure, prompting pacemaker insertion. At postmortem examination, vacuoles were present in cardiac and skeletal muscle. Muscle imaging showed considerable involvement of gastrocnemius and soleus muscles at a younger age. However, later in the course, proximal muscles were affected with mild to moderate fatty degeneration and atrophy of gluteus maximus, hamstring, vastus medialis, and lateralis muscles. In addition there was severe end-stage replacement in gastrocnemius lateralis, soleus, lateral peroneal, and anterior compartment muscles, with relatively preserved deep long toe flexors and the tibialis posterior muscles.

There were no conclusive mutations in titin or other genes noted in the original English-Finnish cases (27), however the pathology was compatible with MFM. Sequencing of the myotilin and Z-band alternatively spliced PDZ-motif-containing protein (*ZASP*) genes led to detection of a mutation in *ZASP* at A165V in originally affected family members (12), the penetrance of which was 100% by age 60 years. Immunohistochemical studies reveal strong accumulation of myotilin, αB-crystallin, and desmin in affected muscle fibers. As with myotilinopathy, abnormal myotilin aggregation was more prominent than abnormal excessive expression of desmin, αB-crystallin and ZASP. Although occasional punctate aberrant cytoplasmic labeling is observed, dystrophin C-terminus does not consistently localize to the accumulated aggregates. Cardiomyopathy is not a regular feature since different isoforms are predominantly expressed in cardiac and skeletal muscle.

NONAKA DISTAL MYOPATHY: EARLY ADULT ONSET, TYPE 1, DISTAL MYOPATHY WITH RIMMED VACUOLES

Patients with early adult-onset autosomal recessive (AR) distal muscular dystrophy were reported in Japanese families (33, 34), although unappreciated until later (35–37). Similar patients were later seen in the United States (38–40), South America (41), and Italy (42, 43). Distal myopathy with rimmed vacuoles (DMRV), or Nonaka myopathy, (NM) is characterized by the unique distribution of muscular weakness and wasting, beginning late in the second or third decade at the average age of 26 years, in the hamstring and TA muscles leading to foot drop and steppage gait, sparing the quadriceps even at late stages of the disease. Finger and hand muscles are not as involved as the legs. Over time, weakness progresses to the neck and proximal arm and leg muscles. The degree of progression is more aggressive in non-Japanese cases. Weakness remained distal in the Japanese cases, whereas non-Japanese cases eventually developed significant proximal weakness in the legs, arms, and neck muscles with loss of ambulation (38), rarely but sometimes noted in Japanese patients (44). Disability occurs after 10 to 20 years of illness. Symptomatic complete heart block can occur, producing syncope and prompting pacemaker insertion (45).

The serum CK level is increased up to fivefold. Electodiagnostic studies, including needle EMG studies, reveal fibrillation potentials at rest and myopathic MUP. Although the usefulness of MRI in the diagnosis of DMRV would seem apparent, there are few if any published studies. Muscle biopsy in Japanese and non-Japanese patients demonstrates dystrophic myopathy and rimmed vacuoles owing to the deposition of granular material that demonstrate basophilia with hematoxylin and eosin (H&E), purple-red with the modified Gomori trichrome, and positively with acid phosphatase (Figure 2A and B). Autophagic vacuoles that have nuclear and cytoplasmic 15- to 18-nm filamentous inclusions on EM (44, 46, 47) and were originally considered characteristic of IBM, also occur in WDM and DMRV or NM (48). Rare patients can have inflammation similar to sporadic, but not to hereditary inclusion body myopathy (hIBM) (49, 50).

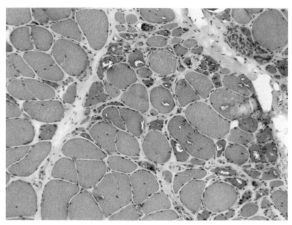

(A)

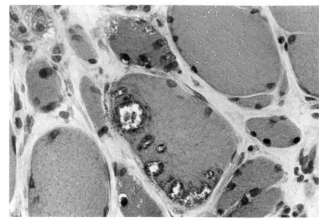

(B)

FIG. 2. Nonaka distal myopathy (early adult onset type 1). **(A)** Muscle fiber size variability and rimmed vacuoles (H&E). From reference 11, with permission.) **(B)** Multiple rimmed vacuoles at periphery of fiber (H&E). From reference 11, with permission.

Almost all cases of DMRV are caused by mutations in the UDP-N-acetylglucosamine 2-epimerase/N-acetylmannosamine kinase gene (*GNE*) located within a 1.5-Mb region between markers D9S2178 and D9S1791 on chromosome 9 (51) and allelic to AR hIBM2. Several mutations in the 9p1-q1 have been detected, including the most common one at M712T, in early-onset Jewish hIBM type 2 (52), the most form of hIBM, originally described in Persian-Jewish families with distal leg onset in the second-to-third decade. Weakness and atrophy progresses proximally, with relative sparing of the quadriceps (53, 54). A homozygous T- to- C substitution at nucleotide position 2186 in the *GNE* gene converting methionine to threonine at codon 712 was found in all Middle Eastern families of both Jewish and non-Jewish descent, whereas affected individuals of other ethnicities were usually compound heterozygous or homozygous for different mutations (55). *GNE* mutations were identified in patients with distal myopathy with rimmed vacuoles also known as Nonaka myopathy (56). In Japanese patients, Nonaka myopathy is most commonly associated with V572L homozygous or compound heterozygous mutation. The identification of the causative gene defect has allowed recognition of phenotypic variants of this disorder in the age of onset, degree of progression of symptoms, and distribution of muscle weakness. For example, a minority of patients lack distal weakness or have distinctive quadriceps involvement, as well as patients with unusual facial weakness (57). Two DMRV patients were postulated to have mutations in the non-coding and intron sites, abnormal transcription or translation of the *GNE* gene, or in other genes with a similar role (52). A *GNE* mutation detected in a non-DMRV patient showed predominant involvement of proximal leg muscles sparing the TA and gastrocnemius. Autosomal dominant inheritance, late onset, severe cardiac involvement, and proximal leg muscle involvement distinguishes DMRV from other myopathies with prominent rimmed vacuoles. Genetic analysis was instrumental in confirming the diagnosis of DMRV in two Japanese patients with the unusual feature of inflammation in muscle biopsy and otherwise typical DMRV (49). Both patients had compound heterozygous mutations in the *GNE* gene, one at V572L, the most prevalent mutation in Japanese DMRV, and the other at I472T, less common among Japanese.

To safely correct *GNE* gene function, one patient with severe HIBM2 was treated with intravenous infusion of seven doses of liposomal wild-type *GNE* gene (58). Quadriceps muscle expression of the delivered GNE, plasmid, and RNA was observed and sialic acid-related proteins were increased with stabilization in the decline of muscle strength. Further assessment of *GNE* gene lipoplex through phase I trial in less advanced HIBM cases is planned. Malicdan and colleagues (59) demonstrated that oral supplementation with sialic acid metabolites in *GNE* knockout mice resulted in an increase of sialic acid in muscle to a nearly normal level and prevented development of the muscle phenotype. Sialic acid metabolite-treated mice showed increased strength, muscle mass, mean muscle fiber cross-sectional area, body weight, and overall survival compared to untreated control littermates. A study of the safety and pharmacokinetics of sialic acid in patients with hIBM is ongoing (http://clinicaltrials.gov/ct2/show/NCT01359319).

MIYOSHI DISTAL MYOPATHY: EARLY ADULT ONSET, TYPE 2

Miyoshi and colleagues (60–62) and others (63–67) described AR gastrocnemius weakness sparing the anterior compartment of the leg, beginning at age 15 to 25 years. Affected patients notice difficulty in walking on toes

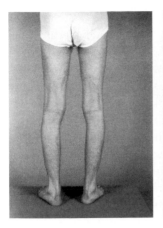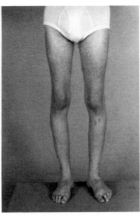

FIG. 3. Miyoshi distal myopathy (early adult onset type 2). Distal tapering with posterior compartment (gastrocnemius) atrophy. From reference 57, with permission.

or climbing stairs, with myalgia of the calves followed by hypertrophy, wasting, and loss of deep tendon reflexes (DTR) of the ankles (Figure 3), with later involvement of the anterior compartment of the legs, arms and hands, selectively involving the biceps brachii muscles (68, 69).

The serum CK, which may be elevated 10- to 150-fold normal, may be a prelude to the disease in asymptomatic patients (64); needle EMG reveals myopathic MUP and recruitment pattern. Examination of the gastrocnemius muscle typically demonstrates high amplitude long-duration polyphasic MUP with a discrete recruitment pattern. Muscle MRI confirms selective involvement of the posterior compartment muscles of the legs (66). A diamond-on-quadriceps sign was present in two-thirds of more of patients with dysferlinopathy, LGMD2B, and MM, with uniform texture and smooth surface at rest, and clinical and radiographic bulging toward the anterolateral aspect at midthigh upon contraction (70).

Gastrocnemius muscle biopsy typically shows end-stage changes of fibrosis, fatty replacement, with few if any myofibers, compared to that of a relatively uninvolved quadriceps muscle that shows minimal myopathic changes of variable

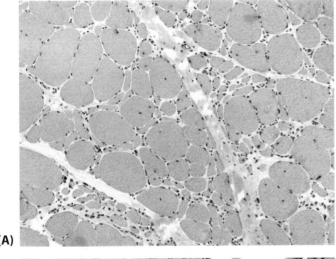

(A)

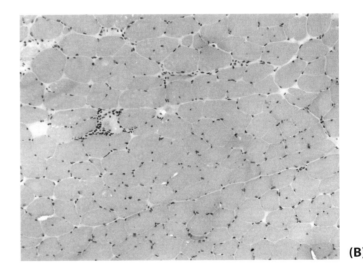

(B)

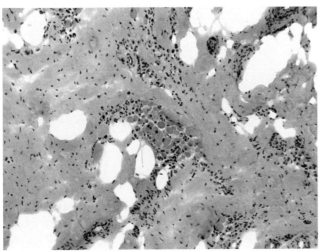

(C)

FIG. 4. Miyoshi distal myopathy (early adult onset type 2). **(A)** Lateral gastrocnemius. Extensive fiber loss with replacement by connective and adipose tissue (H&E). From reference 11, with permission. **(B)** Vastus lateralis. Slight muscle size variability and a single necrotic fiber undergoing phagocytosis (H&E). From reference 11, with permission. **(C)** Biceps femoris. Changes intermediate to A and B, with variable muscle size, groups of small round fibers, and central nuclei (H&E). From reference 11, with permission.

myofiber, size, and internalized myonuclei. Biopsy of the biceps femoris muscle shows the expected histopathologic features (Figure 4A–C) that include lack of staining for dysferlin of the muscle membrane by indirect immunofluorescence (71). Perimysial and perivascular inflammation are common findings in MM, but not vacuoles (72). The genes for both MM and LGMD2B map to the 2p12-14 locus of the dysferlin (*DYSF*) gene (73), comprised of 55 exons, >150 kb, and a gene product of 2,080 amino acids. Both MM and LGMD2B begin in late childhood or early adulthood with marked elevation in serum CK and slow progression of proximal muscle weakness in the latter disease (74) that accounts for up to 25% of all LGMD cases, further suggested by patterns of dysferlin staining in muscle biopsy tissue (75).

Although the function of dysferlin is not well understood, the predicted cytoplasmic component contains calcium-binding motifs homologous to C2 domains believed to trigger calcium-signaled membrane fusion and trafficking (76), suggesting a role in the mediation of calcium-mediated myofiber membrane fusion and repair (77).

LAING DISTAL MYOPATHY: EARLY ONSET, TYPE 3

Laing and colleagues (78) described affected and unaffected members of a three-generation English and Welsh family with AD distal myopathy with age at onset of 4 to 25 years, and selective weakness of toe and ankle extensor and neck flexor muscles. This was followed years later by progressive weakness of the finger extensor muscles and, to a lesser degree, hip and shoulder muscles facilitating hip adduction and external rotation, and shoulder abduction, sparing finger flexor and intrinsic hand muscles. Ambulation was typically preserved for up to 25 years after disease onset. Affected patients demonstrated preservation of DTR, and serum CK levels were normal or minimally elevated. Electrodiagnostic studies showed normal NCS, with occasional fibrillation potentials and positive sharp wave discharges at rest, myopathic MUP with many polyphasic units, and full recruitment of low amplitude MUP and interference patterns at submaximal effort. Quadriceps muscle biopsy showed occasional necrotic and regenerative fibers, excessive variation in fiber size, and central myofiber nuclei without vacuoles or fiber type grouping. Hyaline inclusions stained light green with the Gomori trichrome stain and ultrastructural examination showed 15 to 20 nm intranuclear tubulo-filamentous inclusions. Biopsy of the TA muscle showed end-stage myopathy with normal dystrophin and desmin immunohistochemistry. Muscle MRI studies in another cohort showed increased signal intensity and variable atrophy of both TA, EHL, extensor digitorum longus, and gastrocnemius and sartorius muscles (79). The disorder

has been linked to mutations at the 14q11.2-q13 locus, in the region of two linked genes, alpha and beta cardiac myosin *MYH6* and *MYH7*. Further analysis revealed five novel heterozygous mutations in the light meromyosin (LMM) regions of the MYH7 tail in six of seven families from the Netherlands, Western Australia, Italy, Germany, Austria, and England (80–84) encoding the isoform of myosin present in slow type 1 skeletal muscle fibers in skeletal and cardiac ventricle muscle, mutations of which were associated with hypertrophic cardiomyopathy (HCM). Although the latter was not present in the study cohort (80), atrophy, grouping, and occasionally depletion of type 1 myofibers were noted in muscle biopsy tissue of four families. Mutation in the MYH7 rod domain at chromosome 14q has been linked to hyaline body myopathy (HBM), a rare congenital disorder characterized by AD early nonprogressive proximal and distal weakness with significant wasting and loss of subcutaneous fat, or early progressive scapuloperoneal weakness with loss of ambulation by late teens (84), and subsarcolemmal inclusions known as hyaline inclusion bodies (HB) exclusively in type 1 fibers. Mutation in the rod and light meromyosin (LMM) domain of slow myosin heavy chain (MyHC) gene underlies HBM (85).

MYOFIBRILLAR MYOPATHY

Myofibrillary myopathy (MFM) refers to pathological patterns of myofibrillary dissolution and degradation on EM leading to the accumulation of myotilin, desmin, and αB-crystallin (αBC) (11, 86). Myotilin is a Z-disk-associated protein that cross-links actin filaments and binds to α-actinin and γ-filamin (87, 88). Desmin is an intermediate filament protein of skeletal, cardiac, and some smooth muscles cells that links Z-bands with the plasmalemma and nucleus. αBC is a member of the small heat-shock protein (HSP) family and a molecular chaperone. MFM shares

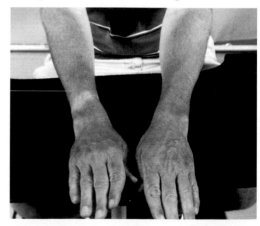

FIG. 5. Myofibrillary myopathy with abnormal foci of desmin. Note atrophy of the extensor forearm muscles.

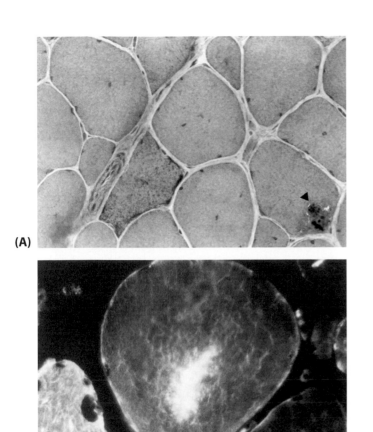

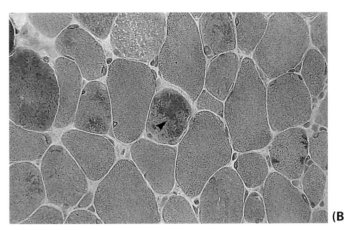

FIG. 6. Myofibrillary myopathy with abnormal foci of desmin. **(A)** Focal granular cytoplasmic bodies and early vacuole formation (arrowhead) (modified TrichromeX460). **(B)** Dark green smudgy amorphous region (arrowhead) (modified TrichromeX460). **(C)** Focal nodular accumulations of desmin (immunofluorescence stain for desminX800).

pathologic similarities with spheroid body myopathy, cytoplasmic body myopathy, Mallory body myopathy, and myopathy with granulofilamentous inclusions (89).

First recognized for desmin-reactive inclusions, its surrounding material and missense mutations of αBC (90–93), the resulting clinical manifestations of MFM include progressive adult-onset myopathy with or without signs of cardiac involvement (94, 95), the latter of which may be the leading (91) or exclusive manifestation (96), with cardiomyopathy, congestive heart failure, heart block and arrhythmias leading to pacemaker insertion. Most patients develop in the third to fifth decade beginning at about age 40 in the distal upper arms (90) (Figure 5), with others presenting in the sixth decade, rarely in the second or third decade. (11). The serum CK may be normal or increased up to sevenfold-normal. Electrodiagnostic studies may show normal or abnormal NCS consistent with polyneuropathy (11), particularly among those with longstanding diabetes. Needle EMG shows myogenic and high amplitude long-duration MUP with occasional fibrillation potentials, positive sharp wave and complex repetitive and rare myotonic discharges.

Muscle biopsy (Figure 6A–C) demonstrates variability in fiber size, increased internalized nuclei, type 1 fiber predominance, and a few rimmed vacuoles. The disorder should be suspected in the setting of characteristic histopathology

consistent with the expected phenotypic and genotypic correlation of desmin (*DES*) and *CRYAB* mutation wherein the abnormal fiber regions are often smaller, less conspicuous, and fewer in immunoflorescent congophilic deposits. Walter and colleagues (97) identified an R350P desmin (*DES*) gene mutation in a large adult-onset, multigeneration kindred of scapuloperoneal syndrome similar to that of four unrelated German families, with variable patterns of distal and proximal weakness that included proximal leg involvement alone or associated with distal leg weakness, proximal and distal arm, or proximal arm weakness, or normal arm strength, in addition to variable cardiac and respiratory involvement, facial weakness, dysphagia, and gynecomastia. Muscle biopsy histology and immunohistochemistry in several patients so studied showed a spectrum of abnormalities including neurogenic atrophy and rimmed vacuoles, and degenerative myopathy, with or without rimmed vacuoles, and accumulation of desmin and desmin-positive staining of inclusions.

Molecular genetic analysis of MFM has implicated mutations in *ZASP* (allelic with Markesbery-Griggs TMD2b), *MYOT* (allelic with LGMD 1A), filamin C (*FLNC*), BCL2-associated athanogene 3 (*BAG3*), Selenoprotein N (*SEPN1*), and four-and-a-half-LIM protein 1 (*FHL1*) (Table 2). A Mayo clinic series (11) identified two of 63 MFM patients

Table 2. Classification of Myofibrillar Myopathy

Type	Inheritance Pattern	Gene Localization	Initial Weakness	CK Level	Muscle Biopsy Findings
MFM1	AD or AR	2p13 DES	Hands or legs	<5-fold increased	Myopathy, occasional rimmed vacuoles, sub-sarcolemmal granules, and desmin bodies
MFM2	AD or AR	11q22 CRYAB	Proximal and distal	Mild elevation	myopathy, and increased desmin
MFM3	AD or sporadic	5q31.2 TTID	Proximal or distal, and dysarthria	NL to 15-fold increased	Myofibrillar myopathy, rimmed vacuoles, hyaline and rod inclusions
MFM4	AD	10q23.2 ZASP	Proximal or distal	NL or mild increased	Myofibrillar myopathy, small vacuoles, and desmin aggregates
MFM5	AD	7q32.1 FLNC	Proximal and respiratory	2 to 8-fold increased	Myopathy, hyaline mass, vacuoles, rods and desmin aggregates
MFM6	AD	10q25.2-q26.2 BAG3	Proximal > distal, cardiac	3 to 15-fold increased	Myopathy, congophilia, desmin accumulation, and small vacuoles
Scapuloperoneal myopathy	AD	Xq26 FHL1	Distal legs and scapular winging	1.5 to 10-fold increased	Myopathy, hyaline bodies with focal desmin inclusions
Congenital musculardystrophy with desmin inclusions	AR	1p36.11 SEPN1	Proximal, rigid spine, and cardiac	NL or mild increase	Myopathy, vacuoles, and desmin inclusions

that carried truncation mutations the in the *CRYAB* gene and four patients with four missense mutations in the head or tail region of *DES*, followed by a later report (98) that identified 32 of 85 patients with mutations in *CRYAB*, *DES*, *MYOT*, *ZASP*, or *FLNC* and *BAG3*.

Excessive desmin accumulation was noted in cardiac muscle of patients with associated cardiomyopathy (99). Desmin accumulation may be seen in X-linked myotubular myopathy, spinal muscular atrophy, nemaline body myopathy, IBM as well as regenerating muscle fibers (100). Besides desmin, patients with MFM may demonstrate overexpression of dystrophin, αBC, gelsolin, ubiquitin, and N terminus of β-amyloid precursor protein (βAPP), in addition to cell division cycle 2 kinase and cyclin-dependent kinase (CDK) 2, 4 and 7 (11, 101). Neural cell adhesion molecule (NCAM) may be overexpressed in nonhyaline lesions with depletion of actin, α-actinin, myosin, titin and nebulin (Table 3), and reaction of hyaline structures to actin, α-actinin, filamin C,

myosin and desmin, respectively composed of thick and thin filament remnants. Immunostaining may reveal positivity to αBC (MFM1, MFM2, MFM4, MFM6 and SEPN1), myotilin (MFM2, MFM4, MFM5 and MFM6), filamin C (MFM5 and SEPN1), BAG3, and geloslin (MFM6) in specific subtypes of MFM.

Electron microscopy, which shows foci of myofibrillar destruction and hyaline structures that appear as spheroidal bodies, may reveal foci of myofibrillary destruction consisting of disrupted myofilaments, Z-disk-derived bodies, dappled dense structures of Z-disk origin, and streaming of the Z-disk with spheroidal bodies composed of compacted and degraded remnants of thick and thin filaments (89). Some authorities have demonstrated the accumulation of 8- to 10-nm filaments (102). Among 19 patients with different genetically-proven MFM, nine were due to mutation in *DES*, five *CRYAB*, three *ZASP*, and two in *MYOT* (103). Ultrastructural analysis demonstrated

Table 3. Classification of Less Common Distal Myopathies

Type	Inheritance Pattern	Gene Localization	Initial Weakness	CK Level	Muscle Biopsy Findings
Myopathy with anterior leg sparing	AD	7q32 *FLNC*	Calves and hands	Normal or variable	Myopathy
Myopathy with Paget disease and dementia	AD	9p13 *VCP*	Proximal and distal legs	Normal to 8-fold increased	Myopathy with vacuoles
Distal myopathy with vocal cord and pharyngeal weakness (MPD2)	AD	5q31.2 *MATR3*	Legs, hands, and vocal cords	Normal to 8-fold increased	Myopathy with vacuoles
Miyoshi-like myopathy 3	AR	11p14.3 *ANO5*	Posterior legs	3 to 100-fold increased	Myopathy with sarcolemmal lesion
Distal nebulin myopathy	AR	2q21.2-q22 *NEB*	Toes and finger extensors	NL	Myopathy with small rods
LGMD 2G	AR	17q12 *TCAP*	Proximal and anterior legs	3 to 17-fold increased	Myopathy with rimmed vacuoles
Distal myopathy type 3 (MPD3)	AD	8p22-q11	Asymmetric distal legs and hands	NL or mild increase	Myopathy with vacuoles

accumulation of 15- to 18-nm diameter tubulofilamentous inclusions and filamentous bundles in the sarcoplasm and nuclei of the myotilinopathies. Similar finding were seen in desminopathy and αB-crystallinopathy, wherein electron-dense granulofilamentous accumulations, reticular material and sandwich formations of granulofilamentous material deposited parallel to or facing the Z-lines with mitochondria at both sides alongside the deposits. Desminopathy and αB-crystallinopathy differ in the occurrence of early apoptotic nuclear changes noted in the latter, in which ZASP-related myopathy was characterized instead by myotilin antibody-labeled filamentous bundles and floccular accumulations of thin filamentous material.

The variability in age onset of weakness in MFM is exemplified by recessively-inherited SEPN1, which begins in infancy or childhood (Table 2) as syndromes of congenital muscular dystrophy with spinal rigidity (104, 105) multi-minicore disease (106), congenital fiber-type disproportion myopathy (107), and desmin-related myopathy with Mallory body-like inclusions (MB-DRM) (108), the latter of which demonstrates muscle inclusions immunoreactive

to desmin, dystrophin, and ubiquitin (109) with rimmed vacuoles (110). Onset was in childhood for a newly identified rare severe AD MFM6, also known as Bcl-associated athanogene-3 (Bag3) myopathy (96). A severe childhood onset phenotype was described in three patients, all with respiratory insufficiency in the teens and hypertrophic or restrictive cardiomyopathy, and rigid spine in two. An adult-onset isolated dilated cardiomyopathy phenotype was noted in others with mutation of *BAG3*, a member of the anti-apoptotic BAG protein family, and Z-disk-associated protein that binds heat shock protein (HSP) 70, serving as a co-chaperone factor controlling the chaperone activity of Hsp70 (111).

UNCLASSIFIED DISTAL MYOPATHY SYNDROMES

Mahnjeh and colleagues (112, 113) designated *MPD3* to describe a syndrome of frequently asymmetric late-onset distal myopathy with intrinsic hand weakness and clumsi-

Table 4. Approach to the Patient with a Myopathic Disorder: The 6 Key Questions

1. Does the patient have "negative" or "positive" symptoms and signs?
   "Negative"
      Weakness
      Fatigue
      Atrophy
   "Positive"
      Pain (myalgia)
      Cramps
      Contractures
      Stiffness/inability to relax
      Hypertrophy
2. Temporal questions about weakness, pain, stiffness
   Constant or episodic?
   Monophasic or relapsing?
   Acute, subacute, chronic?
   Age at onset?
   Lifelong (congenital)?
   Progressive or nonprogressive?
3. What is the distribution of the weakness?
   Proximal arms/legs
   Distal arms/legs:
      Leg anterior compartment
      Leg posterior compartment
      Finger flexors
      Finger extensors
   Proximal and distal
   Neck
   Cranial
      Ocular—ptosis, ocular motility
      Pharyngeal—dysarthria/dysphagia
      Facial
   Atrophy/hypertrophy
4. Are there triggering events for episodic weakness, pain, stiffness?
   During or immediately after exercise?
   After brief or prolonged exercise?
   After exercise followed by rest?
   After carbohydrate meal?
   Relieved by exercise?
   Drugs/toxins?
   Temperature (internal/external)?
5. Is there a family history of a myopathic disorder?
   X-linked
   Autosomal dominant
   Autosomal recessive
   Maternal transmission (mitochondrial)
6. Are there associated medical conditions?
   Rash
   Baldness
   Fever
   Dark/red urine
   Dysmorphic features
   Cardiac
   Pulmonary
   Arthritis, other connective tissue disease findings
   Cataracts
   Mental retardation/CNS
   Skeletal contractures
   Skeletal deformities
   Neuropathy
   Gastrointestinal

ness, AD inheritance in Finnish patients age 32 to 45 years and earlier in men than women. Later, there was glutei, distal anterior and posterior leg muscle involvement followed by infraspinatus, triceps, forearm, and proximal leg muscle involvement. Muscle MRI in one patient showed fatty degeneration, and muscle biopsy revealed frequent rimmed vacuoles and dystrophic changes. Linkage was established at the 8p22-q11 and 12q13-q22 in the candidate genes *MLC1SA* and *ANK1*, respectively encoding myosin light chain 1 slow-twitch muscle A and the muscle specific isoform of ankyrin 1.

Feit and colleagues (114) reported a southeastern Tennessee family with similar AD inheritance of hand, foot and ankle weakness in members age 35 to 57 years. There was occasional asymmetrical peroneal emphasis, with inversion of the ankles, unsteady gait, and sparing of the gastrocnemius muscles and characteristic extensor hand weakness involving the abductor pollicus brevis muscles. Several members had voice changes and others had initial vocal cord and pharyngeal muscle involvement, as did others with asymmetric shoulder weakness and ptosis. Serum CK was normal in one-third of individuals, and elevated two- to eightfold in the others. Electrodiagnostic studies of the vocal and pharyngeal muscles showed myopathic potentials. Muscle biopsy in one-half of the cases disclosed chronic non-inflammatory myopathy with subsarcolemmal rimmed vacuoles. The syndrome of vocal cord and pharyngeal weakness with AD distal myopathy (VCPDM), so termed, mapped to chromosome 5q and, in keeping with earlier precedents (78), was designated MPD2. Autosomal dominant distal atrophy with vocal cord paralysis occurs in association with spinal muscular atrophy (SMA) and in neuronal forms of Charcot-Marie-Tooth (CMT) disease, as well as in LGMD2F at 5q33-34 and LGMD1A, both within the linkage interval of VCPDM. In the originally reported North American family and an unrelated Bulgarian family, Senderek and coworkers (115) identified a heterozygous C-to-G transversion at nucleotide 254 in exon 2 that resulted in a change from serine to cysteine at codon 85 of the matrin 3 (*MATR3*) gene, encoding an internal nuclear matrix protein belonging to the family of nuclear matrins, a group of proteins present in the nuclear matrix of a variety of mammalian tissues and cells (Table 3).

Two large Italian families with AD adult-onset vacuolar distal myopathy with linkage to the 19p13.3 locus were described (116, 117), with age at diagnosis of 27 to 73 years, mild scapular and distal leg weakness with normal CK levels. Severely affected individuals demonstrate marked dorsiflexor, neck flexor, shoulder and finger muscle weakness, wasting, and a 2-fold elevation in the serum CK. Needle EMG in the latter revealed myopathic MUP of proximal and distal limb muscles, more severe

Table 5. Phenotypic Patterns of Muscle Disorders

Pattern 1
  Proximal "limb-girdle" weakness
    Acute/subacute—acquired
      Inflammatory (polymyositis/dermatomyositis)
      Endocrine
      Toxic drugs
    Chronic/congenital/painless—hereditary
      Muscular dystrophy
      Myofibrillar myopathy
      Hereditary inclusion body myopathy (IBMPFD)
      Congenital myopathies
      Myotonic dystrophy type 2
      Mitochondrial
      Pompe disease
      Carnitine deficiency

Pattern 2
  Distal weakness
    Distal muscular dystrophies
      Late adult onset (Welander, Markesbery-Griggs, Udd)
      Early adult onset (Nonaka, Miyoshi, Laing)
    Myofibrillar myopathy
    Myotonic dystrophy type 1
    Congenital myopathy
    Hereditary inclusion body myopathy (HIBM2, HIBM3, and IBMPFD)

Pattern 3
  Proximal arm/distal leg weakness (scapuloperoneal)
    Facioscapulohumeral dystrophy with facial weakness
    Scapuloperoneal myopathy
    Emery-Dreifuss dystrophy
    Pompé
    Congenital myopathy
    IBMPFD

Pattern 4
  Distal arm/proximal leg weakness
    Sporadic inclusion body myositis (IBM)
      Sporadic non-hereditary
      Common presentation
        Finger and wrist flexor weakness
        Knee extensor weakness
      Asymmetric

Pattern 5
  Ptosis/ophthalmoplegia
    Ptosis without ophthalmoplegia
      Myotonic dystrophy
      Congenital myopathies
    Ptosis with ophthalmoplegia
      Oculopharyngeal dystrophy
      Oculopharyngodistal muscular dystrophy
      Mitochondrial myopathy

Neuromuscular junction disorders (myasthenia gravis, Lambert-Eaton myasthenic syndrome, botulism)
HIBM3

Pattern 6
  Prominent neck extensor weakness
    Isolated neck extensor myopathy (INEM)
    Myasthenia gravis
    IBM/PM/DM
    IBMPFD
    Myotonic dystrophy 2
    FSH dystrophy
    Congenital myopathy
    Carnitine deficiency
    Hyperparathyroidism

Pattern 7
  Bulbar weakness—tongue/pharyngeal (dysarthria, dysphagia)
    Myasthenia gravis, Lambert-Eaton syndrome
    Oculopharyngeal dystrophy

Pattern 8
  Episodic pain, weakness, myoglobinuria with trigger
    Related to exercise
      Glycogenoses (McArdle disease)
      Lipid disorders (carnitine palmityl transferase deficiency)
    Unrelated to exercise
      Malignant hyperthermia
      Drugs/toxins
      Trauma (crush injury)
      Viral/bacterial infections

Pattern 9
  Episodic weakness delayed or unrelated to exercise
    Periodic paralysis (PP)
      Na$^+$ channelopathies (hyperkalemic)
      Ca^{++} channelopathies (hypokalemic)
      Andersen syndrome
      Secondary PP (thyrotoxicosis)

Pattern 10
  Stiffness/decreased ability to relax
    Improves with exercise
      Myotonia—Na$^+$ or Cl$^-$ channelopathies
    Worsens with exercise/cold sensitivity
      Paramyotonia—Na$^+$ channelopathies
      Brody disease
    With fixed weakness
      Myotonic dystrophy (DM1)
      Proximal myotonic myopathy (DM2)
      Myotonia congenita
      Paramyotonia congenita

Table 6. Muscle Disorders with Rimmed Vacuoles

Inclusion body myositis
Hereditary inclusion body myopathy (h-IBM)
   h-IBM2 or Nonaka type distal myopathy (GNE)
   hIBM with Paget disease and frontotemporal demen-
      tia[*] (VCP)
   h-IBM3 (myosin heavy chain IIa)[*]
Distal muscular dystrophies
   Welander type[*]
   Markesbery-Griggs type (ZASPopathy)[*]
   Udd type (titinopathy)[*]
Myofibrillar myopathy
   Myotilinopathy (LGMD1A)[*]
   Zaspopathy[*]
   Desminopathy[*]
   Filaminopathy[*]
   Bag3-opathy[*]
   αB-crystallin[*]
   SEPN1
Other muscular dystrophies/myopathies
   Reducing body myopathy (FHL1-opathy)
   Emery-Dreifuss (emerinopathy, laminopathy[*])
   LGMD2G (telethoninopathy)
   Oculopharyngeal muscular dystrophy
      (PABP2-GCG triplet)[*]
   Oculopharyngodistal muscular dystrophy
   Pompe disease (acid maltase deficiency)
   Danon disease (LAMP-2)
   X-linked myopathy with excessive autophagy (VMA21)

*Autosomal dominant

Table 7. Other Neuromuscular Disorders
with Distal Weakness

Myotonic dystrophy facioscapulohumeral dystrophy
Scapuloperoneal syndrome
Oculopharyngeal dystrophy
Oculopharyngodistal myopathy
Emery-Dreifuss humeroperonal dystrophy
Inflammatory myopathy
   Inclusion body myositis
   Polymyositis
Metabolic myopathy
   Debrancher deficiency
   Acid-maltase deficiency
Phosphorylase b Kinase
   Mitochondrial myopathy
Congenital myopathy
   Nemaline myopathy
   Central core myopathy
   Centronuclear myopathy type 2
Nephropathic cystinosis
Myasthenia gravis
Cytoplasmic body myopathy Hyperthyroid myopathy
Hereditary inclusion body myopathy

in the legs. Muscle biopsy showed myopathic changes and rimmed vacuoles in all so studied, clustered mainly along myofibers surfaces, with basophilic granular material that stained positive for acid phosphatase, sarcolemmal protein, laminin alpha 2-chain, and negative for thioflavin-S, Congo red, beta amyloid, and tau protein. Ubiquitin was abnormally present at the surface of myofibers and in the lumen of vacuoles, especially at the fiber surface. Positivity was also noted for the 19 and 20S subunits of proteasome complex on most vacuole surfaces. These findings suggested an endolysosomal origin of the vacuoles caused by abnormality in the lysosomal degradation pathway.

Autosomal dominant distal myopathy was reported in association with mutation in the caveolin-3 (*CAV3*) gene (118), mutations of which cause LGMD1C, sporadic hyper-CKemia and rippling muscle disease (119, 120). Felice and coworkers (121) studied a family with AD adult-onset distal myopathy without linkage to known loci, in whom weakness commenced in distal anterior leg muscles resulting in foot drop with mild proximal leg involvement. Serum CK

was 2- to 6-fold normal, disease progression was slow, and muscle biopsy showed mild myopathic features.

A very late onset AD distal myopathy was described (122) in which serum CK was normal or slightly elevated, and muscle biopsy revealed numerous rimmed and non-rimmed vacuoles accompanied by aggregates of desmin and dystrophin labeling in parts of the cytoplasm of defective fibers. Chinnery and colleagues (123) described a British family with AD distal anterior compartment weakness of the legs and early respiratory muscle involvement, with age at onset of 32 to 75 years, and nighttime hypoventilation resulting from diaphragmatic muscle involvement. Progression of disease was variable with loss of ambulation in one individual after seven years, and similarly in another affected member after 20 years. Serum CK values were normal or slightly elevated. Needle EMG showed myopathic dystrophic features and occasional rimmed vacuoles with some congophilic eosinophilic, desmin, beta-amyloid, and phosphorylated tau immunoreactivity. Linkage was excluded for all known distal myopathy loci.

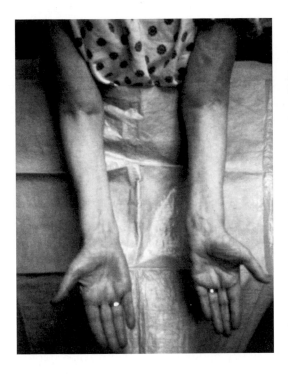

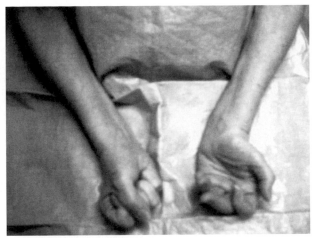

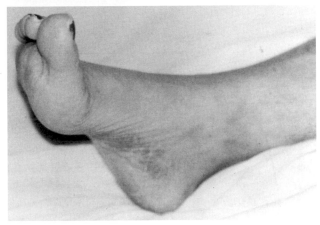

FIG. 7. Inclusion body myositis. **(A)** Note bilateral atrophy of the flexor forearm muscles. **(B)** Same patient as in A. Note inability to flex fingers completely in the left hand. **(C)** Pseudo-Babinski sign with chronic toe extension due to weakness of toe flexors.

Mitsuhashi and coworkers (124) described multiple minicores and preferential involvement of type 1 fibers in a 52-year-old man with distally-predominant, slowly progressive muscle weakness beginning at age 36 years. Muscle CT showed fatty replacement of the soleus, anterior tibial, and paraspinal muscles, with clinical sparing of the quadriceps femoris, gastrocnemius, and arm and hand muscles. A novel heterozygous nucleotide change c.5869T > A at p.S1957T was identified in the *RYR1* gene. Although pathogenicity was not confirmed, this nucleotide change was absent in 100 control DNA.

Other unclassified distal myopathies (Table 7) include childhood-onset distal myopathy described in infants with AD inheritance of foot drop, finger, and hand weakness, and very slow progression (125–127). Affected patients demonstrate myopathic muscle biopsy tissue and needle EMG, the former without vacuolization, and persistence of ambulation into adulthood.

A large Dutch family with AD juvenile-onset distal myopathy with age at onset of 5 to 15 years (128) was associated with very slow progression of flexor and extensor distal leg muscles, such that affected members remain functional and active during their adult life. Myopathic and neuropathic features were found on muscle biopsy and postmortem examination. Although the reports of childhood-onset distal myopathy preceded desmin immunostaining of skeletal muscle tissue, there were no clues on light microscopy to suggest excessive desmin.

Weakness of distal muscle groups was prominent in some forms of muscular dystrophy, including myotonia dystrophica type 1 (DM1) (129, 130), facioscapulohumeral (FSH) dystrophy (131, 132), myopathic scapuloperoneal syndrome (133), X-linked Emery-Dreifuss disease (134), and oculopharyngeal muscular dystrophy (OPMD) (135–137) as well as polymyositis (138, 139) sporadic IBM (140–144) (Figures 7 and 8 A–C), deficiency of debrancher enzyme (145) and acid maltase (146), the lysosomal storage disorder nephropathic cystinosis (147, 148), nemaline rod (147, 148) central core (149), and centronuclear myopathy (150), and a minority of patients with myasthenia gravis (MG).

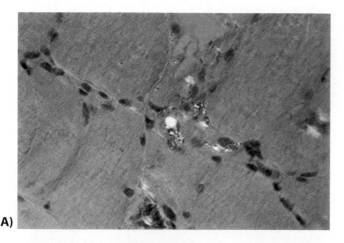

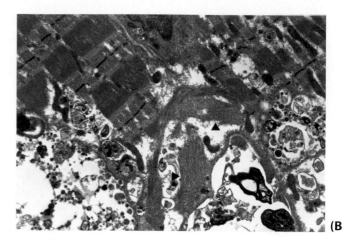

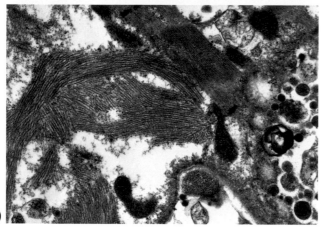

FIG. 8. Inclusion body myositis. **(A)** Apple green birefringence indicating amyloid deposition (Congo red under polarized lightX675). **(B)** Electron microscopy showing the edge of a vacuole (with adjacent normal sarcomeres) containing cytoplasmic debris and 15- to 18-nm filaments (arrowheads) X10,800. Courtesy of Dennis Burns, MD. **(C)** Higher magnification of 15- to 18-nm filaments (X20,000). Courtesy of Dennis Burns, MD.

REFERENCES

1. Gowers WR. A lecture on myopathy and a distal form: delivered at the National Hospital for the Paralysed and Epileptic. *Br Med J* 1902; 2:89–92.

2. Dejerine J, Thomas A. Un cas de myopathie à topographie type Aran-Duchenne suivi d'autopsie. *Rev Neurol* 1904; 12:1187–1190.

3. Campbell CM. A case of muscular dystrophy affecting hands and feet. *Rev Neurol Psychiatry* 1906; 4:192–202.4.

4. Spiller WG. Myopathy of the distal type and its relation to the neural form of muscular atrophy (Charcot-Marie-Tooth type). *J Nerv Ment Dis* 1907; 34:14–30.

5. Welander L. Myopathia distalis tarda hereditaria. *Acta Med Scand* Suppl 1951; 265:1–124.

6. Barohn RJ, Watts GD, Amato AA. A case of late-onset proximal and distal muscle weakness. *Neurology* 2009; 73:1592–1597.

7. Udd B. 165th ENMC International Workshop: distal myopathies 6–8th February 2009 Naarden, The Netherlands. *Neuromuscular Disorders* 2009; 19:429–438.

8. Griggs R, Vihola A, Hackman P, et al. Zaspopathy in a large classic late-onset distal myopathy family. *Brain* 2007; 130:1477–1484.

9. Selcen D, Engel AG. Mutations in ZASP define a novel form of muscular dystrophy in humans. *Ann Neurol* 2005; 57:269–276.

10. Selcen D, Engel AG. Mutations in myotilin cause myofibrillar myopathy. *Neurology* 2004; 62:1363–1371.

11. Selcen D, Ohno K, Engel AG. Myofibrillar myopathy: clinical, morphological and genetic studies in 63 patients. *Brain* 2004; 127:439–451.

12. Watts GD, Wymer J, Kovach MJ, et al. Inclusion body myopathy associated with Paget disease of bone and frontotemporal dementia is caused by mutant valosin-containing protein. *Nat Genet* 2004; 36: 377–381.

13. Stojkovic T, Hammouda el H, Richard P, et al. Clinical outcome in 19 French and Spanish patients with valosin-containing protein myopathy associated with Paget's disease of bone and frontotemporal dementia. *Neuromuscul Disord* 2009; 19:316–323.

14. Hübbers CU, Clemen CS, Kesper K, et al. Pathological consequences of VCP mutations on human striated muscle. *Brain* 2007; 130:381–393.

15. Ahlberg G, von Tell D, Borg K, et al. Genetic linkage of Welander distal myopathy to chromosome 2p13. *Ann Neurol* 1999; 46:399–404.

16. von Tell D, Somer H, Udd B, et al. Welander distal myopathy outside the Swedish population: phenotype and genotype. *Neuromuscul Disord* 2002; 12:544–547.

17. Borg K, Borg J, Lindblom U. Sensory involvement in distal myopathy (Welander). *J Neurol Sci* 1987; 80:323–332.

18. Borg K, Tomé FM, Edström L. Intranuclear and cytoplasmic filamentous inclusions in distal myopathy (Welander). *Acta Neuropathol* 1991; 82:102–106.

19. Lindberg C, Borg K, Edström L, et al. Inclusion body myositis and Welander distal myopathy: a clinical, neurophysiological and morphological comparison. *J Neurol Sci* 1991; 103:76–81.

20. Borg K, Ahlberg G, Borg J, et al. Welander's distal myopathy: clinical, neurophysiological and muscle biopsy observations in young and middle aged adults with early symptoms. *J Neurol Neurosurg Psychiatry* 1991; 54:494–498.

21. Edström L. Histochemical and histopathological changes in skeletal muscle in late-onset hereditary distal myopathy (Welander). *J Neurol Sci* 1975; 26:147–157.

22. Mahjneh I, Lamminen AE, Udd B, et al. Muscle magnetic resonance imaging shows distinct diagnostic patterns in Welander and tibial muscular dystrophy. *Acta Neurol Scand* 2004; 110:87–93.

23. Borg K, Solders G, Borg J, et al. Neurogenic involvement in distal myopathy (Welander). Histochemical and morphological observations on muscle and nerve biopsies. *J Neurol Sci* 1989; 91:53–70.

24. Dahlgaard E. Myopathia distalis tarda hereditaria. *Acta Psychiatr Scand* 1960; 35:440–447.

25. Barrows HS, Duemler LP. Late distal myopathy. Report of a case. *Neurology* 1962; 12:547–550.

26. Sumner D, Crawfurd MD, Harriman DG. Distal muscular dystrophy in an English family. *Brain* 1971; 94:51–60.

27. Markesbery WR, Griggs RC, Leach RP, et al. Late onset hereditary distal myopathy. *Neurology* 1974; 24:127–134.

28. Udd B, Partanen J, Halonen P, et al. Tibial muscular dystrophy. Late adult-onset distal myopathy in 66 Finnish patients. *Arch Neurol* 1993; 50:604–608.

29. Partanen J, Laulumaa V, Paljärvi L, et al. Late onset foot-drop muscular dystrophy with rimmed vacuoles. *J Neurol Sci* 1994; 125:158–167.

30. Udd B, Kääriänen H, Somer H. Muscular dystrophy with separate clinical phenotypes in a large family. *Muscle Nerve* 1991; 14:1050–1058.

31. Hackman P, Vihola A, Haravuori H, et al. Tibial muscular dystrophy is a titinopathy caused by mutations in TTN, the gene encoding the giant skeletal-muscle protein titin. *Am J Hum Genet* 2002; 71:492–500.

32. Udd B, Bushby K, Nonaka I, et al. 104th European Neuromuscular Centre (ENMC) International Workshop: distal myopathies, 8–10th March 2002 in Naarden, The Netherlands. *Neuromuscul Disord* 2002; 12:897–904.

33. Murone I, Sato T, Shirakawa K, et al. Distal myopathy: a case of non-hereditary distal myopathy. *Clin Neurol* (Tokyo) 1963; 3:387–393.

34. Sasaki K, Mori H, Takahashi K, et al. Distal myopathy—report of four cases. *Clin Neurol* (Tokyo) 1969; 9:627–637.

35. Nonaka I, Sunohara N, Ishiura S, et al. Familial distal myopathy with rimmed vacuole and lamellar (myeloid) body formation. *J Neurol Sci* 1981; 51:141–155.

36. Nonaka I, Sunohara N, Satoyoshi E, et al. Autosomal recessive distal muscular dystrophy: a comparative study with distal myopathy with rimmed vacuole formation. *Ann Neurol* 1985; 17:51–59.

37. Sunohara N, Nonaka I, Kamei N, et al. Distal myopathy with rimmed vacuole formation: a follow-up study. *Brain* 1989; 112:65–83.

38. Markesbery WR, Griggs RC, Herr B. Distal myopathy: electron microscopic and histochemical studies. *Neurology* 1977: 27:727–735.

39. Miller RG, Blank NK, Layzer RB. Sporadic distal myopathy with early adult onset. *Ann Neurol* 1979; 5:220–227.

40. Krendel DA, Gilchrist JM, Bossen EH. Distal vacuolar myopathy with complete heart block. *Arch Neurol* 1988; 45:698–699.

41. Isaacs H, Badenhorst ME, Whistler T. Autosomal recessive distal myopathy. *J Clin Pathol* 1988; 41:188–194.

42. Scoppetta C, Vaccario ML, Casali C, et al. Distal muscular dystrophy with autosomal recessive inheritance. *Muscle Nerve* 1984; 7:478–481.

43. Somer H. Distal myopathies. 25th ENMC International Workshop, 18–20 November 1994, Naarden, The Netherlands. *Neuromuscul Disord* 1995; 5:249–252.

44. Mizusawa H, Kurisaki H, Takatsu M, et al. Rimmed vacuolar distal myopathy: a clinical, electrophysiological, histopathological and computed tomographic study of seven cases. *J Neurol* 1987; 234:129–136.

45. Sunohara N, Nonaka I, Kamei N, et al. Distal myopathy with rimmed vacuole formation. A follow-up study. *Brain* 1989; 112:65–83.

46. Kumamota T, Fukuhara N, Nagashima M, et al. Distal myopathy: histochemical and ultrastructural studies. *Arch Neurol* 1982; 39:367–371.

47. Matsubara S, Tanabe H. Hereditary distal myopathy with filamentous inclusions. *Acta Neurol Scand* 1982; 65:363–368.

48. Jongen PJ, Laak HJ, Stadhouders AM. Rimmed basophilic vacuoles and filamentous inclusions in neuromuscular disorders. *Neuromuscul Disord* 1995; 5:31–38.

49. Yabe I, Higashi T, Kikuchi S, et al. GNE mutations causing distal myopathy with rimmed vacuoles with inflammation. *Neurology* 2003; 61:384–386.

50. Krause S, Schlotter-Weigel B, Walter MC, et al. A novel homozygous missense mutation in the GNE gene of a patient with quadriceps-sparing hereditary inclusion body myopathy associated with muscle inflammation. *Neuromuscul Disord* 2003; 13:830–834.

51. Asaka T, Ikeuchi K, Okino S, et al. Homozygosity and linkage disequilibrium mapping of autosomal recessive distal myopathy (Nonaka distal myopathy). *J Hum Genet* 2001; 46:649–655.

52. Tomimitsu H, Shimizu J, Ishikawa K, et al. Distal myopathy with rimmed vacuoles (DMRV): new GNE mutations and splice variant. *Neurology* 2004; 62:1607–1610.

53. Argov Z, Yarom R. "Rimmed vacuole myopathy" sparing the quadriceps. A unique disorder in Iranian Jews. *J Neurol Sci* 1984; 64:33–43.

54. Askanas V, Engel WK. Sporadic inclusion-body myositis and hereditary inclusion-body myopathies: current concepts of diagnosis and pathogenesis. *Curr Opin Rheumatol* 1998; 10:530–542.

55. Eisenberg I, Avidan N, Potikha T, et al. The UDP-N-acetylglucosamine 2-epimerase/N-acetylmannosamine kinase gene is mutated in recessive hereditary inclusion body myopathy. *Nat Genet* 2001; 29:83–87.

56. Nishino I, Noguchi S, Murayama K, et al. Distal myopathy with rimmed vacuoles is allelic to hereditary inclusion body myopathy. *Neurology* 2002; 59:1689–1693.

57. Argov Z, Eisenberg I, Grabov-Nardini G, et al. Hereditary inclusion body myopathy: the Middle Eastern genetic cluster. *Neurology* 2003; 60:1519–1523.

58. Nemunaitis G, Jay CM, Maples PB, et al. Hereditary inclusion body myopathy: single patient response to intravenous dosing of GNE gene lipoplex. *Hum Gene Ther* 2011; 22:1331–1341.

59. Malicdan MC, Noguchi S, Hayashi YK, et al. Prophylactic treatment with sialic acid metabolites precludes the development of the myopathic phenotype in the DMRV-hIBM mouse model. *Nat Med* 2009; 15:690–695.

60. Miyoshi K, Saijo K, Kuryu Y, et al. Four cases of distal myopathy in two families. *Jpn J Hum Genet* 1967; 12:113.

61. Miyoshi K, Tada Y, Iwasa M, et al. Autosomal recessive distal myopathy observed characteristically in Japan. *Jpn J Hum Genet* 1975; 20:62–63.

62. Miyoshi K, Kawai H, Iwasa M, et al. Autosomal recessive distal muscular dystrophy as a new type of progressive muscular

dystrophy. Seventeen cases in eight families including an autopsied case. *Brain* 1986; 109:31–54.

63. Kuhn E, Schröder JM. A new type of distal myopathy in two brothers. *J Neurol* 1981; 226:181–185.

64. Galassi G, Rowland LP, Hays AP, et al. High serum levels of creatine kinase: asymptomatic prelude to distal myopathy. *Muscle Nerve* 1987; 10:346–350.

65. Barohn RJ, Miller RG, Griggs RC. Autosomal recessive distal dystrophy. *Neurology* 1991; 41:1365–1370.

66. Meola G, Sansone V, Rotondo G, et al. Computerized tomography and magnetic resonance muscle imaging in Miyoshi's myopathy. *Muscle Nerve* 1996; 19:1476–1480.

67. Linssen WH, Notermans NC, Van der Graaf Y, et al. Miyoshi-type distal muscular dystrophy. Clinical spectrum in 24 Dutch patients. *Brain* 1997; 120:1989–1996.

68. Fallon KE, Collins SJ, Purdam C. Miyoshi myopathy—an unusual cause of calf pain and tightness. *Clin J Sport Med* 2004; 14:45–47.

69. Rosales XQ, Gastier-Foster JM, Lewis S, et al. Novel diagnostic features of dysferlinopathies. *Muscle Nerve* 2010; 42:14–21.

70. Pradhan S. Clinical and magnetic resonance imaging features of 'diamond on quadriceps' sign in dysferlinopathy. *Neurol India* 2009; 57:172–175.

71. Soares CN, de Freitas MR, Nascimento OJ, et al. Myopathy of distal lower limbs: the clinical variant of Miyoshi. *Arq Neuropsiquiatr* 2003; 61:946–949.

72. Shaibani A, Harati Y, Amato A, et al. Miyoshi myopathy with vacuoles. *Neurology* 1997; 47[Suppl]:A195.

73. Liu J, Aoki M, Illa I, et al. Dysferlin, a novel skeletal muscle gene, is mutated in Miyoshi myopathy and limb girdle muscular dystrophy. *Nat Genet* 1998; 20:31–36.

74. Aoki M, Liu J, Richard I, et al. Genomic organization of the dysferlin gene and novel mutations in Miyoshi myopathy. *Neurology* 2001; 57:271–278.

75. Piccolo F, Moore SA, Ford GC, et al. Intracellular accumulation and reduced sarcolemmal expression of dysferlin in limb-girdle muscular dystrophies. *Ann Neurol* 2000; 48:902–912.

76. Rizo J, Südhof TC. C2-domains, structure and function of a universal Ca2+- binding domain. *J Biol Chem* 1998; 273:15879–15882.

77. Matsuda C, Aoki M, Hayashi YK, et al. Dysferlin is a surface membrane-associated protein that is absent in Miyoshi myopathy. *Neurology* 1999; 53:1119–1122.

78. Laing NG, Laing BA, Meredith C, et al. Autosomal dominant distal myopathy: linkage to chromosome 14. *Am J Hum Genet* 1995; 56:422–427.

79. Mastaglia FL, Phillips BA, Cala LA, et al. Early onset chromosome 14-linked distal myopathy (Laing). *Neuromuscul Disord* 2002; 12:350–357.

80. Meredith C, Herrmann R, Parry C, et al. Mutations in the slow skeletal muscle fiber myosin heavy chain gene (MYH7) cause Laing early-onset distal myopathy (MPD1). *Am J Hum Genet* 2004; 75:703–708.

81. Voit T, Kutz P, Leube B, et al. Autosomal dominant distal myopathy: further evidence of a chromosome 14 locus. *Neuromuscul Disord* 2001; 11:11–19.

82. Zimprich F, Djamshidian A, Hainfellner JA et al. An autosomal dominant early adult-onset distal muscular dystrophy. *Muscle Nerve* 2000; 23:1876–1879.

83. Hedera P, Petty EM, Bui MR, et al. The second kindred with autosomal dominant distal myopathy linked to chromosome 14q: genetic and clinical analysis. *Arch Neurol* 2003; 60:1321–1325.

84. Scoppetta C, Casali C, La Cesa I, et al. Infantile autosomal dominant distal myopathy. *Acta Neurol Scand* 1995; 92:122–126.

85. Bohlega S, Abu-Amero SN, Wakil SM, et al. Mutation of the slow myosin heavy chain rod domain underlies hyaline body myopathy. *Neurology* 2004; 62:1518–1521.

86. Goldfarb LG, Vicart P, Goebel HH, et al. Desmin myopathy. *Brain* 2004; 127:723–734.

87. Salmikangas P, van der Ven PF, Lalowski M, et al. Myotilin, the limb-girdle muscular dystrophy 1A (LGMD1A) protein, cross-links actin filaments and control sarcomere assembly. *Hum Mol Genet* 2003; 12:189–203.

88. van der Ven PF, Wiesner S, Salmikangas P, et al. Indications for a novel muscular dystrophy pathway. gamma-filamin, the muscle-specific filamin isoform, interacts with myotilin. *J Cell Biol* 2000; 151:235–248.

89. Nakano S, Engel AG, Waclawik AJ, et al. Myofibrillar myopathy with abnormal foci of desmin positivity. I. Light and electron microscopy analysis of 10 cases. *J Neuropathol Exp Neurol* 1996; 55:549–562.

90. Edström L, Thornell LE, Eriksson A. A new type of hereditary distal myopathy with characteristic sarcoplasmic bodies and intermediate (skeletin) filaments. *J Neurol Sci* 1980; 47:171–190.

91. Goldfarb LG, Park KY, Cervenáková L, et al. Missense mutations in desmin associated with familial cardiac and skeletal myopathy. *Nature Genet* 1998; 19:402–403.

92. Vicart P, Caron A, Guicheney P, et al. A missense mutation in the αB-crystallin chaperone gene causes a desmin-related myopathy. *Nat Genet* 1998; 20:92–95.

93. Selcen D, Engel AG. Myofibrillar myopathy caused by novel dominant negative alpha B-crystallin mutations. *Ann Neurol* 2003; 54:804–810.94.

94. Dalakas MC, Park KY, Semino-Mora C, et al. Desmin myopathy, a skeletal myopathy with cardiomyopathy caused by mutations in the desmin gene. *N Engl J Med* 2000; 342:770–780.

95. Dalakas MC, Dagvadorj A, Goudeau B, et al. Progressive skeletal myopathy, a phenotypic variant of desmin myopathy associated with desmin mutations. *Neuromuscul Disord* 2003; 13:252–258.

96. Li D, Tapscoft T, Gonzalez O, et al. Desmin mutation responsible for idiopathic dilated cardiomyopathy. *Circulation* 1999; 100:461–464.

97. Walter MC, Reilich P, Huebner A, et al. Scapuloperoneal syndrome type Kaeser and a wide phenotypic spectrum of adult-onset, dominant myopathies are associated with the desmin mutation R350P. *Brain* 2007; 130:1485–1496.

98. Selcen D, Muntoni F, Burton BK, et al. Mutation in BAG3 causes severe dominant childhood muscular dystrophy. *Ann Neurol* 2009; 65:83–89.

99. Muntoni F, Catani G, Mateddu A, et al. Familial cardiomyopathy, mental retardation and myopathy associated with desmin-type intermediate filaments. *Neuromuscul Disord* 1994; 4:233–241.

100. Goebel HH. Desmin-related neuromuscular disorders. *Muscle Nerve* 1995; 18:1306–1320.

101. De Bleecker JL, Engel AG, Ertl BB. Myofibrillar myopathy with abnormal foci of desmin positivity. II. Immunocytochemical analysis reveals accumulation of multiple other proteins. *J Neuropathol Exp Pathol* 1996; 55:563–577.

102. Porte A, Stoeckel ME, Sacrez A, et al. Unusual familial cardiomyopathy with storage of intermediate filaments in the cardiac muscular cells. *Virchows Arch A Pathol Anat Histol* 1980; 386:43–58.

103. Claeys KG, Fardeau M, Schröder R, et al. Electron microscopy in myofibrillar myopathies reveals clues to the mutated gene. *Neuromuscul Disord* 2008; 18:656–666.

104. Moghadaszadeh B, Petit N, Jaillard C, et al. Mutations in SEPN1 cause congenital muscular dystrophy with spinal rigidity and restrictive respiratory syndrome. *Nat Genet* 2001; 29:17–18.

105. Lescure A, Gautheret D, Carbon P, et al. Novel selenoproteins identified in silico and in vivo by using a conserved RNA structural motif. *J Biol Chem* 1999; 274:38147–38154.

106. Ferreiro A, Quijano-Roy S, Pichereau C, et al. Mutations of the selenoprotein N gene, which is implicated in rigid spine muscular dystrophy, cause the classical phenotype of multiminicore disease: reassessing the nosology of early-onset myopathies. *Am J Hum Genet* 2002; 71: 739–749.

107. Clarke NF, Kidson W, Quijano-Roy S, et al. SEPN1: associated with congenital fiber-type disproportion and insulin resistance. *Ann Neurol* 2006; 59:546–552.

108. Ferreiro A, Ceuterick-de Groote C, Marks JJ, et al. Desmin-related myopathy with Mallory body-like inclusions is caused by mutations of the selenoprotein N gene. *Ann Neurol* 2004; 55:676–686.

109. Fidziańska A, Ryniewicz B, Barcikowska M, et al. A new familial congenital myopathy in children with desmin and dystrophin reacting plaques. *J Neurol Sci* 1995; 131:88–95.

110. Fidziańska A, Goebel HH, Osborn M, et al. Mallory body-like inclusions in a hereditary congenital neuromuscular disease. *Muscle Nerve* 1983; 6:195–200.

111. Takayama S, Xie Z, Reed JC. An evolutionarily conserved family of Hsp70/Hsc70 molecular chaperone regulators. *J Biol Chem* 1999; 274:781–786.

112. Mahjneh I, Haravuori H, Paetau A, et al. A distinct phenotype of distal myopathy in a large Finnish family. *Neurology* 2003; 61:87–92.

113. Haravuori H, Siitonen HA, Mahjneh I, et al. Linkage to two separate loci in a family with a novel distal myopathy phenotype (MPD3). *Neuromuscul Disord* 2004; 14:183–187.

114. Feit H, Silbergleit A, Schneider LB, et al. Vocal cord and pharyngeal weakness with autosomal dominant distal myopathy: clinical description and gene localization to 5q31. *Am J Hum Genet* 1998; 63:1732–1742.

115. Senderek J, Garvey SM, Krieger M, et al. Autosomal-dominant distal myopathy associated with a recurrent missense mutation in the gene encoding the nuclear matrix protein, matrin 3. *Am J Hum Genet* 2009; 84:511–518.

116. Servidei S, Capon F, Spinazzola A, et al. A distinctive autosomal dominant vacuolar neuromyopathy linked to 19p13. *Neurology* 1999; 53:830–837.

117. Di Blasi C, Moghadaszadeh B, Ciano C, et al. Abnormal lysosomal and ubiquitin-proteasome pathways in 19p13.3 distal myopathy. *Ann Neurol* 2004; 56:133–138.

118. Tateyama M, Aoki M, Nishino I, et al. Mutation in the caveolin-3 gene causes a peculiar form of distal myopathy. *Neurology* 2002; 58:323–325.

119. Fee DB, So YT, Barraza C, et al. Phenotypic variability associated with Arg26Gln mutation in caveolin 3. *Muscle Nerve* 2004; 30:375–378.

120. Sotgia F, Woodman SE, Bonuccelli G, et al. Phenotypic behavior of caveolin-3 R26Q, a mutant associated with hyperCKemia, distal myopathy, and rippling muscle disease. *Am J Physiol Cell Physiol* 2003; 285:C1150–C1160.

121. Felice KJ, Meredith C, Binz N, et al. Autosomal dominant distal myopathy not linked to the known distal myopathy loci. *Neuromuscul Disord* 1999; 9:59–65.

122. Pénisson-Besnier I, Dumez C, Chateau D, et al. Autosomal dominant late adult onset distal leg myopathy. *Neuromuscul Disord* 1998; 8:459–466.

123. Chinnery PF, Johnson MA, Walls TJ, et al. A novel autosomal dominant distal myopathy with early respiratory failure: clinico-pathologic characteristics and exclusion of linkage to candidate genetic loci. *Ann Neurol* 2001; 49:443–452.

124. Mitsuhashi S, Nonaka I, Wu S, et al. Distal myopathy in multiminicore disease. *Intern Med* 2009; 48:1759–1762.

125. Magee KR, DeJong RN. Hereditary distal myopathy with onset in infancy. *Arch Neurol* 1965; 13:387–390.

126. Does de Willebois AE VA, Meyer AE, Simons AJ, et al. Distal myopathy with onset in early infancy. *Neurology* 1968; 18:383–390.

127. Bautista J, Rafel E, Castilla JM, et al. Hereditary distal myopathy with onset in early infancy. Observation of a family. *J Neurol Sci* 1978; 37:149–158.

128. Biemond A. Myopathia distalis juvenilis hereditaria. *Acta Psychiatr Neurol Scand* 1955; 30:25–38.

129. Morgenlander JC, Massey JM. Myotonic dystrophy. *Semin Neurol* 1991; 11:236–243.

130. Schotland DL, Rowland LP. Muscular dystrophy. Features of ocular myopathy, distal myopathy, and myotonic dystrophy. *Arch Neurol* 1964; 10:433–445.

131. Tawil R, McDermott MP, Mendell JR, et al. Facioscapulohumeral muscular dystrophy (FSHD): design of natural history study and results of baseline testing. FSH-DY Group. *Neurology* 1994; 44:442–446.

132. Wijmenga C, Padberg GW, Moerer P, et al. Mapping of facioscapulo|humeral muscular dystrophy gene to chromosome 4q35-qter by multipoint linkage analysis and in situ hybridization. *Genomics* 1991; 9:570–575.

133. Thomas PK, Schott GD, Morgan-Hughes JA. Adult onset scapuloperoneal myopathy. *J Neurol Neurosurg Psychiatry* 1975; 38:1008–1015.

134. Rowland LP, Fetell M, Olarte M, et al. Emery-Dreifuss muscular dystrophy. *Ann Neurol* 1979; 5:111–117.

135. Satoyoshi E, Kinoshita M. Oculopharyngodistal myopathy. *Arch Neurol* 1977; 34:89–92.

136. Fukuhara N, Kumamoto T, Tsubaki T, et al. Oculopharyngeal muscular dystrophy and distal myopathy. Intrafamilial difference in the onset and distribution of muscular involvement. *Acta Neurol Scand* 1982; 65:458–467.

137. Vita G, Dattola R, Santoro M, et al. Familial oculopharyngeal muscular dystrophy with distal spread. *J Neurol* 1983; 230:57–64.

138. Hollinrake K. Polymyositis presenting as distal muscle weakness. A case report. *J Neurol Sci* 1969; 8:479–484.

139. Van Kasteren BJ. Polymyositis presenting with chronic progressive distal muscular weakness. *J Neurol Sci* 1979; 41:307–310.

140. Dimachkie MM, Barohn RJ. Idiopathic inflammatory myopathies. *Front Neurol Neurosci* 2009; 26:126–146.

141. Griggs RC, Askanas V, DiMauro S, et al. Inclusion body myositis and myopathies. *Ann Neurol* 1995; 38:705–713.

142. Mendell JR, Sahenk Z, Gales T, et al. Amyloid filaments in inclusion body myositis. Novel findings provide insight into nature of filaments. *Arch Neurol* 1991; 48:1229–1234.

143. Dimachkie MM. Idiopathic inflammatory myopathies. *J Neuroimmunol* 2011; 231:32–42.

144. Larue S, Maisonobe T, Benveniste O, et al. Distal muscle involvement in granulomatous myositis can mimic inclusion body myositis. *J Neurol Neurosurg Psychiatry* 2011; 82:674–677.

145. DiMauro S, Hartwig GB, Hays A, et al. Debrancher deficiency: neuromuscular disorder in 5 adults. *Ann Neurol* 1979; 5:422–436.

146. Barohn RJ, McVey AL, DiMauro S. Adult acid maltase deficiency. *Muscle Nerve* 1993; 16:672–676.

147. Hausmanowa-Petrusewicz I, Fidziańska A, Badurska B. Unusual course of nemaline myopathy. *Neuromuscul Disord* 1992; 2:413–418.

148. Laing NG, Majda BT, Akkari PA, et al. Assignment of a gene (NEM1) for autosomal dominant nemaline myopathy to chromosome 1. *Am J Hum Genet* 1992; 50:576–583.

149. Kratz R, Brooke MH. Distal myopathy. *Handb Clin Neurol* 1980; 40:471–483.

150. Moxley RT 3rd, Griggs RC, Markesbery WR, et al. Metabolic implications of distal atrophy. Carbohydrate metabolism in centronuclear myopathy. *J Neurol Sci* 1978; 39:247–259.

151. Nations SP, Wolfe GI, Amato AA, et al. Clinical features of patients with distal myasthenia gravis. *Neurology* 1997; 48[Suppl]:A64.

152. Greenberg SA, Salajegheh M, Judge DP, et al. Etiology of limb girdle muscular dystrophy 1D/1E determined by laser capture microdissection proteomics. *Ann Neurol* 2012; 71:141–145.

CHAPTER 22

The Channelopathies

David S. Younger, Michael Rose, Robert C. Griggs

There has been a virtual explosion in the recognition of disorders of membrane ion channels or channelopathies. Ion channel function may be modulated by changes in voltage (voltage-gated), chemical interaction (ligand-gated), or by mechanical perturbation. Channelopathies can affect both the peripheral (PNS) and central nervous system (CNS) and may be inherited or acquired.

Disturbance of muscle ion channel function may result in muscle membrane hyperexcitability leading to myotonia as the dominant feature, or muscle membrane inexcitability resulting in weakness so noted in periodic paralysis. The myotonias are divided into non-dystrophic and dystrophic disorders, the former of which are further separable into sodium (Na+) and chloride (Cl-) types, manifesting myotonia due to muscle membrane channelopathy as a prominent symptom. The dystrophic myotonias are genetically related disorders distinguished by myotonia, weakness, and wasting.

Classical myotonic dystrophy, or Steinert disease, is linked to chromosome 19q and designated DM1, while proximal myotonic myopathy (PROMM) and proximal myotonic dystrophy (PDM) are linked to 3q and designated DM2. In DM1 and DM2, the myotonic element of these multisystem disorders is believed to result from the primary gene mutation on chloride channel function. Other types of DM not linked to either 19q or 3q await designation as their genetic basis becomes known.

The Schwartz-Jampel syndrome (SJS) of chondrodystrophic myotonia has distinctive clinical features with prominent and severe continuous motor activity. Neurophysiology shows heterogeneous features with a neurogenic origin for the continuous motor activity, at least in some cases, which are, therefore, not true myotonia. In others, physiologic and genetic studies suggest a muscle sodium channel defect.

The periodic paralyses have been traditionally divided into disorders associated with high or normal serum potassium (K+) levels, termed hyperkalemic periodic paralysis (HYPP), and those with a low serum potassium concentration or hypokalemic periodic paralysis (HOKPP). In both, the serum potassium concentration is more a consequence than the cause of the periodic paralysis. This traditional separation has been validated by the demonstration that they are due to disorders of different ion channels with HYKK being due to disturbed sodium channels, and HOKPP, calcium (Ca++)-channel related, and a minority being due to a sodium channel involvement. Acquired periodic paralyses results from disorders that change K+ concentration, and although not primary channelopathy in nature, they merit inclusion because they are important in the differential diagnosis of primary periodic paralysis. Andersen syndrome is a separate familial periodic paralysis with cardiac dysrhythmias and distinctive facial features that is due to a potassium channel gene defect in the majority of cases.

The muscle channelopathies mentioned thus far result from defects of voltage-gated channels, the mechanically regulated defect of which may be responsible for rippling muscle syndrome.

At the neuromuscular junction, defects in a ligand-gated channel, such as the nicotinic acetylcholine receptor (AChR), leads to acquired autoimmune and congenital myasthenia gravis (MG). Autoimmune antibodies that affect voltage-gated presynaptic calcium channels (VGCC) cause Lambert-Eaton Myasthenic Syndrome (LEMS). The ryanodine receptor, a ligand-gated calcium release channel that facilitates the release of calcium from the sarcoplasmic reticulum into the cytoplasm, may be mutated, resulting in malignant hyperthermia and some forms of congenital myopathy.

Along the peripheral nerve, channelopathies can cause nerve hyperactivity, a feature of neuromyotonia or Isaacs syndrome, and myokymia. In Isaacs syndrome, where neuromyotonia is a major feature, most cases are sporadic and usually on an autoimmune basis. Myokymia is also a feature of episodic ataxia type 1, which is due to mutations of a potassium channel gene. The marine toxin ciguatoxin, ingested from contaminated fish or shellfish, is a potent sodium channel blocker that causes a rapid onset of numbness, intense paraesthesia, dysesthesia, and muscle weakness.

SODIUM CHANNELOPATHIES

These are disorders of the α1 subunit of the muscle sodium channel, allelic abnormalities of which result in paramyotonia congenita (PMC), HYPP, normokalemic periodic paralysis, and sodium channel myotonias. The sodium channel myotonias phenotypically resemble myotonia congenita but have atypical features distinguished by worsening of the myotonia with potassium challenge, hence their alternative name of potassium aggravated myotonias. There are a number of variants, including myotonia permanens, myotonia fluctuans, and acetazolamide-sensitive myotonia. Surprisingly, a small proportion of patients with hypokalemic periodic paralysis are also due to a sodium channel mutation.

The predominant symptoms of PMC are paradoxical myotonia, usually present from birth and persisting throughout life, and cold-induced weakness. The myotonia is paradoxical because, unlike classic myotonia, it increases with repetitive movements. The myotonia of PMC is exacerbated by cold exposure, particularly affecting the face, neck, forearms and, less so, the legs. Myotonia may be relieved spontaneously or upon warming although variable degrees of weakness can persist for hours. In a warm environment, patients may have no symptoms at all. Pain and muscle hypertrophy are usually not seen. In some affected families there is a tendency for attacks of paralysis to be independent of the myotonia and of the cold; these can be precipitated by potassium ingestion in much the same way as HYPP. Such symptoms of episodic non-temperature-provoked weakness tend to occur in adolescence, if at all.

As with PMC, HYPP appears in infancy or early childhood with frequent episodes of paralysis that are generally brief and mild and last 15 minutes to four hours. Attacks are often precipitated by a period of rest after exercise or the administration of potassium. They also commonly start in the morning before breakfast. Stress tends to make the attacks more easily provoked. Attacks can be diminished or aborted by carbohydrate intake or exercise. Weakness is mainly proximal, but distal muscles can be involved. There is usually no ocular or respiratory weakness. Examination during an attack reveals a flaccid tetraparesis with absent reflexes and normal sensa-

tion. Serum potassium concentrations may rise during the attack but not necessarily above the upper limit of normal range and rarely into levels that cause cardiac dysrhythmia. So-called normokalemic periodic paralysis may be a sodium channelopathy and merely part of the spectrum of HYPP. At least one family with normokalemic periodic paralysis can have the same Thr704Met sodium channel mutation commonly seen in HYPP. Between attacks, patients maintain normal strength, but in a few cases there is persistent mild weakness. The frequency of attacks may decline as the patient gets older. In some families with HYPP, there is coexistent myotonia that may be subclinical and only detected on electromyography (EMG). If symptomatic it is usually mild. In these patients, cooling may provoke weakness but does not provoke myotonia.

The sodium channel myotonias or potassium aggravated myotonia group of disorders of recently classified myotonias have been shown to be due to sodium channel gene mutations but not have the features of PMV or episodes of periodic paralysis.

Myotonic permanens is characterized by permanent very severe myotonia. One patient was originally diagnosed as having SJS, and another had myotonia severe enough to impair breathing.

In myotonia fluctuans, myotonia fluctuates on a daily basis, being undetectable on some days. When present, myotonia mainly affects eye closure, chewing, swallowing, and hand grip and show a warm-up phenomenon. The myotonia may worsen after exercise, typically after a delay of 20 to 40 minutes, and sometimes to the point of causing immobility. Such exacerbations may persist for 30 minutes to two hours. Exercise after cooling of the forearm may lead to worsening of the myotonia in some, but weakness is uncommon. It is not aggravated by cold. Potassium loading worsens the myotonia but does not cause episodes of weakness.

Acetazolamide-responsive myotonia is characterized by painful myotonia that responds to acetazolamide, both of which are atypical for myotonia congenita. In some patients, myotonia is worsened by cold but is unassociated with weakness or decrease in the compound muscle action potential (CMAP) as seen in PMC. Potassium loading worsens the painful myotonia but does not cause weakness as in HYPP. Fixed interictal weakness does not occur.

All of the aforementioned disorders result from allelic point mutations at the 17q23.3 locus of the sodium channel gene (SCN4A), resulting in amino acid substitutions in conserved portions of the gene, encoding the adult isoform of the skeletal muscle sodium channel α1 subunit. These mutations are all inherited in an autosomal dominant (AD) pattern. The effects of these mutations can be measured by electrical recording of sodium currents in dissociated fibers of muscle biopsies obtained from patients and in cultured myotubules and fibroblasts transfected with cDNA coding for mutant channels. All mutations so studied show abnormalities of voltage gating, causing slowing of fast inactivation of the sodium channel. This finding is consistent with the sites of these mutations that are either situated in the intracellular loop, which is believed to inactivate the channel by occluding the inner mouth of the pore, or else line the inner vestibule of the ion-conducting pore to which the inactivation gate binds. *In vitro* disruption of fast inactivation of just 2% of sodium channels using a specific toxin has shown that the resulting small persistent sodium current is sufficient to cause delayed relaxation of muscle twitch. A prolonged current pulse elicits a train of repetitive action potentials that persists beyond the duration of the current pulse. These effects are analogous to that seen in myotonia. The self-sustained train of discharges occurring after the stimulus depends on an intact T-tubule system. This is thought to occur partly by excess potassium accumulation in T tubules. Hayward and colleagues (1) introduced a missense substitution corresponding to the human M1592V mutation into the mouse *SCN4A* gene, and found that few homozygous mutant (m/m) mice survived and those that did had fixed-limb weakness, atrophy, and abnormal muscle morphology.

The *SCN4A* gene is only expressed in significant levels in skeletal muscle, thus explaining the lack of cardiac or CNS involvement in these disorders (2). Each point mutation has been correlated with a predominant phenotype. However, the various mutations are not distributed along the gene in an obvious way that correlates with the phenotype. Indeed, even adjacent mutations can cause different phenotypes. The Met1592val mutation caused a myotonic, non-dystrophic form of HYPP in six families, whereas an almost adjacent Val1589met mutation causes cold-induced potassium-aggravated myotonia (3, 4). Thr704Met and the Met1592val mutations account for 60% and 30%, respectively, of the genotyped families with HYPP. Those having the Thr704Met mutation were more likely to have fixed progressive weakness and myotonia. The Thr1313Met mutation occurs in 45% of patients with PMC, whereas the Arg1448cys accounts for 35% of patients. There is some overlap of phenotype with the Met1360val, Ser804Phe, Ala1156thr, and Val1592met mutations showing features of HYPP and paramyotonia in some families (5). Matthews and colleagues (6) identified mutations in the *CACNA1S* or *SCN4A* gene in 74/83 (90%) patients with HOKPP2, all of which, including three novel ones, affected arginine residues in the S4 voltage sensing region in1 of the transmembrane domains of each gene.

The phenotypic expression of an *SCN4A* mutation depends on the nature of the amino acid switch, as well as the site of the mutation. An elegant explanation for the descending severity of the myotonia with these mutations is that it appears to relate to decreasing length of the side chain of the substituted amino acid; glutamine has a large side chain, valine has an intermediate-length side chain, whereas alanine has a small one. The glycine at position 1306 is highly conserved and occupies the cytoplasmic loop between domains III and IV at the proposed site of the "hinge" for the "lid" occluding the ion channel pore. Glycine, having no side chains, confers a high degree of flexibility at the hinge that is compromised by its substitution by amino acids having side chains. The restriction of the hinge increases with the length of the side chains and causes increasing impairment of channel inactivation and thus worsening myotonia (7). One family with apparent HYPP was described in which there was no linkage to the *SCN4A* locus, suggesting genetic heterogeneity (8).

The Role of Sodium Channels in Pain

The diversity of sodium channels is illustrated in the diversity of their function, structure, and distribution. Sodium channel polypeptides are not expressed by a single gene but occur as multigene families, the individual products of which are known as isoforms. There are at least nine distinct sodium channel types, designated Nav1.1 to Nav1.9 and Nav2.x, widely distributed in the PNS and heart, encoded by the *SCN1A* to *SCN11A* genes (9).

The reason for the inherent diversity of sodium channel isoforms appears to reside in the need for excitation differences required for the different cell types they subserve; for example, fast channel kinetics for the transmission of high frequency of action potentials in myelinated fibers, or slow kinetic gating of certain other isoforms for long-duration action potentials of skeletal smooth muscle or cardiac tissue. Further amino acid sequence variations may encode signals that allow channel isoforms to be selectively localized to different membrane areas of specialized structures such as the nodes of Ranvier, neuronal dendrites, or muscle T-tubules.

Certain isoforms, such as Nav1.7, Nav1.8, and Nav1.9 are selectively expressed in PNS pain pathways, localized dominantly in peripheral sensory ganglia C-fiber nerve endings and nociceptive fields of the skin, teeth, and cornea that also contain substance P. Isoforms of sodium channels are selectively expressed in peripheral nociceptive pathways (10) where they appear to be functionally important in inflammatory and neuropathic pain (11–13).

Chronic pain appears to be associated with remodeling and altered expression of sodium channel isoforms in human and experimental animal models of chronic demyelination and conditions. Therein myelin fails to form developmentally (14, 15) such that the formation of sodium channel clusters, prompted by demyelination and guided by myelinating glial cells, provide important responses associated with pain. Such occurs in acute demyelinating insults along new nodes of Ranvier or chronically, wherein large numbers of amorphous and enlarged channel clusters form on demyelinated axons at sites of neuromas (9). Improvements in pain therapy might be achieved through development of compounds that specifically inhibit selectively expressed isoforms and sodium channel cluster formations (16–18).

CHLORIDE CHANNELOPATHIES

Three forms of myotonia congenital, Thomsen (THD), myotonia levior, and Becker disease are inherited in AD and autosomal recessive (AR) fashion. The main symptom of THD is painless generalized myotonia, perceived as muscle stiffness, which usually appears in the first and second decade of life, provoked by exertion after rest and demonstrated by asking the patient to rise from a seated position after a period of rest. Myotonia improves with exercise, and affected patients have well-developed muscles with particular hypertrophy of the legs, giving them an athletic appearance. Muscle strength can be normal, possibly even stronger than normal, giving them advantage in power sports where speed is not a requirement. They have normal deep tendon reflexes, with evocable eyelid, grip, and percussion-induced myotonia.

Becker disease is clinically similar to THD; however, myotonia comes on later in life but can be more severe and, in addition, to severe myotonic stiffness, affected patients may also have disabling transient weakness not seen in THD. Their muscles are initially strong and rapidly weaken with a period of activity before full strength returns. The length of time for strength to recover can be 30 minutes or longer, resulting in severe and incapacitating weakness and a misdiagnosis of muscular dystrophy or periodic paralysis. Untreated patients can become wheelchair confined. As in THD, there may be hypertrophy of leg and buttock muscles with spinal hyperlordosis.

Myotonia levior may be considered a mild form of THD. In one affected family (19), myotonia began at five years of age in two affected siblings, was worse with exercise, and the mother had a similar degree of myotonia. Examination showed absence of muscle hypertrophy and weakness. Lid lag, percussion- and grip-induced myotonia with warm-up phenomenon were present, but not aggravated by cooling nor by potassium loading.

The characteristic feature in both forms of myotonia congenita is reduced muscle membrane chloride conductance. This results in muscle membrane hyperexcitability with after-depolarization and repetitive firing leading to the myotonia. Similar abnormal physiology can be reproduced in normal muscle by chloride channel blockers or by the substitution of impermeable ions for chloride. Normal physiologic activity in muscle results in accumulation of potassium in the T-tubules. Where chloride conductance is normal, the depolarizing effect of this accumulated potassium is limited and has no significant consequence. If chloride conductance falls below 30% of the total membrane conductance, the accumulated potassium results in significant after-depolarization and repetitive, self-triggering electrical muscle activity.

All three allelic non–dystrophic skeletal muscle disorders are caused by mutation at the 7q34 locus of the CLCN1 gene encoding skeletal muscle chloride channel-1. Dupre and colleagues (20) described French Canadian kindred of four unrelated families with AD myotonia caused by heterozygous CLCN1 mutations. The mean age of onset was 13 years, and the commonest clinical features were percussion and hand-grip myotonia, warm-up phenomenon, generalized hypertrophy and muscle stiffness, and exacerbation with cold.

Myotonia levior is considered a low expressivity variant of THD. Dupre and colleagues (20) also described 27 French-Canadian patients with AR myotonia associated with biallelic CLCN1 mutations, of mean age at onset of 10 years, with lid lag, lid myotonia, lingual myotonia, and myotonia evoked by percussion and handgrip, with transient weakness, generalized hypertrophy, stiffness, myalgia, and exacerbation with cold temperature.

At least 18, mostly missense, mutations have been described in association with Becker disease (21). The F413X mutation is the most common Becker disease mutation. In one survey, three mutations (R894X, F413C, and the 14bp deletion in exon 13) accounted for nearly one–third of mutations seen in Becker disease (21).

A family with myotonia levior had a gln552arg mutation (19). Because a CLCN1 mutation can be either AR or AD, it becomes difficult to predict the phenotype and inheritance from mutational data alone unless the functional effects of the mutation are known.

Some previously described pathologic AR mutations were demonstrated to be non–pathogenic polymorphisms (21). Dominant mutations do not interfere with protein translation or turnover but when coexpressed 1:1 with wild-type chloride channels in the Xenopus oocyte expression system result in a reduction of the chloride current to 30% to 40% of normal (22). Using the same expression system, AR mutations result in lesser degrees of impairment of chloride conductance. Some mutations exert only a mild dominant negative effect. This may result in AD inheritance pattern with reduced penetrance as seen with the G239E mutation (22), or the mutation may be inherited in either AD or AR fashion as seen with the R894X mutation (21, 23).

Recessive mutations are either homozygous or may exist as compound heterozygotes. In some cases of AR Becker disease, no second mutation was found. Disease expression in true cases of single recessive mutations may be influenced by polymorphisms or the expression levels of other channels. The AR or AD expression of mutations exerting a mild dominant negative effect may also be dependent on similar influences of genetic background.

CALCIUM CHANNELOPATHIES

Type 1 HOKPP is the commonest familial periodic paralyses with an estimated prevalence of between 0.4 and l.25 per 100,000 (24). It is an AD inherited disorder with variable penetrance in women and thus appears to be more common in males. Sporadic cases, accounting for one–third of affected patients, represent new mutations and can transmit the disease to succeeding generations. Attacks usually start in adolescence with 60% occurring before age 16 years. Onset is invariably before age 30 years. Attacks may occur spontaneously, often at night, so that patients awake with a variable degree of weakness. They are most commonly precipitated by carbohydrate intake and rest after exercise but may also be provoked by cold exposure, alcohol, or emotional stress. The frequency of attacks is generally less than that seen in HYPP and can vary from daily or only one or two in a lifetime. The frequency of attacks may diminish with age. Normally, attacks last between one and four hours, but they can occasionally persist for up to three days. Patients are often unaware of the presence of attacks of moderately severe weakness. Prodromal symptoms of muscle stiffness, heavy limbs, or sweating may be followed by proximal lower limb weakness that evolves into tetraparesis. Although respiratory failure is rare, this and hypokalemia-induced cardiac dysrhythmias can cause fatality. Oliguria can result from the sequestration of intracellular water. In younger subjects, the only interictal abnormality may be eyelid myotonia, but older subjects, despite having fewer attacks, may have persistent and sometimes fluctuating weakness. Fixed inter-attack weakness occurs in most patients with frequent attacks. During attacks there is a flaccid, areflexic weakness. Ocular or bulbar involvement and respiratory failure rarely occur.

In HOKPP1, the weakness results from an abnormality of muscle membrane excitability. There is an influx of potassium into the muscle fiber with an accompanying influx of extracellular water that accounts for the oliguria that may be part of the attacks. There is increased sensitivity to the effect of insulin on the movement of potassium into cells independent of its glucopenic action. This may account for the precipitation of hypokalemic periodic paralysis with large carbohydrate meals. In contrast to normal muscle fibers, the influx of potassium in hypokalemic periodic paralysis causes the muscle fibers to become depolarized and inexcitable.

The disorder is caused by heterozygous mutation at the 1q32.1 locus of the dihydropyridine (DHP) receptor (CACNL1A3) gene. Matthews and colleagues (6) identified mutations in the CACNA1S gene in patients with HOKPP, the most common of which were R528H affecting residue arg528, R1239H and R1239G affecting arg1239, supporting the hypothesis (25) that loss of positive charge in S4 voltage sensors was important to the pathogenesis of the disorder.

The dihydropyridine receptor has a primary role in electrocontraction coupling with opening of the calcium channels of the sarcoplasmic reticulum, allowing an influx of calcium into the muscle sarcoplasm and triggering muscle contraction. Although the mutations described in HOKPP lead to a loss of function of the DHP receptor, it is not clear how this results in the abnormal response of muscle fibers to insulin with the consequent hypokalemia and weakness.

Patients with the arg1239his mutation have been younger and have lower potassium levels during attacks compared with those having the arg528His mutation (26); one kindred with the arg528his mutation had coexisting cardiac dysrhythmia, and incomplete penetrance in females is a characteristic of the arg528his mutation. Two disorders, susceptibility to thyrotoxic periodic paralysis (TTPP) and susceptibility to malignant hyperthermia (MHS), are allelic disorders. The former, a frequent complication of thyrotoxicosis among Chinese men, was associated with 12 single-nucleotide polymorphisms (SNP) in Cav1.1 (CACNA1S), three of which were novel, at or near a thyroid hormone–responsive element (TRE), making it possible that it affected binding affinity of the TRE and modulating the stimulation of thyroid hormone on the CAV1.1 gene. A susceptibility to MH, which previously corresponded to mutation in the skeletal ryanodine receptor (RYR1) gene, was ascertained in a mutation in the CACNL1A3 gene that segregated with the disorder in a large French family (27), that localized to a different region of the alpha-1 subunit of the human skeletal muscle L-type voltage-dependent calcium channel (VDCC), suggesting a direct interaction between the skeletal muscle VDCC and the ryanodine receptor in the skeletal muscle endoplasmic reticulum.

Faced with a patient having their first attack of paralysis, the differential diagnosis should include other causes of a flaccid areflexic tetraparesis without sensory involvement. The metabolic causes of hypercalcemia, hypocalcemia, hypophosphatemia, hypomagnesemia, and rhabdomyolysis should be excluded. Guillain-Barré syndrome (GBS), LEMS, and acute poliomyelitis can also produce this picture. In many patients, the history and associated features will point to the correct diagnosis.

Secondary HOKPP usually results from intracellular potassium depletion from renal, endocrine, or gastrointestinal potassium loss. These underlying conditions are usually obvious, but sometimes this is not the case, and the recurrent episodes of transient weakness can then be difficult to distinguish from HOKPP1. An onset after age 25 years should raise a strong suspicion of secondary rather than primary HOKPP1. This includes a susceptibility to TTPP, which results from an alteration of muscle membrane permeability and is more common in Asians but also occurs in Caucasians, the clinical presentation of which is indistinguishable HOKPP1.

ANDERSEN–TAWIL SYNDROME

Andersen and coworkers (28) described two patients with the triad of periodic paralysis, primary cardiac dysrhythmia unrelated to potassium concentration, and dysmorphic features. Tawil and colleagues (29) later employed the designation Andersen syndrome for the clinical trial of potassium-sensitive periodic paralysis, ventricular ectopy, and dysmorphic features, and showed that the syndrome was distinct from other forms of potassium–sensitive periodic paralysis. All patients so studied had potassium–sensitive periodic paralysis.

Attacks of periodic paralysis during the first two decades varied in frequency from one attack ever to one every five weeks, usually lasting a few hours. A recognized precipitant was rest after exercise. Fixed proximal weakness was seen in some cases. Provocative potassium challenges, particularly hypokalemic ones, are not advisable in the presence of preexisting cardiac dysrhythmia. Dysmorphic features included hypertelorism, low-set ears, broad nose, small mandible, clinodactyly, syndactyly high-arched palate, and scoliosis. The facial features were often subtle and better described as distinctive rather than dysmorphic.

Andersen-Tawil syndrome results from heterozygous AD mutation at the 17q24.3 locus of the *KCNJ2* gene that encodes the inwardly rectifying potassium (Kir), which is an important regulator of resting membrane potential and cell excitability (30). Some mutated channels do not co-assemble with wild type channels at the membrane; others interfere with trafficking of the channels to the membrane, and others do co-assemble and co-localize to the membrane but exert dominant-negative suppression of the Kir2.1 channel function (31). The short QT syndrome-3 (SQT3), which was identified in a missense mutation in the *KCNJ2* gene, is an allelic disorder, which in functional studies shows a significant increase in the outward component of the I-V relation of I(K1) (32).

THE DYSTROPHIC MYOTONIAS

Dystrophic Myotonia Type 1

This is the commonest adult-onset muscular dystrophy with an overall estimated prevalence of one in 8,000 (33). It shows AD inheritance with high penetrance and intrafamily phenotypic variation. It is characterized clinically mainly by myotonia, muscular dystrophy, cataracts, hypogonadism, frontal balding, and electrocardiographic abnormalities. Myotonia is rarely symptomatic but is an important diagnostic feature, with evidence thereof, in percussion of the tongue, thenar eminence, forearm extensor and muscles of hand grip, which diminishes with repeated contrac-

tions, the so-called warm-up phenomenon. Muscle wasting affects the temporalis, masseter, and sternocleidomastoid muscles, which along with frontal balding and ptosis, conveys a characteristic appearance. Distal muscle weakness, prominent at first in finger flexor, extensor, and intrinsic hand muscles, and foot extensors, is followed by proximal muscle involvement, although distal emphasis persists.

Nasal voice and dysarthria result from palatal, pharyngeal, and tongue involvement and may be complicated by respiratory insufficiency due to diaphragmatic and intercostal muscle weakness, reduced central respiratory drive, and hypersensitivity to sedating medication, depolarizing blockers, and general anesthetic agents.

Cardiac abnormalities including first-degree heart block or more extensive cardiac conduction defects occur, prompting prophylactic pacemaker insertion. Sudden death is more common in those with tachycardia.

Gastrointestinal symptoms include dysphagia and constipation due to megacolon and reflex myotonic contraction of the anal sphincter. Diabetes mellitus is uncommon despite the evidence of peripheral insulin resistance and increased insulinemia after glucose challenge. Testicular atrophy may be combined with reduced androgen and elevated gonadotropin levels, making infertility more common in both sexes. There is a high rate of fetal loss, and due to uterine smooth muscle involvement, delivery may be delayed, quite apart from any additional delay due to hypotonia in an affected fetus.

Personality change is common with paranoia, apathy, and lack of drive, often accentuated by hypersomnolence. Structural changes in the brain are infrequent, but brain scans may show cerebral atrophy, hydrocephalus, and white matter changes. Cataracts occur, especially in older patients where they may be the only feature of the disease, characteristically iridescent, multicolored crystalline flecks in the posterior subcapsular part of the lens, sometimes necessitating slit-lamp examination to visualize them. Meibomian cysts are common, and some patients may be found to have retinopathy and ophthalmoparesis.

Congenital dystrophia myotonica is a distinct phenotype of DM1 occurring in the offspring of some affected women, some of whom may not have been diagnosed, or unappreciated until after an affected infant is born. Intrauterine fetal hypotonia, often associated with reduced fetal movements, polyhydramnios, and delayed delivery, can render the infant floppy, necessitating ventilator support. Jaw and facial weakness gives a tented appearance to the mouth, causing feeding and sucking difficulty. Myotonia is not evident at this age. Those that survive have mental retardation and delayed motor milestones. DM1 is caused by heterozygous (CTG)n repeat expansion in the 3-prime untranslated region of the dystrophia myotonica protein kinase (*DMPK*) gene at the 19q13.32 chromosome locus. The normal CTGn repeat number, which ranges from 5 to 37, varies from 50 to thousands of repeats in affected individuals; a repeat length exceeding 50 CTG repeats is pathogenic (33).

Age at onset and severity of the disease correlate with repeat expansion size that tends to increase with successive generations, the largest of which are maternally transmitted, providing the molecular basis for anticipation. Replenishment of the gene pool is thought to be due to preferential expansion of the CTGn repeat by healthy individuals having alleles containing greater than 19 repeats. In heterozygous individuals, the allele with CTGn >19 is preferentially transmitted. Enlargement of the abnormal CTGn expansion with successive generations is correlated with the expansion size for both paternal and maternal transmission where the repeat size is less than 0.5 kilobases (kb). When the repeat size exceeds 0.5 kb, intergeneration enlargement of the expansion size is more likely for maternal transmission. Paternal transmission of alleles with expansion size greater than 1.5 kb results in contraction of the expansion size, and thus paternal transmission of congenital DM1 is a very rare but not unheard of event (34). There is a broad correlation between CTGn expansion size and the age at onset and the severity of the disease. A better correlation between tissue involvement and expansion size might, therefore, be found if the expansion size was measured in the affected tissue. Within a given tissue there may be a variation in expansion size, suggesting mitotic instability for the expansion. The smallest size expansion appears to be the original inherited allele that is, therefore, increasing with age, explaining the progressive nature of DM1. The smallest repeat length in blood is the one that correlates best with age at onset.

Wang and colleagues (35) generated an inducible and heart-specific mouse model of DM1 that expressed expanded human DMPK CUG-repeat RNA and recapitulated pathologic features of the human disorder, including dilated cardiomyopathy, arrhythmias, and systolic and diastolic dysfunction. Koshelev and colleagues (36) expressed human CUG triplet repeat RNA binding protein 1 (CUGBP1) in an adult mouse heart, up-regulation of which was sufficient to reproduce molecular, histopathologic, and functional changes observed in a DM1 mouse that expressed expanded CUG RNA repeats (35).

Dystrophic Myotonia Type 2

Heatwole and colleagues recently summarized the clinical and laboratory features of DM2 (37). Although originally described as two disorders, DM2 and PROMM are now referred to collectively as DM2 (38). Affected patients present between age 20 years and 60 years with myalgia, stiffness, myotonia, progressive weakness, male hypogonadism, arrhythmias, diabetes mellitus, and early cataracts, as well as hypersomnia, cognitive dysfunction, tremor, and hear-

ing loss. There is as yet no clear evidence of a neonatal presentation of DM2.

Muscle pain, unrelated to the myotonia, is a distinctive presenting feature often described as an unpleasant, intrusive, sore aching pain present at rest, resistant to aspirin and nonsteroidal anti-inflammatory medication. It can vary in intensity, sometimes disappearing for days at a time, without obvious explanation. Patients may have undue sensitivity to local muscle trauma.

The myotonia of DM2 seems to be associated with a distinctive jerky relaxation phase, particularly of the thumb and index finger, and shows a warm-up phenomenon; however, it may also be as mild and intermittent as to be clinically inapparent. Fluctuations in the severity of myotonia, pain, and weakness was related to temperature in two siblings who described worsening of symptoms in warm temperature accompanied by sparse myotonic discharges at room temperature that became more profuse on needle EMG as the muscle was warmed (39). Weakness is more often proximal than distal, particularly affecting the legs, however distal weakness occurs in the deep flexor muscles of the thumb and the lateral fingers and in the sternocleidomastoid weakness. There may be variability over hours or days with episodes of weakness, unrelated to exercise or to rest after exercise, and transient improvement for one-half hour after exercise.

Cardiac conduction defects occur in DM2 (40), and cataracts are common before age 50 years, indistinguishable from those seen in DM 1. Hypogonadism, insulin resistance and hypogammaglobulinemia are features common to both DM2 and DM1 (40–42) and one reported family had deafness (43). Three patients suffered stroke-like events, including one completed stroke, and two adult-onset epileptic seizures (44). Brain magnetic resonance imaging (MRI) showed white matter changes in six patients (44). Although initial reports stressed the lack of mental changes of the sort seen in DM1, apathy, hypersomnia, Parkinsonian features, and dystonia can all occur. Cognitive impairment and cerebral blood flow abnormalities have been described (45, 46). There can be phenotypic variation within families with some having asymptomatic cataracts or weakness. Anticipation occurs, but not as prominently as for DM1 (47).

Muscle tissue from patients with DM2 shows normal resting potential and normal chloride conductance. Spontaneous activity in isolated muscle fibers reduces with increased extracellular potassium concentration, the converse of that seen with most myotonias (48). Myotonic discharges were reduced on muscle cooling and increased with muscle warming, again the converse of what is seen in several other myotonic syndromes (39). Repetitive stimulation caused a decrement in the CMAP amplitude, particularly in proximal muscles, and this may relate to the development of weakness or its variability (39).

DM2 is caused by heterozygous expansion of a CCTG repeat in intron 1 of the zinc finger protein-9 (*ZNF9*) gene at the 3q21.3 chromosomal locus. Normal *ZNF9* alleles have up to 30 repeats, while pathological alleles contain 75 to 11,000 repeats (49). The literature cites patients with dystrophic myotonia without 19q CTG or 3q CTTG expansion mutations (50–53), making it likely that they were due to other genetic loci yet described.

SCHWARTZ-JAMPEL SYNDROME

In SJS, typical onset is after birth and usually before age three with severe continuous motor activity and muscle stiffness, particularly in the face. Patients have an unusual mask-like face with continuous motor activity of the chin and lips. Eye closure provokes blepharospasm, whereas excitement can cause worsening of muscle contraction and even laryngeal spasm. Hypertrophy of the shoulder muscles with shortening of the neck can occur, as can hypertrophy of thigh muscles. The voice may be high-pitched. They may have a variety of skeletal malformations, including contractures and short stature. Patients show a slow progression sometimes halting or even showing mild improvement in their teens (54).

The diagnosis should be based upon onset after birth and the presence of skeletal malformation on bone radiographs, with EMG evidence of myotonia (54), thus separating classic SJS from more severe neonatal phenotypes that are not genetically linked, those where facial features are due to severe myotonia rather than skeletal malformations, and others with similar skeletal abnormalities without myotonia. Although EMG activity can be continuous or interspersed by periods of electrical silence, it can be abolished by curare, suggesting neurogenic origin, whereas in others the discharges continue and would therefore be of muscle origin. These heterogeneous EMG findings may be explained by the fact that not all reported patients are classic SJS type. The application of stricter clinical criteria for SJS, backed by genetic confirmation, may help clarify the EMG characteristics of the myotonia. The disorder is caused by missense and splicing mutations at the 1p36.12 locus of the *HSPG2* gene encoding perlecan, which has a role in the maintenance of cartilage integrity, but presumably also in regulating muscle excitability (54, 55). Neonatal SJS2, also known as Stuve-Wiedmann syndrome (STWS), is genetically distinct, with a more severe phenotype due to mutation in the *LIFR* gene on chromosome 5p13.

INVESTIGATION OF THE MYOTONIAS AND PERIODIC PARALYSES

Myotonias

The serum creatine kinase (CK) is usually normal, but there may be borderline elevations in THD and Becker disease reflecting the degree of muscle hypertrophy. EMG shows spontaneous myotonic discharges, but in PMC and myotonic dystrophy, provocation by cooling of the examined limb may be required to demonstrate this. Myotonic discharges may not be apparent in children with myotonic dystrophy who are under the age of five years. There is also decrement in the CMAP with exercise or with high-frequency 30-Hz stimulation, particularly in cases of myotonia congenita. The decrement in the CMAP amplitude is particularly marked in Becker disease, and this may be the substrate for the transient weakness seen in that condition. Myopathic EMG features may be seen in both DM1 and DM2, however muscle biopsy tissue may show little abnormality or the expected myopathic features of myofiber size variation, hypertrophy, and increased central nuclei. In DM1 and DM2 there may be selective type-1 fiber atrophy, whereas in myotonia congenita there may be a lack of 2B fibers. Ring fibers and sarcoplasmic masses may be seen in myotonic dystrophy, but muscle fiber necrosis and increased connective tissue are uncommon. In PMC with HYKK, vacuolated fibers and necrotic fibers may be seen.

Study of family members may be valuable because there may be clinical or EMG evidence of disease in apparently asymptomatic individuals, which clarifies the mode of inheritance. Slit-lamp examination may be valuable for carrier detection and diagnosis in myotonic dystrophies. ECG is strongly advisable in cases of myotonic dystrophy.

Clinically it is possible to distinguish PMC from other sodium channel myotonias as PMC is characterized by a marked worsening of myotonia by cold and by the presence of clear episodes of weakness. By contrast, the other sodium channel myotonias are characterized by the absence of episodic weakness but may have myotonia that is cold sensitive.

Chloride channel myotonias may be distinguishable from sodium channel myotonias by the presence of warm-up phenomenon, the absence of paradoxical myotonia, the infrequent occurrence of eyelid myotonia, minimal or absent sensitivity to cold, and transient weakness (56). Where there is clinical overlap, as with some forms of sodium channel myotonia and dominant chloride channel myotonia, detailed neurophysiology assessment may be helpful. These rely on assessing the reduction in CMAP area following a short exercise test for 10 to 20s with and without cooling, and the reduction of CMAP during the long exercise test for three to five minutes with three patterns of response recognized.

Pattern I is a gradual and prolonged decrement in CMAP after exercise most often seen with PMC. This decrement is exacerbated with repeat testing and muscle cooling reflecting the clinically observed cold- and exercise-induced weakness. Pattern II, in which there is an immediate CMAP decrement after exercise that recovers quickly and diminishes with repetition, is most commonly seen in recessive chloride channel myotonia and reflects the transient weakness observed clinically. Pattern III, normal responses to all provocative tests with EMG myotonia as usually the only positive electrophysiological finding is the characteristic finding in sodium channel myotonia (56, 57).

Periodic Paralysis

During an episode, blood tests should be examined for potassium, calcium, magnesium, phosphate, and CK to exclude other causes of myopathic disease. The potassium level may be normal during HYKK and occasionally elevated in HOKPP. Potassium levels should be monitored every 15 to 30 minutes to determine the direction of change at the time when muscle strength is either worsening or improving. An ECG may show changes consistent with hypo- or hyperkalemia and may also forewarn of cardiac complications. EMG shows reduced CMAP amplitudes proportionate to the degree of weakness. Nerve conduction studies, which are otherwise normal, can exclude other causes of paralysis, including GBS, MG, and LEMS.

Patients seen between attacks should undergo investigations to exclude causes of secondary hypokalemia. EMG may be helpful in showing evidence of myotonia that favors HYKK, and in those with fixed weakness, the EMG may be myopathic. Patients with an initially normal EMG may demonstrate a characteristic decrement of the CMAP amplitudes with 30-Hz stimulation or after repetitive muscle contraction. Muscle biopsy is often abnormal between attacks of HOKPP with pathognomonic changes of large central vacuoles and occasional necrotic fibers. In HYKK, smaller vacuoles may be present and tubular aggregates may be seen. Provocative testing may be required to confirm the diagnosis. This must be performed with careful supervision, including monitoring of the potassium and the ECG. A hypokalemic challenge can be performed by administering intravenous glucose with or without insulin. Hyperkalemic challenge can be performed by giving repeated small doses of oral potassium.

TREATMENT OF THE MYOTONIAS AND PERIODIC PARALYSES

There are four clinical symptoms that demand treatment in the myotonia and periodic paralyses including attacks of weakness, persistent fixed weakness, muscle stiffness, and muscle pain. Satisfactory treatment is now available for all symptoms, with the exception of attacks of weakness. There is inadequate controlled data to defend a specific treatment regimen.

Myotonias

Myotonia can be exacerbated by certain muscle relaxant drugs and by anticholinesterase drugs; in addition, anesthesia for these patients needs to be appropriately planned. Potassium administration can exacerbate myotonia, particularly sodium channel disorders, and thus potassium supplementation should only be given where necessary and with caution. Although it has been stated that there is an association between myotonias and malignant hyperthermia necessitating anesthetic precautions, the documentation of this statement is not sufficient to warrant pretreatment with dantrolene.

The treatment of myotonia congenita relies on membrane stabilizing drugs such as procainamide and quinine, and these can be used intermittently on an as-needed basis. Phenytoin is more useful for chronic administration and is less likely to have cardiac side effects. Occasional cases of myotonia, particularly sodium channel myotonia, are responsive to acetazolamide. Mexilitine is useful for both the myotonia and the weakness associated with PMC and Becker myotonia.

A randomized, controlled trial (58) compared 150 mg of mexiletine three times daily with placebo in 20 subjects with DM1 who had grip or percussion myotonia using a cross-over design with seven-week treatment periods separated by a four- to eight-week washout period. It showed a significant reduction in the time for isometric grip force to relax from 90% to 5% of peak force after a three-second maximum grip contraction. There were no serious adverse events and the ECGs did not show prolongation of the PR or QTc intervals or of QRS duration. The same trial design also tested mexiletine at a dose of 200 mg 3 times daily with the same favorable outcome.

Periodic Paralysis

Attacks of HOKPP may be partially prevented by a low carbohydrate and low sodium diet. Acetazolamide was initially noted to be effective in preventing paralytic attacks and improving residual weakness between attacks. A randomized, controlled trial of dichlorphenamide showed efficacy in the treatment of HOKPP (59). Hypokalemic periodic paralysis secondary to thyrotoxicosis should be likewise treated, however interim management includes of the paralytic attacks and persistent weakness can be very effectively treated with α-adrenergic blocking agents. During acute attacks of HOKPP, emergency parenteral potassium treatment may be required, but the preference is very much in favor of oral potassium in these patients.

Supportive therapy may be required for respiratory impairment, and the ECG should be carefully monitored for any cardiac dysrhythmia. In HYPP, attacks are usually mild but are still worth treating to prevent the onset of permanent weakness. Thiazide diuretics are usually effective treatment. During acute attacks, treatment is rarely needed, but carbohydrate-containing food and fluid may aggravate the weakness and potassium-containing foods should be avoided. Inhaled β-adrenergic agonists such as salbutamol are effective treatments but may be contraindicated if there is a coexisting cardiac dysrhythmia (60).

NEUROMYOTONIA

Isaacs Disease

This is a syndrome in which neuromyotonia or hyperexcitability of peripheral nerves results in spontaneous and continuous muscle activity. Although some are inherited, most are acquired. The syndrome is rare, and assessment of its frequency and definitive clinical features is hampered by the variable names given to it in the past.

Typical patients have muscle stiffness, cramps, myokymia, and pseudomyotonias. They may also have generalized weakness and sweating. Onset can be any time during life, and the condition tends to be chronic. Motor features are most prominent in the limbs and trunk. Respiratory muscle involvement can cause breathing difficulty and laryngeal involvement can cause stridor. Examination may reveal mild weakness with reduced or absent tendon reflexes and evidence of myokymia with occasional muscle hypertrophy as a result. The continuous electrical discharges may originate anywhere along the length of the peripheral nerve. EMG confirms the presence of neuromyotonia in the form of doublets, triplets, or multiplet spontaneous motor unit discharges that may be present even in the absence of visible myokymia. Nerve and muscle biopsies show nonspecific features. In a few cases of Isaacs disease, oligoclonal IgG was found in the cerebrospinal fluid.

There is an association between Isaacs disease and autoimmune disease, and it is believed that the acquired varieties are in fact autoimmune, due to antibodies against potassium channel (61, 62). Anticonvulsant medication such as phenytoin and carbamazepine are first line therapy, while plasma exchange and immunosuppressive agents may be appropriate when there is an evident autoimmune etiology.

SUSCEPTIBILITY TO MALIGNANT HYPERTHERMIA

Susceptibility to malignant hyperthermia is an hereditary skeletal muscle disease, characterized by a hypercatabolic reaction of muscle to anesthetic agents or to physical or emotional stress. It has a worldwide distribution with an incidence of one in 12,000 anesthetic incidents in children and one in 50,000 anesthetic events in adults. However, it is possible that many mild cases go unrecognized and are mistaken for other anesthetic complications. Males are more affected than females, and there is a peak incidence at the age of 30 years, after which the incidence declines such that cases are virtually unheard of beyond the age of 75 years.

The most common precipitating event is that of halothane general anesthesia. The muscle relaxant succinylcholine is a milder trigger of attacks when used alone but a more potent one when combined with halothane. The likelihood of triggering an attack with these agents is increased if the patient has been exercising vigorously beforehand or is under stress at the time of anesthetic induction. In between attacks, patients rarely have any muscle symptoms, although some muscle diseases are associated with attacks of malignant hyperthermia. In up to 50% of patients, previous anesthesia had no complication. Attacks often start with jaw spasm followed by generalized muscle spasm and rigidity. This is associated with hyperventilation, tachycardia, and an unstable blood pressure. A mottled, flushed, and cyanotic skin rash may appear, and after an interval of 15 to 60 minutes, the body temperature may start to rise precipitously. Metabolic and respiratory acidosis, hypoxemia, generalized vasoconstriction, and an increased cardiac output then occur. The serum potassium and CK may rise, the latter up to 100-fold. Consequent complications of myoglobinuria and disseminated intravascular coagulation may occur, either of which can lead to renal failure. During recovery, patients may have a further relapse.

The central event in MHS appears to be an increase in the calcium concentration that results in continuous activation of the actin-myosin contraction apparatus and sustained muscle contraction. This increase in calcium level is due to an increased release of calcium from the sarcoplasmic reticulum of the muscle together with a reduction in calcium re-uptake. The continuous muscle activity results in the muscle rigidity, muscle necrosis, hyperpyrexia, and hypermetabolism. One form, MHS1, is caused by heterozygous mutation at the 19q13.2 locus of the *RYR1* receptor gene, a calcium-released channel involved in calcium homeostasis. During the acute illness, the main emphasis of the evaluation is monitoring possible hyperkalemic, cardiac, respiratory, or renal complications so that appropriate measures can be taken.

Evaluation of well patients thought to be at risk of developing malignant hyperthermia can be difficult. Only a few have a raised serum CK. The genetic heterogeneity and the fact that even the recognized point mutations only cover a small percentage of the patients at risk limit the value of genetic testing. A variety of in vivo tests have been purported to highlight at-risk individuals, but these are not particularly reliable. The recognized screening test is the *in vitro* caffeine and halothane contracture test in which one looks for an exaggerated response to caffeine or halothane in freshly isolated muscle. This test is performed only in specialized centers. Even so the overlap between normal and affected individuals is such that false-positive tests, are invariable.

Preventive measures include the avoidance of precipitating agents, namely halothane and succinylcholine. Patients should be advised to wear medical alert bracelets to warn of their susceptibility to malignant hypothermia. Narcotics, barbiturates, benzodiazepines, nitrous oxide, and depolarizing muscle relaxants are safe to use. Acute management consists of the removal of the triggering agents and supportive measures as required. Rapid measures to produce body cooling may be required in response to the hyperpyrexia that, if allowed to continue, aggravates metabolic derangements. Dantrolene is the mainstay of treatment and, given intravenously, results in reversal of the abnormalities. The improved recognition of this complication and better supportive measures with the availability of dantrolene have resulted in a dramatic drop in mortality from 65% to 2%.

RIPPLING MUSCLE DISEASE

Patients with rippling muscle disease (RMD) notice rippling of the muscles or complain of muscle spasms, but these are rarely troublesome. The rippling may be self-induced, especially after a period of rest or in the cold. Percussion of the muscle may cause painless contraction, swelling, or mounding of the muscle that may then roll across the limb over a 10-second period. There is no associated muscle wasting or weakness. There may be modest elevations of the CK. Needle EMG shows no abnormality, and the rippling itself is electrically silent. Muscle biopsy shows nonspecific features of variation in fiber size and scatter atrophic fibers. One patient's muscle tissue showed selective type I fiber atrophy (63). Familial AD, AR, and sporadic cases have been described (63, 64).

The cause of the rippling remains unclear. It has been speculated that it may be due to slow propagation of an internal sarcoplasmic action potential. The mechanical sensitivity could be due to activation of stretch-sensitive channels. One sporadic case of rippling muscles also developed MG and both remitted with immunotherapy, leading to speculation of an autoimmune basis for rippling muscles (64). Familial cases are genetically heterogeneous with RMD2 demonstrating mutations at the 3p25.3 locus of the *CAV3* gene encoding caveolin-3 (65), and RMD1 mapping to chromosome 1q41 (66).

REFERENCES

1. Hayward LJ, Kim JS, Lee M-Y, et al. Targeted mutation o mouse skeletal muscle sodium channel produces myotonia and potassium-sensitive weakness. *J Clin Invest* 2008; 118:1437–1449.

2. Trimmer JS, Cooperman SS, Tomiko SA, et al. Primary structure and functional expression of a mammalian skeletal muscle sodium channel. *Neuron* 1989; 3:33–49.

3. Heine R, Pika U, Lehmann-Horn F. A novel SCN4A mutation causing myotonia aggravated by cold and potassium. *Human Molecular Genetics* 1993; 2:1349–1353.

4. Kelly P, Yang WS, Costigan D, et al. Paramyotonia congenital and hyperkalemic periodic paralysis associated with a new met1592-to-val substitution in the skeletal muscle sodium channel alpha-subunit-a large kindred with a novel phenotype. *Neuromuscul Disord* 1997; 7:105–111.

5. Lehmann-Horn F, Rudel R, Ricker K. Workshop report; nondystrophic myotonias and periodic paralyses. *Neuromuscul Disord* 1993; 3:161–168.

6. Matthews E, Labrum R, Sweeney MG, et al. Voltage sensor charge loss accounts for most cases of hypokalemic periodic paralysis. *Neurology* 2009; 72:1544–1547.

7. Lerche H, Heine R, Pica U, et al. Human sodium channel myotonia: slowed channel inactivation due to substitutions for a glycine within the III–IV linker. *J Physiology* 1993; 470:13–22.

8. Wang J, Zhou J, Todorovic SM, et al. Molecular genetic and genetic correlations in sodium channelopathies: lack of founder effect and evidence for a second gene. *Am J Hum Genet* 1993; 52:1074–1084.

9. Levinson SR, Luo S, Henry MA. The role of sodium channels in chronic pain. *Muscle Nerve* 2012; 46:155–165.

10. Dib-Hajj DS, Cummins TR, Black JA, et al. From genes to pain: Nav1.7 and human pain disorders. *Trends Neurosci* 2007; 30:555–563.

11. Krafte DS, Bannon AW. Sodium channels and nociception: recent concepts and therapeutic opportunities. *Curr Opin Pharmacol* 2008; 8:50–56.

12. Gold MS. Na (+) channel blockers for the treatment of pain: context is everything, almost. *Exp Neurol* 2008; 210:1–6.

13. Dib-Hajj SD, Cummins TR, Black JA, et al. Sodium channels in normal and pathological pain. *Annu Rev Neurosci* 2010; 33:325–347.

14. Henry MA, Freking AR, Johnson LR, et al. Increased sodium channel immunofluorescence at myelinated and demyelinated sites following an inflammatory and partial axotomy lesion of the rat infraorbital nerve. *Pain* 2006; 124:222–233.

15. Luo S, Perry GM, Levinson SR, et al. Pulpitis increases the proportion of atypical nodes of Ranvier in human dental pulp axons without a change in Nav 1.6 sodium channel expression. *Neuroscience* 2010; 169:1881–1887.

16. Priest BT. Future potential and status of selective channel blockers for the treatment of pain. *Curr Opin Drug Discov Devel* 2009; 12:682–692.

17. Priest BT, Kaczorowski GJ. Subtype-selective sodium channel blockers promise a new era of pain research. *Proc Natl Acad Sci USA* 2007; 104:8205–8206.

18. Zuliani V, Patel MK, Fantini M, et al. Recent advances in the medicinal chemistry of sodium channel blockers and their therapeutic potential. *Curr Top Med Chem* 2009; 9:396–415.

19. Lehmann-Horn F, Mailander V, Heine R, et al. Myotonia levior is a chloride channel disorder. *Human Molecular Genetics* 1995; 4:1397–1402.

20. Dupre N, Christian N, Bouchard J-P, et al. Clinical, electrophysiologic, and genetic study of non-dystrophic myotonia in French-Canadians. *Neuromusc Disord* 2009; 19:330–334.

21. Meyer-Kleine C, Steinmeyer K, Ricker K, et al. Spectrum of mutations in the major human skeletal muscle chloride channel gene (CLCN1) leading to myotonia. *Am J Hum Genet* 1995; 57:1325–1334.

22. Steinmeyer K, Lorenz C, Pusch M, et al. Multimeric structure of ClC-1 chloride channel revealed by mutations in dominant myotonia congenita (Thomsen). *EMBO Journal* 1994; 13:737–743.

23. George AL, Jr., Sloan-Brown K, Fenichel GM, et al. Nonsense and missense mutations of the muscle chloride channel gene in patients with myotonia congenita. *Human Molecular Genetics* 1994; 3:2071–2072.

24. Kantola IM, Tarssanen LT. Familial hypokalemic periodic paralysis in Finland. *J Neurol Neurosurg Psychiatry* 1992; 55:322–324.

25. Sokolov S, Scheuer T, Catterall WA, et al. Gating pore current is an inherited ion channelopathy. *Nature* 2007; 446:76–78.

26. Elbaz A, Vale-Santos J, Jurkat-Rott K, et al. Hypokalemic periodic paralysis and the dihydropyridine receptor (CACNL1A3): genotype/phenotype correlations for two predominant mutations and evidence for the absence of a founder effect in 16 Caucasian families. *Am J Hum Genet* 1995; 56:374–380.

27. Monnier N, Procaccio V, Stieglitz P, et al. Malignant-hyperthermia susceptibility is associated with a mutation of the alpha-1-subunit of the human dihydropyridine-sensitive L-type voltage-dependent calcium-channel receptor in skeletal muscle. *Am J Hum Genet* 1997; 60:1316–1325.

28. Andersen ED, Krasilnikoff PA, Overvad H. Intermittent muscular weakness, extrasystoles, and multiple developmental anomalies. A new syndrome? *Acta Paediatrica Scandinavica* 1971; 60:559–564.

29. Tawil R, Ptacek LJ, Pavlakis SG, et al. Andersen's syndrome: potassium-sensitive periodic paralysis, ventricular ectopy, and dysmorphic features. *Ann Neurol* 1994; 35:326–330.

30. Davies NP, Imbrici P, Fialho D, et al. Andersen-Tawil syndrome: new potassium channel mutations and possible phenotypic variation. *Neurology* 2005; 65:1083–1089.

31. Bendahhou S, Donaldson MR, Plaster NM, et al. Defective potassium channel Kir2.1 trafficking underlies Andersen-Tawil syndrome. *J Biol Chem* 2003; 278:51779–51785.

32. Priori SG, Pandit SV, Rivolta I, et al. A novel form of short QT syndrome (SQT3) is caused by a mutation n the KCNJ2 gene. *Circ Res* 2005; 96:800–807.

33. Musova Z, Mazanec R, Krepelova A, et al. Highly unstable sequence interruptions of the CTG repeat in the myotonic dystrophy gene. *Am J Med Genet* 2009; 149A:1365–1374.

34. Nakagawa M, Yamada H, Higuchi I, et al. K. A case of paternally inherited congenital myotonic dystrophy. *J Medical Genetics* 1994; 31:397-400.

35. Wang G-S, Kearney DL, De Biasi M, et al. Elevated of RNA-binding protein CUGBP1 is an early event in an inducible heart-specific mouse model of myotonic dystrophy. *J Clin Invest* 2007; 117:2802–2811.

36. Koshelev M, Sarma S, Price RE, et al. Heart-specific overexpression of CUGBP1 reproduces functional and molecular abnormalities of myotonic dystrophy type 1. *Hum Molec Genet* 2010; 19:1066–1075.

37. Heatwole C, Johnson N, Goldberg B, et al. Laboratory abnormalities in patients with myotonic dystrophy type 2. *Arch Neurol* 2011; 68:1180–1184.

38. Udd B, Meola G, Krahe R, et al. Report of the 115th ENMC workshop: DM2/PROMM and other myotonic dystrophies. 3rd Workshop, 14–16 February 2003, Naarden, The Netherlands. *Neuromuscul Disord* 2003; 13:589–596.

39. Sander HW, Tavoulareas GP, Chokroverty S. Heat-sensitive myotonia in proximal myotonic myopathy. *Neurology* 1996; 47:956–962.

40. Day JW, Ricker K, Jacobsen JF, et al. Myotonic dystrophy type 2: molecular, diagnostic and clinical spectrum. *Neurology* 2003; 60:657–664.

41. Savkur RS, Philips AV, Cooper TA. Aberrant regulation of insulin receptor alternative splicing is associated with insulin resistance in myotonic dystrophy. *Nat Genet* 2001; 29:40–47.

42. Savkur RS, Philips AV, Cooper TA, et al. Insulin receptor splicing alteration in myotonic dystrophy type 2. *Am J Hum Genet* 2004; 74:1309–1313.

43. Udd B, Krahe R, Wallgren-Pettersson C, et al. Proximal myotonic dystrophy—a family with autosomal dominant muscular dystrophy, cataracts, hearing loss and hypogonadism: heterogeneity of proximal myotonic syndromes? *Neuromusc Disord* 1997; 7:217–228.

44. Hund E, Jansen O, Koch MC, et al. Proximal myotonic myopathy with MRI white matter abnormalities of the brain. *Neurology* 1997; 48:33–37.

45. Meola G, Sansone V, Perani D, et al. Executive dysfunction and avoidant personality trait in myotonic dystrophy type 1 (DM-1) and in proximal myotonic myopathy (PROMM/DM-2). *Neuromusc Disord* 2003; 13:813–821.

46. Meola G, Sansone V, Perani D, et al. Reduced cerebral blood flow and impaired visual-spatial function in proximal myotonic myopathy. *Neurology* 1999; 53:1042.

47. Schneider C, Ziegler A, Ricker K, et al. Proximal myotonic myopathy: Evidence for anticipation in families with linkage to chromosome 3q. *Neurology* 2000; 55:383–388.

48. Ricker K, Koch MC, Lehmann-Horn F, et al. Proximal myotonic myopathy: a new dominant disorder with myotonia, muscle weakness, and cataracts. *Neurology* 1994; 44:1448–1452.

49. Todd PK, Paulson HL. RNA-mediated neurodegeneration in repeat expansion disorders. *Ann Neurol* 2010; 67:291–300.

50. Bonsch D, Neumann C, Lang-Roth R, et al. PROMM and deafness: exclusion of ZNF9 as the disease gene in DFNA18 suggests a polygenic origin of the PROMM/DM2 phenotype. *Clin Genet* 2003; 63:73–75.

51. Kress W, Mueller-Myhsok B, Ricker K, et al. Proof of genetic heterogeneity in the proximal myotonic myopathy syndrome (PROMM) and its relationship to myotonic dystrophy type 2 (DM2). *Neuromuscul Disord* 2000; 10:478–480.

52. Wieser T, Bonsch D, Eger K, et al. A family with PROMM not linked to the recently mapped PROMM locus DM2. *Neuromuscul Disord* 2000; 10:141–143.

53. Le B, I, Martinez M, Campion D, et al. A non-DM1, non-DM2 multisystem myotonic disorder with frontotemporal dementia: phenotype and suggestive mapping of the DM3 locus to chromosome 15q21–24. *Brain* 2004; 127:1979–1992.

54. Nicole S, Topaloglu H, Fontaine B. 102nd ENMC International Workshop on Schwartz-Jampel syndrome, 14–16 December, 2001, Naarden, The Netherlands. *Neuromuscul Disord* 2003; 13:347–351.

55. Nicole S, Davoine CS, Topaloglu H, et al. Perlecan, the major proteoglycan of basement membranes, is altered in patients with Schwartz-Jampel syndrome (chondrodystrophic myotonia). *Nat Genet* 2000; 26:480–483.

56. Matthews E, Fialho D, Tan SV, et al. The non-dystrophic

myotonias: molecular pathogenesis, diagnosis and treatment. *Brain* 2010; 133:9–22.

57. Tan SV, Matthews E, Barber M, et al. Refined exercise testing can aid DNA-based diagnosis in muscle channelopathies. *Ann Neurol* 2011; 69:328–340.

58. Logigian EL, Martens WB, Moxley RT, et al. Mexiletine is an effective antimyotonia treatment in myotonic dystrophy type 1. *Neurology* 2010; 74:1441–1448.

59. Griggs RC, Tawil R, Brown R, et al. Dichlorphenamide is effective in the treatment of hypokalemic periodic paralysis. *Ann Neurol* 1997; 42:428.

60. Hanna MG, Stewart J, Schapira AH, et al. Salbutamol treatment in a patient with hyperkalaemic periodic paralysis due to a mutation in the skeletal muscle sodium channel gene (SCN4A). *J Neurol Neurosurg Psychiatry* 1998; 65:248–250.

61. Hart IK, Waters C, Vincent A, et al. Autoantibodies detected to expressed K+ channels are implicated in neuromyotonia. *Ann Neurol* 1997; 41:238–246.

62. Shillito P, Molenaar PC, Vincent A, et al. Aquired neuromytonia: evidence for autoantibodies directed against K+ channels of peripheral nerves. *Ann Neurol* 1995; 38:714–722.

63. Burns RJ, Bretag AH, Blumbergs PC, et al. Benign familial disease with muscle mounding and rippling. *J Neurol Neurosurg Psychiatry* 1994; 57:344–347.

64. Ansevin CF, Agamanolis DP. Rippling muscles and myasthenia gravis with rippling muscles. *Arch Neurol* 1996; 53:197–199.

65. Betz RC, Schoser BGH, Kasper D, et al. Mutations in CAV3 cause mechanical hyperirritability of skeletal muscle in rippling muscle disease. *Nature Genet* 2001; 28:218–219.

66. Stephan DA, Buist NR, Chittenden AB, et al. A rippling muscle disease gene is localized to 1q41: evidence for multiple genes. *Neurology* 1994; 44:1915–1920.

CHAPTER 23

Facioscapulohumeral Muscular Dystrophy

David S. Younger

Facioscapulohumeral muscular dystrophy (FSHD), also known as FSHD1, is the third most common autosomal dominant (AD) hereditary myopathy after the dystrophinopathies and myotonic muscular dystrophy, with variable onset from infancy to adulthood, and characteristic clinical involvement of facial, scapula, foot dorsiflexor, and hip girdle muscles. In contrast to most monogenic disorders in which the genetic lesion typically affects the structure or function of a specific disease gene, current evidence suggests that FSHD is caused by a complex epigenetic mechanism involving the contraction of the D4Z4 subtelomeric macrosatellite repeat. Spatiotemporal–restricted transcription control of one or more disease genes is perturbed as a result of repeat-contraction-mediated chromatin alterations (1). In essence, each 3.3 kb D4Z4 macrosatellite repeat unit contains a double homeobox 4 (DUX4) gene that is activated at a distance due to the induction of chromatin remodeling of the 4qter region. Permissive FSHD haplotypes, each associated with a polyadenylation signal located immediately distal of the last D4Z4 unit, are expressed as a result of DUX4 mRNA transcripts and protein from the most distal DUX4 unit in FSHD myocytes, the latter of which induces significant cellular toxicity (2).

HISTORICAL ASPECTS

Landouzey and Dejerine (3) first described FSHD in a family of four generations. Tyler and Stephens (4) and Tyler (5) reported 17 additional families between 1950 and 1953 followed by Justin-Besancon and colleagues (6) who added three generations to those previously described by Landouzey and Dejerine (3). Small (7) described four siblings with FSHD and bilateral retinal exudative telangiectasia, termed Coats disease, in addition to sensorineural deafness and mental retardation, many features of which were later seen in FSHD patients reported by Taylor (8) and Voit and colleagues (9).

Peripheral retinal capillary abnormalities were further documented in FSHD by Fitzsimons (10), and Padberg and coworkers (11). Restrictive pulmonary disease and cor pulmonale were reported by Yasukohchi and coworkers (12), as was epilepsy in others described by Miura and colleagues (13). Bodensteiner and Schochet (14) identified the supraspinatus muscle as the choice for biopsy. Shen and Madsen (15) described the necessity of atrial pacing in a woman with severe FSHD and symptomatic atrial tachycardia.

EPIDEMIOLOGY

Morton and Chung (16) estimated the frequency of FSHD to be about 2 to 4 per million births, with a prevalence of 4 to 10 persons per 100,000 population. The penetrance of the FSHD gene is probably less than 5% for age up to 4 years, 21% for age 5 to 9 years, and 58% for those 10 to 14 years, increasing to 86% for age 15 to 19, and 95% in those age 20 years or older (17). A study of 34 Brazilian families concluded that at least one-third of cases arose as new mutations (18).

The excess number of affected men has been explained by a greater proportion of asymptomatic women, and a significantly greater number of affected sons than daughters of asymptomatic mothers. The penetrance by age 30 was 95% for men and only 69% for women. Anticipation in FSHD, originally suggested by Zatz and colleagues (18) and substantiated by Tawil and colleagues (19), may in fact be

433

related more to gender differences in penetrance wherein affected male offspring of affected mothers are likely to be more severely affected.

CLINICAL ASPECTS

The disorder should be suspected in those with onset typically by age 20 years and weakness of the face, scapular stabilizers, and foot dorsiflexor muscles. Onset of the disease is variable with more than 90% of affected patients presenting by age 20, although some patients with severe infantile FSHD have weakness at birth. Others, by comparison, with mild disease may remain asymptomatic.

The weakness is typically of the lower facial muscles with inability to purse lips or close the lids tightly. The shoulders tend to slope forward with straightened clavicles and scapular winging and preferential upward movement when attempting to flex or abduct the arms, however there is often prominent asymmetry of limb and scapular weakness. The deltoid muscles may remain minimally affected with selective involvement of the biceps and triceps leading to preferential atrophy of the upper arm and sparing of forearm muscles leading to so-called Popeye arms. Abdominal muscle weakness leads to protuberance of the abdomen and an exaggerated lordosis. There is frequent peroneal muscle involvement with or without pelvifemoral weakness. Sensation is typically preserved and tendon reflexes are absent.

Other manifestations include sensorineural hearing loss, retinal telangiectasia, microaneurysms, and atrial tachyarrhythmia. Retinal telangiectasia compatible with Coats disease, with or without closure, leakage, and microaneurysmal formation, and most often asymptomatic and found only at ocular screening after the diagnosis of FSHD has been established, may be the initial manifestation of FSHD (20). Scapular winging may be the presenting feature of FSHD, however, a history of sleeping with eyes open may be ascertained. Disease progression is typically slow and continuous. Up to 20% of patients eventually require a wheelchair.

MOLECULAR GENETICS

In a linkage study of FSHD families, Upadhyaya and coworkers (21) found three recombinants in a total of 140 meioses for linkage with a hypervariable DNA probe on 4q. Wijmenga and colleagues (22) noted linkage of FSHD to D4S139 that mapped to 4q35-qter. Mathews and colleagues (23, 24) defined the localization of FSHD at 4q35 using a probe with a breakpoint X;4 translocation at 4q35. D4S139, D4S163, and D4S171 were most closely linked with FSHD, with D4S139 being the closest proximal marker (25, 26).

All patients with a confirmed diagnosis of FSHD had

chromosomal rearrangement in the subtelomeric region of 4q35, the latter of which was composed mainly of a 3.3-kb polymorphic repeat designated D4Z4 (26). In that regard, FSHD was found to be associated with contraction of a tandem repeat rather than an expansion as may occur in other disorders such myotonic muscular dystrophy. Southern blot, FISH, and isolation of cDNA and genomic clones led to identification of the D4Z4 tandem repeat locus (27).

Although D4Z4 did not encode a protein per se, the association between documented causative deletions within this locus and FSHD was highly significant and formed the basis for later disease mutational analysis; and the postulate that deletion of D4Z4 produced a position effect involved in the pathogenesis of the disease.

Gabellini and coworkers (28) noted the overexpression of FRG1, FRG2, and ANTI genes in muscle located upstream from D4Z4 on 4q35, with an element that specifically bound to a multiprotein complex consisting of transcriptional repressor YYI, HMGB2, and nucleolin, which in vitro and in vivo mediated transcriptional repression of the 4q35 gene. These authors proposed that a deletion in D4Z4 led to the inappropriate transcriptional derepression of 4q35 genes such that deletion of an integral number of D4Z4 repeats that reduced the number of bound repressor complexes and consequently decreased or abolished transcriptional repression.

Van Overveld and colleagues (29) showed that contraction of the D4Z4 repeat array caused marked hypomethylation of the contracted D4Z4 allele in individuals with FSHD. The methylation signal at H3K9 of histone H3 at lysine-9, as well as at proximal D4Z4 repeat regions, marking transcriptionally permissive euchromatin, was significantly decreased in myoblasts and fibroblasts derived from FSHD cell lines (30).

In the same period, the DUX4 gene initially thought to be nonfunctional, was instead a candidate gene, within the D4Z4 repeat, and was overtly toxic to mouse myoblasts at both high and low expression (31, 32). Patients with FSHD carried specific single-nucleotide polymorphisms in the chromosomal region distal to the last D4Z4 repeat, creating a polyadenylation signal, named 4A polyadenylation signal (4APAS) for stabilized distal DUX4 transcripts leading to FSHD through a toxic gain of function (33). Accordingly, full-length DUX4 (DUX4-fl) transcripts were aberrantly expressed in 5 of 10 FSHD muscle biopsy specimens, but not normal muscle, and similarly, only 0.1% of FSHD muscle nuclei expressed abundant DUX4-fl mRNA and protein (34).

DIAGNOSIS

There may be difficulty a priori in the exclusion of other disorders including myofibrillar myopathy, polymyositis, inclusion body myositis, mitochondrial encephalomyopathy, acid maltase deficiency, limb girdle muscular dystrophy, and myotonic muscular dystrophy, scapuloperoneal syndrome, and congenital myopathy. Like FSHD, the aforementioned may demonstrate a several-fold elevation of the serum creatine kinase (CK), primary myogenic change on electromyography (EMG) and muscle biopsy, including occasional foci of inflammatory cell infiltration.

Molecular genetic testing employs deletion testing and haplotype analyses. Commercially available deletion testing is performed using the restriction enzyme EcoRI that recognizes the *D4Z4* locus on chromosomes 4 and 10. Normal alleles in the *D4Z4* locus demonstrate 11 to 100 repeat units, whereas borderline ones show 10 or 11 repeats, and FSHD-associated alleles demonstrate 1 to 10 repeat units. Up to 5% of symptomatic patients may have unidentified *D4Z4* deletions.

The diagnosis of FSHD can be challenging even in the presence of a clinically compatible phenotype that included AD inheritance, asymmetric weakness in facial, shoulder girdle, anterior foreleg muscles, and myopathic pattern on electrodiagnostic testing. Of 16 patients so studied by Sacconi and colleagues (35), four patients had expected molecular genetic genotypic and phenotypical concordance, two had masking of the *D4Z4* contraction due to complex rearrangement or mosaicism in the FSHD locus, six were later diagnosed as having FSHD2, owing to 45- to 95-kb 4A161 allele and marked hypomethylation of the *D4Z4* locus; two had a valosin-containing protein (VCP)-related myopathy, and two had no identifiable genetic defect.

Conversely, one large-scale population study (36) noted that 3% of healthy Italian and Brazilian controls carried alleles with 4 to 8 *D4Z4* repeats on chromosome 4q, whereas only 50% of 253 unrelated patients with FSHD carried alleles with 1 to 8 *D4Z4* repeats. The remaining FSHD probands instead carried different haplotypes or alleles with a greater number of repeats, challenging the unique genetic signature of FSHD.

MANAGEMENT

Most FSHD treatments involve attempts to physically improve functional impairment (37). Orthotics can improve foot drop and there are surgical procedures to fix the scapula to the chest to improve range of motion of the arms; however, the gains may be offset by further progression of weakness. Pharmacological treatment with 12 weeks of prednisone in those with inflammation on muscle biopsy showed no improvement (38), although albuterol, a beta adrenergic agent, showed a statistically significant improvement in lean body mass and strength after 12 weeks (39). A phase I/II treatment trial using the neutralizing antibody MYO-029 to the muscle growth inhibitor myostatin in adult subjects with muscular dystrophies including FSHD showed no improvement in muscle strength or function (40).

One other logical therapeutic approach that showed promise in experimental FSHD mice (2) was to employ antisense strategies against specifically activated target genes, including RNA interference against the *FRG1* mRNA employing *FRG1*-specific mRNA and shRNA. *DUX4* is a potent transcription factor in the etiopathogenesis of FSHD and retains the capacity to induce a deregulation cascade when fused with existing myofibers. Its estimated presence in only about 0.1% of cells in myoblast culture highlights the challenge of targeting *DUX4* to block the fusion and induction of the deregulation cascade with existing myofibers and those newly produced by the regenerative process.

GENETIC COUNSELING

Genetic counseling and prenatal testing are commercially available and rely upon analysis of DNA extracted from fetal cells obtained through chorionic villus sampling at 10 to 12 weeks or amniocentesis at 16 to 18 weeks gestation.

REFERENCES

1. van der Maarel SM, Frants RR. The D4Z4 repeat-mediated pathogenesis of facioscapulohumeral muscular dystrophy. *Am J Hum Genet* 2005; 76:375–386.
2. Richards M, Coppee F, Thomas N, et al. Facioscapulohumeral muscular dystrophy (FSHD): an enigma unraveled? *Hum Genet* 2012; 131:325–340.
3. Landouzy L, Dejerine J. De la myopathie atrophique progressive. *Rev Med Franc* 1885; 5:81.
4. Tyler FH, Stephens FE. Studies in disorders of muscle II. Clinical manifestations and inheritance of facioscapulohumeral dystrophy in a large family. *Ann Intern Med* 1950; 32:640–660.
5. Tyler FH. The inheritance of neuromuscular disorders. *Res Publ Assoc Res Nerv Ment Dis* 1953; 33:283–292.
6. Justin-Besancon L, Pequignot H, Contamin F, et al. Myopathie du type Landouzy-Dejerine. Rapport d'une observation historique. *Sem Hop Paris* 1964; 40:2990–2999.
7. Small RG. Coats' disease and muscular dystrophy. *Trans Am Acad Ophthal Otolaryng* 1968; 72:225–231.
8. Taylor DA, Carroll JE, Smith ME, et al. Facioscapulohumeral dystrophy associated with hearing loss and Coats syndrome. *Ann Neurol* 1982; 12:395–398.
9. Voit T, Lamprecht A, Lenard HG, et al. Hearing loss in facioscapulohumeral dystrophy. *Eur J Pediatr* 1986; 145:280–285.
10. Fitzsimmons RB, Gurwin EB, Bird AC. Retinal vascular abnormalities in facioscapulohumeral dystrophy: a general association with genetic and therapeutic implications. *Brain* 1987; 110:631–648.

11. Padberg G, Brouwer OF, de Keizer RJW, et al. Retinal vascular disease and sensorineural deafness are part of facioscapulohumeral muscular dystrophy. *Am J Hum Genet* 1992; 51(Suppl):A104.

12. Yasukohchi S, Yagi Y, Akabane T, et al. Facioscapulohumeral dystrophy associated with sensorineural hearing loss, tortuosity of retinal arteries, and an early onset and rapid progression of respiratory failure. *Brain Dev* 1988; 10:319–324.

13. Miura K, Kumagai T, Matsumoto A, et al. Two cases of chromosome 4q35-linked early onset facioscapulohumeral muscular dystrophy with mental retardation and epilepsy. *Neuropediatrics* 1998; 29:239–241.

14. Bodensteiner JB, Schochet SS. Facioscapulohumeral muscular dystrophy: the choice of a biopsy site. *Muscle Nerve* 1986; 9:544–547.

15. Shen EN, Madsen T. Facioscapulohumeral muscular dystrophy and recurrent pacemaker lead dislodgement. *Am Heart J* 1991; 122:1167–1169.

16. Morton NE, Chung CS. Formal genetics of muscular dystrophy. *Am J Hum Genet* 1959; 11:360–379.

17. Lunt PW, Upadhyaya M, Sarfarazi M, et al. Linkage studies in facioscapulohumeral disease. *Cytogenet Cell Genet* 1989; 51:1036.

18. Zatz M, Marie SK, Passos-Bueno MR, et al. High proportion of new mutations and possible anticipation in Brazilian facioscapulohumeral muscular dystrophy families. *Am J Hum Genet* 1995; 56:99–105.

19. Tawil R, Forrester J, Griggs RC, et al. Evidence for anticipation and association of deletion size with severity in facioscapulohumeral muscular dystrophy. The FSH-DY Group. *Ann Neurol* 1996; 39:744–748.

20. Shields CL, Zahler J, Falk N, et al. Neovascular glaucoma from advanced Coats disease as the initial manifestation of facioscapulohumeral dystrophy in a 2-year-old child. *Arch Ophthal* 2007; 125:840–842.

21. Upadhyaya M, Lunt PW, Sarfarazi M, et al. A closely linked DNA marker for facioscapulohumeral disease on chromosome 4q. *J Med Genet* 1991; 28:665–671.

22. Wijmenga C, Sandkuijl LA, Moerer P, et al. Genetic linkage map of facioscapulohumeral muscular dystrophy and five polymorphic loci on chromosome 4q35-qter. *Am J Hum Genet* 1992; 51:411–415.

23. Mathews KD, Mills KA, Leysens NJ, et al. Characterization of the facioscapulohumeral dystrophy locus on 4q35. *Am J Hum Genet* 1991; 49(Suppl):350.

24. Mathews KD, Mills KA, Bosh EP, et al. Linkage localization of facioscapulohumeral muscular dystrophy (FSHD) in 4q35. *Am J Hum Genet* 1992; 51:428–431.

25. Weiffenbach B, Bagley R, Falls K, et al. Linkage analysis of five chromosome 4 markers localizes the facioscapulohumeral muscular dystrophy (FSHD) gene to distal 4q35. *Am J Hum Genet* 1992; 416–423.

26. Weiffenbach B. Dubois J, Storvick D, et al. Mapping the facioscapulohumeral muscular dystrophy gene is complicated by chromosome 4q35 recombination events. *Nature Genet* 1993; 4:165–169.

27. Hewitt JE, Lyle R, Clark LN, et al. Analysis of the tandem repeat locus of D4Z4 associated with facioscapulohumeral muscular dystrophy. *Hum Molec Genet* 1994; 3:1287–1295.

28. Gabellini D, Green MR, Tupler R. Inappropriate gene activation in FSHD: a repressor complex binds a chromosomal repeat deleted in dystrophic muscle. *Cell* 2002; 110:339–348.

29. van Overveld PGM, Lemmers RJFL, Sandkuijl LA, et al. Hypomethylation of D4Z4 I n4q-linked and non-4q-linked facioscapulohumeral muscular dystrophy. *Nature Genet* 2003; 35:315–317.

30. Zeng W, de Greef JC, Chen Y-Y, et al. Specific loss of histone H3 lysine 9 trimethylation and HP1-gamma/cohesion binding at D4Z4 repeats is associated with facioscapulohumeral dystrophy (FSHD). *PLoS Genet* 2009; 5:e1000559.

31. Dmitriev P, Lipinski M, Vassetsky YS. Pearls in the junk: dissecting the molecular pathogenesis of facioscapulohumeral dystrophy. *Neuromuscul Disord* 2008; 19:17–20.

32. Bosnakovski D, Xu Z, Gang EJ et al. Anisogenic myoblast expression screen identifies DUX4-mediated FSHD-associated molecular pathologies. *EMBO J* 2008; 27:2766–2779.

33. Lemmers RJLF, van der Vliet PJ, Klooster R, et al. A unifying genetic model for facioscapulohumeral muscular dystrophy. *Science* 2010; 329:1650–1653.

34. Snider L, Geng LN, Lemmers RJLF, et al. Facioscapulohumeral dystrophy: incomplete suppression of a retrotransposed gene. *PLoS Genet* 2010; 6:e1001181.

35. Sacconi S, Camano P, de Greef JC, et al. Patients with a phenotype consistent with facioscapulohumeral muscular dystrophy display genetic and epigenetic heterogeneity. *J Med Genet* 2012; 49:41–46.

36. Scionti I, Greco F, Ricci G, et al. Large-scale population analysis challenges the current criteria for the molecular diagnosis of facioscapulohumeral muscular dystrophy. *Am J Hum Genet* 2012; 90:628–635.

37. Tawil R. Facioscapulohumeral muscular dystrophy. *Neurotherapeutics* 2008; 5:601–606.

38. Tawil R, McDermott MP, Pandya S, et al. A pilot trial of prednisone in facioscapulohumeral muscular dystrophy. FSH-DY Group. *Neurology* 1997; 48:46–49.

39. Kissel JT, McDermott MP, Natarajan R, et al. Pilot trial of albuterol in facioscapulohumeral muscular dystrophy. FSH-DY Group. *Neurology* 1998; 50:1402–1406.

40. Wagner KR, Fleckenstein JL, Amato AA, et al. A phase I/II trial of MYO-029 in adult subjects with muscular dystrophy. *Ann Neurol* 2008; 63:561–571.

CHAPTER 24

Myalgia, Fibromyalgia, Fasciculation, and Cramps

David S. Younger

Patients are frequently seen in neuromuscular clinics because of muscle complaints. Over the past decade, awareness of neuromuscular disease has probably been most influenced by the recognition of the postulated forms of myotoxicity of statin drugs, ranging from myalgia to rhabdomyolysis, than any other single public relations phenomenon (1–4). The true incidence of neuromuscular involvement associated with statin drugs remains poorly understood, sorely overrated, and overlitigated, spurring a generation of cardiologists and rheumatologists turned myologists, with few if any guidelines to assist physicians in determining whether such effects are the result of statin-related myotoxicity or an underlying neuromuscular disorder (5). Myalgia, cramps, fasciculation, and other spasms are important to recognize in the evaluation of disorders of the peripheral and central nervous system (PNS and CNS), further separable by a detailed history, examination, and electrophysiological and histopathological testing.

MYALGIA

Myalgia means discomfort of muscle, which can involve a single muscle or muscle group, especially in the setting of injury. It is one of the most common complaints that compel patients to seek medical attention. In population-based studies, 20% of patients complained of persistent localized muscle discomfort, and up to 10% complained of widespread muscle pain (6). One-third of 109 consecutive patients received a specific diagnosis to explain the syndrome of myalgia (7). The classification of myalgia is shown in Table 1.

Hereditary myopathy should be considered in all patients with complaints of myalgia. Episodic recurrent exercise intolerance with cramps, myalgia, and myoglobinuria occurs in muscle glycogenosis due to phosphorylase (type V), phosphofructokinase (VII), phosphorylase kinase (VIII), phosphoglycerate kinase (IX), phosphoglycerate mutase (X), lactate dehydrogenase (XI), aldolase (XII), and B-enolase enzyme deficiency (XIII) syndromes, as well as in disturbances of lipid metabolism due to deficiency of carnitine palmitoyltransferase II, very-long chain acyl-CoA and short-chain 3-hydroxyacyl-CoA dehydrogenases, and trifunctional protein, each further separable by the clinical, serum creatinine kinase (CK) levels, and the findings on molecular genetic analysis and muscle biopsy (8–13).

Lack of a muscle-specific isoform of AMP deaminase causes a metabolic myopathy with exercise-induced myalgia, cramps, and early fatigue, found in about 2 to 3% of all muscle biopsies making it probably the most common muscle enzyme defect (14, 15). Patients with proximal myotonic myopathy (PROMM), an autosomal dominant (AD) hereditary multisystemic disorder, may present with myalgia, myotonia, and proximal muscle weakness due to a genetic defect on chromosome 3q21, but an overall less serious course compared with myotonic dystrophy (16).

Rippling muscle disease is a rare AD muscle disorder characterized by exercise-induced myalgia, stiffness, and cramps due to mutations in the caveolin-d (CAV3) gene (17). Myalgia and fatigue during prolonged physical exercise may be the presenting symptoms of primary carnitine deficiency that resolves with oral therapy with L-carnitine (18). Similarly, limb-girdle muscular dystrophy type 2I linked to chromosome 19q13.3 caused by mutation in the fukutin-related protein (FKRP) gene can have a variable phenotype from prominent exercise-induced myalgia to a limb-girdle syndrome with weakness and wasting of the

Table 1. Classification of Myalgia

HEREDITARY MYOPATHY
Muscle glycogenoses
    Type V: phosphorylase deficiency
    Type VII: phosphofructokinase deficiency
    Type VIII: phosphorylase kinase deficiency
    Type IX: phosphoglycerate kinase deficiency
    Type X: phosphoglycerate mutase deficiency
    Type XI: lactate dehydrogenase deficiency
    Type XII: aldolase deficiency
    Type XIII: B-enolase deficiency
Disorders of lipid metabolism
    Carnitine palmitoyltransferase II deficiency
    Very-long-chain acyl-CoA dehydrogenase deficiency
    Trifunctional protein deficiency
    Short-chain 3-hydroxyacyl-CoA dehydrogenase
        deficiency
    Myoadenylate deaminase deficiency
    Proximal myotonic myopathy
    Caveolin-3 gene mutation-rippling muscle disease
    Carnitine deficiency
    Fukutin gene mutation-Limb girdle muscular dystrophy
    Dystrophinopathy of myalgia and cramps syndrome
    Tubular aggregates
    Multicore disease
    Congenital fiber type disproportion myopathy

INFLAMMATORY MYOPATHY
    Polymyositis
    Dermatomyositis
    Inclusion body myositis
    Esosinophilic perimyositis

SYSTEMIC DISORDERS
    Lupus erythematosus, drug-induced lupus
    Rheumatoid arthritis
    Sjogren syndrome
    Polymyalgia rheumatica
    Temporal arteritis
    Wegener granulomatosis
    Microscopic polyangiitis
    Polyarteritis nodosa
    Churg Strauss syndrome
    Sarcoidosis
    Scleroderma
    Mixed connective tissue diseases
    Eosinophilic fasciitis
    Anti-synthetase syndrome
    Crohn disease
    Coeliac disease
    Cholesterol embolism
    Familial Mediterranean fever
    Hyperimmunoglobulin D period fever syndrome
    Tumor necrosis factor receptor-associated period
        syndrome
    Pheochromocytoma

    Inflammatory liver pseudotumor
    Still disease
    Chronic eosinophilic perimyositis
    Hypereosinophilia

METABOLIC DISTURBANCES
    Estrogen deficiency
    Hypothyroidism
    Autoimmune thyroiditis
    Thyrotoxic periodic paralysis
    Alcohol
    Scurvy
    Caffeine

INFECTIOUS AGENTS
Bacteria
    Staphylococcus
    Streptococcus
    Meningococcus
    Borrelia
    Leptospira
    Rickettsia
    Ehrlichia
    Orientia tsutsugamushi
    Mycoplasma
    Mycobacteria
    Legionnella
    Francisella
    Coxiella
    E. Coli
    Chlamydia
    Brucella
Parasites
    Plamodia
    Trichinella
Fungi
    Histoplasma capsulatum
    Anthrax
Viruses
    Aseptic meningitis
    Enterovirus
    Influenza A and B
    Dengue fever
    Cytomegalovirus
    Severe acute respiratory syndrome (SARS)
    Coxsackie B virus
    Japanese encephalitis virus
    Hepatitis C virus
    Coronavirus
    Ebola virus
    Ross River
    Barmah forest
    Human immunodeficiency virus (HIV)

MEDICATIONS
Colchicine
Ibuprofen
Vasopressin
Oseltamivir
Zanamivir
Isotretinoin
Quinine
Cocaine
Ephedrine
AZT
Minocycline
Desloratadine
Succinylcholine
Lidocaine
L-tryptophan
5-hydroxytryptophan
Hydralazine
Captopril
Enalapril
Growth hormone
Mycophenylate mophetil
Cyclosporine
Interferon beta
Tioguanine
Zoledronic bisphosphonate
Statins
Ramipril
Chloroquine
Alefacept
Irbesart
Tadalafil
Sildenafil citrate
Chemotherapeutic agents
Gemcitabine
Letrozole
Vinorelbine, methotrexate, fluorouracil
Marimastat, captopil, fragmin
Carboplatin, paclitaxel
Exatecan mesylate (DX-8951f)
Imatinib
Trastuzumab, paclitaxel
Squalamine
Bryostatin-1
Letrozole
Tirapazamine, carboplatin, paclitaxel
Filgrastim, platinum
Antineoplaston A10 and AS2-1
Immunotoxins: RFT5.dgA and Ki-4

Humanized A33 (huA33; IgG1)
α-Interferon
Difluorodeoxycytidine
Cryptophycin
TAC-101
Mitomycin C, vinblastin
B43-Genistein
Vincristine
Roquinimex
ε-aminocaproic acid

OTHER THERAPIES
Electroconvulsive therapy
Breast implantation
Platelet concentrate transfusion
Allogenic bone marrow transplantation

VACCINATION
Hepatitis B, granulocyte macrophage colony stimulating
    factor augmented vaccine
Pneumococcal vaccine
Influenza vaccine
Meningococcal group C conjugate vaccine
Smallpox vaccination
Measles vaccine
Lyme disease vaccination
Rubella virus vaccine

TOXINS AND VENOMS
Tricholoma equestre
Crotalus durissus snakebite
Latrodectus tredecimguttatus spider
Ciguatera
Viobrio vulnificus oyster
Capnocytophaga canimorsus
Lead
Toxic oil syndrome
Polymer fume fever

INJURY
Muscle sprain, strain, tear
Trapezius myalgia
Pectoral girdle myalgia
Seizure

IDIOPATHIC MYALGIC CONDITIONS
Myofascial pain syndrome
Fibromyalgia

shoulder girdle muscles, and calf hypertrophy (19). One large Spanish family presented with myalgia and cramps, with evidence of deletion of the dystrophin gene involving exons 45 to 52 (20). Exercise-related myalgia and fatigue may be the presenting feature of AD myopathy with tubular aggregates composed of closely packed vesicles and tubules filled with electron dense material or one to several smaller tubules in muscle tissue (21). Myalgia may be the main clinical manifestation of multicore disease and congenital fiber type disproportion myopathy, although these disorders are more commonly recognized by hypotonia and muscle weakness in early life (22).

Dermatomyositis, polymyositis, and inclusion body myositis are the major idiopathic inflammatory myopathies further separable by distinctive clinical, electrophysiological, serological, histopathological features, and associated systemic features, that can nonetheless present with fatigue, myalgia, and weakness at onset (23, 24).

Diverse systemic autoimmune vasculitic disorders can present with, or have prominent associated skeletal muscle involvement with myalgia (Table 1) (25, 26). The most common musculoskeletal symptoms of systemic lupus erythematosus (SLE) are arthralgia, arthritis, and myalgia, noted in 70% of patients (27). Myalgia in Sjogren syndrome, another systemic autoimmune disorder associated with SSA and SSB (Ro and La) antibodies was ascribed to subnormal secretion of cytokines by peripheral blood mononuclear cells and increased IL-18 secretion (28). Serum amyloid A levels was a useful index of disease activity and myalgia in polymyalgia rheumatica (PMR) (29). Skeletal muscle involvement has been well documented in polyarteritis nodosa, usually with diffuse weakness, myalgia, and elevated serum CK levels, at times mimicking polymyositis (30).

Biopsy of a symptomatic muscle with the demonstration of necrotizing arteritis can be helpful in establishing the diagnosis and prompting early effective treatment. Churg-Strauss syndrome or allergic granulomatosis and angiitis is another vasculitic disorder found in adults and, rarely, in children, with myalgia, fever, weight loss, esosinophilia, sinusitis, asthma, arthralgia, and pulmonary infiltrates; muscle biopsy shows necrotizing arteritis with eosinophilic infiltrates (31, 32). Vertigo, serous otitis, polyneuropathy, crescentic glomerulonephritis, hilar adenopathy, and retro-orbital granulomatous inflammation with pulmonary infiltrates were present in a patient with prominent myalgia due to an overlap of Cogan syndrome and Wegener granulomatosis (33). Polyarthritis accompanied by myalgia, fever, and anxiety were the presenting features of a patient with Coeliac disease, which responded to gluten-free dietary management (34). Patients with sarcoidosis may present with early myalgia as a constitutional symptom or as a result of skeletal muscle involvement in up to 13% of patients (35). Scleroderma and scleroderma variant syndromes, including eosinophilic fasciitis, scler-

edema, and scleromyxedema can be associated with myalgia (36, 37). The anti-synthetase syndrome, which includes myositis, idiopathic interstitial lung disease, polyarthritis, and Raynaud phenomenon, is characterized by the presence of autoantibodies directed against aminoacyl-tRNA synthetases (38). Localized gastrocnemius myositis, proposed as gastrocnemius myalgia syndrome, as evidenced by pain and tenderness in the calves associated with pyrexia and neurotrophilic leukocytosis, and antibodies to anti-neutrophilic cytoplasma antibodies, is a rare extraintestinal manifestation of Crohn disease (39). The neurological symptoms of cholesterol emboli syndrome include myalgia, neuropathic pain, and mental change with a short term of 60 to 80% (40).

Familial Mediterranean fever (FMF), hyperimmunoglobulin D period fever syndrome (HIDS), and tumor necrosis factor receptor-associated period syndrome (TRAPS) are hereditary period fever syndromes with prominent symptoms of myalgia (41–43). FMF is caused by mutations in the Mediterranean fever gene, HIDS by mutations in the mevalonat-kinase gene, and TRAPS by mutations in the TNF-receptor superfamily 1A gene. Impaired function of the encoded proteins, pyrin in FMF, mevalonatkinase in HIDS, and p55 TNF-receptor in TRAPS induce a dysregulated cytokine balance with symptoms of relapsing fever, serositis, arthralgia, myalgia, and rash.

Hemorrhagic necrosis of a pheochromocytoma can be recognized by the development of myalgia, high fever, abdominal pain followed by cardiogenic pulmonary edema, and shock (44). Inflammatory pseudotumor of the liver is an unusual tumor-like condition that leads to nonspecific fever, arthralgia, myalgia, and liver mass, recognition of which is vital in differentiating it from a malignant lesion (45). Adult-onset Still disease is a prominent cause of fever of unknown origin (FUO), the clinical findings of which also include arthralgia, rash, sore throat, myalgia, splenomegaly, anemia, adenopathy, and leukocytosis (46). Chronic eosinophilic perimyositis presents with persistent myalgia and results from hypereosinophilia, the diagnosis of which is confirmed by histopathological examination of muscle tissue (47).

There are notable metabolic causes of myalgia (Table 1). It is seen in up to three-quarters of patients with estrogen deficiency in pre-, and perimenopause, postmenopause, surgical menopause, and premature ovarian failure (48). Hypothyrodism leads to a clinical syndrome of myalgia, muscular fatigue, and elevated serum CK levels due to thyroidectomy, and central causes including autoimmune thyroiditis, pituitary adenoma, Sheehan syndrome, and struma ovarii resection (49–51). Excessive alcohol ingestion leads to selective atrophy of type II myofibers, with reduction in muscle mass, weakness, and subjective symptoms of myalgia, cramps, and gait difficulty (52). Scurvy, which results from deficiency of vitamin C, occurs in disadvantaged groups such as alcoholics, elderly, and institutionalized individuals recognized by lethargy, purpura, myalgia, and bleeding of the gums (53). Chills, fever, myalgia, and cephalea have been reported after challenge with caffeine with cross-reactivity to theophylline, but not pentoxifylline (54).

There are diverse bacterial, parasitic, fungi, and infectious viral etiologies for myalgia that can occur in the prodromal period or as a result of the direct or indirect skeletal muscle involvement later in the infective process. Bacteria infectious pathogens that lead to infectious illnesses that may display prominent myalgia include staphylococcus-related toxic shock syndrome and pyomyositis in immunocompetent and incompetent individuals (55), streptococcus-related polyarthritis and tenosynovitis (56), myositis in meningococcal disease (57), neuroborreliosis (58, 59). Weil disease, Boutonneuse fever, and leptospirosis caused by leptospires (60–62). Rickettsioses-zoonotic bacterial infections transmitted to human by arthropods can lead to a African tick bite fever or a benign travelers febrile illness (63, 64), human granulocytic ehrlichiosis (65, 66), scrub typhus caused by the bite of chiggers infected with *Orientia tsutsugamushi* (67), the extrapulmonary complications of mycoplasma pneumoniae (68), polymyositis pattern of disease complicating myobacterial tuberculosis infection (69), infections with Legionella species (70), Tularemia caused by *Francisella tularensis* that resides in wild and domestic animals (71), Q fever caused by infection with *Coxiella burnetii* (72, 73), psittacosis caused by *Chlamydia psittaci* organisms (74), and Brucellosis (75). Two parasitic infectious organisms that predispose to myalgia include *Plasmodium falciparum* that leads to malaria, and contamination of food products with Trichinella (76, 77). Two fungal infections that also lead to prominent myalgia include histoplasmosis and anthrax (78, 79).

The prodrome of aseptic or viral meningitis, especially enteroviruses, can also lead to viral prodromes of photophobia, myalgia, and fatigue (80, 81). Influenza A and B viral outbreaks can lead to cough, fever, myalgia and weakness, and at time pyomyositis (82–84). Epidemic dengue and hemorrhagic dengue fever include myalgia (85), as does cytomegalovirus infection (86). The major features of severe acute respiratory syndrome (SARS) include fever, chills, myalgia, malaise, dry cough, headache, and dyspnea (87); the corona virus has been implicated in its etiopathogenesis (88). Coxsackie viruses belong to the enteroviruses with prominent myalgia (89). Japanese encephalitis virus leads to fever, headache, myalgia, rash, and diarrhea (90). Frequent extrahepatic manifestations of hepatitis C virus infection include myalgia, arthralgia, and sicca syndrome resembling a connective tissue disorder (91). The human Ebola virus leads to fever, chills, myalgia, abdominal pain, diarrhea, vomiting, rash, and headache (92). Ross River virus and Barmah Forest viruses are mosquito-borne viruses that cause diseases characterized by arthralgia, arthritis, and myalgia (93). The Hantavirus pulmonary syndrome includes acute respiratory insufficiency as well as myalgia (94). Primary human immunodeficiency virus (HIV) infection and the acute retroviral syndrome includes myalgia (95).

There has been an awareness of the adverse effects of therapeutic agents on the structure and function of muscle with resulting clinical syndromes varying from mild to profound myalgia with weakness and myoglobinuria. The so-called toxic myopathies that result are generally reversible if recognized promptly and the offending medication withdrawn (96). Diverse medications that can cause myalgia are shown in Table 1. Colchicine induces a vacuolar myopathy with resultant myalgia, the serum level of which rises with renal insufficiency (97, 98). Ibuprofen induces a transient antinuclear antibody (ANA) and anti-histone positive leukocytoclastic vasculitis with resulting myalgia (99). Intravenous vasopressin can lead to myoglobinuria due to overreactive vasoconstriction and resulting myonecrosis (100). Oseltamivir phosphate and zanamivir, administered for naturally acquired influenza A and B infection, leads to myalgia (101, 102). Isotretinoin, a retinoid employed in the treatment of acne, can have a synergistic effect on exercise leading to elevated CK levels and myalgia (103). Quinine induces hepatotoxicity within the first 24 hours of ingestion of the first dose with accompanying myalgia (104). Myalgia, tremor, and cramps occur after the use of ephedrine (105). Although zidovudine (AZT) leads to myalgia and myopathy, 2',3'-dideoxyinosine (ddI) does not have an adverse effect on muscle tissue (106).

Immunoallergic reactions can be seen with minocycline leading to hepatitis, arthralgia, myalgia, and widespread pruritus (107). Desloratadine, the principal metabolite of loratadine, is itself an orally active nonsedating peripheral histamine receptor antagonist with potential myalgia side effect (108). Succinylcholine-induced myalgia syndrome is reduced with lidocaine pretreatment (109). Tryptophan and 5-hydroxytryptophan, administered as natural alternatives to traditional antidepressants, led to potentially fatal eosinophilia myalgia syndrome (110). Drug-induced lupus erythematosus, which shares symptoms and laboratory characteristics with idiopathic systemic (SLE), was first described in hydralazine (111). Myalgia and arthralgia is associated with enalapril and ramipril (112). Recombinant human growth hormone (hGH) leads to an increased frequency of arthralgia, myalgia, and paresthesias (113).

Myalgia is an uncommon and underestimated side effect of mycophenolate mophetil, used to prevent rejection of organ allograft transplantation (114). Cyclosporine for SLE can be associated with arthralgia, myalgia, and fatigue (115). Betaseron and Avonex used for the treatment of multiple sclerosis is accompanied by fever, chills, and myalgia

(116). Tioguanine, used in Crohn disease intolerant and resistant to azathioprine and mercaptopurine, can also lead to myalgia (117). Intravenous zoledronic acid is indicated in postmenopausal women with low bone mineral density, and has myalgia and fever as the major side effects (118). A spectrum of disease from myalgia to myoglobinuria exists as the classic side effects of lipid lowering drugs, mainly statins (3-hydroxy-3-methylglutaryl coenzyme A reductase inhibitors), although the mechanism of myofiber injury is not well understood (119, 120). Chloroquine, which is used in the treatment of uncomplicated malaria, leads to fever, headache, malaise, myalgia, nausea, and vertigo in the first week of treatment (121). Alefacept, which is given intravenously and by intramuscular injection for the treatment of chronic plaque psoriasis and other T-cell mediated disorders, acts by inducing selective T-cell apoptosis, a side effect of which is transient myalgia (122). The angiotensin II antagonist irbesart is administered to children with chronic kidney disease to reduce arterial pressure and pathological proteinuria; however, there can be mild abdominal pain, constipation, diarrhea, fatigue, headache, insomnia, and myalgia (123). Tadalafil and sildenafil citrate are both used to treat erectile dysfunction, however frequent side effects are headache and myalgia (124, 125).

Chemotherapy agents commonly cause a variety of side effects including myalgia. Vasculitis results from gemcitabine that is used in the treatment of small cell lung cancer with resultant myonecrosis (126). Letozole is a nonsteroidal third-generation aromatase inhibitor that is effective in the treatment of postmenopausal early- and advanced-stage hormone-sensitive breast cancer, however arthralgia, myalgia, and arthritis can complicate its use (127). Several combination chemotherapy regimens can lead to myalgia, including vinorelbine, methotrexate and fluorouracil (VMF) as first-line therapy for metastatic breast cancer (128); marimastat, captopril, and fragmin combination antiangiogenesis therapy for renal cancer (129); carboplatin and paclitaxol as induction for patients with biopsy-proven stage IIA N2 non-small cell lung cancer (130), bryostatin-1 and paclitaxel in advanced non-small cell lung cancer (131), carboplatin and paclitaxel for advanced stage IIB and IV non-small cell lung cancer (132), intravenous exatacan mesylate (SX-8951f) for metastatic breast cancer (133), imatinib for chornic myeloid leukemia (134), bryostatin-1 for recurrent epithelial ovarian cancer (135), letrozole in postmenopausal women after tamoxifen therapy for early-stage breast cancer (136), tirapazamine and carboplatin and paclitaxel for malignant solid tumors (137), ricin A-chain immunotoxins for Hodgkin lymphoma (138), humanized monoclonal antibody A33 for colon cancer and interferon alfa-NL as adjuvant treatment for respectable renal cell carcinoma (139), cryptophycin analog LY355703 for malignant solid tumors (140), TAC-101 a novel retinoic acid

receptor alpha selective retinoid for advanced cancer (141), mitomycin C and vinblastine in anthracycline-resistant metastatic breast cancer (142), apoptosis-inducing CD19-directed tyrosine kinase inhibition for leukemia (143), vincristine for a variety of solid tumors (144), roquinimex for myelodysplastic syndrome (145), and ε-aminocaproic acid for chronic granulocytic leukemia (146).

A number of other well recognized therapies pose a possible risk for the development of significant myalgia. Breast implantation patients complain of joint pain and myalgia, presumably due to reaction to silicone (147). Recurrent myositis was reported to acute allogenic bone marrow transplantation for myelodysplasia (148). Fatal septic shock and myoglobinuria occurred after transfusion of platelet concentrates contaminated with streptococcus pneumonia preceded by chest and back pain, and myalgia (149). Muscular injury and myalgia occur after electroconvulsive therapy (150).

Vaccination may be complicated by myalgia as a significant side effect, including the granulocyte macrophage colony-stimulating factor augmented hepatitis B vaccine for rapid seroconversion (151), pneumococcal vaccine (152), influenza vaccine (153), meningococcal C conjugate vaccine (154), smallpox vaccination (155), Lyme disease vaccine (156), measles vaccine (157), and rubella immunization (158).

A variety of toxins and venoms can lead to significant myalgia (Table 1). After ingestion of the mushroom Tricholoma equestre, fatigue, myalgia, weakness, loss of appetite, nausea, and profuse sweating develops with elevation of the serum CK consistent with acute myoglobinuria (159). A bite by the rattlesnake Crotalus durissus leads to prominent neuromuscular manifestations including ptosis, myalgia, and weakness with elevation of the serum CK, also suggestive of myoglobinuria (160). Intoxication by spider venom from Latrodectus tredecimguttatus leads to myalgia, weakness, headache, dizziness, fever, and vomiting (161).

Ciguatera poisoning is associated with human ingestion of large carnivorous fish that harbour the bioaccumulated ciguatoxins of the photosynthetic dinoflagellate Gambierdiscus toxicus, with associated arthralgia, myalgia, pruritis, and dental pain (162). Infection with Vibrio vulnificus leads to septicemia with associated fever, nausea, myalgia, and abdominal cramps (163). Capnocytophaga canimorsus septicemia related to dog bites leads to the common initial complaints of fever, malaise, myalgia, vomiting, diarrhea, abdominal pain, dyspnea, confusion, headache and skin manifestations (164). Lead exposure leads to the general symptoms of colic, headache, paresthesias, myalgia, and dizziness (165). The toxic oil syndrome is a multisystemic disease related to intake of rapeseed cooking oil sold in bulk characterized by pulmonary edema, rash, eosinophilia, and myalgia (166). Polymer fume fever is a self-limiting condition with influenza-like symptoms of fever, headache, dry cough, dyspnea, and myalgia caused by inhalation of toxic products released by the combustion of fluorocarbon polymers (167).

Focal muscle injury, including muscle and tendinous sprains, strains, and tears, can lead to regional myalgia. The work-related myalgias trapezious myalgia (168) and pectoral girdle myalgia (169) and are poorly understood but may be related to tissue hypoxia and other local factors (170). Seizures are another cause of transient myalgia, usually in association with muscle injury and sustained contraction.

FIBROMYALGIA

Patients with muscle aches, pain, and fatigue have long been known to medicine. The roots of fibromyalgia can be traced to Gowers (171) who used fibrositis, muscular rheumatism, and lumbago interchangeably to describe pain in lumbar muscles with contraction or extension, which differed from myalgia in the absence of spontaneous occurrence and in its referral along the fibrous connective tissues that encircled the muscles, in continuity with tendinous sheaths.

Although an inflammatory basis was suggested, Gowers reduced the significance of establishing the etiopathological basis, saying, "These diseases have little gravity so far as concerns the mechanisms by which life is ended. The processes that cause death absorb attention, and minor maladies which coexist are naturally disregarded." Gowers acknowledged the relative infectiveness of aspirin used for articular rheumatism and suggested intramuscular injection much like those currently performed for trigger points. "A local measure that often does good is the deep hypodermic injection of cocaine reported daily for two or three weeks. It unquestionably promotes the subsidence of the sensitiveness, provided the ease obtained is not abused by increased exertion."

Following the lead of Gowers, physicians continued to study muscle pain and its origin. Thomas Lewis (172), who had made his reputation describing fatigue, exhaustion, palpitation, breathlessness, and pain with other slight exertion in soldiers during the First World War with so called "effort syndrome," studied the referral of pain along interspinal ligaments induced by the injection of saline, and described the occurrence of tender points in areas of reflex muscle contraction. During the Second World War, physicians diagnosed fibrositis in more than three quarters of soldiers attending military hospitals, often with similar non-specific complaints and symptomatology. Psychogenic rheumatism, including fibrositis, was proposed by the United States military in 1943 (173) as the most frequent cause of disability in 450 consecutive recruits of which 11% overall were diagnosed with fibrositis, citing that "many patients complaining of stiffness and aching in the muscles and joints,

who are considered to have fibrositis, are actually victims of psychogenic rheumatism. In light of our experience, we find difficulty in accepting the incidence of fibrositis in soldiers as reported by certain English physicians." Traut (174) nonetheless continued the terminology of Gowers, introducing the concept of trigger points and nodular indurations at common sites, such as along the neck, shoulder, elbow, wrist, palms, low back, and at times in a more generalized distribution. Therapy included administration of analgesics, immobilization of the affected areas, infiltration of trigger points with procaine and corticosteroids, local heat, massage, and postural exercises. McCarty (175) introduced the dolorimeter or algesiometer, a quasi-objective device to rate articular and, later local muscle tenderness.

Other investigators noted the concordance of alpha rhythms in non-rapid-eye-movement (NREM) sleep electroencephalogram recordings termed α-δ sleep (176) in association with musculoskeletal and mood disturbances comparable to that seen chronically (177); however, such findings were frequently difficult to reliably replicate. Smythe and Moldofsky (178) proposed the demonstration of 12 or more tendon points from 14 typical sites of deep tenderness in clinically affected patients with fibrositis, hoping to differentiate them from those with other soft tissue pain syndromes, malingering, and rheumatic disorders.

The terms fibrositis and fibromyalgia became interchangeable in the 1980s by investigators in rheumatology (179). Yet even before the American College of Rheumatology (180) and the *Lancet* (181) established fibromyalgia syndrome as a distinctive diagnosis, extending the criteria for tender points to 11 of 18 or the presence of widespread pain of at least three months duration, there was continuing parallel interest in the emotional aspects, as exemplified by the increased comorbid risk of medical and psychiatric disorders, including migraine, irritable bowel syndrome, chronic fatigue syndrome, major depression, and panic disorder that suggested a common basis in the spectrum of major affective disorders (182, 183). It soon became evident that pathophysiological insight was lacking in the fibromyalgia syndrome and that circular reasoning argued the evidence on which the diagnosis was based, since its very nature was only valid in the sense that it included virtually all possibilities (184, 185) despite poor reproducibility of trigger and tender points even among experts (186). It is still not certain whether a routine neuromuscular evaluation really contributes anything to patients with classic fibromyalgia; nonetheless, since current data on prevalence suggests that up to two percent of the adult population of the United States are affected (187), and the cost of health care and disability for this segment of the population continues to rise, neurologists and neuromuscular experts should esteem to avoid denying its existence, and attempt to contribute their expertise to their care.

FASCICULATION

Fasciculation are visible involuntary twitches of the muscle (188). A single fasciculation may be as small as a flicker of the surface of the muscle, or large enough to move a small part of the body such as a finger. Electrophysiologically, they correspond to a spontaneous discharge of the motor unit with activation of some or all of the myofibers. Fasciculation occur in 70 percent of normal individuals exacerbated by extreme exercise, cold temperature, hyperventilation, stress, excessive caffeine and alcohol intake, metabolic derangements, and prescription medication, as well as diverse progressive and non-progressive neuromuscular disorders wherein they may provide a clue to diagnosis. The origin for pathological fasciculation is assumed to be commensurate with the localization of the corresponding pathological process as, for example, the peripheral nerve fiber in multifocal motor neuropathy, the ventral root in compressive radiculopathy, and the perikarya in anterior horn cell disease.

The disorders associated with fasciculation are heterogenous with respect to etiopathogenesis, localization in the motor unit, and prognosis (Table 2). There are two benign fasciculation disorders, including benign fasciculation and cramps and fasciculation syndrome (189). Fasciculation can accompany disturbances of calcium homeostasis in hyper- and hypoparathyroid and thyroid disease, occasionally resembling amyotrophic lateral sclerosis (ALS). When localized to myotomal segments, they may be the presenting signs of poliomyelitis, compressive root disease, chronic inflammatory demyelinating polyradiculoneuropathy (CIDP), myelomatosis, and neurolymphomatosis. When accompanied by focal weakness, wasting, and frank lower motor neuron clinical and electrophysiological involvement, in association with the upper motor neuron signs of hyperreflexia, Hoffman, Babinski signs, and clonus, the diagnosis of ALS is likely. There are reported patients with inclusion body myositis (IBM) that clinically resemble motor neuron disease (MND) with predominant upper or lower motor findings reminiscent, respectively, of ALS or spinal muscular atrophy (SMA). Anticholinesterase drug overdose and cholinomimetics drugs induce fasciculation in normal individuals, as can inhalation of isoflurane gas, which depresses end-plate depolarization and inhibits fasciculation caused by succinylcholine.

Fasciculation may be limited to muscles innervated by individual motor nerves in multifocal motor neuropathy with or without conduction block or elevated titers of GM1 antibodies. Fasciculation may also be limited to individual nerve territories in the setting of compression and entrapment as, for example, along the ulnar nerve around the elbow, or the peroneal nerve at the fibular head or knee. Radiation therapy can lead to focal MND when portions of

Table 2. Classification of Fasciculation

Benign
    Benign fasciculation
    Cramp fasciculation syndrome
Systemic Disorders
    Electrolyte disturbances
    Endocrinopathy
    Paget disease
    Ciguatera infection
Post-irradiation
    Motor neuron disease
    Plexopathy
Peripheral Nervous System Disorders
    Inclusion body myositis
    Plexopathy
    Radiculopathy
    Motor neuropathy
Central Nervous System Disorders
    Poliomyelitis
    Post-poliomyelitis
    Amyotrophic lateral sclerosis
    Spinal muscular atrophy

the spinal cord are incompletely shielded during treatment of a contiguous intramedually glioma or schwannoma, as may brachial plexopathy and lumbosacral plexopathy when these structures are included in the field of radiation as, for example, in the treatment of an apical lung tumor or malignant tumor of the plexus. Paget disease of the high cervical cord can lead to basilar invagination and cervical cord compression resulting in the syndrome of segmental weakness, wasting, fasciculation, and hyperreflexia reminiscent of ALS. Finally, fasciculation occurs in diverse progressive inherited neurological disorders among them Machado-Joseph disease (Azorean disease), pallido-luysio-nigral atrophy, myelofibrosis, multisystem atrophy syndrome, gangliosidosis, and olivopontocerebellar atrophy.

When recorded by needle electromyography (EMG), fasciculation potentials fire irregularly with the configuration of motor unit potentials (MUP) generally signifying irritability or denervation depending upon the associated etiopathogenesis and associated disorder. Their firing frequency varies from a few per minute to one per second. It is possible to differentiate fasciculation potentials from abnormal chronic spontaneous activity of other causes that lead to focal movement of the surface of muscle by careful electrophysiological testing by observation of the firing rate, configuration, and synchronicity of the abnormal MUP.

Myotonia, myokymia, and cramps may present diagnostic challenges. Myotonic discharges are action potentials of single muscle fibers that occur in trains, with a firing frequency and amplitude that continuously changes, a feature that leads to their pitch variation reminiscent of a dive bomber airplane. They are a frequent associated finding in muscle membrane disorders and channelopathies, resulting from disturbances of muscle ion channel function and membrane excitability, as in myotonic muscle dystrophy, periodic paralysis, neuromyotonia, malignant hyperthermia, episodic ataxia, and hereditary rippling muscle disease. Myokymic discharges are composed of two or more grouped repetitive discharges that can also vary in number and firing frequency. They can accompany facial undulating movements due to multiple sclerosis or pontine gliomas. Myokymic movements may also be encountered in radiation-induced plexopathy, multifocal motor neuropathy, CIDP, and gold intoxication. Whereas benign fasciculation are generally uniform and simple in appearance, those seen in ALS are distinguished by their tendency for more complex and varied EMG appearance, especially in areas of subtle and minor clinical wasting and their frequent association with fibrillation and positive sharp waves, especially in advanced disease.

Patients with clinical and electrophysiological fasciculation should be carefully evaluated with the goal of identifying the underlying genetic, metabolic, compressive, or degenerative etiopathogenesis, and ascertainment of a coexisting primary muscle, neuromuscular junction, peripheral nerve, root, or perikaryal localization. Blood studies should be set for parathyroid, calcium levels, thyroid function, detailed electrodiagnostic studies, and appropriate neuroimaging studies if there is suspicion of inflammatory, degenerative, or compressive disease, plexopathy, radiculopathy, or spinal cord involvement. While there is no effective therapy for benign or symptomatic fasciculation, attention to potential provocative factors is useful.

CRAMPS

Cramps are transient, painful, involuntary contractions of a muscle or group of muscles that ordinarily last a few seconds or up to a minute or more, provoked by contraction of an already shortened muscle. They occur most often during or after vigorous exercise. Noctural cramps cause forceful painful flexion of the ankles and toes, and typically the calves (190). Most individuals experience cramps at some time in their lives and at any age. The frequency of cramps in children is 7% compared with 50% in those over age 65 years, with greater occurrence in women, pregnancy, and peripheral vascular disease (191).

The classification of disorders associated with cramps is shown in Table 3. There is a syndrome of cramps and benign fasciculation. They occur in neuromyotonia or Isaacs syndrome accompanied by myokymia, abnormal postures, pseudomyotonia, and hyperhydrosis. Cramps may be the first sign of a metabolic myopathy occurring with myo-

adenylate deaminase deficiency, phosphorylase deficiency, phosphofructokinase deficiency, phosphoglycerate kinase deficiency, dystrophinopathy, myotonia congenital, and in Brody syndrome of calcium ATPase reuptake deficiency of type II fibers. Noctural leg cramps are especially common in restless leg syndrome, sleep-induced myoclonus, sleep paralysis, and bruxism and occur mainly during rapid eye movement (REM) sleep, and in stage 1 through 3 of non-REM sleep. Noctural leg cramps with a known genetic predisposition are usually accompanied by myoclonic jerks and frequently are painful. They are statistically more common with dehydration, hyperhidrosis, thyrotoxicosis, hypothyroidism, uremia, hypomagnesemia, hypokalemia, hypocalcemia, uremia, gout, cirrhosis, stingray injury, and excessive ingestion of licorice. Frequent cramps may be the first clue to underlying peripheral neuropathy and spinal root compression. Dystonia, MND, Parkinson disease, stiff man syndrome, poliomyelitis, post-polio syndrome, and drug ingestions may all predispose to frequent cramps. Possible offending drugs include beta blockers, anticholinesterases, dihydroergotamine, caffeine, statin medication, cimetidine, chemotherapy agents, diuretics, lithium, hexacarbon agents, nifedepine, phenothiazines, terbutaline, theophyllines, and alcohol.

Table 3. Classification of Cramps

Idiopathic
  Noctural leg cramps
  Sleep disorders
  Pregnancy
Systemic Disorders
  Dehydration
  Electrolyte disturbances
  Arthritis
  Peripheral vascular disease
Peripheral Nervous System Diseases
  Neuromyotonia (Isaacs syndrome)
  Stiff-man syndrome
  Metabolic myopathy
  Progressive muscular dystrophy
  Myotonia congenita
  Peripheral neuropathy
  Radiculopathy
Central Nervous System Diseases
  Poliomyelitis
  Post-polio syndrome
  Tropical spastic paraparesis
  Motor neuron disease
Drug Induced
  Albuterol, anticholinesterases, beta blockers, ergotamines, caffeine, statins, chemotherapy agents, diuretics, lithium, hexacarbons, phenothiazines, theophyllines, alcohol

The EMG findings of a cramp consist of high-frequency 200 to 300 Hz repetitive MUP beginning with single potentials, followed by doublets or more. The activity generally spreads synchronously to adjacent areas of muscle and displays more than a single discharge at sites innervated sequentially, that waxes and wanes, continuing for several minutes until it abates. Muscle stretching can interrupt the discharge or render it asynchronous, and eventually stops it altogether. A similar benefit occurs with repetitive nerve stimulation at 10 to 40 Hz for several seconds. Afterward, the muscle may appear irritable, exhibiting spontaneous MUP discharges for several minutes.

Although the exact mechanism of cramps remains unknown, they likely derive from a common expression of several mechanisms in many diverse clinical settings. The experimental application of local anesthetic along a peripheral nerve blocks the electrical discharge of a cramp potential and the severe pain associated therein more effectively than spinal anesthesia, general anesthesia, and intravenous diazepam. The pain that accompanies cramps may be influenced by several factors, including excitation of pain-sensitive nerve terminals in response to mechanical stimulation, local production of lactic acid, accumulation of potassium, creatine, and inflammatory cell infiltration associated with myalgia, swelling, and local injury.

Infrequent calf cramps ordinarily should not lead to inordinate concern, however more persistent ones should prompt general medical and neurological evaluation, blood studies for systemic disorders including serum CK and EMG and nerve conduction studies for muscle, peripheral nerve disorders, and MND, followed by muscle and nerve biopsy if warranted. Noctural cramps that fragment sleep may warrant further investigation with polysomnography with concomitant need EMG recording.

Passive lengthening of the calf muscle by forceful flexion of the foot, standing, and walking on the affected leg lessen the cramp. Prevention may follow discontinuation of the offending drug or correction of a metabolic deficiency. Quinine salts, tonic water, bitter lemon beverages, verapimil hydrochloride, gabapentin, aspirin, roloxifene, and B vitamin supplements may all lead to a reduction in cramps. Trigger point injections with 0.5% to 1% xylocaine hydrochloride and botulinum toxin may also be considered in refractory situations.

REFERENCES

1. Abd TT, Jacobson TA. Statin-induced myopathy: a review and update. *Expert Opin Drug Saf* 2011; 10:373–387.
2. Dalakas MC. Toxic and drug-induced myopathies. *J Neurol Neurosurg Psychiat* 2009; 80:832–838.
3. Sirvent P, Mercier J, Lacampagne A. New insights into mechanisms of statin-associated myotoxicity. *Curr Opin Pharmacol* 2008; 8:333–338.
4. Thompson PD, Clarkson P, Karas Rh. Statin-associated myopathy. *JAMA* 2003; 289:1681–1690).
5. Echaniz-Iaguna A, Mohr M, Tranchant C. *N Engl J Med* 2010; 362:564–565).
6. Kissel JT, Miller R. Muscle pain and fatigue. In: Schapira AHV, Griggs RC, eds. *Muscle diseases.* Woburn, MA: Butterworth-Heinemann, 1999; 33–58).
7. Mills KR, Edward RHT. Investigative strategies for muscle pain. *J Neurol Sci* 1983; 58:73–88).
8. Vorgerd M, Zange J. Carbohydrate oxidation disorders of skeletal muscle. *Curr Opin Clin Nutr Metab Care* 2002; 5:611–617.
9. Deschauer M, Wieser T, Zierz S. Muscle carnitine palmitoyltransferase II deficiency: clinical and molecular genetic features and diagnostic aspects. *Arch Neurol* 2005; 62:37–41.
10. DiMauro S, Lamperti C. Muscle glycogenoses. Muscle Nerve 2001; 24:984–999.
11. Bak H, Cordato D, Carey WF, et al. Adult-onset exercise intolerance due to phosphorylase b kinase deficiency. *J Clin Neurosci* 2001; 8:286–287.
12. Bruno C, Bertini E, Santorelli FM, et al. HyperCKemia as the only sign of McArdle's disease in a child. *J Child Neurol* 2000; 15:137–138.
13. Poulton Kr, Khan AA, Rossi ML, et al. Muscle phosphoglycerate Mutase deficiency: a study of a family with metabolic myopathy. *Functl Neurol* 1994; 9:47–58.
14. Gross M. Clinical heterogeneity and molecular mechanisms in inborn muscle AMP deaminase deficiency. *J Inherit Metab Dis* 1997; 20:186–192.
15. Pantoja-Martinez J, Navarro Fernandez-Balbuena C, Gormaz-Moreno Quintans-Castro B, et al. Myoadenylate deaminase deficiency in a child with myalgias induced by physical exercise. *Rev Neurol* 2004; 39:431–434.
16. Tieleman AA, van der Velden MP. Visser MC, et al. Four family members with proximal myotonic myopathy. *Ned Tijdschr Geneeskd* 2004; 148:948–952.
17. Van der Bergh PY, Gerard JM, Elosegi JA, et al. Novel missense mutation in the caveolin-3 gene in a Belgian family with rippling muscle disease. *J Neurol Neurosurg Psychiatry* 2004; 75:1349–1351.
18. Vielhaber S, Feistner H, Weis J, et al. Primary carnitine deficiency: adult onset lipid storage myopathy with a mild clinical course. *J Clin Neurosci* 2004; 11:919–924.
19. Krasnianski M, Neudecker S, Deschauer M, et al. The clinical spectrum of limb-girdle muscular dystrophies type in cases of a mutation in the "fukutin-related-protein"—gene. *Nervenerzt* 2004; 75:770–775.
20. Sanchez-Arjona MB, Rodriguez-Uranga JJ, Giles-Lima M, et al. Spanish family with myalgia and cramps syndrome. *J Neurol Neurosurg Psychiatry* 2005; 76:286–289.
21. Martin JJ, Ceuterick C, Van Goethem G. On a dominantly inherited myopathy with tubular aggregates. *Neuromuscul Disord* 1997; 7:512–520.
22. Sobreira C, Marques W Jr, Barreira AA. Myalgia as the revealing symptom of multicore disease and fibre type disproportion myopathy. *J Neurol Neurosurg Psychiatry* 2003; 74:1317–1319.
23. Dalakas MC. Autoimmune inflammatory myopathies. *Handb Clin Neurol* 2007; 86:273–301.
24. Hachulla E. Dermatomyositis and polymyositis: clinical aspects and treatment. *Ann Med Interne* (Paris) 2001; 152:455–464.

25. Younger DS, Younger APJ. Vasculitis and connective tissue disorders. In, Kalman B, Brannagan TH III, eds. *Neuroimmunology in Clinical Practice*. Wiley-Blackwell, 2008.

26. Younger DS. Neurovasculitis. Am Academy Neurology. *Continuum-Internal Medicine* 2005.

27. Blakaran BN, Roberts LA, Ramcharan J. Systematic lupus erythematosus in Trinidadian children. *Ann Trop Paediatr* 2004; 24:241–244.

28. Eriksson P, Andersson C, Ekerfelt C, et al. Sjogren's syndrome with myalgia is associated with subnormal secretion of cytokines by peripheral blood mononuclear cells. *J Rheumatol* 2004; 31:729–735.

29. Yamane T, Yamauchi H, Imaizumi Y, et al. 3 cases of polymyalgia rheumatica (PMR), in which serum amyloid A was useful index of the disease activity. *Ryumachi* 2001; 41:756–762.

30. Plumley SG, Rubio R, Alasfar S, et al. Polyarteritis nodosa presenting as polymyositis. *Semin Arthritis Rheum* 2002; 31:377–383.

31. Louthrenoo W, Norasetthada A, Khunamornpong S, et al. Childhood Churg-Strauss syndrome. *J Rheumatol* 1999; 26:1387–1393.

32. Bodenseh A, Klepzig C, Schon D. Chrug-Strauss syndrome. *Dtsch Med Wochenschr* 1994; 119:581–584.

33. Gran JT, Nordvag BY, Storesund B. An overlap syndrome with features of atypical Cogan syndrome and Wegener's granulomatosis. *Scand J Rheumatol* 1999; 28:62–64.

34. Bagnato GF, Quattrocchi E, Guilli S, et al. Unusual polyarthritis as a unique clinical manifestation of coelia disease. *Rheumatol Int* 2000; 20:29–30.

35. Gupta SK. Sarcoidosis: a journey through 50 years. *Indian J Chest Dis Allied Sci* 2002; 44:247–253.

36. Mori Y, Kahari VM, Varga J. Scleroderma-like cutaneous syndromes. *Curr Rheumatol Rep* 2002; 4:113–122.

37. Wojas-Pelc A, Wielowwieyska-Szybinska D, Lipko-Godlewska S. Eosinophilic fasciitis—current database. *Pol Merkuriusz Lek* 2004; 16:585-588).

38. Hengstman GJ, van Venrooij WJ, van den Hoogen FH, et al. The anti-synthetase syndrome: muscle disease and multisystem disorder at the same time. *Ned Tijdschr Geneeskd* 2003; 147:1485–1489).

39. Hengstman GJ, van Venrooij WJ, van den Hoogen FH, et al. The anti-synthetase syndrome: muscle disease and multisystem disorder at the same time. *Ned Tijdschr Geneeskd* 2003; 147:1485–1489.

40. Bendixen B, Younger DS, Hair L, et al. Cholesterol emboli syndrome: a patient with peripheral neuropathy. *Neurology* 1992; 42:428–430.

41. Lamprecht P, Moosig F, Adam-Klages S, et al. Small vessel vasculitis and relapsing panniculitis in tumour necrosis factor receptor associated periodic syndrome (TRAPS). *Ann Rheum Dis* 2004; 63:1518–1520;

42. Kotevoglu N, Sahin F, Ozkiris SO, et al. Protracted febrile myalgia of familial Mediterranean fever. *Clin Exp Rheumatol* 2004; 22(Suppl 34):S69–S70.

43. Lamprecht P, Timmann C, Ahmadi Simab K, et al. Hereditary periodic fever. *Internist* (Berl) 2004; 45:904–911.

44. Mohamed HA, Aldakar MO, Habib N. Cardiogenic shock due to acute hemorrhagic necrosis of a pheochromocytoma: a case report and review of the literature. *Can J Cadiol* 2003; 19:573–576).

45. Koea JB, Broadhurst GW, Rodgers MS, et al. Inflammatory pseudotumor of the liver: demographics, diagnosis and the case for nonoperative management. *J Am Coll Surg* 2003; 196:226–235.

46. Mert A, Ozaras R, Tabak F, et al. Fever of unknown origin: a review of 20 patients with adult-onset Still's disease. *Clin Rheumatol* 2003; 22:89–93.

47. Zivkovic SA, Lacomis D, Clemens PR. Chronic eosinophilic perimyositis with persistent myalgias. *Muscle Nerve* 2002; 25:461–465.

48. Pongsatha S, Morakote N, Sribanditmongkol N, et al. Symptoms of estrogen deficiency in nursing personnel in Mahar Nakorn Chiang Mai Hospital. *J Med Assoc Thai* 2004; 87:405–409).

49. Punzi L, Betterle C. Chronic autoimmune thyroiditis and rheumatic manifestations. *Joint Bone Spine* 2004; 71:275–283.

50. Carvalho JP, Carvalho FM, Lima de Oliveira FF, et al. Hypothyroidism following struma ovarii tumor resection: a case report. *Rev Hosp Clin Fac Med Sao Paulo* 2002; 57:112–114.

51. Djrolo F, Houngbe F, Attolou V, et al. Hypothyroidism: clinical and etiological aspects in Cotonou (Republic of Benin). *Sante* 2001; 11:245–249.

52. Adachi J, Asano M, Ueno Y, et al. Alcoholic muscle disease and biomembrane perturbations. *J Nutr Biochem* 2003; 14:616–625.

53. Pimentel L. Scurvy: historical review and current diagnostic approach. *Am J Emerg Med* 2003; 21:328–332.

54. Daroca P, Rodriguez J, Reano M, et al. Fever from caffeine. *Allergy* 1996; 51:189–191.

55. Lang C, Behnke H, Bitterohl J, et al. Special features of intensive care of toxic shock syndrome. Review and case report of a TSST-1 associated toxic-shock syndrome with adult respiratory distress syndrome and multiple organ failure from a staphylococcal panaritium. *Anaesthesist* 2003; 52:805–813.

56. Balderramo DC, Bertoli AM, Paganini MA, et al. Severe polyarthritis and tenosynovitis due to Streptococcus agalactiae in a patient with functional hyposplenia. *Medicine* (B Aires) 2002; 62:337–338.

57. Carrol ED, Thomson AP, Mobbs KJ, et al. Myositis in children with meningococcal disease: a role for tumor necrosis factor-alpha interleukin-8. *J Infect* 2002; 44:17–21.

58. Montiel NJ, Baumgarten JM, Sinha AA. Lyme disease—part II: clinical features and treatment. *Cutis* 2002; 69:443–448.

59. Weinstein A, Britchkov M. Lyme arthritis and post Lyme disease syndrome. *Curr Opin Rheumatol* 2002; 14:383–387.

60. Karande S, Satam N, Kulkarni M, et al. Leptospiral pneumonia. *Indian J Pediatr* 2005; 72:86.

61. Lablebicioglu H, Sencan I, Sunbul M, et al. Weil's Disease: report of 12 cases. *Scand J Infect Dis* 1996; 28:637–639.

62. Ahuja SR, Karande S, Naik S, et al. Boutonnuese fever in a child: a case report and overview. *J Indian Med Assoc* 2004; 102:170–171, 173.

63. Jensenius M, Fournier PE, Raoult D. Rickettsioses and the international traveler. *Clin Infect Dis* 2004; 39:1493–1499.

64. Jensenius M, Fournier PE, Kelly P, et al. African tick bite fever. *Lancet Infect Dis* 2003; 3: 557–564.

65. Weinstein RS. Human ehrlichiosis. *Am Fam Physician* 1996; 54:1971–1976;

66. Lotric-Furlan S, Petrovec M, Avsic-Zupanc T, et al. Epidemiological, clinical and laboratory distinction between human granulocytic Ehrlichiosis and the initial phase of tick-bone encephalitis. *Wien Klin Wochenschr* 2002; 114:636–640.

67. Thap LC, Supanaranond W, Treeprasertsuk S, et al. Septic shock secondary to scrub typhus: characteristic and complications. *Southeast Asian J Trop Med Public Health* 2002; 33:780–786.

68. Bjorn AM, Lebeech AM. Extrapulmonary complications of Mycoplasma pneumoniae infections. *Ugeskr Laeger* 2002; 164:1805–1809.

69. Ndiaye M, Hane AA, Dieng MT, et al. Sharp syndrome complicating pulmonary tuberculosis: appropo of a case. *Dakar Med* 1999; 44:236–239.

70. Lieberman D, Lieberman D, Shmarkov O, et al. Serological evidence of Legionella species infection in acute exacerbation of COPD. *Eur Respir J* 2002; 19:392–397.

71. Senol M, Ozcan A, Karincaoglu Y, et al. Tularemia: a case transmitted from a sheep. *Cutis* 1999; 63:49–51.

72. Marrie TJ. Coxiella burnetti(Q Fever) pneumonia. *Clin Infect Dis* 1995 Dec; 21 Suppl 3:S253–64.

73. Stevens H, Beeres MP, Meijer JG, et al. Q fever: not just in sheep. *Ned Tijdschr Geneeskd* 2000; 144:1297–1300.

74. Matsushima H, Takayanagi N, Ubukata M, et al. A case of fulminant psittacosis with rhabdomyolysis. *Nihon Kokyuki Gakkai Zasshi* 2002; 40:612–616.

75. Kittang BR, Chelsom J, Jenum PA, et al. Brucellosis—a rare zoonosis. *Tidsskr Nor Laegeforen* 2003; 123:2705–2707.

76. Apanova VI, Badmaev BE, Boloshinov AB, et al. Trichinosis in the Republic Buriatiia. *Med Parazitol* (Mosk) 2004; 34–35.

77. Lopez Hernandez B, Velazquez de Castro MT, Galicia MD, et al. Outbreak of Trichinella britovi infection in Granada in the spring of 2000. *Rev Esp Salud Publica* 2001; 75:467–473.

78. Erkens K, Lademann M, Tinelnot K, et al. Histoplasmosis group disease in bat researchers returning from Cuba. *Dtsch Med Wochenschr* 2002; 127:21–25.

79. Friedlander AM. Clinical aspects, diagnosis and treatment of anthrax. *J Appl Microbiol* 1999; 87:303).

80. Welt S, Ritter G, William C Jr, et al. Phase I study of anticolon cancer humanized antibody A33. *Clin Cancer Res* 2003; 9:1338–1346.

81. Lamonte M, Silberstein SD, Marcelis JF. Headache associated with aseptic meningitis. *Headache* 1995; 35:520–526.

82. Kawai N, Iwaki N, Kawashima T, et al. Clinical symptoms of influenza infection in the 2002–2003 season. *Kansenshogaku Zasshi* 2004; 78:681–689.

83. Brotherton JM, Delpech VC, Gilbert GL, et al. Cruise Ship Outbreak Investigation Team. A large outbreak of influenza A and B on a cruise ship causing widespread morbidity. *Epidemiol Infect* 2003; 130:263–271.

84. Kohno M, Koike Y, Hojo N, et al. A case of pyomyositis following influenza virus infection. *Kansenshogaku Zasshi* 2003; 77:505–509.

85. Casali CG, Pereira MR, Santos LM, et al. The epidemic of dengue and hemorrhagic dengue fever in the city of Rio de Janerio, 2001/2002. *Rev Soc Bras Med Trop* 2004; 37:296–299.

86. Nigro G, Anceschi MM, Cosmi EV; Congenital Cytomegalic Disease Collaborating Group. Clinical manifestations and abnormal laboratory findings in pregnant woman with primary cytomegalovirus infection. *BJOG* 2003; 110:572–577.

87. Leung CW, Chiu WK. Clinical picture, diagnosis treatment and outcome of severe acute respiratory sybdrome (SARS) in children. *Pediatr Respir Rev* 2004; 5:275–288.

88. Peris JS, Lai ST, Pon LL, et al. SARS rudy study group. Coronavirus as a possible cause of severe acute respiratory syndrome. *Lancet* 2003; 361:1319–1325.

89. Brunner J, Litwicki A, Aliani S, et al. Coxsackie virus B 4 encephalitis in a 7-year-old boy. *Klin Padiatr* 2004; 216:297–299.

90. Watt G, Jongsakul K. Acute undifferentiated fever caused by infection with Japanese encephalitis virus. *Am J Trop Med Hyg* 2003; 68:704–706.

91. Perlemuter G, Cacoub P, Sbai A, et al. Hepatitis C virus infection in systematic lupus erythematosus: a case-control study. *J Rheumatol* 2003; 30:1473–1478.

92. Formenty P, Hatz C, Le Guenno B, et al. Human infection due to Ebola virus, subtype Cote d'Ivoire: clinical and biological presentation. *J Infect Dis* 1999; 179(Suppl 1):S48–53.

93. Flexman JP, Smith DW, Mackenzie JS, et al. A comparison of the diseases caused by Ross River virus and Barmah Forest virus. *Med J Aust* 1998; 169:159–163.

94. Mendes WS, Aragao NJ, Santos HJ, et al. Hantavirus pulmonary syndrome in Anajatuba, Maranhao, Brazil. *Rev Inst Med Trop Sao Paulo* 2001; 43:437–440.

95. Rossenberg E, Cotton D. Primary HIV infection and the acute retroviral syndrome. *AIDS Clin Care* 1997; 9:19, 23–25.

96. Sieb JR, Gillessen T. Iatrogenic and toxic myopathies. *Muscle Nerve* 2003; 27:142–156.

97. Caglar K, Safali M, Yavuz I, et al. Colchicine-induced myopathy with normal creatine phosphokinase level in a renal transplant patient. *Nephron* 2002; 92:922–924.

98. Caglar K, Odabasi Z, Safali M, et al. Colchicine-induced myopathy with myotonia in a patient with chronic renal failure. *Clin Neurol Neurosurg* 2003; 105:274–276.

99. Clenin GE, van Rooijen MM, Braathen LR. Ibuprofen-induced, transient ANA- and anti-histone positive leukocytoclastic vasculitis. *Hautarzt* 2000; 51:678–681.

100. Hino A, Mitsui T, Yoneda K, et al. A case of rhabdomyolysis with administration of intravenous vasopressin. *Rinsho Shinkeigaku* 1995; 35:911–913.

101. Li L, Cai B, Wang M, et al. A double-blind, randomized, placebo-controlled multicenter students of oseltamivir phosphate for treatment of influenza infection in China. *Chin Med J* (Engl) 2003; 116:44–48.

102. Bricaire F, Cohen JM, Jacquet M, et al. Committee Journee d' Actualities Grippe. Patient perspective on zanamivir in the treatment of influenza. *Int J Clin Pract* 2002; 56:7–10.

103. Landau M, Mesterman R, Ophir J, et al. Clinical significance of markedly elevated serum creatine kinase levels in patients with acne on isotretinoin. *Acta Derm Venereol* 2001; 81:350–352.

104. Farver DK, Lavin MN. Quinine-induced hepatotoxicity. *Ann Pharmacother* 1999; 33:32–34.

105. Gonzalez Rodriguez JL, Mateos Arribas MT. Tremors, cramps, and myalgia after the use of ephedrine. *Rev Esp Anestesiol Reanim* 2002; 49:501–502.

106. Pedrol E, Masanes F, Fernandez-Sola J, et al. Lack of muscle toxicity with didanosine(ddI). Clinical and experimental studies. *J Neurol Sci* 1996; 138:42–48.

107. Pavese P, Sarrot- Reynauld F, Bonadona A, et al. Immunoallergic reaction with hepatitis induced by minocycline. *Ann Med Interne* (Paris) 1998; 149:521–523.

108. Murdoch D, Goa KL, Keam SJ. Desloratadine: an update of its efficacy in the management of allergic disorders. *Drugs* 2003; 63:2051–2077).

109. Lee TL, Aw TC. Prevention of succinylcholine-induced myalgia with lidocaine pretreatment. *J Anesth* 1991; 5:239–246).

110. Shaw K, Turner J, Del Mar C. Tryptophan and 5-hydroxytryptophan for depression. *Cochrane Database Syst Rev* 2002; CD003198).

111. Atzeni F, Marrazza MG, Sarzi-Puttini P, et al. Drug-induced lupus erythematosus. *Reumatismo* 2003; 55:147–154.

112. Peppers MP. Myalgia and arthralgia associated with enalapril and ramipril. *Am J Health Syst Pharm* 1995; 52:203–204.

113. Chipman JJ, Attanasio AF, Birkett MA, et al. The safety profile of GH replacement therapy in adults. *Clin Endocrinol* 1997; 46:473–81.

114. Piccoli GB, Rossetti M, Guarena C, et al. Myalgia: an uncommon or underestimated side effect of mycophenolate mophetil after transplantation? *Nephrol Dial Transplant* 2004; 19:1940–1942.

115. Morton SJ, Powell RJ. An audit of cyclosporine for systemic lupus erythematosus and related overlap syndromes: limitations of its use. *Ann Rheum Dis* 2000; 59:487–489.

116. William GJ, Witt PL. Comparative study of the pharmacodynamic and pharmacological effects of Betaseron and AVONEX. *J Interferon Cytokine Res* 1998; 18:967–975.

117. Bonaz B, Boitard J, Marteau P, et al. Tioguanine in patients

with Crohn's disease intolerant of resistance to azathioprine/mercaptopurine. *Aliment Pharmacol Ther* 2003; 18:401–408).

118. Reid IR, Brown JP, Burckhardt P, et al. Intravenous zoledronic acid in postmenopausal women with low bone mineral density. *N Engl J Med* 2002; 346:653–661.

119. Thompson PD, Clarkson P, Karas RH. Statin-associated myopathy. *JAMA* 2003; 289:1681–1690.

120. Franc S, Dejager S, Bruckert E, et al. A comprehensive description of muscle symptoms associated with lipid-lowering drugs. *Cardiovasc Drugs Ther* 2003; 17:459–465.

121. Baker SK, Baird JK, Tiwari T, Martin GJ, et al. Chloroquine for the treatment of uncomplicated malaria in Guyana. *Ann Trop Med Parasitol* 2002; 96:339–348.

122. Vaishnaw AK, TenHoor CN. Pharmacokinetics, biologic activity, and tolerability of alefacept intravenous and intramuscular administration. *J Pharmacokinetic Pharmacodyn* 2002; 29:415–426.

123. Franscini LM, Von Vigier RO, Pfister R, et al. Effectiveness and safety of the angiotensin II antagonist irbesart in children with chronic kidney diseases. *Am J Hypertens* 2002; 15:1057–1063).

124. Porst H, Padma-Nathan H, Giuliano F, et al. Efficacy of tadalafil for the treatment of erectile dysfunction at 24 and 36 hours after dosing: a randomized controlled trial. *Urology* 2003; 62:121–126.

125. Osegbe RN, Shittu OB, Aghaji AE, et al. Sildenafil citrate (Viagra) for the treatment of erectile dysfunction in Negerian men. *Int J Impot Res* 2003; 15(Suppl1):S15–S18.

126. Voorburg AM, van Beck FT, Slee PH, et al. Vasculitis due to gemcitabine. *Lung Cancer* 2002; 36:203–205.

127. Simpson D, Curran MP, Perry CM. Letrozole: a review of its use in postmenopausal women with breast cancer. *Drugs* 2004; 64:1213–1230.

128. Elomaa I, Joensuu H, Blomqvist C. Vinorelbine, methotrexate and fluorouracil (VMF) as first-line therapy in metastatic breast cancer: a randomized phase II trial. *Ann Oncol* 2003; 14:699–703.

129. Jones PH, Christodoulos K, Dobbs N, et al. Combination antiangiogenesis therapy with marimastat captop and fragmin in patients with advanced cancer. *Br J Cancer* 2004; 91:30–36.

130. O'Brien ME, Splinter T, Smit EF, et al. EORTC Lung Cancer Group. Carboplatin and paclitaxol (Taxol) as an induction regimen for patients with biopsy-proven stage IIIA N2 non-small cell lung cancer. an EORTC phase II study (EORTC 08958). *Eur J Cancer* 2003; 39:1416–1422.

131. Winegarden JD, Mauer AM, Gajewski TF, et al. A Phase II study of bryostatin-1 and paclitaxel in patients with advanced non-small cell lung cancer. *Lung Cancer* 2003; 39:191v196.

132. Hensing TA, Peterman AH, Schell MJ, et al. The impact of age on toxicity, response rate, quality of life, and survival in patients with advanced, Stage IIIB or IV nonsmall cell lung carcinoma treated with carboplatin and paclitaxel. *Cancer* 2003; 98:779–788.

133. Esteva FJ, Rivera E, Cristofanilli M, et al. A Phase II study of intravenous exatecan mesylate (DX-8951f) administered daily for 5 days every 3 weeks to patients with metastatic breast carcinoma. *Cancer* 2003; 98:900–907.

134. (Lou FD, Lu XC. The early efficacy of imatinib in the treatment of 54 cases of chronic myeloid leukemia. *Zhonghua Nei Ka Za Zhi* 2003; 42:571–573.

135. Clamp AR, Blackhall FH, Vasey P, et al. Cancer Research UK Phase I/II Committee. A phase II trial of a bryostatin-1 administered by weekly 24-hour infusion in recurrent epithelial ovarian carcinoma. *Br J Cancer* 2003; 89:1152–1154.

136. Goss PE, Ingle JN, Martino S, et al. A randomized trial of letrozole in postmenopausal women after five years of tamoxifen therapy for early-stage breast cancer. *N Engl J Med* 2003; 349:1793–1802.

137. D'Alessandro D, Ciriminna S, Rossini A, Bossa MC, Fara GM. Requests of medical examinations after pneumococcal & influenza vaccination in the elderly. *Indian J Med Res* 2004; 119 (Suppl):108–114.

138. Schnell R, Borchmann P, Staak JO, et al. Clinical evaluation of ricin A-chain immunotoxins in patients with Hodgkin's lymphoma. *Ann Oncol* 2003; 14:729–736.

139. Messing EM, Manola J, Wilding G, et al. Eastern Cooperative Oncology Group/Intergroup trial. Phase III study of interferon alfa-NL as adjuvant treatment for resectable renal cell carcinoma: an Eastern Cooperative Oncology Group/Intergroup trial. *J Clin Oncol* 2003; 21:1214–1222.

140. Sessa C, Weigang-Kohler K, Pagani O, et al. Phase I and pharmacological studies of the cryptophycin analog LY355703 administered on a single intermittent or weekly schedule. *Eur J Cancer* 2002; 38:2388–2396.

141. Rizvi NA, Marshall JL, Ness E, et al. Initial clinical trial of oral TAC-101, a novel retinoic acid receptor-alpha selective retinoid, in patients with advanced cancer. *J Clin Oncol* 2002; 20:3522–3532.

142. Kalofonos HP, Onyenadum A, Kosmas C, et al. Mitomycin C and vinblastine in anthracycline-resistant metastatic breast cancer: a phase II study. *Tumori* 2001; 87:394–397.

143. Uckun FM, Messinger Y, Chen CL, et al. Treatment of therapy-refractory B lineage acute lymphoblastic leukemia with an apoptosis-including CD19-directed tyrosine kinase inhibitor. *Clin Cancer Res* 1999; 5:3906–3913.

144. Chae L, Moon HS, Kim SC. Overdose of vincristine: experience with a patient. *J Korean Med Sci* 1998; 13:334–338.

145. Rosenfeld CS, Zeigler ZR, Shadduck RK, et al. Phase II study of rquinimex in myelodysplastic syndrome. *Am J Clin Oncol* 1997; 20:189–192.

146. Seymour BD, Rubinger M. Rhabdomyolysis induced by epsilon-aminocaproic acid. *Ann Pharmacother* 1997; 31:56–58.

147. Kulick M, Daneshmand H. Breast implantation and the incidence of upper extremity somatic complaints. *Aesthetic Plast Surg* 1997; 21:105–109.

148. Sato N, Okamoto S, Mori T, et al. Recurrent acute myositis after allogeneic bone marrow transplantation for myelodysplasia. *Hematology* 2002; 7:109–112.

149. Katayama T, Kamiya M, Hoshina S, et al. Fatal septic shock and rhabdomyolysis following transfusion of platelet concentrates contaminated with Streptococcus pneumoniae. *Rinsho Ketsueki* 2003; 44:381–385.

150. Werawatganon T, Kyokong O, Charuluxananan S, et al. Muscular injury after succinylcholine and electroconvulsive therapy. *Anesth Analg* 2004; 98:1676–1679.

151. Krishnamurthy K, John GT, Abraham P, et al. Granulocyte macrophage colony stimulating factor augmented hepatitis B vaccine protocol for rapid seroprotection in voluntary kidney donors. *Indian J Med Res* 2004; 119:162–164.

152. D'Alessandro D, Ciriminna S, Rossini A, et al. Requests of medical examinations after pneumococcal and influenza vaccination in the elderly. *Indian J Med Res* 2004; 119(Suppl):108–114.

153. Callado AB, Ponte Cameiro TG, da Cunha Parahyba CC, et al. Rhabdomyolysis secondary to influenza A H1N1 vaccine resulting in acute kidney injury. *Travel Med Infect Dis* 2012 Dec. 3 pii: S1477–8939(12)00126-3 [Epub ahead of print].

154. Ruggeberg J, Hearth PT. Safety and efficacy of meningococcal group C conjugate vaccine. *Expert Opin Drug Saf* 2003; 2:7–19.

155. Cono J, Casey CG, Bell DM. Centers for Disease Control and Prevention. Smallpox vaccination and adverse reactions. Guidance for clinicians. *MMWR Recomm Rep* 2003; 52:1v2.

156. Lathrop SL, Ball R, Haber P, et al. Adverse event reports following vaccination for Lyme disease: December 1988–July 2000. *Vaccine* 2002; 20:1603–1608.

157. Amurao GV, Gottwald LD, Duggan J, et al. Vaccine era measles in an adult. *Cutis* 2000; 66:337–340.

158. Tingle AJ, Mitchell LA, Grace M, et al. Randomised double-blind placebo-controlled study on adverse effects of rubella immunization in seronegative women. *Lancet* 1997; 349:1277–1281.

159. Chodorowski Z, Waldman W, Sein Anand J. Acute poisoning with Tricholoma equestre. *Przegl Lek* 2002; 59:386–387.

160. Bucaretchi F, Herrera SR, Hyslop S, et al. Snakebites by Crotalus durissus ssp in children in Campinas Sau Paulo, Brazil. *Rev Inst Med Trop Sao Paulo* 2002; 44:133–138.

161. Vutchev D. A case of intoxication after a bite by Latrodectus Tredecimguttatus. *Scand J Infect Dis* 2001; 33:313–314.

162. Pearn J. Neurology of ciguatera. *J Neurol Psychiatry* 2001; 70:4–8).

163. Vibrio vulnificus infections associated with eating raw oysters—LosAngeles, 1996. *MMWR Morb Mortal Wkly Rep* 1996; 45:621–624.

164. Pers C, Garhn-Hansen B, Frederiksen W. Capnocytophaga canimorsus septicemeia in Denmark, 1982–1995 review of 39 cases. *Clin Infect Dis* 1996; 23:71–75.

165. Calderon-Salinas JV, Valdez Anaya B, Mazuniga-Charles, et al. Lead exposure in a population of Mexican children. *Hum Exp Toxicol* 1996; 15:305–311.

166. Alonso-Ruiz A, Calabozo M, Perez-Ruiz F, et al. Toxic oil syndrome. A long term follow-up of a cohort of 332 patients. *Medicine* 1993; 72:285–295.

167. Ellingsen CL. Polymer fume fever. *Tidsskr Nor Laegeforen* 1998; 118:1223–1224.

168. Rosendal L, Larsson B, Kristiansen J, et al. Increase in muscle nociceptive substances and anaerobic metabolism in patients with trapezius myalgia: microdialysis in rest and during exercise. *Pain* 2004; 112:324–334.

169. Ryan EL. Pectoral girdle myalgia in women: a 5-year study in a clinical setting. *Clin J Pain* 2000; 16:298–303.

170. Larsson B, Bjork J, Kadi F, et al. Blood supply and oxidative metabolism in muscle biopsies of female cleaners with and without myalgia. *Clin J Pain* 2004; 20:440–446.

171. Gowers WR. Lumbago: its lessons and analogues. *Brit Med J* 1904; 1:117–121.

172. Hollman A. Sir Thomas Lewis: clinical scientist and cardiologist, 1881–1945. *J Medical Biography* 1994; 2:63–70.

173. Boland EW, Corr Col. WP. Psychogenic rheumatism. *JAMA* 1943; 123:805–809.

174. Traut EF. *J Am Med Ger Soc* 1968; 16:531–538.

175. McCarty D, Gatter RA, Phelps P. A dolorimeter for quantification of articular tenderness. *Arthrit Rheumat* 1965; 8:551–559.

176. Hauri P, Hawkins DR. Alpha-delta sleep. *Electroenceph Clin Neurophysiol* 1973; 34:233–237.

177. Moldofsky H, Scarisbrick P, England R, et al. Musculoskeletal symptoms and non-REM sleep disturbance in patients with "fibrositis syndrome" and healthy subjects. *Psychosomatic Med* 1975; 37:341–351.

178. Smyth HA, Moldofsky H. Two contributions to understanding of the "fibrositis" syndrome. *Bulletin of Rheumatic Diseases* 1977; 28:928–931.

179. Yunus M, Masi AT, Calabro JJ, et al. Primary fibromyalgia (fibrositis): clinical study of 50 patients with matched normal controls. *Semin Arthritis Rheum* 1981; 11:151–171.

180. Wolfe F, Smythe H, Yunus M, et al. The American College of Rheumatology 1990 criteria for the classification of fibromyalgia: report of the multicenter criteria committee. *Arthritis Rheumat* 1990; 33:160–173.

181. Anon. Fibromyalgia: the Copenhagen declaration. *Lancet* 1992; 340:663–664.

182. Hudson JI, Hudson MS, Pliner LF, et al. Fibromyalgia ad major affective disorders: a controlled phenomenology and family history study. *Am J Psychiat* 1985; 142:441–446.

183. Hudson JI, Golderberg DL, Pope Jr, HG. Comorbidity of fibromyalgia with medical and psychiatric disorders. *Am J Med* 1992; 363–367.

184. Cohen ML, Quintner JL. Fibromyalgia syndrome, a problem of tautology. *Lancet* 1993; 342:906–909.

185. Bohr T. Problems with myofascial pain syndrome and fibromyalgia syndrome. *Neurology* 1996; 46:593–597.

186. Wolfe F, Simons DG, Fricton J, et al. The fibromyalgia and myofascial pain syndromes: a preliminary study of tendon points and trigger points in persons with fibromyalgia, myofascial pain syndrome, and no disease. *J Rheumatol* 1992; 19:944–951.

187. Kissel JT. The problem of fibromyalgia. *Muscle Nerve* 2002; 25:473–476.

188. Desai J, Swash M. Fasciculation: what do we know of their significance? *J Neurol Sci* 1997; 152:S43–S48.

189. de Carvalho M, Swash M. Cramps, muscle pain, and fasciculations: not always benign? *Neurology* 2004; 63:721–723.

190. Leung AK, Wong BE, Chan PY, et al. Nocturnal leg cramps in children: incidence and clinical characteristics. *J Natl Med Assoc* 1999; 91:329–332.

191. Sawaya R, Kanaan N. Nocturnal leg cramps. Clinically mysterious and painful—but manageable. *Geriatrics* 2001; 56:34–42.

CHAPTER 25

Myasthenia Gravis and Myasthenic Syndromes

Mark B. Bromberg

The neuromuscular junction (NMJ) has a complex anatomy and physiology but functions with extraordinary reliability. Its uniqueness is apparent in the expression of clinical disease that results when junctional transmission fails.

This chapter reviews the normal and clinically relevant anatomy and physiology of the NMJ, along with essential features of the clinical and laboratory diagnosis, pathology, therapy, and prognosis of acquired autoimmune myasthenia gravis (MG) including juvenile and neonatal MG, congenital MG, and Lambert Eaton myasthenic syndrome (LEMS).

THE MOTOR UNIT

The motor unit consists of a motor neuron, its peripheral axon process, and the muscle fibers it innervates (Figure 1). The motor axon ends in an arborization of terminal branches, each one making synaptic contact with muscle fibers at the NMJ, the number of which varies from 20 to 1,500. With rare exception, each muscle fiber is innervated by a single motor axon terminal branch. However, a small percentage of extraocular muscle fibers are multiply innervated. The NMJ is located midway along the length of an individual fiber in the region called the innervation zone, which extends over a wide area at the muscle motor point.

The associated weakness of an NMJ disorder results from failure of muscle fiber activation. Symptoms can at times be highly regional among muscle groups, within a muscle, and within motor units. Those from neighboring muscle fibers within a motor unit may show stable, variable, or absence of transmission.

NEUROMUSCULAR JUNCTION ANATOMY

Presynaptic

Terminal branches of the motor axon remain covered by Schwann cells until they lose their myelin covering end over a region of the muscle fiber called the end plate with specialized presynaptic and postsynaptic features (Figure 1). There the axon expands into synaptic boutons comprised of many organelles including mitochondria and enzymes for synthesis and release of acetylcholine (ACh) contained in synaptic vesicles along specialized areas of the presynaptic membrane called *active zones* in association with calcium channels where vesicular release occurs.

ACh is synthesized from acetylCoA and choline by the enzyme choline acetyltransferase. Each vesicle contains about 5,000 molecules of Ach and there are a large number of synaptic vesicles in each bouton. The boutons cluster in rows along specialized regions of the presynaptic membrane that facilitate the secretion of ACh called active zones, where vesicles fuse and ACh is released by exocytosis. Exocytosis is a complex process that depends on the influx of calcium into the presynaptic terminal (Figure 2). The active zone also includes rows of large particles thought to be the calcium channels. To prevent an increase in presynaptic membrane area by fusion of the membrane-bound vesicles, there is a recycling of excess membrane.

Postsynaptic

The presynaptic and postsynaptic membranes are separated by a gap of about 20 nm. The postsynaptic membrane is also highly specialized, thrown into deep folds that lie

451

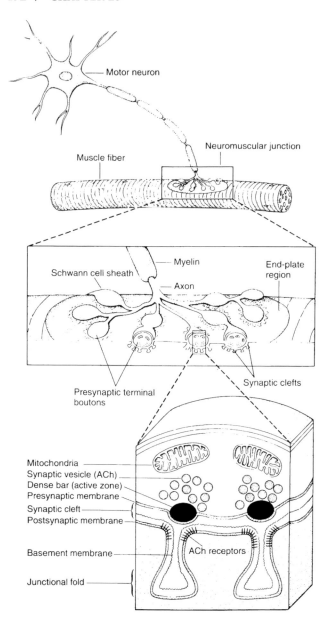

below presynaptic active zones. The shoulders of the folds contain approximately 10,000 ACh receptors (AChR)/μm^2, as well as extrajunction ACh receptors distributed along the membrane in low numbers that have no role in NMJ function. Voltage-sensitive sodium channels are situated beneath them. Clusters of molecules of acetylcholinesterase (AChE) are located in the depths of the folds. The primary mechanism of ACh inactivation occurs via rapid hydrolysis of ACh into choline and acetate by AChE, with lesser amounts by diffusion away from receptor sites. Fifty percent of the choline in ACh is recycled by an active presynaptic re-uptake mechanism.

ACh receptors are pentomeric protein complexes consisting of $\alpha 2$, β, γ, and δ subunits (Figure 3). The receptor complex spans the postsynaptic membrane, and the subunits form a pore, which is the ion channel of the action potential (AP) along the muscle fiber. A constriction in the pore opens when ACh binds to the external portions of the α subunits, allowing sodium, potassium, or chlo-

FIG. 1. Schematic diagram of the motor unit and neuromuscular junction. Only a single terminal branch of the motor unit is shown. (From, Kandel E, Schwartz J, Jessell T. *Principles of Neural Science,* 3rd ed. Norwalk, CT: Appleton & Lange, 1991, with permission.)

FIG. 2. Schematic diagram of the role of calcium on the release and mobilization of synaptic vesicles in the presynaptic terminal. A: Vesicles from the immediately available pool are docked at the active zone. Calcium channels are closed. B: The nerve action potential opens voltage sensitive channels and the calcium influx facilitates vesicular release and mobilization of bound vesicles. (From, Kandel E, Schwartz J, Jessell T. *Principles of Neural Science,* 3rd ed. Norwalk, CT: Appleton & Lange, 1991, with permission.)

A Resting state

B After Ca²⁺ influx

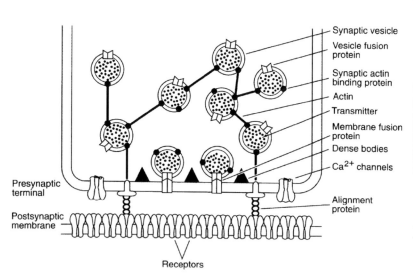
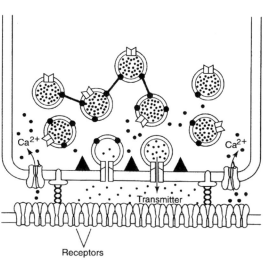

ride to pass. The density of ACh receptors falls off from the endplate region. Between the end-plate and the non-junctional muscle fiber membrane, there is a perijunctional region that contains a mixture of AChR and voltage-gated sodium channels where the muscle fiber AP is initiated. The muscle fiber membrane contains voltage-dependent sodium channels that participate in the propagation of the AP along the muscle fiber.

NEUROMUSCULAR JUNCTION PHYSIOLOGY

Presynaptic

Presynaptic membrane voltage-gated calcium channels in the vicinity of the active zone initiate the process of NMJ transmission that begins with a motor nerve fiber AP (Figure 2). Experimentally, graded degrees of terminal depolarization result in graded influxes of calcium into the presynaptic terminal. The release of ACh is in turn dependent upon, and proportional, to the concentration of calcium in the terminal, and normally there is ample influx of calcium. The release of ACh is not smoothly graded but occurs in quantal units the number of which reside in a single vesicle.

The postsynaptic response includes the number of vesicles released and the nature of the interaction of ACh with the receptors. The number of vesicles released with each motor fiber AP is in turn related to the probability of release. The role of calcium in the presynaptic terminal is to enhance the probability of ACh release, and the magnitude of release is exponential with the concentration of calcium. The spontaneous release of vesicles produces a miniature endplate potential (MEPP), which can be recorded during routine needle electromyography (EMG) studies as endplate noise when the electrode tip is by chance in the vicinity of a NMJ.

Calcium is required for the fusion of vesicles to the presynaptic membrane at the active zone and contributes to the dilation of the fusion pore between the vesicle and membrane, allowing release of ACh into the synaptic cleft (Figure 2), and is also involved in the mobilization of vesicles.

The available vesicles of ACh are distributed among several pools, including one that is immediately available in the active zone, and another pool bound to the cytoskeleton, which can be mobilized. The influx of calcium frees the vesicles from a binding protein, making the latter available to move to the active zone for subsequent fusion and release.

Molecules of AChE float in the clefts like a tethered balloon with competition between the AChR and AChE. Initially, high concentration of ACh favor binding to the receptor, but as molecules of ACh diffuse away from the receptor, enzyme hydrolysis activity dominates instead. The presynaptic membrane takes up approximately 50% of the

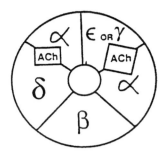

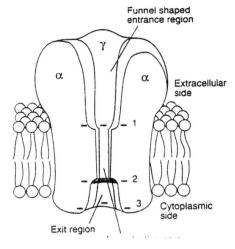

FIG. 3. Schematic diagram of the acetylcholine receptor complex. Top diagram shows the pentomeric structure of the receptor complex and binding sites for acetylcholine molecules to the a-subunits. Bottom diagram shows the transmembrane position of the receptor and the ion pore or channel. (From, Kandel E, Schwartz J, Jessell T. *Principles of Neural Science,* 3rd ed. Norwalk, CT: Appleton & Lange, 1991; and Kaminski H, Suarez J, Ruff R. Neuromuscular junction physiology in myasthenia gravis: isoforms of the acetylcholine receptor in extraocular muscles and the contribution of sodium channels to the safety factor. *Neurology* 1997; 48(Suppl 5):S8–S17, with permission.)

choline. During a motor nerve AP, the concentration of calcium rises a thousand-fold within several hundred microseconds at the active zone where calcium channels are most dense. Limited presynaptic terminal calcium buffering systems results in repeated influx of calcium that follows a train of high-frequency AP, saturating the system and leading to a calcium buildup, increasing the probability of vesicular release when the next nerve AP arrives, underlying the phenomena of post-tetanic potentiation, the process of which is blocked by high serum concentrations of magnesium.

Postsynaptic

The α subunits are the sites where ACh attaches to open the receptor channel. One ACh molecule binds to each of the

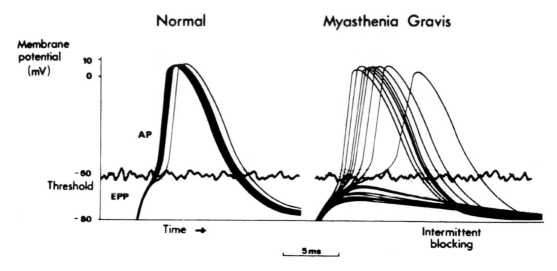

Normal   **Myasthenia Gravis**

Membrane potential (mV)

AP

EPP

Threshold

Time →

Intermittent blocking

5 ms

FIG. 4. Schematic diagram of an intracellular muscle fiber recording showing the generation of end plate potentials (EPP) and muscle fiber action potential (AP). On the left, normal neuromuscular junction function ensures that the rise time and amplitude of successive EPP are sufficient to generate AP. Note the fluctuating threshold for generating an AP and resultant variability of the AP latency. This is normal jitter. On the right, in myasthenia gravis, there are insufficient acetylcholine receptors and the EPP rise times and amplitudes vary markedly. This results in increased jitter and at times failure to initiate an AP. This is called blocking. From, Stalberg E, Trontelj JV. *Single fiber electromyography*, 2nd Ed. New York: Raven Press, 1994, with permission.

2 subunits bringing about a conformational change in the AChR that increases the diameter of the pore or channel (Figure 3). The concentration gradients of sodium, potassium, and chloride are such that sodium is the predominant ion flowing into the muscle fiber at the endplate region. Normally, there is a rapid release of ACh from the presynaptic terminal that results in a near synchronous opening of approximately 20,000 receptor channels. The resultant endplate current causes an EPP that depolarizes the endplate membrane (Figure 4). The ACh concentration in the synaptic cleft falls rapidly due to hydrolysis by AChE and diffusion, and within a millisecond the channels close, causing a fall off of endplate current flow. The EPP decays more slowly due to passive membrane properties of the muscle; with repeated stimuli, there is cyclic activation of different active zones to prevent receptor desensitization (1).

Under normal conditions the rising phase of the EPP reaches threshold, upon which voltage dependent sodium channels open and a muscle fiber AP is initiated (Figure 4). A number of factors govern endplate current flow and the shape of the EPP. The rising phase of the EPP that depends on the nearly simultaneous opening of a large number of AChR channels is largely determined by the concentration of ACh and the number of AChR. Consequently, the rise time and amplitude of the EPP depends on the probability of release of ACh and the total number of receptors available. This results clinically in a normal degree of discharge-

to-discharge temporal variability for the EPP to reach threshold, measured in microseconds, and called neuromuscular jitter. The AP is propagated along the muscle fiber membrane to the ends of the fiber, leading to muscle fiber shortening and the development of force via excitation–contraction coupling.

Muscle fiber AP are clinically and electrodiagnostically important for two reasons. First, they are prerequisites for the development of force and shortening in a muscle. Second, electrodiagnostic studies record the extracellular AP as the compound muscle action potential (CMAP) during nerve conduction studies (NCS) or as the motor unit action potential (MUAP) during needle EMG. Routine electrodiagnostic testing detects abnormalities of the NMJ only if there is a failure to initiate the muscle fiber AP and only if there is an appreciable number of failing NMJ. More subtle abnormalities at the NMJ are assessed by recording increased discharge-to-discharge temporal variability using special electrodiagnostic techniques such as single fiber EMG (SFEMG) or variation thereof employing a small concentric EMG needle.

General Considerations

There are various mechanisms within the complexity of the NMJ that assure a safety factor for NMJ transmission (1) including overabundance of ACh in the presynaptic

Table 1. Model of the Dynamics of Normal NMJ Transmission with Low Frequency RNS*

Stimulus number	ACh pool	Available ACh quanta	ACh quanta released	Resultant EPP amplitude (mV)	Action potential threshold reached
1	Immediate	1,000	200	60	Yes
2	Immediate	800	160	48	Yes
3	Immediate	640	128	38	Yes
4	Mobilizable	>640	>128	>38	Yes
5	Mobilizable	>640	>128	>38	Yes

Two ACh pools (immediately available and mobilizable) are under the influence of the influx of calcium into the presynaptic terminal. Mobilization of ACh ensures the release of an adequate number of ACh quanta. Because there are normal numbers of ACh receptors, each EPP exceeds the threshold for generating an action potential.

In this model, the EPP amplitude must be greater than 30 mV to reach threshold for generation of a muscle fiber action potential.

RNS, Repetitive nerve stimulation

NMJ, Neuromuscular junction; ACh, acetylcholine; EPP, endplate potential

*Adapted from, Albers JW, AAEM Workshop on Repetitive Stimulation.

terminals and more than adequate numbers of postsynaptic receptors, the immediately releasable pool of ACh in vesicles along the active zone, and another pool of vesicles bound to the cytoskeleton that can be freed by calcium and mobilized to the active zone. Even when the reuptake of choline is blocked experimentally by hemicholinium and the NMJ is activated to functional depletion of ACh, approximately 20% of the total ACh store still remains in a pool unavailable for release. The number of vesicles and the amount of ACh released varies, but activation of the various pools ensures a sufficient amount to depolarize the postsynaptic membrane to threshold. Within an NMJ there are a number of boutons that can be cyclically activated to prevent AChR desensitization (1).

Calcium has a leading role in the release of ACh and in mobilization of ACh pools. Depolarization of the presynaptic terminal opens voltage-sensitive calcium channels with a linear relationship between terminal calcium concentration and the amount of presynaptic ACh released. Under normal circumstances, raising the terminal calcium concentration increases the amount of presynaptic ACh released but does not augment NMJ transmission (Table 1). There are maneuvers that increase calcium availability, important in the diagnosis and treatment of NMJ disorders such as a rapid train of nerve impulses that overcomes the removal of calcium and increases ACh release. The postsynaptic AChR interact with varying amounts of ACh. Under normal conditions there is always a sufficient amount of ACh to ensure depolarization of the endplate to threshold with the generation of an AP (Figure 4). The variability in the time to reach threshold in microseconds, which is of little clinical significance, can be measured by SFEMG.

MYASTHENIA GRAVIS

Clinical Spectrum

MG is an autoimmune disorder of the postsynaptic portion of the NJM that results from a reduction in the number or functioning AChR, leading to easy fatigability and weakness, primarily of ocular, bulbar, truncal, or proximal limb muscles. The weakness ordinarily fluctuates over days, weeks, months, and years, resulting in exacerbations and remissions, and the distribution and severity varies among individuals. The first useful clinical classification system was developed by Osserman (2) (Table 2) and modified afterward (3).

Ocular MG presents with ptosis and diplopia, however bulbar symptoms of dysphagia and dysphonia may occur early in the course or follow generalized limb involvement. The onset may be sudden or insidious, with mild symptoms that wax and wane. Early symptoms, such as double vision or mild ptosis, may be so subtle as to escape detection for years. With increasing involvement over time there may be generalization leading to involvement of limb and bulbar muscles. A crisis, defined as a the need for mechanical ventilatory support, rarely occurs without other manfestations of severe generalized disease and oropharyngeal involvement. Occasional patients present with isolated vocal cord paralysis.

Natural History

Untreated, the natural history of MG is difficult to determine because many current therapies, such as corticosteroids, were available as the clinical features were being fully

Table 2. Osserman Clinical Classification of MG*

Stage	Symptoms
Neonatal	Transient symptoms from myasthenic mother
Juvenile	
Adult group I	Localized, usually ocular only
Adult group II	Generalized, both bulbar and generalized
Adult group III	Acute fulminating, bulbar and generalized with respiratory failure
Adult group IV	Late severe, evolving from groups I and II
Adult group V	With muscle atrophy, evolving from group II

*Adapted from reference 2, with permission.

recognized (4). Early investigations showed that about one-third of patients progressively worsened, with another one-third relapsing and remitting, and the remaining one-third improved for long periods of time.

The introduction of positive pressure ventilation and respiratory critical care units reduced mortality and morbidity due to myasthenic crisis and permitted safe performance of thymectomy. The extent and severity of weakness in most patients is revealed during the first 3 to 5 years of their illness, such that ocular MG that does not progress to the generalized disease in that time period will unlikely do so afterward (5).

Pathology

The pathologic alterations at the postsynaptic membrane include simplification of the postsynaptic endplate region with fewer and shallower folds, and reduced numbers of

AChR, resulting largely from antibody attachment to the receptors with complement activation and receptor lysis by membrane attack complex (MAC). In normal individuals, the halflife of the AChR is approximately 12 days, but 3 days in MG.

The various types of AChR antibodies in MG are operationally defined and based on laboratory testing procedures, with most demonstrated by radioimmunoprecipitation or ELISA assays (6). Binding antibodies are detected by reaction of the patient serum with soluble human skeletal muscle AChR. Modulating antibodies are detected by reactivity with AChR on living muscle and may be positive when the binding antibody is negative. Blocking antibodies are detected by binding of sera at or near the neurotransmitter-binding site on soluble human AChR. There is a hierarchy of testing based on the frequency of occurrence (Table 3), yet despite testing for the three available types, only 80 to 86% of patients are seropositive, with few false positives, and high specificity for MG.

Seronegative patients are believed to have an autoimmune pathogenesis similar to the seropositive cases because defects in NMJ transmission can be passively transferred to experimental animals by serum or by the IgG fraction, but the diagnosis can be problematic because 50% can have ocular symptoms alone and diagnostic tests may be equivocal.

Autoantibodies against the muscle-specific receptor tyrosine kinase (MuSK) are identified in 35% to 50% of seronegative patients, with differences in the frequency of anti-MuSK antibodies among different populations and little or no overlap among those with antibodies to the ACh and MuSK receptors (7, 8). The mechanism by which anti-MuSK antibodies affect transmission is not well understood, but both the mechanism and resulting clinical aspects differ from seropositive MG. Most patients are women, often with neck, bulbar, and respiratory muscle involvement, with normal or mildly abnormal repetitive nerve stimulation

Table 3. Muscle-Specific Autoantibodies Associated with MG*

ACh receptor antibody type	Percentage positive	Clinical features	False-positive conditions
Binding	86	71% ocular MG	Thymoma, LEMS, small-cell lung cancer, d-penicillamine
Modulating	86	71% ocular MG. Helpful when AChR binding antibodies are negative	May be caused by extraneous causes
Blocking	52	30% ocular MG	When curare-like agents are used

ACh, acetylcholine; MG, myasthenia gravis; LEMS, Lambert-Eaton myasthenic syndrome.

*Adapted from, Howard F, Lennon V, Finley J, et al. Clinical correlations of antibodies that bind, block, or modulate human acetylcholine receptors in myasthenia gravis. *Ann NY Acad Sci* 1987; 505:526–538.

(RNS) and SFEMG investigations, and variable response to medical therapy.

Advanced serology investigations, not readily available, demonstrate that sera of up to 60% of sera negative for AChR antibodies, showed MuSK reactivity, binding to clusters of AChR on cell surfaces and activate complement (9).

Other organ-specific autoantibodies occur at a higher-than-expected frequency in patients with MG, including those to thyroid microsomes, thyroglobulin, and gastric parietal cells. Such antibodies may provide supportive evidence of an autoimmune MG in clinically affected patients.

Autoimmune Features

The etiopathogenesis of this prototypic autoantibody-mediated disease commences with the breakdown of Tcell immune tolerance in the thymus gland. The initial exposure of T cells to AChR myoid cells or other endemic antigens leads to the breakdown of self tolerance in the trimolecular complex involving autoreactive T-cells, antigen, main histocompatibility complex (MHC) and other genetic influences. The result is activation of B-cells and the production of specific autoantibodies. Once begun, immune mechanisms that regulate T-cell activity affect the production of specific autoantibodies.

Pathophysiology

The pathophysiologic abnormality in MG results from a reduced number and function of AChR with fewer available sodium channels and resultant EPP of slower rising phase with reduced amplitude that fail to depolarize endplate membranes to threshold, generate an AP, or produce myofiber contraction (Table 4) (1).

The quantal release of ACh can be physiologically increased by raising the concentration of calcium in the presynaptic terminal by the application of high-frequency trains of presynaptic AP delivered electrically at ~50Hz or by 5 to 10 seconds of maximal voluntary contraction of the muscle under observation. A second method reduces the rate of ACh hydrolysis by inhibiting the enzyme AChE available as short-acting edrophonium (Tensilon®) or the longer-acting preparation pyridostigmine (Mestinon®). The effect of increasing the ACh concentration on a model of NMJ transmission can be seen in Table 4.

Diagnosis

Clues to the diagnosis of MG can be obtained in the history and neurological examination that indicate fluctuating weakness and fatigue of ocular, bulbar, and proximal limb muscles or a combination thereof, with demonstratble fatigability upon sustained eye gaze or forced limb postures for one to two minutes. Electrodiagnostic studies differentiate presynaptic and postsynaptic NMJ defects, while elevated titers of AChR antibodies, highly correlated with MG, rarely occur in LEMS and when present, are considered a non-pathologic epiphenomenon and not a coexistence of both disorders.

Edrophonium Test

The injection of up to 10 mg of edrophonium briefly corrects the defects in NMJ transmission due to blockage of the action AChE, lasting several minutes, during which improvement is clinically apparent to both the patient and investigator. However, it is important to examine unequivocally weak muscles, not just the lids or oculomotor function, due to the propensity for false positive and negative results. There are protocols for performing the Tensilon

Table 4. Model of the Dynamics of Abnormal NMJ Transmission with Low-Frequency RNS in MG

Stimulus number	ACh pool	Available ACh quanta	ACh quanta released	Resultant EPP amplitude (mV)	Action potential[a] threshold reached
1	Immediate	1,000	200	36	Yes
2	Immediate	800	160	28	No
3	Immediate	640	128	24	No
4	Mobilizable	>640	>128	>30	Yes
5	Mobilizable	>640	>128	>30	Yes

The effects of higher calcium concentration on the release of ACh are normal in MG. However, there are fewer functioning ACh receptors and the resultant EPP is lower than normal. The greater amount of ACh released with mobilization has some effect on the EPP amplitude, resulting in a greater likelihood of an EPP reaching threshold for an action potential. Numbers representing ACh quanta are approximate.

[a]In this model, the EPP amplitude must be greater than 30 mV to reach threshold for generation of a muscle fiber action potential.

NMJ, neuromuscular junction; ACh, acetylcholine; EPP, endplate potential.

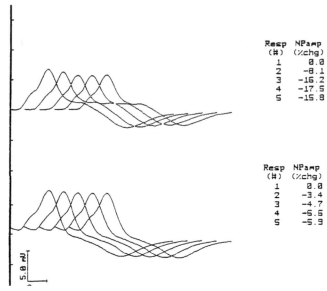

Resp	NPamp
(#)	(%chg)
1	0.0
2	-8.1
3	-16.2
4	-17.5
5	-15.8

Resp	NPamp
(#)	(%chg)
1	0.0
2	-3.4
3	-4.7
4	-6.5
5	-5.9

FIG. 5. Response to 3-Hz repetitive stimulation in a patient with myasthenia gravis. Top trace illustrates the decremental response with a maximal decrement of 17.5% with the fourth response. Bottom trace illustrates partial repair after 10 seconds of maximal muscle activation with a maximal decrement of 5.9%.

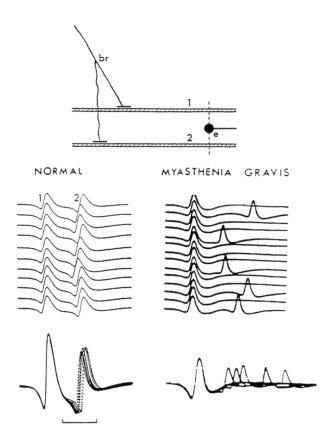

FIG. 6. Schematic diagram of single fiber electromyography (SFEMG) recording technique and illustrative responses. Top diagram shows two muscle fibers (1 and 2) from the same motor unit. The SFEMG electrode, e, is positioned to record single fiber action potentials from each fiber. The higher amplitude of action potential 1 is used as the trigger potential. Lower traces show jitter from a normal and myasthenia gravis (MG) neuromuscular junction. Jitter is extreme in MG, with blocking of action potential 2. Adapted from, Stalberg E, Trontelj JV. *Single fiber electromyography*, 2nd ed. New York: Raven Press, 1994, with permission.

test in a double-blinded, placebo-controlled manner (10). A positive Tensilon test does not distinguish between various forms of presynaptic and postsynaptic NMJ transmission failure.

Repetitive Motor Nerve Stimulation

Repetitive motor nerve stimulation (RNS) assesses the postsynaptic defect of NMJ transmission by measurement of five consecutive CMAP responses stimulated at 2 to 4 Hz. The observed decremental response is considered positive when the CMAP amplitude evoked by the third shock falls by more than 12% due to depletion of the immediate pool of ACh, the magnitude of which reflects the number of failing NMJ. An increase in the release of the readily mobilized pool of ACh after the third shock leads to the characteristic U- or J-shaped curvature (Figure 5) due to restoration of NMJ transmission at failed junctions as a result of increased presynpatic calcium concentrations, similarly evident by asking the patient to voluntarily activate the muscle under investigation for five to ten seconds.

The progressive failure of NMJ transmission demonstrable as a precipitous increase in the CMAP decremental response obtained with RNS performed at one minute intervals for up to five minutes after brief maximal exercise is termed *post-tetanic exhaustion* (Figure 5).

Notwithstanding the security factor for NMJ transmis-

sion, several factors explain the possible occurrence of a decremental response in normal individuals. One is a stimulation train that results in artifactual results due to movement of the limb under investigation, a factor that can be minimized by using stimulus intensities of 150% of maximum and immobilizing the limb. A second is the system of amplitude measurement of the tracing. Whereas peak-to-peak measurements of CMAP amplitude is less susceptible to measurement errors, most EMG machines automatically calculate the decrement from the peak negative CMAP amplitude, while others use the isolectric line that precedes the first CMAP as the baseline for amplitude measurcment, leading to calculation errors with inadvertent movement. It is necessary to add a proximal system to RNS such as the trapezius muscle and accessory nerve when weakness is purely ocular or mild in the arms, to avoid false negative results from the abductor pollicus-median nerve or abductor digiti minimi muscle-ulnar nerve system alone. The ways to reduce false-positive decremental responses include careful examination of the waveform response for the expected U, or J-shaped pattern; making certain that results are reproducible, measurement of peak-to-peak CMAP amplitudes to calculate decrement, and demonstration of the physiological response to 10 seconds of brief exercise that produces an increase in presynaptic terminal calcium and futher reduces the amount of decrement.

Single Fiber and Concentric Needle EMG

This electrophysiologic technique analyzes the variability of NMJ transmission as discharge-to-discharge variability in timing of the AP of single or small groups of myofibers (11) (Figure 6). The measured variability termed *jitter*, is measured in microseconds, reflecting slow EPP rise times and delayed generation of muscle fiber AP, while EPP that fail to reach threshold are blocked. While RNS and SFEMG both detect blocking, only the latter detect abnormal jitter without blocking. It can be performed utilizing a special concentric EMG needle with the exposed active electrode surface along the side of the needle, and computer software to measure the variability, while concentric needle EMG (CNEMG) can also be performed utilizing a non-specialized small-diameter facial or pediatric-size concentric needle electrodes with the same software (12). The SFEMG process can be initiated by having the patient produce weak voluntary contractions with measurement of the co-variability of two NMJ recording. Alternatively, transmission can be initiated by electrical stimulation of motor nerve branches with recording of the variability of one NMJ. The normal values of jitter values have been determined for age, and those that are abnormal are similar for both SFEMG and CNEMG techniques (12, 13) Although abnormal jitter does not distinguish presynaptic and postsynaptic defects of NMJ transmission, the discharge frequency at which maximal jitter occurs may offer additional clues.

Comparison of Diagnostic Techniques

Diagnostic specificity for MG comes close to 100% when ACh receptor antibody titers are present, although their absence does not exclude the diagnosis. While specific for the defect in NMJ transmission, the results of edrophonium testing and RNS depend upon the distribution and severity of symptoms, and may be equivocal in purely ocular and mild generalized MG, as compared to SFEMG because the latter detects abnormalities that do not cause blocked transmission. When comparisons are made between the three studies (Table 5), SFEMG was 89 to 90% sensitive, more so in ocular than generalized involvement, while RNS and serological testing yielded the greatest sensitivity in those with generalized disease (14).

Mediastinal Imaging

Approximately 10% of patients with MG have thymoma detected on computed tomography (CT) of the chest. Whether clinically silent or pathogenic, up to 40% of thymoma are associated with MG, and their presence is neither predicted by clinical features nor by magnetic resonance imaging (MRI), making it imperative to screen all suspected patients.

TREATMENT

Concepts

MG is a chronic disease without known cure, and the goal of treatment is sustained remission, defined as the absence of symptoms and signs without medication. For many patients, complete remission may be elusive, and partial remission is a more practical goal. Therapy is divided into medication that improves NMJ transmission and symptoms of weakness but does not affect the course of the disease, including the AChE inhibitors; procedures that affect the immune system over a limited time period but probably

Table 5. Comparison of Diagnostic Studies Performed in 550 patients with MG*

	SFEMG in any muscle		SFEMG ext dig com		Rep stim in any muscle		Acetylcholine receptor antibody at any time	
	Gen MG	Ocular MG	Gen MG	Ocular MG	Gen MG	Ocular MG	Gen MG	Ocular MG
Percent abnormal	99	97	89	60	76	48	80	55

Gen MG, generalized weakness; Ext dig com, extensor digitorum communis muscle, commonly used studied with SFEMG; Ocular MG, weakness restricted to ocular muscles; SFEMG, single fiber electromyogram; Rep stim, repetitive stimulation.
*Adapted from reference 14.

do not affect the natural history of the disease, such as plasmapheresis and intravenous immunoglobulin (IVIg); and medication or procedures that modify the course of MG such as the immunosuppressants, and thymectomy.

Quantitative Testing

It may be difficult a priori to determine if a particular therapeutic regimen is effective since some patients who report worsening of symptoms may have unchanged or improved strength, making quantitative assessment and objective clinical and electrophysiological comparisons more helpful than self-reporting. However, it is important to try to carry out such measurements at the same time of the day or in proximity to the time of the last dose of pyridostigmine. One frequently encountered problem is differentiation of steroid myopathy from myasthenic exacerbation when weakness contemporaneously advances at onset or in the course of therapy (4). Unchanged or improved serial RNS is more suggestive of steroid myopathy in such instances, emphasizing the importance of establishing baseline electrodiagnostic values in those being actively treated with agents with a propensity to worsen underlying weakness.

Quantitative Scales

Clinically meaningful quantitative scales have been developed to objectify MG status to aid treatment decisions including the Quantitative MG (QMG) (15), Myasthenia Gravis Activities of Daily Living (MG-ADL) (16) and MG Composite scale (17) scales, each with individual strengths and interrelated concordance.

Acetylcholinesterase Inhibitors

Pyridostigmine is the most commonly used AChE inhibitor that reversibly binds to AChE. The result is a slowing of hydrolysis of ACh that raises the concentration of ACh at the junctional folds, increasing the probability of ACh remaining attached to functional AChR, and leading to EPP with more rapid rise time, higher amplitude, and greater likelihood of generating AP in previously blocked muscle fibers. It reaches peak serum concentrations in 90 to 120 minutes and has a similar half-life. Although doses of 60 to 120 mg every three to four hours are most effective, the dose and frequency can be increased in accordance with the level of activity. In the end, anticipated side effects of increased salivation, sweating, cramping, and diarrhea become dose-limiting factors, such that most patients strive for more definitive therapy (10).

Plasmapheresis and Intravenous Immunoglobulin

Plasmapheresis and IVIg are temporary immune regulatory therapies with equal effectiveness but differences in the proposed actions, making them complementary therapies in MG. Plasmapheresis removes pathogenic NMJ antibodies as well as other soluble plasma proteins that modulate the immune system. The response to plasmapheresis occurs over hours to days and is useful to treat or abort myasthenic crisis, but requires special equipment and highly trained personnel. A therapeutic trial consists of 4 to 6 exchanges on alternate days and despite being generally well tolerated, it requires adequate venous access and potential placement of a large-bore venous catheter that can incur secondary complications.

In comparison, IVIg consists of pooled exogenous antibodies from up to a thousand healthy donors, and while the precise mechanisms of the action are not well understood, exogenous antibodies interact at several different sites with autoantibody binding at idiotypic antigen sites and to T-cells, modulating the immune response. Infusions of IVIg can be performed at home by a nurse without the need for special equipment. The recommended total monthly dose is 2 grams per kilogram (g/kg) in five daily doses per month, administered no faster than 10 grams per hour to avert rate-related side effects. With a half-life of four weeks, it is repeat maintenance doses of 1 g/kg are satisfactory with the goal of slowly tapering the frequency in accordance with clinical responsivness, which is typically evident after two to four weeks. Two randomized controlled trials, one prematurely stopped because of insufficient IVIg inventory, showed a positive trend (18), while the other showed efficacy (19).

Corticosteroids

Corticosteroids occupy a central role in the treatment of MG because of their effectiveness and reliability in initiating and maintaining prolonged remission (4). Although they impact the immune system at several different levels, the mechanism of action in MG is not well understood. Prednisone in the United States and prednisolone in other countries are the most widely used oral agents, administered at initial doses of 40 to 60 mg daily for three to six weeks and slowly tapered after a beneficial response is obtained. For unclear reasons, up to 80% of patients can experience temporary worsening of weakness that sometimes culminates in crisis after high initial doses, such that patients should be cautioned about this possibility and monitored in a hospital setting when commencing high-dose therapy. Alternatively, low doses can be started and slowly increased weekly to the desired level. Tapering schedules, which can follow many different protocols, have the common goal of converting daily therapy toward alternate-day dosing early in the course of treatment to avert anticipated weight gain, hyperglycemia, osteopenia, gastric and duodenal erosion, and cataract side effects (4). An alternative approach utilizes a brief course of 2 g of pulse intravenous methylprednisolone followed by a second infusion five days later, but this has never been formally studied.

Azathioprine

Azathioprine (Imuran®) is recommended for patients with poor responsiveness, intolerance, and frequent relapses with corticosteroids, and although it is less effective than prednisone as monotherapy, it has usefulness as a corticosteroid-sparing agent to reduce the long-term side effects (20). Dosage varies, but an expected elevation in the mean corpuscular volume (MCV) and drop in the white blood cell (WBC) count with progressive increase in the daily dose toward the target of 2 to 3 mg/kg/day assures a safe tolerable daily dose. There are several caveats to consider. The first is the anticipated long delay in the onset of action, typically up to 24 months for the anticipated clinical response. Second, idiosynchratic side effects occur in about 10% of patients, including flu-like symptoms such as nausea, fever, chills, arthralgia, and gastrointestinal complaints that promptly resolve with cessation of therapy. The third is the anticipated bone marrow suppression in all patients, but with careful monitoring, it is rarely a reason to stop therapy. The fourth is the concern for an increased risk for lymphoproliferative cancer after 10 to 20 years of continued treatment.

Mycofenolate Mofetil

Mycofenolate mofetil (CellCept®) selectively blocks purine synthesis in T and B lymphocytes, inhibiting their proliferation. Two randomized controlled trials (21, 22) failed to demonstrate efficacy as a corticosteroid-sparing agent or equivalent efficacy to prednisone when assessed over 12 to 36 weeks. However, there was concern that the period of observation was too short to demonstrate efficacy, suggesting instead 6 to 24 months of observation (23). The general consensus is that 1 to 1.5 grams of mycofenolate mofetil administered twice daily is a reasonable alternative to azathioprine.

Rituximab

Rituximab is a monoclonal antibody that targets the CD20 antigen in B cells. While there are isolated reports indicating responsiveness in refractory AChR and MuSK seropositive patients, one study with a mean follow-up period of 31 months demonstrated long-lasting benefit employing 375mg/m² of rituximab with MuSK seropositive patients benefitting most (24).

Thymectomy

Historically, the earliest transsternal thymectomies for MG were performed for the removal of thymic tumors. However, the beneficial results of thymectomy in non-thymomatous patients were appreciated afterward. It has been difficult to judge the efficacy of thymectomy for several reasons. First, the only placebo-controlled trial that has yet to be completed, randomized patients to corticosteroids or thymectomy. Second, there is no certainty as to the efficacy of the available cervical, transsternal, combined cervical and transsternal, and thoracoscopic approaches, or the relative extent of thymic resection needed to achieve a clinical response. Third, while there is little consensus as to the timing of surgery, most authorities agree that thymectomy carries the best assurance of sustained long-term remisssion. Although it is unclear whether all thymic tissue needs to be removed to guarantee the best outcome, the transsternal approach offers the widest exposure of resectable thymic tissue in the chest and should be considered as initial and primary therapy of patients with generalized limb and bulbar involvement, with both younger and older patients responding equally well. Preoperative plasmapheresis improves the clinical status and later immediate postoperative course, especially in those with bulbar weakness, reduced expiratory pressure, and impaired cough at risk for prolonged postoperative intubation. Maximal thymectomy with exenteration of chest and neck thymic implants was associated with sustained remission in up to 90% of patients for up to seven years (25).

Cyclosporine

This T-cell inhibitor, which is generally employed to prevent tranplantation rejection, has been used in the treatment of MG, however the associated side effects, including renal insufficiency, hypertension, headache, and hirsuitism, make it a less desirable routine therapy.

JUVENILE MYASTHENIA GRAVIS

Clinical Features

Juvenile MG is an immune-mediated disorder with onset before age 20 years. Although similar to the adult disorder, there are several differences, including seronegative ocular presentations in prepubertal children, and generalized seropositive involvement in postpubertal patients. The latest facilitates separation from congenital MG and is attributed to the maturing immune system. Disease severity and long-term prognosis improves with prepubertal onset.

Treatment

Spontaneous remission rates are higher in juveniles compared to adults with or without treatment (26). However myasthenic treatment is simlar in juvenile and adult patients, in spite of the challenges inherent in plasmapheresis given the reduced blood volumes, and concerns of growth retardation and lymphoproliferative cancers respectively, in the use of corticosteroids and azathioprine. Even though thymomas are distinctly uncomon in children, thymectomy is still an option in clinically appropriate candidates, with inherent racial differenes in outcome that imparts a somewhat lower remission rate in African-American children.

NEONATAL MYASTHENIA GRAVIS

Clinical Features

Neonatal MG is a transient disorder of NMJ transmission failure due to the passive transfer of maternal antibodies across the placenta. Symptoms include a poor suck, weak-cry, facial weakness, dysphagia, and hypotonia. Clues to the diagnosis *in utero* are the presence of reduced fetal movements, and severe weakness including respiratory failure at birth. Weakness *in utero* leads to joint contractures such that neonatal MG is included in the differential diagnosis of arthrogryposis, the latter of which can demonstrate fetal AChR subunits synthesis. And although the overall probability of neonatal MG is low, it occurs in up to 10% of myasthenic maternal births, including mothers in remission. The neonatal antibody type may differ from the mother, suggesting infant synthesis. Host factors appear to be important in determining whether an individual infant becomes symptomatic, as well as the occurance of neonatal MG in prior childbirths, making it imperative to expectantly monitor each infant born to a myasthenic mother for signs of neonatal MG for up to 10 days, after which the likelihood of developing the disorder becomes negligible. Any sign of weakness should be diagnosed appropriately with a test dose of edrophonium and RNS. In the absence of respiratory failure, the course of the disease is usually self-limited.

Treatment

Treatment depends upon the severity of symptoms, with pyridostigmine and plasmapheresis offering the best option for prompt relief unless the need for respiratory support supervenes.

CONGENITAL MYASTHENIA

Congenital MG represents a spectrum of disorders of NMJ transmission, each due to a unique genetic defect, eventually found in up to 60% of patients so studied (27) (Table 6). By definition, antibodies to the ACh receptor are not present.

The disorder is characterized clinically by early and relatively fixed facial, limb, and variable oropharyngeal and weakess, with clinical exacerbations that culminate in myasthenic crisis. Weakness or hypotonia in early childhood may erroneously be ascribed to other genetic or birth problems, or present so mildly as to escape appreciation until childhood or adulthood. Under such circumstances, a diagnosis of immune-mediated MG may later be entertained.

Affected patients respond poorly to pyridostigmine or not at all to immunomodulating therapy. Ephedrine administered at the dose of 15 mg orally three times daily and 3,4-diaminopyrodine (3,4-DAP) are effective treatment (28), prolonging the presynaptic terminal action potential by blocking potassium channels and enhancing the release of ACh by increasing the calcium concentration in the ter-

Table 6. Classification of Genetic Myasthenic Syndromes*

Presynaptic defects (~6%)
    Choline acetyltransferase (~5%)
    Paucity of synaptic vesicles (very rare)
    Congenital Lambert-Eaton-like syndrome (very rare)

Synpatic Basal Lamina (~14%)
    Endplate AChE deficiency (13%)
    beta-2 laminin deficiency (very rare)

Postsynaptic defects (~68%)
    AChR deficiency with/without kinetic abnormality (~34%)
    Primary kinetic abnormality with/without AChR deficiency (~18%)
    Rapsyn deficiency (~15%)
    Pectin deficiency (very rare)
    Sodium channel deficiency (very rare)

Defects in mechanisms governing endplate development and maintenance (~12%)
    Dok-7 myasthenic (~10%)
    Glutamine-fructose-6-phosphate transamine deficiency (rare)
    Myasthenic syndrome associated with centronuclear myopathy (very rare)

Percentages based on 321 unrelated index patients investigated at the Mayo Clinic.

ACh, acetylcholine; AChE, acetylcholinesterase; AChR, acetylcholine receptor; LEMS, Lambert-Eaton myasthenic syndrome.
*Adapted from reference 27.

minal, particularly those with *DOK7* mutations. Fluoxetine may be effective in those with slow channel mutations.

The diagnosis of congenital MG should be entertained in any child with a diagnosis of MG that is refractory to the usual modes of therapy. Further support for the diagnosis comes from inspection of early childhood photos, looking for ptosis or hyperextension of the neck to optimize forward gaze, and a history of other affected family members. Routine electrodiagnostic testing does not differentiate immune-mediated from congenital-onset patients. However, certain presynaptic forms of congenital MG may show facilitation after exercise. Two forms, one due to endplate AChE deficiency and the other resulting from a slow channel syndrome, show a repetitive discharge after the CMAP following a single shock (Table 6). The meaningful investigation of these syndromes requires sophisticated *in vitro* electrophysiologic studies to assess the quantal release of ACh and morphology of the NMJ, available at only a few centers with a specific interest in these disorders.

LAMBERT-EATON MYASTHENIC SYNDROME

The association of small cell lung cancer (SCLC) and a myasthenic syndrome known as the LEMS, is a prototypical antibody mediated paraneoplastic disease.

Clinical Features

Up to 60% of patients with LEMS have an associated SCLC, although other tumors have been described (29, 30). The disorder can thus be divided into those with or without a detectable cancer (29), with the latter of generally younger age, although most patients with LEMS are older than age 40 years at onset, and males predominate in the tumor-related group.

The most common symptoms of LEMS are proximal leg and truncal weakness, less commonly ptosis and bulbar muscle weakness and, rarely respiratory failure (30). An apparent warming-up phenomena, whereby the first portion of a repetitive movement is more difficult than later ones, leads to near-normal strength and fatiguability in manual muscle testing. Tendon reflexes are first absent, then later obtained after brief agonist muscle contraction. Autonomic symptoms of impotence, dry mouth, constipation, and urinary retention are common.

Natural History

The symptoms of LEMS generally progress rapidly over months from proximal to distal muscles in association with a cancer, but more slowly in the absence thereof (30). The most common initial diagnosis is MG (29). Among those with an associated cancer, the prognosis is largely determined by

tumor progression and response to tumor treatment. Three-quarters of patients with a cancer died within a year compared with 80% of those without a cancer who were alive seven years after diagnosis (29). Nonetheless, an occult cancer may not be diagnosed for up to four years after onset of neurological symptoms, emphasizing the importance of aggressively searching for an occult cancer at the time of initial diagnosis.

Pathophysiology

The disorder is due to autoantibodies directed against presynaptic P/Q voltage-gated calcium channels (VGCC) or related structures affecting the regulation of channels in those both with and without an associated cancer (31). The antibodies are of the IgG class and are heterogeneous in their specificity against the several types of calcium channels. The etiology of antibodies in patients without an associated cancer is unclear, but there is likely antigenic similarity between presynaptic VGCC and those on tumors cells. Those with SCLC-related antibody production are triggered by the tumor, and reduce both the influx of calcium into the presynaptic terminal and the amount of ACh released, in turn decreasing the size of EPP and the likelihood of reaching threshold for a given muscle fiber AP (Table 7). The result is a low CMAP amplitude in most muscles that is also a measure of the severity of NMJ blockade. Similar calcium channels present on autonomic presynaptic nerve parasympathetic and sympathetic terminals account for the associated autonomic symptoms.

Diagnosis

Electrodiagnostic testing demonstrates an initial low CMAP amplitude, often less than 10% of the lower limit of normal in most nerves tested (Figure 7), and RNS at 2 to 4 Hz shows a decrement as in MG. However, high frequency RNS at rates of 50Hz, and 10 seconds of exercise, leads to marked facilitation, at last restoring it to normal, potentially reaching 10,000-fold when the initial CMAP is extremely small (29).

A positive serological assay for P/Q or N-type VGCC is infrequently detected except in LEMS or in other paraneoplastic neurological disorders (31). About 60 to 70% of patients with LEMS have an SCLC and a detectable P/Q-related VGCC antibody, while 10 to 15% lack detectable antibodies, suggesting that they are present at either undetectable titers or directed to other epitopes (30). There is an association between LEMS and both organ-specific and non-organ-specific autoantibodies in patients with LEMS.

Treatment

The treatment of choice is 25 mg of 3,4-DAP which enhances synaptic transmission and increases ACh release by blocking potassium channels, thereby prolonging nerve

Table 7. Model of the Dynamics of Abnormal NMJ Transmission With RNS in LEMS

Stimulus number	ACh pool	Available ACh quanta	ACh quanta released	Resultant EPP amplitude (mV)	Action potential threshold reached
Before exercise					
1	Immediate	1,000	80	18	No
2	Immediate	··800	72	12	No
3	Immediate	··640	58	8	No
4	Mobilizable	>640	>58	>8	No
5	Mobilizable	>640	>58	>8	No
After exercise					
1	Immediate	1,000	200	36	Yes
2	Immediate	··800	160	28	No
3	Immediate	··640	128	24	No
4	Mobilizable	>640	>128	>30	Yes
5	Mobilizable	>640	>128	>30	Yes

Top of table shows the effects of reduced influx of calcium leading to a small number of ACh released. This results in lower amplitude EPPs that fail to elicit muscle fiber action potentials. Bottom of table shows how increased ACh released through enhanced calcium influx will facilitate transmission to normal. Numbers representing ACh quanta are approximate.

*In this model, the EPP amplitude must be greater than 30 mv to reach threshold for generation of a muscle fiber action potential.

NMJ, neuromuscular junction; LEMS, LambertEaton myasthenic syndrome; ACh, acetylcholine; EPP, end plate potential.

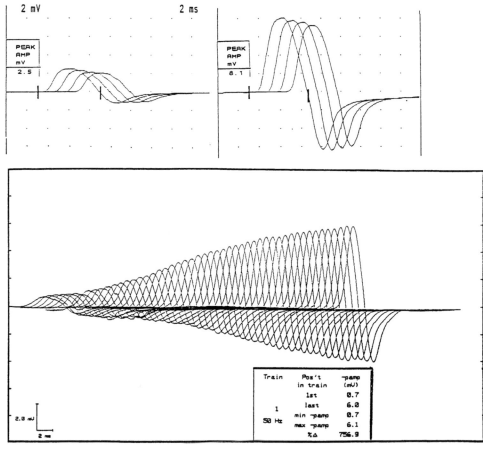

FIG. 7. Responses to repetitive stimulation in LEMS. **Top:** Left trace shows low amplitude response to 3 Hz repetitive stimulation; right trace shows 245% facilitation after 10 seconds of maximal muscle activation. **Bottom:** Facilitation of the response to 50 Hz repetitive stimulation with a 750% increase in amplitude.

AP and the activation of VGCC (32). Mild side effects include perioral and acral paresthesia, epigastric distress, and, rarely, seizures. The CMAP amplitude is a useful prognostic and therapeutic marker. Patients with LEMS may benefit from AChE drugs in doses used for MG, although the improvement in strength is likely to be mild. A trial of plasmapheresis may be effective especially in the absence of an associated cancer. The IgG fraction collected from

the plasma separation of such patients passively transfers symptoms of LEMS to experimental animals (33). Treatment with IVIg in doses of 2 g/kg over two days led to temporary benefit among LEMS patients without cancer in a placebo-controlled crossover trial (34), similar to prednisone that showed efficacy in small cohorts with or without cancer (35). The efficacy of azathioprine monotherapy has not been formally assessed (33).

REFERENCES

1. Ruff RL. Endplate contributions to the safety factor for neuromuscular transmission. Muscle Nerve 2011; 44:854–861.
2. Osserman K. Myasthenia gravis. New York: Grune & Stratton, 1958.
3. Task Force of the Medical Scientific Advisory Board of the Myasthenia Gravis Foundation of America, Jaretzki A, Barohn R, Ernstoff R, et al. Myasthenia gravis: Recommendations for clinical research standards. Neurology 2000; 55:16–23.
4. Bromberg MB, Carter O. Corticosteroid use in the treatment of neuromuscular disorders: empirical and evidence-based data. Muscle Nerve 2004; 30:20–37.
5. Grob D, Brunner N, Namba T, et al. Lifetime course of myasthenia gravis. Muscle Nerve 2008; 37:141–149.
6. Leite MI, Waters P, Vincent A. Diagnostic use of autoantibodies in myasthenia gravis. Autoimmunity 2010; 43:371–379.
7. Hoch W, McConville J, Helms S, et al. Auto-antibodies to the receptor tyrosine kinase MuSK in patients with myasthenia gravis without acetylcholine receptor antibodies. Nature Medicine 2001; 7:365–368.
8. Liyanage Y, Hoch W, Beeson D, et al. The agrin/muscle-specific kinase pathway: New targets for autoimmune and genetic disorders at the neuromuscular junction. Muscle Nerve 2002; 25:4–16.
9. Leite MI, Jacob S, Viegas S, et al. IgG1 antibodies to acetylcholine receptors in 'seronegative' myasthenia gravis. Brain 2008; 131:1940–1952.
10. Riggs J. Pharmacologic enhancement of neuromuscular transmission in myasthenia gravis. Clinical Neuropharmacology 1982; 5:277–29.
11. Stålberg E, Trontelj JV, Sanders DB. Single Fiber EMG, 3rd ed. Fiskebackskil: Edshagen Publishing House, 2010.
12. Stalberg EV, Sanders DB. Jitter recordings with concentric needle electrodes. Muscle Nerve 2009; 40:331–339.
13. Bromberg M, Scott D, and the Ad Hoc committee of the AAEM Single Fiber Special Interest Group. Single fiber EMG reference values. Muscle Nerve 1994; 17:820–821.
14. Sanders D. Electrophsiological and pharmacological tests in neuromuscular junction disorders. In R. Lisak ed. Handbook of Myasthenia Gravis and Myasthenic Syndromes. New York: Marcel Dekker, 1994.
15. Barohn RJ, McIntire D, Herbelin L, et al. Reliability testing of the quantitative myasthenia gravis score. Ann NY Acad Sci 1998; 841:769–772.
16. Wolfe GI, Herbelin L, Nations SP, et al. Myasthenia gravis activities of daily living profile. Neurology 1999; 52:1487–1489.
17. Burns TM, Conaway M, Sanders DB. The MG Composite: A valid and reliable outcome measure for myasthenia gravis. Neurology 2010; 74:1434–1440.
18. Wolfe G, Barohn R, Foster G, et al. Randomized, controlled trial of intravenous immunoglobulin in myasthenia gravis. Muscle Nerve 2002; 26:549–552.
19. Zinman L, Ng E, Bril V. IV immunoglobulin in patients with myasthenia gravis: a randomized controlled trial. Neurology 2007; 68:837–841.
20. Bromberg M, Wald J, Forshew D, et al. Randomized trial of azathioprine or prednisone for initial immunosuppressive treatment of myasthenia gravis. J Neurol Sci 1997; 150:59–62.
21. Sanders DB, Hart IK, Mantegazza R, et al. An international, phase III, randomized trial of mycophenolate mofetil in myasthenia gravis. Neurology 2008; 71:400–406.
22. Group MS. A trial of mycophenolate mofetil with prednisone as initial immunotherapy inmyasthenia gravis. Neurology 2008; 71:394–399.
23. Hehir MK, Burns TM, Alpers J, et al. Mycophenolate mofetil in AChR-antibody-positive myasthenia gravis: outcomes in 102 patients. Muscle Nerve 2010; 41:593–598.
24. Diaz-Manera J, Martinez-Hernandez E, Querol L, et al. Long-lasting treatment effect of rituximab in MuSK myasthenia. Neurology 2012; 78:189–193.
25. Jaretzki A, Penn A, Younger D, et al. "Maximal" thymectomy for myasthenia gravis. J Thorac Cardiovasc Surg 1988; 95:747–757.
26. Chiang LM, Darras BT, Kang PB. Juvenile myasthenia gravis. Muscle Nerve 2009; 39:423–431.
27. Engel AG. Current status of the congenital myasthenic syndromes. Neuromuscul Disord 2012; 22:99–111.
28. Chaouch A, Beeson D, Hantai D, et al. 186th ENMC International Workshop: Congenital myasthenic syndromes 24–26 June 2011, Naarden, The Netherlands.
29. O'Neill J, Murray N, Newsom-Davis J. The Lambert-Eaton myasthenic syndrome: A review of 50 cases. Brain 1988; 111:577–596.
30. Titulaer MJ, Lang B, Verschuuren JJ. Lambert-Eaton myasthenic syndrome: from clinical characteristics to therapeutic strategies. Lancet Neurology 2011; 10:1098–1107.
31. Lennon V, Kryzer T, Griesmann G, et al. Calcium-channel anitbodies in the Lambert-Eaton syndrome and other paraneoplastic syndromes. N Engl J Med 1995; 332:1467–1474.
32. McEvoy K, Windebank A, Daube J, et al. 3,4 diaminopyridine in the treatment of Lambert-Eaton myasthenic syndrome. N Engl J Med 1989; 321:1567–1571.
33. Newsom-Davis J, Murray N. Plasma exchange and immunosuppressive drug treatment in the Lambert-Eaton myasthenic syndrome. Neurology 1984; 34:480–485.
34. Bain P, Motomura M, Newsom-Davis J, et al. Effects of intravenous immunoglobulin on muscle weakness and calcium-channel autoantibodies in the Lambert-Eaton myasthenic syndrome. Neurology 1996; 47:678–683.
35. Ingram D, Davis G, Schwartz M, et al. Cancer-associated myasthenic (Eaton-Lambert) syndrome. Distribution of abnormality and effect of treatment. J Neurol Neurosurg Psychiatry 1984; 47:806–812.

CHAPTER 26

Entrapment Neuropathies

David S. Younger

The entrapment neuropathies are distinctive clinical neuropathic sensory and motor syndromes caused by physical compression or irritation of named nerves. Specific sites along the limbs, such as the neck, wrists, elbows, shoulders, pelvis, knees, and ankles, are more likely to be associated with peripheral nerve entrapment due to the presence of bony prominences, demarcated canals, muscle insertions, fibrous and ligamentous attachments, and anatomic vulnerability. In some instances there may be associated compression of blood vessels, leading to impaired circulation. Clinical, electrodiagnostic, and treatment aspects of the entrapment neuropathies can be found in other general references (1, 2).

GENERAL APPROACH TO DIAGNOSIS AND MANAGEMENT

The patient with an entrapment neuropathy typically complains of pain at the site of compression. Gentle tapping or manipulation elicits a discharge of neuritic pain that radiates along distal nerve fibers. Neurological examination of the sensory and motor peripheral nervous system will reveal the extent of nerve injury due to entrapment, with sparing of uninvolved nerves in the same limb. Normal peripheral sensory innervation of the body has been well studied (3) (Figures 1–4). Autonomic or focal signature sensory loss of a more circumscribed territory follows injury to individual nerves (4) (Figures 5–7). The territories of sensory and motor innervation and the deficits caused by entrapment and injury have been extensively reviewed elsewhere (5).

Blood studies for coexisting metabolic, endocrinologic, rheumatoid, and infectious disorders may reveal diabetes, parathyroid, thyroid disease, rheumatoid arthritis, gout,

Lyme disease, or other disorders that may contribute to the expression and severity of nerve entrapment. Electrodiagnostic studies confirm the physical findings and site of compression, and enable determination of the extent of injury (6). Focal slowing of nerve conduction velocities (NCV) and reduction in the amplitude of the compound muscle action potential (CMAP) and sensory nerve action potential (SNAP) across a site of compression employing nerve conduction studies (NCS) may be indicative of focal conduction block, commensurate with the degree of weakness, numbness, paresthesia, reduced pain, temperature sensation, and sweating. There may be superimposed axonopathic damage, evidenced by acute or chronic denervation potentials on needle EMG, with reduced recruitment and high-amplitude long-duration motor unit action potentials (MUAP) (7). The determination of distal motor and sensory latencies is imperative in the diagnosis of entrapment, wherein prolongation thereof infers focal demyelination across the site of compression (8). Plain radiographs are useful in demonstrating areas of abnormal bone structure at the proposed site of compression; however, magnetic resonance (MR) neurography (9) and ultrasound (10) employing standard protocols for nerve entrapment reveals structural abnormalities and is complementary to electrodiagnosis.

Treatment generally consists of joint and muscle mobilization and physiotherapy and occupational therapy to reduce tissue injury and swelling, sustain function, and promote recovery. Splinting of the wrist is an exception to reduce repeated trauma to the wrist that occurs passively at night during sleep. Oral and injectable steroidal and non-steroidal anti-inflammatory medications can be administered to reduce focal swelling at the site of entrapment, as

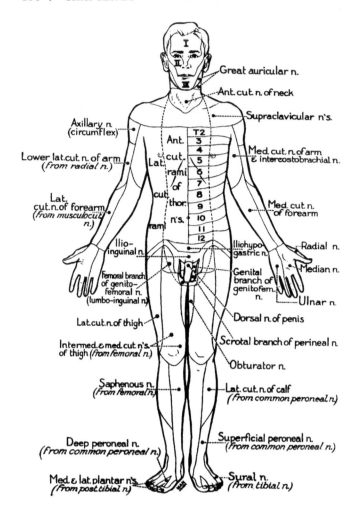

FIG. 1. Anterior view of the cutaneous distribution of the peripheral nerves of the body. From, reference 3, with permission.

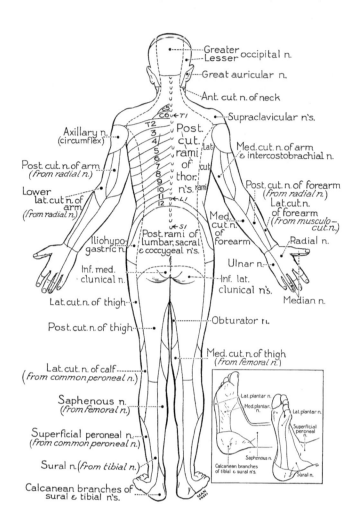

FIG. 2. Posterior view of the cutaneous distribution of the peripheral nerves of the body. From, reference 3, with permission.

will cold or warm compresses. Surgery is definitive treatment in certain entrapment disorders when the proposed procedure has a high likelihood of restoring function and alleviating pain.

INDIVIDUAL PERIPHERAL NERVE DISORDERS

Long Thoracic Nerve

The long thoracic nerve (Figure 8) is a pure motor nerve providing innervation exclusively to the serratus anterior muscle. It forms from the union of branches exiting C5 and C6 root after leaving their respective intervertebral foramina proximal to the middle scalene muscle, where they are joined after traversing this muscle by a branch from the C7 root. The nerve passes posterior to the clavicle, angu-

lated as it enters the axilla, where it runs posterior to the brachial plexus; and then passes over the first and second ribs prior to descending superficially along the thoracic wall to innervate the serratus anterior muscle. This muscle protracts, anchors, and stabilizes the scapula and shoulder girdle during movement. Injury to the long thoracic nerve produces scapular winging that can be accentuated by having the patient flex the arm anteriorly by pushing against a wall. Several potential mechanisms of entrapment based upon cadaveric dissections include scalenus muscle spasm, angulation of the nerve trunk as it crosses the second rib and overlying heavy musculature, trapping of the nerve between the coracoid process and the second rib when the scapula is forced medially, and inflammation of the bursae with which the nerve may be associated, causing nerve compression (11). Other contributing factors may include carrying heavy backpacks, direct blows to the shoulder or lateral thoracic wall during sports, or an accidental fall.

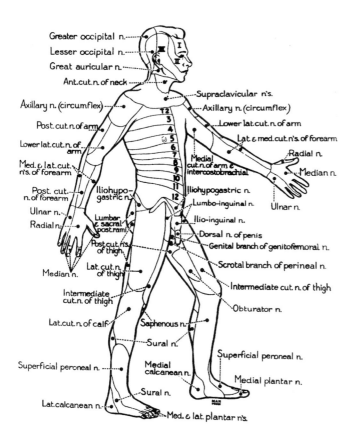

FIG. 3. Lateral view of the cutaneous distribution of the peripheral nerves of the body. From, reference 3, with permission.

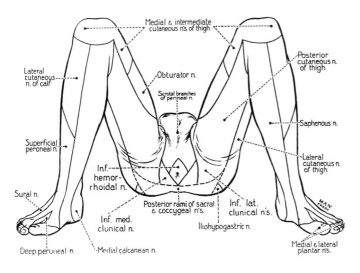

FIG. 4. The cutaneous distribution of the peripheral nerves of the perineum and lower extremities. From, reference 3, with permission.

Electrodiagnostic studies should be performed to confirm the diagnosis (12, 13) and to exclude brachial plexopathy and polyradiculopathy.

The outcome of long thoracic nerve palsy is generally favorable with conservative and, if necessary, surgical treatment (14). A variety of surgical procedures have been used to replace serratus anterior muscle function via transposition of the pectoralis major, minor, rhomboids or teres major muscles. Scapulothoracic fusion eliminates winging at the expense of reduced scapulothoracic motion. There are orthotic devices to maintain the scapula against the thorax but they are largely ineffective.

Accessory Nerve

During its extracranial course, the accessory nerve receives branches from the 2nd cervical nerve and pierces and innervates the sternocleidomastoid muscle. After entering the posterior cervical triangle at a point slightly above the mid-part of the posterior border of the latter muscle, it is joined by nerve fibers derived from the 3rd and 4th cervical nerves, and forms a sort of plexus beneath the trapezius muscle that it innervates. Lesion of the peripheral accessory nerve leads to trapezius palsy with limitation of abduction and elevation of the arm, a lower appearance of the shoulder, and weakness or paralysis of the trapezius muscle with scapular winging. While it has been suggested that branches from the cervical nerves are mainly afferent in nature, Fahrer (15) found electrophysiological evidence of motor fibers provided by the 3rd and 4th cervical nerves to portions of the trapezius muscle. Among a cohort of 16 patients with trapezius palsy who later underwent detailed electrodiagnostic studies and were followed clinically (16) ten had undergone surgical procedures in the posterior neck triangle, three had a history suggestive of brachial neuritis, and three were of uncertain cause. The accessory nerve was stimulated just above the midpoint of the posterior border of the sternocleidomastoid muscle where the nerve becomes superficial. CMAP were recorded from the upper, middle, and lower portions of the trapezius muscle, with latency measurements to the onset of the recorded response and distances measured via obstetric calipers. The range of motor latencies was 2.2 ms to 6.3 ms along distances of 75 mm to 305 mm, similar to those obtained by stimulating of Erb's point and recording from shoulder-girdle and arm muscles (17, 18). In every subject so studied, it was possible to evoke responses from all three sites simultaneously with latencies determined to the upper part in nine, to the middle in eight, and to the lower part in five using simultaneous three channel recordings. Among ten patients selected for detailed analysis, four patients had complete lesions of the accessory nerve at first examination one to three months after injury, and subsequent NCS showed rein-

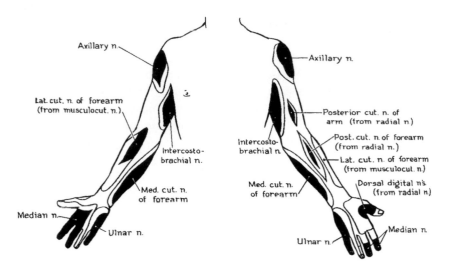

FIG. 5. Sensory deficit following interruption of individual nerve trunks of the upper limb. The black areas represent the autonomous zones and the surrounding lines indicate the approximate border of tactile anesthesia and thermoanesthesia. From, reference 3, with permission.

nervation after Wallerian degeneration, as did 4 others so studied two to five months after accessory nerve injury. The electrophysiological findings were consistent with nerve regeneration after complete axonal degeneration, a premise predicated on the viability and availability of supporting tissue for axonal regeneration, which in the case of accessory nerve injury, implied that in many patients, exploration of the nerve should be delayed until sufficient time has elapsed to allow for spontaneous recovery. Follow-up of patients 11 months to 8 years following accessory nerve injury of the cohort described by Petrera and Trojaborg (16) showed incomplete clinical recovery in all so studied.

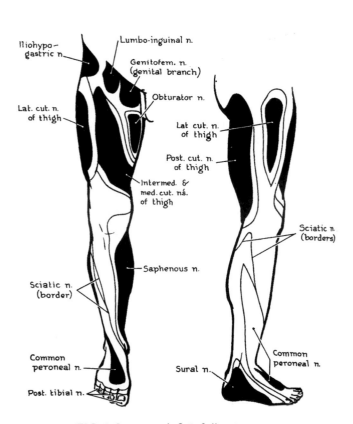

FIG. 6. Sensory deficit following interruption of individual nerve trunks of the lower limb. The pattern has the same significance as in figure 5. From, reference 3, with permission.

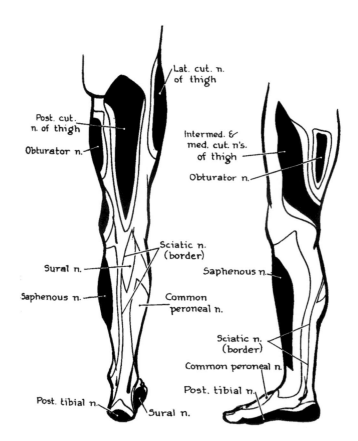

FIG. 7. Sensory deficit following interruption of individual nerve trunks of the lower limb. The pattern has the same significance as in figure 5. From, reference 3, with permission.

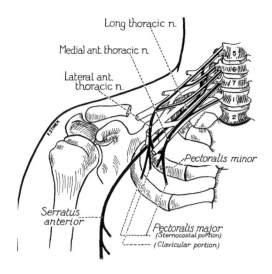

FIG. 8. The course and distribution of the long thoracic nerve. From, reference 3, with permission.

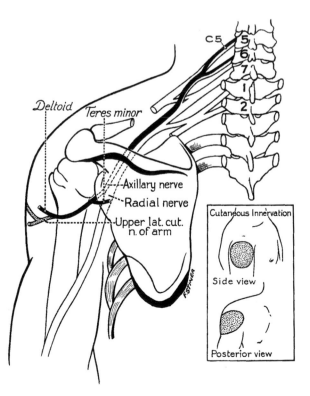

FIG. 9. The course and distribution of the suprascapular and dorsal scapular nerves. From, reference 3, with permission.

Suprascapular Nerve

The suprascapular nerve (Figure 9) is a mixed peripheral nerve that originates from C5 and C6 roots and the upper trunk of the brachial plexus. It provides sensory innervation to the shoulder joint and motor innervation to the supraspinatus and infraspinatus muscles. The motor nerve components innervate the supra- and infraspinatus muscles, whereas the sensory component supplies the posterior capsule of the shoulder joint. Suprascapular nerve compression has been well studied (19, 20). Compressive lesions of the nerve produce weakness and atrophy of the supra- and infraspinatus muscles and a poorly defined aching pain along the posterior aspect of the shoulder and adjacent scapula. After taking origin from the upper trunk of the brachial plexus, the suprascapular nerve crosses the posterior triangle of the neck. It runs parallel to the inferior belly of the omohyoid muscle and runs under the trapezius muscle through the suprascapular notch or foramen below the suprascapular ligament into the supraspinous fossa to innervate the supraspinatus muscle where it is first prone to entrapment. Nearly three-quarters of the notch is bound by bone; the suprascapular ligament converts the suprascapular notch into a foramen rather than a tunnel because of its short distance as compared with the carpal tunnel, which measures 2–3cm as compared with 2–3mm for the suprascapular foramen. Cadaveric studies have demonstrated that opposition, angulation, and kinking of the nerve against the sharp inferior margin of ligament at the foramen that occurs with depression, retraction, and hyperabduction of the shoulder, designated, the "sling effect," especially in marginal or inadequate-sized foramina, is the likely cause of injury at the foraminal level. After supplying the supraspinatus muscle, the suprascapular nerve curves around the lateral border of the spine through the spinoglenoid notch into the infraspinatus fossa where it innervates the infraspinatus muscle, with a risk of further entrapment. Entrapment at the suprascapular notch results in shoulder pain diffusely localized to the posterior aspect of the shoulder joint and adjacent scapula region resulting from compression of the articular branches to the glenohumeral and acromioclavicular joints, in association with weakness and atrophy of the supraspinatus and infraspinatus muscles, often to the same degree, although less perceptible in the supraspinatus because it is essentially subcutaneous and covered by the trapezius muscle. Entrapment at the spinoglenoid notch results in a distal nerve lesion characterized by shoulder pain and isolated infraspinatus weakness (21, 22). Suprascapular neuropathy may be associated with trauma of the shoulder and glenohumeral joint cyst.

The clinical differentiation of suprascapular neuropathy from rotator cuff injury and brachial plexopathy requires detailed study (23). On inspection, patients with either of the other disorders may demonstrate impaired shoulder abduction and visible parascapular muscle atrophy; however, those with suprascapular neuropathy will have restriction of the deficit to the supraspinatus and infraspinatus muscles. Electrodiagnostic studies are highly diagnostic in suprascapular neuropathy. Nerve conduction studies demonstrate prolongation of the distal motor latency from Erb's point to the supraspinatus muscle on affected side using needle recording when compared to age-matched normal controls and the clinically normal contralateral side, accompanied by active and chronic spontaneous activity at rest and neurogenic recruitment pattern in the supraspinatus and infraspinatus muscles. Patients with tears of the supraspinatus and infraspinatus muscles fail to demonstrate abnormalities of nerve conduction or spontaneous activity at rest in the absence of nerve injury, although there may be a neurogenic recruitment pattern due to disuse atrophy. Those with brachial plexus lesions, especially involving the upper trunk, will demonstrate variable involvement of the musculocutaneous and axillary nerves on mixed nerve conduction studies, with neurogenic recruitment and spontaneous activity at rest, depending upon whether the lesion is demyelinative and axonal in type, in the deltoid and deltoid muscles. Magnetic resonance imaging (MRI) of the shoulder and brachial plexus are useful adjunctive studies in all patients with suprascapular nerve, shoulder, and plexus injury. Arthrography and cinefluoroscopy are useful presurgical adjunctive studies in patients contemplating reparative shoulder surgery. Excision of the suprascapular ligament releases the suprascapular nerve, generally without the necessity of dissection in the suprascapular notch or that of the nerve from the surrounding fat tissue.

Axillary Nerve

The axillary nerve (Figure 10) contains motor and sensory fibers that arise from the C5 and C6 roots and traverse the upper trunk, posterior divisions, and posterior cord to innervate the deltoid and teres minor muscles and cutaneous sensation of the lateral aspect of the upper arm. At its origin, the nerve joins the posterior circumflex humeral artery at the anterior inferior border of the subscapularis muscle and together they turn posteriorly to exit the axilla through the quadrilateral space where entrapment can occur (24–26). The inferior border of the teres minor muscle is bound to the space superiorly laterally by the neck of the humerus, medially by the long head of the triceps, and inferiorly by the teres major muscle. Distal to the quadrilateral space the axillary nerve supplies the motor branch to the teres minor, where the nerve then separates into three branches; an anterior one to the anterior and middle portions of the deltoid muscle; a posterior branch to the pos-

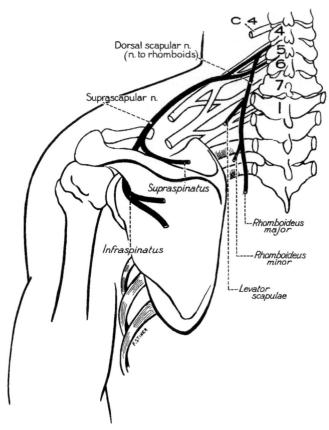

FIG. 10. The course and distribution of the axillary nerve. From, reference 3, with permission.

terior deltoid muscle; and a sensory branch to the superior lateral brachial cutaneous nerve, which supplies the skin overlying the deltoid.

Nerve conduction studies demonstrate prolongation of the distal motor latency along the axillary nerve following stimulation at Erb's point and recording with a concentric needle in the deltoid muscle, sparing other proximal nerves along upper cervical roots, brachial plexus, and forearm and their muscles, and leads to the diagnosis of axillary neuropathy and possible entrapment. Fibrotic bands compressing the axillary and posterior humeral circumflex artery in the quadrilateral space occurs, especially in young active adults, leading to vague discomfort in the shoulder, with intermittent paresthesia of the arm during flexion, abduction, and external rotation, often without weakness. Axillary nerve involvement is also common in neuralgic amyotrophy, and especially with trauma caused by dislocation of the shoulder and humeral fracture because of the short course of the nerve around the humeral neck, which puts it at risk for traction injury with forward humeral displacement. Treatment of axillary nerve entrapment is usually conservative but neurolysis through a posterior approach may lead to relief of symptoms.

Musculocutaneous Nerve

The musculocutaneous nerve (Figure 11) is a mixed motor nerve that innervates the biceps, brachialis, and coracobrachialis muscles and provides cutaneous sensation along the lateral forearm. It receives contributions from C5 to C7 roots via the upper and middle trunks, and anterior divisions and lateral cord of the brachial plexus at the level of the anterior cervical triangle. It innervates the coracobrachialis at the level of the axilla, pierces this muscle where it is first prone to entrapment and injury, and runs in the fascial plane between the biceps and brachialis muscles which it innervates. It exits the deep fascia at the elbow where it is again prone to entrapment, to continue as the lateral antebrachial cutaneous nerve along the lateral forearm.

Rupture of the biceps tendon that presents with forearm weakness, and lateral cord lesions that extend beyond the musculocutaneous nerve usually present little challenge to diagnosis; however, occasional patients with cervical polyradiculopathy, isolated lesions of the upper trunk and lateral cord of the brachial plexus, lateral epicondylitis or tennis elbow, and carpal tunnel syndrome may be misdiagnosed before electrodiagnostic studies are performed.

The electrodiagnostic evaluation of suspected patients includes sensory conduction along the forearm lateral cutaneous sensory nerve, distal motor latency determination along the motor musculocutaneous nerve to the biceps muscle using concentric needle recording after surface stimulation at Erb's point, followed by needle examination of the biceps, coracobrachialis, and brachialis muscles. Trojaborg (18) described the findings of detailed motor and sensory NCS along segments of the musculocutaneous nerve and noted that maximum motor conduction velocities between the anterior cervical triangle and the axilla were similar to those of the radial nerve between the supraclavicular fossa and the elbow (27), as between the axilla and elbow (28). Sensory fibers of the musculocutaneous nerve conducted at the same maximal velocity as motor fibers, the maximal velocities of which were similar along proximal and intermediate segments to those of the median, ulnar, and radial nerves (29). The maximal motor and sensory conduction velocities and SNAP amplitudes diminished with age, respectively, at a rate of 2 µV and 2m/s per decade as in the median nerve (30), whether recorded at the axilla or at Erb's point. Proximal stretch injury of the musculocutaneous nerve occurs with biceps rupture, trauma of the upper arm, and dislocation of the shoulder, and fracture of the clavicle treated with transposition of the coracoid process onto the clavicle. Entrapment of the nerve at the coracobrachialis muscle occurs after heavy lifting, violent extension of the forearm with an accidental fall, and after surgical procedures that require abduction and external rotation of the arm. Entrapment of the sensory nerve occurs along the lateral free margin of the

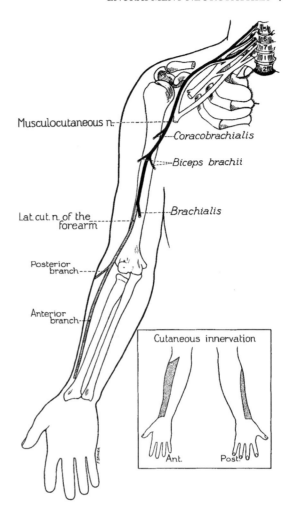

FIG. 11. The course and distribution of the musculocutaneous nerve. From, reference 3, with permission.

biceps aponeurosis with full pronation of the forearm, and with repetitive movements as may occur with tennis, inserting screws, compressive straps, handbags, waitress trays, and traumatic venipuncture. Traumatic avulsion of the C5 root from the spinal cord in one reported patient (18), led to formation of a traumatic meningocele, with preservation of sensory conduction and absent motor conduction, and absent musculocutaneous motor response one month after injury with denervation of the deltoid and brachial biceps muscles clinically and electromyographically, consistent with Wallerian degeneration and the contribution of C6 fibers to the motor root injury. Two years later, sensory conduction along the musculocutaneous nerve was unchanged, even when the motor NCV along the musculocutaneous nerve was 65% of normal. EMG at that time showed discrete activity in the brachial biceps with a voluntary motor unit action potential (MUAP) amplitude of 9mV and mean duration increased by 60%, with few denervation potentials indicative of reinnervation. Isolated involvement of the musculocutaneous nerve was a rare occurrence among 28 cases of World War I injures cited by Sunderland (31), with only one such patient. Most isolated musculocutaneous injuries are self-limited and respond to conservative management, however severe proximal injuries may be treated with nerve grafting or neurotization techniques.

Median Nerve

The median nerve (Figure 12) is derived from the union of the C5 to T1 roots and the lateral and medial cords of the brachial plexus, respectively innervating the forearm and hand. The nerve trunk descends along the medial aspect of the arm in the medial bicipital sulcus lying on the medial intermuscular septum. At the elbow, the nerve lies behind the biceps aponeurosis, and in the forearm between the two heads of the pronator teres, from whence it passes deep in the tendinous arch of the two heads of the flexor digitorum superficialis, and then deep to the muscle in its fascial sheath. Muscular branches are given to the pronator teres, flexor carpi radialis, palmaris longus, and the flexor digitorum superficialis high in the forearm under the bicipital aponeurosis and between the heads of the pronator teres. The anterior interosseus nerve provides innervation to the flexor pollicis longus, the lateral portion of the flexor digitorum profundus, and pronator quadratus. The main median nerve then reaches the wrist whereupon it approaches the surface to lie at the ulnar side of the flexor carpi radialis tendon. After giving off a sensory palmar cutaneous branch to the thenar eminence and proximal radial portion of the palm, the nerve passes through the carpal canal deep to the flexor retinaculum with the tendons of the superficial and deep flexors of the fingers and then divides into its terminal branches. These include a muscular branch to the abductor pollicis brevis, opponens pollicis, and flexor pollicis brevis, and sensory palmar and posterior digital aspects of the thumb, index, middle, and one half of the ring finger, and the palm overlying the metacarpophalangeal joints.

The median nerve may sustain compressive injury at four points along the arm (Figure 13). The most proximal site of entrapment of the median nerve occurs under the ligament of Struthers, 4 to 6 cm proximal to the medial epicondyle, where it fastens to a bony prominence along the anteromedial surface of the humerus. Compression therein leads to pain in the elbow and involvement of the median nerve from above the pronator teres to the hand, reminiscent of more distal lesions. The second site of entrapment occurs along the proximal nerve between the hypertrophied superficial and deep heads of the pronator teres, or under a fibrous band within its substance. These result in characteristic pain along the proximal forearm exacerbated by repetitive elbow movements and dysesthesia that is worse with wrist movements or at night as typically occurs in the carpal tunnel syndrome. The third site of median nerve compression

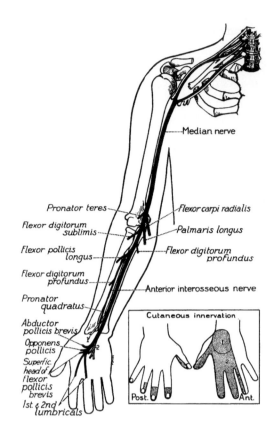

FIG. 12. The course and distribution of the median nerve. From, reference 3, with permission.

occurs distal to the two heads of the pronator teres affecting the anterior interosseus (motor) nerve leading to weakness of the flexor pollicis longus, flexor digitorum profundus digits 3 and 4, and the pronator quadratus. Such patients complain of deep aching pain in the forearm and wrist-sparing sensation. The fourth and clinically most common site of entrapment occurs at the wrist under the transverse in the carpal tunnel. Affected patients complain of pressure sensation, numbness, paresthesia, pain, stiffness, swelling along the median digits, particularly the thumb and index finger, through the wrist to the forearm to the axilla, particularly during sleep (32). Examination shows sensitivity over the wrist with evocation of paresthesia and pain after tapping of the median nerve at the wrist (Tinel sign), passive flexion of the wrist (Phalen sign), weakness, and wasting of the abductor pollicis brevis.

Electrodiagnostic studies are the only means of establishing the site of entrapment with certainty in a given patient, which classically includes prolongation of the distal motor and sensory latencies, low amplitude CMAP and SNAP, slow sensory velocity across the wrist, and a borderline or normal forearm motor velocity with prolonged F- response latency. According to detailed studies reported in the literature (33), there were no significant differences in NCV when stimulating with needle and surface electrodes; how-

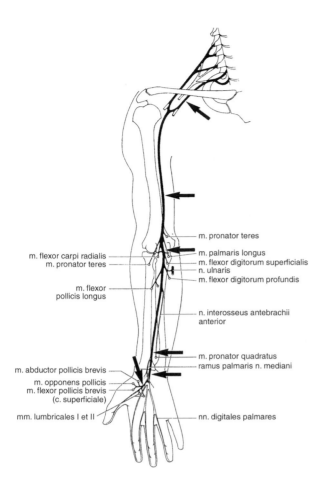

m. flexor carpi radialis
m. pronator teres

m. flexor
pollicis longus

m. abductor pollicis brevis
m. opponens pollicis
m. flexor pollicis brevis
(c. superficiale)

mm. lumbricales I et II

m. pronator teres

m. palmaris longus
m. flexor digitorum superficialis
n. ulnaris
m. flexor digitorum profundis

n. interosseus antebrachii
anterior

m. pronator quadratus
ramus palmaris n. mediani

nn. digitales palmares

FIG. 13. Site of entrapment along the course of the median nerve as marked by arrows respectively, from top to bottom, at the axilla to elbow, distal to the pronator teres, proximal to the wrist joint, at the carpal tunnel and thenar eminence. From, reference 5, with permission.

ever, there was significant slowing of NCV of 18% when comparing distal to proximal segments attributable to a decrease in fiber diameter from the proximal to distal part of the nerve, with an average variation from side to side of 5 to 10%. Among 117 consecutive patients with carpal tunnel syndrome (CTS) and 11 with compression of the median nerve at the elbow, median ulnar motor and sensory NCS and quantitative EMG were compared with findings in 190 normal age-matched controls. In 25% of those with CTS in whom motor NCS and EMG were normal, the lesion was located from abnormalities in sensory NCS, ascertained by detection of moderate slowing from digit to palm, severe slowing across the flexor retinaculum, and normal NCS from wrist to elbow indicative of demyelinating across the site of compression. Up to 15% of patients with CTS had clinical and electrophysiological evidence of ulnar involvement, while ulnar NCS were normal in 100 other patients so studied. Compression at the elbow, which may be due to involvement of the main trunk or the anterior interosseus branch only, was most commonly revealed by electromyo-

graphic abnormalities, including reduced interference pattern and fibrillation potentials in the deep flexor muscles innervating the distal phalanx of digits I, II, and often III.

A practice parameter of the American Association of Neuromuscular and Electrodiagnostic Medicine (AANEM) (34), formerly the American Association of Electrodiagnostic Medicine (AAEM), American Academy of Neurology (AAN) and the American Academy of Physical Medicine and Rehabilitation (AAPMR) for the electrodiagnostic studies of carpal tunnel syndrome, based upon pooled sensitivities and specificities and literature review (35), recommended the initial performance of a median sensory NCS across the wrist with a conduction distance of 13 cm to 14 cm, associated with an anticipated diagnostic sensitivity of 65% and specificity of 98%. If abnormal, comparison of the result to one other adjacent nerve in the symptomatic limb was performed. If the initial conduction employing a distance greater than 8 cm, showed normal results, then additional comparisons could be made with anticipated increased sensitivity and specificity. Comparisons of radial sensory nerve conduction between the wrist and thumb, median motor nerve conduction between the wrist and palm, median and ulnar mixed-nerve conduction between wrist and palm, and median sensory and mixed- nerve conduction between wrist and palm showed minimally increased gains in sensitivity, increasing gradually in sensitivity from 65% to 74%, while decreasing in specificity from 99% to 97%. The comparison of median and ulnar sensory conduction between wrist and ring finger, and comparison of median sensory and mixed-nerve conduction to forearm or digit segments, yielded sensitivities of 85% and specificity of 97% to 98%. Further recommendations included needle EMG sampling of muscles innervated by the C5 to T1 spinal roots, including a thenar muscle innervated by the median nerve of the symptomatic limb. Other maneuvers not recommended due to low anticipated sensitivity and specificity included multiple median F-wave parameters, median motor nerve residual latency, and sympathetic skin response.

In practice, median sensory nerve distal latencies should be measured and compared to either the ulnar or radial sensory latencies in the same hand (36). Five maneuvers enhance the sensitivity of median NCS including comparisons of median motor and sensory conduction studies to ipsilateral ulnar motor and sensory and radial sensory studies, comparison to contralateral median studies, which should be less than 1 msec, digit 4 stimulation, which is invested with both median and ulnar innervation and shows a double peak; median inching techniques across the wrist; and comparison of median digit-to-palm, and palm-to-wrist latencies. Predisposing factors for carpal tunnel syndrome include pregnancy, rheumatoid arthritis, amyloidosis, renal failure, hypothyroidism, diabetes, and ganglionic cyst. One systematic review of pregnancy-related carpal tunnel syndrome (PRCTS) suggested that variations in the reported incidence, which varied from 31% to 62%, persisting in more than 50% of patients after one year, and in about 30% after three years, depended upon the methods used to detect the syndrome. An evidenced-based guideline for the use of neuromuscular ultrasound in the diagnosis of CTS (10) found that the technique of measurement of median nerve cross-sectional area at the wrist was accurate and complementary to electrodiagnostic studies in the diagnosis of CTS, especially in screening for structural abnormalities at the wrist. Regardless of etiology, MRI in CTS (37) demonstrates swelling of the median nerve best evaluated at the pisiform bone level, flattening of the nerve at the hamate level, palmar bowing of the flexor retinaculum, and increased T_2 signal in the median nerve. In addition, MRI can discern atypical features such as a large adductor pollicus muscle, persistent median artery, and excessive fat in the carpal tunnel, ganglion cysts, and synovial hypertrophy due to rheumatoid arthritis. Kleindienst and colleagues (38) noted three features of early CTS including isolated prestenotic and intracarpal swelling of the median nerve, absence of significant median nerve flattening, and a generalized increase in signal intensity retrograde to the distal radius.

The treatment of CTS includes wrist splinting, injection of long active corticosteroids into the wrist in the vicinity of the median nerve and transverse carpal ligament, and arthroscopic and open release of compression by severing the transverse carpal ligament. Four widely used endoscopic techniques that vary primarily in the use of one or two ports (39) give similar complication and success rates to the standard open-release approach, however patients undergoing endoscopic surgery return to work sooner and develop less pain and debilitation (2). A comparison of prognosis with different modes of treatment showed complete cure or only trivial residual symptoms in 75% of patients after surgery, 70% after local corticosteroid injection, 30% after splinting, and 20% without treatment; local corticosteroid injections led to 50% relapses after one year (40). A relatively poorer prognosis was indicated by advanced disease and atypical clinical features, including normal NCS, atypical hand diagram, and symptoms in digit V; coexistence of diabetes, peripheral neuropathy, and arthritis; longer duration; advanced age; alcohol use; smoking; and heavy manual occupation.

Ulnar Nerve

The ulnar nerve (Figure 14) derives from the C8 and T1 roots and is the principal branch of the medial cord of the brachial plexus. The ulnar nerve first descends in the medial bicipital sulcus and then pierces the medial intermuscular septum in the mid-upper arm to descend between the septum and the medial head of the triceps muscle toward the medial epicondyle of the humerus along the antebrachial fascia and ulnar collateral ligament, which forms a tight roof over the sulcus on the epicondyle. It then passes beneath the medial epicondyle and the olecranon, which connects the two heads of the flexor carpi ulnaris and passes deep to enter the anterior portion of the forearm. Distal to the elbow the nerve gives off muscular branches to the flexor carpi ulnaris and the medial part of the flexor digitorum profundus. In the mid-forearm the ulnar nerve gives off a sensory branch to the dorsum of the hand and a sensory palmar cutaneous branch that arises distal to the dorsal branch that perforates the antebrachial fascia in the lower third of the forearm and supplies the skin overlying the medial and palmar portion of the wrist. The main ulnar nerve continues into the palm and, opposite the pisiform bone, gives off a superficial muscular branch to the palmaris brevis muscle, sensory branches to the medial palm and to the fourth and fifth fingers. The remaining deep motor branch gives off muscular branches to the abductor digiti minimi, flexor digiti minimi, and opponens digiti minimi, and arches across the metacarpal bones to the third and fourth lumbricals, all four of the interossei muscles, adductor pollicis, and deep head of the flexor pollicis brevis muscle.

There are four clinically significant sites of entrapment of the ulnar nerve in the arm (Figure 15). The nerve is first subject to entrapment and repeated trauma in the ulnar groove, between the medial epicondyle and the olecranon with repeated flexion, extension, and in the course of arthritic flares. Second, the ulnar nerve may be entrapped somewhat distally in the cubital tunnel as the nerve passes under the aponeurosis of the flexor carpi ulnaris. In both conditions, affected patients complain of paresthesia, hypesthesia, especially frequent with repetitive movement or pressure upon the elbow, with cramping or aching along the ulnar forearm to the hand. Examination shows tenderness of the nerve either in the ulnar groove or in the region of the flexor carpi ulnaris with radiation into the fourth and fifth digits after percussion, with variable distal affliction as evidenced by atrophy of ulnar intrinsic hand muscles, and sensory loss in the medial palmar fourth digit, fifth digit, and along the dorsum of the medial dorsum of the hand. The third site of entrapment occurs at the wrist in Guyon canal, where the ulnar nerve divides into deep motor and superficial palmar sensory and digital branches, distal to the dorsal cutaneous sensory branch. The fourth site of injury occurs in the mid-palm in those subject to repeated trauma, such as in operators of jackhammers, leading to distal thenar and interossei motor involvement.

Although MR neurography (41) provides excellent discrimination of ulnar neuropathy at the elbow from a normal finding, and is useful in assessing mild from severe involvement, electrodiagnostic studies are the most

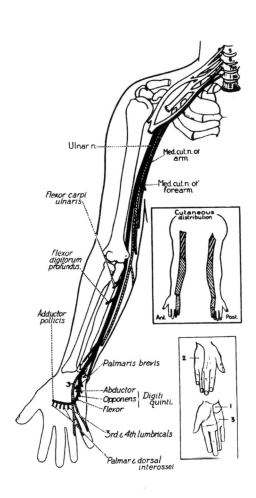

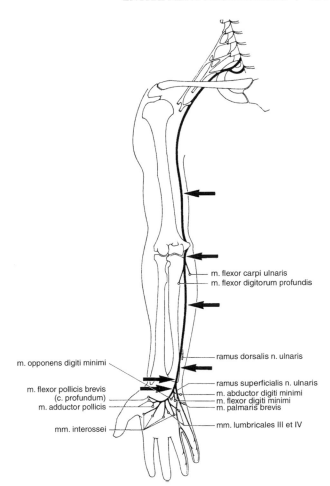

FIG. 14. The course and distribution of the ulnar nerve. From, reference 3, with permission.

FIG. 15. Sites of entrapment along the course of the ulnar nerve as marked by arrows respectively, from top to bottom, at the ulnar sulcus, upper third of forearm, lower third of forearm, immediately proximal to the wrist joint, at the pisiform bone, and slightly distal to the pisiform bone. From, reference 5, with permission.

essential method of accurate diagnosis of ulnar entrapment at all potential sites of compression (42, 43). Nerve conduction studies include recording over the abductor digiti minimi with stimulation at the wrist, above and below the elbow in a flexed position. A drop in the velocity of greater than 15% between the forearm and around the elbow segments indicates focal demyelination. Furthermore, a greater than 20% reduction in the CMAP amplitudes between the two segments, especially with inching techniques, confirms the demyelinating focus as a conduction block. A Practice Parameter of the AANEM, AAN, and the AAPMR (44) recommends that if ulnar sensory or motor NCS are abnormal, then further NCS should be carried out to exclude a diffuse process, that the elbow position be 70 degrees to 90 degrees in flexion from the horizontal plane with distance across the elbow in the range of 10 cm, and avoidance of stimulation more than 3 cm distal to the medial epicondyle to prevent stimulation of the nerve, which may be deep to the flexor carpi ulnaris muscle. The findings suggestive of a focal elbow lesion

included an absolute motor NCV from above elbow (AE) -to-below elbow (BE) of <50 m/s, a decrease in the CMAP negative peak amplitude from BE-to-AE greater than 20%, indicative of conduction block or temporal dispersion due to focal demyelination, and a significant change in CMAP configuration at the AE-to-BE site. In the setting of inconclusive ulnar motor NCS after stimulation of the wrist, AE and BE, other procedures that may be of benefit include NCS recording from the first dorsal interosseus, inching studies for changes in CMAP amplitude, area, and configuration, and NCS to forearm flexor muscles. Needle EMG should always include the FDI muscle and ulnar innervated forearm flexor muscles, and if abnormal, the examination should be extended to non-ulnar C8/medial cord/lower trunk muscle to exclude brachial plexopathy and cervical paraspinal muscles to exclude radiculopathy.

Although the cubital tunnel, which is literally the aponeurosis between the two heads of the flexor carpi ulnaris muscle and contains the ulnar nerve, and is a common site of entrapment, lies distal to the medial epicondyle of the humerus. Some consider the entire area as part of the cubital tunnel, or if not, refer to ulnar nerve entrapment at the elbow as a cubital tunnel syndrome if there is an appropriate symptom complex.

O'Driscoll and colleagues (45) noted that the roof of the cubital tunnel, formed from the cubital tunnel retinaculum in cadaveric studies, derived from a remnant of the anconeus epitrochlear muscle, extended anatomically from the medial epicondyle to the olecranon, forming a band of varying tension. Complete ulnar decompression at the elbow, followed by restoration of the nerve to a safe and unkinked location, is the goal of surgery. There is ongoing controversy as to the relative benefit of simple decompression by freeing the nerve from compressive adhesions and bands alone throughout its course across the elbow

into the cubital tunnel, and decompression with transposition under the flexor muscle mass, which is a currently preferred but is a more involved procedure (2). Simple decompression by opening the cubital tunnel and releasing the nerve from the epicondylar groove alone without placing it anterior to the epidonyle or dissection of the flexor muscle mass was associated with an 89% initially favorable, and 79% long-term outcome, that compares favorably with more extensive transposition (46). There was no difference between simple decompression and transposition of the ulnar nerve for both clinical improvement and neurophysiological improvement (47); however, transposition carried a greater risk of wound infection.

Radial Nerve

The radial nerve (Figure 16) derives from C5 to C8 nerve roots and is the continuation of the posterior cord of the brachial plexus. In the axilla, the radial nerve gives rise to

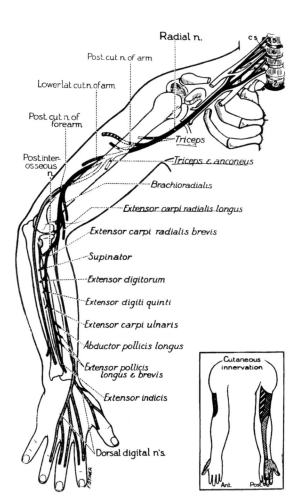

FIG. 16. The course and distribution of the radial nerve. From, reference 3, with permission.

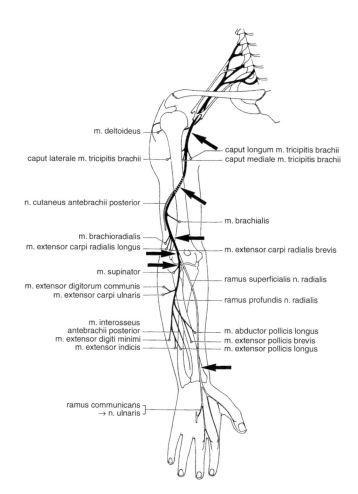

FIG. 17. Sites of entrapment along the course of the radial nerve as marked by arrows respectively, at the axilla, middle of upper arm, at the furrow between the brachioradialis and brachialis muscles, along the cubital fossa, and at the level of the supinator muscle. From, reference 5, with permission.

the posterior cutaneous nerve of the arm to supply the skin of the arm as far down as the olecranon. The main nerve reaches the long and medial heads of the triceps muscle whereupon it gives muscular branches to the triceps before reaching the sulcus for the radial nerve in the mid-shaft of the humerus. In the sulcus, the nerve winds spirally around the bone in contact with it to reach the lateral side of the upper arm where it penetrates the lateral intermuscular septum. The posterior cutaneous nerve of the forearm arises from the main nerve in the middle of the arm to innervate the skin of the extensor portion of the forearm as far as the wrist. After penetrating the septum, the main nerve lies in the intermuscular furrow between the brachioradialis and the lateral border of the brachialis where it gives off branches to the lateral extensor muscles, including the brachioradialis, brachialis, extensor carpi radialis longus, and extensor carpi radialis brevis, and then passes to the cubital fossa. Here is divides above the head of the radius into its terminal branches, the superficial branch and the deep motor branch. The former passes at the junction of the middle and distal thirds of the forearm behind the tendon of the brachioradialis to reach the back of the hand and dorsum of the first four fingers. The deep motor branch passes through the supinator muscle, which it supplies, and goes around the radius to the back of the forearm, where it divides into its terminal branches to innervate the extensor digitorum, extensor carpi ulnaris, extensor digiti minimi, extensor pollicis longus and brevis, abductor pollicis longus, and extensor indicis.

The radial nerve is subject to entrapment at five sites along the arm (Figure 17). The radial nerve is first subject to compression in the axilla, resulting in axillary nerve and triceps involvement. A second site of entrapment occurs in the spiral groove where the nerve wraps around the humerus descending toward the elbow. This leads to paralysis of wrist and finger extension, supination, and elbow flexion, sparing elbow extension, with loss of sensation along the lateral dorsum of the hand and digits in the territory of the superficial radial sensory nerve. A third site of entrapment occurs distal to the elbow where the posterior interosseus motor nerve branch enters the supinator muscle under the arcade of Frohse to supply most of the extensor muscles of the wrist and fingers. This site of entrapment spares the brachioradialis and extensor carpi radialis muscles with partial affliction of wrist strength, and no sensory loss. A fourth site of compression affects superficial radial sensory nerve fibers at the wrist as a result of tight handcuffs, termed *chirurgical paresthetica*.

Electrodiagnostic studies are important in the localization and prognostication of radial nerve lesions early in the course of an acquired lesion and in the course of recovery. Trojaborg (48) described 29 patients with Saturday-night radial palsy, in which the radial nerve was compressed during sleep, assumed to occur at the lateral border of the humerus where the radial nerve pierces the lateral intermuscular septum, or just below this, where the nerve is placed superficially and closely related to the humerus. Compression therein caused paresis of the wrist and fingers, and sensory loss, which was expected to be limited to the dorsum of the wrist, hand, thumb and 2½ fingers as far as the phalanx, so noted in only 10 of 29 patients. In 12 other patients, the clinical findings pointed to injury at a higher level due to involvement of the posterior cutaneous nerve of the forearm or to a lower level with sparing of the brachioradialis muscle. Variations of the expected pattern were ascribed to differing susceptibility of motor and sensory branches to pressure, position of the fibers in the nerve, and anatomical variation. The electrodiagnostic findings of Saturday-night radial palsy showed normal distal motor latency and sensory conduction velocities between the wrist and elbow below the site of the lesion, and 50% of normal values between the axilla and elbow, which is across the compressed segment, during the first two weeks, with return to normal in about seven weeks. Electromyographic findings included prominent single oscillations of motor units in most of the patients, and in one-third, there was no voluntary activity in the brachioradialis and extensor digitorum, or both in the first study, with amplitude of the interference pattern at full effort of less than 50% of normal in nearly one-half of muscles showing voluntary activity. Spontaneous discharges in the form of fibrillation potentials were found in about 80% of brachioradialis and extensor digitorum muscles so studied, which persisted for up to two weeks. These findings were consistent with transient block and neuropraxia secondary to ischemia.

Among 29 additional patients with radial nerve palsy with fracture of the shaft of the humerus and blunt injury, the site of injury of the radial nerve corresponded to the osseous spiral groove and there was total interruption of motor function distal to this point, with decreased sensation to testing by pinprick and cotton wool limited to the dorsum of the hand, and one, two, or all three radial fingers with additional involvement of a small area of the dorsal aspect of the forearm in one-half the patients. Overall, 21 patients presented instead with paralysis to moderate weakness and wasting of the brachioradialis and extensors of the wrist and fingers, and all but three patients had sensory loss of hand and forearm, or both. Among the remaining 11 patients, only the extensors of the wrist and fingers were affected and three had hypoesthesia and hyperalgesia of the appropriate part of the hand; the brachial triceps muscle was spared in all but one patient. Electrodiagnostic studies confirmed the clinical findings due to absence of motor-evoked responses in the brachioradialis and extensor muscles of the wrist and fingers, and sensory potentials after stimulation of the nerve. The rate of recovery was equal in comparable lengths of motor and sensory fibers, using the extensor indicis as an indicator of return of motor function. When it was possible to evoke a motor response, a sensory action potential could also be recorded. The earliest time at which motor fiber showed signs of reinnervation was 3½ months after the time of injury, and 12 to 15 months for sensory fibers when motor fibers to the extensor indicis muscle also conducted impulses. Electromyographic findings, which showed no voluntary activity corresponding to the brachioradialis and extensor digitorum communis muscles, was accompanied by spontaneous activity of fibrillation potentials.

Surgical exploration in one patient showed an intact nerve and electrical stimulation thereof elicited contraction in the brachioradilais but not in the extensor digitorum communis. Electrophysiological studies 150 days later in that patient showed single motor units, polyphasic poten-

tials and a low-voltage polyphasic response in the extensor digitorum communis following radial nerve stimulation at the elbow, with absence of the SNAP. Fifteen months later, motor conduction velocity to the brachioradialis and extensor digitorum communis between the axilla and elbow was 35% of normal, and that to the extensor indicis 50%, reduced. Similarly, sensory conduction velocity between the wrist and elbow was reduced by 50% and between the elbow and axilla by 30%. It was postulated that nerve damage affected mainly axons in blunt injury and humeral fracture, with little or no injury to the myelin sheaths, and sparing of the fastest conducting fibers.

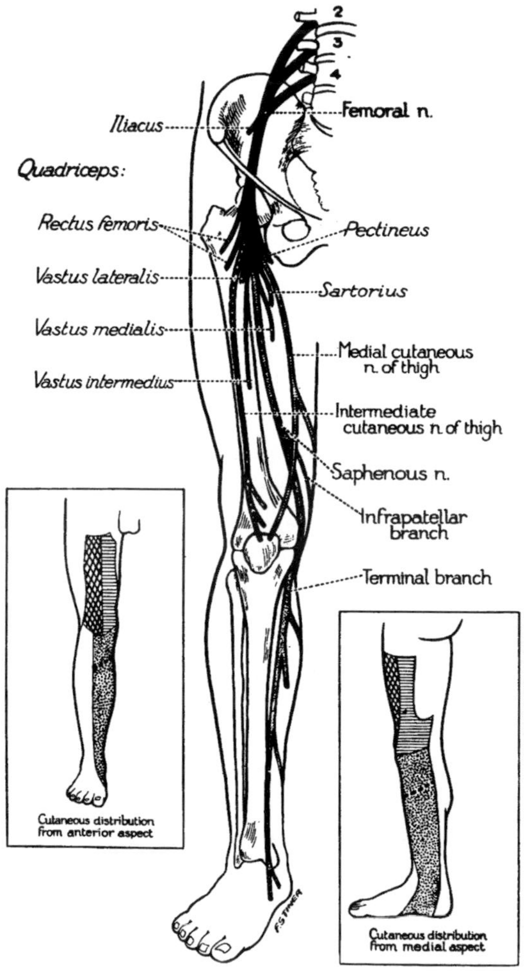

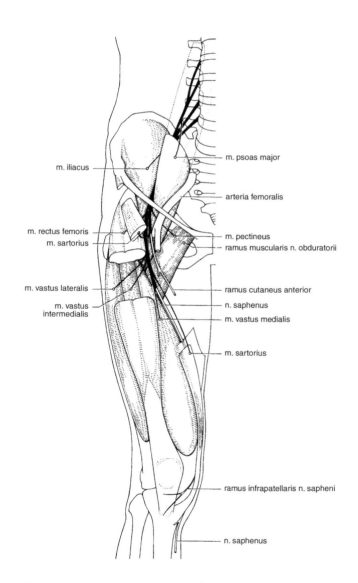

FIG. 18. The course and distribution of the femoral nerve. From, reference 3, with permission.

FIG. 19. Site of nerve entrapment along the course of the femoral nerve. The descent of the femoral mixed nerve from the pelvis between the iliacus and psoas muscles, where it lies at the lateral border of the latter, passing behind the inguinal ligament where it divides into terminal branches. From, reference 5, with permission.

The posterior interosseus nerve, which branches from the radial nerve proper immediately distal to the elbow joint, giving a branch to the extensor carpi radialis longus before turning and entering the supinator muscle can be entrapped along a fibrous ring region called the arcade of Frohse, before continueing distally to innervate the supinator and extensor muscles of the wrist and fingers. Other rare adhesions between the brachialis and brachioradialis muscles, the edge of the extensor carpi radialis brevis, fibrous bands associated with the supinator muscle and a set of vascular branches sometimes termed the *leash of Henry*, are additional sites of entrapment as the nerve exits the supinator muscle (2).

There are various surgical approaches for posterior interosseus nerve entrapment, which presents variably as painless palsy or painful tennis-like elbow, lateral epicondylitis or radial tunnel syndrome typically after strenuous use of the forearm, following blunt injury, or insidiously without provocation. Dissection of the brachialis and brachioradialis is performed until the radial nerve is found with identification of the posterior antebrachial cutaneous nerve and motor branches to the brachioradialis. This is followed by the release of the arcade of Frohse, to free the nerve where it penetrates the supinator muscle up to the extensor carpi radialis muscle until no firm edges can be felt up to the extensor carpi radialis muscle (2). High-resolution MR neurography is a useful intervention to image preoperative nerve anatomy and various possible structural pathologies associated with entrapment (49, 50).

Femoral Nerve

The femoral mixed nerve (Figure 18) derives from the L1 to L4 roots, and descends in the pelvis through the lumbar plexus between the iliacus and psoas muscles, along their border to which it sends motor branches. It passes in the lacuna musculorum going behind the inguinal ligament, where it divides into the terminal branches, namely those to the pectineus, sartorius, and quadriceps femoris muscles, and sensory cutaneous branches to the medial and anterior thigh and knee. The nerve then continues along with the femoral artery in the adductor canal where it pierces the deep fascia at the level of the tibial tuberosity, and runs together with the greater saphenous vein. This nerve supplies the medial knee and infrapatellar branch, and continues down the entire medial portion of the leg to the malleolus.

Femoral nerve entrapment occurs at two sites (Figure 19), most notably under the inguinal ligament such as following inguinal and hip surgery, femoral angiography, and aortofemoral bypass surgery and with prolonged pressure along the medial part of the knee where the saphenous nerve pierces the deep fascia, leading to sensory loss along the medial leg.

Electrodiagnostic studies are essential in the evaluation of femoral entrapment. The femoral nerve is stimulated above the inguinal ligament, and distal motor latencies are recorded to the quadriceps muscle and saphenous sensory conduction is performed according to standard technique and both compared to the contralateral side and published results in normal control or laboratory subjects. CT of the abdomen and pelvis excludes mass lesions, hematoma, and compression in the inguinal canal. MRI of the knee is useful in detecting local trauma and compression along its medial border. Treatment is directed toward the offending injury.

Lateral Femoral Cutaneous Nerve

This purely sensory nerve (Figure 20) derives from L2 to L3 dorsal roots and runs along the inner wall of the pelvis, near the caecum and the lower pole of the kidney in the direction of the anterior superior iliac spine, which serves as a bony landmark located approximately 0.7 cm from the nerve trunk. It passes medially between fibrous fascicles in an aponeurotic fascial tunnel, beginning at the iliopubic tract and ending posteriorly under the inguinal ligament, composed of two laminae between which the lateral femoral cutaneous nerve courses. Within the first 3 cm of leaving the pelvis, the lateral femoral cutaneous nerve is found deep to the tensor fascia lata under which it travels before turning caudally at an angle of nearly 90 degrees and bifurcating into anterior and posterior branches. In the typical pattern the anterior branch innervates the skin of the anterolateral region of the thigh and divides into medial and lateral branches, and the posterior branch distributes to the skin of the cranial half of the lateral surface of the thigh. In about one-third of individuals, there is no posterior branch, and symptoms of entrapment are then limited to the anterior branch region. An accessory nerve is noted also in about a third of cases.

Continuous trauma to the nerve at the boundary between the pelvis and femoral portions, usually several millimeters proximal to the inguinal ligament, where angulation is more prominent, facilitates development of pseudoneuromas at this location (51). The inguinal ligament has most frequently been suggested as the determinant of entrapment. Lateral femoral cutaneous neuralgia also appears to result from compression by the iliopubic tract and the anterior lamina of the iliac fascia between the iliopubic tract and inguinal ligament, notably in obese individuals wherein gravity, due to the erect stance, acts on viscera and adipose tissue of the anterior abdomen, favoring greater traction of the anterior lamina of the iliac fascia. Entrapment at these levels produces burning, paresthesia, and numbness of the lateral upper thigh with tenderness on pressure of the nerve trunk.

Nerve conduction studies are performed orthodromically using signal averaging, with bipolar stimulation placed 11 to 16 cm directly inferior to the anterior iliac spine, and pickup surface electrodes placed 1 cm medial to the antero-

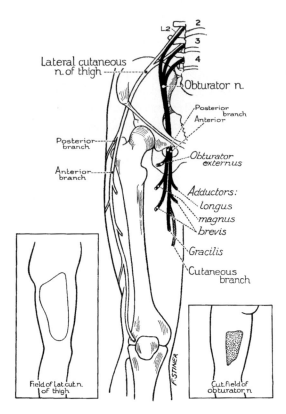

FIG. 20. Course and distribution of the lateral cutaneous nerve of the thigh and the obturator nerve. From, reference 3, with permission.

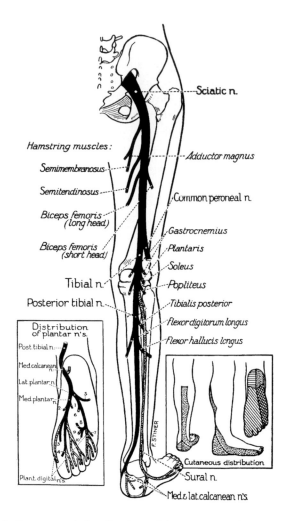

FIG. 21. Course and distribution of the sciatic and posterior tibial nerve. From, reference 3, with permission.

superior iliac spine, with comparison to the asymptomatic side or normal controls (52). Treatment is generally supportive and includes the use of medications such as gabapentin and tricyclic antidepressants to control symptoms. The difficulty in locating and decompressing the nerve are the likely determinants of surgical failure.

Sciatic Nerve

The sciatic nerve (Figure 21) originates from the fourth and fifth lumbar, and first to third ventral and dorsal sacral roots. They combine to form a flat ribbon-like nerve that measures almost three-quarters of an inch in diameter at the anterior border of the great sciatic foramen where it passes from the pelvis into the thigh, descending midway between the greater trochanter of the femur and the ischial tuberosity to its lower third. The upper part of the nerve gives off articular branches to the hip joint, perforating the posterior part of its fibrous capsule, and the lower portion of the sciatic nerve beneath the biceps femoris muscle gives off muscular branches to flexor muscles of the thigh, namely the biceps, semitendinous, semimembranous, and adductor magnus, whereupon the nerve then divides into the peroneal and tibial terminal nerves. All along its path, the sciatic nerve can be considered as the combination of two nerves

predictably organized in the same sheath, including a tibial portion derived, respectively, from the anterior divisions of the lumbosacral plexus located internally in the sheath, and the fibular component so derived from posterior divisions of the lumbosacral plexus and located more laterally.

Compressive lesions of the sciatic nerve (Figure 22) may be partial or complete, involving some or all of the flexor thigh muscles alone, or those of the individual terminal branches separately or together, with variable sensory loss of the foot (53). Lesions of the sciatic nerve with a fibular emphasis show unmistakable paresis of extensor foot muscles with foot drop and steppage gait, along with sensory loss of the lateral calf and the small web space adjacent to the big toe. Involvement of the tibial component of the sciatic nerve that leads to weakness of ankle plantar flexion and intrinsic foot muscles and sensory loss along the heel and sole, may sometimes go unnoticed except with careful examination because of the contribution of gravity to muscle function and the variable pattern of sensory loss (Figure 23).

The pathogenesis of sciatic nerve entrapment varies

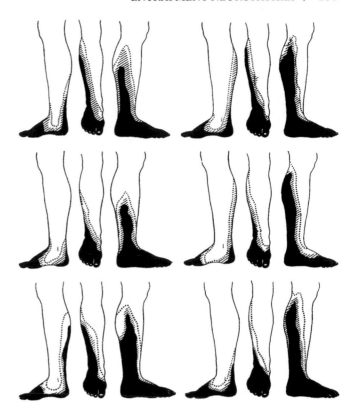

FIG. 23. Variable patterns of sensory loss due to sciatic lesion. From, reference 3, with permission.

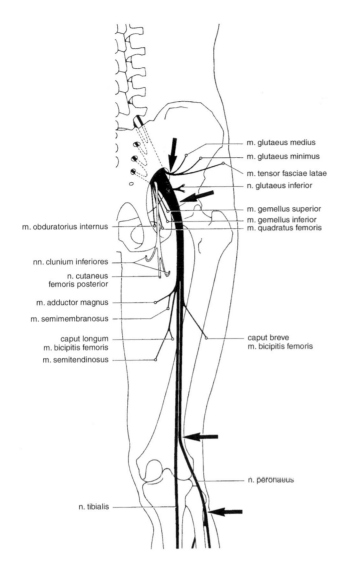

FIG. 22. Sites of entrapment of the sciatic nerve as marked by arrows respectively, through the greater sciatic notch in the supra-, and infrapiriformis foramina of the gluteal region, in the lower thight distal to the origin of flexor muscles of the knee, and passing on to the back of the head of the sibula. From, reference 5, with permission.

according to the site and etiology of the injury (54, 55). Its proximity to the trochanter and ischial tuberosity in the pelvis makes it prone to injury in the setting of total hip arthroplasty, hip fracture, dislocation, gluteal injection, and acute compression during a drug overdose, with prolonged sitting, and coma in the intensive care unit. Sciatic nerve compression also occurs with stretch injury, contusion, and compression along the edges of the greater sciatic foramen in association with mass lesions, arterial aneurysm, myositis ossificans, and compartment syndrome in association with hematoma, as well as in the course of vasculitis, radiation, femoral popliteal artery bypass, tuberculosis infection, and upon compression by the tendon or fibrosis bands in the vicinity of the piriformis muscle. There is a progressive

idiopathic sciatic mononeuropathy in young people, but little is known of its pathogenesis (55). The evaluation of a given patient with sciatic neuropathy should include MRI or CT of the lumbar spine, hip, pelvis, thigh, and sciatic notch, depending upon suspected area of entrapment or injury. Electrophysiological studies are necessary to establish the diagnosis and prognosis of sciatic nerve lesions.

Gassel and Trojaborg (56) determined conduction velocities and distal latencies along the sciatic nerve in 24 normal subjects, and the patterns of involvement and localization in two patients with traumatic lesions of the sciatic nerve in the upper thigh. Both patients presented with foot drop, which developed shortly after injections of barbital and aprobarbital into the upper posterior thigh. Electrodiagnostic studies were performed employing sciatic nerve stimulation in the gluteal region or upper thigh and in the upper popliteal region. One patient demonstrated polyphasic potentials in the tibialis anterior on stimulation of the upper thigh along the sciatic nerve, and less polyphasia on stimulation in the popliteal fossa, with conduction velocity reduced to 37 m/s; no response was obtained from the wasted extensor digitorum brevis muscle. Responses were, however, normal in muscles innervated by the posterior tibial nerve. The other patient had an absent response from the extensor digitorum brevis and tibialis anterior muscles at any level of sciatic motor stimulation, and responses were normal in muscles supplied by the posterior tibial nerve. There were pronounced signs of denervation in the biceps femoris, and reduced amplitude potential elicited in that muscle on stimulation of the sciatic nerve. The findings of both patients were consistent with lesions of the sciatic nerve in the upper thigh. Among the two normal subjects, there was a 20% to 22% higher conduction velocity in the nerve to the leg muscles than to the foot muscles without differences among velocities to the nerves to the leg muscles, such as the tibialis anterior, soleus, or gastrocnemius, consistent with the demonstration that the diameters of fibers in the nerves to these muscles do not show pronounced differences. In comparison to traumatic lesions of the sciatic nerve, sciatica presents diagnostic challenges, particularly when there are equivocal or normal imaging studies despite clinical suspicion of a radiculopathy. While it can be stated that the sensitivity is higher if a number of electrophysiological tests are added, Albeck and colleagues (57) found a high predictive value for the H-reflex examination, but not for electromyography, F-wave latencies, or motor and sensory NCS in monoradicular (S1) sciatica. The H-reflex, which has the advantage of testing both sensory and motor function, is unfortunately only applicable to S1 radiculopathy and mono-radicular sciatica, limiting its usefulness in the lumbar region.

The *piriformis syndrome* remains controversial (58–61).

It has been considered a form of sciatica affecting one or both buttocks with compression of the sciatic nerves by the piriformis muscle with resultant buttock pain, tingling and numbness along the nerve, sometimes down the leg, often worsening with sitting for long periods, climbing stairs, walking, or running. Several criteria, rarely seen in a given patient, should ideally be met before accepting the diagnosis as conclusive (59). Symptoms, signs, and electrophysiological criteria of sciatic nerve damage should be present, and paraspinal EMG should be normal to exclude radiculopathy. There should be normal neuroimaging of the lumbar spine, pelvis, and sciatic notch. Symptoms should be relieved with surgical decompression upon division of the piriformis muscle, tendon, or associated fibrous bands. Nonetheless, four clinical maneuvers are helpful in the clinical diagnosis of piriformis syndrome. The Freiberg maneuver of forceful internal rotation of the extended thigh elicits pain by stretching the piriformis muscle. The Pace maneuver of abduction of the legs in the seated position elicits pain due to contraction of the piriformis muscle. A third maneuver is performed with the patient lying with painful side up, the painful leg flexed, and the knee resting on the table in which deep buttock pain is produced when the patient lifts and holds the knee several inches off the table, due to contraction of the piriformis muscle. A fourth maneuver combines prolongation of the electrophysiological H reflex with hip flexion, adduction, and internal rotation. Prognosis is usually good

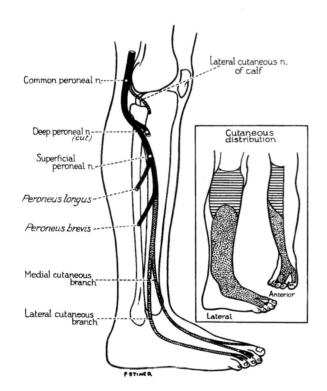
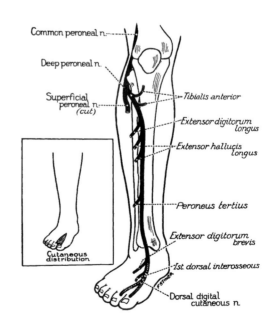

FIG. 24. The course and distribution of the fibular nerve: **(A)** superficial branch, and **(B)** deep motor branch. From, reference 3, with permission.

in most patients treated conservatively with physiotherapy and injection of corticosteroids, with only rare patients ever undergoing surgery for diagnostic or therapeutic purposes, so raising the question of its validity as a diagnostic entity of such a presumed common occurrence.

Common Fibular Nerve

The common fibular nerve (Figure 24 A, B) is a mixed nerve that derives from the L4 to S1 roots and descends though the lateral angle of the popliteal fossa and, after becoming subcutaneous, passes along the back of the fibula head where it is prone to entrapment. It then enters the substance of the peroneus longus muscle on the lateral side of the neck of the fibula where is divides into its terminal branches, the superficial and deep fibular nerves. The superficial fibular nerve descends along the anterior intermuscular septum together with the anterior tibial artery in the extensor compartment of the leg, supplying the muscles located therein, including the extensor digitorum longus, tibialis anterior, extensor hallucis longus, and peroneus tertius. The terminal branch of the deep fibular nerve passes under the inferior extensor retinaculum, where it is prone to compression, termed *anterior tarsal tunnel syndrome*. This nerve then divides into two terminal branches, the lateral branch, which innervates the extensor digitorum brevis muscle, and the medial cutaneous branch, which distributes to the skin of the first interosseus space and adjacent portions of the great and second toes.

Entrapment of the fibular nerve occurs at three sites (Figure 25). Compression of the common fibular nerve at the fibula head combines the deficits of the deep and superficial fibular nerves, leading to impairment of dorsiflexion and eversion of the foot and extension of the toes, and hypoesthesia to touch and pain in the lower two-thirds of the lateral leg and dorsum of the foot. Risk factors for common fibular nerve compression included anesthesia, weight loss, habitual leg crossing, prolonged squatting, tight knee cast or ankle foot orthosis, anti-thrombotic stockings, and trauma to the knee. Compression of the deep fibular nerve, such as in anterior compartment syndrome with sparing of the superficial branch, spares sensory loss along the lateral calf and weakness of foot eversion. Distal compression of the deep fibular nerve under the inferior extensor retinaculum spares involvement of foot extensor muscles; a common complaint of affected patients is pain and numbness of the feet with trophic changes of the metatarsal bones reminiscent of distal peripheral neuropathy, or even undefined pain of the dorsum of the foot and anterolateral leg. The commonest causes of this entrapment include compression of the nerve by tight shoe straps, high shoes edges, stretch injuries incurred during Islamic prayer postures, as well as osteophytes in bony structures, synovial pseudocysts, and ganglia. Electrodiag-

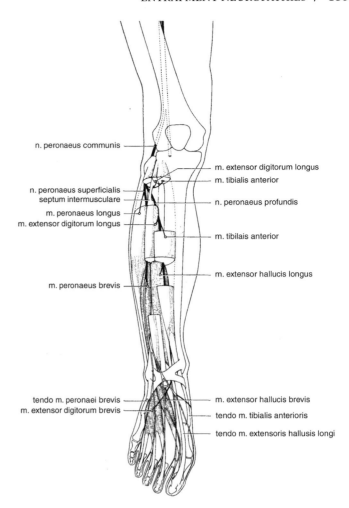

FIG. 25. Sites of entrapment of the fibular nerve from top to bottom respectively, as it rounds the head of the fibula, in the substance of the peroneus longus muscle, along a gap in the anterior intermuscular septum in the extensor compartment, and on the dorsum of the foot. From, reference 5, with permission.

nosis should confirm the clinical diagnosis, localization, and prognosis of virtually all fibular nerve lesions (62, 63).

Treatment of fibular nerve entrapments is usually supportive. Ankle foot orthosis temporarily improves gait and prevents contracture and ankle sprain if the deficit is severe and active foot exercises are not feasible. Surgical intervention is indicated in acute anterior compartment compression, and in the release of anterior tarsal tunnel entrapment.

Tibial Nerve

The tibial nerve (Figure 21) is a mixed nerve that derives from L4 to S3 roots, mainly L5 and S1, and traverses the popliteal fossa wherein it gives off the medial sural cutaneous nerve that innervates the skin of the calf and joins the lateral sural cutaneous nerve, a branch of the common fibular nerve, at the level of the Achilles tendon to form the sural nerve that supplies sensory innervation to the lateral aspect of the foot, including the 5th toe, heel, and ankle. In the distal part of the popliteal fossa, the tibial nerve sends motor branches to the gastrocnemius and soleus muscle and to the plantaris and popliteus muscles, the principal flexors of the foot. The tibial nerve passes between the two heads of the gastrocnemius, deep to the fibrous arch of the soleus and into the flexor compartment, wherein it gives off branches to the tibialis posterior, flexor hallucis, and digitorum longus muscles. The tibial nerve passes along with the respective tendon and the posterior tibial artery and venous concomitants behind the medial malleolus under the flexor retinaculum of the deep leg fascia that forms the tarsal tunnel, and the site of most frequent entrapment. Shortly before entering the tarsal tunnel, the nerve gives off the median calcaneal sensory branch to the medial aspect of the heel and, in the tunnel, the tibial nerve divides into the two mixed terminal nerve branches, the medial and laeral plantar nerves.

Entrapment of the tibial nerve (Figure 26) in the tarsal tunnel (64–66) results in usually non-localizing plantar pain, and numbness sensation over the median and lateral plantar aspect of the foot, with decreased pinprick sensation along the sole of the foot, sparing the lateral border, sole, and heel. There is weakness of small muscles of the foot, in particular the big toe, which cannot be abducted, and of spreading function of the toes due to weakness of the lumbricals and interossei muscles, in addition to burning causalgic pain, especially during walking and prolonged standing. A positive Tinel sign behind the medial malleolus at the site of entrapment can be elicited. The symptoms and signs of tarsal tunnel syndrome can be aggravated by passive eversion and dorsiflexion with maximal metatarsophalangeal joint dorsiflexion held in position for five to ten seconds (65).

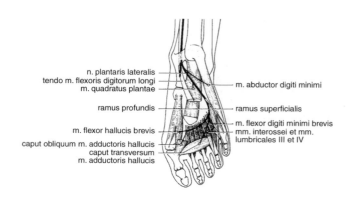

FIG. 26. Sites of entrapment of the tibial nerve at the tarsal tunnel as it passes from behind the medial malleolus underneath the flexor retinaculum where it thence divides into its two mixed terminal brances, the medial and lateral plantar nerves. From, reference 5, with permission.

Although most cases are idiopathic, ankle trauma, ankle sprain, fracture, arthritis, and tenosynovitis, tight-fitting footwear and valgus foot deformity may be precipitating factors of tarsal tunnel syndrome. Electrodiagnostic studies are important in the assessment of tarsal tunnel syndrome and include stimulation surface or near nerve needle sensory nerve conduction studies of digital nerves of the medial and lateral plantar nerves with the recording electrode placed over the posterior tibial nerve at the medial malleolus above the flexor retinaculum, and comparison to the contralateral side and normal control values (67).

Most patients are treated with injection of long-acting corticosteroids, orthotic shoe inserts to promote heel valgus and varus and, if necessary, surgical release of the flexor retinaculum.

REFERENCES

1. Nakano KK. The entrapment neuropathies. *Muscle Nerve* 1978; 1:264–279.
2. Arle JS, Zager EL. Surgical treatment of common entrapment neuropathies in the upper limbs. *Muscle Nerve* 2000; 23:1160–1174.
3. Haymaker W, Woodhall B. *Peripheral nerve injuries*. WB Saunders: Philadelphia, 1953.
4. Foerster O. Die symptomatologie der schussuerletzungen der peripherin nerven. In Lewandowsky M. *Handbuch der Neurologie, Erganzungbd*, 2. Teil, 1929, 975–1508.
5. Mumenthaler M. Topographic diagnosis of peripheral nerve lesions. *Handb Clin Neurol* 1978; 2:15–51.
6. Buchtal F, Kuhl V. Nerve conduction, tactile sensibility and electromyogram after suture or compression of peripheral nerve: a longitudinal study in man. *J Neurol Neurosurg Psychiatry* 1979; 42:436–445.
7. Trojaborg W. Peripheral conduction block with axonal degeneration. *J Neurol Neurosurg Psychiatry* 1977; 40:50–57.
8. Kraft GH. Axillary, musculocutaneous, and suprascapular nerve latency studies. *Arch Phys Med Rehabil* 1972; 53:383–87.
9. Baumer P, Dombert T, Staub F, et al. Ulnar neuropathy at the elbow: MR neurography-nerve T2 signal increase and caliber. *Radiology* 2011; 260:199–206.
10. Cartwright MS, Hobson-Webb LD, Boon AJ, et al. Evidence-based guideline: neuromuscular ultrasound for the diagnosis of carpal tunnel syndrome. *Muscle Nerve* 2012; 46:287–293.
11. Horowitz MT, Tocantins LJ. Isolated paralysis of the serratus anterior muscle. *J Bone Joint Surg* 1955; 37:567–576.
12. Kaplan PE. Electrodiagnostic confirmation of long thoracic nerve palsy. *J Neurol Neurosurg Psychiatry* 1980; 43:50–52.
13. Petera JE, Trojaborg W. Conduction studies of the long thoracic nerve in serratus anterior palsy of different etiology. *Neurology* 1984; 34:1033–1037.

14. Auppaila LI, Vstamaki M. Iatrogenic serratus anterior palsy: long term outcome in 26 patients. *Chest* 1996; 109:31–34.

15. Fahrer H, Ludin HP, Mumenthaler M, et al. The innervation of the trapezius muscle. An electrophysiological study. *J Neurol* 1974; 207:183–188.

16. Petrera JE, Trojaborg W. Conduction studies along the accessory nerve and follow-up of patients with trapezius palsy. *J Neurol Neurosurg Psychiatry* 1984; 47:630–636.

17. Gassel MM. A test of nerve conduction to muscles of the shoulder girdle as an aid in the diagnosis of proximal neurogenic and muscular disease. *J Neurol Neurosurg Psychiatry* 1964; 27:200–205.

18. Trojaborg W. Motor and sensory conduction in the musculocutaneous nerve. *J Neurol Neurosurg Psychiatry* 1976; 39:890–899.

19. Freehill MT, Shi LL, Tompson JD, et al. Suprascapular neuropathy: diagnosis and management. *Phys Sports Med* 2012; 40:72–83.

20. Aiello I, Serra G, Traina GC, et al. Entrapment of the suprascapular nerve at the glenoid notch. *Ann Neurol* 1982; 12:314–316.

21. Henlin JL, Rousselot JP, Monnier G, et al. Syndrome canalaire du nerf sus-scapulaire dans le defile spino-glenoidien. *Rev Neurol* 1992; 5:362–367.

22. Post M, Mayer J. Suprascapular nerve entrapment. Diagnosis and treatment. *Clin Orthop* 1987; 223:126–136.

23. Kirby JF, Jr., Kraft GH. Entrapment neuropathy of anterior branch of axillary nerve: review and case. *Arch Phys Med Rehabil* 1972; 53:338–40.

24. Johnson EW. Axillary nerve injury. Arch Neurol 1984; 41:1022.

25. Lester B, Jeong GK, Weiland AJ, et al. Quadrilateral space syndrome: diagnosis, pathology, and treatment. *Am J Orthop* 1999; 28:718–722.

26. Liveson JA. Nerve lesions associated with shoulder dislocation: An electrodiagnostic study of 11 cases. *J Neurol Neurosurg Pyschiatry* 1984; 47:742–744.

27. Gassel M, Diamantopoulos E. Pattern of conduction times in the distribution of the radial nerve. A clinical and electrophysiological study. *Neurology* 1964; 14:222–231.

28. Trojaborg W, Sindrup EH. Motor and sensory conduction in different segments of the radial nerve in normal subjects. *J Neurol Neurosurg Psychiatry* 1969; 32:354–359.

29. Buchtal F, Rosenfalck A. Evoked action potentials and conduction velocity in human sensory nerves. *Brain Research* 1966; 3:1–122.

30. Buchtal F, Rosenfalck A. Sensory potentials in polyneuropathy. *Brain* 1971; 94:241–262.

31. Sunderland S. *Nerves and nerve injuries.* Livingstone: Edinburgh, 1968, 1161.

32. Buchtal F, Rosenfalck A, Trojaborg W. Electrophysiological findings in entrapment of the median nerve at wrist and elbow. *J Neurol Neurosurg Psychiatry* 1974; 37:340–360.

33. Trojaborg W. Motor nerve conduction velocities in normal subjects with particular reference to the conduction in proximal and distal segments of median and ulnar nerve. *Electroenceph Clin Neurophysiol* 1964; 17:314–321.

34. American Association of Neuromuscular and Electrodiagnostic Medicine, American Academy of Neurology, and American Academy of Physical Medicine and Rehabilitation. Practice parameter for electrodiagnostic studies in carpal tunnel syndrome: summary statement. *Muscle Nerve* 2002; 25:918–922.

35. Jablecki CK, Andary MT, Floeter MK, et al. Second literature review of the usefulness of nerve conduction studies and electromyography for the evaluation of patients with carpal tunnel syndrome. *Muscle Nerve* 2002; Published online 1 June 2002 in Wiley InterScience (www.interscience.wiley.com). DOI 10.1002/mus.10215.

36. Werner RA, Andary M. Electrodiagnostic evaluation of carpal tunnel syndrome. *Muscle Nerve* 2011; 44:597–607.

37. Mesgarzadeh M, Schneck CD, Bonakdarpour A, et al. Carpal tunnel: MR imaging. Part II. Carpal tunnel syndrome. *Radiology* 1989; 171:749–754.

38. Kleindienst A, Hamm B, Lanksch WB. Carpal tunnel syndrome: staging of median nerve compression by magnetic resonance imaging. *J Magn Reson Imaging* 1998; 8:1119–1125.

39. Jimenez DF, Gibbs SR, Clapper AT. Endoscopic treatment of carpal tunnel syndrome-a critical review. *J Neurosurg* 1998; 88:817–826.

40. Bland JDP. Treatment of carpal tunnel syndrome. *Muscle Nerve* 2007; 36:167–171.

41. Baumer P, Dombert T, Staub F, et al. Ulnar neuropathy at the elbow: MR neurography-nerve T2 signal increase and caliber. *Radiology* 2011; 260:199–206.

42. Kincaid JC. The electrodiagnosis of ulnar neuropathy at the elbow. *Muscle Nerve* 1988; 11:1005–1015.

43. Lo YL, Ratnagopal P, Leoh TH, et al. Clinical and electrophysiological aspects of distal ulnar neuropathy. *Acta Neurol Scand* 2002; 105:390–394.

44. American Association of Neuromuscular and Electrodiagnostic Medicine, American Academy of Neurology, and American Academy of Physical Medicine and Rehabilitation. Practice parameter: Electrodiagnostic studies in ulnar neuropathy at the elbow. *Neurology* 1999; 52:688–690.

45. O'Driscoll SW, Horii E, Carmichael SW, et al. The cubital tunnel and ulnar neuropathy. *J Bone Joint Surg* 1991; 73:613–617.

46. Kim DH, Han K, Tiel RL, et al. Surgical outcomes of 654 ulnar nerve lesions. *J Neurosurg* 2003; 98:993–1004.

47. Caliandro P, La Torre G, Padua R, et al. Treatment for ulnar neuropathy at the elbow. *Cochrane Database Syst Rev* 2012 Jul 11; 7:CD006839.

48. Trojaborg W. Rate of recovery in motor and sensory fibers of the radial nerve. Clinical and electrophysiological aspects. *J Neurol Neurosurg Psychiatry* 1970; 33:625–638.

49. Faridian-Aragh N, Chalian M, Soldatos T, et al. High-resolution 3T MR neurography of radial neuropathy. *J Neuroradiol* 2011; 38:265–274.

50. Kara M, Tiftik T, Yetisgin A, et al. Ultrasound in the diagnosis and treatment of posterior interosseus nerve entrapment; a case report. *Muscle Nerve* 2012; 45:299–300.

51. Dias Filho LC, Valenca MM, Guimaraes Filho FAV, et al. Lateral femoral cutaneous neuralgia: an anatomical insight. *Clinical Anatomy* 16:309–316.

52. Sarala P, Nishihara T, Joong S. Meralgia paresthetica: electrophysiological study. *Arch Phys Med Rehabil* 1979; 60:30–31.

53. Pollack LJ, Davis L. Peripheral nerve injuries: the sciatic nerve. *Am J Surg* 1932; 18:176–193.

54. Yuen EC, So YT, Olney RK. The electrophysiologic features of sciatic neuropathy in 100 patients. *Muscle Nerve* 1995; 18:414–420.

55. Yuen EC, Olney RK, So YT. Sciatic neuropathy: clinical and prognostic features in 73 patients. *Neurology* 1994; 44:1669–1674.

56. Gassel MM, Trojaborg W. Clinical and electrophysiological study of the pattern of conduction times in the distribution of the sciatic nerve. *J Neurol Neurosurg Psychiatry* 1964; 27:351–357.

57. Albeck MJ, Taher G, Lauritzen M, et al. Diagnostic value of electrophysiological tests in patients with sciatica. *Acta Neurol Scand* 2000; 101:249–254.

58. Beatty RA. The piriformis muscle syndrome: a simple diagnostic maneuver. *Neurosurg* 1994; 34:512–514.

59. Stewart JD. The piriformis is overdiagnosed. *Muscle Nerve* 2003; 28:644–646.

60. Fishman LM, Schaefer MP. The piriformis syndrome is underdiagnosed. *Muscle Nerve* 2003; 28:646–649.

61. Fishman LM, Dombi GW, Michaelsen C, et al. Piriformis syndrome: diagnosis, treatment, and outcome in a 10-year study. *Arch Phys Med Rehabil* 2002; 83:295–301.

62. Katiriji MB, Wilbourn AJ. Common peroneal neuropathy: a clinical and electrophysiological study of 116 lesions. *Neurology* 1988; 38:1723–1728.

63. Smith T, Trojaborg W. Clinical and electrophysiological recovery from peroneal palsy. *Acta Neurol Scand* 1986; 74:328–335.

64. Akyuz G, Us O, Turan B, et al. Anterior tarsal tunnel syndrome. *Electromyogr Clin Neurophysiol* 2000; 40:123–128.

65. Kinoshita M, Iluda R, Morikawa J, et al. The dorsiflexion–eversion test for diagnosis of tarsal tunnel syndrome. *J Bone Joint Surg* 2001; 83:1835–1839.

66. De Lisa JA, Saeed MA. The tarsal tunnel syndrome. *Muscle Nerve* 1983; 6:664–670.

67. Oh SJ, Kwon KH, Hah JS, et al. Lateral plantar neuropathy. *Muscle Nerve* 1999; 22:1234–1238.

CHAPTER 27

Plexus Disorders

David S. Younger

Plexus disorders are an important consideration in motor disorders because of their propensity to involve motor nerve axons of the arms and legs. This chapter reviews localization of the site of plexus lesions and the etiopathogenesis of common plexus disorders.

GENERAL CONSIDERATIONS

Embryogenesis

During early embryological development, the spinal nerve roots, plexus, and peripheral nerves originate from afferent and efferent axons of primitive neural crest located in the developing dorsal root ganglia (DRG). Efferent axons innervate segmental muscles while afferent branches enter the primitive neural tube forming the dorsal spinal roots. The afferent fibers are joined by efferent fibers growing from the basal lamina of the developing spinal cord as ventral spinal roots, and both ventral and dorsal spinal roots merge to form the nerve root proper. In humans, an inherently strict segmental pattern present at the level of a given root coincides with the development of limb buds as reflected in the enlargement of the spinal cord and spinal roots of the cervical and lumbar region to accommodate the added number of nerve fibers. The anterior primary rami (APR) of C1 to C4, and those of C5 to T1, respectively, populate the cervical and brachial plexus. The anterior and posterior roots of L1 to L4, and those of L4 to S3, along with the undivided rami of the sacral region, respectively, comprise the lumbar and sacral regions of the lumbosacral plexus.

Segmental Innervation

Fully developed, a given segmental spinal nerve contains a posterior primary division that innervates dorsal paraspinous musculature and related spinal dermatomes, a communicating ramus to sympathetic ganglion, and an anterior primary division that innervates the segmental limb myotomal muscles and the remaining dermatomes of the limbs. The segmental sensory innervation of the body, which is the body dermatomes (1) (Figures 1–5), reflects the combination of segmental truncal and limb innervation of somatic sensory structures located primarily in the skin that travel in lateral and medial branches of anterior and posterior primary rami that traverse mixed spinal nerves along with motor fibers that enter divergent posterior roots at each segmental level. The motor fibers of a segmental nerve of the trunk traverse lateral branches of the posterior primary ramus to innervate longitudinal muscles of the axial skeleton in a predictable myotomal pattern adjacent to spinal nerves of the same root segment (Figure 6). Myotomal motor innervation of limb muscles is more complicated due to segregation and rearrangement of fibers in the plexus, which has practical implications for disease. To illustrate, motor fibers from the C5 spinal segment extend through the corresponding anterior root, mixed spinal nerve, and undivided primary ramus to traverse the upper trunk of the plexus, its anterior and posterior divisions, and subsequently the lateral and posterior cords, en route to one of several emergent peripheral nerves, each carrying C5 fibers (Figure 7). While a very proximal lesion of the root results in near total loss of peripheral myotomal innervation, a less proximal lesion, for example, in the upper trunk, results in loss of only a part of the myotome, and an even more distal lesion, beyond the emergence of the motor branches, will be of less widespread consequence.

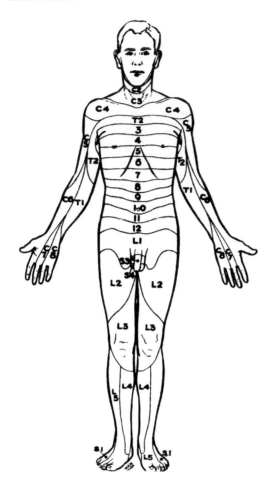

FIG. 1. Dermatomes of the body from the anterior aspect. From, reference 1, with permission.

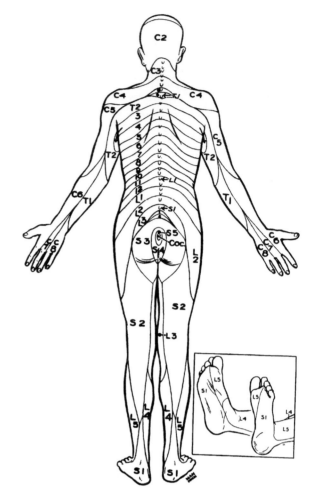

FIG. 2. Dermatomes of the body from the posterior view. From, reference 1, with permission.

CERVICAL PLEXUS

Anatomy

The cervical plexus resembles a series of loops (2) (Figure 8) the motor components of which are arranged in a characteristic pattern that can assist in the localization of a lesion (Figure 9). The descending ramus of the hypoglossal nerve, derived from rootlets of C1, unites with branches of those from C2 and C3 to form the ansa hypoglossi, which innervates strap muscles of the neck below the hyoid, namely the omohyoid, sternohyoid, sternothyroid, geniohyoid, and thyrohyoid muscles. The phrenic nerve forms from the union of motor fibers derived from the APR of the C3 to C5 roots that descend to innervate the diaphragm, while those from C3 and C4 innervate the middle scalene and levator scapular muscles. The cervical plexus is closely related to the accessory nerve, which arises from cells in the lateral part of the anterior horn of the first four cervical segments, and ascends in a common trunk entering the skull through the foramen mag-

num. The nerve joins bulbar rootlets of the vagus nerve and the two together leave the skull through the jugular foramen. Accessory nerve filaments separate from the vagus nerve and form the major motor supply to the sternocleidomastoid muscle and the upper one-third to one-half of the trapezius muscles, however, before innervating these muscles, the nerves receive branches from the APR of the C2 to C4 roots.

The sensory components of the cervical plexus are also characteristic in their distribution to the head and neck. There is no dorsal root or sensory contribution to C1. The lesser and greater occipital nerves arise from the C2 root and provide sensation to the mastoid process, skin of the scalp, and the posterior aspect of the scalp. The greater auricular nerve and the transverse cervical nerve arise from the loops of C2 and C3. These two nerves extend beyond the occipital nerve territory to the skin of the mandible, lower portion of the pinna, and the upper anterior part of the neck to below the ear. The union of C3 and C4 gives rise to the posterior, middle, and anterior supraclavicular nerves, which innervate the skin surface cranial to the clavicle.

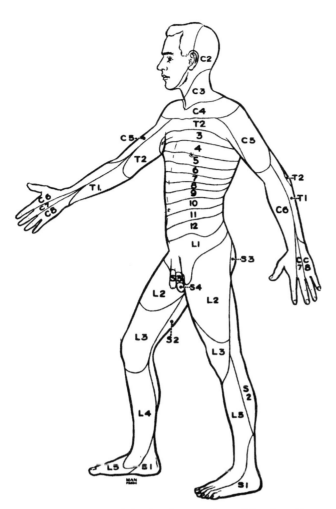

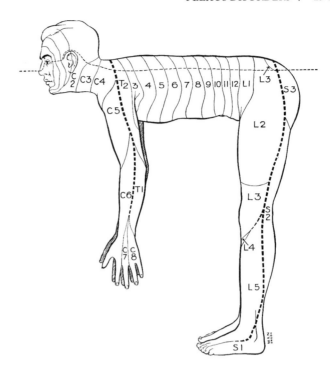

FIG. 5. Alignment of the dermatomes in the quadriped position. From, reference 1, with permission.

FIG. 3. Dermatomes of the body seen in a side view. From, reference 1, with permission.

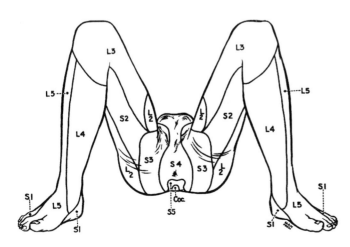

FIG. 4. Dermatomes of the perineum and limbs. From, reference 1, with permission.

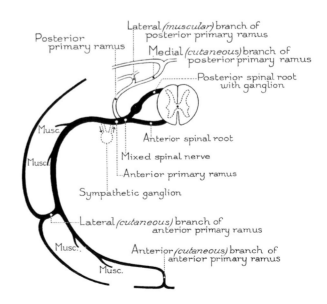

FIG. 6. Composition of a segmental nerve. From, reference 1, with permission.

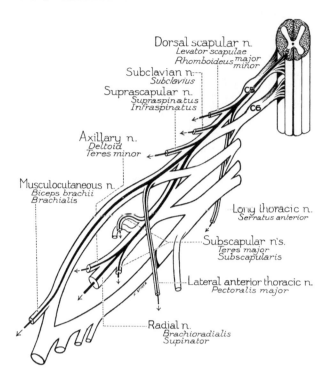

FIG. 7. Myotomal distribution of motor fibers of the fifth cervical segment. From, reference 1, with permission.

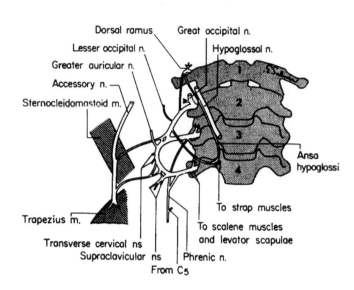

FIG. 8. Diagramatic representation of the cervical plexus. From, reference 1, with permission.

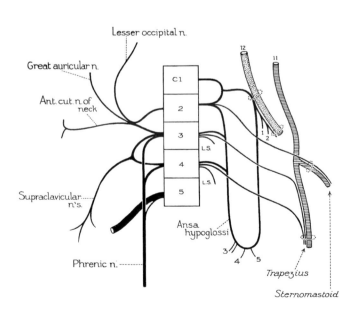

FIG. 9. Anatomical representation of the cervical plexus and its branches. From, reference 1, with permission.

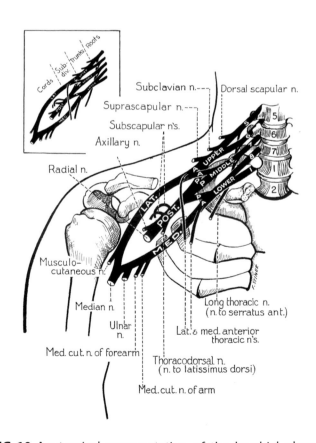

FIG. 10. Anatomical representation of the brachial plexus showing its various components. From, reference 1, with permission.

Lesions

The cervical plexus is most often injured by compression such as by enlarged cervical lymph nodes, the direct effects of local surgery and radiotherapy. The localization of plexus injury can generally be ascertained by combining areas of altered sensation due to one or more of the sensory branches, and by demonstration of weakness and denervation in the distribution of named muscles of the lateral and anterior flexors of the neck as previously described. Weakness and paralysis of the diaphragm caused by injury of the phrenic nerve or the subservient roots may cause few or no symptoms if unilateral, or there may be elevation of the hemidiaphragm and weakness when analyzed by inspiration and expiration chest radiography and fluoroscopy.

BRACHIAL PLEXUS

Anatomy

The brachial plexus is divided into five elements from proximal to distal, including the roots, trunks, divisions, and cords and peripheral nerves (Figure 10). The APR from C5 to T1 combine to form the upper, middle, and lower trunks. The upper trunk is composed of the APR of C5 and C6, and exceptionally the C4 root. The middle trunk is a continuation of the APR of the C7 root. The lower trunk is formed by the combination of the APR of C8, T1, and exceptionally the T2 root. Each trunk divides into an anterior and posterior division. The three posterior divisions combine to form the posterior cord. The anterior divisions of the upper and middle trunk unite to form the lateral cord; and the anterior division of the lower trunk continues as the medial cord. Numerous named motor, sensory and mixed nerves emerge from the plexus to innervate muscle and skin areas.

Lesions

Application of anatomical considerations will assist in localization of many brachial plexus lesions. Lesions along the C4 and C5 roots proximal to the origin of the dorsal scapular nerve lead to weakness of the rhomboid muscle; a branch from C5 also contributes to the phrenic nerve. Branches from the APR of C5 to C7 form the long thoracic nerve, which supplies the serratus anterior muscle. A lesion proximal to the origin of this branch causes scapular winging. Localization of a lesion along the first thoracic root should be suspected with ipsilateral ptosis, elevation of the lower lid, papillary meiosis, and anhidrosis indicative of interruption of preganglionic sympathetic nerve fiber interruption. The localization of brachial plexus lesions along the trunks and cords are best approached by careful consideration of the origin and composition of its major nerve branches. Several branches leave the superior trunk of the plexus, including the suprascapular nerve to the supraspinatus and infraspinatus muscles, which initiate abduction and external rotation of the arm, respectively. Several nerves originate from the anterior divisions of the plexus, including the lateral pectoral nerve from the upper and middle trunks, and the medial pectoral nerve from anterior divisions of the lower trunk, both of which supply the pectoralis major muscle. Before the posterior cord continues into the axilla, four branches emerge, including one each via the subscapular nerve to innervate the subscapularis and teres major muscles, one to the thoracodorsal nerve to the latissimus dorsi muscle, and a fourth to the axillary nerve to innervates the deltoid muscle and a small patch of skin to the lower lateral third of the deltoid. Prior to joining the medial cord to form the median nerve, the lateral cord gives off the musculocutaneous nerve, a mixed nerve that supplies the biceps and brachioradialis muscles and sensory innervation to the lateral forearm via the lateral antebrachial cutaneous nerve. Thus, injury to the lateral cord should be suspected with lesions of both the musculocutaneous nerve and the forearm portion of the median nerve. The medial cord has four branches, including one to the medial brachial cutaneous nerve that carries sensation from the skin of the medial aspect of the upper arm and a second to the medial antebrachial cutaneous nerve that supplies sensation to the medial aspect of the forearm. The medial cord then divides into a third branch comprising the ulnar mixed nerve, and a fourth branch to the median nerve that unites with a branch of the lateral cord to provide motor and sensory innervation to the hand.

Brachial Plexus Neuritis

First described by Spillane (3) and later by Turner and Parsonage (4), and Magee and DeJong (5), there is acute onset of severe aching and boring pain in the neck, shoulder, or upper arm that leads to early maximal weakness and pain with occasional intensification for a day or two that tapers over several weeks. The most frequently affected muscles are the deltoid, supraspinatus, infraspinatus, and biceps. Objective sensory impairment commonly occurs in the cutaneous distribution of the axillary nerve but may extend further along the arm or hand.

The diagnosis of brachial plexopathy, so suggested by pain, weakness, sensory loss, and reflex asymmetry in a given patient, and confirmed by motor and sensory nerve conduction studies (NCS) and needle electromyography (EMG). Compound muscle action potentials (CMAP) and distal motor latencies are recorded using a concentric needle in selected muscles innervated by motor nerve fibers that traverse the trunks, divisions, and nerves of the plexus with overlapping territories, as well as NCS along distal peripheral nerve segments. For example, in suspected C5 radiculopathy or upper trunk plexopathy, electrodiagnostic studies are performed along the musculocutaneous, axillary or suprascapular motor nerves by stimulation at Erb's point, and recording via concentric needle in the biceps brachialis, deltoid, supraspinatus, or infraspinatus muscle following stimulation at Erb's point employing standard techniques (6, 7). The available sensory components of the mixed musculocutaneous nerve and radial nerve, namely the lateral cutaneous nerve of the forearm and the radial sensory nerve, contribute additional information because alteration of their sensory nerve action potential (SNAP) is consistent with a pre-ganglionic and possible plexus nerve fiber injury. Finally, the distribution of active denervation on needle EMG and the pattern of recruitment in weak muscles add the necessary complimentary information to make the diagnosis definite, after which other studies may be warranted to explain the etiopathogenesis.

There may be a history of otherwise innocuous trauma, upper respiratory tract infection, flu illness, neuroborreliosis, obstetrical delivery, recent anesthesia, mononucleosis, hepatitis, immunization, malabsorption syndrome, poliomyelitis, diabetes mellitus, allergy, rheumatoid arthritis, vasculitis, treatment for breast or lung carcinoma, tuberculosis, or drug reaction which will dictate further serological or radiographic testing. Brachial neuralgia should raise suspicion of possible spinal or apical lung tumor, cervical spondylosis, intervertebral disc herniation, intrinsic shoulder disease, and a mass lesion or focal inflammatory process of the plexus prompting further studies, including magnetic resonance imaging (MRI) of the brachial plexus, shoulder, cervical spine and cord, and plain radiographs and computed tomography (CT) of the chest.

The natural history of brachial plexus neuropathy remains excellent overall despite the severity of the lesion, with improvement beginning one to two months in those with less severe involvement, especially as inferred by electrodiagnostic studies, and for up to three years in those with more severe damage (8). Those with pure unifocal or multifocal demyelinative changes and conduction block on electrodiagnostic studies appear to have the best recovery of motor, sensory, and joint function, while those with corresponding axonal damage (9) are likely to develop fixed weakness and wasting, with a more guarded prognosis. Notwithstanding, an aggressive program with oral analgesics and physiotherapy may lessen restriction of joint mobility from tendon shortening leading to adhesive capsulitis.

Hereditary Brachial Plexopathy

There are two autosomal dominant (AD) disorders of recurrent brachial plexus neuropathy. The first is the syndrome of *hereditary neuropathy with liability to pressure palsies* (HNPP), which results from point mutation and deletion at the 17p12 locus of the *PMP22* gene encoding peripheral myelin protein-22, stoichiometric alterations of which determine the phenotype of HNPP (10). Duplications in the *PMP22* gene instead cause Charcot-Marie-Tooth disease type 1 A (CMT1A). The deletion breakpoints in HNPP map to the same intervals in which the CMT1A duplication breakpoints map, such that the rearranged HNPP and CMT1A chromosomes are reciprocal products of an unequal crossover during germ cell meiosis. Attacks of acute demyelinating nerve palsy commence during adolescence and are characterized by numbness, weakness, and atrophy with associated peroneal palsies, carpal tunnel syndrome, brachial plexus neuropathy, and other entrapments, frequently after minor trauma. Motor and sensory nerve conduction velocities (NCV) are mildly reduced in clinically affected nerves as well as in asymptomatic gene carriers. In the Australian family described by Li and colleagues (10), the mean age at onset was 15 years, and all 11 patients reported transient episodes of focal weakness or sensory loss, nine of whom had mild neurological abnormalities in the feet. Electrophysiological studies showed a pattern similar to HNPP resulting from a classic *PMP22* deletion with accentuated slowing at sites subject to nerve compression, while several older members demonstrated length-dependent axonal loss. The expected pathological changes in a cutaneous nerve biopsy include segmental demyelination and tomaculous swellings on teased nerve fiber studies.

Hereditary neuralgic amyotrophy (HNA), which is due to mutation at the 17q25.2-q25.3 locus of the *SEPT9* gene, presents in childhood with acute recurrent episodes of brachial plexus neuropathy preceded by severe pain in the affected arm followed by weakness and atrophy of the brachial region. Laccone and colleagues (11) described dysmorphic features, including hypertelorism, upslanting palpebral fissures, thinned down slanting eyebrows, deep-set eyes, and blepharophimosis in an affected brother and sister with heterozygous mutations in the *SEPT9* gene. Other dysmorphic features include epicanthal folds, cleft palate, syndactyly, small mouth, short and stubby fingers, pectus excavatum, cleft palate, as well as, IgG hypergammaglobulinema, aminoaciduria, long skull bone contour, small orbits, hypoplastic atlas, metacarpal and wrist bone anomalies. Diagnostic guidelines for HNA were elucidated by the European CMT consortium (12) that included pertinent exclusion criteria of absence of pain before or during attacks, signs of a generalized neuropathy, and presence of mutations in the *PMP22* gene, separating it from HNPP. Electrodiagnostic studies reveal axonal involvement with often normal or mildly impaired motor and sensory velocities in the affected limbs. Pathological studies in affected patients demonstrate axonal degeneration and tomaculous changes in nerve biopsies. The prognosis for partial or complete recovery is generally good.

Birth Trauma

Injury during childbirth results in upper, lower, and pan-plexus paralysis. Although first recognized more than 200 years ago, obstetrical paralysis was brought to full attention by Duchenne (13), Erb (14), and Klumpke (15). Classically affected patients have flaccid paralysis of the arm that hangs limp at the side, with elbow extended, forearm pronated, and the arm inwardly rotated after a difficult forceps delivery, or with extreme lateral flexion of the neck, or traction on the shoulders and arms during delivery. Upper arm plexopathy or Erb palsy (14) involves the C5 and C6 roots leading to suprascapular nerve involvement with paralysis of the upper arm sparing the supinators. A less common lower arm paralysis or Klumpke plexopathy (15) results from stretching and over-extension of the plexus in those born by facial presentation, and injury of the lower cords derived from APR of the C7, C8, and T1 roots, the latter of which engenders inequality of the pupils due to injury of sympathetic fibers along the deep cervical ganglionic plexus.

The various forms of obstetrical plexus injury were reviewed by Sever (16) in 1,100 cases. Pathological changes of affected infant plexuses followed stretching and tearing, resulting in hemorrhage and edema of the nerve sheaths, with occasional rupture of the perineural sheath, separation of nerve fibers, and focal scarring. The most severe cases of the upper arm type showed partial or complete division of the fifth and sixth cervical roots, leading to a more permanent form of paralysis and a more extensive area of scar tissue. Postmortem dissection of affected infantile cadavers showed that traction and forcible separation of the head and shoulder place the upper cords and C5 and C6 roots under tension (17). Any sudden force applied to the subject with the head bent to the side and the shoulder held injured the cords. Forcible abduction and elevation of the arm and shoulder places the lower cords of the plexus and the C8 and T1 roots in a stretched position, whereas further force leads to tearing and rupture of these segments.

Affected patients with an upper plexus syndrome demonstrate adduction and medial rotation of the shoulder extension and supination of the elbow, with flexion of the wrist and extension of the fingers, figuratively described as the policeman's tip position. Examination shows weakness of the deltoid, biceps, brachioradialis muscles, and dorsiflexors of the wrist; sensory deficits, often less noticeable, occur along the lateral aspect of the upper arm and radial border, with decreased or absent biceps and brachioradialis tendon reflexes. Weakness of external rotators of the shoulder and forced internal rotation can lead to dislocation of the head of the humerus if the arm is not immobilized in an abducted and externally rotated position. Those with a lower trunk C8 and T1 root syndromes demonstrate weakness and atrophy of intrinsic hand muscles with a claw-hand deformity, altered sensation along the ulnar forearm and medial aspect of the upper arm, in addition to ipsilateral meiosis and ptosis. Sever (16) described upper trunk brachial palsy in about 80% of patients, and lower plexus and total paralysis in the remainder.

Early views of causation included local pressure of poorly applied forceps or the obstetrician's finger applied over the clavicle region. Experimental cadaveric studies by Adson (18) showed that traction on the brachial plexus in stillborn and adults so studied caused lesions near the point of exit of the nerve roots from the intervertebral canal proximal to the trunks of the plexus. The only exception to this rule occurred when a downward and backward force was applied to the arm. In these instances, damage to the cords of the plexus exceeded that of the roots. Injuries varied from slight laceration of the fascia about the root to completely separated roots or avulsion of the roots from the cord. It is important to recognize childbirth plexus injury at an early stage to prevent the development of contractures, which undiagnosed and therefore untreated, can seriously impair subsequent arm function. The tendency to develop contractures results from holding the shoulder in an adducted and internally rotated position. Various reconstructive procedures can be performed in infancy or when the child reaches adult life. One group (19) reported excellent functional results far superior to conservative management in 152 of 357 infants with brachial plexus paralysis following delivery, with 82% reaching strength versus resistance and gravity at three years, in the biceps and 50% recovery in the deltoid muscle after surgical exploration. Adduction contractures can be corrected by subscapularis release, but prevention is the best method of management with early institution of passive movements.

Bullet Injury

Brachial plexus injury due to bullet injury has been described in wartime since the American Civil War but only in the past century with the emergence of modern surgical techniques have these injured been explored surgically. In 1949, Brooks (20) noted that exploration of bullet injuries to the plexus in 54 patients showed division of neural elements in 16, of which 11 could be repaired. It remains wise to explore all cases of possible plexus injury if there is any doubt as to the state of the nerves, especially if there is vascular damage.

Postoperative Plexopathy

Faulty positioning of the arm for surgery is another cause of brachial plexus injury. Ewing (21) studied brachial plexopathy after surgery among several patients and in three cadaveric subjects to directly visualize the brachial plexus and how the nerves lay in different positions of the arm. When the shoulders were placed in abduction and lateral rotation, with the elbow in extension, there was prominence of the humeral head in the axilla around which the nerve trunks of the brachial plexus seemed to be stretched, especially the musculocutaneous nerve closely applied to the subscapularis cushion. With forcible caudal motion of the acromion, the plexus and nerve trunks became as tight as bow strings. Wide abduction of the arm for long periods should be avoided during any operation, and the arm should not be secured in extension. Patients under the influence of alcohol, drugs, and those who have spent hours or days unconscious, lying on an arm, are at similar risk for brachial plexus injury due to direct pressure, but have an equally good prognosis for full spontaneous recovery since there is no disruption of the neural sheath.

Accidental Traction Injury

This form of injury is typified by injury incurred by motorcycles, an arm caught in heavy machinery, and with vigorous sports, when there is forcible separation of the arm and neck from the trunk (22). If the arm is by the side and sharply pulled away from the trunk, the upper roots of the plexus are damaged. When the arm is above the head at the moment of impact, as in climbing accidents, the lower trunks are most at risk. When the injury is severe in a high-speed injury with a high velocity of impact, the natural protective mechanism of the brachial plexus fails and all five roots can be avulsed from the spinal cord. As in motorcycle injury, the cyclist hits an oncoming car, and momentarily his body moves off the vehicle while the arms lay on the handlebars with severe stretch injury of the plexus. The cyclist is then thrown against the oncoming vehicle or onto the road and the lesion is aggravated by the impact of the ground.

Traction injury of the brachial plexus can result in one or more characteristic pathological findings. A traction lesion can occur in continuity in which the axis cylinders are disrupted but the nerve sheath is intact, so-called axonotmesis. There may be rupture of the upper portion of the nerve root where it is secured along the transverse process of the corresponding vertebra with discontinuity of the nerve distal to the intervertebral foramen. Finally, there may be avulsion or tearing of the nerve root from the spinal cord during or after which the corresponding dorsal root ganglia are seen freely in the supraclavicular fossa upon surgical exploration.

Several anatomical considerations impact upon the upper and lower brachial plexus during the course of traction and stretch injury. The upper roots of C5 to C7 are anchored to the transverse processes by strong spiral ligaments that do not exist for the C8 and T1 roots. Therefore, the proximal anchorage point for the upper roots is the transverse process, and for the lower roots it is the spinal cord. Second, the upper roots have a caudal inclination as they emerge, whereas the T1 root is virtually horizontal. Third, the upper roots are about twice as long as the C8 and T1 roots. Other factors help to explain the relative motor disability of most accidental traction injuries. The dorsal roots are less susceptible than the anterior roots because of their relative thickness and the relatively greater stress on the anterior roots during injury. The effects of traction on the dorsal roots are dispersed over synapses in the spinal cord, whereas in the anterior roots, the force is transmitted directly to the nerve bodies. This explains the somewhat puzzling feature of total motor paralysis of all five roots of the brachial plexus with sparing of a considerable degree of sensation.

Investigation and Management of Traumatic Brachial Plexopathy

The investigation and management of brachial plexus injury has evolved over the past century with improved diagnostic and surgical techniques and rehabilitation. Neuroimaging employing MRI of the cervical spine and brachial plexus has replaced CT and myelography to evaluate the integrity of the cervical roots and proximal components of the plexus for stretch injury, root rupture, and avulsion. Root avulsion, the most serious, leads to meningocele, obliteration of the root pouch, exaggeration of the size of the root pouch, diminution in the size or absence of the root shadow, and cystic accumulation of cerebrospinal fluid (CSF) in the spinal canal. Surgical laminectomy of traumatic meningocele does not always confirm true root avulsion; conversely, unsuspected roots avulsed at high or lower levels may not be seen radiographically. Dorsal root avulsion spares the ventral root, leading to disturbed sensation with intact motor function. The major practical point of electrodiagnostic studies employing nerve NCS and concentric needle EMG is to assess the site of the nerve injury as pre- or postganglionic. A normal sensory nerve response in the anesthetic area indicative of continuity of the axon as high up as the level of the dorsal root ganglia (23). If the damage to the plexus is preganglionic, there is less prospect for spontaneous recovery or with surgery, whereas a postganglionic lesion with rupture of the root is generally accessible to nerve repair. Sensory evoked potential analysis allows further investigation of the plexus and roots by the demonstration of localized near-field N9 potential when recording averaged responses from mixed nerve sensory stimulation and recording at Erb point near the trunks, along the proximal roots, and at the cervical enlargement. If the clinical and electrophysiological feature of a given patient who has sustained injury suggests a repairable lesion, and the vascular supply to the limb is adequate, then surgical exploration may be advised.

Fifty years ago, only 10% of cases of presumed avulsion were reparable when surgically explored (20). Decades later, Narakas (24) showed that up to one-third of patients with severe traction injury have repairable lesions, including those due to rupture of the upper trunks distal to the intervertebral foramen treated by insertion of suitable grafts, usually from the sural nerve, or in the case of avulsion of the lower trunks, by the ulnar nerve. The correct time to operate is as soon after injury as possible because it enables as correct a diagnosis of the extent and type of plexus injury as possible, and establishes a clear prognosis, as for example in the cases of discovering that all five roots of the plexus are avulsed, as compared with rupture of the upper roots, which can then be grafted, or if the trunks are noted to be stretched without discontinuity, warranting a singularly good prognosis without surgical manipulation. Individuals who should not be considered for surgical exploration because of other serious injuries will come to evaluation some months afterward. Reconstructive surgery has been used to provide active muscle function to a weak limb. These include various procedures to move the origin of flexors and extensors of the forearm further proximally along the humerus and procedures to transfer the latissimus dorsi or triceps muscle with its own innervation to the biceps to facilitate elbow flexion. Management of pain is an important element in the recovery of plexus injury that generally requires the input of a pain management specialist for the prescription of oral, parenteral, and dermal patches of medications, and transcutaneous stimulation procedures when necessary.

Cancer-Related Plexopathy

Between 1924 and 1940, Pancoast (25, 26), and later Moersch and colleagues (27), established the entity of lower arm plexopathy in association with posterior shoulder, axillary, and upper arm, and medial lower arm pain, ulnar intrinsic muscle wasting, Horner syndrome, and variable destruction of the upper ribs and vertebra due to a superior pulmonary sulcus or apical tumor. Pancoast (24–26) postulated a location of the tumor in the region of the common trunk at the convergence of the anterior and posterior roots of the eighth cervical and first thoracic vertebra before the emergence of the sympathetic ganglia, to account for the neurological presentation and the frequent association with epidural spread of the tumor along the transverse processes and into the intervertebral foramen. Thomas (28), Kori

(29), Stoll (30), and Match and coworkers (31) studied the clinical characteristics of brachial plexopathy caused by either tumor infiltration or local radiation. It has become clear that a clinical definition of cancerous involvement of the plexus requires strict criteria, including surgical exploration and documentation of locally invasive or metastatic extension to the plexus, or new distant metastases, especially to the adjacent lung, clavicle, or vertebral bodies. The clinical definition of radiation injury to the plexus suffices if surgical exploration fails to reveal tumor, and if follow-up for several years does not reveal tumor recurrence. The commonest primary tumors of the brachial plexus are lung and breast, followed by schwannoma and lymphoma.

Severe and persistent pain is the most common presenting symptom of cancerous involvement, present in almost 90% of proven cases, compared with 20% of those with radiation injury. Although metastases elsewhere in the body suggest a concurrent plexus lesion, lack thereof does not rule out tumor infiltration of the plexus. A plexus lesion may rarely be the singular evidence of tumor. Epidural deposits of metastatic tumor are found in two-thirds of patients so studied, suggesting a high frequency of epidural extension and this should be considered in the presence of severe plexus pain (32). Neuroimaging for epidural metastasis is indicated when there is metastatic plexopathy, because there is a higher frequency of epidural cord compression which when treated early, yields better results and allows delineation of appropriate radiation ports (33, 34). The higher frequency of lower plexopathy in cancerous plexopathy is explained by the more frequent proximity of metastatic axillary lymph nodes to the divisions of the lower trunk of the plexus, unlike the upper trunk and its divisions that remain essentially free of lymph nodes and are instead involved predominantly in radiation plexopathy.

Radiotherapy for cancer leads instead to dose-related damage to connective tissues and blood supply of the nerve rather than the axon or myelin tissue, with low dose of <4,000 rads posing the least risk, and moderate doses of 4,000 to 5,000 rads, and severe doses of >5,000 rads, leading to higher rates of complication. A short source-to-skin distance, especially less than 80 cm, produce steep dose gradients in the body and a higher dose anterior or posterior to the midplane and complex field arrangements with multiple abutting portals that increase the opportunity for overlap and a resulting unsuspected high-dose region. The reported incidence of radiation plexopathy at moderate to high-radiation doses varied between 15 and 75% in a European study (30) and 1% in a subsequent American study (28).

Practically, the diagnosis of radiation-induced plexopathy and locally invasive, metastatic, or continuously spreading neoplasm is difficult, if not impossible, without surgical exploration. Local skin changes, arm edema, shoulder stiffness, pneumonitis, and mediastinitus precede delayed onset of painless paresthesia, weakness, and reflex changes after irradiation, with a severity related to the dosage level. Cancerous plexopathy, on the other hand, is usually extremely painful. Both radiation and cancerous plexopathy can follow a progressive downhill course; however, those with radiation plexopathy have overall good prognosis and do not succumb to the underlying neoplasm. There is limited available information on the pathological alterations in radiation-induced plexopathy; however, postmortem analysis of two patients showed marked fibrosis of the nerves of the plexus with demyelination (30).

Thoracic Outlet Syndrome

Although, strictly speaking, the anatomic thoracic outlet refers to the inferior aspect of the thoracic cage covered by the diaphragm, it has become synonymous instead with the thoracic inlet of the upper thoracic cage, wherein the brachial plexus, subclavian artery, and subclavian vein traverse, in sequential order, the interscalene triangle delimited by the anterior and middle scalene muscles and first rib, the costoclavicular space between the first thoracic rib and the clavicle, and the subcoracoid or subpectoral space beneath the pectoralis minor tendon (35) (Figures 11, 12). The first rib can be divided further into three portions. The first segment extends from the head of the rib to its neck. The second portion contains attachments for the middle scalene, serratus anterior, and muscles of the first intercostal space. The third part contains the scalene tubercle and serves as a site of attachment for the anterior scalene and subclavian muscle, and costoclavicular ligaments (36). Both the subclavian vein, which is located anterior to the anterior scalene muscle, and the subclavian artery, which lies between the anterior and middle scalene muscles, are situated anteriorly, in proximity to the lower trunk of the brachial plexus.

Neurovascular compression can occur in one of the three aforementioned predisposed anatomic areas (37). Muscles of the interscalene space or triangle, delineated anteriorly by the anterior scalene muscle, posteriorly by the middle scalene muscle, and inferiorly by the first rib function to raise the first rib during respiration, and bend and rotate the neck, with overlapping or intermingling insertions on the first rib leading to a narrow V- or U-shaped space that the brachial plexus and subclavian artery traverse wherein compression occurs. A cervical rib, varying from a small bony exostosis to a full-grown rib with ligamentous, cartilaginous, and bony attachment to the first rib contributes to interscalene compression.

A second site of compression occurs in the costoclavicular space. This triangular area is bordered anteriorly by the medial portion of the clavicle and underlying subclavian muscles, its tendon, and costocoracoid ligament; posteromedially by the first rib and the insertion of both the anterior and middle scalene muscles; and posterolaterally by the upper border of

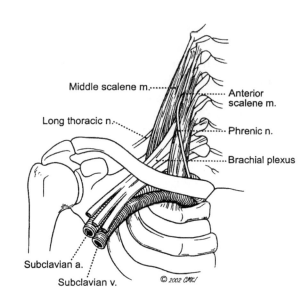

FIG. 11. Anatomic representation of the thoracic outlet. From, reference 35, with permission.

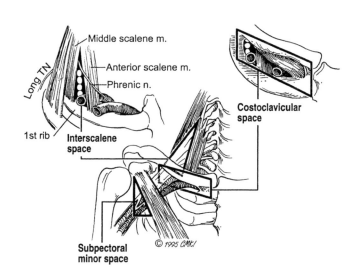

FIG. 12. Anatomic representation of thoracic outlet areas prone to entrapment. From, reference 35, with permission.

the scapula. Compression in this space occurs as a result of acquired changes to the first rib and clavicle due to trauma, structural changes in the subclavian muscle and tendon, or the costocoracoid ligament; a horizontally situated first rib and straight clavicle with lack of anterior curvature so minimizing the space the plexus traverses. Patients with droopy, sagging shoulders caused by poor posture or disabling illness are prone to narrowing of the costoclavicular space. Individuals with this nature of compression have exacerbation of symptoms with traction of the arm downward and relief thereof by movements of the opposite direction.

A third site of thoracic outlet compression occurs in the subpectoralis space, just below the pectoralis muscle and its insertion upon the coracoid process. Clinical symptoms occur upon hyperabduction with backward and upward motion of the clavicle leading to primarily compression of neurovascular structures under taut pectoralis muscle. A hyperabduction syndrome is observed in short muscular men whose jobs require them to keep their hands and arms above the shoulders and head, with incipient weakness, numbness, and tingling.

Ferrante (36) divided thoracic outlet syndrome (TOS) into five categories depending upon the primary source of brachial plexus compression. The first two, venous-, and arterial-vascular TOS attribute neurological sequela to primary vascular involvement. Venous-vascular TOS begins with a scarred segment of vessel near the origin of the subclavian vein in an area of anomalous compression variably between the first rib and a hypertrophic scalene or subclavius tendon, the two tendons themselves, along the clavicle and a cervical rib, or a congenital web. This progresses to complete venous thrombosis with secondary neurological and plexus involvement.

Arterial-vascular TOS, is characterized instead by an anatomic obstruction to blood flow along the subclavian artery variably between the anterior scalene muscle and a large bony anomaly, a fully formed cervical rib, protuberant supernumerary bony process, or deformed first thoracic rib, leading to intimal arterial damage, poststenotic dilatation, turbulent blood flow, aneurysm and even thrombus formation, with secondary neurological and plexus involvement.

The third type is traumatic neurovascular TOS typically associated with clavicular trauma, most commonly a remote mid-shaft fracture, leading to both secondary neurological and vascular sequel. A fourth category, termed nonspecific TOS, results from traction and compression of the brachial plexus resulting from an inherited congenital anomaly, trauma, or abnormal posture or body habitus.

Tandem compression of neurovascular structures leads to a variety of symptoms, including neck, shoulder and arm pain, numbness, tingling, weakness, and vasomotor changes, the intensity of which depends upon the severity and duration of compression, compression of nerve fibers, particularly along the lower trunk and medial cord of the brachial plexus. The latter leads to visible atrophy and weakness of muscles of the thenar and hypothenar eminence, with numbness and tingling along the ulnar forearm to the last digit and medial palm. One provocative maneuver, the scalene test, considered to be of diagnostic value in the section of patients for surgical release of the insertion of the anterior scalene muscle (38), later gained importance in the selection of patients for more complicated surgical procedures (39), and in the initial diagnosis of TOS, nonetheless without prospective confirmation. It is performed by palpation of the radial pulse while the

patients inspires while maintaining the symptomatic extremity at the side, neck hyperextended, and the head rotated toward the symptomatic side.

The fifth category, true neurogenic TOS, occurs in association with taut fibrous bands originating from the body of the T1 vertebra, the tip of the transverse process of C7, cervical rib, and the neck of the first rib, leading to focal compression of nerve fibers composing the T1 APR, which tend to be angulated and stretched more than those composing the C8 APR. Affected patients present with accentuated involvement of thenar eminence muscles, hand weakness and wasting, and a lesser degree of sensory function that is more apparent along the medial forearm compared to the hand, with a combination of intermittent aching and paresthesia of the medial arm and forearm. The evaluation of suspected patients includes imaging studies to identify responsible taut bands and the bony anomalies from which they originate. CT and MRI offer no advantage over plain films of the cervical spine and thoracic cage in identifying bony anomalies and bilateral cervical ribs, the smaller of which is usually on the symptomatic side. Magnetic resonance angiography (MRA) and venography (MRV), and selective venous and arterial catheterization utilizing intravenous dye may be indicated in selected patients considered for surgical intervention.

Electrodiagnostic studies are important in examining the degree of neurogenic involvement to localize the site of the lesion and to exclude other syndromes that can give rise to pain and weakness of small hand muscles. Smith and Trojaborg (40) studied ten patients with unilateral wasting of hand muscles and sensory symptoms who were diagnosed as TOS and operated on for it. The SNAP recorded from digit 5 was reduced in amplitude in eight patients and those from digit 3 in three patients. Sensory and motor NCV were normal in all ten patients. Quantitative EMG studies of ulnar and median innervated small hand muscles showed chronic partial denervation. The combination of chronic partial denervation of small hand muscles, decreased SNAP amplitude from digit 5 and sometimes from digit 3, and normal motor and sensory NCV, was compatible with compression of the C-8 and T-1 roots or the lower trunk of the brachial plexus. Radiographic studies disclosed bony abnormalities in all patients, nine of whom had rudimentary cervical ribs, bilaterally in four and an enlarged C-7 transverse process in one patient. All patients underwent surgical exploration by a supraclavicular approach.

Whereas some authors suggested that NCS across the thoracic outlet region in the area of supposed compression would be the best objective test of nerve impingement (41, 42), this has not turned out to be the case for three reasons. First, the normal range for median and ulnar NCV across this area may vary according to different authors and in the different limb position, from 52 to 88 m/s (40, 43). Second, comparisons between left and right sides does not solve the problem as the differences between the two arms in the same subject can be as much as 11 m/s, twice as much as encountered for the elbow-to-wrist segment (40, 44). Third, the reliability of motor NCS across the thoracic outlet can be questioned, as has empiric surgical decompression thereof. Urshell and Razzuk (39) asserted the reliability of motor NCV along proximal and distal segments of the ulnar nerve according to the technique described by Caldwell and colleagues (41) employing supramaximal stimulation at the supraclavicular fossa, mid-upper arm, below the elbow and the wrist in the diagnosis of TOS, and the selection of patients for surgical resection of the first rib. In a cohort of preoperative patients so studied, the average motor NCV was 53 m/s across the outlet with a range of 32 to 65 m/s, compared to controls with a respective average ulnar motor NCV of 72 m/s and range of 68 to 75 of 68, and those postoperatively, respectively, with a mean of 70 m/s, and range of 58 to 85 m/s (39). Wilbourne and Lederman (45) questioned the reliability and objectivity of this technique and its usefulness in the selection of surgical patients more than a decade later, asserting that the slowing, demonstrated in a polaroid-constructed image labeled Figure 2B of stacked tracings of ulnar motor NCS (39). The portrayed slowing across the thoracic outlet in a patient with TOS, specifically the supraclavicular fossa/fourth response, seemed markedly delayed as compared with the mid-upper arm/third response, "appearing to be nothing more than a repeat of the mid-upper-arm tracing recorded at twice the sweep speed used for all the other tracings shown" (45) and thus artifactual. The uncontested response from Urschel (45) included a paraphrase from Dr. Caldwell, who indicated that the figure in question, performed on modified electrodiagnostic equipment in which a given sweep tracing was difficult to mark, had been altered during stimulation at the supraclavicular fossa and so constructed for illustrative purposes.

Surgical treatment for TOS performed at the turn of the nineteenth century, which included cervical rib dissection followed by scalenectomy and later claviculectomy, were often disfiguring. In the past several decades, first rib resection using posterior, supraclavicular, infraclavicular, and transaxillary approaches have been reintroduced. Scalenectomy has been refined to treat recurrent thoracic outlet compression following first rib resection, and those after injury of the neck and shoulder region. Patients carefully chosen after detailed clinical, radiographic, and electrodiagnostic evaluation may benefit from a combined approach that utilizes a transaxillary first rib resection followed immediately by a transcervical and medial scalenectomy, to achieve total decompression of the thoracic outlet. Uniform improvement of vascular compression symptoms in those with primary vascular compromise is contrasted to those with predominant nerve compression, in whom two surgical outcome groups with differing rates of improvement were described

(39). Those with classical manifestations of ulnar neuralgia-like symptoms, loss or diminution of the radial pulse elicited by the Adson test, and reduced ulnar motor NCV to 53 m/s, showed improvement in 95% of patients so studied, whereas those with atypically distributed pain, without pulse changes by compression tests, and in whom the average ulnar motor NCV was only reduced to 60 m/s, showed variable responses to surgery, experiencing both poor and fair, as well as improved status. It is therefore evident that unnecessary surgical exploration of patients with uncertain evidence of TOS, with removal of the first rib, are at risk of uncertain benefit from surgery and even unfortunate side effects, including brachial plexopathy (46, 47).

LUMBOSACRAL PLEXUS

Anatomy

The anatomy of the lumbar and sacral plexus has been recognized for over a century (48–50) (Figures 13, 14). Two anatomical structures are important in understanding the relationship of the lumbosacral plexus to the pelvis. The first is the linea terminalis that divides the pelvis major and minor. The second are the major and minor pelvis outlets. The major pelvic outlets include the inguinal canal, lacuna musculorum and vasculorum, and the superior aperture of the minor pelvis. The minor pelvic outlets include the obturator canal, and the supra- and infrapiriform foramina. The main nerves that arise from the lumbosacral plexus include the iliohypogastric, ilioinguinal, genitofemoral, lateral femoral cutaneous sensory nerves, and the mixed motor and sensory pudendal, femoral, obturator, and sciatic nerves. Ventral APR of the lumbar plexus from T12 to L5 remain cephalad to the terminal linea except for the lumbosacral trunk, composed of L4 to L5 roots, that enter the minor pelvis through its superior aperture and contribute to the sacral plexus and the obturator nerve, composed of APR of L2 to L4 segments, passes through the obturator canal to the anterior femoral region. The nerve to the iliopsoas muscle, in which the lumbar plexus is embedded, and the nerves to the thoracic and ventrolateral abdominal wall muscles exit the pelvis through the lacuna musculorum and vasorum to the anterior femoral region. The nerves to the cremaster muscle and skin of the inguinal and pudendal region traverse the inguinal canal. The nerves of the sacral plexus, composed of APR of L4 to S4, and the parasympathetic pelvic splanchnic nerves, inclusive of the S2 to S4 rami, reside in the minor pelvis caudal to the terminal linea. The nerves to the floor of the pelvic cavity and structures related to the external genitals, and the internal obturator muscle exit via the infrapiriform foramen to re-enter the pelvis via the ischiorectal fossa and Alcock pudendal canal. The superior

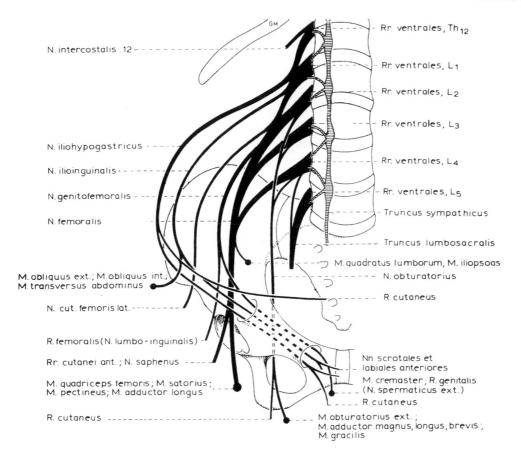

N. intercostalis 12
N. iliohypogastricus
N. ilioinguinalis
N.genitofemoralis
N. femoralis
M. obliquus ext.; M.obliquus int.;
M. transversus abdominus
N. cut. femoris lat.
R. femoralis (N. lumbo-inguinalis)
Rr. cutanei ant.; N. saphenus
M. quadriceps femoris; M. satorius;
M. pectineus; M. adductor longus
R. cutaneus

Rr. ventrales, Th₁₂
Rr. ventrales, L₁
Rr. ventrales, L₂
Rr. ventrales, L₃
Rr. ventrales, L₄
Rr. ventrales, L₅
Truncus sympathicus
Truncus lumbosacralis
M.quadratus lumborum, M.iliopsoas
N. obturatorius
R.cutaneus
Nn. scrotales et labiales anteriores
M. cremaster; R. genitalis (N. spermaticus ext.)
R. cutaneus
M.obturatorius ext.; M. adductor magnus, longus, brevis; M. gracilis

FIG. 13. Anatomic representation of the lumbar plexus. From, reference 48, with permission.

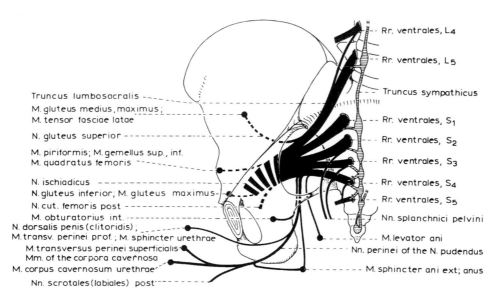

Truncus lumbosacralis
M. gluteus medius, maximus; M. tensor fasciae latae
N. gluteus superior
M. piriformis; M. gemellus sup., inf. M. quadratus femoris
N. ischiadicus
N. gluteus inferior; M. gluteus maximus
N. cut. femoris post
M. obturatorius int.
N. dorsalis penis (clitoridis);
M. transv. perinei prof.; M. sphincter urethrae
M. transversus perinei superficialis
Mm. of the corpora cavernosa
M. corpus cavernosum urethrae
Nn. scrotales (labiales) post

Rr. ventrales, L₄
Rr. ventrales, L₅
Truncus sympathicus
Rr. ventrales, S₁
Rr. ventrales, S₂
Rr. ventrales, S₃
Rr. ventrales, S₄
Rr. ventrales, S₅
Nn. splanchnici pelvini
M. levator ani
Nn. perinei of the N. pudendus
M. sphincter ani ext; anus

FIG. 14. Anatomic representation of the sacral plexus. From, reference 48, with permission.

gluteal nerve, composed of L4 to S1, exits the suprapiriform foramen for the gluteal region. The other major portions of the sacral plexus, composed of L4 to S2 segments, pass through the infrapiriform foramen to the gluteal, posterior femoral, and crural regions to the leg. The plexus is supplied by five lumbar arteries, which originate from the abdominal aorta: the deep circumflex iliac artery, which is a branch of the external iliac artery; and the iliolumbar and gluteal branches of the internal iliac artery (51). Although there is a rich anastomotic blood supply, the middle and distal intrapelvic portions are nonetheless prone to ischemia.

Lesions

The etiopathogenesis of lumbosacral plexopathy includes acquired disorders such as lumbosacral plexus neuritis, parainfectious, and diabetic-associated forms; genetic plexopathy syndromes; plexus injury due to local intragluteal injections, drug abuse, pelvic trauma, and surgery; compression during delivery, by expanding aortic aneurysms, hematomas, and other mass lesions; cancerous disorders due to locally invasive tumor and metastases, and the secondary effects of radiation and chemotherapy.

Idiopathic Lumbosacral Plexopathy

Painful lumbosacral plexus neuritis or plexopathy was first recognized by both Sanders (52) and Evans and coworkers (53) as a distinct entity analogous to brachial plexus neuritis. Acute onset of pain in one or both legs is followed by weakness, loss of stretch reflexes, and variable atrophy of affected muscles, along individual nerves or parts of the plexus, as demonstrated clinically and by electrodiagnostic studies with generally normal spinal imaging, serum studies, and cerebrospinal fluid, and improved without specific treatment usually within a month (54, 55). The laboratory evaluation of a suspected patient with lumbosacral plexopathy should be directed first toward confirming the diagnosis, and then to uncovering the most likely etiopathogenesis. Electrodiagnostic studies, including motor and sensory NCS and concentric needle EMG, localizes the disorder to the lumbar plexus or in its constituent nerves in symptomatic cases, regardless of the duration of illness. Typical findings include asymmetrically reduced SNAP and CMAP amplitudes and NCV that reflect the number of functioning axons, variably prolonged F responses, and patchy active and chronic denervation potentials sparing paraspinal muscles, with neurogenic recruitment pattern of high amplitude MUP upon maximal voluntary effect reflective of the degree of limb weakness. Contrast abdomen and pelvis CT and MRI should be performed in all patients, especially those with seemingly innocuous trauma and suspected cases of possible retropelvic tumor, hematoma,

aneurysm, or abscess. Neuroimaging of the lumbar plexus employing MRI and, when necessary, CT-myelographic imaging of the lumbar spine, can be performed to discern infiltrative disease of the plexus, incidental and contributory spine disease. Serum should be sent as deemed appropriate for connective tissue studies, Lyme neuroborreliosis, viral serologies, parasitic mycobacterial studies, and other postulated source of infection; as well as HgA1c and fasting glucose levels for diabetes mellitus, and molecular genetic studies for HNPP. Lumbar puncture for CSF analysis may provide useful information in the setting of infectious, inflammatory, and known carcinomatous disease.

Infection

One of the four patients reported by Sanders (52) had preceding immunization, and one each of the patients reported by Sanders (52) and Evans (53) had preceding upper respiratory infections before onset of lumbosacral plexopathy. Typical painful lumbosacral plexus neuritis has been reported in association with *Borrelia burgdorferi* infection (56–58), Epstein Barr virus infection (59), and pulmonary tuberculosis (60). Peripheral nerve biopsy in the patient with Lyme neuroborreliosos and lumbar plexopathy (56) showed infiltration by CD8 T cells with activation of C5b-9 membrane attack complex (MAC) and improved with a second course of intravenous antibiotics for persistent *Borrelia burgdorferi* infection. Psoas muscle abscess can also lead to lumbosacral plexopathy due to contiguous infection resulting in increased pressure under the muscle aponeurosis, with concomitant compression.

Diabetic Lumbosacral Radiculoplexus Neuropathy

There is a spectrum of diabetic-related neurological disorders with primary or overlapping clinicopathologic involvement of the lumbosacral plexus (61–75). Diabetic lumbrosacral radiculoplex neuropathy (DLSRPN) commences with painful asymmetrical radicular involvement of the legs and progresses to bilateral acute, subacute, or chronic weakness, muscular atrophy, and sensory loss, disturbing gait and balance. Initial electrophysiological studies are generally consistent with multiple mononeuropathy, although later findings lead to difficulty in differentiation from lumbosacral plexopathy. Femoral intermedius, superficial peroneal sensory, and sural nerve biopsy specimens frequently reveal lymphocytic inflammatory cell infiltration around (perivasculitis) or in the wall (microvasculitis) of epineurial blood vessels. Detailed morphological studies in addition may show multifocal axon degeneration and loss, segmental demyelination, perineurial degeneration and scarring, neovascularization, fragmentation of vascular smooth muscle, microscopic hemorrhages with hemosiderin deposition, and activation of C5b-9 MAC, indicative of an ischemic autoimmune neuropathy. There is typically no evidence of true vasculitis. Further, it is distinctly rare for either diabetic neuropathy or lumbosacral plexopathy to accompany true vasculitis. Occasional spontaneous improvement occurs often with residual disability. However, treatment with intravenous gammaglobulin has led to dramatic recovery in many patients anecdotally studied. Dyck and colleagues (76, 77) noted equally significant improvement in primary outcome measures of 49 patients with DLSRPN randomized to 1 gram three times weekly of intravenous methylprednisolone for 12 weeks, compared to 26 patients with DLSRPN who received placebo when analyzed at 52 weeks (77) and 104 weeks (76). However, the methylprednisolone treated patients reported a greater degree of symptom improvement as judged by changes in a neuropathy symptom change subscore for pain. A randomized, double-blind, placebo-controlled trial of IVG on recovery time of patients with proximal diabetic neuropathy and EMG evidence of proximal lower limb plexus or radicular denervation that commenced in 1999 (78) is no longer recruiting patients and has yet to publish its findings. More recently, Younger (79) described the clinicopathologic aspects of DLSRPN in a postmortem studied patient.

Relapsing Lumbosacral Plexopathy

Two adolescents were described by Awerbuch and colleagues (80) with relapsing lumbosacral plexus neuropathy. A girl, age 16, developed severe lancinating pain radiating into the left thigh followed by weakness of the leg, diminished femoral sensory nerve sensation, and focal reflex asymmetry of the left patellar reflex. Needle EMG showed active denervation in muscle supplied by the femoral nerve sparing lumbosacral paraspinal muscles, with normal motor and sensory NCS. She improved in three months, with recurrence three years later in a similar distribution, and six years later only in pain without disturbance of strength. A 17-year-old girl developed similar lancinating pain in the left anterior thigh and leg, followed by weakness, with diminished peripheral femoral nerve sensory loss and patellar reflex asymmetry. There was acute denervation in femoral-innervated thigh muscles sparing lumbosacral paraspinal muscles, with normal motor and sensory NCS. She improved in three months, with recurrence six years later. A 59-year-old man with recurrent idiopathic lumbosacral plexopathy reported by Yee (81) developed sudden onset of burning pain, numbness, and tingling sensation in the low back with radiation down the anterior right leg, followed by weakness, with emphasis of weakness in the thigh compared to the lower leg, diminished sensation over the anteromedial part of the right calf, and absent patellar reflex. Needle EMG showed active denervation in femoral-innervated muscles, sparing lumbosacral

paraspinal muscles, and normal motor and sensory NCS. He improved over three months but symptoms recurred three years later in a similar pattern in the other leg. The cause of relapsing lumbosacral plexopathy is not well understood. Few if any patients with HNPP or HNA present with pure syndrome of relapsing lumbosacral plexopathy. Nerve biopsy tissue was not obtained to examine for tomaculous swellings, and in one patient so studied, there was no molecular genetic evidence of HNPP (81).

Direct Injury

The lumbosacral plexus, which is located deep in the pelvis along the posterior abdominal wall, lies close to bony and soft tissues, and other organs, making it susceptible to local injury. The constituent nerves are susceptible to compression especially as they exit the bony pelvis as, for example, in pregnancy, following expansion of an aortic aneurysm, retroperitoneal hematoma, and other mass lesions. The bony ridge of the linea terminalis crossed by the lumbosacral trunks and the obturator nerve, and the edge of the major ischiatic incisure crossed by the superior gluteal nerve, are common sites of compression. The proximity of the nerves leaving the infrapiriform foramen, such as the sciatic nerve, makes them prone to injury as, for example, with local intragluteal injections.

Pregnancy

Maternal obstetrical lumbar plexopathy results from trauma of the lumbosacral trunk by the fetal head or instruments. The patients reported by Cole (82) had radiographic features of a shortened posterior ilium and a flattened sacral promotorium, as well as shallow anterior cavities of the sacral alae. All of the patients so studied exhibited primipara, prolonged and difficult forceps delivery, and disproportion of the fetal head and maternal pelvis. In mild cases, pain and paresthesia are the only complaint, with palsy occurring during or after delivery. Motor and sensory deficits result from increased pressure leading to trauma of the lumbosacral pelvis or the proximal portion of the sciatic nerve. This leads to palsy of foot and toe dorsiflexors, and occasionally the hamstrings and gluteal muscles, with diminished or absent ankle reflex, and sensory disturbance along the fifth lumbar dermatome, but that may vary. Pain can persist for weeks or months, but typically subsides days after delivery.

Intragluteal Injection

Lumbosacral plexopathy rarely, if ever, results from direct needle injury. More likely, lumbosacral plexopathy in such instances results from the inadvertent injection of angiotoxic medication into the inferior gluteal, ipsilateral iliac, or aortic bifurcation vessels, which lead to thrombosis and arteritis of the internal and external iliac artery, and ischemic neuropathy (83). Intragluteal injection, which can promote vascular spasm, occurs with crystalline medication and microembolism with partial or complete segmental arterial stenosis and necrosis. Affected patients note severe pain and swelling at the site of intragluteal injection that extends into the upper leg, followed by numbness and paralysis within a few hours, bluish discoloration of the skin, and impaired circulation in the leg. An analogous disorder in newborns results from injection of vasotoxic medication into the umbilical artery, a branch of the internal iliac, with resultant gangrene of the buttock and sciatic nerve palsy. Vascular thrombosis of the inferior gluteal artery in adults after intragluteal injection most often leads to sciatic nerve involvement, whereas thrombosis that extends into the iliac arteries leads to lumbar and sacral plexus injury. The restriction of intragluteal injections to the upper outer part of the buttock, and aspiration of the syringe before injecting any substance reduces the risk of this disorder.

Abdominal Aortic Aneurysm

Lumbosacral plexopathy due to expansion of an abdominal aortic aneurysm (84–86) should be considered in instances of sciatic or femoral pain. Pain is the initial manifestation of an aneurysm prior to rupture, often located in the back, legs, and in the distribution of cutaneous nerves emanating from the lumbar plexus, often associated with a pulsatile mass. It should be contemplated in instances of sciatica or femoral pain, often with only part of the plexus, but in case of rupture, the entire plexus may be involved due to a combination of compression and retroperitoneal hemorrhage. The aneurysm usually originates from the abdominal aorta, common and internal iliac arteries, or their branching vessels. Compression of the iliohypogastric and ilioinguinal nerves lead to referred pain in the lower abdomen and inguinal area. Pressure on the genitofemoral nerve produces pain in the inguinal area, testicle, and anterior thigh. Involvement of the L5 to S2 nerve trunks that lie directly posterior to the hypogastric artery may also give rise to sciatica. Most aneurysms compressing the lumbar and sacral plexus are false or pseudo-aneurysms originating from the aorta or iliac arteries due to rupture of an atherosclerotic true aneurysm, whereas those originating from the gluteal vessels are most often post-traumatic. The diagnosis of aneurysm is most often missed and only shown at autopsy in up to one-half of those who die from bleeding. Palpation and auscultation of the upper and lower abdomen and the gluteal region, followed by CT or MRI, should be performed in those with a spinal origin of radiating pain to exclude an expanding aneurysm. Surgery is the best option for survival and to partially or completely alleviate the neurological syndrome.

Trauma

Lumbosacral plexopathy is associated with fracture of the sacrum, sacroiliac joint, femur, and acetabulum. The reported frequency varies from less than 1% (87) to 46% (88) in clinical series, and 48% in postmortem analysis of accident victims (89). This discrepancy is difficult to explain, however several factors may be contributory. First, there have been only a small number of clinically and electrodiagnostically studied cases compared to the large number of trauma cases, which translates into a low calculated incidence. Kutsy (87) diagnosed 22 patients with lumbosacral plexopathy during a five-and-one-half-year period among 3,000 patients with pelvic trauma, for an expected frequency of 0.7%. Second, the unexpected low incidence of lumbosacral plexopathy may be influenced by the inherent difficulty in performing an adequate clinical neurological study at a time when stabilization of bodily trauma is of primary importance. Those with undiagnosed lumbosacral plexopathy may not come to attention until the nerve deficits become evident weeks after severe trauma when physiotherapy and ambulation are attempted. Third, some patients and physicians may delay or resist the performance of detailed electrophysiological studies, especially when the deficit is improving. This may lead to erroneous assumptions as to causation and prognosis as, for example, in those with post-traumatic superior gluteal, obturator, and femoral neuropathies that are incorrectly ascribed to compressive mononeuropathy simplex or multiplex rather than to lesions of the lumbosacral plexus.

Weis (90) noted an overall frequency of 39% of electrophysiological abnormalities reflective of lumbosacral plexopathy after acetabular, pelvic, and sacral bone fractures. Sacral and sacroiliac injuries were associated with a 64% frequency of EMG abnormalities compared with 24% for acetabular fractures and femoral fractures. Similar findings were noted by Kutsy (87) who found electrophysiologic abnormalities reflective of lumbosacral plexopathy in 68% of patients with sacral fractures and sacroiliac joint separation, as compared to 14% with acetabular and 9% with femoral fractures (9%) after detailed evaluation. Patients with acetabular and femoral fractures are more likely to suffer injury to multiple proximal nerves originating from the lumbosacral plexus, including the sciatic, inferior gluteal, and superior gluteal nerves, than injury to the plexus itself.

Signs of nerve injury were noted in 20 of 42 (48%) autopsied victims of lethal pelvic fracture injury (88). The fracture patterns were separable into those of the anterior pelvic ring involving the pubic rami and symphysis, and unilateral and bilateral fractures with or without dislocation of the posterior pelvic ring affecting the sacrum, sacroiliac joint, and juxta-articular area. In order of frequency, injuries of the lumbosacral plexus were divisible into traction, rupture, and compressive injuries, most often affecting the lumbosacral trunk, followed by the superior gluteal nerve, roots of the cauda equina, the first three sacral nerves, obturator nerve, and fifth lumbar nerve. Components of the lumbosacral plexus were often affected by more than one type or location of injury, and combined nerve injuries were commoner than singular ones. Traction injuries noted in 21 autopsied cases, most often affecting the lumbosacral trunk, superior gluteal nerve, and obturator nerve, frequently in association with dislocation of the hemipelvis, which changed the course of the nerve and so stretched them. Rupture injuries noted in 15 of 42 autopsied cases, most commonly affected the roots of the cauda equina, superior gluteal nerve, obturator nerve, and anterior primary ramus of the fifth lumbar nerve and corresponding rami of the three upper sacral nerves. Compression injury, noted in four of 42 cases, most often affected the primary anterior rami of the sacral nerves, especially with comminuted fractures of the pelvis, which caused narrowing of the sacral foraminal spaces where they were most vulnerable to injury.

Among 27 patients with traumatic lumbosacral plexopathy described by Stoehr (91), the most severe clinical motor involvement was noted in the common fibular nerve and gluteal nerves, with less severe involvement of the tibial and femoral nerves. Sensory involvement was slight in one-third of patients, and severe in two-thirds, especially affecting the skin area of the posterior femoral cutaneous and sciatic nerves.

The occurrence of lumbosacral plexopathy after acetabular and femoral fracture results in large part from stretch and traction injury alone with milder reversible deficits. However, lumbosacral plexus deficits after severe injuries, typified by unstable combined fractures of the anterior and posterior pelvic ring, sacroiliac separation, pelvic hemidislocation, crush injury of neighboring structures, retroperitoneal hematoma, and damage to genital and genitourinary organs, alone or in combination, results from the combination of traction, nerve rupture, and compression injury.

Pelvic Surgery

Lumbosacral plexopathy has been reported in association with kidney transplantation surgery and abdominal hysterectomy (92–96). In retrospect, Winkelman (96) first described six patients who awoke with extensive intrapelvic injury to fibers of the femoral nerve following total abdominal hysterectomy in five patients, and exploratory laparotomy with appendectomy in another patient. All six presented with flexion motor weakness of the hip and marked loss or absence of strength in knee extension of the leg with absent patellar reflex, sensory loss along the medial and anterior aspects of the thigh, and the medial aspect of the leg and foot, with recovery afterward. Although lik-

ened to the femoral damage that occurred in obstetrical cases during delivery, the author suggested an influence of anesthesia upon the plexus as the cause for the injury. Luzzio (95) described a patient with lumbosacral plexopathy after kidney transplantation attributed to an aneurysm of the internal iliac artery. Hefty (93) described four women with insulin-dependent diabetes mellitus who underwent cadaveric kidney transplantation in whom the internal iliac artery was used for revascularization of the renal allograft with ligation of the anterior and posterior divisions. All four patients developed ipsilateral buttock pain, numbness of the leg, and weakness below the knee within 24 hours of surgery consistent with acute lumbosacral plexopathy, two of whom were confirmed by electrophysiological testing. At follow-up, one patient died of infectious complications two months postoperatively, and three others had incomplete return of motor and sensory function consistent with postulated pervasive ischemic injury. Ligation of the internal iliac artery performed in the course of renal transplantation is usually well tolerated because of multiple sources of collateral blood flow through the contralateral vesical arteries, inferior mesenteric, medial femoral circumflex, lateral sacral, and iliac circumflex artery, but predisposes the lumbosacral plexus to ischemic injury in the setting of extensive small vessel disease because of reduced flow through the obturator, umbilical, and gluteal vessels.

Dhillon (92) described a diabetic patient who underwent dual renal transplantation with extensive vascular reconstruction associated with placement of both donor kidneys on the same side, followed postoperatively by ipsilateral lumbosacral plexopathy. There was anastomosis of the right common iliac artery to the renal artery of the left donor kidney, right external iliac artery to the renal artery of the right donor kidney, anastomosis of the renal vein of the left donor kidney to the inferior vena cava, and the renal vein of the right donor kidney to the external iliac vein of the recipient. After surgery the patient complained of right leg paresthesia with flail function throughout the leg, and loss of tendon reflexes without disturbance of bladder function or anal tone. Initial electrophysiological study showed absence of motor and sensory responses, and an inconclusive EMG. A second study performed one month later showed denervation in the distribution of the femoral, obturator, posterior tibial, and peroneal nerves without paraspinal denervation consistent with severe lumbosacral plexopathy, ipsilateral to the surgery. He later died of the complications of an infected sacral decubitus ulcer without autopsy.

Luzzio (95) described a patient with lumbosacral plexopathy ipsilateral to a second renal transplant in which there was arterial anastomosis to the bifurcation of the left common iliac artery. Twelve months after the procedure he complained of back and leg pain, and progressive foot drop. Electrodiagnostic studies showed acute and chronic lumbosacral plexopathy. Neuroimaging of the lumbosacral plexus employing MRI and, later, arteriography, revealed a large saccular pseudoaneurysm arising from the internal iliac artery extending posteromedially, with compression of the left lumbosacral plexus, resection of which led to immediate improvement.

Alsever (94) reported a young woman with multiple laparoscopies, laparotomy, and later hysterectomy for endometriosis. Immediately postoperatively she noted low back pressure and pain, hyperesthesia of the ipsilateral abdominal wall and anteromedial thigh, without weakness, presumed to be due to traction injury of the intrapelvic portions of the iliohypogastric, ilioinguinal, and genitofemoral nerves during surgery.

Hemorrhage

Apart from accidental and postoperative bleeding, aneurysmal leaks and rupture, lumbosacral plexopathy may also follow retroperitoneal bleeding in association with hemophilia, anticoagulant therapy, and acquired coagulopathy. In 1966, DeBolt (97) first drew attention to spontaneous hemorrhage associated with intramuscular injection of heparin in two patients treated for acute myocardial infarction and another with an impending infarct. In both patients, heparin was administered every eight hours for three to five days in the flank area just above the iliac crests. According to the authors, the injections were probably inadvertently placed into the muscular layers of the lateral abdominal wall rather than into subcutaneous fatty tissue before onset of the neurological disorder. Their second patient typified the syndrome of acute retroperitoneal hemorrhage with acute pain in the right inguinal area with weakness in the femoral innervated muscles; sensory loss was impaired in the distribution of the right femoral and ilioinguinal nerves. The first patient, who differed from the second due to involvement of the lateral femoral cutaneous nerve and color changes suggestive of involvement of lumbosacral sympathetic nerve fibers, was similar in sparing of the obturator nerve. A palpable mass was felt above the right inguinal ligament with ecchymosis and tenderness along the right flank. The patient held his right thigh flexed and resisted attempts to extend the thigh because of severe inguinal and thigh pain. The hematocrit was noted to drop 11 points with associated hypotension. Postmortem examination showed a large hematoma of freshly clotted blood in the right retroperitoneal area, right flank, and right anterior abdominal wall.

One year later, in 1967, Goodfellow (98) described hematomas of the iliopsoas muscle in 23 hemophiliacs and one non-hemophilic patient on anticoagulant therapy. Insidious or sudden groin pain extending to the back and thigh followed the onset of the joint crisis. Affected patients assumed a flexed posture while lying laterally rotated in bed to alleviate the pain, differentiating it from suppurative arthritis and hemiarthrosis of the hip. A tender mass was palpable deep in the iliac fossa extending along the iliac crest. Pain subsided in several weeks, but full power of the paralyzed femoral muscles and sensation along the thigh and leg returned more slowly, typically over several months to a year or more.

A decade later, Chiu (99) described five patients with retroperitoneal hemorrhage and lumbar plexopathy several days after initiation of therapeutic anticoagulation with intravenous heparin therapy in four patients, and in another patient soon after addition of warfarin, four of whom underwent electrodiagnostic studies to document lumbar plexopathy. In such cases, blood typically collects along the iliopsoas muscle and extends under the iliac fascia to the inguinal ligament where it forms a dense and indistensible tunnel enclosing the lower portions of the iliacus and psoas muscles. This leads to entrapment of the mixed femoral and obturator nerves, and femoral cutaneous nerves from their site of origin in the paravertebral area to their destination in the thigh. Symptoms of nerve entrapment appear within several hours of the onset of lumbar, abdominal, or inguinal pain, which typically radiates into the thigh and is soon followed by weakness, sensory loss, and reflex loss in the distribution of the affected components of the lumbar plexus. Some patients may demonstrate involvement of the sacral plexus. Symptoms and signs worsen with increasing size and consolidation of the hematoma. The hematoma may not be readily palpable in acute stages because of severe guarding, but soon after there is ecchymosis through the femoral canal when hemorrhage migrates through the inguinal canal. Retroperitoneal hematomas are readily discerned by contrast CT-imaging of the abdomen and pelvis because they obscure the normal concavity of the inner aspect of the wing of the ilium. Apart from the mechanical compressive or disruptive effects of a hematoma on the lumbosacral plexus, there may be a toxic effect of blood and its degradation products on the nerves. Early surgical decompression of retroperitoneal and iliac hematomas, but not psoas muscle hematomas, should be considered in those with progressive or fixed nerve deficits.

Cancer

Systemic and local cancer presents certain challenges to the etiopathogenesis, diagnosis, and management of lumbosacral plexopathy because of the frequent association with external radiation and radioactive implants (100, 101), and the adverse effects of intra-arterial chemotherapy, metastasis and contiguous tumor spread (102, 103).

Radiation Plexopathy

The peripheral nervous system (PNS) has generally been thought to be relatively resistant to damage by ionizing radiation. As with brachial plexopathy induced by radiation, the latter mainly damages connective tissues and blood supply of the nerve, rather than the axon or myelin tissue. Radiation effects are related to the biologically effective dose delivered with an increasing risk of neurologic injury as the dose increased, with low doses of <4,000 rads posing the least risk, and moderate doses of 4,000 to 5,000 rads to severely elevated doses of >5,000 rads, associated with higher risks of complication. A short source-to-skin distance, especially less than 80 cm, produces steep dose gradients in the body and a higher dose anterior or posterior to the midplane and complex field arrangements with multiple abutting portals that increase the opportunity for overlap and a resulting unsuspected high-dose region.

Thomas (101) studied 20 patients with lumbosacral plexopathy resulting from radiation treatment. Painless bilateral weakness occurred after a symptom-free interval of one to five years after radiation therapy. There was an emphasis of proximal and distal L2 to S1 root distribution with lesser distal predominance than proximal emphasis, and slow indolent progression. Stretch reflexes were almost always abnormal at the knees and ankles. Electrodiagnostic studies show myokymic discharges recognized as spontaneous grouped discharges due to spontaneous activity of a single axon by local membrane abnormalities. There is no effective treatment for radiation plexopathy. At follow-up ranging from one to 16 years after onset of the neurological disorder, only one patient died of an unrelated process; all the others were alive, and among the remaining 16, 12 were worse, 4 were unchanged, and one was improved.

Intraarterial chemotherapy injected through the internal iliac artery for treatment of pelvic cancer can also induce lumbosacral plexopathy and is reminiscent of radiation-induced cases in the absence of severe pain, but it differs in onset directly after, similar to radiation plexopathy in the infrequent absence of pain and typical onset of injection of the medication (102).

Direct Cancerous involvement

Although there is no relation between the histological type of malignancy, Hodgkin and non-Hodgkin lymphoma, colorectal cancers, and retroperitoneal and pelvic sarcomas most frequently involve the lumbosacral plexus, along with less common types, including acute myelogenous leukemia; multiple myeloma; breast, uterine and cervical cancer; testicular and genitourinary cancers; prostate, colonic, rectal, and stomach cancer, squamous cell carcinoma; and osteosarcoma. Jaeckle and workers (103) studied 85 patients with cancer and lumbosacral plexopathy and a documented pelvis tumor by CT or biopsy. Three clinical syndromes emerged: a lower plexopathy involving the L4 to S1 segments, seen in 51% of patients; upper lumbar plexopathy involving the L1-L4 segments, seen in 31% of patients; and pan-plexopathy involving the L1 to S3 segments, encountered in the remaining 18% of patients. Clinical signs of lumbosacral plexopathy developed within three months of onset of symptoms in one-half of patients, and within a year in 90% of patients, notably the insidious onset of pelvic or radicular leg pain, followed weeks to months later by sensory symptoms and weakness. The combination of leg pain, weakness, edema, rectal mass, and hydronephrosis suggested plexopathy due to cancer. Up to one-third of patients developed lumbosacral plexopathy due to tumor invasion demonstrable by CT, and the remainder by laparotomy. In 15% of cases so studied, symptoms of typical lumbosacral plexopathy preceded discovery of an occult pathogenic tumor demonstrable by contrast CT. The addition of myelography demonstrated epidural metastasis usually below the conus medullaris in 45% of patients studied.

Direct extension from an intra abdominal neoplasm to the plexus occurred in three-quarters of patients, as did metastasis from an extra-abdominal tumor in the remainder (103). Direct infiltration of the lumbosacral plexus by neoplasm occurs in about three-quarters of patients with a pelvic tumor, and via osteogenic or paravertebral or para-aortic lymph node metastasis in the remaining one-quarter of patients. The primary tumor most frequently involved in metastatic lumbosacral plexopathy is carcinomas of the breast, melanoma, and lung cancer. Hematogenous spread to the PNS is improbable, with the exception of the dorsal root ganglia, because of its fenestrated vascular endothelium. Nearly two-thirds of patients with lumbosacral plexus involvement by metastases have lower plexopathy clinically due to direct sacral involvement; conversely, less than one-half of patients with direct extension of an intra abdominal or pelvis tumor have lower plexopathy, with proportionately more having upper or pan-plexopathy. For unknown reasons, lumbosacral plexopathy is more often left-sided than right. Lymphomatous involvement leads to unilateral plexopathy, whereas breast cancer more frequently causes a bilateral syndrome. The location of the pelvic or retropelvic tumor also correlated with the clinical neurological signs. For example, upper plexopathy- associated tumors were most often located posteromedially in the paravertebral gutter extending into the true pelvis, wherein close examination often shows lack of contact with sacral roots. Patients with tumor extension above the pelvic brim complained of lumbar and flank pain. Patients with suprapelvic upper paravertebral tumor extension on CT demonstrated a positive reverse straight leg raising test (RSLRT). Patients with lower plexopathy generally have a tumor placed posteriorly in the true pelvis with erosion of the sacrum and abdominal extension. Although posterior radicular leg pain is most common with tumor extension to the pelvic sidewall, there may be flank, groin, and anterior thigh pain. Lateral extension of tumor leads to lower lumbar root involvement clinically. Low plexus tumors are most often bilateral in contrast with the unilateral involvement of upper plexus lesions. Sidewall extension of the tumor leads to positive RSLRT with sidewall extension. Those with pan-plexopathy often have a posterior medial massive tumor with extension from the true pelvis into the lower abdomen and frequent crossing of the midline.

Thomas (101) studied 30 patients with plexus damage from pelvic malignancy and compared them with 20 patients with plexopathy following radiation treatment. Pain marked the onset of tumor plexopathy, which was followed later by indolent unilateral weakness in all 30 patients. The level of plexus involvement could be inferred by the observed gait. For example, a rigid knee extension type of ambulation accompanied by difficulty rising from a sitting position suggests L2 to L3 or femoral nerve involvement associated with upper lumbosacral plexopathy, whereas lower plexopathy most often leads to footdrop gait suggestive of lumbosacral trunk lesion or pelvis tilt due to superior gluteal nerve involvement, and pelvic hyperlordosis consistent with an inferior gluteal nerve lesion. Jaeckle and coworkers (103) found epidural extension most commonly in those with pan-plexopathy and lower plexopathy. Early and prompt diagnosis of epidural metastasis may be suggested by vertebral or sacral erosion on plain radiographs, as well as abnormal pelvic, sacral, or vertebral uptake on whole body bone scan. If a patient with cancer develops lumbosacral plexopathy, the first diagnostic procedures should be MRI and CT of the pelvis and spine to provide information about tumor extent, epidural extension, and hydronephrosis. Electrophysiological studies should be performed in all patients with suspected lumbosacral plexopathy to confirm the diagnosis. Patients with lumbosacral plexopathy and intrapelvic tumor must choose from among the available treatments of radiotherapy, surgery, and chemotherapy, on the basis of responsiveness of the tumor to the specific therapy and the anticipated side effects. Pettigrew (102) studied six patients with lumbosacral plexopathy secondary to metastatic cancer, including two each with radiation-, or intra-arterial chemotherapy induced-plexopathy, and one patient with plexopathy due to a second primary cancer. Of the six patients with malignant extension to the lumbosacral plexus, two received radiotherapy alone, two received systemic chemotherapy with high-dose cytarabine, and one received a combination of radiation and systemic chemotherapy with cisplatin. Pain improved in all six, and there was mild to moderate improvement of weakness in three patients.

In the series by Jaeckle and colleagues (103) of cancer-related plexopathy, only 28% of patients had objective response on CT with concerted treatment, and 17% by examination and at the end of the study; the remainder died or were lost to follow-up, with an overall median survival of 5.5 months after treatment. Similar results were reported by Thomas and coworkers (101), who noted 86% mortality despite treatment within 3½ years of onset of plexopathy. Treatment of pain alone should rarely, if ever, be justification for use of chemotherapy since pain overall worsens in up to two-thirds of patients afterwards. Long-term survival after successful treatment with chemotherapy and radiotherapy remains about 40% effective overall, with a median duration of improvement of both CT and neurological examination of only 15 months, and a range of median survival from the time of diagnosis to death of one to 34 months.

REFERENCES

1. Haymaker W, Woodhall B. Peripheral nerve injuries. *Principles of Diagnosis*. WB Saunders: Philadelphia, 1953.
2. Feringa ER. Plexus syndromes. *Handbook of Clin Neurol* 1969; 2:128–156.
3. Spillane JD. Localized neuritis of the shoulder girdle: a report of 46 cases in the MEF. *Lancet* 1943; 532–535.
4. Turner AJW, Personage MJ. Neuralgic amyotrophy (paralytic brachial neuritis): with special reference to prognosis. *Lancet* 1957; 1:209–212.
5. Magee KR, DeJong RN. Paralytic brachial neuritis: discussion of clinical features with review of 23 cases. *JAMA* 1960; 112–116.
6. Kraft GH. Axillary, musculocutaneous, and suprascapular nerve latency studies. *Arch Phys Med Rehabil* 1972; 53:383–387.
7. Gassel MM. A test of nerve conduction to muscles of the shoulder girdle as an aid in the diagnosis of proximal neurogenic and muscular disease. *J Neurol Neurosurg Psychiatry* 1964; 27:200–205.
8. Tsairis P, Dyck PJ, Mulder DW. Natural history of brachial plexus neuropathy. *Arch Neurol* 1972; 27:109–117.
9. Trojaborg W. Peripheral conduction block with axonal degeneration. *J Neurol Neurosurg Psychiatry* 1977; 40:50–57.
10. Li J, Ghandour K, Radovanovic D, et al. Stoichiometric alteration of PMP22 protein determines the phenotype of hereditary neuropathy with liability to pressure palsies. *Arch Neurol* 2007; 64:974–978.
11. Laccone F, Hannibal MC, Neeson J, et al. Dysmorphic syndrome of hereditary neuralgic amyotrophy associated with a SEPT9 gene mutation—a family study. *Clin Genet* 2008; 74:279–283.
12. Kuhlenbaumer G, Stogbauer F, Timmerman V, et al. Diagnostic guidelines for hereditary neuralgic amyotrophy or heredofamilial neuritis with brachial plexus predilection. *Neuromusc Disord* 2000; 10:515–517.
13. Duchenne GBA. *De l'electrisation localisee, et de son application a la pathologie et a la therapeutique.* 3rd ed, Paris: TB Bailliere and Fils, 1872; 353–367.

14. Erb WB. Uber eine eigentumliche localization von Lahmungen im Plexus brachialis. *Verb naturh med Ver zu Heidelberg* 1874–1876; 1:130–137.

15. Klumpke A. Contributino a l'etude des paralysies radiculaires du plexus brachial. Paralysies radiculaires totales. Paralysies radiculaires inferieurs. De la participation des filets sympathetiques oculopupillaires dans ces paralysies. *Rev Medecine* 1885; 5:591–616.

16. Sever JW. Obstetrical paralysis: report of eleven hundred patients. *JAMA* 1925; 138:1862–1865.

17. Sever JW. Obstetrical paralysis—An orthopedic problem. *Am J Orthop Surg* 1916; 14:456–475.

18. Adson AW. The gross pathology of brachial plexus injuries. *Surg Gynecol Obstet* 1922; 34:351–357.

19. Gilbert A, Tassin JL. Obstetrical palsy. *Chirurgie* 1984; 110:70–75.

20. Brooks DM. Open wounds of the brachial plexus. *J Bone Jt Surg Ser B* 1949; 31:17–33.

21. Ewing MR. Postoperative paralysis in the upper extremity: report of five cases. *Lancet* 1950; 1:101–103.

22. Wynn Parry CB. Brachial plexus injuries. *Handbook of Clin Neurol* 1987; 51:143–155.

23. Bonney G, Gilliat RW. Sensory nerve conduction after traction lesions of the brachial plexus. *Proc R Soc Med* 1958; 57:365–367.

24. Narakas A. Indications et resultats du traitement chirugical direct dans les lesions par elongation du plexus brachial. *Rev Chir Orthop Repar Appar Mot* 1977; 63:88–106.

25. Pancoast HK. Importance of careful roentgen-ray investigations of apical chest tumors. *JAMA* 1924; S3:1407.

26. Pancoast HK. Superior pulmonary sulcus tumor. *JAMA* 1932; 99:1391–1396.

27. Moersch HJ, Hinshaw HC, Wilson IH. Apical lung tumors or so-called superior pulmonary sulcus tumors. *Minn Med* 1940; 23:221–226.

28. Thomas JE, Colby MY. Radiation-induced or metastatic brachial plexopathy. *JAMA* 1972; 222:1392–1395.

29. Kori SH, Foley KM, Posner JB. Brachial plexus lesions in patients with cancer: 100 cases. *Neurology* 1981; 31:45–50.

30. Stoll BA, Andrews JT. Radiation-induced peripheral neuropathy. *Brit Med J* 1966; 1:834–837.

31. Match RM. Radiation-induced brachial plexus paralysis. *Arch Surg* 1975; 110:384–386.

32. Ray BS. The management of intractable pain by posterior rhizotomy. *Res Publ Assoc Res Nerv Men Dis* 1943; 23:391–407.

33. Gilbert RW, Kim JH, Posner JB. Epidural spinal cord compression from metastatic tumor: diagnosis and treatment. *Ann Neurol* 1978; 3:40–51.

34. Posner JB. Spinal cord compression—a neurological emergency. *Clin Bull* 1971; 1:65–71.

35. Atasoy E. Thoracic outlet syndrome: anatomy. *Hand Clin* 20:7–14.

36. Ferrante MA. The thoracic outlet syndromes. *Muscle Nerve* 2012; 45:780–795.

37. Roos DB, Wilbourn AJ. Issues and opinions: thoracic outlet syndrome. *Muscle Nerve* 22, 1999; 126–138.

38. Adson AW. Cervical ribs: symptoms, differential diagnosis and indications for section of the insertion of the scalenus anticus muscle. *J Int Coll Surg* 1951; 16:546–559.

39. Urschel HC Jr., Razzuk MA. Management of the thoracic-outlet syndrome. *N Engl J Med* 1972; 286:1140–1143.

40. Smith T, Trojaborg W. Diagnosis of thoracic outlet syndrome. Value of sensory and motor conduction studies and quantitative electromyography. *Arch Neurol* 1987; 44:1161–1163.

41. Caldwell JW, Crane CR, Krusen EM. Nerve conduction studies: An aid in the diagnosis of the thoracic outlet syndrome. *South Med J* 1971; 64:210–212.

42. Urschel HC Jr, Razzuk MA, Wood RE, et al. Objective diagnosis (ulnar nerve conduction velocity) and current therapy of the thoracic outlet syndrome. *Ann Thorac Surg* 1971; 12:608–620.

43. London GW. Normal ulnar nerve conduction velocity across the thoracic outlet: comparison of two measuring techniques. *J Neurol Neurosurg Psychiatry* 1975; 38:756–760.

44. Yiannikas C, Walsh JC. Somatosensory evoked responses in the diagnosis of thoracic outlet syndrome. *J Neurol Neurosurg Psychiatry* 1983; 46:234–240.

45. Wilbourn AJ, Lederman RJ. Evidence for conduction delay in thoracic outlet syndrome is challenged, and Urschel HC Jr. Reply. *N Engl J Med* 1984; 310:1052–1053.

46. Cherington M, Happer I, Machanic B, et al. Surgery for thoracic outlet syndrome may be hazardous to your health. *Muscle Nerve* 1986; 9:632–634.

47. Wilbourne AJ. Thoracic outlet surgery causing severe brachial plexopathy: clinical and EMG features in five cases. *Muscle Nerve* 1985; 8:612–613.

48. Paterson AM. The origin and distribution of the nerves to the lower limb. *J Anat Lond* 1894; 28:84–95;169–193.

49. Buruma GJS, Maat GJR. Lumbosacral plexus lesions. *Handb Clin Neurol* 17:157–170.

50. Webber RH. Some variations in the lumbar plexus of the nerves in man. *Acta Anat* 1961; 44:336–345.

51. Day MH. The blood supply of the lumbar and sacral plexuses in the human foetus. *J Anat* 1964; 98:105–116.

52. Sander JE, Sharp FR. Lumbosacral plexus neuritis. *Neurology* 1981; 31:470–473.

53. Evans BA, Stevens JC. Dyck PJ. Lumbosacral plexus neuropathy. *Neurology* 1981; 31:1327–1330.

54. Hinchey JA, Preston DC, Logigian EL. Idiopathic lumbosacral neuropathy: a cause of persistent leg pain. *Muscle Nerve* 1996; 19:1484–1486.

55. Van Alfen N, Van Engelen BGM. Lumbosacral plexus neuropathy: a case report and review of the literature. *Clin Neurol Neurosurg* 1997; 99:138–141.

56. Younger DS. Rosoklija G, Hays AP. Lyme polyradiculoneuritis: immunohistochemical findings in sural nerve. *Muscle Nerve* 1995; 18:359–360.

57. Garcia-Monco JC, Beldarrain MG, Estrade L. Painful lumbosacral plexitis with increased ESR and Borrelia burgdorferi infection. *Neurology* 43, 1993; 1269.

58. Vallat JM, Hugon J, Lubeau M. Tick-bite meningoradiculoneuritis: clinical, electrophysiologic, and histologic findings in 10 cases. *Neurology* 1987; 37:749–753.

59. Sharma KR, Sriram S, Fries T. Lumbosacral radiculopathy as a manifestation of Epstein-Barr virus infection. *Neurology* 1993; 43:2550–2554.

60. Stoeckli TC, Mackin GA, De Groote MA. Lumbosacral plexopathy in a patient with pulmonary tuberculosis. *Clin Infect Dis* 2000; 30:226–227.

61. Garland H, Taverner D. Diabetic myelopathy. *Br Med J* 1953; 1:1405–1408.

62. Garland H. Diabetic amyotrophy. *Br Med J* 1961; 15:9–13.

63. Garland H. Diabetic amyotrophy. *Br Med J* 1955; 2:1287–1290.

64. Raff MC, Sangalang V, Asbury AK. Ischemic mononeuropathy multiplex associated with diabetes mellitus. *Arch Neurol* 1968; 18:487–499.

65. Raff MC, Asbury AK. Ischemic mononeuropathy and mononeuropathy multiplex in diabetes mellitus. *N Engl J Med* 1968; 279:17–21.

66. Asbury AK. Proximal diabetic neuropathy. *Ann Neurol* 1977; 2:179–180.

67. Bradley WG, Chad D, Verghese JP. Painful lumbosacral

plexopathy with elevated erythrocyte sedimentation rate: a treatable inflammatory syndrome. *Ann Neurol* 1984; 15:457– 464.

68. Johnson PC, Doll SC, Cromey DW. Pathogenesis of diabetic neuropathy. *Ann Neurol* 1986; 450–457.

69. Barohn RJ, Sahent Z, Warmolts JR. The Bruns-Garland syndrome (diabetic amyotrophy): revisited 100 years later. *Arch Neurol* 1991; 48:1130–1135.

70. Said G, Goulon-Goeau C, Lacroix C. Nerve Biopsy findings in different patterns of proximal diabetic neuropathy. *Ann Neurol* 1994; 35:559–569.

71. Dyck PJB, Norell JE, Dyck PJ. Microvasculitis and ischemia in diabetic lumbosacral radiculoplexis neuropathy. *Neurology* 1999; 53:2113–2121.

72. Dyck PJ, Engelstad J, Norell J. Microvasculitis in non-diabetic lumbosacral radiculoplexus neuropathy (LSRPN): similarity to the diabetic variety (DLSRPN). *J Neuropathol Exp Neurol* 2000; 59:525–538.

73. Younger DS, Rosoklija G, Hays AP, et al. Diabetic peripheral neuropathy: a clinical and immunohistochemical analysis of sural nerve biopsies. *Muscle Nerve* 1996; 19:722–727.

74. Younger DS. Diabetic Neuropathy: A clinical and neuropathological study of 107 patients. Neurol Res International, 2010, Article ID 140379:1–4.

75. Younger DS. Diabetic lumbosacral radiculoplexus neuropathy: a postmortem studied patient and review of the literature. *J Neurol* 2011; 258:1364–1367.

76. Dyck PJB, O'Brien PC, Bosch P, et al. The multi-center double-blind controlled trial of IV methylprednisolone in diabetic lumbosacral radiculoplexus neuropathy. *Neurology* 2006; 66(Suppl 2):A191.

77. Dyck PJB, O'Brien PC, Bosch P, et al. Results of a controlled trial of IV methylprednisolone in diabetic lumbosacral radiculoplexus neuropathy (DLRPN): a preliminary indication of efficacy. *J Periph Nerv Syst* 2005; 101:21.

78. Windebank A. Study Chair. Randomized study of intravenous immunoglobulin (IVIg) in patients with subacute proximal diabetic neuropathy. FDA Office of Orphan Products Development. Mayo Clinic, clinicaltrials.gov/show/NCT 00004407.

79. Awerbuch GI, Nigro MA, Sandyk R. Relapsing lumbosacral plexus neuropathy: report of two cases. *Eur Neurol* 1991; 31:348–351.

80. Yee T. Recurrent idiopathic lumbosacral plexopathy. *Muscle Nerve* 2000; 23:1439–1442.

81. Cole JT. Maternal obstetric paralysis. *Am J Obstet Gynaecik* 1946; 52:372–385.

82. Kleinberg S. Maternal obstetrical sciatic paralysis. *Surg Gynaecol Obstet* 1927; 45:61–64.

83. Stöhr M, Dichans J, Dörstelmann. Ischaemic neuropathy of the lumbosacral plexus following intragluteal injection. *J Neurol Neurosurg Psychiatry* 1980; 43:489–494.

84. Levy-Valensi J, Delvaille. Nevralgie sciatique par compression anevrismale: rupture de l'anevrisme: mort. *Sem Hop Paris* 1927; 3:115.

85. Lodder J, Cheriex E, Oostenbroek R, et al. Ruptured abdominal aortic aneurysms presenting as radicular compression syndromes. *J Neurol* 1982; 227:121–124.

86. Kubacz GJ. Femoral and sciatic compression neuropathy. *Br J Surg* 1971; 58(8):580–582.

87. Kutsy, R, Robinson LR, Routt ML. Lumbosacral plexopathy in pelvic trauma. *Muscle Nerve* 2000; 23:1757–1760.

88. Huittinen VM, Slatis P. Nerve injury in double vertical pelvic fractures. *Acta Chir Scand* 1972; 138:571–575.

89. Huittinen VM. Lumbosacral nerve injury in fracture of the pelvis. *Acta Chir Scand* 1972; 429 (Suppl 1):1–43.

90. Weis EB. Subtle neurological injuries in pelvic fractures. *J Trauma* 1984; 24:983–985.

91. Stoehr M. Traumatic and postoperative lesions of the lumbosacral plexus. *Arch Neurol* 1978; 35:757–760.

92. Dhillon SS, Sarac E. Lumbosacral plexopathy after dual kidney transplantation. *Am J Kidney Dis* 2000; 36:1045–1048.

93. Hefty TR, Nelson KA, Hatch TR, et al. Acute lumbosacral plexopathy in diabetic women after renal transplantation. *J Urol* 1990; 143:107–109.

94. Alsever JD. Lumbosacral plexopathy after gynecologic surgery: case report and review of the literature. *Am J Obstet Gynecol* 1996; 174:1769–1778.

95. Luzzio CC, Waclawik AJ, Gallagher CL, et al. Iliac artery pseudoaneurysm following renal transplantation presenting as lumbosacral plexopathy. *Transplantation* 67; 1077–1078.

96. Winkelman NW. Femoral nerve complications after pelvic surgery. A report of six cases. *Am J Obst Gynec* 1958; 75:1063–1065.

97. DeBolt WL, Jordan JC. Femoral neuropathy from heparin hematoma. *Bull Los Angeles Neurological Societies* 1966; 31:45–50.

98. Goodfellow J, Fearn BD, Matthews JM. Iliacus haematoma. A common complication of haemophilia. *J Bone Joint Surg* 1967; 49B:748–756.

99. Chiu WS. The syndrome of retroperitoneal hemorrhage and lumbar plexus neuropathy during anticoagulant therapy. *Southern Med J* 1976; 69:595–599.

100. Aho K, Sainio K. Late irradiation-induced lesions of the lumbosacral plexus. *Neurology* 1983; 33:953–955.

101. Thomas JE. Cascino TL, Earle JD. Differential diagnosis between radiation and tumor plexopathy of the pelvis. *Neurology* 1985; 35:1–7.

102. Pettigrew LC, Glass JP, Maor M, et al. Diagnosis and treatment of lumbosacral plexopathies in patients with cancer. *Arch Neurol* 1984; 41:1282–1285.

103. Jaeckle KA, Young DF, Foley KM. The natural history of lumbosacral plexopathy in cancer. *Neurology* 1985; 35:8–15.

CHAPTER 28

Diabetic Neuropathy

David S. Younger

Diabetes mellitus (DM) is a chronic disease character-ized by persistent hyperglycemia. Patients with insulin dependent DM (IDDM) demonstrate relatively little insu-lin secretion by pancreatic beta cells, whereas those with non-IDDM (NIDDM) have normal or increased insulin secretion related to peripheral tissue receptor resistance. A clinically significant neuropathy manifested by weakness and sensory changes occurs in about 10% of all patients with diabetes and is one of the most common neuropathies worldwide. Although the pathogenesis of diabetic periph-eral neuropathy is unknown, it is generally ascribed to a complex interaction of genetic, metabolic, microvascular, and autoimmune factors related to chronic hyperglycemia. The result is a spectrum of distinct neuropathy types, with variable motor and sensory involvement, including distal symmetrical polyneuropathy (DSPN), diabetic lumbosa-cral radiculoplexus neuropathy (DLSRPN), mononeuropa-thy multiplex (MNM), and diabetic autonomic neuropathy. Cranial and entrapment neuropathies, as well as chronic inflammatory demyelinating polyradiculoneuropathy (CIDP), all occur in DM with increased frequency com-pared to the general population.

This chapter reviews the historical aspects, epidemiol-ogy, clinical presentation, laboratory diagnosis, pathology, etiopathogenesis, and treatment of diabetic peripheral neu-ropathy with an emphasis on the motor sequela.

HISTORICAL ASPECTS AND BACKGROUND

The earliest reported patients with diabetic neuropathy had prominent motor involvement in association with variable pain and sensory involvement. In 1887, Pryce (1) described

a patient with clinical and pathological evidence of a painful distal leg weakness. Charcot (2) coined the term "diabetic paraplegia" to describe a patient with ataxia resembling tabes dorsalis with profound leg weakness. Pryce (3) later suggested separation of the diabetic neuropathic syndromes into motor or paralytic, and sensory or ataxic types. Bruns (4), and later Garland and Taverner (5), described a painful, predominantly motor disorder of asymmetrical weakness and wasting, with Babinski signs, without sensory changes, so-termed "diabetic myelopathy." Garland (6) termed the same disorder "diabetic amyotrophy" in consideration of the presumed clinical spinal cord and anterior horn cell and root involvement. Early investigations of diabetic neu-ropathy utilized nerve trunks obtained from diseased limbs obtained at surgical amputation and postmortem examina-tion (7–9). However, such patients had long-standing diabe-tes that tended to increase the likelihood of arteriosclerosis, and Renaut corpuscles, a feature of peripheral neuropathy, were probably misinterpreted as infarcts.

Decades later, investigations of peripheral nerve microvessels stained by periodic acid Schiff (PAS) showed thickening of the walls of endoneurial blood vessels (10) that was subsequently found to be reduplication of the basal lamina, a change also common to retinopathy and nephropathy. Other investigators (11–14) were unable to validate the correlation between so-called microangiopa-thy and neuropathy, and attention focused on metabolic alterations in nerve elements (15). A variety of inter-changeable descriptive terms evolved to emphasize the often proximal nature of the illness, including ischemic mononeuropathy multiplex, diabetic proximal amyotro-phy, subacute proximal diabetic neuropathy, painful lum-bosacral plexopathy, proximal diabetic neuropathy, and femoral sciatic neuropathy (16–18), and most recently DLRPN or the equivalent abbreviation DLSRPN (19, 20).

With the availability of ultrastructural and biochemical analysis of nerve biopsy specimens from affected patients, it appeared that metabolic derangements played important roles in the pathogenesis of diabetic neuropathy (21, 22). The earliest morphological alterations in epineurial and endoneurial blood vessels inferred local hypoxia, cellular disturbances, and changes in vascular permeability. Some investigators (23, 24) attempted to correlate chronic hyperglycemia with metabolic derangements, particularly in the polyol pathway responsible for the conversion of glucose to sorbitol by aldose reductase and sorbitol to fructose. Such were associated with alterations of intrinsic nerve lipids, alcoholic sugars, and a series of biochemical consequences leading to altered protein synthesis, abnormal glycosylation, slowed axon transport, axoglia dysjunction, osmotic swelling and thickened axolemmal and endoneurial basement membranes.

EPIDEMIOLOGY

Estimates of the prevalence of diabetic peripheral neuropathy vary widely in the literature, largely because of the discrepancy in diagnostic criteria, methods of patient selection, and assessment. The consensus statement of the San Antonio conference on diabetic peripheral neuropathy proposed guidelines for epidemiologic studies (25). Thirty percent of 1184 subjects with type I DM, of mean age 47 years and duration of disease of 26 years, screened by the Michigan Neuropathy Screening Instrument (MNSI), had confirmed neuropathy employing neurological examination and nerve conduction studies (NCS) (26) compared to 10.5% of 1414 subjects with newly diagnosed DM, comprising 17.5% of the cohort, and the remainder with known DM, employing vibration pressure thresholds (27). Although increasing age is an independent risk factor for diabetic neuropathy, others such as longer duration of DM, retinopathy, and nephropathy are generally considered to correlate with a higher frequency of neuropathy as well.

CLINICAL PRESENTATION

Patients with DSPN present with distal leg weakness and wasting, in association with neuropathic pain, paresthesias, hyperesthesia, proprioceptive defect, weakness, atrophy, gait disturbance, imbalance, hyporeflexia, and impaired autonomic function. In its most advanced form, it can resemble tabes dorsalis as there may be Charcot foot joint deformity and ulceration. The presence of fasciculation should lead to the suspicion of CIDP. Patients with DLSRPN have prominent

pelvifemoral pain followed by weakness, beginning focally in the upper leg or thigh with spread to the contralateral limb, and variable weight loss (20). Those with MNM present with a stepwise pattern of neuropathic motor and sensory loss and weakness in the distribution of named peripheral nerves, especially in the femoral, sciatic, and upper limb nerves accompanied by asymmetrical weakness, wasting and, at a later stage, by the coalescence of lesions resembling severe DSPN. Diabetic autonomic neuropathy may be subclinical or clinically evident, with cardiovascular, ocular, gastrointestinal, genitourinary, sudomotor, and hypoglycemic symptoms. Carpal tunnel syndrome and other entrapment neuropathies may go unheeded because of an elevated threshold to ischemic pain. Oculomotor nerve palsy occurs with the abrupt onset of ocular pain, and headache, followed by partial paralysis of eye movement, with papillary sparing. Some patients develop truncal radiculopathy manifested by girdle-like pain, abdominal wall weakness, and hyperesthesia due to root infarction, which when combined with a neurogenic bladder, can raise suspicion of cord compression by a ruptured thoracic disc. When manifested in lumbar segments, affected patients may similarly be thought to harbor lumbar root entrapment or compression by a ruptured disc with radicular weakness, hyporeflexia, and dermatomal sensory loss. Generalized weakness may accompany acute painful neuropathy and diabetic neuropathic cachexia, manifested by precipitous and profound weight loss, followed by severe and unremitting cutaneous pain due to primarily small nerve fiber involvement, often with superimposed large fiber disease and dysautonomia. Symptoms of autonomic neuropathy in the order of frequency at occurrence, include nausea, incomplete bladder emptying, urinary frequency, orthostatic dizziness, impotence, hyperhydrosis, and early satiety.

CLINICAL AND LABORATORY EVALUATION

The assessment of patients with diabetic neuropathy of any type should begin with a thorough history and examination. All new patients should have baseline and serial fasting serum glucose and glycosylated hemoglobin levels to assess glycemic control. Since up to 10% of diabetic patients may have an alternative cause for the neuropathy, various other potential pathogenic causes or associated contributory condition should be considered as appropriate for a given patient. Those with prominent motor involvement should be evaluated for B12 deficiency, heavy metal intoxication, malnutrition, uremia, occult cancer and lymphoproliferative disease, including benign and malignant plasma cell dyscrasia, systemic vasculitis, thyroid disease, human immunodeficiency virus (HIV)-1 neuropathy, serologically specific connective tissue disorders, anti-GM1 ganglioside and anti-myelin-associated glycoprotein (MAG) neuropathies. The determination of such disorders should be approached systematically by obtaining serum and serological studies, imaging of the body by computed tomography (CT) after adequate hydration and determination of renal function, and appropriate urinary studies, all of which are generally relatively inexpensive and informative from the outset. Determination of heart rate by auscultation and electrocardiography (ECG) may reveal a resting tachycardia in patients with autonomic cardiac parasympathetic neuropathy, whereas those with both parasympathetic and sympathetic involvement may have slightly less rapid rates. Whereas autonomic cardiac neuropathy contributes to the mortality of diabetes by heightening the risk of malignant ventricular arrhythmia due to prolongation of the QTc interval of the resting electrocardiogram (EKG), and to sudden cardiac death following general anesthesia or after use of medications that suppress baroreceptors, autonomic neuropathy heightens the risk of orthostatic intolerance (OI) with the ensuing propensity for syncope. The secondary retinal, peripheral vascular and renal complications of diabetes also confer independent long-term morbidity and mortality in a given patient. Those with retinopathy should undergo full ophthalmological testing, including retinography. Patients with occlusive vascular disease, as suggested by absence of distal leg pulsations, should undergo Doppler studies. Diabetic patients with clinical and laboratory evidence of nephropathy should undergo measurement of total urinary protein and creatinine, with 24-hour clearance of the latter before exposure to contrast dye or IVIG, and those with known paraproteinemia should have urine electrophoresis for Bence Jones proteinuria. Cerebrospinal fluid (CSF) analysis should be considered in patients with suspected CIDP.

All newly diagnosed patients should undergo electrodiagnostic studies employing baseline NCS along the median, ulnar, fibular, tibial, and femoral mixed nerves for motor parameters, and along corresponding sensory nerve branches using standard surface recording techniques at skin temperature of 34 degrees centigrade. Since compression of the median nerve at the wrist and the ulnar nerve at the elbow are frequent occurrences in diabetics and in the general population with age, the radial nerve is probably the most useful determinant of motor and sensory function in the arms. Femoral nerve motor and saphenous sensory studies are useful in confirming or excluding clinically significant DLSRPN. When the distal fibular motor responses are not obtainable, proximal conductions along the fibular nerve at the fibula head and knee, while recording to the tibialis anterior muscle can provide an accurate estimate of nerve velocity. Patients with conduction block, segmental motor nerve slowing, and excessive temporal dispersion should be suspected of CIDP. Concentric needle electromyography (EMG) is the most sensitive measure of focal or asymmetrical

lesions and of active motor axonal degeneration, and assists in the confirmation of demyelinating neuropathy. Quantitative sensory testing (QST) by computer-assisted techniques, and quantitative autonomic testing (QAT) for determination of the heart-rate response to Valsalva maneuver, deep breathing, and erect stance; and blood pressure changes with head-up tilting (HUT), and the quantitative sudomotor axon reflex testing (QSART) all amplify conventional electrophysiology and bedside testing.

Peripheral nerve and muscle biopsy are useful in selected patients with progressive, disabling symptoms, especially when electrodiagnostic studies suggest a possible alternative or coexisting diagnosis with morphologically distinctive findings such as hereditary neuropathy, vasculitis, and CIDP. Contrary to popular belief, diabetics probably have no greater risk of healing or complications after nerve and muscle biopsy. However, such procedures should be undertaken at centers with an experienced neuropathologist able to process and evaluate paraffin, frozen, and epoxy-embedded tissue for histologic, histochemical, ultrastructural, morphometric, and teased nerve fiber analysis, necessary to address all of the possible diagnoses, including diabetes. Similarly, the neurologist or surgeon performing the biopsy should be skilled in biopsy techniques to reduce morbidity, provide optimal specimens adequate for analysis, and reduce handling artifacts. Nerve biopsy is the only means of providing an accurate assessment of the density of myelinated fibers, the presence of multifocal fiber loss, state of myelination of large and small fibers, cellular infiltration, and nerve fiber degeneration and regeneration. Immunohistochemistry, useful in elucidating the different patterns of humoral and cell-mediated immunity in selected patients, can be performed on snap-frozen tissue using a battery of monoclonal and polyclonal antibodies against antigens specific for T and B cells, macrophages, cytokines, immunoglobulin classes, and complement components (28). Skin biopsy obtained by a simple 3-mm punch can be placed in cold paraformaldehyde and picric acid solution, thick-sectioned, and immunologically stained for epidermal nerve fiber (ENF) density, histology, and amyloidosis employing Congo red stain (29).

NEUROPATHOLOGY

There are few modern series of diabetic neuropathy confirmed by nerve tissue obtained at biopsy or postmortem examination available to allow examination of the different neuropathic syndromes. In 1996, Younger and coworkers (30) reported the clinicopathologic and immunohistochemical findings of sural nerve biopsy in a cohort of 20 patients with diabetic neuropathy. That series was continued to a total of 107 patients (31), the detailed clinicopath-

Table 1. Clinicopathological Findings in 107 Patients with Diabetic Neuropathy

	Number	Percentage
Study Cohort		
(Mean age 64.7 years)		
(Range 31 to 95 years)		
Women	36	34
Men	71	66
Clinical Neuropathic Syndrome		
MNM	1	1
DLSRPN	35	33
DSPN	71	66
Histologic Severity of Neuropathy		
Normal	1	1
Mild	17	16
Moderate	54	50
Severe	35	33
Teased Fiber/Semithin Section Analysis		
Normal	1	1
Axonopathy	45	65
Myelinopathy	23	34
Cellular Response		
Perivasculitis	26	23
Microvasculitis	3	3
Necrotizing vasculitis	3	3
Complement Immuno-fluorescence		
C3 deposition	70	67
C5b-9	65	62
Other Findings		
Onion bulb formations	10	9
Epineurial vascular thrombosis	5	5

ological findings of which are summarized (Table 1). Two patients had juvenile-onset DM, and the remainder had type 1 and 2 DM in equal ratio. One patient had MNM, and the remainder had DSPN and DLSRPN in a 2:1 ratio. Five patients (4%) had minor wound infection at the incision site that responded to antibiotics and 4% had short-lasting postoperative causalgia. The severity of neuropathy was mild in 17%, moderate in 50%, and severe in 33%, based upon the degree of myelinated fiber degeneration and loss in transverse paraffin and epoxy sections. Two-thirds of nerves showed primary axonopathy and one-third primary myelinopathy after analysis of semithin epoxy sections and teased nerve fiber preparations. Altogether, 3% and 23% of nerves, respectively, revealed microvasculitis (MV) and

perivasculitis (PV) (Figures 1 A, B), defined respectively, as mononuclear cellular infiltration in or around the walls of peripheral nerve microvessels. Necrotizing arteritis was detected in nerve biopsy tissue in two patients with DSPN and in one with DLSRPN, although absent in postmortem tissue of the latter patient in whom femoral, sciatic nerve, and lumbar plexus instead showed PV of the epineurium, perineurium, and endoneurium (32).

IMMUNE ETIOPATHOGENESIS OF DIABETIC NEUROPATHY

In the past several years, several lines of investigations have suggested the importance of altered humoral and cell-mediated immunity in the pathogenesis of diabetic microangiopathy. Diabetes itself appears to be caused by autoimmune mechanisms directed against the insulin-producing beta cells of the pancreas, and a variety of autoantibodies have been detected in patients with IDDM, including anti-islet-cell cytoplasmic autoantibodies, present in up to 80% of newly diagnosed patients (33), and glutamic acid decarboxylase antibodies, also present in patients with stiff-man syndrome (34). The pancreas of newly diagnosed IDDM patients showed insulitis consisting predominantly of CD8+ T cells with variable numbers of CD4+ T cells, killer cells, and expression of major histocompatibility class I molecules (35), as did the pancreas' of two children who died rapidly of cerebral edema after apparent onset of juvenile IDDM, in addition to membrane-bound superantigen (36). IDDM occurs with increased frequency in several other autoimmune disorders, including Grave disease, pernicious anemia, Hashimoto thyroditis, myasthenia gravis, anti-phospholipid antibody syndrome, and Addison disease. Investigators have reported mononuclear cell infiltration, first employing light microscopic analysis of paraffin sections stained with hematoxylin and eosin (H&E) (7–9, 17, 37, 38), and later with cell-marker immunocytochemistry (39) and immunofluorescence microscopy demonstrating perineurial deposition of immunoglobulins and complement (40). Other patients with diabetic neuropathy were noted to have multifocal ischemia without vascular occlusion in peripheral nerve biopsy specimens (37).

Two disorders of known autoimmune etiopathogenesis, CIDP and LSRPN, have now been well studied in diabetics. Stewart (41), Haq, and coworkers (42) described the clinical, electrophysiological, and histopathologic findings of a small series of patients with DM who met formal criteria for CIDP, the associated features of which did not discriminate diabetics from non-diabetics. Dyck and colleagues (43) compared 57 patients with LSRPN alone or with diabetes in 33 other patients, with regard to natural history variables, electrophysiological features, quantita-

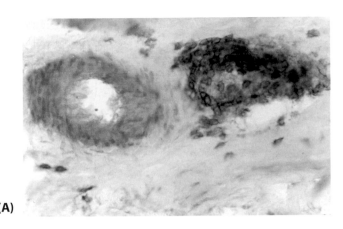 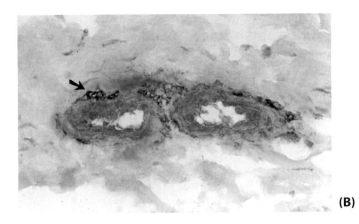

FIG. 1. Inflammatory changes in diabetic nerve biopsies.
(A) Microvasculitis is seen on the left with invasion of the vessel wall.
(B) Perivasculitis is seen on the right characterized by inflammation around the vessel wall.
(Immunoperoxidase staining technique using monoclonal antibodies that recognize CD3+ cells; reproduced from reference 30, with permission).

tive sensory and autonomic analysis, histopathology, and outcome. None of the indices differentiated diabetic from non-diabetic patients, but MV was noted in the cutaneous sensory nerves of two patients, and PV noted in all 33 cutaneous nerves in DLSRPN, of which 15 (45%) infiltrated the vessel wall, suggesting even a higher frequency of MV, consistent with a mechanism of ischemic nerve injury due to microscopic vasculitis.

TREATMENT

The prevention and amelioration of the secondary complications of diabetes has been an important focus of therapy, with theoretical importance in neuropathy. The significance of early intervention and tight glycemic control has been amply examined (44). Tight control reduced the adjusted mean risk of clinical neuropathy by 60%, however there was a two- to three-fold increase in symptomatic hypoglycemic episodes and weight gain. Patients with NIDDM for whom diet, exercise, and oral hypoglycemic therapy are usually first-line treatments, who then commence right glycemic control, appeared to have a heightened risk of macrovascular complications and increased morbidity due to symptomatic hypoglycemia (45). Aldose reductase inhibitor drugs, given to ameliorate the presumed biochemical and morphological abnormalities of diabetic neuropathy in randomized controlled trials, did not demonstrate consistent benefit (46). Pancreatic transplantation achieves normoglycemia and prevents or halts the progression of peripheral neuropathy (47); however, acceptable candidates should have end-stage renal disease as little argument can be made against the addition of islet cell transplantation to a renal allograft recipient who is already obligated to chronic

immunosuppression to prevent rejection. Nonuremic diabetic candidates should be so labile and have such extreme secondary complications as to outweigh the anticipated side effects of chronic immunosuppression to achieve normoglycemia and control of the neuropathy.

A team approach combining the expertise of neuromuscular and vascular specialists, physiatrist, podiatrist, occupational and physical therapist, and orthotist should be available to all patients to improve gait and balance, encourage independence in daily activities, and prevent complications. Regular foot examinations should be performed to assess foot deformity, integument, circulation, and sensation, and detect indolent infection, pressure sores, and small ulcers. More than half of all leg amputations are caused by neuropathy and impaired circulation, and may be preventable by attentive foot care.

Symptomatic pain management begins with the use of topical and oral medications. The American Academy of Neurology has published guidelines for the treatment of painful diabetic neuropathy (48). Pregabalin, an established and effective medication for relief of pain should be offered first, followed by capsaicin and isosorbide spray; Lidoderm patches; the antidepressants venlafaxine, duloxetine, and amitriptyline; the anticonvulsants gabapentin and valproate; and the opioids morphine sulfate, tramadol, and controlled-release oxycodone, all of which are probably effective. Other treatments, such as electrical stimulation, magnetic field treatment, low-intensity laser therapy, and Reiki therapy are not recommended.

When there is progressive motor disability, symptomatic treatment is rarely helpful and consideration should be given instead to stronger therapies. High-dose intravenous immunoglobulin (IVIg) therapy, which is administered with the expectation of improving motor function by modulating the humoral and cellular immune system, was effective therapy in 16 diabetic patients who fulfilled the most restrictive criteria for CIDP as judged by the Neuropathy Impairment Score (49), as was similar high-dose IVIg therapy in patients with painful multifocal, but not DSPN, as judged by the Visual Analog Scale, suggesting the multifactorial nature and heterogeneous causes of pain (50), and in LSRPN, the endpoint of which was improved Medical Research Council

(MRC) graced strength that enabled ambulation. (51). A randomized controlled trial of one gram three times weekly of intravenous methylprednisolone for 12 weeks led to equally significant objective improvement in primary outcome measures of 49 patients with DLSRPN compared to 26 patients with DLSRPN who received placebo when analyzed at 52 (52) and 104 weeks (53).

REFERENCES

1. Pryce TD. Perforating ulcers of both feet associated with diabetes and ataxic symptoms. *Lancet* 1887; 2:11–12.

2. Charcot M. Sur un cas de paraplegie diabetique. Lecon du 13 Decembre 1889. In, Guinon G, ed. *Clinique des maladies du system nerveu*. Paris: Progres Medical 1891; 1:257–284.

3. Pryce TD. On diabetic neuritis, with a clinical and pathological description of three cases of diabetic pseudo-tabes. *Brain* 1893; 16:416–424.

4. Bruns L. Ueber neuritische Lahmungen beim diabetes mellitus. *Berl Klin Wochenschr* 1890; 27:509–515.

5. Garland H, Tavener D. Diabetic myelopathy. *Br Med J* 1953; 1:1405–1408.

6. Garland H. Diabetic amyotrophy. *Br Med J* 1955; 2:1287–1290.

7. Dolman CL. The morbid anatomy of diabetic neuropathy. *Neurology* 1963; 13:135–142.

8. Raff MC. Sangalang V, Asbury AK. Ischemic mononeuropathy multiplex associated with diabetic mellitus. *Arch Neurol* 1968; 18:487–499.

9. Woltman HW, Wilder RM. Diabetes mellitus: pathological changes in the spinal cord and peripheral nerves. *Arch Intern Med* 1929; 44:576–605.

10. Fagerberg SE. Diabetic neuropathy-a clinical and histological study on the significance of vascular affections. *Acta Med Scand* 1959; 164(Suppl 345):1–97.

11. Dolman CL. The morbid anatomy of diabetic neuropathy. *Neurology* 1963; 13:135–142.

12. Greenbaum D, Richardson PC, Salmon MV, et al. Pathological observations on six cases of diabetic neuropathy. *Brain* 1964; 87:201–214.

13. Thomas PK, Lascelles RG. The pathology of diabetes mellitus. *Q J Med* 1966; 35:489–501.

14. Chopra JS, Fannin T. Pathology of diabetic neuropathy. *J Pathol* 1971; 104:175–184.

15. Thomas PK, Lascelles RG. Schwann-cell abnormalities in diabetic neuropathy. *Lancet* 1965; 1:1355–1357.

16. Raff MC, Sangalang V, Asbury AK et al. Ischemic mononeuropathy multiplex associated with diabetes mellitus. *Arch Neurol* 1968; 18:487–499.

17. Bradley WG, Chad D, Verghese JP, et al. Painful lumbosacral plexopathy with elevated erythrocyte sedimentation rate: a treatable inflammatory syndrome. *Ann Neurol* 1984; 15:457–464.

18. Asbury AK. Proximal diabetic neuropathy. *Ann Neurol* 1977; 2:179–180.

19. Dyck PJB, Norell JE, Dyck PJ. Microvasculitis and ischemia in diabetic lumbosacral radiculoplexus neuropathy. *Neurology* 1999; 53:2113–2121.

20. Younger DS. Diabetic lumbosacral radiculoplexus neuropathy: a postmortem studied patient and review of the literature. *J Neurol* 2011; 258:1364–1367.

21. Dyck PJ, Karnes JL, O'Brien P, et al. Fiber loss in primary and multifocal in sural nerves in diabetic polyneuropathy. *Ann Neurol* 1986; 19:425–439.

22. Gianini C, Dyck PJ. Ultrastructural morphometric abnormalities of sural nerve endothelial microvessels in diabetes mellitus. *Ann Neurol* 1994; 36:408–415.

23. Yasuda H, Dyck PJ. Abnormalities of endoneurial microvessels and sural nerve pathology in diabetic neuropathy. *Neurology* 1987; 37:20–28.

24. Sima AFF, Lattimer SA, Yagihashi S, et al. Axo-glial dysjunction: a novel structural lesion that accounts for poorly reversible slowing of nerve conduction in spontaneous diabetic BB-rat. *J Clin Invest* 1986; 77:474–484.

25. American Diabetes Association, American Academy of Neurology, Consensus Statement. Report and recommendations of the San Antonio conference on diabetic neuropathy. *Diabetes Care* 1988; 11:592–597.

26. Herman WH, Pop-Busul R, Braffett BH, et al. Use of the Michigan Neuropathy Screening Instrument as a measure of distal symmetrical peripheral neuropathy in type 1 diabetes; results from the Diabetes Control and Compliations Trial/Epidemiology of Diabetes Interventions and Compucations. *Diabet Med* 2012; Mar 14 [Epub ahead of print],

27. Raman R, Gupta A, Krishna S, et al. Prevalence and risk factors for diabetic microvascular complications in newly diagnosed type II diabetes mellitus. Sankara Nethralaya Diabetic Retinopathy Epidemiology and Molecular Genetic Study (SN-DREAMS, report 27). *J Diabetes Complications* 2012; March 23 [Epub ahead of print].

28. Younger DS, Rosoklija G, Hays AP. Peripheral nerve immunohistochemistry in diabetic neuropathy. *Semin Neurol* 1996; 16:139–142.

29. Vickova-Moravcova E, Bednarik J, Du Sek L, et al. Diagnostic validity of epidermal nerve fiber densities in painful sensory neuropathies. *Muscle Nerve* 2008; 37:50–60.

30. Younger DS, Rosoklija G, Hays AP, et al. Diabetic peripheral neuropathy: a clinicopathologic and immunohistochemical analysis of sural nerve biopsies. *Muscle Nerve* 1996; 19:722–727.

31. Younger DS. Diabetic neuropathy: a clinical and neuropathological study of 107 patients. *Neurology Research International* 2010, Article ID 140379.

32. Younger DS, Hays AP. Diabetic lumbosacral radiculoplexus neuropathy (DLRPN): case report of nerve biopsy and postmortem findings. *Neurology;* 70(Suppl1):A38.

33. Atkinson MA, Caclaren NK. The pathogenesis of insulin-dependent diabetes mellitus. *N Engl J Med* 1994; 331:1428–1436.

34. Grimaldi LME, Mertini G, Braghi S, et al. Heterogeneity of autoantibodies in stiffman syndrome. *Ann Neurol* 1993; 34:57–64.

35. Hanninen A, Jolkanen S, Salmi M, et al. Macrophages, T cell receptor usage, and endothelial cell activation in the pancreas at the onset of insulin-dependent diabetes mellitus. *J Clin Invest* 1992; 90:1901–1910.

36. Conrad B, Weidmann E, Trucco G, et al. Evidence for superantigen involvement in insulin-dependent diabetes mellitus aetiology. *Nature* (Letter) 1994; 371:351–355.

37. Johnson PC, Doll SC, Cromez DW. Pathogenesis of diabetic neuropathy. *Ann Neurol* 1986; 19:450–457.

38. Said G, Goulon-Golau C, Lacroix C, et al. Nerve biopsy findings in different patterns of proximal diabetic neuropathy. *Ann Neurol* 1994; 35:559–569.

39. Cornblath DR, Griffin DE, Welch D, et al. Quantitative analysis of endoneurial T-cells in human sural nerve biopsies. *J Neuroimmunol* 1990; 26:113–118.

40. Graham AR, Johnson PC. Direct immunofluorescence findings in peripheral nerve from patients with diabetic neuropathy. *Ann Neurol* 1985; 17:450–545.

41. Stewart JD, McKelvey R, Durcan L, et al. Chronic inflammatory demyelinating polyneuropathy (CIDP). *J Neurol Sci* 1996; 142:59–64.

42. Haq RU, Pendlebury WW, Fries TJ, et al. Chronic inflammatory demyelinating polyradiculoneuropathy in diabetic patients. *Muscle Nerve* 2003; 27:465–470.

43. Dyck PJ, Norell JE, Dyck PJ. Non-diabetic lumbosacral radiculoplexus neuropathy: natural history, outcome and comparison with the diabetic variety. *Brain* 2001; 124:1197–1207.

44. The Diabetes Control and Complications Trial Research Group. The effect of intensive treatment of diabetes on the development and progression of long-term complications in insulin dependent diabetes mellitus. *N Engl J Med* 1993; 329:977–986.

45. Lasker RD. The diabetes control and complications trial. Implications for policy and practice (editorial). *N Engl J Med* 1993; 329:1035–1036.

46. Dyck PJ, Zimmerman BR, Vilen TH, et al. Nerve glucose, fructose, sorbitol, myo-inositol, and fiber degeneration and regeneration in diabetic neuropathy. *N Engl J Med* 1988; 319:542–548.

47. Sutherland DER. Pancreatic transplantation: State of the art. *Transplant Proc* 1992; 24:762–766.

48. Bril V, England J, Franklin GM, et al. Evidence-based guideline: Treatment of painful diabetic neuropathy. Report of the American Academy of Neurology, the American Association of Neuromuscular and Electrodiagnostic Medicine, and the American Academy of Physical Medicine and Rehabilitation. *Neurology* 2011; 76:1758–1765.

49. Jann S, Branerio MA, Facchetti D, et al. Intravenous immunoglobulin is effective in patients with diabetes and with chronic inflammatory demyelinating polyneuropathy: long term followup. *J Neurol Neurosurg Psychiatry* 2009; 80:70–73.

50. Kawagashira Y, Watanabe H, Morozumi S, et al. Differential response to intravenous immunoglobulin (IVIg) therapy among multifocal and polyneuropathy types of painful diabetic neuropathy. *J Clin Neurosci* 2010; 17:1003–1008.

51. Varma A, Bradley WG. High-dose intravenous immunoglobulin therapy in chronic progressive lumbosacral plexopathy. *Neurology* 1994; 44:248–250.

52. Dyck PJB, O'Brien PC, Bosch EP, et al. Results of a controlled trial of IV methylprednisolone in diabetic lumbosacral radiculoplexus neuropathy (DLRPN): a preliminary indication of efficacy. *J Periph Nerv Syst* 2005; 101:21.

53. Dyck PJB, O'Brien P, Bosch P, et al. The multi-center double-blind controlled trial of IV methylprednisolone in diabetic lumbosacral radiculoplexus neuropathy. *Neurology* 2006; 66(Suppl2):A191.

CHAPTER 29

Multifocal Motor Neuropathy

Suraj A. Muley, Gareth J. Parry

INTRODUCTION

Parry and Clarke (1, 2) described a clinical lower motor neuron (LMN) syndrome of weakness, wasting, cramps, fasciculation, and preserved tendon reflexes, that differed both from motor neuron disease (MND) clinically by the presence of multifocal motor conduction block (MCB), and from multifocal demyelinating neuropathy (3), also characterized by MCB and absence of objective sensory involvement. Recognition of so-called multifocal motor neuropathy (MMN) is important because it responds to immunotherapy (4).

CLINICAL FEATURES

The essential clinical feature of MMN is slowly progressive multifocal distal limb weakness in the distribution of individual peripheral nerves, rather than that of individual myotomes as in MND. Cramps, fasciculation, and myokymia are common associated features, however cranial (5, 6) and respiratory muscle (7) involvement rarely occurs. Although CB may be found at almost any site along the length of an affected nerve, the resulting weakness is usually most severe distally in the arms. There may be palpable enlargement of tumor-like swellings of the nerve corresponding to sites of MCB and onion bulb formations on nerve ultrasonography (8), and magnetic resonance imaging (MRI) shows abnormal signal intensity changes (9). There may be vague sensory complaints such as numbness and paresthesias without objective sensory loss, and hypo- and areflexia in severely weak and wasted muscles. The disorder, which typically begins in the third to fourth decade, also occurs in childhood and older age, and shows slow and insidious progression such that patients may not recall when the weakness first began, or there can be rapid progression resulting in quadriplegia (10). Patients remain ambulatory and functional after years of progression; fatality from the disease is uncommon.

The similarity between the disorder and MND may be over-exaggerated with lingering uncertainty as to whether a given patient has been mistakenly diagnosed with ALS and will eventually prove to have MMN after detailed electrophysiological studies for MCB. The differences outweigh their similarities and MMN should rarely, if ever, be mistaken for frank ALS on clinical grounds alone. Bulbar involvement and frank upper motor neuron (UMN) signs, including Babinski, Hoffman signs, and clonus, commonly noted in MND, are not expected features of MMN. Moreover, severe weakness without severe wasting in the distribution of individual nerves as a result of MCB, and slow indolent progression over years to decades so commonly observed in MMN, is rarely if ever seen in MND, which always follows an inexorably fatal course.

LABORATORY EVALUATION

The general laboratory investigation of a patient with MMN is seldom helpful as there is typically no associated systemic illness. While serum protein electrophoresis and immunofixation electrophoresis are typically negative for monoclonal paraproteinemia, and systemic illness including cancer, are uncommon, one patient had motor neuropathy with MCB in association with chronic lymphocytic leukemia and IgG-κ paraproteinemia (11). A significant number of patients with MMN have detectable antibodies to glycolipid determinants.

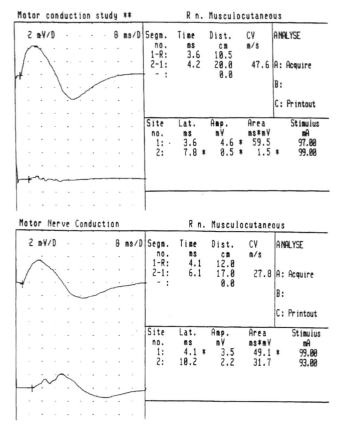

FIG. 1. The motor NCS along the musculocutaneous nerve shows severe CB between axilla and supraclavicular fossa (upper tracing). Following treatment with several courses of high-dose IVIg therapy, there is partial resolution of the CB (lower tracing). From, reference 41, with permission.

Electrodiagnostic Studies

Motor Nerve Conduction Studies

The diagnosis of MMN rests upon the finding of MCB (Figure 1) confined to motor axons (2, 12), which is most often detected along forearm and distal nerve segments of the arms, but can occur at any level or along the length of a single nerve. Clinical weakness emerges when the block reaches 80%, although lesser degrees of block can be noted in asymptomatic nerves. Although maximal conduction velocity through blocked segments is severely slowed when measured over short segments of 3 to 10 centimeters in length (13), when evaluated over longer lengths of nerve by conventional NCS, the block may be less severe and nerve conduction velocity (NCV) may even be normal, suggesting highly focal slowing. Some patients with typical clinical aspects of MMN may not have identifiable MCB (14). So-called MMN without conduction block (MMNWOCB) (15, 16) is postulated to have very proximal or distal MCB that require more advanced electrophysiological techniques such as the triple stimulation technique to uncover MCB (17).

Sensory Nerve Conduction Studies

Sensory conduction was normal distal to, and through, blocked mixed nerve segments ranging from 90% (2) to complete MCB (18). Moreover, there was no difference in sensory nerve action potential (SNAP) amplitudes across segments of severe motor block in patients with MMN compared to controls (13).

Electromyography

Needle electromyography (EMG) shows denervation in weak muscles and a paucity of fibrillation and fasciculation potentials with reduced voluntary motor unit potential (MUP) recruitment that varies depending upon the degree and duration of MCB and distal axonal degeneration. Myokymia, when present, is an important clue to demyelination.

CONDUCTION BLOCK

Conduction Block in Acute Demyelination

There is normally a small drop in the amplitude of the compound muscle action potential (CMAP) along adjacent segments due to physiologic temporal dispersion that does not exceed 15% to 20% along the wrist-to-elbow segment. A drop in the CMAP amplitude greater than 20% is strongly suggestive of MCB provided that temporal dispersion does not exceed 15% to 20%. When demyelinating neuropathy progresses for more than a few days, the range of conduction velocities increases and abnormal temporal dispersion develops, resulting in decreased CMAP amplitudes. Therefore amplitude reduction alone is insufficient to define conduction block. The electrodiagnostic features of acute conduction block due to pure demyelination were classically examined by injecting antibodies to galactocerebroside, a component of myelin into rat sciatic nerve (19). Entirely normal proximal CMAP amplitude progressively fell to a nadir in three hours, without temporal dispersion and with preservation of segmental conduction velocities.

Pathogenesis of Pure Motor Block

It is not known why conduction block in MMN is confined to motor axons. One explanation is the difference between the antigenic properties of motor and sensory nerve myelin, which differs in ceramide composition of gangliosides imparting antigenic differences (20). Another explanation is the greater safety factor for impulse transmission in sensory axons that leads to preferential conduction block in motor fiber alone (21). However, this is unlikely since the largest diameter axons have the most secure conduc-

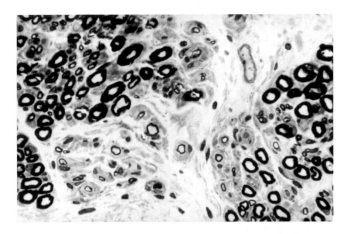

FIG. 2. Ulnar nerve biopsy from the axilla at a site of conduction block. There is an area of demyelination in the center, but adjacent fascicles are spared. From, reference 30, with permission.

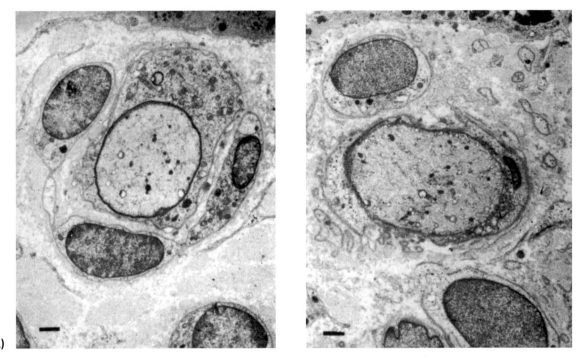

(A)   (B)

FIG. 3. Electron microscopy of a biopsy taken from the medial pectoral nerve adjacent to a site of conduction block in the medial cord of the brachial plexus. **(A)** A thinly myelinated large-diameter axon surrounded by a small onion bulb. Bar, 1 m. **(B)** A large-diameter axon entirely devoid of myelin. Bar=1 μm. From, reference 31, with permission.

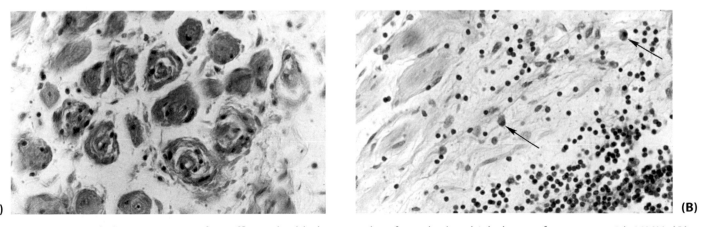

(A)   (B)

FIG. 4. Low-power light microscopy of paraffin-embedded nerve taken from the brachial plexus of a woman with MMN. **(A)** There is exuberant onion bulb formation and a marked increase in the endoneurial interstitial space. **(B)** Prominent endoneurial mononuclear cell infiltration with occasional macrophages (arrows). From, reference 32, with permission.

tion and motor axons are clearly the largest. Demyelination might be confined to motor fascicles within the nerve trunk, whereas the sensory fascicles are spared. Variation in the extent of the demyelination seen in different fascicles is observed in chronic inflammatory demyelinating polyradiculoneuorpathy (CIDP), and the differences may occasionally be striking (22).

Role of Antiglycolipid Antibodies

Patients with MMN and serum IgG and IgM antibodies to GM1 gangliosides have been described (23, 24). Three groups were discerned, one with distal weakness and proximal conduction block, the majority of which had high anti-GM1 ganglioside antibody titers, and two others, presenting with either distal or proximal weakness without MCB. Two-thirds of those with distal involvement, without MCB also had elevated anti-GM1 ganglioside antibodies. Since then, increased titers of anti-GM1 ganglioside antibodies have been noted regardless of the motor neuron or concomitant neuropathic disorder. The prevalence of anti-GM1 ganglioside antibodies in MMN varies from 20% to 85%, in part because there is no consensus on the most reproducible assay for this antibody (25). Elevated anti-GM1 ganglioside antibodies are also elevated in MMNWOCB wherein they provide a useful marker of the disorder. Patients with MMN and anti-GM1 ganglioside antibodies have more severe weakness, disability, and axon loss than those without such antibodies, suggesting a role for them in MMN pathogenesis (26), however this remains an unproven hypothesis since initial reports of anti-GM1 ganglioside antibody-mediated focal demyelination and sodium channel blockade (27) were contradicted by subsequent studies (28). Moreover, MCB can be successfully induced by sera from patients with MMN having no anti-GM1 ganglioside antibodies, suggesting instead that soluble disease mediators other than anti-GM1 ganglioside antibodies play the key pathogenic role in MMN (25, 29).

PATHOLOGY

Motor Nerve

The motor nerve pathology of MMN, derived from biopsies of mixed nerves in affected patients (30) showed patchy demyelination, many thinly myelinated axons, including some with onion bulb formations, suggesting repeated demyelination and remyelination without inflammatory cell infiltration (Figure 2). Biopsy of a medial pectoral nerve (31) (Figures 3A and B) showed non-inflammatory multifocal enlargements of the brachial plexus that correlated with severe MCB on intraoperative NCS across the site of enlargement. In addition, there were large diameter axons

with very thin myelin sheaths on electron microscopy (EM), including some devoid of myelin surrounded only by Schwann cell processes and redundant basal lamina forming rudimentary onion bulbs, increased endoneurial space, and thickening of the perineurium. Biopsy of a supraclavicular mass (32) (Figures 4A and B) in a patient with MMN showed exuberant onion bulb formation with increased endoneurial space, and mononuclear inflammatory cell infiltration concentrated around endoneurial venules, extending into the general endoneurial compartment. Fascicular nerve biopsy in another patient with MMN (33) showed a predominance of multifocal fiber degeneration without segmental demyelination or onion bulb formation due instead to presumed antibody-mediated attack on the axolemma at the node of Ranvier.

Sensory Nerve

The only quantitative study of sensory nerves in MMN (34) showed mild demyelination in all 11 nerves so studied, consisting of an increased number of thinly myelinated fibers, miniature onion bulbs, rare demyelinated fibers, and active macrophage-mediated demyelination, without endoneurial edema or inflammatory cell infiltration.

TREATMENT

Consensus guidelines of the European Federation of Neurological Societies and Peripheral Nerve Society for the treatment of MMN (35) concluded that after defining MMN by clinical and electrophysiological criteria, high dose intravenous immune globulin (IVIg) was first-line therapy with other immunosuppressant drugs as possible alternative modes of therapy.

Intravenous Immunoglobulin

High dose IVIg was recommended by the Therapeutics and Technology Assessment Subcommittee of the American Academy of Neurology (AAN) (36), with up to 80% of the patients favorably responding. In a natural history analysis (37), and three randomized, placebo-controlled trials (38–40), there was significant short-term improvement in up to 94% of patients, with contrasting results of long-term efficacy which appeared to be influenced by the duration of untreated disease, degree of axonal loss, and faulty nerve regeneration. Neither MCB nor anti-GM1 ganglioside antibody status were reliable predictors of treatment responsiveness. One of three patients so treated (41) had improvement in MCB that paralleled the clinical response demonstrated in Figure 1, the rapidity of which could only be explained by reversal of MCB. The inability to document reversal of conduction block in some cases probably reflects sites of MCB technically difficult to evaluate, such as nerve roots and proximal nerve trunks. Segmental amplitude ratios may not improve with treatment because of the slowly conducting components, giving rise to dispersed responses that occur too late to contribute to the CMAP amplitude. Subcutaneous administration (SCIG), advocated as an alternative to IVIg therapy in MMN (42), was associated with a small increase in follow-up muscle strength in a two-year tolerability trial, without major side effects.

Cyclophosphamide

Cyclophosphamide is employed in severely impaired patients with MMN that are refractory or intolerant of IVIg. Although efficacy was first established with a single 3 g/m² intravenous dose over 8 days followed by oral therapy for 10 months (23), a similar result was achieved by pretreating for two days with plasma exchange that allowed a 50% to 70% reduction in the intravenous dose (23, 43) and a one- to two-year period of sustained improvement after cessation of treatment.

Azathioprine

There are anecdotal reports of improvement or stabilization of MMN when treating with azathioprine alone or in combination with IVIg (44).

Rituximab

Rituximab (RTX) is a monoclonal antibody that depletes greater than 90% of circulating B-lymphocytes and has been used with varying success in MMN. It was administered to three patients with MMN who had become increasingly less responsive to IVIg and showed sustained improvement following RTX monotherapy (45). Although RTX was later employed in an open-label trial and administered safely to six patients with MMN, it did not reduce the concomitant dose of IVIg (46). It was also successfully administered as long-term complementary treatment to an elderly patient who developed severe quadriparesis while being treated with IVIg therapy that was previously unresponsive to azathioprine, mycophenolate mofetyl, and cyclophosphamide. However, in the end, he remained dependent upon IVIg.

Interferon-beta 1A

Nine patients with MMN were treated with interferon-(INF)-beta1A who had previously responded favorably to IVIg without any additional effect in six, and improvement in three patients (47). Three other patients with MMN were given INF-beta-1A as an adjunctive measure to enhance the effect of IVIg leading to a prolonged interval of IVIg infusions in one patient. After discontinuation of INF–beta1A there was no measurable changes in muscle strength, neuropathy cause and treatment (NCAT) score, quality of life, or electrophysiological parameters (48).

Corticosteroids and Plasma Exchange

Corticosteroids are not recommended for MMN (35) However, plasma exchange was employed to increase the efficacy of a smaller dose of parenteral cyclophosphamide (43), and as adjunctive therapy to a patient with resolving tetraplegia on IVIg to ameliorate the ability to walk (49).

REFERENCES

1. Parry GJ, Clarke S. Pure motor neuropathy with multifocal conduction block masquerading as motor neuron disease. *Muscle Nerve* 1985; 8:167.
2. Parry GJ, Clarke S. Multifocal acquired demyelinating neuropathy masquerading as motor neuron disease. *Muscle Nerve* 1988; 11:103–107.
3. Lewis RA, Sumner AJ, Brown MJ, Asbury AK. Multifocal demyelinating neuropathy with persistent conduction block. *Neurology* 1982; 32:958–964.
4. Vlam L, van der Pol WL, Cats EA, et al. Multifocal motor neuropathy: diagnosis, pathogenesis and treatment strategies. *Nat Rev Neurol* 2011; 8:48–58.
5. Magistris MR, Roth G. Motor neuropathy with multifocal persistent conduction blocks. *Muscle Nerve* 1992; 15:1056–1057.
6. Kaji R, Shibasaki H, Kimura J. Multifocal demyelinating motor neuropathy: cranial nerve involvement and immunoglobulin therapy. *Neurology* 1992; 42:506–509.
7. Van den Bergh P, Logigian EL, Kelly JJ Jr. Motor neuropathy with multifocal conduction blocks. *Muscle Nerve* 1989; 11:26–31.
8. Beekman R, van den Berg LH, Franssen, H, et al. Ultrasonography shows extensive nerve enlargements in multifocal motor neuropathy. *Neurology* 2005; 65:305–307.
9. Van den Berg-Vos RM, Franssen H, Wokke JH, et al. Multifocal motor neuropathy: diagnostic criteria that predict the response to immunoglobulin treatment. *Ann Neurol* 2000; 48:919–926.
10. Roth G, Rohr J, Magistris MR, Ochsner F. Motor neuropathy with proximal multifocal persistent conduction block, fasciculations and myokymia. Evolution to tetraplegia. *Eur Neurol* 1986; 25:416–423.
11. Younger DS, Rowland LP, Hays AP, et al. Lymphoma, motor neuron diseases, and amyotrophic lateral sclerosis. *Ann Neurol* 1991; 29:78–86.
12. Pestronk A, Cornblath DR, Ilyas AA, et al. A treatable multifocal motor neuropathy with antibodies to GM1 ganglioside. *Ann Neurol* 1988; 24:73–78.
13. Krarup C, Stewart MB, Sumner AJ, Pestronk A, Lipton SA. A syndrome of asymmetric limb weakness with motor conduction block. *Neurology* 1990; 40:118–127,
14. Pakiam AS, Parry GJ. Multifocal motor neuropathy without overt conduction block. *Muscle Nerve* 1998; 21:243–245.

15. Delmont E, Azulay JP, Giorgi R, et al. Multifocal motor neuropathy with and without conduction block: a single entity? *Neurology* 2006; 67:592–596.

16. Menkes DL. Multifocal motor neuropathy with and without conduction block: a single entity? *Neurology* 2007; 68:1161–1162.

17. Deroide N, Uzenot D, Verschueren A, et al. Triple-stimulation technique in multifocal neuropathy with conduction block. *Muscle Nerve* 2007; 35:632.

18. Pouget J, Azulay J-P, Bile-Turc F, et al. Sensory function study in 15 cases of multifocal motor neuropathy. *Muscle Nerve* 1994; 17: S237.

19. Sumner AJ, Saida K, Saida T, Silberberg DH, Asbury AK. Acute conduction block associated with experimental antiserum-mediated demyclination of peripheral nerve. *Ann Neurol* 1982; 11:469–477.

20. Ogawa-Goto K, Funamoto N, Abe T, Nagashima K. Different ceramide compositions of gangliosides between human motor and sensory nerves. *J Neurochem* 1990; 55:1486–1493.

21. Sumner AJ. Separating motor neuron diseases from pure motor neuropathies. Multifocal motor neuropathy with persistent conduction block. *Adv Neurol* 1991; 56:399–403.

22. Nukada H, Pollock M, Haas LF. Is ischemia implicated in chronic multifocal demyelinating neuropathy? *Neurology* 1989; 39, 9:106–110.

23. Pestronk A, Cornblath DR, Ilyas AA, et al. A treatable multifocal motor neuropathy with antibodies to GM1 ganglioside. *Ann Neurol* 1988; 24:73–78.

24. Pestronk A, Chaudhry V, Feldman EL, et al. Lower motor neuron syndromes defined by patterns of weakness, nerve conduction abnormalities, and high titers of antiglycolipid antibodies. *Ann Neurol* 1990; 27:316–326.

25. Gooch CL, Amato AA. Are anti-ganglioside antibodies of clinical value in multifocal motor neuropathy? *Neurology* 2010; 75:1950–1951.

26. Cats EA, Jacobs BC, Yuki N, et al. Multifocal motor neuropathy. Association of anti-GM1 antibodies with clinical features. *Neurology* 2010, 75:1961–1967.

27. Uncini A, Santoro M, Corbo M, et al. Conduction abnormalities induced by sera of patients with multifocal motor neuropathy and anti-GM1 antibodies. *Muscle Nerve* 1993; 16:610–615.

28. Harvey G, Toyka K, Zielasek J, et al. Failure of anti-GM-1 IgG or IgM to induce conduction block following intraneural transfer. *Muscle Nerve* 1995; 18:388–394.

29. Roberts M, Willison H, Vincent A, et al. Multifocal motor neuropathy human sera block motor nerve conduction in mice. *Ann Neurol* 1995; 38:111–118.

30. Auer RN, Bell RB, Lee MA. Neuropathy with onion bulb formations and pure motor manifestations. *Can J Neurol Sci* 1989; 6:194–197.

31. Kaji R, Oka N, Tsuji T, et al. Pathological findings at the sites of conduction block in multifocal motor neuropathy. *Ann Neurol* 1993; 33:152–158.

32. Midani H, Parry GJ, Day JW: Electrophysiology and brachial plexus pathology in a woman misdiagnosed as HMSN-I. *Muscle Nerve* 1993; 16:1103A.

33. Taylor BV, Dyck P.J, Engelstad J, et al. Multifocal motor neuropathy: pathologic alterations at the site of conduction block. *J Neuropathol Exp Neurol* 2004; 63:129–137.

34. Corse AM, Chaudhry V, Crawford TO, et al. Sensory nerve pathology in multifocal motor neuropathy. *Ann Neurology* 1996; 39:319–325.

35. European Federation of Neurological Societies: Peripheral Nerve Society, van Schaik IN, Bouche P, Illa I, et al. European Federation of Neurological Societies/Peripheral Nerve Society guidelines on management of multifocal motor neuropathy. *Eur J Neurol* 2006; 13:802–808.

36. Patwa HS, Chaudhry V, Katzberg H, et al. Evidence-based guideline: intravenous immunoglobulin in the treatment of neuromuscular disorders: Report of the Therapeutics and Technology Assessment Subcommittee of the American Academy of Neurology. *Neurology* 2012; 78:1009–1015.

37. Taylor BV, Wright RA, Harper CM, et al. Natural history of 46 patients with multifocal motor neuropathy with conduction block. *Muscle Nerve* 2000; 23:900–908.

38. Cats EA, van der Pol WL, Piepers S, et al. Correlates of outcome and response to IVIg in 88 patients with multifocal motor neuropathy. *Neurology* 2010; 75:818–825.

39. Slee M, Selvan A, Donaghy M. Multifocal motor neuropathy: the diagnostic spectrum and response to treatment. *Neurology* 2007; 69:1680–1687.

40. Leger JM, Viala K, Cancalon F, et al. Intravenous immunoglobulin as short- and long-term therapy of multifocal motor neuropathy: a retrospective study of response to IVIg and of its predictive criteria in 40 patients. *J Neurol Neurosurg Psychiatry* 2008; 79:93–96.

41. Parry GJ. AAEM Case Report #30: Multifocal motor neuropathy. *Muscle Nerve* 1996;19:269–276.

42. Harbo T, Andersen H, Jakobsen J. Long-term therapy with high doses of subcutaneous immunoglobulin in multifocal motor neuropathy. *Neurology* Oct 2010; 75(15)1377–1380.

43. Pestronk A, Lopate G, Kornberg AJ, et al. Distal lower motor neuron syndrome with high-titer serum IgM anti-GM1 antibodies: improvement following immunotherapy with monthly plasma exchange and intravenous cyclophosphamide. *Neurology* 1994; 44:2027–2031.

44. Hausmanova-Petrusewicz I, Rovisnka-Marchinska K, Kopec K. Chronic acquired demyelinating motor neuropathy. *Acta Neurol Scand* 1991; 84:40–45.

45. Stieglbauer K, Topakian R, Hinterberger G, et al. Beneficial effects of rituximab monotherapy in multifocal motor neuropathy. *Neuromuscul Disord* 2009; 19:473–475.

46. Chaudhry V, Cornblath DR. An open-label trial of rituximab (Rituxan® in multifocal motor neuropathy. *J Peripher Nerv Syst* 2010; 15:196–201.

47. Van den Berg-Vos RM, Van den Berg LH, Franssen H, et al. Treatment of multifocal motor neuropathy with interferon-beta 1A. *Neurology* 2000; 54:1518–1521.

48. Radziwill AJ, Botex SA, Novy J, et al. Interferon beta-1a as adjunctive treatment for multifocal motor neuropathy: an open label trial. *J Peripher Nerv Syst* 2009; 14:201–202.

49. Claus D, Specht S, Zieschang M. Plasmapheresis in multifocal motor neuropathy: a case report. *J Neurol Neurosurg Psychiatry* 2000; 68:533–535.

CHAPTER 30

Charcot-Marie-Tooth Disorders

Gregory M. Pastores, David S. Younger

Charcot-Marie-Tooth disease (CMT) disorders refers to inherited peripheral neuropathies named for the three investigators who described them in the late 19th century. It affects approximately one in 2,500 individuals and is the commonest inherited neurological disorder. The majority of affected patients display autosomal dominant (AD) inheritance, although X-linked (XL) dominant and autosomal recessive (AR) forms occur, however sporadic cases occur as new mutations. The majority of CMT neuropathies are demyelinating, although up to one-third have a primary axonal basis. The typical CMT phenotype occurs in childhood or early adulthood with distal weakness, sensory loss, pes cavus, hammertoes, steppage gait, and areflexia. Some patients develop severe disability in infancy while others develop few if any symptoms of disease. At least 40 separate causal genes encoding protein components of the axonal cytoskeleton, Schwann cells homeostasis, and neuronal function affect peripheral nerves (1), leading to an intersection of dysfunction and overlapping phenotypes. (2, 3) (Table 1).

CLASSIFICATION

Historically, the classification of CMT disease commenced with an assumption that it was possible to classify the different clinically and genetically distinct forms into two groups, type 1 with slow NCV and type 2, with normal or near-normal NCV (4). Recognizing the bimodal distribution of NCV in genetic polyneuropathies, the threshold of 38 meters per second (m/s) appeared to further separate patients into the two categories of demyelinating and axonal polyneuropathy (5). With the advent of histochemical studies to evaluate peripheral cutaneous nerve biopsy tissue, it

was possible to confirm the presence of primary demyelinating and axonal neuropathology. In demyelinating CMT forms, the presumed genetic defect affects Schwann cells first, which tightly communicate with axons to regulate their development, function, and maintenance, and failing this interaction due to Schwann cell damage, there is denser axonal neurofilaments with consequent secondary axonal damage and degeneration typified by demyelinating CMT. By contrast, axonal forms of CMT result from disturbances in axonal transport causing subsequent axonal degeneration. Although the optimal fashion of classifying CMT disease would be to classify disease-causing genes on the basis of altered function contributing to the primary insult to the peripheral nerve or perikaryon, this becomes complicated since each of the more than 30 known CMT disease-causing genes usually can have more than one function, and the attributed molecular mechanisms of injury to each gene remains speculative at best. With a steady increase in the number of CMT forms, it has been useful to subcategorize them by the intersection of inheritance pattern and underlying electrophysiology and pathology, including demyelinating AD (CMT1) and AR (CMT4), axonal AD and AR (CMT2), AD intermediate (CMTDI) with intermediate median motor NCV, XL (CMTX) forms wherein the primary pathology resides in the peripheral nerve process; hereditary motor neuronopathy (HMN) wherein the primary pathology resides in the motor perikaryon.

There are six recognized CMT1 genes and associated chromosomal loci that lead to clinically indistinguishable subtypes due to mutation or sequence changes separately in the peripheral myelin protein (PMP) 22 gene (CMT1A and CMT1E); myelin protein zero (MPZ) gene (CMT1B); small integral membrane protein of lysosome late endosome/lipopolysaccharide-induced necrosis alpha factor (*LITAF/SIM-PLE*) gene (CMT1C); early growth response 2 (*EGR2*) gene (CMT1D); and intermediate filament protein (*NEFL*) gene (CMT1F). Affected children with a classic CMT1 phenotype present in the first or second decade with a delay in the onset of walking before or after 15 months, depending upon the clinical severity and degree of uniform NCV slowing in nerve conduction studies (NCS), which is typically between 15 and 25 m/s, in association with palpable hypertrophic nerves, pes cavus foot deformity, and bilateral extensor foot weakness. The clinical progression is typically slow, with fewer than 5% of patients becoming wheelchair dependent.

There are 15 chromosomal loci of CMT2 (CMT2A1 and 2; 2B, B1, B2, 2C-L and N) that correspond to mutations in the kinesin-like protein (*KIF1B*) and mitofusin-2 (*MFN2*) genes (CMT2A1 and 2), Ras-related protein Rab-7 (*RAB7A*) gene (CMT2B), lamin A/C (*LMNA*) and mediator of RNA polymerase II transcription subunit 25 (*MED25*) genes (CMT2B1 and 2); in the transient receptor potential cation channel subfamily V member 4 (*TRPV4*) gene (CMT2C), glycyl-tRNA synthase (*GARS*) gene (CMT2D), neurofilament light polypeptide (*NEFL*) gene (CMT2E), heat-shock protein beta-1 (*HSPB1*) gene (CMT2F), ganglioside-induced differentiation-associated protein-1 (*GDAP1*) gene (CMT2H and K), *MPZ* gene (CMT2I and J), *HSPB8* gene (CMTL), and alanyl-tRNA synthetase, cytoplasmic (*AARS*) gene (CMT2N). Patients affected with CMT2 present with pes cavus foot deformity, axonal peripheral neuropathy characterized by less disabling distal muscle weakness, wasting, less prominent sensory loss, normal or near-normal motor NCV, non-hypertrophic nerves, and less prominent footdrop than those with CMT1.

There are four recognized chromosomal loci and four genes associated with AD intermediate CMT (CMTDI), including 10q24.1-q25.1 (CMTDIA), dynamin 2 (*DNM2*) (CMTDIB), tyrosyl-tRNA synthetase (*YARS*) (CMTDIC), and *MPZ* (CMTDID). Patients affected with CMTDI display a relatively typical CMT phenotype with clinical and pathological evidence of both a myelinopathy and axonopathy, with motor NCV intermediate between those of CMT1 and CMT2.

There are nine chromosomal loci of CMT4 and 8CMT4 subtypes (CMT4A, B1, B2, C-F, H, J) that correspond to mutations in the ganglioside-induced differentiation-associated protein 1 (*GDAP1*) gene (CMT4A), myotubularin-related protein 2 (*MTMR2*) gene (CMT4B1), myotubularin-related protein 13 (*SBF2*) gene (CMT4B2), SH3 domain and tetratricopeptide repeats-containing protein 2 (*SH3TC2*) gene (CMT4C), *NDRG1* gene (CMT4D), *ERG2* (CMT4E), periaxin (*PRX*) gene (CMT4F), *FYVE*, *RhoGEF* and PII domain-containing protein 4 (*FGD4*) gene (CMT4H), and in the phosphatidylinositol 3, 5 biphosphate (*FIG4*) gene (CMT4J). Originally described as hypertrophic polyneu-

ropathy, the clinical features of affected infants and children born to unaffected parents manifest pes cavus, ataxia, pes cavus, kyphoscoliosis, distal sensory and motor deficits, and muscular atrophy predominating in the legs, progressing in a length-dependent patter, with palpably hypertrophic nerves, Argyll-Robertson pupils, very slow motor NCV, elevated cerebrospinal fluid (CSF) protein, and onion bulb formation.

There are five chromosomal loci of XL CMT (CMTX1-5) respectively localized to the gap junction beta-1 protein (connexin 32) (*GJB1*) gene (CMTX1), Xp22.2 (CMTX2), Xp26 (CMTX3), Xq24-q26.1 (CMTX4), and the ribose-phosphate pyrophosphokinase 1 (*PRPS1*) gene (CMTX5). CMTX presents in male children from infancy to early childhood with delayed motor development, sensorineural hearing loss, tremor, pathologic fractures, and transient CNS disturbances. Axon loss is reflected in low compound muscle action potentials (CMAP) amplitudes, while carrier females show abnormal neurologic or neurophysiologic features of a lesser degree.

Finally, there are five genes and four other designated genetic loci for distal HMN, respectively, including HSPB8 (HMN2A), *HSPB1* (HMN2B), *HSPB3* (HMN2C), *GARS* and *BSCL2* (HMN5), and 7q34-q36 (HMN1), 11q13 (HMN3 and 4), 2q14 (HMN7A), 2p13.1 (HMN7B). The growing number of genes attests to the complexity of pathways and purported mechanisms that contribute to CMT etiopathogenesis making genetic testing ever more important in understanding the pathogenetic mechanisms. The latter include disturbances in transcriptional regulation, protein turnover, protein synthesis, stress responses, apoptosis, Schwann cell-axonal interactions, axonal transport, and mitochondrial dysfunction.

CHARCOT-MARIE-TOOTH TYPE 1 DISORDERS

CMT1A

First noted by Lupski (6), CMT1A is caused by duplication or mutation at the 17p12 locus of the *PMP22* gene encoding PMP22 (Table 1). Patel and colleagues (7) later showed that the *PMP22* gene was located entirely within the CMTA1 duplication and that *PMP22* was duplicated and not disrupted in CMT1A. Chance and colleagues (8) identified an interstitial deletion of distal 17p11.2 that included the *PMP22* gene in patients with hereditary neuropathy with liability to pressure palsies (HNPP). Roa and colleagues (9) identified point mutations in the *PMP22* gene. PMP22 is a major component of myelin expressed in the compact portion of essentially all myelinated fibers of the peripheral nervous system (PNS) and produced by Schwann cells. CMT1A is the most common form of CMT occuring in approximately 70% of CMT1 patients with this duplication. The *PMP22* gene

TABLE 1. The Genetic Basis of Charcot-Marie-Tooth Disorders

CMT	Inheritance Pattern	Neuropathy Pattern	Gene Symbol	Gene Locus	GENE OMIM No.	Gene Product	Phenotype OMIM No.
CMT1A	AD	Demyelinating	PMP22	17p12	601097	Peripheral myelin protein 22	118220
CMT1B	AD	Demyelinating	MPZ	1q23.3	159440	Myelin P0 protein	118200
CMT1C	AD	Demyelinating	LITAF	16p13.13	603795	Liposaccharide-induced tumor necrosis factor- alpha factor	601098
CMT1D	AD	Demyelinating	EGR2	10q21.3	129010	Early growth response protein 2	607678
CMT1E	AD	Demyelinating	PMP22	17p12	601097	Peripheral myelin protein 22	118300
CMT1F	AD	Demyelinating	NEFL	8p21.2	162280	Neurofilament light polypeptide	607734
HNPP	AD	Demyelinating	PMP22	17p12	601097	Peripheral myelin protein 22	162500
CMTX1	XL	Axonal/ demyelinating	GJB1	Xq13.1	304040	Gap junction beta-1 protein (connexin 32)	302800
CMTX2	XL	Axonal/ demyelinating	-	Xp22.2	-	-	302801
CMTX3	XL	Axonal/ demyelinating	-	Xq26	-	-	302802
CMTX4	XL	Axonal/ demyelinating	-	Xq42-q26.1	-	-	310490
CMTX5	XL	Axonal/ demyelinating	PRPS1	Xq22.3	311850	Ribose-phosphate pyrophosphokinase 1	311070
CMT2A1	AD	Axonal	KIF1B	1p36.22	605995	Kinesin-like protein KIF1B	118210
CMT2A2	AD	Axonal	MFN2	1p36.22	608507	Mitofusin-2	609260
CMT2B	AD	Axonal	RAB7	3q21.3	602298	Ras-related protein Rab-7	600882
CMT2B1	AR	Axonal	LMNA	1q22	150330	Lamin A/C	603588
CMT2B2	AR	Axonal	MED25	19q13.13	610197	Mediator of RNA polymerase II transcription subunit 25	605589
CMT2C	AD	Axonal	TRPV4	12q24.11	605427	Transient receptor potential cation channel subfamily V member 4	606071
CMT2D	AD	Axonal	GARS	7p14.3	600287	Glycyl-tRNA synthetase	601472
CMT2E	AD	Axonal	NEFL	8p21.2	162280	Neurofilament light polypeptide	607684
CMT2F	AD	Axonal	HSPB1	7q11.23	602195	Heat-shock protein beta-1	606595
CMT2G	AD	Axonal	-	12q12-q13.3	-	-	608591
CMT2H	AR	Axonal	-	8q21.3	-	-	-
CMT2I	AD	Axonal	MPZ	1q23.3	159440	Myelin P0 protein	607677
CMT2J	AD	Axonal	MPZ	1q23.3	159440	Myelin P0 protein	607736
CMT2K	AR	Axonal	GDAP1	8q21.11	606598	Ganglioside-induced differentiation-associated – protein-1	607831
CMT2L	AD	Axonal	HSPB8	12q24.23	608614	Heat-shock protein beta-8	608673
CMT2N	AD	Axonal	AARS	16q22.1	601065	Alanyl-tRNA synthetase, cytoplasmic	613287
CMT2O	AD	Axonal	DYNC1H1	14q32.31	600112	Cytoplasmic dynein 1 heavy chain 1	614228
CMT4A	AR	Demyelinating	GDAP1	8q21.11	606598	Ganglioside-induced differentiation-associated protein-1	214400
CMT4B1	AR	Demyelinating	MTMR2	11q21	603557	Myotubulurin-related protein 2	601382
CMT4B2	AR	Demyelinating	SBF2	11p15.4	607697	Myotubularin-related protein 13	604563
CMT4C	AR	Demyelinating	SH3TC2	5q32	608206	SH3 domain and tetratrico-peptide repeats-containing protein 2	601596
CMT4D	AR	Demyelinating	NDRG1	8q24.22	605262	Protein NDRG1	601455
CMT4E	AR	Demyelinating	MPZ	159440	1q23.3	Myelin P0 protein	605253
			EGR2	129010	10q21.3	Early growth response protein 2	605253

Abbreviations: AD, autosomal dominant; AR, autosomal recessive; XL, X-linked
OMIM, Online Mendelian Inheritance in Man, OMIM®. McKusick-Nathans Institute of Genetic Medicine, Johns Hopkins University (Baltimore, MD), [1/2/13]. World Wide Web URL:http://omim.org

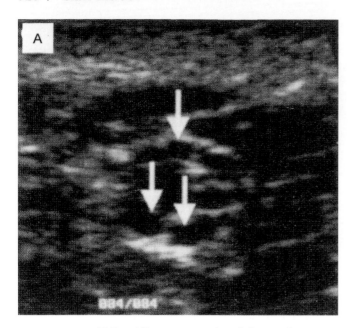
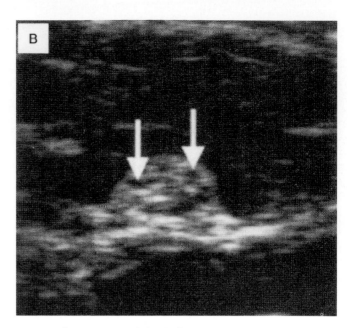

FIG. 1. Ultrasonography of the median nerve in a patient with CMT1A. With high-frequency transducers, peripheral nerves show a typical fascicular structure in longitudinal sections. In CMT1A, the nerve and the fascicles (arrows) appear enlarged compared to those from a normal control.

encodes an integral membrane protein that is a major component of myelin in the PNS. Missense mutations in *PMP22* cause the Trembler (Tr) and TremblerJ, (TrJ) naturally occurring mouse models of CMT1. CMT1A represents the typical CMT phenotype. Patients are slow runners in childhood, develop foot problems in their teenage years due to high arches and hammer toes, and often require orthotics for ankle support as adults. Variable degrees of hand weakness occur, typically lagging about ten years behind the development of

foot weakness. Sensory loss is variable and affects large nerve fiber modalities of vibration and proprioception, and small nerve fiber modalities of pain and temperature sensation. Almost all patients with CMT1A have absent deep tendon reflexes. Enlarged nerve trunks may be palpated in the arm. While the combination of weak ankles and decreased proprioception often leads to problems with balance, the vast majority of patients remain ambulatory throughout their life, which is not shortened by their disease. Additional features

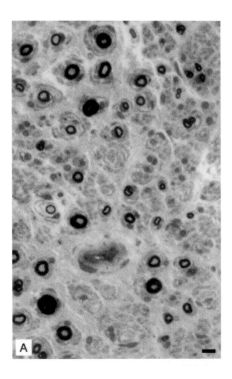
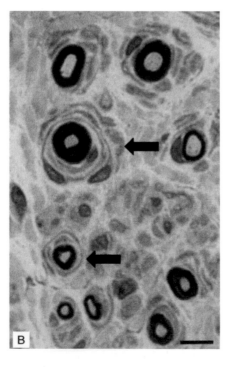

FIG. 2. Sural nerve biopsy from a patient with CMT1A. The density of the myelinated fibers is decreased from normal. Onion bulbs (arrows) made by concentric proliferation of Schwann cell cytoplasm around normally or thinly myelinated fibers are frequently observed. Semithin section, Toluidine blue; bars = 10 μm.

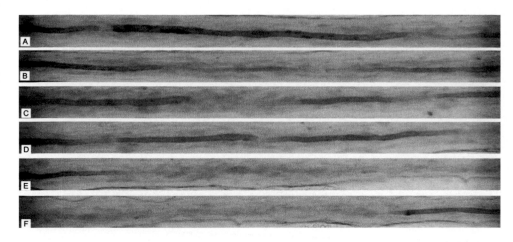

FIG. 3. Sural nerve biopsy from a patient with CMT1A. Teased fiber preparation. Several internodes lacking myelin (demyelinated internodes) can be seen along a single fiber (A–F) O.T. 2%

include postural tremor in the Roussy-Levy syndrome, and muscle cramps. Occasionally, patients develop a severe phenotype in infancy while others develop minimal disability throughout life. Since phenotypic variability occurs within the same generation and in the same family, it is not possible to predict who will have more disabling forms of the disease. Nerve biopsy in association with PMP22-duplication shows both axonal loss evidenced by reduced myelinated fiber densities ranging from moderate to severe, normal, or mildly reduced unmyelinated fiber density, and increased transverse fascicular area so suggested by non-invasive ultrasonography (Figure 1) (10), as well as onion bulb formations comprised of concentric layers of Schwann cell cytoplasm surrounding thinly or near normally myelinated axons so noted in up to 85% of tissue specimens (Figure 2) (11). Some onion bulbs may contain several myelinated or unmyelinated axons, suggesting that the axons are regenerating nerve sprouts. The presence of large axons devoid of a myelin sheath and surrounded by an onion bulb formation further confirms the demyelinating nature of the pathological process, and is even more evident in teased nerve fiber preparations wherein most fibers show segmental demyelination and remyelination (Figure 3). Morphometric studies show that larger fibers are more affected than smaller ones. The mean internodal length is less than in normal nerves, demonstrating that remyelination is also prominent in nerve fibers of CMT1A patients. The presence of myelinated fibers with reduced axon diameter compared to myelin thickness again suggests the presence of an associated axonal impairment The relevance of axonal atrophy in CMT1A nerves was demonstrated in xenografts of sural nerves from CMT1A patients into nude mice sciatic nerves (12).

The relatively rare neuropathies caused by *PMP22* missense mutations are often clinically more severe than those caused by *PMP22* gene duplication as are the pathological changes although genotype-phenotype correlations can be discordant. Inflammatory cell infiltrates may be observed in sural nerve biopsy tissue in CMT1A (13, 14) suggesting a concomitant inflammatory process. Combining features of motor NCV and phenotype in a cohort of 527 patients led to the molecular diagnosis of CMT in 67% of patients, 55% of whom had CMT1A (15). The management of CMT1A is generally supportive with a view toward monitoring progression. Shy and colleagues (16) described a CMT Neuropathy Score (CMTNS) and the Neuropathy Impairment Score (NIS) to monitor disease progression. Videler and coworkers (17) found that loss of motor axons was the cause of progressive hand dysfunction and loss of fine motor skills. A double-blind, randomized, placebo-controlled trial found that subcutaneous nerve growth factor neurotrophin-3 (NT3) promoted peripheral nerve regeneration and sensory improvement in several patients with CMT1A compared to untreated patients (18) similar to that observed in two CMT1A mouse models due to a common *PMP22* duplication or point mutation.

The related disorder HNPP, also known as bulb-diggers palsy because of the capacity of peroneal palsies to occur after prolonged kneeling, was later distinguished by tomacula in motor and sensory nerves. Chance and colleagues (19) demonstrated a large intersitital deletion in distal 17p11.2 among affected persons with HNPP from three unrelated pedigrees that spanned 1.5 Mb and included all markers known to be duplicated in CMT1A, that uniformly appeared in all pedigrees, and included the *PMP22* gene. Affected patients typically present with transient episodes of focal weakness or sensory loss that lasts hours, days, or months (20). Some patients have also been reported to develop symptoms of length-dependent neuropathy, although that is an unusual occurrence. Neurological examination between episodes is often normal or only minimally abnormal. Occasionally, a painless brachial plexopathy may be the presenting symptom. The most common abnormality observed in nerve biopsy are tomacula (Figure 4), found in both internodal and paranodal regions of approximately 40 to 250 um in length (21). Analysis of longitudinal sections and teased fiber preparations is sometimes needed to

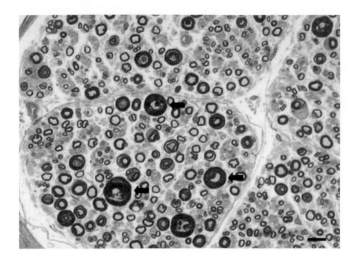

FIG. 4. Sural nerve biopsy from a patient with HNPP. The density of myelinated fibers is within normal limits. Several focal thickenings of the myelin sheath or tomacula (arrows) may be seen. (Toludine blue, bar=10µm)

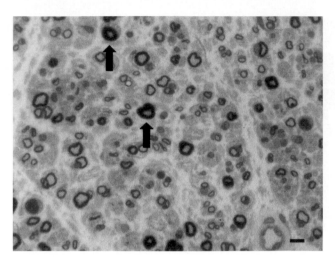

FIG. 5. Sural nerve biopsy from a patient with HNPP. Teased fiber preparation. Several thickenings of the myelin sheath (tomacula) may be seen along the fibers. O.T. 0.2%.

identify these peculiar myelin abnormalities (Figure 5). At the electron microscopic (EM) level, tomacula appear as redundant loops of myelin with irregularly folded lamellae, and have been observed in other hereditary neuropathies, including those with *MPZ* mutations (22). The density of myelinated fibers may be normal or slightly reduced, however axonal loss is not as pronounced as in CMT forms, and onion bulb formations are a frequent occurrence.

CMT1B

CMT1B is caused by heterozygous mutation at the 1q23.3 locus of the *MPZ* gene (Table 1) (23) encoding the MPZ protein, a member of the immunoglobulin superfamily. Apart from the three other major components of the myelin, including myelin back protein (MBP), PLP1, and myelin-associated glycoprotein (MAG), the MPZ protein accounts for more than 50% of the protein present in the myelin sheath of peripheral nerves, the expression of which is restricted to Schwann cells. MPZ is believed to link adjacent myelin lamellae and stabilize their assembly. In the PNS, it is a necessary constituent in the adhesion of concentric myelin wraps along internodes. Mutations in the *MPZ* gene can produce other sensorineural neuropathies including CMTDID, CMT2I, CMT2J, DSD, congenital hypomyelinating neuropathy (CHN), and Russe syndrome. Inoue and colleagues (24) presented evidence suggesting that truncating mutations in the 5-prime end of the gene resulted in milder clinical phenotypes than in those in the 3-prime end of the gene, such that those associated with the normal phenotype were located in an internal exon and resulted in a decrease in mutant mRNA compared to those associated with severe disease located in the last exon and were not followed by an intron, resulting in a larger accumulation of mutant mRNA.

Although patients with CMT1B were thought to have the typical CMT1 phenotype with more pronounced calf wasting, it is now recognized that *MPZ* mutations cause a wide range of phenotypes, including very severe forms with congenital hypomyelination presenting *in utero*, infancy, and milder still in adulthood. The type and location of the mutation on the *MPZ* coding region appears to determine the severity of the neuropathy, although genotype-phenotype correlations are imperfect. Many neuropathies caused by *MPZ* mutations tend to cluster with very early onset, usually presenting prior to one year of age, or as late-onset neuropathy presenting well into adulthood (23).

Abnormalities of myelin are the prominent feature of nerve biopsy from early-onset patients evidencing a loss of myelinated axons with demyelination, remyelination, and onion bulb formations on semithin plastic sections stained with toluidine blue and teased fiber preparation in most patients. Electron microscopy (EM) identified two ultrastructural abnormalities, including extensive areas of uncompacted myelin and numerous areas of focally folded myelin or tomaculae that appear to be mutually exclusive (25). Axonal degeneration, prominent in those with late-onset disease with less evident demyelination, is associated with marked loss of myelinated fibers of all calibers, numerous clusters of regenerating axons, abnormal compaction, and tomacula formation, compared to those with early-onset disease.

CMT1C

CMT1C is caused by mutation at the 16p13.13 locus of the *SIMPLE/LITAF* gene (Table 1). Chance and colleagues

(26) studied seven pedigrees that segregated AD CMT1 without linkage to CMT1A or 1B on chromosomes 17, representing a third genetic locus in the slow NCV type, termed CMT1C, later mapped to the 16p13.1-p12.3 locus in two families (27), later identifying three missense mutations in *LITAF*, the causal gene (28). The encoded transcription factor, first identified as a regulator of TNF-alpha gene expression, is an early endosomal membrane protein that is highly expressed in the peripheral nerves and Schwann cells, and interacts with proteins of the lysosomal degradation pathway. Two transcripts encoding different proteins, SIMPLE and LITAF, have been reported from the same gene. Affected patients develop distal muscle weakness and atrophy, sensory loss, and slow nerve conduction velocities in the range of 20 to 25 m/sec (28). The neuropathological abnormalities are suggestive of a hypertrophic demyelinating neuropathy, like CMT1A. In particular, myelin loss and onion bulbs similar to those observed in CMT1A have been reported in one large family with CMT1C (28).

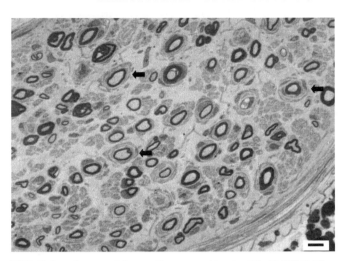

FIG. 6. Sural nerve biopsy from a patient with CMT1D. The density of myelinated fibers is moderately decreased. Several onion bulbs (arrows) may be seen surrounding thinly myelinated fibers. (Seminthin section, Toludine blue; bar-10 µm)

CMT1D

First reported by Warner and colleagues (29) and specifically referred to by Street and coworkers (28), CMT1D is due to mutation at the 10q21.3 locus of the *EGR2* gene (Table 1), involved in the transcription of genes involved in Schwann cell mediated myelination (30). It is associated with variable phenotypes, depending on the site and nature of the specific mutation, accounting for not only CMT 1D, but DSD and CHN. Affected patients demonstrate a typical CMT1 phenotype and display neuropathological changes ranging from a severe to relatively mild loss of myelinated fibers in nerve biopsy, depending on the particular patient. Onion bulbs, although present, are not as prominent as in CMT1A (Figure 6). Fibers showing a reduced axonal diameter compared to myelin thickness were observed in a CMT1D family consistent with axonal atrophy and demyelination (29).

CMT1E

Hamiel and colleagues (31) described a variant of CMT that included sensorineural deafness in early childhood and infancy excluding linkage to CMT1A and 1B; Korvach and coworkers (32) later described a point mutation in the *PMP22* gene in a large family reported by Kousseff and colleagues (33) that included 82 persons in seven generations with onset of deafness and weakness of peroneal muscles in childhood, eventuating in distal involvement of the arms and legs resulting in clawing, pes cavus, and hammertoes. CMT 1E is caused by mutation at the 17p12 locus of the *PMP22* gene (Table 1).

CMT1F

Jordanova (34) and Abe and colleagues (35) described heterozygous mutations in the *NEFL* gene with severe infantile and childhood-onset of dominant CMT1, some of whom had been clinically diagnosed with DSS. CMT1F is caused by mutation at the 8p21.2 locus of the *NEFL* gene (Table 1), of which nonsense mutations were postulated to result in loss of function in contrast to missense mutations, which resulted in toxic gain-of-function, concluding that homozygous nonsense mutations in the *NEFL* gene caused a recessive phenotype. Mutant NEFL proteins, which cause *CMT1F* and 2E, disrupt both neurofilament assembly and axonal transport of cytoskeletal neurofilaments in cultured mammalian cells and neurons. Accumulation of neurofilaments, a pathological feature of several neurodegenerative disorders, including amyotrophic lateral sclerosis (ALS), Parkinson disease (PD), dementia with Lewy bodies, and diabetic neuropathy, and implicate defective neurofilament metabolism in the pathogenesis of human neurodegenerative disease in which they are found (36).

X-LINKED CHARCOT-MARIE-TOOTH DISORDERS

CMTX1

This XL dominant form of CMT presents electrophysiologically, with more severely slow NCV in men, and mildly slow or normal NCV in women. Phillips (37) and Hahn and colleagues (38) reported multigenerational families with XL dominant, early-onset CMT severely affecting men, and mild or subclinical involvement in women. Birouk and colleagues (39) described the clinical and electrophysiological features of ten CMTX families confirmed by mutation analysis and concluded that it was an axonal neuropathy rather than demyelinating, similar to the findings of Yiu and colleagues (40), who retrospectively reviewed 17 affected children with proven pathogenic mutations in whom nerve biopsies showed a reduction in myelinated fiber density, thin myelin sheaths, and onion bulb formations (Figure 7). CMTX1 is due to hemizygous or heterozygous mutation at the Xq13.1 locus of the *GJB1* gene (Table 1) encoding connexin 32 expressed in myelinated peripheral nerve fibers at the nodes of Ranvier and Schmidt-Lanterman incisures, forming gap junctions that connect the folds of Schwann cell cytoplasm, allowing the transfer of nutrients, ions, and molecules to the innermost myelin layers (41).

CMTX2

Ionasescu and colleagues (42, 43) reported linkage to DNA markers Xp22.2 (Table 1) in one family with XL recessive CMT, characterized by infantile onset of leg weakness, wasting, areflexia, and pes cavus in boys, several of whom had mental retardation and electrophysiology consistent with both demyelination and axonal degeneration.

CMTX3

Two of the families studied by Ionasescu and colleagues (42, 43) demonstrated linkage to Xq26 markers, as did another large Austrian family with XL CMT that mapped to Xq26.3-Xq27.1 in the CMTX locus, haplotype analysis of which delineated a 5.7-Mb region between DXS1041 and DXS8106. A second large Austrian family with CMTX3, studied by Huttner and colleagues (44), mapped to the CMTX3 locus. Reexamination of an American family studied by Ionasescu and colleagues (42), shared the distal portion of the haplotype, suggesting a common founder mutation. CMTX3 is caused by mutation at the Xq26 locus (Table 1).

CMTX4

Cowchock and colleagues (45) described an XL recessive infantile-onset motor sensory neuropathy associated with deafness and mental retardation, with minor clinical features in female carriers, the preliminary molecular genetics of which were summarized by Sladky and Brown (46), Fischbeck (47), and Priest and colleagues (48) who characterized the unique clinical and molecular genetics, mapping it to the Xq24-q26.1 locus (Table 1).

CMTX5

Rosenberg and Chutorian (49) described the triad of early-onset hearing loss, polyneuropathy, and optic atrophy, later characterized and designated CMT5X by Kim and colleagues (50, 51) due to mutation at the Xq22.3 locus of the *PRPS1* gene encoding phosphoribosyl pyrophosphate synthetase (Table 1), necessary in purine and pyrimidine synthesis.

CHARCOT-MARIE-TOOTH TYPE 2 DISORDERS

CMT2A

Saito and colleagues (52) reported a Japanese family with four members in three generations with CMT2A1. The proband developed running difficulty at age 7, and at age 11, bilateral pes cavus, hammertoes, and mild lordosis were evident, with anterior tibial, fibular, and posterior tibial compartment weakness and wasting, and normal sensation. However, sural sensory response was not obtained and nerve biopsy showed decreased myelinated fibers. Zhao and colleagues (53) identified a loss-of-function mutation in the *KIF1B* gene. CMT 2A patients have typical CMT clinical presentations with sensorimotor peripheral neuropathies. CMT2A1 is caused by mutation at the 1p36.22 locus of the *KIF1B* gene encoding an N-terminal-type motor protein (Table 1) that functions as a monomeric motor for anterograde transport of mitochondria.

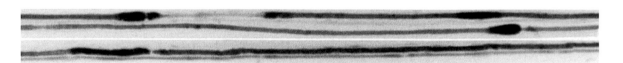

FIG. 7. Sural nerve biopsy from a patient with CMTX1. The density of myelinated fibers is moderately decreased. Several clusters of thinly myelinated fibers (arrows) are seen. Fibers with thin myelin sheaths, occasionally surrounded by concentric layers of Schwann cell cytoplasm forming small onion bulbs are occasionally present (arrowheads). (Semithin section, Toluidine blue, bar = 10 μm)

CMT2A2

Zuchner and colleagues (54) identified mutations in the *MFN2* gene in several affected members of previously reported CMT2A2 families (52, 55, 56), characterized clinically by typical signs and symptoms of axonal CMT and range of age of onset from 4 to 20 years. Several members had corticospinal tract (CST) signs, impaired distal pain and vibratory sensation, deafness, spinal deformities, and as many as one-quarter were asymptomatic. CMT2A2 results from heterozygous mutation at the 1p36.22 locus of the *MFN2* gene encoding MFN2 (Table 1), which in culture has vasoactive antiproliferative effects, tethering endoplasmic reticulum (ER) to mitochondria in juxtaposition for efficient mitochondrial calcium uptake.

CMT2B

Verhoeven and colleagues (57) performed molecular genetic analysis of several previously reported families (58; 59), refining the CMT2B locus to a 2.5-cM region and reporting missense mutations in the *RAB7* gene, identifying the same mutation in other affected members in a family described by Auer-Grumbach and colleagues (60). A common feature was distal sensory loss affecting all modalities resulting in calluses, non-healing ulcers, osteomyelitis, and auto-amputation, accompanied by pes cavus, pes planus, and hammertoes, with occasional distal weakness and wasting. Moor and sensory NCV were typically normal or showed axonal degeneration. CMT2B is caused by a mutation at the 3q21.3 locus of the *RAB7* gene (Table 1) encoding a 207-amino acid protein related to endocytic endosome pathways, mutations in which can interfere with endosomal transport mechanisms within axons.

CMT2B1

Bouhouche and colleagues (61) studied a large consanguineous Moroccan AR CMT2 family with nine affected sibs, with onset in the second decade, distal weakness, wasting, and areflexia, with normal or slightly reduced NCV reflecting an axonal process. A genome-wide search showed linkage of the disorder to 1q21.2-q21.3. De Sandre-Giovannoli and colleagues (62) identified a homozygous mutation in the *LMNA* gene. AR axonal CMT type 2B1 can be caused by homozygous mutation at the 1q22 locus of the *LMNA* gene encoding lamin A/C (Table 1). The structural protein components of the nuclear lamina underlying the inner nuclear membrane contributes to its shape and size.

CMT2B2

Leal and colleagues (63) reported a consanguineous family from a single town in the province of Alajuela, Costa Rica, with AR adult-onset CMT characterized by symmetrical weakness, wasting, stocking sensory loss, and normal or slightly reduced motor NCV indicative of axonal degeneration. Linkage was found to 19q13.3. Further investigations (64) identified a homozygous A335V mutation in the *MED25* gene. CMT2B2 is caused by mutation at the 19q13.33 locus of the *MED25* gene (Table 1) which is expressed in a coordinated fashion with *PMP22* in murine CMT (64).

CMT2C

Dyck and colleagues (65), and later Klein (66, 67), and Landoure and coworkers (68) described two kindred with AD CMT characterized by limb, vocal cord, and intercostal muscle weakness, and minimally symptomatic sensory loss beginning in infancy or childhood, with life expectancy decreased due to respiratory failure and significant intrafamilial clinical variability. Linkage was noted to a region at 12q23-q24, and Auer-Grumbach and colleagues (69) identified heterozygous R315W mutation in the *TRPV4* gene, also present in distal and scapuloperoneal forms of spinal muscular atrophy (SMA). CMT2C is caused by heterozygous mutation at the 12q24.11 locus of the *TRPV4* gene (Table 1) that encodes a cation channel mediating calcium influx.

CMT2D

Ionasescu and coworkers (70) described a three-member pedigree, 14 of whom presented in late childhood and early adulthood with weakness and wasting of the hands and moderate involvement of the feet with absent arm- and hypoactive leg deep-tendon reflexes, and sensory involvement with variable pes cavus and hammertoes. Motor NCV were normal and EMG showed evidence of active denervation, and there was linkage to chromosome 7p14. Antonellis and colleagues (71) identified a mutation in the *GARS* gene. CMT2D is caused by a mutation at the 7p13.3 locus of the *GARS* gene encoding glycyl-tRNA synthetase (Table 1), essential in protein synthesis by catalyzing the esterification of glycine to its cognate tRNA.

CMT2E

Meriyanova and colleagues (72) described a six-generation Russian family with AD CMT with onset in the second and third decade with gait disturbance due to weakness and wasting of the legs, with variable pes cavus and hyperkeratosis, suggesting the designation of CMT2E. Fabrizi and colleagues (73) reported similar large Southern Italian kindred with CMT2E due to mutation in the *NEFL* gene. Sural nerve biopsy showed a mild decrease in large fiber diameter density, and several fibers demonstrate small axon calibers compared to the myelin thickness (Figure 8). CMT2E is caused by mutation at the 8p21.2 locus of the *NEFL* gene (Table 1). Since the NEFL protein is an important constituent of the neurofilaments used in axonal transport systems, and neurofilament phosphorylation is known to be abnormal in demyelinating forms of CMT, CMT2E may provide important clues into mechanisms of axonal damage, not only in CMT2 but also in CMT1 (74). Giant axons in a nerve biopsy of a child with CMT2E suggested primary axonal neuropathy despite decreased motor NCV in his mother indicative of a primary demyelinating neuropathy with a Pro22Ser mutation of *NEFL* (73).

CMT2F

Ismailov and colleagues (75) reported a six-generation family with AD CMTI in whose onset of symmetrical progressive weakness and wasting of the legs, resulting in footdrop and steppage gait, with weakness, wasting, and clawing of the hands, with hypoactive- or absent deep-tendon reflexes occurred in the second or third decade with slow progressive worsening. Electrophysiologic studies were consistent with axonal neuropathy. The disorder was linked to chromosome 7q11-q21. Further investigations in the same family by Evgrafov and colleagues (76) identified a S135F mutation in the *HSPB1* gene; a second mutation was noted in a Belgian family with CMT2F. CMT2F is caused by

mutation at the 7q11.23 locus of the *HSPB1* gene encoding the 27-kD heat-shock protein 1 stress protein (Table 1) that antagonize the induction of reactive oxygen species contributing to cell death.

CMT2G

Berciano (77) and Nelis and colleagues (78) characterized a large family of 14 affected members with a wide-range of onset from childhood to adulthood and AD inheritance characterized clinically by foot deformity, gait difficulty, and very slow progression, and normal or mildly decreased motor NCV consistent with an axonopathy. The disorder was assigned the CMT2G on chromosome 12q12-q13.3 (Table 1).

CMT2H

Barhoumi and colleagues (79) reported a large Tunisian family of 13 affected members with AD axonal CMT and CST signs, and onset in the first decade. The genetic defect mapped to a region overlapping the *GDAP1* gene involved in signal transduction pathways of neuronal development. CMT2H is caused by mutation at the 8q21.3 locus (Table 1).

CMT2I

Marrousu (80), Senderek (81), Boerkoel (82) and Auer-Grumbach and coworkers (83) reported unrelated families with AD CMT2 characterized clinically by late onset distal leg weakness, wasting, foot deformity, sensory loss, hyporeflexia, and normal or mildly decreased motor NCV consistent with axonopathy. CMTZ is caused by mutation in the 1q23.3 locus of the *MPZ* gene (Table 1).

CMT2J

CMT2 with hearing loss and pupillary abnormalities in a Belgian family was described by De Jonghe and coworkers, (84) with onset in the fourth to fifth decade associated with variable sensory and hearing deficits, normal or slightly reduced motor NCV, and clusters of remyelinating axons in nerve biopsy consistent with axonopathy. Chapon and colleagues (85) reported a French family with three generation of CMT2 characterized by pupillary deficits, dysphagia, and deafness, and axonal electrophysiology and nerve biopsy tissue findings. Misu and coworkers (86) reported a novel pro105thr mutation in the *MPZ* gene, similar to a two-generation family reported by Kabzinski and colleagues (87) in a 57-year old woman discussed by Triggs and coworkers (88). Misu and coworkers (86) noted had an asp75val mutation as well in the *MPZ* gene. Late-onset CMT2J, associated with hearing loss and pupillary abnormalities, is caused by mutation at the 1q23.3 locus of the *MPZ* gene (Table 1).

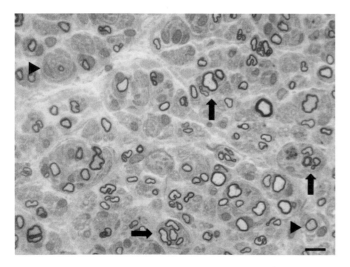

FIG. 8. Sural nerve biopsy from a patient with CMT2. The density of myelinated fibers is slightly decreased, particularly for large diameter fibers. Several fibers have small axonal calibers compared to their myelin thickness (arrows). (Semithin section, Toluidine blue; bar = 10 μm)

Pupillary abnormalities are attributed to autonomic nervous system (ANS) dysfunction.

CMT2K

Birouk and colleagues (89) reported a Moroccan family with AR axonal CMT with onset before age three years, with hypotonia, delayed motor development, and milestones, and later arm, gait involvement, foot deformity, kyphoscoliosis, distal limb weakness and wasting, areflexia, and diminished sensation, as did siblings from a consanguineous Amish family with AR CMT2K, described by Xin and colleagues (90) with childhood onset of distal leg weakness and borderline NCV slowing consistent with axonal degeneration. Chung (91) and Crimella and colleagues (93) respectively, reported Korean and Italian probands with late- and early onset AD CMT2K with less severe onset than the AR phenotypes. CMT2K is caused by mutation at the 8q21.11 locus of the *GDAP1* gene encoding GDAP proteins (Table 1). The *GDAP1* gene functions in the signal transduction of neuronal development.

CMT2L

Tang and colleagues (93, 94) reported a Chinese family with AD CMT designated CMT2L, affected members of which showed linkage to chromosome 12q24, and after sequencing all known candidate genes in the 12q24 region, identified a lys141- to-asn substitution (K141N) in the *HSPB8* gene (Table 1), the function of which is to reduce the chaperone activity of the encoded protein, a decrease of which contributes to neuropathies (95).

CMT2M

CMT2M and forms of dominant intermediate CMT shared a common genetic basis due to mutation at the 19p13.2 in the *DNM2* gene encoding dynamin-2 in a mother and two daughters with an axonal form of CMT characterized by progressive gait unsteadiness, foot deformities, pes cavus, toe clawing, hand weakness, sensory loss, areflexia, and onset in the first decade of life. A form of axonal CMT designated CMT2M by Gallardo and colleagues (96), was similar genetically and phenotypically to a family with CMT2M reported by Fabrizi and colleagues (97). CMT2M, like CMTDIB, are caused by mutations at the 19p13.2 locus of the *DNM2* gene encoding dynamin-2 (Table 1). The dynamin-2 protein plays a role in endocytosis and interacts with microtubules. Mutations in DNM2 alter microtubule dynamics that are essential to axonal transport (98).

CMT2N

Latour and colleagues (99) reported a five-generation French family with CMT characterized clinically by mild to moderate leg weakness at a mean age of 28 years without significant disability in later years, and a mean motor NCV of 41 m/s, similar to a Taiwanese family with AD CMT2N described by Lin and coworkers (100). There was marked variability in age at onset, slowly progressive leg weakness, and mild weakness and wasting of intrinsic hand muscles. An Australian family described by McLaughlin and colleagues (101) manifested heterozygous mutations between R329H and N71Y at the 16q22.1 locus of the *AARS* gene encoding alanyl-tRNA synthetase (Table 1) catalyzing the attachment of alanine to the appropriate tRNA. The folding of mRNA, which is influenced by the presence of single-nucleotide polymorphisms, and the activity of amino acid synthetase, governs a wide range of biological events such as mRNA splicing, processing, and translational control and regulation, which may be an important determinant in neurological disease.

CMT2O

Weedon and colleagues (102) reported a four-generation family with AD CMT clinically characterized by delayed motor milestones and abnormal gait, slowly progressive leg weakness and wasting, pes cavus, and, less common, upper limb involvement, with normal range of motor NCV and sural nerve biopsy pathology consistent with axonopathy. Heterozygous mutation (H306R) in CMT2O was detected at the 14q32.31 locus of the *DYNC1H1* gene (Table 1). The encoded cognate dynein protein binds to the multisubunit complex dynactin-1 critical for microtubule-mediated fast axonal transport. A murine model of CMT2O implicates mutations in the *DYNC1H1* gene in neuropathic disease. (103).

CMT2P

Guernsey and colleagues (104) described a multiply consanguineous Canadian family with seven affected members with AD CMT clinically characterized by distal leg and hand weakness and wasting, muscle cramping, pes cavus, areflexia, and onset in early adult years. A splice site mutation was detected in the *LRSAM1* gene with unaffected heterozygous carriers. Weterman and colleagues (105) described a three-generation family with AD CMT consistent with CMT2P and frameshift mutations in the *LRSAM1* gene. CMT2P is caused by homozygous or heterozygous mutation at the 9q33.3 locus of the *LRSAM1* gene (Table 1) encoding LRSAM1, a multifunctional RING finger protein that selectively regulates cell adhesion molecules, has ubiquitin liagase activity, and plays a role in receptor endocytosis and viral budding (106, 107).

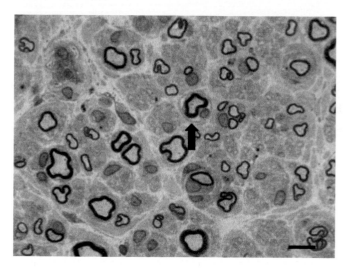

FIG. 9. Sural nerve biopsy from a patient with CMT4A. The density of myelinated fibers is decreased. Several thinly myelinated fibers are seen, occasionally surrounded by concentric layers of the Schwann cell cytoplasm, forming a small onion bulb (arrow). (Semithin section, Toluidine blue; bar = 10 μm)

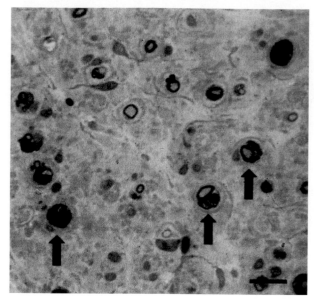

FIG. 10. Sural nerve biopsy from a patient with CMT4B. The density of myelinated fibers is severely decreased. The majority of fibers demonstrate the typical CMT4B abnormalities of the myelin sheath, which is redundant and irregularly folded myelin (arrows). (Semithin section, Toluidine blue; bar = 10 μm)

CHARCOT-MARIE-TOOTH TYPE 4 DISORDERS

CMT4A

Ben Othmane and colleagues (108) designated CMT4A in a severe Tunisian family of AR demyelinating CMT characterized clinically by onset before age two years of rapidly progressive distal weakness and wasting, leading to loss of walking by late adolescence, with normal cerebrospinal fluid (CSF) protein, severely depressed motor NCV and hypomyelination on cutaneous nerve biopsy. Baxter and colleagues (109) identified the *GDAP1* gene as the site of three different mutations in CMT4A. Nerve biopsy in CMT4A shows thinly myelinated axons surrounded by Schwann cell processes concentrically organized to form small onion bulbs (Figure 9). CMT4A is caused by mutation at the 8q21.11 locus of the *GDAP1* gene encoding ganglioside-induced differentiation-associated protein-1 (Table 1), anchored to the mitochondrial outer membrane and involved in a signal transduction pathway in neuronal development, the mutation of which leads to perturbed axonal transport and impaired energy production.

CMT4B1

Quattrone (110) and Bolina and colleagues (111, 112) reported large consanguineous southern Italian families with AR demyelinating CMT distinguished pathologically by focally folded myelin sheaths in nerve biopsy specimens (Figure 10), identifying pathogenic homozygosity and compound homozygous mutations at the 11q21 locus in the *MTMR2* gene (Table 1). It has been postulated that lack of a functional MTMR2 protein results in constitutive phosphorylation or an unknown substrate leading to Schwann cell proliferation with overgrowth of myelin sheaths. Affected patients become symptomatic early, with an average age of onset of 34 months, and unlike most forms of CMT, proximal as well as distal weakness are prominent, with severely slow, temporally dispersed motor NCS and absent sensory nerve action potentials (SNAP) on electrodiagnostic studies, and segmental demyelination in nerve biopsy.

CMT4B2

Senderek and colleagues (113) described a Turkish family with early onset beginning age five years, of severe AR CMT, clinically characterized by distal leg weakness, wasting, foot deformities, pes cavus, hammertoes, steppage gait, areflexia, and very slow motor NCV of 16 m/s, with focally folded myelin protrusions on cutaneous nerve biopsy. Homozygous in-frame deletions of exons 11 and 12 at the 11p15.4 locus of the *SBF2* gene (Table 1) and splice site mutations were later discerned.

CMT4C

Kessali and colleagues (114) reported two large Algerian families with AR demyelinating CMT, with mean age at onset of five years, with foot deformities, scoliosis, severely decreased motor NCV, and cutaneous nerve biopsy that showed Schwann cell proliferation with multiple small onion bulbs. Senderek and colleagues (113) described 17 additional patients from 11 families with onset from infancy to 12 years, median motor NCV of 23 m/s, and cutaneous nerve biopsy that showed demyelination, onion bulb formation, and extended Schwann cell processes. Segregation analysis showed AR inheritance and 11 different mutations in the *SH3TC2* gene of which eight were protein-truncating and 3 missense. Azzedine and colleagues (115) described 10 families with CMT4C from Europe and North Africa with onset from two to ten years with scoliosis, kyphoscoliosis, foot deformities, and compound heterozygous and homozygous mutations in the *SH3TC2* gene, a total of ten different, including eight novel including one recurrent R954X. Lupski (116), Lassuthova and colleagues (117) determined that the R954X mutation accounted for 63% of mutant *SH3TC2* Czech alleles overall. CMT4C is caused by homozygous or compound heterozygous mutations at the 5q32 locus of the *SH3TC2* gene (Table 1) encoding a protein expressed in Schwann cells of peripheral nerves, localized to the plasma membrane and perinuclear endocytic recycling compartments, suggesting a role in myelination in regions of axoglial interactions (118).

CMT4D

Kalaydjieva and colleagues (119) described AR CMT4D among 14 affected individuals from the Gypsy community of Lom, Bulgaria, characterized clinically by distal leg weakness, wasting, foot and hand deformities, sensory loss, areflexia, severely reduced motor NCV, and onset in the first decade of life with severe disability by the fifth decade. Molecular genetic analysis identified a founder *HMSNL* gene mutation, consisting of a premature-termination codon at the 148 position of the *NDRG1* gene. Cutaneous nerve biopsy shows demyelination, remyelination, severe axonal loss, and hypertrophic onion bulb formation in younger patients that regresses, with hypomyelinated axons, partial ensheathment of axons by Schwann cells, uncompacted myelin, accumulation of pleomorphic material in adaxonal Schwann cell cytoplasm, with intraaxonal accumulation of irregular arranged curvilinear profiles (120). CMT4C is caused by mutation at the 8q24.22 locus of the *NDRG1* gene (Table 1), which is highly expressed in Schwann cells and has been implicated in growth arrest and cell differentiation (121).

CMT4E

CMT4E or CHN is characterized clinically by early onset of hypotonia, areflexia, distal weakness, markedly slow NCV, with hypomyelination of most or all of nerve fibers. Warner and colleagues (122) reported a hypotonic patient with CHN manifesting distal weakness and diminished muscle bulk who at age 7 ambulated with a walker and wore ankle-foot orthoses for bilateral footdrop. Electrodiagnostic studies showed low amplitude CMAP amplitudes, markedly slow velocities and prolonged motor latencies with absent sensory responses. Nerve biopsy showed profound demyelination and relative axonal preservation. A heterozygous mutation was identified in the *MPZ* gene. Warner and colleagues (123) later identified a heterozygous mutation in the *ERG2* gene in patients with infantile hyptonia, motor developmental delay, and ambulation after age two. CMT4E is caused by mutations at the 1q23.3 locus of the *MPZ* gene, and at the 10q21.3 locus of the *EGR2* gene (Table 1).

CMT4F

The original patients described by Dejerine and Sottas (124) included two sibs of presumably unaffected parents, one affected in infancy and the other at age 14, with clubfoot, kyphoscloliosis, generalized weakness, wasting, fasciculation, sensory loss, areflexia with Romberg sign, miosis, decreased pupillary reactivity, and nystagmus. Delague and colleagues (125) reported a large inbred Lebanese family with AR demyelinating CMT referred to at CMT4F in which nerve biopsy revealed absence of L-perivaxon from the myelin sheath. Linkage was established to 19q13.1-q13.2, and Guilbot and colleagues (126) identified a mutation in the *PRX* gene which cosegratated with the family studied by Delague and colleagues (125). Timmerman and colleagues (127), who described two additional patients with CMT4F in whom heterozygous mutation in the alpha-helix domain of the first zinc finger of *EGR2* gene, described severe demyelination, classic onion bulbs, and focally myelin sheaths in affected patients. Similar patients with MPZ and PMP22 gene mutation were respectively described by Hayasaka (128) and Roa and colleagues (129). CMT4F is caused by mutations at the 1q23.3 locus of the *MPZ* gene, at the 17p12 locus of the *PMP22* gene, at the 19q13.2 locus of the *PRX* gene, and at the 10q21.3 locus of the *EGR2* gene (Table 1).

CMT4G

De Sandre-Giovannoli and colleagues (130) identified linkage at chromosome 10q22-q23 for which the corresponding gene had not yet been cloned. Affected Romany Gypsy family members described by Rogers and colleagues (131) presented with severe disabling CMT disease, as did others reported by Thomas and coworkers (132), who developed several generalized weakness and sensory loss and neuropathic joint degeneration. CMT4G is caused by mutation at the 12p11.21 locus (Table 1).

CMT4H

De Sandre-Giovannoli (130), Delague (133), and Stendel and colleagues (134) identified homozygous mutations in the FDG4 gene among Lebanese and Algerian individuals with CMT4G clinically characterized by delayed walking, unsteady gait, arcflexia, scoliosis, foot deformities, and severely reduced motor and sensory NCV. Sural nerve biopsy showed severe loss of myelinated fibers, onion bulb formations, and features of CHM with myelin outfoldings similar to patients with MTMR2 and MTMR13 mutations (135). CMT4H is caused by mutations as the 12p11.21 locus of the FGD4 gene encoding frabin (Table 1), which induces Cdc42-mediated cell-shape changes in transinfected Schwann cells and has a role in Rho GTPase signaling, essential for proper myelination of the PNS.

CMT4J

Chow and colleagues (136) described five patients from four families, two of whom were quadriplegic or wheelchair-bound due to severe AR CMT and mutations in the FIG4 gene. Cutaneous nerve biopsy showed profound axonal loss, thinly myelinated fibers, and evidence of remyelination and demyelination. CMT4J is caused by mutation at the 6q21 locus of the FIG4 gene (Table 1) which encodes a protein involved in phosphatidylinositol metabolism. The pale tremor mouse develops multiorgan CNS and PNS neuronopathy and diluted pigmentation (136). FIG4 gene mutations have has been implicated in genetic forms of amyotrophic lateral sclerosis (ALS11) and primary lateral sclerosis (PLS).

AUTOSOMAL DOMINANT INTERMEDIATE CHARCOT-MARIE-TOOTH DISORDERS

CMTDIA

Rossi and colleagues (137) studied a large Italian family with CMTDIA, characterized by walking difficulty from age six years, with leg weakness beginning in the second decade, and slow progression thereafter until the sixth decade wherein patients developed severe weakness and atrophy of the arms and legs, steppage gait, and pes cavus. Crutches were needed to walk in the eighth decade. NCV were slowed in proportion to the clinical deficit. Cutaneous nerve biopsy showed demyelinating features including

onion bulbs and uncompacted myelin lamellae, and signs of axonal degeneration. Verhoeven and coworkers (138) mapped the gene for CMTDIA to a 10.7-Mb interval on chromosome 10q24.1-q25.1 (Table 1) between tandem repeat markers D10S1795 and D10S1795.

CMTDIB

Salisachs (139) described families with a dominant intermediate form of CMT based upon electrophysiological and neuropathological criteria. Davis and colleagues (140) proposed the term intermediate CMT. Kennerson and coworkers (141) described a large Austrian family with a classic CMT phenotype in which motor NCV overlapped the division between CMT1 and CMT2 ranging from 24 to 54 m/s, and cutaneous nerve biopsy showed axonal degeneration, loss of large diameter fibers, rare segmental demyelination, and remyelination, with onion bulb formations. Linkage was demonstrated to the short arm of chromosome 19. Speer and coworkers (142) reduced the candidate interval to a 9-cM interval spanned by two markers. Zhu and colleagues (143) performed haplotype analysis of the family described by Kennerson and coworkers (141), further narrowing the candidate region for CMTDIB. Mutations in the DNM2 gene encoding dynamin-2 at the 19p13.2-p12 locus were later identified among families reported by Kennerson (141), Speer (142), Zhu and colleagues (143) with CMTDI. CMTDIB is caused by mutation at the 19p13.2 locus of the DNM2 gene encoding dynamin-2 (Table 1).

CMTDIC

Jordanova and coworkers (144) described two unrelated American families, one of German and Polish descent, and the other from Bulgaria, with a variable range at onset from the first to sixth decade of a classical CMT phenotype, motor NCV ranging from 30 to 40 m/s, and cutaneous nerve biopsy showing clusters of regenerating fibers and reduction in fiber density and myelin thickness, without onion bulb formations. Different missense mutations were found in the YARS gene as well as an in-frame deletion. CMTDIC, caused by mutation at the 1p35.1 locus of the YARS gene encoding tyrosyl-tRNA synthetase (Table 1), linking protein-synthesizing complex to neurodegeneraiton.

CMTDID

Mastaglia and colleagues (145) described a four-generation Macedonian family with symmetrical pattern of distal leg weakness and sensory impairment, with intermediate NCV, and cutaneous nerve biopsy that showed axonal degeneration, areas of segmental demyelination and remyelination without onion bulb formation, and mutation in the *MPZ* gene. CMTDID is caused by mutations at the 1q23.3 locus of the *MPZ* gene (Table 1).

CMTDIE

Boyer and colleagues (146) described 12 index patients with CMTDIE clinically characterized by variable classical AD CMT phenotype with mean age at onset of 13 years, associated with proteinuria often before, concomitant, or after onset of neurological symptoms. Cutaneous nerve biopsy showed axonal loss and onion bulb formation, and electrodiagnostic studies were intermediate in severity. Nine novel heterozygous mutations were detected in the *INF2* gene. CMTDIE is caused by mutation at the14q32.33 locus in the *INF2* gene (Table 1) that was predicted to disrupt actin dynamics in peripheral Schwann cells leading to disturbed myelin formation and maintenance.

DISTAL HEREDITARY MOTOR NEURONOPATHY DISORDERS

HMN1

Gopinath and colleagues (147) reported a family of 10 affected members with AD HMN1 previously considered to have juvenile ALS, with age at onset in the first or second decade, and presenting features of gait difficulty, weakness, wasting of the legs, pes cavus, hammertoes, and frequent Babinski signs, without sensory involvement. Cutaneous nerve biopsy showed chronic axonal neuropathy. The disorder was mapped to chromosome 7q34-q36 (Table 1).

HMN2A

Timmerman and investigators (148) described a six-generation kindred with AD weakness of the foot and legs beginning at age 21 years, slow progression to complete paralysis of distal leg muscles and mild weakness of the arms and thighs, and preserved deep tendon reflexes (DTR). Some of the older patients required walking or wheelchair assistance. NCV were normal but electromyography (EMG) showed chronic neurogenic changes. Linkage was obtained to a region on chromosome 12q24. Irobi and colleagues (149) identified heterozygous mutations in several additional families, including that of Timmerman and colleagues (148) in the same codon of the *HSPB8* gene. HMN2A is caused by mutation at the 12q24.23 locus of the *HSPB8* gene (Table 1), and is allelic to CMT2L with an overlapping phenotype.

HMN2B

Houlden and investigators (150) reported five families with very slow AD progressive weakness and wasting of the legs, with involvement of the arms, and depressed DTR, in association with four different heterozygous mutations in the *HSPB1* gene, including one patient with a homozygous mutation that had AR inheritance. An animal model of distal HMN expresses the P182L *HSPB1* mutation (151). HMN2A is caused by mutation at the 7q11.23 locus of the *HSPB1* gene (Table 1).

HMN2C

Kolb and coworkers (152) reported two sisters with slowly progressive distal arm and leg weakness and wasting beginning in the third decade, in whom electrodiagnostic studies suggested axonal neuropathy. Genetic analysis identified a heterozygous mutation in the *HSPB3* gene. HMN2C is caused by mutation at the 5q11.2 locus of the *HSPB3* gene (Table 1).

HMN4

Viollet and colleagues (153, 154) who described Lebanese kindred in which both HMN3 and HMN4, suggested the same gene was involved in both phenotypes. One patient described in infancy was normal at birth until two months when found to have hip subluxation and at age nine months, poor movement of the legs and hypotonia. By six years of age there was generalized weakness and a high right hemediaphram on chest radiography. HMN3 and HMN4 both have juvenile onset and differ only by less severe involvement in the former. The disorder has been linked to chromosome 11q13.3 (Table 1).

HMN5

Antonellis and investigators (155) reported mutations in the *GARS* gene in an Algerian Sephardic Jewish family with AD inheritance of hand weakness and wasting particularly affecting the thenar and dorsal interosseus muscles, with normal motor and sensory NCV. Similar patients were presented by Christodoulou and colleagues (156). Auer-Grumbach and colleagues (157) identified a heterozygous mutation in the *SDCL2* gene in other similar Austrian kindred. HMN5 is caused by mutation at the 7p14.3 locus of the *GARS* gene as well as mutation at the 11q12.3 locus of the *BSCL2* gene (Table 1).

HMN7A

Young and Harper (158) and later Boltshauser and colleagues (159) described large kindred with AD SMA-like weakness and wasting, vocal cord paralysis, and variable hearing impairment. The disorder showed linkage to 2q14 (Table 1).

HMN7B

Puls and colleagues (160) described AD slowly progressive motor neuron disease without sensory involvement, associated with breathing and vocal cord paralysis, progressive facial and hand weakness, and wasting, and later distal leg involvement. There was linkage to 2p13 and a mutation in the *DCTN1* gene. HMN7B is caused by mutation at the 2p13.1 locus of the *DCTN1* gene (Table 1).

DIAGNOSIS

There are several steps in diagnosing an inherited neuropathy. The first is establishing whether the patient has symptoms and examination findings of length-dependent weakness and sensory loss in a symmetrical pattern. The neurological examination typically reveals weakness of foot dorsiflexion and eversion that is out of proportion to plantar flexion and inversion weakness. Patients often have abnormalities with dorsiflexion of their fingers and performing fine movements of their hands. Muscle wasting in feet and hands is frequent. Tendon reflexes are often, but not always, decreased. Foot abnormalities, such as pes cavus, and scoliosis are frequent. Nerve conduction studies have an important role in characterizing CMT disorders, with their initial use in separating CMT1 from CMT2 by conduction velocity.

Whereas most patients with inherited neuropathy have uniformly slow NCV, those with acquired demyelinating neuropathy have asymmetric slowing with abnormal temporal dispersion (161). The pattern of slowing can thus be used, along with the family pedigree, to distinguish between inherited and acquired neuropathies. Over the past decade, this approach has been further qualified. Most CMT1 patients, particularly those with CMT1A, have uniformly slow conduction velocities of about 20 meters (m)/sec, although 38 m/sec is used as a "cut off" value (6). Conduction velocities in CMT1B tend to cluster at less than 10 m/sec in early onset cases and over 30 m/sec in late-onset cases with only occasional examples in the range of 20 m/sec (23). Asymmetric slowing is characteristic of HNPP, and also may be found in patients with missense mutations in *PMP22*, *MPZ*, *EGR-2* and *GJB1* (162). Since all of these disorders may present without a clear family history of neuropathy, one must be cautious in using conduction velocity to distinguish acquired from inherited demyelinating neuropathies. The distinction between demyelinating and axonal features is particularly confusing in CMTX wherein NCV are faster than in most patients with CMT1, often with prominent reductions in

CMAP and SNAP amplitudes (163). CMTX was described as an axonal neuropathy, but analysis of NCS reveals primary demyelinating features caused by mutations in the *GJB1* gene expressed in the myelinating Schwann cell. The results of NCV, which in men are usually between 30 and 40m/ sec, would be considered intermediate between CMT1 and CMT2 while distal motor and F-wave latencies are usually prolonged (161, 164) consistent with demyeination. Female carriers usually have normal conduction velocities, but some have slowed velocities, probably due to inactivation of the mutant X chromosome.

It is important to appreciate that although hereditary neuropathies are classified as demyelinating and axonal, all forms, including CMT1A, have axonal loss. Patient disability correlates better with axonal loss than with NCV(165). Reduced CMAP and SNAP amplitudes were found in most CMT1 patients and in a series of 43 CMT1A patients, 34 of whom had unobtainable fibular CMAP, and 41 others with unobtainable sural SNAP (165). Whereas NCV are essential to determine which patients are likely to have forms of demyelinating neuropathy, it is also important to evaluate NCS for subtle signs of demyelination, such as prolonged distal motor latencies or F-wave latencies in determining whether the underlying cause is likely to be axonal or demyelinating. While sural nerve biopsy is invaluable for research studies, investigating pathogenic mechanisms of disease, their role in clinical practice has diminished with the increasing availability of genetic testing.

Typically, inherited neuropathies are chronic diseases with symptoms extending back into childhood, although some atypical forms can have their onset in adulthood. Obtaining a careful pedigree is critical in the diagnosis of inherited neuropathies, not only to determine that there is an inherited neuropathy but also to determine who is at risk for developing the neuropathy. Careful pedigrees require going back at least three generations. Identifying male-to-male transmission excludes XL inheritance. Caution should be taken in interpreting negative pedigrees, since some families with a dominant disorder can start in a given individual as a *de novo* or spontaneous event, while other family histories with recessive disorders will often be negative. In other circumstances, testing is necessary to determine the genetic cause of the neuropathy and to predict at-risk family members. Genetic testing has become an important tool in the diagnosis of CMT. A full characterization of the neuropathy is critical for determining if a genetic test will be informative. The diagnostic yield is higher for cases wherein NCV are slow. However, mutations in myelin genes may have relatively normal conduction velocities. When one family member with CMT1 has been genotyped, it is usually not necessary to test other family members, and they can be screened by clinical examination and NCS.

Genes known to cause CMT were sequenced in 1,607

United Kingdom patients, of whom 425 patient attended an Inherited Neuropathy Clinic. Of 1,182 patients in whom DNA was received for genetic testing, molecular diagnosis was achieved in 62.6% of patients, among them, 80.4% had CMT1 and 25.2%, CMT2 (166). Mutations or rearrangements in *PMP22*, *GJB1*, *MPZ*, and *MFN2* accounted for over 90% of the molecular diagnoses while mutations in all other genes tested were rare. These observations suggested that testing could be more selective based on likelihood of a positive result. A patient with an unusual CMT phenotype without mutation in one of the four preceding genes should be referred for expert evaluation to maximize the chance of reaching a molecular diagnosis.

PATHOGENESIS

While it is not yet possible to arrive at a unified genetic cause of CMT disease, extraordinary progress has been achieved in elucidating the contribution of known disease-causing genes according to shared or interactive function. As defects in myelination are a major cause of CMT neuropathy, mutations in a number of different genes involved in myelination have been recognized, leading to the classical demyelinating CMT phenotype, including *PMP22*, which encodes a small protein expressed primarily in Schwann cells and a major component of the myelin sheath. Duplication, deletion, or point mutations of the *PMP22* gene causes CMT1A, CMT1E, and HNPP. The *MPZ* gene, which encodes the major integral membrane protein of peripheral nerve myelin, is mutated in CMT1B, CMT2I and CMT2J. *MED25*, a component of the mediator complex that recruits RNA polymerase II to specific gene promotors, is mutated in CMT2B2, leading to classical axonal neuropathy. Other genes involved in myelination that are defective in CMT include *EGR2* mutation which causes inhibition of myelin gene expression associated with CMT1D, CMT4E, and CHN. Mutation of the *GJB1* gene is associated with CMTX1, and those of *PRX* lead to altered myelination and ensheathing of regenerating axons so noted in CMT4F.

Mutations in several CMT disease genes encoding proteins directly or indirectly involved in the regulation of intracellular trafficking, a complex network of pathways and diverse cytoskeletal cellular machinery involved in biogenesis, motility, transport, and cargo sorting of cellular vesicles, as well as the components essential for vesicular tethering, docking, and fusion, have assumed importance in axonal forms of CMT and in distal HMN. Disturbances in membrane trafficking, which has important consequences on different key cellular processes such as signal transduction, proliferation, migration, apoptosis, and mitosis, contribute to the pathogenesis of CMT disease. According to the concept of disturbed intracellular trafficking in CMT (167, 168)

genetically mediated disturbances of the PNS cytoskeleton and transport mechanisms along peripheral nerve axon, which can extend up to one meter from the neuronal perikaryon to its target, can result in progressive neurodegeneration. Mutations in *NEFL*, a member of the neurofilament family expressed exclusively in neurons and a prominent element in the axonal cytoskeleton, occur in CMT2E and CMT1F where they cause disruption of the neurofilament network and aggregation. The *MFN2* gene encoding mitofusion-2, a protein located in the outer membrane of mitochondrial, which serves as an adaptor to dock mitochondria to motor proteins, is mutated in CMT2A2. One mitochondrial protein encoded by the *GDAP1* gene, ganglioside-induced differentiation-associated protein-1, plays a role in mitochondrial fusion and fission and causes mitochondrial fragmentation associated with CMT4A. Small vesicles transported along the axonal microtubules are partially controlled by a GTPase encoded by *RAB7A* involved in membrane traffic and vesicular transport to late endosomes and lysosomes in the endocytic pathway, mutation of which leads to CMT2B. The *DNM2* gene encoding dynamin-2, which plays a role in endocytosis and regulates vesicle budding, when defective in CMTDIB, leads to prominent decoration of microtubules and alters microtubule dynamics necessary for correct axonal transport. Two other motor proteins, dynein encoded by *DYNC1H1*, and dynactin 1 encoded by *DCTN1*, act together for microtubule-mediated fast axonal transport and are deficient, respectively, in CMT2O and HMN7B. *KIF1B*, which controls vesicle motility in microtubules, is mutated in CMT2A1. The *TRPV4* gene, which encodes a calcium permeable non-selective channel that contributes to the regulation of systemic osmotic pressure, is mutated in CMT2C, the excitotoxic effects of which appear to be deleterious to axonal transport. Mutations in the three HSP molecular chaperones encoded by the *HSPB8*, *HSPB1*, and *HSPB3* genes, implicated in the regulation of the assembly of cytoskeletal structures such as actin and intermediate neurofilaments, are respectively associated with HMN2A, HMN2B, and HMN2C. *LITAF/SIMPLE* gene function that participates in the endocytic pathway regulating protein degradation is mutated in CMT1C. The myotubularin-related proteins, MTMR2 and MTMR13, and FIG4, which regulate polyphosphoinositide metabolism at the level of early endosomes, are respectively mutated in CMT4B1 and CMT4B2. Mutation in the *LMNA* gene encoding lamin, constituting a two-dimensional matrix next to the inner nuclear membrane, is associated with CMT2B1. Although it is unclear whether defective nuclear proteins contribute to neuropathy, inhibition of extranuclear lamin B2 is associated with axonal degeneration (169). The *SCHTC2* gene, which regulates endosomal recycling, and *NDRG1*, which regulates membrane trafficking, are respectively mutated in CMT4C and CMT4D.

MANAGEMENT

There are no specific cures for inherited neuropathies and current management consists of rehabilitation, orthotics, symptomatic treatment of pain, physical and occupational therapy, foot care, and surgical correction of foot and hand deformities (170). When done effectively, they help patients ambulate independently throughout their lives. Difficulties with fine movements of the fingers are frequent, and occupational therapy can help with techniques to aid in buttoning, zippering, and other hand movements requiring dexterity.

Treatment with progesterone (171) and ascorbic acid (172) were studied in the context of demyelinating CMT. The former promotes myelination of the PNS and stimulates *PMP22* and *MPZ* gene expression. The latter has ameliorative effects on collagen and laminin-containing extracellular matrix in promoting Schwann cell myelination. However, neither is routinely prescribed outside of a clinical trial setting.

The characterization of mutant *HSPB1*-expressing mice that phenocopy human CMT2 and distal HMN (173) due to defective mitochondrial transport, is associated with a reduction in acetylated tubulin levels in peripheral nerves isolated from symptomatic animals. This prompted treatment with HDAC6 inhibitors resulting in an increase in acetylated tubulin in symptomatic mutant HSPB1-expressing mice. The restoration of axonal transport defects and reversal of some key symptoms in mice suggested that reinnervation occurred after HDAC6 administration, a potentially useful future strategy for CMT2 in humans (167, 174). Medications known to cause neurotoxicity, such as vincristine or cis platinum should be avoided in CMT because they are likely to exacerbate already existing neuropathy.

REFERENCES

1. Gentil BJ, Cooper L. Molecular basis of axonal dysfunction and traffic impairments in CMT. *Brain Res Bull* 2012; 88:444–453.
2. Niemann A, Berger P, Suter U. Pathomechanisms of mutant proteins in Charcot-Marie-Tooth disease. *Neuromolecular Med* 2006; 8:217–242.
3. Dierick I, Baets J, Irobi J, et al. Relative contribution of mutations in genes for autosomal dominant distal hereditary motor neuropathies: a genotype-phenotype correlation study. *Brain* 2008; 131:1217–1227.
4. Dyck PJ, Lambert EH. Lower motor and primary sensory neuron diseases with peroneal muscular atrophy. 1. Neurologic, genetic, and electrophysiologic findings in hereditary polyneuropathies. *Arch Neurol* 1968; 18:603–618.
5. Harding AE, Thomas PK. The clinical features of hereditary motor and sensory neuropathy types I and II. *Brain* 1980; 103:259–280.
6. Lupski JR, de Oca-Lusa RM, Slaugenhaupt S, et al. DNA duplication associated with Charcot-Marie-Tooth disease type 1A. *Cell* 1991; 66:219–23.
7. Patel PI, Roa BB, Welcher AA, et al. The gene for the peripheral myelin protein PMP-22 is a candidate for Charcot-Marie-Tooth disease type 1a. *Nature Genet* 1992; 1:159–165.
8. Change PF, Alderson MK, Leppig KA, et al. DNA deletion associated with hereditary neuropathy with liability to pressure palsies. *Cell* 1993; 72:143–151.
9. Roa BB, Dyck PJ, Marks HG, et al. Dejerine-Sottas syndrome associated with point mutation in the peripheral myelin protein 22 (PMP22) gene. *Nature Genet* 1993; 5:269–273.
10. Martinoli C, Schenone A, Bianchi S, et al. Sonography of the median nerve in Charcot-Marie-Tooth disease. *AJR Am J Roentgenol* 2002; 178:1553–1556.
11. Hattori N, Yamamoto M, Yoshihara T, et al. Demyelinating and axonal features of Charcot-Marie-Tooth disease with mutations of myelin-related proteins (PMP22, MPZ and Cx32): a clinicopathological study of 205 Japanese patients. *Brain* 2003; 126:134–151.
12. Sahenk Z, Chen L, Mendell JR. Effects of PMP22 duplication and deletions on the axonal cytoskeleton. *Ann Neurol* 1999; 45:16–24.
13. Ginsberg L, Malik O, Kenton AR, et al. Coexistent hereditary and inflammatory neuropathy. *Brain* 2004; 127:193–202.
14. Vital A, Vital C, Lagueny A, et al. Inflammatory demyelination in a patient with CMT1A. *Muscle Nerve* 2003; 28:373–376.
15. Saporta ASD, Sottile SL, Miller LJ, et al. Charcot-Marie-Tooth disease subtypes and genetic testing strategies. *Ann Neurol* 2011; 69:22–33.
16. Shy ME, Chen L, Swan ER, et al. Neuropathy progression in Charcot-Marie-Tooth disease type 1A. *Neurology* 2008; 70:378–383.
17. Videler AJ, van Dijk JP, Beelen A, et al. Motor axon loss is associated with hand dysfunction in Charcot-Marie-Tooth disease 1a. *Neurology* 2008; 71:1254–1260.
18. Sahenk Z, Nagaraja HN, McCracken BS, et al. NT-3 promotes nerve regeneration and sensory improvement in CMT1A mouse models and in patients. *Neurology* 2005; 65:681–689.
19. Chance PF, Alderson MK, Leppig KA, et al. DNA deletion associated with hereditary neuropathy with liability to pressure palsies. *Cell* 1993; 72:143–151.
20. Li J, Krajewski K, Lewis RA, et al. Loss-of-function phenotype of hereditary neuropathy with liability to pressure palsies. *Muscle Nerve* 2004; 29:205–210.
21. Windebank A. Inherited recurrent focal neuropathies. In: Dyck PJ TP, Griffin JW, Low PA, Poduslo JF, ed. *Peripheral Neuropathy*. Philadelphia: WB Saunders, 1993; 1137–1148.
22. Fabrizi GM, Taioli F, Cavallaro T, et al. Focally folded myelin in Charcot-Marie-Tooth neuropathy type 1B with Ser49Leu in the myelin protein zero. *Acta Neuropathol* 2000; 100:299–304.
23. Shy ME, Jani A, Krajewski KM, et al. Phenotypic Clustering in MPZ mutations. *Brain* 2004; 127:371–384.
24. Inoue K, Khajavi M, Ohyama T, et al. Molecular mechanisms for distinct neurological phenotypes conveyed by allelic truncating mutations. *Nature Genet* 2004; 36:361–369.
25. Gabreels-Festen AA, Hoogendijk JE, Meijerink PH, et al. Two divergent types of nerve pathology in patients with different P0 mutations in Charcot-Marie-Tooth disease. *Neurology* 1996; 47:761–765.
26. Chance PF, Bird TD, O'Connell P, et al. Genetic linkage and heterogeneity in type 1 Charcot-Marie-Tooth disease (hereditary

motor and sensory neuropathy type 1). *Am J Hum Genet* 1990; 47:915–925.

27. Street VA, Goldy JD, Golden AS, et al. Mapping of Charcot-Marie-Tooth disease type 1C to chromosome 16p identifies a novel focus for demyelinating neuropathies. *Am J Hum Genet* 2002; 70:244–250.

28. Street VA, Bennett CL, Goldy JD, et al. Mutation of a putative protein degradation gene LITAF/SIMPLE in Charcot-Marie-Tooth disease 1C. *Neurology* 2003; 60:22–26.

29. Warner LE, Mancias P, Butler IJ, et al. Mutations in the early growth response 2 (EGR2) gene are associated with hereditary myelinopathies. *Nat Genet* 1998; 19:382–384.

30. Safka Brožková D, Nevšímalová S, Mazanec R, et al. Charcot-Marie-Tooth neuropathy due to a novel EGR2 gene mutation with mild phenotype. Usefulness of human mapping chip linkage analysis in a Czech family. *Neuromuscul Disord* 2012. Epub ahead of print.

31. Hamiel OP, Raas-Rothschild A, Upadhyaya M, et al. Hereditary motor-sensory neuropathy (Charcot-Marie-Tooth disease) with nerve deafness: a new variant. *J Pediat* 1993; 123:431–434.

32. Kovach MJ, Lin J-P, Boyadjiev S, et l. A unique point mutation in the PMP22 gene is associated with Charcot-Marie-Tooth disease and deafness. *Am J Hum Genet* 1999; 64:1580–1593.

33. Kousseff BG, Hadro TA, Treiber DL, et al. Charcot-Marie-Tooth disease with sensorineural hearing loss-an autosomal dominant trait. *Birth Defects Orig Art Ser* 1982; 18:223–228.

34. Jordanova A, De Johghe P, Boerkoel CF, et al. Mutations in the neurofilament light chain gene (NEFL) cause early onset severe Charcot-Marie-Tooth disease. *Brain* 2003; 126:590–597.

35. Abe A, Numakura C, Saito K, et al. Neurofilament light chain polypeptide gene mutations in Charcot-Marie-Tooth disease: nonsense mutation probably causes a recessive phenotype. *J Hum Genet* 2009; 54:94–97.

36. Brownlees J, Ackerley S, Grierson AJ, et al. Charcot-Marie-Tooth disease neurofilament mutations disrupt neurofilament assembly and axonal transport. *Hum Mol Genet* 2002; 11:2837–2844.

37. Phillips LH, Kelly TE, Schnatterly P, et al. Hereditary motor-sensory neuropathy (HMSN): possible X-linked dominant inheritance. *Neurology* 1985; 35:498–502.

38. Hahn AF, Brown WF, Koopman WJ, et al. X-linked dominant hereditary motor and sensory neuropathy. *Brain* 1990; 113:1511–1525.

39. Birouk N, LeGuern E, Maisonobe T, et al. X-linked Charcot-Marie-Tooth disease with connexin 32 mutations: clinical and electrophysiological study. *Neurology* 1998; 50:1074–1082.

40. Yiu EM, Geevasinga N, Nicholson GA, et al. A retrospective review of X-linked Charcot-Marie-Tooth disease in childhood. *Neurology* 2011; 76:461–466.

41. Bergoffen J, Scherer SS, Wang S, et al. Connexin mutations in X-linked Charcot-Marie-Tooth disease. *Science* 1993; 262:2039–2042.

42. Ionasescu VV, Trafatter J, Haines JL, et al. Heterogeneity in X-linked recessive Charcot-Marie-Tooth neuropathy. *Am J Hum Genet* 1991; 48:1075–1083.

43. Ionasescu VV, Trofatter J, Haines JL, et al. X-linked recessive Charcot-Marie-Tooth neuropathy: clinical and genetic study. *Muscle Nerve* 1992; 15:368–373.

44. Huttner IG, Kennerson ML, Reddel SW, et al. Proof of genetic heterogeneity in X-linked Charcot-Marie-Tooth disease. *Neurology* 2006; 67:2016–2021.

45. Cowchock FS, Duckett SW, Streletz LJ, et al. X-linked motor-sensory neuropathy type-II with deafness ad mental retardation: a new disorder. *Am J Med Genet* 1985; 20:307–315.

46. Sladky JT, Brown MJ. Infantile axonal polyneuropathy with X-linked inheritance. *Ann Neurol* 1984; 16:402.

47. Fischbeck KH, Ritter A, Shi Y, et al. Linkage studies of X-linked neuropathy and spinal muscular atrophy. *Cytogenet Cell Genet* 1987; 46:614.

48. Priest JM, Fischbeck KH, Nouri N, et al. A locus for axonal motor-sensory neuropathy with deafness and mental retardation maps to Xq24-q26. *Genomics* 1995; 29:409–412.

49. Rosenberg RN, Chutorian A. Familial opticoacoustic nerve degeneration and polyneuropathy. *Neurology* 1967; 17:827–832.

50. Kim HJ, Hong SH, Ki C-S, et al. A novel locus for X-linked recessive CMT with deafness and optic neuropathy maps to Xq21.32-q24. *Neurology* 2005; 64:1964–1967.

51. Kim HH, Sohn KM, Shy ME, et al. Mutations in PRPS1, which encodes the phosphoribosyl pyrophosphage synthetase enzyme critical for nucleotide biosynthesis, cause hereditary peripheral neuropathy with hearing loss and optic neuropathy (CMT5X). *Am J Hum Genet* 2007; 81:552–558.

52. Saito M, Hayashi Y, Suzuki T, et al. Linkage mapping of the gene for Charcot-Marie-Tooth disease type 2 to chromosome 1p (CMT2A) and the clinical features of CMT2A. *Neurology* 1997; 49:1630–1635.

53. Zhao C, Takita J, Tanaka Y, et al. Charcot-Marie-Tooth disease type 2A caused by mutation in a microtubule motor KIF1B-beta. *Cell* 2001; 105:587–597.

54. Zuchner S, Mersiyanova IV, Muglia M, et al. Mutations in the mitochondrial GTPase mitofusin 2 cause Charcot-Marie-Tooth neuropathy type 2A. *Nat Genet* 2004; 36:449–451.

55. Bissar-Tadmouri N, Nelis E, et al. Absence of KIF1B mutation in a large Turkish CMT2A family suggests involvement of a second gene. *Neurology* 2004; 62:1522–1525.

56. Muglia M, Zappia M, Timmerman V, et al. Clinical and genetic study of a large Charcot-Marie-Tooth type 2A family from southern Italy. *Neurology* 2001; 56:100–103.

57. Verhoeven K, De Jonghe P, Coen K, et al. Mutations in the small GTP-ase late endosomal protein RAB7 cause Charcot-Marie-Tooth type 2B neuropathy. *Am J Hum Genet* 2003; 72:722–727.

58. Kwon JM, Elliott JL, Yee WC, et al. Assignment of a second Charcot-Marie-Tooth type II locus to chromosome 3q. *Am J Hum Genet* 1995; 57:853–858.

59. De Jonghe P, Timmerman V, FitzPatrick D, et al. Mutilating neuropathic ulcerations in a chromosome 3q13-q22 linked Charcot-Marie-Tooth disease type 2B family. *J Neurol Neurosurg Psychiatry* 1997; 62:570–573.

60. Auer-Grumbach M, De Johghe P, Wagner K, et al. Phenotype-genotype correlations in a CMT2B family with refined 3q13-q22 locus. *Neurology* 2000; 55:1552–1557.

61. Bouhouche A, Benomar A, Birouk N, et al. A locus for an axonal form of autosomal recessive Charcot-Marie-Tooth disease maps to chromosome 1q21.2-q21.3. *Am J Hum Genet* 1999; 65:722–727.

62. De Sandre-Giovannoli A, Chaouch M, Kozlov S, et al. Homozygous defects in LMNA, encoding lamin A/C nuclear-envelope proteins, cause autosomal recessive axonal neuropathy in human (Charcot-Marie-Tooth disorder type 2) and mouse. *Am J Hum Genet* 2002; 70:726–736.

63. Leal A, Morera B, Del Valle G, et al. A second locus for an axonal form of autosomal recessive Charcot-Marie-Tooth disease maps to chromosome 19q13.3. *Am J Hum Genet* 2001; 68:269–274.

64. Leal A, Huehne K, Bauer F, et al. Identification of the variant Ala335Val of MED25 as responsible for CMT2B2: molecular data, functional studies of the SH3 recognition motif and correlation between wild-type MED25 and PMP22 RNA levels in CMT1A animal models. *Neurogenetics* 2009; 10:275–287.

65. Dyck PJ, Litchy WJ, Minnerath S, et al. Hereditary motor and

sensory neuropathy with diaphragm and vocal cord paresis. *Ann Neurol* 1994; 35:608–615.

66. Klein CJ, Cunningham JM, Atkinson EJ, et al. The gene for HMSN2C maps to 12q23-24: a region of neuromuscular disorders. *Neurology* 2003; 60:1151–1156.

67. Klein CJ, Shi Y, Fecto F, et al. TRPV4 mutations and cytotoxic hypercalcemia in axonal Charcot-Marie-Tooth neuropathies. *Neurology* 2011; 76:887–894.

68. Landouré G, Zdebik AA, Martinez TL, et al. Mutations in TRPV4 cause Charcot-Marie-Tooth disease type 2C. *Nat Genet* 2010; 42:170–174.

69. Auer-Grumbach M, Olschewski A, Papic L, et al. Alternations in the ankyrin domain of TRPV4 cause congenital distal SMA, scapuloperoneal SMA and HMSN2C. *Nat Genet* 2010; 42:160–164.

70. Ionasescu V, Searby C, Sheffield VC, et al. Autosomal dominant Charcot-Marie-Tooth axonal neuropathy mapped on chromosome 7p (CMT2D). *Hum Molec Genet* 1996; 5:1373–1375.

71. Antonellis A, Ellsworth RE, Sambuughin N, et al. Glycyl tRNA synthetase mutations in Charcot-Marie-Tooth disease type 2D and distal spinal muscular atrophy type V. *Am J Hum Genet* 2003; 72:1293–1299.

72. Meriyanova IV, Perepelov AV, Polyakov AV, et al. A new variant of Charcot-Marie-Tooth disease type 2 is probably the result of a mutation in the neurofilament-light gene. *Am J Hum Genet* 2000; 67:37–46.

73. Fabrizi GM, Cavallaro T, Angiari C, et al. Giant axon and neurofilament accumulation in Charcot-Marie-Tooth disease type 2E. *Neurology* 2004; 62:1429–1431.

74. Kamholz J, Menichella D, Jani A, et al. Charcot-Marie-Tooth disease type 1: molecular pathogenesis to gene therapy. *Brain* 2000; 123:222–233.

75. Ismailov SM, Fedotov VP, Dadali EL, et al. A new locus for autosomal dominant Charcot-Marie-Tooth disease type 2 (CMT2F) maps to chromosome 7q11-q21. *Eur J Hum Genet* 2001; 9:646–650.

76. Evgrafov OV, Mersiyanova I, Irobi J, et al. Mutant small heat-shock protein 27 causes Charcot-Marie-Tooth disease and distal hereditary motor neuropathy. *Nat Genet* 2004; 36:602–606.

77. Berciano J, Combarros O, Figols J, et al. Hereditary motor and sensory neuropathy type II: clinicopathological study of a family. *Brain* 1986; 109:897–914.

78. Nelis E, Berciano J, Verpoorten N, et al. Autosomal dominant axonal Charcot-Marie-Tooth disease type 2 (CMT2G) maps to chromosome 12q12-q13.3. *J Med Genet* 2004; 41:193–197.

79. Barhoumi C, Amouri R, Ben Hamida C, et al. Linkage of a new locus for autosomal recessive axonal form of Charcot-Marie-Tooth disease to chromosome 8q21.3. *Neuromuscul Disord* 2001; 11:27–34.

80. Marrosu MG, Vaccargiu S, Marrosu G, et al. Charcot-Marie-Tooth disease type 2 associated with mutation of the myelin protein zero gene. *Neurology* 1998; 50:1397–1401.

81. Senderek J, Hermanns B, Lehmann U, et al. Charcot-Marie-Tooth neuropathy type 2 and P0 point mutations: two novel amino acid substitutions (Asp61Gly; Tyr119Cys) and a possible "hotspot" on Thr124Met. *Brain Path* 2000; 10:235–248.

82. Boerkoel CF, Takashima H, Garcia CA, et al. Charcot-Marie-Tooth disease and related neuropathies: mutation distribution and genotype-phenotype correlation. *Ann Neurol* 2002; 51:190–201.

83. Auer-Grumbach M, Strasser-Fuchs S, Robl T, et al. Late onset Charcot-Marie-Tooth 2 syndrome caused by two novel mutations in the MPZ gene. *Neurology* 2003; 61:1435–1437.

84. De Jonghe P, Timmerman V, Ceuterick C, et al. The Thr124Met mutation in peripheral myelin protein zero (MPZ) gene is associated with a clinically distinct Charcot-Marie-Tooth phenotype. *Brain* 1999; 122:281–290.

85. Chapon F, Latour P, Diraison P, et al. Axonal phenotype of Charcot-Marie-Tooth disease associated with a mutation in the myelin protein zero gene. *J Neurol Neurosurg Psychiatry* 1999; 66:779–782.

86. Misu K, Yoshihara T, Shikama Y, et al. An axonal form of Charcot-Marie-Tooth disease showing distinctive features in association with mutations in the peripheral myelin protein zero gene (Thr124Met or Asp75Val). *J Neurol Neurosurg Psychiatry* 2000; 69:806–811.

87. Kabzinska D, Korwin-Piotrowska T, Dreschsler H, et al. Late-onset Charcot-Marie-Tooth type 2 disease with hearing impairment associated with a novel Pro105Thr mutation in the MPZ gene(Letter). *Am J Med Genet A* 2007; 143A:2196–2199.

88. Triggs WJ, Brown RH Jr, Menkes DL. Case Records of the Massachusetts General Hospital. Case 18-2006: a 57-year-old woman with numbness and weakness of the feet and legs. *N Engl J Med* 2006; 354:2584–2592.

89. Birouk N, Azzedine H, Bubourg O, et al. Phenotypical features of a Moroccan family with autosomal recessive Charcot-Marie-Tooth disease associated with the S194X mutation in the GDAP1 gene. *Arch Neurol* 2003; 60:598–604.

90. Xin B, Puffenberger E, Nye L, et al. A novel mutation in the GDAP1 gene is associated with autosomal recessive Charcot-Marie-Tooth disease in an Amish family. *Clin Genet* 2008; 74:274–278.

91. Chung KW, Kim SM, Sunwoo IN, et al. A novel GDAP1 Q218E mutation in autosomal dominant Charcot-Marie-Tooth disease. *J Hum Genet* 2008; 53:360–364.

92. Crimella C, Tonelli A, Airoldi G, et al. The GST domain of GDAP1 is a frequent target of mutations in the dominant form of axonal Charcot-Marie-Tooth type 2K. *J Med Genet* 2010; 47:712–716.

93. Tang BS, Luo W, Xia K, et al. A new locus for autosomal dominant Charcot-Marie-Tooth disease type 2 (CMT2L) maps to chromosome 12q24. *Hum Genet* 2004; 114:527–533.

94. Tang BS, Zhao GH, Luo W, et al. Small heat-shock protein 22 mutated in autosomal dominant Charcot-Marie-Tooth disease type 2L. *Hum Genet* 2005; 116:222–224.

95. Carra S, Sivilotti M, Chávez Zobel AT, et al. HspB8, a small heat shock protein mutated in human neuromuscular disorders, has in vivo chaperone activity in cultured cells. *Hum Mol Genet* 2005; 14:1659–1669.

96. Gallardo E, Claeys KG, Nelis E, et al. Magnetic resonance imaging findings of leg musculature in Charcot-Marie-Tooth disease type 2 due to dynamin 2 mutation. *J Neurol* 2008; 255:986–992.

97. Fabrizi GM, Ferrarini M, Cavallaro T, et al. Two novel mutations in dynamin-2 cause axonal Charcot-Marie-Tooth disease. *Neurology* 2007; 69:291–295.

98. Sidiropoulos PN, Miehe M, Bock T, et al. Dynamin 2 mutations in Charcot-Marie-Tooth neuropathy highlight the importance of clathrin-mediated endocytosis in myelination. *Brain* 2012; 135:1395–1411.

99. Latour P, Thauvin-Robinet C, Baudelet-Méry C, et al. A major determinant for binding and aminoacylation of tRNA(Ala) in cytoplasmic alanyl-tRNA synthtase is mutated in dominant axonal Charcot-Marie-Tooth disease. *Am J Hum Genet* 2010; 86:77–82.

100. Lin KP, Soong BW, Yang CC, et al. The mutational spectrum in a cohort of Charcot-Marie-Tooth disease type 2 among the Han Chinese in Taiwan. *PLoS One* 2011; 6:e29393.

101. McLaughlin HM, Sakaguchi R, Giblin W, et al. A recurrent los-of-function alanyl-tRNA synthetase (AARS) mutation in

patients with Charcot-Marie-Tooth disease type 2N (CMT2N). *Hum Mutat* 2012; 33:244–253.

102. Weedon MN, Hastings R, Caswell R, et al. Exome sequencing identifies a DYNC1H1 mutation in a large pedigree with dominant axonal Charcot-Marie-Tooth disease. *Am J Hum Genet* 2011; 89:308–312.

103. Hafezparasat M, Klocke R, Ruhrberg C, et al. Mutations in dynein link motor neuron degeneration to defects in retrograde transport. *Science* 2003; 300:808–812.

104. Guernsey DL, Jiang H, Bedard K, et al. Mutation in the gene encoding ubiquitin ligase LRSAM1 in patients with Charcot-Marie-Tooth disease. *PLoS Genet* 2010; 6:e1001081.

105. Weterman MA, Sorrentino V, Kasher PR, et al. A frameshift mutation in LRSAM1 is responsible for a dominant hereditary polyneuropathy. *Hum Mol Genet* 2012; 21:358–370.

106. Amit I, Yakir L, Katz M, et al. Tal, a Tsg101-specific E3 ubiquitin ligase, regulates receptor endocytosis and retrovirus budding. *Genes Dev* 2004; 18:1737–1752.

107. Li B, Su Y, Rydel J, et al. RIFLE: a novel finger-leucine-rich repeat containing protein regulates select cell adhesion molecules in PC12 cells. *J Cell Biochem* 2003; 90:1224–1241.

108. Ben Othmane K, Hentati F, Lennon F, et al. Linkage of a locus (CMT4A) for autosomal recessive Charcot-Marie-Tooth disease to chromosome 8q. *Hum Mol Genet* 1993; 2:1625–1628.

109. Baxter RV, Ben Othmane K, Rochelle JM, et al. Ganglioside-induced differentiation-associated protein-1 is mutant in Charcot-Marie-Tooth disease 4A/8q21. *Nat Genet* 2002; 30:21–22.

110. Quattrone A, Gambardella A, Bono F, et al. Autosomal recessive hereditary motor and sensory neuropathy with focally folded myelin sheaths: clinical, electrophysiologic, and genetic aspects of a large family. *Neurology* 1996; 46:1318–1324.

111. Bolino A, Brancolini V, Bono F, et al. Localization of a gene responsible for autosomal recessive demyelinating neuropathy with focally folded myelin sheaths to chromosome 11q23 by homozygosity mapping and haplotype sharing. *Hum Mol Genet* 1996; 5:1051–1054.

112. Bolina A, Muglia M, Conforti FL, et al. Charcot-Marie-Tooth type 4B is caused by mutations in the gene encoding myotubularin-related protein-2. *Nat Genet* 2000; 25:17–19.

113. Senderek J, Bergmann C, Weber S, et al. Mutation of the SBF2 gene, encoding a novel member of the myotubularin family, in Charcot-Marie-Tooth neuropathy type 4B2/11p15. *Hum Mol Genet* 2003; 12:349–356.

114. Kessali M, Zemmouri R, Guilbot A, et al. A clinical, electrophysiologic, neuropathologic, and genetic study of two large Algerian families with an autosomal recessive demyelinating form of Charcot-Marie-Tooth disease. *Neurology* 1997; 48:867–873.

115. Azzedine H, Ravisé N, Verny C, et al. Spine deformities in Charcot-Marie-Tooth 4C caused by SH3TC2 gene mutations. *Neurology* 2006; 67:602–606.

116. Lupski JR, Reid JG, Gonzaga-Jauregui C, et al. Whole-genome sequencing in a patient with Charcot-Marie-Tooth neuropathy. *N Engl J Med* 2010; 362:1181–1191.

117. Lassuthová P, Mazanec R, Vondráček P, et al. High frequency of SH3TC2 mutations in Czech HMSN I patients. *Clin Genet* 2011; 80:334–345.

118. Arnaud E, Zenker J, de Preux Charles A-S, et al. SH3TC2/KIAA1985 protein is required for proper myelination and the integrity of the node of Ranvier in the peripheral nervous system. *Proc Nat Acad Sci* 2009; 106:17528–17533.

119. Kalaydjieva L, Gresham D, Gooding R, et al. N-myc downstream-regulated gene 1 is mutated in hereditary motor and sensory neuropathy-Lom. *Am J Hum Genet* 2000; 67:47–58.

120. King RHM, Tournev I, Colomer J, et al. Ultrastructural changes in peripheral nerve in hereditary motor and sensory neuropathy-Lom. *Neuropathol Appl Neurobiol* 1999; 25:306–312.

121. Hunter M, Bernard R, Freitas E, et al. Mutation screening of the N-myc downstream-regulated gene 1 (NDRG1) in patients with Charcot-Marie-Tooth Disease. *Hum Mutat* 2003; 22:129–135.

122. Warner LE, Hilz M, Appel SH, et al. Clinical phenotypes of different MPZ (P0) mutations may include Charcot-Marie-Tooth type 1B, Dejerine-Sottas, and congenital hypomyelination. *Neuron* 1996; 17:451–460.

123. Warner LE, Mancias P, Butler IJ, et al. Mutations in the early growth response 2 (ERG2) gene are associated with hereditary myelinopathies. *Nature Genet* 1998; 18:382–384.

124. Dejerine J, Sottas J. Sur la nevrite interstitielle hypertrophique et progressive de l'enfance. *Comp Rend Soc Biol* 1893; 45:63–96.

125. Delague V, Bareil C, Tuffery S, et al. Mapping of a new locus for autosomal recessive demyelinating Charcot-Marie-Tooth disease to 19q13.1-13.3 in a large consanguineous Lebanese family: exclusion of MAG as a candidate gene. *Am J Hum Genet* 2000; 67:236–243.

126. Guilbot A, Williams A, Ravisé N, et al. A mutation in periaxin is responsible for CMT4F, an autosomal recessive form of Charcot-Marie-Tooth disease. *Hum Mol Genet* 2001; 10:415–421.

127. Timmerman V, De Jonghe P, Ceuterick C, et al. Novel missense mutation in the early growth response 2 gene associated with Dejerine-Sottas syndrome phenotype. *Neurology* 1999; 52:1827–1832.

128. Hayasaka K, Himoro M, Sawaishi Y, et al. De novo mutation of the myelin P0 gene in Dejerine-Sottas disease (hereditary motor and sensory neuropathy type III). *Nat Genet* 1993; 5:266–268.

129. Roa BB, Dyck PJ, Marks HG, et al. Dejerine-Sottas syndrome associated with point mutation in the peripheral myelin protein 22 (PMP22) gene. *Nat Genet* 1993; 5:269–273.

130. De Sandre-Giovannoli A, Delague V, Hamadouche T, et al. Homozygosity mapping of autosomal recessive demyelinating Charcot-Marie-Tooth neuropathy (CMT4H) to a novel locus on chromosome 12p11.21-q13.11 (Letter). *J Med Genet* 2005; 42:260–265.

131. Rogers T, Chandler D, Angelicheva D, et al. A novel locus for autosomal recessive peripheral neuropathy in the EGR2 region on 10q23. *Am J Hum Genet* 2000; 67:664–671.

132. Thomas PK, Kalaydjieva L, Youl B, et al. Hereditary motor and sensory neuropathy-russe: new autosomal recessive neuropathy in Balkan Gypsies. *Ann Neurol* 2001; 50:452–457.

133. Delague V, Jacquier A, Hamadouche T, et al. Mutations in FGD4 encoding the Rho GDP/GTP exchange factor FRABIN cause autosomal recessive Charcot-Marie-Tooth type 4H. *Am J Hum Genet* 2007; 81:1–16.

134. Stendel C, Roos A, Deconinck T, et al. Peripheral nerve demyelination caused by a mutant Rho GTPase guanine nucleotide exchange factor, frabin/FGD4. *Am J Hum Genet* 2007; 81:158–164.

135. Fabrizi GM, Taioli F, Cavallaro T, et al. Further evidence that mutations in FGD4/frabin cause Charcot-Marie-Tooth disease type 4H. *Neurology* 2009; 72:1160–1164.

136. Chow CY, Zhang Y, Dowling JJ, et al. Mutation of FIG4 causes neurodegeneration in the pale tremor mouse and patients with CMT4J. *Nature* 2007; 448:68–72.

137. Rossi A, Paradiso C, Cioni R, et al. Charcot-Marie-Tooth disease: study of a large kinship with an intermediate form. *J Neurol* 1985; 232:91–98.

138. Verhoeven K, Villanova M, Rossi A, et al. Localization of the gene for the intermediate form of Charcot-Marie-Tooth

to chromosome 10q24.1-q25.1. *Am J Hum Genet* 2001; 69:889–894.

139. Salisachs P. Wide spectrum of motor conduction velocity in Charcot-Marie-Tooth disease: an anatomico-physiologial interpretation. *J Neurol Sci* 1974; 23:25–31.

140. Davis CJ, Bradley WG, Madrid R. The peroneal muscular atrophy syndrome: clinical, genetic, electrophysiological and nerve biopsy studies I. Clinical, genetic and electrophysiological findings and classifications. *J Genet Hum* 1978; 26:311–349.

141. Kennerson ML, Zhu D, Gardner RJ, et al. Dominant intermediate Charcot-Marie-Tooth neuropathy maps to chromosome 19p12-p13.2. *Am J Hum Genet* 2001; 69:883–888.

142. Speer MC, Graham FL, Bonner E, et al. Reduction in the minimum candidate interval in the dominant-intermediate form of Charcot-Marie-Tooth neuropathy to D19S586 to D19S432. *Neurogenetics* 2002; 4:83–85.

143. Zhu D, Kennerson M, Merory J, et al. Refined localization of dominant intermediate Charcot-Marie-Tooth neuropathy and exclusion of seven known candidate genes in the region. *Neurogenetics* 2003; 4:179–183.

144. Jordanova A, Irobi J, Thomas FP, et al. Disrupted function and axonal distribution of mutant tyrosyl-tRNA synthetase in dominant intermediate Charcot-Marie-Tooth neuropathy. *Nat Genet* 2006; 38:197–202.

145. Mastaglia FL, Nowak KJ, Stell R, et al. Novel mutation in the myelin protein zero gene in a family with intermediate hereditary motor and sensory neuropathy. *J Neurol Neurosurg Psychiatry* 1999; 67:174–179.

146. Boyer O, Nevo F, Plaisier E, et al. INF2 mutations in Charcot-Marie-Tooth disease with glomerulopathy. *N Engl J Med* 2011; 365:2377–2388.

147. Gopinath S, Blair IP, Kennerson ML, et al. A novel locus for distal motor neuron degeneration maps to chromosome 7q34-q36. *Hum Genet* 2007; 121:559–564.

148. Timmerman V, De Jonghe P, Simokovic S, et al. Distal hereditary motor neuropathy type II (distal HMNII): mapping of a locus to chromosome 12q24. *Hum Mol Genet* 1996; 5:1065–1069.

149. Irobi J, De Johghe P, Timmerman V. Molecular genetics of distal hereditary motor neuropathies. *Hum Mol Genet* 2004; 13:R195–R202.

150. Houlden H, Laura M, Wavrant-De Vrieze F, et al. Mutations in the HSP27 (HSPB1) gene cause dominant, recessive, and sporadic distal HMN/CMT type 2. *Neurology* 2008; 71:1660–1668.

151. d'Ydewalle C, Krishnan J, Chiheb DM, et al. HDAC6 inhibitors reverse axonal loss in a mouse model of mutant HSPB1-induced Charcot-Marie-Tooth disease. *Nature Med* 2011; 17:968–974.

152. Kolb SJ, Snyder PJ, Poi EJ, et al. Mutant small heat shock protein B3 causes motor neuropathy: utility of a candidate gene approach. *Neurology* 2010; 74:502–506.

153. Viollet L, Barois A, Rebeiz JG, et al. Mapping of autosomal recessive chronic distal spinal muscular atrophy to chromosome 11q13. *Ann Neurol* 2002; 51:585–592.

154. Viollet L, Zarhrate M, Maystadt I, et al. Refined genetic mapping of autosomal recessive chronic distal spinal muscular atrophy to chromosome 11q13.3 and evidence of linkage disequilibrium in European families. *Eur J Hum Genet* 2004; 12:483–488.

155. Antonellis A, Ellsworth RE, Sambuughin N, et al. Glycyl tRNA synthetase mutations in Charcot-Marie-Tooth disease type 2D and distal spinal muscular atrophy type V. *Am J Hum Genet* 2003; 72:1293–1299.

156. Christodoulou K, Kyriakides T, Hristova AH, et al. Mapping of a distal form of spinal muscular atrophy with upper limb predominance to chromosome 7p. *Hum Mol Genet* 1995; 4:1629–1632.

157. Auer-Grumbach M, Loscher WN, Wagner K, et al. Phenotypic and genotypic heterogeneity in hereditary motor neuronopathy type V: a clinical, electrophysiological and genetic study. *Brain* 2000; 123:1612–1623.

158. Young ID, Harper PS. Hereditary distal spinal muscular atrophy with vocal cord paralysis. *J Neurol Neurosurg Psychiatry* 1980; 43:413–418.

159. Boltshauser E, Lang W, Spillmann T, et al. Hereditary distal muscular atrophy with vocal cord paralysis and sensorineural hearing loss: a dominant form of spinal muscular atrophy? *J Med Genet* 1989; 26:105–108.

160. Puls I, Jonnakuty C, La Monte BH, et al. Mutant dynactin in motor neuron disease. *Nat Genet* 2003; 33:455–456.

161. Lewis RA, Sumner AJ. The electrodiagnostic distinctions between chronic familial and acquired demyelinative neuropathies. *Neurology* 1982; 32:592–596.

162. Lewis RA, Sumner AJ, Shy ME. Electrophysiological features of inherited demyelinating neuropathies: A reappraisal in the era of molecular diagnosis. *Muscle Nerve* 2000; 23:1472–1487.

163. Lewis RA, Shy ME. Electrodiagnostic findings in CMTX: a disorder of the Schwann cell and peripheral nerve myelin. *Ann N Y Acad Sci* 1999; 883:504–507.

164. Nicholson G, Nash J. Intermediate nerve conduction velocities define X-linked Charcot-Marie-Tooth neuropathy families. *Neurology* 1993; 43:2558–2564.

165. Krajewski KM, Lewis RA, Fuerst DR, et al. Neurological dysfunction and axonal degeneration in Charcot-Marie-Tooth disease type 1A. *Brain* 2000; 123:1516–1527.

166. Murphy SM, Laura M, Fawcett K, et al. Charcot-Marie-Tooth disease: frequency of genetic subtypes and guidelines for genetic testing. *J Neurol Neurosurg Psychiatry* 2012; 83:706–710.

167. Ydewalle C, Benoy V, Van Den Bosch L. Charcot-Marie-Tooth disease: Emerging mechanisms and therapies. *Int J Biochem Cell Biol* 2012; 44:1299–1304.

168. Bucci C, Bakke O, Progida C. Charcot-Marie-Tooth disease and intracellular traffic. *Prog Neurobiol* 2012, doi:10.1016/j.pneurobio.2012.03.003

169. Yoon BC, Jung H, Dwivedy A, et al. Local translation of extranuclear lamin B promotes axon maintenance. *Cell* 2012; 148:752–764

170. Reilley MM, Shy ME. Diagnosis and new treatments in genetic neuropathies. *J Neurol Neurosurg Psychiatry* 2009; 80:1304–1314

171. Désarnaud F, Do Thi AN, Brown AM, et al. Progesterone stimulates the activity of the promoters of peripheral myelin protein-22 and protein zero genes in Schwann cells. *J Neurochem* 1998; 71:1765–1768.

172. Pareyson D, Reilly MM, Schenone A, et al. Ascorbic acid in Charcot-Marie-Tooth disease type 1A (CMT-TRIAAL and CMT-TRAUK): a double-blind randomised trial. *Lancet Neurol* 2011; 10:320–328.

173. d'Ydewalle C, Krishnan J, Chiheb DM, et al. HDAC6 inhibitors reverse axon loss in a mouse model of mutant HSPB1-induced Charcot-Marie-Tooth disease. *Nature Medicine* 2011; 17:968–974

174. Almeida-Souza L, Timmerman V, Janssens S. Microtubule dynamics in the peripheral nervous system: A matter of balance. *Bioarchitecture* 2011; 1:267–270.

CHAPTER 31

Acute Inflammatory Demyelinating Polyneuropathy

Mazen M. Dimachkie, Richard J. Barohn

The commonest acute inflammatory demyelinating poly-neuropathy (AIDP), known as Landry-Guillain-Barré-Strohl, Guillain-Barré-Strohl, or simply Guillain-Barré syndrome (GBS) was described a century ago by French investigators among three prototypical patients with radic-ulopathic neuropathy, absent reflexes, and albuminocyto-logic dissociation of the cerebrospinal fluid (CSF) (1, 2). A recent review has been published (3).

EPIDEMIOLOGY

With an estimated worldwide incidence of 0.6 to 2.4/100,000 (4–6), the reported incidence ranges from 0.89 to 1.89 (median, 1.11) per 100,000 person-years, with a mean age at onset of 40 years, and occurrence in men slightly more than women. The incidence increases with age with an estimated overall incidence of 0.34 to 1.34/100,000 in childhood to 1.7/100,000 to 3.3/100,000 after age 50 (7), an increase of 20% with every 10-year rise in age from the first decade of life (8). Up to 70% of patients have an antecedent infection consisting of an upper respiratory tract infection or diarrhea. Whereas most patients have sporadic GBS, an axonal variant occurs in summer epidemics of *Campylobacter jejuni* (*C. jejuni*) infection in Northern China, compared to 5% of similar patients in North America and Europe (9). *C. jejuni* was the most frequently identified infectious agent associated with subsequent development of GBS in a meta-analysis (10) with an estimated 0.25 to 0.65 per 1,000 cases of *C. jejuni* infection, and 0.6 to 2.2 per 1,000 cases of primary cytomegalovirus infection (CMV), with other associated agents including Epstein-Barr virus (EBV), varicella-zos-ter virus (VZV), and *Mycoplasma pneumonia* (11–14).

CLINICAL PRESENTATION

Guillain-Barré Syndrome

The clinical aspects of GBS have been well-described (15). Table 1 lists the diagnostic criteria for GBS. Although the commonest initial symptom of GBS is numbness, tin-gling, pain, and paresthesia of the legs, objective sensory is typically mild and demonstrable later in the course of the disease. Within days of paresthesia, weakness follows a symmetric ascending pattern involving first proximal and distal leg muscles before spreading to the arms and progressing over a period of 12 hours to 28 days before a plateau is reached (16), followed by generalized hypo-reflexia or areflexia, which may be delayed for up to a week. Although distinctly inconsistent, GBS may be associated with normal or hyperactive reflexes and other supportive features present (17). Pain, a common and often severe fea-ture, described as moderate to severe in virtually all GBS including its variants (18) was reported as persistent pain at two weeks in more than one-third of patients, with two-thirds throughout the acute phase, and continuing for more than one year in a third of the latter. A descending pattern of weakness with onset in the face or arms is less commonly encountered, and selected patients present with leg or arm weakness alone. Facial nerve involvement occurs in up to 70% of patients, with lesser oropharyngeal, oculomotor involvement, or ptosis. Less frequent findings include hear-ing loss, papilledema and vocal cord paralysis. Up to 50% of patients reaching a nadir of weakness by two weeks, 80% by three weeks, and 90% by four weeks; further symptom progression for up to eight weeks is consistent with sub-acute inflammatory demyelinating polyradiculoneuropathy

Table 1. Diagnostic Criteria for GBS

Required	Supportive	Features casting Doubt	Exclusionary
Progressive weakness of >1 limb	Progression <4 weeks	Marked asymmetry	Other causes (toxins, botulism, porphyria, diphtheria)
Hyporeflexia or areflexia	Symmetric weakness	Onset with or persistence of bladder/bowel dysfunction	
	Sensory symptoms or signs	>50 lymphocytes/mm3 in CSF	
	Cranial nerve involvement especially VII	Polys in CSF	
	Autonomic dysfunction	Sensory level	
	CSF protein elevation		
	CSF cell count <20/mm3		
	Electrophysiologic features of demyelination		
	Recovery		

(SIDP), and afterward, chronic inflammatory demyelinating polyradiculoneuropathy (CIDP). Some patients have mild weakness while others progress to flaccid quadriplegia, with up to 30% of patients overall requiring mechanical ventilator support. Dysautonomia affects 65% of patients overall, the commonest manifestations of which include resting sinus tachycardia, bradycardia, labile blood pressure, orthostatic hypotension, cardiac arrhythmias, neurogenic pulmonary edema, sweating disturbances, urinary retention due to neurogenic bladder, constipation, ileus, gastric distension, diarrhea, and fecal incontinence due to gastrointestinal autonomic dysfunction.

While GBS typically follows a monophasic course and typically does not recur (3), two or more episodes were reported in 7% of patients with a mean interval of seven years (19). Relapsing-remitting CIDP should be considered as an alternate diagnosis in relapsing cases (20). When the first relapse is delayed by more than two months following an acute attack, or the number of relapses exceeds two instances, either should raise suspicion for CIDP (21). Further clues favoring CIDP in relapsing cases include maintaining the ability to ambulate independently at nadir, absence of cranial nerve dysfunction, and markedly demyelinating electrophysiology. Two-thirds of patients are unable to ambulate

independently when maximal weakness is reached (22) and respiratory dependency occurs in up to one-quarter of patients with other major complications, including pneumonia, sepsis, pulmonary embolism, and gastrointestinal bleeding in up to 60% of intubated patients (23).

Guillain-Barré Syndrome Variants

The Miller-Fisher syndrome (MFS) presents with ophthalmoplegia, ataxia, and areflexia without weakness (24) with most patients qualifying for two or three of the requisite features, in addition to increased CSF protein content. Whereas MFS occurs in up to 10% of all Western hemisphere patients with GBS cases, it accounts for up to 25% of Asian patients (25). Affected patients overlap with, and even progress to, otherwise typical GBS. Conversely, opthlamoplegia occurs in up to 5% of patients with typical GBS. About 10% of MFS patients have Bickerstaff brainstem encephalitis (BBE) (26), manifesting alteration in consciousness, hyperreflexia, ataxia, and ophthalmoplegia (27), with up to 92% demonstrating antecedent infection, 59% increased CSF protein content, 66% elevated anti-GQ1b antibody titer (28), and 30% demonstrating brain magnetic resonance imaging (MRI) abnormalities (29). A paraparetic

GBS variant affects the legs, mimicking an acute spinal cord lesion associated with back pain (30).

There are two axonal variants, acute motor axonal neuropathy (AMAN) (31, 32) and acute motor-sensory axonal neuropathy (AMSAN) (33), described largely from northern China, both of which are associated with *C. Jejuni* enteritis, which is a poor prognostic factor (34). Patients with AMAN have faster progression of weakness to an earlier nadir than those with GBS, resulting in prolonged paralysis and respiratory failure over a few days (35). The variant of acute motor conduction block neuropathy, which also follows *C. Jejuni* enteritis and presents with symmetric proximal and distal weakness in association with transient partial motor conduction block in intermediate and distal nerve segments, and normal clinical and electrophysiologic sensory function, can have elevated serum IgG GD1a and GM1 antibody titers (36). Other GBS variants include pharyngeal-cervical-brachial weakness with ptosis that mimics botulism, ptosis without opthalmoplegia, those characterized by either facial nerve diplegia or sixth cranial nerve palsy with paresthesia, and pure sensory and pan-autonomic dysfunction (30, 37).

IMMUNOPATHOLOGY

The classical histopathologic findings in AIDP are lymphocytic infiltration and intense macrophage-associated segmental demyelination of spinal nerve roots and proximal nerve segments. Insight into the autoimmune pathogenesis of GBS derived from the animal model of experimental allergic neuritis (EAN) (38) induced by immunization with peripheral-nerve proteins or transferred to animals by T-cells sensitized to these proteins. EAN resembles demyelinating GBS clinically and pathologically (39) and is caused by T-cell-mediated immunity to myelin proteins and humoral antibodies to myelin glycolipids.

However, EAN may not be a valid model after all, as autoreactive T-cells and autoantibodies do not occur in all patients (3). Antibody-mediated, early complement activation, and binding to the outer surface of the Schwann cell membrane, not myelin sheaths, in affected patients with GBS, leads to vesicular paranodal myelin degeneration and retraction (40), and recruitment of macrophages that strip off myelin lamellae with bystander axon loss detected in spinal roots, as well as in large and small motor and sensory nerves (41), especially with severe inflammation (42). Affected patients harbor antibodies to peripheral nerve myelin and myelin glycolipids, the titer of which correlates with clinical status. Unlike GBS, AMAN is characterized by the paucity of lymphocytic infiltration, sparing of dorsal nerve roots, dorsal root ganglia (DRG), and peripheral sensory nerves. Two early histopathologic changes in

AMAN are reversible, lengthening of the nodes of Ranvier that leads to impaired electrical impulse transmission due to absence of sodium channels, and complement activation that results in macrophage recruitment to the nodal region (43). Recruited macrophages distort paranodal axons and myelin sheaths, separating myelin from the axolemma and inducing condensation of axoplasm, with only the most severely damaged nerves demonstrating aspects of Wallerian degeneration.

ANTECEDENT EVENTS

Although most of the antecedent infectious events are upper respiratory infections (URI) without a specific identified organism, known viral precipitants in up to 6% of patients are attributed to EBV, CMV, and VZV, which affects younger patients with severe disease and a higher likelihood of respiratory failure. Antecedent human immunodeficiency virus type-1 (HIV-1) infection occurs at the time of seroconversion or early in the disease, and when suspected, is proven by measurement of HIV-1 viral load through a polymerase chain reaction (PCR), which is more sensitive than circulating antibodies.

Bacterial infections include *Mycoplasma pneumonia* and *Borrelia burgdorferi* infection. *C. jejuni* enteritis, the commonest identifiable antecedent infection, precedes GBS by up to nine days in about one-third of patients, when stool cultures for *C. jejuni* may be negative although serologic evidence of the infection persists. GBS occurs in one per 1,000 with antecedent *C. jejuni* enteritis each year in the United States (US), usually with an appropriate genetic susceptibility and human leukocyte antigen (HLA), haplotype (44, 45). During a 1976 mass immunization against A/New Jersey/1976/H1N1(3) swine influenza (flu) in the US, people receiving the vaccine were at increased risk of GBS (46), with an excess of ten affected GBS patients per million vaccinations (47); however, in the 1992 to 1993 and 1993 to 1994 flu seasons, there was an estimated excess of one GBS patient per million immunizations, based upon an adjusted relative risk of 1.7 within six weeks of influence vaccine administration (48). The concern about the swine flu vaccine risk resurged during the 2009 to 2010 H1N1 immunization campaign wherein the Centers for Disease Control and Prevention (CDC) (49) determined the risk to be similar to that for seasonal influenza immunization. The 2009 H1N1 flu virus epidemic was associated with a hospitalization rate of 222 per one million and a death rate of 9.7 per one million. Therefore, the risk of this illness outweighs the risk of the vaccines. Anyone with a history of GBS, as well as elderly persons or those with a serious illness should consider prophylactic vaccination. Patients recovering from GBS during the three- to six-month convalescent period should be cautious when considering any vaccine for fear of relapse of GBS. However, cases associated with influenza vaccination are at an estimated risk of 3.5% for GBS relapse (50). Besides influenza, the hepatitis vaccine and others alike have been associated with GBS, although less often than the flu vaccine (51). A comprehensive study (52) showed that about one-third of patients with GBS, and up to 18% of those with MFS, were seropositive for recent C. jejuni infection (53). Other anecdotal antecedent events of GBS include surgery, epidural anesthesia, concurrent Hodgkin lymphoma, and vaccinations.

LABORATORY EVALUATION

Electrophysiologic Studies

When GBS is suspected, electrophysiologic studies, including nerve conduction studies (NCS) and needle electromyography (EMG), are essential to confirm the presence, pattern, and severity of the neuropathy and exclude disorders that may mimic it. Such studies have been essential for the research definition of the disease (54). The electrophysiologic criteria for GBS are shown in Table 2. The finding of multifocal demyelination on early and serial electrodiagnostic studies is extremely helpful in confirming the diagnosis of AIDP with a high sensitivity and specificity in demyelinating GBS, and also increases the yield of axonal Guillain-Barré syndrome, which may be later evident (55).

Needle EMG is non-specific as it demonstrates reduced recruitment initially and fibrillations potentials at three to four weeks after onset. The earliest findings in AIDP are prolonged F-wave latencies or poor F-wave repeatability due to demyelination of the nerve roots. This is followed by prolonged distal latencies due to distal demyelination, and temporal dispersion or conduction block. Slowing of nerve conduction velocities (NCV) is less helpful as it tends to appear two to three weeks after the onset. However, the sensitivity of NCS, based on reported criteria, may be as low as 22% in early AIDP (54), rising to 87% at five weeks into the illness (56). The reasons for the limited sensitivity of NCS in AIDP include first, the common sites of demyelination being at the level of the nerve roots, most distal nerve segments, and at sites of entrapment. The nerve root is outside the reach of routine NCS, and such sites are usually excluded when assessing the diagnosis of AIDP. However, slowing of NCV at multiple common entrapment sites is unusual in an otherwise normal young adult and may, therefore, support the clinical impression of GBS. Second, the number of motor nerves studied or those with an elicited response may be inadequate and finding prolongation of blink reflex latencies may be helpful. Finally, changes in the sensory NCS lag behind the motor abnormalities. How-

ever, a potential clue is the preservation of a normal sural nerve response when median or ulnar sensory potentials are reduced in amplitude (56). A variety of motor NCS criteria have been published in an attempt to optimize sensitivity while maintaining specificity. A recent comparison of 10 published sets of criteria in 53 patients with AIDP, amyotrophic lateral sclerosis, and diabetic polyneuropathy controls, yielded 72% sensitivity and 100% specificity (57). Clinicians should not expect each AIDP patient to meet strict research criteria for demyelination, particularly early in the course.

In AMAN, compound muscle action potential (CMAP) amplitudes are significantly reduced in the first few days and then become absent (58). It is difficult in AMAN to ascertain if the absence of CMAP is due to axon loss, conduction block due to sodium channel dysfunction distal to the most distal stimulation site, or an immune attack on the nodes of Ranvier. For this reason, fibrillation potentials may occur early on in the course of AMAN and needle electrode examination is helpful. The sensory responses are normal and demyelinating conduction findings are lacking. However, in AMSAN the sensory potentials are reduced in amplitude and often absent (59). While sensory and motor NCS are often normal, H-reflexes are absent in 75% of MFS and BBE cases (26).

Cerebrospinal Fluid

CSF analysis is essential in all GBS cases revealing albuminocytologic dissociation with protein content that may reach 1,800 mg/dl (60) with 10 or less white cells/mm^3 in the majority of patients. About one-half of patients with GBS can have a normal CSF protein in the first week but that proportion declines to 10% when repeated one week later (1). Those with MFS and up to one-half of others with BBE demonstrate albuminocytologic dissociation (26). If there are more than 50 cell/mm3 up to two weeks after the onset of symptoms, consideration should be given to early HIV infection, leptomeningeal carcinomatosis, CMV polyradiculitis, and sarcoidosis. In HIV, GBS occurs at the time of seroconversion or early in the disease. The serum creatine kinase (CK) level may be mildly and non-specifically elevated.

Anti-ganglioside Antibodies

Gangliosides, composed of a ceramide attached to one or more hexoses, contain sialic or N-acetylneuraminic acid linked to an oligosaccharide core, and are important compounds of the peripheral nerves, four of which, termed GM1, GD1a, GT1a, and GQ1b, differ with respect to the number and position of their sialic acids (3). With the demonstration of molecular mimicry between GM1 and bacterial lipo-oligosaccharide of C. jejuni isolated from affected patients with GBS, disease models for GBS have

Table 2. Electrophysiological Criteria for GBS

Electro-physiologic criteria for GBS	Percent conduction velocity slowing			Percent distal latency prolongation			Percent F-wave latency prolongation			Amplitude conduction block		Abnormal temporal dispersion		
	≥80% of LLN	<80% of LLN	No. of nerves	≥80% of LLN	>80% of LLN	No. of nerves	≥80% of LLN	<80% of LLN	No. of nerves	%	No. of nerves	%	No. of nerves	Abnormal parameters required
Albers, 1985 (56)	>5	>15	2	>10	>20	2	>20	>20	2	>30	2	>30	1	1
Albers, 1989 (58)	>10	>20	2	>15	>25	2	>25	>25	1	>30	1	>30	1	3
Asbury, 1990 (54)	>20	>30	2	>25	>50	2	>20	>50	2	>20*	1	>15	1	3
Hadden 1998 (9)	>10¶	>15	2	>10	>20°	2	>20	>20	2	>50†	2	—	—	1
Van den Bergh, 2004 (57)	>30	>30	2	> 50	>50	2	>25	>50	2	>50†	2‡	>30	2	1

LLN, lower limit of normal
† distal amplitude >20% of LLN
‡ alternatively one finding with another NCS abnormality
*by area or amplitude
¶ distal amplitude >50% LLN
° distal amplitude <LLN

been developed produced by sensitization with GM1 or GM1-like lipo-oligosaccharides illustrating the autoimmune nature of GBS (61), which when cross-reactive with GM1, explain the etiopathogenesis of neuropathy due to bacterial-mediated molecular mimicry (62). Antibodies to GM1 gangliosides, described more frequently in AMAN, are associated with greater functional disability at six months after onset of the disease (63). Bacterial isolates from patients with GBS and antecedent infection with *C. jejuni* bear GM1-like or GD1a-like lipo-oligosaccharides, while those from patients with MFS have lipo-oligosaccharides mimicking GQ1b (64, 65). Similar findings of a *Hemophilus influenza* isolate from another patient with MFS were found to have GQ1b-mimicking lipo-oligosaccharides (66). While serum antibodies to GM1 or GD1b may not necessarily mediate the extensive axonal damage seen in severely affected patients, IgG antibodies to GD1a are highly associated with AMAN, detectable in 60% of affected patients, and in 4% of those with AIDP (67). GD1a antibodies correlate with the presence of bulbar signs and symptoms and are seen with BBE in addition to GQ1b antibodies. Compared to GBS, routine screening of anti-ganglioside antibodies in MFS is the notable exception wherein antibodies to GQ1b (68, 69) are highly sensitive and specific to MFS, although noted in other patients with GBS and marked ophthalmoparesis, and in up to 66% of patients with BBE (70).

Neuroimaging Studies

Gadolinium-enhanced magnetic resonance imaging (MRI) of the lumbosacral region shows cauda equina nerve root enhancement in affected patients with AIDP (71, 72). Moreover, in patients with the paraparetic variant of GBS, MRI may reveal the site of the lesion.

Microbial Testing

The isolation of *C. jejuni* from the stool of an affected patient with diarrhea, and later development of GBS, is near-certain proof of the association of *C. jejuni* enteritis. Although it is usually self-limited and requires no specific treatment, antimicrobial therapy hastens the clearance of *C. jejuni* from the stool (73) and may indicate a relatively poorer prognosis.

TREATMENT

General Supportive Care

Evidence in support of the general management of GBS is derived from observational studies and expert opinion consensus (74). Since respiratory failure may be inevitable in some patients, supportive care is the most important element of management. GBS patients are admitted to the neurological intensive care unit or an intermediary care telemetry unit to allow for close monitoring of respiratory, bulbar and autonomic function. A rapid decline of the expiratory forced vital capacities (FVC) to <15cc/kg of ideal body weight adjusted for age, or the negative inspiratory force (NIF) to <60 cm H_2O, indicate the need for urgent intubation and mechanical ventilation before hypoxemia supervenes. This is often associated with marked weakness of neck muscles and inability to count out loud to 20. Patients with severe dysphagia may require nasogastric or feeding tubes. Intubation should also be considered for patients who cannot handle their secretions or who have an ineffective cough. After two weeks of intubation, tracheostomy should be considered in those without improved pulmonary mechanics. In those intubated but with improved pulmonary parameters at two weeks, an additional week of intubation may be judicious to allow for successful weaning from the ventilator (74). When managing autonomic instability, it is potentially deleterious to aggressively control blood pressure fluctuations, and the use of long-acting antihypertensives is contraindicated.

Those with radicular back and neuropathic pain refractory to acetaminophen and non-steroidal anti-inflammatory agents (NSAIDS) should be given a trial of tricyclic antidepressants, gabapentin, carbamazepine, tramadol, or mexiletene (74). Bedridden patients should have deep venous thrombosis prophylaxis with compressive hose and anticoagulants in the form of subcutaneous heparin or enoxaprin. Bedside passive range of motion can help prevent muscle contractures in paralyzed patients. It is important to be mindful that these patients are most often alert and cognitively intact. A means for communication must be established for patients who are on mechanical ventilation. Vigilance toward infections is important since most severe cases develop urinary or pulmonary infections. Treatment with plasma exchange (PE) and intravenous immune globulin (IVIg) is indicated for patients with weakness-impairing function or any respiratory involvement. Patients and their families should be educated about the fact that it takes an average of two to three months for patients to walk without aids, no matter what therapy is used.

Immunotherapy

Plasma Exchange

Plasma exchange (PE) directly removes humoral factors such as autoantibodies, immune complexes, complement, cytokines, and other nonspecific inflammatory mediators and was the first treatment shown to be effective in GBS based on two randomized controlled-trials (75, 76). In both studies, PE performed within two weeks from onset con-

sistently demonstrated a statistically significant reduction in the time to weaning from the ventilator by 13 to 14 days and time to walk unaided by 32 to 41 days. In addition, the French Cooperative Group (75) showed a reduction in the proportion of patients who required assisted ventilation, a decrease in the time to onset of motor recovery, and a reduction in time to walk with assistance. The Guillain-Barré syndrome Study Group (76) identified similar benefits with more PE recipients improved at four weeks, with one grade of improvement occurring three weeks earlier. The French Cooperative Group on Plasma Exchange in Guillain-Barré syndrome (77) showed, in addition, that patients with mild GBS on admission who could walk with or without aid, but not run, as well as those able to stand unaided, benefitted from two exchanges whereas in those with moderate involvement limiting the ability to stand unaided, four exchanges were more beneficial; six exchanges were no more beneficial than four exchanges in patients with severe disease or on ventilator assistance. Those with mild ambulatory GBS reach a clinical nadir within a mean of eight days.

Intravenous Immunoglobulin

The Dutch Guillain-Barré Study Group (78) compared the efficacy of IVIg to PE in 147 patients, demonstrating that IVIg showed greater efficacy than PE in inducing one improvement grade at four weeks. The Plasma Exchange and Sandoglobulin Guillain-Barré Syndrome Trial Group (79) subsequently showed no difference in outcomes with IVIg and PE. The salutary benefit of IVIg is related to interference with costimulatory molecules involved in antigen presentation, antibody modulation, cyotokines, and adhesion molecules production, as well as macrophage Fc receptor activity, modulation of complement activation and membrane attack complex formation (80). Sialylated IgG Fc fragments, important in the *in vivo* activity of IVIg (81), initiate an anti-inflammatory cascade through the lectin receptors SIGN-R1 and DC-SIGN, leading to upregulation of the surface expression of the inhibitory Fc gamma receptor IIb (FCgRIIb) on inflammatory cells attenuating autoantibody-initiated inflammation. The total dose of IVIg is 2gm/kg administered over two to five days. Mild reactions include headache, nausea, chills, myalgia, chest discomfort, and back pain in up to 10% of treated patients, most of which improve with slowing the infusion rate and are preventable by pre-medication with acetaminophen, diphenhydramine, methylprednisolone and hydration.

Rare reactions include chemical meningitis, neutropenia, and delayed red, macular skin reaction of the palms, soles, and trunk with desquamation. Acute renal failure is related to patient dehydration and the sucrose or maltose diluent. Other severe, rare reactions include anaphylaxis, stroke, myocardial infarction, and pulmonary emboli due to hyperviscocity syndrome. Relapse of GBS can occur after effective therapy with IVIg (82, 83) or PE (76). The French Cooperative Group (77) noted a relapse rate of 5.5% compared to 1% for the control group. The weight of all available clinical evidence indicates it is better to treat GBS patients than not to. Both PE and IVIg are equally effective, but in the hemodynamically unstable patient, PE is contraindicated. Further, IVIg is more often readily available in most hospitals. The Plasma Exchange and Sandoglobulin Guillain-Barré (PSGBS) study group (84) that examined PE, IVIg monotherapy and PE followed by IVIg, noted no significant differences in outcome.

Corticosteroids

Corticosteroids are probably not of benefit in the treatment of GBS as steroid-treated patients do worse than controls (85). In one randomized British study (86), 124 patients received 500 mg of methylprednisolone for five days within 15 days of onset and 118 patients received placebo, and about one-half of patients in both groups received PE. There was no difference between the two groups in the degree of improvement at four weeks or in secondary outcome measures, concluding that a short course of high-dose methylprednisolone given early in GBS was ineffective. A Dutch open-label pilot study (87) suggested that 25 patients receiving intravenous methylprednisolone and IVIg did better than patients who received IVIg alone. A double-blind, placebo-controlled multicenter trial (88) of 116 and 117 Dutch patients, respectively, who were unable to walk independently and treated within 14 days of weakness-onset with IVIg additionally received 500 mg per day of intravenous methylprednisolone or placebo for five days, the primary outcome of which was improvement from baseline in GBS disability score of 1 or more grades four weeks after randomization. The study showed that the GBS disability scores decreased by one grade or more in 68% of patients in the methylprednisolone group and in 56% of controls (p=0.06), concluding that there was no significant difference between treatment with methylprednisolone and IVIg, or IVIg alone. Thus, intravenous corticosteroids at the present time are not recommended therapy for GBS.

An AAN practice parameter (89) concluded that PE should be considered for non-ambulatory adult patients with GBS within four weeks of the onset of symptoms, and that PE should also be considered for ambulatory patients examined within two weeks of the onset of symptoms. IVIg was recommended for non-ambulatory adult patients with GBS within two or possibly four weeks of the onset of neuropathic symptoms. Neither sequential treatment of PE or immunoabsorption followed by IVIg nor corticosteroids were recommended for GBS, however both PE and IVIg are treatment options for severe childhood GBS.

PROGNOSIS

Most patients with GBS recover spontaneously beginning at 28 days with a mean time to complete recovery of 200 days in 80% of patients; however, many (65%) have minor residual signs or symptoms, making recovery less than complete (1). Major residual neurologic deficits affect 10 to 15% of patients. In a study of 79 patients examined one year after the onset of GBS (90), 8% all >age 60 years had died, 4% were bedbound or ventilator-dependent, 9% were unable to walk unaided, 17% were unable to run, and 62% were in complete or almost complete recovery, not uncommonly with some functionally significant residual deficits. Among a cohort of patients studied a mean of seven years after the acute GBS illness and compared to 40 healthy control subjects (91), residual neuropathy affecting large- and medium-sized myelinated fibers was present in approximately one-half of patients, leading to motor and sensory dysfunction, with self-reported impaired physical health status. Other long-term studies demonstrated similar functionally relevant neurological deficits for up to seven years after the acute GBS attack, predominantly in the lower extremities, in some instances affecting autonomic function (92, 93). Slowed recovery and a reduced likelihood of walking unaided at six months was attributed to a suboptimal increase in IgG levels at two weeks after IVIg infusion (21). A retrospective study in 174 GBS patients enrolled in randomized, controlled clinical trials (21) showed that patients with a minor increase of serum IgG level two weeks after a single dose of IVIg recovered significantly slower, and fewer of the patients reached the ability to walk unaided at six months, indicating that a small increase in serum IgG level at two weeks should be followed by a higher dosage or second course thereafter.

Four factors associated with a poor prognosis in the North American GBS study (94) were age >50 to 60 years, a rapid onset prior to presentation within seven days, the need for mechanical ventilation, and severely reduced distal motor amplitudes to 20% or less of the lower limit of normal; a preceding diarrheal illness due to C. jejuni or CMV may be added to this list (95).

Variations in the rate and extent of recovery make prognostication difficult (3) however, there are validated scoring systems, one of which incorporates age, presence or absence of antecedent diarrhea, and disease severity to predict whether a patient will be able to ambulate independently at one, three, or six months (96, 97), and another that employs the number of days between onset of weakness and hospital admission, the presence or absence of facial or bulbar weakness, and severity of limb weakness to predict respiratory insufficiency (98). One (96) was derived from data of 388 patients enrolled in two randomized controlled trials and a pilot study.

Although most patients with AMAN have a more

delayed recovery than with AIDP (99), some do recover quickly, presumably due to reversible changes of the sodium channels at nodes of Ranvier or by degeneration followed by regeneration of motor nerve terminals and intramuscular axons (100). Among 28 untreated MFS, all returned to normal activities in a median period of 32 days between neurologic onset and the disappearance of ataxia, with a median period of 88 days for ophthalmoplegia (101). IVIg hastens amelioration of ophthalmoplegia and ataxia. Altogether, 96% of patients were free of all symptoms and signs one year after onset of neurologic symptoms, whether or not treatment was given. Among 62 patients with BBE, with or without limb weakness, treated with immunotherapy including corticosteroids, PE, and IVIg (102) two-thirds showed complete remission without residual symptoms.

REFERENCES

1. Ropper AH. The Guillain-Barré syndrome. *N Engl J Med* 1992; 326:1130–1136.

2. Guillain G, Barré JA, Strohl A. Sur un syndrome de radilculonévrite avec hyperalbuminose du liquid céphalo-rachidien sans reaction cellulaire. Remarques sur les catactères cliniques et graphiques de reflexes tendineux. *Bull Soc Med Hosp Paris* 1916; 40:1462–1470.

3. Yuki N, Hans-Peter Hartung. Guillain-Barré syndrome. *N Engl J Med* 2012; 366:2294–2304.

4. Hughes RA, Cornblath DR. Guillain-Barré syndrome. *Lancet* 2005; 366:1653–1666.

5. Van Koningsveld R, Van Doorn PA, Schmitz PI, Ang CW, et al. Mild forms of Guillain-Barré syndrome in an epidemiologic survey in The Netherlands. *Neurology* 2000; 54:620–625.

6. Govoni V, Granieri E. Epidemiology of the Guillain-Barré syndrome. *Curr Opin Neurol* 2001; 14:605–613.

7. McGrogan A, Madle GC, Seaman HE, et al. The epidemiology of Guillain-Barré syndrome worldwide. A systematic literature review. *Neuroepidemiology* 2009; 32:150–163.

8. Sevjar JJ, Baughman AI, Wise M, et al. Population incidence of Guillain-Barré syndrome: a systematic review and meta-analysis. *Neuroepidemiology* 2011; 36:123–133.

9. Hadden RD, Cornblath DR, Hughes RA, et al. Electrophysiological classification of Guillain-Barré syndrome: clinical associations and outcome. Plasma Exchange/Sandoglobulin Guillain-Barré Syndrome Trial Group. *Ann Neurol* 1998; 44:780–788.

10. Poropatich KO, Walker CI, Black RE, et al. Quantifying the association between Campylobacter infection and Guillain-Barré syndrome: a systematic review. *J Health Popul Nutr* 2010; 28:545–552.

11. Jacobs BC, Rothbarth PH, van der Meche PGA, et al. The spectrum of antecedent infections in Guillain-Barré syndrome: a case-control study. *Neurology* 1998; 51:1110–1115.

12. Kang JH, Sheu JJ, Lin HC. Increased risk of Guillain-Barré syndrome following; recent Herpes zoster: a population-based study across Taiwan. *Clin Infect Dis* 2010; 51:525–530.

13. Hadden RDM, Karch H, Hartung HP, et al. Preceding infections, immune factors, and outcomes in Guillain-Barré syndrome. *Neurology* 2001; 56:758–765.

14. Orlikowski D, Porcher R, Sivadon-Tardy V, et al. Guillain-Barré syndrome following primary cytomegalovirus infection: a prospective cohort study. *Clin Infect Dis* 2011; 52:837–844.

15. Barohn RJ, Saperstein DS. Guillain-Barré syndrome and chronic inflammatory demyelinating polyneuropathy. *Semin Neurol* 1998; 18:49–61.

16. Sejvar JJ, Kohl KS, Gidudu J, et al. Guillain-Barré syndrome and Fisher syndrome: case definitions and guidelines for collection, analysis, and presentation of immunization safety data. *Vaccine* 2011; 29:599–612.

17. Yuki N, Nokubun N, Kuwabara S, et al. Guillain-Barré syndrome associated with normal or exaggerated tendon reflexcs. *J Neurol* 2012; 259:1181–1190.

18. Ruts L, Drenthen J, Jongen JL, et al. Pain in Guillain-Barré syndrome: a long-term follow-up study. *Neurology* 2010; 75:1439–1447.

19. Kuitwaard K, van Koningsveld R, Ruts L, et al. Recurrent Guillain-Barré syndrome. *J Neurol Neurosurg Psychiatry* 2009; 80:56–59.

20. Ruts L, Drenthen J, Jacobs BC, et al. Dutch GBS Study Group. Distinguishing acute-onset CIDP from fluctuating Guillain-Barré syndrome: a prospective study. *Neurology* 2010; 74:1680–1686.

21. Kuitwaard K, de Gelder J, Tio-Gillen AP, et al. Pharmacokinetics of intravenous immunoglobulin and outcome in Guillain-Barré syndrome. *Ann Neuro* 2009; 66:597–603.

22. Hughes RAC, Swan AV, Raphael JC, et al. Immunotherapy for Guillain-Barré syndrome: a systematic review. *Brain* 2007; 130:2245–2257.

23. Hughes RAC, Wijdicks EF, Benson E, et al. Supportive care for patients with Guillain-Barré syndrome. *Arch Neurol* 2005; 62:1194–1198.

24. Fisher CM. An unusual variant of acute idiopathic polyneuritis (syndrome of ophthalmoplegia, ataxia and areflexia). *N Engl J Med* 1956; 255:57–65.

25. Overell JR, Hsieh ST, Odaka M, et al. Treatment for Fisher syndrome, Bickerstaff's brainstem encephalitis and related disorders. *Cochrane Database Syst Rev* 2007; 1:CD004761.

26. Ito M, Kuwabara S, Odaka M, et al. Bickerstaff's brainstem encephalitis and Fisher syndrome form a continuous spectrum: clinical analysis of 581 cases. *J Neurol* 2008; 255:674–682.

27. Bickerstaff E, Cloake P. Mesencephalitis and rhombencephalitis. *Br Med J* 1951; 2:77–81.

28. Odaka M, Yuki N, Yamada M, et al. Bickerstaff's brainstem encephalitis: clinical features of 62 cases and a subgroup associated with Guillain Barré syndrome. *Brain* 2003; 126:2279–2290.

29. Odaka M, Yuki N, Yamada M, et al. Bickerstaff's brainstem encephalitis: clinical features of 62 cases and a subgroup associated with Guillain Barré syndrome. *Brain* 2003; 126:2279–2290.

30. Ropper AH. Unusual clinical variants and signs in Guillain-Barré syndrome. *Arch Neurol* 1986; 43:1150–1152.

31. Feasby TE, Gilbert JJ, Brown WF, et al. An acute axonal form of Guillain-Barré polyneuropathy. *Brain* 1986; 109:1115–1126.

32. McKhann GM, Cornblath DR, Griffin JW, et al. Acute motor axonal neuropathy: a frequent cause of acute flaccid paralysis in China. *Ann Neurol* 1993; 33:333–342.

33. Griffin JW, Li CY, Ho TW, et al. Pathology of the motor-sensory axonal Guillain-Barré syndrome. *Ann Neurol* 1996; 39:17–28.

34. Ho TW, Mishu B, Li Cy, et al. Guillain-Barré syndrome in northern China. Relationship to Campylobacter jejuni infection and anti-glycolipid antibodies. *Brain* 1995; 118:597–605.

35. Hiraga A, Mori M, Ogawara K, et al. Differences in patterns of

progression in demyelinating and axonal Guillain-Barré syndromes. *Neurology* 2003; 61:471–474.

36. Capasso M, Caporale CM, Pomilio F, et al. Acute motor conduction block neuropathy: another Guillain-Barré syndrome variant. *Neurology* 2003; 61:617–622.

37. Ropper AH. Further regional variants of acute immune polyneuropathy. Bifacial weakness or sixth nerve paresis with paresthesia lumbar polyradiculopathy and ataxia with pharyngeal-cervical-brachial weakness. *Arch Neurol* 1994; 51:671–675.

38. Waksman BH, Adams RD. Allergic neuritis: experimental disease rabbits induced by the injection of peripheral nervous tissue and adjuvants. *J Exp Med* 1955; 102:213–236.

39. Willison HJ. Biomarkers in experimental models of antibody-mediated neuropathies. *J Peripher Nerv Syst* 2011; 16(Suppl1):60–62.

40. Hafer-Macko CE, Sheikh KA, Li CY et al. Immune attack on the Schwann cell surface in acute inflammatory demyelinating polyneuropathy. *Ann Neurol* 1996; 39:625–635.

41. Asbury AK, Arnason BG, Adams RD, et al. The inflammatory lesion in idiopathic polyneuritis: its role in pathogenesis. *Medicine* 1969; 48:173–215.

42. Hafer-Macko C, Sheikh KA, Li CY, et al. Immune attack on the Schwann cell surface in acute inflammatory demyelinating polyneuropathy. *Ann Neurol* 1996; 39:625–635.

43. Griffin JW, Li CY, Macko C, et al. Early nodal changes in the acute motor axonal neuropathy pattern of the Guillain-Barré syndrome. *J Neurocytol* 1996; 25:33–51.

44. Allos BM. Association between Campylobacter infection and Guillain-Barré syndrome. *J Infect Dis* 1997; 176:S25–S127.

45. Magira EE, Papaioakim M, Nachamkin I, et al. Differential distribution of HLA-DQ beta/DR beta epitopes in the two forms of Guillain-Barré syndrome, acute motor axonal neuropathy and acute inflammatory demyelinating polyneuropathy (AIDP): identification of DQ beta epitopes associated with susceptibility to and protection from AIDP. *J Immunol* 2003; 170:3074–4080.

46. Lehmann HC, Hartung HP, Kieseier BC, et al. Guillain-Barré syndrome after exposure to influenza virus. *Lancet Infect Dis* 2010; 10:643–651.

47. Schonberger LB, Bregman DJ, Sullivan-Bolyai JZ, et al. Guillain-Barré syndrome following vaccination in the National Influenza Immunization Program, United States, 1976–1977. *Am J Epidemiol* 1979; 110:105–123.

48. Lasky T, Terracciano GJ, Magder L, et al. The Guillain-Barré syndrome and the 1992–1993 and 1993–1994 influenza vaccines. *N Engl J Med* 1998 17; 339:1797–1802.

49. CDC) surveillance data indicated an excess GBS risk of 0.8 cases per million vaccinations (Centers for Disease Control and Prevention. Preliminary Results: Surveillance for Guillain-Barré Syndrome After Receipt of Influenza A (H1N1) 2009 Monovalent Vaccine-United States, 2009–2010. *Morbidity and Mortality Weekly Report* (MMWR) June 2, 2010/59(Early Release); 1–5. Accessed at http://www.cdc.gov/mmwr/preview/mmwrhtml/mm59e0602a1.htm?s_cid=mm59e0602a1_e).

50. Pritchard J, Mukherjee R, Hughes RA. Risk of relapse of Guillain-Barré syndrome or chronic inflammatory demyelinating polyradiculoneuropathy following immunization. *J Neurol Neurosurg Psychiatry* 2002; 73:348–349.

51. Souayah N, Nasar A, Suri MF, et al. Guillain-Barré syndrome after vaccination in United States a report from the CDC/FDA Vaccine Adverse Event Reporting System. *Vaccine* 2007; 25:5253–5255.

52. Koga M, Yuki N, Takahashi M, et al. Close association of IgA anti-ganglioside antibodies with antecedent Campylobacter jejuni infection in Guillain-Barré and Fisher's syndromes. *J Neuroimmunol* 1998; 81:138–143.

53. Koga M, Gilbert M, Li J, et al. Antecedent infections in Fisher syndrome: a common pathogenesis of molecular mimicry. *Neurology* 2005; 64:1605–1611.

54. Asbury AK, Cornblath DR. Assessment of current diagnostic criteria for Guillain-Barré syndrome. *Ann Neurol* 1990; 27(Suppl):S21–S24.

55. Tsang TY, Umapathi T, Yuki N. Serial electrodiagnostic studies increases the diagnostic yield of axonal Guillain-Barré syndrome. *Clin Neurophysiol* 2012; 124:210–210.

56. Albers JW, Donofrio PD, McGonagle TK. Sequential electrodiagnostic abnormalities in acute inflammatory demyelinating polyradiculoneuropathy. *Muscle Nerve* 1985; 8:528–539.

57. Van den Bergh PY, Piéret F. Electrodiagnostic criteria for acute and chronic inflammatory demyelinating polyradiculoneuropathy. *Muscle Nerve* 2004; 29:565–574.

58. Albers JW, Kelly JJ Jr. Acquired inflammatory demyelinating polyneuropathies: clinical and electrodiagnostic features. *Muscle Nerve* 1989; 12:435–451.

59. Griffin JW, Li CY, Ho TW, et al. Pathology of the motor-sensory axonal Guillain-Barré syndrome. *Ann Neurol* 1996; 39:17–28.

60. Wiederholt WC, Mulder DW, Lambert EH. The Landry-Guillain-Barré-Strohl Syndrome or Polyradiculoneuropathy: Historical review, report on 97 patients, and present concepts. *Mayo Clin Proc* 1964; 39:427–451.

61. Yuki N. Guillain-Barre syndrome and anti-ganglioside antibodies: a clinician-scientists journey. *Ro Jpn Acad Ser B Phys Biol Sci* 2012; 88:299–326.

62. Oomes PG, Jacobs BC, Hazenberg MP, et al. Anti-GM1 IgG antibodies and Campylobacter bacteria in Guillain-Barré syndrome: evidence of molecular mimicry. *Ann Neurol* 1995; 38:170–—.

63. Kuwabara S, Yuki N, Koga M, et al. IgG anti-GM1 antibody is associated with reversible conduction failure and axonal degeneration in Guillain-Barré syndrome. *Ann Neurol* 1998; 44:202–208.

64. Kusunoki S, Kaida K. Antibodies against ganglioside complexes in Guillain-Barré syndrome and related disorders. *J Neurochem* 2011; 116:828–832.

65. Yuki N, Taki T, Inagaki F, et al. A bacterium lipopolysaccharide that elicits Guillain-Barré syndrome has a GM1 ganglioside-like structure. *J Exp Med* 1993; 178:1771–1775.

66. Houliston RS, Koga M, Li J. Haemophilus influenza strain associated with Fisher syndrome expresses a novel disialylated ganglioside mimic. *Biochemistry* 2007; 46:8164–8171.

67. Ho TW, Willison HJ, Nachamkin I, et al. Anti-GD1a antibody is associated with axonal but not demyelinating forms of Guillain-Barré syndrome. *Ann Neurol* 1999; 45:168–173.

68. Willison HJ, Veitch J, Paterson G, et al. Miller Fisher syndrome is associated with serum antibodies to GQ1b ganglioside. *J Neurol Neurosurg Psych* 1993; 56:204–206.

69. Yuki N, Sato S, Tsuji S, et al. Frequent presence of anti-GQ1b antibody in Fisher's syndrome. *Neurology* 1993; 43:414–417.

70. Overell JR, Hsieh ST, Odaka M, et al. Treatment for Fisher syndrome, Bickerstaff's brainstem encephalitis and related disorders. *Cochrane Database Syst Rev* 2007; 1:CD004761.

71. Morgan GW, Barohn RJ, Bazan C, et al. Nerve root enhancement with MRI in inflammatory demyelinating polyradiculoneuropathy. *Neurology* 1993; 43:618–620.

72. Gorson KC, Ropper AH, Muriello MA, et al. Prospective evaluation of MRI lumbosacral nerve root enhancement in acute Guillain-Barré syndrome. *Neurology* 1996; 47:813–817.

73. Anders BJ, Lauer BA, Paisley JW, et al. Double-blind placebo

controlled trial of erythromycin for treatment of Campylobacter enteritis. *Lancet* 1982; 1:131–132.

74. Hughes RA, Wijdicks EF, Benson E, et al. Multidisciplinary Consensus Group. Supportive care for patients with Guillain-Barré syndrome. *Arch Neurol* 2005; 62:1194–1198.

75. French Cooperative Group on Plasma Exchange in Guillain-Barré syndrome. Efficiency of plasma exchange in Guillain-Barré syndrome: role of replacement fluids. *Ann Neurol* 1987; 22:753–761.

76. The Guillain-Barré Syndrome Study Group. Plasmapheresis and acute Guillain-Barré syndrome. *Neurology* 1985; 35:1096–1104.

77. French Cooperative Group on Plasma Exchange in Guillain-Barré syndrome. Appropriate number of plasma exchanges in Guillain-Barré syndrome. *Ann Neurol* 1997; 41:298–306.

78. Van der Meché FG, Schmitz PI, and the Dutch Guillain-Barré Study Group. A randomized trial comparing intravenous immune globulin and plasma exchange in Guillain-Barré syndrome. *N Engl J Med* 1992; 326:1123–1129.

79. Plasma Exchange and Sandoglobulin Guillain-Barré Syndrome Trial Group. Randomized trial of plasma exchange, intravenous immunoglobulin and combined treatments in Guillain-Barré syndrome. *Lancet* 1997; 349:225–230.

80. Dalakas MC. Intravenous immunoglobulin in autoimmune neuromuscular diseases. *JAMA* 2004 May; 291:2367–2375.

81. Anthony RM, Ravetch JV. A novel role for the IgG Fc glycan: the anti-inflammatory activity of sialylated IgG Fcs. *J Clin Immunol* 2010; 30:S9–S14.

82. Irani DN, Cornblath DR, Chaudhry V, et al. Relapse in Guillain-Barré syndrome after treatment with human immune globulin. *Neurology* 1993; 43:872–875.

83. Castro LH, Ropper AH. Human immune globulin infusion in Guillain-Barré syndrome: worsening during and after treatment. *Neurology* 1993; 43:1034–1036.

84. Hughes RA. Plasma exchange versus intravenous immunoglobulin for Guillain-Barré syndrome. *Ther Apher* 1997; 1:129–130.

85. Hughes RA, Newsom-Davis JM, Perkin GD, Pierce JM. Controlled trial prednisolone in acute polyneuropathy. *Lancet* 1978; 2:750–753.

86. Guillain-Barré Syndrome Steroid Trial Group. Double-blind trial of intravenous methylprednisolone in Guillain-Barré syndrome. *Lancet* 1993; 341:586–590.

87. The Dutch Guillain-Barré Study Group. Treatment of Guillain-Barré syndrome with high-dose immune globulins combined with methylprednisolone: a pilot study. *Ann Neurol* 1994; 35:749–752.

88. Van Koningsveld R, Schmitz PI, Meché FG, et al. Effect of methylprednisolone when added to standard treatment with intravenous immunoglobulin for Guillain-Barré syndrome: randomised trial. *Lancet* 2004; 363:192–196.

89. Hughes RA, Wijdicks EF, Barohn R, et al. Quality Standards Subcommittee of the American Academy of Neurology. Practice parameter: immunotherapy for Guillain-Barré syndrome: report of the Quality Standards Subcommittee of the American Academy of Neurology. *Neurology* 2003; 61:736–740.

90. Rees JH, Thompson RD, Smeeton NC, et al. Epidemiological study of Guillain-Barré syndrome in south east England. *J Neurol Neurosurg Psychiatry* 1998; 64:74–77.

91. Dornonville de la Cour C, Jakobsen J. Residual neuropathy in long-term population-based follow-up of Guillain-Barré syndrome. *Neurology* 2005; 64:246–253.

92. Vedeler CA, Wik E, Nyland H. The long-term prognosis of Guillain-Barré syndrome. Evaluation of prognostic factors including plasma exchange. *Acta Neurol Scand* 1997; 95:298–302.

93. Koeppen S, Kraywinkel K, et al. Long-term outcome of Guillain-Barré syndrome. *Neurocrit Care* 2006; 5:235–242.

94. McKhann GM, Griffin JW, Cornblath DR, et al. Plasmapheresis and Guillain-Barré syndrome: analysis of prognostic factors and the effect of plasmapheresis. *Ann Neurol* 1988; 23:347–353.

95. The Dutch Guillain-Barré Study Group. Prognostic factors of Guillain-Barré syndrome after intravenous immunoglobulin or plasma exchange. *Neurology* 1999; 53:598–604.

96. Van Koningsveld R, Steyerberg EW, Hughes RAC, et al. a clinical prognostic scoring system for Guillain-Barré syndrome. *Lancet Neurol* 2007; 6:589–594.

97. Walgaard C, Lingsma HF, Ruts L, et al. Early recognition of poor prognosis in Guillain-Barré syndrome. *Neurology* 2011; 76:968–975.

98. Walgaard C, Lingsma HF, Ruts L, et al. Prediction of respiratory insufficiency in Guillain-Barré syndrome. *Ann Neurol* 2010; 67:781–787.

99. Ho TW, Li CY, Cornblath DR, et al. Patterns of recovery in the Guillain-Barré syndromes. *Neurology* 1997; 48:695–700.

100. Ho TW, Hsieh ST, Nachamkin I, et al. Motor nerve terminal degeneration provides a potential mechanism for rapid recovery in acute motor axonal neuropathy after Campylobacter infection. *Neurology* 1997; 48:717–724.

101. Mori M, Kuwabara S, Fukutake T, et al. Intravenous immunoglobulin therapy for Miller Fisher syndrome. *Neurology* 2007; 68:1144–1146.

102. Odaka M, Yuki N, Yamada M, et al. Bickerstaff's brainstem encephalitis: clinical features of 62 cases and a subgroup associated with Guillain-Barré syndrome. *Brain* 2003; 126:2279–2290.

CHAPTER 32

Chronic Inflammatory Demyelinating Polyradiculoneuropathy and Related Disorders

Mazen M. Dimachkie, Richard J. Barohn

GENERAL CONSIDERATIONS AND HISTORICAL BACKGROUND

The first case of recurrent neuritis was published by Eichhorst in 1890 (1). In 1958, Austin (2) described steroid responsiveness, recurrence and cerebrospinal fluid (CSF) protein elevation. Dyck and colleagues (3) described the clinicopathological findings of monophasic progression, steady deterioration, stepwise progression and recurrence, with histologic peripheral nervous system (PNS) inflammation, and demyelination. Dyck and Arnason (4) termed the disorder *chronic inflammatory demyelinating polyradiculoneuropathy* (CIDP), which accounted for 21% of initially undiagnosed patients with peripheral neuropathy at the Mayo Clinic (5), and 13 to 20% of cases of immune-mediated neuropathy referred to in academic centers worldwide (6).

EPIDEMIOLOGY

With an estimated incidence of CIDP in Olmstead County, Minnesota, of 1.6/100,000/year and prevalence of 8.9/100,000 (7), the disease occurs at virtually any age with a mean age at onset of 48 years, and higher prevalence in men than women (8). The prevalence of CIDP in 70- to 79-year-old males ranges from 0.15 per 100,000 to 10 in 100,000 individuals (8). Although a relapsing course occurs most often between the second and fourth decade, a chronic nonrelapsing course is more common between the fifth and the seventh decades (8).

CLINICAL PRESENTATION

The disorder typically presents with chronic progressive, stepwise progressive, or relapsing weakness for two or more months, with a peak age of onset in the third decade, whereas a progressive form is more typical in older individuals. The overwhelming majority of patients over the age of 65 have a chronic insidious course. Weakness can vary in severity but is typically symmetric and characteristically involves proximal and distal muscles. Facial and neck flexor muscle weakness may occur but the extraocular muscles are rarely involved. Papilledema and clinical central nervous system (CNS) involvement rarely occurs. Sensory manifestations consist of numbness and tingling but painful paraesthesia is not uncommon. Most patients have some degree of sensory involvement, but pure motor presentations may occur. Most patients describe gait imbalance. Muscle stretch reflexes are usually depressed or absent. Autonomic and respiratory insufficiency occurs infrequently compared with the Guillain-Barré syndrome (GBS). Up to 18% of patients with CIDP presented acutely and follow a relapsing course (9), and with few exceptions, early in the course of illness, the relapsing form of CIDP was virtually indistinguishable from GBS (10, 11). Those with CIDP were more likely to have prominent sensory signs and less likely to manifest autonomic involvement, facial weakness, preceding infectious illness, or to need mechanical ventilation than those with GBS. Treatment-related fluctuation or relapses of GBS first occurred within eight weeks from the onset of weakness, with lessening over time. Patients with acute presentations of CIDP are more likely to remain able to walk independently, without cranial nerve dysfunction, or display full electrophysiologic features of the disease.

557

DIAGNOSTIC APPROACH

Cerebrospinal fluid examination, motor nerve conduction studies (NCS), and biopsy of a cutaneous nerve are the most important studies that support the diagnosis of CIDP; however, of the three studies, CSF evaluation was the most sensitive, demonstrating elevation in up to 94% of patients reflecting proximal nerve root involvement (3, 12), typically presenting with albuminocytologic dissociation. A CSF white blood cell count >10/mm3 should lead to consideration of human immunodeficiency virus type 1 (HIV-1), sarcoidosis, Lyme neuroborreliosis, lymphomatous, and leukemic nerve root infiltration. Oligoclonal bands (OCB) are identified in up to 65% of patients (13). Few blood tests, with the exception of serum protein electrophoresis and immunofixation, are required in patients with typical CIDP for the detection of monoclonal paraproteinemia, which if detected, should prompt a search for lymphoproliferative disease. Antibodies to myelin P0 protein, detected in up to 29% of patients (14, 15), is of little diagnostic value. Magnetic resonance imaging (MRI) may provide support of the diagnosis of CIDP by demonstrating enlargement and increased T_2-signal intensity of spinal nerve roots with enhancement after administration of intravenous contrast.

ELECTRODIAGNOSTIC CRITERIA

CIDP is characterized by slow motor nerve conduction velocities (NCV), prolonged distal motor latencies, prolonged F-wave latencies, conduction block, and abnormal temporal dispersion. Less than 70% of cases met the Barohn criteria (12) for demyelination demonstrating 30% slowing of motor NCV. An ad hoc subcommittee of the American Academy of Neurology (AAN) later proposed research criteria (16) that distinguished CIDP from GBS, although highly specific to CIDP, they were quite stringent with a sensitivity of 39 to 43%, and failed to recognize up to 89% of CIDP cases (17). Up to 16 different diagnostic criteria for typical CIDP have been proposed or employed (9, 17, 18–24). Despite the plethora of proposed criteria, each with its own merits, none has solved the challenge of infallibly elucidating the diagnosis in partially treated patients in whom some, but not all, of the requisite electrodiagnostic features would be present, nor provide clinically useful evidenced-based criteria, that would aptly apply to patients outside of clinical trials. The most current useful research criteria stemmed from the recognition that it would be advantageous for a group of experts to validate the most appropriate criteria for research studies and for clinical use at the time (25), the results of which (17) served as the basis for derived distal latency, conduction velocity, and F-wave response parameters, which when applied to 75% or more of the studied nerves in 117 analyzed CIDP literature cases (16, 22, 26), resulted in a sensitivity of 83% and specificity of 97%. The first report of the Joint Task Force of the European Federation of Neurological Societies (EFNS) and the Peripheral Neuropathy Society (PNS) in 2005 (27) demonstrated criteria with 34% sensitivity and 99% specificity for the diagnosis of CIDP. The first revision in 2010 (24, 28) has served as the most current set of clinical and electrodiagnostic criteria for definite demyelination (Table 1) and CIDP (Table 2) as well as, in the selection of subjects into clinical trials. Moreover, health insurance providers have utilized these criteria (24, 28) in determining the diagnosis of CIDP in the approval process of various medical therapies such as intravenous immune globulin (IVIg), plasma exchange (PE), and other potentially expensive or innovative therapies.

Table 1. *Electrodiagnostic Criteria for Peripheral Nerve Demyelination**

Definite: At least one of the following:

Motor distal latency: ≥50% above ULN in two nerves (excluding median neuropathy at the wrist from carpal tunnel syndrome), or

Motor conduction velocity: ≥30% below LLN in two nerves, or

F-wave latency: ≥30% above ULN in two nerves (≥50% if amplitude of distal negative peak CMAP <80% of LLN values) or absent in two nerves if these nerves have distal negative peak CMAP amplitudes ≥20% of LLN + at least one other demyelinating parameter in at least 1 other nerve, or

Partial motor conduction block: 50% or more reduction in the amplitude of the proximal negative peak CMAP relative to distal, if distal negative peak CMAP ≥20% of LLN, in two nerves, or in one nerve + one other demyelinating parameter in another nerve, or

Abnormal temporal dispersion: >30% duration increase between the proximal and distal negative peak of the CMAP in ≥two nerves or distal CMAP duration (interval between onset of the first negative peak and return to baseline of the last negative peak) increase in 1≥ nerves (median = 6.6 ms, ulnar = 6.7 ms, peroneal = 7.6 ms, tibial = 8.8 ms) and ≥one other demyelinating parameter in ≥1 nerves.

Probable:
≥30% amplitude reduction of the proximal negative peak CMAP relative to distal, excluding the posterior tibial nerve, if distal negative peak CMAP ≥20% of LLN value, in two nerves, or in one nerve + at least one other demyelinating parameter in at least 1 other nerve.

Possible:
As in Definite, but in only one nerve.

*Adapted from references 24 and 28, with permission.

Table 2. Nerve Conduction Study Values Needed to Be Considered Demyelinating

	NCV (m/sec)				DL (msec)			F-WAVES (msec)		
	LLN	<80%[1]	<70%[2]	ULN	>125%1	>150%2	ULN	>120%[1]	>150%[2]
Median	49	39.2	34.3	4.5	5.6	6.7	31.0	37.2	46.5
Ulnar	50	40.0	35.0	3.6	4.5	5.4	32.0	38.4	48.0
Fibular	41	32.8	28.7	6.6	8.2	9.9	58.0	69.6	87.0
Tibial	41	32.8	28.7	6.0	7.5	9.0	58.0	69.6	87.0

[1] = If Amp >80% LLN
[2] = If Amp <80% LLN

If: Median CMAP LLN 4.5 mV; then 80% LLN = 3.6 mV
Ulnar CMAP LLN 5.0 mV; then 80% LLN = 4 mV
Fibular CMAP LLN 2.0 mV; then 80% LLN = 1.6 mV
Tibial CMAP LLN 4.0 mV; then 80% LLN = 3.2 mV

A sensory conduction velocity <80% of lower limit of normal (LLN) (<70% if SNAP amplitude, <80% of LLN) was supportive of CIDP according the 2010 EFNS revision (24, 28); however, Rajabally and Samarasekera (29) found that sensory NCV were significantly slower for median and sural nerves in 19 CIDP patients, but Receiver Operating Characteristic (ROC) curves did not demonstrate cut-offs with useful sensitivities and specificities when compared to 26 control patients with distal large fiber sensory axonal neuropathy. Median sensory conduction block (CB) along the forearm and dispersion of the distal median or sural sensory nerve action potentials (SNAP) and ROC curve analysis showed that the 67% cut-off value for median sensory conduction block had a sensitivity of 42% for CIDP, with a specificity of 100%. In addition, cut-offs for median (2.85 ms) and sural (2.48 ms) SNAP duration offered a sensitivity of 52.6% and 42.9%, with specificities of 96.2% and 100%, respectively. The presence of a normal sural potential with absence of, or abnormal median SNAP, the so-called sural-sparing pattern, which occurred in 28% of patients with CIDP, compared to 39% of those with GBS (39%), 23% in diabetic neuropathy, 22% with motor neuron disease (MND), and 3% of control subjects, was not predictive of CIDP (17). A comparison of patients with CIDP to cryptogenic sensory neuropathy, in which a sural sparing pattern was revealed in 8% of patients with CIDP likewise showed equally poor specificity (30). The combination of an abnormal radial sensory response with sural-sparing in a comparison of patients with CIDP to axonal polyneuropathy and myopathy patient controls (31) yielded a diagnostic sensitivity of 25% for CIDP and 100% specificity for axonal neuropathy. The 2010 EFNS guidelines (24, 28) suggest that the pattern of a normal sural response, combined with an abnormal median or radial SNAP, supports the diagnosis of CIDP. Other ancillary electrophysiological studies may contribute to the diagnosis of CIDP.

For example, 17 of 20 patients had abnormal blink reflexes, and 12 of 20 had prolonged distal facial motor latencies, supportive of the diagnosis of CIDP in the proper clinical setting (32). Cervical root stimulation (CRS) in 21 healthy controls (33, 34) increased the sensitivity of the Nicolas (21), Hughes (22), and Saperstein and colleagues (26) criteria by 72%. Somatosensory evoked potentials (SSEP) may add evidence of sensory disturbances, particularly in those with normal SNAP and typical CIDP or sensory CIDP variant syndromes without CNS disturbances.

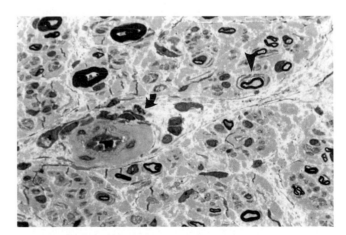

FIG. 1. Sural nerve biopsy from a patient with chronic inflammatory demyelinating polyradiculoneuropathy. Thinly myelinated nerve fibers have excessive Schwann cell process proliferation ("onion bulbs," arrowhead). The number of large myelinated fibers is decreased. A few mononuclear inflammatory cells surround an endoneurial blood vessel (curved arrow). (Toluidine blue stain.) From, Brey RL, Barohn RJ and Tami JA. Neuroimmunology: clinical and therapeutic approach. *Neurologist* 1996; 2:25–52, with permission.

HISTOPATHOLOGICAL ASPECTS

Biopsy of a cutaneous nerve such as the sural nerve, in spite of the extensive available normative data, is probably least useful in establishing the diagnosis of CIDP (35, 36), as it does not improve the accuracy of the diagnosis when the clinical features, CSF and NCS, are already consistent with CIDP. The histopathologic aspects of CIDP include macrophage-mediated demyelination, hypomyelination, and onion bulb formation, which while detectable by conventional light microscopic techniques, may be a feature of other types of primary demyelinating neuropathy. Foci of endoneurial and perivascular inflammatory cell infiltrates were noted in 11% to 18% of biopsied cutaneous nerves (12), and prominent in four nerves (37). Since inflammatory changes are slight and often difficult to distinguish from normal controls, cell marker immunocytochemistry with lymphocyte flow cytometry is necessary to identify inflammatory cell infiltrates typically comprised of macrophages and CD8+ T-cells and, to a lesser extent, CD4+ lymphocytes (38). However, these findings are not specific to CIDP as infiltrating endoneurial T-cells may be seen in sural nerves from patients with a wide variety of peripheral neuropathies (39), including CIDP (40), so noted in 26% of CIDP nerve biopsies compared to those with the diagnosis of chronic idiopathic axonal polyneuropathy and normal controls. The presence of three or more macrophages clustered around an endoneurial microvessel was considered a useful marker to support the histopathologic diagnosis of CIDP (41). Teased nerve fiber analysis revealed primary myelinopathy in 48% of affected nerves so studied, 21% of which demonstrated axonopathy, 18% indefinite, and 13% mixed axonopathy and myelinopathy in one analysis (12), compared to another analysis that showed 68% primary myelinopathy, 20% mixed myelinopathy and axonopathy, and 5% primary axonopathy (37).

There was a considerable overlap in the microscopic aspects of nerve demyelination, axonal neuropathy, and inflammatory cell infiltration among 21 nerves affected by CIDP compared to 13 with chronic idiopathic axonal polyneuropathy (CIAP) patients (36). Electron microscopy, combined with immunofluorescence, improved the detection of chronic demyelination in a study of superficial fibular sensory nerve biopsies in patients with CIDP compared to CIAP and normal controls (42). Multiple alterations in the nodal and paranodal regions were detected that predominated in Schwann cells among those with CIDP as compared to the axons of others with CIAP. Paranodin/Caspr immunofluorescence was more widespread in the nerves affected by CIDP, extending along the axon at internodes where it appeared intense. While cutaneous nerve biopsy is not mandatory in the diagnosis of CIDP, a Practice Parameter of the AAN (43) recommended cutaneous nerve biopsy in the evaluation of atypical forms of CIDP, and in equivocal clinical instances of CIDP, wherein demonstration of demyelination and inflammation may be necessary to guide further therapy.

PATHOGENESIS

The pathogenesis of CIDP is ascribed to a combination of cell- and humoral immune-mediated mechanisms that result in the active stripping of myelin lamella from nerve roots and peripheral nerves. Infiltrating epineurial and endoneurial T-cells express activation markers, chemokines, and chemokine receptors notably CXCR-3 (44), and secrete matrix metalloproteinase-2 and -9 (45) in response to native peripheral nerve myelin antigens. The immune attack on the Schwann cell surface is mediated by macrophages (46) that invade the Schwann cell basement membrane (38). The resultant antibody-mediated complement attack against peripheral nerve myelin leads to myelin stripping and phagocytosis.

Humoral immune mechanisms are suggested by at least three observations. First, the development of peripheral demyelination in experimental animals that received passive transfer of sera and immunoglobulin G antibodies transfer from patients with CIDP (47, 48) that impairs nerve conduction by increasing the permeability of the blood-nerve barrier. Second, the observed increase in circulating serum complement levels, with activation of the terminal components of complement and immunoreactive C3d present on the surface of myelin sheaths (49, 50), and serum autoantibodies to components of peripheral nerve myelin and neuronal antigens, including P0 found in up to 20% of patients with CIDP (51). Third, the effectiveness of PE in patients with CIDP irrespective of detectable serum antibodies; and suppressor T-cell function, which is defective in CIDP and enhanced *in vivo* by prednisone and PE in conjunction with clinical improvement (52).

Several lines of evidence offer clues to the loss of self-tolerance and alteration of cell-mediated immune responses in CIDP. The percentage of circulating regulatory FoxP3+CD4+ CD25+ T-cells is reduced in patients with CIDP in comparison to normal control subjects (53). Inhibitory Fc-gamma receptor (FcγR) IIB, expressed on myeloid and B cells, appears to play a critical role in the balance of tolerance and autoimmunity (54), such that treatment-naive active CIDP patients show a lower expression of FcγIIB levels on naive B-cells and fail to upregulate or maintain upregulation of FcγIIB, as they progress from the naive to the memory compartment. Patients with CIDP and systemic lupus erythematosus each share the increased representation of a polymorphism in the promoter for the gene that controls expression of the Fcγ receptor IIB (55). Comic and colleagues (56) found that defective Fas function, associated with a death receptor present on activated lymphocytes and involved in switching-off the immune response, was correlated with the development of CIDP development and its aggressive evolution. Fas function was lower in patients with CIDP than those with AIDP and in control subjects, especially when there was a progressive disease course and secondary axonal damage than that of a relapsing-remitting course associated with pure demyelination.

CIDP AND CONCURRENT SYSTEMIC DISORDERS

Two concurrent systemic disorders, monoclonal paraproteinemia and diabetes mellitus, contribute to the development of CIDP in some patients. Up to 20% of patients with CIDP may harbor a monoclonal paraprotein of unknown significance (CIDP-MGUS). All such patients should probably undergo radiographic skeletal surveys and hematologic evaluation including bone marrow studies to exclude a lymphoproliferative process, such as lymphoma, osteosclerotic myeoloma and plasmacytoma. The latter two account for about 3% of patients with multiple myeloma, differ from the former in the absence of bone pain, often initial presentation of peripheral neuropathy, and the excretion of lambda light chains, termed Bence-Jones protein. Such occurs in the patients with IgG and IgA monoclonal proteins even when the serum concentration is reduced, and can be missed by serum protein electrophoresis as an M protein, and detectable by immunofixation alone (57, 58). The combination of osteosclerotic myeloma, polyneuropathy, organomegaly, endocrinopathy, M-protein, and skin changes constitutes the POEMS syndrome, the etiopathogenesis of which appears to be related to vasoactive endothelial growth factor (VEGF) production, which is used as a diagnostic marker even in patients with partial elements of the syndrome (59, 60). Skeletal survey is more sensitive than nuclear bone scan in the detection of osteoslerotic lesions (58). Radiation and surgical removal of the plasmacytoma is effective treatment for osteosclerotic myeloma and neuropathy, as is autologous stem cell transplantation, which normalizes serum VEGF levels (61, 62). Among nine thalidomide patients so treated, six had concomitant improvement in peripheral neuropathy, and three remained clinically stable (63). Patients with CIDP and IgM paraprotein usually, but not invariably, present with predominant distal involvement that is less responsive to immunotherapy, especially in those with the DADS phenotype.

Patients with diabetes mellitus may have an increased risk of developing demyelinating neuropathy and elevated CSF protein content suggestive of CIDP (64–66), but they also may be features of diabetes and not a result of concomitant CIDP especially when conduction block is absent. An Olmsted County epidemiologic study (67) showed that diabetes mellitus occurred no more frequently in CIDP when compared to normal controls. Only 4% of those with CIDP had diabetes mellitus compared to 12% of controls. However, there are reported patients with diabetes mellitus and a classical phenotype of CIDP that respond to standard mode of therapy for CIDP (68, 69), including intravenous immune globulin IVIg (70) and prednisone (71) suggesting a common autoimmune-mediated etiopathogeneis.

CIDP may follow treatment with the tumor necrosis factor-alpha (TNF-α) antagonists (72–75), among them tacrolimus (76–79), that responds to discontinuation of therapy, administration of IVIg and immunosuppressive therapy (74).

TREATMENT

First Line Therapy

Randomized controlled trials have confirmed the efficacy of prednisone (80), PE (81, 82), and IVIg (83–85) in the treatment of CIDP. Recognizing the need for specialized facilities for providing outpatient PE makes that therapy somewhat less appealing. Moreover, recognizing the potential adverse side effects of long-term corticosteroids, IVIg emerged as the preferred initial therapy for CIDP.

Corticosteroids

A multicenter, randomized, double-blind, crossover trial (22) that compared the outcome of six weeks of tapering prednisolone from 60 mg to 10 mg daily to 2.0 g/kg of IVIg administered over one to two days in CIDP to 24 of the 32 eligible subjects, showed no significant differences in outcome, however, IVIg led to more rapid improvement. When treating CIDP with prednisone, it is usual practice to commence therapy at 100 mg orally once daily in the morning and when improvement begins, typically in two to four weeks, the patient is switched to alternate day therapy. Upon evidence of significant recovery of strength and function, the dose of prednisone is gradually tapered by 5 mg per week to four weeks, to the lowest possible dose that maintains normal function, over a period that typically lasts five to six months. A minority of patients will be successfully tapered off of prednisone, but others may relapse, the latter requiring initiation of a steroid-sparing agent such as azathioprine or mycophenolate mofitel to facilitate successful further tapering of prednisone. Baseline studies for diabetes, lipid panel, PPD skin testing, bone density measurements, and ophthalmologic examinations for cataracts are all recommended before commencement of prednisone, as well as oral supplementation of calcium, 500 mg to 600 mg two to three times daily with vitamin D 400 IU to 800 IU, to avert development of osteopenia, osteoporosis, and consequent compression fractures. Prophylactic alendronate can be given to those at risk for compression fracture, H2-blockers or proton pump inhibitors to patients at risk for gastrointestinal ulcer, and dietary modification to avoid electrolyte imbalance and incipient hypertension. Lopate and colleagues (86) found that various regimens of high-dose pulse IV methylprednisolone was equivalent therapy overall to IVIg and oral prednisone in improving strength six months after initiation of therapy, and led to less weight gain and Cushingoid features than treatment with daily oral prednisone. An open-label prospective study of oral weekly pulse methylprednisolone, (87) in ten patients with CIDP followed by oral methylprednisolone 500 mg once weekly for three months with needed dose adjustments, was well-tolerated with only short-lasting side effects, and subsequent remission in 60% so treated, allowing discontinuation of therapy.

Intravenous Immune Globulin

Mendell and colleagues (84) established superiority of IVIg compared over placebo and demonstrated efficacy, employing measures of strength and functionality in newly diagnosed and untreated patients with CIDP. The beneficial effects of IVIg in isokinetic strength, gait velocity, and hand function were rapid in onset and typically noticeable by the fifth day of therapy, peaking by day 10 (88). The INCAT group found IVIg and prednisolone to be equivalent therapy (22). While Harbo and colleagues (88) and Hughes and coworkers in the INCAT Trial (22) analyzed the therapeutic effects of IVIg at six weeks, a subsequent study by Hughes and colleagues of the ICE Study Group (85) established efficacy of IVIg in a long-term, randomized, double-blind, placebo-controlled, response-conditional crossover trial of 117 patients with CIDP who met INCAT criteria (22) for study inclusion, and received caprylate-chromatography purified 10% immune globulin intravenous or placebo every three weeks for up to six months. Overall, 54% of patients treated with IVIg showed improvement in the adjusted INCAT disability score through week 24 compared to 21% of subjects who received placebo (p=0.0002), as well as in recorded grip strength. During the 24-week extension phase, participants who continued to receive IVIg had a longer time to relapse than did patients treated with placebo (p=0.011). A post-hoc finding was the improvement in CMAP amplitudes of proximal nerves and those most severely affected (89). In comparison to the 2005 EFNS/PNS CIDP Guidelines (27, 90) the most recent treatment recommendations (28) upgraded use of IVIg to Level A, rendering it first-line

therapy for CIDP while maintaining the Level A status for PE when IVIg and corticosteroids were ineffective.

Although there can be acceptable dosing and frequency adjustments for individual patients, it is accepted practice to commence therapy at 2 g/kg over two to five days, infusing no faster than 150 to 200 cc/hr or more than 10 grams per hour, tapering to a monthly maintenance dose of 0.4 g/kg once sustained benefit in strength and function is seen. The complications of IVIg, which occur in 10% to 26%, can be classified as mild, moderate, and severe, wherein mild side effects include headache, nausea, chills, myalgia, chest discomfort, and back pain, all of which may be improved with slowing of the infusion rate and prevented by hydration and premedication with acetaminophen, Benadryl and, if needed, IV methylprednisolone. Moderate and more uncommon reactions include chemical meningitis and delayed red macular skin rash of the palms, soles, and trunk with desquamation. More severe, often preventable side effects through the careful selection of patients for treatment include acute renal-related dehydration and reaction to sucrose or maltose diluents, anaphylaxis in IgA-deficient patients; and stroke, myocardial infarction, pulmonary embolism and thrombophlebitis associated with hyperviscocity. Subcutaneous infusion of immunoglobulins (SCIg) is an effective alternative to IVIg therapy in CIDP but the administered daily dose typically does not exceed 15 grams (91).

The salutary effects of IVIg in CIDP are ascribed to the modulation and inhibition of pathogenic autoantibodies, suppression of proinflammatory cytokines, blocking of Fc receptors, and increase of macrophage colony stimulating factor and monocyte chemotactant protein-1 levels, alteration in T-cell function, and a reduction in circulating CD54 lymphocytes, and inhibition of cellular transmigration into skeletal muscle. Fc core polysaccharide sialylation contributes to the anti-inflammatory properties the IVIg (92). Moreover, the precise IgG Fc fragment N-linked glycan requirements for the observed *in vitro* anti-inflammatory property of IVIg associated with a 2, 6 sialylated IgG Fc recombinant molecule is observed at a much reduced dose than unfractionated IVIG (93). Sialylated Fc fragments require a specific C-type lectin, (SIGN-R1), specifically ICAM-3 grabbing non-integrin-related 1 expressed on macrophages in the splenic marginal zone (94). IVIg mediated the suppression of inflammation through a novel T helper type 2 (TH2) cell pathway in transgenic mice (95). Administration of Fc fragments with glycans terminating in α2, 6 sialic acids results in the production of IL-33, which, in turn, induces expansion of IL-4-producing basophils that promote increased expression of the inhibitory type IIB Fc-gamma receptor (FcγRIIB) in effector cells, the modulation of which may be a potentially promising therapeutic approach in CIDP. The systemic administration of IVIg therapy, like that of TH2 cytokines, IL-33 and IL-4, upregulates FcγRIIB and partially restores its expression on naïve B-cells and monocytes that are already low in untreated patients with CIDP compared to demographically-matched healthy controls, after administration of IVIg (96). Single nucleotide polymorphisms in transient axonal glycoprotein 1(TAG 1), a crucial molecule in IVIg responsiveness in Japanese CIDP patients CIDP (97), influences the favorable response to IVIg.

Plasma Exchange

Plasma exchange, demonstrated to be more effective than sham PE in CIDP (81, 82), is typically employed in severely weak patients maintained in an intensive care setting who relapse or are unresponsive to prednisone and IVIg. The risks of PE relate to the placement and maintenance of an indwelling central venous catheter, hypotension, allergic reactions to albumin and citrate toxicity, hypocalcemia, anemia, and thrombocytopenia. A therapeutic course of PE includes five to ten treatments performed over two to four weeks however there are no benchmark goals as to the total volume of blood needed to be exchanged affects a therapeutic effect. The effects of PE are transient, usually lasting four to eight weeks, but sometimes only one to two weeks; therefore, unless another immunomodulatory treatment such as prednisone is given, PE would need to be performed long-term, something that is rarely pursued for logistical reasons.

Overall, 66% of patients with CIDP responded to prednisone, IVIg or PE, and 35% improved with a second agent in one analysis (98), as did 87% of those fulfilling 2005 EFNS/PNS criteria (27) for a definite diagnosis of CIDP, with an equal efficacy of prednisone and IVIg, including one-quarter of patients with severe disease (9); however, 40% of patients remained dependent on long-term treatment for IVIg and prednisone, respectively, in 55% and 18% of those so treated.

Second and Third Line Therapy

Patients who fail to respond or cannot tolerate prednisone, PE, or IVIg, may be considered for treatment with the second-tier agents, azathioprine, mycophenolate mofetil, and methotrexate alone or in combination with one of the first-tier agents (99–101), or other therapies from among available tertiary agents including cyclophosphamide, cyclosporine, interferon (INF)-α and INF-β, autologous stem cell transplantation, and monoclonal antibodies targeting B-cells in patients with malignant and non-malignant disorders associated with CIDP (102–109). A small controlled-trial of patients randomly assigned to azathioprine 2 mg/kg and prednisone showed no difference in outcome than assigned to prednisone alone (110). One retrospective analysis of patients treated with mycophenolate mofetil allowed tapering of corticosteroids and IVIg but only 30% showed this overall improvement (101), and in another series (111), with treatment with mycophenolate mofetil led to overall improvement in the average Neuropathy Impairment Score (NIS), with the majority so treated able to discontinue or reduce the dose of frequency, respectively, of corticosteroids or IVIg by 50% or more. However, one-third of patients so treated developed potentially fatal opportunistic infection (112). More than one-half of patients administered methotrexate reduced the weekly dose of corticosteroids or IVIg by up to 20%. Treatment with 30 micrograms once, twice, or three times weekly of INFb-1a, did not show significant benefit in reduction of the dose of IVIg during the four-month period of treatment (113).

High-dose cyclophosphamide without stem cell rescue can lead to long-term remission with refractory CIDP and improved quality of life (102). In isolation, the latter therapy is rarely employed and associated with potentially serious adverse events such as neutropenic septicemia, and pneumonia. The chimeric monoclonal antibody rituximab, which binds to the CD20 antigen expressed from pre- to mature B-cell stages in normal and malignant B-cells, and reduces peripheral B-lymphocyte counts by 90% within three days, and showed recovery in 90 days, acts as a cellular decoy (109). Its salutary mechanism of action in CDIP results from the formation of rituximab-IgG molecules to B cells, and cellular immune complexes that efficiently attract and bind Fcγ receptor-expressing effector cells, in turn reducing B-cell substrates for tissue inflammation A retrospective, observational and multicenter trial of four consecutive weekly doses of 375 mg/m^2 of intravenous rituximab in 13 patients with CIDP, eight of whom had hematologic malignancies (114), led to improvement in nine patients so treated, with a clinical response that typically began two months after commencement of therapy and was sustained for up to one year. Alemtuzumab, a monoclonal antibody, was administered to seven severe IVIG-dependent CIDP cases refractory to conventional immunosuppression (115), and was associated with a 26% reduction in the required dose IVIG to sustain benefit, as well as prolonged remission in two patients and partial in two others with the remaining three patients unchanged. However, toxicity, like that of rituximab, limits its more widespread use.

OUTCOME OF TREATMENT

The natural history of CIDP has gradually improved with more prompt initiation of immunosuppressant therapy. Three decades ago (3), 60% of patients with CIDP improved following immunosuppressant therapy and were able to return to work, 4% achieved remission status, 8% were ambulatory but unable to work, and 28% were bedridden, wheelchair-bound, or died of their disease or a concomitant illness. A decade later (12), 90% of patients experienced improvement following initial management with immunosuppressive therapy, and 30% in sustained remission. With one-half of patients experiencing a clinical relapse, the longer patients were followed the more likely a relapse occurred. The current response rate to immunotherapy is 63% to 76% (83, 84), with symptoms of less than one year predicting a beneficial response to IVIg therapy in those so treated (83). The overall mortality rate has decreased to about one percent and only seven percent of treated patients are likely to be wheelchair-bound, with a progressive course, CNS involvement, a higher proportion of nerve fibers showing active demyelination on nerve biopsy, and overall degree of axonal loss, all correlated with greater disability. Early, aggressive therapy prevents secondary axon loss and improves prognosis (37).

CHILHOOD CIDP

CIDP is an unusual cause of childhood neuropathy. It was diagnosed in only 8.8% of one biopsy series (116) and 11% of a clinical series of polyneuropathy unassociated with a more widespread neurological disorder (117). A comparison of 15 children with idiopathic CIDP with 69 adults (118) demonstrated similarities and differences between the two cohorts. Similar to adults, antecedent events were uncommon in children. Weakness, areflexia, sensory loss were common, and pain and cranial neuropathies were uncommon. CSF protein content was elevated. Not all children satisfied strict electrodiagnostic criteria for CIDP. Moreover, children differed in more precipitous onset of symptoms, more frequent gait abnormalities, and other neurological dysfunction, and initial response to immunomodulatory therapy was excellent. Long-term follow-up of 12 children with CIDP demonstrated a more rapidly fluctuating and relapsing course than adults, with generally full recovery from each episode of deterioration. Multiple courses of IVIg given for episodes of relapse showed continued efficacy with an overall excellent prognosis (119).

CIDP VARIANTS

The spectrum of disorders included in the chronic acquired demyelinating polyneuropathies (CADP) and their relation to CIDP continues to be more precisely defined. In addition to classic CIDP, characterized by symmetrical proximal and distal weakness and sensory loss, a number of different entities can be placed under the heading of CIDP, the subtypes or variant syndromes of which share both basic similarities and important differences. Three well-understood CADP syndromes include multifocal motor neurop-

athy (MMN), multifocal acquired demyelinating sensory and motor (MADSAM) neuropathy or Lewis-Sumner syndrome, and distal acquired demyelinating symmetric (DADS) neuropathy.

It is uncertain whether a sensory CIDP variant truly exists (26). The former includes subsets of patients with clinically predominant sensory syndromes (8, 120–124), others with emergence of late motor involvement (125), sensory ataxic forms of CIDP (126), cryptogenic sensory polyneuropathy (127) or minimal CIDP (128). Demyelinating features were evident in motor NCS, but not sensory NCS, in patients with CADP utilizing near nerve studies indicative of sensory nerve fiber loss compared to demyelination along motor nerves, suggesting different pathophysiological mechanisms in sensory and motor dysfunction. Moreover, motor NCS in reported patients with sensory CIDP (122, 123, 125, 129) have often revealed evidence of demyelinating of motor fibers preceding weakness.

Multifocal Motor Neuropathy

First described by Parry and Clarke (130) as a disorder masquerading as motor neuron disease (MND), MMN was later associated with anti-GM1 serum antibodies and motor CB (MCB) (131) that improved with systemic immunosuppressant therapy (132) and IVIg (133–135). Affected patients present with asymmetric distal limb weakness affecting the arm more frequently than the leg, usually in the distribution of individual peripheral nerves with limited or no sensory symptoms. Although the lack of atrophy in muscles weakened by MCB should prompt consideration of MMN, the presence of atrophy may develop with denervation associated with secondary axonal loss. Deep tendon reflexes may be diminished but are often normal in unaffected nerves. The CSF protein content, which is generally normal, should prompt an alternate diagnosis when significantly elevated (136). Although most patients do not have a serum M-protein, polyclonal IgM GM1 antibodies are detected in the sera of 40% to 80% of affected patients (132, 137–142). Very high titers appear to be specific for MMN, but the sensitivity of standard anti-GM1 antibody testing, which is 50% at best (143–146), is increased using a specialized enzyme-linked immunosorbent assay (ELISA) (147), while lower titers of anti-GM1 antibodies are detected in other neuropathies (148, 149). Serum IgM binding to NS6S heparin dissacharide correlated with distally predominant asymmetric arm weakness due to MCB, so noted in the majority of patients (150). High titers (> or = 7,000) of serum NS6S or GM1 antibody in motor neuropathy increased sensitivity from 43% based on GM1 antibody positivity, to 64% when either antibody is detected. Although MCB has been considered the electrophysiologic hallmark of MMN, there are patients with otherwise typical MMN without detectable

MCB (151), presumably due to activity-dependent MCB or a very proximal location of the blocks. The electrophysiological features of MMN include prolongation of distal motor latencies, temporal dispersion, slow motor conduction velocity, and delayed or absent F-waves (144). Conduction block is not essential to the diagnosis of MMN if other features of demyelination are detected (144, 152). MCB was present in 31% of patients with MMN and temporal dispersion in 44%, with other features of frank demyelination in 94% (144), without a difference in response to treatment with or without MCB (144, 153), so noted by other investigators who administered cyclophosphamide (154) or IVIg (155). Cervical root stimulation established the diagnosis of MMN among 13 patients with possible or definite MMN (34), augmenting the sensitivity of 46% of consensus criteria for MMN (151). Although predicted to be normal in MMN (151), a variable degree of sensory loss was described in patients with otherwise typical MMN (156, 157) with a mean time to appearance of objective sensory signs in several patients with MMN more likely than MADSAM and seropositivity for anti-GM1 IgM antibodies, of 7.2 years, being preceded by intermittent paraesthesia in the same nerve territories as motor involvement. Moreover, a significant reduction in the amplitude of at least one SNAP was noted in 62% of MMN patients followed for at least three years (157) and comparisons of MMN patients with or without minor sensory abnormalities showed no significant differences among variables of gender, age at onset, number of involved motor nerves, CSF protein content, anti-GM1 serum antibody titer, or response to IVIg. The revised guidelines of the EFNS/PNS for MMN (158) allows only minor vibration sense abnormalities in the lower legs and the development of sensory signs and symptoms in the course of the illness. While the clinical and electrodiagnostic changes are typically found in multiple motor nerves, three affected patients had involvement of the median, fibular, or ulnar nerves alone, with improvement after IVIg therapy (159). Similarly, 50% of patients with an MMN phenotype and axonal electrodiagnostic changes, with so-called multifocal acquired motor axonopathy (MAMA), improved with immunotherapy (160) as did the majority of patients in another cohort of MAMA (161). Sensory cutaneous nerve biopsies in patients with MMN are usually unrevealing (162, 163), however demyelination without inflammatory cell infiltration and multifocal axonal degeneration without demyelination were found at presumed sites of MCB (164, 165), presumably due to caused by antibody-mediated attack against components of axolemma at the nodes of Ranvier. T_2-weighted MRI of involved brachial plexus showed increased signal intensity associated with diffuse nerve swelling (166).

While corticosteroids and PE are generally ineffective in MMN (167, 168), the efficacy of IVIg was demonstrated in two randomized, controlled trials (169, 170), with the therapeutic response occurring after several days after single course of treatment, and the salutary effects lasting weeks to months afterward, with some exhibiting long-term benefit or maintenance IVIg therapy (171–173). However, over time, axon loss and disability may accrue (174). Effective therapy leads to resolution of MCB in some, but not all, nerves with occasional appearance of axonal loss. Most of the observed improvement in patients treated regularly for up to eight years was noted in the first several months of therapy, with strength slightly decreasing over time, although still significantly improved compared to the most recent prior follow-up visit (33). Among ten patients with MMN treated with IVIg for up to 12 years (175), two patients maintained maximal improvement and eight showed worsening, with the decline manifested between three to seven years into the therapy. A cross-sectional descriptive study of 88 MMN patients (134) showed a 94% response rate to IVIg. Independent determinants of non-responsiveness to IVIg were longer duration of disease and electrodiagnostic features of concomitant axon loss. Early IVIg treatment may postpone axonal degeneration and permanent deficits. A recently concluded 15-month multicenter cross-over trial of the efficacy of 10% IVIg among 44 subjects with MMN across three stabilization and two blinded phases has yet to be published but the results were compelling enough for the FDA to approve Gammagard liquid 10% as a treatment for MMN in June 2012.

Other methods of therapy for refractory MMN are available including rituxamib (176–180), the largest study of which concluded a two-year open-label trial (177) in which quantitative strength testing improved by 13% to 22% as well as a 45% reduction in anti-GM1 antibody titers in the rituximab-treated group at one and two years, compared to unchanged clinical status in control subjects. Those with initial benefit, followed by recurrent weakness in the first year after treatment, received a second course of treatment and maintained benefit. Patients with significant deficits unresponsive to IVIg or rituximab should be considered for treatment with 0.5 to 1.0 mg/m² pulse intravenous cyclophosphamide, which was associated with clinical efficacy in >70% of patients (132, 142, 181). Short-term SCIg leads to preservation of muscle strength for several months (182), the side effects of which consist of mild and transient local skin reactions. An analysis of five patients with MMN treated with SCIg equivalent to a maintenance dose of IVIg led to stable muscle strength over a six-month follow-up (183). An open-label multicenter study of eight patients with MMN (184) concluded that SCIg was an efficacious and safe therapy in the transition from IVIg to SCIg over a six-month period. A randomized, controlled-trial of 28 patients with MMN and an initial response to IVIg, randomized to two grams per day of oral mycophenolate mofetil or placebo with appropriate dose reduction in IVIg over the ensuing 12 months (185), showed that adjunctive treatment with mycophenolate mofitel was not effective in dose reduction of IVIg, nor did it lead to changes in serum anti-GM1 antibody titers.

Multifocal Acquired Demyelinating Sensory and Motor Neuropathy

Oh and colleagues (186) described the CIDP variant MADSAM neuropathy (187), or multifocal inflammatory demyelinating neuropathy (188). MADSAM neuropathy is a multifocal variant of CIDP, and both diseases are distinct from MMN. Affected patients have a chronic sensorimotor MMN with insidious onset, slow progression and initial involvement in the arms, with later spread to the distal legs. Lesions in single nerves become confluent, leading to the appearance of symmetrical distal involvement. Deep tendon reflexes are diffusely reduced or absent, and the CSF protein content is raised in the majority of patients, with electrophysiological features of MCB, temporal dispersion, prolonged distal latencies, slow NCV and delayed or absent F-waves in one or more motor nerves. In contrast to MMN, sensory NCS are also abnormal at onset. Up to one-half of patients with MADSAM evolve into a clinical pattern of generalized CIDP (189). Cranial neuropathy occurs, including optic neuritis, as well as oculomotor, trigeminal, and facial palsy. Unlike MMN, MADSAM neuropathy is not associated with elevated anti-GM1 antibody titers. Sensory cutaneous nerve biopsy shows prominent demyelinating features with many thinly myelinated large-diameter fibers, scattered demyelinating fibers, and onion bulbs similar to the findings in CIDP. Teased nerve fiber preparations show evidence of demyelination or remyelination with asymmetric pathologic findings within and between fascicles (190, 191). Retrospective studies demonstrate improvement in response to IVIg treatment in more than 70% of affected patients (187, 188). However, in contrast to MMN, those with MADSAM neuropathy show a demonstrably favorable response to corticosteroid treatment, making it important to separate this disorder from MMN as the former is steroid-responsive while the latter is not.

Distal Acquired Demyelinating Symmetric Neuropathy

Men are affected more often than women with DADS, especially in the sixth decade or later, with sensory symptoms and weakness confined to the toes, ankles, fingers, and wrists. In two-thirds of patients a monoclonal protein, especially IgM-κ, is detected, so termed M-DADS. Profound sensory loss is associated with gait unsteadiness and tremor. Motor NCS demonstrate widespread symmetric slowing, most accentuated in distal sensory and motor

nerves without CB. In most patients, distal latencies are dramatically prolonged, resulting in a short terminal latency index (TLI), which is a hallmark of anti-MAG neuropathy (192–193). A short TLI reliably distinguished patients with anti-MAG neuropathy from other chronic demyelinating neuropathies (160, 192). The CSF protein content is elevated in most patients. Cutaneous sensory nerve biopsy shows the characteristic finding of widely spaced myelin outer lamellae on EM, in addition to deposits of IgM and complement along myelinated nerve fibers. Epidermal nerve fiber (ENF) studies of the skin show IgM deposits on dermal myelinated fibers with a greater prevalence along the distal leg and reduced ENF density consistent with axonal loss (194). Serum antibodies reactive against IgM myelin-associated glycoprotein (MAG) are present in two-thirds of DADS-M neuropathy patients (160). Other DADS-M patients may be of the IgM-MGUS type. Those with DADS-M neuropathy respond poorly to IVIg, prednisone, PE, and cyclophosphamide. Only 30% of patients in one series (160) improved, most with only sensory manifestations, making objective assessments of treatment responses challenging. Although most IgM-MGUS literature patients lack sufficient clinical description, demonstration of demyelinating electrophysiology, and serological assessment, there is general consensus that IgM-MGUS and MAG-positive patients do not respond or poorly respond to immune therapies (195–199). In 3 randomized, placebo-controlled trials assessing immunomodulatory therapies in IgM-MGUS polyneuropathy, PE was no better than sham PE in IgM-MGUS; however, active treatment produced a superior response among those with IgG- and IgA-MGUS (197). Dalakas and colleagues (200) found a response rate of 18% for IVIg in IgM-MGUS patients; moreover, there was no benefit for INF-α in a placebo-controlled trial (201), nor benefit in open-label administration of rituximab in DADS-M (30, 176, 177, 202–204), although Benedetti and colleagues (205) detected significant improvement in the mean INCAT (22) sensory sum score at one year in those with anti-MAG neuropathy. Among 17 patients with polyneuropathy and IgM monoclonal gammopathy (206), rituximab induced an improvement of 1 or more points on an overall disability sum score in two patients, and improvement of 5% or more in the distal Medical Research Council (MRC) motor sum score in four others, similarly in the sensory sum score of nine patients so studied. The presence of anti-MAG antibody and disease duration <10 years predicted a positive treatment response. A randomized, placebo-controlled trial of rituximab in 26 anti-MAG neuropathy patients (207) showed no statistical significance employing a primary endpoint measure of the change of ≥1 point in the INCAT leg disability scale score (22) at eight months. Since the clinical deficit in most patients with IgM-MGUS polyneuropathy is primarily sensory, and significant progression over time may be minimal even without treatment, the risks of aggressive management should be weighed against the relatively benign course (198). Recent guidelines jointly issued by the EFNS/PNS (208) advocate withholding immunomodulatory therapy from DADS-M patients without significant disability due to the slow disease progression and likelihood of incurred side effects. Those with IgG and IgA monoclonal gammopathy and neuropathy are clinically different (209). Patients with IgM monoclonal are more likely to have predominantly sensory clinical manifestations, ataxia, and distal demyelination on motor NCS, essentially confirming the DADS phenotype, while IgA/IgG cohorts are heterogeneous with regard to axonal and demyelinating features. Isoardo and colleagues (210) showed that patients with anti-MAG antibodies were more likely to have a sensory phenotype with severe distal demyelinating electrophysiology on motor NCS.

The one-third of patients with the DADS phenotype without an M-protein, referred to as idiopathic DADS neuropathy (DADS-I), do not manifest features of male predominance or older age so noted in DADS-M, and their response to immune therapy is intermediate between DADS-M and CIDP (160). Some patients corresponding to DADS-I, and labeled sensory CIDP because of sensory symptoms or signs alone, despite demyelinating motor electrophysiology (121, 122, 124), respond to immunomodulatory therapy, but assessment of efficacy has been difficult.

Citak and colleagues (211) described a patient with chronic, progressive, distally severe sensory impairment and mild distal weakness, with slightly increased CSF protein content, and normal sensory NCS and sural nerve biopsy pathology. Later renamed chronic inflammatory sensory polyradiculopathy (CISP), it was considered to be CIDP restricted to sensory roots even though such patients did not fulfill strict electrodiagnostic criteria for CIDP (212). Similar patients were reported by Sinnreich and colleagues (212) with paraesthesia, gait ataxia, large fiber sensory loss, frequent falls, normal limb strength, CSF protein elevation, normal motor and sensory NCS and needle EMG. SSEP studies were consistent with sensory root involvement. MRI showed enlargement and enhancement of lumbar nerve roots on post-gadolinium MRI. Sensory root biopsy shows decreased density of large myelinated fibers, segmental demyelination, onion-bulb formation, and endoneurial inflammation. Among six patients treated with immunomodulatory therapy, all had marked improvement, with four returning to normal ambulation. Such patients were termed progressive sensory radiculopathy (211) and chronic sensory polyradiculopathy (CISP) (212). A related syndrome of chronic inflammatory lumbosacral polyradiculopathy (213) was described in two patients with chronic sensory disturbances, proximal leg weakness, normal motor and sensory NCS and EMG, and SSEP and neuroimaging that similarly suggested a process involving the lumbosacral roots likened to CISP, both of whom responded favorably to IVIg, but neither of whom met strict diagnostic criteria for CIDP. Two of 146 patients in a French CIDP series (9), neither of whom were described electrophysiologically, were purported to have a similar clinical presentation of chronic inflammatory lumbosacral polyradiculopathy.

Patients with chronic ataxic neuropathy, ophthalmoparesis, IgM paraproteinemia, cold agglutinins, and disialosyl ganglioside antibodies (CANOMAD) (214) present instead with slowly progressive or relapsing ataxia, ocular, sensory, bulbar, and motor, and rarely, respiratory involvement. Disialosyl groups containing the sequence NeuNAC (a2-8) NeuNAc (a2-3) Gal are common to the gangliosides GD1b, GT1b, GQ1b, and GD3, densely located in the neurons of dorsal root ganglia of humans and within the oculomotor cranial nerves. Evidence that such antibodies are pathogenic is suggested by the fact that immunization of rabbits with GD1b antibodies induced a sensory neuropathy and sensory neuronal degeneration (215–217). The majority of patients demonstrate demyelinating changes on NCS, with elevation of the CSF protein content, and white matter lesions on brain neuroimaging with absent oligoclonal bands. Although there may be a response to IVIg and PE, up to one-third of affected patients can remain wheelchair bound. Two patients with CANOMAD (218) presented with severe ataxic neuropathy and minimal weakness that progressed over a several-year period, later developing opthalmoplegia, IgM paraproteinemia, and anti-disialosyl antibodies. Both patients had reduction in SNAP amplitudes associated with demyelinating or axonal changes on cutaneous nerve biopsy, and both responded to treatment with IVIg.

REFERENCES

1. Eichhorst H. Beitrage zur pathologie der nerven und muskeln. *Cor Kl Schweiz Aertze* 1890; 20:59–71.

2. Austin JH. Recurrent polyneuropathies and their corticosteroids treatment. *Brain* 1958; 8:157–92.

3. Dyck PJ, Lais AC, Otha M, et al. Chronic inflammatory polyradiculoneuropathy. *Mayo Clin Proc* 1975; 50:621–637.

4. Dyck PJ, Arnason BG. Chronic inflammatory demyelinating polyradiculoneuropathy. In: Dyck PJ, Thomas PK, Lambert EH, Bunge R, editors. *Peripheral neuropathy.* 2nd ed. Philadelphia: WB Saunders, 1984:2101–2114.

5. Dyck PJ, Oviatt KF, Lambert EH. Intensive evaluation of referred unclassified neuropathies yields improved diagnosis. *Ann Neurol* 1981; 10:222–226.

6. Barohn RJ. Approach to peripheral neuropathy and neuronopathy. *Semin Neurol* 1998; 18:7–18.

7. Laughlin RS, Dyck PJ, Melton LJ 3rd, et al. Incidence and prevalence of CIDP and the association of diabetes mellitus. *Neurology* 2009; 73:39–45.

8. McCombe PA, Pollard JD, McLeod JG. Chronic inflammatory demyelinating polyradiculoneuropathy. A clinical and electrophysiological study of 92 cases. *Brain* 1987; 110:1617–1630.

9. Viala K, Maisonobe T, Stojkovic T, et al. A current view of the diagnosis, clinical variants, response to treatment and prognosis of chronic inflammatory demyelinating polyradiculoneuropathy. *J Peripher Nerv Syst* 2010; 15:50–56.

10. Dionne A, Nicolle MW, Hahn AF. Clinical and electrophysiological parameters distinguishing acute-onset chronic inflammatory demyelinating polyneuropathy from acute inflammatory demyelinating polyneuropathy. *Muscle Nerve* 2010; 41:202–207.

11. Ruts L, Drenthen J, Jacobs BC, et al, and the Dutch GBS Study Group. Distinguishing acute-onset CIDP from fluctuating Guillain-Barré syndrome: a prospective study. *Neurology* 2010; 74:1680–1686.

12. Barohn RJ, Kissel JT, Warmolts JR, et al. Chronic inflammatory polyradiculoneuropathy. Clinical characteristics, course, and recommendations for diagnostic criteria. *Arch Neurol* 1989; 46:878–884.

13. Dalakas M, Houff SA, Engel WK, et al. CSF "monoclonal" bands in chronic relapsing polyneuropathy. *Neurology* 1980; 30:864–867.

14. Yan WX, Archelos JJ, Hartung HP, et al. P0 protein is a target antigen in chronic inflammatory demyelinating polyradiculoneuropathy. *Ann Neurol* 2001; 50:286–292.

15. Allen D, Giannopoulos K, Gray I, et al. Antibodies to peripheral nerve myelin proteins in chronic inflammatory demyelinating polyradiculoneuropathy. *J Peripher Nerv Syst* 2005; 10:174–180.

16. Ad Hoc Subcommittee of the American Academy of Neurology AIDS Task Force. Research criteria for diagnosis chronic inflammatory demyelinating polyneuropathy. *Neurology* 1991; 41:617– 618.

17. Koski CL, Baumgarten M, Magder LS, Derivation and validation of diagnostic criteria for chronic inflammatory demyelinating polyneuropathy. *J Neurol Sci* 2009; 277:1–8.

18. Bromberg MB. Review of the electrodiagnostic criteria for chronic inflammatory polyradiculoneuropathy. *Muscle Nerve* 2011; 780–794.

19. Thaisetthawatkul P, Logigian EL, Herrmann DN. Dispersion of the distal compound muscle action potential as a diagnostic criterion for chronic inflammatory demyelinating polyneuropathy. *Neurology* 2002; 59:1526–1532.

20. Rotta FT, Sussman AT, Bradley WG, et al. The spectrum of chronic inflammatory demyelinating polyneuropathy. *J Neurol Sci* 2000; 173:129–139.

21. Nicolas G, Maisonobe T, Le Forestier N, et al. Proposed revised electrophysiological criteria for chronic inflammatory demyelinating polyradiculoneuropathy. *Muscle Nerve* 2002; 25:26–30.

22. Hughes R, Bensa S, Willison H, et al. Randomized controlled trial of intravenous immunoglobulin versus oral prednisolone in chronic inflammatory demyelinating polyradiculoneuropathy. *Ann Neurol* 2001; 50:195–201.

23. Isose S, Kuwabara S, Kokubun N, et al. Tokyo Metropolitan Neuromuscular Electrodiagnosis Study Group. Utility of the distal compound muscle action potential duration for diagnosis of demyelinating neuropathies. *J Peripher Nerv Syst* 2009; 14:151–158.

24. Joint Task Force of the EFNS and the PNS. European Federation of Neurological Societies/Peripheral Nerve Society Guideline on management of chronic inflammatory demyelinating polyradiculoneuropathy: Report of a joint task force of the European Federation of Neurological Societies and the Peripheral Nerve Society, 1st rev. *J Peripher Nerv Syst* 2010; 15:1–9.

25. Koski CL, Study Group for the Validation of CIDP Criteria. Development and validation of diagnostic criteria for chronic inflammatory demyelinating polyneuropathy. *J Peripher Nerv Syst* 2005; 10 (Suppl):45–46.

26. Saperstein DS, Katz JS, Amato AA, et al. Clinical spectrum of chronic acquired demyelinating polyneuropathies. *Muscle Nerve* 2001; 24:311–324.

27. Joint Task Force of EFNS and the PNS. European Federation of Neurological Societies/Peripheral Nerve Society Guildline on management of chronic inflammatory demyelinating polyradiculoneuropathy. Report of a joint task force of the European Federation of Neurological Societies and the Peripheral Nerve Society. *J Peripher Nerv Syst* 2005; 10:220–228.

28. Members of the Task Force: Van den Bergh PYK, Hadden RDM, Bouche P, et al. European Federation of Neurological Societies/ Peripheral Nerve Society Guideline on management of chronic inflammatory demyelinating polyradiculoneuropathy: Report of a joint task force of the European Federation of Neurological Societies and the Peripheral Nerve Society-First revision. *Eur J Neurol* 2010; 17:356–363.

29. Rajabally YA, Samarasekera S. Electrophysiological sensory demyelination in typical chronic inflammatory demyelinating polyneuropathy. *Eur J Neurol* 2010; 17:939–944.

30. Dimachkie MM, Anderson HS, Gronseth GS, et al. How common is sural nerve sparing in chronic inflammatory demyelinating polyneuropathy? 2008 Meeting of the Inflammatory Neuropathy Consortium. *J Peripher Nerv Syst* 2008; 13:166a.

31. Rajabally YA, Narasimhan M. The value of sensory electrophysiology in chronic inflammatory demyelinating polyneuropathy. *Clin Neurophysiol* 2007; 118:1999–2004.

32. Kokubun N, Hirata K. Neurophysiological evaluation of trigeminal and facial nerves in patients with chronic inflammatory demyelinating polyneuropathy. *Muscle Nerve* 2007; 35:203–207.

33. Vucic S, Cairns KD, Black KR, et al. Cervical nerve root stimulation. Part I: technical aspects and normal data. *Clin Neurophysiol* 2006; 117:392–397.

34. Vucic S, Black K, Siao Tick Chong P, et al. Cervical nerve root stimulation. Part II: findings in primary demyelinating neuropathics and motor neuron disease. *Clin Neurophysiol* 2006; 117:398–404.

35. Molenaar DS, Vermeulen M, de Haan R. Diagnostic value of sural nerve biopsy in chronic inflammatory demyelinating polyneuropathy. *J Neurol Neurosurg Psychiatry* 1998; 64:84–89.

36. Bosboom WM, Van den Berg LH, Franssen H, et al. Diagnostic value of sural demyelination in chronic inflammatory demyelinating polyneuropathy. *Brain* 2001; 124:2427–2438.

37. Bouchard C, Lacroix C, Plante V, et al. Clinicopathologic findings and prognosis of chronic inflammatory demyelinating polyneuropathy. *Neurology* 1999; 52:498–503.

38. Matsummuro K, Izumo S, Umehara F, et al. Chronic inflammatory demyelinating polyneuropathy: Histological and immunopathological studies in biopsied sural nerves. *J Neurol Sci* 1994; 127:170–178.

39. Cornblath DR, Griffin DE, Welch D, Griffin JW, et al. Quantitative analysis of endoneurial T-cells in human sural nerve biopsies. *J Neuroimmunol* 1990; 26:113–118.

40. Bosboom WM, Van den Berg LH, De Boer L, et al. The diagnostic value of sural nerve T cells in chronic inflammatory demyelinating polyneuropathy. *Neurology* 1999; 53:837–845.

41. Sommer C, Koch S, Lammens M, Gabreels-Festen A, et al. Macrophage clustering as a diagnostic marker in sural nerve biopsies of patients with CIDP. *Neurology* 2005; 65:1924–1929.

42. Cifuentes-Diaz C, Dubourg O, Irinopoulou T, et al. Nodes of Ranvier and Paranodes in Chronic Acquired Neuropathies. PLoS ONE 2011; 6(1): e14533. doi:10.1371/journal.pone.0014533.

43. England JD, Gronseth GS, Franklin G, et al. American Academy of Neurology. Practice Parameter: evaluation of distal symmetric polyneuropathy: role of autonomic testing, nerve biopsy, and skin biopsy (an evidence-based review). Report of the American Academy of Neurology, American Association of Neuromuscular and Electrodiagnostic Medicine, and American Academy of Physical Medicine and Rehabilitation. *Neurology* 2009; 72:177–184.

44. Kieseier BC, Tani M, Mahad D, et al. Chemokines and chemokine receptors in inflammatory demyelinating neuropathies: a central role for IP-10. *Brain* 2002; 125:823–834

45. Leppert D, Hughes P, Huber S, et al. Matrix metalloproteinase upregulation in chronic inflammatory demyelinating polyneuropathy and nonsystemic vasculitic neuropathy. *Neurology* 1999; 53:62–70.

46. Hafer-Macko CE, Sheikh KA, Li CY, et al. Immune attack on the Schwann cell surface in acute inflammatory demyelinating polyneuropathy. *Ann Neurol* 1996; 39:625–635.

47. Yan WX, Taylor J, Andrias-Kauba S, Pollard JD. Passive transfer of demyelination by serum or IgG from chronic inflammatory demyelinating polyneuropathy patients. *Ann Neurol* 2000; 47:765–775.

48. Hartung HP, Kieseier BC, Meyer zu Horste G, et al. From bench to bedside – experimental rationale for immune-specific therapies in the inflamed peripheral nerve. *Nat Clin Pract Neurol* 2007; 3:198–221.

49. Koski CL, Sanders ME, Swoveland PT, et al. Activation of terminal components of complement in patients with Guillain-Barre syndrome and other demyelinating neuropathies. *J Clin Invest* 1987; 80:1492–1497.

50. Hays AP, Lee SS, Latov N, et al. Immune reactive C3d on the surface of myelin sheaths in neuropathy. *J Neuroimmunol* 1988; 18:231–244.

51. Allen D, Giannopoulos K, Gray I, et al. Antibodies to peripheral nerve myelin proteins in chronic inflammatory demyelinating polyradiculoneuropathy. *J Peripher Nerv Syst* 2005; 10:174–180.

52. De Luca G, Lugaresi A, Iarlori C, et al. Prednisone and plasma exchange improve suppressor cell function in chronic inflammatory demyelinating polyneuropathy. *J Neuroimmunol* 1999; 95:190–194.

53. Chi LJ, Wang HB, Wang WZ. Impairment of circulating CD4+CD25+ regulatory T cells in patients with chronic inflammatory demyelinating polyradiculoneuropathy. *J Peripher Nerv Syst* 2008; 13:54–63.

54. Nimmerjahn F, Lünemann JD. Expression and function of the inhibitory Fcγ-receptor in CIDP. *J Peripher Nerv Syst* 2011; 16(Suppl 1):41–44.

55. Tackenberg B, Jelcic I, Baerenwaldt A, et al. Impaired inhibitory Fcgamma receptor IIB expression on B cells in chronic inflammatory demyelinating polyneuropathy. *Proc Natl Acad Sci USA* 2009; 106:4788–4792.

56. Comic C, Gaviani P, Leone M, et al. Fas-mediated T-cell apoptosis is impaired in patients with chronic inflammatory demyelinating polyneuropathy. *J Peripher Nerv Syst* 2006; 11:53–60.

57. Kelly JJ, Kyle RA, Miles JM, et al. Osteosclerotic Myeloma and Peripheral Neuropathy. *Neurology* 1983; 33:202–210.

58. Dispenzieri A, Kyle RA, Lacy MQ, et al. POEMS syndrome: definitions and long-term outcome. *Blood* 2003; 101:2496–2506.

59. Watanabe O, Maruyama I, Arimura K, et al. Overproduction of vascular endothelial growth factor—Vascular permeability factor is causative in Crow-Fukase (POEMS) syndrome. *Muscle Nerve* 1998; 21:1390–1397.

60. Watanabe O, Arimura K, Kitajima I, et al. Greatly raised vascular endothelial growth factor (VEGF) in POEMS syndrome. *Lancet* 1996; 347:702.

61. Kuwabara S, Misawa S, Kanai K, et al. Autologous peripheral blood stem cell transplantation for POEMS syndrome. *Neurology* 2006; 66:105–107.

62. Mahdi-Rogers M, Kazmi M, Ferner R, et al. Autologous peripheral blood stem cell transplantation for chronic acquired demyelinating neuropathy. *J Peripher Nerv Syst* 2009; 14:118–124.

63. Kuwabara S, Misawa S, Kanai K, et al. Thalidomide reduces serum VEGF levels and improves peripheral neuropathy in POEMS syndrome. *J Neurol Neurosurg Psychiatry* 2008; 79:1255–1257.

64. Sharma KR, Cross J, Farronay O, et al. Demyelinating neuropathy in diabetes mellitus. *Arch Neurol* 2002; 59:758–765.

65. Wilson JR, Park Y, Fisher MR. Electrodiagnostic criteria in CIDP: comparison with diabetic neuropathy. *Electromyogr Clin Neurophysiol* 2000; 40:181–185.

66. Barohn RJ, Sahenk Z, Warmolts JR, et al. The Bruns-Garland syndrome (diabetic amyotrophy). Revisited 100 years later. *Arch Neurol* 1991; 48:1130–1135.

67. Laughlin RS, Dyck PJ, Melton LJ 3rd, et al. Incidence and prevalence of CIDP and the association of diabetes mellitus. *Neurology* 2009; 73:39–45.

68. Gorson KC, Ropper AH, Adelman LS, et al. Influence of diabetes mellitus on chronic inflammatory demyelinating polyneuropathy. *Muscle Nerve* 2000; 23:37–43.

69. Sharma KR, Cross J, Ayyar DR, et al. Diabetic demyelinating polyneuropathy responsive to intravenous immunoglobulin therapy. *Arch Neurol* 2002; 59:751–757.

70. Jann S, Bramerio MA, Facchetti D, et al. Intravenous immunoglobulin is effective in patients with diabetes and with chronic inflammatory demyelinating polyneuropathy: long term follow-up. *J Neurol Neurosurg Psychiatry* 2009; 80:70–73.

71. Kalita J, Misra UK, Yadav RK. A comparative study of chronic inflammatory demyelinating polyradiculoneuropathy with and without diabetes mellitus. *Eur J Neurol* 2007; 14:638–643.

72. Stübgen JP. Tumor necrosis factor-alpha antagonists and neuropathy. *Muscle Nerve* 2008; 37:281–292.

73. Hooper DR, Tarnopolsky MA, Baker SK. Lewis-Sumner syndrome associated with infliximab therapy in rheumatoid arthritis. *Muscle Nerve* 2008; 38:1318–1325.

74. Lozeron P, Denier C, Lacroix C, Long-term course of demyelinating neuropathies occurring during tumor necrosis factor-alpha-blocker therapy. *Arch Neurol* 2009; 66:490–497.

75. Alshekhlee A, Basiri K, Miles JD, et al. Chronic inflammatory demyelinating polyneuropathy associated with tumor necrosis factor-alpha antagonists. *Muscle Nerve* 2010; 41:723–727.

76. Younger DS, Orsher S, Appel G, et al. Progressive demyelinating nuropathy after renal transplantion. *Muscle Nerve* 2012. Abstracts, 46:621–679.

77. Wilson JR, Conwit RA, Eidelman BH, et al. Sensorimotor neuropathy resembling CIDP in patients receiving FK506. *Muscle Nerve* 1994; 17:528–532.

78. Echaniz-Laguna A, Battaglia F, Ellero B, et al. Chronic inflammatory demyelinating polyradiculoneuropathy in patients with liver transplantation. *Muscle Nerve* 2004; 30:501–504.

79. Labate A, Morelli M, Palamara G, et al. Tacrolimus-induced polyneuropathy after heart transplantation. *Clin Neuropharmacol* 2010; 33:161–162.

80. Dyck PJ, O'Brien PC, Oviatt KF, Dinapoli RP, Prednisone improves chronic inflammatory demyelinating polyradiculoneuropathy more than no treatment. *Ann Neurol* 1982; 11:136–141.

81. Dyck PJ, Daube J, O'Brien P, Plasma exchange in chronic inflammatory demyelinating polyradiculoneuropathy. *N Engl J Med* 1986; 314:461–465.

82. Hahn AF, Bolton CF, Pillay N, et al. Plasma-exchange therapy in chronic inflammatory demyelinating polyneuropathy: A double-blind, sham-controlled, cross-over study. *Brain* 1996; 119:1055–1066.

83. Hahn AF, Bolton CF, Zochodne D, et al. Intravenous immunoglobulin treatment in chronic inflammatory demyelinating polyneuropathy: A double-blind, placebo-controlled, cross-over study. *Brain* 1996; 119:1067–1077.

84. Mendell JR, Barohn RJ, Freimer ML, et al. and the Working Group on Peripheral Neuropathy: Randomized controlled trial of IVIg in untreated chronic inflammatory demyelinating polyradiculoneuropathy. *Neurology* 2001; 56:445–449.

85. Hughes RA, Donofrio P, Bril V, et al. and the ICE Study Group. Intravenous immune globulin (10% caprylate-chromatography purified) for the treatment of chronic inflammatory demyelinating polyradiculoneuropathy (ICE study): A randomised placebo-controlled trial. *Lancet Neurol* 2008; 7:136–144.

86. Lopate G, Pestronk A, Al-Lozi M. Treatment of chronic inflammatory demyelinating polyneuropathy with high-dose intermittent intravenous methylprednisolone. *Arch Neurol* 2005; 62:249–254.

87. Muley SA, Kelkar P, Parry GJ. Treatment of chronic inflammatory demyelinating polyneuropathy with pulsed oral steroids. *Arch Neurol* 2008; 65:1460–1464.

88. Harbo T, Andersen H, Jakobsen J. Acute motor response following a single IVIG treatment course in chronic inflammatory demyelinating polyneuropathy. *Muscle Nerve* 2009; 39:439–447.

89. Bril V, Banach M, Dalakas MC, et al, and the ICE Study Group. Electrophysiologic correlations with clinical outcomes in CIDP. *Muscle Nerve* 2010; 42:492–497.

90. Members of the Task Force: Hughes RAC, Bouche P, Cornblath DR, et al. European Federation of Neurological Societies/Peripheral Nerve Society guideline on management of chronic inflammatory demyelinating polyradiculoneuropathy: report of a joint task force of the European Federation of Neurological Societies and the Peripheral Nerve Society. *Eur J Neurol* 2006; 13:326–332.

91. Lee DH, Linker RA, Paulus W, et al. Subcutaneous immunoglobulin infusion: A new therapeutic option in chronic inflammatory demyelinating polyneuropathy. *Muscle Nerve* 2008; 37:406–409.

92. Kaneko Y, Nimmerjahn F, Ravetch JV. Anti-inflammatory activity of immunoglobulin G resulting from Fc sialylation. *Science* 2006; 313:670–673.

93. Anthony RM, Nimmerjahn F, Ashline DJ, et al. Recapitulation of IVIG anti-inflammatory activity with a recombinant IgG Fc. *Science* 2008; 320:373–376.

94. Anthony RM, Wermeling F, Karlsson MC, et al. Identification of a receptor required for the anti-inflammatory activity of IVIG. *Proc Natl Acad Sci USA* 2008; 105:19571–19578.

95. Anthony RM, Kobayashi T, Wermeling F, et al. Intravenous gammaglobulin suppresses inflammation through a novel TH2 pathway. *Nature* 2011; 475:110–113.

96. Tackenberg B, Nimmerjahn F, Lünemann JD. Mechanisms of IVIG efficacy in chronic inflammatory demyelinating polyneuropathy. *J Clin Immunol* 2010; 30(Suppl 1):S65–69.

97. Iijima M, Tomita M, Morozumi S, et al. Single nucleotide polymorphism of TAG-1 influences IVIg responsiveness of Japanese patients with CIDP. *Neurology* 2009; 73:1348–1352.

98. Gorson KC, Allam G, Ropper AH. Chronic inflammatory demyelinating polyneuropathy: clinical features and response to treatment in 67 consecutive patients with and without a monoclonal gammopathy. *Neurology* 1997; 48:321–328.

99. Chaudhry V, Cornblath DR, Griffin JW, et al. Mycophenolate mofetil: a safe and promising immunosuppressant in neuromuscular diseases. *Neurology* 2001; 56:94–96.

100. Mowzoon N, Sussman A, Bradley WG. Mycophenolate (CellCept) treatment of myasthenia gravis, chronic inflammatory polyneuropathy and inclusion body myositis. *J Neurol Sci* 2001; 185:119–122.

101. Gorson KC, Amato AA, Ropper AH. Efficacy of mycophenolate mofetil in patients with chronic immune demyelinating polyneuropathy. *Neurology* 2004; 63:715–717.

102. Brannagan TH III, Pradham A, Heiman-Patterson T, et al. High-dose cyclophosphamide without stem-cell rescue for refractory CIDP. *Neurology* 2002; 58:1856–1858.

103. Pavesi G, Cattaneo L, Marbini A, et al. Long-term efficacy of interferon-alpha in chronic inflammatory demyelinating neuropathy. *J Neurol* 2002; 249:777–779.

104. Vallat JM, Hahn AF, Leger JM, et al. Interferon beta 1a as an investigational treatment for CIDP. *Neurology* 2003; 60(Suppl 3):S23–S28.

105. Fialho D, Chan YC, Allen DC, et al. Treatment of chronic inflammatory demyelinating polyradiculoneuropathy with methotrexate. *J Neurol Neurosurg Psychiatry* 2006; 77:544–547.

106. Vermeulen M, Van Oers MH. Successful autologous stem cell transplantation in a patient with chronic inflammatory demyelinating polyneuropathy. *J Neurol Neurosurg Psychiatry* 2002; 72:127–128.

107. Oyama R. Sufit Y, Loh L et al. Nonmyeloablative autologous hematopoietic stem cell transplantation for refractory CIDP. *Neurology* 2007; 69:1802–1803.

108. Mahdi-Rogers M, Kazmi M, Ferner R, et al. Autologous peripheral blood stem cell transplantation for chronic acquired demyelinating neuropathy. *J Peripher Nerv Syst* 2009; 14:118–124.

109. Taylor RP, Lindorfer MA. Drug insight: the mechanism of action of rituximab in autoimmune disease—the immune complex decoy hypothesis. *Nat Clin Pract Rheumatol* 2007; 3:86–95.

110. Dyck PJ, O'Brien PC, Swanson C, et al. Combined azathioprine and prednisone in chronic inflammatory-demyelinating polyneuropathy. *Neurology* 1985; 35:1173–1176.

111. Bedi G, Brown A, Tong T, Chronic inflammatory demyelinating polyneuropathy responsive to mycophenolate mofetil therapy. J Neurol Neurosurg Psychiatry 2010; 81:634–636.

112. Rowin J, Amato AA, Deisher N, et al. Mycophenolate mofetil in dermatomyositis: is it safe? Neurology 2006; 66:1245–1247.

113. Hughes RA, Gorson KC, Cros D, et al. Avonex CIDP Study Group.Intramuscular interferon beta-1a in chronic inflammatory demyelinating polyradiculoneuropathy. Neurology 2010; 74:651–657.

114. Benedetti L, Briani C, Franciotta D, et al. Rituximab in patients with chronic inflammatory demyelinating polyradiculoneuropathy: a report of 13 cases and review of the literature. J Neurol Neurosurg Psychiatry 2011; 82:306–308.

115. Marsh EA, Hirst CL, Llewelyn JG, et al. Alemtuzumab in the treatment of IVIG-dependent chronic inflammatory demyelinating polyneuropathy. J Neurol 2010; 257:913–919.

116. Ouvrier RA, McLeod JG. Chronic peripheral neuropathy in children: an overview. Aust Paediatr J 1988; Suppl:80–82.

117. Sladky JT, Brown JM, Berman PH. Chronic inflammatory demyelinating polyneuropathy of infancy: a corticosteroid-responsive disorder. Ann Neurol 1986; 20:76–81.

118. Simmons Z, Wald JJ, Albers JW. Chronic inflammatory demyelinating polyradiculoneuropathy in children: I. Presentation, electrodiagnostic studies, and initial clinical course, with comparisons to adults. Muscle Nerve 1997; 20:1008–1015.

119. Simmons Z, Wald JJ, Albers JW. Chronic inflammatory demyelinating polyradiculoneuropathy in children: II. Long-term followup, with comparison to adults. Muscle Nerve 1997; 20:1569–1575.

120. Dyck PJ, Lais AC, Ohta M, et al. Chronic inflammatory polyradiculoneuropathy. Mayo Clin Proc 1975; 50:621–637.

121. Oh SJ, Joy JL, Sunwoo IN, et al. A case of chronic sensory demyelinating neuropathy responding to immunotherapies. Muscle Nerve 1992; 15:255–256.

122. Oh SJ, Joy JL, Kuruoglu R. Chronic sensory demyelinating neuropathy—chronic inflammatory demyelinating polyneuropathy presenting as a pure sensory neuropathy. J Neurol Neurosurg Psychiatry 1992; 55:677–680.

123. Berger AR, Herskovitz S, Kaplan J. Late motor involvement in cases presenting as chronic sensory demyelinating polyneuropathy. Muscle Nerve 1995; 18:440–444.

124. Simmons Z, Tivakaran S. Acquired demyelinating polyneuropathy presenting as pure sensory syndrome. Muscle Nerve 1996; 19:1174–1176.

125. Van Dijk GW, Notermans NC, Franssen H, et al. Development of weakness in patients with chronic inflammatory demyelinating polyneuropathy and only sensory symptoms at presentation: A long-term follow-up study. J Neurol 1999; 246:1134–1139.

126. Ohkoshi N, Harada K, Nagata H, et al. Ataxic form of chronic inflammatory demyelinating polyradiculoneuropathy: Clinical features and pathological study of the sural nerves. Eur Neurol 2001; 45:241–248.

127. Chin RL, Latov N, Sander HW, et al. Chronic inflammatory demyelinating polyneuropathy presenting as cryptogenic sensory polyneuropathy. J Peripher Nerv Syst 2004; 9:128–133.

128. Uncini A, Di Muzio A, De Angelis MV, et al. Minimal and asymptomatic chronic inflammatory demyelinating polyneuropathy. Clin Neurophysiol 1999; 110:694–698.

129. Krarup C, Trojaborg W. Sensory pathophysiology in chronic acquired demyelinating neuropathy. Brain 1996; 119:257–270.

130. Parry GJ, Clarke S. Multifocal acquired demyelinating neuropathy masquerading as motor neuron disease. Muscle Nerve 1988; 11:103–107.

131. Krarup C, Stewart JD, Sumner AJ, et al. A syndrome of asymmetric limb weakness with motor conduction block. Neurology 1990; 40:118–127.

132. Pestronk A, Cornblath DR, Ilyas AA. A treatable multifocal motor neuropathy with antibodies to GM1 ganglioside. Ann Neurol 1988; 24:73–78.

133. Van den Berg-Vos RM, Franssen H, Wokke JHJ, et al. Multifocal motor neuropathy: long-term clinical and electrophysiological assessment of intravenous immunoglobulin maintenance treatment. Brain 2002; 125:1875–1886.

134. Cats EA, van der Pol WL, Piepers S, et al. Correlates of outcome and response to IVIg in 88 patients with multifocal motor neuropathy. Neurology 2010; 75:818–825.

135. Patwa HS, Chaudhry V, Katzberg H, et al. Evidence-based guideline: intravenous immunoglobulin in the treatment of neuromuscular disorders: Report of the Therapeutics and Technology Assessment Subcommittee of the American Academy of Neurology. Neurology 2012; 78:1009–1015.

136. Joint Task Force of the EFNS and the PNS. European Federation of Neurological Societies/Peripheral Nerve Society Guideline on management of multifocal motor neuropathy. Report of a joint task force of the European Federation of Neurological Societies and the Peripheral Nerve Society. J Peripher Nerv Syst 2006; 11:1–8.

137. Kaji R, Hirota N, Oka N, Anti-GM1 antibodies and impaired blood-nerve barrier may interfere with remyelination in multifocal motor neuropathy. Muscle Nerve 1994; 17:108–110.

138. Kornberg AJ, Pestronk A. The clinical and diagnostic role of anti-GM1 antibody testing. Muscle Nerve 1994; 17:100–104.

139. Lange DJ, Trojaborg W, Latov N, Hays AP, et al. Multifocal motor neuropathy with conduction block: is it a distinct clinical entity? Neurology 1992; 42:497–505.

140. Parry GJ. Anti-ganglioside antibodies do not necessarily play a role in multifocal motor neuropathy. Muscle Nerve 1994; 17:97–99.

141. Sadiq SA, Thomas FP, Kilidireas K, The spectrum of neurologic disease associated with anti-GM1 antibodies. Neurology 1990; 40:1067–1072.

142. Tan E, Lynn DJ, Amato AA, et al. Immunosuppressive treatment of motor neuron syndromes. Attempts to distinguish a treatable disorder. Arch Neurol 1994; 51:194–200.

143. Kuntzer T, Radziwill AJ, Lettry-Trouillat R, et al. Interferon-B1a in chronic inflammatory demyelinating polyneuropathy. Neurology 1999; 53:1364–1365.

144. Katz JS, Wolfe GI, Bryan WW, Jackson CE, et al. Electrophysiologic findings in multifocal motor neuropathy. Neurology 1997; 48:700–707.

145. Taylor BV, Gross L, Windebank AJ. The sensitivity and specificity of anti-GM1 antibody testing. Neurology 1996; 47:951–955.

146. Van Schaik IN, Bossuyt PMM, Brand A. Vermeulen M. Diagnostic value of GM1 antibodies in motor neuron disorders and neuropathies: a meta-analysis. Neurology 1995; 45:1570–1577.

147. Pestronk A, Choksi R. Multifocal motor neuropathy. Serum IgM anti-GM1 ganglioside antibodies in most patients detected using covalent linkage of GM1 to ELISA plates. Neurology 1997; 49:1289–1292.

148. Sadiq SA, Thomas FP, Kilidireas K, et al. The spectrum of neurologic disease associated with anti-GM1 antibodies. Neurology 1990; 40:1067–1072.

149. Pestronk A, Chaudhry V, Feldman EL, et al. Lower motor neuron syndromes defined by patterns of weakness, nerve conduction abnormalities, and high titers of anti-glycolipid antibodies. Ann Neurol 1990; 27:316–326.

150. Pestronk A, Chuquilin M, Choksi R. Motor neuropathies and serum IgM binding to NS6S heparin disaccharide or GM1 ganglioside. J Neurol Neurosurg Psychiatry 2010; 81:726–730.

151. Olney RK, Lewis RA, Putnam TD, et al, and the American Association of Electrodiagnostic Medicine. Consensus criteria for the diagnosis of multifocal motor neuropathy. *Muscle Nerve* 2003; 27:117–121.

152. Pakiam AS, Parry GJ. Multifocal motor neuropathy without overt conduction block. *Muscle Nerve* 1998; 21:243–245.

153. Chaudhry V, Corse AM, Cornblath DR, et al. Multifocal motor neuropathy: electrodiagnostic features. *Muscle Nerve* 1994; 17:198–205.

154. Azulay JP, Attarian S, Pouget J. Effect of cyclophosphamide in multifocal motor neuropathies with or without conduction block. *Neurology* 1999; 52(Suppl 2):A550–A55.

155. Ellis CM, Leary S, Shaw J, et al. Use of human intravenous immunoglobulin in lower motor neuron syndromes. *J Neurol Neurosurg Psychiatry* 1999; 67:15–19.

156. Lambrecq V, Krim E, Rouanet-Larriviere M, et al. Sensory loss in multifocal motor neuropathy: a clinical and electrophysiological study. *Muscle Nerve* 2009; 39:131–136.

157. Lievens I, Fournier E, Viala K, et al. Multifocal motor neuropathy: a retrospective study of sensory nerve conduction velocities in long-term follow-up of 21 patients. *Rev Neurol* (Paris) 2009; 165:243–248.

158. Joint Task Force of the EFNS and the PNS. European Federation of Neurological Societies/Peripheral Nerve Society guideline on management of multifocal motor neuropathy. Report of a joint task force of the European Federation of Neurological Societies and the Peripheral Nerve Society, 1st rev. *J Peripher Nerv Syst* 2010; 15:295–301.

159. Felice KJ, Goldstein J. Monofocal motor neuropathy: improvement with intravenous immunoglobulin. *Muscle Nerve* 2002; 25:674–678.

160. Katz JS, Barohn RJ, Kojan S, et al. Axonal multifocal motor neuropathy without conduction block or other features of demyelination. *Neurology* 2002; 58:615–620.

161. Fisher D, Grothe C, Schmidt S, et al. On the early diagnosis of IVIg-responsive chronic multifocal acquired motor axonopathy. *J Neurol* 2004; 251:1204–1207.

162. Bouche P, Moulonguet A, Younes-Chennoufi AB, et al. Multifocal motor neuropathy with conduction block: a study of 24 patients. *J Neurol Neurosurg Psychiatry* 1995; 59:38–44.

163. Corse AM, Chaudhry V, Crawford TO, et al. Sensory nerve pathology in multifocal motor neuropathy. *Ann Neurol* 1996; 39:319–325.

164. Kaji R, Oka N, Tsuji T, et al. Pathological findings at the site of conduction block in multifocal motor neuropathy. *Ann Neurol* 1993; 33:152–158.

165. Taylor BV, Pyck PJ, Engelstad J, et al. Multifocal motor neuropathy; pathologic alterations at the site of conduction block. *J Neuropathol Exp Neurol* 2004; 63:129–137.

166. Van Es HW, Van den Berg LH, Franssen H, et al. Magnetic resonance imaging of the brachial plexus in patients with multifocal motor neuropathy. *Neurology* 1997; 48:1218–1224.

167. Carpo M, Cappellari A, Mora G, et al. Deterioration of multifocal motor neuropathy after plasma exchange. *Neurology* 1998; 50:1480–1482.

168. Donaghy M, Mills KR, Boniface SJ, et al. Pure motor demyelinating neuropathy: deterioration after steroid treatment and improvement with intravenous immunoglobulin. *J Neurol Neurosurg Psychiatry* 1994; 57:778–783.

169. Azulay JP, Blin O, Pouget J, et al. Intravenous immunoglobulin treatment in patients with motor neuron syndromes associated with anti-GM1 antibodies: A double-blind, placebo-controlled study. *Neurology* 1994; 44:429–432.

170. Van den Berg LH, Kerkhoff H, Oey PL, et al. Treatment of multifocal motor neuropathy with high dose intravenous immunoglobulins: A double blind, placebo controlled study. *J Neurol Neurosurg Psychiatry* 1995; 59:248–252.

171. Chaudhry V, Corse A, Cornblath D, et al. Maintenance immune globulin therapy for multifocal motor neuropathy: Results of long-term follow-up. *Ann Neurol* 1996; 40:513–514.

172. Azulay JP, Rihet P, Pouget J, et al. Long term follow up of multifocal motor neuropathy with conduction block under treatment. *J Neurol Neurosurg Psychiatry* 1997; 62:391–394.

173. Biessels GJ, Franssen H, Van den Berg LH, et al. Multifocal motor neuropathy. *J Neurol* 1997; 244:143–152.

174. Taylor BV, Wright RA, Harper CM, et al. Natural history of 46 patients with multifocal motor neuropathy with conduction block. *Muscle Nerve* 2000; 23:900–908.

175. Terenghi F, Cappellari A, Bersano A, et al. How long is IVIg effective in multifocal motor neuropathy? *Neurology* 2004; 62:666–668.

176. Levine TD, Pestronk A. IgM antibody-related polyneuropathies: B-cell depletion chemotherapy using Rituximab. *Neurology* 1999; 52:1701–1704.

177. Pestronk A, Florence J, Miller T, et al. Treatment of IgM antibody associated polyneuropathies using rituximab. *J Neurol Neurosurg Psychiatry* 2003; 74:485–489.

178. Ruegg SJ, Fuhr P, Steck AJ. Rituximab stabilizes multifocal motor neuropathy increasingly less responsive to IVIg. *Neurology* 2004; 63:2178–2179.

179. Gorson TG, Natarajan N, Ropper AH, et al. Rituximab treatment in patients with IVIg-dependent immune polyneuropathy: a prospective pilot trial. *Muscle Nerve* 2007; 35:66–69.

180. Stieglbauer K, Topakian R, Hinterberger G, et al. Effect of rituximab monotherapy in multifocal motor neuropathy. *Neuromuscul Disord* 2009; 19:473–475.

181. Feldman EL, Bromberg MB, Albers JW, et al. Immunosuppressive treatment in multifocal motor neuropathy. *Ann Neurol* 1991; 30:397–401.

182. Harbo T, Andersen H, Hess A, et al. Subcutaneous versus intravenous immunoglobulin in multifocal motor neuropathy: A randomized, single-blinded cross-over trial. *Eur J Neurol* 2009; 16:631–638.

183. Eftimov F, Vermeulen M, de Haan RJ, et al. Subcutaneous immunoglobulin therapy for multifocal motor neuropathy. *J Peripher Nerv Syst* 2009; 14:93–100.

184. Misbah SA, Baumann A, Fazio R, et al. A smooth transition protocol for patients with multifocal motor neuropathy going from intravenous to subcutaneous immunoglobulin therapy: An open-label proof-of-concept study. *J Peripher Nerv Syst* 2011; 16:92–97.

185. Piepers S, Van den Berg-Vos R, Van der Pol WL, et al. Mycophenolate mofetil as adjunctive therapy for MMN patients: A randomized, controlled trial. *Brain* 2007; 130:2004–2010.

186. Oh SJ, Claussen GC, Dae SK. Motor and sensory demyelinating mononeuropathy multiplex (multifocal motor and sensory demyelinating neuropathy): A separate variant of chronic inflammatory demyelinating polyneuropathy. *J Periph Nerv Syst* 1997; 2:362–369.

187. Saperstein DS, Amato AA, Wolfe GI, et al. Multifocal acquired demyelinating sensory and motor neuropathy: the Lewis-Sumner syndrome. *Muscle Nerve* 1999; 22:560–566.

188. Van den Berg-Vos RM, Van den Berg LH, Franssen H, et al. Multifocal inflammatory demyelinating neuropathy: A distinct clinical; entity? *Neurology* 2000; 54:26–32.

189. Viala K, Renié L, Maisonobe T, et al. Follow-up study and response to treatment in 23 patients with Lewis-Sumner syndrome. *Brain* 2004; 127:2010–2017.

190. Gibbels E, Behse F, Kentenich M, et al. Chronic multifocal neuropathy with persistent conduction block (Lewis- Sumner

syndrome). A clinico-morphologic study of two further cases with review of the literature. *Clin Neuropathol* 1993; 12:343–352.

191. Nukada H, Pollock M, Haas LF. Is ischemia implicated in chronic multifocal demyelinating neuropathy? *Neurology* 1989; 39:106–110.

192. Kaku DA, England JD, Sumner AJ. Distal accentuation of conduction slowing in polyneuropathy associated with antibodies to myelin-associated glycoprotein and sulphated glucuronyl paragloboside. *Brain* 1994; 117:941–947.

193. Trojaborg W, Hays AP, van den BL, et al. Motor conduction parameters in neuropathies associated with anti-MAG antibodies and other types of demyelinating and axonal neuropathies. *Muscle Nerve* 1995; 18:730–735.

194. Lombardi R, Erne B, Lauria G, Pareyson D, et al. IgM deposits on skin nerves in anti-myelin-associated glycoprotein neuropathy. *Ann Neurol* 2005; 57:180–187.

195. Kissel JT, Mendell JR. Neuropathies associated with monoclonal proteins. *Neuromuscl Disord* 1995; 6:3–18.

196. Yeung KB, Thomas PK, King RH, et al. The clinical spectrum of peripheral neuropathies associated with benign monoclonal IgM, IgG and IgA paraproteinaemia. Comparative clinical, immunological and nerve biopsy findings. *J Neurol* 1991; 238:383–391.

197. Dyck PJ, Low PA, Windebank AJ, et al. Plasma exchange in polyneuropathy associated with monoclonal gammopathy of undetermined significance. *N Engl J Med* 1991; 325:1482–1486.

198. Nobile-Orazio E, Meucci N, Baldini L, et al. Long-term prognosis of neuropathy associated with anti-MAG IgM M-proteins and its relationship to immune therapies. *Brain* 2000; 123:710–717.

199. Pollard JD, Young GAR. Neurology and the bone marrow. J Neurol Neurosurg Psychiatry 1997; 63:706–718.

200. Dalakas MC, Quarles RH, Farrer RG, et al. A controlled study of IVIg in demyelinating neuropathy with IgM gammopathy. *Ann Neurol* 1996; 40:792–795.

201. Mariette X, Brouet JC, Chevret S, et al. A randomised double blind trial versus placebo does not confirm the benefit of alpha-interferon in polyneuropathy associated with anti-MAG monoclonal IgM. *J Neurol Neurosurg Psychiatry* 2000; 69:279–280.

202. Briani C, Zara G, Zambello R, et al. Rituximab-responsive CIDP. *Eur J Neurol* 2004; 11:788.

203. Renaud S, Gregor M, Fuhr P, et al. Rituximab in the treatment of polyneuropathy associated with anti-MAG antibodies. *Muscle Nerve* 2003; 27:611–615.

204. Renaud S, Fuhr P, Gregor M, et al. High-dose rituximab and anti-MAG-associated polyneuropathy. *Neurology* 2006; 66:742–744.

205. Benedetti L, Briani C, Grandis M, et al. Predictors of response to rituximab in patients with neuropathy and anti-myelin associated glycoprotein immunoglobulin. *J Peripher Nerv Syst* 2007; 12:102–107.

206. Niermeijer JM, Eurelings M, Lokhorst HL, et al. Rituximab for polyneuropathy with IgM monoclonal gammopathy. *J Neurol Neurosurg Psychiatry* 2009; 80:1036–1039.

207. Dalakas MC, Rakocevic G, Salajegheh M, et al. Placebo-controlled trial of rituximab in IgM anti-myelin-associated glycoprotein antibody demyelinating neuropathy. *Ann Neurol* 2009; 65:286–293.

208. Joint Task Force of the EFNS and the PNS. European Federation of Neurological Societies/Peripheral Nerve Society Guideline on management of paraproteinemic demyelinating neuropathies. Report of a joint task force of the European Federation of Neurological Societies and the Peripheral Nerve Society. *J Peripher Nerv Syst* 2006; 11:9–19.

209. Magy L, Chassande B, Maisonobe T, et al. Polyneuropathy associated with IgG/IgA monoclonal gammopathy: a clinical and electrophysiological study of 15 cases. *Eur J Neurology* 2003; 10:677–685.

210. Isoardo G, Migiaretti G, Ciaramitaro P, et al. Differential diagnosis of chronic dysimmune demyelinating polyneuropathies with and without anti-MAG antibodies. *Muscle Nerve* 2005; 31:52–58.

211. Citak KA, Dickoff DJ, Simpson DM. Progressive sensory radiculopathy responsive to corticosteroid therapy. *Muscle Nerve* 1993; 16:679–680.

212. Sinnreich M, Klein CJ, Daube JR, et al. Chronic immune sensory polyradiculopathy: A possibly treatable sensory ataxia. *Neurology* 2004; 63:1662–1669.

213. Caporale CM, Staedler C, Gobbi C, et al. Chronic inflammatory lumbosacral polyradiculopathy: A regional variant of CIDP. *Muscle Nerve* 2011; 44:833–837.

214. Willison HJ, O'Leary CP, Veitch J, et al. The clinical and laboratory features of chronic sensory ataxic neuropathy with anti-disialosyl IgM antibodies. *Brain* 2001; 124:1968–1977.

215. Kusunoki S, Shimizu J, Chiba A, et al. Experimental sensory neuropathy induced by sensitization with ganglioside GD1b. *Ann Neurol* 1996; 39:424–431.

216. Kusunoki S, Hitoshi S, Kaida K, et al. Monospecific anti-DG1b IgG is required to induce rabbit ataxic neuropathy. *Ann Neurol* 1999; 45:400–403.

217. Ohsawa T, Miyatake T, Yuki N. Anti-B-series gangliosides-recognizing autoantibodies in an acute sensory neuropathy patient cause cell death of rat dorsal root ganglia neurons. *Neurosci Lett* 1993; 157:167–170.

218. Kam C, Balaratnam MS, Purves A, et al. Canomad presenting without opthalmoplegia and responding to intravenous immunoglobulin. *Muscle Nerve* 2011; 44:829–833.

CHAPTER 33

Lyme Neuroborreliosis

David S. Younger

Lyme neuroborreliosis (LNB) is the preferred term for the neurological complications of Lyme disease, caused worldwide by *Borrelia burgdorferi* (*Bb*) *sensu lato* world and *Borrelia burgdorferi* (*Bb*) *sensu stricto* (1), hereafter referred to as *B. burgdorferi*, the vector of Lyme disease in North America. Central nervous system (CNS) manifestations result from involvement of the brain and spinal cord that presents as meningitis, encephalitis, and encephalopathy. Peripheral nerve system (PNS) manifestations result from involvement of large caliber, named peripheral nerves that present as cranial neuritis, radiculoneuritis, mononeuritis multiplex (MNM), distal polyneuropathy (DPN), and painful small-fiber neuropathy (SFN). Autonomic nervous system (ANS) manifestations result from autonomic neuropathy and ganglioneuritis that presents as orthostatic intolerance (OI) and postural orthostatic tachycardia syndrome (POTS).

HISTORICAL ASPECTS

Even before recognition of the responsible spirochete, European investigators described erythema chronicum migrans (EM) in 1922 (2) and, a year later, the neurological triad of meningitis, cranial neuritis, and painful radiculitis (3). European physicians familiar with the disorder emphasized both neurological and rheumatic involvement (4) and routinely treated it with penicillin. In 1977, EM rash was later described in the United States in conjunction with childhood arthritis in near epidemic proportions in towns surrounding Lyme, Connecticut (5). Detailed epidemiological studies demonstrated that the disorder occurred in children with a history of *Ixodes* tick bites and EM. Two years later,

a triad of neurological sequelae was described similar to those in Europe years before (6). Subsequent studies in the United States (7–9) and Europe (10, 11) led to the isolation and identification of the causative *Borrelia* spirochete and the neurological sequelae thereof.

EPIDEMIOLOGY

With an incidence of one in 2719 persons, and involvement of the nervous system in 12 to 15% of individuals infected by *B. burgdorferi* in the United States (12), reported cases of Lyme disease have been rising steadily for the past three decades. This underreported disease has a 15-year mean annual rate for all states ranging from less than .01 cases per 100,000 persons of Montana and Colorado, to 74 cases per 100,000 in Connecticut. The vast majority of statistically affected individuals are white, children of age less than 15 years, and adults of either gender of more than 30 years of age. Since the responsible spirochete is transmitted almost exclusively by the bite of infected hard-shell back legged *Ixodes* ticks that occur in specific locations in which appropriate hosts are available, residence in or visitation to endemic areas during the spring and summer months are useful in determining the likelihood of contracting the illness.

ETIOLOGY

The life cycle of the causative *Borrelia* spirochete is well understood. Larval ticks transmitted by the bite of infected Ixodes ticks hatch uninfected and feed upon small mammals such as white-footed field mice, catbirds, squirrels, opossum, and other small mammals, and then mature into nymphs. If the initial host is infected so will be the nymph tick, which can transmit the disease. For the second host, perhaps human, two other conditions must be met before contraction of the disease. First, spirochetes must proliferate in the tick gut, prompted by ingestion of blood with subsequent dissemination to tick salivary glands. Second, the infected tick must attach to the host for a relatively prolonged period, typically 24 to 48 hours. Endemic cycles have been established in discrete areas of North America, Europe, and Asia. Along the eastern coast of the United States from Maryland to Massachusetts, infected *Ixodes scapularis* ticks, known colloquially as "deer ticks" for the preferred host of the adult forms, are widely prevalent. The same ticks are also found in Minnesota and Wisconsin where they are known as "bear ticks." In general, causative ticks live where animal hosts are widespread, habitats both in underdeveloped areas to wealthy exurban regions beyond the suburbs of a city. Some mammalian species are poor Lyme disease hosts because they infect few of the ticks that bite them, or kill the ticks when they groom their fur. Habitats high in biodiversity lead to an overall reduced risk of Lyme disease to its inhabitants because ticks feed both upon efficient hosts such as field mice and less efficient ones such as squirrels and opossum.

CLINICAL MANIFESTATIONS

Clinical manifestations of this infection are said to differ in other parts of the world. In Europe, most studies have emphasized cutaneous abnormalities, including some rather unusual dermatological entities known an acrodermatitis chronica atrophicans and lymphocytoma cutis, which have rarely been recognized in the United States. Joint symptoms appear to be less frequent in European reports, as are cardiac and rheumatologic, while neurological involvement is usually said to be more frequent in Europe.

Several factors appear to contribute to these apparent differences, including bias of ascertainment, and significant differences in the prevalent strains of infecting *Borrelia* organisms in different parts of the world, each with tropisms for different organ involvement leading to clinical differences, the broad group of which is now known collectively as *B. burgdorferi sensu lato*. Bias of ascertainment may be influenced by rheumatologists who have traditionally treated the disease in the United States, while in Europe it has been historically treated by neurologists. While the predominant North American spirochete known as *B. burgdorferi sensu stricto* also occurs in Europe, other more common strains include *B. garinii*, responsible for most neurological diseases, and *B. afzelii* which causes acrodermatitis as "sheep ticks." There are differences in tick vec-

tor species around the world with *Ioxides ricinus* noted in Europe, and *Ioxides persulcatus* predominating in Asia.

Although the causative pathogen has only been characterized within the past three decades, many of the clinical disorders it causes have been well known for many years. After acute exposure via prolonged tick attachment, most but not all patients develop a characteristic EM rash. This slowly enlarging erythroderm, which may reach many inches in diameter, typically develops over days to weeks at the site of the tick bite and attachment, which may be unapparent. One prospective study noted occurrence of an EM rash in up to 90% of affected children (13). In some patients the spirochetes disseminate early and cause multifocal EM. There is often concomitant fever, arthralgia, malaise, and flu-like illness but not so in the sense of a typical upper respiratory or gastrointestinal infection. However, as both the tick bite and rash may be asymptomatic and occur on parts of the body not easily seen, affected patients may be unaware of either.

Three neurological disorders clearly attributed to Lyme disease are lymphocytic meningitis, painful meningoradiculoneuritis, and encephalomyelitis. Lymphocytic meningitis is clinically indistinguishable from viral or aseptic meningitis, occurs several weeks after the skin rash, and is characterized by varying degrees of headache, neck stiffness, and photophobia. Radicular involvement, especially evident in painful polyradiculoneuritis, is typically asymmetric, of sudden onset, and localized close to the bite with a burning quality and nocturnal exacerbation (14). Weakness appears over several days with cranial nerve involvement, especially the facial nerve, although this may occur as part of the PNS disorder in the absence of meningitis (15, 16), and tendon reflexes, which may be reduced or absent, suggesting Guillain-Barre syndrome. Lyme encephalomyelitis (17–19), which occurs in 0.1% or fewer of untreated patients in Europe and North America with a presentation of symptoms and signs appropriate to the site of inflammatory focal white matter brain and spinal cord involvement, typically manifests focal cerebral deficits or progressive gait disorder with sphincter dysfunction.

DIAGNOSTIC TESTING

The systematic approach to the investigation of the CNS, PNS, and ANS function in LNB employing strict CDC criteria for case selection has been described (20).

Serology

A two-tier approach to active disease and previous infection with demonstration of significant changes in IgM and IgG antibody responses to *B. burgdorferi* in paired acute and convalescent-phase serum samples, including diagnostic levels of IgM and IgG antibodies, and isolation of *B. burgdorferi* from CSF, is recommended by most authorities (21–23) including the Centers for Disease Control and Prevention (CDC) to improve diagnostic accuracy of serological testing in Lyme disease. However, the sensitivity and specificity of the serological diagnosis of Lyme disease has not been determined in any given cohort. First-tier screening is performed by an enzyme-linked immunoassay (ELISA), which should be performed in all suspected patients that becomes informative 3 to 4 weeks after initial exposure, when Lyme-specific IgM serology is also detectable, followed months later by a Lyme-specific IgG response.

During the early phase of exposure, serological testing may be uninformative and falsely negative. Second-tier confirmatory Lyme IgM and IgG Western blots (WB) should be obtained with borderline and reactive first-tier test results. The Lyme IgM WB response is the first to appear after initial exposure to *B. burgdorferi* and is comprised of specific and non-specific bands. This is followed by the Lyme IgG WB response of specific and non-specific band reactivity months later.

Consensus criteria have been developed for WB confirmation which have very high specificity, wherein a positive Lyme WB IgG provides compelling confirmation that an acute disorder may indeed be due to *B. burgdorferi* infection, and a positive Lyme WB IgG provides strong support of more long-standing infection. However, neither IgM nor IgG have very high sensitivity. Early treatment may lead to falsely negative serological test results as may also occur in immune-compromised individuals and immune-competent patients with true infection that are tested before a Lyme IgM WB immune response is mounted. Baseline serology at the onset of antibiotic treatment may provide documentation of a favorable response to therapy with improvement in the number of specific reactive bands.

Cerebrospinal Fluid

A spinal tap for CSF studies should be considered in all patients with CNS involvement for routine studies and paired serum for *B.burgdorferi* serology, including diagnostic levels intrathecal Lyme specific IgM and IgG antibodies, and isolation studies for *B. burgdorferi* culture by DNA using a polymerase chain reaction (PCR) methodology with comparison to a paired serum specimen.

Common CSF findings in LNB include elevated protein content, normal glucose, lymphocytic pleocytosis, and humoral immune response composed of intrathecal immunoglobulins that depend upon the stage and activity of the disorder (24). There may rarely be CSF lymphoid pleocytosis suggestive of cerebral or cerebromeningeal malignancy due to activation and transformation of T- and B-lymphocytes as a result of antigenic stimulation by *B. burgdorferi*

(25). CXCL13 is a very sensitive specific chemokine biomarker of acute untreated LNB that appears in the early stages of the disease when *B. burgdorferi*-specific antibody index A1 is still negative. Stromal cell-derived factor-1α, a ligand of the chemokine receptor CXCR4 known as fusin, also appeared to be expressed in CSF and blood of patients with various stages of Lyme disease.

Neuroimaging

Magnetic resonance imaging (MRI) of the brain and spinal cord should be considered in all patients with suspected LNB employing T_1- and T_2-weighted sequences to quantify the structural integrity of the brain and search for white matter change (WMC) and gray matter (GM) atrophy, as well as other disease-associated lesions. Conventional MRI shows subcortical white matter lesions indistinguishable from multiple sclerosis (MS) in T_2 and fluid-attenuated inversion recovery (FLAIR) imaging. Muliparametric magnetization transfer and diffusion tensor MRI demonstrate multiple brain and cervical spinal cord T_1- and T_2-weighted WMC on conventional MRI unassociated with structural damage, distinguishing them from MS lesions (26). High-field 3-D ^{1}H-MR spectroscopy (MRS), coupled with metabolic analysis (27) employed in a case control treatment of various stages of LNB did not show significant changes in WMC on T_2/FLAIR MRI, whole brain N-acetylaspartate (NAA) levels, or anomalies of the tissue fraction inside the volume-of-interest (VOI) tissue fractions, compared to healthy age- and sex-matched controls (28).

Nuclear medicine cerebral perfusion with single photon emission computed tomography (SPECT) reveals various patterns of potentially reversible cortical hypoperfusion in various stages of LNB and encephalopathy (29, 30). Brain proton-emission tomography (PET), used experimentally in an analysis of Lyme encephalopathy, shows global cerebral blood flow and metabolic rate measurements that do not differ from controls except after hypercapneic challenge (31).

Electrophysiological Studies

Nerve conduction studies (NCS) and electromyography (EMG) of the affected limbs and regions employing standard techniques should be considered in clinically symptomatic patients to investigate large fiber PNS function. Such studies can discern the type, duration, severity, and likely histological basis of the underlying neuropathic disorder from among the likely disorders associated with LNB, including radiculopathy, plexopathy, MNM, and DPN that typically presents with involvemenat of named peripheral nerves, patchy radicular and distal sensory disturbances characterized as stiffness, numbness, tingling, prickling, aching, or jabbing sensations, with little or minimal frank motor involvement. Quantitative sensory testing (QST) for heat pain perception thresholds screens for SFN, often reported as burning or shooting sensations in association with coldness of the limbs, which can be later confirmed by epidermal nerve fiber (ENF) studies of the thigh and calf. Quantitative sudomotor axon reflex testing, beat-to-beat blood pressure (BP) and heart rate (HR) responses to head-up tilt, deep breathing, and Valsalva maneuver, with calculation of a composite autonomic scoring scale screens for ANS dysfunction, the symptoms of which typically consist of palpitation, dizziness, headache, and lightheadedness in association with OI and POTS.

PATHOPHYSIOLOGY

The mechanisms of the etiopathogenesis of nervous system damage in LNB are not well understood but are likely related to aspects of the infectious process and post-infectious autoimmune host factors; the two processes may overlap in a given patient. The factors that influence the infectious process include tropism of the *B. burgdorferi* pathogen for particular areas of the CNS and PNS, the duration of tick attachment, dose of spirochete inoculum, the particular organism strain, and persistent atypical cystic and granular spirochete forms. The factors that influence the host response to *B. burgdorferi* infection may include a prior history of infection, the status of host immune competence, the innate host major histocompatibility complex, (MHC) or human leukocyte antigen (HLA) system that resides on chromosome 6, encoding antigen-presenting proteins and other essential elements of cell-mediated and humoral immune host responses. Moreover there may be concomitant tick-borne opportunistic infection with Bartonella, Chlamydia, Babesia, Mycoplasma, Herpes simplex, Varicella zoster virus, and tick-borne viral encephalitis viral infection. The possible mechanisms of inflammation in LNB have been reviewed (32).

Non-human primate models offer some clues to the etiopathogenesis of parenchymal CNS disease with *B. burgdorferi*. Immune suppressed non-human primates inoculated with the N40 strain of *B. burgdorferi* developed infection of multiple tissues, including the CNS and PNS (33) with higher numbers of spirochetes than immune-competent and uninfected controls along the leptomeninges, nerve roots and dorsal root ganglia, but not CNS parenchyma, suggesting spirochete tropism for those areas (34). Although frank CNS inflammation is not observed, one reported primate model of LNB (35) demonstrated *B. burgdorferi* penetration into freshly collected slices with increased overall expression of inflammatory intermediates and their transcripts employing DNA microarray analysis, as well as increased expression of TNF-α, interleukin (IL)-

6, IL-8, and CXCL13 in glial cells *in situ* by immunoflourescent staining and confocal microscopy. Mitogen-activated protein kinase (MAPK), which inhibits p38 and Erk1/2 MAPK and diminishes TNF-α production in primary rhesus macaques monkey astrocyte cultures infected with *B. burgdorferi,* may be one strategy to control inflammation and apoptosis in CNS LNB (36). The expression of toll-like receptor (TLR), in particular TLR 1, -2, and -5, that play a major role in innate immune responsiveness against microbial pathogens and recognize a variety of highly conserved structural motifs and pathogen-associated molecular pattern (PAMO), was enhanced in the phagocytosis of B. burgdorferi in primary cultures of rhesus microglia and astrocytes (37). Three patients with neuropathologically confirmed LNB demonstrated atypical and cystic spirochete forms with nuclear fragmentation and apoptosis of infected astrocytes employing deoxynuclerotidyltranferase (TdT)-mediated dUTP nick end labeling (TUNEL), induced *in vivo,* and *in vitro* by following infection of primary chicken and rat neurons, as well as rat and human astrocytes (38).

Lyme meningoradiculoneuritis, which combines aspects of direct spirochete infection with host autoimmunity, offers additional clues to the etiopathogenesis of injury in LNB. Reported patients develop early CNS and PNS involvement related 18 days to two months after EM manifested, respectively, by transient encephalopathy, and objective distal sensory involvement in a radicular or diffuse sensory neuropathy type (11). Cerebrospinal fluid analysis in such patients shows lymphocytic pleocytosis of up to a few hundred cells, with mildly elevated protein and normal glucose content, with isolation *of B. burgdorferi,* the causative pathogen, in up to 10% of CSF cultures (39) and demonstrable intrathecal antibody in up to 90% of CSF specimens (40). Sural nerve biopsy in such patients confirms axonal and secondary demyelination mediated by endoneurial and epineurial lymphocytic invasion forming perivascular cuffs, in agreement with tandem electrophysiological studies (11, 14). In other patients, autoimmune mechanisms related to *B. burgdorferi* infection were associated instead with vasculitic MNM (9).

Lyme encephalomyelitis and the far more common chronic Lyme encephalopathy, originally considered a peculiarly American phenomenon, was later observed in European patients (41). Both demonstrate abnormalities on neuroimaging studies and CSF studies, including intrathecal antibody production, and responsiveness to antimicrobial therapy (42, 43). Affected patients with serologically proven and previously treated late LNB, manifest neurophysiological abnormalities, including DPN and MNM with minimally abnormal sural nerve histopathology of mild axonopathy and secondary demyelinating, that resolves with higher doses or a more prolonged regimen of parenteral penicillin and ceftriaxone, suggesting insensitivity of the spirochete or inadequate antibiotic penetration across the blood-brain and blood-nerve barriers (44). Moreover, affected patients with chronic polyneuropathy and detectable *B. burgdorferi* DNA by PCR amplification have demonstrable C5b-9 membrane attack complex (MAC) deposits in biopsied sural nerve tissue, and show improvement of neuropathic symptoms after parenteral ceftriaxone (45), suggesting induction of immune injury by *B. burgdorferi* even in the late stages of LNB. One other patient with serologically proven LNB and polyradiculoneuritis had demonstrable CD8+ suppressor T cell infiltrates in association with MAC deposits in biopsied sural nerve tissue and improved with a second course of parenteral ceftriaxone (14) suggesting participation of both cell- and humoral-mediated immune injury as a likely consequence of *B. burgdorferi* infection. A variety of candidate antigens that cross-react with constituent peripheral nerve molecules were found in sera and peripheral nerves of affected patients with LNB (46, 47). Acquired autonomic neuropathy in association with LNB, in which autonomic fibers are selectively or disproportionately affected leading to OI and other dysautonomic syndromes, are also presumably of autoimmune cause (20, 48) as suggested by the occurrence of autonomic neuropathy after Lymerix and the Connaught vaccination (49, 50).

TREATMENT

In general, once the suspected diagnosis of *B. burgdorferi* infection is ascertained in affected patients, antibiotics therapy should commence. For LNB with objective brain and spinal cord involvement, there is good evidence and consensus that parenteral antibiotics, including ceftriaxone, cefotaxime, and penicillin are all safe and effective. For LNB without brain or spinal cord involvement there is good evidence and consensus that oral doxycycline is probably safe and effective but this medication should not be used in children under the age of eight or in pregnant women. Recommendations of the Quality Standards Subcommittee of the American Academy of Neurology (AAN) (51) include treatment with parenteral antibiotics for syndromes associated with meningitis, encephalomyelitis, encephalopathy, and any neurological syndrome with CSF pleocytosis (Table 1). Similarly, severe neuropathic disease syndromes, particularly those deemed oral antibiotic treatment failures, warrant treatment with parenteral therapy, including peripheral nerve radiculopathy, diffuse neuropathy, MNM, and cranial neuropathy. The recommendation guidelines were based upon an aggregated analysis of treatment data from 300 patients with definite LNB from among eight studies conducted in the United States and Europe (where strains of *borrelia*-causing Lyme disease differ slightly), between 1988

Table 1. Suggested Treatments[1]

Disorder

Meningitis: IV ceftriaxone or cefotaxime or penicillin G
Encephalomyelitis: IV ceftriaxone or cefotaxime or penicillin G
Encephalopathy: treat as encephalomyelitis if CSF abnormal; IV or PO antibiotics if CSF normal
PNS radiculopathy, neuropathy, MNM, cranial neuritis: Oral antibiotics or IV if treatment failure or severe

[1]Adapted from reference 52, with permission.

Table 2. Treatment Regimens[1]

First Line

Oral adult regimen: Doxycycline 100–200 mg bid
Parenteral adult regimen: Ceftriaxone 2 g IV daily
Oral pediatric regimen (> or = 8 year olds): Doxycycline 4–8 mg/kg/d in divided doses.
Parenteral pediatric regimen: Ceftriaxone 50–75 mg/kg/d in 1 dose.

Second Line

Oral adult regimen (when Doxycycline is contraindicated): Amoxicillin 500 mg TID
Parenteral adult regimen: Cefotaxime 2 g IV Q8H
Oral pediatric regimen (when Doxycycline is contraindicated): Amoxicillin 50 mg/kg/d in 3 divided doses.
Parenteral pediatric regimen: Cefotaxime 150–200 mg/kg/d in 3–4 divided doses.

Third Line

Oral adult regimen (when Doxycycline is contraindicated): Cefuroxine axetil 500 mg BID
Parenteral adult regimen: Penicillin G 18-24 MU/d, divided doses Q4H.
Oral pediatric regimen (when Doxycycline is contraindicated): Cefuroxine axetil 30 mg/kg/d.
Parenteral pediatric regimen: Penicillin G 200-400U/kg/d in divided doses Q4H.

[1]Adapted from reference 51, with permission.

and 2005 (52–59). While there is a general reluctance in the United States to treat CNS *B.burgdorferi* infection with oral regimens, the response rate among those treated with oral doxycycline or parenteral beta lactam antibiotics is quite similar. This did not apply to other oral agents. Notwithstanding, since there have not been Class I studies of Lyme disease employing prospective randomized controlled clinical trials with masked outcome assessment, the treatment of LNB with parenteral beta lactam antibiotics seems reasonable. Most authorities agree with a one month course of antibiotic therapy for LNB with reassessment. However, treatment should ultimately be individualized. Recommended first-, second-, and third-line treatment options are shown in Table 2. The role of immunomodulatory therapy in the treatment of various syndromes of LNB is not well understood. However, two serologically confirmed reported patients appeared to benefit from treatment with intravenous immunoglobulin (IVIg), including one with acute Lyme radiculoneuritis (60), and another with chronic encephalopathy, neuropathy, and dysautonomia (20).

CONCLUSIONS

Lyme disease, a spirochete that has been the subject of extensive study in the past three decades, frequently affects the CNS and PNS, and occasionally ANS, with aspects related to the infectious and post-infectious autoimmune processes. The abrupt onset of acute meningoradiculoneuritis with CSF pleocytosis and a triad of meningitis, radiculitis, and cranial neuritis in an affected patient, weeks to months after a spreading erythroderm, so-called Garin's triad, should prompt a vigorous search for the causative agent B. burgdorferi. Occasional patients present with CNS involvement, including encephalopathy long after initial treatment that may be due to mild encephalitis. Non-human primate models have contributed to our understanding of the etiopathogenesis of nervous system injury and clues to the complexity of clinical presentation in humans. Experimental primate models demonstrate spirochete tropism for leptomeninges, nerve roots, and dorsal root ganglia, and up-regulation of proinflammatory intermediates and apoptosis in CNS parenchyma, suggesting tandem autoimmune mechanisms of injury. Accurate diagnosis of CNS infection requires paired serum and CSF specimens, measurement not just of CSF anti-*borrelia* antibody but actual intrathecal antibody production. When the diagnosis is secure, antimicrobial therapy is usually successful.

REFERENCES

1. Burgdorferi W, Barbour AG, Hayes SF, et al. Lyme disease: a tick borne spirochetosis? *Science* 1982; 216:1317–1319.

2. Afzelius A. Erythema chronicum migrans. *Acta Derm Venereol* 1921; 2:120–125.

3. Garin C, Bujadoux A. Paralysie par les tiques. *J Med Lyon* 1922; 71:765–767.

4. Bannwarth A. Chronische lymphocytare meningitis, entzundliche polyneuritis und "rheumatismus." *Arch Psychatra Nervenkr* 1941; 113:284–376.

5. Steere AC, Malawista SE, Hardin JA, et al. Erythema chronicum migrans and Lyme arthritis. The enlarging clinical spectrum. *Ann Intern Med* 1977; 86:685–698.

6. Reik L, AC Steere NH Bartenhagen, et al. Neurological abnormalities of Lyme disease. *Medicine* 1979; 58:281–294.

7. Benach JL, Bosler EM, Hanrahan JP, et al. Spirochetes isolated from the blood of two patients with Lyme disease. *N Engl J Med* 1983; 308:740–742.

8. Steere AC, Grodzicki RL, Kornblatt AN, et al. The spirochete etiology of Lyme disease. *N Engl J Med* 1983; 308:733–740.

9. Pachner AR, Steere AC. The triad of neurological manifestations of Lyme disease. *Neurology* 1985; 35:47–53.

10. Asbrink E, Hederstedt B, Hovmark A. The spirochete etiology of acrodermatitis chronica atrophicans Herxheimer. *Acta Derm Venereol* 1984; 64:506–512.

11. Vallat JM, Hugon M, Lubeau M, et al. Tick bite meningoradiculoneuritis. *Neurology* 1987; 37:749–753.

12. Lyme disease-United States, 2001-2002. *Morb Mortal Wkly Rep* 2004; 53:365–369.

13. Gerber MA, Shapiro ED, Burke GS, et al. Pediatric Lyme Disease Study Group. Lyme disease in children in southeastern Connecticut. *N Engl J Med* 1996; 335:1270–1274.

14. Younger DS, Rosoklija G, Hays AP. Lyme polyradiculoneuritis. Immunohistochemical findings in sural nerve. *Muscle Nerve* 1995; 18:359–360.

15. Halperin JJ, Luft BJ, Volkman DJ, et al. Lyme neuroborreliosis-peripheral nervous system manifestations. *Brain* 1990; 113:1207–1221.

16. Halperin JJ. Facial nerve palsy associated with Lyme disease. *Muscle Nerve* 2003; 28:516–517.

17. Ackermann R, Rehse KB, Gollmer E, et al. Chronic neurologic manifestations of erythema migrans borreliosis. *Ann NY Acad Sci* 1988; 539:16–23.

18. Halperin JJ, Pass HL, Anand AK, et al. Nervous system abnormalities in Lyme disease. *Ann NY Acad Sci* 1988; 539:24–34.

19. Broderick JP, Sandok BA, Mertz LE. Focal encephalitis in a young woman 6 years after onset of Lyme disease. *Mayo Clin Proc* 1987; 62:313–316.

20. Younger DS, Orsher ST. Lyme neuroborreliosis: Preliminary results from an urban referral center employing strict CDC criteria for case selection. *Neurology Research International* 2010; Hindawi Publ Corp, Article ID 525206.

21. Centers for Disease Control and Prevention. Recommendations for test performance and interpretation from the Second National Conference on Serological Diagnosis of Lyme disease. MMWR *Morbidity and Mortality Weekly Rep* 1995; 44:590–591.

22. Dressler F, Whalen JA, Reinhardt BN, et al. Western blotting in the serodiagnosis of Lyme disease. *J Infect Dis* 1993; 167:392–400.

23. Dattwyler RJ, Volkman DJ, Luft BJ, et al. Seronegative Lyme disease. Dissociation of specific T- and B-lymphocyte responses to *Borrelia burgdorferi*. *N Engl J Med* 1988; 319:1441–1446.

24. Sindern E, Malin JP. Phenotypic analysis of cerebrospinal fluid over the course of Lyme meningoradiculitis. *Acta Cytol* 1995; 39:73–75.

25. Kieslich M, Fiedler A, Hernaiz Driever P, et al. *Brain and Development* 2000; 22:403–406.

26. Agosta F, Rocca MA, Beneditti B, et al. MR imaging assessment of brain and cervical cord damage in patients with neuroborreliosis. *AJNR* 2006; 27:892–894.

27. Rigotti DJ, Inglese M, Gonen O. Whole-brain N-acetylaspartate as a surrogate marker of neuonral damage in diffuse neurological disorders. *AJNR* 2007; 28:1843–1849.
28. Younger DS, Wu WE, Hardy C, et al. Lyme neuroborreliosis and proton MR spectroscopy: Preliminary results from an urban referral center employing strict CDC criteria for case selection [Abstract]. *Neurology* 2012; 78:ID 166864.
29. Logigian EI, Johnson KA, Kijewski MF, et al. Reversible cerebral hypoperfusion in Lyme encephalopathy. *Neurology* 1997; 49:1661–1670.
30. Samiya H, Kobayashi K, Mizukoshi C, et al. Brain perfusion SPECT in Lyme neuroborreliosis. *J Nucl Med* 1997; 38:1120–1122.
31. Fallon BA, Lipkin RB, Corbera KM, et al. Regional cerebral blood flow and metabolic rate in persistent Lyme encephalopathy. *Arch Gen Psychiatry* 2009; 66:554–563.
32. Fallon BA, Levin ES, Schweitzer PJ, et al. Inflammation and central nervous system Lyme disease. *Neurobiol Dis* 2010; 37:534–54.
33. Pachner AR, Delaney E, O'Neill T, et al. Inoculation of nonhuman primates with the N40 strain of *Borrelia burgdorfei* leads to a model of Lyme neuroborreliosis faithful to the human disease. *Neurology* 1995; 45:165–172.
34. Cadavid D, O'Neill T, Schaefer H, et al. Localization of *Borrelia burgdorferi* in the nervous system and other organs in a nonhuman primate model of Lyme disease. *Lab Invest* 2000; 80:1043–1054.
35. Ramesh G, Borda JT, Dufour J, et al. Interaction of the Lyme disease spirochete *Borrelia burgdorferi* with brain parenchyma elicits inflammatory mediators from glial cells as well as glial and neuronal apoptosis. *Am J Pathol* 2008; 173:1415–1427.
36. Ramesh G, Philipp MT. Pathogenesis of Lyme neuroborreliosis: mitogen-activated protein kinases Erk1, Erk2, and p38 in the response of astrocytes to Borrelia burgdorferi lipoproteins. *Neuroscience Letters* 2005; 384:112–116.
37. Bernardino ALF, Myers TA, Alvarez X, et al. Toll-like receptors: insights into their possible role in the pathogenesis of Lyme neuroborreliosis. *Infection and Immunity* 2008; 76:4385–4395.
38. Miklossy J, Kasas S, Zurn AD, et al. Persisting atypical and cystic forms of *Borrelia burgdorferi* and local inflammation in Lyme neuroborreliosis. *Journal Neuroinflammation* 2008; 5:40.
39. Karlsson M, Hovind HK, Svenungsson, et al. Cultivation and characterization of spirochetes from cerebrospinal fluid of patients with Lyme borreliosis. *J Clin Microbiol* 1990; 28:473–479.
40. Halperin JJ, Luft BJ, Anand AK, et al. Lyme neuroborreliosis: central nervous system manifestations. *Neurology* 1989; 39:753–759.
41. Benke T, Gasse T, Hittmair-Delazer M, et al. Lyme encephalopathy: long-term neuropsychological deficits after acute neuroborreliosis. *Acta Neurol Scand* 1995; 91:353–367.
42. Fallon BA, Keilp JG, Corbera KM, et al. A randomized, placebo-controlled trial of repeated IV antibiotic therapy for Lyme encephalopathy. *Neurology* 2008; 70:992–1003.
43. Krupp LB, Masur D, Schwartz J, et al. Cognitive functioning in late Lyme borreliosis. *Arch Neurol* 1991; 48:1125–1129.
44. Halperin JJ, Little BW, Coyle PK et al. Lyme disease: cause of a treatable peripheral neuropathy. *Neurology* 1987; 37:1700–1706.
45. Maimone D, Villanova M, Stanta G, et al. Detection of *Borrelia burgdorferi* DNA and complement membrane attack complex deposits in the sural nerve of a patient with chronic polyneuropathy and tertiary Lyme disease. *Muscle Nerve* 1997; 20:969–975.
46. Garcia-Monco JC, Seidman RJ, Benach JL. Experimental immunization with Borrelia burgdorferi induces development of antibodies to gangliosides. *Infection and Immunity* 1995; 63:4130–4137.
47. Rupprecht TA, Elstner M, Weil S, et al. Autoimmune-mediated polyneuropathy triggered by borrelial infection? *Muscle Nerve* 2008; 37:781–785.
48. Burman M, Nguten HL, Murthy V, et al. Severe orthostatic hypotension in a diabetic patient may not be due to diabetic autonomic neuropathy. *Clin Med* 2011; 3:290–291.
49. Magda P, Younger DS. Assessment for dysautonomia in patients with neurologic symptoms following LYMErix vaccination. *Neurology* 2007; 68:A295.
50. Magda P, Younger DS, Tanji K, et al. Painful small and large fiber and autonomic polyneuropathy after Connaught Lyme disease vaccination. *Neurology* 2008; 70:A40.
51. Halperin JJ, Shapiro ED, Logigian E, et al. Practice parameter: treatment of nervous system Lyme disease (an evidence-based review). Report of the Quality Standards Subcommittee of the American Academy of Neurology. *Neurology* 2007; 69:91–102.
52. Skoldenberg B, Stiernstedt G, Karlsson M, et al. Treatment of Lyme borreliosis with emphasis on neurological disease. *Ann NYU Acad Sci* 1988; 539:317–323.
53. Kohlepp W, Oschmann P, Mertens H, et al. Treatment of Lyme borreliosis. Randomized comparison of doxycycline and penicillin G. *J Neurol* 1989; 236:464–469.
54. Karlsson M, Hammers-Berggren S, Lindquist I, et al. Comparison of intravenous penicillin G ad oral doxycycline for treatment of Lyme neuroborreliosis. *Neurology* 1994; 44:1203–1207.
55. Borg R, Dotevall L, Hagberg L, et al. Intravenous ceftriaxone compared with oral doxycycline for the treatment of Lyme neuroborreliosis. *Scand J Infect Dis* 2005; 37:449–454.
56. Berglund J, Stjernberg L, Ornstein K, et al. 5-year Followup study of patients with neuroborreliosis. *Scand J Infect Dis* 2002; 34:421–425.
57. Wahlberg P, Granlund H, Nyman D, et al. Treatment of late Lyme borreliosis. *J Infect* 1994; 29:255–261.
58. Krbkova L, Stanek G. Therapy of Lyme borreliosis in children. *Infection* 1996; 24:170–173.
59. Thorstrand C, Belfrage F, Bennet R, et al. Successful treatment of neuroborreliosis with ten day regimens. *Pediatr Infect Dis J* 2002; 21:142–145.
60. Crisp D, Ashby P. Lyme radiculoneuritis treated with intravenous immunoglobulin. *Neurology* 1996; 46:1174–1175.

CHAPTER **34**

Motor Neuropathy and Monoclonal Gammopathy

Thomas H. Brannagan III, Norman Latov

Motor neuropathy is manifested by weakness, wasting, fasciculation, and normal sensations; thus, it resembles motor neuron disease (MND) clinically (1–3). It can be generalized or involve one or more individual nerves, with acute, subacute, or slowly progressive onset. Motor nerve axons are primarily affected, not the perikaryon. Motor neuropathy is often immunologically mediated and, in contrast to MND, may respond to immunosuppressive therapy.

Laboratory investigations can aid in the diagnosis of motor neuropathy and provide clues as to its etiology. Electrophysiologic studies often reveal conduction abnormalities, including conduction block. Serologic studies may reveal high titers of anti-GM1 or GD1a ganglioside autoantibodies, sometimes in association with an IgM paraprotein. This chapter reviews aspects of motor neuropathy due to monoclonal gammopathy.

CLINICAL FEATURES

Motor neuropathy begins at almost any age from the second to eighth decade, with a predilection for men. The neuropathy can be generalized or involve only one or several nerves, and is frequently asymmetric. The arms are more frequently involved than the legs (4, 5), and unlike MND, bulbar involvement and respiratory failure are rare (6, 7). It is usually slowly progressive, sometimes over 20 years or more (7, 8). Deep tendon reflexes (DTR) may be absent or hypoactive but are sometimes active in weak and wasted limbs (9-11); Babinski signs are never a feature of motor neuropathy, and myokymia rarely occurs (12, 13).

ELECTRODIAGNOSTIC STUDIES

Electrophysiological studies in both motor neuropathy and MND show reduced compound motor action potentials (CMAP) amplitudes, with fibrillation and fasciculation activity, and long-duration neurogenic motor unit potentials on needle electromyography (EMG) consistent with axonal degeneration and denervation. There may be associated demyelinating features that help distinguish it from MND, including slowing of motor nerve conduction velocities, prolongation of distal motor and F-wave latencies into a demyelinating range, with temporal dispersion, and motor conduction block (MCB). Some patients with motor neuropathy exhibit minimal conduction abnormalities in life and thus may be difficult to diagnose.

Multifocal demyelinating neuropathy with persistent conduction block (CB), first described electrophysiologically in 1982 by Lewis et al. (14) among several patients with chronic sensorimotor demyelinating polyneuropathy, was clinically characterized by mononeuritis multiplex (MNM) and electrophysiologically defined by persistent MCB. The latter was similarly detected in 1985 by Parry and Clark (15, 16) among several patients with a clinical MND syndrome, and normal sensory nerve conduction studies (NCS). Persistent MCB unequivocally identifies a patient with neuropathy, although its demonstration may be technically difficult. Paranodal and internodal demyelination, which increases the transverse capacitance and reduces the resistance at the internode, is associated with increased outward leakage current, prolonging the time that the internal longitudinal current must flow to generate an impulse at the next node of Ranvier. If the transverse current leakage is excessive, then insufficient current

583

will be available to depolarize the next node of Ranvier and impulse transmission may block (17, 18).

The demonstration of a drop in the CMAP amplitude from proximal to distal stimulation is insufficient in itself to conclude the presence of CB because similar findings can result from submaximal stimulation along sites where the nerve trunk is deep to the skin as occurs at Erb point (19). Interphase shift and cancellation of the negative phase of the motor unit action potential with the positive phase of another motor unit potential leads to a significant drop in amplitude, particularly with chronic partial denervation.

There is no definitive consensus as to the required amplitude or area loss for the block in multifocal motor neuropathy (MMN), with published figures ranging from 20 to 50% (4, 5, 13, 20–28). However, an amplitude loss of up to 41% and area loss of 29% can be seen in normal subjects (29). Computer modeling indicates that normal temporal dispersion in patients with chronic neurogenic disorders can result in a drop in amplitude of greater than 50%, but a drop in the area of greater than 50% is due to CB (30). The analysis of short nerve segments is most helpful in demonstrating CB because a gradual change in amplitude is also likely to be caused by temporal dispersion (31).

Motor CB may be verified by comparing the partially blocked CMAP with the surface-recorded potential obtained during maximal volitional effort. This is accomplished by triggering on the largest peak of the recruitment pattern during maximal effort (32). If the volitional summated potential is larger than the proximal CMAP, then true CB has not occurred and the reduced proximal amplitude may be due to submaximal stimulation.

Patients with motor neuropathies diagnosed by presence of CB and elevated titers of anti-GM1 antibodies frequently exhibit other conduction abnormalities. In nine patients with MCB, features of demyelination included temporal dispersion in five, slowed motor nerve conduction velocity (NCV) in seven, and prolonged distal motor latencies in four. All had prolonged F waves in at least one nerve (21). In a study of 16 patients with MMN including nine with elevated anti-GM1 antibodies and five with MCB, 15 patients had other features of demyelination including five with prolonged distal motor latencies, seven with abnormal temporal dispersion, eight with prolonged F waves not explained by distal slowing, and 13 with slow of NCV. In addition, eight patients had at least one nerve with pure axonal features with others meeting demyelinating criteria. The one patient that did not meet formal criteria for demyelinating neuropathy instead had a prolonged F-wave latency and a 31% drop in the median CMAP area across the forearm.

Two-thirds each of patients treated with intravenous immunoglobulin (IVIg), with or without CB, improved (33). Sensory NCS across the site of motor conduction block should have been normal (16, 26), but that would have required special techniques to prove isolated pure MCB was present (34, 35).

PATHOLOGIC STUDIES

Non-inflammatory demyelination was noted at the site of CB in two patients with anti-GM1 antibodies (36). Similar findings were noted in the peripheral nerves of other patients, although not at the site of CB (22, 37). Deposits of IgM at the nodes of Ranvier were observed in the sural nerve of a patient with MMN and anti-GM1 antibodies (23). However, other reported patients were normal (25, 38) or showed minimal abnormalities (38, 39).

While pathological specimens at the site of MCB may show signs of demyelination, they usually do not (36, 40). The mean regenerative cluster density of nerves from patients with motor neuropathy was $75.4/mm^2$ compared to a mean cluster density in MND of $13.6/mm^2$. The commonest finding that separates patients with motor neuropathy from MND is an increase in regenerative clusters. Whereas signs of demyelination, remyelination, and IgM, and complement deposition are noted in a minority of motor neuropathy biopsies, it is generally absent from those with MND (37, 41, 42).

There are limited postmortem examination data of patients with motor neuropathy. However, four patients (24, 43–45) with a lower motor neuron (LMN) syndrome resembling spinal muscular atrophy (SMA) included one with motor neuropathy and IgM monoclonal gammopathy without known CB or elevated GM1 antibody titers as reported by Rowland and coworkers (43), that had central chromatolysis of anterior horn cells (AHC) accompanied by severe loss of nerve fibers in the ventral roots. A second patient with motor neuropathy and IgM polyclonal gammopathy was found to have endoneurial perivascular lymphocytic infiltration (44). A third patient with elevated anti-GM1 antibodies revealed immunoglobulin deposits on myelin sheaths and predominant involvement of the anterior roots highlighting the lack of correlation between distal CB and the distribution or severity of weakness (24). A fourth patient with motor neuropathy and absent anti-GM1 antibodies or CB instead had perineurial perivascular mononuclear inflammation of peripheral motor nerves (45).

The differentiation of motor neuropathy and MND can be challenging even after extensive evaluation as clinical features that distinguish motor neuropathy from MND include multifocal or asymmetric involvement and a prolonged time course. Moreover, electrophysiology may show persistent multifocal MCB (16), other features of demyelination (21, 33), and high titers of anti-GM1 and anti-GD1a antibodies often seen in motor neuropathy are rarely found in MND (11, 46).

Although motor neuropathy can be difficult to distinguish from motor forms of CIDP, both may respond to immunotherapy (47, 48). Unlike CIDP, motor NCV in motor neuropathy are typically normal between regions of CB as are sensory NCS, and cerebrospinal fluid (CSF) protein levels are not commonly elevated. Corticosteroids and plasmapheresis, frequently helpful in CIDP, are not in MMN (49–52).

MOTOR NEUROPATHY AND MONOCLONAL GAMMOPATHY

Monoclonal gammopathy results from the abnormal proliferation of monoclonal B-cells that secrete excessive IgM, IgG, or IgA antibodies (53), detected by serum protein immunoelectrophoresis (SPEP) as M-proteins or paraproteins, or more fully characterized by immunofixation electrophoresis (IFE). While they may be autoreactive and cause autoimmune disease, up to 1% of normal adults can have serum M-proteins and monoclonal gammopathy that may be coincidental and unrelated to motor neuropathy.

With an estimated incidence of IgM monoclonal gammopathy in peripheral neuropathy of 5 to 50% (54–57), the monoclonal gammopathy is typically non-malignant, and the M-proteins display autoantibody activity reactive with oligosaccharide determinants of glycolipids, glycoproteins, or glycoconjugates concentrated in peripheral nerve. There may be associated Waldenström macroglobulinemia, B-cell lymphoma, or chronic lymphocytic leukemia.

Structure of Glycolipids

Glycosphingolipids are composed of the long-chain aliphatic amine sphingosine, and an acylated ceramid attached to one or more sugars. Gangliosides are complex glycosphingolipids containing sialic acid, the latter of which is a generic term for N-acylneuraminic acid. Gangliosides are designated G for ganglioside followed by M, D, T, or Q for mono, di, tri, or quad, respectively, referring to the number of sialic acids. Arabic numbers and lowercase letters follow and refer to the sequence of migration by thin-later chromatography (58, 59).

IgM Monoclonal Gammopathy

In 1968, Peters and Clatanoff (60) described a patient with SMA and IgM monoclonal gammopathy who improved upon treatment with chlorambucil. However, the patient probably had a motor neuropathy rather than MND. The first documented patient with motor neuropathy and IgM monoclonal gammopathy was reported by Rowland and colleagues in 1982 (43). That patient presented with progressive weakness, wasting, and fasciculation, and had an IgM-κ monoclonal gammopathy. Motor NCS showed slow velocities, however sensory NCS were normal.

Motor Neuropathy and Anti-GM1 Antibodies

In 1986, Freddo and colleagues (61) described a patient with SMA clinically, anti-GM1 antibodies, and IgM monoclonal gammopathy. A second similar patient improved with intravenous cyclophosphamide therapy (62). In 1988, Pestronk and coworkers (20) demonstrated high titers of IgM anti-GM1 antibodies in patients with MMN and MCB. In 1990, Yuki and colleagues (63) reported IgG anti-GM1 antibodies in patients with the Guillain-Barré syndrome (GBS) variant of acute motor axonal neuropathy (AMAN). With an estimated frequency of increased titers of IgM anti-GM1 antibody in patients with MMN ranging from 18 to 84% (11, 64), they are most often polyclonal although some are monoclonal, and the total serum IgM concentration is generally increased.

In a review of 14 patients chosen for the presence of highly elevated anti-GM1 antibody titers, five had a single site of CB, four had MCV, one had diffusely slowed motor NCV, and the remainder had normal motor NCS. In most patients, the anti-GM1 antibodies recognize the Gal(B1-3) GalNAc determinant shared by asialo-GM1 (aGM1) and the ganglioside GDLB. The same determinant is also present on some glycoproteins and is recognized by the lectin peanut agglutinin. Some of the antibodies, however, are highly specific for GM1 or recognize internal determinants shared by GM2 (65–68). Although GM1 and other Gal(B1-3)Gal-NAc-bearing glycoconjugates are highly concentrated and widely distributed in the central and peripheral nervous systems, they are generally cryptic and unavailable to the antibodies. Anti-GM1 antibodies bind to spinal cord gray matter and to GM1 on the surface of isolated bovine spinal motor neurons, but not to dorsal root ganglia (DRG) neurons (69). In peripheral nerve, GM1 ganglioside and Gal(B1-3)GalNAc–bearing glycoproteins are expressed at the nodes of Ranvier (70, 71). Two glycoproteins were identified as the oligodendroglial-myelin glycoprotein in paranodal myelin and a versican-like glycoprotein in the nodal gap (72). The antibodies also bind to the presynaptic terminals at the motor end-plate in skeletal muscle, where they might also exert an effect (62, 73).

It is not known whether the anti-GM1 antibodies cause or contribute to the disease or whether they are only an associated abnormality. The binding to motor but not sensory neurons correlates with the clinical syndrome. GM1 is highly enriched in myelin sheaths of motor nerves and differs in its ceramides in comparison with sensory nerves (74, 75). This might render the anterior roots more susceptible to the autoantibody effects. In one study, rabbits immunized with GM1 or Gal(1-3)GalNAc-BSA developed conduction abnormalities with immunoglobulin deposits at the nodes of Ranvier (76), as did sera from a patient with increased titers of anti-GM1 antibodies and IgM deposits at the nodes of Ranvier that produced demyelination and CB after injection into rat sciatic nerve (77). Human anti-GM1 antibodies bind to, and kill, mammalian spinal motor neurons in culture (78) and at the motor end-plate (79). Sera from patients with MMN, with and without anti-GM1 antibodies, block nerve conduction in the mouse phrenic nerve-diaphragm preparation (80). Anti-GM1 antibodies alter potassium current and, in the presence of complement, block sodium channels in rat myelinated nerve fibers (81). Based on the persistence of the MCB and the pathologic findings of axons devoid of myelin and only minimal onion bulbs, Kaji and colleagues (82) suggested that anti-GM1 antibodies impaired remyelination. The variable regions of anti-GM1 antibodies from normal individuals and patients with neuropathy that exhibit multiple somatic mutations in their hypervariable regions suggests initial derivation from a process of antigenic stimulation (83, 84).

Immune reactivity to gangliosides is associated with neuropathy in experimental animals (85). However, alone, anti-ganglioside antibodies may not be sufficient to cause the neuropathy as T-cell reactivity or breakdown of the blood-nerve barrier may be necessary for their pathogenicity (86, 87). In contrast to the IgM anti-GM1 antibodies of patients with chronic motor neuropathies, increased titers of polyclonal IgG and IgA anti-GM1 antibodies are associated with AMAN and occur after infection with *Campylobacter jejuni* (*C. jejuni*) (63, 88–91), which bears GM1-like oligosaccharides (92-94), or after parenteral injection of GM1-containing gangliosides (95–98). Postmortem studies in patients with Guillain-Barré syndrome (GBS) who died after *C. jejuni* infection showed non-inflammatory degeneration of the anterior roots and chromatolytic changes in spinal motor neurons (90) similar to the chronic disease associated with IgM anti-GM1 antibodies.

IgM Anti-GD1a Autoantibodies

Several patients with motor neuropathy and anti-GD1a antibodies have been described (99, 100). The first patient (99) was a 73-year-old man with three years of leg weakness, IgM-κ monoclonal gammopathy, and absent leg and reduced arm DTR. Cerebrospinal fluid (CSF) examination was normal, and NCV were slow. He did not progress while receiving two years of melphalan and corticosteroids (99). Two other patients (100) had high titers of anti-GD1a IgM antibodies, including a 66-year-old woman with eight months of progressive weakness and wasting in distal muscles of the arms and legs; and a 63-year-old woman with six months of asymmetric weakness who was unable to walk

or use her arms. Sensation was normal in both, and DTR were absent with the exception of reduced ankle DTR in the second patients. Cerebrospinal fluid analysis revealed one to three white blood cells, (WBC)/mm³, and a total protein level of 60 to 78 mg/dL. The amplitudes of CMAP and motor NCV were reduced in the latter patient to the demyelinating range. While some sensory responses were abnormal in the first patient, the same parameters were normal in the other patients. The first patient responded to IVIg and oral cyclophosphamide, and there was slight definite improvement with prednisone leading to the ability to stand and walk with a cane. The other patient improved with IVIg and rapidly deteriorated later despite prednisone and plasma exchange, however, reinstitution of IVIg and oral cyclophosphamide led to ultimate improvement. In both patients with IgG anti-GD1a antibodies and GBS so treated (100), clinical improvement was accompanied by a corresponding decline in anti-GD1a titers (100).

IgG and IA Monoclonal Gammopathy

Patients with motor neuropathies and non-malignant IgA monoclonal gammopathy have also been described (101, 102), including several with IgA monoclonal gammopathy (103–105). One patient had motor neuropathy with an IgG-κ paraprotein and the Crow-Fukase syndrome of gynecomastia, hypertrichosis, leg edema, impotence, and raised CSF protein content (106). It is not known whether the monoclonal gammopathy in these patients was coincidental or related to the neuropathy.

TREATMENT

The treatment of choice for motor neuropathy is IVIg, which has been shown to be effective in placebo-controlled trials (4, 107–109). A favorable response to IVIg was noted in 67 to 100% of patients (110, 111), including reduction in the degree of CB and increase in the CMAP amplitude (21), however the effect was transient, and prolonged therapy was often required. Sustained remission lasting up to four years was reported with and without therapy (110, 112). Patients occasionally have diminished responses to prolonged treatment (110, 113), and among patients with motor neuropathy and anti-GM1 antibodies, those with CB had the best response to IVIg (4) while anti-GM1 antibodies and MMN was associated with a more favorable therapeutic response (110). Patients without anti-GMI antibodies or CB similarly respond to IVIg (33, 37).

The mode of action of IVIg in motor neuropathy is probably multifactorial. Although titers of anti-GM1 antibodies remain unchanged after IVIg treatment, it probably exerts anti-idiotypic activity (114, 115), blocks Fc-receptor-mediated recruitment of macrophages, and inhibits complement activation and the action of various cytokines, as suggested in other autoimmune diseases (116–118). Patients in remission status with MMN after treatment with IVIg were successfully switched to maintenance therapy with subcutaneous Ig (119, 120), which assuming equal efficacy, has the advantage of ease of administration, flexibility, and improved tolerability.

Motor neuropathy is also responsive to the chemotherapeutic agent chlorambucil (62), cyclophosphamide (20, 34, 49) and fludarabine (121), both of which lower autoantibody titers and serum IgM concentrations with less dependency on IVIg. Rituximab, a monoclonal antibody against the

B-cell marker CD20 (122–125) is effective in some patients, including those with a suboptimal response to IVIg (125, 126). While studies of beta-interferon for MMN have been promising (126–128), corticosteroids, oral cyclophosphamide, and plasmapheresis (6, 36) were generally ineffective and treatment with corticosteroids and plasmapheresis were associated with disease exacerbations (49–52).

Rare patients with motor neuropathy without NCS abnormalities suggesting demyelination also responded to immunotherapy with chlorambucil (62); plasmapheresis followed by cyclophosphamide (129); IVIg (130, 131), and plasmapheresis, dexamethasone or cyclophosphamide (44).

REFERENCES

1. Rossi O. La neurite sistematizzata motrice. *Rassegna Clin Sci* 1928; VI: 3–7.

2. Hyland HH, Russell WR. Chronic progressive polyneuritis, with report of a fatal case. *Brain* 1930; 53:278–289.

3. Wilson SAK. Motor neuritis. In: AN Bruce, ed. *Neurology*. Baltimore: Williams & Wilkins, 1940; 305–307.

4. Azulay JP, Blin O, Pought J, et al. Intravenous immunoglobulin treatment in patients with motor neuron syndromes associated with anti-GM1 antibodies: a double-blind, placebo-controlled study. *Neurology* 1994; 44:429–432.

5. Lange DJ, Trojaborg W, Latov N, et al. Multifocal motor neuropathy with conduction block. is it a distinct clinical entity? *Neurology* 1992; 42:497–505.

6. Kaji R, Shibasaki H, Kimura J. Multifocal demyelinating motor neuropathy: cranial nerve involvement and immunoglobulin therapy. *Neurology* 1992; 42:506–509.

7. Magistris M, Roth G. Motor neuropathy with multifocal persistent conduction blocks [Letter]. *Muscle Nerve* 1992; 9:1056–1057.

8. Parry GJG. Motor neuropathy with multifocal persistent conduction blocks [reply]. *Muscle Nerve* 1992; 1057.

9. Evangelista T, Carvalho M, Conceicao I, et al. Motor neuropathies mimicking amyotrophic lateral sclerosis/motor neuron disease. *J Neurol Sci* 1996; 139:95–98.

10. Kaji R, Mezaki T, Hirota N, et al. Multifocal motor neuropathy with exaggerated deep tendon reflexes. *Neurology* 1994; 44:A180 (Abstract).

11. Kinsella LJ, Lange DJ, Trojaborg W, et al. Clinical and electrophysiologic correlates of elevated anti-GM1 antibody titers. *Neurology* 1994; 44:1278–1282.

12. Roth G, Rohr J, Magistric MR, Ochsner F. Motor neuropathy with proximal multifocal persistent conduction block, fasciculations, and myokymia. Evolution to tetraplegia. *Eur Neurol* 1986; 25:416–423.

13. Bouche P, Moulonguet A, Younes-Chennoufi AB, et al. Multifocal motor neuropathy with conduction block: a study of 24 patients. *J Neurol Neurosurg Psychiatry* 1995; 59:38–44.

14. Lewis RA, Sumner AJ, Brown MJ, Asbury AK. Multifocal demyelinating neuropathy with persistent conduction block. *Neurology* 1982; 32:958–964.

15. Parry GJ, Clarke S. Pure motor neuropathy with multifocal conduction block masquerading as motor neuron disease. *Muscle Nerve* 1985; 8:617 (abstract).

16. Parry GJ, Clarke S. Multifocal acquired demyelinating neuropathy masquerading as motor neuron disease. *Muscle Nerve* 1988; 11:103–107.

17. Brown WF. Acute and chronic inflammatory demyelinating neuropathies. In: Brown WF, Bolton CF, Eds. *Clinical electromyography*, 2nd ed. Boston: Butterworth Heinemann, 1993.

18. Koles ZJ, Rasminsky M. A computer simulation of conduction in demyelinated nerve fibers. *J Physiol* 1972; 227:351–364.

19. Cornblath DR, Sumner AJ. Conduction block in neuropathies with necrotizing vasculitis. *Muscle Nerve* 1991; 2:185–186.

20. Pestronk A, Cornblath DR, Ilyas AA, et al. A treatable multifocal motor neuropathy with antibodies to GM1 ganglioside. *Ann Neurol* 1988; 24:73–73.

21. Chaudhry V, Corse AM, Cornblath DR, et al. Multifocal motor neuropathy: electrodiagnostic features. *Muscle Nerve* 1994; 17:198–205.

22. Auer RN, Bell RB, Lee MA. Neuropathy with onion bulb formations and pure motor manifestations. *Can J Neurol Sci* 1989; 16:194–197.

23. Santoro M, Thomas FP, Fink ME, et al. IgM deposits at nodes of Ranvier in a patient with amyotrophic lateral sclerosis, anti-GM1 antibodies, and multifocal motor conduction block. *Ann Neurol* 1990; 28:273–377.

24. Adams D, Kuntzer T, Steck AJ, et al. Motor conduction block and high titers of anti-GM1 ganglioside antibodies: pathological evidence of a motor neuropathy in a patient with lower motor neuron syndrome. *J Neurol Neurosurg Psychiatry* 1993; 56:982–987.

25. Van Den Bergh P, Logigian EL, Kelly JJ. Motor neuropathy with multifocal conduction blocks. *Muscle Nerve* 1989; 12:26–31.

26. Krarup C, Stewart JD, Sumner AJ, et al. A syndrome of asymmetrical limb weakness and motor conduction block. *Neurology* 1990; 40:118–127.

27. Olney RK, Lewis RA, Putnam TD, et al. American Association of Electrodiagnostic Medicine. Consensus criteria for the diagnosis of multifocal motor neuropathy. *Muscle Nerve* 2003; 27:117–121.

28. Cappellari A, NobileOrazio E, Meucci N, et al. Criteria for early detection of conduction block in multifocal motor neuropathy (MMN): a study based on control populations and follow-up of MMN patients. *J Neurol* 1997; 244:625–630.

29. Oh SJ, Kim DE, Kuruoglu HR. What is the best diagnostic index of conduction block and temporal dispersion. *Muscle Nerve* 1994; 17:489–4983.

30. Rhee EK, England JD, Sumner AJ. A computer simulation of conduction block: effects produced by actual block versus interphase cancellation. *Ann Neurol* 1990; 28:146–156.

31. Cornblath DR, Sumner AJ, Daube J, et al. Conduction block in clinical practice. *Muscle Nerve* 1991; 14:869–871.

32. Lange DJ, Trojaborg W, McDonald TD, et al. Persistent and transient conduction block in motor neuron diseases. *Muscle Nerve* 1993; 16:896–903.

33. Katz JS, Wolfe GI, Bryan WW, et al. Electrophysiologic findings in multifocal motor neuropathy. *Neurology* 1997; 48:700–707.

34. Krarup C, Sethi RK. Idiopathic brachial plexus lesion with conduction block of the ulnar nerve. *Electroencephalogr Clin Neurophysiol* 1989; 72:259–267.

35. Parry GJG. Motor Neuropathy with multifocal conduction block. In, Dyck PJ, Thomas PK, et al, eds. *Peripheral neuropathy*, 3rd ed. Philadelphia: WB Saunders, 1993; 1343–1353.

36. Kaji R, Oka N, Tsuji T, et al. Pathological findings at the site of conduction block in multifocal motor neuropathy. *Ann Neurol* 1993; 33:152–158.

37. Corbo M, Abouzahr MK, Latov N, et al. Motor nerve biopsy studies in motor neuropathy and motor neuron disease. *Muscle Nerve* 1997; 20:15–21.

38. Hays AP. Separation of Motor Neuron diseases from pure motor neuropathies: pathology. In: Rowland LP, ed. *Amyotrophic lateral sclerosis and other motor neuron diseases*. New York: Raven Press, 1991; 385–398.

39. Corse AM, Chaudry V, Crawford TO, et al. Sensory nerve pathology in multifocal motor neuropathy. *Ann Neurol* 1996; 3:319–325.

40. Taylor BV. Dyck PJ. Engelstad J. et al. Multifocal motor neuropathy: pathologic alterations at the site of conduction block. *J Neuropathol Exp Neurol* 2004; 63:129–37.

41. Riva N, Iannaccone S, Corbo M et al. Motor nerve biopsy: clinical usefulness and histopathological criteria. *Ann Neurol* 2011; 69:197–201.

42. Riva N, Gallia F, Iannaccone S et al. Chronic motor axonal neuropathy. *J Periph Nerv Sys* 2011; 16:341–346.

43. Rowland LP, Defendini R, Sherman W, et al. Macroglobulinemia with peripheral neuropathy simulating motor neuron disease. *Ann Neurol* 1982; 11:532–536.

44. Parry GJ, Holtz SJ, Ben-Zeev D, et al. Gammopathy with proximal motor axonopathy simulating motor neuron disease. *Neurology* 1986; 36:273–276.

45. Ropper AH, Gorson KC. Autopsy of chronic inflammatory axonal motor radiculoneuropathy resembling motor neuron disease. *Neurology* 1997; 48:A226(abstract).

46. Taylor BV, Gross L, Windebank AJ. The sensitivity and specificity of anti-GM1 antibody testing. *Neurology* 1996; 47:951–955.

47. Krendal DA. Biopsy findings link multifocal motor neuropathy to chronic inflammatory demyelinating polyneuropathy. *Ann Neurol* 1996; 40:948–950 (Letter).

48. Brannagan TH III. Current treatments of chronic immune-mediated demyelinating neuropathies. *Muscle Nerve* 2009; 39:363–378.

49. Feldman EL, Bromberg MB, Albers JW, et al. A. Immunosuppressive treatment in multifocal motor neuropathy. *Ann Neurol* 1991; 30:397–401.

50. Donaghy M, Mills KR, Boniface SJ, et al. Pure motor demyelinating neuropathy: deterioration after steroid treatment and improvement with intravenous immunoglobulin. *J Neurol Neurosurg Psychiatry* 1994; 57:778–783.

51. Thomas PK, Claus DJ, Workman JM, et al. Focal upper limb demyelinating neuropathy. *Brain* 1996; 119:765–774.

52. Carpo M, Cappellari A, Mora G, et al. Deterioration of multifocal motor neuropathy after plasma exchange. *Neurology* 1998; 50:1480–1482.

53. Latov N. Pathogenesis and therapy of neuropathies associated with monoclonal gammopathies. *Ann Neurol* 1995; 37:S32–S42.

54. Logothetis J, Silverstein P, Coe J. Neurological aspects of Waldenström's macroglobulinemia. *Arch Neurol* 1960; 3:564–573.

55. Harbs H, Arfmann M, Frick E, et al. Reactivity of sera and isolated monoclonal IgM from patients with Waldenström's macroglobulinemia with peripheral nerve myelin. *J Neurol* 1985; 232:43–48.

56. Kyle RA, Garton JP. The spectrum of IgM monoclonal gammopathy in 430 cases. *Mayo Clin Proc* 1987; 62:719–731.

57. Nobile-Orazio E, Marmiroli P, Baldini L, et al. Peripheral neuropathy in macroglobulinemia: incidence and antigen specificity of M-proteins. *Neurology* 1987; 37:1506–1514.

58. Svennerholm L. Designation and schematic structure of gangliosides and allied glycosphingolipids. *Progr Brain Res* 1994; 101:11–14.

59. Willison HJ. Antiglycolipid antibodies in peripheral neuropathy: fact or fiction? *J Neurol Neurosurg Psychiatry* 1994; 57:1303–1307.

60. Peters HA, Clatanoff DV. Spinal muscular atrophy secondary to macroglobulinemia: reversal of symptoms with chlorambucil therapy. *Neurology* 1968; 18:101–108.

61. Freddo L, Yu RK, Latov N, et al. Gangliosides GM1 and Gd1b are antigens for IgM M-protein in a patient with motor neuron disease. *Neurology* 1986; 36:454–458.

62. Latov N, Hays AP, Donofrio PD, et al. Monoclonal IgM with a unique specificity to gangliosides GM1 and GD1b and to lacto-N-tetraose associated with human motor neuron disease. *Neurology* 1988; 33:763–768.

63. Yuki N, Yoshino H, Sato S, et al. Acute axonal polyneuropathy associated with anti-GM1 antibodies following Campylobacter enteritis. *Neurology* 1990; 40:1900–1902.

64. Carpo M, Allaria S, Scarlato G, Nobile-Orazio E. Marginally improved detection of GM1 antibodies by Covalink ELISA in multifocal motor neuropathy. *Neurology* 1999; 53:2207–2207.

65. Ilyas AA, Willison HJ, Dalakas M, Whitaker JN, Quarles RH. Identification and characterization of gangliosides reacting with IgM paraproteins in three patients with neuropathy and biclonal gammopathy. *J Neurochem* 1988; 51:851–858.

66. Kusunoki S, Shimizu T, Matsumura K, Maemura K, Mannen T. Motor dominant neuropathy and IgM paraproteinemia: the IgM M-protein binds to specific gangliosides. *J Neuroimmunol* 1989; 21:177–181.

67. Baba H, Daune GC, Ilyas AA, et al. Anti-GM1 ganglioside antibodies with differing specificities in patients with multifocal motor neuropathy. *J Neuroimmunol* 1989; 25:143–150.

68. Sadiq SA, Thomas FP, Kilidireas K, et al. The spectrum of neurological disease associated with anti-GM1 antibodies. *Neurology* 1990; 40:1067–1072.

69. Corbo M, Quattrini A, Lugaresi A, et al. Patterns of reactivity of human anti-GM1 antibodies with spinal cord and motor neurons. *Ann Neurol* 1992; 32:487–493.

70. Corbo M, Quattrini A, Latov N, Hays AP. Localization of GM1 and Gal(B1-3)GalNAc antigenic determinants in peripheral nerve. *Neurology* 1993; 43:809–816.

71. Sheikh KA, Deerinck TJ, Ellisman MH, et al. The distribution of ganglioside-like moieties in peripheral nerves. *Brain* 1999; 122:449–460.

72. Apostolski S, Sadiq SA, Hays A, et al. Identification of Gal(B1-3)GalNAc bearing glycoproteins at the nodes of Ranvier in peripheral nerve. *J Neurosci Res* 1994; 38:134–141.

73. Thomas FP, Adapon PH, Goldberg GP, et al. Localization of neural epitopes that bind to IgM monoclonal autoantibodies (M-proteins) from two patients with motor neuron disease. *J Neuroimmunol* 1989; 21:31–39.

74. Ogawa-Goto K, Funamoto N, Abe T, Nagashima K. Different

ceramide compositions of gangliosides between human motor and sensory nerves. *J Neurochem* 1990; 55:1486–1492.

75. Ogawa-Goto K, Funamoto N, Ohta Y, et al. Myelin gangliosides of human peripheral nervous system: an enrichment of GM1 in the motor nerve myelin isolated from cauda equina. *J Neurochem* 1992; 59:1844–1848.

76. Thomas FP, Trojaborg W, Nagy C, et al. Experimental autoimmune neuropathy with anti-GM1 antibodies and immunoglobulin deposits at the nodes of Ranvier. *Acta Neuropathol* 1991; 82:278–383.

77. Santoro M, Uncini A, Corbo M, et al. Experimental conduction block induced by serum from a patient with anti-GM1 antibodies. *Ann Neurol* 1992; 31:385–390.

78. Heiman-Patterson T, Krupa T, Thompson P, et al. Anti-GM1/GDLB M-proteins damage human spinal cord neurons cocultured with muscle. *J Neurol Sci* 1991; 30:38–45.

79. Willison HJ, Roberts M, O'Hanlon G, et al. Human monoclonal anti-GM1 ganglioside antibodies interfere with neuromuscular transmission. *Ann Neurol* 1994; 36:289.

80. Roberts M, Willison HJ, Vincent A, Newsom-Davis J. Multifocal motor neuropathy human sera block distal motor nerve conduction in mice. *Ann Neurol* 1995; 38:111–118.

81. Takigawa T, Yasuda H, Kikkawa R, et al. Antibodies against GM1 ganglioside affect K+ and Na+ currents in isolated rat myelinated nerve fibers. *Ann Neurol* 1995; 37:436–442.

82. Kaji R, Hirota N, Oka N, et al. Anti-GM1 antibodies and impaired blood-nerve barrier may interfere with remyelination in multifocal motor neuropathy. *Muscle Nerve* 1994; 17:108–110.

83. Weng NP, Yu-Lee LY, Sanz I, et al. Structure and specificities of anti-ganglioside autoantibodies associated with motor neuropathies. *J Immunol* 1992; 149:2518–2529.

84. Marcus DM, Went N. The structure of human anti ganglioside antibodies. *Progr Brain Res* 1994; 101:289–293.

85. Susuki K, Nishimoto Y, Yamada M, et al. Acute motor axonal neuropathy rabbit model: immune attack on nerve root axons. *Ann Neurol* 2003; 54:383–388.

86. Lee G, Jeong Y, Wirguin I, et al. Induction of human IgM anti-GM1 antibodies in transgenic mice in response to lipopolysaccharide from Campylobacter jejuni. *J Neuroimmunol* 2004; 146:63–75.

87. Sheikh KA, Zhang G, Gong Y, et al. An anti-ganglioside antibody-secreting hybridoma induces neuropathy in mice. *Ann Neurol* 2004; 56:228–239.

88. Walsh FS, Cronin M, Koblar S, et al. Association between glycoconjugate antibodies and Campylobacter infection in patients with Guillain-Barré syndrome. *J Neuroimmunol* 1991; 34:43–51.

89. Van den Berg LH, Marrink J, de Jager AEJ, et al. Anti-GM1 antibodies in patients with Guillain-Barré syndrome. *J Neurol Neurosurg Psychiatry* 1992; 55:6–11.

90. McKhann GM, Cornblath DR, Griffin JW, et al. Acute motor axonal neuropathy: a frequent cause of acute flaccid paralysis in China. *Ann Neurol* 1993; 33:333–342.

91. Kornberg A, Pestronk A, Bieser K, et al. The clinical correlates of high-titer IgG anti-GM1 antibodies. *Ann Neurol* 1994; 35:234–237.

92. Aspinall GO, McDonald AG, Raju TS, et al. Serological diversity and chemical structure of Campylobacter jejuni low-molecular weight lipopolysaccharides. *J Bacteriol* 1992; 174:1324–1332.

93. Yuki N, Handa S, Taki T, et al. Cross-reactive antigen between nervous tissue and bacterium elicits Guillain-Barré syndrome: molecular mimicry between ganglioside GM1 and lipopolysaccharide from Penner's serotype 19 of Campylobacter jejuni. *Biomed Res* 1992; 13:451–453.

94. Wirguin I, Suturkova-Milosevic LJ, Della-Latta P, et al. Monoclonal IgM antibodies to GM1 and asialo-GM1 in chronic neuropathies cross-react with Campylobacter jejuni lipopolysaccharides. *Ann Neurol* 1994; 35:698–703.

95. Latov N, Koski CL, Walicke PA. Guillain-Barré syndrome and parenteral gangliosides [letter]. *Lancet* 1991; 338:757.

96. Nobile-Orazio E, Carpo M, Meucci N, et al. Guillain-Barré syndrome associated with high titers of anti-GM1 antibodies. *J Neurol Sci* 1992; 109:200–206.

97. Landi G, D Alessandro R, Dossi BC, et al. Guillain-Barré syndrome after exogenous gangliosides in Italy. *BMJ* 1993; 307:1463–1464.

98. Illa I, Ortiz N, Gallard E, et al. Acute axonal Guillain-Barré syndrome with Ig antibodies against motor axons following parenteral gangliosides. *Ann Neurol* 1995; 38:218–224.

99. Bollensen E, Schipper HI, Steck AJ, et al. Motor neuropathy with activity of monoclonal IgM antibody to GD1a ganglioside. *J Neurol* 1989; 236:353–355.

100. Carpo M, Nobile-Orazio E, Neucci N, et al. Anti-GD1a ganglioside antibodies in peripheral motor syndromes. *Ann Neurol* 1996; 39:539–543.

101. Yeung KB, Thomas PK, King RHM, et al. The clinical spectrum of peripheral neuropathies associated with benign monoclonal IgM, IgG, IgA paraproteinaemia. Comparative clinical, immunological and nerve biopsy findings. *J Neurol* 1991; 238:383–391.

102. Chazot G, Berger B, Carrier H, et al. Manifestations neurologiques des gammapathies monoclonales. *Rev Neurol* 1976; 132:195–212.

103. Bosch EP, Ansbacher LE, Goeken JA, et al. Peripheral neuropathy associated with monoclonal gammopathy. Studies of intraneural injections of monoclonal immunoglobulin sera. *J Neuropathol Exp Neurol* 1982; 41:446–459.

104. Nemni R, Mamoli A, Fazio R, et al. Polyneuropathy associated with IgA monoclonal gammopathy: a hypothesis of its pathogenesis. *Acta Neuropathol* 1991; 81:371–376.

105. Hemachudha T, Phanuphak P, Phanthumchinda K, et al. Proximal motor neuropathy, IgA paraproteinaemia and anti-myelin-associated glycoprotein reactivity. *Postgrad Med J* 1989; 65:662–664.

106. Berkovic SF, Scarlett JD, Symington GR, et al. Proximal motor neuropathy, dermato-endocrine syndrome, and IgGk paraproteinemia. *Arch Neurol* 1986; 43:845–848.

107. Van den Berg LH, Kerkhoff H, Oey PL, et al. Treatment of multifocal motor neuropathy with high dose intravenous immunoglobulins: a double blind, placebo controlled study. *J Neurol Neurosurg Psychiatry* 1995; 59:248–252.

108. Federico P, Zochodne DW, Hahn AF, et al. Multifocal motor neuropathy improved by IVIg—Randomized, double-blind, placebo-controlled study. *Neurology* 2000; 55:1256–1262.

109. Leger JM, Chassande B, Musset L, et al. Intravenous immunoglobulin therapy in multifocal motor neuropathy: A double-blind, placebo-controlled study. *Brain* 2001; 124:145–153.

110. Azulay J, Rihet P, Pouget J, et al. Long term follow up of multifocal motor neuropathy with conduction block under treatment. *J Neurol Neurosurg Psychiatry* 1997; 62:391–394.

111. Chaudhry V, Corse AM, Cornblath DR, et al. Multifocal motor neuropathy: Response to human immune globulin. *Ann Neurol* 1993; 33:237–242.

112. Chad DA, Hammer K, Sargent J. Slow resolution of multifocal weakness and fasciculation: a reversible motor neuron syndrome. *Neurology* 1986; 36:1260–1263.

113. Elliott JL, Pestronk A. Progression of multifocal motor neuropathy during apparently successful treatment with human immunoglobulin. *Neurology* 1994; 44:967–968.

114. Yuki N, Miyagi F. Possible mechanism of intravenous

immunoglobulin treatment on anti-GM1 antibody-mediated neuropathies. *J Neurol Sci* 1996; 139:160–162.

115. Mali U, Oleksowicz L, Latov N, et al. Intravenous g-globulin inhibits binding of anti-GM1 to its target antigen. *Ann Neurol* 1996; 39:136–139.

116. Kurlander RJ. Reversible and irreversible loss of Fc receptor function of human monocytes as a consequence of interaction with immunoglobulin G. *J Clin Invest* 1980; 66:776–781.

117. Basta M, Dalakas MC. High-dose intravenous immunoglobulin exerts its beneficial effect in patients with dermatomyositis by blocking endomysial depostition of activated complement fragments. *J Clin Invest* 1994; 94:1729–1735.

118. Abe Y, Horiuchi A, Miyake M, et al. Anti-cytokine nature of natural human immunoglobulin; one possible mechanism of the clinical effect of intravenous immunoglobulin therapy. *Immunol Rev* 1994; 139:5–19.

119. Eftimov F, Vermeulen M, de Haan RJ, et al. Subcutaneous immunoglobulin therapy for multifocal motor neuropathy. *J Peripher Nerv Syst* 2009; 14:93–100.

120. Harbo T, Andersen H, Jakobsen J. Long-term therapy with high doses of subcutaneous immunoglobulin in multifocal motor neuropathy. *Neurology* 2010; 75:1377–80.

121. Sherman WH, Latov N, Lange D, et al. Fludarabine for IgM antibody mediated neuropathies. *Ann Neurol* 1994; 36:326.

122. Levine TD, Pestronk A. IgM antibody-related polyneuropathies: B-cell depletion chemotherapy using Rituximab. *Neurology* 1999; 52:1701–1704.

123. Pestronk A, Florence J, Miller T, et al. Treatment of IgM antibody associated polyneuropathies using rituximab. *J Neurol Neurosurg Psychiatry* 2003; 74:485–489.

124. Stieglbauer K, Topakian R, Hinterberger G, et al. Beneficial effect of rituximab monotherapy in multifocal motor neuropathy. *Neuromuscul Disord* 2009; 19:473–475.

125. Rheug SJ, Fuhr P, Steck AJ. Rituximab stabilizes multifocal motor neuropathy increasingly less response to IVIg. *Neurology* 2004; 63:2178–2179.

126. Van den Berg-Vos RM, van den Berg LH, Franssen H et al. Treatment of multifocal motor neuropathy with interferon-beta1A. *Neurology* 2000; 54:1518–1521.

127. Martina IS, van Doorn PA, Schmitz PI, et al. Chronic motor neuropathies: response to interferon beta 1a after failure of conventional therapies. *J Neurol Neurosurg Psychiatry* 1999; 66:197–201.

128. Radziwill A, Botez SA, Novy J, et al. Interferon beta-1a as adjunctive treatment for multifocal motor neuropathy: an open label trial. *J Periph Nerv Syst* 2009; 14:201–202.

129. Pestronk A, Lopate G, Kornberg AJ, et al. Distal lower motor neuron syndrome with high-titer serum IgM anti-GM1 antibodies: improvement following immunotherapy with monthly plasma exchange and intravenous cyclophosphamide. *Neurology* 1994; 44:2027–2031.

130. Van den Berg LH, Franssen H, Van Doorn PA, et al. Intravenous immunoglobulin treatment in lower motor neuron disease associated with highly raised anti-GM1 antibodies. *J Neurol Neurosurg Psychiatry* 1997; 63:674–677.

131. Katz JS, Barohn RJ, Kojan S, et al. Axonal multifocal motor neuropathy without conduction block or other features of demyelination. *Neurology* 2002; 58:615–620.

CHAPTER 35

Critical Illness Disorders

David S. Younger

Weakness of limb and respiratory muscles is a serious and increasingly common problem in adult and pediatric intensive care units (ICU). Its management frequently demands consideration of neurologic consultation, creatine kinase (CK) measurement, detailed electrodiagnostic and neuroimaging studies and muscle and nerve biopsy to elucidate the etiopathogenesis of the weakness due to a causative lesion in the central or peripheral nervous system (CNS or PNS). This chapter describes the general approach to the evaluation of neuromuscular disorders in the ICU. There are several recent reviews of pediatric and adult neurological critical illness and ICU disorders (1–5).

NOMENCLATURE

The primary myopathic and neuropathic disorders that occur during critical illness, respectively termed critical illness myopathy (CIM) and polyneuropathy (CIP), include acute quadriplegic myopathy (AQM), thick myosin filament myopathy, necrotizing myopathy, combined thick filament and necrotizing myopathy; and primarily motor and sensory demyelinating and axonal neuropathies, further separable by detailed electrophysiological studies and histopathological analysis of muscle and nerve tissue obtained by biopsy or at postmortem examination as noted in the literature (6–17).

NEUROMUSCULAR EVALUATION IN CRITICALLY ILL AND INJURED PATIENTS

History

If the child or adult patient is alert and able to write, an adequate history can be obtained by having the patient respond by handwriting. If limb paralysis precludes this, the patient may respond by nodding or shaking the head for yes or no answers. If the patient is stuporous, confused, or comatose, the history of neuromuscular symptoms can generally be obtained from the referring physician, emergency room or ICU physician, hospital chart, relatives, friends, or an employer.

Spinal and radicular pain, bulbar and limb weakness, breathing difficulty, impaired sensation, bladder dysfunction, muscle cramping, fasciculation, and fatigability may be a clue to underlying neuromuscular disorder. The neuromuscular problem may follow a major surgical procedure; for example, surgery on the thoracic aorta that may accompany spinal cord ischemia and resulting paraplegia. Neuromuscular blocking agents, even short-acting ones such as vecuronium, can have an action of several hours in the setting of renal failure. It is important to recognize the reasons for intubation and mechanical ventilation, whether for airway protection or weakness of the respiratory muscles, and the type of mechanical ventilation, frequency of intermittent mandatory ventilation, degree of pressure support, blood gas results, and the ability to breathe while off the ventilator.

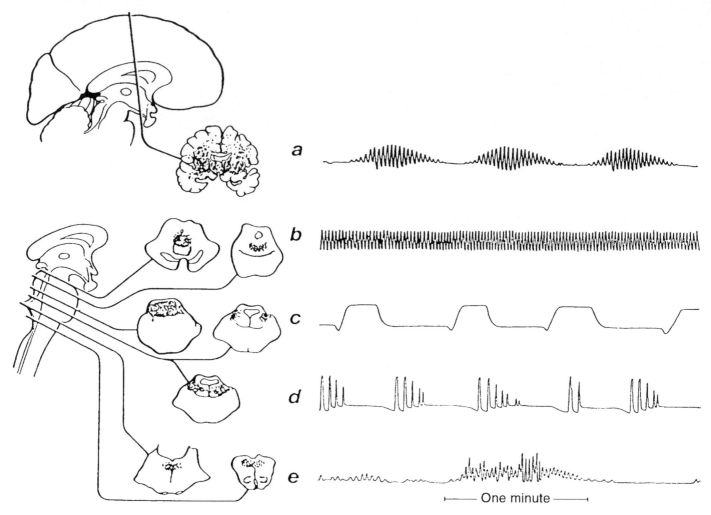

FIG. 1. Abnormal respiratory patterns associated with pathologic lesions (shaded areas) at various locations in the brain. **(A)** Cheyne-Stokes respiration; **(B)** Central neurogenic hyperventilation; **(C)** Apneusis; **(D)** Cluster breathing; **(E)** Ataxic breathing. Respiratory movements were recorded with a chest-abdomen pneumograph.

Physical Examination

General inspection of the skin may reveal localized edema and redness at sites of compression that are likely to occur in patients with drug-induced coma lasting hours. Pressure at the site of an underlying peripheral nerve can cause mononeuropathy. Signs of sympathetic insufficiency, such as increased temperature, redness, and dry skin in a paretic lower limb compared with the opposite limb, suggest a lesion of the lumbar plexus because sympathetic fibers bypass the caudal nerve roots.

Ptosis, asymmetric ocular palsies, and facial weakness require exclusion of a neuromuscular transmission defect. The response to a tracheal tug on the endotracheal tube assesses the ability to swallow and cough. Abnormalities of this type are seen in motor neuron disease (MND), Guil-lain-Barré syndrome (GBS), and disorders of the neuromuscular junction (NMJ).

Assessment of the respiratory system should be done in the presence of the intensivist and, if necessary, assisted by the respiratory technologist. The ability to breathe independently is assessed by discontinuing or altering mechanical ventilation by stopping intermittent mandatory ventilation while keeping the patient on pressure support or continuous positive airway pressure to overcome airway/ventilator resistance; a maximum of 15 minutes maintains reasonable oxygenation. Mechanical ventilation is warranted when there is respiratory distress, arterial oxygen saturation of <90% based on an oximeter reading, or a significant rise in breath rate or blood pressure. Needle electromyography (EMG) of the diaphragm can accurately assess the pattern of respiration by observing the bursts of motor unit poten-

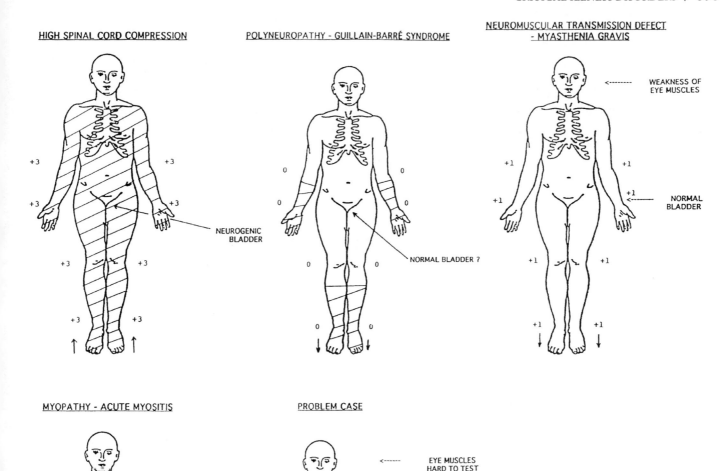

FIG. 2. Typical physical findings in sites of nervous system dysfunction that may cause the syndrome of acute limb and respiratory weakness are illustrated top to bottom and left to right. Numbers, briskness of deep tendon reflexes; arrows, plantar responses; lateral lines, areas of sensory loss. Problem case illustrates these typical signs may be absent or difficult to interpret.

tials (MUP) with each inspiration and may be of localizing value as shown in Figure 1. The overall strength and rate of respiratory effort should be ascertained. The signs of reduced movement of chest wall muscles on attempted inspiration with forced outward movement of the abdominal muscles as the diaphragm descends are important clinical clues of an underlying NMJ disorder.

Generalized or focal muscle wasting is difficult to deter-

mine in the presence of limb edema. An affected patient can have voluntary or partial voluntary movements in bulbar and limb muscles in a pattern that suggests hemiplegia, quadriplegia, or paraplegia. If there are no such movements, compression of the nailbeds with a pencil may induce one of several involuntary motor responses. Simple flexion movement of the stimulated ipsilateral or contralateral limbs occurs on a reflex basis at the level of the spinal cord level and even in brain death. More complex movements of a voluntary nature require intact cerebral function. If the opposite hand accurately moves in a coordinated way to attempt to remove the painful stimulus, reasonable function of that limb must be present. In addition, the patterns of limb movement may offer further clues as to the presence or absence of coexisting neuromuscular disease. Painful stimulation that induces vigorous facial grimacing without limb movement implies normal afferent and efferent cranial conduction of the painful stimulus along PNS and CNS pathways. Similar findings are often seen in high cervical cord lesions, but because severe pain impulses are not transmitted through the spinal cord, facial grimacing is not present. Vigorous upward movement of the great toe on plantar stimulation may be absent on the side of a fibular nerve palsy. There may be focal absence of deep tendon reflexes (DTR), suggesting lumbosacral plexopathy with particular involvement of the femoral nerve.

Laboratory Evaluation

Clues to diagnosis of a critical illness involving the CNS and PNS can be inferred by the associated findings as shown in Figure 2.

Neuroimaging, preferably brain and spinal cord magnetic resonance imaging (MRI), should be performed immediately in all patients suspected of acute spinal cord dysfunction, trauma, ischemia, infection, and spinal shock.

Electrophysiological studies are important in the evaluation of patients with critical illness associated weakness (18, 19). Serial nerve conduction studies (NCS) and conventional EMG should be obtained in all patients and timed to allow for maturation of the proposed lesion, but never postponed so as to delay timely diagnosis. Only precipitous weakness will be promptly recognized by physicians and staff in the ICU, whereas most other affected patients will certainly have a less well-documented onset and duration of their neuromuscular condition as a result of prolonged unconsciousness and limb restraints. NCS and EMG may fail to distinguish between neuropathy and myopathy since both disorders may be characterized by low amplitude of the compound muscle action potential (CMAP) and either can show spontaneous activity in the form of fibrillation potentials and positive sharp waves. Voluntary MUP evaluation is often problematic because of poor patient cooperation. The differentiating feature may rest on the presence of normal sensory nerve action potentials (SNAP), but these too may be unreliable when there is leg edema.

Quantitative electromyography is useful in distinguishing neuropathy from myopathy in the ICU. Whenever possible, 20 different MUP are collected by random insertion of a concentric needle electrodes into several regions of the muscle under examination. The mean duration and amplitude of the collected MUP from each muscle are compared to normal age-matched values, and the duration expressed as a percentage deviation from normal age-matched values for all collected MUP, with even greater accuracy obtained by selection of non-polyphasic MUP for analysis.

Peripheral neuropathy severe enough to caused marked weakness should be indicated by alteration in motor unit number estimation, whereas the latter is unaltered in myopathy using standard techniques. However, technical challenges to EMG can arise in the ICU due to electrical interference from adjacent machines, poorly grounded plug-ins, inadequate shielding of cables, and other electrical devices. The skin should be adequately prepared to reduce resistance. The 60-cycle notch filter on the EMG machine may have to be used. It may not be possible to electrically stimulate certain nerves due to the presence of intravascular lines, surgical wounds and dressings, casts, and splints. Cardiac arrhythmias may be induced if an electrical stimulus is applied along a limb with an intravascular line that resides distally in the heart, in which case it may be wise to test the opposite side. The ground electrode should be on the same side of the body that is being stimulated to avoid transmission of the electrical impulse through the heart. Virtually all EMG studies, including those of the diaphragm, are quite safe. In our experience, these various technical challenges can be easily overcome, and a complete electrophysiologic assessment can almost always be achieved.

Muscle and nerve biopsy should be considered in all patients with critical illness neuropathy and myopathy, regardless of the duration of weakness. Properly performed in the operating room by a neurologist or surgeon experienced in these techniques at a center with experienced neuropathology, there is a high likelihood of reaching a categorical diagnosis with few side effects. The histopathological findings of critical illness myopathy include prominent myofibrillar degeneration and atrophy of myofibers, chiefly histochemical type 2, accompanied by focal reduction or absence of myosin ATP staining at ph 9.4 in small fibers, and necrotic and regenerative fibers. Electron microscope (EM) studies confirm the prominent myofibrillar disarray and demonstrate selective loss of thick myosin filaments. The diagnosis of CIM can be confirmed by quantification of the myosin/actin ratio performed by densitometry and horizontal pore gradient sodium dodecyl sulfate (SDS) electrophoresis on muscle tissue. A mean myosin/actin ratio of 1.37 ± 0.21 and 0.37 ± 0.17 was noted in patients with CIM (20).

Peripheral nerve biopsy should be performed in patients with suspected critical illness polyneuropathy. Patients with CIP demonstrate evidence of axonal or demyelinat-

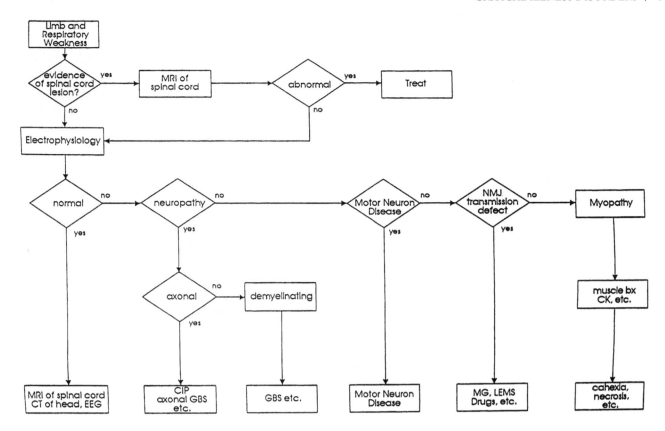

FIG. 3. An algorithm to guide the approach to the investigation of ICU patients with limb and respiratory muscle weakness. Positive serology or stool culture for C. jejuni may be the earliest warning of the axonal form of GBS. Abbreviations: MRI: magnetic resonance imaging, NMJ: neuromuscular junction; Bx: biopsy; CK: creatine kinase; CT: computed tomography; CIP: critical illness polyneuropathy; GBS: Guillain-Barré syndrome; MG: myasthenia gravis; LEMS: Lambert-Eaton myasthenic syndrome.

ing lesions depending upon the severity and duration of the lesions. Patients with sensory CIP may also present clinically and histopathologically with sensory cutaneous nerve involvement alone, sparing muscle tissue.

ACUTE LIMB AND RESPIRATORY WEAKNESS DEVELOPING BEFORE ADMISSION TO THE ICU

Some patients present with rapidly developing paralysis of limb and respiratory muscles, requiring endotracheal intubation and mechanical ventilation. Their course may be so rapid that time is insufficient for an accurate diagnosis or screening diagnostic studies before admission to the ICU. In this acutely developing situation, clinical signs may be confusing. The differential diagnosis should be systematically and the relevant conditions eliminated as shown in Figure 3.

Spinal Cord Compression

Acute disorders of the high cervical spinal cord may be due to compression by neoplasm, infection, and acute transverse myelitis, in which the traditional signs of localized spinal cord disease may be absent. Hyperreflexia is usually abolished by spinal shock, and the sensory level may be difficult to determine, particularly in high cervical lesions, thus warranting emergency MRI of the spinal cord. Motor NCS may show decreased CMAP amplitudes due to anterior horn cell injury if five days have elapsed since the injury. If sensory NCS are normal and if clinical sensory loss is present, the lesion lies proximal to the dorsal root ganglion, usually indicating a myelopathy. Needle EMG abnormalities appear 10 to 20 days afterward in direct relation to the distance from the site of injury to the muscle examined. The pattern of denervation on needle EMG assists in localization of the segmental level, although it may not be precise due to considerable overlap of paraspinal muscle innervation. Scalp somatosensory evoked potential (SSEP) recordings can also assist in diagnosis as when the peripheral nerve and T-12 responses are normal, so localizing the lesion to above the T-12 level, or when the T-12 responses are absent or delayed, instead indicating localization to the cauda equina or lumbosacral plexus. However, SSEP results may be normal even in large spinal cord lesions if the sensory tracts are spared.

Motor Neuron Disease

Respiratory involvement may be the first clue to MND. The combination of clinical upper (UMN) and lower motor neuron (LMN) signs, including hyperreflexia, Babinski, Hoffman, and ankle clonus combined with focal weakness, wasting and fasciculation make the diagnosis of amyotrophic lateral sclerosis (ALS) inescapable. Lingual involvement may be overlooked in an intubated patient. Electrophysiologic studies confirm the diagnosis and exclude motor neuropathy with multifocal conduction block (MCB).

Guillain-Barré Syndrome

Polyneuropathy is generally suspected by the presence of weakness, hyporeflexia, and distal sensory loss. The clinical and electrophysiologic features of GBS reflect peripheral nerve demyelination. In the initial stages, conduction velocities are mildly depressed or normal, F waves are prolonged or absent, and there may be evidence of conduction block and rapidly firing MUP without spontaneous needle activity. Electrodiagnostic studies of the diaphragm are particularly valuable in establishing the type and severity of phrenic nerve and diaphragm involvement. Serial electrophysiologic studies are valuable in following the course of the disease and response to treatment, after plasmapheresis, intravenous immunoglobulin (IVIg), and corticosteroids. Symptomatic improvement generally precedes electrophysiologic improvement.

The acute motor and sensory axonal variants of GBS progress rapidly and reach completion over hours and necessitate prompt admission to the ICU for ventilator assistance. With varying severity, all muscles of the body, including cranial musculature, are susceptible to paralysis. At the worst extreme, it can simulate brain death, however the electroencephalogram is normal. The peripheral cranial nerves may be unresponsive to high-voltage and long-duration electrical stimulation, and SNAP and CMAP are reduced or absent.

Acute axonal GBS in children and adults is separable from CIP by clinical, electrophysiological, serological, and CSF analysis (21). Axonal GBS is the primary neurological reason for admission to the ICU, whereas CIP develops during a patient's stay therein. Axonal GBS often presents and an infectious symptom prodrome accompanied

by fever and diarrhea. The clinical presentation of axonal GBS is symmetrical ascent over days with normal sensation with loss of DTR. Electrophysiologic studies reveal motor axonopathy. There is often serological evidence of residual Campylobacter jejuni in the stool, and as weakness is evident, elevation of GM1, GM1b, GD1a, and GalNac-GD1serum gangliosides. Both axonal GBS and CIP may present with significant respiratory involvement, raised protein content without pleocytosis on lumbar CSF analysis, reduced CMAP amplitudes with normal distal motor latencies and SNAP responses on NCS, varying amounts of active denervation on concentric needle EMG, and slow steady recovery. Acute porphyria, Lyme disease, and concurrent human immunodeficiency virus (HIV) type 1 infection should be considered in patients with the syndrome of axonal GBS.

Chronic Inflammatory Demyelinating Polyradiculoneuropathy

Patients with chronic inflammatory demyelinating polyradiculoneuropathy (CIDP) can have rapid deterioration of respiratory function. In addition to the more typical clinical and electrophysiologic signs of these polyneuropathies, phrenic NCS and needle EMG of the diaphragm confirm the neuropathic basis of the respiratory insufficiency.

Efforts to devise sets of clinical and electrodiagnostic criteria to distinguish primary demyelination from primary axonal neuropathies have been elusive, and despite modifications, established guidelines continue to be of limited sensitivity and likely related to a wide range of clinical, electrophysiological, and histopathological changes among patients with CIDP (22).

Neuromuscular Transmission Defects

Myasthenia gravis and Myasthenic Syndromes

Disorders due to defects in NMJ transmission can be challenging to diagnose. Respiratory insufficiency occurs in myasthenia gravis (MG) and Lambert-Eaton myasthenic syndrome (LEMS) (23), accompanied by weakness in swallowing and breathing muscles. While the mortality associated with myasthenic crisis has dropped from 50% to less than 3% in over five decades since institution of prompt pulmonary ICU care, the incidence of crisis has remained constant at about 16% (24) with many patients presenting for the first time with crisis. The unequivocal diagnosis of MG rests on the presence of fluctuation of weakness in eye, facial, and limb muscles, a positive edrophonium test, decremented response of sequential CMAP with 3 per second supramaximal stimulation, and elevated titers of acetylcholine receptor (AChR) antibodies. Immunomodulating therapy improves all aspects of MG, including respiratory muscles (25). LEMS, hypocalcemia, hypermagnesemia, organophosphate poisoning, and wound botulism may affect presynaptic neuromuscular transmission and may be identifiable on electrophysiologic studies.

Myopathy

Patients with chronic myopathy may require intubation and admission to the ICU because of respiratory muscle weakness, although the diagnosis is usually evident, as in the case of muscular dystrophy. In more acute myopathies, such as necrotizing myopathy with myoglobinuria, the diagnosis is later evident because of high serum levels of CK, myoglobinuria, and necrosis on a muscle biopsy.

ACUTE LIMB AND RESPIRATORY WEAKNESS DEVELOPING AFTER ADMISSION TO THE INTENSIVE CARE UNIT

Up to one-half of patients in medical and surgical ICU have significant involvement of the nervous system, and neuromuscular problems are much more frequent than generally recognized, with sepsis and multiple organ failure occurring in up to half of patients and CIP in up to 70% of patients. Neuromuscular blocking agents and steroids may cause further distinctive neuromuscular syndromes. The difficulty in clinically evaluating patients with neuromuscular problems, often with difficulty in weaning from the ventilator, has led to increased reliance on electrophysiologic studies and occasionally muscle and nerve biopsy.

Myelopathy

Myelopathy in the ICU setting is usually due to trauma, compression by neoplasm, hemorrhage, or infection in the epidural space or infarction of the spinal cord secondary to surgical procedures on the aorta. In most instances the myelopathy occurs before admission to the ICU.

Critical Illness Polyneuropathy

Patients with CIP are included in the syndrome termed *systemic inflammatory response syndrome* (SIRS) that occurs in response to both infection and several forms of trauma, including major surgery and burns.

The earliest neurological manifestation of SIRS is generally septic encephalopathy characterized by inattention and disorientation. Affected patients slip into coma, usually without focal signs, seizures, myoclonus, or asterixis. The electroencephalogram (EEG) is a sensitive indicator of the presence and severity of septic encephalopathy. Computed

tomography (CT) and MRI of the brain and serial neurologic examinations are usually unremarkable.

Treated specifically with antibiotics, surgical drainage of an infected focus, inotropic drugs, and fluid replacement, the encephalopathy improves rapidly, but difficulty in weaning from the ventilator often persists. Critical illness polyneuropathy is the most common neuromuscular cause of ventilator dependency after cardiac and pulmonary etiologies have been excluded. Clinical signs of polyneuropathy are present in about half of patients. Electrophysiologic studies are therefore necessary to firmly establish the diagnosis of CIP.

Central respiratory drive may be assessed by decreasing ventilatory support from 5 to 8 cm H_2O pressure support or continuous positive airway pressure to overcome airway and ventilator resistance for a maximum of 15 minutes. Mechanical ventilation is restored if there is evidence of respiratory distress, arterial oxygen saturation less than 90% based on a pulse oximeter reading, or a significant rise in heart rate or blood pressure. This is done at the time of needle EMG of the diaphragm.

The earliest electrophysiologic sign, usually within a week, is reduction in the amplitude of the CMAP with little or no change in distal latencies indicative of axonal damage. Voluntary evoked MUP when present, often appear normal or somewhat low in amplitude with increased polyphasia suggestive of primary involvement of muscle by sepsis. These electrophysiologic changes are also consistent with primary myopathy. Hence, it is important to demonstrate depression of SNAP amplitudes before a firm diagnosis of CIP is made. Repetitive motor nerve stimulation may be abnormal if neuromuscular blocking agents have been given, and their effects may persist beyond several hours to a number of days if the patient is in renal or liver failure. Phrenic NCS and needle EMG of the chest wall and diaphragm are useful in showing that CIP is the probable proximate cause of difficulty in weaning from the ventilator (26).

Knowledge of the presence of CIP aids ventilator management and signals that the patient has a neuromuscular problem which may prolong the ICU stay. If the disorder is mild, recovery can occur over weeks, but when severe, it can take several months and/or remain incomplete. Physiotherapy and rehabilitation should be tailored to the severity of the polyneuropathy. Other than management of the septic syndrome, there is no specific treatment of CIP.

The morphologic aspects of CIP have been examined in peripheral nerve and muscle biopsies and in postmortem studies of the CNS and PNS, revealing evidence of a noninflammatory motor and sensory axonopathy. Muscle tissue shows acute and chronic denervation, with scattered grouped atrophic myofibers and occasional necrotic myofibers, suggesting associated primary myopathy as well. The only CNS manifestation is central chromatolysis of anterior horn cells and loss of dorsal root ganglion neurons, secondary to the axonopathy.

Acute Motor Neuropathy Associated with Competitive Neuromuscular Blocking Agents

Patients with forms of this polyneuropathy have generally been in the ICU for days to weeks and have received competitive neuromuscular blocking agents, such as pancuronium bromide, or the shorter acting agent vecuronium for 48 hours or more, and occasionally for days or weeks to ease mechanical ventilation. When the agents are discontinued, difficulty weaning from the ventilator and limb paralysis ensues. The serum CK level is mild or moderately elevated. There is electrophysiologic evidence of severe primary motor axonopathy, with or without a defect in neuromuscular transmission with repetitive motor nerve stimulation. Muscle biopsy shows varying degrees of denervation atrophy and myofiber necrosis.

The mechanism of the neuropathy is unknown, but sepsis appears to be an underlying factor in most patients. When various contributing systemic complications are successfully treated, the neuromuscular condition itself improves and rapid recovery sometimes occurs. Neuromuscular blocking agents have not been implicated as a causative factor in CIP.

Neuromuscular Transmission Disorders

Transient neuromuscular blockade, thick filament myopathy, cachectic myopathy, and acute necrotizing myopathy, in the order of their severity, may be the cause of difficulty in weaning from the ventilator in critical illness and injury.

Competitive neuromuscular blocking agents, often used to ease mechanical ventilation, are metabolized or cleared by the liver and kidney. In the presence of multiorgan failure, neuromuscular blockage may be prolonged for days after discontinuation. Decremented response of sequential CMAP correctly identifies the defect in NMJ transmission; however, by the time of testing, many patients will already have developed underlying CIP. Recovery may occur over a short period of time but may be prolonged for weeks or even months in severe cases.

Myopathy

Thick filament myopathy and AQM occur in children and adults during exacerbations of severe asthma and after organ transplantation. Endotracheal intubation and ventilator support for several days is usually necessary, accompanied by high-dose corticosteroids and neuromuscular blocking agents to ease mechanical ventilation. On attempted weaning from the ventilator, the patient is found to have severe neuromuscular respiratory insufficiency and limb weakness; ophthalmoplegia may also be present. Serum CK levels are considerably increased. Repetitive motor nerve stimulation and sensory NCS are usually normal however motor NCS reveal low CMAP amplitudes. Voluntary MUP are generally low in amplitude and short in duration, with excessive polyphasia indicative of primary myopathy. Direct electrical stimulation of the muscle membrane may reveal inexcitability. Muscle biopsy shows central pallor of muscle fibers due to destruction of thick myosin filaments. The administration of corticosteroids may activate an ATP–ubiquitin-dependent proteolytic system that leads to myosin degradation. One etiopathogenic mechanism is proteolysis due to increased expression of calpain resulting from alteration of calcium metabolism. Clinical recovery may occur rapidly. The clinical and electrophysiologic features are usually so distinctive that muscle biopsy is often not necessary.

Cachectic myopathy, disuse atrophy, and catabolic myopathy are interchangeable terms used to describe the syndrome of muscle weakness and wasting. Motor and sensory NCS, needle EMG, and CK levels are all generally normal. Muscle biopsy may be normal or show nonspecific type 2 muscle fiber atrophy.

Necrotizing myopathy of intensive care is a rare disorder precipitated by a wide variety of infective, chemical, and metabolic insults that enters in the differential diagnosis of acute myoglobinuria. It presents with severe weakness, high serum CK levels, and myoglobinuria. Electrophysiologic studies were consistent with severe myopathy, and muscle biopsy showed widespread fiber necrosis. Rapid and spontaneous recovery occurs in mild cases, but less so in more severe ones. The disorder is associated with a reduction in bioenergetic reserves, as measured by ^{31}P nuclear MR spectroscopy (MRS) so noted as very low ratios of phosphocreatine/inorganic phosphate that return toward normal as recovery from the critical illness and polyneuropathy ensues.

Plexopathy

Lumbosacral or brachial plexopathies may be secondary to direct trauma, usually from motor vehicle accidents or surgery. Insertion of catheters into the iliac arteries or aorta may dislodge thrombi, and the resulting embolization impairs vascular supply to nerves and in this manner, induces focal ischemic plexopathy. Direct surgical trauma to vessels may also induce vascular insufficiency. Motorcycle accidents commonly traumatize the brachial plexus, proximal lesions of which are suggested by Horner syndrome, winging of the scapular, and diaphragm paralysis. Electrophysiologic studies performed within three weeks of injury will further help localize the lesion. MRI provides unequivocal evidence of root avulsion, which when present, precludes attempts at operative nerve repair. Fractures of the pelvis can lead to varying patterns of damage to the lumbosacral plexus. Observations of focal weakness on reflex or voluntarily induced movement, plus abnormalities of the deep tendon reflexes, may provide an initial clue to the presence of such damage. Weakness of hip adduction and flexion, knee extension, and an absent DTR suggests damage of the L2 to L4 roots of the lumbosacral plexus. Electrophysiologic studies can localize the lesion to the brachial or lumbosacral plexus.

Focal neuropathy and mononeuropathy also present diagnostic challenges, the etiopathogenesis of which may be due to direct injury, entrapment, autoimmune palsy, or infarction. If the primary reason for admission to the ICU was the postoperative state, the initial surgery may be the cause. Weakness of wrist and fiber dorsiflexion and an absent brachioradialis reflex suggests radial nerve damage in the spinal groove of the humerus by fracture or direct compression. Phrenic nerves, either bilaterally or unilaterally, may be damaged at the time of surgery by direct trauma or by the application of cold, as occurs in the hypothermia associated with cardiac surgery. Distal nerves may be damaged as a result of impairment of nutrient blood supply and distal embolization, as for example in the occurrence of femoral or sciatic neuropathy after cardiac or vascular surgery. Electrophysiologic studies show a relatively pure axonopathy affecting motor and sensory fibers.

Anticoagulated patients are at risk of hemorrhage due to a sudden rise in tissue pressure leading to compartment syndrome and severe compression resulting in nerve ischemia. The compartments most commonly involved are the iliopsoas and gluteal, producing acute femoral or sciatic neuropathies. Fractures and soft tissue trauma can be the proximate cause of a compartment syndrome, and should prompt immediate body CT imaging to discern the location of the hematoma, surgical decompression of which may be necessary for full neurological recovery. In this situation, which is so acute and emergent, electrophysiologic studies need not be obtained when the suspected nerves have a troncal rather than limb location.

PATHOPHYSIOLOGY OF CRITICAL ILLNESS NEUROPATHY AND MYOPATHY

The microcirculation is disturbed in sepsis as shown in Figure 3. Blood vessels supplying the peripheral nerves lack autoregulation, rendering these vessels susceptible to such disturbances. Moreover, cytokines that are secreted in sepsis have histamine-like properties that may increase microvascular permeability, the result of which is hypoxia, endoneurial edema, and an increase in intercapillary distance. Severe energy deficits can induce a primarily distal axonal degeneration if highly energy-dependant systems involve axonal transport of structural proteins. The pre-

dominantly distal involvement may explain why recovery in some patients can be surprisingly short, conforming to the short length of nerve through which axonal regeneration takes place.

The molecular chain of events leading to myofiber involvement in critical illness is not well understood, however ubiquitin-mediated proteolysis, cytoplasmic calpain-related lysosomal-dependent, and cathespin-mediated proteolysis pathways have been elucidated in patients with critical illness myopathy, and in vivo and in vitro animal models (27–29). Lack of muscle excitability due to sodium channel inactivation was described in affected patients and an animal model of AQM (30, 31). Gene expression changes in animal models of AQM and CIM showed regression of specific Na+ channels and induction of proteolysis at the RNA transcription level (32, 33)

Giovanni and colleagues (34) described apoptotic features in atrophic fibers in human muscle biopsies from patients with AQM, as shown by DNA fragmentation in situ by terminal deoxynucleotidyltransferase-mediated dUTP nick end labeling (TUNEL), and nuclear margination and condensation by EM. Many myofibers showed strong expression of calpain, cathespin B, and caspase-3, not seen in muscle tissue from patients with neurogenic myofibers atrophy syndromes, suggesting stimulation of proapoptotic pathways underlying the pathogenesis of AQM. Acute stimulation of the proapoptotic transforming growth factor (TGF)-β/MAPK pathway that underlies myogenic atrophy and the muscle-specific Skp1-Cullin-F-box protein SCF ubiquitin ligase component, atrogin-1protesosome pathway, is strongly induced in AQM (35). The combination of cellular stress, inactivity of muscle, and corticosteroid drug stimulation could all appear to converge on the TGF-β/MAPK and atrogin-1 pathways, leading to acute stimulation of apoptosis and myofilament loss. Friedrich and coworkers (36) showed that sera from patients with CIM affected membrane excitability and the excitation-contraction coupling process at the level of sarcoplasmic reticulum mediated calcium release in mammalian myofibers.

The increased proliferation of proinflammatory cytokines and cell adhesion molecules can induce dysfunction in the endothelial barrier of microvessels in various organs, including muscle and nerve, may explain the enhanced effects of neuromuscular blocking agents and corticosteroids. Increased capillary permeability induced by sepsis and neuromuscular blocking agents such as vecuronium or its metabolite, 3 desacetyl-vecuronium, can have a direct toxic effect on peripheral nerve axons, presumably due to functional denervation.

Antibiotics, particularly aminoglycosides, can lead to CIP by gaining access to the peripheral nerve as a result of increased capillary permeability. However, there has been no statistical proof that antibiotics cause peripheral nerve dysfunction in sepsis.

TREATMENT AND OUTCOME

There are only a few prospective, systematic follow-up studies in children and adult patients with CIM and CIP to judge the timing and effects of neurological and rehabilitative intervention (37, 38). They demonstrated motor and sensory deficits, and variable persistent chronic partial denervation on EMG testing indicative of residual disease, respectively, in 59% and 95% of patients so studied. Critical illness neuromuscular disorders in children occur infrequently, but pose unique challenges. Acute quadriplegia, noted in 14 (1.7%) of 830 pediatric ICU admissions, was ascribed to myopathy in all affected children, many of whom underwent detailed electrophysiological studies and muscle biopsy evaluation (39). In eight (57%) children, solid organ and bone marrow transplantation preceded multiple organ failure, sepsis, pulmonary insufficiency, and prolonged machine ventilation, leading up to the neurological disorder. Three (21%) children died, and among 11 surviving children available for follow-up, only three (27%) children obtained normal strength and variable endurance.

There are no specific therapies available to treat critical illness neuromuscular disorders. Although most authorities agree with early preventive medical management to reduce its occurrence and lessen severity, at least three obstacles impede our ability to promptly intercede in all cases. First, standardized screening for weakness in the ICU is not routinely performed. Second, critical care physicians are under pressure to move patients out of the unit after restoration of independent ventilation, relegating the neurological evaluation to other medical services. Third, most patients diagnosed with myopathy and neuropathy are typically well into their medical recovery, receiving intensive rehabilitation weeks to months after onset of the neuromuscular disorder, too late to envision a therapeutic medical intervention for critical illness mediated weakness.

Intensive glucose management is accepted therapy in critically ill patients, and should be considered for all those at risk for critical illness neuromuscular disease. Until there are specific modalities to treat neuromuscular disorders associated with critical illness, the judicious use of conventional immunotherapies, including IVIg and plasmapheresis, as well as immunosuppressive agents other than corticosteroids, should be offered to patients with polymyositis, dermatomyositis, GBS, CIDP, and MG, to hasten recovery and achieve long-lasting remission.

REFERENCES

1. Chawla J, Gruener G. Management of critical illness polyneuropathy and myopathy. *Neurol Clin* 2010; 28:961–977.
2. Hermans G, Vanhorebeek I, Derde S, et al. Metabolic aspects of critical illness polyneuromyopathy. *Crit Care Med* 2009; 37 (Suppl 10):S391–397.
3. Zink W, Kollmar R, Schwab S. Critical illness polyneuropathy and myopathy in the intensive care unit. *Nat Rev Neurol* 2009; 5:372–379.
4. Pati S, Goodfellow JA, Iyadural S, et al. Approach to critical illness polyneuropathy and myopathy. *Postgrad Med J* 2008; 84:354–360.
5. Williams S, Horrocks IA, Ouvrier RA, et al. Critical illness polyneuropathy and myopathy in pediatric intensive care: a review. *Pediatr Crit Care Med* 2007; 8:18–22.
6. Bolton CF. Critical illness polyneuropathy. A useful concept. *Muscle Nerve* 1999; 419–422.
7. Bolton CF. Closing remarks and brief historical review. *Muscle Nerve* 2000; 9:S63–S65.
8. Bolton CF, and Young GB. Critical illness polyneuropathy. *Curr Treat Options Neurol* 2000; 2:489–498.
9. Lacomis D. Critical illness myopathy. *Current Rheumatology Reports* 2002; 4:403–408.
10. Tabarki B, Coffinieres A, Van den Bergh P, et al. Critical illness neuromuscular disease: clinical, electrophysiological, and prognostic aspects. *Arch Dis Child* 2002; 86:103–107.
11. Banwell BL, Mildner RJ, Hassall AC, et al. Muscle weakness in critically ill children. *Neurology* 2003; 61:1779–1782.
12. Hund E. Neurological complications of sepsis: critical illness polyneuropathy and myopathy. *J Neurol* 2001; 248:929–934.
13. Hund E. Critical illness polyneuropathy. *Curr Opin Neurol* 2001; 14:649–653.
14. Lacomis D, Zochodne DW, Bird SJ. Critical illness myopathy. *Muscle Nerve* 2000; 23:1785–1788.
15. Deconinck N, Van Parijs V, Beckers-Bleukx G, et al. Critical illness myopathy unrelated to corticosteroids or neuromuscular blocking agents. *Neuromuscul Disord* 1998; 8:186–192.
16. Gutmann L, Gutmann L. Critical illness neuropathy and myopathy. *Arch Neurol* 1999; 56:527–528.
17. Hudson LD, Lee CM. Neuromuscular sequelae of critical illness. *N Engl J Med* 2003; 348:745–747.
18. Latronico N, Shehu I, Guarneri B. Use of electrophysiological testing. *Crit Care Med* 2009; 37(Suppl 10):S316–320.
19. Trojaborg W, Weimer LH, Hays AP. Electrophysiological studies in critical illness associated weakness: myopathy or neuropathy-a reappraisal. *Clin Neurophysiol* 2001; 112:1586–1593.
20. Stibler H, Edstrom L, Ahlbeck K, et al. Critical illness polyneuromyopathy: the electrophysiological components of a complex entity. *Intensive Care Med* 2003; 29:1515–1527.
21. De Letter MACJ, Visser LH, Ang W et al. Distinctions between critical illness polyneuropathy and axonal Guillain-Barre syndrome. *J Neurol Neurosurg Psychiatry* 2000; 68:388–399.
22. Bromberg MB. Review of the evolution of electrodiagnostic criteria for chronic inflammatory demyelinating polyradiculopathy. *Muscle Nerve* 2011; 43:780–794.
23. Younger DS, Braun NMT, Jaretzki A, et al. Myasthenia gravis: determinants for independent ventilation after transsternal thymectomy. *Neurology* 1984; 34:336–340.
24. Cohen M, Younger DS. Aspects of the natural history of myasthenia gravis: crisis and death. *Ann NY Acad Sci* 1981; 377:670–677.
25. Younger DS, Worall BB, Penn AS. Myasthenia gravis: historical perspective and overview. *Neurology* 1997; 48(Suppl 5):S1–S7.
26. Sander HW, Saadeh PB, Chandswang D, et al. Diaphragmatic

denervation in intensive care unit patients. *Electromyogr Clin Neurophysiol* 1999; 39:3–5.

27. Matsumoto N, Nakamura T, Yasui Y, et al. Analysis of muscle proteins in acute quadriplegic myopathy. *Muscle Nerve* 2000; 23:1270–1276.

28. Bodine SC, Latres E, Baunhueter S, et al. Identification of ubiquitin ligases required for skeletal muscle atrophy. *Science* 2001; 294:1704–1708.

29. Glass DJ. Signalling pathways that mediate skeletal muscle hypertrophy and atrophy. *Nat Cell Biol* 2003; 5:87–90.

30. Rich MM, Pinter MJ. Sodium channel inactivation in an animal model of acute quadriplegic myopathy. *Ann Neurol* 2001 50:26–33.

31. Rich MM, Pinter MJ. Crucial role of sodium channel fast inactivation in muscle fibre inexcitability in a rat model of critical illness myopathy. *J Physiol* 2003; 547:555–566.

32. Jagoe RT, Lecker SH, Gomes M, et al. Patterns of gene expression in atrophying skeletal muscles: response to food deprivation. *FASEB J* 2002; 16:1697–1712.

33. Childs TE, Spangenburg EE, Vyas DR, et al. Temporal alterations in protein signaling cascades during recovery from muscle atrophy. *Am J Physiol Cell Physiol* 2003; 285:C391–C398.

34. Di Giovanni S, Mirabella M, D'Amico A, et al. Apoptotic features accompany acute quadriplegic myopathy. *Neurology* 2000; 55:854–858.

35. Di Giovanni S, Molon A, Broccolini A, et al. Constitutive activation of MAPK cascade in acute quadriplegic myopathy. *Ann Neurol* 2004; 55:195–206.

36. Friedrich O, Hund E, Weber C, et al. Critical illness myopathy serum fractions affect membrane excitability and intracellular calcium release in mammalian skeletal muscle. *J Neurol* 2004 251:53–65.

37. Fletcher SM, Kennedy DD, Ghosh IR, et al. Persistent neuromuscular and neurophysiological abnormalities in long-term survivors of prolonged critical illness. *Crit Care Med* 2003; 31:1012–1016.

38. Murphy S. Pediatric neurocritical care. *Neurotherapeutics* 2012; 9:3–16.

39. Banwell BL, Mildner RJ, Hassall AC, et al. Muscle weakness in critically ill children. *Neurology* 2003; 61:1779–1782.

PART III

Spinal Cord Diseases

CHAPTER 36

Rupture of an Intervertebral Disk and Related Disorders

David S. Younger

The peripheral nerve roots, thecal sac, and spinal cord are susceptible to injury by the rupture of an intervertebral disk. The clinical neurological sequela include mono- and polyradiculopathy, and compression syndromes of the spinal cord and cauda equina, influenced by the location and severity of the disk rupture, coexistent spinal disease, systemic disorders, and genetic influences. This chapter reviews historical background of intervertebral disc rupture, normal and pathological anatomical factors of the spine and intervertebral disk, followed by the epidemiology, clinical presentation, laboratory diagnosis, and medical and surgical management of cervical, thoracic, and lumbar intervertebral disk ruptures. The past several years have witnessed increased reliance upon evidence-based guidelines and randomized clinical trials (RCT), when available, to guide clinical decisions regarding the decision to proceed to cervical (1) and lumbar spine (2) surgery, and in the application of interventional techniques of chronic spinal pain management (3).

HISTORICAL

Goldthwait (4) reported a 39-year-old man who presented with severe back pain, paraplegia, sensory loss, and sphincter incontinence one day after carrying a heavy suitcase for half a mile. The patient underwent exploratory surgery by Dr. Harvey Cushing for possible spinal tumor with surgical removal of the spinous processes of the L1 vertebra through the mid-sacrum for narrowing of the spinal canal; however, the proposed clinical diagnosis was traumatic L5-S1 spondylolisthesis and superimposed rupture of the intervertebral disk at L5-S1.

Three months later, Middletown and Teacher (5) described a 38-year-old man with severe back pain, paraplegia, sensory loss below the knees, and sphincter involvement occurring several hours after lifting a heavy metal plate. Death ensued 16 days after the accident due to urosepsis. Postmortem examination showed rupture of a large intervertebral disk fragment in the canal adjacent to the lumbar cord enlargement, however the exact disc designation could not be further specified because the disc was not noticed until the day after the postmortem examination; however, from the portion of the injury to the cord it was proposed to originate from the T12-L1 level. The mechanism of disk rupture was described as follows:

"With regard to the mechanism of the injury, it can be inferred from the history of the case that the man, at the moment at which he felt the "crack" in his back, must have had his back more of less bent forward, with the lumbar and abdominal muscles in full action. This would cause powerful compression of the intervertebral discs, with the anterior margins of the vertebrae approximated to one another, and, therefore, in a favourable position for displacement of the pulp of the intervertebral disc backwards, if that were possible."

To test this theory, the authors applied pressure via a carpenter's wooden vice to the first three vertebra of the spinal column with the cord and nerves cut out, leaving the dura in situ. A prior, the intervertebral disks were slightly bulged inward toward the canal, but after pressure a rounded swelling appeared at the L1-2 interspace corresponding to protrusion of the disc, which with greater pressure led to rupture of the soft pulp through the inner and outer fibrous layers of the disc. For two more decades, additional patients were reported under the rubric of chondroma of the intervertebral disk.

In 1929, Dandy (6) provided convincing case histories of intervertebral disc rupture among two men, one age 47, and another age 61, with attacks of lumbar pain 10 to 12 weeks before onset of radiating pain into the legs, with progressive paralysis, sensory loss, and retention of urine and feces. In each case, surgery was prompted by the possibility of a spinal tumor leading to laminectomy in the first patient at L3-4, and in the second patient at L4-5, with discovery of large fragments of dorsally bulging intervertebral cartilage compressing the thecal sac of the cauda equina. Both patients made a full recovery after surgery.

Four years later, in 1934, Mixter and Barr (7) described a 25-year-old man with a syndrome of extreme back strain and examination that showed absence of the ankle jerk and tenderness in the sciatic notch. He was first treated conservatively; however, the finding of a cerebrospinal fluid (CSP) protein of 108 mg/dL and a negative lipidol myelographic examination prompted laminectomy from L2 to the first sacral vertebra, searching for a malignancy. However, an intervertebral disc mass occupying the region of the neural formen of the fifth lumbar root was found and removed with full recovery. This lesion was first classified as a chrondroma and then reclassified as an intervertebral disc rupture. More importantly, the authors concluded that herniation of the nucleus pulposus into the spinal canal was a not uncommon cause of sciatic pain, ending the tendency to classify them as chondromata, and indicating the benefit of surgery as treatment thereof. In a discussion of the paper, Barr (8) refined the concepts of the disorder:

"If the annulus is injured, either from trauma or degeneration so as to produce a break in its continuity or weakening of the wall, the nucleus pulposus will herniated or extrude. If the extrusion takes place posteriorly into the vertebral canal or either intervertebral foramen, symptoms of spinal cord or root pressure are thus produced."

The historical literature on cervical spine surgery with respect to the development of surgical approaches, management of degenerative disk disease, and methods to treat segmental instability is reviewed elsewhere.

ANATOMY

The spine is a flexible column formed by 33 vertebrae including 7 cervical, 12 thoracic, 5 lumbar, 5 sacral, and 4 coccygeal; however, the number may be increased or decreased in the lower spine, and those found in the sacral and coccygeal area are united as the sacrum and coccyx (Figure 1). Each vertebra contains an anterior solid body and a posterior arch, the latter formed by 2 pedicles and 2 lamina supporting 7 processes, including 4 articular, 2 transverse, and 1 spinous process surrounding the vertebral foramen. The vertebrae are stacked for the support of the cranium and

trunk, comprising a vertical spinal canal for passage of the spinal cord and thecal sac. The bodies articulate one to the other via articular processes and intervertebral ligaments.

Thirty-one pairs of spinal nerves, 8 cervical, 12 thoracic, 5 lumbar, 5 sacral and 1 coccygeal, exit through intervertebral foramina formed by the union of 2 intervertebral notches located above and below neighboring pedicles (Figure 2). Excluding the C8 root, which lacks a similarly numbered vertebra, other cervical roots exit superiorly to the related vertebra and disk. For example, the C5 root exits between C4 and C5 alongside the C4 disc, whereas the C8 root leaves the intraspinal canal between C7 and T1. Inferior thoracic and lumbar roots exit below the corresponding numbered vertebra, adjacent to the same numbered disk. For example, the L5 root passes between L5 and S1 adjacent to the L5 disk. Caudal spine roots of the lumbar spine descend alongside and then beyond the conus medullaris as the cauda equina, both sensory and motor fibers, the former of which are preganglionic and situated between the spinal cord and dorsal root ganglia (DRG). The boundaries of the intervertebral foramina include adjacent pedicles, facet and uncovertebral joints, intervertebral disk, and the adjacent vertebra.

Root and vertebral designations may be a source of confusion in the assessment of root disease or radiculopathy. Some physicians may refer to root involvement in terms of intervertebral or disc levels, whereas others may be concerned about a specific root affliction as, for example, a C5-6 lesion leading to C6 radiculopathy owing to compression at the level. Furthermore, more than one root can be affected at a single intervertebral level depending upon the location of the compressive disk. Whereas the majority of disc herniation occurs between the L4 and L5 vertebra, far lateral disk herniation may injure the L4 root, whereas more central ruptures will compress S1 to S4 roots yet to emerge.

The cervical vertebrae are smaller, denser, and readily distinguished by foramina in the transverse process for vertebral arteries. Their pedicles direct outward and backward, and the spinous processes are short and bifid. The articular and transverse processes are flat and oblique. The narrow lamina encloses a triangular spinal canal which when combined with degenerative arthritis, can place individuals at heightened risk for cord compression. The first and second cervical vertebrae or atlas and axis, accommodate movement of the head. The spinous process of the seventh vertebra is easily palpable under the skin, and the anterior root of the transverse process sometimes exists as a separate bone known as a cervical rib. Unique features of the cervical spine lend it particularly susceptible to entrapment and compression of the exiting spinal nerve roots. The shape of the cervical intervertebral foramina approximate a funnel, with the entrance zone being the narrowest part, and the root sleeves conical, with their takeoff points from the cen-

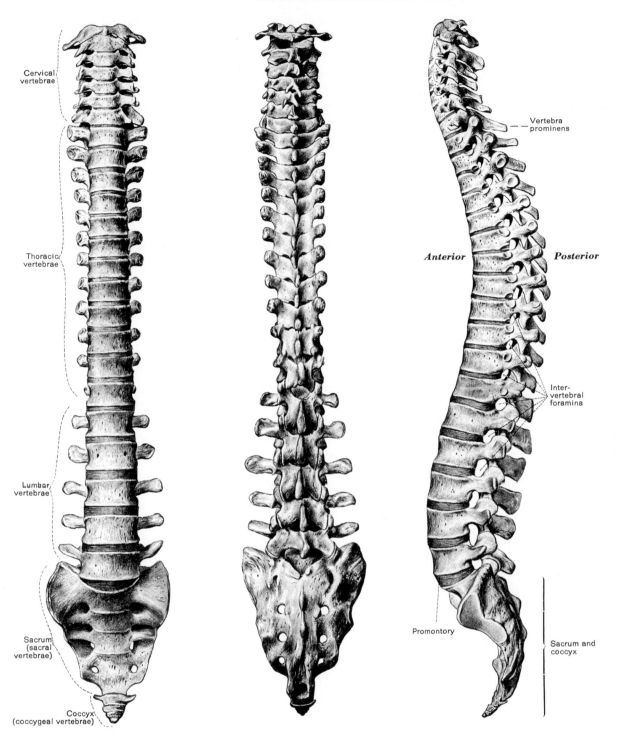

FIG. 1. Anterior, posterior, and lateral views of the human spine. From, Clemente CD. *Anatomy. A regional atlas of the human body*. Philadelphia: Lea and Febiger, 1975; with permission.

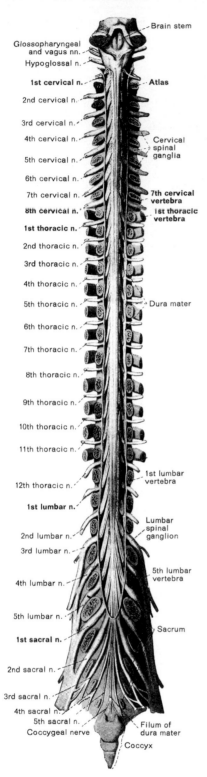

Brain stem

Glossopharyngeal and vagus nn.

Hypoglossal n.

1st cervical n. — Atlas

2nd cervical n.

3rd cervical n.

4th cervical n. — Cervical spinal ganglia

5th cervical n.

6th cervical n.

7th cervical n. — **7th cervical vertebra**

8th cervical n. — **1st thoracic vertebra**

1st thoracic n.

2nd thoracic n.

3rd thoracic n.

4th thoracic n.

5th thoracic n. — Dura mater

6th thoracic n.

7th thoracic n.

8th thoracic n.

9th thoracic n.

10th thoracic n.

11th thoracic n.

12th thoracic n. — 1st lumbar vertebra

1st lumbar n.

2nd lumbar n. — Lumbar spinal ganglion

3rd lumbar n.

4th lumbar n. — 5th lumbar vertebra

5th lumbar n.

1st sacral n. — Sacrum

2nd sacral n.

3rd sacral n.

4th sacral n.

5th sacral n. — Filum of dura mater

Coccygeal nerve

Coccyx

FIG. 2. Anatomic representation of the spinal nerves. From, Clemente CD. *Anatomy. A regional atlas of the human body.* Philadelphia: Lea and Febiger, 1975; with permission.

tral dural sac being the largest part. A reduction of 20 to 30% of the foramina area occurs after only 1 mm narrowing of the intervertebral disk spaces. With further encroachment of the foramina with progressive narrowing of the intervertebral disk space, leading, ultimately, to frank compression of the exiting nerve root with collapse of the intervertebral disk space. This has been attributed to settling and sliding of the inferior facets of the upper cervical vertebra down upon the superior facets of the subjacent lower vertebra and is reproducible with computer assisted simulation.

The thoracic vertebrae are recognized by facets and half-facets for the articulation of the ribs. The pedicles are directed backward and inferiorly, and lamina overlap, delineating a more circular spinal canal. The spinous processes are triangular in appearance and are directed obliquely downward. The articular processes are flat and nearly vertical and the transverse processes appear thickened.

The lumbar vertebrae are the largest segments of the movable vertebral column, and can be distinguished by absence of foramina in the transverse processes, facets on the side of the body, broader pedicles and lamina, and quadrilateral spinous processes. The spinal canal is triangular, larger than the thoracic but smaller than in the cervical region. The superior and inferior articular processes are well defined and respectively project upward and downward from the junctions of the pedicles and lamina. The facets on the superior processes are concave and look backward and medial, while the inferior ones are convex and direct forward and lateral. In the adult, the sacral and coccygeal vertebrae consist of nine united pieces. The sacrum articulates with four bones, the last lumbar vertebra above, the coccyx below, and the hip bones of either side. The female sacrum is shorter and wider than in the male, and the lower half forms a greater angle and curvature than the upper portion, which is relatively straight. It is also directed more obliquely backward, increasing the size of the pelvic cavity and accentuating the sacrovertebral angle. The sacral and coccyx are less prone to the development of intervertebral disk disease.

The spine presents several curves including a convex cervical curve that spans the axis of the odontoid process to the middle of the second thoracic vertebra. The thoracic curvature is concave forward from the second to the middle of the twelfth thoracic vertebra. The lumbar curve spans from the twelfth thoracic to the sacral vertebral angle, with an anterior convexity that is much more pronounced for the third to fifth lumbar vertebra than the upper two. The pelvic curvature commences at the sacral vertebral articulation and ends at the coccyx.

The articulations of the spine consist of slightly movable amphiarthrodial joints between pairs of vertebral bodies. The latter are connected by flattened disks of fibrocartilage which allows for considerable movement when summated over the full entire length of the spinal column, and freely movable diarthrodal joints between neighboring vertebral arches. The anterior and posterior longitudinal ligaments and the intervertebral disks are important in the maintenance of the articulation of the spine. The longitudinal ligaments extend from the anterior and posterior surfaces of the bodies of the vertebrae, from the axis to the sacrum, and broader caudally, thicker in the thoracic region, and opposite the vertebral bodies than against the intervertebral disks. The joints between the articular processes of the vertebrae are enveloped by synovial membranes while the lamina, spinous and transverse processes are connected by the supra-spinal, inter-transverse, inter-spinal ligaments, and ligament flavum, which are thickest in the lumbar region and, through their marked elasticity, preserve the upright posture and enable movement.

The principal muscles that produce flexion of the spine include the sternocleidomastoid, longus capitus, longus coli, scalene, abdominal, and psoas muscles. Extension is possible through the action of intrinsic back muscles assisted by the splenius, semi-spinales, and multifidus. Lateral motion is executed by the instrinsic back muscles assisted by the scalene, quadratus lumborum, and psoas major. Rotation follows contraction of the sternocleidomastoid, longus capitus, scalene, multifidus, semi-spinalis capitis, and abdominals. The articulation of the fifth lumbar vertebra with the sacrum is similar to that of the movable segments of the vertebral column mediated by the anterior and posterior longitudinal ligaments, the intervertebral fibrocartilage disk, and ligament flavum uniting the fifth lumbar to the first sacral vertebra, interspinal, supraspinal, and iliolumbar ligaments.

The intervertebral fibrocartilaginous discs are interposed between adjacent vertebral bodies that vary in shape, size, and thickness, depending upon the vertebra they subserve. Although uniform in a given region, they constitute about one-fourth of the length of the vertebral column. They are adherent to thin layers of hyaline cartilage that cover the upper and under surfaces of the vertebral bodies, and closely apposed to the anterior and posterior longitudinal ligaments. Each disk is circumscribed by lamina of fibrous tissue and fibrocartilage forming the annulus fibrosis. At its center, a soft, pulpy, high-elastic substance, the nucleus pulposus functions as an important shock absorber, which under pressure, becomes flatter and broader, pushing the most resistant fibrous lamina in all directions.

The intervertebral disk functions as a hydrostatic load-bearing structure, with fluid confined in the nucleus pulposus by the inner lamella of the annular fibrosis. The nucleus therein converts axial loading into tensile strain onto annular fibers and the cartilaginous end-plates, although less effectively when the disk begins to degenerate. This hydrostatic property results from a high water composition of 85%. Proteoglycans, enmeshed in a collagen network with its fixed negative charge, imbibes water. The nucleus is richer in proteoglycans than the annulus, inclusive of chondroitin-6-sulfate, keratan sulphate, hyaluronic acid and chrondroitin-4-sulfate.

INFLUENCE OF AGE AND DEGENERATION

The conspicuous changes in disk structure with progressive age, and in experimental disk herniation in animals, include a decrease in water content, increase in the proportion of annular type 1 collagen in the annulus, and a decrease in nuclear proteoglycans. In early childhood, the nucleus pulposus is a gelatinous structure that is sharply demarcated from the surrounding annulus fibrosis, while the annulus consists of inner and outer layers, respectively, of densely packed fibers and fibrocartilage. With age, first the nucleus and annulus become more fibrous with a progressive loss of sharp distinction between the two. Second, fibers of the inner annulus invade the nucleus at the equator of the disk. Third, the outer annulus remains densely fibrous. Fourth, the inner annulus and nucleus form a large central mass devoid of fibrocartilage. Fifth, the water content of the nucleus pulposus and annulus both fall to 70%. Sixth, proteoglycans and collagen, both important disc constituents along with water, also change with increasing age. Type 1 collagen, found in the outermost part of the annulus, increases with age and type 2 collagen increases in content with its greater resistance to compression, especially along the posterior portion of the annulus. The proportion of chondroitin sulfate to keratin sulfate, which is increased in young disks, reverses with age. The proteoglycan content of the nucleus pulposus, which is more than five-fold higher than in the annulus in childhood, decreases with age, with an increase in the ratio of keratan sulphate to chondroitin sulphate. Acid and neutral metalloproteinases that digest proteoglycans in osteoarthritic patellar cartilage due to reduced levels of tissue inhibitor of metalloproteinase, may contribute to the degeneration of human intervertebral disks in some individuals with aging.

Correlative changes using magnetic resonance imaging (MRI) reveal high intensity signals on T_2-weighted images in the nucleus pulposus and a sharp demarcation from the annulus, which classifies it as an immature, type I disk (9). With maturation, this demarcation becomes less distinct and the fibrocartilage of the nucleus and inner annulus becomes less distinct, and the fibrocartilage of both can be differentiated from the low signal of the outer annulus. Transitional or so-called type II disks of adolescence are demarcated by the presence of a fibrous band in the equator of the maturing disk derived from the inner annulus. Adult or type III disks, which predominate after age 20 to 30 years, demonstrates high signal fibrocartilage of the nucleus and inner annulus accompanied by central fibrous tissue degeneration, and low intensity outer annulus signal. Even with aging over eight decades, there is little difference in signal intensities of sequential disk levels unless pathological degeneration supervenes due to injury, leading to changes in the signal intensity accompanied by radial tears, loss of disk space height, stability, and eventual bulging. Posterior annular tears recognized by MRI as high-intensity zones on sagittal T_2-weighted spin echo imaging represent inflammation in the annulus. Full-thickness (Grade 5) and lesser grade annular tears that enhance with intravenous gadolinium, correlate with painful disk degeneration (10, 11). Cryomicrotome sections and MRI imaging of cadaveric specimens have provided additional understanding of disk degeneration (12, 13). Immature (type I) disks reveal that nucleus pulposus and annular fibrosus lack any tears. The transitional (type II) disk reveals occasional concentric tears of the annulus. Adult (type III) disks more commonly have annuli with concentric or transverse tears sparing the nucleus. An early degenerated nucleus pulposus is almost always associated with a radial tear and other types as well. Severely degenerated nucleus pulposus is associated with complete disruption of the annulus. Such findings suggest that not only do disks progress from immature through transitional and adult types as previously discussed, but that radial tears of the annulus and progressive loss of cartilage from the nucleus are the hallmarks of disk degeneration. In the early state, disk height is lost, whereas in late stages, fibrocartilage in the disk is replaced with fluid and dense, disorganized fibrous tissue.

Studies of the relationship of disk degeneration to pain have led to enhanced understanding of the innervation of normal and degenerated disks. Normally, the intervertebral disks are surrounded by a continuous network of interlacing nerve fibers, ventrally by the nerve plexus of the anterior longitudinal ligament and dorsally by the nerve plexus of the posterior longitudinal ligament. At the level of the intervertebral foramina, the anterior and posterior nerve plexuses are interconnected by branches directed medioventrally and mediodorsally termed rami communicants, which overly the lateral border of the disk (14). Contributions to the ventral nerve plexus are delivered by the sympathetic trunk, its rami communicants, and perivascular nerve plexuses of segmental arteries. Cervical sinuvertebral nerves, connected to both the spinal nerve and the sympathetic trunk and its rami communicants, supply the disk at their level of entry as well as the disk above (15). Nerve endings are found in the longitudinal ligaments and in the most superficial layers of the annulus fibrosis. Innervation of the disk has been found to extend as deep as the outer third of the annulus fibrosis Immunohistochemical studies have shown the centripetal growth of nerve fibers in the disk, which provide a morphological basis for true discogenic pain (16). Sensory and autonomic nerve terminals in

herniated lumbar disc tissue that may be involved in the elaboration of pain-specific peptides and inflammatory, tissue repair processes (17).

The inflammatory propensity of nucleus pulposus has been studied in operative specimens removed at surgery (18) and in experimental animals (19). Several patients with symptomatic back pain who underwent anterior spinal fusion and histological analysis of the subjacent vertebral specimens and intervertebral disks, had inflammatory changes in all such specimens. Homogenized autogenous nucleus pulposus was injected into the lumbar epidural space in dogs through an indwelling catheter. Microscopic analysis of the dural sac, spinal cord, and roots showed inflammatory changes which were absent in the control group that received normal saline. In another experimental animal model, the adverse effects on neurophysiological testing, but not histological analysis in animals that received epidural transplants of nucleus pulposus, was reduced by high-dose methylprednisolone (20).

TERMINOLOGY

Rupture of an intervertebral disk, herniation of the nucleus pulposus, lumbar disk prolapse, and slipped disk are equivalent terms for the commonest cause of nerve root pain. The resulting clinical syndromes depend upon the ultimate location of the displaced disk material. Rupture of the disk into the vertebral body endplate leads to a Schmorl node, the most common non-intervertebral disk abnormality, which is generally an incidental finding on MRI, unassociated with focal neurological disease in up to 19% of asymptomatic subjects (21). Extension of the disk material symmetrically and circumferentially beyond the interspace, or focally and asymmetrically with the base of the generally abutting into the canal with a base against the disk of origin broader than any other dimension of the disk extension, defines disk bulge and protrusion. Both can be either pathogenic or incidental findings, respectively, in 52% and 27% of asymptomatic subjects on MRI (22), with increasing defects reported with increasing age in other studies of the cervical and lumbar spine when studied by MRI and computed tomography (23, 24) of questionable significance. Extrusion of an intervertebral disk, which is found in only 1% of individuals without back pain, is virtually always clinically significant (25). It is defined as a more severe extension of the disk material beyond the interspace with the base against the disk of origin narrower than the diameter of the extruding material itself and generally with or without connection to the disk of origin such as occurs with free fragments. Lateral lumbar disk herniation can lead to individual root compression by impingement of the exiting root along the neural foramen with focal radiculopathy. Larger space-occupying extruded disks, and fragments thereof, can compromise the spinal canal and neural foramina with impingement of the thecal sac, spinal cord, and descending roots. The parts of the spine most liable to intervertebral disk rupture include the mid- to lower cervical spine from C5 to C7 at the fulcrum of the cervical curvature above the fixed thoracic region, and in the lower lumbar region at L4-5 and L5-S1 where the leverage is greatest.

Epidemiology

The most detailed epidemiologic data is available for lumbar spine disorders, less so than in disorders of the cervical and thoracic spine. The lifetime prevalence of lumbar spine disease is approximately 80%, and it is the number two reason that patients seek medical attention after the common cold. Overall, the rate of disability from low back pain and related lumbar spine disorders has increased by 14-fold the rate of population growth. In comparison, it is estimated that one patient in a million experiences thoracic disk herniation (26) or 0.2 to 5% of all intervertebral disks are attributable to thoracic disk rupture (27), with only 24 and 17% of reported patients experiencing sensory or motor changes, respectively (28). A number of variables correlate specifically with spinal disorders, including poor general health, obesity, angina pectoris, calf pain, breathlessness on exertion, smoking, physical activity at work and during leisure time, feelings of worry and tension, fatigue at the end of the day, and perception of stress although their causal role is inconclusive (29, 30). Four variables, calf pain on exertion, smoking, high physical activity at work, and worry and tension appear to have the strongest association with later spinal disorders (29). Hard physical work, in particular, frequent lifting and postural stress, are the most likely lifestyle issues to result in disk degeneration, low back pain, and sciatica (30). Most intervertebral disk ruptures occur when activity is at its height, uncommonly before age 20 and/or after age 70 years, unless there is a history of significant trauma. Among 600 intervertebral postmortem specimens from infancy to 90 years of age, graded from normal (grade I) to the earliest (grade II) or progressively severe macroscopic changes in the nucleus pulposus and annular fibrosus (grade III and IV) (disks from men were more degenerated overall than those from women across the second, fifth, sixth, and seventh decades. On average, L4-5 and L3-4 level disks were the most degenerated (31), however, clinical experience suggests preferential involvement at the L5-S1 level. The onset of low back disorders commences in men almost a decade before women, peaking at about 27 years.

Clinical Presentation

Acute cervical disk rupture is generally suggested by the presence of stiff neck and muscle spasm that prevents normal turning of the head, with pain and paresthesia that radiates upward to the temples, down one or both arms, and across the chest in a radicular manner. Symptoms worsen with voluntary movement of the neck toward the side of the disk rupture due to further narrowing the neural foramen. Although reports may vary regarding the incidence of each root, most authorities agree that C7 radiculopathy accounts for up to 70% of all cervical lesions, with an incidence of 25% for C6, 10% for C8, and 5% for C5. The clinical expression of an individual root lesion conforms to recognized patterns of myotomal muscular weakness, dermatomal sensory loss, and segment referred pain, and hypoactive tendon stretch reflexes.

Rupture of an intervertebral thoracic disk is uncommon with a frequency of 0.75% of all herniated disks, with peak incidence in the fourth decade, and most occurring below T8. Pain, often intractable at times and localized to the back and torso, is the most common initial symptom followed by sensory and motor disturbance. By the time of diagnosis, almost 90% of patients have signs of spinal cord compression, however, that depends upon the level of occurrence in the thoracic column. In the upper third of the thoracic spine, T1-2 disk herniation is the most common level with a lateral disk location responsible for T1 radiculopathy and central disk location leading to myelopathy. The clinical features of T1 radiculopathy differ from C8 root compression in the involvement of intrinsic hand muscles, hand paresthesia, medial arm and shoulder pain, Horner syndrome of oculo sympathetic paralysis, and diminished sensation in the axilla. The heterogeneity of thoracic disk rupture is particularly evident at the thoracic-lumbar junction wherein those with T10-11 and T11-12 disk herniation manifest moderate lower extremity weakness, increased patellar tendon reflexes, and sensory disturbances of the entire leg, with bowel and bladder dysfunction due to upper motor involvement associated with spinal cord, conus, and cauda equina compression.

Lumbar radiculopathy due to intervertebral disk rupture is typically episodic with remissions and exacerbations. Sciatica, defined as pain along the distribution of the sciatic nerve from the buttock along the leg to the heel, big toe or ankle associated with prior physical trauma, is aggravated by Valsalva maneuver, coughing, sneezing, straining on the toilet, heavy lifting, excessive bending and twisting. Most patients equate the time of disk rupture with the onset of intense pain, sensory and motor symptoms, and even a popping sound in the spine. Muscular spasm and root irritation leads to muscular spasm often without a comfortable position. Neurological examination shows loss of the normal lumbar curve, asymmetrical long erector muscle spasm, and splinting. There is reduced flexion and rotation at the waist, and limited passive straight leg that evokes back and leg pain on the affected side. Palpation of the spine may reveal tenderness and erythema along the spine and discomfort with firm pressure over the sciatic notch. Fasciculation is common in a myotomal distribution, and paresthesia, numbness, and sensory loss occur in a dermatomal distribution, even though the dorsal root and ganglia are not directly compressed.

History and Examination

The history should be directed toward identifying the onset and precipitants of disk rupture, concomitant medical and psychosocial factors that may prolong pain and disability, including depression, narcotic and other substance abuse, contemplated or active litigation, disability compensation, work dissatisfaction, social withdrawal, and the expectation of benefit from passive rather than active treatment and intervention (32). Even though many individuals will identify a suspected injury, potentially serious and rare medical disorders occur in those at high risk, leading to a more serious spinal disorder. Concomitant cancer may be suggested by a history of cancer, unexplained weight loss, advanced age, and lymphadenopathy. Concomitant infection is supported by fever, chills, recent infection, immunosuppression, and intravenous injections. Inflammatory arthritis should be suspected at any age with morning stiffness, gradual onset, and slow improvement with exercise. Painful bone fractures occur with advanced age, significant trauma, history of osteoporosis, and corticosteroid use (32). It is useful to consider the presence of a predisposing or contributing genetic disorder such as achondroplasia, osteochondritis juvenilis, and Marfan syndrome with widespread skeletal abnormalities. The sequela of osteoarthritis, including facet arthropathy, spondylosis, spondylolisthesis, annular defects, and stenosis of the central canal and neural foramen, namely, may contribute but rarely simulates, rupture of an intervertebral disk.

The examination should focus on identifying focal motor, sensory, and reflex dysfunction and the presence and level of myotomal and dermatomal root involvement. Several maneuvers can be performed with the intended usefulness of screening for nerve root irritation such as the crossed, uncrossed, and reverse straight-leg raising test and femoral tension sign.

Lesions of the C5 and C6 roots which resemble lesions of the upper trunk and lateral cord of the brachial plexus, may be mistaken for neuralgic amyotrophy when there is involvement of one or more proximal and distal peripheral nerves, including the supra-scapular, axillary, dorsal scapular, and musculocutaneous nerves with referred pain. Intervertebral disk disease involving the C6 and C7 roots can be mistaken for middle trunk, posterior cord, or carpal tunnel syndromes, depending upon the relative contribution of radial or median middle trunk fibers, which diverge in the posterior or lateral cord to innervate distal, radial, and forearm median muscles, respectively. A C8 radiculopathy may resemble a lower trunk, medial cord lesion, or neurogenic thoracic outlet syndrome due to an abnormal cervical rib, as can ulnar mononeuropathy and combined lesions of the median and ulnar nerves, further elucidated by detailed electrodiagnostic studies. Non-neuropathic disorders simulating cervical radiculopathy include supra-spinatus tendonitis, acromio-clavicular joint disease, ipsilateral rotator cuff tear, and focal injury of myotomal muscles and their ligaments.

The differential diagnosis of lumbar radiculopathy depends upon the level of proposed involved roots. Lesions of L2, L3 and L4 have extensive overlap and motor weakness is typically encountered in the quadriceps, thigh adductors, and iliacus, also innervated by the lumbar plexus, femoral and obturator nerves. Both L5 and S1 radiculopathy occur in association with traumatic sacral plexopathy, sciatic mononeuropathy, and ischemic mononeuropathy multiplex, all of which may be exquisitely painful at onset. An L5 root disorder may be confused with common fibular neuropathy at the fibular head as a cause of footdrop due to axonal loss or, less often, demyelinating conduction block further distinguished by detailed electrodiagnostic studies. Finally, the hallmark of lumbar stenosis is neurogenic intermittent claudication, often associated with disabling back pain, spasm, and stiffness in the hips, thighs, and legs after walking a short distance, relieved by sitting or flexing the lumbar spine, often with variable electrodiagnostic features and a coexisting pathogenic or incidental multilevel disk herniation, spondylolisthesis, and arthritic disease.

LABORATORY EVALUATION

Neuroimaging

Plain radiographs with anteroposterior and lateral views of the spine are appropriate in patients with back pain due to spinal fracture; however, they are not useful in the diagnosis of rupture of an intervertebral disk. Suspected patients should undergo advanced neuroimaging. In years past, myelography with CT was the procedure of choice for the diagnosis of disk rupture because it allowed examination of the entire spinal canal, and dynamic changes that occur with standing, flexion, and extension, as well as analysis of CSF. Most neuroradiologists favor MRI as the best screening procedure in disorders of the spine based upon its superior ability to detect paravertebral soft tissue abnormalities, osteomyelitis, intradural and root pathology, and most inflammatory, malignant, and vascular etiologies of back pain (33). Notwithstanding, a consequence of the high sensitivity of advanced neuroimaging procedures is the high prevalence of abnormalities, even in asymptomatic individuals, which may then lead to confusion.

ELECTRODIAGNOSTIC STUDIES

Conventional electromyography (EMG) and nerve conduction studies (NCS) are indispensable in the localization and prognosis of radiculopathy due to rupture of an intervertebral disk (34). With the exception of H responses, the sensory axons of most roots are unavailable for study with conventional NCS and are, therefore, typically normal. Significant alteration of evoked compound muscle action potential (CMAP) are infrequent, even in an affected myotome because of collateral sprouting and the innervation of most muscles by more than one segment. Weakness in conjunction with intervertebral disc rupture is classically recognized by demyelinative conduction block, axonal degeneration, or both. Paraspinal spontaneous activity in adjacent paraspinal muscles, the finding of which adds precision to the localization of the involved roots, especially single root lesions (35), also increases in prevalence with advancing age among asymptomatic subjects (36).

Nerve Root Stimulation

Direct stimulation of the cervical and lumbar roots is performed in selected patients, especially those with mild radicular lesions when routine EMG and NCS are normal or equivocal. The cervical roots are stimulated by monopolar needles inserted into paraspinal muscles, and recording CMAP in the biceps, triceps, abductor digiti minimi muscles. Among 16 subjects with symptoms but no signs of radiculopathy, EMG was abnormal in 31% and cervical root stimulation was abnormal in 56% (37). Conduction in the fourth and fifth lumbar and first sacral nerve roots has been performed for more than three decades (38). Similar to cervical root stimulation, a concentric needle electrode is inserted into the spinal canal and directed away from the midline of the back to rest extrathecally, either between the spinal processes of L3 and L4 to stimulate the fourth lumbar nerve root or between L4 and L5 to evoke the fifth lumbar root. Similarly a needle electrode inserted between L5 and S1 to evoke a response from the first sacral nerve, recording respectively from the tibialis anterior, extensor hallicus longus, and the soleus-gastrocnemius muscles.

Somatosensory Evoked Potentials

Cutaneous nerve and dermatomal somatosensory evoked responses of the arms and legs at stimulation sites chosen to most closely approximate activation of a single dermatome often show normal latency with abnormal amplitude reduction reflecting conduction block in sensory fibers when sensory deficits predominate in affected individuals (39). However, the observed morphological and amplitude changes are often difficult to quantify owing to the excessive normal variability, making the studies of questionable usefulness in the routine electrophysiological evaluation of radiculopathy. Somatosensory evoked potentials have been used intraoperatively for the presence of certain near field responses, which when altered, may guide surgery involving the proximal roots.

Magnetic Stimulation

Surface stimulation by a magnetic coil is a potentially useful technique for non-invasive evaluation of the cervical and lumbosacral roots (40). A reduction of CMAP amplitudes after proximal stimulation suggests conduction block at the proximal level. However, the drawbacks include the difficulty in failing to locate the roots with sufficient precision and the inherent inaccuracy of distance measurements between sites of stimulation and recording, making latency measurements to the onset of the evoked CMAP in the appropriate muscles more reliable than conduction velocity. One study noted no statistical differences between magnetic stimulation and electrical stimulation of cervical spinal nerves among six normal volunteers; however, there was increased discomfort with magnetic stimulation, especially at C5-6, when compared with monopolar needle stimulation (41).

TREATMENT

Conservative Management

Physicians must decide the management of patients with rupture or herniation of an intervertebral disk from among the many available conservative and invasive therapeutic measures. Most authorities agree that as long as there is no evidence of neurological compromise, most patients can be managed conservatively with oral analgesics, muscle relaxants, steroidal, and non-steroidal anti-inflammatory medications to reduce pain, inflammation, and muscle spasm. At the same time, an effort should be undertaken to initiate a multidisciplinary program combining physical rehabilitation, psychological, behavioral, and education interventions. Nonsteroidal anti-inflammatory drugs, acetaminophen, and cyclo-oxygenase-2-selective agents are all equally effective in the initial treatment of low back pain (42), although the latter have fewer side effects. Individuals with pain caused by acute disk rupture will generally require the addition of a muscle relaxant such as cyclobenzaprine, 10 mg twice daily, and a narcotic analgesic for clearly defined periods, typically up to two weeks. Although there is a clear scientific rationale for the use of six-day tapering methylprednisolone administered as a six-day tapering dose pack, the evidence in support of it is still mainly circumstantial and anecdotal. Although bedrest remains a common recommendation for those with acute radicular pain from a disk rupture, more proactive approaches have emerged (43) that incorporate low-stress, aerobic activity early in the course such a walking, avoidance of sitting or standing postures, and taking care to rise or sit down slowly (44). A referral to physical therapy is often met with increased levels of patient satisfaction compared with strict physician-directed care (45, 46). Specific back exercises should be reserved for the prevention of future episodes, and may worsen symptoms during the acute period of disk rupture (47). There is additionally no evidence to support the regular use of lumbar supports, braces, corsets, spinal traction, acupuncture, or transcutaneous electrical nerve stimulation for acute pain associated with disk rupture with or without radicular involvement.

Anesthetic and Corticosteroid Injections

Anesthetic and corticosteroid medication can be injected under fluoroscopy, delivering a higher concentration of medication in a relatively smaller volume to the site of anticipated pathology at the interface of the posterior annulus of the disk and the ventral aspect of the nerve root sleeve. A curved 25-gauge 6-inch spinal needle is advanced in the direction of a triangular area delineated on top by the pedicle, at the base along the exiting nerve root, and along the lateral border by the vertebral body. One to 2 cc of contrast can be injected to check for free flow before injection of the anesthetic corticosteroid mixture. Epidural corticosteroid injections should have little expectation of providing more than short-term benefit at best in the pain associated with mechanical root compression due to disk extrusion (48). Overall, up to 75% of patients can be expected to experience greater than 50% sustained improvement in pain. Selected patients with refractory cervical disk may be candidates for epidural steroid injection; however, the expected long-term outcome of less than 50% relief in pain by six months suggests that it offers no more assurance of benefit than a six-day oral methylprednisolone dose pack.

Surgical Interventions

Forty RCT and two quasi-RCT have assessed the effect of surgical intervention for the treatment of lumbar disk prolapse (49). The primary rationale of any form of disk surgery is to relieve nerve root irritation or compression due to herniated disk material, but the results should be balanced against the likely natural history, and the long-term impact which is unclear. The absolute indications for surgery include altered bladder function and progressive muscle weakness, however surgical intervention may also be considered in those with large compressive disc ruptures. Painful radiculopathy refractory to conservative management, in association with persistent weakness, sensory loss, and reflex change due to focal root or cauda equina compression are surgical indications because the risk of permanent neurological deficit increases if left untreated. Notwithstanding, most patients and physicians proceed to surgery to provide rapid relief of pain and disability in the minority of patients whose recovery is unacceptably slow. Of the available techniques open discectomy performed with or without an operating microscope is probably the most common, with automated percutaneous discectomy and arthroscopic microdiscectomy to promote faster patient recovery and earlier hospital discharge (50, 51). A trial of discectomy in the treatment of sciatica due to intervertebral disk herniation found discectomy was significantly better than conservative management at one year, without significant differences in outcome at four and ten years (52). The multicenter Spine Patient Outcomes Research Trial (53) comparing open discectomy with nonoperative treatment individualized to the patient, favored surgery however, treatment effects on primary outcome measures were small and statistically insignificant. Fusion, in addition to discectomy, offered no advantage over discectomy alone (54).

Most cervical disk herniations regress with time without the need for surgical resection. A prospective study with repeat MRI showed regression of cervical intervertebral disk herniation in 12 of 13 patients who presented with cervical radiculopathy in whom pain was controlled by epidural corticosteroid injection and analgesic medication (55). Surgical intervention should be avoided with adequate pain control allowing the herniation time to regress. Maigne and coworkers (56) investigated cervical radiculopathy due to intervertebral disk herniation among 21 patients with CT at the first onset of the disorder, and at followup one to 30 months later. All 21 disk herniations demonstrated relative decrease in size, with the larger herniation showing the greatest tendency to decrease in size. When surgery is deemed necessary, modified microsurgical discectomy, with removal of all compressive disk fragments and osteophytes and only partial removal of the posterior ligament, is the procedure of choice for symptomatic intervertebral disk disease (57). Cervical spondylotic myelopathy (CSM) warrants special consideration as to the role and timing of surgery (58), with patients younger than age 75 and stable, mild-to-moderate CSM managed conservatively. Abnormal low signal on T_1-weighted MRI and high signal on T_2-weighted images suggesting cord atrophy on preoperative scanning are an indication of poor outcome.

With over 90% of thoracic disk herniation classified as contralateral, the transpedicular and transfacet pedicle-sparing approaches are simpler than anterolateral transthoracic and lateral extracavitary approaches, facilitating a true lateral exposure (59). Extensive muscle dissection, thoracotomy, rib removal, chest tube placement, significant postoperative pain, and vascular compromise to the spinal cord resulting from possible disruption of the artery of Adamkiewicz can occur when the contents of the neural foramina, including the major radicular artery, are disrupted and sacrificed. Nonetheless, the overall outcome of surgery is favorable in the majority of patients, with improvement noted in 87% of radicular pain, 95% in spasticity, 84% in sensory changes, 76% in bowel and bladder dysfunction, and 58% in muscle strength. Lumbar discectomy continues to be the preferred procedure for uncomplicated intervertebral disk rupture, however, fusion may be inadequate when there is more than one level, complicating degenerative factors, revision surgery, or spinal stenosis.

RFERENCES

1. Fehlings MG, Arvin B. Surgical management of cervical degenerative disease: the evidence related to indications, impact, and outcome. *J Neurosurg Spine* 2009; 11:97–100.
2. Gibson JN, Waddell G. Surgical interventions for lumbar disc prolapse. *Spine* 2007; 32:1735–1747.
3. Manchikanti L, Boswell MV, Singh V, et al and ASIPP-IPM. Comprehensive evidence-based guidelines for interventional techniques in the management of chronic spinal pain. *Pain Physician* 2009; 12:699–802.
4. Goldthwait JE. The lumbosacral articulation: an explanation of many cases of "lumbago," "sciatica," and paraplegia. Boston. *M&SJ* 1911; 164:365–372.
5. Middletown GS, Teacher JH. Injury of the spinal cord due to rupture of an intervertebral disk during muscular effort. *Glasgow MJ* 1911; 76:1–6.
6. Dandy WE. Loose cartilage from intervertebral disk simulating tumor of the spinal cord. *Arch Surg* 1929; 19:660–672.
7. Mixter WJ, Barr JS. Rupture of the intervertebral disc with involvement of the spinal canal. *N Engl J Med* 1934; 211:210–215.
8. Denaro V, Di Martino A. Cervical spine surgery. An historical perspective. *Clin Orthop Relat Res* 2011; 469:639–648.
9. Sether LA, Yu Shiwei, Haughton VM. Intervertebral disk: normal age-related changes in MR signal intensity. *Radiology* 1990; 177:385–388.
10. Saifuddin A, Braithwaite I, White J, et al. The value of lumbar spine magnetic resonance imaging in the demonstration of annular tears. *Spine* 1998; 23:453–457.
11. Aprill C, Bogduk N. High-intensity zone: a diagnostic sign of painful lumbar disc on magnetic resonance imaging. *British Journal of Radiology* 1992; 65:361–369.
12. Yu S, Haughton VM, Sether LA, et al. Criteria for classifying normal and degenerated lumbar intervertebral disks. *Radiology* 1989; 170:523–526.
13. Yu S, Haughton VM, Lynch KL, et al. Fibrous structure in the intervertebral disk: correlation of MR appearance with anatomic sections. *AJNR* 1989; 10:1105–1110.
14. Groen GH, Baljet B, Drukker J. Nerves and nerve plexuses of the human vertebral column. *Am J Anat* 1990; 188:282–296.
15. Bogduk N, Windsor M, Inglis A. The innervation of the cervical intervertebral discs. *Spine* 1988; 13:2–8.
16. Coppes MH, Marani E, Thomeer RTWM, et al. Innervation of "painful" lumbar discs. *Spine* 1997; 22:2342–2350.
17. Palmgren T, Gronblad M, Virri J, et al. Immunohistochemical demonstration of sensory and autonomic nerve terminals in herniated lumbar disc tissue. *Spine* 1996; 21:1301–1306.
18. Jaffray D, O'Brien JP. Isolated intervertebral disc resorption. A source of mechanical and inflammatory back pain? *Spine* 1986; 11:397–401.
19. McCarron RF, Wimpee MW, Hudkins PG, et al. The inflammatory effect of nucleus pulposus. A possible element in the pathogenesis of low-back pain. *Spine* 1987; 760–764.
20. Olmarker K, Gyrod G, Cornefjord M, et al. Effects of methylprednisolone on nucleus pulposus-induced nerve root injury. *Spine* 1994; 19:1803–1808.
21. Jensen MC, Brant-Zawadzki MN, Obuchowski N, et al. Magnetic resonance imaging of the lumbar spine in people without back pain. *N Engl J Med* 1994; 331:69–73.
22. Jensen MC, Brant-Zawadzki MN, Obuchowski N, et al. Magnetic resonance imaging of the lumbar spine in people without back pain. *N Engl J Med* 1994; 331:69–73.
23. Boden SD, McCowin PR, Davis DO, et al. Abnormal magnetic-resonance scans of the cervical spine in asymptomatic subjects. *J Bone Joint Surg* 72:1178–1184.
24. Boden SD, Davis DO, Dina TS, et al. Abnormal magnetic-resonance scans of the lumbar spine in asymptomatic subjects. *J Bone Joint Surg* 1990; 72:403–408.
25. Jensen MC, Brant-Zawadzki MN, Obuchowski N, et al. Magnetic resonance imaging of the lumbar spine in people without back pain. *N Engl J Med* 1994; 331:69–73.
26. Carson J, Gumbert J, Jefferson A. Diagnosis and treatment of thoracic intervertebral disc protrusions. *J Neurosurg* 1971; 34:68–77.
27. Stone J, Lichtor T, Banerjee S. Intradural thoracic disc herniation. *Spine* 1994; 19:1281–1284.
28. Arce CA, Dohrmann GJ. Herniated thoracic discs. *Neurosurg Clin* 1985; 3:338–392.
29. Svensson H-O, Vedin A, Wilhelmsson C, et al. Low-back pain in relation to other diseases and cardiovascular factors. *Spine* 1983; 8:277–293.
30. Heliovaara M. Risk factors for low back pain and sciatica. *Ann Med* 1989; 21:257–264.
31. Miller JAA, Schmatz C, Schultz AB. Lumbar disc degeneration: correlation with age, sex, and spine level in 600 autopsy specimens. *Spine* 1988; 13:173–178.
32. Atlas SJ, Nardin RA. Evaluation and treatment of low back pain: an evidence-based approach to clinical care. *Muscle Nerve* 2003; 27:265–284.

33. Modic MT, Masaryk T, Boumphrey F, Goormastic M, et al. Lumbar herniated disk disease and canal stenosis: prospective evaluation by surface coil MR, CT, and myelography. *AJR* 1986; 147:757–765.

34. Wilbourne AS, Aminoff MJ. AAEM minimonograph 32: The electrodiagnostic examination in patients with radiculopathies. *Muscle Nerve* 1998; 1612–1631.

35. Levin KH, Maggiano HJ, Wilbourn AS. Cervical radiculopathies: comparison of surgical and EMG localization of single-root lesions. *Neurology* 1996; 46:1022–1025.

36. Date ES, Mar EY, Bugola MR, et al. The prevalence of lumbar paraspinal spontaneous activity in asymptomatic subjects. *Muscle Nerve* 1996; 19:350–354.

37. Berger AR, Busis NA, Logigian EL, et al. Cervical root stimulation in the diagnosis of radiculopathy. *Neurology* 1987; 37:329–332.

38. Peiris OA. Conduction in the fourth and fifth lumbar and first sacral nerve roots: preliminary communication. *NZ Med J* 1974; 80:502–503.

39. Eisen A, Hoirch M, Moll A. Evaluation of radiculopathies by segmental stimulation and somatosensory evoked potentials. *Can J Neurol Sci* 1983; 10:178–182.

40. Chokroverty S, Sachdeo R, Dilullo J, et al. Magnetic stimulation in the diagnosis of lumbosacral radiculopathy. *J Neurol Neurosurg Psychiatry* 1989; 52:767–772.

41. Evans BA, Daube JR, Litchy WJ. A comparison of magnetic and electrical stimulation of spinal nerves. *Muscle Nerve* 1990; 13:414–420.

42. Van Tulder MW, Scholten RJPM, Koes BW, et al. Non-steroidal anti-inflammatory drugs for low back pain. A systematic review within the framework of the Cochrane Collaboration Back Review Group. *Spine* 2000; 25:2501–2513.

43. Bigos SJ, Bower OR, Braen GR, et al. Acute low back problems in adults. *Clinical practice guidelines no. 14.* Rockville, MD: Department of Health and Human Services; 1994 (AHCPR publication number 95-0642).

44. Malmivaara A, Hakkinen U, Aro T, et al. The treatment of acute low back pain-bed rest, exercise, or ordinary activity? *N Engl J Med* 1995; 332:351–355.

45. Carey TS, Garrett J, Jackman A, et al. The outcomes and costs of care for acute low back pain among patients seen by primary care practitioners, chiropractors, and orthopedic surgeons. *N Engl J Med* 1995; 333:913–917.

46. Cherkin DC, Deyo RA, Battie M, et al. A comparison of physical therapy, chiropractic manipulation, and provision of an educational booklet for the treatment of patients with low back pain. *N Engl J Med* 1998; 339:1021–1029.

47. Malmivaara A, Hakkinen U, Aro T, et al. The treatment of acute low back pain-bed rest, exercise, or ordinary activity? *N Engl J Med* 1995; 332:351–355.

48. Carette S, Leclaire R, Marcoux S, et al. Epidural corticosteroid injections for sciatica due to herniated nucleus pulposus. *N Engl J Med* 1997; 336:1634–1640.

49. Gibson JNA, Waddell G. Surgical interventions for lumbar disc prolapse. *Spine* 2007; 32:1735–1747.

50. Onik G, Mooney V, Maroon JC, et al. Automated percutaneous discectomy: a prospective multi-institutional study. *Neurosurgery* 1990; 2:228–233.

51. Kambin P, Vaccaro A. Arthroscopic microdiscectomy. *Spine* 2003; 3(Suppl 1):60S–64S.

52. Weber H. Lumbar disk herniation: a controlled, prospective study with ten years of observation. *Spine* 1983; 8:131–140.

53. Weinstein JN, Tosteson TD, Lurie JD, et al. Surgical vs nonoperative treatment for lumbar disk herniation. The Spine Outcomes Research Trial (SPORT): a randomized trial. *JAMA* 2006; 296:2451–2459.

54. Turner JA, Ersek M, Herron L, et al. Patient outcomes after lumbar spinal fusions. *JAMA* 1992; 268:907–911.

55. Bush K, Chaudhuri R, Hillier S, et al. The pathomorphological changes that accompany the resolution of cervical radiculopathy. A prospective study with repeat magnetic resonance imaging. *Spine* 1997; 22:183–187.

56. Maigne J-Y, Delingne L. Computed tomographic follow-up study of 21 cases of nonoperatively treated cervical intervertebral soft disc herniation. *Spine* 1994; 19:189–191.

57. Savolainen S, Rinne J, Hernesniemi J. A prospective randomized study of anterior single level disc operations with long-term follow-up: surgical fusion is unnecessary. *Neurosurgery* 1998; 43:51–55.

58. Fehlings MG, Arvin B. Surgical management of cervical degenerative disease: the evidence related to indications, impact, and outcome. *J Neurosurg Spine* 2009; 11:97–100.

59. Stillerman CB, Chen TC, Couldwell WT, et al. Experience in the surgical management of 82 symptomatic herniated thoracic discs and review of the literature. *J Neurosurg* 1998; 88:623–633.

CHAPTER 37

Vitamin B12 (Cobalamin) Deficiency

David S. Younger

Since its first description 150 years ago, deficiency of vitamin B12 or cobalamin is an important cause of treatable neurological injury affecting the brain, spinal cord, and peripheral nerves with prominent motor dysfunction. This chapter reviews the historical, epidemiological, clinical, and histopathologic aspects, followed by a discussion of the etiopathogenesis and management of B12 deficiency in neurological disease.

HISTORICAL ASPECTS

In 1822, Combe (1) described the first case of idiopathic anemia. From 1849 to 1855, Addison associated pallor and asthenia due to pernicious anemia (PA) in 2 papers (2, 3), mentioning only fatty degeneration of a portion of the semilunar ganglion of the solar plexus. In 1872, Biermer (4) employed the term progressive PA for the first time, emphasizing its invariably progressive and lethal course and referred to weakness, giddiness, and palpitation, and capillary hemorrhages in the brain and retina. There was little interest in cases of PA in the Anglican literature until a November 1876 *Medical Times and Gazette* editorial was published or approved entitled, "Pernicious Anaemia, a New Disease." Soon after it became an international pastime to identify new cases, report old ones, and exclude others based on different criteria. Kaher and Pick (5) were credited by Henneberg (6) for pathological description of the long fiber tracts in the posterior and lateral columns leading to combined degeneration in 1878. In 1880, Little (7) described mental depression, neuralgic pains, and muscular weakness in association with PA. In 1884, Lichtenstern (8) reported two patients with progressive PA in tabes,

later described by Gowers in 1886 (9) as ataxic paraplegia, separating it from PA. It was suggested that Lichtenstern's patients may in fact have had PA, not tabes (10). In 1887, Lichtheim (11) reported several patients with anemia, ataxia, and paresthesia due to spinal cord disease associated with anemia. By 1991, Dana (12), Putnam (13), Von Noorden (14), and Stewart (15) published the clinical and pathological features of quite similar patients with mental, sensory, and motor deficits that eventuated in enfeeblement, spastic paralysis, and profound anemia. Postmortem examination showed lateral and posterior sclerosis and softening of the cervicothoracic spinal cord. Russell (16) hesitated in separating the patients with pernicious anemia and spinal pathology associated with tabes, primary lateral sclerosis, and Friedreich ataxia that also manifested combined degeneration of posterior and lateral columns, a view that was later amended (17) by affixing the term *subacute*, to *combined degeneration*, and emphasizing the different time course of PA.

Several influential publications at the turn of the century described the clinical and histopathologic changes in the central nervous system (18–23), including some that emphasized symptoms and signs implicating lesions in the brain (24, 25) and peripheral nerves (10, 17, 26–28).

Several important advances ushered in modern understanding of PA, subacute combined degeneration, and B12 deficiency. First, Ehrlich and colleagues (29) discovered the value of aniline dyes for staining blood smears and bone marrow specimens that was later applied to the detection of megaloblastic changes in nucleated red cells in patients with PA. Later, Hurst (30) recognized the etiological role of achylia gastrica in PA and emphasized the constancy of a lack of hydrochloric acid in the stomach and its persistence during spontaneous clinical remissions. This was followed by dramatic successes in some patients with hematological and neurological sequela of PA to liver feeding that suggested some type of nutritional or metabolic defect (31–35).

In a series of experiments, Castle and coworkers (36–38) identified intrinsic factor (IF) secreted by active normal gastric mucosa, not present in detectable amounts in the gastrointestinal tract of patients with PA. If interacted with an extrinsic factor present in beef muscle leading to clinical improvement and reticulocytosis as noted previously with liver feeding. There was an equivalent efficacy in red blood cell formation of purified injectable liver extract given by mouth as 1 ug of cyanocobalamin in 10 ml of gastric juice, but not to a similar extent as the same amount given by injection, demonstrating vitamin B12 as the extrinsic factor. It was inferred that the essential physiological action of IF was to enhance the assimilation of extrinsic factor in the form of B12 (39).

One other important milestone was the availability of radioactive B12 and the enhanced absorption of radioactive B12 (40) that could be demonstrated, whether or not the patient was anemic. The distal ileum was the site of assimilation of vitamin B12 complex with intrinsic factor (41), and explained its deficiency with ileal resection.

ETIOPATHOGENESIS

Concurrent with the explosion of immunological methodology, Taylor and colleagues (42, 43) reported circulating antibodies to IF and gastric parietal cells and their reactive antigens. As presently understood, PA is the end stage of type A chronic atrophic autoimmune gastritis that results from a humoral and T-cell-mediated attack on the 100-kh catalytic alpha subunit of gastric parietal cells, and the 60 to 90-kh glycoprotein beta unit of the enzyme H+/K+-ATPase, which regulates secretion of hydrogen ions by parietal cells (44, 45, 46, 47).

The chemical pathophysiology depends upon the action of two enzymes, methyl cobalamin and adenosyl cobalamin, which are essential, for the synthesis of methionine and succinyl-coenzyme A. Disruption of the cytoplasmic enzymatic reaction involved in methionine synthesis results in a disturbance in *de novo* synthesis of DNA leading to impaired hematopoiesis resulting in the hematologic manifestations of B12 deficiency, as well as abnormalities of gastrointestinal endothelium. Impairment of the mitochondrial succinyl coenzyme A enzymatic reaction leads to alternation in the generation of fatty acids necessary for peripheral nerve myelin metabolism.

MURINE MODEL OF PERNICIOUS ANEMIA

Recognition of experimental autoimmune gastritis in mice led to some interesting speculations regarding the etiopathogenesis of PA in humans (48–51). Thymectomy or cyclosporine treatment of two- to-four day old BALB/c mice, thymectomy of adult mice combined with cyclophosphamide treatment or irradiation, or immunization of adult mice with gastric H+/K+-ATPase resulted in autoimmune gastritis. Like the human counterpart, there was submucosal infiltration of mononuclear cells extending into the lamina propria with loss of acid secreting gastric parietal cells, and pepsinogen-secreting zymogenic cells. The mononuclear cells in early lesions were predominantly macrophages and CD4 T-cells producing a mixture of Th1-type and Th2-type cytokines, and reactive to H+/K+-ATPase present in regional gastric lymph nodes. Serum autoantibodies to gastric H+/K+-ATPase were present, and transfer of infiltrating CD4 T-cells into native mice resulted in gastritis and serum autoantibodies to gastric H+/K+-ATPase, whereas autoantibodies and CD8 T-cells did not appear to be fundamental to the genesis of gastritis. Interestingly, transgenic expression of the beta subunit of the gastric H+/K+-ATPase in the thymus of BALB/c mice prevented the development of experimental gastritis, suggesting that pathogenic T-cells could be rendered tolerant after encountering the beta subunit in the thymus. Murine autoimmune gastritis only occurs when pathogenic T-cells are transferred to immunocompromised mice. Pathogenic T-cells, therefore, appear to be resting; and the mechanisms that govern their activation and expansion and homing to the stomach in normal individuals remains unknown.

CLINICAL PRESENTATION OF B12 DEFICIENCY

Cole (52), Healton and coworkers (53) extensively reviewed the neurological manifestations of B12 deficiency. Six well-described neurological syndromes associated with B12 deficiency occur alone or together, including peripheral neuropathy, myelopathy, alteration of mental status, optic neuropathy, paresthesia without abnormal neurological findings on examination, and symptoms due to either myelopathy or neuropathy. In general, PA accounts for more than three- quarters of patients with B12 deficiency, followed by tropical sprue, gastric and ileal resection, jejunal diverticula and dietary deficiency.

Paresthesia and numbness are the commonest initial symptoms noted in up to one-half of patients, followed by gait ataxia, leg weakness, impaired dexterity, memory loss, and dysautonomic bladder, rectal, and orthostasis. At first presentation, the syndrome of B12 deficiency may be mistaken for spinal cord compression, amyotrophic lateral sclerosis, diabetic, alcoholic and idiopathic peripheral neuropathy, and Alzheimer disease.

Symptoms and signs attributable to neuropathy or myelopathy were the most common neurological syndrome so noted in 41% of patients in the series by Healton and colleagues (53), clinically characterized by impaired proprioceptions, non-segmental diminished vibratory sensation, postural hypotension, urinary and fecal incontinence, and impotence. Peripheral neuropathy, so noted in 25% of patients, manifested variable non-segmental distal cutaneous sensory loss, limb weakness, and hypo- or areflexia. Paresthesia without abnormal neurological examination was noted in 14% of patients reported as prickling, tingling, burning, and numbness of the feet. Myelopathy, so noted in 12% of patients, typically presented with spastic paraparesis accompanied by Babinski signs, hyperreflexia, and dysautonomia. One patient had optic neuropathy, evidenced by central visual impairment without optic atrophy. Altered mental status, cognitive impairment, or dementia was present in up to 47% of patients as determined by standardized neuropsychological and bedside tests of mental function. Other symptoms of reversible dyautonomia, include symptomatic bronchospasm, bladder disturbances, and cardiac arrhythmias leading to frank autonomic failure.

LABORATORY DIAGNOSIS

All patients with suspected B12 deficiency should undergo detailed hematological evaluation with peripheral blood smear and bone marrow examination prior to vitamin therapy for anemia, increased macrocytosis, and hypersegmented neutrophils. Serial hematological studies may bear no relation to the onset of neurological symptoms. The mean corpuscular volume (MCV) may remain normal, remain unchanged, or worsen for months and years before anemia develops. Folic acid treatment leads to hematological improvement while neurological symptoms progress. A serum cobalamin level of less than 200 pg/ml by microbiologic and radioassay is strongly associated with neurological involvement. Lindenbaum and coworkers (54) noted involvement of the nervous system and hematopoietic system despite normal cobalamin levels in 5.2% of patients with recognized cobalamin deficiency, as evidenced by neurotrophic hypersegmentation, macro ovalocytes, megaloblastic bone marrow changes in an aspirate specimen, significantly increased MCV, elevated serum methylmalonic acid and total homocysteine concentrations, and clinical and laboratory response to therapy. Not infrequently, patients with cobalamin deficiency may be encountered in whom only one of the two metabolite concentrations are high. Although the serum methylmalonic acid generally correlates well with serum total homocysteine; however, both may be elevated by renal failure and intravascular volume depletion. The metabolic byproduct, proprionic acid, derived from enteric microflora, can contribute to the total amount of methylmalonic acid that is generated in association with cobalamin deficiency. Suppression of gut flora can lower serum cobalamin levels and necessitate parenteral therapy in patients at risk for intestinal malabsorption.

Serological studies are invaluable in the diagnosis and management of patients with PA. Serum antibodies to gastric parietal cells can be detected in about 90% of patients with PA, as well as by indirect immunofluorescence in 30% of non-anemic first-degree relatives, and in those with autoimmune endocrinopathy. There are two types of antibodies to IF: type I autoantibodies that block the binding of vitamin B12 to IF, demonstrable in 70% of patients with PA, and type II that bind to a site remote from the B12 binding site, detected in about 35 to 40% of patients, rarely though in the absence of the first type. Both types of antibodies can be detected more frequently in gastric juice than in the serum. Serum gastrin may be elevated due to sparing of the antrum and stimulation of gastrin-producing cells by achlorhydria. A low serum pepsinogen I concentration results from destruction of chief cells of the stomach.

Neurological diagnostic studies should be appropriate to the neurological syndrome but not so restrictive when the diagnosis of cobalamin deficiency is known as to exclude an alternative underlying pathogenic process such as autoimmune peripheral neuropathy, multiple sclerosis, compressive spinal disease, occult neoplasm, infection, and endocrinopathy. In addition, PA may be associated with autoimmune endocrinopathies and anti-receptor autoimmune diseases, including chronic autoimmune Hashimoto thyroiditis, insulin-dependent diabetes mellitus, Addison disease, primary ovarian failure, primary hyperparathyroidism, Graves' disease, vitiligo, myasthenia gravis, and the Lambert-Eaton myasthenic syndrome, all of which have specific clinical and laboratory features.

Electromyography and nerve conduction studies (EMG-NCS) should be obtained in all patients with sensory symptoms to establish the presence or absence of neuropathy. Peripheral neuropathy is usually sensorimotor of either acute or insidious onset, with predominant axonal features in three-quarters of patients and demyelinating in one-quarter (55), or isolated sensory axonal (56). An evidenced-based review (57) suggested mandatory screening for B12 with its metabolite methylmalonic acid, with or without hemocyteine, in any patient with distal symmetric polyneuropathy. Autonomic neurophysiological studies should be performed in those with suspected autonomic dysfunction and abnormal hemodynamics (58, 59). Lumbar cerebrospinal fluid (CSF) analysis is generally unrevealing in subacute combined degeneration.

Magnetic resonance imaging (MRI) of the spine in patients with cobalamin deficiency reveals variable abnormalities, including increased T_2-weighted signal in the posterior columns of the cervical and thoracic cord, swelling on T_1-weighted images, enhancement of posterior columns and lateral columns on post-contrast T_1-weighted imaging, and increased signal on T_2-weighted imaging in the posterior columns, with variable involvement of the lateral and anterior columns (60). Complete partial resolution and improvement of MRI abnormalities have all been described, suggesting the presence of reversible demyelination and irreversible axonal degeneration in spinal lesions (61, 62, 63, 64). T_2-weighted MRI of the brain in one reported patient (65) showed extensive areas of high-intensity signal in the periventricular white matter. Although there is no precedent for other studies, there may be a rationale for consideration of electroencephalography, cerebral MR angiography, brain single photon emission computed tomography (SPECT) and positron emission tomography (PET) in carefully selected patients. Recent studies (66) suggest a correlation between brain MRI measures of total brain volume (TBV) and white matter hyperintensity volume (WMHV), and global cognition in multiple domains in relation to vitamin B12 status, but not in relation to cerebral infarcts. These findings lend support to the contention that poor vitamin B12 status is a risk factor for brain atrophy and possibly WMHV, which in turn may contribute to cognitive impairment. Mini Mental State Examination (MMSE) is a useful bedside tool to assess cognitive impairment in B12 deficiency, which typically includes impairment of attention span, memory, abstraction, fund of knowledge, and alteration of mood and behavior (67).

Gastrointestinal evaluation includes gastric biopsy to detect type A chronic atrophy gastritis, direct assay for pentagastrin-resistant total achlorhydria, and screening for intestinal and gastric cancer. The risk of adenocarcinoma increases with biopsy-proven intestinal metaplasia, as does carcinogenic nitrosoamines in association with achlorhydria and intestinal overgrowth. There is an increased risk of gastric carcinoma, as well as gastric carcinoid tumors due to hypergastrinemia and the trophic action of gastrin. The estimated risk of gastric carcinoma in Sweden among those with pernicious anemia increased three-fold, while that of gastric carcinoid tumors was 13-fold higher than the general population (68).

Genetic factors may contribute to congenital and acquired PA. A genetic predisposition has been suggested by the clustering of the disease and gastric autoantibodies in pedigrees, and the association of the disease and gastric antibodies with autoimmune endocrinopathy, which may also be related to human leukocyte antigens (HLA) on chromosome 6. About 20% of the relatives of patients with PA have a similar affection. These relatives, especially first-degree women, also have a higher incidence of gastric auto-antibodies. Concordance with respect to PA was observed in 12 sets of monozygotic twins (69). There are also patients with juvenile PA with onset in late childhood or adolescence and clinical findings identical to those of adults (70). There is an isolated lack of IF secretion unassociated with lack of acid and pepsin, and without histological evidence of gastritis or anti-parietal cell or anti-IF antibodies (70, 71).

Nonetheless, except for its rare advent in adolescence (70), the onset of PA and the neurological complications is usually delayed until middle or later life, reflecting the increased incidence of achlorhydria, chronic gastritis, and parietal cell antibody after middle age.

NEUROPATHOLOGY

The neuropathological features of PA were reported in detail by Pant and coworkers (72). The degree of anemia does not correlate with the severity or rapidity of progression of the neurological disease, which may be insidious, rapidly progressive, or episodic with remissions and exacerbations, even without treatment. Nonetheless, the spinal cord disease correlates with the severity of the clinical disease in most cases.

Pathological changes are frequently encountered in the brain, but are most often the result of conditions other than pernicious anemia, especially in an older patient with cerebrovascular disease. Nonetheless, there may be lesions in periventricular white matter, centrum semiovale, and elsewhere in the deep white matter, often in association with severe myelopathy. Gliotic lesion can occur in the optic nerve and tracts.

In the spinal cord, the histological event that precedes all others is swelling of myelin sheaths, which in early lesions appears as a thin rim of myelin encircling a clear vacuolar space, with each vacuole representing a single axon. Large myelinated axons appear to be preferentially affected. With time, myelinated fiber breakdown appears in the form of lipid-laden macrophages. There is some astrocytic activation and proliferation in early lesions, and a dense isomorphic fibrillary gliosis in chronic lesions. Larger visible lesions result from the coalescence of smaller lesions. Lesions mainly occupy the upper thoracic and lower cervical cord. The posterior columns are affected in every patient, and in some restricted to them, with secondary degeneration in segments of the cord not directly affected by the disease, indicating that axons as well as myelin sheaths have been injured.

The posterior roots show selective fiber loss, with swelling of myelin sheaths similar to the white matter of the cord, with otherwise normal anterior roots and entry zones. The peripheral nerves show variable and patchy large and small myelinated fiber loss. Skeletal muscle can show denervation atrophy. The dorsal root ganglia typically show accumulation of lipofuscin consistent with aging in older patients, without central chromatolysis, cell loss, or residual nodules of Nageotte.

MANAGEMENT

The standard treatment for confirmed PA and cobalamin deficiency is the parenteral administration of adequate amount of vitamin B12 to correct the vitamin deficiency, neurological complications, and anemia, followed by regular monthly intramuscular injection of 1000 ug of vitamin B12.

REFERENCES

1. Combe JS. History of a case of anaema. *Trans Med Chir Soc Edin* 1822; 1:194–204.
2. Addison T. Anaemia, disease of the suprarenal capsules. *London Med Gazette* 1849; 8:517–518.
3. Addison T. Idiopathic anaemia: *On the constitutional and local effects of disease of the suprarenal capsules.* London: Samuel Highley, 1855.
4. Biermer A. Uber eine form von progressiver pernicioser anamie. *Cbl Schweiz Arzte* 1872; 2:15–18.
5. Kahler, Pick. Ueber kombinierte system erkrankung des ruckenmarks. *Arch f Psychiat* 1878; 8:251.
6. Hennenberg R. Die funikulare myelitis und die anamische fokale keukomyelitis. In, *Lewandowsky M. Hanbuch der Neurologie,* Berlin, Julius Springer, 1911; 2:769.
7. Little HW. Progressive pernicious anemia, a disease of the vasomotor system. *Med Rec* 1880; 16:313–315.
8. Lichtenstern O. Progressive perniciose anamie bei tabeskranken. *Keutsch Med Wchnschr* 1884; 10:849.
9. Gowers WD. Clinical lecture on ataxic paraplegia. *Lancet* 1886; 2:1–3, 61–63, 130–131.
10. Hamilton AS, Nixon CE. Sensory changes in the subacute combined degeneration of pernicious anemia. *Arch Neurol Pyschiatry* 1921; 6:1–31.
11. Lichtheim L. Zur kermtoriss der perniciosen anaemie. *Munch Med Wschr* 1887; 34:300–306.
12. Dana CL. Progressive spastic ataxia (combined fascicular sclerosis) and the combined scleroses of the spinal cord. *NY Med Rec* 1887; 32:1–11.
13. Putnam JJ. A group of cases of system sclerosis of the spinal cord, associated with diffuse collateral degeneration occurring in enfeebled persons past middle life, and especially in women; studied with particular reference to etiology. *J Nerv Ment Dis* 1891; 16:69–110.
14. Von Noorden C. Untersuchung über schwere anamie. *Charite Ann* 1891; 16:217–266.
15. Stewart G. Notes on a case probably referable to a recently described form of spinal disease. *Brit M J* 1891; 1:1219–1220.
16. Russell JSR. The relationship of some forms of combined degeneration of the spinal cord to one another and to anaemia. Lancet 1898; 2:4–14.
17. Russell JSR, Batten FE, Collier J. Subacute combined degeneration of the spinal cord. *Brain* 1900; 23:39–110.
18. Brown MA, Langdon FW. Combined sclerosis of Lichtman-Putnam-Dana type accompanying pernicious anemia. *JAMA* 1901; 552–554.
19. McAlpine D. A review of the nervous and mental aspects of pernicious anemia. *Lancet* 1929; 2:643–647.
20. Billings F. The changes in the spinal cord and medulla in pernicious anemia. The Shattuck Lecture. *Boston Med Surg J* 1902; 147:225–233, 257–263.
21. Bowman HM. On the association of disease of the spinal cord with pernicious anemia. *Brain* 1894; 17:198–213.
22. Bramwell B. Clinical studies. II-On the association of pernicious anaemia with subacute combined degeneration of the spinal cord. *Edinburgh Med Jour* 1915; 14:260–276.
23. Greenfield JG. Subacute combined degeneration and pernicious anemia. *Lancet* 1933; 2:62–63.
24. Woltman HW. Brain changes associated with pernicious anemia. *Arch Int Med* 1918; 21:791–843.
25. Pfeiffer JAF. The neuropathological findings in a case of pernicious anemia with psychical implication. *J Nerv Ment Dis* 1915; 42:75–93.
26. Woltman HW. The nervous symptoms in pernicious anemia. *AJ Med Sci* 1919; 157:400–409.
27. Foster DB. Degeneration of peripheral nerves in pernicious anemia. *Arch Neurol Psychiatry;* 102–109.
28. Greenfield JG, Carmichael EA. The peripheral nerves in cases of subacute combined degeneration of the cord. *Brain* 58:483–491.
29. Ehrlich P, Lazarus A. Progressive, pernicious anemia. In: *Nothnagel's Encyclopedia of Medical Practice, American edition: Diseases of the Blood.* Philadelphia: WB Saunders, 1905; 227–336.
30. Hurst AF. Addison's (pernicious) anaemia and subacute combined degeneration of the spinal cord. *Br Med J* 1924; 1:93–100.
31. Elders C. Tropical sprue and pernicious anemia: aetiology and treatment. *Lancet* 1925; 1:75–77.
32. Davison C. Subacute combined degeneration of the cord. Changes following liver therapy; a histopathological study. *Arch Neurol Psychiatry* 1936; 36:1195–1219.
33. Minot GR, Murphy WP. Treatment of pernicious anemia by a special diet. *JAMA* 1926; 87:470–476.
34. Hyland HH, Farquharson RF. Subacute combined degeneration of the spinal cord in pernicious anemia. Results of treatment in seventy-four consecutive cases with certain clinical observations. *Arch Neurol Psychiatry,* 1166–1205;
35. Farquharson RF, Graham D. Liver therapy in the treatment of subacute combined degeneration of the cord. *Can Med Assoc J* 1930; 23:237–244).
36. Castle WB. Observations on the etiologic relationship of achylia gastrica to pernicious anemia. Part 1. The effect of the administration to patients with pernicious anemia of the contents of the normal human stomach recovered after the ingestion of beef muscle. *Am J Med Sci* 1929; 178:748–764.
37. Castle WB, Townsend WC. Observations on the etiologic relationship of achylia gastrica to pernicious anemia. Part II. The effect of the administration to patients with pernicious anemia of beef muscle after incubation with normal gastric juice. *Am J Med Sci* 1929; 178:764–777.
38. Castle WB, Townsend WC, Heath CW. Observastion on the etiologic relationship of achylia gastrica to pernicious anemia. Part III. The nature of the reaction between normal human gastric juice and beef muscle leading to clinical improvement

and increased blood formation similar to the effect of liver feeding. *Am J Med Sci* 1930; 180:305–335.

39. Castle WB. Development of knowledge concerning the gastric intrinsic factor and its relation to pernicious anemia. *N Engl J Med* 1953; 249:603–614.

40. Schilling R. The effect of gastric juice on the urinary excretion of radioactivity after the oral administration of radioactive B12. *J Lab Clin Med* 1953; 42:860–866.

41. Booth CC, Mollin DL. The site of absorption of vitamin B12 in man. *Lancet* 1959; I:18-21.

42. Taylor KB. Inhibition of intrinsic factor by pernicious anemia sera. *Lancet* 1959; 2:106–108.

43. Taylor KB, Roitt IM, Doniach D, et al. Autoimmune phenomena in pernicious anemia: gastric antibodies. *BMJ* 1962; 2:1347–1352.

44. Karlson FA, Burman P, Loof L, et al. Major parietal cell antigen in autoimmune gastritis with pernicious anemia is the acid-producing H+,K+-adenosine triphosphatase of the stomach. *J Clin Invest* 1988; 81:475–479.

45. Goldhorn I, Gleeson PA, Toh B-H. Gastric parietal cell antigens of 60–90, 92, and 100–120 kDa associated with autoimmune gastritis and pernicious anemia: role of N-glycons in the structure and antigenicity of the 60-90 kDa component. *J Biol Chem* 1989; 264:18768–18774.

46. Gleeson PA, Toh B-H. Molecular targets in pernicious anemia. *Immunology Today* 1991; 12:233–238.

47. Toh B-H, van Driel IR, Gleeson PA. Pernicious anemia. *N Engl J Med* 1997; 337:1441–1448.

48. Barrett SP, Toh BH, Alderuccio F, et al. Organ-specific autoimmunity induced by adult thymectomy and cyclophosphamide-induced lymphopenia. *Eur J Immunol* 1995; 25:238–244.

49. Martinelli TM, van Driel IR, Alderuccio F, et al. Analysis of mononuclear cell infiltrate and cytokine production in murine autoimmune gastritis. *Gastroenterology* 1996; 110:1791–1802.

50. Suri-Payer E, Kehn PJ, Cheever AW, et al. Pathogenesis of post-thymectomy autoimmune gastritis: identification of anti-H/K adenosine triphosphate-reactive T cells. *J Immunol* 1996; 157:1799–1805.

51. Jones CM, Callaghan JM, Gleeson PA, et al. The parietal cell autoantigens recognized in neonatal thymectomy-induced murine gastritis are the alpha and beta subunits of the gastric proton pump. *Gastroenterology* 1991; 101:287–294.

52. Cole M. Neurological manifestations of vitamin B12 deficiency. *Handb Clin Neurol* 1998; 26:367–405.

53. Healton EB, Savage DG, Brust JCM, et al. Neurological aspects of cobalamin deficiency. *Medicine* 1991; 70:229–245.

54. Lindenbaum J, Savage DG, Stabler SP, et al. Diagnosis of cobalamin deficiency: II. Relative sensitivities of serum cobalamin, methylmalonic acid, and total homocysteine concentrations. *Am J Hematol* 1990; 34:99–107.

55. Huang C-R, Chang W-N, Tsai N-W, et al. Serial nerve conduction studies in vitamin nB12 deficiency-associated polyneuropathy. *Neurol Sci* 2011; 32:183–186.

56. Torre CD, Lucchetta M, Cacciavillani M, et al. Reversible isolated sensory axonal neuropathy due to cobalamin deficiency. *Muscle Nerve* 2012; 45:428–430.

57. England JD, Gronseth GS, Franklin G, et al. Evaluation of distal symmetrical polyneuropathy: the role of laboratory and genetic testing (an evidence based review). *Muscle Nerve* 2009; 39:116–125.

58. Beitzke M, Pfister P, Fortin J, et al. Autonomic dysfunction and hemodynamics in vitamin B12 deficiency. *Auton Neurosci* 2002; 97:45–54.

59. Puntambekar P, Basha MM, Zak IT, et al. Rare sensory and autonomic disturbances associated with vitamin B12 deficiency. *J Neurol Sci* 2009; 287:285–287.

60. Pittock SJ, Payne TA, Harper CM. Reversible myelopathy in a 34-year-old man with vitamin B12 deficiency. *Mayo Clin Proc* 2002; 77:291–294.

61. Berger JR, Quencer R. Reversible myelopathy with pernicious anemia: clinical/MR correlation. *Neurology* 1991; 41:97–948.

62. Timms SR, Cure JK, Kurent JE. Subacute combined degeneration of the spinal cord: MR findings. *AJNR* 1993; 14:1224–1227.

63. Murata S, Naritomi H, Sawada T. MRI in subacute combined degeneration. *Neuroradiology* 1994; 36:408–440.

64. Locatelli ER, Laureno R, Ballard P, et al. MRI in vitamin B12 deficiency myelopathy. *Can J Neurol Sci* 1999; 26:60–63.

65. Scherer K. Neurologic manifestations of vitamin B12 deficiency. *N Engl J Med* 2003; 348:2208.

66. Tangney CC, Aggarwal NT, Li H, et al. Vitamin B12, cognition, and brain MRI measures. *Neurology* 2011; 77:1276–1282.

67. Kalita J, Misra UK. Vitamin B12 deficiency neurological syndromes: correlation of clinical, MRI and cognitive evoked potentials. *J Neurol* 2008; 255:353–359.

68. Hsing AW, Hansson LE, McLaughlin JK. Pernicious anemia and subsequent cancer: a population-based cohort study. *Cancer* 1993; 71:745–750.

69. Delva PL, MacDonell JE, MacIntosh OC. Megaloblastic anemia occurring simultaneously in white female monozygotic twins. *Can Med Assoc J* 1965; 92:1129–1131.

70. McIntyre OR, Sullivan LW, Jeffries GH, et al. Pernicious anemia in childhood. *N Engl J Med* 1965; 272:981–986.

71. Grasbeck R, Gordin R, Kantero I, et al. Selective vitamin B12 malabsorption and proteinuria in young people. A syndrome. *Acta Med Scand* 1960; 167:289–296.

72. Pant SS, Asbury AK, Richardson EP. The myelopathy of pernicious anemia. A neuropathological reappraisal. *Acta Neurologica Scand* 1968; 44 (Suppl35):8–32.

CHAPTER 38

Hereditary Spastic Paraplegia

David S. Younger

Hereditary spastic paraplegia (HSP) denotes syndromes of familial spastic paraplegia that are definable clinically, pathologically, and genetically by the presence of progressive spasticity of the arms and legs, and heterogeneous in mode of inheritance, pattern of neurological presentation and severity, gene localization, and molecular gene defect. There are autosomal dominant (AD), autosomal (AR) and X-lined (XL) forms. Progressive spasticity occurs alone as a pure (pHSP) upper motor neuron (UMN) disorder, or in conjunction with additional neurologic or non-neurologic features including dementia, retardation, extrapyramidal involvement, ataxia, incontinence, deafness, ichthyosis, retinopathy, neuropathy, and amyotrophy in otherwise complicated (cHSP) UMN syndromes. The postmortem findings of pHSP and cHSP include degeneration of crossed and uncrossed CST, with variable similar involvement of other long tracts such as the dorsal columns and spinocerebellar tracts. There are 19 genetically distinct pHSP loci and related phenotypes (Table 1) enumerated spastic paraplegia (SPG) 3–8, 10–13, 19, 28, 31, 33, 34, 37, 41, and 42; and 30 cHSP catalogued as SPG1, 2, 9, 14–18, 20, 11, 23, 24, SPAX1, SACS, ALDH3A2, 25–27, 29, 30, 32, 35, 36, 38, 39, 44, 45–48 (Table 2). This topic has been previously reviewed (1–4).

EPIDEMIOLOGY

It is difficult to estimate the frequency of HSP in patients with spastic paraparesis of diverse cause, wherein mostly index cases will be found. The overall prevalence of HSP is estimated at 9.6 per 100,000 population, with 70 to 80% of patients displaying AD inheritance, and the remainder AR and X-linked forms. The reported prevalence of AD pHSP in Ireland was 1.27 per 100,000 population (5).

PURE HEREDITARY SPASTIC PARAPLEGIA

SPG3

Zhao et al (6) analyzed five AD pHSP kindred showing linkage to chromosome 14q at the 14q11-q21 locus, identifying disease-specific missense mutations in a novel gene from SPG3A linked kindred. The SGP3A variety was characterized by the onset of progressive leg weakness and spasticity between ages 5 to 10 years. The peptide encoded in SPG3A showed significant homology with the GTPase guanylate-binding protein-1. Muglia (7) described an Italian family with HSP and a mutation in the SPG3A gene which resulted in an arg217-to-gln substitution in a conserved area of GTPase. Ivanova and coworkers (8) identified 12 different heterozygous *ATL1* mutations in European and Australian SPG3A probands, seven of which were novel and three *de novo*. Rainier and colleagues (9) opinioned that SPG3A accounts for about 10% of dominantly inherited pSPG and can present as childhood cerebral palsy. The cause of SPG3A is now known to be due to pathogenic mutations at the 14q22.1 locus of the *ATL1* gene encoding atlastin (Table 1).

SPG4

Svenson (10) screened the spastic gene for mutations in 15 families showing linkage to the SPG4 locus and identified 11 mutations, 10 of which were novel. In 15 of 76 unrelated individuals with AD pHSP, Meijer (11) found five previ-

Table 1. Pure Hereditary Spastic Paraplegia

SPG Type/Gene Symbol	Inheritance	Chromosome Locus	Gene Protein	Phenotype OMIM#
SPG3A/*ATL1*	AD	14q22.1	Atlastin	182600
SPG4/*SPAST*	AD	2p22.3	Spastin	182601
SPG5A/*CYP7B1*	AR	8q12.3 α–hydroxylase	Oxysterol 7-	270800
SPG5B/*SPG5*	AR	8p		600146
SPG6/ *NIPA1*	AD	15q11.2	NIPA1	600363
SPG7/*PGN*	AR	16q24.3	Paraplegin	607259
SPG8/*K1AA0196*	AD	8q24.13	Strumpellin	603563
SPG10/*KIF5A*	AD	12q13.3	KIF5A	604187
SPG11/*SPG11*	AR	15q21.1	Spatacsin	604360
SPG12/*RTN2*	AD	19q13.32	Reticulon 2	604805
SPG13/*HSPD1*	AD	2q33.1	HSP60	605280
SPG19/*SPG19*	AD	9q		607152
SPG28/*SPG28*	AR	14q21.3-q22.3		609340
SPG31/*REEP1*	AD	2p11.2	REEP1	609139
SPG33/*ZFYVE27*	AD	10q24.2	Protrudin	610244
SPG34/*SPG34*	XL	Xq24-q25		300750
SPG37/*SPG37*	AD	8p21.1-q13.3		611945
SPG41/*SPG41*	AD	11p14.1-p11.2		613364
SPG42/*SLC33A1*	AD	3q25.31	ACATN	612539

OMIM: Online Mendelian Inheritance in Man, OMIM®. McKusik Institute of Genetic Medicine, Johns Hopkins University (Baltimore, MD), World Wide Web URL:http://omin.org

ously reported mutations and eight novel ones in the SPG4 gene locus. Among families with AD pHSP linked to the SPG4 locus on chromosome 2, the age of onset ranged from infancy to 63 years, with a clinical expression of asymptomatic to mildly affected spastic gait and otherwise independent ambulation to severe weakness and wheelchair state. Depienne and colleagues (12) identified 19 different sporadic mutations in the SPG4 gene, as did Crippa and colleagues (13), who noted 12 different mutations, eight of which were novel, none of which were noted in 10 additional patients with cHSP. The cause of SPG4 is now known to be pathogenic mutation at the 2p22.3 locus of the *SPAST* gene encoding spastin (Table 1).

SPG5A

Linkage analysis of four Italian families with AR pHSP was accompanied by posterior column sensory impairment and bladder dysfunction, with age of onset between 8 and 40 years, so enabling Muglia (14) to refine the candidate SPG5A locus to an 11–cM region on 8q. This locus was further refined by Wilkinson (15) in a large consanguineous English family with six affected sibs, to a 23.6–cM interval between markers D8S1833 and D8S285 on chromosome 8q11.1-q21.2. Tsaousidou and colleagues (16) identified

homozygous mutations in the *CYP7B1* gene. Goizet and colleagues (17) identified eight different mutations, including six novel ones in the *CYP7B1* gene among 82 unrelated kindred with AR SPG and three of 90 individuals with sporadic SPG. All presented with gait difficulties and developed severe spastic paraplegia of the legs after a mean duration of 28 years, 69% of whom displayed severe handicap, 38% wheelchair bound, and the majority sensory impairment. Other features in affected patients include bladder dysfunction, mild cerebellar signs, retinitis pigmentosa, optic atrophy, mental retardation, dysarthria, glossopharygneal, vagus, and hypoglossal nerve involvement. The cause of SPG5A is due to pathogenic mutation at the 8q12.3 locus of the *CYP7B1* gene (Table 1).

SPG5B

Hentati and colleagues (18) noted linkage of the disease locus to the pericentric region of chromosome 8. The onset of symptoms among affected individuals of five kindred ranged in age from 1 to 20 years, and the clinical presentation characterized by lower leg spasticity, hyperreflexia, mild loss of vibratory and position sensation, without amyotrophy, cerebellar or cognitive involvement.

SPG6

Rainer (19) analyzed a large kindred of AD pHSP linked to the SPG6 locus, and studied four unique candidate genes, including locus 1 of the NIPA1 protein wherein a nucleotide substitution at position 159 resulted in an amino acid substitution at position 45 of the *NIPA1* protein in each of 28 affected subjects. The clinical features of SPG6 includes late teenage to early adult symptom onset of insidiously progressive spastic leg weakness associated with urinary urgency and mild vibratory sensation impairment of the feet. The molecular pathogenesis of *NIPA1* T45R missense mutations in HSP is poorly understood. Chai (20) observed that the *NIPA1* gene encoded putative polypeptides with nine transmembrane domains suggesting function as a receptor or transporter, and phylogenetic analyses showed that it was highly conserved among vertebrate species, with ancestral members in invertebrates and plants. Patients with Prader-Willi and Angelman syndrome, two imprinted genetic disorders, demonstrate 15q class 1 deletions although such individuals do not exhibit progressive SPG. The cause of SPG6 is a pathogenic mutation at the 15q11.2 locus of the *NIPA1* gene (Table 1).

SPG7

DeMichele (21) reported a large family pedigree from southern Italy in which the locus of AR pHSP was identified in a region spanning about 6 cM on chromosome 16q terminus at the 16q24.3 locus. Their disease was characterized as age at onset of greater than 25 years, although without obvious clinical peculiarities; the most severely affected patients showed dysarthria, vibratory sensation loss in the legs, urinary urgency, pes cavus, and mild axonal neuropathy.

Other disorders mapped to the telomeric region of chromosome 16q include the gene responsible for Fanconi anemia, the cellular adhesion regulator molecule gene involved in suppression of tumor invasion and melanocyte-stimulating hormone receptor. Casari (22) found that patients from a chromosome 16q24.3-linked pHSP family were homozygous for a 9.5 kb deletion involving a gene encoding a novel protein, named paraplegin, that was highly homologous to the yeast mitochondrial ATPases, AFGC3, RCA1, and YME1, with both proteolytic and chaperone-like activities at the inner mitochondrial membrane. Immunofluorescence analysis and import experiments showed protein localized to mitochondria. Analysis of needle muscle biopsies from two affected patients showed ragged red fibers, electron microscopy (EM) of which showed mitochondria of bizarre shape, hyperplastic cristae, and subsarcolemmal paracrystalline inclusions consistent with a mitochondrial etiopathogenesis. Elleuch and colleagues (23) identified compound heterozygosity for two mutations in the SPG7 gene. The cause of this disorder is now known to be caused by pathogenic mutation at the 16q24.3 locus of the *PGN* gene (Table 1).

SPG8

Hedera (24) demonstrated a new locus for AD pHSP on 8q in European kindred of 15 subjects characterized by onset at age 25 to 49 years of severe disability resulting in a wheelchair bound state, and only a single asymptomatic member. The chromosome 8q23-q24 gene locus, which spanned 6.2 cM, was proposed as the gene locus for SPG8. Rocco (25) described non-consanguineous kindred of 16 affected subjects with linkage to the SPG8 locus and a less severe clinical course with onset between 18 and 26 years. The gene, which had not yet been characterized, mapped to the SPG8 region on chromosome 8q23-24 (25). Valdmanis and colleagues (26) later identified three mutations in the *KIAA0196* gene which mapped to the SPG8 locus, one of which segregated in three large North American families of European ancestry. The cause of SPG8 is a pathogenic mutation at the 8q24.13 locus of the *KIAA096* gene (Table 1).

SPG10

Reid (27) studied 45 members from two families with AD pHSP with markers on chromosome 12q that allowed them to assign a new locus for SPG10 to a 9.2-cM region on chromosome 12q13. All affected members had symptomatic gait abnormality with an age range of onset of five to 40 years. Reid (28) later identified the missense mutation in the motor domain of the neuronal kinesin heavy chain gene, *KIF5A*. Fichera (29), Blair (30), Lo Giudice and workers (31) later described affected adult and later-onset patients, the latter of whom presented with a four-generation pedigree of gait, urinary, CST signs associated with pes cavus and weakness in the legs, sparing the arms and without sensory involvement. The KIF5A protein belongs to the superfamily of kinesins, which are molecular motor proteins responsible for major microtubule-dependent transport pathways in neuronal and non-neuronal cells. The cause of SPG10 is due to pathogenic mutations at the 12q13.3 locus of *KIF5A* (Table 1).

SPG11

Martinez Murillo (32) performed linkage analysis of eight AR HSP families of Puerto Rican, North American, and Italian descent and characterized the locus for SPG11 at 15q13-q15. Although most families had a pHSP phenotype, two North American and Italian families had sibs with either mental retardation or abnormalities of the corpus callosum, including atrophy, thinning, agenesis, and ventricular dilatation on brain magnetic resonance imaging (MRI). Stevanin and colleagues (33) identified 10 nonsense or insertion or deletions leading to frameshift mutations in the *KIAA1840* or *SPG11* gene encoding spastacsin consistent with loss of function mechanism. Among four unrelated families described by Orlen (34), affected patients presented in the third to fourth decade with limb spasticity, hyperreflexia, sphincter disturbances, amyotrophy of the hands and calves, thin corpus callosum, cerebral atrophy, and periventricular white matter changes on brain MRI, and some degree of cognitive dysfunction or mental retardation, and central retinal degeneration in some older patients reminiscent of SPG15. It is now known that SPG11 is caused by homozygous or compound heterozygous mutations at the 15q21.1 locus of the *SPG11* gene encoding spastacsin (Table 1).

SPG12

Reid (35) screened a Welsh family of 28 members with AD pHSP in which early age at onset and severe progression mapped to chromosome 19q. Haplotype construction and analysis of recombination events narrowed the SPG12 locus to a 16.1cM region at 19q13. Ashley-Koch (36) evaluated seven families segregating AD pHSP linkage to the 19q13 locus, and narrowed the candidate gene region to a 5cM region. Orlacchio (37) performed linkage studies in 16 members of a large Italian family with AD pHSP of early onset, rapid progression, and indolent sensory involvement, and further narrowed the SPG12 locus to the 3.3 cM region between D19S416 and D19S220. Fourteen of the 16 had sensory involvement, 13 of 16 were wheelchair bound, six had urinary difficulty, and three had sexual dysfunction. A decrease in the age of onset and worsening over the four generations suggested genetic anticipation. Montenegro and colleagues (38) identified heterozygous truncating mutations in the endoplasmic reticulum-shaping protein reticulon (*RTN2*) gene in affected members of the families reported by Reid (35) and Orlacchio (37) and colleagues. The *RTN2* gene encodes a member of the reticulon family of prototypic ER-shaping proteins, mutation of which leads to frameshift alterations forming a highly truncated protein. The latter combined with ATPase-defective versions of spastin leads to the inability to severe microtubules and profound tabulation of the ER implicating spastin as an ER morphogen (38). Mutations causing SPG11 are found at the 19q13.32 locus of the *RTN2* gene (Table 1).

SPG13

Fontaine (39) described the gene locus for this disease at chromosome 2q24-q34 for SPG13 among 28 members of a French family with AD pHSP, however detailed clinical information was not provided. It was contemplated at the time that AR symmetrical spastic cerebral palsy, which also

mapped to chromosome 2q24-25, might be allelic. Henson (40) presented genetic data from the French family studied by Fontaine (39), indicating that SPG13 is associated with mutation in the gene encoding the human mitochondrial chaperonin heat shock protein (Hsp) 60. It is now known that SPG13 is caused by a pathogenic mutation at the 2q33.1 locus of *HSPD1* gene (Table 1).

SPG19

Valente (41) mapped a novel AD pHSP locus for SPG19 on chromosome 9q33-q34 in a large family from central Italy. The age of onset appeared to be higher in SPG19 than for other forms of pHSP, with an age range of onset of 36 to 55 years, slow progression, and relatively benign course. Only one of 14 patients were wheelchair bound and two walked with the aid of a cane even after 20 to 30 years of disease. A characteristic feature of SPG19 was urgency and incontinence, reported in nearly all affected individuals, and a low incidence of muscle weakness, wasting, pes cavus, hyperreflexia, mild paresthesia, and diurnal fluctuation of spasticity. Candidate genes were mapped to the dense region surrounding the gene locus for SPG19, including *LOC92391* that encodes for a putative protein similar to frataxin precursor, and others putatively involved in intracellular trafficking (*RAB9P40*), in maintenance of cytoskeleton structure (GAPCENA), protein folding, and degradation via the HSPA5 and PSMD5 proteasome pathway. An AD form of amyotrophic lateral sclerosis (ALS4) maps to a 3 cM interval within the SPG19 region characterized by onset in the second decade with progressive gait difficulty, weakness, wasting, and spasticity that may represent an allelic mutation. The cause of SPG19 is due to pathogenic mutation at the 9q locus of the *SPG19* gene (Table 1).

SPG28

Bouslam and colleagues (42) described affected patients with this AR pHSP in a Moroccan family characterized by progressive spastic gait during childhood with assistance in walking up until the fifth decade, often accompanied by distal sensory loss, pes cavus and scoliosis. Candidate disease loci were noted between markers D14S58 and D14S1064 at the chromosome locus 14q21.3-q22.3 in the *SGP28* gene (Table 1).

SPG31

Zuchner and colleagues (43, 44) identified mutations in the *REEP1* gene causing SPG31 in 6.5% of patients in their sample, making it the third most common HSP gene after *SPAST* and *ATL1*. Widely expressed and localized to mitochondria, such findings highlight the potential importance of mitochondrial dysfunction in HSP. Hewamadduma (45) described families with genetically confirmed SPG31, including heterozygous mutations in the *REEP1* gene in up to 2.3% of their cohort, of ages 15 to 30 years at onset. There was associated pes cavus, severe gait disturbance, amytrophy, and disturbance of joint position and vibration sensation. All were wheelchair bound by age 35 years, and one proband had severe spastic tetraparesis with bulbar dysfunction. Beetz and coworkers (46) identified 16 mutations, including 14 novel ones, in the *REEP1* gene, most commonly small frameshift type. The cause of SPG31 is due to pathogenic mutation at the 2p11.2 locus of the *REEP1* gene (Table 1).

SPG33

Mannan and colleagues (47) described a five-generation German kindred with SPG33 characterized by pHSP and mutation in the zinc finger fyve domain-containing protein 27 (*ZFYVE27)* or protrudin. This spastin-interacting protein colocalized with the endosomal marker EEA1 and the endoplasic reticulum marker RTN1. Down-regulation of protrudin in turn regulates Rab11-dependent membrane cycling that promotes directional membrane trafficking required for neurite formation (48). The cause of SPG33 is due to pathogenic mutation at the 10q24.2 locus of the *ZFYVE27* gene encoding protrudin (Table 1).

SPG34

Starling and coworkers (49) provided linkage analysis of a large Brazilian pedigree reported earlier by Zatz and colleagues (50), evidence of a fourth gene that mapped to Xq24-q25 (Table 1), causing XL pHSP. Inheritance was XL recessive and onset was in late childhood or adolescence with very slow progression and no additional features. Macedo-Souza and colleagues (51) provided follow-up of the family reported by Zatz and colleagues (50), and provided linkage analysis identifying the *SPG34* candidate locus.

SPG37

Hanein and colleagues (52) described a four-generation French kindred with AD pHSP and incomplete penetrance of mild to moderate pure spastic paraparesis, an a candidate disease locus on chromosome 8p21.1-q13.3 for the *SPG37* gene (Table 1) and another region at 10q22.3-q23.31 that segregated with all affected patients that was postulated to be a possible gene modifier.

SPG41

Zhao and colleagues (53) described a 4-generational kindred of AD pHSP, some of whom had involvement of small

hand muscles or urinary urgency without other neurological signs, in whom linkage analysis defined a possible region between the D11S1324 and D11S1993 markers at the 11p14.1-p11.2 locus of the *SPG41* gene (Table 1).

SPG42

Lin and coworkers (54) described 20 or more Chinese individuals with AD pHSP. Onset was in the first two decades of life with pes cavus, none of whom were wheelchair bound, and without other neurological involvement. Linkage analysis mapped the disorder to chromosome 3q24-q26 and identified heterozygous mutation in the solute carrier family 33 acetyl-CoA transporter member 1 (*SLC33A1*) gene postulating haplo-insufficiency. Schlipf and others (55) did not defect similar pathogenic mutations in the *SLC33A1* gene among 220 patients of German, French and Norweigian descent negative for the *SPAST* gene. Mutation at the 3q25.31 of the *SLC33A1* gene, which is involved in the process of O-acetylation, is the candidate gene for SPG42 (Table 1) and AR congenital cataracts, hearing loss, and neurodegeneration (CCHLND), which maps to the same chromosomal locus.

COMPLICATED HEREDITARY SPASTIC PARAPLEGIA

SPG1

The complexity of the scope of SPG1 as a syndrome of cHSP can be appreciated by reviewing the steps that led to its delineation. The syndrome of mental retardation, adducted thumbs, shuffling gait due to spastic paraplegia, and aphasia or slow speech development (MASA) was reported as a new entity by Biachine and colleagues (56). A family with XL mental retardation was described as having spastic paraplegia (57), which in turn was determined to have a clinical semblance and genetic linkage to MASA at the Xq28 locus (58). The chromosomal locus for congenital hydrocephalus due to acqueductal stenosis abbreviated HSAS, which varied clinically from lethal *in utero* and to early infancy with later mental retardation, spastic paraplegia, and adducted thumbs, was established at Xq28.

The demonstration of mutation in the L1 cell adhesion molecule (*L1CMA*) gene in X-lined hydrocephalus suggested that a mutation in the same gene might be responsible for MASA syndrome and this was indeed the case. Scharander-Stumpel and colleagues (59, 60) referred to the HSAS/MASA spectrum in attributing common linkage to Xp28 in kindred with cHSP, MASA syndrome, and XL hydrocephalus. Virtually all affected members were boys or men with rare lethal obligate female carriers and others that survived with incomplete syndromes of learning

Table 2. Complicated Hereditary Spastic Paraplegia

SPG Type/Gene Symbol	Inheritance	Chromosome Locus	Gene Protein	Phenotype OMIM#
SPG1/*LICAM*	X-linked	Xq28	L1CAM	303350
SPG2/*PLP1*	X-linked	Xq22.2	PLP1	312920
SPG9/*SPG9*	AD	10q23.3-q24.1		601162
SPG14/*SPG14*	AR	3q27-q28		605229
SPG15/*ZFYVE26*	AR	14q24.1	Spastizin	270700
SPG16/*SPG16*	XL	Xq11.2		300266
SPG17/*BSCL2*	AD	11q12.3	Seipin	270685
SPG18/*ERLIN2*	AR	8p11.23		611225
SPG20/*SPG20*	AR	13q13.3	Spartin	275900
SPG21/*ACP33*	AR	15q22.31	Maspardin	248900
SPG23/*SPG23*	AR	1q24-q32		270750
SPG24/*SPG24*	AR	13q14		607584
SPG25/*SPG25*	AR	6q23-q24.1		608220
SPG26/*SPG26*	AR	12p11.1-q14		609195
SPG27/*SPG27*	AR	10q22.1-q24.1		609041
SPG29/*SPG29*	AD	1p31.1-p21.1		609727
SPG30/*SPG30*	AR	2q37.3		610357
SPG32/*SPG32*	AR	14q12-q21		611252
SPG35/*FA2H*	AR	16q23.1	FA2H	612319
SPG36/*SPG36*	AD	12q23-q24		613096
SPG38/*SPG38*	AD	4p16-p15		612335
SPG39/*PNPLA6*	AR	19p13.2	NTE	612020
SPG44/*GJC2*	AR	1q42.13	Connexin47	613206
SPG45/*SPG45*	AR	10q24.3-q25.1		613162
SPG46/*SPG46*	AR	9p21.2-q21.12		614409
SPG47/*AP4B1*	AR	1p13.2		614066
SGP48/*KIAA0415*	AR	7p22.1		613647
SPAX1/*SAX1*	AD	12p13		108600
SACS/*SACS*	AR	13q12.12	Sacsin	270550
SLS/*ALDH3A2*	AR	17p11.2	ALDH3A2	270200

problems, mild mental retardation, and adducted thumbs. Hydrocephalus was present in 60% of documented MASA patients and in 50% of surviving HSAS cases. All but one member had mild to severe mental retardation, with intelligence quotients lower in those of older age. Spastic paraplegia and adducted thumbs were equally present in 85 to 90% of members with or without manifest hydrocephalus. Agenesis of the corpus callosum was an X-linked feature of MASA/HASA spectrum.

The phenotypic variability in families with an L1CAM mutation is extensive. Since spastic paraplegia was not always a feature of MASA, the acronym CRASH was proposed by Fransen and colleagues (61) for corpus callosum hypoplasia, retardation, adducted thumbs, spastic paraplegia, and hydrocephalus. The various functions of *LICAM* include neurite outgrowth in development, neuronal cell migration and cellular survival, axon bundling, myelination, synaptogenesis, and long-term potentiation were

reviewed by Kenwrick and colleagues (62). Up to 14 different mutations have been described in XL HSAS/MASA syndrome kindred at the Xq28 locus of the *LICAM* gene (Table 2).

SPG2

This type of cHSP, clinically described in kindred that developed spastic paraplegia in association with nystagmus, dysarthria, sensory disturbance, mental retardation, optic atrophy, muscle wasting, joint contracture, and wheelchair dependency in early adult life (63), was associated pathologically with degeneration of CST and spinocerebellar tracts (64). Keppen (65) described a similar kindred with XL recessive pHSP without complicated features. Both cHSP and cHSP forms of this disease (63, 65) narrowed the genetic interval containing the disease-producing gene in other large kindred with SGP2 so designated, to the Xq21-

q22 region. Bonneau and colleagues (66) located the SPG2 locus at Xq21, suggesting variable clinical expression of the single gene locus accounting for both c-, and pHSP. Mutant proteolipid protein 1 (PLP1) or lipophilin, the primary constituent of myelin in the CNS, assembles into stable ER oligomers as in wild type forms, with a postulated gain-of-function effect overwhelming ER degradation machinery and causing cellular toxicity (67). Mutation of the *PLP* gene, which also occurs in the XL childhood demyelinating disorder Pelizaeus-Merzbacher disease (PMD), shares the clinical features of nystagmus, cerebellar ataxia, and spasticity. Two disorders can be distinguished by delayed onset of nystagmus, predominant gait difficulty, and absence of large hyperintense white matter changes in SPG2 in contrast to PMD, indicating the variable phenotypic expression of allelic mutations of the *PLP* gene. Pathogenic mutations in the Xq22.2 locus of the *PLP1* gene are the cause of SPG2 (Table 2), the associated clinical severity of which correlate with the nature of the mutation.

SPG9

Slavotinek (68) reported a large kindred in which affected individuals had cataracts, motor axonal neuropathy, short stature, developmental delay, skeletal deformities including delayed bone age, shallow acetabulum, small carpal bones, skull base dysplasia, and clindodactyly. There was AD inheritance with anticipation, rare instances of male-to-male transmission, and age at onset from the first to the fourth decade of life. Seri and colleagues (69) in addition recognized variable expressivity of cHSP, with pes cavus, gastroesophageal reflux, and hiatal hernia, and mapped the disorder to the 10q23.3-q24.2 gene region, as did Slavotinek and colleagues (68) to the 10q23.2-q24.2 locus in a 12 cM region. Electrodiagnostic studies in affected patients showed axonal motor neuropathy. Two other neurological disorders mapped to the same region, including infantile-onset spinocerebellar ataxia (IOSA) and progressive external ophthalmoplegia (PEO). The cause of SPG9 is now known to be a result of pathogenic mutations at the 10q23.3-q24.1 locus (Table 2).

SPG14

Vazza (70) studied a consanguineous Italian family with AR HSP associated with mental retardation, motor neuropathy, and onset in the fourth decade with slow progression. A sural nerve biopsy in the index patient was normal. Neuropsychological studies showed visual agnosia, short- and long term memory impairment, preservation, and confabulation. None of the affected individuals showed abnormalities on electroencephalographic (EEG) testing, and results of computed tomography (CT) and MRI were normal in the index patient. Using homozygosity mapping, the disorder mapped to chromosome 3q27-q28, which was deemed to be the *SPG14* gene locus (Table 2).

SPG15

Hughes (71) described two Irish families with slowly progressive HSP and onset of slow intellectual development in the second decade. Several had pigmentary maculopathy, with a mild decrease in visual acuity and all had distal amyotrophy. The clinical features of the affected cases were similar to those reported by Kjellin (72) with the differences of earlier age of onset, fecal and urinary incontinence, dysarthria, cerebellar ataxia, and progressive intellectual deterioration. Brain MRI of affected patients showed diffuse atrophy of the cerebral hemispheres, corpus callosum, and brainstem. Evidence was obtained for linkage to a locus on chromosome 14q, narrowing it to a 19-cM interval flanked by D14S1038 and D14S61 at 14q22-q24.

Hanein and colleagues (73) identified six different homozygous mutations in the zinc finger *FYVE* domain-containing protein 26 (*ZFYVE26*) gene in the families described by Hughes (71), Elleuch (74), Casali (75), and Boukhris and colleagues (76). The SPG15 interval contains 57 other known genes, including the one for presenilin 1 (PS 1), which has been implicated in early onset familial Alzheimer disease. This is of particular interest given the report of a family affected with spastic paraplegia and Alzheimer-like dementia in which a deletion of exon 9 of PS-1 was found (77). The cause of SPG15 is due to pathogenic mutations at the 14q24.1 locus of the *ZFYVE26* gene encoding spastizin (Table 2).

SPG16

Claes (78) studied large kindred with XL recessive slowly progressive HSP, and mental retardation with facial hypotonia, strabismus, maxillary hypoplasia, and MASA-like habitus. Although the gene locus had not been firmly established, Tamagaki (79) found a faintly stained variant X chromosome gap at Xq11.2, which stained nucleolus organizer (NOR) positive, C-banding negative, FISH analysis positive, and α-satellite FISH analysis negative. The gap, therefore, represented an insertion of the NOR derived from the short arm of an acrocentric chromosome. The cause of SPG16 is due to pathogenic mutation at the Xq11.2 locus of the *SPG16* gene (Table 2).

SPG17

Silver (80) reported two families with progressive AD HSP and amyotrophy of thenar and dorsal interosseus muscles, foot deformity, and vibratory sensory loss in the legs. Patel and coworkers (81) linked so called Silver syndrome variant of cHSP to chromosome 11q12-q14. Recombination events positioned the locus, which the authors designated SPG17, to a 13cM interval flanked by two markers, that was later narrowed to a 5.9 cM gene interval. Windpassinger and colleagues (82) confirmed linkage of phenotypically characteristic Silver syndrome to the SGP17 locus in 16 kindred, and identified heterozygous mutations in the *BSCL2* gene in a family with distal hereditary motor neuropathy type V (DSMAV) reported earlier by Auer-Grumbach and coworkers (83). Causative mutations in the *BSCL2* gene encoding seipin, the protein product localized mainly to the ER membrane (84), included ser90 to leu and asn88 to ser, glycosylated seipin resulting in aggregate formation and neurodegeneration. Silver syndrome and DSMAV were considered extreme phenotypes resulting from mutations in the same *BSCL2* gene. The cause of SPG17 is due to pathogenic mutation at the 11q12.3 locus of the *BSCL2* gene encoding seipin (Table 2).

SPG18

Al-Yahyaee and colleagues (85) described two unrelated consanguineous Omani families with AR cHSP with age of onset in the first two years of life in one family, all with spastic paraparesis, including some with arm involvement, mental retardation, agenesis of hypoplasia of the corpus callosum, and epilepsy, the latter despite normal CT and mental development. A later consanguineous Saudi family reported by Alazami and colleagues (86) included a 30-month-old proband who developed spasticity of the legs followed by the legs rendering him wheelchair bound by age four years, associated with delayed motor development, impaired cognition, and generalized spike and slow-wave abnormalities on EEG. A homozygous 20-kb deletion was detected on chromosome 8, the interval of which spanned the protein-coding endoplasmic reticulum lipid raft-associated protein 2 (*ERLIN2*) gene involved in the ER degradation pathway, loss of which was postulated to result in persistent activation of IP3 signaling and neuronal channel activity. Pathogenic mutation at the 8p11.23 locus of the *ERLIN2* is the cause of SPG18 (Table 2).

SPG20

Cross and McKusick (87) studied an Amish kindred with 20 cases of AR HSP and distal muscle wasting, designated Troyer syndrome for the surname of many of the affected persons. The disorder has onset in early childhood with dysarthria, atrophy of thenar, hypothenar, and dorsal interosseus muscles, gait difficulty, drooling, and cerebellar involvement. Patel and colleagues (88) identified a homozygous 1-bp deletion in the *SPG20* gene consistent with a founder effect.

In affected members of a large Omani kindred with *SPG20*, Manzini and coworkers (89) identified a homozygous truncating mutation in the *SPG20* gene and expression at modest levels in fetal and adult human brains, including amygdala, cortex, thalamus, less so in hippocampus and cerebellum. The cause of SPG20 is causative mutations at the 13q13.3 locus of the *SPG20* gene encoding the spastic paraplegia autosomal recessive Troyer syndrome protein, abbreviated spartin (Table 2). The latter shares sequence similarity with the N-terminal region of spastic as well as other proteins involved in the morphology and membrane trafficking of endosomes. A mechanism for endosomal transportation that involves microtubules appears to be disturbed by cells that overexpress spastin mutants leading to redistribution of microtubule array.

SPG21

Cross and McKusick (90) described 20 patients with an AR form of presenile dementia, which they termed MAST syndrome, with onset in late teens, slow progression of spastic paraparesis, and basal ganglia involvement. Simpson (91) investigated 29 additional family members from the extended Amish pedigrees originally studied by Cross and McKusick (87), of whom 14 were affected with MAST syndrome. Affected members were generally normal in teenage years and early adulthood, with later decline in ambulation and mental function associated with developmental delay and personality disturbance, including bipolar disease, paranoid ideation, and psychosis. Other neurological involvement, which included swallowing difficulty, extrapyramidal and pyramidal motor disturbance, incoordination, oromandibular dyskinesia, and athetoid movements, had onset in the third decade, less often in the fourth to fifth decades. Brain MRI showed thin corpus callosum and white matter abnormalities. The disorder, which mapped to the 15q22.31 locus, encompassed three genes, showed transcripts in all 14 affected patients that were homozygous for a 1-bp insertion in the acid cluster protein of 33kDa (*ACP33*) gene. The MAST syndrome is caused by pathogenic mutations at the 15q22.31 locus of the *ACP33* gene that encodes the 33-kD acidic cluster protein, termed *maspardin*, for Mast syndrome, spastic paraplegia, AR, and dementia. The homozygous 1-bp insertion in the *ACP33* gene so noted (91) presumably leads to a frameshift and premature termination of the maspardin protein involved in protein transport and sorting. The cause of SPG 21 is due to pathogenic mutation at the 15q22.31 locus of the *ACP33* gene (Table 2).

SPG23

Abdallat (92) reported a consanguineous Jordanian family in which siblings from first-cousin parents had AR

HSP, peripheral neuropathy, vitiligo, hyperpigmentation, numerous lentigines, and premature graying beginning in the first decade of life. A 13-year-old Arab proband from another affected family, reported by Mukamel and coworkers (93), had microcephaly, café au lait spots, freckles, spastic paraplegia, and white hair present from birth. A similarly affected 18-year-old European girl had acquired hypopigmentation, vitiligo, diffuse lentigines, spastic gait, kyphoscoliosis, small stature, and normal intelligence (94). Linkage of the disorder in an Arab family was detected along a 25-cM region on chromosome 1q24-q32 (93). Haplotype analysis showed allelic homozygosity in all affected members. SPG23 is caused by pathogenic mutation at the 1q24-q32 locus in the *SPG23* gene.

SPG24

Hodgkinson and coworkers (95) reported consanguineous Saudi Arabian kindred in which several sibs had AR HSP. Symptoms of spasticity evidenced by disturbed standing, with later scissoring gait, tiptoe walking, and frank spasticity, became evident in the teenage years. Affected individuals remained ambulatory until the third decade. Three of five affected sibs, and two carrier individuals, had sensorineural deafness without other complicating features. Metabolic and biochemical investigations, and MRI of the brain and spinal cord, as well as EEG and somatosensory evoked potentials were normal. Genome analysis showed linkage of SPG24 to a 1.8 Mb region of chromosome 13q14 flanked by FLJ11712 and D13S270 markers. GPG23 is caused by a pathogenic mutation at the 13q14 locus of the *SPG24* gene (Table 2).

SPG25

Zortea and colleagues (96) described an Italian family with AD adult-onset HSP associated with painful spinal disc herniation and minor spondylosis and linkage to chromosome 6q23.3-q24.1 between the markers D6S1699 and D6s314. The cause of SPG25, also known as disc herniation with spastic paraplegia, is due to causative mutation at the 6q23-q24.1 locus in the *SPG25* gene (Table 2)

SPG26

Farag and colleagues (97) described a consanguineous Kuwaiti family of five sibs with cHSP with progressive spastic paraparesis associated with pes cavus and small hand muscle wasting, Wilkinson and coworkers (98) reported associated intellectual impairment in affected patients. Follow-up studies of both families (97, 98) identified a putative 22.8-cM disease locus on chromosome 12p11.1-q14 for the *SPG26* gene (Table 2).

SPG27

Meijer and colleagues (99) described a French Canadian family with progressive onset of spastic paraplegia and distal vibration sensory impairment, which after detailed analysis identified a putative disease locus designated *SPG27* at chromosome locus 10q22.1-q24.1 (Table 2).

SPG29

Orlacchio and colleagues (100) described a Scottish family in which 19 members were affected with progressive AD HSP with an onset age of 15 years, and associated sensorineural hearing loss, pes cavus, and neonatal hyperbilirubinemia. There was anticipation manifested by earlier age at onset and increasing disease severity in subsequent generations. Affected members shared a common disease haplotype located in a 22.3-cM locus designated *SPG29* at 1p31.1-p21.1 (Table 2).

SPG30

Klebe and colleagues (101) described a consanguineous Algerian family of cHSP in whom the mean age of onset was about 17 years of age, with associated features of distal pinprick sensation, saccadic ocular movements and cerebellar signs. Brain imaging in one patient showed diffuse midline cerebellar atrophy. Patients remained ambulatory for up to 15 years.

Ehrlich and coworkers (102) reported three Palestinian sibs with early childhood onset progressive spastic paraplegia. By homozygosity mapping, exone sequencing, and examination of candidate genes, a homozygous mutation was noted in the *KIF1A* gene. The cause of SPG30 results from pathogenic mutations in the 2q37.3 locus of the *SPG30* gene (Table 2).

SPG32

Stevanin and colleagues (103) described a consanguineous Portuguese family with slowly progressive AR spastic paraplegia complicated by pes cavus, mild mental retardation, thin corpus callosum, cortical and cerebellar atrophy, and pontine dysgraphia on brain MRI. A 30-cM interval on 14q12-q21, positioned between D14S264 and D14S978, was noted on haplotype analysis in a candidate locus termed *SPG32* (Table 2).

SPG35

Dick and colleagues (104) described a large consanguineous Omani family of seven affected individuals with spastic paraplegia ranging in age from 6 to 11 years with foot drop, gait difficulty, cognitive decline, and rapid progression of spasticity over two to four years first affecting the legs, then arms, resulting in complete dependence, usually by age 25 years. Dick and coworkers (105) later reported a Pakistani family with complicated SPG35, identifying two different homozygous mutations in the *FA2H* gene. Brain MRI was normal in one patient studied in the first family, and showed parietal and occipital periventricular, and subcortical T_2 hyperintensities, in an affected individual of the second cohort. Edvardson and coworkers (106) identified a homozygous mutation in the *FA2H* gene among two sisters from a consanguineous Arab Muslim family with gait difficulty, ataxia, dystonia, cognitive decline, and white matter abnormalities on brain MRI, commencing at age four and six years. Kruer and coworkers (107) identified two different homozygous mutations in the *FA2H* gene in affected members of two unrelated families with progressive spastic paraplegia, associated with brain iron accumulation in the globus pallidus, and noted the *FA2H* gene mapped to chromosome 16q23.1 (Table 2) encoding fatty acid 2-hydroxylase. FA2H catalyzes the hydroxylation of the 2 position of the N-acyl chain modifying the ceramide moiety of central nervous system (CNS) sphingolipids (108).

SPG36

Schule and investigators (109) described a three-generation German kindred with AD spastic paraplegia complicated by electrophysiological evidence of peripheral neuropathy, without evidence of associated neuropsychological or brain MRI abnormalities. Two of the individuals became wheelchair-dependent. Linkage analysis detected a 15.8-cM region on chromosome 12q23-q24, the locus of which was designated *SPG36* (Table 2).

SPG38

Orlacchio and coworkers (110) described two large Italian families, designated RM-36 and RM-51, showing cardinal clinical features of Silver syndrome, a disabling form of AD cHSP characterized by amyotrophy and weakness of small hand muscles in addition to lower limb spasticity. The RM-36 family, which contained 19 definitely affected individuals and AD mode of inheritance, spanned four generations with age at onset early both in the legs and arms typically 16 years, with spastic gait presenting in all patients with additional weakness in foot extensor muscles. The RM-51 family also spanned 4 generations with AD mode of inheritance, and age of onset from 9 to 35 years, with typical presentation of leg followed by arm spasticity, an impression of anticipation supported by an increase in the severity of disease in successive generations, and intrinsic hand muscle weakness most severe in the thenar eminence. Addi-

tional fibular nerve related muscle wasting and weakness was noted in severe patients, including impaired vibration sensation, pes cavus, temporal lobe epilepsy, and cognitive dysfunction. Electrophysiological studies in both families showed chronic neurogenic features on NCS evidencing low compound muscle action potentials with normal or mild slowing, sparing sensory nerve involvement. In addition, central motor conduction times in the RM-36 family to the first dorsal interosseus muscle was normal in all but one patient. A genome-wide survey in the RM-36 family detected a novel locus termed *SPG38* within a 13.1cM interval on chromosome 4p16-p15 between D4S432 and D4S1599 (Table 2). The RM-51 family was linked to the *SPG4* locus at 2p21-p24, sequence analysis of which disclosed a novel frameshift mutation at p.Asp321GlyfsX6 indicating allelism of the novel locus of *SPG38* to *SPG4*. The diagnosis of HSP was more likely than familial ALS or primary lateral sclerosis (PLS) in the two families for several reasons. In the case of the former, there was no cranial nerve involvement; second, the clinical course was relatively benign as none of the patients were bedridden due to weakness; third, none had active spontaneous activity on needle EMG, or clinical fasciculation. Moreover, PLS was differentiated by AD inheritance, chronic neurogenic features on needle EMG in association with frank wasting, and early onset (111). Involvement of motor neurons in addition to other cortical neuronal populations is reminiscent of presenilin 1 (PS1) of familial Alzheimer disease accompanied by spastic paraplegia (112). Spastin and PS1 are expressed ubiquitously and spastin has a critical biological role in the regulation of microtubule severing since it assembles into a hexamer containing pore loops, which recognize the extreme C terminus of its target protein tubulin. Animal models of *SPG4*-HSP and neuronal expression of both spastin RNA interference and mutant spastin showed conformational changes of the pore loops or absence of hexamer leading to altered stabilization of microtubules and dysfunctional severing (113).

SPG39

Rainier and coworkers (114) evaluated consanguineous kindred of Ashkenzai Jewish ancestry, and a genetically unrelated non-consanguineous family of northern European ancestry in which affected subjects developed childhood onset of insidiously progressive spastic leg weakness and progressive wasting of distal arm and leg muscles. Electrophysiological studies were consistent with a motor axonopathy affecting the arms and legs. Brain MRI demonstrated spinal cord atrophy most severe in the thoracic region. The affected phenotype in each family conformed both to organophosphate compound-induced delayed neuropathy (OPIDN) and Troyer syndrome or, AR SPG20, associated with spartin gene mutation, in whom affected patients exhibit additional neurologic ad systemic features of delayed milestone acquisition, skeletal abnormalities; cerebellar, extrapyramidal, and cognitive impairments not observed in the those described by Rainier with SPG39 (114). Analysis of the SPG20/spartin gene coding sequence showed no mutations. A genome-wide linkage analysis in the consanguineous family suggested linkage to a 22cM homozygous locus at chromosome 19p13 to which neuropathy target esterase (NTE) had been mapped, and was a candidate locus because of its role in OPIDN and the similarity of the patients to those with OPIDN. Affected subjects in the consanguineous kindred were furthermore homozygous for disease-specific NTE mutation c.3034A to G that disrupted an interspecies conserved residue M1012V in the NTE catalytic domain. Affected non-consanguineous family were compound heterozygote, with one allele c.2669G to A mutation, which disrupted an interspecies conserved residue in the catalytic domain of NTE at R890H, and the other allele manifesting the insertion c.2946_2947insCAGC, causing frameshift and protein truncation at p.5982fs1019. These disease-specific non-conserved NTE mutations in unrelated motor neuron disease (MND) patients indicated the importance of NTE in maintaining the integrity of the CST and peripheral motor axons. The finding that NTE mutations underlie CSF and peripheral motor axon degeneration raises the possibility that other NET polymorphisms or genetic variations in factors that regulate or interact with NET, could contribute to other MND, including ALS and PLS. The two NTE mutations were the likely cause of AR MND closely resembling OPIDN and sufficient to cause the disorder even in the absence of apparent exposure to OP compounds. It is now known that SPG39 results from pathogenic mutations at the 19p13.2 locus of the *PNPLA6* gene encoding NTE.

SPG44

Orthmann-Murphy and colleagues (115) described three patients from one family with late-onset slowly progressive spastic paraplegia with near normal psychomotor development and preserved walking through adulthood. Brain MRI and magnetic resonance spectroscopy (MRS) were consistent with a hypomyelinating leukoencephalopathy. All three patients were found to possess a novel recessively inherited mutation in the GAP junction protein, gamma-2 (*GJC2*) gene at 99C>G, that predicted an Ile>Met amino acid substitution at 133M encoding the gap junction protein connexin47 (Cx47). Gap junction proteins are members of a large family of homologous connexins, comprising four transmembrane, two extracellular, and three cytoplasmic domains, and have been identified in a broad range of mammalian tissues, with most expressing more than one connexin protein. Whereas Cx47 is expressed specifically in oligodendrocytes and is regulated in parallel with other myelin genes (116), Cx47 and Cx43 are partially colocalized in oligodendrocytes, which together with Schwann cells synthesize multilamellar myelin membranes in the CNS. The causative mutation at 133M presumably forms overlapping gap junction plaques and functional channels with Cx43. However, 133M/Cx43 channels open only when a large voltage difference is applied to paired cells, and probably do not function under physiological conditions, suggesting disruption of Cx47/Cx43 channels between CNS astrocytes and oligodendrocytes similar to the allelic hypomyelinating leukodystrophy, Pelizaeus-Merzbacher-like disease (PMLD), clinically characterized by nystagmus, psychomotor delay, progressive spasticity, and cerebellar involvement. SPG44 is caused by pathogenic mutation at the 1q42.13 locus of the *GJC2* gene (Table 2) encoding Cx47.

SPG45

Durson and coworkers (117) described five individuals born to parents of known consanguinity or from the same Turkish village. All patients' parents were unaffected and were ambulatory, reportedly walked from five to eight years of age, and had clinical findings of spastic paraplegia accompanied by leg contractures and mental retardation. Ophthalmological examination showed variable myopia, optic atrophy, and bilateral congenital pendular nystagmus. Mapping designated a new AR-HSP locus, termed *SPG45*, within a 4.6-Mb region on chromosome 10q24.3-q25.1 containing 87 genes, one of which, at *MRPL43* stood out as the best candidate, being a mitochondrial ribosome protein, the substrate for paraplegia encoded by SPG7, the gene responsible for the most frequent form of AR-HSP after *SPG11* encoding spatacsin. Another candidate gene, *SORCS3*, a member of the vacuolar protein sorting 10 domain-containing receptor proteins, was considered unlikely since only the first two exons were within the gene locus.

SPG46

Boukhris and colleagues (118) assessed 73 affected patients from 33 apparently unrelated southern Tunisian families of Arab origin, of whom 19 patients from eight families met the criteria for diagnosis of AR HSP with thinning of the corpus callosum (TCC) by brain MRI, mental impairment, and exclusion of other disorders. Onset occurred at a mean age of 10 years and presenting symptoms were gait abnormality with the appearance of stiffness and weakness of the legs. Cognitive decline occurred in all but one affected patient who evolved over only seven years. Additional signs included pseudobulbar dysarthria, bladder dysfunction, and non-pyramidal cerebellar ataxia, amyotrophy of the legs, cataracts, and impaired vibratory sensation. Brain MRI at mean age of 26 years that showed TCC was most prominent in the rostrum, genu, and body and associated with cerebellar and cerebral atrophy, with white matter changes in two-thirds of patients, including hyperintense T_2-weighted lesions restricted to the occipital, frontal, and diffuse periventricular regions. Linkage to either SPG11 or SPG15 was suggested by haplotype reconstruction and positive logarithm of odds score values for microsatellite markers in seven of the eight families, but not for the other family, suggesting another genetic form. Later analysis by Boukhris and colleagues (119) identified a single chromosome region on chromosome 9p21.2-q21.12 linkage in the TUN35 family, segregating at the homozygous state, termed SPG46 (Table 2), the candidate region of which narrowed down to a 45-Mb (15cM) region containing 183 genes. They included the CNTFR gene encoding ciliary neurotophic factor, DNAJB5 encoding a member of the HSP40 protein family, and FBXO10 encoding F-box, an arginine methyl-only protein, all possibly relevant for HSP pathology. However, no disease-causing alteration was found in any of the affected patients of the TUN35 family. Mutations in non-coding sequences, unknown exons, or duplications might nonetheless have escaped detection. SPG46 is caused by pathogenic mutation at the 9p21.2-q21.12 locus of the SPG46 gene (Table 2).

SPG47

Abou Jamra and colleagues (120) described eight affected Israeli-Arab individuals from three consanguineous families with severe intellectual disability, absent speech, shy character, stereotypic laughter, microcephaly, and hypotonia that progressed to spastic paraplegia, foot deformity, and amyotrophy of the legs, inability to walk, and growth retardation. Linkage analysis resulted in significant linkage peaks at 1p13.2-q21.2 for one family, 14q11-q12 for another, and 15q21.1-q25.1 for the third, at critical intervals, respectively, of 34Mb, 9.1Mb, and 32.9 Mb. After screening eight genes, mapping to the 1p13.1-q21.2 chromosomal locus, one mutation in each of three genes encoding adaptor complex 4 (AP4) subunits: a nonsense mutation in AP4S1, frameshift mutation in AP4B1, and a splice mutation in APE1 were identified. The AP1-4 complexes are ubiquitously expressed and evolutionarily conserved heterotetrameric complexes that mediate different types of vesicle formation and selection of cargo molecules for inclusion into the vesicles. Two of the mutations at AP4M1 and AP4EI are known to cause cerebral palsy associated with severe intellectual disability. Blumkin and colleagues (121) found linkage to a 7.3-Mb region on chromosome 1p13.2-1p12 locus for AR-HSP-TCC in two siblings from an Arabic consanguineous family with slowly progressive spastic paraparesis, mental

retardation, seizures, TCC and periventricular white matter abnormalities. Using exome sequencing, Bauer and coworkers (122), the novel AP4B1 frameshift mutation c.664delC at 1p13.2 was delineated (Table 2) that differed from Abou Jamra (120) who described a another family with a different AP4B1 mutation, c.487_488insTAT, but similar phenotype, in a consanguineous Arabic family with two affected siblings with progressive spastic paraplegia, intellectual disability, seizures, periventricular white matter changes and TCC. AP4 interacts with α-amino-3-hydroxy-5-methyl-4-isoxazolepropionic acid (AMPA) glutamate receptors to selectively transport them from the trans-Golgi network to the postsynaptic somatodendritic domain (123), and may contribute to axonal degeneration of the terminal portions of the CTS and ascending dorsal column pathways in HSP due to disruption of axonal transport of macromolecules, organelles, and other cargo. SPG47 is caused by pathogenic mutation at the 1p13.2 locus of the AP4B1 gene (Table 2).

SPG48

Stabicki and colleagues (124) employed a genome-scale DNA endoribonuclease-prepared short interfering RNA (esiRNA) screen for the genes involved in homologous recombination DNA double-strand break repair (HR-DSBR). One previously uncharacterized gene, KIAA0415, was found to interact with SPG11 and SPG15, and associated with HSP-TCC. Sequencing in 166 unrelated patients, including 38 and 64 patients respectively with AR and AD inheritance and 64 sporadic patients, identified 7 known and 15 new variants, most of which were not considered causative because they did not affect protein sequence, and were not predicted to alter correct splicing or found frequently in control samples. However, a homozygous mutation was found in two French siblings who were not detected in Caucasian or North African chromosome controls, comprising a complex indel in exon 2 that generated a frameshift and a stop codon following amino acid 29. The insertion was an imperfect quadruplication of the sequence CTGTAA (A) suggesting DNA polymerase slippage during DNA synthesis as the mechanism for introduction of the mutation. Both affected patients had progressive HSP associated with urinary incontinence since age 50 and 49 years, respectively. Brain MRI was normal in one, and cervical spine MRI in the other showed C3-4 and C7 cord hyperintensities. Their parents originated from two neighboring villages without consanguinity. A comparison of drug sensitivity in lymphoblast cell lines established, from a patient carrying the KIAA0415 gene mutation, showed that KIAA0415 mutant cells were significantly more sensitive to mitomycin C and bleomycin treatments than the mutation from the patient with SPG15. Taken together, these experiments identified

KIAA0415 as a novel gene which was mutated in HSP and implicated a link between HSP and DNA repair. SPG48 is caused by pathogenic mutation at the 7p22.1 locus of the *KIAA0415* gene (Table 2).

Spastic Ataxia 1

Meijer (125) described AD spastic paraplegia, so-called spastic ataxia 1 or SPAX1, among three Newfoundland kindred with severe spasticity, dysarthria, dysphagia, ocular movement abnormalities including slow saccades, impaired vertical gaze, and lid retraction, in addition to involuntary head jerking, dystonia, pes cavus, ptosis, and decreased vibration sensation. The severity of the phenotype varied greatly within and among the families, and age at onset ranged from 10 to 20 years. Neuropathologic findings included degeneration of CST and posterior columns. A genome-wide scan performed in one family revealed linkage to a novel locus for HSP on chromosome 12p13 in the SAX1 gene locus. Haplotype construction with 13 polymorphic markers revealed that all three families shared the disease haplotype with key recombinants and overlapping haplotypes that refined to a 5-cM region flanked by the markers D12S93 and GATA151H05. The detections of a shared disease haplotype suggested the origin from a common ancestor. The cause of SPAX1 is due to pathogenic mutation at the 12p13 locus of the *SAX1* gene (Table 2).

SACS

ARSACS, or SACS, were named for the region of Quebec where one in 22 individuals carrying the gene was first described among 42 French Canadians in 24 sibships (126). The incidence at birth of this disorder has been estimated at 1 in 1932 persons, giving a carrier frequency of 1 in 21 persons for the period 1941 to 1985 (127). It is likely to be the result of a founder effect, and unique mutation accounts for most, if not all, of the ARSACS cases in these regions. None of the patients ever walked normally; the oldest patient was 52 years old and the disorder had a long course with little progression over 20 years from early childhood. Clinical features included ataxia, dysarthria, spasticity, distal atrophy, nystagmus, defective conjugate ocular pursuit, retinal striation, mitral valve prolapse; slow nerve conduction velocities with evidence of denervation on needle electromyography, diffuse abnormalities on EEG, low intelligence quotient, and atrophy of the vermal and anterior lobes of the cerebellum (128, 129).

Breckpot and colleagues (130) reported a Belgian patient who was found to be compound heterozygous for a point mutation in the *SACS* gene and a *de novo* 1.54-Mb microdeletion on chromosome 13q12.12 involving six genes, including the *SACS* gene. Baets and coworkers (131) identi-

fied homozygous and compound heterozygous mutations in the *SACS* gene in 13% of 85 index patients with suggestive ARSACS phenotypes, among them 11 missense, five frameshift, one nonsense, and one in-frame deletion.

The disorder presumably stems from two ancestral haplotypes of the gene for ARSACS located on chromosome 13q11. The gene for ARSACS encodes the protein sacsin. The gene is highly conserved in humans and mice and encodes a single gigantic exon, which is the largest to be identified in any vertebrate organism. Sacsin is comprised of three large segments with sequence similarity to each other, two of which have domains similar to the N-terminal of the heat shock protein Hsp90 class of heat shock proteins. Truncation of sacsin by frameshift and nonsense mutations in the putative gene causes ARSACS. Sacsin possesses both the N-terminal domain of Hsp90 and a DnaJ domain, which are involved in ATP-dependent folding of target proteins. The yeast DnaJ gene, YDJi, has specific effects on Hsp70 and Hsp90 heterocomplexes known as foldosomes, which function in chaperone-mediated protein folding. The high expression of mRNA seen in granular cell layer of experimental rat cerebellum, and the reduced thickness of the granular layer in affected patients so studied at postmortem, similarly indicate a unique role for sacsin in the CNS and neural function. The cause of SACS is due to pathogenic mutations at the 13q12.12 locus in the *SACS* gene encoding the sacsin protein (Table 2).

Sjogren-Larsson Syndrome

Sjogren and Larsson (132, 133) described the disorder named for them among kindred from Northern Sweden thought to be derived from the same mutation. It has been postulated that 1.3% of the population in that region is heterozygous for a mutation in the causative gene that leads to deficient fatty aldehyde dehydrogenase (FALDH) enzyme located at 17p11.2. The Sjogren-Larsson syndrome (SLS) is usually evident at birth due to generalized ichthyosis, ecchymosis, macular dystrophy, pigmentary degeneration of the retina, and photophobia. Failure to achieve normal cognitive, motor, and growth milestones is evident during the first and second year of life, with later progression of mental retardation, spastic di- and tetraplegia, short stature, photophobia, leg contractures, and seizures. The latter improves with fat restriction and supplementation of medium chain triglycerides. Cultured skin fibroblasts from SLS patients show impaired hexadecanol oxidation due to fatty alcohol: NAD-oxidoreductase deficiency, a complex enzyme that sequentially catalyzes the oxidation of fatty alcohol to fatty aldehyde by fatty alcohol dehydrogenase (FADH) and then to fatty acid by FALDH, which is selectively deficient in SLS cells. The latter is reduced to 50% of normal activity in obligate SLS heterozygote. The cause of

SLS is due to pathogenic mutation at the 17p11.2 locus of the aldehyde dehydrogenase, family 4, subfamily A member 2 (*ALDH3A2*) gene (Table 2), encoding FALDH.

DIFFERENTIAL DIAGNOSIS AND DIAGNOSTIC WORKUP

The differential diagnosis and laboratory evaluation of HSP is summarized in Table 3, guided by systemic evaluation of suspected kindred or index cases of HSP of possible alternative genetic and non-genetic disorders. Patients with presumed AD pHSP should be distinguished from Machado-Joseph spinocerebellar ataxia, Salla disease, and dopamine-sensitive dystonia because of the potential dramatic response to levodopa therapy in such cases.

Index cases of possible AR p-, and cHSP should be screened for Friedrich AR spinocerebellar ataxia, Krabbe and metachromatic leukodystrophy, Tay-Sachs, Sandhoff, Refsum disease, abeta-lipoproteinemia, arginase deficiency, and cerebrotendinous xanthomatosis.

Those with X-linked forms of HSP should undergo assay for long-chain-fatty acids for adrenoleukodystrophy (ALD) and adrenomyeloneuropathy (AMN), including possible heterozygote females with the AMN complex, but not kindred with male-to-male transmission (134). The gene for AMN encodes a peroxisomal membrane protein that has been mapped to Xq28, and the disease is diagnosed by the demonstration of abnormally high levels of plasma very-long-chain fatty acids (135). The clinical presentation of AMN varies widely, and the diagnosis may be missed with as many as 50% of patients demonstrating normal adrenal function (136). Identification of females with AMN complex who are carriers for X-linked ALD can be particularly challenging because adrenal function is normal in 99%, and plasma very-long-chain fatty acid levels are normal in approximately 20%. Mutational analysis (137) is the most reliable method for the identification of women who are carriers for ALD. Approximately 50% of carriers develop

an AMN-like syndrome in middle age or later. X-linked HSP syndromes are allelic with Pelizaeus-Merzbacher disease. It is likely that considered together, these three entities account for a significant proportion of X-linked familial spastic paraparesis.

The differential diagnosis of sporadic spastic paraparesis is extensive with most cases due to non-genetic causes such as cerebral palsy, human immunodeficiency virus type 1 associated tropical spastic paraparesis, multiple sclerosis, sporadic and hereditary ALS, lathyrism, chronic communicating hydrocephalus, B12 deficiency, compression of the base of the brain and spinal cord by Arnold-Chiari malformation, arteriovenous malformation, neoplasm, cervical spondylosis, or the rupture of a cervical or thoracic disk with subsequent myelopathy, as well as bilateral cerebral strokes, CNS syphilis, and PLS, the latter of which is a diagnosis of exclusion (138).

THERAPY AND COUNSELING

The important aspects of therapy are the general supportive and rehabilitative measures. Specific therapies are available for a few of the disorders, such as dietary therapy for Refsum disease, levodopa for dopamine responsive dystonia, and bone marrow transplantation for the adult form of Krabbe leukodystrophy.

Genetic counseling is of great importance and can be specific and accurate for AMN, SLS, Krabbe and metachromatic leukodystrophy, and the disorders cited above in which the gene defects and mutations have been identified. Counseling for HSP, in which the gene or metabolic defects have not yet been defined, continues to represent a challenge. In respect to the AD pHSP syndromes, it should be noted that most of these disorders are compatible with personally and professionally satisfactory quality of life and can be helped by rehabilitative measures.

REFERENCES

1. Schule R, Schols L. Genetics of hereditary spastic paraplegias. *Semin Neurol* 2011; 31:484–493.
2. de Bot ST, van de Warrenburg BPC, Kremer HPH, et al. Child neurology: hereditary spastic paraplegia in children. *Neurology* 2010; 75:e75–e79.
3. Fink JK. Hereditary Spastic Paraplegia Overview. In, Pagon RA, Bird TD, Dolan DR, et al., eds. *GeneReviews* [Internet], Seattle (WA): University of Washington, Seattle. Bookshelf ID: NBK1509, PMID: 20301662.
4. Salinas S, Proukakis C, Crosby A, et al. Hereditary spastic paraplegia: clinical features and pathogenetic mechanisms. *Lancet Neurol* 2008; 7:1127–1138.
5. McMonagie P, Webb S, Hutchinson M. The prevalence of "pure" autosomal dominant hereditary spastic paraparesis in the island of Ireland. *J Neurol Neurosurg Psychiatry* 2002; 72:43–46.
6. Zhao X, Alvarado D, Rainier S, et al. Mutations in a newly identified GTPase gene cause autosomal dominant hereditary spastic paraplegia. *Nature Genet* 2001; 29:326–331.
7. Muglia M, Magariello A, Nicoletti G, et al. Further evidence that SPG3A gene mutations cause autosomal dominant hereditary spastic paraplegia. *Ann Neurol* 2002; 51:794–795.
8. Ivanova N, Claeys KG, Deconick T, et al. Hereditary spastic paraplegia 3A associated with axonal neuropathy. *Arch Neurol* 2007; 64:706–713.

9. Rainier S, Sher C, Reish O, et al. De novo occurrence of novel SPG3A/atlastin mutation presenting as cerebral palsy. *Arch Neurol* 2006; 63:445–447.

10. Svenson IK, Ashley-Koch AE, Gaskell PC, et al. Identification and expression analysis of spastin gene mutations in hereditary spastic paraplegia. *Am J Hum Genet* 2001; 68:1077–1085.

11. Meijer IA, Hand CK, Cossette P, et al. Spectrum of SPG4 mutations in a large collection of North American families with hereditary spastic paraplegia. *Arch Neurol* 2002; 59:281–286.

12. Depienne C, Tallaksen C, Lephay JY, et al. Spastic mutations are frequent in sporadic spastic paraparesis and their spectrum is different than that observed in familial cases (Letter). *Med Genet* 2006; 43:259–265.

13. Crippa F, Panzeri C, Martinuzzi A, et al. Eight novel mutations in SPG4 in a large sample of patients with hereditary spastic paraplegia. *Arch Neurol* 2006; 63:750–755.

14. Muglia M, Criscuolo C, Magariello A, et al. Narrowing of the critical region in autosomal recessive spastic paraplegia linked to the SPG5 locus. *Neurogenetics* 2004; 5:49–54.

15. Wilkinson PA, Crosby AH, Turner C, et al. A clinical and genetic study of SPG5A linked autosomal recessive hereditary spastic paraplegia. *Neurology* 2003; 61:235–238.

16. Tsaousidou MK, Ouahchi K, Warner T, et al. Sequence alterations within CYP7B1 implicate defective cholesterol homeostasis in motor-neuron degeneration. *Am J Hum Genet* 2008; 82:510–515.

17. Goizet C, Boukhris A, Durr A, et al. CYP7B1 mutations in pure and complex forms of hereditary spastic paraplegia type 5. *Brain* 2009; 132:1589–1600.

18. Hentati A, Pericak-Vance MA, Hung W-Y, et al. Linkage of 'pure' autosomal recessive familial spastic paraplegia to chromosome 8 markers and evidence of genetic locus heterogeneity. *Hum Mol Genet* 1994 3:1263–1267.

19. Rainer S, Chai JH, Tokarz D, et al. NIPA1 gene mutations cause autosomal dominant hereditary spastic paraplegia (SPG6). *Am J Hum Genet* 2003; 73:967–971.

20. Chai JH, Locke DP, Greally JM, et al. Identification of four highly conserved genes between breakpoint hotspots BP1 and BP2 of the Prader-Willi/Angelman syndromes deletion region that have undergone evolutionary transposition mediated by flanking duplicons. *Am J Hum Genet* 2003; 73:898–925.

21. De Michele G, De Fusco M, Cavalcanti F, et al. A new locus for autosomal recessive hereditary spastic paraplegia maps to chromosome 16q24.3. *Am J Hum Genet* 1998; 63:135–139.

22. Casari G, DeFusco M, Ciarmatori S, et al. Spastic paraplegia and OXPHOS impairment caused by mutations in paraplegin, a nuclear-encoded mitochondrial metalloprotease. *Cell* 1998; 93:973–983.

23. Elleuch N, Depienne C, Benomar A, et al. Mutation analysis of the paraplegin gene (SPG7) in patients with hereditary spastic paraplegia. *Neurology* 2006; 66:654–659.

24. Hendera P, Rainer S, Alvarado D, et al. Novel locus for autosomal dominant hereditary spastic paraplegia, on chromosome 8q. *Am J Hum Genet* 1999; 64:563–569.

25. Rocco P, Vainzof M, Froehner SC, et al. Brazilian family with pure autosomal dominant spastic paraplegia maps to 8q: analysis of muscle beta 1 syntrophin. *Am J Med Genet* 2000; 92:122–127.

26. Valdmanis PN, Meijer IA, Reynolds A, et al. Mutations in the KIAA0196 gene at the SPG8 locus cause hereditary spastic paraplegia. *Am J Hum Genet* 2007; 80:152–161.

27. Reid E, Dearlove AM, Rhodes M, et al. A new locus for autosomal dominant "pure" spastic hereditary paraplegia mapping to chromosome 12q13, and evidence for further genetic heterogeneity. *Am J Hum Genet* 1999; 65:757–763.

28. Reid E, Kloos M, Ashley-Koch A, et al. A kinesin heavy chain (KIF5A) mutation in hereditary spastic paraplegia (SPG10). *Am J Hum Genet* 2002; 71:1189–1194.

29. Fichera M, Lo Giudice M, Falco M et al. Evidence of kinesin heavy chain (KIF5A) involvement in pure hereditary spastic paraplegia. *Neurology* 2004; 63:1108–1110.

30. Blair MA, Ma S, Hedera P. Mutation in KIF5A can also cause adult-onset hereditary spastic paraplegia. *Neurogenetics* 2006; 7:47–50.

31. Lo Giudice M, Neri M, Falco M, et al. A missense mutation in the coiled-coil domain of the KIF5A gene and late-onset hereditary spastic paraplegia. *Arch Neurol* 2006; 63:284–287.

32. Martinez Murillo F, Kobayashi H, Pegoraro E, et al. Genetic localization of a new locus for recessive familial spastic paraparesis to 15q13-15. *Neurology* 1999; 53:50–56.

33. Stevanin G, Montagna G, Azzedine H, et al. Spastic paraplegia with thin corpus callosum: description of 20 new families, refinement of the SPG11 locus, candidate gene analysis and evidence of genetic heterogeneity. *Neurogenetics* 2006; 7:149–156.

34. Orlen H, Melberg A, Raininko R, et al. SPG11 mutations cause Kjellin syndrome, a hereditary spastic paraplegia with thin corpus callosum and central retinal degeneration. *Am J Med Genet B Neuropsychiat Genet* 2009; 150B:984–992.

35. Reid E, Dearlove AM, Osborne O, et al. A locus for autosomal dominant "pure" hereditary spastic paraplegia maps to chromosome 19q13. *Am J Hum Genet* 2000; 66:728–732.

36. Ashley-Koch A, Bonner ER, Gaskell PC, et al. Fine mapping and genetic heterogeneity in the pure form of autosomal dominant familial spastic paraplegia. *Neurogenetics* 2001; 3:91–97.

37. Orlacchio A, Kawarai T, Rogaeva E, et al. Clinical and genetic study of a large Italian family linked to SPG12 locus. *Neurology* 2002; 59:1395–1401.

38. Montenegro G, Rebelo AP, Connell J, et al. Mutations in the ER-shaping protein reticulon 2 cause the axon-degenerative disorder hereditary spastic paraplegia type 12. *J Clin Invest* 2012; 122:538–544.

39. Fontaine B, Davoine CS, Durr A, et al. A new locus for autosomal dominant pure spastic paraplegia, on chromosome 2q24-q34. *Am J Hum Genet* 2000; 66:702–707.

40. Hansen JJ, Durr A, Cournu-Rebeix I, et al. Hereditary spastic paraplegia SPG13 is associated with a mutation in the gene encoding the mitochondrial chaperonin Hsp60. *Am J Hum Genet* 2002; 70:1328–1332.

41. Valente EM, Brancati F, Caputo V, et al. Novel locus for autosomal dominant pure hereditary spastic paraplegia (SPG19) maps to chromosome 9q33-q34. *Ann Neurol* 2002; 51:681–685.

42. Bouslam N, Benomar A, Azzedine H, et al. Mapping of a new form of pure autosomal recessive spastic paraplegia (SPG28). *Ann Neurol* 2005; 57:567–571.

43. Zuchner S, Kail ME, Nance MA, et al. A new locus for dominant hereditary spastic paraplegia maps to chromosome 2p12 (Letter). *Neurogenetics* 2006; 7:127–129.

44. Zuchner S, Wang G, Tran-Viet KN, et al. Mutation in the novel mitochondrial protein REEP1 cause hereditary spastic paraplegia type 31. *Am J Hum Genet* 2006; 79:365–369.

45. Hewamadduma C, McDermott C, Kirby J, et al. New pedigrees and novel mutation expand the phenotype of REEP1-associated hereditary spastic paraplegia (HSP). *Neurogenetics* 2009; 10:105–110.

46. Beetz C, Schule R, Deconirck T, et al. REEP1 mutation spectrum and genotype/phenotype correlation in hereditary spastic paraplegia type 31. *Brain* 2008; 131:1078–1086.

47. Mannan AU, Krawen P, Sauter SM, et al. ZFYVE27 (SPG33),

a novel spastin-binding protein, is mutated in hereditary spastic paraplegia. *Am J Hum Genet* 2006; 79:351–357.

48. Shirane M, Nakayama KI. Protrudin induces neurite formation by directional membrane trafficking. *Science* 2006; 314:818–821.

49. Starling A, Rocco P, Cambi F, et al. Further evidence for a fourth gene causing X-linked pure spastic paraplegia. *Am J Med Genet* 2002; 111:152–156.

50. Zatz M, Penha-Serrano C, Otto P, et al. X-linked recessive type of pure spastic paraplegia in a large pedigree: absence of detectable linkage with Xg. *J Med Genet* 1976; 13:217–222.

51. Macedo-Souza LI, Kok F, Santos S, et al. Reevaluation of a large family defines a new locus for X-linked recessive pure spastic paraplegia (SPG34) on chromosome Xq25. *Neurogenetics* 2008; 9:225–226.

52. Hanein S, Durr A, Ribai P, et al. A novel locus for autosomal dominant "uncomplicated" hereditary spastic paraplegia maps to chromosome 8p21.1-q13.3. *Hum Genet* 2007; 122:261–273.

53. Zhao G, Hu Z, Shen L, et al. A novel candidate locus on chromosome 11p14.1-p11.2 for autosomal dominant hereditary spastic paraplegia. *Chin Med J* 2008; 121:430–434.

54. Lin P, Liu Q, Mao F, et al. A missense mutation in SLC33A1, which encodes the acetyl-CoA transporter, causes autosomal-dominant spastic paraplegia (SPG42). *Am J Hum Genet* 2008; 83:752–759.

55. Schlipf NA, Beetz C, Schule R, et al. A total of 220 patients with autosomal dominant spastic paraplegia do not display mutations in the SLC33A1 gene (SPG42). *Eur J Hum Genet* 2010; 18:1065–1067.

56. Bianchine JW, Lewis RC Jr. The MASA syndrome: a new heritable mental retardation syndrome. *Clin Genet* 1974; 5:298–306.

57. Kenwrick S, Ionasescu G, Ionasescu V, et al. Linkage studies of X-linked recessive spastic paraplegia using DNA probes. *Hum Genet* 1986; 73:264–266.

58. Winter RM, Davies KE, Bell MV, et al. MASA syndrome: further clinical delineation and chromosomal localisation. *Hum Genet* 1989; 82:367–370.

59. Schrander-Stumpel C, Meyer H, Merckx D, et al. The spectrum of "complicated spastic paraplegia, MASA syndrome, and X-linked hydrocephalusz": Contribution of DNA linkage analysis in genetic counseling of individual families. *Genet Counsel* 1994; 5:1–10.

60. Schrander-Stumpel C, Howeler C, Jones M, et al. Spectrum of X-linked hydrocephalus (HSAS), MASA syndrome, and complicated spastic paraplegia (SPG1): Clinical review with six additional families. *Am J Med Genet* 1995; 57:107–116.

61. Fransen E, Lemmon V, Van Camp G, et al. CRASH syndrome: clinical spectrum of corpus callosum hypoplasia, retardation, adducted thumbs, spastic paraparesis, and hydrocephalus due to mutation in one single gene, L1. *Eur J Hum Genet* 1995; 3:273–284.

62. Kenwrick S, Watkins A, De Angelis E. Neuronal cell recognition molecule L1: relating biological complexity to human disease mutations. *Hum Molec Genet* 2000; 9:879–886.

63. Johnston AW, McKusick VA. A sex-linked recessive form of spastic paraplegia. *Am J Hum Genet* 1962; 14:83–94.

64. Ginter DN, Konigsmark BW, Abbott MH. X-linked spinocerebellar degeneration. *Birth Defects Orig Art Ser* 1974; 10:334–336.

65. Keppen LD, Leppert MF, O'Connell P, et al. Etiological heterogeneity in X-linked spastic paraplegia. *Am J Hum Genet* 1987; 4:933–943.

66. Bonneau D, Rozet J-M, Bulteau C, et al. X linked paraplegia (SPG2): clinical heterogeneity at a single gene locus. *J Med Genet* 1993; 30:381–394.

67. Swanton E, Holland A, High S, et al. Disease-associated

mutations cause premature oligomerization of myelin proteolipid protein in the endoplasmic reticulum. *Proc Nat Acad Sci USA* 2005; 102:4342–4347.

68. Slavotinek AM, Pike M, Mills K, et al. Cataracts, motor system disorder, short stature, learning difficulties, and skeletal abnormalities: a new syndrome? *Am J Med Genet* 1996; 62:42–47.

69. Seri M, Cusano R, Forabosco P, et al. Genetic mapping to 10q23.3-q24.2, in a large Italian pedigree, of a new syndrome showing bilateral cataracts, gastroesophageal reflux, and spastic paraparesis with amyotrophy. *Am J Hum Genet* 1999; 64:586–593.

70. Vazza G, Zortea M, Boaretto F, et al. A new locus for autosomal recessive spastic paraplegia associated with mental retardation and distal motor neuropathy, SPG14, maps to chromosome 3q27-q28. *Am J Hum Genet* 2000; 67:504–509.

71. Hughes CA, Byrne PC, Webb S, et al. SPG15, a new locus for autosomal recessive complicated HSP on chromosome 14q. *Neurology* 2001; 56:1230–1233.

72. Kjellin K. Familial spastic paraplegia with amyotrophy, oligophrenia, and central retinal degeneration. *Arch Neurol* 1959; 1:133–140.

73. Hanein S, Martin E, Boukhris A, et al. Identification of the SPG15 gene, encoding spastizin, as a frequent cause of complicated autosomal-recessive spastic paraplegia, including Kjellin syndrome. *Am J Hum Genet* 2008; 82:992–1002.

74. Elleuch N, Bouslam N, Hanein S, et al. Refinement of the SPG15 locus candidate interval and phenotypic heterogeneity in three large Arab families. *Neurogenetics* 2007; 8:307–315.

75. Casali C, Valente EM, Bertini E, et al. Clinical and genetic studies in hereditary spastic paraplegia with thin corpus callosum. *Neurology* 2004; 62:262–268.

76. Boukhris A, Feki I, Denis E, et al. Spastic paraplegia 15: linkage and clinical description of three Tunisian families. *Mov Disord* 2008; 23:429–433.

77. Crook R, Verkkoniemi A, Periz-Tur J, et al. A variant of Alzheimer's disease with spastic paraparesis and unusual plaques due to deletion of exon 9 of presenilin 1. *Nat Med* 1998; 4:452–455.

78. Claes S, Devriendt K, Van Goethem G, et al. Novel syndromic form of X-linked complicated spastic paraplegia. *Am J Med Genet* 2000; 94:1–4.

79. Tamagaki A, Shima M, Tomita R, et al. Segregation of a pure form of spastic paraplegia and NOR insertion into Xq11.2. *Am J Med Genet* 2000; 94:5–8.

80. Silver JR. Familial spastic paraplegia with amyotrophy of the hands. *Ann Hum Genet* 1966; 30:69–75.

81. Patel H, Hart PE, Warner TT, et al. The Silver syndrome variant of hereditary spastic paraplegia maps to chromosome 11q12-q14, with evidence for genetic heterogeneity within this subtype. *Am J Hum Genet* 2001; 69:209–215.

82. Windpassinger C, Auer-Grumbach M, Irobi J, et al. Heterozygous missense mutations I BSCL2 are associated with distal hereditary motor neuropathy and Silver syndrome. *Nature Genet* 2004; 36:271–276.

83. Auer-Grumbach M, Loscher WN, Wagner K, et al. Phenotypic and genotypic heterogeneity in hereditary motor neuronopathy type V: a clinical, electrophysiological and genetic study. *Brain* 2000; 123:1612–1623.

84. Ito D, Suzuki N. Seipinopahy: a novel endoplasmic reticulum stress-associated disease. *Brain* 2009; 132:8–15.

85. Al-Yahyaee S, Al-Gazali LI, De Jonghe P, et al. A novel locus for hereditary spastic paraplegia with thin corpus callosum and epilepsy. *Neurology* 2006; 66:1230–1234.

86. Alazami AM, Adly N, Al Dhalaan H, et al. A nullimorphic ERLIN2 mutation defines a complicated hereditary spastic paraplegia locus (SPG18). *Neurogenetics* 2011; 12:333–336.

87. Cross HE, McKusick VA. The Troyer syndrome: A recessive form of spastic paraplegia with distal muscle wasting. *Arch Neurol* 1967; 16:473–485.

88. Patel H, Cross H, Proukakis C, et al. SPG20 is mutated in Troyer syndrome, an hereditary spastic paraplegia. *Nat Genet* 2002; 31:347–348.

89. Manzini MC, Rajab A, Maynard TM, et al. Developmental and degenerative features in a complicated spastic paraplegia. *Ann Neurol* 2010; 67:516–525.

90. Cross HE, McKusick VA. The Mast syndrome: a recessively inherited form of presenile dementia with motor disturbances. *Arch Neurol* 1967; 16:1–13.

91. Simpson MA, Cross H, Proukakis C, et al. Maspardin is mutated in mast syndrome, a complicated form of hereditary spastic paraplegia associated with dementia. *Am J Hum Genet* 2003; 73:1147–1156.

92. Abdallat A, Davis SM, Farrage J, McDonald WI. Disordered pigmentation, spastic paraparesis and peripheral neuropathy in three siblings: a new neurocutaneous syndrome. *J Neurol Neurosurg Psychiatry* 1980; 43:962–966.

93. Mukamel M, Weitz R, Metzker A, Varsano I. Spastic paraparesis, mental retardation, and cutaneous pigmentation disorder: A new syndrome. *Am J Dis Child* 1985; 139:1090–1092.

94. Bamforth JS. Vitiligo-spasticity syndrome; new case. *Clin Dysmorphol* 2003; 12:137–139.

95. Hodgkinson CA, Bohlega S, Abu-Amero SN, et al. A novel form of autosomal recessive pure hereditary spastic paraplegia maps to chromosome 13q14. *Neurology* 2002; 59:1905–1909.

96. Zortea M, Vettori A, Trevisan CP, et al. Genetic mapping of a susceptibility locus for disc herniation and spastic paraplegia on 6q23.3-q24.1). *J Med Genet* 2002; 39:387–390.

97. Farag TI, El-Badramany MH, Al-Sharkawy S. Troyer Syndrome: report of the first "non-Amish" sibship and review (Letter). *Am J Med Genet* 1994; 53.383–385.

98. Wilkinson PA, Simpson MA, Bastaki L, et al. A new locus for autosomal recessive complicated hereditary spastic paraplegia (SPG26) maps to chromosome 12p11.1-12q14 (Letter). *Med Genet* 2005; 42:80–82.

99. Meijer IA, Cossette P, Roussel J, et al. A novel locus for pure recessive herditary spastic paraplegia maps to 10q22.1-10q24.1. *Ann Neurol* 2004; 56:579–582.

100. Orlacchio A, Kawarai T, Gaudiello F, et al. New locus for hereditary spastic paraplegia maps to chromosome 1p31.1-1p21.1. *Ann Neurol* 2005; 58:423–429.

101. Klebe S, Azzedine H, Durr A, et al. Autosomal recessive spastic paraplegia (SPG30) with mild ataxia and sensory neuropathy maps to chromosome 2q37.3. *Brain* 2006; 129:1456–1462.

102. Erlich Y, Edvardson S, Hodges E, et al. Exome sequencing and disease-network analysis of a single family implicate a mutation in K1F1A in hereditary spastic paraparesis. *Genome Res* 2011; 21:658–664.

103. Stevanin G, Paternotte C, Coutinho P, et al. A new locus for autosomal recessive spastic paraplegia (SPG32) on chromosome 14q12-q21. *Neurology* 2007; 68:1837–1840.

104. Dick KJ, Al-Mjeni R, Baskir W, et al. A novel locus for an autosomal recessive hereditary spastic paraplegia (SPG35) maps to 16q21-q23. *Neurology* 2008; 71:248–252.

105. Dick KJ, Eckhardt M, Paisan-Ruiz C, et al. Mutation of FA2H underlies a complicated form of hereditary spastic paraplegia (SPG35). *Hum Mutat* 2010; 31:E1251–E1260.

106. Edvardson S, Hama H, Shaag A, et al. Mutations in the fatty acid 2-hydroxylase gene are associated with leukodystrophy with spastic paraparesis and dystonia. *Am J Hum Genet* 2008; 83:643–648.

107. Kruer MC, Paisan-Ruiz C, Boddaert N, et al. Defective FA2H leads to a novel form of neurodegeneration with brain iron accumulation (NBIA). *Ann Neurol* 2010; 68:611–618.

108. Alderson NL, Rembiesa BM, Walla MD, et al. The human FA2H gene encodes a fatty acid 2-hydroxylase. *J Biol Chem* 2004; 279:48562–48568.

109. Schule R, Bonin M, Durr A, et al. Autsomal dominant spastic paraplegia with peripheral neuropathy maps to chr12q23-24. *Neurology* 2009; 72:1893–1898.

110. Orlacchio A, Patrono C, Gaudiello F, et al. Silver syndrome variant of hereditary spastic paraplegia: a locus to 4p and allelism with SPG4. *Neurology* 2008; 70:1959–1966.

111. Single MA, Statland JM, Wolfe GI, et al. Primary lateral sclerosis. *Muscle Nerve* 2007; 35:291–302.

112. Rogaeva E, Bergeron C, Sato C, et al. Alzheimer's disease family with spastic paraplegia: the search for a gene modifier. *Neurology* 2003; 61:1005–1007.

113. White SR, Evans KJ, Lary J, et al. Recognition of C-terminal amino acids in tubulin by pore loops in Spastin is important for microtubule severing. *J Cell Biol* 2007; 176:995–1005.

114. Rainier S, Bui M, Mark E, et al. Neuropathy target esterase gene mutations cause motor neuron disease. *Am J Hum Genet* 2008; 82:780–785.

115. Orthmann-Murphy JL, Salsano E, Abrams CK, et al. Hereditary spastic paraplegia is a novel phenotype for GJA12/GJC2 mutations. *Brain* 2009; 132:426–438.

116. Menichella DM, Goodenough DA, Sirkowski E, et al. Connexins are critical for normal myelination in the CNS. *J Neurosci* 2003; 23:5963–5973.

117. Dursun U, Koroglu C, Orhan EK, et al. Autosomal recessive spastic paraplegia (SPG45) with mental retardation maps to 10q24.3-q25.1. *Neurogenetics* 2009; 10:325–331.

118. Boukhris A, Stevanin G, Feki I, et al. Hereditary spastic paraplegia with mental impairment and thin corpus callosum in Tunisia. SPG11, SPG15, and further genetic heterogeneity. *Arch Neurol* 2008; 65:393–402.

119. Boukhris A, Feki I, Elleuch N, et al. A new locus (SPG46) maps to 9p21.2-q21.12 in a Tunisian family with a complicated autosomal recessive hereditary spastic paraplegia with mental impairment and thin corpus callosum. *Neurogenetics* 2010; 11:441–448.

120. Abou Jamra RA, Philippe O, Raas-Rothschild A, et al. Adaptor protein complex 4 deficiency causes severe autosomal-recessive intellectual disability, progressive spastic paraplegia, shy character, and short stature. *Am J Hum Genet* 2011; 88:788–795.

121. Blumkin L, Lerman-Sagie T, Lev D, et al. A new locus (SPG47) maps to 1p13.2-1p12 in an Arab family with complicated autosomal recessive hereditary spastic paraplegia and thin corpus callosum. *J Neurol Sci* 2011; 305:67–70.

122. Bauer P, Leshinsky-Silver E, Blumkin L, et al. Mutation in the AP4B1 gene cause hereditary spastic paraplegia type 47 (SPG47). *Neurogenetics* 2012; 13:73–76.

123. Moreno-De Luca A, Helmers SL, Mao H, et al. Adaptor protein complex-4 (AP-4) deficiency causes a novel autosomal recessive cerebral palsy syndrome with microcephaly and intellectual disability. *J Med Genet* 2011; 48:141–144.

124. Slabicki M, Theis M, Krastev DB, et al. A genome-scale DNA repair RNAi screen identifies SPG48 as a novel gene associated with hereditary spastic paraplegia. *PLoS Biol* 2010; 8:1000408.

125. Meijer IA, Hand CK, Grewal KK, et al. A locus for autsomal dominant hereditary spastic ataxia, SAX1, maps to chromosome 12p13. *Am J Hum Genet* 2002; 70:763–769.

126. Bouchard J, Barbeau A, Bouchard R, et al. Autosomal recessive spastic ataxia of Charlevoix-Saguenay. *Canad J Neurol Sci* 1978; 5:61–69.

127. De Braekeleer M, Gauthier S. Autosomal recessive disorders

in Saguenay-Lac-Saint-Jean (Quebec, Canada): a study of inbreeding. *Ann Hum Genet* 1996; 60:51–56.

128. Langelier R, Bouchard JP, Bouchard R. Computed tomography of posterior fossa in hereditary ataxias. *Canad J Neurol Sci* 1979; 6:195–198.

129. Bouchard JP, Barbeau A, Bouchard R, et al. Electromyography and nerve conduction studies in Friedrich's ataxia and autosomal recessive spastic ataxia of Charlevoix-Saguenay (ARSACS). *Canad J Neurol Sci* 1979; 6:191–194.

130. Breckpot J, Takiyama Y, Thienpont B, et al. A novel genomic disorder: a deletion of the SACS gene leading to spastic ataxia of Charlevoix-Saguenay. *Eur J Hum Genet* 2008; 16:1050–1054.

131. Baets J, Deconinck T, Smets K, et al. Mutations in SACS cause atypical and late-onset forms of ARSACS. *Neurology* 2010; 75:1181–1188.

132. Sjogren T. Oligophrenia combined with congenital ichthyosiform erythrodermia, spastic syndrome and macular retinal degeneration: a clinical and genetic study. *Acta Genet Statist Med* 1956; 6:80–91.

133. Sjogren T, Larsson T. Oligophrenia in combination with congenital ichthyosis and spastic disorders; a clinical and genetic study. *Acta Psychiatr Neurol Scand* Suppl 1957; 32:1–112.

134. Maris GT, Androlidakis J, Tzagournissakis M, et al. X-linked adrenoleukodystrophy presenting as neurologically pure familial spastic paraparesis. *Neurology* 1995; 45:1101–1104.

135. Moser AB, Kreiter N, Bezman L, et al. Plasma very long chain fatty acids in 3,000 perixosomal disease patients and 29,000 controls. *Ann Neurol* 1999; 45:100–110.

136. Brennemann W, Kohler W, Zierz S, et al. Occurrence of adrenocortical insufficiency in adrenomyeloneuropathy. *Neurology* 1996; 47:605.

137. Boehm CD, Cutting GR, Lachtermacher MB, et al. Accurate DNA-based diagnostic carrier testing for X-linked adrenoleukodystrophy. *Mol Genet Metab* 1999; 66:128–136.

138. Younger DS, Chou S, Hays AP, et al. Primary lateral sclerosis: a clinical diagnosis reemerges. *Arch Neurol* 1988; 45:1304–1307.

CHAPTER 39

Tropical Myeloneuropathies

Gustavo C. Román

INTRODUCTION

The pattern of neurologic disease in the tropics is determined primarily by socioeconomic factors rather than by geography or climate (1–3). In fact, tropical diseases such as malaria and cysticercosis were common in Europe and North America a century ago. Lack of proper environmental sanitation, potable water, overcrowding, malnutrition, and exposure to neurotoxins are some of the determinants of spinal cord and peripheral nerve diseases in the tropics (4).

TROPICAL MYELOPATHY

Acute Tropical Myeloneuropathy

Schistosomiasis, or bilharziasis, is the commonest cause of acute adult myelopathy in the tropics due to spinal cord involvement by *Schistosoma haematobium*, particularly in Africa and the Middle East, and by *S. mansoni* in the Caribbean, Venezuela, and Brazil. Bilharziasis is a major health problem in the tropics, with an estimated 600 million people at risk (1, 2, and 5). It occurs when cercariae, released from a freshwater intermediate snail host, pierce and penetrate human skin or mucosal surfaces with invasion of the bloodstream, usually while the human host swims in a pond or a river. Magnetic resonance imaging (MRI) shows abnormal hyperintense lesions due to parasitic involvement in the region of the conus medullaris. An enzyme-linked immunosorbent assay (ELISA) confirms the causative organism. Praziquantel is the drug of choice in uncomplicated cases, but corticosteroids and decompressive laminectomy may be necessary in those with severe compression or cerebrospinal fluid (CSF) block on myelogram.

Transverse Myelitis

Acute transverse myelitis is the commonest cause of back pain in children presenting with a spinal cord syndrome that evolves over hours or days after a viral infection or vaccination, the differential diagnosis of which is with nucleus pulposus embolism (6). Corticosteroids are recommended treatment for this condition. Human rabies likewise presents as a postviral transverse myelitis following the bite of a rabid bat. African children that survive on a diet of cassava are at risk for konzo, a form of acute spastic paraplegia due to excessive cyanide consumption and poor dietary intake of sulphur-containing amino acids (7).

Multiple sclerosis (MS) is rare in the tropics; however a number of well-documented patients have been reported from Africa and Latin America. Devic disease or neuromyelitis optica, which includes bilateral optic neuritis and transverse myelitis, is the commonest form of MS in India, Japan, and the Caribbean. Subacute myelo-optic neuropathy (SMON), due to consumption of clioquinol and the related halogenated quinolones, present in plants of the *Annonaceae* family and in herbal teas of the Caribbean, cause a similar disease (8).

Chronic Tropical Myelopathy

Tropical Spastic Paraparesis

Infection with the human T-lymphotropic virus type I (HTLV-I) is the cause of tropical spastic paraparesis, the commonest late-onset spastic paraplegia in the tropics (9). It is also the cause of adult T-cell leukemia-lymphoma. Cases occur endemically in South America, the Caribbean, Seychelles Islands in the Indian Ocean, Africa, and non-tropical areas of Japan. It presents clinically with leg stiffness and cramps accompanied by incapacitating gait difficulty due to proximal weakness of the legs, urinary frequency, constipation, and impotence in men. Serum and CSF shows typical segmented leukocytes or flower cells, and high titers of anti-HTLV-I antibodies. Rare patients with HTLV-II-associated tropical spastic paraparesis have been described that bears striking resemblance to amyotrophic lateral sclerosis (ALS) because of muscle weakness, wasting, and fasciculation in distal hand, shoulder, and tongue muscles.

Symptomatic treatment of HTLV-I myelitis includes anti-spasticity agents such as baclofen and tizanidine, along with physical therapy and bladder catheterization. Pentoxifylline (Trental®) appeared to be safe and moderately effective in open-label trials. This medication has immuno-modulatory effects such as increase in levels of interleukin (IL)-4 and IL-10, and a decrease in interferon-γ gamma levels. Other suggested treatments include oral prednisolone, high-dose methylprednisolone, azathioprine, high-dose vitamin C, and danazole. Short-term benefit with plasma exchange has been reported. Interferon-alpha (IFN)-α may have beneficial effects as does high-dose zidovudine at a dose of 2 grams per g/day. The nucleoside reverse-transcriptase inhibitors, including lamivudine (3-TC), zalcitabine (ddC), didanosine (ddI), and stavudine (d4T) have also been administered.

TROPICAL NEUROPATHY

Peripheral neuropathy is relatively common in the tropics (4). In addition to leprosy, other etiologies of neuropathy include diabetes mellitus, genetic disorders, alcoholism, inflammatory, post-infectious, neurotoxic, and nutritional micronutrient deficiencies (Table 1).

According to the World Health Organization (WHO) leprous neuropathy due to infection by *Mycobacterium leprae* had an estimated global prevalence of 10 to 12 million persons in the 1980s, that fell to 2.4 million persons in the 1990s, due to widespread use of combined antimicrobial therapy (2). With an occurrence throughout the tropics and subtropics of Southeast Asia, Africa, Central and South America, the western Pacific, the eastern Mediterranean, Japan, Korea, China, Hawaii, Florida, and Louisiana, the tuberculoid, lepromatous, and borderline forms are all characterized by palpable nerve thickening accompanied by skin areas of anesthesia. Multi-drug treatment includes dapsone, rifampicin, and clofazimine. Corticosteroids and thalidomide are often required for the treatment of erythema nodosum leprosum and other reactions to the treatment. Prevention of eye complications, joint erosion, and deformities is mandatory.

Table 1. Tropical Peripheral Neuropathy

Inflammatory and Postinfective Neuropathies
- Leprosy
- Guillain-Barré syndrome
  - Acute demyelinating neuropathy
  - Acute motor axonal neuropathy (Chinese paralytic syndrome)
  - Postrabies vaccine paralysis
- Other postinfectious neuropathies
- Neuropathies of infectious diseases
  - *Campylobacter jejuni*
  - Rabies
  - Diphtheria
  - Mycoplasma
  - Lyme borreliosis (Bannwarth's syndrome)
  - HIV (AIDS)
  - HTLV-I/II

Toxic Neuropathy
- Heavy metals
  - Arsenic
  - Lead
  - Thalium
- Insecticides
  - Organophosphorous esters
  - Plant poisons
  - *Manihot* (cassava)
  - *Karwinskia humboldtiana*
  - *Gloriosa superba*
  - *Podophyllum pelatum*
- Animal poisons
  - Ciguatoxin
  - Paralytic shellfish poisoning (saxitoxin)
  - Tick-bite paralysis

Systemic Disease
- Diabetes mellitus
- Amyloidosis
- Uremia
- Sarcoidosis
- Myxedema
- Connective tissue diseases
- Acute intermittent porphyria
- Critical illness neuropathy

Nutritional Neuropathy
- Beriberi and other B-group vitamin deficiencies
- Strachan's syndrome
- Tropical malabsorption-malnutrition
- Alcoholic neuropathy

Disorders of Neuromuscular Transmission
- Myasthenia gravis
- Botulism
- Animal poisons
  - Neurotoxic snake bite
  - Marine neurotoxins
  - Dart-poison frogs (South America)
  - Tick-bite paralysis
- Plant Poisons
  - Curare
- Insecticide intoxication (intermediate syndrome)
- Other etiologies
- Trauma, neoplasia, genetic neuropathies

Modified from Román GC. Tropical neuropathies. *Baillière's Clin Neurol* 1995; 4:469–487.

With the decline of poliomyelitis as a cause of acute flaccid paralysis, Guillain-Barré syndrome (GBS) is the most frequent cause of acute childhood tropical paralysis with an incidence that exceeds that of developed countries. In Central America, poisoning with *Karwinskia calderoni* and *K. humboldtiana* resembles GBS. Clusters of affected GBS patients occur in association with swine flu vaccination, poliomyelitis vaccination, and after exposure to rabies vaccination in Latin America, India, and Thailand. Infectious agents believed to play a role in cases of GBS in the tropics include cytomegalovirus (CMV), Epstein-Barr virus (EBV), the human immunodeficiency virus type-1 (HIV-1), dengue, varicella-zoster virus (VZV), measles, and *Mycoplasma pneumoniae*. Rabies may present as an ascending or descending paralysis identical to GBS, with typical hydrophobia and aerophobia mistaken for bulbar and respiratory paralysis.

A seasonal syndrome resembling GBS in China, manifested clinically by pure motor axonopathy, was associated with *Campylobacter* infection. Neuropathologic changes in fatal cases from Mexico, Colombia, and Cuba, were similar to those observed in China. Other conditions presenting with acute tropical flaccid paralysis include botulism, elapid snake envenoming, and epidemic paralysis from dietary consumption of gossypol, a phenolic compound present in cottonseed oil leading to renal loss of potassium, and licorice (*Glycyrrhiza glabra*).

Nutritional deficiency is a proximate cause of axonal neuropathy including beriberi due to thiamine or vitamin B1 deficiency, and subacute combined degeneration due to cyanocobalamin or vitamin B12 deficiency. Less well-defined nutritional sensory neuropathies, often accompanied by optic, auditory, and spinal cord involvement, have been clinically classified under the broad term of Strachan syndrome. Vitamin B and vitamin E have experimentally been shown to cause predominant axonal neuropathy that rarely occurs in isolation in tropical conditions because most instances of human malnutrition are due instead to overall dietary deficiency however malabsorption may be an important contributory role in decreasing the availability of vitamins.

Nutritional neuropathy, endemic in subpopulations of Africa, Asia, and Latin America, results from chronically deficient diets and widespread malnutrition, however, the number of patients seeking medical attention is relatively low. When a population precariously at risk is exposed to an added factor that precipitates the expression of marginally asymptomatic patients, epidemic outbreaks occur. There may be an interaction between toxic and nutritional factors such as in superimposed alcoholic neuropathy, tobacco–alcohol amblyopia, and those associated with the consumption of cyanide-producing tropical foodstuffs, such as cassava. Precipitating factors include pregnancy and lactation, infectious diarrhea, malaria, and the increased metabolic requirements for thiamine leading to increased carbohydrate intake and intense physical activity under hot and humid weather conditions. Neurologic involvement in nutritional disorders, which may occur relatively late, is often due to severe chronic deficiency of essential or protective nutrients such as sulfur-containing amino acids and the antioxidant carotenoid lycopene which can selectively effect elements of the peripheral nervous system (PNS) including dorsal root ganglia (DRG) neurons, large myelinated distal axons, bipolar retinal and cochlear neurons.

Strachan Syndrome

First recognized by Strachan in Jamaica, this syndrome includes orogenital dermatitis, painful sensory neuropathy, amblyopia, and deafness (10). With regional variations, Strachan syndrome occurs in malnourished populations of Africa, India, and the Caribbean, and most recently in Cuba, with an estimated prevalence of 50,000 persons (11–13). It was observed during World War II in prisoners-of-war in tropical camps under conditions of dietary restriction and forced labor (14). African patients are relatively young with a mean age of 35 years, and generally come from low socioeconomic environments in sub-Saharan Africa. Sensory neuropathy, decreased vision, and hearing loss, along with sensory ataxia and spastic paraparesis, are the predominant presenting features. In about one-fourth of patients, malnutrition is evident, with skin and mucosal pellagroid changes. Women are the most affected, with pregnancy precipitating up to one-third of patients. Gastrointestinal problems were frequent, including chronic diarrhea, gastric achlorhydria or hypochlorhydria, as well as, abnormal liver biopsy, and normal CSF studies. Slow fibular motor nerve conduction velocities (NCV) were found in all patients. Sural nerve biopsy has shown histological features consistent with axonal neuropathy. Up to 65% of patients improve with parenteral vitamin B-complex treatment.

In India, patients have a predominantly sensory neuropathy associated with chronic malnutrition, alcohol abuse, and pellagra, in addition to low blood levels of thiamine, riboflavin, nicotinic acid, pantothenic acid, pyridoxine, and folic acid. Absorption and levels of vitamin B12 are generally normal. Withdrawal of alcohol, balanced diet, and vitamin B-group treatment leads to neurologic improvement. Traditionally, the neuropathy and myelopathy of pernicious anemia have been rare in the tropics, even among strict vegetarians or vegans. However, such patients are probably underdiagnosed and underreported since Indian vegan patients affected by megaloblastic anemia so studied in England were found to be dietary B12 deficiency, including some with overt pernicious anemia.

In the Caribbean, a cluster of nutritional neuropathies have been observed in Cuba (11). This epidemic neuropathy, which affected 50,862 patients between 1992 and 1993, had an incidence of 462 per 100,000 persons, with most occurring in those age 25 to 64 years, wherein children, adolescents, pregnant women, and the elderly were rarely affected. The highest rates of occurrence were found in the tobacco-growing province of Pinar del Río (11–13). Clinical manifestations include retrobulbar optic neuropathy, sensorineural deafness, sensory and autonomic neuropathy, and dorsolateral myelopathy, less often dysphonia and dysphagia, and spastic paraparesis, which occurs in mixed forms. Neurologic symptoms are preceded by weight loss, anorexia, chronic fatigue, lack of energy, irritability, sleep disturbances, and difficulties with concentration and memory. Optic neuropathy, consisting of blurred vision, photophobia, central and cecocentral scotomata, deficit of color vision for red and green, and loss of axons in the maculopapillary bundle with temporal disc pallor, is noted in advanced cases (11, 15, 16). Approximately one-third of patients have skin and mucous membrane lesions, peripheral nerve and spinal cord involvement, and 20% have hearing loss. Neuropathic symptoms include painful and burning dysesthesia of the soles and palms, numbness, cramps, paresthesiae, and hyperhidrosis (11). The peripheral nerves are sensitive to pressure, and motor involvement is minimal. Objective sensory signs are mild and include stocking and glove vibratory, light touch, and pinprick sensory loss, with decreased or absent Achilles tendon reflexes. Motor NCV are generally normal, and sensory nerve action potentials (SNAP) are decreased in severe cases. Sural nerve biopsy shows axonal neuropathy with predominant loss of large myelinated fibers (17).

Patients with dorsolateral myelopathy (11) present with sensory gait ataxia due to proprioceptive loss, imbalance, and proximal leg weakness, brisk knee reflexes, and crossed adductor responses despite decreased or absent ankle reflexes, Babinski signs, and frank spasticity. Sensorineural deafness was usually symmetric, with high-pitch tinnitus and deafness. Pure tone audiometry demonstrates 4 to 8 kHz hearing loss. There are no associated vestibular symptoms. Affected patients are generally farmers of lower income with less education compared to healthy control subjects. The use of tobacco, in particular at least four cigars per day, was the factor most associated with the highest risk of optic neuropathy (12, 13). Other contributing factors include lack of food for several days, eating lunch less than 5 days per week, and eating breakfast less than once per week. Protective factors include relatives overseas that can purchase supplementary food, raising chickens at home for the ingestion of B-group vitamins, and sulfur-containing amino acids. High levels of lycopene, a non-vitamin A carotenoid antioxidant found in tomatoes, guavas, watermelons, and other red fruits, conferred the strongest protection, in addition to the antioxidant riboflavin (13). Marked improvement of vision was obtained with parenteral B-group vitamins and folic acid. Despite absence of overt malnutrition in Cuba, a deficit of B-group vitamins,

mainly cobalamin and thiamine, compounded by lack of essential sulfur-amino acids in the diet, was the cause of the outbreak. The relative absence of cases in children, pregnant women, and the elderly, those so often affected by nutritional neuromyelopathies in the tropics, was explained by the availability of nutritional supplements.

Beriberi

Until early in this century, beriberi was a major public health problem in China, Japan, Indonesia, the Philippines, and Africa and among populations dependent on polished rice for their staple diet. Food supplementation with thiamine practically eliminated beriberi around the world. Most cases are currently observed in alcoholic patients and in the elderly on poor diets, however beriberi continues to occur in the tropics when conditions of low thiamine intake, high carbohydrate diet, and high energy expenditure are met (4). So-called wet beriberi presents clinically with dysesthesia and foot drop. The more prominent systemic illness is cardiac failure, suggested by pedal edema that accounts for the high fatality rate. Typical lesions in the heart include myocardial edema, central necrosis of fibers, and mitochondrial lesions. Sural nerve biopsy shows axonopathy. The diagnosis is confirmed by low serum levels of thiamine and thiamine pyrophosphate activity. The dietary history usually reveals low intake of thiamine in the diet or consumption of thiaminase present, for example, in raw fish. There is no effective body storage of thiamine, and dietary deficiency leads to symptoms in a month or two. Thiamine plays a central role in energy production, and thiamine requirements depend on the metabolic rate of the body. High energy expenditures in the hot and humid conditions of the tropics and a diet based on complex carbohydrates contribute to outbreaks of beriberi. It responds rapidly to parenteral thiamine.

Toxic Neuropathy

A large number of industrial or environmental products selectively affect the nerves. In the tropics, widespread and indiscriminate use of toxic pesticides, compounded by a lack of education on their proper handling and storage, increases the problem of toxic exposure. This is amplified by inherent malnutrition, infection, and genetic susceptibility (18, 19). The commonest heavy metal compounds that cause peripheral neuropathy are arsenic, lead, and thallium (20). Pharmacologic products (21), such as isoniazid, ethambutol, sulfonamides, nitrofurantoin, metronidazole, chloroquine, clioquinol, chloramphenicol, dapsone, and aromatic diamines, used in the treatment of leishmaniasis and trypanosomiasis cause peripheral nerve disease in the tropics. Neurotoxic industrial agents include n-hexane, methyl-n-butyl ketone, carbon disulfide, acrylamide, and trichloroethylene (20).

Tri-ortho-cresyl phosphate intoxication is the cause of Jamaica ginger paralysis. Epidemics have occurred in Morocco, Durban, Bombay, and Sri Lanka due to contamination or adulteration of food or cooking oils with the intoxicant. The clinical disorder includes symmetric weakness and wasting of distal muscles of the arms with claw-hand deformity, wrist drop, minimal sensory abnormalities, and late corticospinal tract signs (CST) signs.

Organophosphorous pesticides produce a delayed distal axonopathy. A postsynaptic neuromuscular junction (NMJ) disorder occurs two to three days after toxic exposure. Ocular toxicity, or Saku disease, occurs with fenthion, dichlorovos, fenitrothion, malathion, parathion, and methyl-parathion exposure.

Neurologic Disorders Associated with Dietary Cyanide Intoxication

Staple foods in the tropics contain large amounts of cyanogenic glycosides including cassava, yams, sweet potatoes, corn, millet, bamboo shoots, and beans, particularly small black lima beans, which grow wild in Puerto Rico and Central America. Inhaled tobacco smoke contains 150 to 300 mg of cyanide per cigarette. The hydrolysis of plant glycosides also releases cyanide in the form of hydrocyanic acid. Intoxication occurs by rapid cyanide absorption through the gastrointestinal tract or the lungs. Detoxification, mainly due to thiocyanate, is a reaction mediated by a sulfur-transferase or rhodanase, which converts thiosulfate into thiocyanate and sulfite. Thiocyanate is a goitrogenic agent that may be responsible for endemic cretinism in some tropical areas. The sulfur-containing essential amino acids cystine, cysteine, and methionine provide the sulfur for these detoxification reactions.

Cassava is a root crop consumed in large quantities throughout the tropics and constitutes the major source of calories for some 300 million people. It contains linamarin, a cyanogenic glycoside. Cassava is the staple diet in western Nigeria, Zaire, Tanzania, Senegal, Uganda, and Mozambique wherein a number of neurologic disorders have been associated with high dietary intake of cassava in association with depletion of sulfur-containing amino acids. However, these disorders are uncommon in Latin America, even though cassava consumption in countries such as Brazil is among the highest in the world.

The clinical syndromes associated with chronic cyanide intoxication include tropical ataxic neuropathy (TAN), a form of spastic paraparesis known as konzo; tropical amblyopia, and nerve deafness. TAN was first observed in Nigeria, in areas where the diet depended almost exclusively on cassava (22), and reached an estimated prevalence of 18 to 26 per 1,000 persons with equal sex distribution. Recent studies by Oluwole and colleagues (23, 24) showed the persistence of TAN in areas with high exposure to cyanide from cassava foods. However, not all affected patients haved high cyanide levels, suggesting another contributing associated cause etiological factor (23, 24). Onset is usually in the third to fourth decade with chronic, slowly progressive predominantly sensory polyneuropathy, and posterior column involvement of the spinal cord, with optic atrophy and sensorineural deafness. Affected patients complain of distal painful burning paresthesia, numbness, and cramps. Other symptoms include blurring of vision due to bilateral optic atrophy in over 80% of patients, tinnitus followed by bilateral nerve deafness in more than one-third, and skin and mucosal lesions suggestive of vitamin deficiency occur in 40% of patients. Examination reveals impaired stocking vibratory sensory loss with areflexia in the legs. About two-thirds of patients have incoordination and a broad-based ataxic gait, in addition to weakness and atrophy of distal leg muscles, especially of the peroneal group. In other African countries such as Senegal, similar syndromes have been observed in malnourished populations, although not necessarily in association with high cassava intake; with less frequent involvement of visual loss in 19%, deafness in 13%, and mucocutaneous lesions in 15%, than in patients from Nigeria.

Konzo is the traditional name given in Kwango, Zaire, to a form of epidemic spastic paraparesis described during droughts and famine in cassava-staple areas (7); epidemics have also occurred in rural areas of Mozambique, Tanzania, Zaire, and the Central African Republic. It occurs in up to two-thirds of children and lactating women with a prevalence of 29 to 34 per 1,000 persons. Affected women and children eat raw and sun-dried uncooked bitter cassava, whereas men are unaffected because their food is normally well-cooked. Traditional methods of cassava preparation in Africa include soaking, fermentation, and sun drying, which leaves substantial amounts of cyanogenic glycosides in the cassava meal. Affected patients develop signs of acute cyanide intoxication followed by sudden, non-progressive spastic paraparesis followed later by flexion hamstring muscle and Achilles tendon contractures, with scissoring gait, toe-walking, and the need for a stick or two to walk. Tone is increased in the legs with hyperreflexia, ankle clonus, and Babinski signs without light touch and pinprick sensory loss, however rapid movement are impaired and reflexes are increased in the arms, and nystagmus and dysarthria may occur. There is minimal recovery with a nutritious diet and vitamin therapy. Despite major advances in the understanding of the natural history of konzo, the disease continues to occur in Africa. A recent outbreak in the Democratic Republic of Congo (25) included 237 patients, mainly in children and women, the latter especially after childbirth. In Mozambique, Cliff and colleagues (26, 27) found 27 new patients with konzo, and up to 22% of school children had ankle clonus associated with higher urinary thiocyanate (26, 27). Essential sulfur-containing amino acids in the cassava flour consumed by children is used up to detoxify cyanide to thiocyanate. The depletion of methionine and cystine may lead to protein deficiency and may contribute to the onset of konzo (28).

Tropical amblyopia has been described in association with chronic cassava intake (29). Tobacco amblyopia, variously known as tobacco-alcohol amblyopia, West Indian amblyopia, and Jamaican optic neuropathy, is similar to patients observed in Cuba and recently described in Tanzania in association with peripheral neuropathy (30). All are probably clinically identical to the retrobulbar neuropathy

of pernicious anemia due to vitamin B12 deficiency and to the nutritional amblyopia described above. The common element is an underlying deficiency of micronutrients, in particular, B-group vitamins, folic acid, and sulfur amino acids. For these reasons, the term nutritional or deficiency amblyopia is preferred. The differential diagnosis includes methyl alcohol intoxication, a common cause of epidemic blindness in the tropics resulting from consumption of adulterated alcohol. As with tropical amblyopia, sensorineural deafness was commonly found in patients from Nigeria in association with cassava intake and micronutrient deficiencies (22), also probably primarily nutritional in origin.

REFERENCES

1. Román GC. Tropical myeloneuropathies revisited. *Curr Opin Neurol* 1998; 11:539–544.
2. Román GC. Neurology in public health. In: Detels R, Holland WW, McEwen J, Omenn GS, eds. *Oxford textbook of public health*, 3rd ed. Oxford: Oxford University Press, 1997; 1195–1223.
3. Toro G, Román GC, *Navarro de Román LI. Neurologia tropical.* Bogota: Printer, 1983.
4. Román GC. Tropical neuropathies. *Baillière's Clin Neurol* 1995; 4:469–487.
5. Shakir RA, Newman PK, Poser CM, eds. *Tropical neurology.* London: WB Saunders, 1996.
6. Toro G, Román GC, Navarro-Román L, et al. Cantillo J, Serrano B, Vergara I. Natural history of spinal cord infarction caused by nucleus pulposus embolism. *Spine* 1994; 19:360–366.
7. Tylleskär T. The causation of konzo. Studies on a paralytic disease in Africa. *Acta Univ Upsaliensis* 1994; 43:1–67.
8. Caparros-Lefebre D, Charpentier D, Joseph H, et al. High prevalence of SMON after use of tropical herbal medicine. Other etiologies: Trauma, neoplasia, genetic neuropathies. *Neurology* 1997; 48[Suppl 2]:A95.
9. Román GC, Vernant JC, Osame M. *HTLV-I and the nervous system.* New York: Liss, 1989.
10. Omán GC. Epidemic neuropathies of Jamaica. *Trans Stud Coll Phys Philadelphia Med Hist* 1985; 7:261–274.
11. Román GC. An epidemic in Cuba of optic neuropathy, sensorineural deafness, peripheral sensory neuropathy and dorsolateral myeloneuropathy. *J Neurol Sci* 1994; 127:11–28.
12. Centers for Disease Control and Prevention. Epidemic neuropathy-Cuba, 1991–1994. *MMWR Mortal Morb Wkly Rep* 1994; 43:183–192.
13. Cuba Neuropathy Field Investigation Team. Epidemic optic neuropathy in Cuba-clinical characterization and risk factors. *N Engl J Med* 1995; 333:1176–1182.
14. Román GC, Spencer PS, Schoenberg BS. Tropical myeloneuropathies: The hidden endemics. *Neurology* 1985; 35:1158–1170.
15. Newman NJ, Torroni A, Brown D, et al. Epidemic neuropathy in Cuba not associated with mitochondrial DNA mutations found in Leber's hereditary optic neuropathy patients. *Am J Ophthalmol* 1994; 118:158–168.
16. Sadun AA, Martone JF, Muci-Mendoza R, et al. Epidemic optic neuropathy in Cuba: eye findings. *Arch Ophthalmol* 1994; 112:691–699.

17. Borrajero I, Pérez JL, Domínguez C, et al. Epidemic neuropathy in Cuba: morphological characterization of peripheral nerve lesions in sural nerve biopsies. *J Neurol Sci* 1994; 127:68–76.
18. Senanayake N, Román GC. Disorders of neuromuscular transmission due to natural environmental toxins. *J Neurol Sci* 1992; 107:1–13.
19. Senanayake N, Román GC. Toxic neuropathies in the tropics. *J Trop Geograph Neurol* 1991; 1:3–15.
20. Ludolph AC, Spencer PS. Toxic neuropathies and their treatment. *Baillière's Clin Neurol* 1995; 4:505–527.
21. Windebank AJ. Drug-induced neuropathies. *Baillière's Clin Neurol* 1995; 4:529–573.
22. Osuntokun BO. An ataxic neuropathy in Nigeria: a clinical, biochemical and electrophysiological study. *Brain* 1968; 91:215–248.
23. Oluwole OS, Onabolu AO, Link H, Rosling H. Persistence of tropical ataxic neuropathy in a Nigerian community. *J Neurol Neurosurg Psychiatry* 2000; 69:96–101.
24. Oluwole OS, Onabolu AO, Cotgreave IA, et al. Rosling H, Persson A, Link H. Incidence of endemic ataxic polyneuropathy and its relation to exposure to cyanide in a Nigerian community. *J Neurol Neurosurg Psychiatry* 2003; 74:1417–1422.
25. Bonmarin I, Nunga M, Perea WA. Konzo outbreak, in the south-west of the Democratic Republic of Congo, 1996. *J Trop Pediatr* 2002; 48:234–238.
26. Cliff J, Lundqvist P, Martensson J, et al. Rosling H, Sorbo B. Association of high cyanide and low sulphur intake in cassava-induced spastic paraparesis. *Lancet* 1985; 2:1211–1213.
27. Cliff J, Nicala D, Saute F, et al. Givragy R, Azambuja G, Taela A, Chavane L, Gani A. Ankle clonus and thiocyanate, linamarin, and inorganic sulphate excretion in school children in communities with Konzo, Mozambique. *J Trop Pediatr* 1999; 45:139–142.
28. Paula Cardoso A, Ernesto M, Nicala D, et al. Mirione E, Chavane L, N'zwalo H, Chikumba S, Cliff J, Paulo Mabota A, Rezaul Haque M, Howard Bradbury J. Combination of cassava flour cyanide and urinary thiocyanate measurements of school children in Mozambique. *Int J Food Sci Nutr* 2004; 55:183–190.
29. Osuntokun BO, Osuntokun O. Tropical amblyopia in Nigerians. *Am J Ophthalmol* 1971; 71:708–716.
30. Plant GT, Mtanda AT, Arden GB, et al. An epidemic of optic neuropathy in Tanzania: characterization of the visual disorder and associated peripheral neuropathy. *J Neurol Sci* 1996; 145:127–140.

CHAPTER 40

Motor Dysfunction in Multiple Sclerosis

Jonathon E. Howard

Multiple sclerosis (MS) is a chronic, immune-mediated, demyelinating disease of the central nervous system (CNS), characterized pathologically by plaques of inflammation, demyelination, and gliosis disseminated in time (DIT) and space (DIS). The signs and symptoms depend on the location of the lesions within the brain and spinal cord. Motor dysfunction, which includes spasticity, weakness, tremor, and ataxia, is the commonest disabling aspect of MS. Multiple sclerosis and related disorders have been recently reviewed (1).

EPIDEMIOLOGY AND ETIOPATHOGENIC FACTORS

The prevalence of MS is estimated to be two per 100,000 in Japan, to 100 or more persons per 100,000 in northern Europe and North America (2, 3), with the disease twice as common in temperate regions than in the tropics. Although the etiology is unknown, three factors enhance the occurrence of MS. The first is genetic vulnerability, the second factor is yet-to-be identified environmental exposures, and the last is the host immune system that damages the CNS.

Genetic predisposition is an important risk factor in MS (4) with siblings of affected patients having a 2% to 5% lifetime risk, and parents and children of MS patients having a 1% lifetime risk. Monozygotic twins have a 30% risk, whereas dizygotic twins have a risk similar to that of another sibling (5, 6). Linkage studies implicate the major histocompatibility complex and other immunoregulatory genes as important determinants of this hereditary risk (7).

Migration studies suggest that a critical environmental exposure occurs before age 15 (8, 9). Patients who reside further from the equator and are exposed to less sunlight have lower vitamin D levels, placing them at increased risk of MS (10). The association of MS with latent Epstein-Barr virus (EBV) infection is more controversial, with evidence of immune activation of latent EBV in active MS lesions of some patients (11), and absence of EBV in the brain and CSF in other patients (12, 13). Women are affected twice as often as men, and whites have a much higher incidence rate than other races. The incidence of MS peaks in the fourth decade of life, but the disease commonly presents between age 15 and 60 years. Childhood onset occurs but is uncommon. Overall, MS is the third commonest cause of disability in the United States in 15-, to 50-year-old individuals after trauma and musculoskeletal disease (14).

Both T- and B-cells are active in immune processes in MS, with circulating T-cells binding to specific receptors on the endothelium of the blood-brain barrier, and then passing into the parenchyma where they are stimulated by microglia to proliferate, recruiting more cells from the circulation, destroying myelin, activating B-cells, and stimulating secretion of cytokines. Increased levels of Th1–like cytokines in the cerebrospinal fluid (CSF) of patients with MS have been associated with progression of disease, as have cytokines released from activated T cells that amplify the immune response within the CNS, promoting the expression of adhesion molecules on adjacent blood vessels, and up-regulating T-cells through interaction with main histocompatibility (MHC) class II molecules. A variety of inflammatory mediators, including tumor necrosis factor (TNF), oxygen radicals, nitric oxide, and other cytokines may modulate axonal conduction and synaptic transmission and contribute to structural myelin damage. Pathogenic B-cell activation is suggested by elevated CSF oligoclonal bands (OCB), increased levels of CSF immunoglobulin-G (IgG) and anti-myelin-associated glycoprotein (MAG) antibody in affected patients.

PATHOLOGY

A yet defined activating process triggers the immune response against one or more myelin antigens, including myelin basic protein (MBP), proteolipid protein (PLP), myelin/oligodendrocyte glycoprotein, MAG, and gangliosides. Plaques occur throughout the CNS, but are particularly common in the optic nerves, cerebral periventricular white matter, brainstem, and spinal cord tracts. The histological lesions in MS lesions are classified as active, chronically active, and chronically inactive. Acute lesions have marked perivascular inflammatory cell infiltrates, comprised predominantly of mononuclear cells, T lymphocytes, and macrophages, with occasional B cells and plasma cells. As the lesion progresses, demyelination ensues, with phagocytosis of myelin debris by macrophages and microglial cells. Oligodendrocytes, the myelin-producing cells, proliferate but are destroyed as infiltration and astrocytic gliosis progresses, and demyelination cause symptoms through slowed axonal conduction, conduction block, and ectopic signal transmission (15). Remyelination is activated by oligodendrocyte progenitor cells and not the surviving oligodendrocytes in the areas of demyelination. When the process of demyelination is more severe and longstanding, axonal loss may be evident. Axonal degeneration is responsible for the irreversible neurologic disability in MS patients. The extent of axonal injury is associated with the inflammation in active MS lesions, and later disability, even in clinically silent lesions. Involvement of the subpial gray matter early in the course of the disease process is a feature of MS and a contributor to disability (16).

PATHOPHYSIOLOGY

Motor dysfunction is manifested by clinical spasticity, weakness, tremor, and ataxia. Spasticity, defined as a velocity-dependent increase in muscular tone, is caused by the loss of inhibitory inputs from the corticospinal tracts (CST) and other descending motor pathways to g-motor neurons and interneuron networks that participate in spinal cord reflex arcs, as are hyperreflexia, muscle spasms, and other upper motor neuron (UMN) signs. Weakness and impairment of fine motor control are due more specifically to interruption of input to α-motor neurons (MN). Rarely, muscle atrophy and other lower motor neuron (LMN) signs may be present, though this is likely due to chronic disuse of the muscle rather than from the underlying disease process. Tremor and ataxia are related to lesions of the cerebellum and cerebellar pathways through the brainstem, red nucleus, thalamus, and basal ganglia, specifically in Mollaret triangle, comprising the dentate nucleus of the cerebellum, inferior olive, and red nucleus. In some patients, proprioceptive loss may be the primary cause for impairment. The neural circuitry involved in the pathogenesis of tremor is complex and variable, as evidenced by the mixed results of ablative procedures such as thalamotomy (17). Fatigue, defined as a loss of force-generating capacity during sustained motor activity, contributes to motor dysfunction and disability in patients without other signs of motor dysfunction.

DIAGNOSIS

The classical approach to the diagnosis of MS includes clinical and laboratory assessments aimed at demonstrating two or more lesions DIT and DIS, while excluding alternative diagnoses. Initial criteria defined the certainty of MS for the purposes of epidemiologic studies and clinical trials (18). The McDonald criteria of the International Panel on Diagnosis of MS (19, 20) emphasized that although the diagnosis could be made on clinical grounds alone, magnetic resonance imaging (MRI) of the CNS could support, supplement, or even replace some clinical criteria, resulting in earlier detection of MS with a high degree of specificity and sensitivity in clinically isolated syndromes (CIS) (21), in the early conversion to clinically definite MS (CDMS) (22), in predicting response to immunotherapy including interferon beta-1a (23), and in documenting the first demyelinating episode (24). Revisions to the McDonald criteria (25) incorporated criteria for demonstration of DIS (26, 27) and those of Montalban and colleagues for demonstration of DIT (28). Recognizing the special diagnostic needs of primary progressive (spinal) MS (PPMS), the 2010 McDonald criteria maintained (20, 29) two of three MRI or CSF findings for PPMS, replacing previous brain imaging criteria for DIS (26). The final criteria for PPMS was one year of retrospective or prospective disease progression, plus two of the three following criteria: one or more T2-weighted lesions in at least one area characteristic for MS (periventricular, juxtacortical, or infratentorial), two or more T2-weighted lesions in the cord, or positive CSF isoelectric focusing evidence of oligoclonal bands and elevated IgG index. Gadolinium enhancement of lesions was not required.

Recognizing that spinal cord abnormalities on MRI are frequently found in patients with CDMS, spinal cord lesions became increasingly important, and now have the same weight as brain lesions in the 2010 revisions (25). Among 121 patients who underwent MRI of the brain and spinal cord shortly after monofocal relapsing onset CIS of the brain (58 patients) and spinal cord (63 patients), 36 fulfilled McDonald criteria (25) for CDMS by brain imaging only and 6 additional patients met criteria for CDMS with spinal cord imaging (30).

Magnetic resonance spectroscopy (MRS) has been studied extensively in MS and differs from MRI because the signal does not derive from protons in water but instead from organic molecules contained in living tissue. The most relevant metabolites available for study, reflecting the integrity of neurons, are creatine (Cr), N-acetyl aspartate (NAA), choline, and my-inositol, wherein changes in NAA, specifically localized to the neuronal compartment, and Cr, present in both neurons and glial cells, or their relative ratio, respectively correlate with neuronal loss, neuroaxonal injury, and disability both in cross-sectional and longitudinal studies (31).

Lymphocytic CSF pleocytosis of five to 50 cells/mm^3 is noted in up to two-thirds of MS patients, and OCB in over 90% of patients. While not specific for MS, OCB may not appear until several years after onset of MS, persisting thereafter though not indicative of active disease. It is seen also in other inflammatory nervous system disorders, including encephalitis, meningitis, Guillain-Barré syndrome, and even cerebral infarction.

Evoked responses are useful in detecting subclinical lesions and in confirming the relation of questionable symptoms and signs to a CNS process (33). Trimodal evoked responses are commonly employed in clinical practice for the detection of clinical and subclinical demyelinating lesions. Visual evoked responses (VER) evidencing prolongation of the P100 latency, and an inter-eye latency difference greater than 12 ms, with preserved amplitude, likely have prechiasmal optic nerve conduction block due to focal demyelination, so noted in 80 to 95% of patients with optic neuritis, while others have less specific reduced amplitude. Brainstem auditory evoked responses (BAER) show prolonged interpeak latencies in up to two-thirds of patients with clinically definite lesions, mainly wave III to IV, and disappearance of wave V. By comparison, somatosensory evoked responses (SSER) recording from the tibial and median mixed nerve show a sensitivity of 86% in clinically definite MS, due to the increased length of CNS long tracts that can be studied, from the lumbar or cervical enlargement to sensory cortex. Patients with spinal cord MS lesions can have significantly delayed motor evoked responses after transcutaneous magnetic stimulation of the brain (34), although the overall utility of this technique for detecting subclinical motor deficits is relatively low compared with trimodal evoked responses.

Finally, optical coherence tomography (OCT), which utilizes near-infrared light to generate cross-sectional images of the retina yielding highly quantitative anatomic data of retinal nerve fiber layer (RNFL) thinning that occurs throughout the natural history of MS, is proving to be a useful adjunctive methodology to address mechanisms of injury, inflammation, and efficacy of therapeutic interventions (32).

MS VARIANTS AND DIFFERENTIAL DIAGNOSIS

Neuromyelitis optica (NMO) or Devic syndrome and MS can have phenotypic similarities at disease onset and can present a relapsing clinical course (35). The discovery of circulating IgG1 antibodies against the astrocyte water channel protein aquaporin 4 (AQP4) and evidence that AQP4-IgG is involved in the development of NMO revolutionized present understanding of this disorder (36, 37). This rare inflammatory and demyelinating autoimmune CNS disorder is characterized by recurrent attacks of optic neuritis and longitudinally extensive transverse myelitis, which is distinct from MS.

Guidelines for the diagnosis and management of NMO were recently proposed (38). NMO-IgG determination is crucial in detecting patients who will develop NMO; however, its value as a routine test in patients with symptoms of CIS of the type seen in MS is low and should be reserved for those in which the initial diagnosis is unclear (39). New drug candidates have emerged, including the non-pathogenic antibody blocker of AQP4-IgG binding drug aquaporumab, the neutrophil elastase inhibitor sivelestat, and the complement inhibitor eculizumab (40). Important unanswered questions remain including the cause of AQP4-IgG-negative disease, how astrocyte mediated damage leads to demyelination, the role of T-cells, why peripheral AQP4-expressing organs are undamaged, and how circulating AQP4-IgG enters NMO lesions (40).

Acute disseminated encephalomyelitis (ADEM) is a monophasic, immune-mediated CNS demyelinating disorder that predominates among children following specific viral infections including measles, rubella, and mumps, especially in the spring and winter months, and after vaccine immunization. Milder versions of the disease have been described in adults.

The diagnosis of ADEM is based on the acute onset of neurological symptoms that may include fever, vomiting, headache, gait disturbance, and generalized seizures, with signs of altered sensorium, nystagmus, diplopia, and isolated facial nerve or multiple cranial nerve involvement, speech, dystonia, chorea, bladder disturbances, para-, and quadriparesis (41). Optic neuritis occurs in up to one-third, and CSF pleocytosis in up to two-thirds of patients. Neuroimaging employing MRI shows multifocal demyelinating lesions in subcortical white matter, midbrain, pons, corpus callosum, basal ganglia, medulla, and cerebellum, with up to one-third of lesions in the spinal cord. Outcome is associated with remission in up to 70% of patients within a week of commencing corticosteroids, with residual symptoms in the remaining one-third.

Diverse autoimmune, post-infectious, genetic and metabolic CNS disorders can mimic MS (42, 43), including systemic lupus erythematosus, Sjögren syndrome, Behçet syndrome, sarcoidosis, CNS vasculitis, and infectious disorders such as syphilis, tuberculosis, and Lyme borreliosis, human T-lymphotropic virus type I, cytomegalovirus, herpes simplex virus, and varicella zoster virus, and the neurologic hereditary disorders, metabolic disorders, adrenoleukodystrophy, Refsum disease, spinocerebellar degeneration, and cerebral autosomal dominant arteriopathy with subcortical infarcts and leukoencephalopathy (CADASIL), all further separable by individually distinctive clinical and laboratory features after detailed evaluation.

CLINICAL MANIFESTATIONS

Symptoms and signs in MS reflect the location of demyelinating CNS lesions. Affected patients commonly present with afferent pupillary defect, visual loss, and diplopia related to optic neuritis; internuclear ophthalmoplegia, facial weakness and numbness, and vertigo resulting from brainstem lesions; ataxia from cerebellar lesions; bowel and bladder urgency, frequency, and retention due to autonomic lesions; and paresthesia and hyperesthesia due to sensory tract lesions. Cognitive deficits, including slowed information processing, loss of executive function, and impaired short-term memory, appear to be related to the overall burden of subcortical white matter lesions. Seizures occur in up to 5% of patients, coinciding with an active lesion near the cerebral cortex. Fatigue and depression are common throughout the disease course but do not clearly relate to specific CNS lesions.

Spastic paraparesis, the most common UMN abnormality, is associated with stiffness, cramps, weakness, and motor fatigability, and flexor, extensor, and painful adductor spasms provoked by active or passive movements. Motor deficits may also be quite asymmetric, with isolated monoparesis and hemiparesis related to focal demyelinating lesions. The cutaneous reflexes, such as the superficial abdominal, may be absent as an early sign of spinal cord involvement, with loss of tendon stretch reflexes later in the course as a correlate of demyelination at the dorsal root entry zone.

Gait difficulty is probably the most common and disabling consequence of motor dysfunction in MS. Patients have measurable deficits in walking speed and endurance. Among a cohort of 237 ambulatory MS patients (44) 78% took more than five seconds to walk 8 m (range, 2.6 to 185.1 seconds), compared to healthy control subjects, with one-half unable to walk 100 to 500 m despite support. An Expanded Disability Status Scale (EDSS) based on ambulatory impairment (45) classically rates disability status in MS. Motor function worsens with exercise, fever, sun exposure, and hot bath so characteristically that the latter is considered a diagnostic inference of MS, the underlying mechanism of which presumably involves worsening of conduction block in partially demyelinated pathways.

CLINICAL COURSE AND PROGNOSIS

The course of MS is quite variable but can be divided into a relapsing-remitting pattern of distinct attacks and relatively symptom-free or stable periods, and a chronic progressive course of worsening disease without clear attacks, with one-half of those with relapsing-remitting course evolving into steadily progressive disease termed secondary progressive MS (46). Early prognostic features of the later course of MS include sensory symptoms at the onset which correlate with an ultimately benign course (47), whereas motor and cerebellar signs, early relapse, and onset after age 40 predict an ultimately more aggressive and rapid course (48–50). Men presenting after age 40 with progressive myelopathy exhibit a steadily worsening paraparesis with variable involvement of the arms and few deficits related to the cerebral subcortical white matter.

TREATMENT

Treatments for MS can be divided into four categories, including agents that modulate the immune system, improve conduction through demyelinated pathways, enhance remyelination, and render symptomatic improvement without directly impacting the underlying pathological process. Immune modulatory therapy interferes with activation and proliferation of immune cells, reduces migration of immune cells into the CNS, enhances suppressor activity within the immune system, and limits the destruction caused by activated immune cells and their inflammatory mediators. In most instances, these agents alter the natural history of the disease. Since the immune process in MS is fairly constant and similar in various stages of the disease, more than one type of immunosuppressive agent can be used, each with a unique mode of action.

Corticosteroids are commonly administered during an acute exacerbation, enhancing the resolution of symptoms and signs, without significantly affecting the ultimate outcome of an exacerbation. However, the optimal dose and regimen remains uncertain. Pulse therapy with corticosteroids is associated with temporary insomnia, irritability, fluid retention, increased appetite, weight gain, hyperglycemia, hypertension, dyspepsia, depression, psychosis, bone fractures, and osteoporosis. Interferon (INF) beta-1b (Betaseron, Berlex™) and INF beta-1a (Avonex, Biogen™) reduce the number of exacerbations occurring in patients prone to relatively frequent exacerbations and may prevent worsening disability.

Serial MRI shows a dramatic decrease in the incidence of new lesions and less increase in overall lesion burden during treatment. Efficacy has not been well established in patients with progressive disease, and studies thus far have not provided clear guidance for the role of INF therapy in progressive MS. In patients with newly diagnosed MS and low disease activity, the consensus is to start treatment as soon as possible to influence the frequency of relapses, stabilize disease activity, and lessen long-term disability. Side effects include flu-like symptoms, injection-site reactions, leukopenia, elevated liver function studies, thrombocytopenia, headache, depression and low sustained adherence (51).

Neutralizing antibodies develop in more than one-third of patients taking INF beta-1b and in about 10% of those taking INF beta-1a. The clinical significance of these antibodies remains uncertain, but experience suggests that they may seriously compromise efficacy. Glatiramer acetate or copolymer-1 (Copaxone, Teva™), was equally efficacious in a similar patient population (52). Direct comparisons between INF beta-1a with glatiramer acetate failed to show an advantage to either as did a direct comparison between INF beta-1b and glatiramer acetate (53, 54).Comparisons between every-other-day INF beta-1b and once-weekly INF beta 1-a showed a lower relapse rate and fewer active lesions on MRI with the use of INF beta-1b (55, 56). However, adherence rates may be higher with once-weekly INF beta 1-a (57).

Natalizumab (Tysabri, Biogen™) is a monoclonal antibody that binds to a 4-integrin on lymphocytes, and in turn, prevents lymphocyte binding to the VCAM1 receptor on vascular endothelium needed for lymphocytes to cross the blood-brain barrier and enter the CNS. Natalizumab, administered as an intravenous infusion every 28 days, reduced the annualized relapse rate (ARR) by 68% compared to placebo (ARR natalizumab 0.26, placebo 0.81), and the risk of sustained disability progression for three months by 42% compared to placebo (58). The combination of natalizumab and once-weekly INF beta 1-a reduced ARR from 0.82 compared with 0.34 with once-weekly INF beta 1-a alone, with a significant reduction in disability progression (59). The use of natalizumab has been associated with the development of progressive multifocal leukoencephalopathy cause by infection with the JC virus, a common, though not ubiquitous, polyomavirus often acquired in childhood. The overall incidence of PML in patients treated with natalizumab is estimated to be 1 in 1000 persons. A reliable and validated assay for detection of JC virus antibodies in patients with MS has been developed and, thus far, no patient who tested negative for the antibody later developed PML (60). Other risk factors for the development of PML include prior treatment with immunosuppression and over 24 infusions of natalizumab (61). In patients who test positive for the JC virus antibody, and have both a history of immunosuppression and received over 24 infusions of natilizumab the risk of PML may be as high as 1 in 85 persons (62). The use of natilizumab in patients at high risk for PML should be reserved for patients with active disease unresponsive to the platform agents.

Fingolimod (Gilyena™) was the first oral medication for MS to receive approval from the Food and Drug Administration (FDA). It is derived from a fungus that interacts with the sphingosine-1-phosphate receptor to prevent lymphocyte egress from lymph nodes into the periphery. It is thought that because the lymphocytes are still active within the lymphatic system, the integrity of immune function in the rest of the body is maintained. The medication was studied in two doses, 1.25mg and .5mg once daily. The ARR was 0.18 with 0.5 mg of fingolimod, 0.16 with 1.25 mg of fingolimod, and 0.40 with placebo (P<0.001 for either dose vs. placebo). Both doses reduced the risk of disability progression over the 24-month period of the trial (63). In comparison with intramuscular INF, the ARR was 0.20 and significantly lower in the group receiving 1.25 mg fingolimod (95% confidence interval [CI], 0.16 to 0.26) and 0.16 (95% CI, 0.12 to 0.21) in the 0.5-mg group, than in the INF group (0.33; 95% CI, 0.26 to 0.42; P<0.001 for both comparisons) (64). There were two fatalities from infections in this study, one from a primarily varicella-zoster virus (VZV) infection and the other from herpes encephalitis, that occurred with the 1.25mg dose of the medicine. Only the 0.5mg fingolimod dose received FDA approval. The medication was also associated with reversible macular edema and transient bradycardia during the administration of the first dose, requiring patients to be monitored for six hours after their ingestion of the first pill. From December 2011 to the present, over 30,000 patients have taken the medication, and in post-marketing there have been several fatalities with fingolimod wherein cardiac arrhythmias have been suspected as the cause of death.

A number of other oral agents, including dimethyl fumarate (BG-12), teriflunomide, and laquinimod have shown efficacy is reducing relapses in MS, without serious safety concerns (65, 66). Dimethyl fumarate and teriflunomide are currently under review by the FDA.

Nonspecific immunosuppression has been employed in MS with variable results (67). The efficacy of azathioprine and cyclophosphamide has never truly been clearly established, although they continue to be administered. Weekly oral methotrexate showed less progression of deficits after treatment for two years (68). However, it can cause stomatitis, diarrhea, nausea, anemia, liver transaminitis and rash, and the poorly quantified risk of malignancy limits the use of this treatment to more severely affected patients. Cladribine, mitoxantrone, antilymphocyte globulins, cyclosporine, and tacrolimus are chemotherapeutic agents with use as semi-specific suppressors of MS disease activity. Plasmapheresis, total lymphoid irradiation, and intravenous immunoglobulin (IVIg) have proposed immunomodulatory actions of potential benefit in MS. Several peptides that interfere with binding in the trimolecular complex, comprised of the T-cell receptor, antigen, and an MHC class II molecule (69) should lead to more specific agents to decrease the activity of the disease and prevent further CNS damage with minimal systemic immunosuppression.

Other agents with proposed benefit in improving conduction through demyelinated pathways, or enhance remyelination, include 4-aminopyridine (4-AP) and 3, 4-diaminopyridine (3,4-DAP), both potassium channel blockers that increase the amplitude and duration of action potentials. Preliminary studies using 4-AP found improvement in a variety of subjective and semi-quantitative measures of neurologic function; however, a multicenter, double-blind, placebo-controlled, parallel study failed to show an effect on EDSS (70). Optimal administration of these agents is limited by the risk of seizures and encephalopathy with elevated peak serum levels (71).

Symptomatic therapy may be contemplated for the management of residual symptoms with agents that do not directly affect the underlying disease process (72), including antidepressants and anticonvulsants for paresthesia, anticholinergic and β-blocker medications to improve bladder function, and amantadine and CNS stimulants to minimize fatigue. There are no available treatments to improve strength. However physical therapy can minimize motor components related to disuse, and adaptive equipment such as ankle-foot orthoses (AFO) can be fitted to improve foot-drop dysfunction, as may other adaptive accessories including canes, walkers, and wheelchairs to foster mobility. Spasticity, muscle cramps, and spasms respond to stretching and gradually increasing doses of the CNS-active anti-spasticity medications baclofen, tizanidine, benzodiazepines, dantrolene, and botulinum toxin. Refractory patients can consider intrathecal baclofen administered by an implantable subcutaneous pump, alcohol block, and dorsal root rhizotomy. Tremor may respond to propranolol, primidone, isoniazid, buspirone, trazadone, baclofen, carbamazepine, gabapentin, benzodiazepines, and unilateral thalamotomy.

REFERENCES

1. Rizvi SA, Coyle PK, eds. Clinical neuroimmunology. *Multiple sclerosis and related disorders.* New York: Springer, 2012.
2. Baum HM, Rothschild BB. The incidence and prevalence of reported MS. *Ann Neurol* 1981; 10:420–428.
3. Rosati G. Descriptive epidemiology of multiple sclerosis in Europe in the 1980s: a critical overview. *Ann Neurol* 1994; 36:S164–174.
4. Ebers GC. Genetics and multiple sclerosis: an overview. *Ann Neurol* 1994; 36:S12–S14.
5. McFarland HF, Greenstein F, McFarlin DE, et al. Family and twin studies in multiple sclerosis. *Ann NY Acad Sci* 1985; 436:118–124.
6. Ebers GC, Bulman DE, Sadovnick AD, et al. A population based study of multiple sclerosis in twins. *N Engl J Med* 1986; 3 15:1638–1642.
7. Hillert J. Human leukocyte antigen studies in multiple sclerosis. *Ann Neurol* 1994; 36:S15–S17.
8. Kurtzke JF, Beebe GW, Norman JE. Epidemiology of multiple sclerosis in U.S. veterans. 1. Race, sex, and geographic distribution. *Neurology* 1979; 29:1228–1235.
9. Kurtzke JF, Beebe GW, Norman JE. Epidemiology of multiple sclerosis in U.S. veterans. 3. Migration and the risk of MS. *Neurology* 1985; 35:672–678.
10. Cantorna MT. Vitamin D and multiple sclerosis: an update. *Nutrition Reviews* 2008; 66(Suppl 2):5135–5138.
11. Tzartos JS, Khan G, Vossenkamper A, et al. Association of innate immune activation with latent Epstein-Barr virus in active MS lesions. *Neurology* 2012; 78:15–23.
12. Willis SN, Stadelmann C, Rodig SJ, et al. Epstein-Barr virus infection is not a characteristic feature of multiple sclerosis brain. *Brain* 2009; 132:3318–3328.
13. Sargsyan SA, Shearer AJ, Ritchie AM, et al. Absence of Epstein-Barr virus in the brain and CSF of patients with multiple sclerosis. *Neurology* 2010; 74:1127–1135.
14. Smith CR, Scheinberg LC. Clinical features of multiple sclerosis. *Semin Neurol* 1985; 5:85–93.
15. Waxman SG. Membranes, myelin, and the pathophysiology of multiple sclerosis. *N Engl J Med* 1982; 306:1529–1533.
16. Popescu BF, Lucchinetti CF. Meningeal and cortical grey matter pathology in multiple sclerosis. *BMC Neurology* 2012; 12:11.
17. Whittle IR, Haddow LJ. CT guided thalamotomy for movement disorders in multiple sclerosis: problems and paradoxes. *Acta Neurochir* 1995; 64:S13–S16.
18. Poser CM, Paty DW, Scheinberg L, et al. New diagnostic criteria for multiple sclerosis: guidelines for research protocols. *Ann Neurol* 1983; 13:227–231.
19. McDonald WI, Compston A, Edan G, et al. Recommended diagnostic criteria for multiple sclerosis: guidelines from the International Panel on the diagnosis of multiple sclerosis. *Ann Neurol* 2001; 50:121–127.
20. Polman CH, Reingold Edan G, et al. Diagnostic accuracy for multiple sclerosis: 2005 revisions to the McDonald Criteria." *Ann Neurol* 2005; 58:840–846.
21. Dalton CM, Brex PA, Miszkiel KA, et al. Application of the new McDonald criteria to patients with clinically isolated syndromes suggestive of multiple sclerosis. *Ann Neurol* 2002; 52:47–53.
22. CHAMPS Study Group. MRI predictors of early conversion to clinically definite MS in the CHAMPS placebo group. *Neurology* 2002; 59:998–10005.
23. Barkhof F, Rocca M, Francis G, et al. Validation of diagnostic magnetic resonance imaging criteria for multiple sclerosis and response to interferon beta-1a. *Ann Neurol* 2002; 53:718–724.
24. Tintore M, Rovira A, Rio J, et al. New diagnostic criteria for multiple sclerosis: application in first demyelinating episode. *Neurology* 2003; 60:27–30.
25. Polman CH, Reingold SC, Banwell B, et al. Diagnostic criteria for multiple sclerosis: 2010 revisions to the McDonald criteria. *Ann Neurol* 2011; 69:292–302.
26. Swanton JK, Rovira A, Tintore M, et al. MRI criteria for multiple sclerosis in patients presenting with clinically isolated syndromes: a multicenter retrospective study. *Lancet Neurol* 2007; 6:677–686.
27. Swanton JK, Fernando K, Dalton CM, et al. Modification of MRI criteria for multiple sclerosis in patients with clinically isolated syndromes. *J Neurol Neursurg Psychiatry* 2006; 77:830–833.
28. Montalban X, Tintore M, Swanton J, et al. MRI criteria for MS in patients with clinically isolated syndromes. *Neurology* 2010; 74:427–434.
29. McDonald WI, Compston A, Edan G, et al. Recommended diagnostic criteria for multiple sclerosis: guidelines from the

International Panel on the diagnosis of multiple sclerosis. *Ann Neurol* 2001; 50:121–127.

30. Sombekke MH, Wattjes MP, Balk LJ, et al. Spinal cord lesions in patient with clinically isolated syndrome. *Neurology* 2013; 80:69–75.

31. Kirov II, Tal A, Babb JS, et al. Serial proton MR spectroscopy of gray and white matter in relapsing-remitting MS. *Neurology* 2013; 80:39–46.

32. Ratchford JN, Saidha S, Sotirchos ES, et al. Active MS is associated with accelerated retinal ganglion cell/inner plexiform layer thinning. *Neurology* 2013; 80:47–54.

33. Hume AL, Waxman SG. Evoked potentials in suspected multiple sclerosis: diagnostic value and prediction of clinical course. *J Neurol Sci* 1988; 83:191–210.

34. Ingram DA, Thompson AJ, Swash M. Central motor conduction in multiple sclerosis: evaluation of abnormalities revealed by transcutaneous magnetic stimulation of the brain. *J Neurol Neurosurg Psychiatry* 1988; 51:487–494.

35. Rubiera M, Rio J, Tintore M, et al. Neuromyelitis optica diagnosis in clinically isolated syndromes suggestive of multiple sclerosis. *Neurology* 2006; 66:1568–1570.

36. Lennon VA, Wingerchuk DM, Kryzer TJ, et al. A serum auto-antibody marker of neuromyelitis optica: distinction from multiple sclerosis. *Lancet* 2004; 364:2106–2112.

37. Weinshenker BG, Wingerchuk DM, Pittock SJ, et al. NMO-IgG: a specific biomarker for neuromyelitis optica. *Dis Marker* 2006; 22:197–206.

38. Sellner J, Boggild M, Clanet M, et al. EFNS guidelines on diagnosis and management of neuromyelitis optica. *Eur J Neurol* 2010; 17:1010–1032.

39. Costa C, Arrambide G, Tintore M, et al. Value of NMO-IgG determination at the time of presentation as CIS. *Neurology* 2012; 78:1608–1611.

40. Papadopoulos MC, Verkman A. Aquaporin 4 and neuromyelitis optica. *Lancet Neurol* 2012; 11:535–544.

41. Jayakrishnan MP, Krishnakumar P. Clinical profile of acute disseminated encephalomyelitis in children. *J Pediatr Neurosci* 2010; 5:111–114.

42. Younger DS, Younger APJ. Vasculitis and connective tissue disorders. In, Kalman B, Brannagan TH III, eds. *Neuroimmunology in Clinical Practice*. Wiley-Blackwell, 2008.

43. Younger DS, Younger APJ. CNS vasculitis. In, P Coyle and S Rivzi, eds. *Clinical Neuroimmunology: Multiple Sclerosis and Related Disorders*. Springer, 2011.

44. Schwid SR, Goodman AD, Mattson DH, et al. The measurement of ambulatory impairment in multiple sclerosis. *Neurology* 1997; 49:1419–1424.

45. Kurtzke JF. Rating neurologic impairment in multiple sclerosis: an expanded disability status scale (EDSS). *Neurology* 1983; 33:1444–1452.

46. Lublin FD, Reingold SC. Defining the clinical course of multiple sclerosis: results of an international survey. *Neurology* 1996; 6:907–911.

47. McAlpine D. The benign form of multiple sclerosis: a study based on 241 cases seen with three years of onset and followed up until the tenth year or more of the disease. *Brain* 1961; 84:185–203.

48. Detels R, Clark VA, Valdiviezo NL, et al. Factors associated with a rapid course of multiple sclerosis. *Arch Neurol* 1982; 39:337–341.

49. Poser S, Kurtzke JF, Poser W, Sclaf G. Survival in multiple sclerosis. *J Clin Epidemiol* 1989; 42:159–168.

50. Runmarker B, Andersen O. Prognostic factors in a multiple sclerosis incidence cohort with twenty-five years of follow-up. *Brain* 1993; 116:117–134.

51. Wong J, Gomes T, Mamdani M, et al. Adherence to multiple sclerosis disease-modifying therapies in Ontario is low. *Can J Neurol Sci* 2011; 38:429–433.

52. Johnson KP, Brooks BR, Cohen JA, et al. Copolymer 1 reduces relapse rate and improves disability in relapsing-remitting multiple sclerosis: results of a phase III multicenter, double-blind, placebo controlled trial. *Neurology* 1995; 45:1268–1276.

53. Mikol DD, Barkhof F, Chang P, et al on behalf of the REGARD study group. Comparison of subcutaneous interferon beta-1a with glatiramer acetate in patients with relapsing multiple sclerosis (the REbif vs Glatiramer Acetate in Relapsing MS Disease [REGARD] study): a multicentre, randomized, parallel, open-label trial. *Lancet Neurol* 2008; 7:903–914.

54. O'Connor P, Filippi M, Arnason B, et al, for the BEYOND Study Group. 250 ug or 500 ug interferon beta-1b versus 20 mg glatiramer acetate in relapsing-remitting multiple sclerosis: a prospective, randomized, multicenter study. *Lancet Neurol* 2009; 8:889–897.

55. Durelli L, Verdun E, Barbero P, et al, and Independent Comparison of Interferon (INCOMIN) Trial Study Group. Every-other-day interferon beta-1b versus once-weekly interferon beta-1a for multiple sclerosis: results of a 2-year prospective randomized multicentre study (INCOMIN). *Lancet* 2002; 359:1453–1460.

56. Barbero P, Bergui M, Versino E, et al, and the INCOMIN Trial Study Group. Every-other-day interferon beta-1b versus once-weekly interferon beta-1a for multiple sclerosis (INCOMIN Trial) II: analysis of MRI responses to treatment and correlation with Nab. *Multiple Sclerosis* 2006; 12:72–76.

57. Arroyo E, Grau C, Ramo-Tello C, et al, on behalf of the GAP Study Group. Adherence to disease-modifying therapies in Spanish patients with relapsing multiple sclerosis: two-year interim results of the global adherence project. *Eur Neurol* 2011; 65:59–67.

58. Polman CH, O'Connor PW, Havrdova E, et al, for the AFFIRM Investigators. A randomized, placebo-controlled trial of natalizumab for relapsing multiple sclerosis. *N Engl J Med* 2006; 354:899–910.

59. Rudick RA, Stuart WH, Calabresi PA, et al., for the SENTINEL investigators. Natalizumab plus interferon beta-1a for relapsing multiple sclerosis. *N Engl J Med* 2006; 354:911–923.

60. Plavina T, Berman M, Njenga M, et al. Multi-site analytical validation of an assay to detect anti-JCV antibodies in human serum and plasma. *J Clin Virol* 2012; 53:65–71.

61. Gorelik L, Lerner M, Bixler S, et al. Anti-JC virus antibodies: implications for PML risk stratification. *Ann Neurol* 2010; 68:295–303.

62. Fox RJ, Rudick RA. Risk stratification and patient counseling for natalizumab in multiple sclerosis. *Neurology* 2012; 78:436–437.

63. Kappos L, Radue EW, O'Connor P, et al., for the FREEDOMS Study Group. A placebo-controlled trial of oral fingolimod in relapsing multiple sclerosis. *N Engl J Med* 2010; 362:387–401.

64. Cohen JA, Barkhof F, Comi G, et al, for the TRANSFORMS Study Group. Oral fingolimod or intramuscular interferon for relapsing multiple sclerosis. *N Engl J Med* 2010; 362:402–415.

65. O'Connor P, Wolinsky JS, Confavreux C, et al., for the TEMSO Trial Group. Randomized trial of oral teriflunomide for relapsing multiple sclerosis. *N Engl J Med* 2011; 365:1293–1303.

66. Comi G, Jeffery D, Kappos L, et al., for the ALLEGRO Study Group. Placebo-controlled trial of oral laquinimod for multiple sclerosis. *N Engl J Med* 2012; 366:1000–1009.

67. Carter JL, Rodriguez M. Immunosuppressive treatment of multiple sclerosis. *Mayo Clin Proc* 1989; 64:664–669.

68. Goodkin DE, Rudick RA, Medendorp S, et al. Low dose oral

methotrexate reduces the rate of progression in chronic progressive multiple sclerosis. *Ann Neurol* 1994;37:30–40.

69. Vandenbark AA, Chou YK, Whitham R, et al. Treatment of multiple sclerosis with T-cell receptor peptides: results of a double-blind pilot trial. *Nat Med* 1996; 2:1109–1115.

70. van Diemen HAM, Polman CH, van Dongen TM, et al. The effect of 4-aminopyridine on clinical signs in multiple sclerosis: a randomized, placebo-controlled, double-blind, crossover study. *Ann Neurol* 1992; 32:123–130.

71. Bever CT, Young D, Anderson PA, et al. The effects of 4-aminopyridine in multiple sclerosis patients: Results of a randomized, placebo-controlled, double-blind, concentration-controlled, crossover trial. *Neurology* 1994; 44:1054–1059.

72. Schapiro RT. Symptom management in multiple sclerosis. *Ann Neurol* 1994; 3 6:S123–124S.

CHAPTER 41

Hereditary Cerebellar Ataxia

David S. Younger

Since the last writing of this chapter in 2005, extraordinary progress has continued in the elucidation of the hereditary cerebellar ataxia syndromes, which has expanded from seven autosomal dominant (AD) and three autosomal recessive (AR), and rare X-linked (XL) spinocerebellar ataxia (SCA) subtypes, to dozens more syndromes, making them easily discernable. This chapter will review advances in the etiopathogenesis, classification, neurological and molecular genetic diagnosis, and treatment of hereditary cerebellar ataxia.

AUTOSOMAL RECESSIVE HEREDITARY ATAXIAS

The AR subtypes of hereditary cerebellar include Friedrich ataxia (FRDA), Marinesco-Sjogren syndrome (MSS), mitochondrial DNA depletion syndrome-7, Joubert syndrome (JS), ataxia-oculomotor apraxia-1 (AOA1), AOA2, ataxia-telangiectasia (AT), ataxia with vitamin E deficiency (AVED), and AR spastic ataxia of Charlevoix-Saguenay (ARSACS), primary coenzyme Q_{10} deficiency 1 (COQ10D1), cerebro-tendinous xanthomatosis (CTX), and adult Refsum disease (Table 1).

Friedreich Ataxia

Friedreich ataxia was recently reviewed (1). It is the commonest AR early-onset ataxia with an estimated prevalence of one per 50,000, and a carrier rate of one in 120 in the United States (US) compared to one in 2,2000,000 in Cuba wherein the carrier rate is one in 745 suggesting that it is rare on the island (2). Boys and girls are equally affected, and parents of an affected proband are asymptomatic, with

rates of consanguinity of 5.6 to 28%, leading to the risk for siblings of 25%. The patient may be the only affected member of a small family. The diagnosis is ascertained by a high clinical suspicion and confirmatory molecular genetics. McCleod (3) regarded the triad of hypoactive knee and ankle deep tendon reflexes (DTR), progressive cerebellar dysfunction, and preadolescent onset as sufficient for clinical diagnosis. However, age at onset, rate of progression, and associated signs may vary within and between families and according to the genetic defect. The onset of progressive gait and limb ataxia typically occurs in childhood before age 25, typically at a mean of six years of age, accompanied by absent leg deep tendon reflexes (DTR) in association with cardiomyopathy, visual-field impairment, dysarthria, corticospinal tract (CST) weakness, stocking proprioceptive loss, scoliosis, and diabetes mellitus.

The most common molecular abnormality is a GAA trinucleotide repeat expansion at the 9q21.11 locus of the frataxin (*FXN*) gene encoding frataxin (Table 1). Most FRDA patients are homozygous for an unstable GAA trinucleotide expansion in the first intron of X25, a non-coding region. There are 10 to 36 copies of the GAA repeat in normal chromosomes, but between 120 and 1,700 or more GAA repeats are present in greater than 95% of FRDA chromosomes. The longer normal alleles of greater than 27 GAA repeats are interrupted by the hexanucleotide repeat GAGAA (4). Less than 5% of FRDA patients are compound heterozygote, with a GAA expansion of one allele and a missense or nonsense point mutation in the other allele (5). Compound heterozygotes have atypical clinical findings. About 20% of patients with homozygous GAA expansions, especially of the Acadian variant, have atypical FRDA characterized by an older age at presentation, usually up to age 51 years, and present DTR (6). Larger GAA expansions correlate with earlier age at onset and shorter time to immobility. The smaller GAA expansion of each pair of alleles is the main determinant of disease phenotype and severity. The smaller of the two GAA expansions correlates with an increased frequency of cardiomyopathy, diabetes mellitus, and areflexia (7). Meiotic instability shows a sex bias, with paternally transmitted alleles tending to decrease and maternally inherited alleles increasing or decreasing (8). The expression of X25 is highest in the primary sites of degeneration in FRDA, including heart, liver, skeletal muscle, pancreas, spinal cord, cerebellum, and cerebrum. There is germline and somatic instability with varied GAA lengths in different tissues. The expanded GAA repeat results in a massive number of consecutive AG splice acceptor sites and a consequent loss of function. It can interfere in frataxin nuclear RNA processing and cause an absence of a mature message in the cytoplasm (9).

Patients with FRDA have undetectable or extremely low levels of X25 mRNA; thus, the disease is probably caused by a loss of function of frataxin. Frataxin, which localizes to mitochondria, is associated with mitochondrial membranes and crests and has a homology to genes in distant species such as *Caenorhabiditis elegans* and *Saccharomyces cerevisiae*. Moreover, a yeast homolog of frataxin involved in iron homeostasis and respiratory function, raises the intriguing possibility that abnormal iron mitochondrial metabolism in FRDA produces toxic-free radicals (10–12).

Marinesco-Sjogren Syndrome

First described by Marinesco and colleagues in four Romanian twins (13) and later by Sjogren (14), MSS is an early onset cerebellar ataxia that also includes congenital cataracts, mental retardation, and delayed development with short stature. Hypotonia and muscular weakness are common findings with a range of changes on muscle biopsy from pure myopathy to a neurogenic pattern. Zimmer and colleagues (15) reported neuropathy with lysosomal changes in skeletal muscle and conjunctiva biopsy tissue. Labier-Tourenne and colleagues (16) described homozygous mapping of MSS to 5q31.

Anttonen and colleagues (17) identified four disease-associated, predicted loss-of-function mutations in *SIL1*, which encodes a nucleotide exchange factor for the endoplasmic reticulum (ER) resident, heat-shock protein 70 (HSP70) chaperone HSPA5. Together with the similar spatial and temporal patterns of tissue expression of *SIL1* and HSPA5, it suggests disturbed *SIL1*-HSPA5 interaction and protein folding as the primary pathology in MSS. Anttonen and colleagues (17) described novel *SIL1*, mutations, including the first missense substitution p.Leu457Pro in MSS. Takahata and coworkers (18) described two novel mutations in a Japanese pedigree with MSS, instead with array comparative genomic hybridization and quantitative PCR analyses, indicating that some patients with MSS without base alterations in the *SIL1* gene may be caused by deletions rather than locus heterogeneity. MSS is caused by homozygous or compound heterozygous mutation at the 5q31.2 locus of the *SIL1* gene encoding SIL1 (Table 1).

Table 1. Autosomal Recessive Cerebellar Ataxia

HGNC Disease	Inheritance Pattern	Gene Designation	Gene Locus	Gene OMIM#	Gene Product	Phenotype OMIM#
FRDA	AR	*FXN*	9q21.11	606829	Frataxin	229300
MSS	AR	*SIL1*	5q31.2	608005	SIL1	248800
IOSCA	AR	*C10orf2*	10q24.31	606075	Twinkle, twinky	271245
JS-3	AR	*AHI1*	6q23.3	608894	Jouberin	608629
AOA1	AR	*APTX*	9p21.1	606350	Aprataxin	208920
AOA2	AR	*SETX*	9q34.13	608465	Senataxin	606002
AVED	AR	*TTPA*	8q12.3	600415	alpha-tocopherol transfer protein	277460
AT	AR	*ATM*	11q22.3	607585	Ataxia telangiectasia mutated protein	208900
ARSACS	AR	*SACS*	13q12.12	604490	Sacsin	270550
CoQ10D1	AR	*COQ2*	4q21.23	609825	Parahydroxybenzoate polyprenyltransferase	607426
CTX	AR	*CYP27A1*	2q35	606530	Sterol 27-hydroxylase	213700
Adult Refsum	AR	*PEX7*	6q23.3	601757	Peroxin-7	266500
		PHYH	10p13	602026	Phytanoyl-CoA hydroxylase	266500

OMIM: Online Mendelian Inheritance in Man, OMIM®. McKusik Institute of Genetic Medicine, Johns Hopkins University (Baltimore, MD) World Wide Web URL:http://omin.org

Mitochondrial DNA Depletion Syndrome-7

This disorder was originally classified as infantile onset spinocerebellar ataxia (IOSCA) in Finnish patients by Koshinen and colleagues (19). It is the second commonest inherited ataxia in Finland, with a carrier frequency of more than one in 230 individuals (20). Finnish patients presented between 1 to 2 years of age with clumsiness, gait ataxia, athetosis, muscle hypotonia, and areflexia. By school age, ophthalmoplegia and hearing loss developed, while sensory neuropathy developed in adolescence. Acute status epilepticus was a later manifestation. Laboratory studies showed abnormal nerve conduction studies (NCS) and progressive loss of myelinated fibers on sural nerve tissue biopsy. Brain magnetic resonance imaging (MRI) showed severe cerebellar atrophy often missed on brain computed tomography (CT).

The oldest studied patients were in their thirties with an expected shortened lifespan. Similar patients were described by Nikali and colleagues (20) who identified a founder mutation at the 10q24.31 locus of the *C10orf2* gene at Y508C encoding twinkle and twinky proteins (Table 1). Compound heterozygous mutations in *C10orf2* are generally more severe than homozygous ones. Hakonen and coworkers (21) observed mtDNA depletion in the brain and liver of postmortem tissue samples from several patients with *C10orf2*-associated IOSCA concluding that IOSCA could be considered an mtDNA-depletion syndrome. Lonneqvist and colleagues (22) reported long-term follow-up in 21 patients with IOSCA homozygous for the Y508C mutation in *C10orf2*, noting a more severe epileptic encephalopathy in patients progressing after childhood.

Disorders Characterized by Ataxia-Oculomotor Apraxia

Oculomotor apraxia is a disorder characterized by limitation of ocular movements on command dissociated from movements of pursuit. It occurs in a variety of syndromes, including JS, AOA1, AOA2 and AT.

Joubert syndrome is characterized by agenesis of the cerebellar vermis, ataxia, hypotonia, oculomotor apraxia, neonatal breathing abnormalities, and mental retardation. More than 15 different pathogenic mutations at the 6q23.3 locus of the *AHI1* gene encoding the Jouberin protein cause specific forms of JS-related disorders (Table 1) (23). The Jouberin protein, expressed strongly in embryonic hindbrain and forebrain, is required for human cerebellar and cortical development.

Ataxia-oculomotor apraxia-1 is the most frequent cause of AR ataxia in Japan, and is second only to FRDA in Portugal. It shares neurological features with ataxia-telangiectasia, including early onset ataxia, oculomotor apraxia, and cerebellar atrophy, along with hypoalbuminemia, hypercholesterolemia, and axonal motor neuropathy. Mutations in the

APTX gene at the 9p21.1 locus encoding aprataxin cause AOA1 (Table 1) (24). The disorder is the fourth commonest form of AR cerebellar ataxia in Alsace, France, following FRDA, AOA2, and MSS (25). Aprataxin is a nuclear protein with a role in DNA repair. Accordingly, *APTX*-defective cell lines are sensitive to agents that cause single-strand breaks and exhibit an increased incidence of inducted chromosomal aberrations; neurological disorders associated with *APTX* mutation may be caused by gradual accumulation of unrepaired DNA strand breaks resulting from abortive DNA ligation events (26).

Ataxia-oculomotor apraxia-2, which is instead due to mutation at the 9q34.13 locus of the senataxin (*SETX*) gene (Table 1) (27) presents between age 10 to 22 years with cerebellar atrophy, axonal sensorimotor neuropathy, oculomotor apraxia, and elevated serum concentration of α-fetoprotein. The senataxin-interacting proteins play a role in coordinating transcriptional events and DNA repair (28).

The clinical features of AT include ataxia, telangiectasia, dystonia, tremor, myoclonus, cellular and humoral immune deficiencies, growth retardation, progeria, high serum α-fetoprotein, chromosomal instability, predisposition to lymphoreticular malignancy, and sensitivity to ionizing radiation. The gene for ataxia telangiectasia was mapped to chromosome 11 (29), cloned, and named *ATM* for ataxia telangiectasia mutated gene (30). The disorder is caused by pathogenic mutations at the 11q22.3 locus of the *ATM* gene encoding the ATM protein (Table 1). The stable association of the ATM repair protein with chromatin is a likely critical step in triggering, amplifying and maintaining the DNA damage repair signal even in the absence of DNA lesions (31).

Familial Vitamin E Deficiency

Vitamin E deficiency (VED) occurs as an isolated abnormality unassociated with fat malabsorption. Except for cardiomyopathy, ataxia with vitamin E deficiency (AVED) in some patients is very similar or identical to those of FRDA. Neurological symptoms included ataxia, dysarthria, hyporeflexia, and decreased proprioceptive and vibratory sensations. Electrophysiological and pathological examinations point to the central axons of dorsal root ganglia (DRG) and the retina at the major areas of involvement, followed by peripheral sensory nerves, optic nerve, and CST. Oral administration of vitamin E halted progression of visual and neurological symptoms. Familial VED, which results from pathogenic frameshift and missense point mutations at the 8q12.3 locus of the α–tocopheral transfer protein *TTPA* gene encoding α-tocopheral transfer protein (Table 1), leads to impaired incorporation of α–tocopherol into very-low-density lipoprotein required for efficient vitamin E recycling.

Autosomal Recessive Spastic Ataxia of Charlevoix-Saguenay (HRSACS)

This spastic ataxia unique to Charlevoix-Saguenay was identified more than two decades ago by Bouchard and coworkers (32). It was a frequent cause of inherited spastic ataxia, with an estimated carrier frequency of the gene of one in 22 persons in the Saguenay-Lac-Saint-Jean population during 1941 to 1985 (33). All ARSACS patients exhibit signs of spasticity in the legs with a tendency to fall, especially at the onset of gait initiation from 12 to 18 months of age when there is little sign of cerebellar dysfunction. Speech is slightly dysarthria in childhood and becomes explosive in adulthood. Early non-progressive signs include bilateral Babinski signs, saccadic alteration of smooth ocular pursuit, and prominent myelinated fibers radiating from the optic disc, embedding the retinal vessels at fundoscopy. Children of elementary school age are generally slow to learn and even more so to write, with more than half dropping out of school.

The disease progresses more obviously in the teens and twenties with progressive increase in muscle tone, DTR, jerky scissoring gait, and discrete to marked distal amyotrophy. Progression to the wheelchair state occurred at a mean of 41 years of age, with a mean age at death of 51 years, and some surviving into the eighth decade. Brain CT and MRI show atrophy of the cerebellar vermis, progressive atrophy of the cerebellar hemispheres and of the cervical spinal cord. Electrodiagnostic (EMG) studies reveal absent sensory nerve action potentials, and low motor conduction velocities, with signs of severe denervation in distal muscles. Electroencephalographic abnormalities include bursts of generalized slow waves of subcortical origin, with rare epileptic activity, although up to 7% have clinical seizures. The disorder is caused by pathogenic mutations at the 13q12.12 locus of the *SACS* gene encoding the sacsin protein (Table 1), which is most highly expressed in large neurons, including cerebellar Purkinje cells, wherein integration of ubiquitin-proteasome Hsp70 protects against polyglutamine-expanded ataxin-1 (34).

Coenzyme Q_{10} Deficiency 1

Musumeci and coworkers (35) described the most common phenotype of CoQ_{10} or ubiquinone deficiency, in muscle associated with childhood-onset cerebellar ataxia and atrophy, variably associated with neuropathy, seizures, mental retardation, muscle weakness, hypogonadism, and low levels of CoQ_{10} in fibroblasts that respond to CoQ_{100} supplementation. The concentration of muscle CoQ_{10} ranged from 26 to 35% while that of fibroblasts varied from 54 to 71%, both significantly lower than controls. Pathogenic mutation at the 4q21.23 locus of the COQ_2 gene leads to disturbance in the biosynthesis of CoQ or ubiquinone due to a defect in para-hydroxybenzoate-polyprenyl transferase, a redox carrier in the mitochondrial respiratory chain and lipid-soluble antioxidant (Table 1). Quinzii and colleagues (36) described a homozygous missense mutation in COQ_2 encoding para-hydroxybenzoate-polyprenyl transferase in a previously studied 33-month-old boy with infantile encephalomyopathy, nephropathy, and CoQ_{10} deficiency (37).

An A to G transition at nucleotide 890 changed a highly conserved tyrosine to cysteine at amino acid 297 within a predicted transmembrane domain. Radioisotope assays confirmed a severe defect of CoQ_{10} biosynthesis in fibroblasts of one patient so studied. Lagier-Tourenne (38) and Mollet and colleagues (39) described mutations in *ADCK3 CABC1* associated with CoQ_{10} deficiency in individuals with juvenile-onset cerebellar ataxia, while others described similar mutations in *CABC1/ADCK3* and progressive cerebellar ataxia and atrophy but without mention of CoQ_{10} levels (40). The *ADCK3* gene encodes the yeast homolog of CoQ_8 which is involved in CoQ_{10} synthesis. Other presentations of CoQ_{10} deficiency syndromes (41) include AOA1 due to mutation in *APTX* (42), severe infantile multisystemic disease presentation with cardiofaciocutaneous syndrome due to mutation in the *BRAF* gene (43), and isolated mitochondrial myopathy associated with muscle coenzyme Q_{10} deficiency associated with exercise intolerance, recurrent myoglobinuria, developmental delay, ataxia, and seizures due to mutation in the *ETFDH* gene (44, 45). Two patients with late-onset cerebellar ataxia, beginning at ages 35 and 39 years, with hypogonadism and muscle coenzyme Q_{10} deficiency, described by Gironi and colleagues (46), improved with high-dose CoQ_{10} supplementation, stressing the importance of considering the diagnosis in the differential diagnosis of cerebellar ataxia, even when onset is relatively late in life.

Cerebrotendinous Xanthomatosis

Van Bogaert and colleagues (47) described affected cousins with onset at age 12 and 13 years with spastic ataxia, palatal myoclonus, mental impairment, cataracts, xanthelasmata, and xanthomata of the tendons. At postmortem examination there were white matter cerebral and cerebral peduncle deposits. Menkes and colleagues (48) speculated that the metabolic defect concerned transport of cholesterol out of cells. Cali and coworkers (49, 50) identified mutations at the 2q35 locus of the *CYP27A1* gene, cloning cDNA for the encoded protein product, sterol 27-hydroxylase (Table 1). Bile acid production in CTX1 is subnormal, yet the activity of cholesterol 7-α-hydroxylase, the rate-limiting enzyme of bile acid synthesis, is elevated. Cholestanol, the 5-α-dihydro derivative of cholesterol, is enriched related to cholesterol in the serum and tendons of affected individuals, with low normal plasma cholesterol levels. Oral administration of chenodeoxycholic acid, which is virtually absent from the bile in CTX, produces a substantial reduction in cholestanol synthesis and lowers serum levels.

Adult Refsum Disease

This inborn error of lipid metabolism, first described by Refsum (51), classically presents with retinitis pigmentosa, peripheral neuropathy, cerebellar ataxia, and acellular CSF with increased protein levels. Milhalik and colleagues (52) noted that individuals with Refsum disease were homozygous for inactivating mutations in the *PHYH* gene, while Braverman and colleagues (53) demonstrated mutations in the *PEX7* gene. The cause of adult Refsum disease is ascribed to pathogenic mutations at the 10p13 locus of the *PHYH* gene encoding phytanoyl-CoA hydroxylase, a peroxisomal protein that catalyzes the first step in the α-oxidation of phytanic acid, and other mutations at the 6q23.3 locus of the *PEX7* gene, the receptor for type 2 peroxisomal targeting signal (PTS2) encoding peroxin-7, one of a set of peroxisomal assembly proteins required for import of matrix proteins into peroxisomes (Table 1).

X-LINKED HEREDITARY ATAXIAS

XL SCA is a clinically and genetically heterogeneous disorder with five recognized subtypes, abbreviated SCAX1-5.

SCAX1

A relatively pure of form of olivopontocerebellar degeneration was described by Lutz and colleagues (54) that had the clinical features of infantile onset of cerebellar ataxia, very slow progression, mental retardation, and neuroimaging evidence of olivary and pontine involvement. Muscle biopsy performed for infantile hypotonia and ataxia in infancy in one patient was normal. Illarioshkin and colleagues (55) mapped a locus for XL recessive congenital ataxia in large Russian kindred to Xp11.21-q24, as did Bertini and colleagues (56), who narrowed the interval to another critical region at Xp11.21-q21.3.

SCAX2

Early-onset of cerebellar ataxia with extrapyramidal features was described by Malamud and Cohen (57) in a family of affected males related through females, with head tremor, spasticity, rigidity, unilateral sixth nerve palsy, and mental retardation. Postmortem examination showed severe cerebellar atrophy with absence of Purkinje cells, pale inferior olives, and intact pons.

SCAX3

Ataxia and deafness were described by Schmidley and colleagues (58) among six affected males in five sibships connected through carrier females in three successive generations. Infantile onset hypotonia was associated with ataxia, sensorineural deafness, developmental delay, esotropia, and optic atrophy leading to death in childhood. Postmortem examination showed neuronal loss and gliosis in the dentate nucleus and inferior olive, red nucleus, dorsal motor nucleus of the vagus, and central auditory pathways, with less conspicuous involvement of the cerebellar cortex.

SCAX4

Ataxia and adult-onset dementia was described by Farlow and colleagues (59) in men of a three-generation kindred connected through female carriers. Initial symptoms of delayed walking and tremor were evident by two to three years, with mild progressive ataxia and CST signs during teenage years, followed by memory disturbance in the third decade, culminating in death by the sixth decade.

SCAX5

Neonatal hypotonia, delayed motor development, nonprogressive ataxia, nystagmus, and dysarthria appearing in the first year of life, that tended to improve with age and all eventually walked without support in a large American family was described by Zanni and coworkers (60). The candidate locus termed SCAX5 mapped to Xq25-q27.

Sideroblastic Anemia and Ataxia

Sideroblastic anemia is a heterogeneous disorder characterized by hypochromic microcytic erythrocytes and iron accumulation in the mitochondria of bone marrow erythrocyte precursors. Pathogenic mutation at the Xp11.21 locus of the erythroid tissue-specific *ALAS2* gene encoding delta-aminolevulinate synthase 2 (ALAS), which catalyzes 5-aminoleulinic acid from glycine and succinyl-coenzyme A in a pyridoxal 5-phosphate-dependent manner, is the cause of XL sideroblastic anemia (XLSA) (61).

The clinical phenotype for XLSA is microcytic, hypochromic anemia with iron accumulation and severity ranging widely depending upon the amount of residual enzymatic activity, and onset in youth but ranging from birth to the ninth decade. Probands are frequently males because of hemizygosity of the XL defect, but females are occasionally affected because of skewed chromosomal inactivation sparing the mutant allele. A distinct form of sideroblastic anemia and spinocerebellar syndrome that segregated together in an XL pattern in several males with

dysfunction and that PQBP1 was involved in the pathology of SCA1. Xia and coworkers (80) targeted ataxin-1 as a therapeutic use of RNA interference for the intracerebellar delivery of viral vectors expressing short hairpin RNA. The treated mice showed reduced ataxin-1 expression in Purkinje cells, resolution of intracellular ataxin-1 inclusions in the cerebellum, and improved motor performance. Serra and colleagues (81) showed that delaying postnatal expression of mutant human ATXN1 until completion of cerebellar maturation led to a substantial reduction in disease severity in adults compared with early postnatal expression of mutant ATXN1.

The worldwide frequency of SCA1 as determined by the CAG repeat has been assessed. Pareyson and colleagues (82) found that SCA1 was the most common SCA phenotype, present in 41% of patients and 30 families. Storey and colleagues (83) examined the frequency of SCA types 1, 2, 3, 6, and 7 in southeastern Australia. Of 63 genetically confirmed pedigrees, 30% had SCA1. Zhou and colleagues (84) reported SCA1 in 5 of 75 or 7% of Chinese families, all heterozygous for alleles, with CAG repeat numbers ranging from 51 to 64 with a control of 26 to 35 repeats, and significant negative correlation between age of disease onset and number of CAG repeat. Other investigators have reported a frequency of SCA1 of 3 to 50%, depending on geographic and ethnic background and clinical and familial criteria for inclusion. The largest United States (US) series reported that only 3% of 149 dominant kindred were SCA1 (85). SCA1 rarely, if ever, underlies ataxia in singular cases or in those that appear to be AR.

SCA2

Individuals from a homogeneous population in the Holguin province of Cuba who descended from an Iberian founder age 2 to 65 years, with limb and gait ataxia, dysarthria, action tremor, cramps, ophthalmoparesis, slowed saccades, hypotonia, hypoactive upper limb reflexes, increased or decreased lower limb reflexes, and rare instances of dementia, were some of the first recognized persons with SCA2 (86). Several additional SCA2 pedigrees of Italian-American (87), Italian (88), Austrian-Canadian, French-Canadian (89), and Tunisian ancestry were subsequently identified (90).

Pathology reveals a pattern of OPCA with severe neuronal loss in the inferior olive, pons, cerebellum and, to a limited degree, the anterior horn cells, with degeneration of the substantia nigra and the dorsal columns (91).

A CAG expansion at the SCA2 locus on chromosome 12q was first identified independently by three groups using different techniques, including positional cloning (92), a specific antibody for polyglutamine repeats (93), and direct identification of repeat expansion and cloning techniques (DIRECT) (94). SCA2 is caused by an expanded CAG

nucleotide repeat at the 12q24.12 locus of the *ATXN2* gene (Table 2). The gene contains 16 exons with the CAG expansion present in exon 1. It encodes a 1,313 amino acid protein of molecular weight 140 kDa, termed *ataxin-2* (93). Normal individuals have 14 to 31 CAG repeats in the open reading frame, and there are one to three CAA within the CAG repeat (95, 96); however, SCA2 patients have CAG expansions of 34 to 59 and no CAA within the repeat. There is an inverse correlation between age at onset and the CAG number, as in the other CAG repeat disorders. Myoclonus, dystonia, chorea, and dementia are more likely to occur when the CAG expansion is large. The CAG expansion is unstable in both paternal and maternal transmission. Anticipation was reported with paternal transmission in one study (95) but not in another (96).

Ueyama and colleagues (97) studied two Japanese kindred with 25 affected members among two families, and a mean age of onset of symptoms of 44 years that included cerebellar ataxia with deep sensory disturbances, and slow saccadic eye movements, especially in those younger than 35 years. Schols and colleagues (69), in addition, noted slow saccades, hyporeflexia, myoclonus, and action tremor. Van de Warrenburg and colleagues (70) found electrodiagnostic evidence of neuronopathy, dorsal root ganglionopathy, and AHC features in three patients so studied. Brain MRI in the two studies showed pontocerebellar atrophy (69, 97). Brain MRI I studies in 20 affected individuals showed olivopontocerebellar atrophy that correlated with CAG repeats but not with infratentorial atrophy or disease duration (98). Brain PET showed reduced dopamine distribution in the caudate and putamen.

There has been considerable interest in the association of central nervous system (CNS) neurodegenerative disorders including Parkinsonism and amyotrophic lateral sclerosis (ALS) and interrupted SCA2 CAG repeat expansions. Ragothaman and coworkers (99) reported a consanguineous Indian family with SCA2 expansions and a complex phenotype of ataxia, Parkinsonism, and retinitis pigmentosa. Two members, both homozygous for SCA2, had dopa-responsive Parkinsonism, with tremor, rigidity, and bradykinesia and age at onset of 15 and 22 years. Charles and colleagues (100) noted SCA2 expansions ranging in size from 37 to 39 repeat interrupted by CAA triplets among 2% of 164 French families with AD Parkinsonism. Elden and coworkers (101) demonstrated genetic, biochemical, and neuropathologic interactions between the ALS protein TDP43 and ATXN2, raising the possibility that the former, localized normally to the nucleus, might be more prone to mislocalize to the cytoplasm under stressful situations due to the genetic influence of *ATXN2* polyQ repeats. To the contrary, Ross and colleagues (102) found no association between intermediate ATXN2 CAG repeat expansions of greater than 30 units in PD among 702 patients with PD and 4,877 controls, nor did Van Damme and colleagues (103).

SCA3

SCA3 or Machado-Joseph disease (MJD) was first described among New England descendants of William Machado, a native of an island in the Portuguese Azores (104). Gait and limb ataxia, dysarthria, and progressive ophthalmoplegia are commonly observed regardless of age at onset, whereas CST signs, dystonia and rigidity, peripheral amyotrophy, facial and lingual fasciculation, and bulging eyes occur with younger age. Shimizu and colleagues (105) estimated the prevalence of SCA in Nagano, Japan, to be 22 per 100,000, with 31 of 86 families or 36% positive for SCA disease-causing repeat expansions, of which SCA3 accounted for 3%, a prevalence lower than other regions in Japan.

The pathologic findings that distinguish MJD from other ADCA include extensive involvement of the spinocerebellar tracts, AHC, and neurons in the dentate, pons, nigra, oculomotor nuclei, and basal ganglia, with sparing of the olivary nuclei and cerebellar cortex.

Takiyama et al. (106) mapped the gene for MJD in several Japanese families to chromosome 14q24.3-32. This locus was confirmed in MJD families of Azorean descent (107), including Azorean families with the unusual phenotype (type 4) of dopa-responsive parkinsonism (108). In 1994, a linkage study of French families implicated the same region, and the locus was numbered SCA3 (109). Since the families were not of Azorean descent and because of several clinical differences, including the lack of dystonia and facial fasciculation, the question remained as to whether MJD and SCA3 were disorders due to different genes, different mutations in the same gene, or in the phenotypic spectrum of the same mutation in individuals with differing ancestry. However, in 1994 an expanded and unstable CAG repeat in the coding region of the MJD gene (MJD1) was identified (110). Subsequent studies of ataxia patients confirmed that all 14q linked families have the same unstable CAG repeat within the MJD gene. SCA3 is caused by a (CAG) trinucleotide repeat expansion in the ataxin-3 (ATXN3) gene at the 14q32.12 locus (Table 2).

Perez and colleagues (111) demonstrated that ataxin-3 adopts a unique conformation when expressed within the nucleus of transfected cells that was not due to proteolysis, instead suggesting that the association with nuclear proteins altered the structure of full-length ataxin-3, exposing the polyglutamate domain. One early event in the pathogenesis of SCA3/MJD may be an altered conformation of ataxin-3 within the nucleus that exposes the polyglutamine domain.

Chai and colleagues (112) presented evidence supporting a central role for protein misfolding in the pathogenesis of the disorder indicating that modulating proteasome activity was a potential approach to altering disease progression. Gaspar and coworkers (113) explored the possibility of frameshift mutations in expanded CAG tracts of ataxin-3 in the generation of polyalanine mutant proteins and the formation of intranuclear inclusions. The results of transfection experiments suggest that frameshifts were more likely to occur in longer CAG repeats, and alanine polymers alone might be harmful to cells. Ishikawa and coworkers (114) reported four patients with MJD confirmed by CAG repeat in the ataxin-3 gene that had symptoms of dementia and delirium and long CAG repeat lengths. Pathological examination of two patients showed cerebrocortical and thalamic neuronal intranuclear inclusions that stained with anti-polyglutamine antibody.

Mueller and coworkers (115) showed that protein casein kinase-2(CK2)-dependent phosphorylation controlled the nuclear localization, aggregation, and stability of ataxin-3. Unlike SCA1 and SCA2, there is a wide difference between normal and affected SCA3 subjects in the number of repeats, with normal ranging from 12 to 40, and from 61 to 89 in disease alleles. Moreover, as in other CAG repeat diseases, there is an inverse relation between the length of the repeat and the age at onset. Almost all affected individuals with the MJD CAG expansion have an AD inheritance pattern with rare sporadic MJD expansions (85). Most of the US MJD cases are of German and not Portuguese extraction (85), and a single founder may account for the French and Brazilian MJD kindred while at least two different founders may account for the Portuguese families, with other mutations accounting for MJD kindred in Algeria, French-Guiana, and Belgium (116).

SCA4

Gardner and (117) described a five-generation Utah family with late-onset ataxia, prominent sensory axonal neuropathy, CST signs, and normal eye movements, with linkage to chromosome 16q24-qter, termed SCA4, that was later reassigned to 16q22.1 (Table 2) (118, 119). The earliest symptoms of SCA4 were unsteadiness of gait typically in the fourth or fifth decade, with a range of age at onset of 19 to 59 years. Absent ankle jerks and decreased sensation were present in all affected individuals, while dysarthria was present in 50%, Babinski signs in 20%, and saccadic pursuit eye movements in 15%. Electrodiagnostic studies were consistent with axonal sensory neuropathy.

SCA5

Ranum and colleagues (120) described a kindred with slowly progressive cerebellar dysfunction, CST signs, and bulbar dysfunction. All four juvenile-onset patients of age 10 to 18 years resulted from maternal transmission, suggesting maternal anticipation bias for SCA5. Linkage analysis mapped the disease locus, designated SCA5, to the centromeric region of chromosome 11. Burk and coworkers (121) narrowed the SCA5 locus to a 5.15-Mb internal between PYGM and D11S4136 at chromosome 11p11-q11 in a large German family in which 15 members spanning four generations with a mean age at onset of 32 years, range of 15 to 50 years, and a tendency toward earlier onset in later generations.

The most consistent clinical feature was downbeat nystagmus, imbalance of stance and gait, dysarthria, intention and resting tremor, impaired smooth muscle pursuit, and gaze-evoked nystagmus. There was a slow progression of symptoms and all patients were ambulatory despite disease duration of up to 31 years. Brain MRI showed cerebellar and hemispheric atrophy. Ikeda and colleagues (122) found a 39-bp deletion in exon 12 of the spectrin beta non-erythrocytic 2 (SPTBN2) gene that caused an in-frame 13 amino acid deletion within the third of 17 spectrin repeats in all 90 affected individuals and 35 presymptomatic carriers from a large 11-generation American kindred, as well as a short in-frame deletion in the same spectrin repeat of the SPTBN2 gene of a French family, and a T-to-C transition in exon 7 of the SPTBN2 gene of a German family that caused a leucine-to-proline change in the calponin homology domain containing the actin/ARP1-binding site. SCA5 is caused by pathogenic mutations at the 11q13.2 locus of SPTBN2 (Table 2) (123).

SCA6

Subramony and colleagues (124) described a family with late-onset progressive cerebellar ataxia. Zhuchenko and colleagues (125) reported several unrelated families with a similar slowly progressive ataxia, dysarthria, nystagmus, vertigo, mild vibratory, and proprioceptive sensory loss. Brain MRI showed isolated cerebellar atrophy. A genotype survey disclosed a CAG repeat expansion in the calcium channel, voltage-dependent, P/Q type, alpha-1A subunit (CACNA1A) gene. Affected patients had 21 to 30 CAG repeats whereas normal individuals had 4 to 20 repeats. SCA6 is due to mutation at the 19p13 locus of the CACNA1A gene encoding the transmembrane pore-forming subunit of the P/Q-type or CaV2.1 voltage-gated channel (VGCC) (Table 2) (126). The latter mediate the entry of Ca^{2+} ions into excitable cells and other Ca^{2+} processes, including muscle contraction, hormonal and neurotransmitter release, and gene expression. Gene expression studies show downregulation of the HSF1-HSPA1A axis as an event in 24-CAG repeat cells that appear to be critical for cellular toxicity consistent with a pathogenesis of SCA6-related polyglutamine disease.

Sinke and colleagues (127) described 24 Dutch families with SCA6 as a late-onset ataxia in which eye movement abnormalities were prominent and early, with some associated with episodic headache and nausea, suggesting overlap with familial hemiplegic migraine and episodic ataxia type 2. In a large Portuese family of over 17 patients spanning four generations, with hemiplegic migraine and progressive SCA6, Alonso and coworkers (128) noted that all affected patients shared a common haplotype and an arg583-to-gln mutation in the CACNA1A gene. Takahashi and colleagues (129) described 140 patients with SCA6 and observed an inverse relation between age at onset and length of the expanded allele. Unsteadiness of gait, vertigo, oscillopsia, and cerebellar signs were detected in nearly all patients; by contrast, extra-cerebellar signs were relatively mild and infrequent. There was a close relationship between down-beating positional nystagmus and positional vertigo, which became more common at later ages. The total number of CAG repeat units in both alleles was a good parameter for assessment of age at onset in SCA6, including homozygous patients.

Fujutake and colleagues (130) described a 55-year-old man, the offspring of first-cousin parents, who presented with cerebellar ataxia, vertical anti-directional nystagmus, and retinitis pigmentosa. Christova and colleagues (131) noted ocular motor abnormalities in four presymptomatic SCA6 patients with CACNA1A mutations, including low-amplitude horizontal gaze-evoked nystagmus, abnormal frequently of square wave jerks, and reduced gain for pursuit tracking.

Van de Warrenburg and colleagues (70) noted no significant electrophysiological evidence of peripheral neuropathy among seven SCA6 patients. Soong and colleagues (132) performed brain PET using labeled glucose on seven patients with SCA6 and seven healthy controls and found significant hypometabolism ranging from 63 to 78% that of controls in the brainstem, cerebellar hemispheres, basal ganglia, and various areas of the cortex.

Takahashi and colleagues (133) described the neuropathological findings in the proband of a Japanese family who developed gait disturbance at age 62 and died five years later due to subarachnoid hemorrhage. There was severe loss of Purkinje cells, predominantly in the dorsal vermis, and absence of neuronal loss of the inferior olives of two affected sisters and an affected father. CAG expansions of 23 CAG in the CACNA1A gene caused both intermittent and a progressive cerebellar dysfunction within the same family, blurring the distinction between SCA6 and EA2 (134).

There are differences between the mutation in SCA6 and those responsible for SCA1, SCA2, SCA3, Huntington disease (HD), DRPLA, and spinobulbar muscular atrophy. First, the expanded mutant alleles in SCA6 were smaller than in any of the other neurodegenerative disorders. Second, the size of normal alleles, up to 20 repeats, was without a gap between the distribution of CAG-repeat numbers on the normal and SCA6 chromosome. Third, the CAG expansion occurred in a gene known to be important for normal Purkinje cell function and survival. Thus, the CAG repeat appeared to result in a loss of function or a dominant negative effect. For example, the transcribed abnormal allele could interfere with transcription and translation of the normal allele rather than the gain of function seen with the polyglutamine stretches in SCA1, SCA2, SCA3, HD, DRPLA, and spinobulbar muscular atrophy (135).

Alonso and colleagues (128) noted a common haplotype and arg583-to-gln mutation in the *CACNA1A* gene, suggesting that episodic ataxia-2, SCA6, and familial hemiplegia migraine were not only allelic, but the same disorder with phenotypic variability.

SCA7

Froment and colleagues (136) described spincoerebellar degeneration in association with retinal degeneration in four affected persons of a three-generation family, noting the variability of the retinopathy that was peripheral in the first generation, macular in the second, and macular and circumpapillary in the third. Whereas SCA7 is considered to be one of the rarest forms of genetically verified ADCA, Jonasson and colleagues (137) noted that it was the most frequent subtype of ADCA in Sweden and Finland.

Michalik and coworkers (138) reviewed the clinical, pathological, and molecular aspects of SCA7. Age at onset averages 30 years, with a range from childhood to the seventh decade. The clinical course varies with age at onset with duration of disease to death averaging six years in those with onset before age six, and 20 years in those with onset after age 10 years.

Early and progressive deterioration of limb and gait ataxia can occur in isolation or precede visual complaints that include abnormal yellow-blue color discrimination, which in the earliest or mildest forms may be asymptomatic. Optic disc pallor, granular and atrophic changes in the macula, slow saccades, and ophthalmoparesis, especially in upgaze, gait and limb ataxia, dysarthria, and pyramidal signs. Parkinsonism and decreased vibration sense may be noted.

Van de Warrenburg and colleagues (70) noted that of four patients with SCA7, and electrophysiological evidence of peripheral nerve involvement, two patients had axonopathy and two had neuronopathy. Neuropathological changes include degeneration of the cerebellum, basis pontis, inferior olive, and retinal ganglion cells.

David and coworkers (139) identified the causative gene, *ATXN7*, a 2,2727-bp open reading frame predicting an 892-amino acid polypeptide, designated ataxin-7 (ATXN7) with a nuclear localization signal and a polyglutamate tract.

SCA7 is caused by an expanded trinucleotide repeat at the 3p14.1 locus of the *ATXN7* gene encoding ataxin-7 (Table 2), a transcription factor that appears to be critically important for chromatin remodeling at the level of histone acetylation and de-ubiquitination and is a core component of 2 different transcription coactivator complexes, the SPT3

acetyltransferase (STAGA) complex, which has histone acetyltransferase activity, and the USP22 de-ubiquitination complex (140). Anticipation occurs with significantly greater male transmission. Gonadal instability is associated with paternal transmission and is greater than in any of the seven neurodegenerative diseases caused by translated CAG repeat expansions (139).

Postmortem examination of an affected 10-year-old boy with genetically confirmed SCA7 showed neuronal inclusions, identified by an antibody directed against the expanded polyglutamine domain in multiple areas of the brain, with inclusions noted most frequently in the inferior olivary complex, lateral geniculate body, and substantial nigra as well as others areas, some of which stained positively for ubiquitin (141). Ansorge and colleagues (142) reported an infant with SCA7 and 180 CAG repeats in the *ATAXN* gene in which symptoms and signs appeared at 9 months of age with developmental delay, failure to thrive, and limb tremor. By 19 months, there was retinal pigmentary degeneration, nystagmus, hypotonia, and cerebellar ataxia, and the patient died at 29 months. Postmortem examination showed severe olivopontocerebellar atrophy and thinning of the spinal cord. Ataxia-7 nuclear inclusions were seen throughout the nervous system, in endothelial cells, cardiac and skeletal muscle, pancreas, and epithelial cells of Brunner glands in the duodenum.

Yvert and coworkers (143) generated transgenic mice which expressed mutant human *ATXN7* in either Purkinje cells or retinal rod photoreceptors. Mice expressing full-length mutant *ATXN7* had deficiencies in motor coordination and vision. A severe degeneration was caused by overexpression of *ATXN7*, whereas a similar overexpression of normal ataxia-7 had no obvious effect. La Spada and colleagues (144) generated a transgenic mouse model of SCA7 that expressed ATXN7 with 92 glutamines in the CNS and retina. They observed a cone-rod dystrophy type of retinal degeneration. Using yeast 2-hybrid studies, ataxin-7 interacted with CRX, a nuclear transcription factor predominantly expressed in retinal photoreceptor cells.

Mutations in the *CRX* gene cause cone-rod dystrophy-2 in humans. Co-immunoprecipitation experiments colocalized ataxin-7 with CRX in nuclear aggregates. Using a rhodopsin promoter-reporter construct, La Spada and colleagues (144) observed that polyglutamine-expanded *ATXN7* suppressed CRX transactivation. With electrophoretic mobility shift assays and PT-PCR analysis, they observed a reduction in CRX binding activity and reductions in CRX-regulated genes in SCA7 transgenic retinas. The data suggested that the SCA7 transgenic mice faithfully recapitulated the process of retinal degeneration observed in human SCA7 patients. The authors hypothesized that *ATXN7*-mediated transcription interference of photoreceptor-specific genes could account for the retinal degeneration in SCA7, and provide an explanation for how cell-type specificity is achieved in this poly-glutamine disorder.

Yoo and colleagues (145) generated a transgenic mouse model of severe infantile SCA7 with 266 CAG repeats. At five weeks of age, the mice demonstrated progressive weight loss, ptosis, ataxia, muscle wasting, kyphosis, and tremor. Electroretinogram showed cone and rod photoreceptor defects, and shortening of the outer segments of the retina with accumulation of mutant ataxin-7. Mutant ataxin-7 accumulated in various neuronal subtypes throughout the brain, suggesting that polyglutamine expansion stabilizes mutant ataxin-7. Accumulation of the mutant protein may cause downstream molecular events that hinder cell function and survival.

SCA8

Koob and colleagues (146) reported eight pedigrees with slowly progressive, severely affected members with nystagmus, spastic and ataxic dysarthria, incoordination, gait ataxia, spasticity, and vibratory sensory loss, with onset from age 18 to 65 years, and a mean age at onset of 40 years, with most non-ambulatory by the fifth decade. Linkage was found at the 13q21 locus in eight pedigrees with CTG repeat expansion in the ataxin-8 opposite strand (ATXN8OS) gene, found to be transcribed into mRNA with an expanded CUG repeat in its 3-prime UTR.

Ikeda and colleagues (147) described six Japanese patients with expanded CTG repeat alleles in the ATXN8OS gene ranging from 89–155 repeats, with 15 to 34 repeats in those age 79 years and older. Brain MRI showed cerebellar vermis and hemispheric atrophy.

Daughter and colleagues (148) showed that the expanded CTG repeat in the ATXN8OS gene was transcribed into mRNA with an expanded CUG repeat causing a toxic gain of function. Moreover, ATXN8OS mRNA containing the expanded repeat accumulated as ribonuclear inclusions and colocalized with an RNA-binding protein in selected cerebellar cortical neurons of human and murine SCA8 brain tissue. Moseley and colleagues (149) detected polyglutamine expansions in IC2-immunoreactive intranuclear inclusions from SCA8 human brain tissue encoded by an expanded CAG repeat in ATXN8 complimentary to the expanded CTG repeat of ATNX8OS on the opposite strand indicating bidirectional transcription with expression of both a polyglutamine protein and a CUG expansion transcript. It is now known that SCA8 is caused by a CTG/CAG trinucleotide repeat expansion at the 13q21.33 locus, with two genes spanning the repeat, expressed in opposite directions, with ATXN8 encoding a nearly pure polyglutamine expansion protein in the CAG direction and ATXN8OS transcribing a noncoding CUG expansion RNA(Table 2). It is speculated that bidirectional transcription at the SCA8

locus of both a polyglutamine protein and CUG expansion transcript may represent a toxin gain of function at both the protein and RNA levels (149). Wu and colleagues (150) reported repeat expansion at the SCA8 locus in 1.5% of patients with typical late-onset levodopa-responsive PD that ranged in size from 75 to 92 repeats.

SCA9

Higgins and colleagues (151) studied an extensive multigenerational American family of more than 1,200 individuals with family origins in the city of London and Durham County of England, the founder couple of whom were early American colonists who immigrated to Maryland after marrying in London in 1685. The phenotypic features included ataxia, ophthalmoplegia, and variable degrees of dysarthria, CST involvement, dopa-responsive Parkinsonism features of shuffling gait, bradykinesia, cogwheel rigidity, bradylalia, and 2 to 6/second tremor. Brain MRI in several patients demonstrated mild degrees of cerebellar atrophy, including one with demyelinating periventricular and subcortical white matter lesions. Exclusion of all known SCA loci by mutational analysis and linkage analysis suggested a new SCA locus.

SCA10

Grewal and colleagues (152) described a four-generation pedigree that segregated a distinct form of SCA characterized by cerebellar ataxia and seizures. Anticipation was observed in available parent-child pairs suggesting that a dinucleotide repeat expansion could be the mutagenic mechanism. A genome-wide search performed by Zu and coworkers (153) identified linkage to a 15-cM region on chromosome 22q13 so designating the SCA10 gene locus.

Ramussen and colleagues (154) reported 18 affected individuals from four Mexican families with gait ataxia, dysarthria, limb ataxia, ocular movement abnormalities, and other features including generalized seizures, partial seizures, CST signs, and sensorimotor polyneuropathy. Grewal and colleagues (155) presented a phenotype-genotype analysis of two large Mexican families originally reported by Grewal and colleagues (152) and Matsuura and coworkers (156) with genetically confirmed SCA10. Of 22 affected individuals, seizures developed in 11; several individuals had mild personality changes and anticipation was present in both families. Matsuura and colleagues (156) described an expansion of a pentanucleotide (ATTCT) repeat in intron 9 of the ataxin 10 (ATXN10) gene, the latter of which consisted of 12 exons spanning 172 kb of genomic DNA.

Teive and colleagues (157) reported five Brazilian families spanning six generations with genetically confirmed SCA10 with gait ataxia, dysarthria, dysmetria, dysdiadochokinesis, and nystagmus. Brain MRI showed cerebellar atrophy. Electrodiagnostic studies were normal. SCA10 accounts for approximately 15% of ADCA in Mexicans (158). SCA 10 is caused by an expanded 5-bp ATTCT repeat at the 22q13.31 locus of the ATXN10 gene encoding ataxin-10 (159) (Table 2). Pathological alleles have 400 to 4,500 repeats while normal alleles have 10 to 29.

SCA11

Worth (160) and Houlden and coworkers (161) described multigenerational British families with relatively benign late-onset slowly progressive cerebellar ataxia, and characterized the causative gene for SCA11, tau tubulin kinase 2 (TTBK2), encoding a protein of 1,244 amino acids. The encoded TTBK2 protein is a member of the casein kinase (CK1) group of protein kinases with an ability to phosphorylate tau and tubulin in vitro. SCA11 is caused by a mutation at the 15q15.2 locus of the TTBK2 gene encoding tau tubulin kinase-2 (Table 2).

SCA12

Holmes and colleagues (162) reported a German pedigree with a novel form of spinocerebellar ataxia, termed SCA12, with variable age of onset typically in the fourth decade of hand and, later, head tremor, dysmetria, dysdiadochokinesis, hyperreflexia, bradykinesia, abnormal eye movements, and in the oldest individuals, dementia. Neuroimaging showed cortical and cerebellar atrophy. A 2.5-kb genomic clone contained an expanded CAG repeat in a brain-specific regulatory subunit of the protein phosphatase PP2A (PPP2R2B) gene.

Among 293 individuals of 77 Indian families with AD spinocerebellar ataxia, Srivastava and colleagues (163) found an expanded SCA12 repeat in six patients and three asymptomatic at-risk individuals from five families, accounting for 7% of patients. Among 20 northern Indian families with SCA12, Bahl and colleagues (164) identified expanded CAG repeats of 51 to 69 triplets, found a common founder in one asymptomatic individual homozygous for an expanded repeat of 52 to 59 triplets and one haplotype that was associated with the disease allele. It was estimated that SC12 accounts for about 16% of ADCA patients in northern India. The cause of SCA12 is an expansion of a CAG repeat at the 5q32 locus in the PPP2R2B gene encoding brain-specific regulatory subunit B of protein phosphatase 2 (PP2A) (Table 2), which has been implicated in a number of cellular functions including modulation of cell cycle progression, tau phosphorylation, and apoptosis.

SCA13

Two articles by Durr, Herman-Bret and colleagues (165, 166) examined the same large French family with ADCA who displayed mental retardation, cerebellar dysarthria, moderate mental retardation in the IQ range of 62 to 76, mild developmental motor delays, as well as horizontal and vertical nystagmus, square wave jerks, and pyramidal signs, generalized bradykinesia, upward gaze palsy, swallowing difficulty, urinary urgency, short stature, slight facial dysmorphia, and petit mal epilepsy. Cerebral MRI showed moderate dorsal cerebellar vermis, and posterior pons and medulla atrophy with enlargement of the fourth ventricle. After exclusion of trinucleotide repeat expansions in the SCA1, 2, 3, 6, 7, 8, and 12 genes and linkage to SCA4, 5, 10 and 11 loci, the authors conducted a genome-wide search and found evidence for linkage to chromosome 19q13.3-q13.4 in an 8cM interval between markers D19S219 and D19S553. SCA is due to heterozygous mutation at the 19q13.33 locus of the KCNC3 gene encoding the potassium voltage-gated channel subfamily C member 3 protein that mediates voltage-dependent potassium ion permeability.

SCA14

Initial evidence for the assignment of the protein kinase C, gamma (PKCG) gene derived from informative RFLP studies (167) and fluorescence in situ hybridization (168). Yamashita and colleagues (169) described a three-generation Japanese family onset of cerebellar ataxia with an age at onset of 27 years or less of cerebellar ataxia and intermittent axial myoclonus. Brain MRI showed cerebellar atrophy. Systematic linkage established a novel mutation and locus to a 10.2-cM interval on chromosome 19q13.4-qter. Brkanac and colleagues (170) later described of a four-generation family of English and Dutch descent of 14 members, 10 of whom available for analysis showed gait ataxia, dysarthria, dysmetria, abnormal eye movement, and onset in the third decade. Chen and colleagues (171) identified three mutations in the PKCG gene, two of which co-segregated with the disorder.

Yabe and coworkers (172) identified a mutation in the PRKCG gene in all 11 affected members of the family reported by Yamashita and colleagues (169) with SCA14, as did Klebe and colleagues (173) who described 6 different mutations, including five novel ones, in the PRKCG gene among 15 affected members of six French families.

Stevanin and colleagues (174) studied a family of French origin with 20 affected members with SCA14 in four generations. Age of onset ranged from childhood to 60 years, with mild to moderate cerebellar signs as well as dysphagia, facial myokymia, decreased vibratory sensation in the feet, chorea of the hands, head tremor and memory and attention deficits. Najmabadi and colleagues (175) identified a frame-shift and missense mutation in the *PRKCG* gene among two separate consanguineous families segregrating SCA14. The cause of SCA14 is due to mutation at the 19q13.42 locus of the *PRKCG* gene encoding protein kinase C gamma type (Table 2), that has a putative role in the regulation of neuronal receptors including synaptic plasticity, synaptogenesis, and excitability of cerebellar neurons.

SCA15

Storey and colleagues (176) described an Australian family in which eight members had slowly progressive cerebellar ataxia, so-termed SCA-15 with linkage to chromosome 3pter-p24.2. Most patients have disabling action and postural tremor, some have CST and dorsal column involvement and gaze palsy; brain imaging shows cerebellar atrophy mainly involving the vermis (177).

Van de Leemput and colleagues (178) identified heterozygous deletions involving the inositol 1, 4, 5-triphosphate receptor type 1 (*ITPR1*) gene in affected members of three unrelated families, including SCA15 families of Australian origin used to map the locus (176, 179), as well as a large deletion removing the first 10 exons of the *ITPR1* gene in the family reported by Knight and colleagues (179). Affected members of two additional families were found to have even larger deletions removing exons 1-44 and 1-40 of the *ITPR1* gene. Accordingly, deletions in the *ITPR1* gene are believed to underlie the SCA15 phenotype. Hara (180) identified a 414-kb deletion of chromosome 3p26, including in the *ITPR1* gene. The cause of SCA15 is heterozygous mutation and deletions at the 3p26.1 locus of the *ITPR1* gene encoding type 1 inositol 1, 4, 5-triphosphate (Table 2) an intracellular second messenger that releases calcium from endoplasmic reticulum (ER) by binding to specific receptors coupled to calcium channels, abundant in neuronal tissues including the cerebellum, particularly the perikaryon of Purkinje cells.

Miyoshi and colleagues (181) identified ADCA in a four-generation Japanese family of nine affected members with onset in the third to seventh decades. All individuals showed cerebellar ataxia, in addition to head tremor in three. Brain MRI showed cerebellar atrophy without brainstem involvement. Mutational analysis by PCR excluded mutations in previously identified genes causing SCA. Although linkage analysis suggested a new locus for SCA16 situated on 8q22.1-q24.1, subsequent studies showed heterozygous deletion of axons 1 to 48 in the *ITPA1* gene.

SCA17

Koide and colleagues (182) described a sporadic patient with cerebellar ataxia, CST signs, and severe intellectual impairments associated with expansion of the CAG repeat in exon 3 of the Tata box-binding protein (*TBP*) gene encoding 63 glutamines, far exceeding the range of 25 to 42 I normal Caucasians or 31 to 42 I Japanese individuals. Zuhlke and colleagues (183) described two German kindred with a multisystemic degenerative disorder comprising cerebellar ataxia, CST and extrapyramidal signs, and autonomic nervous system (ANS) and cognitive involvement. Genetic analysis revealed expanded (CAG)n alleles of the *TBP* gene ranging between 50 and 55 residues in affected individuals. Two affected sisters in one family differed by one trinucleotide repeat which upon transmission to her daughter was elongated by two units and may have contributed to the earlier onset of the disease. In the other family, the (CAG)n element combined with CAA interruptions was not described for CAG expansions in other genes.

Nakamura and coworkers (184) described four Japanese pedigrees with SCA17 evidenced by abnormal (CAG)n expansion in *TBP* to a range of 47 to 55 repeats in association with cerebellar ataxia, bradykinesia, and dementia that commenced from age 19 to 48 years. Postmortem tissue from one patient showed moderate Purkinje cell loss and neuronal intranuclear inclusion bodies reactive to anti-*TBP* antibodies which stained the 1C2 antibody recognizing expanded polyglutamine tracts.

Rolfs and colleagues (185) identified 15 Caucasian patients from four families with cerebellar ataxia, dysarthria, dysphagia, extrapyramidal, and psychiatric involvement associated with repeat expansions of the *TBP* gene. Neuropathological examination of brain tissue from three affected sisters showed Purkinje cell loss and neuronal inclusions with immunoreactive anti-*TBP* and IC2. Stevanin (186), Bauer (187), and Toyoshima and colleagues (188) noted repeat expansions of the TBP gene with a disease phenotype similar to Huntington disease (HD) in addition to cerebellar ataxia, psychiatric disturbances, dementia, and chorea without mutation in the huntingtin (*HTT*) gene. One individual studied by Toyoshima and colleagues (188) was homozygous for 48 trinucleotide *TBP* gene repeats, in whom postmortem analysis showed mild neuronal loss with compaction of cerebral cortex neuropil, with mild loss of striatal neurons, moderate Purkinje cell loss, and many IC2-positive neuronal nuclei in the putamen and cerebellum, and diffuse intranuclear polyglutamine aggregate accumulation in a wide range of CSN regions, even in the absence of neuronal loss.

Filla and coworkers (189) reported a southern Italian kindred with 14 members spanning five generations with onset age of 22 to 53 years with psychiatric features, progressive dementia, ataxia, axial rigidity, dysarthria, dystonia, and generalized seizures, and CAG repeat expansion in the *TBP* gene establishing the diagnosis of SCA17. Brain MRI showed cortical and cerebellar atrophy, with postmortem evidence of severe neuronal loss and gliosis in the striatum, dorsomedial thalamus, and inferior olive, with neuronal intranuclear inclusions autoreactive with anti-TBP and IC2.

Shatunov and colleagues (190) found no mutation in the prion protein gene (PRNP) of a patient thought to have variant Creutzfeldt-Jakob disease (CJD), but instead an expanded allele with excessive CAG/CAA repeats in the TBP gene was identified. SCA17 is caused by heterozygous expansion at the 6q27 locus of the trinucleotide repeat CAG or CAA encoding glutamine in the TBP gene. Wu and colleagues (150) detected 46 trinucleotide repeats in the SCA17 gene in a patient with typical features of abnormal trinucleotide repeat expansion in a patient with levodopa-responsive late-onset idiopathic PD. Expanded repeats in the TBP gene were noted in .3% of Korean patients with ataxia and in 2% of those with chorea (191), and reduced penetrance is seen with 45 to 46 repeats (192).There is a murine model of polyQ-expanded TBP with the characteristic features of neuronal dysfunction, including reduced cell viability and defective neurite outgrowth (193). The function of the TBP gene is not well understood but contrary to the previously hypothesized existence of a family of TBP-related DNA-binding proteins, there is a highly conserved C-terminal DNA-binding domain, which when bound to the TATA box and contacts DNA, interacts with TBP-associated factors (TAF) and positive and negative modulators of basal and activated transcription of class II genes. SCA17 is caused by heterozygous expansion of the CAG/CAA repeat at the 6q27 locus of the TBP gene encoding TAT box-binding protein (Table 2).

SCA18

Brkanac and colleagues (194) described a five-generation American family of Northern European ancestry with AD axonal sensorimotor neuropathy and ataxia (SMNA) in all family members as the earliest sign of the disease, followed later by cerebellar, UMN and LMN involvement, without genetic anticipation, mental retardation, dementia, or overlap with other ADCA and neuropathies. A non-synonymous variant in the human interferon-related developmental regulator gene 1 (IFRD1) as a disease-causing candidate was noted. Sequence conservation, animal models, and protein structure evaluation supported the involvement of IFRD1 in SMNA (195). Linkage evidence supports mapping of SMNA to the 7q22-q32 locus of SCA18 gene (Table 2).

SCA19

Schelhaas and colleagues (196) studied 12 patients in a four-generation Dutch family with early-onset of cerebellar ataxia, intention and postural irregular low frequency tremor, myoclonus, and cognitive impairment, followed by dysarthria, limb ataxia, fine saccadic eye movements, and horizontal nystagmus. Anticipation, as evidenced by earlier age of onset in successive generations was encountered, with disease onset ranging from the first to fourth decade. Electrophysiological studies showed mild axonal polyneuropathy. Myoclonus was accompanied by paroxysmal temporal and parietal lobe slowing on EEG indicative of a cortical basis in one patient, and a spinal epilogue in another. Brain MRI showed marked atrophy of the cerebellar hemispheres, with mild vermian cerebellar and cerebral atrophy. Molecular genetic analysis excluded other known genetic loci for SCA. Verbeek and colleagues (197) mapped and designated SCA19 to chromosome 1p21-q21 (Table 2).

SCA20

Knight and colleagues (198) described a pedigree of Anglo-Celtic origin with dysarthria, variable palatal tremor, spasmodic dysphonia, hypermetric saccades and CST signs. Brain MRI showed dentate nucleus calcification producing a low signal. Linkage analysis mapped to chromosome 11 and repeat explanation detection failed to identify repeat expansions segregating with the disease, excluding all testable SCA mutations except for SCA5, which was considered phenotypically unlikely. A provisional assignment of SCA20 was designated. Cerebellar ataxia with spasmodic cough was later ascribed to the SCA20 gene (199).

Lorenzo and colleagues (200) refined the SCA20 critical region by studying the recombination events, first refining the distal portion of the SCA20 critical region that overlapped the SCA5 locus by designing and analyzing a panel of polymorphic short tandem repeat markers that spanned the overlapping region, as a 23.6-Mb interval from D11S903 to KAD199, using DNA from an affected SCA20 family member reported by Knight and colleagues (198) along with previously reported PCR primers and conditions, amplification and subsequent sequencing of the 37 exons of SPTBN2, analysis of which did not reveal any sequence changes with the exception of single-nucleotide polymorphisms (SNP) that did not change the amino acid sequence of the protein or were located in a position likely to affect splicing, indicating that SCA20 was genetically distinct from SCA5. Single-nucleotide polymorphism genotyping to detect structural alterations in genomic DNA of those with SCA20 detected a 260 kb duplication in the previously linked SCA20 region, later confirmed by quantitative polymerase chain reaction (PCR) and fiber fluorescence in situ hybridization, spanning 10 known and two unknown genes in all affected individuals (201). The critical gene within the duplicated segment was considered to be diacylglycerol lipase α subunit (DAGLA), a neural stem cell-derived dendrite regulator present at the base of Purkinje cell dendritic spine contributing to the modulation of parallel fiber-Purkinje cell synapses. SCA is caused by a heterozgyous 26-kb duplication at the 11q12 locus of the *SCA20* gene (Table 2).

SCA21

Devos and colleagues (202) reported a four-generation French family of 11 members affected with cerebellar ataxia, akinesia, limb ataxia, dysarthria, dysgraphia, rigidity, tremor, hyporeflexia, and cognitive impairment with age at onset from 7 to 30 years. T_1-weighted brain MRI of the index patient, age 69, with a 40-year history of cerebellar and upper limb ataxia, postural and intermittent rest tremor, although still ambulatory unassisted for short distances, showed atrophy of the cerebellum without lesions in the brainstem. Ten parent-child pairs suggested genetic anticipation. Vuillaume and colleagues (203) investigated a French family with gait and limb ataxia, akinesia, hyporeflexia, and mild cognitive impairment, and atrophy of the cerebellum without brainstem lesion or basal ganglia on brain MRI. Genome-wide screening showed evidence for linkage to chromosome 7p21.3-p15.1 (Table 2), tracing the locus by key recombinants and haplotype reconstruction to a 24cM interval flanked by D7S2464 and D7S516. Three contemplated candidate genes due to their known function or pattern of expression included *SCIN*, a Ca++ dependent actin-severing and–capping protein (204); *SP4*, a nuclear transcriptional activator mainly expressed in brain belonging to the SP1 family of zinc-finger protein (205); and *IGFBP3* encoding insulin-like growth factor-binding protein 3, that plays a key role in regulating cell proliferation and apoptosis.

SCA22

Chung and colleagues (206) characterized a four-generation Chinese pedigree with ADCA, the index patient of which had a 23-year history of slowly progressive cerebellar gait and limb ataxia. Hyporeflexia, scanning speech and dysphagia, intermittent microsaccadic pursuits, and gaze-directed horizontal nystagmus were noted without cognitive impairment, CST and dorsal column involvement, myoclonus, tremor, or extrapyramidal signs. Somatosensory (SSER) and brainstem auditory evoked responses (BAER) were abnormal, suggesting impaired brainstem and spinal cord conduction, and T_1-weighted brain MRI showed distinct atrophy of the cerebellar vermis without brainstem or cortical involvement. Molecular genetic analysis mapped the locus to a 43.7-cM interval defined by the flanking markers D1S206 and D1S2878 on chromosome 1p21-q23. The request for a novel SCA locus was submitted to the HUGO Gene Nomenclature Committee (HGNC) in November 2001. At the time, no other

SCA disorders were known to be linked to 1p21-q21. Therefore, an SCA22 assignment was made. Contemporaneously, several novel SCA types, including SCA19, were reserved in HGNC without linkage data or original clinical descriptions. The authors did not retrieve the paper by Schelhaas and colleagues (207) which, according to Schelhass and colleagues (208), described the clinical features of a virtually identical Dutch ADCA family and linkage with marker D1S534 spanning 35 cM on chromosome 1p21-q23, located between markers D1S1588 and D1S1595. In reply, Chung and colleagues (209) asserted that both SCA19 and SCA22 were linked to 1p21-q21, their clinical features were slightly different since the Chinese family with SCA22 did not reveal cognitive impairment, peripheral neuropathy, myoclonus or tremors noted in the Dutch family with SCA19 (207), yet concurring that it was unlikely that there were two different genes within the same 68-Mb region. SCA22 is caused by a pathogenic mutation at the 1p21-q21 locus of the *SCA22* gene (Table 2).

SCA23

Verbeek and colleagues (210) reported five members of a three-generation Dutch family with onset from age 43 to 56 years, with gait or simultaneous cycling difficulties and speech disturbances, often in association with dysarthria, slow saccades, ocular dysmetria, decreased vibratory sensation, and hyperreflexia. Neuropathological examination of the brain in one affected subject showed generalized moderate to severe atrophy, most pronounced in the frontotemporal region, cerebellar vermis, basis pontis, and spinal cord. Pronounced neuronal loss was evident in the Purkinje cell layer, especially the vermis, dentate nuclei, and inferior olives accompanied by gliosis and myelin loss in surrounding white matter. There were ubiquitin-positive, IC2 and ataxin-3 negative intranuclear inclusions in substantial nigra neurons interpreted as Marinesco bodies. The new SCA23 locus was found on chromosome 20p13-p12.3.

Bakalkin and colleagues (211) identified missense mutations in the prodynophin (*PDYN*) gene in the original reported SCA23 family (210) and in three families from a Dutch ataxia cohort. PDYN is the precursor protein for the opioid neuropeptides, α-neoendrophin, and dynophins A (Dyn A) and B (Dyn B). Alterations in Dyn A activity and impairment of secretory pathways by mutant PDYN may lead to glutamate neurotoxicity which may underlie Purkinje cell degeneration and ataxia. Schicks and colleagues (212) did not identify mutation in the *PDYN* gene in 104 German families with ADCA in comparison to the infrequent occurrence of SCA23 in 0.5% of patients in the Netherlands (211). SCA23 is caused by heterozygous mutation at the 20p13 locus of the *PDYN* gene (Table 2).

SCA25

Stevanin and colleagues (213) reported 18 affected members of a large French family in which cerebellar ataxia and prominent sensory neuropathy segregated as a dominant trait, with intrafamilial variability of age at onset that ranged from 17 months to 39 years. Clinical presentation ranged from pure sensory neuropathy with little cerebellar involvement to a phenotype of FRDA. The index case, a 22-year-old man, walked at age 17 months with frequent falls. At age 8 years he was noted to have fatigue, hypotonia, cerebellar signs, nystagmus, and slow eye movements without gaze-paresis. Electrodiagnostic studies showed sensory neuropathy with abnormal sensory nerve action potential (SNAP) amplitudes, normal motor nerve conduction velocities (NCV), abnormal F-wave latencies, and normal needle electromyographic (EMG) findings. Sural nerve biopsy showed a loss of large myelinated fibers. T_2- and T_1-weighted MRI of the brain showed marked atrophy of the vermis with enlargement of the fourth ventricle, and molar tooth appearance of the mesencephalon. Genome-wide search detected linkage of SCA25 to chromosome 2p21-p13, and the new locus was designated *SCA25* after testing of 16 additional markers (Table 2).

SCA26

Yu and colleagues (214) described 50 affected members of a six-generation kindred of Norwegian ancestry that immigrated to North Dakota with ADCA, with age at onset that ranged from 26 to 60 years. The cardinal features were limb ataxia, dysarthria, and irregular visual pursuit movement and none had significant motor, sensory deficits, Babinskši signs, fasciculation, or seizures, and all were of normal intelligence. Brain MRI showed atrophy of the cerebellum sparing the pons and medulla. Linkage was found between markers D19S591 and D19S1034, flanked by markers D19S886 and D19S894, designating the SCA26 gene locus. The genes for recessively inherited Cayman ataxia (215) and *CACNA1A* mutated in EA2 and SCA6, respectively located in the haplotype region or approximately 19cM further centrometric far beyond the haplotype region of SCA26, were excluded. Ataxia families that map to *SCA6* without a *CACNA1A* mutation may be genetically linked to SCA26. The authors suggested that the mutation responsible for the disease was probably a nonsense mutation such as allelic mutations in the PKC gamma or FGF14 gene. The candidate region for their kindred contained about 100 genes several of which were of particular interest included *GRIN3B, BRUNOL5, GNG7,* and *SGTA*. SCA26 is caused by pathogenic mutation at the 19p13.3 locus of the *SCA26* gene (Table 2).

SCA27

Van Swieten and colleagues (216) described a large three-generation Dutch family in which 14 members had trembling of the hands, exacerbated by emotional stress and exercise, beginning in childhood followed by slowly progressive cerebellar gait and upper limb ataxia starting at age 28 to 40 years. Neurological examination from age 24 to 79 years showed dysmetric saccades, disrupted ocular pursuit movements, gaze-evoked nystagmus, cerebellar dysarthria, and small-amplitude high-frequency hand tremor, head tremor, orofacial dyskinesia, hyperreflexia and vibratory sensory loss, and variably impaired cognition, memory, and cortical language disturbances. Brain MRI showed cerebellar hemispheric atrophy on T_1-weighted images.[123] I benzamine single photon emission tomography (IBZM-SPECT) showed reduced dopamine D2-receptor binding of the left striatum. Electrodiagnostic studies showed mild axonal polyneuropathy in two patients so studied. Linkage analysis and recombination analysis in affected individuals demonstrated a critical region on chromosome 13q34 that included the fibroblast growth factor -14 (*FGF14*) gene. Recognizing a murine model of ataxia and paroxysmal dyskinesia (217), led to candidate-gene mutation analysis of *FGF14* and the eventual elucidation of a pathogenic mutation in *FGF14*. A T-to-C transition at position 434 of the FGF14a open reading frame (ORF) results in an amino acid substitution of a serine for a phenylalanine at position 145 (F145S).

Dalski and colleagues (218) reported ataxia in an 18-year-old male with mental retardation, inborn strabismus, red-green vision defect, and normal motor development until age 12 when he developed slowly progressive gait disturbance, memory loss, and depressed mood. Examination showed truncal and gait ataxia, small-amplitude tremor in the hands, gaze-evoked nystagmus, and pes cavus. Electrodiagnostic studies showed mild axonal sensory neuropathy. Brain MRI was normal. The patient's father reportedly had gait disturbances, memory loss, and pes cavus. Genetic analysis revealed six different DNA variations, two of which resulted in amino acid level changes, including a single base pain deletion in exon 4 (c.487delA) creating a frameshift mutation, and DNA polymorphisms in exon 1a, 4 and 5, an amino-acid exchanged at position 124, as well as single-nucleotide polymorphism in the 3′-untranslated region of exon 5 of the *FGF14* gene. The AD *FGF14* mutations were in contrast to the recessive Fgf14 knockout murine model of ataxia and paroxysmal dyskinesia (217).

Miscco and colleagues (219), who reported a daughter and mother with karyotype XXt (5, 13) (q31.2, q33.1) and a translocation breakpoint identical in both patients disrupting the gene encoding the isoform FGF14-1b, showed clinical signs of SCA including early onset in the daughter, with gait ataxia, dysarthria, writing disability, dyskinesia, and titubation, and pes cavus and UMN involvement in both mother and daughter. The authors suggested that truncation of one allele could lead to *FGF14* haplo-insufficiency, in turn, causing SCA27. SCA27 is caused by a mutation at the 13q33.1 locus in the *FGF14* gene encoding FGF14 (Table 2), which appears to function in neuronal signaling, axonal trafficking, and synaptosomal function.

SCA28

Cagnoli and colleagues (220) reported 11 affected members of a four-generation Italian family with cerebellar ataxia and gaze-evoked nystagmus, and age of onset from 12 to 36 years, followed by slow saccades, ophthalmoparesis, ptosis, and CTS without cognitive or sensory impairment. T_1-weighted brain MRI showed cerebellar atrophy particularly involving the superior vermis, and T_2-weighted images showed atrophy of the cerebellar hemispheres. Electrodiagnostic studies, visual (VER), BAER, and SSER, were normal. Electro-oculographic evaluation showed variable hypometric and hypermetric saccades with reduced gain in smooth horizontal pursuit, saccadic breakdown of pursuit, and reduced optokinetic gain. Genetic studies and linkage analysis showed linkage to chromosome 18 markers, and haplotype analysis refined a critical region of 7.9 Mb between markers D18S1418 and D18S1104, identifying a new SCA locus at 18p11.22-q11.2- designated *SCA28*. On the basis of expression profiles in the nervous system, 12 genes were selected by Di Bella and coworkers (221) within the 7.9-megabase critical regions, including the gene encoding the mitochondrial metalloprotease ATPase family gene 3-like 2 (*AFG3L2*), and defined heterozygous missense mutations in the *AFG3L2* gene in five unrelated affected families. AFGL2 is highly and selectively expressed in human cerebellar Purkinje cells, and m-AAA-deficient yeast cells expressing human mutated *AFG3L2* homocomplex show respiratory deficiency, proteolytic impairment, and deficiency of respiratory chain complex IV. Mutations in *AFG3L2* may not only affect AFG3L2 substrate handling but have an essential role in protecting the cerebellum from neurodegeneration. Cagnoli and colleagues (222) found six missense changes in the *AFG3L2* gene in nine unrelated index cases from France and other countries with progressive SCA and a family history thereof, and mean age at onset of 41 years. AFG3L2 is the catalytic subunit of the m-AAA protease, an ATP-dependent proteolytic complex of the mitochondrial inner membrane that degrades misfolded proteins and regulates ribosome assembly (223). SCA28 is caused by heterozygous mutation at the 18p11.21 locus of the *AFGL2* gene (Table 2).

SCA29

Furman and coworkers (224) reported three members of a family with AD inherited early-onset non-progressive syndrome that included cerebellar gait ataxia and spontaneous upbeating nystagmus. Brain MRI showed localized cerebellar vermis atrophy. Fenichel and colleague (225) reported other similar patients with hypoplasia and partial vermal aplasia, but were struck by the more severely affected males, leading them to suggest both XL dominant and AD inheritance.

Dudding and colleagues (226) characterized a four-generation pedigree of congenital non-progressive cerebellar ataxia associated with cognitive impairment, and detected linkage to chromosome 3p (Table 2) between satellite markers D3S1304 and D3S1620, designating the *SCA29* gene region. Jen and colleagues (227) followed the previously reported family (224) and noted ataxic spells and vertical oscillopsia triggered by stress and exercise in older family members.

SCA30

Storey and colleagues (228) described six affected and four unaffected members of an Australian family of Anglo-Celtic ethnicity that manifested pure slowly progressive cerebellar ataxia of mean age at onset of 52 years. All affected members had mild to moderate dysarthria, appendicular and gait ataxia, and slightly impaired visual suppression of the vestibulo-ocular reflex (VOR) with saccadic hypermetria. Brain MRI showed atrophy of superior and dorsal vermis and cerebellar hemispheres with sparing of inferior vermis, brainstem, and supratentorial structures. Linkage analysis, which excluded known SCA, identified a locus termed *SCA30* on chromosome 4q34.3-q35.1 (Table 2), and haplotype analysis delineated a 5-Mb region between rs1397413 and rs2175476. A ranking of 19 genes in the *SCA30* region of interest produced *ODZ3*, a known gene with brain expression as the candidate (229).

SCA31

Nagaoka and colleagues (119) described six Japanese families with pure cerebellar gait and limb ataxia, cerebellar dysarthria, and horizontal gaze nystagmus with average age at onset of 56 years. Brain MRI showed cerebellar atrophy. The disorder mapped to chromosome 16q13.1-q22.1, the same region to which SCA4 maps. Families with 16q-ADCA harbored a common, "founder" haplotype for the 3.8 Mb region between GGAA05 and D16S3095 (230).

Owada and colleagues (231) presented a new kindred with ADCA linked to chromosome 16q22.1 associated with progressive hearing loss, which by haplotype analysis defined a critical region slightly narrowed to three megabase regions between GATA01 and D16S3095. Neuropathological study demonstrated shrinkage of Purkinje cell bodies surrounded by synaptophysin-immunoreactive amorphous material containing calbindin- and ubiquitin-positive granules, indicating that the amorphous material was formed in association both with the degeneration of Purkinje cell processes and the increase of presynaptic terminals innervated from basket cells, inferior olivary neurons, or other neurons. Alteration of calbindin-immunoreactivity in Purkinje cells may have indicated that the intracellular calcium buffering system, which is one of the important roles of calbindin, may be altered in this disorder (231). Sato and colleagues (232) narrowed the critical region down to a 900-kb interval in chromosome 16q22.1 where the disease shows a strong founder effect. Southern blot analysis and BAC- and fosmid-based sequencing isolated two genetic changes segregating with SCA31, one a single nucleotide change in an intron of the thymidine kinase 2 (TK2) gene that did not affect splicing or expression patterns. The other, an insertion from 2.5 to 3.8 kb of complex penta-nucleotide repeats, includes a long (TGGAA)n stretch. The repeat insertion was located in introns of TK2, associated with Nedd4 (BEAN) and expressed in the brain forming RNA foci in nuclei of patients' Purkinje cells.

Ishikawa and colleages (233) showed that SCA31 is associated with diverse pentanucleotide repeats that included the prototypical (TAAAA)n; (TGGAA)n and (TGAAA)n in Japanese, whereas (TACAA)n, (GAAA)n, (TAACA)n, and (TGAAA)n were expressed exclusively in Caucasians, each potentially arising from a single-nucleotide mutation in TAAAA before their expansion. SCA31 is considered one of a growing number of neuromuscular diseases with RNA-mediated gain-of-function mechanism (234). SCA31 is caused by a 2.5 to 3.8-kb insertion containing pentanucleotide repeats, including (TGGAA)n with an intron at the 16q21 locus of the BEAN gene encoding (TGGAA)n mRNA (Table 2).

SCA32

Jiang and colleagues (235) presented preliminary details of a Chinese family with ADCA evidencing cognitive impairment, male infertility, azoospermia, and testicular atrophy. Genome-wide linkage analysis found linkage to a locus termed SCA32 on chromosome 7q32-q33 (Table 2) between rs3847110 and rs2241728, in a critical region that spanned 989 kb.

SCA34

Giroux and Barbeau (236) described a neurocutaneous disorder in 25 members of a five-generation French Canadian family with papulosquamous erythematous plaques soon after birth that disappeared by age 25, sometimes to reappear after age 40, associated with slowly progressive cerebellar ataxia. Turcotte-Gauthier (237) identified a disease locus termed SCA34 by genome-wide linkage analysis of the family described by Giroux and Barbeau (236) on chromosome 6p12.3-q16.2 (Table 2).

SCA35

Wang and colleagues (238) sequenced the whole exome of four patients in a four-generation Chinese SCA family and identified a missense mutation, c.1550t-G transition (L517W), in exon 10 of the transglutaminease 6 (TGM6) gene located at chromosome 20p13-12.2, the same as identified by linkage analysis as the causative SCA gene of this family. A second missense mutation, c.980A-G transition (D327G) in exon 7 of TGM6, was noted in an additional SCA family that co-segregated with the phenotype of late onset, slowly progressive gait, limb ataxia and, in some patients, spasmodic torticollis. SCA35 is caused by heterozygous mutation at the 20p13 locus in the TGM6 gene encoding transglutaminease 6 (Table 2). Hadjivassiliou and colleagues (239) described IgG, and IgA antibodies against transglutaminase 6 (TG6) expressed by a subset of neurons of the CNS, which served as a marker for gluten sensitivity with cerebellar involvement known as gluten ataxia (GA).

SCA36

Ohta and colleagues (240) reported two unrelated patients who showed ataxia as the first symptom followed by late-onset motor neuron disease (MND) resembling amyotrophic lateral sclerosis (ALS). Kobayashi and colleagues (241) undertook a genome-wide linkage analysis and subsequent mapping of five unrelated Japanese families with onset of cerebellar truncal and gait ataxia, ataxic dysarthria, and limb incoordination at a mean age of 53 years, with signs of MND with longer disease duration exhibiting lingual atrophy, fasciculation, skeletal muscle atrophy and fasciculation, and hyperactive reflexes. Electrophysiology showed neurogenic features indicative of LMN involvement typically limited to the tongue, which differentiated it from typical ALS. The disorder was mapped to a 1.8 Mb region on chromosome 20p13 harboring 44 genes. Expansions of the hexanucleotide repeat GGCCTG (rs68063608) were found in intron 1 of NOP56 in all five index cases through the use of a repeat-primer PCR method, and complete segregation of the expanded hexanucleotide was confirmed in all pedigrees. A founder haplotype was found in these cases, and RNA foci formation was detected in lymphoblastoid cells from affected subjects by fluorescence in situ hybridization. Double staining and gel-shift assay showed that (GGCCUG)n bound protein SRSF2, and transcription of *MIR1292*, a neighboring mRNA, was significantly decreased in lymphoblastoid cells of SCA patients. The findings suggested that SCA36 is caused by hexanucleotide repeat expansions through RNA gain-of-function. SCA36 is caused by heterozygous expansion of an intronic GGCCTG hexanucleotide repeat at the 20p13 locus of the *NOP56* gene encoding NOP56-associated preribosomal RNP complex (Table 2). Unaffected individuals carry 3 to 8 repeats, whereas affected patients carry 1,500 to 2,000 repeats (241). The *NOP56* gene functions in an early to middle step in pre-rRNA processing.

Dentatorubral-Pallidoluysian Atrophy

First described by Smith and Gonda in 1958 (242) under the designation *dentatorubropallidoluysian atrophy*. DRPLA occurs almost only in Japanese, and Koide suggesting there may even be a founder effect (243). Onset in the third decade of myoclonic epilepsy, dementia, ataxia, and choreoathetosis was followed by death in the fifth decade (244). The three clinical types of DRPLA include ataxo-choreoathetoid, pseudo-Huntington, and myoclonic epilepsy forms (245). There is anticipation, and paternal transmission is associated with more severe early-onset disease (246). The Haw River syndrome, characterized by development, between 15 and 30 years of age, of ataxia, seizures, choreiform movements, progressive dementia, and death after 15 to 25 years of illness, showed remarkably similar findings of marked dentate neuronal loss, microcalcification of the globus pallidus, neuroaxonal dystrophy of the nucleus gracilis, and demyelination of the centrum semiovale (247).

Koide and colleagues (243) searched a catalogue of gene-identified by Li and colleagues (248) that contained trinucleotide repeats expressed in the human brain, and one of the cDNA, B37 (*ATN1*), known to map to chromosome 12, showed CAG repeat expansion in 22 individuals with DRPLA, with an inverse relationship between repeat size and age at onset. Normal individuals had 7 to 23 repeats, and in affected patients, one allele was expanded from 49 to 75 repeats or more (249). An expanded CAG repeat at the same locus was found in the Haw River syndrome (250). The gene has been sequenced and the cDNA is composed of 4,294 bases encoding a protein of 1,184 amino acids (249, 251). DRPLA is caused by an expanded trinucleotide repeat at the 12p13.31 locus of the *ATN1* gene encoding atrophin1 (Table 2). The (CAG)n repeat that is expanded in patients with DRPLA is located at position 1462 and is predicted to code for a polyglutamine tract. Northern blot analysis reveals a 4.7-kb transcript that is widely expressed in various tissues, including the brain, heart, lung, kidney, placenta, and skeletal muscle. Using antibodies against a synthetic peptide corresponding to the sequence of the

C-terminus of the DRPLA gene product, Yazawa and colleagues (252) identified the DRPLA gene product in normal human brains as a protein of 190 kD and found a larger protein of 205 kD in DRPLA brains in neuronal cytoplasm, demonstrating the existence of the expanded CAG repeat gene product and supporting the possibility that the expanded CAG-encoded polyglutamine stretch participated in the pathological process of similar trinucleotide repeat diseases.

Sato and coworkers (253, 254) generated a DRPLA Q129 mouse resulting from en masse expansion of the 76 CAG repeat in a Q76 mouse breeding program, such that mRNA expression levels of both Q76 and Q129 transgenes were each 80% of that of the endogenous mouse gene. Only the Q129 mice exhibited devastating progressive neurological phenotypes and premature death similar to those of juvenile-onset DRPLA patients with age- and expanded-polyQ-length-dependent massive neuronal intranuclear accumulation (NIA) of mutant proteins had expanded polyglutamine stretches, starting on postnatal day 4. However, Q76 mice appeared later with regional specificity to vulnerable regions of DRPLA. At 14 weeks postnatal, there was specific presynaptic dysfunction in the globus pallidus and cerebellum, atrophy of Purkinje cell primary and dendrites, and a decrease in the number and size of the spines without any obvious neuronal loss. The age-, and expanded-polyQ-length-dependent NIA of mutant proteins without any obvious neuronal loss raised the possibility that such an NI of mutant proteins led to neuronal dysfunction, including synaptic transmissions through transcriptional dysregulation. Neuronal loss may well be the latest event observed in advanced stages. Supporting this concept was that juvenile-onset DRPLA patients initially did not show markedly atrophic changes in the cerebellum in MRI, in contrast to markedly atrophic changes observed in late-adult-onset DRPLA patients (255).

Episodic Ataxia

Episodes of ataxia can be the initial sign of metabolic disorders such as multiple carboxylase deficiency and aminoaciduria. However, the term episodic or paroxysmal ataxia is generally applied to a condition in which the major finding is self-limited episodes of cerebellar dysfunction with little fixed or progressive neurologic dysfunction.

EA1

Episodes of ataxia with myokymia are brief, usually lasting minutes, and provoked by startle, sudden movements, or changes in posture and exercise, especially if excited or fatigued. They can occur 1 to 15 times per day. Onset is in childhood and adolescence. The disorder is not associated with neurologic deterioration, but subtle myokymia around the eyes and in the hands can occur. The Achilles tendons may be shortened, and there may be tremor of the hands. The attacks are often heralded by an aura of weightlessness or weakness, and during attacks there is ataxia, dysarthria, shaking or tremor, and twitching (256). Physical findings among 11 members of three consecutive generations of a kindred described by Van Dyke and colleagues (257) included large calves, normal muscle strength, and widespread myokymia of the face, hands, arms, and legs, with hard posturing resembling carpopedal spasm. Electromyography at rest showed continuous spontaneous activity. Gastrocnemius muscle biopsy showed denervation changes as well as myofiber enlargement. EA1 is caused by heterozygous missense point mutations at the 12p13.32 locus of the postassium channel, voltage-gated, Shaker-related subfamily, member 1 (*KCNA1*) gene encoding potassium-voltage-gated channel subfamily A member 1 (Table 2) (258, 259). *KCNA1* is a member of the Shaker-related subfamily of potassium channel genes. In some families, acetazolamide reduces attack frequency, and anticonvulsants may reduce the myokymia (260).

EA2

Attacks of ataxia and nystagmus last hours to days and are provoked by stress, exercise, fatigue, and alcohol, typically occurring one per day. Age at onset varies from infancy to 40 years, and unlike EA1, there can be mild progressive cerebellar degeneration with ataxia and dysarthria. Among 11 members of a genetically confirmed family with EA2 (261), fever and heat triggered ataxic episodes, headache, weakness, vertigo, nausea and vomiting, and six showed interictal cerebellar deficits. Spacey and colleagues (262) reported two unrelated patients with genetically confirmed EA2 who developed later dystonia considered to be due to degenerative aspects of the disorder. During the attacks, headache, diaphoresis, nausea, vertigo, ataxia, dysarthria, ptosis, and ocular palsy can occur (263). Attacks can be a dramatic response to acetazolamide (256). Litt and colleagues (265) excluded linkage to 12p responsible for EA1, and von Brederlow and coworkers (266) later mapped the disorder to 19p.

Kramer and colleagues (267) suggested two AD forms of EA, EA1 lasting minutes with interictal myokymia that mapped to chromosome 12 and by the candidate gene approach shown to be due to mutation in *KCNA1*, and the second type, EA2, often associated with nystagmus or truncal instability and beneficial response to acetazolamide, that mapped to 19p.

Ophoff and colleages (268) identified two mutations in the brain-specific P/Q-type Ca^{2+} channel, alpha1-subunit gene, *CACNL1A4*, resulting in disrupted reading frame in EA2 and familial hemiplegic migraine (FHM), leading to

a frameshift in the putative translation product with a stop codon in the next exon. Riant (269, 270) described a heterozygous 39.5-kb deletion in the calcium ion channel, voltage-dependent, P/Q type, alpha-1A subunit (*CACNA1A*) gene in three affected members of a family with EA2, and later four different exonic deletions in the *CACNA1A* gene in 14% of patients with EA2, all in whom sequencing analysis was negative for *CACNA1A* mutations. EA2 is caused by mutation at the 19p13.2 locus of the *CACNA1A* gene (Table 2), the 75-kD C-terminal of which is the location of the polyglutamine tract expanded, which when cleaved and in the expanded state from full-length protein and translocated to the nucleus, is cytotoxic (271).

EA3

Steckley and colleagues (272) described a large Canadian kindred of Mennonites with familial episodes of generalized ataxia, vertigo, incoordination, and imbalance. Other findings included frequent bouts of interictal myokymia, mild persistent gait ataxia, congenital nystagmus, seizures and colobomata. EA3 differed from the two forms of ADEA in several respects, including vertigo in their kindred, which accompanied episodic ataxia; many individuals reported tinnitus as another sensation during episodes; age at onset ranged from age one year shortly after the individual started walking, and linkage analysis of markers flanking the EA1 and EA2 loci at 12p13 and 19p13 demonstrated genetic exclusion. Cader and colleagues (273) performed a genome-wide screen of the same kindred segregated with linkage on 1q42, and haplotype analysis and fine mapping indicated a 4-cM region on 1q42 (Table 2) likely to harbor the EA3 gene.

EA4

Damji and colleagues (274) studied two previously described (275, 276) multigenerational North Carolina families with vestibulocerebellar ataxia who resided on the same street in Johnston Country 100 years earlier. Affected members presented with ataxia, marked loss of smooth pursuit, marked gaze-evoked nystagmus, and impaired vestibulo-ocular reflex suppression, in addition to esophoria or tropia. Periodic vestibulocerebellar ataxia or EA4, was deemed to be genetically distinct, excluded from loci linked to EA1 and EA2, and SCA1-5. The authors speculated that the distinctive neuro-ophthalmological findings suggested that the cerebellar flocculus and brainstem neural integrator was the primary site of illness; however, brain neuroimaging did not demonstrate anatomic lesions and there were no neuropathological studies to corroborate that hypothesis.

21. Hakonen AH, Goffart S, Marjavaara S, et al. Infantile-onset spinocerebellar ataxia and mitochondrial recessive ataxia syndrome are associated with neuronal complex 1 defect and mtDNA depletion. *Hum Molec Genet* 2008; 17:3822–3833.

22. Lonnqvist T, Paetau A, Valanne L, et al. Recessive twinkle mutations cause severe epileptic encephalopathy. *Brain* 2009; 132:1553–1562

23. Valente EM, Brancati F, Silhavy JL, et al. AHI1 gene mutations cause specific forms of Joubert syndrome-related disorders. *Ann Neurol* 2006; 59:527–534.

24. Moreira MC, Barbot C, Tachi N, et al. The gene mutated in ataxia-ocular apraxia 1 encodes the new HT/Zn-finger protein Aprataxin. *Nature Genet* 2001; 29:189–193.

25. Anheim M, Fleury M, Monga B, et al. Epidemiological, clinical, paraclinical, and molecular study of a cohort of 102 patients affected with autosomal recessive progressive cerebellar ataxia from Alsace, Eastern France: implications for clinical management. *Neurogenetics* 2010; 11:1–12.

26. Ahel I, Rass U, El-Kharmisy SF, et al. The neurodegenerative disease protein aprataxin resolves abortive DNA ligation intermediates. *Nature* 2006; 443:713–716.

27. Moreira MC, Klur S, Watanabe M, et al. Senataxin, the ortholog of a yeast RNA helicase, is mutant in ataxia-ocular apraxia. *Nature Genet* 2004; 36:225–227

28. Suraweera A, Lim Y, Woods R, et al. Functional role for senataxin, defective in ataxia oculomotor apraxia type 2. In transcriptional regulation. *Hum Molec Genet* 2009; 18:3384–3396.

29. Hanauer A, Chery M, Fujita R, et al. The Friedreich ataxia gene is assigned to chromosome 9q13-q21 by mapping of the tightly linked markers and shows linkage disequilibrium with D9S15. *Am J Hum Genet* 1990; 46:133–137.

30. Savitsky K, Bar-Shira A, Gilad S, et al. A single ataxia telangiectasia gene with a product similar to PI-3 kinase. *Science* 1995; 2 68: 1749–1753

31. Soutoglou E, Misteli T. Activation of the cellular DNA damage response in the absence of DNA lesions. *Science* 2008; 320:1507–1510.

32. Bouchard JP, Barbeau A, Bouchard R, et al. Autosomal recessive spastic ataxia of Charlevoix-Saguenay. *Can J Neurol Sci* 1978; 5:61–69.

33. De Braekeleer M, Giasson F, Mathieu J, et al. Genetic epidemiology of autosomal recessive spastic ataxia of Charlevoix-Saguenay in northeastern Quebec. *Genet Epidemiol* 1993; 10:17–25.

34. Parfitt DA, Michael GJ, Vermeulen EGM, et al. The ataxia protein sacsin is a functional co-chaperone that protects against polyglutamine-expanded ataxin-1. *Hum Molec Genet* 2009; 18:1556–1565.

35. Musumeci O, Naini A, Slonim AE, et al. Familial cerebellar ataxia with coenzyme Q10 deficiency. *Neurology* 2001; 56:849–855.

36. Quinzii C, Naini A, Salviati L, et al. A mutation in para-hydroxybenzoate-polyprenyl transferase (COQ2) causes primary coenzyme Q10 deficiency. *Am J Hum Genet* 2006; 78:345–349.

37. Salviati I, Sacconi S, Murer L, et al. Infantile encephalomyopathy and nephropathy with CoQ10-responsive condition. *Neurology* 2005; 65:606–608.

38. Lagier-Tourenne C, Tazir M, Lopez LC, et al. ADCK$_3$, an ancestral kinase, is mutated in a form of recessive ataxia associated with coenzyme Q10 deficiency. *Am J Hum Genet* 2008; 82:661–672.

39. Mollet J, Delahodde A, Serre V, et al. CABC1 gene mutations cause ubiquitin deficiency with cerebellar ataxia and seizures. *Am J Hum Genet* 2008; 82:623–630.

40. Gerards M, van den Bosch B, Calis C. Nonsense mutations in CABC1/ADCK3 cause progressive cerebellar ataxia and atrophy. *Mitochondrion* 2010; 10:510–515

41. Quinzii CM, Hirano M. Primary and secondary C0Q10 deficiencies in humans. *Biofactors* 2011; 37:361–365.

42. Quinzii CM, Kattah AG, Naini A, et al. Coenzyme Q deficiency and cerebellar ataxia associated with an aprataxin mutation. *Neurology* 2005; 64:539–541.

43. Aeby A, Sznajer Y, Cave H, et al. Cardiofaciocutaneous (CFC) syndrome associated with muscular coenzyme Q$_{10}$ deficiency. *J Inherit Metab Dis* 2007; 30:827.

44. Lalani SR, Vladutiu GD, Plunkett K, et al. Isolated mitochondrial myopathy associated with muscle coenzyme Q$_{10}$ deficiency. *Arch Neurol* 2005; 62:317–320.

45. Horvath R, Schneiderat P, Schoser BG, et al. Coenzyme Q$_{10}$ deficiency and isolated myopathy. *Neurology* 2006; 66:253–255.

46. Gironi M, Lamperti C, Nemni R, et al. Late-onset cerebellar ataxia with hypogonadism and muscle coenzyme Q$_{10}$ deficiency. *Neurology* 2004; 62:518–520.

47. Van Bogaert L, Scherer HJ, Epstein E. *Une forme crebrale de la cholesterinose generalisee* [Thesis]. Paris: Masson et cie, 1937.

48. Menkes JH, Schimschock JR, Swanson PD. Cerebrotendinous xanthomatosis: the storage of cholestanol within the nervous system. *Arch Neurol* 1968; 19:47–53.

49. Cali JJ, Russell DW. Characterization of human sterol 27-hydroxylase: a mitochondrial cytochrome P-450 that catalyzes multiple oxidation reactions in bile acid biosynthesis. *J Biol Chem* 1991; 266:7774–7778.

50. Cali JJ, Hsieh C-L, Francke U, et al. Mutations in the bile acid biosynthetic enzyme sterol 27-hydroxylase underlie cerebrotendinous xanthomatosis. *J Biol Chem* 1991; 266:7779–7783.

51. Refsum S, Salomonsen L, Skatvedt M. Heredopathia atactica polyneuritiformis in children. *J Pediat* 1949; 35:335–343.

52. Mihalik SJ, Morrell JC, Kim D, et al. Identification of PAHX, a Refsum disease gene. *Nature Genet* 1997; 17:185–189.

53. Braverman N, Chen L, Lin P, et al. Mutation analysis of PEX7 in 60 probands with rhizomelic chondrodysplasia punctata and functional correlations of genotype with phenotype. *Hum Mutat* 2002; 20:284–297.

54. Lutz R, Bodersteiner J, Schaefer B, et al. X-linked olivopontocerebellar atrophy. *Clin Genet* 1989; 35:417–422.

55. Illarioshkin SN, Tanaka H, Markova ED, et al. X-linked non-progressive congenital cerebellar hypoplasia: clinical description and mapping to chromosome Xq. *Ann Neurol* 1996; 40:75–83.

56. Bertini E, des Portes V, Zanni G, et al. X-linked congenital ataxia: a clinical and genetic study. *Am J Med Genet* 2000; 92:53–56.

57. Malamud N, Cohen P. Unusual form of cerebellar ataxia with sex-linked inheritance. *Neurology* 1958; 8:261–268.

58. Schmidley JW, Levinsohn MW, Manetto V. Infantile X-linked ataxia and deafness: a new clinicopathologic entity. *Neurology* 1987; 37:1344–1349.

59. Farlow MR, DeMeyer W, Dlouhy SR, et al. X-linked recessive inheritance of ataxia and adult-onset dementia: clinical features and preliminary linkage analysis. *Neurology* 1987; 37:602–607.

60. Zanni G, Bertini F., Bellcross C, et al. X-linked congenital ataxia: a new locus maps to Xq25-q27.1. *Am J Med Genet* 2008; 146A:593–600.

61. Bekri S, May A, Cotter PD, et al. A promoter mutation in the erythroid-specific 5-aminolevulinate synthase [ALAS2] gene causes X-linked siderblastic anemia. *Blood* 2003; 102:698–704.

62. Pagon RA, Bird TD, Detter JC, et al. Hereditary sideroblastic anemia and ataxia: an X linked recessive disorder. *J Med Genet* 1985; 22:267–273.

63. Raskind WH, Wijsman E, Pagon RA, et al. X-linked sideroblastic anemia and ataxia: linkage to phosphoglycerate kinase at Xq13. *Am J Hum Genet* 1991; 48:335–341.

64. Allikmets R, Raskind WH, Hutchinson A, et al. Mutation of a putative mitochondrial iron transporter gene (ABC7) in X-linked sideroblastic anemia and ataxia (XLSA/A). *Hum Molec Genet* 1999; 8:743–749.

65. Nino HE, Noreen HJ, Dubey DP, et al. A family with hereditary ataxia: HLA typing. *Neurology* 1980; 30:12–20.

66. Genis D, Matilla T, Volpini V, et al. Clinical, neuropathologic, and genetic studies of a large spinocerebellar ataxia type I (SCA1) kindred: (CAG)n expansion and early premonitory signs and symptoms. *Neurology* 1995; 45:24–30.

67. Dubourg O, Durr A, Cancel G, et al. Analysis of the SCA1 CAG repeat in a large number of families with dominant ataxia: clinical and molecular correlation. *Ann Neurol* 1995; 37:176–188.

68. Rivaud-Pechoux S, Durr A, Gaymard B, et al. Eye movement abnormalities correlate with genotype in autosomal dominant cerebellar ataxia type 1. *Ann Neurol* 1998; 43:297–302.

69. Schols L, Amoiridis G, Buttner T, et al. Autosomal dominant cerebellar ataxia: phenotypic differences in genetically defined subtypes? *Ann Neurol* 1997; 42:924–932.

70. van Warrenburg BPC, Notermans NC, Schelhaas HJ, et al. Peripheral nerve involvement in spinocerebellar ataxias. *Arch Neurol* 2004; 61:257–261.

71. Zoghbi HY. Spinocerebellar ataxia type 1. *Clin Neurosci* 1995; 3:5–11.

72. Yakura H, Nakisaka A, Fujimoto S, Itakura K. Hereditary ataxia and HLA genotypes. *N Engl J Med* 1974;291:154–155.

73. Orr Ht, Chung M-Y, Banfi S, et al. Expansion of an unstable trinucleotide (CAG) repeat in spinocerebellar ataxia type I. *Nat Genet* 1993; 4:221–226.

74. Banfi S, Servadio A, Chung M, et al. Identification and characterization of the gene causing type 1 spinocerebellar ataxia. *Nature Genet* 1994; 7:513–520.

75. Kurosaki T, Ninokata A, Wang L, et al. Evolutionary scenario for acquisition of CAG repeats in human SCA1 gene. *Gene* 2006; 373:23–27.

76. Jodice C, Malaspina P, Persichetti F, et al. Effect of trinucleotide repeat length and parental sex on phenotypic variation in spinocerebellar ataxia I. *Am J Hum Genet* 1994; 54:959–964.

77. Tong X, Gui H, Jin F, et al. Ataxin-1 and brother of ataxin-1 are components of the Notch signaling pathway. *EMBO Rep* 2011; 12:428–435.

78. Servadio A, Koshy B, Armstrong D, Antalffy B, Orr H, Zoghbi HY. Expression analysis of the ataxin-I protein in tissues from normal and spinocerebellar ataxia type I individuals. *Nat Genet* 1995; 10:94–98.

79. Okuda T, Hattori H, Takeuchi S, et al. PQBP-1 transgenic mice show a late-onset motor neuron disease-like phenotype. *Hum Molec Genet* 2003; 12:711–725.

80. Xia H, Mao Q, Eliason SL, et al. RNAi suppresses polyglutamine-induced neurodegeneration in a model of spinocerebellar ataxia. *Nature Med* 2004; 10:816–820.

81. Serra HG, Duvick L, Zu T, et al. ROR-alpha-mediated Purkinje cell development determines disease activity in adult SCA1 mice. *Cell* 2006; 127:697–708.

82. Pareyson D, Gellera C, Castellotti B, et al. Clinical and molecular studies of 73 Italian families with autosomal dominant cerebellar ataxia type 1: SCA1 and SCA2 are the most common phenotypes. *J Neurol* 1999; 246:389–393.

83. Storey E, du Sart D, Shaw JH, et al. Frequency of spinocerebellar ataxia types 1, 2, 3, 6, and 7 in Australian patients with spinocerebellar ataxia. *Am J Med Genet* 2000; 95:351–357.

84. Zhou Y-X, Qiao W-H, Gu W-H, et al. Spinocerebellar ataxia type 1 in China: molecular analysis and genotype-phenotype correlation in 5 families. *Arch Neurol* 2001; 58:789–794.

85. Ranum LPW, Lundgren JK, Schut LJ, et al. Spinocerebellar ataxia type I and Machado-Joseph disease: incidence of CAG expansions among adult-onset ataxia patients from 311 families with dominant, recessive, and sporadic ataxia. *Am J Hum Genet* 1995; 57:603–668.

86. Orozco-Diaz G, Nodarse-Fleites A, Cordoves-Sagaz R, et al. Autosomal dominant cerebellar ataxia: clinical analysis of 263 patients from a homogenous population in Holquin, Cuba. *Neurology* 1990; 40:1369–1375.

87. Filla A, DeMichele G, Banfi S, et al. Has spinocerebellar ataxia type 2 a distinct phenotype: Genetic and clinical study of an Italian family. *Neurology* 1995; 45:793–796.

88. Lopes-Cendes I, Andermann E, Attiq E, et al. Confirmation of the SCA-2 locus as an alternative locus for dominating inherited spinocerebellar ataxias and refinement of the candidate region. *Am J Hum Genet* 1994; 54:774–781.

89. Belal S, Cancel G, Stevanin G, et al. Clinical and genetic analysis of a Tunisian family with autosomal dominant cerebellar ataxia type I linked to the SCA2 locus. *Neurology* 1994; 44:1423–1426.

90. Pulst SM, Nechiporuk A, Starkuan S. Anticipation in spinocerebellar ataxia type 2. *Nat Genet* 1933; 5:8–10.

91. Orozco-Diaz G, Nodarse-Fleites A, Cordoves-Sagaz R, Auburger G. Autosomal dominant cerebellar ataxia: clinical analysis of 263 patients from a homogenous population in Holquin, Cuba. *Neurology* 1990; 40:1369–1375.

92. Pulst SM, Nechiporuk A, Nechiporuk T, et al. Moderate expansion of a normally biallelic trinucleotide repeat in spinocerebellar ataxia type 2. *Nat Genet* 1996; 14:269–284.

93. Imbert G, Saudou F, Devys D, et al. Cloning of the gene for spinocerebellar ataxia 2 reveals a locus with high sensitivity to expanded CAG/glutamine repeats. *Nat Genet* 1998; 14:237–238.

94. Sanpei K, Takano H, Igarashi S, et al. Identification of the spinocerebellar ataxia type 2 gene using a direct identification of repeat expansion and cloning technique, DIRECT. *Nat Genet* 1996; 14:277–284.

95. Schols L, Gispert S, Vorgerd M, et al. Spinocerebellar ataxia type 2. *Arch Neurol* 1997; 54:1073–1080.

96. Cancel G, Durr A, Didierjean O, et al. Molecular and clinical correlations in spinocebellar ataxia 2: a study of 32 families. *Hum Mol Genet* 1997; 6:709–715.

97. Ueyama H, Kumamoto T, Nagao S, et al. Clinical and genetic studies of spinocerebellar ataxia type 2 in Japanese kindreds. *Acta Neurol Scand* 1998; 98:427–432.

98. Giuffrida S, Saponara R, Restivo DA, et al. Supratentorial atrophy in spinocerebellar ataxia type 2: MRI study of 20 patients. *J Neurol* 1999; 246:383–388.

99. Ragothaman M, Sarangmath N, Chaudhary S, et al. Complex phenotypes in an Indian family with homozygous SCA2 mutations. *Ann Neurol* 2004; 55:130–133.

100. Charles P, Camuzat A, Benammar N, et al. Are interrupted SCA2 CAG repeat expansions responsible for parkinsonism? *Neurology* 2007; 69:1970–1975.

101. Elden AC, Kim H-J, Hart MP, et al. Ataxin-2 intermediate-length polyglutamine expansions are associated with increased risk for ALS. *Nature* 2010; 466:1069–1075.

102. Ross OA, Rutherford NJ, Baker M, et al. Ataxin-2 repeat-length variation and neurodegeneration. *Hum Molec Genet* 2011; 20:3207–3212.

103. Van Damme P, Veldink JH, van Blitterswijk M, et al. Expanded ATXN2 repeats in ALS identifies genetic overlap between ALS and SCA2. *Neurology* 2011; 76:2066–2072.

104. Nakano K, Dawson D, Spence A. Machado disease: hereditary ataxia in Portuguese immigrants to Massachusetts. *Neurology* 1972; 22:49–59.

105. Shimizu Y, Yoshida K, Okano T, et al. Regional features of autosomal-dominant cerebellar ataxia in Nagano: clinical and molecular genetic analysis of 86 families. *J Hum Genet* 2004; 49:610–616.

106. Takiyama Y, Nishizawa M, Tanaka H, et al. The gene for Machado-Joseph disease maps to human chromosome 14q. *Nat Genet* 1993; 4:300–303.

107. St. George-Hyslop PH, Rogaeva E, Hutterer J, et al. Machado-Joseph disease in pedigrees of Azorean descent is linked to chromosome 14. *Am J Hum Genet* 1994; 55:120–125

108. Tuite PJ, Rogaeva EA, St. George-Hyslop PH, et al. Dopa-responsive parkinsonism phenotype of Machado-Joseph disease: confirmation of 14q CAG expansion. *Ann Neurol* 1995; 38:684–687.

109. Stevanin G, LeGuern E, Ravise N, et al. A third locus for autosomal dominant cerebellar ataxia type I maps to chromosome 14q24-3-qter: evidence for the existence of a fourth locus. *Am J Hum Genet* 1994; 54:11–30.

110. Kawaguchi Y, Okamoto T, Taniwaki M, et al. CAG expansions in a novel gene from Machado-Joseph disease at chromosome 14q32.1. *Nat Genet* 1994; 8:221–228.

111. Perez MK, Paulson HL, Pittman RN. Ataxin-3 with an altered conformation that exposes the polyglutamine domain is associated with the nuclear matrix. *Hum Molec Genet* 1999; 8:2377–2385.

112. Chai Y, Koppenhafer SL, Shoesmith SJ, et al. Evidence for proteasome involvement in polyglutamine disease: localization to nuclear inclusions in SCA3/MJD and suppression of polyglutamine aggregation in vitro. *Hum Molec Genet* 1999; 8:673–682.

113. Gaspar C, Jannatipour M, Dion P, et al. CAG tract of MJD-1 may be prone to frameshifts causing polyalanine accumulation. *Hum Molec Genet* 2000; 9:1957–1966.

114. Ishikawa A, Yamada M, Makino K, et al. Dementia and delerium in 4 patients with Machado-Joseph disease. *Arch Neurol* 2002; 59:1804–1808.

115. Mueller T, Breuer P, Schmitt I, et al. CK2-dependent phosphorylation determines cellular localization and stability of ataxin-3. *Hum Molec Genet* 2009; 18:3334–3343.

116. Stevanin G, Cancel G, Didierjean O, et al. Linkage disequilibrium at the Machado-Joseph disease/spinal cerebellar ataxia 3 locus: evidence for a common founder effect in French and Portuguese-Brazilian families as well as a second ancestral Portuguese-Azorean mutation. *Am J Hum Genet* 1995; 57:1247–1250.

117. Gardner K, Alderson K, Galster B, et al. Autosomal dominant spinocerebellar ataxia: clinical description of a distinct hereditary ataxia and genetic localization to chromosome 16 (SCA4) in a Utah kindred. *Neurology* 1994; 44[Suppl 2]:A361.

118. Flanigan K, Gardner K, Alderson K, et al. Autosomal dominant spinocerebellar ataxia with sensory axonal neuropathy (SCA4): clinical description and genetic localization to chromosome 16q22.1. *Am J Hum Genet* 1996; 59:392–399.

119. Nagaoka U, Takashima M, Ishikawa K, et al. A gene on SCA4 locus causes dominantly inherited pure cerebellar ataxia. *Neurology* 2000; 54:1971–1975.

120. Ranum LP, Schut LJ, Lundgren JK, Orr HT, Livingston PM. Spinocerebellar ataxia type 5 in a family descended from the grandparents of President Lincoln maps to chromosome 11. *Nat Genet* 1994; 8:280–284.

121. Burk K, Zuhlke C, Konig IR, et al. Spinocerebellar ataxia type 5: clinical and molecular genetic features of German kindred. *Neurology* 2004; 62:327–329.

122. Ikeda Y, Dick KA, Weatherspoon MR, et al. Spectrin mutations cause spinocerebellar ataxia type 5. *Nature Genet* 2006; 38:184–190.

123. Clarkson YL, Gillespie T, Perkins EM, et al. Beta-III spectrin mutation L253P associated with spinocerebellar ataxia type 5 interfaces with binding to Arp1 and protein trafficking from the Golgi. *Hum Molec Genet* 2010; 19:3634–3641.

124. Subramony SH, Fratkin JD, Manyam BV, et al. Dominantly inherited cerebello-olivary atrophy is not due to mutation at the spincocerebellar ataxia-I, Machado-Joseph disease, or dentate-rubro-luysian atrophy locus. *Mov Disord* 1996; 11:174–180.

125. Zhuchenko O, Bailey J, Bonnen P, et al. Autosomal dominant cerebellar ataxia (SCA6) associated with small polyglutamine expansions in the alpha 1A-voltage-dependent calcium channel. *Nat Genet* 1997; 15:62–69.

126. Lory P, Ophoff RA, Nahmias J. Toward a unified nomenclature describing voltage-gated calcium channel genes. *Hum Genet* 1997; 100: 149–150.

127. Sinke RJ, Ippel EF, Diepstraten CM, et al. Clinical and molecular correlations in spinocerebellar ataxia type 6: a study of 24 Dutch families. *Arch Neurol* 2001; 58:1839–1844.

128. Alonso I, Barros J, Tuna A, et al. Phenotypes of spinocerebellar ataxia type 6 and hemiplegic migraine caused by a unique CACNA1A missense mutation in patients from a large family. *Arch Neurol* 2003; 60:610–614.

129. Takahashi H, Ishikawa K, Tsutsumi T, et al. A clinical and genetic study in a large cohort of patients with spinocerebellar ataxia type 6. *J Hum Genet* 2004; 49:256–264.

130. Fukutake T, Kamitsukasa T, Arai K, et al. A patient homozygous for the SCA6 gene with retinitis pigmentosa. *Clin Genet* 2002; 61:375–379.

131. Christova P, Anderson JH, Gomez CM. Impaired eye movements in presymptomatic spinocerebellar ataxia type 6. *Arch Neurol* 2008; 65:530–536.

132. Soong B, Liu R, Wu L ,et al. Metabolic characterization of spinocerebellar ataxia type 6. *Arch Neurol* 2001; 58:300–304.

133. Takahashi H, Ikeuchi T, Honma Y, et al. Autosomal dominant cerebellar ataxia (SCA6): clinical, genetic and neuropathological study in a family. *Acta Neuropath* 1998; 95:333–337.

134. Jodice C, Mantuano E, Veneziano L, et al. Episodic ataxia type 2 (EA2) and spinocerebellar ataxia type 6 (SCA6) due to CAG repeat expansion in the CACNA1A gene on chromosome 19p. *Hum Mol Genet* 1997; 11:1973–1978.

135. Zhuchenko O, Bailey J, Bonnen P, et al. Autosomal dominant cerebellar ataxia (SCA6) associated with small polyglutamine expansions in the alpha 1A-voltage-dependent calcium channel. *Nat Genet* 1997; 15:62–69.

136. Froment J, Bonnet P, Colrat A. Heredo-degenerations retinienne et spino-cerebelleuse: variants ophtalmoscopiques et neurologiques presentees par trois generations successives. *J Med Lyon* 1937; 153–163.

137. Jonasson J, Juvonen V, Sistonen P, et al. Evidence for a common spinocerebellar ataxia type 7 (SCA7) founder mutation in Scandinavia. *Europ J Genet* 2000; 8:918–922.

138. Michalik A, Martin J-J, Van Broekhoven C. Spinocerebellar ataxia type 7 associated with pigmentary retinal dystrophy. *Europ J Hum Genet* 2004; 12:2–15.

139. David G, Abbas N, Stevanin G, et al. Cloning of the SCA7 gene reveals a highly unstable CAG repeat expansion. *Nature Genet* 1997; 17:65–70.

140. Sopher BL, Ladd PD, Pineda VV, et al. CTCF regulates ataxin-7 expression through promotion of a convergently transcribed, antisense noncoding RNA. *Neuron* 2011; 70:1071–1084.

141. Holmberg M, Duyckaerts C, Durr A, et al. Spinocerebellar

ataxia type 7 (SCA7): a neurodegenerative disorder with neuronal intranuclear inclusions. *Hum Molex Genet* 1998; 7:913–918.

142. Ansorge O, Giunti P, Michalik A, et al. Ataxin-7 aggregation and ubiquintination in infantile SCA7 with 180 CAG repeats. *Ann Neurol* 2004; 56:448–452.

143. Yvert G, Lindenberg KS, Picaud S, et al. Expanded polyglutamines induce neurodegeneration and trans-neuronal alterations in cerebellum and retina of SCA7 transgenic mice. *Hum Molec Genet* 2000; 9:2491–2506.

144. La Spada AR, Fu Y-H, Sopher BL, et al. Polyglutamine-expanded ataxin-7 antagonizes CRX function and induces cone-rod dystrophy in a mouse model of SCA7. *Neuron* 2001; 31:913–927.

145. Yoo SY, Pennesi ME, Weeber EJ, et at. SCA7 knockin mice model human SCA7 and reveal gradual accumulation of mutant ataxin-7 in neurons and abnormalities in short-term plasticity. *Neuron* 2003; 37:383–401.

146. Koob MD, Moseley ML, Schut LJ, et al. An untranslated CTG expansion causes a novel form of spinocerebellar ataxia (SCA8). *Nature Genet* 1999; 21:379–384.

147. Ikeda Y, Shizuka M, Watanable M, et al. Molecular and clinical analyses of spinocerebellar ataxia type 8 in Japan. *Neurology* 2000; 54:950–955.

148. Daughters RS, Tuttle DL, Gao W, et al. RNA gain-of-function in spinocerebellar ataxia type 8. *POoS Genet* 2009; 5:e1000600.

149. Moseley ML, Zu T, Ikeda Y, et al. Bidirectional expression of CUG and CAG expansion transcripts and intranuclear polyglutamine inclusions in spinocerebellar ataxia type 8. *Nature Genet* 2006; 38:758–769.

150. Wu YR, Lin HY, Chen C, et al. Genetic testing in spinocerebellar ataxia in Taiwan: expansions of trinucleotide repeats in SCA8 and SCA17 are associated with typical Parkinson's disease. *Clin Genet* 2004; 65:209–214.

151. Higgins JJ, Pho LT, ide SE, et al. Evidence for a new spinocerebellar ataxia locus. *Mov Disord* 1997; 12:412–417.

152. Grewal RP, Tayag E, Figueroa KP, et al. Clinical and genetic analysis of a distinct autosomal dominant spinocerebellar ataxia. *Neurology* 1998; 51:1423–1426.

153. Zu L, Figueroa KP, Grewal R, et al. Mapping of a new autosomal dominant spinocerebellar ataxia to chromosome 22. *Am J Hum Genet* 1999; 64:594–599.

154. Rasmussen A, Matsuura T, Ruano L, et al. Clinical and genetic analysis of four Mexican families with spinocerebellar ataxia type 10. *Ann Neurol* 2001; 50:234–239.

155. Grewal RP, Achari M, Matsurra T, et al. Clinical features and ATTCT repeat expansion in spinocerebellar ataxia type 10. *Arch Neurol* 2002; 59:1285–1290.

156. Matsuura T, Achari M, Khajavi M, et al. Mapping of the gene for a novel spinocerebellar ataxia with pure cerebellar signs and epilepsy. *Ann Neurol* 1999; 45:407–411.

157. Teive HAG, Roa BB, Raskin S, et al. Clinical phenotype of Brazilian families with spinocerebellar ataxia 10. *Neurology* 2004; 63:1509–1512.

158. Fujigasaki H, Tardieu S, Camuzat A, et al. Spinocerebellar ataxia type 10 in the French population. *Ann Neurol* 2002; 51:408.

159. Wakamiya M, Matsuura T, Liu Y, et al. The role of ataxin 10 in the pathogenesis of spinocerebellar ataxia type 10. *Neurology* 2006; 67:607–613.

160. Worth PF, Giunti P, Gardner-Thorpe C, et al. Autosomal dominant cerebellar ataxia type III: linkage in a large British family to a 7.6-cM region on chromosome 15q14-21.3. *Am J Hum Genet* 1999; 65:420–426.

161. Houlden H, Johnson J, Gardner-Thorpe C, et al. Mutations I

nTTBK2, encoding a kinase implicated in tau phosphorylation, segregate with spinocerebellar ataxia type 11. *Nature Genet* 2007; 39:1434–1436.

162. Holmes SE, O'Hearn EE, McInnis MG, et al. Expansion of a novel CAG trinucleotide repeat in the 5-prime region of PPP2R2B is associated with SCA12. *Nature Genet* 1999; 23:391–392.

163. Srivastava AK, Choudhry S, Gopinath MS, et al. Molecular and clinical correlation in five Indian families with spinocerebellar ataxia 12. *Ann Neurol* 2001; 50:796–800.

164. Bahl S, Virdi K, Mittal U, et al. Evidence of a common founder for SCA12 in the Indian population. *Ann Hum Genet* 2005; 69:528–534.

165. Durr A, Herman A, Stevanin G, et al. Autosomal dominant cerebellar ataxia with mental retardation is linked to chromosome 19q13.3. *Neurology* 2000; 54(Suppl 3):A465–A466.

166. Herman-Bert A, Stevanin G, Nettr J-C et al. Mapping of spinocerebellar ataxia 13 to chromosome 19q13.3-q13.4 in a family with autosomal dominant cerebellar ataxia and mental retardation. *Am J Hum Genet* 2000; 67:229–235.

167. Johnson KJ, Jones PJ, Spurr N, et al. Linkage relationships of the protein kinase C gamma gene which exclude it as a candidate for myotonic dystrophy. *Cytogenet Cell Genet* 1988; 48:13–15

168 Trask B, Fertitta A, Christensen M, et al. Fluorescence in situ hybridization mapping of human chromosome 19: cytogenetic location of 540 cosmids and 70 genes or DNA markers. *Genomics* 19913; 15:133–145.

169. Yamashita I, Sasaki H, Yabe I, et al. A novel locus for dominant cerebellar ataxia (SCA14) maps to a 10.2-cM interval flanked by D19S206 and D19S605 on chromosome 19q13.4-qter. *Ann Neurol* 2000; 48:156–163.

170. Brkanac Z, Bylenok L, Fernandez M, et al. A new dominant spinocerebellar ataxia linked to chromosome 19q13.4-qter. *Arch Neurol* 2002; 59:1291–1295.

171. Chen DH, Brkanac Z, Verlinde CL, et al. Missense mutations in the regularoty domain of PKC-gamma: a new mechanism for dominant nonepisodic cerebellar ataxia. *Am J Hum Genet* 2003; 72:839–849.

172. Yabe I, Sasaki H, Chen D-H, et al. Spinocerebellar ataxia type 14 caused by a mutation in protein kinase C gamma. *Arch Neurol* 2003; 60:1749–1751.

173. Klebe S, Faivre L, Forlani S, et al. Another mutation in cysteine 131 in protein kinase C-gamma as a cause of spinocerebellar ataxia type 14 (Letter). *Arch Neurol* 2007; 64:913–914.

174. Stevanin G, Hahn V, Lohmann E, et al. Mutation in the catalytic domain of protein kinase C gamma and extension of the phenotype associated with spinocerebellar ataxia type 14. *Arch Neurol* 2004; 61:1242–1248.

175. Najmabadi H, Hu H, Garshasbi M, et al. Deep sequencing 50 novel genes for recessive cognitive disorders. *Nature* 2011; 478:57–63.

176. Storey E, Gardner RJM, Knight MA, et al. A new autosomal dominant pure cerebellar ataxia. *Neurology* 2001; 57:1913–1915.

177. Synofzik M, Beetz C, Bauer C, et al. Spincerebellar ataxia type 15: diagnostic assessment, frequency, and phenotypic features. *J Med Genet* 2011; 48:407–412.

178. van de Leemput J, Chandran J, Knight MA, et al. Deletion at ITPR1 underlies ataxia in mice and spinocerebellar ataxia 15 in humans. *PLoS Genet* 2007; 3:e108.

179. Knight MA, Kennerson ML, Anney RJ, et al. Spinocerebellar ataxia type 15 (SCA15) maps to 3p24.23pter: exclusion of the ITPR1 gene, the human orthologue of an ataxic mouse mutant. *Neurobiol Dis* 2003; 13:147–157.

which predisposes to draping of the cord over the anterior spinal elements. Anterior corpectomy accompanied by intervertebral fusion with an allograft, harvesting iliac crest or fibular strut, are effective anterior approach that achieves the goals of decompression via anterior osteophyte removal and stabilization of excessively mobile segments by interbody graft fusion. The factors predictive of a favorable prognosis in CSM with surgical intervention via anterior decompression and fusion have included age younger than 60 years and duration of symptoms less than two years (41). The most widely cited disadvantages of the anterior approach are increased operative time, complexity, and a higher incidence of operative complications (42, 43). In addition, technical and biomechanical considerations may preclude anterior decompression of disease that extends beyond three spinal segments. Complications are typically related to injury of the various vascular, neural, and visceral structures in the anterior neck. One common one is C-5 radiculitis; others include hoarseness due to recurrent laryngeal nerve injury, dysphagia, wound infection, and hematoma, in addition to worsening of the myelopathy. Complications related to fusion include bleeding and infection at the graft donor site and graft extrusion that occur in 3 to 10% of patients.

RECOMMENDATIONS

An analysis of the results reported for anterior and posterior decompressive approaches to CSM provides no clear consensus as to which approach offers optimal results. However, among 84 patients treated with anterior corpectomy or posterior laminectomy and followed a mean of 7.35 years (44), initial improvement was seen in about 70% of patients operated by either approach. Long-term follow-up revealed sustained improvement in 54% of anterior oper-

ated cases and 37% of posterior approaches. At follow-up, 18% of anterior patients and 37% of posterior patients had deteriorated. Posterior approaches were not combined with fusion in this series, and the issue of postoperative instability was not addressed. The risk of late decline strongly correlated with duration of preoperative symptoms, suggesting that some patients with CSM have sustained irreversible cord damage before surgery, a supposition supported by pathologic cord studies. The vascular pathology associated with CSM may be a contributing factor in late deterioration. When evaluating approaches to CSM, a complete evaluation of potential morbidity and mortality should be undertaken. The incidence of reported complications from anterior approaches is extremely variable ranging from 3 to 48%. Complications are somewhat less frequent in posterior decompressive surgery, but the incidence of postoperative deformity is as high as 42%. Mortality for both approaches is 2% or less.

The proposed management of CSM should be guided by a consideration of the risks and benefits of conservative management, followed by a discussion of the indications, advantages, and limitations of a given intended surgical approach (45), incorporating the insights of evidence-based studies (37). The favored surgical approach or approaches will be those that allow removal of the compressive elements most directly, taking into consideration the curvature of the cervical spine, whether lordotic or kyphotic, and the location and extent of compression. For segmental disease over one to three spinal levels, anterior discectomy or corpectomy with interbody fusion (ACDF or ACCF) should be considered. For posteriorly located compressive elements or diffuse disease that extends over more than three levels, a posterior approach is generally preferred. Additionally, posterior fusion and instrumentation may be required to avoid postoperative instability.

REFERENCES

1. Fehlings MG, Jha NK, Hewson SM, et al. Is surgery for cervical spondylotic myelopathy cost-effective? A cost utility analysis based on data from the AOSpine North America prospective CSM study. *J Neurosurg Spine* 2012 (Suppl) 17:89–93.
2. Polly DW Jr. Cervical spondylotic myelopathy. *J Neurosurg Spine* 2012; (Suppl) 17:87–88.
3. Schmorl G, Junghanns H. Gesunde und kranke Wirbelsaule, [etc.]. In: Schmorl G, Junghanns H, eds. *Pathologische-anatomische untersuchungen.* Leipzig: Georg Thieme, 1932.
4. McNab I. The traction spur. An indicator of segmental instability. *J Bone Joint Surg Am* 1971; 53:663–670.
5. Payne EE, Spillane JD. The cervical spine: an anatomico-pathologic study of 70 specimens (using a special technique) with particular reference to the problem of cervical spondylosis. *Brain* 1957; 80:571–596.

6. Wilkinson M. The morbid anatomy of cervical spondylosis and myelopathy. *Brain* 1960; 83:589–617.
7. Barnes MP, Saunders M. The effect of cervical mobility on the natural history of cervical spondylotic myelopathy. *J Neurol Neurosurg Psychiatry* 1984; 47:17–20.
8. Nurick S. The pathogenesis of the spinal cord disorder associated with cervical spondylosis. *Brain* 1972; 95:87–100.
9. Adams CBT, Logue V. Studies in cervical spondylotic myelopathy. II. The movement and contour of the spine in relation to the neural complications of cervical spondylosis. *Brain* 1971; 94:568–586.
10. Cusick JF. Pathophysiology and treatment of cervical spondylotic myelopathy. *Clin Neurosurg* 1991; 37:661–681.
11. Epstein JA, Epstein NE. The surgical management of cervical spinal stenosis, spondylosis, and myeloradiculopathy by means of the posterior approach. In: Sherk HH, Dunn EJ, Eismont FJ, et al., eds. *The cervical spine.* Philadelphia: J.B. Lippincott, 1989:625–643.

12. Ogino H, Tada K, Okada K, et al. Canal diameter, anteroposterior compression ratio, and spondylotic myelopathy of the cervical spine. *Spine* 1983; 8:1–15.

13. Parke WW. Correlative anatomy of cervical spondylotic myelopathy. *Spine* 1988; 13:831–837.

14. Symon L, Lavender P. The surgical treatment of cervical spondylotic myelopathy. *Neurology* 1967; 17:117–127.

15. Epstein JA, Carras R, Hyman RA, et al. Cervical myelopathy caused by developmental stenosis of the spinal canal. *J Neurosurg* 1979; 51:362–367.

16. Nagashima C. Cervical myelopathy due to ossification of the posterior longitudinal ligament. *J Neurosurg* 1972;37:653–660.

17. Panjabi M, White A III. Biomechanics of nonacute cervical spinal cord trauma. *Spine* 1988; 13:838–842.

18. Doppman JL. The mechanism of ischemia in anteroposterior compression of the spinal cord. *Invest Radiol* 1975;10:543–551.

19. Ono K, Ota H, Tada K, et al. Cervical myelopathy secondary to multiple spondylotic protrusions: a clinicopathologic study. *Spine* 1977; 2:109–125.

20. Phillips DG. Surgical treatment of myelopathy with cervical spondylosis. *J Neurol Neurosurg Psychiatry* 1973; 36:879–884.

21. Lees F, Aldren-Turner JW. Natural history and prognosis of cervical spondylosis. *Br Med J* 1963; 2:1607–1610.

22. Nurick S. The natural history and the results of surgical treatment of the spinal cord disorder associated with cervical spondylosis. *Brain* 1972; 95:101–108.

23. Roberts AH. Myelopathy due to cervical spondylosis treated by collar immobilization. *Neurology* 1966;16:951–954.

24. Crandall PH, Batzdorf U. Cervical spondylotic myelopathy. *J Neurosurg* 1966; 25:57–66.

25. Dagi TF, Tarkington MA, Leech JJ. Tandem lumbar and cervical spinal stenosis. Natural history, prognostic indices, and results after surgical decompression. *J Neurosurg* 1987; 66:842–849.

26. Epstein NE, Epstein JA, Carras R, et al. Coexisting cervical and lumbar spinal stenosis: diagnosis and management. *Neurosurgery* 1984; 15:489–496.

27. Rowland LP. Surgical treatment of cervical spondylotic myelopathy: time for a controlled trial. *Neurology* 1992; 42:5–13.

28. Nagata K, Kiyonaga K, Ohashi T, et al. Clinical value of magnetic resonance imaging for cervical myelopathy. *Spine* 1990; 15:1088–1096.

29. Jones JG, Cen SY, Lebel RM, et al. Diffusion tensor imaging correlates with the clinical assessment of disease severity in cervical spondylotic myelopathy and predicts outcome following surgery. *AJNR* 2012 July 19 [Epub ahead of print].

30. Matz PG, Anderson PA, Holly LT, et al. The natural history of cervical spondylotic myelopathy. *J Neurosurg Spine* 2009; 11:104–111.

31. Ito T, Oyanagi K, Takahashi H, et al. Cervical spondylotic myeopathy. Clinicopathologic study on the progression pattern and thin myelinated fibers of the lesions of seven patients examined during complete autopsy. *Spine* 1996; 21:827–833.

32. Kadanka Z, Mares M, Bednanik J, et al. Approaches to spondylotic cervical myelopathy: conservative versus surgical results in a 3-year follow-up study. *Spine* 2002; 27:2205–2210.

33. Kadanka Z, Mares M, Bednarik J, et al. Predictive factors for mild forms of spondylotic cervical myelopathy treated conservatively or surgically. *Eur J Neurol* 2005; 12:16–24.

34. Lee TT, Manzano GR, Green BA. Modified open-door cervical expansive laminoplasty for spondylotic myelopathy: operative technique, outcome, and predictors for gait improvement. *J Neurosurg* 1997; 86:64–68.

35. Cloward R. The anterior approach for the removal of ruptured cervical discs. *J Neurosurg* 1958; 14:602–617.

36. Bohlman HH. Cervical spondylosis with moderate to severe myelopathy: a report of seventeen cases treated by Robinson anterior cervical discectomy and fusion. *Spine* 1977; 2:151–161.

37. Mummaneni PV, Kaiser MG, Matz PG, et al. Cervical surgical techniques for the treatment of cervical spondylotic myelopathy. *J Neurosurg Spine* 2009; 11:130–141

38. Yonenobu K, Fuji T, Ono K, et al. Choice of surgical treatment for multisegmental cervical spondylotic myelopathy. *Spine* 1985; 10:710–716.

39. Gonzalez-Feria L, Peraita-Peraita P. Cervical spondylotic myelopathy: a cooperative study. *Clin Neurol Neurosurg* 1975; 78:19–33.

40. Lunsford LD, Bissonette DJ, Zorub DS. Anterior surgery for cervical disc disease. Part 2: Treatment of cervical spondylotic myelopathy in 32 cases. *J Neurosurg* 1980; 53:12–19.

41. Chagas H, Dominiques F, Aversa A, et al. Cervical spoindylotic myelopathy: 10 years of prospective outcome analysis of anterior decompression and fusion. *Surg Neurol* 2005; 64(Suppl 1):S30–S35.

42. Saunders RL, Bernini PM, Shirreffs TG Jr, et al. Central corpectomy for cervical spondylotic myelopathy: a consecutive series with long-term follow-up evaluation. *J Neurosurg* 1991; 74:163–170.

43. Whitecloud TS III. Anterior surgery for cervical spondylotic myelopathy. Smith-Robinson, Cloward, and vertebrectomy. *Spine* 1988; 13:861–863.

44. Ebersold MJ, Pare MC, Quast LM. Surgical treatment for cervical spondylotic myelopathy. J Neurosurg 1995; 82:745–751.

45. Muthukumar N. Surgical management of cervical spondylotic myelopathy. *Neurol India* 2012; 60:201–209.

CHAPTER 43

Spinal Cord and Foramen Magnum Tumors

David S. Younger, James M. Powers

The past decade has witnessed advances in the classification, diagnosis, and management of tumors of the spinal cord, meningeal and epidural compartments, and vertebral and paravertebral spaces. This chapter reviews aspects of childhood and adult primary tumors of the spinal cord, spinal meninges, and cauda equina.

EPIDEMIOLOGY

The estimated incidence of primary spinal cord tumors, both malignant and nonmalignant combined, was reported as 0.74 per 100,000 person-years, with the highest rates in adults, age 65 to 74 years, and mean age of 51 years at diagnosis. Tumors of the spinal cord and cauda equina accounted for 3% of primary brain and spinal cord tumors overall, among 158,088 patients in The Central Brain Tumor Registry of the United States (CBTRUS), with nerve sheath tumors accounting for 40.5% of 4,838 patients age 20 years and older, followed by ependymomas for 33.6%, meningeal tumors for 6.1%, and astrocytoma or glioblastoma, and lymphoma each for about 4% of patients (1). Among 16 pooled population-based United States cancer registries combining 3,226 primary cord tumors diagnosed between 1998 and 2000 (2), 69% of tumors were benign, among which the spinal cord was the site of the tumor in 70%, spinal meninges in 26%, and cauda equina in 4%. The commonest tumors were meningeal in 29%, nerve sheath in 24%, and ependymal in 23% of patients so studied, with a slight predominance of women over men and non-Hispanic whites over non-Hispanic blacks.

Tumors of the CNS are the most frequent group of malignant solid tumors in pediatric patients, comprising approximately 20% of all tumors in children under age 15 years with a slight overall preponderance in boys, particularly in the first two years of life (3). Employing criteria of the World Health Organization (WHO) (4), spinal cord tumors comprised 5% (5, 6) to 10% (7) of primary CNS pediatric tumors, with three-quarters comprised of pilocytic astrocytoma, followed by anaplastic astrocytoma, ependymoma, primitive neuroectodermal tumors, and ganglioglioma each in 10% (5), 44% of which were intramedullary and 56% extramedullary. Among the latter, ependymomas and schwannomas were the most frequent (7).

It may not be surprising to the inexperienced student that the spinal cord has the full spectrum of primary CNS neoplasia because, like the brain, it contains the full spectrum of elements, including neurons, astrocytes, oligodendrocytes; ependymal cells lining the central canals, blood vessels with endothelium, pericytes, smooth muscle, and a leptomeningeal covering comprised of fibroblasts, blood vessels, and arachnoid meningothelial cells. However, the relative proportion of tumor types found as primary tumors in the spinal cord differs considerably from those reported in the brain. Equally important are the major differences in the reported incidence of various pediatric intramedullary spinal cord tumor types as compared to those in adult patients, unparalleled by the respective incidence in the brain. The attempt to radically surgically remove spinal cord tumors primarily in adult patients (8–10), children (11–13), or both populations (14) resulted in valuable patient series and neuropathological tumor material, rather than small biopsy specimens, from which trends in the observed frequency of spinal cord tumor types were ascertained. Low-grade fibrillary astrocytoma was the commonest intramedullary spinal cord tumor (IMSCT) in pediatric patients, ranging from just under 40% (12, 14)

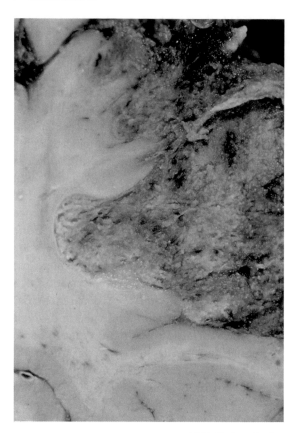

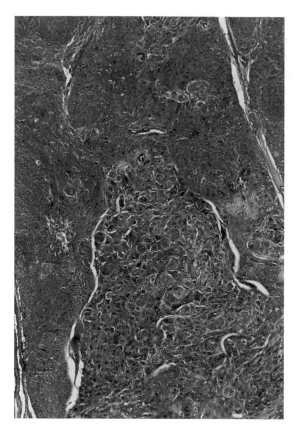

FIG. 3. Atypical meningioma with brain invasion.

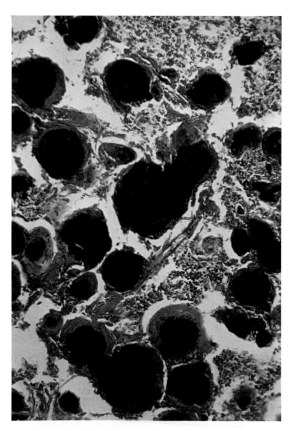

FIG. 4. Psammomatous meningioma with calcified psammoma bodies.

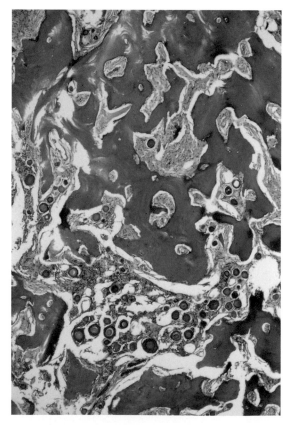

FIG. 5. Bone formation dominating the meningothelial elements (bottom) and simulating a bone tumor on neuroimaging.

(PET-MRI) may offer valuable information in the prospective grading, prognosis, and approach to treatment in a variety of spinal cord neoplasms.

EXTRADURAL INTRAMEDULLARY TUMORS

Meningioma

Meningiomas arise from meningothelial cells of the arachnoid membrane, which are attached to the inner layer of the dura mater (Figure 1). These tumors have been subcategorized by the WHO into at least 15 histological subtypes and graded according to increasing severity, enumerated I to III, according to cytopathologic features and invasiveness (4) (Figure 2). Grade I refers to typical benign lesions (Figure 3), while Grade II corresponds to atypical meningioma when there are increased mitoses and either sheeting architecture, hypercellularity, macronuclei, small cell formation, or parenchymal invasion. Grade III corresponds to anaplastic meningioma that manifests excessive mitotic activity, focal or diffuse loss of light microscopic meningothelial differentiation resulting in a similarity to a sarcoma, carcinoma, or melanoma. Grade I meningiomas, particularly thoracic forms in women, may show extensive calcification (psammomatous) (Figure 4), and even metaplasic ossification (Figure 5), both of which can obscure the underlying meningothelial elements.

A variety of noninvasive neuroimaging modalities applied to meningiomas of the brain can contribute to the diagnosis, WHO classification, grading, and prognostication of spinal cord meningioma (27). MR spectroscopy (MRS) measures the concentrations of various metabolites producing spectral peaks with unique resonance frequency, height, width, and area. Meningiomas display increased intratumoral alanine and pyruvate (28, 29) allowing for the differentiation of meningeal from non-meningeal tumors, and an increase in choline and a decrease in creatine (30), the reciprocal of which characterizes gliomas and metastases (31), along with low to absent N-Acetyl-containing compound lipids. A significant increase in spectral lactate was associated with malignancy among embolized meningiomas (32) as was the lipid/Cr ratio that differentiated the WHO meningioma grades I to III (33). With nearly 85% of spinal cord meningiomas, both intradural and extramedullary, and the thoracic region the most commonly involved area, there may be insidious signs of spinal cord compression leading to asymmetric progressive paralysis and sensory disturbances (34). Perfusion-weighted MRI, employing an exogenous contrast agent or blood coupled with the blood-oxygen-level-dependent (BOLD) principle, in which oxygenated and deoxygenated blood, each with

different paramagnetic effects; or arterial spin labeling to obtain radiofrequency impulses and images representative of regional cerebral blood volume (rCBV), detects hypervascularized tumor foci and areas of hypovascularized necrosis. An increasing grade of meningioma was associated with increased rCBV and differentiated preoperative grade I and II meningiomas (35), and others with grade III tumors, revealing abnormal rCBV in tumoral parenchyma and peritamoral edema in preoperative meningothelial, fibrous, angiomatous, and anaplastic meningiomas (36). The use of PET in the diagnosis, target delineation of radiotherapy, and response to therapy is well described in meningiomas. It shows defects in the tumor-to-gray-matter ratio (TGR) preoperatively in benign and atypical-malignant lesions, the measured value of which was higher in benign lesions and correlated with M1B-1 labeling, mitotic counts, WHO grade, and brain parenchymal invasion (34, 37).

Total surgical resection was obtained in 82% of patients who underwent dorsal microneurosurgery between 1995 and 2009, at a single institution (38), 78% of whom presented with back pain followed by leg weakness and sensory loss. Recurrences noted in 17%, were ascribed to tumor regrowth in those incompletely resected due to a predominantly ventral location.

Nerve Sheath Tumors

Schwannoma

These tumors arise on a segment of the nerve root, usually posterior, after it has penetrated the pia mater. They are firm, well circumscribed, and encapsulated, and in most instances solitary (Figure 6). A microscopic appearance of interwoven bundles of long spindle-shaped bipolar Schwann cells is characteristic of the Antoni A pattern, while the intermingled and pleomorphic Schwann cell pattern embedded in a loose eosinophilic matrix characterizes the Antoni B pattern, both of which display sparse mitotic figures. The parallel alignment of spindle nuclei separated by an eosinophilic matrix, termed the *Verocay body*, is a modification of the Antoni A pattern and is of diagnostic value (Figure 7). Among 187 patients with single or multiple (six patients) schwannomas who underwent partial or total laminectomy to remove the lesions, the commonest presenting features in order of diminishing frequency were radiating pain, local pain, dermatomal sensory deficit, inability to walk due to paraparesis, radicular motor weakness, and bladder paresis.

While most schwannomas occur as isolated lesions, the presence of multiple schwannomas in a single patient is suggestive of schwannomatosis. First described in 1973 (39) as neurofibromatosis type 3, the disorder is characterized by multiple cutaneous neurilemmonas and spinal schwan-

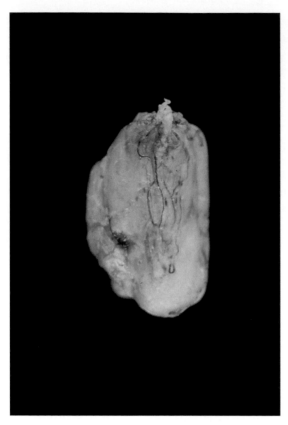

FIG. 6. Soft encapsulated Schwannoma.

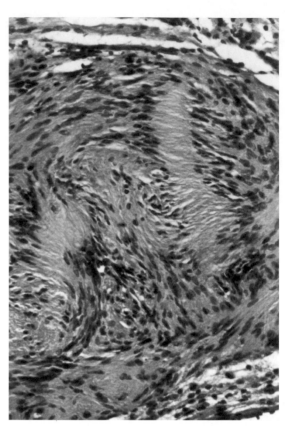

FIG. 7. Schwannoma demonstrating a Verocay body. The parallel alignment of spindle nuclei separated by an eosinophilic matrix is a modification of the Antoni A pattern.

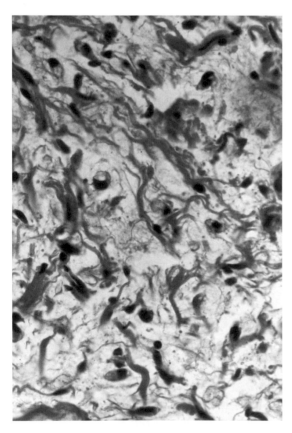

FIG. 8. Neurofibroma demonstrating a loose and haphazard arrangement of nuclei within a collagenous matrix.

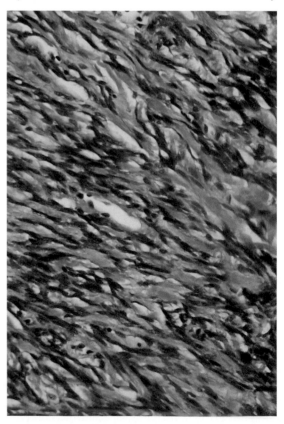

FIG. 9. Solitary fibrous tumor with broad eosinophilic fibers.

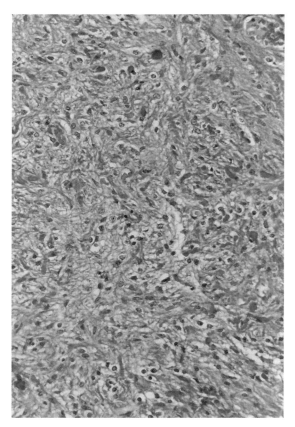

FIG. 10. Pilocytic astrocytoma with numerous scattered bright red Rosenthal fibers.

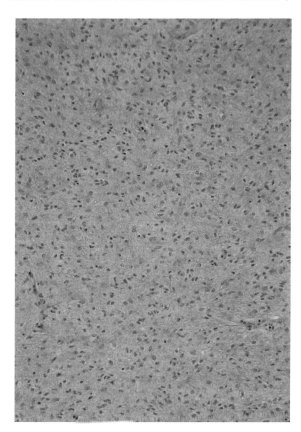

FIG. 11. Diffuse astrocytoma, grade II.

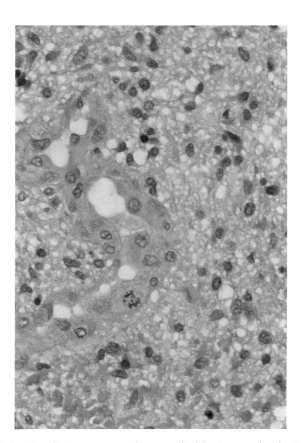

FIG. 12. Grade III area within a glioblastoma displaying endothelial proliferation and a mitosis (bottom center).

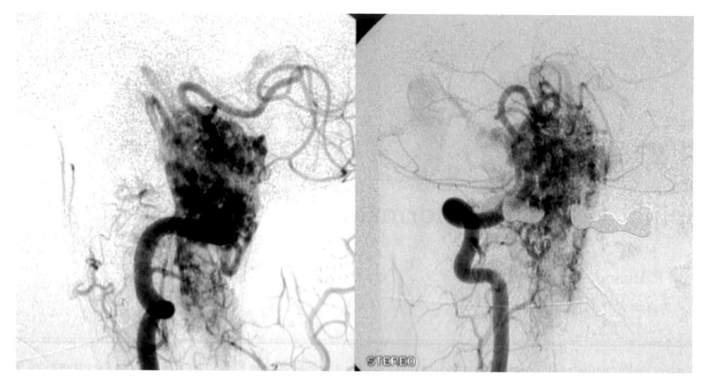

FIG. 1. Intradural dorsal spinal AVF. Anteroposterior spinal angiography demonstrates the lesion at the T6 spinal level. Dilated serpiginous veins can be seen over the dorsal surface of the spinal cord.

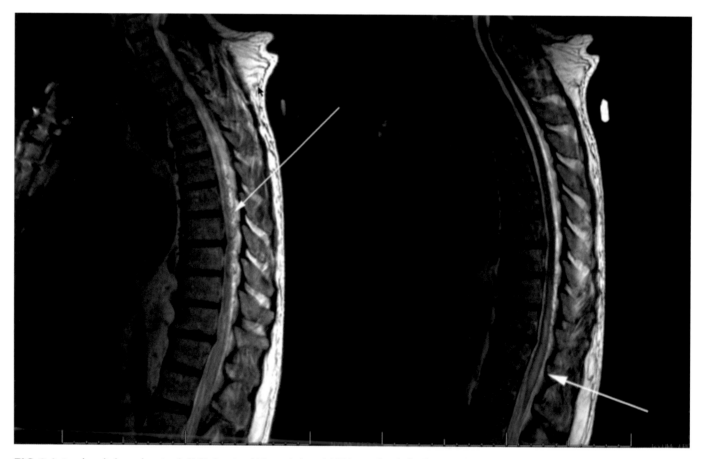

FIG. 2. Intradural dorsal spinal AVF. Sagittal T_2-weighted MRI on the left shows serpiginous flow voids in the dorsal subarachnoid space (arrow). T_2-weighted image on the right shows abnormal signal intensities at the level of the conus (arrow). The patient presented with a progressive myelopathy that improved after surgical ligation of the fistula.

Table 1. Classification of Spinal Vascular Malformations

Spinal arteriovenous fistula (AVF)
    Extradural spinal AVF
    Intradural spinal AVF
        Dorsal location
        Ventral location
Spinal arteriovenous malformation (AVM)
    Extradural-intradural spinal AVM
    Intramedullary spinal AVM
Spinal cavernous malformation

use of spinal angiography, it is now apparent that spinal parenchymal AVM exhibit a discrete nidus that is structurally similar to cerebral AVM. Subsets of spinal vascular lesions exhibit large, tortuous veins without an obvious nidus. The improvement in imaging techniques and use of microcatheters show that the enlarged veins are actually arterialized vessels associated with arteriovenous fistula. Such lesions have been categorized as dural, gliomic, and juvenile. Additional refinements in the classification system, based upon continued improvements in the understanding of the feeding and draining patterns of this heterogeneous group of malformations, had led to the present classification of spinal vascular malformations shown in Table 1.

CLINICAL PRESENTATION

Symptoms from spinal vascular malformations can be attributed to direct compression or mass effect on neuronal structures, elevated venous pressure from an arteriovenous shunt, hemorrhage, and hemodynamic diversion of blood flow causing local ischemia or steal, alone or in combination. The final common pathway is neuronal ischemia which ultimately leads to neuronal injury and neurological dysfunction. Involvement of the spinal cord leads to focal motor or sensory impairment, progressive myelopathy, loss of bowel and bladder control, and sexual dysfunction. Involvement of a nerve root causes focal motor or sensory dysfunction as well as radicular or non-specific pain that may be poorly localized. The absence of a capillary bed allows arterial pressures to be transmitted directly to the venous system, resulting in elevated venous pressures and venous engorgement. Venous hypertension reduces perfusion to the spinal cord resulting in progressive ischemia of the cord. Increased flow through the arteriovenous shunt may redirect normal flow to other areas of the spinal cord leading to ischemia from a vascular steal phenomenon.

The distended vessels can become quite large causing progressive deficits from mass effect on the underlying parenchyma. These processes often develop over a prolonged period of time, resulting in slowly progressive symptoms that can occur over months or years. Hemorrhage into spinal cord parenchymal typically results in sudden and severe neurological deficits, while bleeding into the subarachnoid space leads to localized back pain, headaches, and diffuse meningeal signs.

ARTERIOVENOUS FISTULA

An arteriovenous fistula (AVF) consists of a single or multiple arterial feeding vessel that leads to a common fistula site and draining vein. They are categorized into extradural and intradural fistula, the latter further subdivided into dorsal and ventral types.

Extradural Arteriovenous Fistula

Extradural fistulas demonstrate a direct connection between an extradural artery and vein resulting in engorgement of the epidural venous system (7, 8). The enlarged epidural veins can cause compression on the underlying spinal cord resulting in a progressive myelopathy. High flow fistulas can shunt blood flow away from the spinal cord, resulting in a steal phenomenon with elevation of venous pressure and venous hypertension. The vast majority of the lesions can be treated by closed endovascular techniques and do not require an open operation.

Intradural Arteriovenous Fistula

Dorsal and ventral spinal AVF are located in the subarachnoid space. Dorsal AVF are fed by one or more vascularized pedicles in the dural root sleeve (Figures 1 and 2). Such lesions are often referred to as dural fistulas, suggesting that the fisula is within the dura. Blood flow through these lesions is directed into the higher resistance coronal venous plexus rather than the lower resistance epidural or dural venous system, suggesting that the fistula exists in the subdural rather than dural space (9).

When there is more than one feeding vessel, there is the formation of a common single fistula within the intradural space supporting the premise that the fistula is subdural. Ventral AVF are much less common than dorsal lesions and are located centrally within the subarachnoid space, usually along the ventral surface of the spinal cord.

The lesions originate directly from the anterior spinal artery and have a direct connection to the venous network. Smaller ventral lesions have a relatively slow flow rate and moderate venous engorgement. Larger ventral shunts have progressively higher flow rates, and can develop extremely large, torturous veins.

Spinal AVF rarely present with a hemorrhage. The clinical

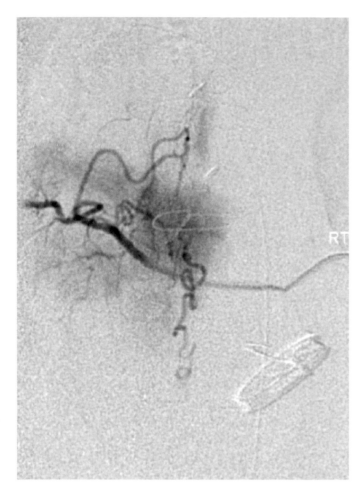

FIG. 3. Spinal intramedullary AVM. Sagittal T$_2$-weighted MRI shows flow voids at the cervical medullary junction.

manifestations are instead, secondary to venous hypertension. Affected patients present in later life with progressive pain, paresthesia, sphincteric dysfunction, and progressive myelopathy, the former suggesting an acquired rather than congenital, etiology. Some patients note exacerbation of symptoms with increased physical activity, likely due to transient elevation of their venous hypertension. The majority of such lesions occur in the thoracic region, leading to predominant leg manifestations.

Many patients also have concurrent lumbar or cervical stenosis from spinal degenerative disease, and initial treatment is sometimes focused unsuccessfully on the spinal stenosis before the true etiology of the symptoms is diagnosed. Ventral fistulas can become quite large and associated with markedly distended veins. Symptoms attributable to progressive vascular steal and spinal cord compression become more pronounced in these larger lesions.

Treatment employing simple obliteration of the fistula is advocated over extensive stripping of the lesions (10–12). The surgical management of dorsal AVF is generally safer and more efficacious than embolization, whereas ventral AVF are

often more difficult to reach surgically and are intimately associated with the anterior spinal artery. Treatment of the latter requires closure of the fistulous connection between the anterior spinal artery and the dilated draining veins for definitive management, a process that can be accomplished by preoperative embolization in large lesions to decrease the flow and turgor of the fistula, rendering them easier to resect surgically. Embolization is not possible for smaller ventral lesions, making surgical management the only reasonable option. Friable giant ventral fistulas with the high risk of associated rupture and vascular injury from surgical manipulation, are best treated with endovascular techniques.

ARTERIOVENOUS MALFORMATIONS

Extradural–Intradural Malformations

Arteriovenous malformations (AVM) are a collection of blood vessels wherein arterial blood flows directly into draining veins without interposed capillary beds. They appear grossly as a tangle of vessels, often with a fairly well circumscribed center or nidus, and arterialized veins. In contrast to AVF, single or multiple dilated arterioles in the AVM connect directly to a vein without a nidus. Extradural-intradural spinal AVM are large, complex malformations with multiple arterial feeders originating from multiple vertebral levels that respect no tissue boundaries and have extensive intramedullary, extramedullary and extraspinal involvement. The occurrence of these lesions is fortunately rare. The presence of multiple large-caliber arterial feeders with tortuous engorged veins renders them susceptible to extensive blood loss, with an overall poor prognosis due to the elevated risk of neurological morbidity and mortality. Treatment is generally comprised of a multiple staged endovascular embolization followed by surgical resection of the residual components.

Intramedullary Malformations

Like cerebral AVM, spinal intramedullary AVM also have a true parenchymal nidus (Figures 3 and 4). These lesions can be supplied by multiple branches of the anterior and posterior spinal arteries, and subsequently drain into the coronal venous plexus, often with associated aneurysms. Spinal intramedullary AVM are usually present with acute headaches, photophobia and meningismus due to subarachnoid hemorrhage and physical activity does not exacerbate the symptoms.

Surgical resection of spinal intramedullary AVM can be challenging because the lesions can be incorporated within the spinal cord, often sharing arterial blood supply. During the resection, each feeding vessel should be preserved

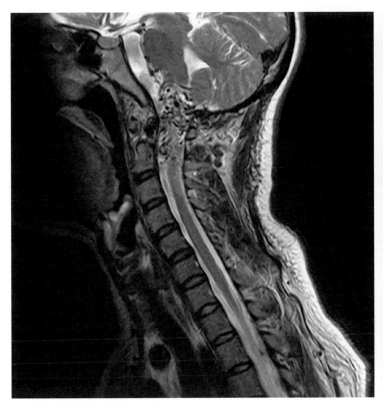

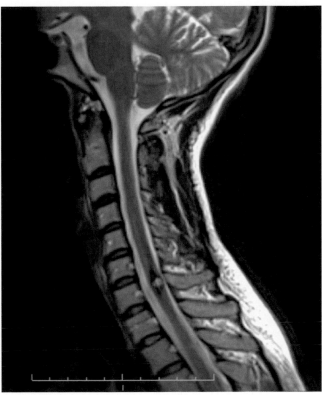

FIG. 4. Spinal intramedullary AVM. Lateral vertebral angiogram on the left side, and anteroposterior view on the right shows the diffuse vascular malformation lesion at the cervicomedullary junction.

FIG. 5. Cavernous spinal malformation. Sagittal T_2-weighted MRI shows abnormal central heterogeneous signal intensity surrounded by a dark rim of hemosiderin.

until certain that it goes only to the AVM nidus and does not contribute to the anterior spinal artery. Manipulation of the surrounding spinal cord should be minimized. Preoperative embolization is employed to reduce flow through the malformation, significantly improving the ease of surgical resection.

CAVERNOUS MALFORMATIONS

Spinal cord cavernous malformations or cavernomas, are well-circumscribed lesions that consist of irregular thick- and thin-walled sinusoidal vascular channels without intervening neural parenchyma, large feeding arteries, or large drainage veins. They can present with an acute deterioration from a large hemorrhage, but more commonly with insidious chronic or progressive deterioration from recurrent small hemorrhages, neither of which result in a cata-strophic event. However relapsing symptoms may coalesce, leading to the erroneous diagnosis of multiple sclerosis.

These angiographically occult lesions are diagnosed with high resolution magnetic resonance imaging (MRI) (Figure 5), appearing as a central area of heterogeneous signal intensity of various age thrombi, surrounded by a thin rim of hemosiderin staining best seen on T_2-weighted or gradient-echo images.

The hemorrhage risk of intracranial cavernomas has been estimated at 0.6% per year (13), such that there is little urgency and perhaps no need for treatment of asymptomatic lesions. Surgical resection is instead, reserved for well-circumscribed symptomatic lesions amenable to a complete resection (14–16). Larger lesions that rise to the pial surface surrounded by a gliotic margin are easier to resect, whereas smaller, ventrally located lesions are associated with higher surgical risks (17). Some symptomatic lesions that exhibit a very benign course (18) can be observed without surgery.

REFERENCES

1. Prestigiacomo CJ, Niimi y, Setton A, et al. Three-dimensional rotational spinal angiography in the evaluation and treatment of vascular malformations. *AJNR* 2003; 24:1429–1435.

2. Si-jia G, Meng-wei Z, Xi-ping L, et al. The clinical application studies of CT spinal angiography with 64-detector row spiral CT in diagnosing spinal vascular malformations. *Eur J Radiol* 2009; 71:22–28.

3. Lv X, Li Y, Yang X, et al. Endovascular embolization for symptomatic perimedullary AVF and intramedullary AVM: a series and a literature review. *Neuroradiology* 2012; 54:349–359.

4. Zuccaro G, Arganaraz R, Villasante F, et al. Neurosurgical vascular malformations in children under 1 year of age. *Childs Nerv Syst* 2010; 26:1381–1394.

5. Rosenblum B, Oldfield EH, Doppman JL, et al. Spinal arteriovenous malformations: a comparison of dural arteriovenous fistulas and intradural AVMs in 81 patients. *J Neurosurg* 1987; 67:795–802.

6. Satran R. Spinal cord infarction. *Stroke* 1988; 19:529–532.

7. Arnaud O, Bille F, Pouget J, et al. Epidural arteriovenous fistula with perimedullary venous drainage: case report. *Neuroradiology* 1994; 36:490–491.

8. Graziani N, Bouillot P, Figarella-Branger D, et al. Cavernous angiomas and arteriovenous malformations of the spinal epidural space: report of 11 cases. *Neurosurgery* 1994; 35:856-863; Discussion 863–854.

9. Spetzler RF, Detwiler PW, Riina HA, et al. Modified classification of spinal cord vascular lesions. *J Neurosurg* 2002; 96:145–156.

10. Mourier KL, Gelbert F, Rey A, et al. Spinal dural arteriovenous malformations with perimedullary drainage. Indications and results of surgery in 30 cases. *Acta Neurochirurgica* 1989; 100:136–141.

11. Oldfield EH, Di Chiro G, Quindlen EA, et al. Successful treatment of a group of spinal cord arteriovenous malformations by interruption of dural fistula. *J Neurosurg* 1983; 59:1019–1030.

12. Ommaya AK, Di Chiro G, Doppman J. Ligation of arterial supply in the treatment of spinal cord arteriovenous malformations. *J Neurosurg* 1969; 30:679–692.

13. Kondziolka D, Lunsford LD, Kestle JR: The natural history of cerebral cavernous malformations. *J Neurosurg* 1995; 83:820–824.

14. Anson JA, Spetzler RF: Surgical resection of intramedullary spinal cord cavernous malformations. *J Neurosurg* 1993; 78:446–451.

15. Vishteh AG, Sankhla S, Anson JA, et al. Surgical resection of intramedullary spinal cord cavernous malformations: delayed complications, long-term outcomes, and association with cryptic venous malformations. *Neurosurgery* 1997; 41:1094–1100; Discussion 1100–1091.

16. McCormick PC, Michelsen WJ, Post KD, Carmel PW, et al. Cavernous malformations of the spinal cord. *Neurosurgery* 1988; 23:459–463.

? Ogilvy CS, Louis DN, Ojemann RG. Intramedullary cavernous angiomas of the spinal cord: clinical presentation, pathological features, and surgical management. *Neurosurgery* 1992; 31:219–229; discussion 229–230.

17. Liang JT, Bao YH, Zhang HQ, et al. Management and prognosis of symptomatic patients with intramedullary spinal cord cavernoma. *J Neurosurgery Spine* 2011; 15:447–456.

18. Kharkar S, Shuck J, Conway J, Rigamonti D: The natural history of conservatively managed symptomatic intramedullary spinal cord cavernomas. *Neurosurgery* 2007; 60:865–872; discussion 865–872.

PART IV

The Neuronal Degenerations

CHAPTER 45

Cerebral Vascular Malformations

Christina Hadzitheodoro, David S. Younger, Paul P. Huang

Cerebral vascular malformations are a heterogeneous group of lesions that include cerebral cavernous malformations (CCM), arteriovenous malformations (AVM), capillary telangiectasias, and cerebral developmental venous anomaly (DVA) (1).

CEREBRAL CAVERNOUS MALFORMATIONS

Cerebral cavernous malformations, which account for about 10 to 15% of all CNS vascular malformations, and occur with a frequency of 1 in 200 to 600 individuals or 0.1 to 0.5% of the general population (2), are comprised of vascular sinusoids lacking smooth muscle cells, elastic lamina, and tight junctions between endothelial cells, rendering then prone to intracerebral hemorrhage (3). Familial CCM (FCCM) is probably underestimated due to the proportion of asyptomatic lesions in affected patients. It is an autosomal dominant (AD) inherited disorder due to mutations in the CCM complex. The latter include CCM1, CCM2, and CCM3, further separable by known pathogenic mutations, respectively, at the 7q21.2 locus of the *KRIT1* gene in 53% of cases; the 7p13 locus of the *MGC4607* gene in 15%, and at the 3q26.1 locus of the *PDCD10* gene in 10% of patients. These genes encode proteins that are involved in junction formation between vascular endothelial cells and alteration of function due to mutation, which leads to development of thin-walled, dilated blood vessels and endothelial cell gaps characteristic of CCM (2).

Of 292 retrospectively studied patients with the diagnosis of CCM (4), 182 (62%) had findings related to the CM, 95 (33%) patients had CM as an incidental radiographic finding on brain computer tomography (CT) or magnetic resonance imaging (MRI), and 15 (5%) presented with symptoms related to the CM. Altogether 74/184 (40%) patients presened with radiographc evidence of acute hemorrhage, of whom 40 (54%) presented with focal clinical neurological deficits on examination; 15 (20%) had one or more seizures, 13 (18%) had headache, and 6 (8%) patients had neurological symptoms without focal clinical deficits (4). In all, 237 of 292 (82%) had a single CM and 55 (18%) had multiple lesions generally between two to four. Overall, 169 (58%) CM were cortical, 40 (14%) supratentorial subcortical, and 84 (28%) infratentorial in location, 63 (22%) of which were associated with a venous angioma that was cortical in location in 60%, supratentorial subcortical in 13.7%, and infratentorial in 83%, 21% of whom were associated with venous angioma (4).

Neuroimaging criteria for the definition of CCM have previously been described (4–6). T_2-weighted gradient-echo MRI identifies CCM as ill-defined lobulated lesions with a central complicated core surrounded by a rim of decreased signal intensity (Figure 1) that appear at a rate of 0.2 to 0.4 lesions per patient per year (2). Computed tomography shows well-circumscribed nodular lesions with juxtaposition of calcifications, hemorrhage, and cystic components. Cerebral angiography may be normal due to low flow.

Histopathologically, CCM appear as well-circumscribed, dark red to purple lesions surrounded by hemosiderin, a blood breakdown product consisting of iron salts. They are often described as having a popcorn or mulberry appearance, which upon closer inspection reveals clusters of capillary-like channels with a single layer of endothelium without intervening brain parenchyma. The lesions are filled with blood at various stages of thrombosis, and their

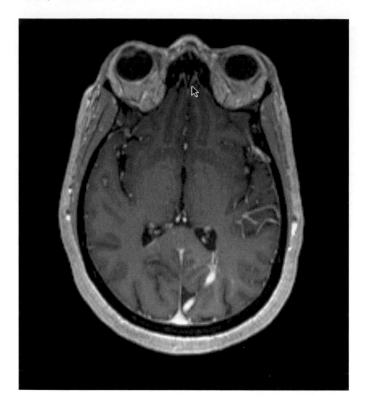

FIG. 1. T_2–weighted magnetic resonance image of a left frontal cavernous malformation.

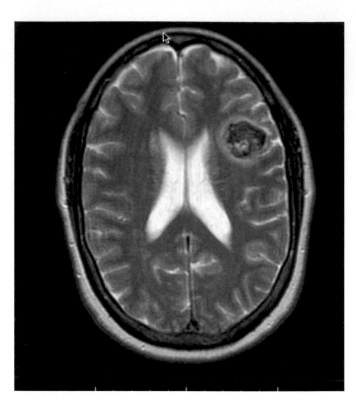

FIG. 2. T_2–weighted magnetic resonance image of a left medial temporal arteriovenous malformation.

size may range from a few millimeters to several centimeters, usually becoming symptomatic when the diameter exceeds one centimeter. The presence of hemosiderin is a sign of previous hemorrhage, even if not clinically overt. Over time, recurrent hemorrhages and thromboses lead to increasing size with eventual mass effect on the surrounding tissue. There are no associated large feeding or draining vessels and low flow maintains intravascular pressure roughly midway between arterial and venous pressures.

The estimated annual rate of prospective hemorrhage of 18% after initial hemorrhage was higher than the observed rates of 2% or less when neurological symptoms at the time of CCM detection were unclear or clearly incidental to radiographic detection of a CCM (4). Moreover, the rate of recurrent hemorrhage of 18% in the first year fell steadily with time to 9% in years 1 to 2; and 1 to 3% during years 2 to 10, with an overall annual rate of 6% of prospective rehemorrhage (4).

With both low rates of prospective hemorrhage in incidentally detected CCM, the steep declining rate of rehemorrhage after two years, and the mild severity of CCM hemorrhage, most clinically asymptomatic patients can generally be assured of the success of conservative management. However, patients with progressive neurological deficits and rehemorrhage may be candidates for micro-

neurosurgical excision or stereotactic radiosurgery, as are those with epilepsy secondary to CCM after extensive evaluation, including electroencephalopathy (EEG), video-EEG, and other studies, such as the Wada test to determine hemispheric dominance; and magnetoencephalography and dedicated brain positron emission tomography (PET) to confirm the localization of epilelpsy and to exclude other epileptogenic lesions. The best outcome of microneurosurgical excision occurs when the lesion is in non-eloquent brain and visible on the pial surface. Radiosurgery was performed with a 201-source cobalt-60 gamma knife unit and 40 mg of methylprednisolone in 82 patients of mean age 37 years, between 1987 and 2000 for surgically inaccesible lesions without unacceptable surgical risk (7). There was a 12% annual hemorrhage rate for the first two years followed by a 0.76% annual rate of hemorrhage per year afterward. New neurological symptoms without hemorrhage after treatment was noted in 13% of patients, suggesting that the treatment be considered in selected younger patients who have sustained a major neurological deficit from their first bleed. A decade later (8), stereotactic radiosurgery (SRS) employing the same technique in 103 patients of mean age 39 years with solitary symptomatic CCM had two or more hemorrhages associated with new neurological deficits rendering them high risk for resection. SAS was associated

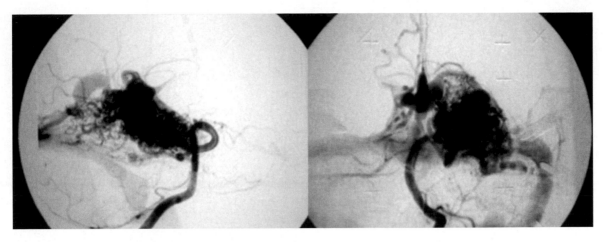

FIG. 3. Lateral and anterioposterior vertebral angiogram of a left medial temporal arteriovenous malformation.

with significant reduction in CCM bleeding rates, especially after a two-year latency interval with a hemorrhage rate of 1% after a two-year latency interval, and minimally lower adverse radiation effects in 11% of patients, leading to worsening of pre-SRS neurological symptoms.

ARTERIOVENOUS MALFORMATIONS

These congenital tangles of abnormal arteries and veins are interconnected by one or more fistulas without an intervening capillary bed. The direct arteriovenous connection results in high-pressure vascular channels, particularly along veins with fibromuscular thickening and incompetent elastic lamina, rendering them at greater risk of rupture (9). The prevalence of sporadic AVM is 0.01 to 0.50% and the incidence is 1 in 100,000, with an estimated 300,000 Americans believed to have intracranial or intraspinal AVM, of which 85% are supratentorial, and 15% are infratentorial. Altogether, AVM represent 10 to 15% of clinically significant cerebral vascular malformations with an estimated yearly.

Clincally apparent AVM are typically diagnosed between age 20 and 40 years, presenting with seizures, headache, and focal neurological deficits in association with intracerebral hemorrhage, stroke, and mass effect from direct compression or swelling related to the AVM. In the absence of bleeding, migraine headaches have been assocaited with AVM. Although the majority of AVM have no known genetic susceptibility, the occurrence of cerebral AVM is increased in several genetic disorders, including hereditary hemorrhagic telangiectasia (HHT) and hereditary neurocutaneous angioma (10). A promoter polymorphism at the 7p15.3 in the *IL6* gene (-174G/C) is associated with susceptibility to intracranial hemorrhage in brain AVM (11). Affected

patients homozygous for the G allele had a 2.62 odds ratio of increased risk of intracranial bleeding compared to carriers of the C allele. The highest IL protein and mRNA levels were associated with the *IL6-174GG* genotype compared to the *GC* and *CC* genotypes (12). It is suggested that *IL6* gene expression may modulate downstream inflammatory and angiocentric targets that contibute to intracranial hemorrhage in brain AVM (12).

Brain AVM are adequately visualized by brain computer tomography (CT), MRI, CT-angiography (CTA), and MR angiography (MRA). While brain CT is sensitive in the detection of acute hemorrhage, CTA provides better information about the vascular detail of the AVM than MRA, whereas the latter and conventional brain MRI permit better information about the relation of the AVM to surrounding cerebral tissue (Figure 2). Functional MRI localizes eloquent areas of the brain, but it is often difficult to interpret because of the high flow rates in the vicinity of the AVM. Despite continued advances in non-invasive imaging modalities, catheter cerebral angiography is the optimal study to examine AVM architecture and to exclude the presence or absence associated aneurysms, obstruction of venous outflow, and the pattern of venous drainage relevent to planning future management (Figure 3).

Most AVM range in size from a few millimeters to the majority of a hemisphere, and pyramidal-shaped with their base at the cortical surface and their apex toward the center of the brain, anywhere in the central nervous system (CNS), although most commonly in the frontal and parietal lobes. The majority present as independent lesions, but occasionally occur with other vascular malformations, making the diagnosis and management more difficult. Arterial feeders to the AVM differ in size and histological composition but share the characteristic of increased luminal diameters and irregular areas of thickening. A single AVM may have one or more arterial feeders that connect directly to anomalous venous loops to form a tangle of vessels or the nidus, which is almost always located subcortically and directs blood flow from feeding arteries into the communicating venules. The latter connect the nidus to surrounding cerebral veins which then converge into one or several major draining veins that distend (Figure 4). The lack of pressure-lowering capillaries between arteries and veins results in high cerebral blood flow through the malformation, often diverting blood away from other regions of the brain leading to ischemic steal phenomena. Pressure exerted by the lesion may cause congestion and edema in the surrounding brain tissue with xanthochromia at the cortical surface from prior hemorrhages.

Hemorrhage occurs in 42 to 72% of clinically inapparent AVM (9, 13) at the annual rate of between 2 to 4% (14), with smaller ones rupturing more often than larger ones (15). Hemorrhage of AVM accounts for approximately 2% of all strokes (16). Brain AVM presenting with hemorrhage, deep venous drainage, and asociated aneurysm have a two-fold greater likelihood of a future hemorrhage (17), each hemorrhage of which may be associated with a 15% mortality and a 30% chance of permanent neurological deficit. Additional risk factors include deep venous drainage, deep location in the basal ganglia, internal capsule, thalamus, and corpus callosum, hypertension, single draining vein, and associated aneurysms (9).

Treatment of AVM includes surgical resection, endovascular embolization, and SRS with the goal of treatment to completlely eliminate the AVM. The Spetzler-Martin grading system for AVM was first introduced in 1986 (18) as a five-tier system based on the size of the AVM, eloquence of the adjacent tissue, and venous draining. It provided a guide to treatment and predictive of outcome. However, perceiving no practical differences within grade I and II or IV and V, the original five-tier system was condensed into a three-tier system with grades I and II condensed to Class A; grade III to Class B, and grades IV and V to Class C (19). Microsurgical removal is the standard for definitive treatment. It is the first line of treatment for Class A or grade I and II AVM, employing microscope-integrated indocyanine green fluorescent angiography during resection to provide immediate high-resolution identification of feeding arteries and draining veins (19, 20). A multimodality approach is employed in grade III or Class B AVM, drawing upon microsurgical, endovascular, and SRS techniques reflecting the complexity and heterogeneity of this Class (20); Class C or grades IV and V AVM, are managed conservatively or by multimodality therapy if not appropriate for observation alone (20). Notwithstanding, there are reports of curative embolization of cerebral AVM (21) employing Onyx, a new liquid embolic material that slowly solidifies and allows for more prolonged and controlled injection, enabling larger

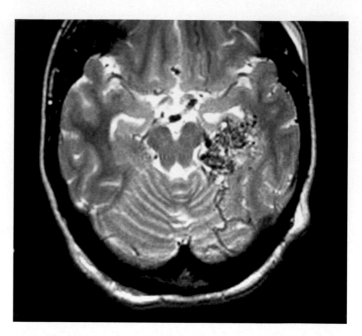

FIG. 4. Intraoperative photograph of a cerebral arteriovenous malformation. The nidus of the AVM is indicated by the black arrow. An arterialized draining vein is indicated by the white arrow.

parts of the malformation to occlude with each micro-catheterization. SRS, which can also produce angiographic and clinical cure in many patients especially those with small AVM, offers no protection from hemorrhage for at least two years, may leave a residual lesion, and carries the risk of radiation necrosis (20).

CAPILLARY TELANGIECTASIAS

Capillary telangiectasias are the most frequent incidental vascular malformations of the pontine brainstem occasionally in the deep periventricular regions of the cerebral hemispheres or spinal cord discovered in neuroradiographic imaging for other reasons or at postmortem examination, with an estimated prevalence of 0.1–0.8%. Up to 50% of patients with symptomatic capillary telangiectasia present after age 30 years, and represent 16 to 20% of all cerebral vascular malformations, although the actual incidence may be higher since the majority are clinically asymptomatic (22). Affected patients present with headache, confusion, weakness, dizziness, visual changes, vertigo, tinnitus, and seizures. In patients presenting with hemorrhage, the cause is most often an associated CCM or AVM (23). They consist of irregular clusters of enlarged, thin-walled vascular channels interposed between normal brain parenchyma and appear as a faint, pink blush on fresh sections of the brain without adjacent gliosis or hemosiderin deposition. Feeding arterioles appear normal, but draining veins from the telangiectasias may be enlarged. The lesions are small, ranging from several millimeters to two centimeters in diameter. Similar to capillaries, telangiectasias are devoid of smooth muscle or elastic fibers and are lined with a single layer of endothelium; however, it is unclear whether the vessels are true capillaries or simply dilated venules. The size of their vascular channels and the presence of intervening parenchyma differentiate capillary telangiectasias from CM. The telangiectasias become more numerous and prominent with age, resulting in recurrent bleeding, which can occur either spontaneously or following minimal trauma. Given their small size, these lesions are best seen only on MRI employing T2-weighted images as isointense or hyperintense areas compared to the normal brain parenchyma, whereas hypointense signal areas reflect the presence of deoxyhemoglobin from slow-flowing blood. Gadolinium-enhanced MRI reveals small radiating venous vessels converging on a small collecting vein. Such small radiating vessels may not resolve the presence of individual vessels, suggesting instead the presence of a homogenous mass.

Hereditary hemorrhagic telangiectasia (HHT) is an AD inherited disorder with high penetrance and a frequency of 1 or 2 in 100,000, that leads to telangiectasia and AVM of the skin, mucosa, liver and brain (24). Clinical diagnostic criteria were suggested (25), including epistaxis, telangiectasia, visceral lesions, and an appropriate family history with a definite diagnosis if three were present, and unlikely if fewer than two. Epistaxis and gastrointestinal bleeding are frequent complications of mucosal involvement, while angiodysplasia are found in the lung, liver, and brain. Two-thirds of patients with HHT are clinically affected by age 16 with epistaxis being the commonest presenting feature. Angiographic studies show arterial aneurysms, arteriovenous communications leading to discrete arteriovenous fistulas, conglomerate masses of angiectasias, phlebectasias, and angiomas. Pulmonary AVM, noted in up to 20% of patients (26), can lead to signfiicant morbidity and mortality by causing heart failure, polycythemia, paradoxical emboli and secondary cerebral infarction, and abscess formation in the brain and elsewhere. Although occasonal patients with HTT have symptomatic cerebral lesions requiring surgical repair (27), up to one-half of HHT carriers fulfill diagnostic criteria for migraine with aura, four-fold the frequency of disease controls and ten-fold the estimated population prevalence (28). Headaches improve in patients who undergo balloon occlusion of pulmonary AVM (29) suggesting the concordance of occult intracranial AVM and the secretion of vasoactive substances, which would normally be removed by the pulmonary vascular bed, instead of reaching the CNS. Reconstruction of cutaneous telangiectases in HTT patients by computer simulation (30) demonstrate that the earliest lesion is focal dilatation of postcapillary venules which continues to enlarge and eventually connect with dilated arterioles through capillaries. With increased vascular size, the capillary segments disappear and a direct arterovenous communication forms associated with perivascular cell infiltration. There are two forms of HHT, HHT1 and HHT2, respectively caused by heterozygous mutations at the 9q34.11 locus of the *ENG* and *ALK1* genes encoding endoglin, a transforming growth factor-beta binding protein, and ALK1, an activin receptor-like kinase. Patients with HHT1 have an earlier onset of epistaxis and telangiectasia than those with HHT2. The latter have more hepatic and dermal involvement, and rare pulmonary AVM.

The differential diagnosis of capillary telangiectasia includes primary or metastatic brain neoplasm such as a cerebral astrocytoma or brainstem glioma, lymphoma, subacute infarction, acute or chronic area of demyelination or inflammation, CM, and the connective tissue disorder, scleroderma manifesting calcinosis, Raynaud syndrome, sclerodactyly, and telangiectasia (CREST). Distinguishing features on neuroimaging suggestive of the diagnosis of capillary telangiectasia include lack of mass effect, unchanging appearance over time, often discernible draining vein, and absence of edema, gliosis, or signs of prior hemorrhage. Given the benign natural history of these lesions, treatment is rarely necessary. However, it is essential to distinguish capillary telangiectasias from other types of vascular malformations that may require further treatment. Typically, capillary telangiectasias are asymptomatic, usually located in the pons, show no mass effect or evidence of previous hemorrhage, and demonstrate no change over time on sequential studies. Once the diagnosis is established, follow-up imaging is not necessary. Treatment is generally conservative in cerebral telangiectasia, with progesterone and estrogen for control of epistaxis and embolotherapy of brain AVM, and pulmonary AVM in HTT1.

DEVELOPMENTAL VENOUS ANOMALIES

The term DVA is a synonym for venous angioma, cerebral venous malformation, and cerebral venous medullary malformation (31). DVA is the most frequently encountered cerebral vascular malformation in both pediatric and adult populations after routine brain and CT and MRI with an incidence of 2.6% (32). This developmentally pure venous structure occurs due to the absence of normal pial or subependymal veins (33). Morphologically, it presents as a cluster of venous radicles that converge into a collecting vein, whether it drains centrifugally toward the cortical surface into cortical veins or the dural venous sinus as an anomalous pathway for the deep venous territory (31, 34), or centripetally toward the network of deep subependymal

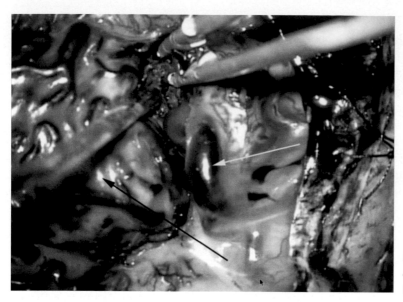

FIG. 5. T_1–weighted magnetic resonance image with contrast showing a developmental venous anomaly located in the left occipital lobe.

veins of the deep venous system from cortical or subcortical venous territorites (33). Histopathologically, it is characterized as hyalinized collecting veins with parietal fibrous thickening, absent elastic lamina, loosely arranged smooth muscle layers, proximal ampullary dilatation or stenosis of the DVA collecting vein at the point of penetration into the draining dural venous sinus (31).

Neuroimaging with CT and MRI demonstrates a typical caput medusae appearance of draining veins into a collecting vein. Digital substration angiography (DSA) captures the hemodynamic behavior of DVA opacifying during the venous phase, with a delayed outflow demonstrating the impairment in drainage whether or not collecting vein stenosis is appreciated (31). Noncontrast brain CT shows an associated hemorrhage, as well as parenchymal dystrophic calcification, cortical atrophy, and white matter lesions in the drainage territory of the DVA (31). Noncontrast T_2-, and T_1-weighted MRI (Figure 5) demonstrates flow voids and phase shift artifact produced by the collecting vein while contrast-enhanced MRI delineates large venous radicles of the caput medusae (31). A so-called arterialized DVA that blushes during the mid-, or late arterial phase of angiography without demonstrable arterial feeders or AVM nidus is termed type 1, whereas type 2 arterialized DVA present with enlarged arterial feeders to the caput medusae without angiographically demonstrable AVM nidus, the latter of which identifies type-3 lesions.

The annual risk of hemorrhage from DVA is estimated to be .22 to .68% (35, 36) although only one-half of the patients were symptomatic. Nineteen separately reported patients with symptomatic DVA and thrombosis of the collecting vein presented with focal and nonfocal neurological deficits attributable to ischemic venous infarction in 53%, parenchymal hemorrhage in 37%, subarachnoid and intraventricular hemorrhage in 5%, and no intraaxial or extraxial lesion in 5%. An overall favorable clinical outcome was noted in 84% of patients, with complete recovery or persistence of mild findings after conservative management in 47%, anticoagulation in 32%, and decompression craniectomy in 21% of patients (31).

Treatment strategies depend upon the presence of parenchymal hemorrhage, characteristics of the neurological eloquence of the lesion, identifiable arterial feeders and an AVM nidus. Incidentally discovered and arterialized DVA without demonstrable arterial feeders or AVM nidus generally do not warrant surgery due to the low risk of hemorrhage. Conversely, care to preserve the collecting vein should be taken when surgically evacuating DVA closer in behavior to AVM to prevent ischemic and hemorrhagic complications, often requiring en bloc resection of the DVA along with surrounding brain tissue, particularly when at a distance from eloquent brain parenchyma (31).

REFERENCES

1. Brown RD, Jr., Flemming KD, Meyer FB, et al. Natural history, evaluation, and management of intracranial vascular malformations. *Mayo Clin Proc* 2005; 80:269–281.

2. Haasdijk RA, Cheng C, Maat-Kievit AJ, et al. Cerebral cavernous malformations: from molecular pathogenesis to genetic counselling and clinical management. *Eur J Hum Genet* 2012; 20:134–140.

3. Al-Shahi Salman R, Murray GD. The next step in understanind the prognosis of cerebral cavernous malformations. *Neurology* 2012; 78:614–615.

4. Flemming KD, Link MJ, Christianson TJH, et al. Prospective hemorrhage risk of intracerebral cavernous malformations. *Neurology* 2012; 78:632–636.

5. Zabramski J, Wascher T, Spetzler R, et al. The natural histoyr of familial cavernous malformations: results of an ongoing study. *J Neurosurg* 1994; 80:422–432.

6. Rigamonti D, Hadley M, Drayer B, et al. Cerebral cavernous malformations: incidence and familal occurrence. *N Engl J Med* 1988; 319:343–347.

7. Hasegawa T, McInerney J, Kondziolka D, et al. Long-term results after stereotactic radiosurgery for patients with cavernous malformations. *Neurosurgery* 2002; 50:1190–1198.

8. Lunsford LD, Khan AA, Niranjan A, et al. Stereotactic radio-surgery for symptomatic solitary cerebral cavernous malformations considered high risk for resection. *J Neurosurg* 2010; 113:23–29.

9. Friedlander RM. Arteriorvenous malformations of the brain. *N Engl J Mcd* 2007, 356.2704–2712.

10. Zaremba J, Stepien M, Jelowicka M, et al. Hereditary neuro-cutaneous angioma: a new clinical entity? *Med Genet* 1979; 16:443–447.

11. Pawlikowska L, Tran MN, Achrol AS, et al. Polymorphisms in genes involved in inflammatory and angiocentric pathways and the risk of hemorrhagic presentation of brain arteriovenous malformations. *Stroke* 2004; 35:2294–2299.

12. Chen Y, Pawlikowska L, Yao JS, et al. Interleukin-6 in brain arteriovenous malformations. *Ann Neurol* 2006; 59:72–80.

13. Brown RD Jr., Wiebers DO, Torner JD, et al. Frequency of intracranial hemorrhage as a presenting symptom and subtype analysis: a population based study of intracranial vascular malformations in Olmsted Count, Minnesota. *J Neurosurg* 1996; 85:29–32.

14. Ponce FA, Spetzler RF, Arteriovenous malformations: classification to cure. *Clin Neurosurgery* 2011; 58:10–12.

15. Duong DH, Younge WL, Vang MC et al. Feeding artery pressure and venous drainage pattern are primary determinants of hemorrhage from cerebral arteriovenous malformations. *Stroke* 1998; 29:1167–1176.

16. Gross CR, Kase CS, Mohr JP, et al. Stroke in south Alabama: incidence and diagnostic features—a population-based study. *Stroke* 1984; 15:249–255.

17. de Costa L, Wallace C, ter Brugge KG, et al. The natural history and predictive features of hemorrhage from brain arteriovenous malformations. *Stroke* 2009; 40:100–105.

18. Spetzler RF, Martin NA. A proposed system for arteriovenous malformations. *J Neurosurg* 1986; 65:476–483.

19. Spetzler RF, Ponce FA. A 3-tier classification of cerebral arteriovenous malformations. *J Neurosurg* 2011; 114:842–849.

20. Ponce FA, Spetzler RF, Arteriovenous malformations: classification to cure. *Clin Neurosurgery* 2011; 58:10–12.

21. Katsaridis V, Papagiannaki C, Aimar E. Curative embolization of cerebral arteriovenous malformations (AVMs) with Onyx in 101 patients. *Neuroradiology* 2008; 50:589–597.

22. Castillo M, Morrison T, Shaw JA, et al. MR imaging and histologic features of capillary telangiectasia of the basal ganglia. *AJNR Am J Neuroradiol* 2001; 22:1553–1555.

23. Van Roost D, Kristof R, Wolf HK, et al. Intracerebral capillary telangiectasia and venous malformation: a rare association. *Surg Neurol* 1997; 48:175–183.

24. Govani FS, Shovlin CL. Hereditary haemorrhagic telangiectasia: a clinical and scientific review. *Eur J Hum Genet* 2009; 17:860–871.

25. Shovlin CL, Guttmacher AE, Buscarini E, et al. Diagnostic criteria for hereditary hemorrhagic telangiectasia (Rendu-Osler-Weber syndrome). *Am J Med Genet* 2000; 91:66–67.

26. Vase P, Holm M, Arendrug H. Pulmonary arteriovenous fistules in hereditary haemorrhagic telangiectasia. *Acta Med Scan* 1985; 218:105–109.

27. Guillen B, Guizar J, de la Cruz, et al. Hereditary hemorrhagic telangiectasia: report of 15 affected cases in a Mexican family. *Clin Genet* 1991; 39:214–218.

28. Steele JS, Nath PU, Burn J, et al. An association between migrainous aura and hereditary haemorrhagic telangiectasia. *Headache* 1993; 33:145–148.

29. White RI Jr., Lynch-Nyhan A, Terry P, et al. Pulmonary arteriovenous malformations: techniques and long-term outcome of embolotherapy. *Radiology* 1988; 169:663–669.

30. Braverman IM, Keh A, Jacobson BS. Ultrastructure and three-dimensional organization of the telangiectases of hereditary hemorrhagic telangiectasia. *J Invest Derm* 1990; 95:422–427.

31. Ruiz DSM, Yilmaz H, Gailloud P. Cerebral developmental venous anomalies: current concepts. *Ann Neurol* 2009; 66:271–283.

32. Sarwar M, McCormick WF. Intracerebral venous angioma. Case report and review. *Arch Neurol* 1978; 35:323–325.

33. Ruiz DSM, Gandhi D. Venous anomaly. *J Neurosurg* 2010; 112:213–214.

34. Lasjaunias P, Burrows P, Planet C. Developmental venous anomalies (DVA).: the so called venous angioma. *Neurosurg Rev* 1986; 9:233–242.

35. Garner TB, Del Curling O Jr., Kelly DL Jr, et al. The natural history of intracranial venous angioma. *J Neurosurg* 1991; 75:715–722.

36. McLaughlin MR, Kondziolka D, Flickinger JD, et al. The prospective ntural history of cerebral venous malformation. *Neurosurgery* 1998; 43:195–200.

CHAPTER 46

Brain Tumors

David S. Younger

The past decade has witnessed significant advances in the classification, diagnosis, and molecular understanding of primary brain tumors. This chapter reviews aspects of childhood and adult primary brain tumors.

GENERAL CONSIDERATIONS

Epidemiology

According to the Central Brain Tumor Registry of the United States (CBTRUS) (1), 62,930 new cases of primary non-malignant and malignant brain and CNS tumors were diagnosed in 2010. With an overall incidence rate of 18.71 cases per 100,000 person-years or 11.52 for nonmalignant contrasted to 7.19 per 100,000 person-years for malignant tumors, the rate of primary nonmalignant and malignant brain and central nervous system (CNS) tumors in women exceeds that of men, respectively 19.88 versus 17.44 per 100,000 person-years.

The pediatric incidence of childhood primary nonmalignant and malignant brain and CNS tumors is considerably less, 4.71 cases per 100,000 person-years, with a rate higher in boys than girls, 4.75 versus 4.66 per 100,000 person-years. An estimated 12,920 deaths were attributed to primary malignant brain and CNS tumors in 2009.

From 1995 to 2006, the five-year survival rate following diagnosis of a primary malignant brain and CNS tumor, including lymphoma, pineal, and olfactory tumors, was 33.6% for men and 37% for women with diminishing rates in successive decades of life. The five-year survival was 72.1% from age 0 to 19 years, compared to 55.9% from age 20 to 44 years, 30.7% from age 45 to 54 years, 16.7% from

age 55 to 64 years, 9.6% from age 65 to 74 years, and 5.2% at age 75 years and older. The commonest tumors were meningeal in 29%, nerve sheath in 24%, and ependymal in 23% of patients so studied, with a slight predominance of women over men and non-Hispanic whites over non-Hispanic blacks; the former comprised 78% of patients, with incidence rates of 79 per 100,000 versus .45 per 100,000 person-years.

Employing criteria of the World Health Organization (WHO) (2), the most frequent histology is the predominantly nonmalignant meningioma, accounting for almost 34% of all tumors, followed by glioblastoma in 17%, pituitary and nerve sheath tumors, respectively, in 13% and 9%, the most common of which are acoustic neuromas, and gliomas in about 32% of all tumors which include astrocytoma, glioblastoma, oligodendroglioma, and ependymoma. Brain tumors are the second commonest malignancy among children, with leukemia being the most common; however, only 7% of all primary brain tumors occurred in children.

Classification

The WHO Classification of Tumors of the Central Nervous System, the universal standard for classifying and grading neoplasms, first published in 1979 (3), established the histological typing of tumors, while the second edition (4) advanced the introduction of immunohistochemistry into diagnostic pathology. The third (5) and current fourth edition (2, 6) incorporated genetic profiles as additional aids to the definition of CNS tumors, and included sections on epidemiology, clinical signs, and symptoms, imaging, prognosis, and predictive factors, and added several new neoplasms and tumor variants.

The International Classification of Diseases for Oncology (ICD-O-3) (7), which serves as an interface between pathologists and cancer registries, provides histological coding for human neoplasms, including topographical codes for spinal cord tumors. An accurate pathological diagnosis is essential to diagnosis and management. To achieve this, the histopathological diagnostic process is rigorously joined with the clinical history, preoperative imaging, any prior pathological diagnoses, as well as the results of tumor biopsy tissue and ancillary studies, including immunohistochemistry, electron microscopy (EM), and molecular studies as may be available (8). The WHO classification of nervous system tumors (2) recognized seven major categories of neoplasms, including 1) *tumors of neuroepithelial tissue,* including astrocytic, oligodendroglial, ependymal, choroid plexus, pineal, and embryonal tumors, the latter of which included medulloblastoma and primitive neuroectodermal tumor (PNET); 2) *tumors of cranial and paraspinal nerves,* among them schwannoma, neurofibroma, perineuroma, and malignant peripheral nerve sheath tumor; 3) *tumors of the meninges,* represented by meningioma, mesenchymal tumors, and primary melanocytic lesions such as melanoma; 4) *lymphomas and hematopoietic neoplasms,* among them primary CNS lymphoma (PCNSL), plasmacytoma, and granulocytic sarcoma; 5) *germ cell tumors,* such as germinant, embryonal carcinoma, and teratoma; 6) *tumors of the sellar region* including craniopharyngioma and pituicytoma; and 7) *metastatic tumors.*

Grading

Histological grading is important in predicting the biological behavior of a tumor, and is an important factor in the choice of therapies, particularly when adjuvant radiation and chemotherapy are contemplated. In 1979, the WHO Classification of CNS tumors (3) included a malignancy or grading scheme across a range of neoplasms rather than a strict histological grading system; however, current grading by the WHO (2) employs a four tier system from grade I to IV. Grade I lesions are generally tumors with low proliferative potential and are likely curable with surgical resection alone. Those designated grade II are generally infiltrative, but despite low proliferative propensity they tend to recur, with some grade II tumors progressing to higher grades as occurs in low-grade astrocytomas that can transform to anaplastic and glioblastoma forms. Grade III neoplasms contain markers of malignancy such as nuclear atypia and brisk mitotic activity. Grade IV tumors show cytologic malignancy, are mitotically active, necrosis-prone, and have a propensity to disseminate craniospinally, examples of which include glioblastoma, embryonal neoplasms, and sarcomas.

SPECIFIC TUMOR TYPES

Astrocytoma

Gliomas arise from glial cells, representing about one-third of all primary brain and CNS tumors by histology. With an annual incidence of five cases per 100,000 people, they represent 70% of the 22,500 new cases of malignant primary brain tumors diagnosed in adults in the United States each year (9). The most common gliomas are astrocytic, oligodendroglioma, ependymoma, and medulloblastoma tumors.

Astrocytic tumors are classified by the WHO (2) into grades I (pilocytic astrocytoma), grade II (diffuse astrocytoma), grade III (anaplastic astrocytoma), and grade IV (glioblastoma). Grades III and IV are considered malignant gliomas. Pilocytic astrocytomas comprise about 6% of all gliomas, and with an overall incidence of about 0.37 per 100,000 persons per year, they are the commonest gliomas in children arising from the glial cells in the cerebellum (1). They are characterized by solid growth of compacted bipolar cells associated with Rosenthal fibers and loose-textured multipolar cells, microcytes, eosinophilic granular bodies, and hyaline inclusions, with little parenchymal entrapment, partial infiltration at the borders, and infrequent malignant anaplastic transformation (Figure 1).

Diffuse infiltrating astrocytoma demonstrates a high degree of cellular differentiation, slow growth, and tends to occur in supratentorial locations. Fibrillary astrocytoma is the most commonly encountered type of diffuse infiltrating astrocytoma, with prototypical cytology of elongated cells, atypical nuclei, and cytoplasmic processes. Anaplastic astrocytoma, which locates hemispherically, is characterized by increased cellularity, nuclear atypia, and mitotic activity.

Glioblastoma is the most frequent and malignant glioma, demonstrating areas of microvascular proliferation, necrosis, or both. Proliferative activity is accompanied by detectable mitoses and angiogenesis is seen in association with sprouting of capillaries from preexisting vessels and necrosis of large areas due to insufficient blood supply. Multiple small irregularly shaped, band-like or serpiginous foci, surrounded by radially oriented densely packed fusiform cells in a pseudopalisading pattern, is considered a hallmark of glioblastoma (Figures 2, 3). Glioblastoma cerebri shows an exceptional extensive infiltration of three or more cerebral lobes and bilateral hemispheric, and not infrequent deep gray matter, brain stem, and cerebellar involvement by malignant astrocytic cells.

There is no unifying clinical presentation for gliomas, which instead depend upon the tissue type, grade, and location of the neoplasm. Relatively circumscribed, slow-growing, deeply situated and often cystic, low-grade astrocytoma typically produces focal neurological deficits or non-localizing signs depending upon the location, often

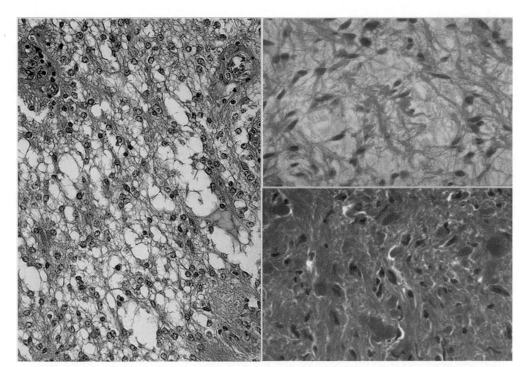

FIG. 1. Pilocytic astrocytoma. There is a compact and spongy pattern of growth with micro-cysts (upper left and lower right. Smear preparation (upper right) shows bipolar cells and Rosenthal fibers.

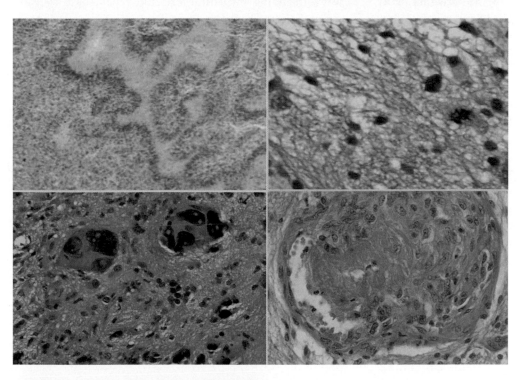

FIG. 2. Glioblastoma. Counter-clockwise from upper left, there is necrosis with pseudopalisading mitotic figures, vascular hyperplasia, and nuclear pleomorphism.

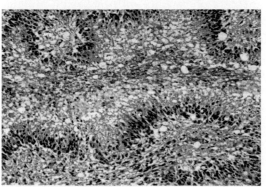

FIG. 3. Glioblastoma. Necrosis with surrounding pseudopalisading and hypoxic cells are the pathological hallmark of glioblastoma.

without seizures. Those that occur in the optic pathways may lead to visual loss or proptosis, while internal capsule localization may lead to initial hemiparesis, and others with cerebellar and brainstem lesions may present with nausea, vomiting, hydrocephalus, clumsiness, or incoordination. Headache, which usually accompanies dural irritation or increased intracranial pressure (ICP), is more common in diffuse astrocytoma and glioblastoma, both of which occur supratentorially. Involvement of the frontal and temporal regions of both children and adults produce seizures, language difficulties, personality and behavioral changes, as well as motor and sensory deficits due to mass effect. Higher grade glioblastoma and gliomatosis cerebri respectively present with less than a three-month history of rapid deterioration, including headache, increased ICP, nausea, vomiting, and papilledema, and seizures in the former, or headache, mental status change, lethargy, dementia, seizures, corticospinal tract (CST) signs, gait disturbance, and multiple cranial nerve deficits in the latter.

Primary brain tumors are usually identified by computed tomography (CT) and magnetic resonance imaging (MRI) employing T_1-weighed, T_2-weighted and gadolinium-enhanced images. These imaging studies typically show a heterogeneous enhancing mass with surround edema. In general, the higher the grade of astrocytoma, the more ill-defined, diffusely infiltrating, and heterogeneous the images will be, with more surrounding T_2 hyperintense signals indicative of vasogenic edema. Accordingly, MRI of glioblastoma in addition shows central areas of necrosis and more extensive peritumoral edema than that associated with anaplastic gliomas (10). Coronal MRI (Figure 4) in a patient with glioblastoma showed an irregularly shaped tumor with central area of necrosis and adjacent ring enhancement that correlated with poorly delineated necrotic tumor tissue at postmortem examination. The classic images of gliobastoma multiforme include central T_1- and T_2-hyperintensities, and a butterfly appearance in the spread of the tumor from one side to the other via the anterior corpus callosum.

There has been important progress in the understanding of the molecular pathogenesis of malignant gliomas, especially in the importance of cancer stem cells (11, 12). The cellular origin of gliomas, which has been ascribed to a small population of neural stem cells and glial progenitor cells in multiple regions of the adult brain, may contribute to the resistance of malignant gliomas to standard therapies. While radioresistance in stem cells generally results from the preferential activation of DNA-damage response pathways (13), chemoresistance results partly from over-expression of O⁶-methylguanine-DNA methyltransferase (MGMT), the upregulation of multidrug resistance genes, and the inhibition of apoptosis (14–16). These cells, which are pluripotent and self-renewing, have been found in the subventricular zone, lining of the ventricles, dendate gyrus, hippocampus, and subcortical white matter, and stain positive for CD133 (14).

Stem cells isolated from ependymoma are consistent with a radial glia phenotype, suggesting them as candidate cells of origin (17). The molecular and cellular events associated with gliomagenesis and malignant transformation appears to result from the sequential accumulation of genetic aberrations and the deregulation of growth-factor signaling pathways (11, 18). This multistep process involves genetic losses and gains on chromosomes, copy number alterations and allelic imbalances (19), with loss of heterozygosity (LOH), evident at distinct loci or in entire copies on chromosome 10, suggesting the concomitant presence of tumor suppressor genes. Other findings include oncogene amplification of the epidermal growth factor receptor (*EGFR*) gene on chromosome 7, amplification of cyclin-dependent kinase 4 (*CDK4*), glioma-associated oncogene (*GL1*) and cyclin D1 (*CCND1*), and a mutator phenotype due to dysfunction of several possible DNA repair pathways, including nucleotide excision repair, base excision repair, mismatch repair, and direct reversal of lesions in recombination (19, 20).

The majority of malignant gliomas including GBM, demonstrate inactivating mutations in either the TP53, a short-lived transcription factor that is upregulated in response to cellular stress, DNA strand breaks, and toxins, and facilitates DNA repair by halting the cell cycle for repair enzymes to work. Others may contribute to cell death by setting the cells apoptotic threshold and inducing transcription of other pathogenic genes (21).

The overall survival of patients with glioblastoma remains exceptionally poor despite progress in the surgical, radiotherapy (RT), and chemotherapy (CTX) management of brain tumors, with less than 20% of patients surviving more than one year and less than 3% living longer than three years (22, 23). Excluding myxopapillary and subependymoma, a poor outcome in ependymoma was correlated with anaplastic changes, mitotic index, proliferative indices, foci of hypercellularity, and less differentiated tumor cells (24). Cerebrospinal dissemination is also associated with a poor prognosis.

Much of the care of patients with malignant gliomas involves general medical management of the commonest problems, including seizures, peritumoral edema, venous thromboembolism, fatigue, and cognitive disturbances (25). Corticosteroids such as dexamethasone are used to treat peritumoral edema, however Cushing syndrome, corticosteroid myopathy, and a propensity for *Pneumocystis jiroveci* pneumonitis, osteoporosis, and compression fractures, may develop in patients who receive prolonged high-dose therapy, the latter of which are preventable with vitamin D, calcium, and bisphosphonate supplements.

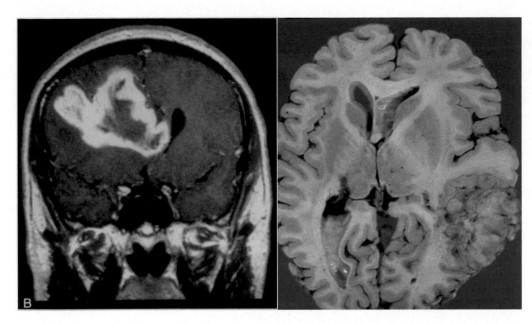

FIG. 4. Glioblastoma. Coronal MRI (left) shows an irregularly shaped tumor with a central area of necrosis and adjacent contrast ring enhancement. A transverse section of the postmortem specimen (right) shows a poorly delineated, gray, necrotic tumor.

Corticotropin-releasing factor, bevacizumab, and VEGFT inhibitors that decrease peritumoral edema, may reduce the needs for corticosteroids (25, 26). While those who present with seizures should be managed with antiepileptic drugs, there is no benefit in the routine use of antiepileptic drugs in newly diagnosed patients with brain tumors who have not had a seizure (27). Other medical considerations include an increased risk of venous thromboembolism with a cumulative incidence of up to 30% (25, 28), the prevention of which with anticoagulation or low-molecular-weight heparin is relatively low compared to the likelihood of an intratumoral hemorrhage.

The standard alternative care of newly diagnosed patients with WHO grade III and IV gliomas (9) is generally maximal feasible resection, followed by RT with concomitant or adjuvant temozolomide (TMZ) (29). Surgical debulking reduces the symptoms from mass effect and provides tissue for definitive diagnosis and molecular studies employing MRI-guided neuro-navigation, intraoperative MRI, functional MRI, intraoperative mapping, and fluorescence-guided surgery (30), and in turn, improves the effectiveness and safety of surgery. Molecular markers have had an important impact on the diagnosis and treatment of gliomas (31). Radiation therapy administered as 60 Gy of partial-field external-beam irradiation is delivered five days per week in fractions of 1.8 to 2.0 Gy in six weeks to the tumor volume with 2 to 3 cm margin (32). Whereas 90% of tumors recur at the original site (33), the addition of surgery to RT increases survival among patients with glioblastoma from four months to up to one year, while newer CTX (34), targeted molecular agents (35), and anti-angiogenic agents (36) further increase the effectiveness of RT. Study endpoints have included overall survival (OS) or survival rate (SR), progression-free survival (PFS), radiographic response rate divided into complete response (CR) and partial response (PR), and progressive disease (PD) (37, 38). The SR at two years among patients who received RT and TMZ was significantly improved compared to those treated with RT alone (26.5% versus 10.4%) (34). Promoter methylation that silences the *MGMT* gene (39) predicts benefit from temozolomide (40).

Oligodendroglioma

With an estimated incidence of 0.27 to 0.35 per 100,000 persons, oligodendroglioma accounts for approximately 6.6% of all primary brain and CNS gliomas, and 2.1% of all primary brain and CNS tumors by histologic subtypes (1). They arise preferentially in the cortex and white matter of the cerebral hemispheres, with the frontal lobe in up to two-thirds of cases, and temporal, parietal, and occipital lobes in decreasing frequency (41, 42). Two-thirds of patients present with seizures, as well as headache, signs of increased ICP, focal neurological deficits, and cognitive or mental changes (43). Oligodendroglioma tumors comprise a spectrum of well-differentiated tumors to frankly malignant tumors. Oligodendroglioma neoplasms are diffusely infiltrating gliomas of moderate cellularity that correspond histologically to WHO grade II, composed of monomorphic cells with clear cytoplasm, uniform round nuclei, and a perinuclear halo, the so-called "fried egg" appearance, and a dense network of branching capillaries (Figure 5). Additional characteristics include microcalcifications and mucoid cystic degeneration. Tumors with significant

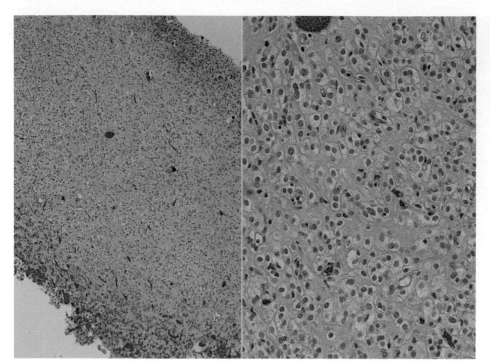

FIG 5. Oligodendroglioma. Low magnification of tumor tissue (left) and higher magnification (right) reveals cells with clear cytoplasm around round nuclei characteristic of the so called "fried-egg" appearance; branching capillaries can be seen.

mitotic activity, prominent microvascular proliferation, and conspicuous necrosis indicate progression to anaplastic oligodendroglioma (AO) (WHO grade III) (2).

While AO and anaplastic oligoastrocytomas (AOA) may be indolent, they are typically incurable despite maximal therapeutics. The role of extensive surgical resection is controversial and the proper timing and sequence of RT and CTX alone or in combination is undefined as established in three randomized phase III trials (44–46). In concept, RT has effective in AO, but patients harboring unbalanced translocation of 19p and 1q respectively in up to 89% and 20% of patients, make them particularly sensitive to chemotherapy with procarbazine/1-[1-[2-chloroethyl]-3-cyclohexyl-1-nitrosourea (CCNU), and lomustine/vincristine (PCV), with response rates of up to 100% compared to those without deletions (44). With the additional risk of delayed RT toxicity, up to 42% of surveyed neuro-oncologists recommended CTX alone in 1p19q codeleted cases, deferring RT until after disease progression (47). Moreover, among CTX regimens, TMZ has largely replaced PCV, at least in part because it is viewed as better tolerated and easier to administer. However, controversy remains as to whether TMZ efficacy is equivalent to that of PCV (48). Among 1,013 adults with OA/AOA treated retrospectively between 1981 and 2007 (49) treatment with CTX+RT sequentially and concurrently at diagnosis lengthened TTP but no OS compared to CTX alone for the overall cohort, likely because the majority of patients who received CTX alone were treated with RT after progression. Unexpectedly, RT alone was associated with inferior TTP and OS. In codeleted cases,

TTP was shorter following CTX than CTX+ RT, but differences in OS did not approach significance. Shorter TTP was observed following RT alone than CTX alone. Deferring RT would have avoided the risk of late RT-induced neurocognitive decline resulting from early RT. Among cases with no 1p or 19q deletion, both TTP and OS were shorter following CTX or RT alone than CTX+RT. In essence, PCV alone afforded better disease control than TMZ alone in 1p19q codeleted cases, with median TTP longer by more than 4 years, a medically and statistically significant difference despite the small sample size for each group (49). Two international trials opened for patients with anaplastic gliomas stratified by 1p19q deletion status, the Codeleted Tumors (CODEL) and Concurrent and Adjuvant TMZ for 1p19q Nondeleted Tumors (CATNON) trials that, respectively, randomized patients with 1p19q codeleted tumors to RT alone, RT with concurrent and adjuvant TMZ, or TMZ alone; or involve combinations of RT with or without TMZ at different time points, may help make more definitive treatment recommendations for OA and AOA tumors.

Ependymoma

Ependymoma are well demarcated from surrounding parenchyma. Ependymal tumors include subependymoma and myoxopapillary ependymoma, both indolent tumors (WHO grade I), ependymoma (WHO grade II), subcategorized into cellular, papillary, clear cell, and tanycytic cell types; and anaplastic ependymoma (WHO grade III). Subependymoma are indolent tumors typically attached to the ventricular wall composed of glial tumor cell clusters. Microcysts have occasional mitoses and much lesser degrees of proliferation than other ependymal neoplasms. Nuclear clusters are usually embedded in abundant dense fibrillary matrix. The myxopapillary variant, which arises in the filum terminale, appears as a vascular ovoid mass with a thin capsule and often adherent nerve roots. Ependymoma are slow-growing tumors of children and young adults, originating from the ventricle wall or spinal canal, composed of neoplastic ependymal cells. The commonest or classic histolopathologic pattern is a papillary architecture of round to oval nuclei, with rare mitoses and the feature of perivascular pseudorosettes and ependymal rosettes that originate from tumor cells arranged radially around blood vessels with perivascular anuclear zones of glial fibrillary protein (GFAP)-rich and fibrillary processes. True rosettes and ependymal canals, formed instead by columnar cells arranged around a central lumen, develop in a minority of cases (2). Occasional non-palisading foci of necrosis may be seen. The tumor and parenchymal interface is typically sharp. The cellular variant is most common in extraventricular locations, and papillary ependymoma typically form linear epithelial-like surfaces along areas of CSF exposure while clear cell tumors display an oligodendroglioma-like appearance with cell perinuclear halos and tanycytic tumors and are most commonly found in the spinal cord.

Anaplastic tumors are characterized by increased cellularity, mitotic activity, microvascular proliferation, necrosis, and pseudopalisading necrosis. Geographic tumor necrosis may be found in all ependymal subtypes. Cytogenic changes in ependymoma include aberrations of chromosome 22 (50). Supratentorial tumors preferentially show loss of chromosome 9 (51) and, unlike other gliomas, the *NF2* gene shows an increased incidence of mutations in intramedullary spinal ependymoma (52).

Management of intracranial ependymoma employing surgery alone (53) as primary treatment in 22 patients with infra- and five patients with supratentorial tumors, 14 of whom had ependymoma (WHO grade II) and 13 with anaplastic ependymoma (WHO grade III), achieved complete tumor resection with the first operation in three-quarters of cases, and primary adjuvant therapy consisting of CTX and RT alone or in combination in the remainder, was associated with a five-year PFT in 80% following a complete surgical resection, and 56% PFS in those with residual tumor. Among 44 patients who underwent postoperative RT following subtotal resection of supratentorial ependymoma lesions (54), age, the extent of surgery, and location were major independent prognostic factors.

Medulloblastoma

Medulloblastoma was recently reviewed (55). It comprises 13% of primary brain and CNS tumors in children age up to 14 years, and 3.9% in those age 15 to 19 years, and with an estimated incidence of 1% of all primary brain and CNS tumors by histology (1). Medulloblastoma, which corresponds histologically to WHO grade IV lesions, has a peak age at presentation of 7 years, with 70% occurring in individuals younger than age 16. In adulthood, 80% arise in the age 21 to 40 groups (56). Different polyomaviruses have been considered as possible causative agents, including the human JC polyomavirus (57) and transgenic mice that express SV40 large T-antigen under the influence of different promoters (58).

More than three-quarters of tumors occur in the cerebellar vermis and project into the fourth ventricle. The main clinical manifestations are cerebellar, including gait ataxia and those of hydrocephalus and increased ICP, present in up to 80% of patients at presentation due to CSF obstruction.

The duration of symptoms before diagnosis ranges from one to three months. Other findings at presentation include head tilt and rigidity of the neck associated with tonsilar herniation, diplopia due to abducens palsy, and other cranial nerve deficits. Infants and young children will manifest open fontanels, enlarging head, vomiting, and irritability, and those with dilatation of the third ventricle may have paralysis of visual upgaze. Other children with rapid growth of expanding lesions may present with alteration of consciousness. Those that occur in the first decade of life are usually located in the midline with the inferior aspect in the fourth ventricle arising from the inferior medullary velum, while others of the second decade lateralize toward the lateral cerebellar hemisphere and the cerebellopontine angle cistern (59).

Medulloblastoma classically appear hypointense to cortex on T_1-, and T_2-weighted and fluid-attenuated inversion recovery (FLAIR) images. However, with administration of intravenous contrast, they demonstrate homogeneous enhancement on T_1-weighted MRI, with low signal of the tumor on FLAIR images, and increased signal on diffusion-weighted imaging (55, 60). The tumors appear hyperintense to the cerebellum on brain CT, reflecting tumor hypercellularity with occasional calcification. The tumors appear histopathologically as densely packed cells with round-to-oval or carrot-shaped hyperchromatic nuclei surrounded by scanty cytoplasm (Figure 6) (2).

There are desmoplastic nodular, anaplastic, and large cell tumor types. Desmoplastic medulloblastoma are composed of ill-defined and rudimentary reticulum-free nodular zones surrounded by densely packed highly proliferative reticulin-rich internodular areas (61). Those with extensive nodularity and advanced neuronal differentiation have little or no intranodular tissue. The large cell, anaplastic types are comprised of sheets and lobules of round cells with pleomorphic nuclei, prominent nucleoli, and more abundant cytoplasm (62). Leptomeningeal dissemination is a common feature of supratentorial medulloblastoma (Figure 7).

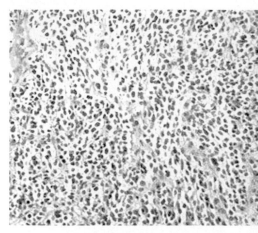 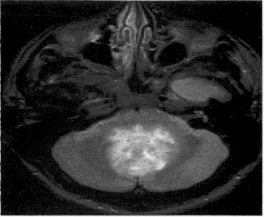

FIG. 6. Medulloblastoma. The tumors are typically highly cellular and contain undifferentiated neoplastic cells (left). Brain MRI (right) shows a heterogeneous enhancing midline cerebellar tumor.

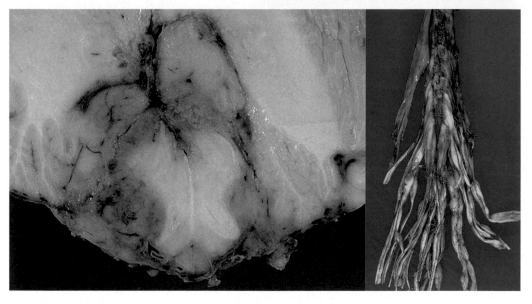

FIG. 7. Medulloblastoma. Leptomeningeal (left) and lumbar region (right) dissemination are common features of medulloblastoma.

The commonest cytogenetic abnormality in medulloblastoma is isochromosome 17q, present in up to 40% of tumors (63) resulting in both loss- and gain-of-function owing to a breakpoint in the short arm and a dicentric resulting structure. The molecular biology of medulloblastoma has been reviewed (64). Medulloblastoma can be caused by germline mutations at the 10q24.32 locus of the *SUFU* gene, at the 13q13.1 locus of the *BRCA2* gene and at the 1p34.1 locus of the *PTCH2* gene. The recognition of multiple signaling pathways in medulloblastoma malignancy (65) has led to therapeutic advances. Berman and colleagues (66) investigated the efficacy of cyclopamine that blocks the hedgehog pathway in preclinical models of malignant childhood medulloblastoma, which blocked proliferation *in vitro* and induced changes in gene expression consistent with initiation of neuronal differentiation and loss of neuronal stem-cell-like character. A patient with metastatic medulloblastoma refractory to multiple therapies had activation of the hedgehog pathway with loss of heterozygosity and somatic mutation of the *PTCH1* gene encoding patched-1, a negative regulator of the sonic hedgehog (SHH) receptor pathway (67).

Treatment with the hedgehog pathway inhibitor GDC-0449 was associated with rapid, although transient, regression of the tumor and reduction of symptoms. A murine model of medulloblastoma is caused by Cre-LoxP-mediated inactivation of Rb and p53 tumor suppressor genes in the cerebellar external granular layer cells (68). The preoperative extent of disease, and the presence of postoperative residual disease, combined with histology and immunohistochemistry and molecular genetic studies have combined to improve the stratification of children and adults.

In general, patients with localized disease resulting from total or near-total resectable tumors without evidence of dissemination on staging studies, and near-total or total postoperative resection, have the lowest risk deemed to be good or average in comparison to high-risk patients with disseminated or subtotal resections (59). The results of histological analysis and molecular genetic studies performed on tissue obtained at the time of surgery adds to the precision of staging, with classical or desmoplastic histology; β-catenin staining; monosomy 6; SHH pathway, loss of 17p 13.3 or i (17q), associated, respectively, with good or average risk. Anaplastic histology, heightened expression of *ERBB2*, *MYCC*, higher surviving expression, and P53 accumulation were associated with poorer prognosis. Other molecular genetic findings such as increased TrkC and catenin expression were associated with improved survival, while overexpressed PDGFRα and upregulated downstream RAS/mitogen-activated protein kinase MAPK signal transduction pathway conveyed a higher stratified risk and poorer prognosis (55, 69). Twenty adult patients with medulloblastoma who received craniospinal RT (70) had a three-year DFS and OS rates of 45% and 50%, respectively. An improved outcome was associated with a higher clinical function, neurologic symptoms for >30 days, lateral tumor location, standard risk, no hydrocephalus, and brain-boosted craniospinal RT field at a dose of 30 Gy or more.

Schwannoma

Although the vast majority of schwannomas occur outside the CNS, intracranial schwannomas show a strong predilection for the eighth cranial nerve in the cerebellopontine angle, particularly in the autosomal dominant (AD) disorder NF2. The disorder occurs with an estimated incidence of one in 25,000 live births and nearly 100% penetrance by age 60 years (71). The tumors arise along a segment of the nerve root, usually posterior, after it has penetrated the pia. The adjacent cochlear division of the eighth nerve is almost never the site of origin. They are firm, well circumscribed, encapsulated and, in most instances, solitary with a microscopic appearance of interwoven bundles of long spindle-shaped bipolar Schwann cells characteristic of the Antoni A pattern. The intermingled and pleomorphic Schwann cell pattern embedded in a loose eosinophilic matrix characterizes the Antoni B pattern, both of which display sparse mitotic figures. The parallel alignment of spindle nuclei separated by an eosinophilic matrix form nuclear palisades or Verocay bodies (Figure 8). Hypercellular, plexiform, or multinodular, and a rare melanotic unencapulated variant containing melanosomes, are encountered.

NF2 has few of the hallmarks of the peripheral or type 1 form of NF (NF1). Gardner and Frazier (72), and later Gardner and Turner (73), described five generations of 38 members who were deaf because of bilateral acoustic neuromas, with average age at onset of 20 years. Mayfrank and colleagues (74) described ten sporadic cases, each due to presumed new mutational events. Among 100 patients of mean age 21 years in whom neurological presentation was attributed to vestibular schwannoma, cranial meningioma, and spinal tumors (75, 76), 44 presented with deafness, 35 of whom were unilateral. Those and others were divided into early, rapid course, and other tumors, and a second type of late onset, benign course, and bilateral vestibular schwan-

noma involvement. The criteria for the diagnosis of both NF1 and NF2 was suggested by bilateral eighth nerve masses seen with CT or MRI, and a first-degree relative with NF2 and either unilateral eighth nerve mass or neurofibroma, meningioma, glioma, schwannoma, or juvenile posterior subscapular lenticular opacity was noted (77). Pastores and colleagues (78) noted that acoustic neuromas measuring less than 8 mm might be missed in presymptomatic individuals at risk by use of gadolinium-enhanced MRI. Parry and colleagues (79) identified mutations in the *NF2* gene in two-thirds of 32 patients assigned 20 different mutations, suggesting that their results confirmed the association between nonsense and frameshift mutations and clinical manifestations compatible with severe disease. Two other mitigating factors which increased the severity of disease were protein-truncating mutations versus single codon alterations, and mutations that led to premature truncation of the NF2 protein. This disorder, which results from mutations at the 22q12.2 locus of the *NF2* tumor suppressor gene encoding neurofibromin-2, also called merlin. Microsurgical resections are considered definitive therapy while stereotactic radiosurgery prevents long-term tumor growth, maintains neurologic function, and prevents new deficits (80).

Meningioma

Meningiomas arise from meningothelial cells of the arachnoid membrane with broad dural attachment and tumor-free margins (Figure 9), while others show invasion through the dura (Figure 10) where there may be invasion into the underlying calvarium cause hyperostosis. Adjacent brain may be compressed but rarely shows parenchymal invasion.

The grading of meningiomas has been reviewed extensively (81). These tumors were subcategorized by the WHO (2) into 15 histological subtypes and graded according to cytopathologic features and invasiveness. Among them, meningothelial, fibrous, and transitional meningiomas are the most common. Criteria used in grading meningiomas by the WHO classification largely followed those outlined by Perry and colleagues (82, 83).

Grade I tumors were characterized by typical morphology and low proliferative activity. Grade II, or atypical meningiomas, were defined as tumors showing increased proliferative activity with four or more mitoses per ten-high power field (HPF), or at least of the features of increased cellularity, sheet-like patternless growth, macronucleoli, small cell change, or spontaneous necrosis unrelated to embolization. Grade III, or anaplastic, was diagnosed when frank histological anaplasia was present as, for example, if the tumor resembled carcinoma, melanoma, or sarcoma, or were in the presence of 20 or more mitoses per 10 HPF. Meningiomas may show progression upon recurrence, and in most tumors multiple

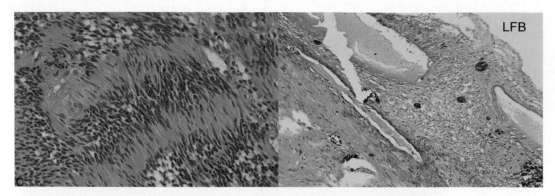

FIG. 8. Schwannoma. Low (right) and high power (left) sections of tumor show elongated tumor cells with slight nuclear polymorphism forming palisades and Verocay bodies. Adjacent nerve fibers are identified a Luxol Fast Blue stain.

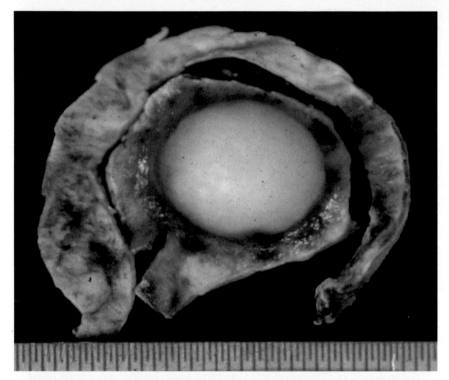

FIG. 9. Meningioma. Macroscopic features include a well demarcated dural based tumor with margin of recession free of tumor.

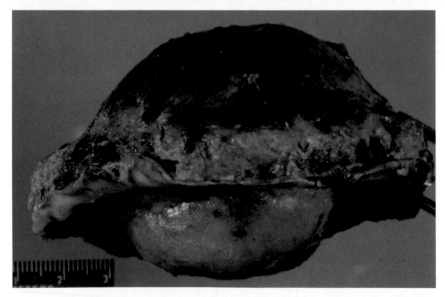

FIG. 10. Meningioma. Macroscopic features include both intra- and extra-calvarial components. These tumors often invade bone.

morphological patterns may be present such that a given subtype should be reserved as the predominant pathology. MIB-1 and p53 labeling, and DNA flow cytometry are helpful adjunctive methods in evaluating the proliferative activity in meningiomas. An MIB-1 index >4% was associated with an increased risk of recurrence, similar to atypical meningiomas (84). The mitosis-specific antibody anti-phosphohistone-H3 (PHH3) recognizes mitotic figures with a higher sensitivity than hematoxylin and esosin (H&E), and facilitates rapid reliable grading of meningiomas according to WHO 2000 criteria (85). The presence of brain invasion in a histologically benign meningioma confers an increased frequency of recurrence similar to that of atypical meningioma (83).

Meningiomas can exhibit a variety of histological appearances. Typical benign meningothelial meningiomas, the commonest subtype, presents with characteristic uniform oval tumor cells and ample tightly clustered cytoplasm, without distinct cell borders, arranged in small lobules. Clearing of nuclei and distinct intranuclear inclusions (Figure 11) are frequent, as are wrapping of cells into whorl formation and psammoma bodies (Figure 12). The vast majority of meningiomas stain for epithelial membrane antigen (EMA) and vimentin positivity is found in all meningiomas (Figure 13). Electron microscopy shows the ultrastructural features that include an abundance of intermediate filaments of vimentin, complex interdigitating cellular processes, and demosomal intercellular junctions (Figure 14). These cell surface specializations, as well as intermediate filaments, are few in fibrous meningiomas, the cells being separated instead by collagen.

Neuroimaging employing T_1-weighted MRI shows the characteristic features of the meningioma dural base, its interface with adjacent brain, and potential mass effects (Figures 15, 16). Magnetic resonance spectroscopy (MRS), which measures the concentrations of various metabolites producing spectral peaks with unique resonance frequency, height, width, and area, facilitates the differentiation of meningeal from non-meningeal tumors and grading (86–88), wherein meningiomas can be distinguished by increased intratumoral alanine, pyruvate, and choline, with a decrease in creatine, the reciprocal of which characterizes gliomas and metastases (89). A significant increase in spectral lactate was associated with malignancy among embolized meningiomas (90), as was the lipid/Cr ratio that differentiated the WHO meningioma grades I to III (91).

Perfusion-weighted MRI, employing an exogenous contrast agent or blood coupled with the blood oxygen level-dependent (BOLD) principle, in which oxygenated and deoxygenated blood, each with different paramagnetic effects; or arterial spin labeling to obtain radiofrequency impulses and images representative of regional cerebral blood volume, detects hypervascularized tumor foci and areas of hypovascularized necrosis. An increasing grade of meningioma was associated with increased rCBV and differentiated preoperative grade I and II meningiomas (92), and others with grade III tumors revealed abnormal rCBV in tumoral parenchyma and peritumoral edema in preoperative meningothelial, fibrous, angiomatous, and anaplastic meningiomas (93). Positron emission tomography (PET), which detects differences in the tumor-to-gray-matter ratio (TGR) preoperatively in benign and atypical-malignant lesions, correlated with M1B-1 labeling, mitotic counts, WHO grade, and brain parenchymal invasion (94, 95). Genetic mutations at the 22q12.2 locus of the *NF2* gene can be found in up to 60% of sporadic meningioma (94).

For the majority of patients presenting with a meningioma, the lesion is benign and a surgical cure is obtained by means of gross-total resection. In contrast to benign meningiomas, atypical and anaplastic meningiomas are associated with shorter overall and PFS (96). Since recurrences are seen in up to one-half of atypical and anaplastic meningiomas, many of these tumors are treated with adjuvant RT and external-beam radiation therapy (EBRT) for recurrences. Retrospective studies of the efficacy of treatment for meningioma WHO Grades II and III attempting to clarify the most efficacious treatment for non-benign meningiomas have been challenged by the 2007 WHO classification that included a more pronounced stratification in prognosis between grade II and III (2, 96).

Primary CNS Lymphoma

The demographics of primary CNS lymphoma (PCNSL) and the impact of the acquired immune deficiency syndrome (AIDS), human immunodeficiency type 1 virus (HIV-1) epidemic, and introduction of highly effective antiviral therapy (HAART) are extensively summarized by Louis and colleagues (2). Altogether, PCNSL comprise an estimated 1.62% of all primary brain and CNS tumors by histology (1). Incidence ranges from 0.8% to 1.5%, up to 6.6% of primary intracranial neoplasms worldwide (97) as a consequence of the impact of the AIDS epidemic. Prior to the introduction of HAART, the incidence of PCNSL in AIDS was 4.7 per 1,000 person-years, about 3,600-fold higher than in the general population (98), with 2 to 12% of AIDS patients developing PCNSL, mainly during the later stages of AIDS (99). HAART reduced the incidence of non-Hodgkin's lymphoma (NHL) to 0.4 for primary and secondary brain lymphomas in AIDS (100). PCNSL affected all ages with a peak incidence in immunocompromised persons during the sixth to seventh decade, with a male-to-female ratio of 3:2. Epstein-Barr virus (EBV) infection plays a major role in immunocompromised patients with PCNSL, the genome of which is present in more than 95% of affected patients.

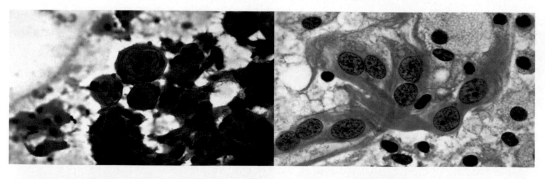

FIG. 11. Meningioma. The smear preparation highlights the whorls (left) and nuclear pseudo-inclusions (right).

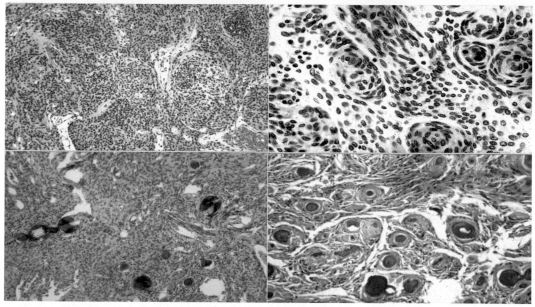

FIG. 12. Meningioma. Hypercellular tissue seen in the bottom left panel is followed left to right in the upper panel by whorl formations and psammoma bodies in the bottom right panel.

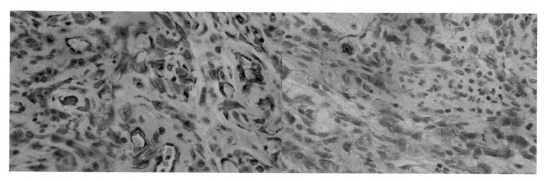

FIG. 13. Meningioma. These tumors are immunoreactive with vimentin (left) and epithelial membrane antigen (right).

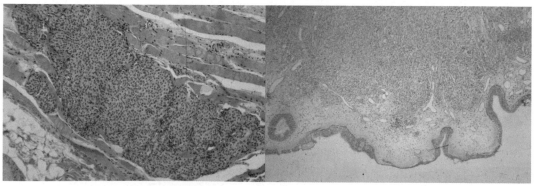

FIG. 14. Meningioma. Ultrastructural analysis reveals desmosomal an intercellular junctional complex composed of specialized cell surfaces as well as intermediate filaments shown in the middle of the electron micrograph.

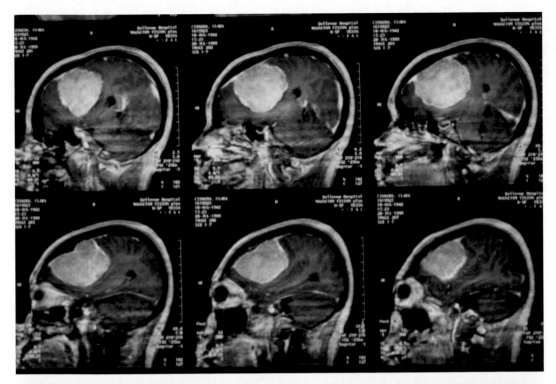

FIG. 15. Meningioma. T_1-weighted MRI after gadolinium showing consecutive images of a dural-based large tumor with a distinct interface that exerts marked mass effect on adjacent brain tissue.

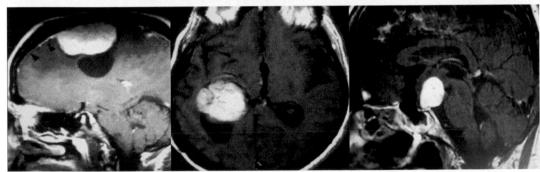

FIG. 16. Meningioma. T_1-weighted MRI after gadolinium showing, respectively, from left to right, convexity, intraventricular and basal large masses, each with bright contrast enhancement. The convexity tumor has both adjacent cysts and obvious dural tails.

Up to two-thirds of PCNSL involve the supratentorial space and up to one-half may be multiple in AIDS and posttransplant patients. Dural and epidural primary tumors are rare. Occult lymphoma occurs in less than 10% of patients presenting with CNS lesions, warranting systemic evaluation. Most patients present with focal neurological deficits, including seizures, and evidence of elevated ICP. MRI has been the most sensitive neuroimaging study to detect PCNSL, which shows isointense to hyperintense lesions on T_2-FLAIR, and diffusion-weighted images that densely enhance with administration of intravenous contrast (101). Corticosteroids may lead to disappearance of lesions, suggesting the diagnosis of PCNSL. ^{18}F-Fluorodeoxyglucose (FDG) PET is a useful noninvasive adjunct to conventional PCNSL, and is more sensitive than conventional body staging, disclosing a systemic site of malignancy in 15% of patients for staging of PCNSL (102). Cytological examination of the CSF is of diagnostic value in up to one-third of patients with PCNSL and in up to 95% of those with metastatic lymphoma. CSF flow cytometry greatly improves diagnostic accuracy, more than twice that of cytomorphology, which should still nonetheless be performed (103).

The probability of meningeal dissemination, present in 16% of patients with PCNSL in a large prospective study (104) is higher in patients with CSF pleocytosis of >5/µL and is associated with a discordant rate of monoclonal polymerase chain reaction (PCR) noted in 32%, and cytomorphological positivity in 8% of cases, rendering them complementary.

Tissue histopathology of PCNSL shows a typical infiltrating angiocentric pattern wherein tumor cells form collars within concentric perivascular cuffs and invade neural parenchyma, evidencing a diffuse growth pattern. Large areas of necrosis. B-cell NHL constitute up to 98% of PCNSL, demonstrating expression of pan-B markers, including CD20, CD79a, and MUM1 (2, 8). T-cell lymphoma is quite rare in the CNS but may be responsible for a higher proportion of Asian cases (105). Extranodal marginal zone B-cell lymphoma is the commonest primary intracranial low-grade B-cell lymphoma (2).

With over 40 prospective clinical trials since 1978, and

calls to undertake more definitive studies to determinate the optimal management of PCNSL, an International Working Group (106) published guidelines for the baseline evaluation and response assessment of PCNSL. Standard therapy in immunologically normal, often older patients with PCNSL is high-dose methotrexate (MTX). High-dose MTX, with or without whole brain radiotherapy, was studied in a phase III randomized trial of HIV-negative PCNSL (107) showed no significance in OS when whole brain irradiation (WBI) was omitted from first-line CTX employing 4 g/m² on day one of six 14-day cycles, thereafter receiving high-dose MTX plus ifosfamide 1.5 g/m² on days three to five of two 14-day cycles. Those not achieving complete response were given high-dose cytarabine as well. Other investigators have defined the role of MTX as a critical CTX agent in the treatment of PCNSL, suggesting that while MTX combined with WBI may achieve superior therapeutic results, the optimal MTX-based combination has not been defined (108). The efficacy of salvage therapy for PCNSL with a combination of rituximab and TMZ was suggested for older patients with progressive disease (109). A retrospective analysis of HIV-associated lymphoma between 2000 and 2010 indicated a poor prognosis, with none surviving two or five years or demonstrating complete response of PCNSL to chemotherapy with rituximab, MTX, procarabazine and vincristine, several of whom received WBI, while up to two-thirds of those with non-HIV-associated PCNSL survived more than two years after diagnosis (110).

ACKNOWLEDGMENT

Dr. David Zagzag provided figures and legends.

REFERENCES

1. *CBTRUS Statistical Report: Primary brain and central nervous system tumors diagnosed in the United States in 2004–2006.* Central Brain Tumor Registry of the United States: Hinsdale, IL.

2. Louis DN, Ohgaki H, Wiestler OD, et al, eds. *World Health Organization classification of tumors of the central nervous system.* 4th ed., Lyon: IARC Press, 2007.

3. Zulch KJ, Ed. *Histological typing of tumours of the central nervous system.* World Health Organization, Geneva, 1979.

4. Kleihues P, Burger PC, Scheithauer BW, eds. *Histological typing of tumours of the central nervous system. World Health Organization international histological classification of tumours.* Heidelberg: Springer, 1993.

5. Kleihues P, Cavenee WK, eds. *World Health Organization classification of tumours. Pathology and genetics of tumours of the nervous system.* Lyon: IARC Press, 2000.

6. Louis DN, Ohgaki H, Wiestler OD, et al. The 2007 WHO classification of tumours of the central nervous system. *Acta Neuropathol* 2007; 114:97–109.

7. *International Classification of Diseases for Oncology.* 3rd ed., (ICD-0-3). WHO, Geneva.

8. Rodriquez FJ, Giannini C. Diagnostic neuropathology of tumors of the central nervous system. *Handb Clin Neurol* 2012; 104:77–107.

9. Wen PY, Kesari S. Malignant gliomas in adults. *N Engl J Med* 2008; 359:492–507.

10. Cha S. Update on brain tumor imaging: from anatomy to physiology. *AJNR* 2006; 27:475–487.

11. Furnari FB, Fenton T, Bachoo RM, et al. Malignant astrocytic glioma: genetics, biology, and paths to treatment. *Genes Dev* 2007; 21:2683–2710.

12. Lee da Y, Gutmann DH. Cancer stem cells and brain tumors: uprooting the bad seeds. *Expert Rev Anticancer Ther* 2007; 7:1581–1590.

13. Bao S, Wu Q, McLendon RE, et al. Glioma stem cells promotes radioresistance by preferential activation of the DNA damage response. *Nature* 2006; 444:756–760.

14. Liu G, Yuan X, Zeng Z, et al. Analysis of gene expression and chemoresistance of CD133+ cancer stem cells in glioblastoma. *Mol Cancer* 2006; 5:67.

15. Galmaggi A, Boiardi A, Gelati M, et al. Glioblastoma-derived tumorospheres identify a population of tumor stem-like cells with angiocentric potential and enhanced multidrug resistance phenotype. *Glia* 2006; 54:850–860.

16. Dean M, Fojo T, Bates S. Tumour stem cells and drug resistance. *Nat Rev Cancer* 2005; 5:275–284.

17. Taylor MD, Poppleton H, Fuller C, et al. Radial glia cells are candidate stem cells of ependymoma. *Cancer Cell* 2005; 8:323–335.

18. Ohgaki H, Kleihues P. Genetic pathways to primary and secondary glioblastoma. *Am J Pathol* 2007; 170:1445–1453.

19. Adamson DC, Rasheed BA, McLendon RE, et al. Central nervous system. *Cancer Biomark* 2010; 9:193–210.

20. Hoeijmakers JH. Genome maintenance mechanisms for preventing cancer. *Nature* 2001; 411:366–374.

21. Ishii N, Maier D, Merlo A, et al. Frequent co-alterations of TP53, p16/CDKN2A, p14ARF, PTEN tumor suppressor genes in human glioma cell lines. *Brain Pathol* 1999; 9:469–479.

22. Ohgaki H, Dessen P, Jourde B, et al. Genetic pathways to glioblastoma: a population based study. *Cancer Res* 2004; 64:6892–6899.

23. Ohgaki H, Kleihues P. Population-based studies on incidence, survival rates, and genetic alterations in astrocytic and oligodendroglial gliomas. *J Neuropathol Exp Neurol* 2005; 64:479–489.

24. Kurt E, Zheng PP, Hop WC, et al. Identification of relevant prognostic histopathologic features in 69 intracranial ependymomas, excluding myxopapillary ependymomas and subependymomas. *Cancer* 2006; 106:388–395.

25. Wen PY, Schiff D, Kesari S, et al. Medical management of patients with brain tumors. *J Neurooncol* 2006; 80:313–332.

26. Batchelor TT, Sorensen AG, di Tomaso E, et al. AZD2171, a pan-VEGF receptor tyrosine kinase inhibitor, normalizes tumor vasculature and alleviates edema in glioblastoma patients. *Cancer Cell* 2007; 11:83–95.

27. Glantz MJ, Cole BF, Forsyth PA, et al. Practice parameter: anticonvulsant prophylaxis in patients with newly diagnosed brain tumors: Report of the Quality Standards Subcommittee of the American Academy of Neurology. *Neurology* 2000; 54:1886–1893.

28. Gerber DE, Grossman SA, Streiff MB. Management of venous thromboembolism in patients with primary and metastatic brain tumors. *J Clin Oncol* 2006; 24:1310–1318.

29. Hau P, Koch D, Hundsberger T, et al. Safety and feasibility of long-term temozolamide treatment in patients with high-grade glioma. *Neurology* 2007; 68:688–690.

30. Stummer W, Pichlmeier U, Meinel T, et al. Fluroescence-guided surgery with 5-aminolevulinic acid for resection of malignant glioma: a randomized controlled multicenter phase III trial. *Lancet Oncol* 2006; 7:392–401.

31. Mason WP, Cairncross JG. Invited article: the expanding impact of molecular biology on the diagnosis and treatment of gliomas. *Neurology* 2008; 71:365–373.

32. Keime-Guibert R, Chinot O, Taillandier L, et al. Radio-therapy for glioblastoma in the elderly. *N Engl J Med* 2007; 356:1527–1535.

33. Hochberg FH, Pruitt A. Assumptions in the radiotherapy of glioblastoma. *Neurology* 1980; 30:907–911.

34. Stupp R, Hegi ME, Gilbert MR, et al. Chemotherapy in malignant glioma: standard of care and future directions. *J Clin Oncol* 2007; 25:4127–4136.

35. Chi AS, Wen PY. Inhibiting kinases in malignant gliomas. *Expert Opin Ther Targets* 2007; 11:473–496.

36. Duda DG, Jain RK, Willett CG. Antiangiogenics: the potential role of integrating this novel treatment modality with chemo-radiation for solid cancers. *J Clin Oncol* 2007; 25:4033–4042.

37. Wen PY, Macdonald DR, Reardon DA, et al. Updated response assessment criteria for high-grade gliomas: response assessment in neuro-oncology working group. *J Clin Oncol* 2010; 28:1963–1972.

38. Quant EC, Wen PY. Response assessment in neuro-oncology. *Curr Oncol Rep* 2011; 13:50–56.

39. Hegi ME, Diserens AC, Gorlia T, et al. MGMT gene silencing and benefit from temozolomide in glioblastoma. *N Engl J Med* 2005; 352:997–1003.

40. Colman H. Aldape K. Molecular predictors in glioblastoma: toward personalized therapy. *Arch Neurol* 2008; 65:877–883.

41. Shaw EG, Scheithauer BW, O'Fallon JR, et al. Oligoden-drogliomas: the Mayo Clinic experience. *J Neurosurg* 1992; 76:428–434.

42. Kros JM, Pieterman H, Van Eden CG, et al. Oligodendrogli-oma: the Rotterdam-Dijkzigt experience. *Neurosurgery* 1994; 34:959–966.

43. Olson JD, Riedel E, DeAngelis LM. Long-term outcome of low-grade oligodendroglioma and mixed glioma. *Neurology* 2000; 54:1442–1448.

44. Intergroup Radiation Therapy Oncology Group Trial 9402, Cairncross G, Berkey B, et al. Phase III trial of chemotherapy plus radiotherapy compared with radiotherapy alone for pure and mixed anaplastic oligodendroglioma: Intergroup Radiation Therapy Oncology Group Trial 9402. *J Clin Oncol* 2006; 24:2707–2714.

45. Van den Bent MJ, Carpentier AF, Brandes AA, et al. Adjuvant procarbazine, lomustine, and vincristine improves progression-free survival but not overall survival in newly diagnosed anaplastic olidodendrogliomas and oligoastrocytomas: a randomized European Organization for Research and Treatment of Cancer phase III trial. *J Clin Oncol* 2006; 24:2715–2722.

46. Wick W, Hartmann C, Engel C, et al. NOA-04 randomized phase III trial of sequential radiochemotherapy of anaplastic glioma with procarbazine, lomustine, and vincristine or temo-zolomide. *J Clin Oncol* 2009; 27:5874–5880.

47. Abrey LE, Louis DN, Paleologos N, et al. Survey of treatment recommendations for anaplastic oligodendroglioma. *Neurooncol* 2007; 9:314–318.

48. DeAngelis LM. Anaplastic glioma: how to prognosticate outcome and choose a treatment strategy. *J Clin Oncol* 2009; 27:5861–5862.

49. Lassman AB, Iwamoto FM, Cloughesy TF, et al. International retrospective study of over 1000 adults with anaplastic oligo-dendroglial tumors. *Neurooncol* 2011; 13:649–659.

50. Hamilton RL, Pollack IF. The molecular biology of ependymo-mas. *Brain Pathol* 1997; 7:807–822.

51. Carter M, Nicholson J, Ross F, et al. Genetic abnormalities detected in ependymomas by comparative genomic hybridisa-tion. *Br J Cancer* 2002; 86:929–939.

52. Birch BD, Johnson JP, Parsa A, et al. Frequent type 2 neurofibro-matosis gene transcript mutations in sporadic intramedullary spinal cord ependymomas. *Neurosurgery* 1996; 39:135–140.

53. Boström A, Boström J, Hartmann W, et al. Treatment results in patients with intracranial ependymomas. *Cent Eur Neurosurg* 2011; 72:127–132.

54. Swanson EL, Amdur RJ, Morris CG, et al. Intracranial epen-dymomas treated with radiotherapy: long-term results from a single institution. *J Neurooncol* 2011; 102:451–457.

55. Packer RJ, Macdonald T, Vezina G, et al. Medulloblastoma and primitive neuroectodermal tumors. *Handb Clin Neurol* 2012; 105:529–548.

56. Giordana MT, Schiffer P, Lanotte M, et al. Epidemiology of adult medulloblastoma. *Int J Cancer* 1999; 80:689–692.

57. Matsuda M, Yasui K, Nagashima K, et al. Origin of the medul-loblastoma experimentally induced by human polyomavirus JC. *J Natl Cancer Inst* 1987; 79:585–591.

58. Fung KM, Trojanowski JQ. Animal models of medulloblasto-mas and related primitive neuroectodermal tumors. A review. *J Neuropathol Exp Neurol* 1995; 54:285–296.

59. Packer RJ, Cogen P, Vezina G, et al. Medulloblastoma: clinical and biologic aspects. *Neurooncol* 1999; 1:232–250.

60. Erdem E, Zimmerman RA, Haselgrove JC, et al. Diffusion-weighted imaging and fluid attenuated inversion recovery imaging in the evaluation of primitive neuroectodermal tumors. *Neuroradiology* 2001; 43:927–933.

61. Katsetos CD, Herman MM, Frankfurter A, et al. Cerebellar desmoplastic medulloblastomas. A further immunohisto-chemical characterization of the reticulin-free pale islands. *Arch Pathol Lab Med* 1989; 113:1019–1029.

62. Giangaspero F, Rigobello L, Badiali M, et al. Large-cell medul-loblastomas. A distinct variant with highly aggressive behavior. *Am J Surg Pathol* 1992; 16:687–693.

63. Griffin CA, Hawkins AL, Packer RJ, et al. Chromosome abnormalities in pediatric brain tumors. *Cancer Res* 1988; 48:175–180.

64. Crawford JR, MacDonald TJ, Packer RJ. Medulloblastoma in childhood: new biological advances. *Lancet Neurol* 2007; 6:1073–1085.

65. Guessous F, Li Y, Abounader R. Signaling pathways in medul-loblastoma. *J Cell Physiol* 2008; 217:577–583.

66. Berman DM, Karhadkar SS, Hallahan AR, et al. Medulloblas-toma growth inhibition by hedgehog pathway blockade. *Science* 2002; 297:1559–1561.

67. Rudin CM, Hann CL, Laterra J, et al. Treatment of medullo-blastoma with hedgehog pathway inhibitor GDC-0449. *N Engl J Med* 2009; 361:1173–1178.

68. Marino S, Vooijs M, van der Gulden H, et al. Induction of medulloblastomas in p53-null mutant mice by somatic inacti-vation of Rb in the external granular layer cells of the cerebel-lum. *Genes Dev* 2000; 14:994–1004.

69. Eberhart CG, Kratz J, Wang Y, et al. Histopathological and molecular prognostic markers in medulloblastoma: c-myc, N-myc, TrkC, and anaplasia. *J Neuropathol Exp Neurol* 2004; 63:441–449.

70. Lai SF, Wang CW, Chen YH, et al. Medulloblastoma in adults: Treatment outcome, relapse patterns, and prognostic factors. *Strahlenther Onkol* 2012; 188:878–886.

71. Asthagiri AR, Parry DM, Butman JA, et al. Neurofibromatosis type 2. *Lancet* 2009; 373:1974–1986.

72. Gardner WJ, Frazier CH. Hereditary bilateral acoustic tumors. *J Hered* 1931; 22:7–8.

73. Gardner WJ, Turner O. Bilateral acoustic neurofibromas: further clinical and pathologic data on hereditary deafness and Recklinghausen's disease. *Arch NeuroPsych* 1940; 44:76–99.

74. Mayfrank L, Wullich B, Wolff G, et al. Neurofibromatosis 2: a clinically and genetically heterogeneous disease? Report on 10 sporadic cases. *Clin Genet* 1990; 38:362–370.

75. Evans DG, Huson SM, Donnai D, et al. A clinical study of type 2 neurofibromatosis. *Quart J Med* 1992; 84:603–618.

76. Evans DG, Huson SM, Donnai D, et al. A genetic study of type 2 neurofibromatosis in the United Kingdom. I. Prevalance, mutation rate, fitness, and confirmation of maternal transmission effect on severity. *J Med Genet* 1992; 29:841–846.

77. Martuza RL, Eldridge R. Neurofibromatosis 2. *N Engl J Med* 1988; 318:684–688.

78. Pastores GM, Michels VV, Jack CR Jr. Early childhood diagnosis of acoustic neuromas in presymptomatic individuals at risk for neurofibromatosis 2. *Am J Med Genet* 1991; 41:325–329.

79. Parry DM, MacCollin MM, Kaiser-Kupfer MI, et al. Germ-line mutations in the neurofibromatosis 2 gene: correlations with disease severity and retinal abnormalities. *Am J Hum Genet* 1996; 59:529–539.

80. Kondziolka D, Lunsford LD, McLaughlin MR, et al. Long-term outcomes after radiosurgery for acoustic neuromas. *N Engl J Med* 1998; 339:1426–1433.

81. Perry A, Stafford SL, Scheithauer BW, et al. Meningioma grading: an analysis of histologic parameters. *Am J Surg Pathol* 1997; 21:1455–1465.

82. Perry A, Scheithauer BW, Stafford SL, et al. "Malignancy" in meningiomas: a clinicopathologic study of 116 patients, with grading implications. *Cancer* 1999; 85:2046–2056.

83. Perry A, Stafford SL, Scheithauer BW, et al. The prognostic significance of MIB-1, p53, and DNA flow cytometry in completely resected primary meningiomas. *Cancer* 1998; 82:2262–2269.

84. Ribalta T, McCutcheon IE, Aldape KD, et al. The mitosis-specific antibody anti-phosphohistone-H3 (PHH3) facilitates rapid reliable grading of meningiomas according to WHO 2000 criteria. *Am J Surg Pathol* 2004; 28:1532–1536.

85. Buhl R, Nabavi A, Wolff S, et al. MR spectroscopy in patients with intracranial meningiomas. *Neurol Res* 2007; 29:43–46.

86. Bendszus M, Warmuth-Metz M, Klein R, et al. Sequential MRI and MR spectroscopy in embolized meningiomas: correlation with surgical and histopathologoical findings. *Neuroradiology* 2002; 44:77–82.

87. Qi ZG, Li Y, Wang YX, et al. Lipid signal in evaluation of intracranial meningiomas. *Clin Med J* (Engl) 2008; 121:2415–2419.

88. Yang S, Law M, Zagzag D, et al. Dynamic contrast-enhanced perfusion MR imaging measurements of endothelial permeability: differentiation between atypical and typical meningiomas. *AJNR* 2003; 24:1554–1559.

89. Zhang H, Rödiger LA, Shen T, et al. Preoperative subtyping of meningiomas by perfusion MR imaging. *Neuroradiology* 2008; 50:835–840.

90. Weber DC, Lovblad KO, Rogers L. New pathology classification, imagery techniques and prospective trials for meningiomas: the future looks bright. *Curr Opin Neurol* 2010; 23:563–570.

91. Lee JW, Kang KW, Park SH, et al. 18F-FDG PET in the assessment of tumor grade and prediction of tumor recurrence in intracranial meningioma. *Eur J Nucl Med Mol Imaging* 2009; 36:1574–1582.

92. Ngwenya LB, Chiocca EA. Editorial: Meningioma and radiotherapy. *J Neurosurg* 2012 Aug 17 [Epub ahead of print].

93. Miller DC, Hochberg FH, Harris NL, et al. Pathology with clinical correlations of primary central nervous system non-Hodgkin's lymphoma. The Massachusetts General Hospital experience 1958–1989. *Cancer* 1994; 74:1383–1397.

94. Coté TR, Manns A, Hardy DR, et al. Epidemiology of brain lymphoma among people with or without acquired immunodeficiency syndrome. AIDS/Cancer Study Group. *J Natl Cancer Inst* 1996; 88:675–679.

95. Camilleri-Broët S, Davi F, Feuillard J, et al. AIDS-related primary brain lymphomas: histopathologic and immunohistochemical study of 51 cases. The French Study Group for HIV-Associated Tumors. *Hum Pathol* 1997; 28:367–374.

96. Sacktor N, Lyles RH, Skolasky R, et al. HIV-associated neurologic disease incidence changes: Multicenter AIDS Cohort Study, 1990–1998. *Neurology* 2001; 56:257–260.

97. Batchelor T, Loeffler JS. Primary CNS lymphoma. *J Clin Oncol* 2006; 24:1281–1288.

98. Mohile NA, Deangelis LM, Abrey LE. The utility of body FDG PET in staging primary central nervous system lymphoma. *Neurooncol* 2008; 10:223–228.

99. Bromberg JE, Breems DA, Kraan J, et al. CSF flow cytometry greatly improves diagnostic accurary in CNS hematologic malignancies. *Neurology* 2007; 68:1674–1679.

100. Fischer L, Martus P, Weller M, et al. Meningeal dissemination in primary CNS lymphoma: prospective evaluation of 282 patients. *Neurology* 2008; 71:1102–1108.

101. Choi JS, Nam DH, Ko YH, et al. Primary central nervous system lymphoma in Korea: comparison of B- and T-cell lymphomas. *Am J Surg Pathol* 2003; 27:919–928.

102. Abrey LE, Batchelor TT, Ferreri AJM, et al. Report of an International Workshop to standardize baseline evaluation and response criteria for primary CNS lymphoma. *J Clin Oncol* 2005; 23:5034–5043.

103. Thiel E, Korfel A, Martus P, et al. High-dose methotrexate with or without whole brain radiotherapy for primary CNS lymphoma (G-PCNSL-SG-1): a phase 3, randomised, non-inferiority trial. *Lancet Oncol* 2010; 11:1036–1047.

104. Gerstner ER, Carson KA, Grossman SA, et al. Long-term outcome in PCNSL patients treated with high-dose methotrexate and deferred radiation. *Neurology* 2008; 70:401–402.

105. Enting RH, Demopoulos A, DeAngelis LM, et al. Salvage therapy for primary CNS lymphoma with a combination of rituximab and temozolomide. *Neurology* 2004; 63:901–903.

106. Gopal S, Martin KE, Richards KL, et al. Clinical Presentation, Treatment, and Outcome Among 65 Patients with HIV-Associated Lymphoma Treated at the University of North Carolina, 2000–2010. *AIDS Res Hum Retroviruses* 2012; 28:798–805.

CHAPTER 47

Childhood Spinal Muscular Atrophy

David S. Younger, Jennifer Werely

HISTORY

Werdnig and Hoffmann, both clinicians and neuropathologists recognized striking atrophy of the ventral nerve roots of the spinal cord on gross postmortem examination of patients who had a previously described form of infantile paralysis, and correlated it with a decreased number of motor neurons of the anterior horns and skeletal myofiber atrophy due to denervation (1). In 1891, Guido Werdnig (2), a retired battalion physician working at the Institute of Anatomy and Physiology of the Central Nervous System at the University of Vienna gave a lecture entitled, "On a case of muscular dystrophy with positive spinal cord findings." One year later, Hoffmann employed the term *spinale muskelatrophie*, (3), which were probably the first references to spinal muscular atrophy (SMA). Their combined observations characterized the clinical and pathologic aspects of infantile SMA that included onset in siblings with normal parents during the first year of life of progressively lethal hypotonia, weakness, and hand tremor, culminating in early childhood (4, 5).

CLASSIFICATION

Hoffmann (5) recognized chronic slowly progressive forms of SMA(5), which were later incorporated into the classification of Byers and Banker (6), and those of observations of Dubowitz (7) that correlated age at onset and disease severity with prognosis. International collaborations beginning in 1991 (8–10) prompted adoption of currently employed nomenclature based upon agent at onset, with type I before age 6 months, type II with onset between 6 and 18 months, and type III after 18 months The three types were further differentiated by the highest achieved motor milestone and mortality. An adult-onset form (11), later termed SMA type IV, described patients older than 18 years who were still walking in adulthood without respiratory involvement. Patients with SMA type I almost never sat after placed without support and with onset before 3 months of age, had a mortality rate of 90%, whereas those with onset after age THREE months survived to adulthood, albeit with severe motor handicap, whereas type III patients ambulated independently for part of their lives with normal life expectancy

EPIDEMIOLOGY

Spinal muscular atrophy are rare inherited disorders with an estimated incidence of 10 per 100,000 live births and a carrier frequency of one in 50 in the United States and Germany (12, 13). It is the most common fatal neuromuscular disease of infancy and the third most common neuromuscular diagnosis seen in children less than 18 years of age. SMA Type I has the highest incidence followed, respectively, by Type II and Type III. Considering the relative mortality rate of SMA type I, it is not surprising that the highest prevalence is for types II and III.

SMA Type I

Infantile onset SMA and Werdnig-Hoffmann disease are synonyms for SMA type I, the most severe form of the autosomal recessive (AR) disease beginning at birth or in the first few months, resulting in death from respiratory failure

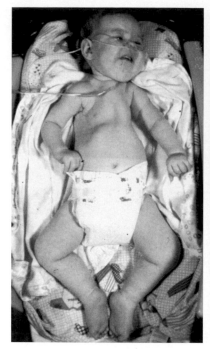

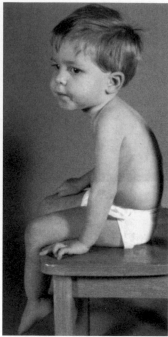

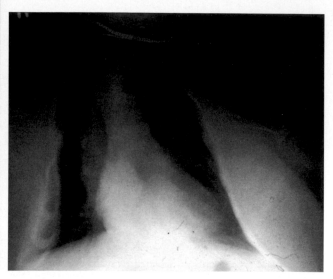

FIG. 1. A 3-month-old infant with SMA I and bell-shaped chest died soon afterward of respiratory failure.

FIG. 2. This 11-month-old boy diagnosed with SMA II learned to sit without support at 12 months of age.

FIG. 3. A chest x-ray from a 14-year-old boy with SMA II had markedly decreased lung volumnes and the rib cage collapsed into a bell-shape.

before age two. Physical examination in the characteristic frog-leg position reveals a relative absence of spontaneous movements except for the hands and feet that show a fine tremor termed *polyminimyoclonus*. Affected infants have severe weakness and profound hypotonia striking discrepancy in the level of social interaction and paucity of motor skills. Tongue fasciculation is superimposed upon lingual wasting and scalloping of its borders. The combination of pectus excavatum combined with bell-shaped deformity of the lower rib cage (Figure 1), weakened intercostal muscles, and diaphragmatic breathing, lead to inefficient respiration, however rare individuals develop frank diaphragm paralysis. Deep tendon reflexes (DTR) are absent while intact sphincter tone and sensation remain intact.

SMA type I infants tire quickly during feeding and, if breast fed, may begin to lose weight before it is evident that they are not taking in appropriate calories. Malnutrition and respiratory insufficiency exacerbate fatigue and cause susceptibility to aspiration. Any minor upper respiratory infection may quickly become a life-threatening crisis. The most common cause of death is respiratory failure, often preceded by several months of subtle changes due to complications associated with weakness.

Spinal Muscular Atrophy Type II

Juvenile SMA, intermediate SMA, and chronic SMA are synonyms for SMA type II. Affected patients usually achieve normal milestones up to 6 to 8 months of age in spite of relative hypotonicity. The legs are weaker than the arms, resulting in paraparesis, and there may be a clubfoot deformity with resulting gait (Figure 2). The DTR are preserved in stronger muscles. Minipolymyoclonus is often combined with fasciculation of intrinsic hand muscles. Infants with SMA type II are able to sit without support when placed in a position during some or all of their life but are rarely able to stand; notwithstanding, it is customary to classify a child who walks at any time as type III. The age for sitting or standing is nearly always delayed. Many children survive to the third and fourth decade. One contributing factor between survivors and non-survivors is adequate pulmonary function and toilet (Figure 3).

Spinal Muscular Atrophy Type III

Wohlfart-Kugelberg-Welander and mild SMA are synonyms for SMA type III, which typically presents in late childhood or adolescence with proximal neurogenic muscular atrophy that may be confused with limb girdle muscular dystrophy (LGMD). The serum creatine kinase (CK) level is typically elevated. Patients with SMA type III remain ambulatory during part or all of their lives with a typical waddling gait, lumbar lordosis, genu recurvatum, and protuberant abdomen or stick-man appearance. Although not always elicited, DTR are almost never hyperactive. Six of eight children described by Byers and Banker (6) stood without assistance from one to two years of age, whereas only two ever walked without assistance. The prognosis for continued independent ambulation is correlated with age at onset of weakness with children showing onset of weakness before age two unlikely to continue ambulating after age 15 years, and those with onset after two years likely to continue ambulating into the fifth decade.

LABORATORY EVALUATION

The laboratory evaluation of SMA has evolved with discovery of the underlying genetic defect since the diagnosis in a suspected patient can be ascertained by DNA analysis for the causative mutation or deletion at the 55q13.2 locus of the survival motor neuron genes SMN1 and SMN2, with SMN1 the primary disease-causing gene. Infants with deletions or truncation of exons 7 and 8 of SMN1 require no further workup. Although most patients have deletions in SMN, rare patients with duplication or heterozygous point mutations have been described. If gene sequencing is normal, a more traditional approach is warranted that includes measurement of serum CK, which is usually normal in types I and II and elevated in type III and nerve conduction studies (NCS) and needle electromyography (EMG) for the anticipated features of motor neuron disease (MND). The electrodiagnostic evaluation of SMA can be challenging because of small-sized limbs in children leading to relatively short distances between stimulus and recording electrodes, and profound muscle wasting that alters the reliability of motor NCS, which in SMA should remain normal (14). Needle EMG shows evidence of acute denervation, including fibrillation potentials and re-innervation in the form of large polyphasic motor units and reduced recruitment. In infants, electromyography may be normal or suggestive of a myopathic process because of small amplitude, short duration, and polyphasic motor unit potentials.

Motor unit number estimation (MUNE), a methodology that assesses the number of motor neurons innervating a muscle group with utility in amyotrophic lateral sclerosis (15), was applied to the ulnar nerve-hypothenar muscle group in 14 patients with SMA due to homozygous deletion in SMN1, including asymptomatic patients from age 16 days to 45 years (16). The results included a fall in MUNE values to low levels early in the progression of weakness. Test-retest reliability showed consistent values, making it a desirable methodology for following disease progression.

The finding of progressive selective degeneration of motor neurons in SMA was similar to experimental mutant mice harboring a deletion at exon 7 in SMN1 (17). Skeletal muscle biopsy is warranted when mutation analysis is uninformative. Skeletal muscle biopsy in affected patients shows group atrophy with large type 1 myofibers and clumps of type 1 hypertrophic fibers by ATPase staining, characteristic of the infantile pattern, and angulated fibers that increase with age from mid-childhood due to reinnervation.

GENETICS

In 1990, Gilliam and colleagues (18) linked SMA to chromosome 5q11.2-q13.3. By 1994, Melki and colleagues (19, 20) had assigned SMAI to 5q12-q13.3 and analyzed allele segregation at the closest genetic loci in more than 200 SMA families. The severe form of SMA was statistically associated with deletion events. One year later, Thompson and colleagues (21) identified several coding sequences unique to the SMA region. Lefebvre and coworkers (22) identified the SMN gene within the SMA candidate region on chromosome 5q13 and demonstrated deletion or disruption of the gene in nearly all SMA patients so studied. That same year, Lefebvre (22), Roy, and colleagues (23) identified a different gene at 5q13.1 encoding neuronal apoptosis inhibitory protein (NAIP) found in the first two coding exons of the gene. The latter was deleted in two-thirds of SMAI patients so studied compared to 2% of normal controls. This suggested that mutations in the latter locus resulted in failure of a normally occurring inhibition of motor neuron apoptosis and contributed to the SMA phenotype. One year later, Matthijs and colleagues (24) identified homozygous deletion of exon 7 of the SMN1 gene in 34 of 38 SMA patients studied, as well as homozygous deletion of exon 8 in 31 patients. Other patients were reported with homozygous deletion of exon 7 but not exon 8 (25). A similar experience of homozygous absence of exons 7 and 8 of SMN1 was found in 90% of several hundred Spanish SMA patients (26). Jedrzejowska and colleagues (27) later reported asymptomatic carriers of biallelic deletion of the SMN1 gene, all whom had four copies of the SMN2 gene, confirming that an increased number of SMN2 copies in healthy carriers of biallelic SMN1 deletion were an important phenotype modifier.

Experimental mutant mice, NSE-Cre+, SMnF7/F7 mice carrying an experimental deletion of the SMN exon 7 generated by crossing smnF7/F7 mice homozygous for the loxP-flanked SMN exon 7 with smnF7/+NSE-cre+ in the Cre recombinase, specifically directed to mature neurons via the neuron specific enolase (NSE), underwent selective degeneration of motor neurons (17). Other experimental animal models, including the wobbler mouse model of amyotrophic lateral sclerosis (28) and autosomal dominant canine SMA (29), were phenotypically similar but molecularly distinct from human SMA.

The SMN1 gene encodes the full-length 294 amino acid protein molecule necessary for LMN function (22) whereas the SMN2 gene encodes a survival motor neuron protein that lacks exon 7, thereby producing a less stable protein.

When full-length SMN (fl-SMN) protein levels approach 23% of normal, motor neuron function is normal, whereas SMA is associated with lower levels rather than complete absence. Thus, individuals with SMAI have as little as 9% fl-SMN; SMA II, 14%, SMA III, 18%; and carriers 45 to 55% of the normal fl-SMN protein. The presence of three or more copies of *SMN2* compensate, leading to small amounts of fl-*SMN* transcripts that can compensate for the lack of *SMN1* expression and lead to the less severe SMAII and SMAIII phenotypes (13).

OTHER FORMS OF SPINAL MUSCULAR ATROPHY

Very Severe SMA

Very severe SMA phenotypes have been described in association with *SMN1* at the 5q13 locus associated with reduced fetal movements *in utero* and severe weakness at birth (30), fetal hypokinesia and asphyxia (31), neurogenic arthrogryposis (32, 33), and multiple contractures and bone fractures (34) at birth, suggesting a relation to SMA. Commenting on the five patients described by MacLeod and colleagues (31), Dubowitz (35) considered the severe cases of SMA an expanding clinical phenotypic spectrum of prenatal onset and intrauterine death, severe asphyxia at birth or early neonatal death that fit into a category of "very severe SMA (type 0)," and an extension to the previous severe SMA (type 1). He suggested the decimal designation of 0.1 to .0.9, depending upon whether there was early intrauterine death or viability at birth (35). The presence of multiple joint contractures has been an exclusionary research criterion for SMA (36).

SMA Plus Types

Even prior to *SMN1* gene analysis, three categories of SMA-plus syndromes were excluded by the International SMA consortium in 1992 because of atypical features or additional organ involvement (37) and, subsequently, none had informative *SMN1* gene findings. Mellins (38), Bertini (39), and colleagues delineated diaphragmatic SMA, a variant of SMA1. In a series of more than 200 patients with early-onset SMA, Rudnik-Schoneborn (40) found that 1% presented with diaphragmatic SMA but did not have a deletion of *SMN* gene at chromosome 5q. Affected infants present with a weak cry, inspiratory stridor, and life-threatening respiratory distress due to diaphragmatic paralysis, followed later by distal weakness and wasting. The disorder, known now as SMA with respiratory distress type 1 (SMARD1), was further characterized by Grohmann et al (41, 42) and demonstrates AR inheritance caused by a mutation at the

11q13.3 locus of the *IGHMBP2* gene encoding immunoglobulin μ-binding protein 2.

A second category of SMA-plus syndromes is X-linked SMA (SMAX) or Kennedy disease (SMAX1) of X-linked spinal and bulbar muscular atrophy. Kennedy and colleagues (43) described non-lethal slowly progressive bulbar and limb weakness, wasting, and fasciculation in men of average age 40 years with gynecomastia, dysphagia, and absent corticospinal, sensory, and cerebellar long tract signs. La Spada and Fischbeck (44) identified an expanded CAG repeat in the first exon of the AR gene at the Xp12 locus. The AR CAG is normally polymorphic, with an average of 22 repeats; however, patients with SMAX1 have 40 to 52 CAG repeats. Further investigation (45) established the relationship between disease severity and CAG repeat length. X-linked arthrogryposis (SMAX2) was the second X-linked SMA disorder described by Greenberg (46) of X-linked hypotonia, areflexia, chest deformity, facial dysmorphic features, and congenital joint contractures, with a disease course similar to SMA1. Later linkage (47) and marker studies (48) of SMAX2 revealed causative deletion, missense, and C-to-T substitutions mutation at the Xp11.23 locus of the *UBE1* gene encoding ubiquitin-activating enzyme-1.

Distal SMA (SMAX3) was the third X-linked disorder described by Takata and colleagues (49) in a Brazilian family that manifested initial pes cavus and varus foot deformity, followed by slowly progressive distal leg weakness and wasting, and later involvement of the hands; gait was maintained into late life without cognitive, corticospinal tract or sensory signs. A three-generation family of SMAX3 manifesting X-linked distal motor neuropathy was described by Kennerson and colleagues (50), allelic to that reported by Takata and coworkers (49), and mapped to the DSMAX locus to chromosome Xq13.1-q21. Kennerson and coworkers (51) later identified disease-causing mutations at the Xq21.1 locus of the ATP7A copper transport gene among affected members of the two families reported by Takata (49) and Kennerson and colleagues (50).

A third SMA-plus category is pontocerebellar hypoplasia with infantile SMA. Pontocerebellar hypoplasia refers to abnormal growth and function of the brainstem and cerebellum, resulting in little or no development. The combination of AR PCH and infantile SMA (PCH1) was first described by Normal (52) and later by Chou (53), Barth (54), Rudnick-Schoneborn (55), and Renbaum and coworkers (56), and most recently by Najmabadi and coworkers (57). Early features include microcephaly, poor suck, lingual fasciculation, swallowing difficulty, and hypotonia, followed by limb ataxia, weakness, hyperreflexia, developmental delay, and mental retardation in surviving children. Neuroimaging discloses cerebellar hypoplasia associated with cisterna magna and midline cerebellar atrophy. The disorder is due to homozygous missense mutation at the 14q32.2 locus of the *VRK1* gene. There are five different types (PCH2 to 6) based on the clinical and pathological changes. Type 1 has central and peripheral motor dysfunction associated with infantile SMA. Other types manifest microcephaly with extrapyramidal dyskinesia (PCH2); hyporeflexia, hyperreflexia, microcephaly, optic atrophy, and seizures (PCH3); hypertonia, joint contractures, olivopontocerebellar hypoplasia and early death (PCH4); second trimester cerebellar and seizures (PCH5); and mitochondrial respiratory chain defects (PCH6) (58).

ETIOPATHOGENESIS OF SMA

The exact function of the SMN protein is not known (59). Reduced amounts of functional SMN protein are found in all cell types of patients with SMA, and mRNA splicing is probably dependent upon the abundance of SMN protein (60). The exact role of the SMN is not well known, however knockdown of the SMN protein in zebrafish causes defects in motor axonal outgrowth and pathfinding (61), and SMN protein has a experimentally protective role for motor neurons against mutant superoxide dismutase 1 (SOD1) by increasing chaperone activity (62).

Substantial progress has been made in understanding the molecular genetic aspects of SMA, prompted by recognition that the disease phenotype is proportional to the amount of full-length SMN, which has prompted clinical investigation into possible drug treatments to improve outcome in SMA by increasing expression of SMN protein levels, enhancing transcriptional activity of SMN2 to increase full-length SMN RNA, translational activation and stabilization of full-length SMN protein, and the administration of neuroprotective or neurotrophic agents (63).

CLINICAL TRIALS

There is yet no proven therapy to slow or arrest disease progression of SMA type I (64) or SMA types II and III (65) including therapeutic trials employing gabapentin (66), phenylbutryrate (67), riluzole (68), valproate and L-carnitine (69, 70). Several laboratories have achieved compelling success in experimental models of SMA using sophisticated methods for targeted delivery, repair, and increased expression of *SMN* that may have meaningful outcomes for patients in the future. Hydroxyurea-treated lymphoblastoid cell lines from patients with SMA led to time-related and dose-dependent increase in the ratio of fl-SMN messenger RNA that correlated with SMA phenotypic severity (71). A similar effect was noted in SMA II and III in patients treated for one week, however there was no functional analysis (72). Neuronal *SMN* expression corrects

spinal muscular atrophy in severe *SMN* mice, suggesting a rationale for increasing the expression of SMN protein levels to modify the clinical phenotype and improve outcome in SMA (73). Postsymptomatic restoration of *SMN* rescued the disease phenotype in a mouse model of severe SMA (74), while prolactin increased *SMN* expression and survival in another mouse model of severe SMA via the STA5 pathway, a member of the STAT family of transcription factors (75), suggests hope for the development of an effective therapy for SMA based upon *SMN* induced through upregulation (76). Moreover, experimental conversion of *SMN2* to *SMN1* has been achieved in human cells (77). Gene therapy for SMA employs RNA technology or oligonucleotides to modify *SMN2* splicing, and viral vectors have been employed to replace *SMN1*, thereby decreasing motor neuron death and increasing SMA mice life span (78, 79). It is hoped that pluripotent (iPSC) and human embryonic stem cells (hESC), particularly iPS-SMA cells, will lead to small molecule drugs to enhance SMN protein output, which can be measured by the number of gems or protein aggregates, inversely related to disease severity (80). Various compounds have been tested on SMA patient fibroblast cells and shown to increase gem numbers and SMN protein levels through stabilization or prevention of exon 7 skipping.

MANAGEMENT

Management consists of the prevention and treatment of the complications of SMA (81), the latter of which include restrictive lung disease, poor nutrition, osteopenia, orthopedic deformities, immobility, and psychosocial problems. Restrictive lung disease results from weakness of intercostal muscles and diaphragm, causing hypoventilation and weak cough. Aggressive prophylaxis against pneumonia and atelectasis may include assisted cough, chest percussion therapy. Intermittent positive pressure breathing can be used together to provide adequate airway clearance. Mechanical in-exsufflation is a safe, well-tolerated, and effective modality for those with impaired cough (82) and in others to maintain adequate pulmonary toilet to prevent progressive atelectasis (83–86). With aggressive ventilator support, the life expectancy and quality of life of children with neuromuscular disease has improved remarkably in the last two decades (82, 87–89). Non-invasive ventilation is successful in children with sleep hypoventilation and hypercapnia (90).

The risk of pneumonia increases as forced vital capacity (FVC) decreases without a significant change in limb or trunk strength. Influenza and pneumococcal vaccination should be offered to all patients. Poor nutrition with failure to thrive occurs as a result of a weak suck, unprotected airway, and easy fatigability. There may be an exacerbation of weakness and fatigue secondary to negative nitrogen balance, however the mechanism is not well understood. A feeding evaluation should be done by a team of occupational and speech therapists and dieticians to adjust the feeding schedule, positioning during feeding, and food textures to maximize caloric intake. If necessary, the child should be examined during a modified barium swallow using several food textures, including liquid, semiliquid, soft, and solid food. If aspiration occurs, a gastrostomy may be necessary for supplemental gastrostomy feedings. Constipation is commonly noted because of immobility, but responds to increasing fluid and fiber intake.

Scoliosis is a serious orthopedic problem in patients with SMA (91) and non-ambulatory children tend to develop spinal deformities earlier than those who are still ambulatory. The goal of spinal surgery is to maximize growth before surgery. Club-foot deformity may be a presenting feature of infantile SMA. Range of motion exercises can prevent such contractures, but need to be done daily and consistently. Walking can be facilitated by lightweight orthoses for the legs, although it will likely be a temporary (92). Power chairs prescribed before the second birthday can provide independent mobility at an appropriate developmental age (93), and the high cognitive function of most patients allows them to maneuver a joy stick (94). School-aged children generally benefit from a full-time aide to assist in toileting, feeding, and maintenance of physical, occupational, and respiratory therapy regimens during the school day. Psychometric evaluation can be performed starting at an early age, even by age 4.

REFERENCES

1. Iannaccone ST, Caneris O. Johann Hoffmann. In: Ashwal S, ed. *Founders of Child Neurology*. San Francisco: Norman Publishing, 1990, 278–284.

2. Groger H. Guido Werdnig. In: Ashwal S, Ed. *The Founders of Child Neurology*. San Francisco: Norman Publishing, 1990, 383–388.

3. Hoffmann J. Ueber familiäre progressive spinale muskelatrophie. *Arch Psych* (Berlin) 1892; 24:644–646.

4. Hoffmann J. Ueber chronische spinale muskelatrophieim kindesalter auf familiärer basis. *Dtsch Zeit Nervenheilk* 1892; 3:427–470.

5. Hoffmann J. Weiterer beitrag zur lehre von der hereditaren progressiven spinalen muskelatrophie im kindesalter nebst bemerkungen Über den fortschreitenden muskelschwund im Allgemeinen. *Dtsch Zeit Nervenheilk* 1896; 10:292–320.

6. Byers RK, Banker BQ. Infantile Muscular Atrophy. *Arch Neurol* 1961; 5:140–164.

7. Dubowitz V. Infantile muscular atrophy A prospective study with particular reference to a slowly progressive variety. *Brain* 1964; 87:707–718.

8. Munsat TL. International SMA Collaboration (Workshop Report). *Neuromusc Dis* 1991; 1(2):81.

9. Dubowitz V. Chaos in the classification of SMA: a possible resolution. *Neuromuscul Disord* 1995; 5:3–4.

10. Zerres K, Davies KE. 59th ENMC International Workshop: Spinal muscular atrophies: recent progress and revised diagnostic criteria. *Neuromuscul Disord* 1999; 9:272–278.

11. Pearn JH, Hudgson P, Walton JN. A clinical and genetic study of spinal muscular atrophy of adult onset. *Brain* 1978; 101:591–603.

12. Thieme A, Mitulla B, Schulze F, et al. Epidemiological datea on Wernig-Hoffman disease in Germany (West-Thuringen). *Hum Genet* 1993; 91:295–297.

13. Mailman MD, Heinz JW, Papp AC, et al. Molecular analysis of spinal muscular atrophy and modification of the phenotype by SMN2. *Genet Med* 2002; 4:20–26.

14. Iijama M, Arasaki K, Iwamoto H, Nakanishi T. Maximal and minimal motor nerve conduction velocities in patients with motor neuron disease: correlation with age of onset and duration of illness. *Muscle Nerve* 1991; 14:1110–1115.

15. Bromberg M. Motor unit estimation: reproducibility of the spike-triggered averaging technique in normal and ALS subjects. *Muscle Nerve* 1993; 16:466–471.

16. Bromberg MB, Swoboda KJ. Motor unit number estimation in infants and children with spinal muscular atrophy. *Muscle Nerve* 2002; 25:445–447.

17. Ferri A, Melki J, Kato AC. Progressive and selective degeneration of motoneurons in a mouse model of SMA. *NeuroReport* 2004; 15:275–280.

18. Gilliam TC, Brzustowicz LM, Castilla LH, et al. Genetic homogeneity between acute and chronic forms of spinal muscular atrophy. *Nature* 1990; 345:823–825.

19. Melki J, Sheth P, Abdelhak S, et al., and the French Spinal Muscular Atrophy Investigators. Mapping of acute (type 1) spinal muscular atrophy to chromosome 5q12-q14. *Lancet* 1990; 336:271–273.

20. Melki J, Lefebvre S, Burglen L, et al. De novo and inherited deletions of the 5q13 regions in spinal muscular atrophies. *Science* 1994; 264:1474–1477.

21. Thompson TG, DiDonato CJ, Simard LR, et al. A novel cDNA detects homozygous microdeletions in greater than 50% of type 1 spinal muscular atrophy patients. *Nature Genet* 1995; 9:56–92.

22. Lefebvre S, Burglen L, Reboullet S, et al. Identification and characterization of a spinal muscular atrophy-determining gene. *Cell* 1995; 80:155–165.

23. Roy N, Mahadevan MS, McLean M, et al. The gene for neuronal apoptosis inhibitory protein is partially deleted in individuals with spinal muscular atrophy. *Cell* 1995; 80:167–178.

24. Matthijs G, Schollen E, Legius E, et al. Unusual molecular findings in autosomal recessive spinal muscular atrophy. *J Med Genet* 1996; 33:469–474.

25. Hahnen E, Schonling J, Rudnik-Schoneborn S, et al. Hybrid survivial motor neuron genes in patients with autosomal recessive spinal muscular atrophy: new insights into molecular mechanisms responsible for the disease. *Am J Hum Genet* 1996; 59:1057–1065.

26. Alias L, Bernal S, Fuentes-Prior P, et al. Mutation update of spinal muscular atrophy in Spain: molecular characterization of 745 unrelated patients and identification of four novel mutations in the SMN1 gene. *Hum Genet* 2009; 125:29–39.

27. Jedrzejowska M, Borkowska J, Zimowski J, et al. Unaffected

patients with a homozygous absence of the SMN1 gene. *Europ J Hum Genet* 2008; 16:930–934.

28. Kaupmann K, Simon-Chazottes D, Guenet J-L, et al. Wobbler, a mutation affecting motoneuron survival and gonadal functions in the mouse, maps to proximal chrosomsome 11. *Genomics* 1992; 13:39–43.

29. Blazej RG, Mellersch CS, Cork LC, et al. Hereditary canine spinal muscular atrophy is pheotypically similar but molecularly distinct from human spinal muscular atrophy. *J Hered* 1998; 89:531–537.

30. MacLeod MJ, Taylor JE, Lunt PW, et al. Prenatal onset spinal muscular atrophy. *Eur J Paediatr Neurol* 1999; 3:65–72.

31. Devriendt K, Lammens M, Schollen E, et al. Clinical and molecular genetic features of congenital spinal muscular atrophy. *Ann Neurol* 1996; 40:731–738.

32. Bingham P, Shen N, Rennert H, et al. Arthrogryposis due to infantile neuronal degeneration associated with deletion of the SMNt gene. *Neurology* 1997; 49:848–851.

33. Burglen L, Spiegel R, Ignatius J, et al. SMN gene deletion in variant of infantile spinal muscular atrophy. *Lancet* 1995; 346:316–317.

34. Garcia-Cabezas MA, Garcia-Alix A, Martin Y, et al. Neonatal spinal muscular atrophy with multiple contracture, bone fractures, respiratory insufficiency and 5q13 deletion. *Acta Neuropathol* 2004; 107:475–478.

35. Dubowitz V. Very severe spinal muscular atrophy (SMA type 0): an expanding clinical phenotype. *Eur J Paediatr Neurol* 1999; 3:49–51.

36. Munsat TL, Davies KE. Meeting report: International SMA Consortium meeting, 26–28 June, 1992, Bonn, Germany *Neuromuscul Disord* 1992; 2:423–428.

37. The International SMA consortium. Meeting Report. *Neuromuscul Disord* 1992; 2:2423–428.

38. Mellins RB, Hays AP, Gold AP, et al. Respiratory distress as the initial manifestation of Werdnig-Hoffmann disease. *Pediatrics* 1974; 53:33–40.

39. Bertini E, Gadisseux JL, Palmieri G, et al. Infantile spinal muscular atrophy associated with paralysis of the diaphragm: a variant of infantile spinal muscular atrophy. *Am J Med Genet* 1989; 33:328–335.

40. Rudnik-Schoneborn S, Forkert R, et al. Clinical spectrum and diagnostic criteria of infantile spinal muscular atrophy: further delineation on the basis of SMN gene deletion findings. *Neuropediatrics* 1996; 27:8–15.

41. Grohman K, Wienker TF, Saar K, et al. Diaphragmatic spinal muscular atrophy with respiratory distress is heterogeneous and one form is linked to chromosome 11q13-q21 (Letter). *Am J Hum Genet* 1999; 65:1459–1462.

42. Grohmann K, Varon R, Stolz P, et al. Infantile spinal muscular atrophy with respiratory distress type 1 (SMARD1). *Ann Neurol* 2003; 54:719–724.

43. Kennedy WR, Alter M, Sung JH. Progressive proximal spinal and bulbar muscular atrophy of late onset: a sex linked recessive trait. *Neurology* 1968; 671–680.

44. (La Spada AR, Fischbeck KH. Androgen receptor gene defect in X-linked spinal and bulbar muscular atrophy (Abstract). *Am J Hum Genet* 1991; 49:20.

45. La Spada AR, Roling DB, Harding AE, et al. Meiotic stability and genotype-phenotype correlation of the trinucleotide repeat in X-linked spinal and bulbar muscular atrophy. *Nature Genet* 1992; 2:301–304.

46. Greenberg F, Fenolio KR, Hejtmancik JF, et al. X-linked infantile spinal muscular atrophy. *Am J Dis Child* 1988; 142:217–219.

47. Baumbach L, Best B, Edwards J, et al. X-linked lethal infantile spinal muscular atrophy: from clinical description to molecular mapping (Abstract). *Am J Hum Genet* 1994; 55(Suppl):A211.

48. Dressman D, Ahearn ME, Yariz KO, et al. X-linked infantile spinal muscular atrophy: clinical definition and molecular mapping. *Genet Med* 2007; 9:52–60.

49. Takata RI, Spect Martins CE, Passosbueno MR, et al. A new locus for recessive distal spinal muscular atrophy at Xq13.1-q21. *J Med Genet* 2004; 41:224–229.

50. Kennerson M, Nocholson G, Kowalski B, et al. X-linked distal hereditary motor neuropathy maps to the DSMAX locus on chromosome Xq13.1-q21. *Neurology* 2009; 72:246–252.

51. Kennerson ML, Nicholson GA, Kaler SG, et al. Missense mutations in the copper transporter gene ATP7A cause X-linked distal hereditary motor neuropathy. *Am J Hum Genet* 2010; 86:343–352.

52. Norman RM. Cerebellar hypoplasia in Werdnig-Hoffmann disease. *Arch Dis Child* 1961; 36:96–101.

53. Chou SM, Gilbert EF, Chun RWM, et al. Infantile olivopontocerebellar atrophy with spinal muscular atrophy (infantile OPCA +SMA). *Clin Neuropath* 1990; 9:21–32.

54. Barth PG. Pontocerebellar hypoplasia: an overview of a group of inherited neurodegenerative disorders with fetal onset. *Brain Dev* 1993; 15:411–422.

55. Rudnik-Schoneborn S, Sztriha L, Aithala GR, et al. Extended phenotype of pontocerebellar hypoplasia with infantile spinal muscular atrophy. *Am J Med Genet* 2003; 117A:10–17.

56. Renbaum P, Kellerman E, Jaron R, et al. Spinal muscular atrophy with pontocerebellar hypoplasia is caused by a mutation in the VRK1 gene. *Am J Hum Genet* 2009; 85:281–289.

57. Najmabadi H, Hu H, Garshasbi M, et al. Deep sequencing reveals 50 novel genes for recessive cognitive disorders. *Nature* 2011; 478:57–63.

58. Graham JM, Spencer AH, Grinberg I, et al. Molecular and neuroimaging findings in pontocerebellar hypoplasia type 2 (PCH2): is prenatal diagnosis possible? *Am J Med Genet* 2010; 152A:2268–2276.

59. Sumner CJ. Molecular mechanisms of spinal muscular atrophy. *J Child Neurol* 2007; 22:979–989.

60. Jablonka S, Rossoll W, Schrank B, et al. The role of SMN in spinal muscular atrophy. *J Neurol* 2000; 247(Suppl1):137–142.

61. McWhorter ML, Monani UR, Burghes AH, et al. Knockdown of the survival motor neuron (Smn) protein in zebrafish causes defects in motor axonal outgrowth and pathfinding. *J Cell Biol* 2003; 162:919–931.

62. Zou T, Ilangovan R, Yu F, et al. SMN protects cells against mutant SOD1 toxicity by increasing chaperone activity. *Biochem Biophysical Res Comm* 2007; 364:850–855.

63. Hirtz D, Iannacone S, Heemskerk J, et al. Challenges and opportunity in clinical trials for spinal muscular atrophy. *Neurology* 2005; 65:1352–1357.

64. Waldman RI, Bosboom WM, van den Berg LH, et al. Drug treatment for spinal muscular atrophy type 1 (Review). *Cochrane Database Syst Rev* 2011 Dec 7; 12:CD006281.

65. Waldman RI, Bosboom WM, van den Berg LH, et al. Drug treatment for spinal muscular atrophy types II and III (Review). *Cochrane Database Syst Rev* 2011 Dec 7; 12:CD006282.

66. Miller TG, Moore DH, Dronsky V, et al. A placebo-controlled trial of gabapentin in spinal muscular atrophy. *J Neurol Sci* 2001; 191:127–131.

67. Mercuri E, Bertini E, Messina S, et al. Randomized, double-blind, placebo-controlled trial of phenylbutyrate in spinal muscular atrophy. *Neurology* 2007; 68:51–55.

68. Russman BS, Iannacone ST, Samaha FJ, et al. A phase 1 trial of riluzole in spinal muscular atrophy. *Arch Neurol* 2003; 60:1601–1603.

69. Swoboda KJ, Scott CB, Crawford TO, et al. SMA CARNI-VAL Trial Part I:Double-blind, randomized, placebo-controlled trial of L-carnitine and valproic acid in spinal muscular atrophy. *PLoS ONE* 5(8):e12140.doi:10.1371/journal.pone.0012140.

70. Kissel JT, Scott CB, Reyna SP, et al. SMA CARNI-VAL Trial Part II: A prospective, single-armed trial of L-carnitine and valproic acid in ambulatory children with spinal muscular atrophy. *PLoS ONE* 6(7): e21296. Doi:10.1371/journal.pone.0021296.

71. Grzeschik SM, Ganta M, Prior TW, et al. Hydroxyurea enhances SMN2 gene expression in spinal muscular atrophy cells. *Ann Neurol* 2005; 58:194–202.

72. Liang WC, You CY, Chang JG, et al. The effect of hydroxyurea in spinal muscular atrophy cells and patients. *J Neurol Sci* 2008; 268:87–94.

73. Gavrilina TO, McGovern VL, Workman E, et al. Neuronal SMN expression corrects spinal muscular atophy in severe SMN mice while muscle-specific SMN expression has no phenotypic effect. *Hum Molec Genet* 2008; 17:1063–1075.

74. Lutz CM, et al. Postsymptomatic restoration of SMN rescues the disease phenotype in a mouse model of severe spinal muscular atrophy. *J Clin Invest* 2011; 121:3029–3041.

75. Farooq F, et al. Prolactin increases SMN expression and survival in a mouse model of severe spinal muscular atrophy via the STAT5 pathway. *J Clin Invest* 2011; 121:3042–3050.

76. Swoboda KJ. Of SMN in mice and men: a therapeutic opportunity. *J Clin Invest* 2011; 121:2978–2981.

77. DiMatteo D, Callahan S, Kmiec EB. Genetic conversion of SNM2 gene to SMN1: a novel approach to the treatment of spinal muscular atrophy. *Experiment Cell Res* 2008; 314:878–886.

78. Baughan T, Shababi M, Coady TH, et al. Stimulation full-length SMN2 expression by delivering bifunctional RNAs via a viral vector. *Mol Ther* 2006; 14:54–62.

79. Azzouz M, Le T, Ralph GS, et al. Lentivector-mediated SMN replacement in a mouse model of spinal muscular atrophy. *J Clin Invest* 2004; 114:1726–1731.

80. Lefebvre S, Burlet P, Liu Q, et al. Correlation between severity and SMN protein level in spinal muscular atrophy. *Nature Genet* 1997; 16:265–269.

81. Eng GD, Binder H, Koch B. Spinal Muscular Atrophy: Experience in Diagnosis and Rehabilitation Management of 60 Patients. *Arch Phys Med Rehabil* 1984; 65:549–553.

82. Miske LJ, Hickey EM, Kolb SM, Weiner DJ, Panitch HB. Use of the mechanical in-exsufflator in pediatric patients with neuromuscular disease and impaired cough. *Chest* 2004 Apr; 125(4):1406–1412.

83. Bach JR. Update and perspectives on noninvasive respiratory muscle aids Part 1: The inspiratory aids. *Chest* 1994; 105:1230–1240.

84. Bach JR. Management of chronic alveolar hypoventilation by nasal ventilation. *Chest* 1990; 97:52–57.

85. Bach JR, Alba AS. Intermittent abdominal pressure ventilator in a regimen of noninvasive ventilatory support. *Chest* 1991; 99:630–636.

86. Wang T-G, Bach JR, Avilla C, Alba AS, Yang G-FW. Survival of individuals with spinal muscular atrophy on ventilatory support. *Am J Phys Med Rehabil* 1994; 73:207–211.

87. Wallgren-Pettersson C, Bushby K, Mellies U, Simonds A. 117th ENMC workshop: ventilatory support in congenital neuromuscular disorders —congenital myopathies, congenital muscular dystrophies, congenital myotonic dystrophy and SMA (II) 4–6 April 2003, Naarden, The Netherlands. *Neuromuscul Disord* 2004 Jan; 14(1):56–69.

88. Eagle M, Baudouin SV, Chandler C, Giddings DR, Bullock R, Bushby K. Survival in Duchenne muscular dystrophy: improvements in life expectancy since 1967 and the impact of home nocturnal ventilation. *Neuromuscul Disord* 2002 Dec; 12(10):926–929.

89. Finder JD, Birnkrant D, Carl J, et al. Respiratory care of the patient with Duchenne muscular dystrophy: ATS consensus statement. *Am J Respir Crit Care Med* 2004 Aug 15; 170(4):456–465.

90. Manzur AY, Muntoni F, Simonds A. Muscular dystrophy campaign sponsored workshop: Recommendation for respiratory care of children with spinal muscular atrophy type II and III. 13th February 2002, London, UK. *Neuromuscul Disord* 2003; 13:184–189.

91. Shapiro F, Specht L. The diagnosis and orthopaedic treatment of childhood spinal muscular atrophy, peripheral neuropathy, Friedreich ataxia, and arthrogryposis. *J Bone Joint Surg* 1993; 75-a:1699–1714.

92. Russman BS, Buncher CR, White M, Samaha FJ, Iannaccone ST, DCN/SMA Group. Function changes in spinal muscular atrophy II and III. *Neurology* 1996; 47:973–976.

93. Siegel IM, Silverman M. Upright Mobility System for Spinal Muscular Atrophy Patients. *Arch Phys Med Rehabil* 1984; 65:418.

94. Whelan TB. Neuropsychological performance of children with Duchenne muscular dystrophy and spinal muscle atrophy. *Devel Med Child Neurol* 1987; 29:212–220.

CHAPTER **48**

Genetic Basis of Familial Amyotrophic Lateral Sclerosis

Paloma Gonzalez-Perez, Robert H. Brown, Jr.

Amyotrophic lateral sclerosis (ALS), the commonest adult-onset motor neuron disease (MND), results from motor neuron degeneration in the motor cortex, brainstem, and spinal cord, and culminates in death, typically from respiratory failure, within three to five years. It has an incidence of one to two per 100,000, and a prevalence of four to six per 100,000, with a lifetime ALS risk of approximately 1/600 (1, 2).

COMMON FAMILIAL ALS GENES

While most ALS cases are sporadic (SALS), approximately 5 to 10% are familial (FALS), transmitted in most pedigrees as an autosomal dominant (AD) trait (3). ALS is typically defined as FALS when it is encountered in more than one first- or second-degree relative within a pedigree. From a clinical perspective, there are no significant differences between typical SALS and FALS, other than a slightly earlier age of onset in FALS as compared to SALS (55–63 years) (4). Rarely, and devastatingly, some patients with FALS show onset in early teen years. As the numbers of causative ALS genes and mutations increase, subtle features are emerging that begin to highlight genotype-phenotype associations. For instance, A4V mutations in the superoxide dismutase 1 (*SOD1*) gene are more frequent in North American ALS patients and are associated with substantially shorter survival of less than two years. P525L FUS gene mutations have been associated with the most aggressive juvenile forms of ALS, starting even before 25 years. While age and male gender are well-documented risk factors for SALS, they do not appear to influence risk of FALS (5).

In recent years, improvements in the technology for gene sequencing have facilitated whole exome and whole genome sequencing, dramatically accelerating identification of familial ALS genes (Figure 1). As outlined in Table 1, at least 14 causative genes of FALS have been identified as denoted by comigration with ALS within individual pedigrees. Genetic variants in at least 12 additional genes may be described as susceptibility factors, based on statistical over-representation in ALS in case-control comparisons. Five additional variants have been described as modifiers of phenotype (survival or age of onset). Overall, we now know the genetic basis in approximately 60% of FALS cases (Figure 2), although this number varies somewhat in different studies because of many factors, including differences in the numbers of FALS patients in each study (large cohorts are expected to yield more accurate and more meaningful small frequency distributions) and over-representation of specific ALS gene mutations in some geographical regions probably due to founder effects. Thus, mutations in optineurin (*OPTN*) account for almost 3% of patients with FALS in Japan, whereas these mutations in other populations are quite rare (6). The following provides a brief review on the most common and best-studied ALS genes, building on the outline provided in Table 1.

Superoxide Dismutase 1

In 1993, a multicenter collaborative study (7) identified 11 missense mutations in 13 FALS pedigrees in the *SOD1* gene. Nearly 20 years later, more than 150 mutations have been identified, distributed throughout all five exons (http://

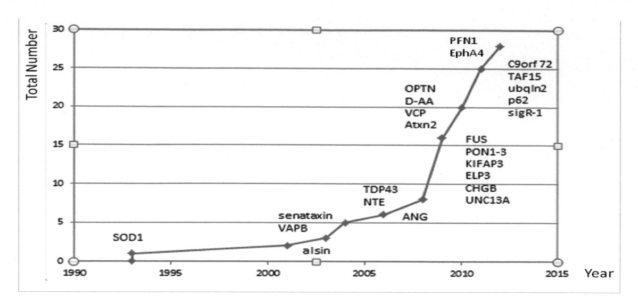

FIG. 1. Time Course of Discovery of ALS Genes. The rate of ALS gene discovery is increasing due in large measure to improved DNA sequencing technologies.

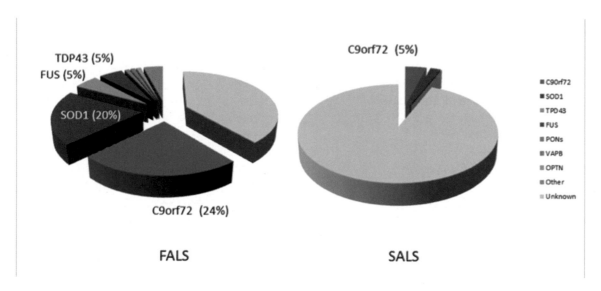

FIG. 2. Distribution of ALS genes in FALS and SALS. These graphs illustrate the frequencies of the major ALS genes in FALS and SALS.

alsod.iop.kcl.ac.uk/). These are overwhelmingly missense mutations, with fewer than 10% involving truncations of the distal-most domains of the protein (encoded by exons 4 and 5). These observations are consistent with the concept that mutant *SOD1* protein is a prerequisite for induction of motor neuron toxicity. In total, *SOD1* mutations account for 15 to 20% of AD FALS cases and 2 to 3% of SALS, the latter of which probably represent incomplete penetrance, incomplete family history information, or (rarely) *de novo* mutations (8). In general, the *SOD1* mutations are clinically quite penetrant, with notable exceptions such as E100K, I113T, and D90A (discussed below) (9).

SOD1 encodes a copper/zinc-binding cytosolic protein of 16 kDa and 153 amino acids that is ubiquitous and abundant. Its enzymatic activity is to catalyze conversion of superoxide anion radicals (O2-) to molecular oxygen (O2) and hydrogen peroxide (H2O2). Because these products can be subsequently metabolized to H_2O and O_2 through the actions of catalase and glutathione peroxidase SOD1 has been viewed as an antioxidant protein. The catalytic activity of SOD1 requires its homodimerization with linking of both 16k Da subunits via two cysteines that form an intrasubunit disulphide bond. Numerous lines of investigation support the hypothesis that the mutant SOD1 protein has acquired one

Gene		Chr	Inheritance	Frequency (%)		Association with FTD	Ref
				FALS	SALS		
Superoxide dismutase	SOD1	21q	AD	15-20%	3-Feb	Rarely I113T	7
Transactive DNA binding protein	TARDBP	1p	AD	up to 5%	up to 5	Sometimes	30
Fused in sarcoma / translocated in liposarcoma	FUS/TLS	16p	AD (AR for H517Q)	up to 5%	0.7	Sometimes	42, 43
Valosin-containing protein	VCP	9p	AD	2%	0	Yes	61
C9orf72	c9orf72	9p	AD	40%	5	Yes	49, 59, 60
Ubiquilin-2	UBQLN2	Xp	X-linked	<1%	<1%	Yes	62
Profilin-1	PFN1	17p	AD	2%	0	No	110
Vesicle-associated membrane protein B	VAPB	20q	AD	Brazilians		No	94
Senataxin	SETX	9q	AD	0-1%		No	95
Dynactin	DCTN1	2p	AD	0-1%		Rarely K17I	96
Alsin	ALSIN	2q	AR	0-1%		No	98
Angiogenin	ANG	14q	AD	Scottish and Irish		Rarely K17I	100
Optineurin	OPTN	10p	AD/AR	up to 3% in Japanese		No	104
Ataxin-2	ATXN2	12q	N/A	6% (vs 4% in controls)		No	107

TABLE 1. ALS Genes Whose Mutations Comigrate with ALS in Pedigrees

Gene		Chr	References
Paroxonases 1-3	PON1,2,3	7q	112
Dipeptidyl-peptidase-6	DPP6	7q	115
Neuropathy target esterase	NTE	19p	118
Elongator protein 3	ELP3	8p	119
FIG4	FIG4	6q	120
Chromogranin B	CHGB	20p	121
Unc13A	UNC13A	19p	72
D-amino acid oxidase	DAO	12q	126
Sequestosome 1	SQSTM1/p62	5q	129
Survival motor neurin	SMN	5q	130

TABLE 2. Genetic Variants that Confer Susceptibility to SALS or FALS

Gene		Chr	References
Ephrin A4	EphA4	2q	111
Kinesin-associated protein 3	KIFAP3	1q	131
Chromogranin B	CHGB	20p	121
Survival motor neuron	SMN	5q	Several reports
Unc13A	UNC13A	19p	125

TABLE 3. Genetic Variants that Modify the ALS Phenotype

or more toxic properties. This view is consistent with dual observations in mice. Mice bearing transgenes that express high levels of mutant SOD1 protein develop a phenotype that clinically and histopathologically mimics human ALS. Conversely, mice in which the SOD1 have been genetically deleted (10). We highlight below some of the most important *SOD1* mutations and their associated phenotypic features.

A4V

In North America, this missense variant accounts for about 50% of ALS patients with mutations in this gene

(11–13). Its phenotype is characterized by rapid disease progression and death, on average occurring at 1.4 years (versus three–five years in ALS patients with other *SOD1* mutations) (14). This mutation occurs on a haplotype that is common in North American and probably of Asian origin (15, 16). The molecular basis for this aggressive phenotype is not clear; our investigations failed to identify any disease-modifying genetic variants within the conserved haplotypic region shared by *A4V* patients. This suggested that the aggressive clinical trajectory in *A4V* ALS reflects the intrinsic properties of the A4V protein (or its RNA, or both) (17). It is notable that other ALS-associated missense mutations affecting this alanine residue also are correlated with rapid disease courses (e.g., A4S and A4T) (18, 19).

I113T

This is the second most common *SOD1* mutation in FALS patients. It is also detected in some apparently sporadic cases, probably because of incomplete penetrance within pedigrees (20). This mutation has been reported to be co-inherited with frontotemporal dementia in some ALS families (21, 22); in general, cognitive impairment is infrequent in ALS cases arising from *SOD1* mutations (23).

G93A

The molecular pathology of this mutation has been widely investigated because mice that express high levels of transgenic G93A-SOD1 develop motor neuron disease with clinical and pathological features that closely mimic human ALS. The phenotype of patients with this mutation is typical of ALS (24), a point that underscores the potential value of ALS in transgenic SOD1G93A mice and rats.

D90A

This mutation has been the subject of considerable attention because in Western Europe and the United States, individuals heterozygous for this variant develop typical ALS while, by contrast, in northern Sweden D90A heterozygotes, which are two top 3% of the population, are normal. In that region, individuals homozygous for the mutation develop atypical motor neuron disease that is slowly progressive with prominent involvement of the corticospinal tracts. These considerations suggest the hypothesis that individuals in northern Scandinavia may possess one or more genetic variants that are neuroprotective, or there is an environmental variable that is similarly protective there (25, 26).

The molecular mechanisms whereby mutations in the SOD1 gene and protein mediate motor neuron degeneration are being intensively investigated; potentially important pathways invoke misfolding and aggregation of the mutant protein, defective axonal transport, altered oxidative status in the central nervous system parenchyma, excitotoxicity within the motor neurons, in part secondary to defective EAAT2 glutamate transporter, or one or more categories of non-cell autonomous cell death (27). Some data argue that, when post-translationally modified, WT SOD1 can mimic the toxicity of mutant SOD1 and that non-Mendelian modifications of SOD1 are involved in the pathogenesis of SALS cases (28).

TAR DNA Binding Protein

In 2006, the 43 kDa transactive response (TAR) DNA-binding protein (TDP-43), a ubiquitous nuclear protein of 414 amino acids involved in transcription regulation and splicing process among other functions, was identified as the major component of the cytosolic ubiquitinated inclusions that are observed in cortical neurons in the vast majority of ALS patients and in patients with tau-negative frontotemporal dementia (FTD) (29). This pathological finding, and the coexistence of ALS and FTD in some patients, underscored the point that diseases are part of the same clinic-pathological spectrum. In 2008, TAR DNA-binding protein 43 (*TARDBP*) mutations were identified in both FALS and SALS (30). All such mutations identified to date map to exon 6, except Asp169Gly in exon 4 (http://alsod.iop.kcl.ac.uk/). Exon 6 encodes a highly conserved region of the C-terminal domain of TDP-43 protein; this domain has been involved in the inhibition of the splicing of the cystic fibrosis transmembrane conductance regulator mRNA (31). This C-terminal domain has been observed in a phosphorylated form in the neuronal cytosolic ubiquitinated inclusions of ALS and FTD patients, together with a TDP-43 nuclear loss, suggesting that cleavage, phosphorylation, and cytoplasmic accumulation of this C-terminal fragment underlie the neurodegenerative process involved in ALS and FTD (29).

The frequency of *TARDBP* mutations in ALS dramatically varies among different studies; the highest frequencies are estimated to be 5 to 6% in both FALS and SALS cohorts (30, 32–38). On the other hand, little is known about phenotype-genotype correlations in patients with *TARDBP* mutations. Only one study (39) investigated the phenotypes of 28 patients with *TARDBP* mutations (nine were SALS) and reviewed the phenotypes of 117 patients with *TARDBP* mutations reported in the literature (21 were SALS). In that report (39), individuals with *TARDBP* mutations had an earlier onset and longer survival than SALS patients without *TARDBP* mutations. Moreover, the site of onset in this group was predominantly upper limb. Additionally, the G298S mutation was associated with shorter survival. Given that ALS and FTD co-exist in some individuals, and that there are cytosolic ubiquitinated TDP43 inclusions in both diseases, it is reasonable to anticipate that *TARDBP* mutations could also account for FTD cases without MND. In fact, one *TARDBP* mutation (N267S) has been reported in a single patient with FTD without MND (40). A more common observation is that *TARDBP* mutations may cause both ALS and FTD in the same individual (41).

Fused in Sarcoma/Translocated in Liposarcoma

Approximately one year after the identification of *TARDBP* mutations in ALS, it was reported that mutations in another

RNA-processing protein, Fused-in-sarcoma/translated-in-liposarcoma (*FUS/TLS*), also accounted for about 5% of FALS cases (42, 43). Although originally mutations in this gene were not found in SALS, later studies have estimated a 0.7% frequency of *FUS* mutations in this group (44–46). All *FUS/TLS* mutations identified to date map within exon 14 and 15 (http://alsod.iop.kcl.ac.uk/).

Over the last three years, several important similarities between *TARDBP* and *FUS/TLS* mutations have emerged (47). First, most of the mutations cluster to the glycine rich region that is present in both proteins. In *FUS/TLS*, another mutational hot spot is the nuclear localization signal (NLS) domain. In the TDP-43 protein, the glycine rich region is contained within the c-terminal fragment of the protein. In the FUS/TLS protein (526 amino acids), the glycine rich region extends from amino acids 165 to 267, whereas the c-terminal domain contains the RNA recognition motif (RRM), Arg-Gly-Gly (RGG) repeat rich, zinc finger, and NLS domains. Second, these similarities in protein structure are paralleled by similarities in the functions of TARDBP and FUS/TLS. Both are RNA-processing proteins that are involved in transcription regulation, splicing, RNA transport, and local translation. Third, postmortem analyses of ALS patients with mutations in either of these genes have revealed cytosolic ubiquitinated inclusions in both brain and spinal cord. In the case of *TARDBP* mutations, these inclusions are TDP-43 positive, while in the case of *FUS/TLS* mutations they are FUS positive. It is important to point out that these pathological hallmarks are not exclusive to ALS patients with *TARDBP* or *FUS/TLS* mutations. Thus, TDP-43 inclusions have been widely observed in ALS and FTD patients without *TARDBP* mutations and in other neurodegenerative diseases. Although less frequent, FUS inclusions have also been observed in some cases of FTLD that are currently grouped under the name of FTLD-FUS. This grouping includes three entities: atypical FTLD with ubiquitinated inclusions (aFTLD-U), neuronal intermediate filament inclusion disease, and basophilic inclusion body disease.

As with *TARDBP* mutations, little has been published about phenotype-genotype correlations in ALS patients with *FUS/TLS* mutations. However, several reports have described quite specific clinical syndromes in patients with mutations in this gene. Thus, R521C, the most common *FUS* mutation to date, has been associated with an atypical ALS phenotype characterized by early onset (before 25 years), proximal limb girdle weakness, dropped head, and short survival (<36 months) (48, 49). Other *FUS* mutations also cause an early onset of the disease as P525L, which has been associated with several instances of rapidly progressive, juvenile-onset ALS (50). As well, a few ALS-FTD patients, and also rare cases of isolated FTD, have been identified as carriers of *FUS* mutations too (51–54).

ALS ASSOCIATED WITH FRONTOTEMPORAL DEMENTIA

The term FTD refers to a clinical syndrome that includes three different clinical variants: the behavioral variant (bvFTD), semantic dementia (SD), and progressive non-fluent aphasia (PNFA). Frontotemporal lobar degeneration (FTLD) is the term most commonly used to designate the different sub-categories of FTD pathologically. FTLD, in which neuronal inclusions are tau-positive, have been labeled as FTLD-tau, while those without tau have been grouped as FTLD-U because their inclusions are positive for ubiquitin. Some cases in this latter group are positive for TDP-43 (FTLD-TDP43) but not FUS, while others are positive for FUS (FTLD-FUS), suggesting that the underlying pathogenic pathways in these two entities are mutually exclusive (55).

FTD is the second most common early-onset dementia in adults. At least 15% of ALS cases have elements of FTD (usually bvFTD). Even without frank FTD, up to 50% of ALS patients reveal some degree of cognitive impairment (56, 57). As many as a third of ALS-FTD cases have a family history of FTD, ALS, or ALS-FTD. For these reasons, an understanding of the molecular pathogenesis of FTD promises to illuminate the pathophysiology of ALS as well. The most frequent genetic cause of this phenotype is a recently identified hexanucleotide (GGGGCC) repeat expansion in the non-coding region of c9orf72 (58–60); these expansions account for the majority of familial cases of ALS-FTD. However, for most of the remaining ALS-FTD cases, no underlying genetic defects have been identified. A small subset is a consequence of mutations in *TARDBP* and *FUS/TLS*, rarely in *SOD1*, and also in *VCP* and *UBQLN2* (21–23, 40, 41, 51–54, 61, 62).

C9orf72

It was recognized several years ago that there are large pedigrees in which ALS, FTD, or (in the same individual) concurrent ALS and FTD migrated as genetically dominant traits. A locus for this was mapped to the pericentric region of chromosome 9 (63–70). It was, therefore, striking that genome-wide association studies (GWAS) in large SALS cohorts yielded highly significant associations of sporadic ALS with single nucleotide polymorphisms (SNP) that also mapped to this region, suggesting that an unique genetic variant accounted for a high proportion of cases of both SALS and FALS (including ALS-FTD) (71–73). A major milestone in this field was the identification by independent laboratories of the offending genetic variant —a hexanucleotide repeat (GGGGCC) in the non-coding region of a largely unstudied gene, *c9orf72*, within ALS-FTD locus on chromosome 9p (58–60). This expansion, sometimes termed c9FTD/ALS, accounts for all 9p-linked

ALS-FTD families and represents around 40% of FALS and 5% of SALS. It is therefore, the most frequent genetic cause of ALS to date. Although the minimum size of the expansion required to trigger neurodegeneration is not yet well defined, it is generally accepted that the normal range spans up to about 30 hexanucleotide repeats. By contrast, in affected cases, Southern blotting methods have identified expansions with more than 600 repeats. The GGGGCC repeat is located between the first two non-coding exons of the c9orf72 gene. These exons are alternatively spliced, thus, the repeat may function as an element of the *c9orf72* promoter that is presumably active when the first exon is spliced out. Little is known about how the hexanucleotide influences either promoter activity (or overall *c9orf72* expression) or the process of alternative splicing of these exons. Preliminary data point to a reduction of the isoform a (full-length transcript) in chromosome 9p-linked FTD and ALS (c9FTD/ALS) carriers (58).

One of the striking aspects of the c9orf72 ALS gene is that its molecular biology is likely to be analogous to that in other non-coding nucleotide repeat disorders such as myotonic dystrophy type 1 (CTG repeats) and myotonic dystrophy type 2 (CCTG repeats) (74). Potential mechanisms for the pathobiology of these repeats have recently been reviewed (75). However, by contrast with the phenomenon of genetic anticipation encountered in myotonic dystrophy, there has thus far been no evidence of anticipation in ALS families with the *c9orf72* GGGGCC expansion (58). Bulbar onset is strikingly over-represented in ALS cases arising from this gene defect (76–78). Technical difficulties in accurately defining the sizes of the enormously expanded alleles have hindered analyses of the impact of expansion size on age of onset or survival.

The profile of pathologies associated with c9FTD/ALS is beginning to be defined. Even prior to the identification of the *c9orf72* mutations, it was evident that one pathological hallmark of the 9p-linked ALS-FTD families was the presence of widespread neuronal cytoplasmic inclusions (NCI) that stained positively for TDP-43, p62, and ubiquitin. Also described are p62 and ubiquitin-positive but TDP-43 negative inclusions in the granular layer of the cerebellum in some cases confirmed to be c9FTD/ALS (79), a finding that may be pathognomonic of this form of ALS (80, 81). Ubiquilin-positive cytoplasmic inclusions are also sometimes detected in the hippocampal molecular layer in c9FTD/ALS cases; this finding may differentiate ALS and FTD patients with expansions from those without this molecular defect (82).

Valosin Containing Protein

Before it was clearly associated with ALS, valosin containing protein (*VCP*) mutations were linked to three dominantly inherited disease traits: inclusion body myopathy (IBM),

Paget disease of the bone, and FTD (IBMPFD) (83, 84). In 2010, studies (61) using whole exome sequencing identified a *VCP* mutation (R191Q) in a family in which some individuals presented clinically with ALS. This finding suggested that ALS was part of the VCP-associated clinical spectrum. Subsequent mutational analysis estimated that as many as 2% of FALS pedigrees may harbor *VCP* mutations. Interestingly, some members of these families were also affected with myopathy, Paget disease of the bone, or FTD, consistent with substantial phenotypic heterogeneity associated with VCP mutations. To date, nine mutations in the *VCP* gene have been identified in ALS families; most of them map to exon 5 and were previously reported in IBMPFD pedigrees (85–91).

UBQLN2

Within the last 18 months, some cases of dominantly inherited, X-linked ALS (and ALS-FTD) have been ascribed to mutations in ubiquilin 2 (*UBQLN2*). *UBQLN2* mutations were originally identified in 2% of potentially X-linked FALS cases (defined by the absence of male-to-male transmission) (62), but their frequency is considerably lower when all FALS are considered irrespective of apparent transmission patterns (92, 93). Nonetheless, *UBQLN2* may have a general role in ALS pathogenesis. That wild-type *UBQLN2* can participate in the pathophysiology of ALS is indicated by the presence of cytosolic, ubiquilin2-positive neuronal inclusions in ALS patients without *UBQLN2* gene mutations (62). The mechanism whereby mutant *UBQLN2* initiates neurodegeneration is not yet known. All *UBQLN2* mutations alter proline residues within a region containing 12 tandem repeats of the three amino acid sequence proline-X-X. While the function of this domain remains unclear, it is likely that these mutations alter the function of ubiquilin 2 protein in the process of protein degradation by the ubiquitin proteasome system.

OTHER ALS-ASSOCIATED GENES

In the last five years, mutations in many other genes have been proposed to cause FALS. Some are associated with ALS that is clinically typical while others trigger forms of motor neuron degeneration with clinical features that are atypical for ALS. In general, these mutant genes are less common in either FALS or SALS than mutations in *c9orf72*, *SOD1*, *TDP43* and *FUS*.

Associated with Typical and Atypical ALS

Vesicle Associated Membrane Protein-Associated Protein B

Mutations in the vesicle associated membrane protein (*VAMP*)/synaptobrevin-associated membrane protein B gene

(*VAPB*), first reported in a large Brazilian ALS family of Portuguese descent, generate at least three phenotypes: a) late-onset spinal muscular atrophy; b) atypical ALS with bulbar onset and slow progression, pyramidal signs, and a distinctive essential tremor; and c) typical ALS. The VAPB protein is involved in the vesicle trafficking in the endoplasmic reticulum and Golgi apparatus (94). *VAPB* gene mutations may perturb protein trafficking and folding in these structures.

Senataxin

Mutations in the senataxin (*SEXT*) gene were first identified as cause of juvenile onset ALS, characterized by severe distal weakness and atrophy, pyramidal signs, and normal life span. Subsequently, other dominantly acting *SEXT* mutations were delineated in other cases of MND characterized by two other phenotypes, hereditary motor neuropathy and ataxia-tremor MND syndrome. Yet another mutant *SEXT* phenotype, ataxia—ocular apraxia 2 (AOA2), is transmitted as a recessive trait. The function of the senataxin protein is incompletely understood. One view is that it is implicated in RNA biogenesis and DNA repair (95).

Dynactin

Mutations in the dynactin (*DCTN1*) gene have been related to a slowly progressive, autosomal dominant lower motor neuron disorder characterized clinically by early onset, vocal cord paralysis, and facial and distal weakness, predominantly in the hands (96). One mutation (R1101K) was identified in an ALS family that was also afflicted with FTD (97). Dynactin is an accessory motor protein that functions in the active transport of organelles in the cell body and in retrograde transport in axons. Accordingly, a leading hypothesis for *DCTN1*-associated MND is that dysfunction in some aspect of retrograde transport underlies the slow demise of motor neurons.

Alsin

The alsin (*ALS2*) gene on chromosome 2p encodes a multifunctional protein. One of its functions is to regulate GTPase signaling that is central to microtubule assembly and membrane trafficking (98, 99). Recessive (loss-of-function) mutations in this gene were first detected in an inbred family in Tunis with juvenile-onset motor neuron disease that was predominantly corticospinal in distribution. Slowly progressive lower motor neuron disease was documented by electrophysiological studies but was only minimally apparent on clinical grounds. In most families subsequently described with alsin mutations, lower motor neuron involvement has rarely been encountered. Thus, in most instances the disorder has been described as a form of

juvenile primary lateral sclerosis or hereditary spastic paraparesis. The alsin gene expresses two ALS2 transcripts. In most cases with the juvenile primary lateral sclerosis phenotype, the mutations lead to deletions in exon 9, selectively affecting the longer of the two transcripts while the shorter transcript remains intact; one view is that this shorter transcript mitigates complete loss of alsin function. By contrast, in the family with combined corticospinal and lower motor neuron dysfunction, the genetic lesion involves exon 3, as a result of which both transcripts are absent or truncated. Presumably this leads to a more complete loss of alsin function and the more severe phenotype.

Angiogenin

Angiogenin (ANG) is a bifunctional ribonuclease protein that is important in tRNA metabolism, and it is (as its name suggests), an angiogenic factor. Heterozygous mutations in the *ANG* gene were first identified in Scottish and Irish ALS cases (100). Both in the initial reports and subsequently, it has been difficult to identify large ALS pedigrees in which these *ANG* mutations robustly co-migrate with ALS. It has, therefore, seemed likely that ANG mutations are incompletely penetrant and thus might best be considered as enhancing ALS susceptibility rather than frankly causing MND. This view was recently supported by a large study again documenting over-representation of heterozygous *ANG* mutations in cohorts of ALS and Parkinson disease compared to controls (101). The association of *ANG* variants has been largely reported with pure ALS, although in one pedigree the *ANG* missense variant K17I was associated with ALS-FTD (102). As observed in *c9orf72*-based ALS, bulbar onset ALS is over-represented in ALS cases bearing *ANG* mutations (100). The pathological hallmarks of *ANG*-related ALS in brain and spinal cord are not yet reported in detailed autopsy series; it is established in a single case with the K171I mutation that there are neuronal, intranuclear, and cytoplasmic inclusions positive for smooth muscle alpha-actin and TDP-43, respectively (103).

Optineurin

Another gene whose mutations have been infrequently linked to ALS is *OPTN*, whose protein product is implicated in activation of transcription and trafficking of membranes and vesicles. While *OPTN* mutations are rare in North America, they may account for as much as 3% of FALS cases in Japan (<1%) (104, 105). In general terms, these mutations have been associated with slow progression and long duration of the disease. Some of these patients also develop primary open angle glaucoma (POAG), another disorder well documented to be caused by OPTN mutations (106). Cytosolic, optineurin-positive inclusions are evident in brain autopsy samples of some *OPTN* mutation cases, but are also detected in ALS patients without *OPTN* mutations, suggesting that (like *UBQLN2*) *OPTN* may participate in the pathogenesis of many types of ALS. These inclusions co-localize with TDP-43 and with SOD1-positive Lewy-body-like hyaline inclusions in SOD1 cases (104). These points notwithstanding, a transparent definition of the role of OPTN in motor neuron death has not yet evolved.

Ataxin 2

It is well established that expansions of a CAG tract (encoding glutamate) in the ataxin-2 (*ATXN2*) gene to more than 34 repeats leads to spinocerebellar ataxia type 2 (SCA2). Clinicians have noted for several years that late in the course of SCA2 there may be evidence of MND. It was therefore intriguing that intermediate length expansions of the same CAG repeat tract to a range of 26–34 repeats were statistically more abundant in ALS cohorts than controls (107, 108). Hopefully, further investigations will elucidate the mechanism whereby polyQ tracts of intermediate length increase the risk of ALS. A relevant finding is that there is a direct interaction between TDP-43 and ataxin 2, suggesting that the mild expansions might in some manner invoke the same molecular events that are activated by mutant TDP-43. In the presence of the expanded ataxin-2 allele, wild type TDP-43 is induced to form aberrant, sometimes skein-like, cytoplasmic foci (107, 109).

Profilin 1 and Ephrin A4

Quite recently, it was reported that loss-of-function mutations in the gene encoding profilin-1 (PFN1) are the likely trigger of ALS in some families (110). Normally, PFN1 regulates the polymerization of actin, a property that influences nuclear events during cell division and both axonal extension and growth cone expansion. Functional studies documented that the PFN1 variants impair growth cone outgrowth. In the recent report, the frequency of *PFN1* mutations in FALS is—2% (110). Also recently reported was the finding that inactivation of Ephrin A4, a cell surface receptor whose ligand interactions trigger an intracellular cascade that probably acts to suppress axon extension, rescues the mutant SOD1 phenotype in zebrafish and prolongs the survival in mice models of ALS (111). One view is that this may entail silencing of the activity of profilin-1, a downstream target of Ephrin A4. Quite strikingly, Robberecht and colleagues (111) reported that the motor axonal phenotype induced in zebrafish by mutant *SOD1* could be attenuated and even entirely blocked by inactivation of Ephrin A4 (111). That these findings are probably relevant to human ALS is suggested by two points. First, as reported by Robberecht and colleagues (111) in a cohort of ALS patients, expression of *EphA4* in circu-

lating mononuclear cells was inversely correlated with age onset; individuals with less EphA4 tended to have later onset. Second, two individuals with loss of function mutations in *EphA4* were identified in a screen of 200 FALS and SALS cases and found to have strikingly prolonged survival. This parallels the observation from the Robberecht team (111) that, in ALS mice, survival is improved by inhibition of the EphA4 human system (by breeding the ALS mice to a line of mice that are hemizygous for EphA4).

Less Definitive ALS-Associated Genes

There are still other genes whose variants have been genetically linked to either FALS or SALS but whose roles in motor neuron degeneration are less definitive. These are enumerated briefly below.

Paraoxonase

The *PON1*, *PON2*, and *PON3* variants in the paraoxonase genes, which have been implicated in the defensive response of tissues to exogenous intoxicants, are significantly over-represented in ALS (112–114).

Dipeptidyl Peptidase 6

The minor allele frequency of a variant in dipeptidyl peptidase 6 (*DPP6*) was the first polymorphism associated with SALS using a genome-wide association study in a European population (115). This association has not been consistently replicated in subsequent studies (116, 117). Among other possible functions, the DPP6 protein influences activity of some potassium ion channels.

Neuropathy Target Esterase

Recessive neuropathy target esterase (*NTE*) mutations have been identified in two unrelated families, one consanguineous. In both families, the motor neuron disease showed childhood onset and slow progression. NTE is a membrane protein that regulates the composition of the cell membrane and cell-signaling. It is the target of some organophosphates and mediates organophosphate-induced delayed neuropathy (OIPDN) (118).

Elongator Protein 3

A microsatellite repeat (D8S1820) that maps to intron 10 of *ELP3* gene was associated with ALS in three independent populations in the United Kingdom, United States, and Belgium. Independently, a mutagenesis screen in Drosophila yielded two mutations in *ELP3* that caused neuronal defects, suggesting that a loss of function of this gene may contribute to neurodegeneration in ALS. The ELP3 protein is a component of the RNA polymerase II complex and therefore is another RNA processing protein involved in neurodegeneration (119).

Figure 4

Recessively-inherited mutations in this gene cause Charcot-Marie-Tooth 4J with motor neuron involvement. In one unconfirmed study, 10 non-synonymous *FIG4* variants were identified in ALS patients with prominent upper motor neuron signs (120).

Chromogranin B

A known polymorphism (P413L) in chromogranin B (*CHGB*) was identified as a genetic risk factor for ALS in three different populations. In addition, ALS patients carrying the P413L variant developed the disease nearly ten years earlier than ALS patients without this variant. Subsequent studies failed to replicate this association (121–123).

UNC13A

A common variant that maps to intron 21 of UNC13A was associated with ALS in two genome-wide scans, one of which was a *UNC13A* polymorphism identified as a modifier of the ALS phenotype (124, 125).

D-Amino Acid Oxidase

A unique D-amino acid oxidase (*DAO*) mutation (R199W) comigrated with ALS in a single pedigree (126). This enzyme degrades D-serine, an agonist of N-methyl-D-aspartate receptors, and accumulates in the spinal cord of ALS patients, suggesting a pathogenic role in motor neuron death.

Sequestosome

Dysfunction in protein degradation by proteasomes and autophagy are implicated in multiple neurodegenerative diseases. The 62-kD protein (p62) protein that shuttles ubiquitinated proteins to the proteasome for degradation is a ligand of the p56-1ck SH2 domain. Histopathological studies have revealed that p62 is present in the neuronal ubiquitinated inclusions of ALS patients and other neurodegenerative diseases (127). It is, therefore, of interest that mutations in SQSTM1 have been reported in ALS patients; like mutations in VCP, those of SQSTM1 have been described in Paget disease of the bone (128, 129).

Survival Motor Neuron

Whether copy number of survival of motor neuron 1 (*SMN1*) and *SMN2* is a risk factor for ALS or a modifier factor of the ALS phenotype remains somewhat controversial.

Recently, a group (130) reported that *SMN1* duplication (SMN1=3 copies) was associated with ALS susceptibility, a finding that remained significant in a meta-analysis of multiple studies.

Kinesin-Associated Protein 3

We identified a variant in the *KIFAP3* gene that correlates with longer survival in SALS patients (131). While other studies based on different populations have failed to replicate this association, the same allele has independently associated with an upper motor neuron-ALS (UMN-ALS) phenotype (132, 133).

TAF15 and SigR-1

Rare ALS-associated variants have been reported in the genes encoding TAF-15, a FUS-associated RNA binding protein, and SigmaR-1, a non-opioid intracellular receptor (134, 135).

CONCLUSIONS

It is quite remarkable that innovative new approaches to gene sequencing have dramatically accelerated the process of identifying and confirming novel ALS genes. Each new gene will potentially provide fresh insights into adverse molecular cascades that lead to motor neuron death. Each new gene defect can potentially be used to generate new ALS models in cells and in mice. Most importantly, each step in these cascades is potentially a novel target for new treatments. These considerations give one considerable hope that with continued progress in the discovery of ALS genes there will emerge treatments that slow or even reverse the relentlessly downward clinical trajectory in ALS.

ACKNOWLEDGMENTS

P.G.-P. is supported by the Alfonso Martin Escudero Foundation. R.H.B. Jr. is supported by the US National Institute for Neurological Disease and Stroke (NINDS) (5RO1-NS050557-05) and NINDS American Recovery and Reinvestment Act Award RC2-NS070-342, and acknowledges generous support from the Angel Fund, the ALS Association, P2ALS, Project ALS, the Pierre L. de Bourgknecht ALS Research Foundation and the ALS Therapy Alliance.

REFERENCES

1. McGuire V, Longstreth WT Jr, Koepsell TD, et al. Incidence of amyotrophic lateral sclerosis in three countries in western Washington State. *Neurology* 1996; 47:571–573.

2. Mitsumoto H, Chad DA, Pioro, EP. *Amyotrophic Lateral Sclerosis.* Oxford Univ. Press. New York 1998.

3. Byrne S, Walsh C, Lynch C, et al. Rate of familial amyotrophic lateral sclerosis: a systematic review and meta-analysis. *J Neurol Neurosurg Psychiatry* 2011; 82:623–627.

4. Haverkamp LJ, Appel V, Appel SH. Natural history of amyotrophic lateral sclerosis in a database population. Validation of a scoring system and a model for survival prediction. *Brain* 1995; 118:707–719.

5. Kurtzke JF. Risk factors in amyotrophic lateral sclerosis. *Adv Neurol* 1991; 56:245–270.

6. Maruyama H, Morino H, Ito H, et al. Mutations of optineurin in amyotrophic lateral sclerosis. *Nature* 2010; 13:223–226.

7. Rosen DR, Siddique T, Patterson D, et al. Mutations in Cu/Zn superoxide dismutase gene are associated with familial amyotrophic lateral sclerosis. *Nature* 1993; 362:59–62.

8. Shaw CE, Enayat Z, Chioza BA, et al. Mutations in all five exons of SOD-1 may cause ALS. *Ann Neurol* 1998; 43:390–394.

9. Felbecker A, Camu W, Valdmanis PN, et al. Four familial ALS pedigrees discordant for two SOD1 mutations: are all SOD1 mutations pathogenic? *J Neurol Neurosurg Psychiatry* 2010; 81:572–577.

10. Gurney ME, Pu H, Chiu AY, et al. Motor neuron degeneration in mice that express a human Cu, Zn superoxide dismutase mutation. *Science* 1994; 264:1772–1775.

11. Cudkowicz ME, Brown RH. An update on superoxide dismutase 1 in familial amyotrophic lateral sclerosis. *J Neuron Sci* 1996; 139(Suppl.):10–15.

12. Juneja T, Pericak-Vance MA, et al. Prognosis in familial amyotrophic lateral sclerosis: progression and survival in patients with glu100gly and ala4val mutations in Cu,Zn superoxide dismutase. *Neurology* 1997; 48:55–57.

13. Radunovic A, Leigh PN. Cu/Zn superoxide dismutase gene mutations in amyotrophic lateral sclerosis correlation between genotype and clinical features. *J Neurol Neurosurg Psychiatry* 1996; 61:565–572.

14. Cudkowicz ME, Mckenna-Yasek D, Sapp PE, et al. Epidemiology of mutations in superoxide dismutase in amyotrophic lateral sclerosis. *Ann Neurol* 1997; 41:210–221.

15. Rosen DR. A shared chromosome-21 haplotype among amyotrophic lateral sclerosis families with the A4V SOD1 mutation. *Clin Genet* 2004; 66:247–250.

16. Broom WJ, Johnson DV, Auwarter KE et al. SOD1 A4V-mediated ALS: absence of a closely linked modifier gene and origination in Asia. *Neurosci Lett* 2008; 430:241–245.

17. Broom WJ, Russ C, Sapp PC, et al. Variants in candidate ALS modifier genes linked to Cu/Zn superoxide dismutase do not explain divergent survival phenotypes. *Neurosci Lett* 2006; 392:52–57.

18. Aksoy H, Dean G, Elian M, et al. A4T mutation in the SOD1 gene causing familial amyotrophic lateral sclerosis. *Neuroepidemiology* 2003; 22:235–238.

19. Nakanishi T, Kishikawa M, Miyazaki A, et al. Simple and defined method to detect the SOD-1 mutants from patients with familial amyotrophic lateral sclerosis by mass spectrometry. *J Neurosci Methods* 1998; 81:41–44.

20. Andersen PM, Restagno G, Stewart HG, et al. Disease penetrance in amyotrophic lateral sclerosis associated with mutations in the SOD1 gene. *Ann Neurol* 2004; 55:298–299.

21. Katz JS, Katzberg HD, Wooley SC, et al. Combined fulminant frontotemporal dementia and amyotrophic lateral sclerosis associated with an I113T SOD1 mutation. *Amyotroph Lateral Scler* 2012 Jun 7 {Epub ahead of print}

22. Lopate G, Baloh RH, Al-Lozi MT et al. Familial ALS with extreme phenotypic variability due to the I113T SOD1 mutation. *Amyotroph Lateral Scler* 2010; 11:232–236.

23. Wicks P, Abrahams S, Al-Chalabi, et al. SOD1 and cognitive dysfunction in familial amyotrophic lateral sclerosis. *J Neurol* 2009; 256:234–241.

24. Synofzik M, Fernández-Santiago R, Maetzler W, et al. The human G93A SOD1 phenotype closely resembles sporadic amyotrophic lateral sclerosis. *J Neurol Neurosurg Psychiatry* 2010; 81:764–767.

25. Andersen PM Forsgren L, Binzer M, et al. Autosomal recessive adult-onset amyotrophic lateral sclerosis associated with homoozygosity for Asp90Ala CuZn-superoxide dismutase mutation. A clinical and genealogical study of 36 patients. *Brain* 1996; 119:1153–1172.

26. Andersen PM, Nilsson P, Ala-Hurula V, et al. Amyotrophic lateral sclerosis associated with homozygosity for an Asp90Ala mutation in CuZn-superoxide dismutase. *Nature Genet* 1995; 10:61–66.

27. Boillee S, Vande Velde C, Cleveland DW. ALS: a disease of motor neurons and their nonneuronal neighbors. *Neuron* 2006; 52:39–59.

28. Bosco DA, Morfini G, Karabacak NM, et al. Wild-type and mutant SOD1 share an aberrant conformation and a common pathogenic pathway in ALS. *Nat Neurosci* 2010; 13:1396–1403.

29. Neumann M, Sampathu DM, Kwong LK, et al. Ubiquitinated TDP-43 in frontotemporal lobar degeneration and amyotrophic lateral sclerosis. *Science* 2006; 3 14:130–133.

30. Sreedharan J, Blair IB, Tripathi VB, et al. TDP-43 mutations in familial ad sporadic Amyotrophic lateral Sclerosis. *Science* 2008; 319:1668–1672.

31. Buratti E, Brindisi A, Giombi M, et al. TDP-43 binds heterogeneous nuclear ribonucleoprotein A/B through its C/terminal tail: an important region for the inhibition of cystic fibrosis transmembrane conductance regulator exon 9 splicing. *J Biol Chem* 2005; 280:37572–37584.

32. Kabashi E, Valdmanis PM, Dion ,P et al. TARDBP mutations in individuals with sporadic and familial amyotrophic lateral sclerosis. *Nature Genetics* 2008; 40:572–574.

33. Van Deerlin VM, Leverenz JB, Bekris LM, et al. TARDBP mutations in amyotrophic lateral sclerosis with TDP-43 neuropathology: a genetic and histopathological analysis. *Lancet Neurol* 2008; 7:409–416.

34. Kühnlein P, Sperfeld AD, Vanmassenhove B, et al. Two German kindreds with familial amyotrophic lateral sclerosis due to TARDBP mutations. *Arch Neurol* 2008; 65:1185–1189.

35. Rutherford NJ, Zhang YJ, Baker M, et al. Novel mutations in TARDBP (TDP-43) in patients with familial amyotrophic lateral sclerosis. *PLoS Genet* 2008; 4(9):e1000193

36. Yokoseki A, Shiga A, Tan CF, et al. TDP-43 mutation in familial amyotrophic lateral sclerosis. *Ann Neurol* 2008; 63:538–542.

37. Daoud H, Valdmanis PN, Kabashi E, et al. Contribution of TARDBP mutations to sporadic amyotrophic lateral sclerosis. *J Med Genet* 2009; 46:112–114.

38. Lemmens R, Race V, Hersmus N, et al. TDP-43 M311V mutation in familial amyotrophic lateral sclerosis. *J Neurol Neurosurg Psychiatry* 2009; 80:354–355.

39. Corcia P, Valdmanis P, Millecamps S, et al. Phenotype and genotype analysis in amyotrophic lateral sclerosis with TARDBP gene mutations. *Neurology* 2012; 78:1519–1526.

40. Borroni B, Bonvicini C, Alberici A, et al. Mutation within TARDBP leads to frontotemporal dementia without motor neuron disease. *Hum Mutat* 2009; 30:E974–E983.

41. Benajiba L, Le Ber I, Camuzat A et al. TARDBP mutations in

motorneuron disease with frontotemporal lobar degeneration. *Ann Neurol* 2009; 65:470–473.

42. Kwiatkowski TJ, Bosco DA, LeClerc L, et al. Mutations in the FUS/TLS gene on chromosome 16 cause familial amyotrophic lateral sclerosis. *Science* 2009; 323:1205–1208.

43. Vance C, Rogelj B, Hortobágyi T, et al. Mutations in FUS, an RNA processing protein, cause familial amyotrophic lateral sclerosis type 6. *Science* 2009; 323:1208–1211.

44. Belzil VV, Valdmanis PN, Dior PA, et al. Mutations in FUS cause FALS and SALS in French and French Canadian populations. *Neurology* 2009; 73:1176–1179.

45. Corrado L, Del Bo R, Castelloti B, et al. Mutations in FUS gene in sporadic amyotrophic lateral sclerosis. *J Med Genet* 2010; 47:190–194.

46. Rademakers R, Stewart H, De Jesus-Hernandez M, et al. FUS gene mutations in familial and sporadic amyotrophic lateral sclerosis. *Muscle Nerve* 2010; 42:170–176.

47. Lagier-Tourenne C, Polymenidou M, Cleveland DW. TDP-43 and FUS/TLS: emerging roles in RNA processing and neurodegeneration. *Hum Mol Genet* 2010; 19(R1):R46–64.

48. Syriani E, Morales M, Gamez J. FUS/TLS gene mutations are the second most frequent cause of familial ALS in the Spanish population. *Amyotroph Lateral Scler* 2011; 12:118–123.

49. Rademakers R, Stewart H, Dejesus-Hernandez M et al. Fus gene mutations in familial and sporadic amyotrophic lateral sclerosis. *Muscle Nerve* 2010; 42:170–176.

50. Conte A, Lattante S, Zollino M et al. P525L FUS mutation is consistently associated with a severe form of juvenile amyotrophic lateral sclerosis. *Neuromuscul Disord* 2012; 22:73–75.

51. Broustal O, Camuzat A, Guillot-Noël L et al. FUS mutations in frontotemporal lobar degeneration with amyotrophic lateral sclerosis. *J Alzheimers Dis* 2010; 22:765–769.

52. Ticozzi N, Silani V, LeClerc AL et al. Analysis of FUS gene mutation in familial amyotrophic lateral sclerosis within an Italian cohort. *Neurology* 2009; 73:1180–1185.

53. Blair IP, Williams KL, Warraich ST et al. FUS mutations in amyotrophic lateral sclerosis: clinical, pathological, neurophysiological and genetic analysis. *J Neurol Neurosurg Psychiatry* 2010; 81:639–645.

54. Van Langenhove T, van der Zee, Sleegers K et al. Genetic contribution of FUS to frontotemporal lobar degeneration. *Neurology* 2010; 74:366–371.

55. Neumann M, Rademakers R, Rueber S et al. A new subtype of frontotemporal lobar degeneration with FUS pathology. *Brain* 2009; 132:2922–2931.

56. Lomen-Hoerth C, Murphy J, Langmore S, et al. Are amyotrophic lateral sclerosis patients cognitively normal? *Neurology* 2003; 60:1094–97.

57. Ringholz GM, Appel SH, Bradshaw M, et al. Prevalence and patterns of cognitive impairment in sporadic ALS. *Neurology* 2005; 65:586–590.

58. Dejesús-Hernández M, Mackenzie IR, Boeve BF, et al. Expanded GGGGCC hexanucleotide repeat in noncoding region of c9orf72 causes chromosome 9p-linked FTD and ALS. *Neuron* 2011; 72:245–256.

59. Renton AE, Majounie E, Waite A, et al. A hexanucleotide repeat expansion in c9orf72 is the cause of chromosome 9p21-linked ALS-FTD. *Neuron* 2011; 72:257–268.

60. Gijselinck I, Van Langenhove T, Van der Zee J, et al. A C9orf72 promoter repeat expansion in a Flanders-Belgian cohort with disorders of the frontotemporal lobar degeneration-amyotrophic lateral sclerosis spectrum: a gene identification study. *Lancet Neurol* 2012; 11:54–65.

61. Johnson JO, Mandrioli J, Benatar M, et al. Exome Sequencing reveals VCP mutations as a cause of familial ALS. *Neuron* 2010; 68:857–864.

62. Deng H-X, Chen W, Hong S-T, et al. Mutations in UBQLN2 cause dominant X-linked juvenile and adult-onset ALS and ALS/dementia. *Nature* 2011; 477:211–215.

63. Boxer AL, Mackenzie IR, Boeve BF, et al. Clinical, neuroimaging and neuropathological features of a new chromosome 9p-linked FTD-ALS family. *J Neurol Neurosurg Psychiatry* 2011; 82:196–203.

64. Momeni P, Schymick J, Jain S, et al. Analysis of IFT74 as a candidate gene for chromosome 9p-linked ALS-FTD. *BMC Neurology* 2006; 13 6:44.

65. Morita M, Al-Chalabi AA, Andersen PM, et al. A locus on chromosome 9p confers susceptibility to ALS and frontotemporal dementia. *Neurology* 2006; 66:839–844.

66. Vance C, Al-Chalabi A, Ruddy D, et al. Familial amyotrophic lateral sclerosis with frontotemporal dementia is linked to a locus on chromosome 9p13.2–21.3. *Brain* 2006; 129:868–876.

67. Valdmanis PN, Dupre N, Bouchard J-P, et al. Three families with amyotrophic lateral sclerosis and frontotemporal dementia with evidence of linkage to chromosome 9p. *Arch Neurol* 2007; 64:240–245.

68. Luty AA, Knok JBJ, Thompson EM, et al. Pedigree with frontotemporal lobar degeneration-motor neuron disease and Tar DNA binding protein-43 positive neuropathology: genetic linkage to chromosome 9. BMC *Neurology* 2008; 29:8:32.

69. Le Ber I, Camuzat A, Berger E, et al. Chromosome 9p-linked families with frontotemporal dementia associated with motor neuron disease. *Neurology* 2009; 72:1669–1676.

70. Hosler BA, Siddique T, Sapp PC, et al. Linkage of familial amyotrophic lateral sclerosis with frontotemporal dementia to chromosome 9q21-q22. *JAMA* 2000; 284:1664–1669.

71. Laaksovirta H, Peuralinna T, Schymick JC, et al. Chromosome 9p21 in amyotrophic lateral sclerosis in Finland: a genome-wide association study. *Lancet Neurol* 2010; 9:978–985.

72. van Es MA, Veldink JH, Saris CGJ, et al. Genome-wide association study identifies 19p13.3 (UNC13A) and 9p21.2 as susceptibility loci for sporadic amyotrophic lateral sclerosis. *Nat Genet* 2009; 41:1083–1088.

73. Shatunov A, Mok K, Newhouse S, et al. Chromosome 9p21 in sporadic amyotrophic lateral sclerosis in the UK and seven other countries: a genome-wide association study. *Lancet Neurol* 2010; 9:986–994.

74. Machuca-Tzili L, Brook D, Hilton-Jones D. Clinical and molecular aspects of the myotonic dystrophies : a review. *Muscle Nerve* 2005; 32:1–18.

75. Todd PK, Paulson HL. RNA-mediated neurodegeneration in repeat expansion disorders. *Ann Neurol* 2010; 67:291–300.

76. Stewart H, Rutherford NJ, Briemberg ,H et al. Clinical and pathological features of amyotrophic lateral sclerosis caused by mutation in the C9orf72 gene on chromosome 9p. *Acta Neuropathol* 2012; 123:409–417.

77. Millecamps S, Boillee S, Le Ber I, et al. Phenotype difference between ALS patients with expanded repeats in C9orf72 and patients with mutations in other ALS-related genes. *J Med Genet* 2012; 49:258–263.

78. Chio A, Borghero G, Restagno G et al. Clinical characteristics of patients with familial amyotrophic lateral sclerosis carrying the pathogenic GGGGCC hexanucleotide repeat expansion of C9orf72. *Brain* 2012; 135:784–793.

79. Pikkarainen M, Hartikainen P, Alafuzoff I. Neuropathologic features of frontotemporal lobar degeneration with ubiquitin-positive inclusions visualized with ubiquitin-binding protein p62 immunohistochemistry. *J Neuropathol Exp Neurol* 2008; 67:280–298.

80. Troakes C, Maekawa S, Wijesekera L, et al. An MND/ALS phenotype associated with c9orf72 repeat expansion: Abundant p62-positive, TDP-43 negative inclusions in cerebral cortex,

hippocampus and cerebellum but without associated cognitive decline. *Neuropathology* 2011; Dec 19. doi: 10.1111/j.1440–1789.2011.01286.x. [Epub ahead of print]

81. Simon-Sanchez J, Dopper EGP, Cohn-Hokke PE, et al. The clinical and pathological phenotype of c9orf72 hexanucleotide repeat expansions. *Brain* 2012; 135:723–735.

82. Brettschneider J, Van Deerlin VM, Robinson JL, et al. Pattern of ubiquilin pathology in ALS and FTLD indicates presence of c9orf72 hexanucleotide expansion. *Acta Neuropathol* 2012; 123:825–839.

83. Kovach MJ, Waggoner B, Leal SM, et al. Clinical Delineation and Localization to Chromosome 9p13.3-p12 of a Unique Dominant Disorder in Four Families: Hereditary Inclusion Body Myopathy, Paget Disease of the Bone, and Frontotemporal Dementia. *Molecular Genetics and Metabolism* 2001; 74:458–475.

84. Watts GD, Wymar J, Kovach MJ, et al. Inclusion body myopathy associated with Paget disease of bone and frontotemporal dementia is caused by mutant valosin-containing protein. *Nat Genet* 2004;3 6:377–381.

85. Haubenberger D, Bittner RE, Rauch-Schorny S, et al. Inclusion body myopathy and Paget disease is linked to a novel mutation in the VCP gene. *Neurology* 2005; 65:1304–1305.

86. Watts GD, Thomasova D, Ramdean SK, et al. Novel VCP mutations in inclusion body myopathy associated with Paget disease of bone and frontotemporal dementia. *Clin Genet* 2007; 72:420–426.

87. Gidaro T, Modoni A, Sabatelli M, et al. An Italian family with inclusion-body myopathy and frontemporal dementia due to mutation in VCP gene. *Muscle Nerve* 2008; 37:111–114.

88. Djamshidian A, Schaefer J, Haubenberger D, et al. A novel mutation in the VCP gene (G157R) in a German family with inclusion body myopathy with Paget disease of bone and frontotemporal dementia. *Muscle Nerve* 2009; 39:389–391.

89. Stojkovic T, Hammouda el H, Richard P, et al. Clinical outcome in 19 French and Spanish patients with valosin-containing proteína myopathy associated with Paget's disease of bone and frontotemporal dementia. *Neuromuscul Disord* 2009; 19:316–323.

90. Kumar KR, Needham M, Mina K, et al. Two Australian families with inclusion body myopathy, Paget's disease of bone and frontotemporal dementia: novel clinical and genetic findings. *Neuromuscul Disord* 2010; 20:330–334.

91. Palmio J, Sandell S, Snominen T, et al. Distinct distal myopathy phenotype caused by VCP gene mutation in a Finnish family. *Neuromuscul Disord* 2011; 21:551–555.

92. Daoud H, Suhail H, Szuto A, et al. UBQLN2 mutations are rare in French and French-Canadian amyotrophic lateral sclerosis. *Neurobiol Aging* 2012; 33:2230.e1-5.

93. Millecamps S, Corcia P, Cazeneuve C, et al. Mutations in UBQLN2 are rare in French amyotrophic lateral sclerosis. *Neurobiol Aging* 2012; 33:839.e1-3.

94. Nishimura AL, Mitne-Neto M, Silva HCA, et al. A mutation in the vesicle-trafficking protein VAPB causes late-onset spinal muscular atrophy and amyotrophic lateral sclerosis. *Am J Hum Genet* 2004; 75:822–831.

95. Chen YZ, Bennett CL, Huynh HM, et al. DNA/RNA helicase gene mutations in a form of juvenile amyotrophic lateral sclerosis (ALS4). *Am J Hum Genet* 2004; 74:1128–1135.

96. Puls I, Jonnakuty C, LaMonte BH, et al. Mutant dynactin in motor neuron disease. *Nat Genet* 2003; 33:455–456.

97. Munch C, Rosenbohm A, Sperfeld AD, et al. Heterozygous R1101K mutation of the DCTN1 gene in a family with ALS and FTD. *Ann Neurol* 2005; 58:777–780.

98. Yang Y, Hentati A, Deng HX, et al. The gene encoding alsin, a protein with three guanine—nucleotide exchange factor domains, is mutated in a form of recessive amyotrophic lateral sclerosis. *Nat Genet* 2001; 29:160–165.

99. Hadano S, Hand CK, Osuga H, et al. A gene encoding a putative GTPase regulator is mutated in familial amyotrophic lateral sclerosis. *Nat Genet* 2001; 29:166–173.

100. Greenway MJ, Andersen PM, Russ C, et al. ANG mutations segregate with familial and sporadic amyotrophic lateral sclerosis. *Nat Genet* 2006; 38(4):411–413.

101. van Es MA, Schelhaas HJ, van Vught PW, et al. Angiogenin variants in Parkinson disease and amyotrophic lateral sclerosis. *Ann Neurol* 2011; 70:964–973.

102. van Es MA, Diekstra FP, Veldink JH, et al. A case of ALS-FTD in a large FALS pedigree with a K17I ANG mutation. *Neurology* 2009; 72:287–288.

103. Seilhean D, Cazeneuve C, Thuri[es V, et al. Accumulation of TDP-43 and alpha/actin in an amyotrophic lateral sclerosis patient with the K17I ANG mutation. *Acta Neuropathol* 2009; 118:561–573.

104. Maruyama H, Morino H, Ito H, et al. Mutations of optineurin in amyotrophic lateral sclerosis. *Nature* 2010; 465:223–226.

105. Sugihara K, Maruyama H, Kamada M, et al. Screening for OPTN mutations in amyotrophic lateral sclerosis in a mainly Caucasian population. *Neurobiol Aging* 2011; 32:1923.e9-10.

106. Allingham RR, Liu Y, Rhee DJ. The genetics of primary open-angle glaucoma: a review. *Exp Eye Res* 2009; 88:837–844.

107. Elden AC, Kim HJ, Hart MP, et al. Ataxin-2 intermediate-length polyglutamine expansions are associated with increased risk for ALS. *Nature* 2010; 466:1069–1075.

108. Ross OA, Rutherford NJ, Baker M, et al. Ataxin-2 repeat-length variation and neurodegeneration. *Hum Mol Genet* 2011; 20:3207–3212.

109. Hart MP, Brettschneider J, Lee VM, et al. Distinct TDP-43 pathology in ALS patients with ataxin 2 intermediate-length polyQ expansions. *Acta Neuropathol* 2012; 124:221–230.

110. Wu CH, Fallini C, Ticozzi N, et al. Mutations in the profilin 1 gene cause familial amyotrophic lateral sclerosis. *Nature* 2012; 488:499–503.

111. Van Hoecke A, Schoonaert L, Lemmens R, et al. EPHA4 is a disease modifier of amyotrophic lateral sclerosis in animal models and in humans. *Nat Med* 2012; Aug 26.doi:10.1038/nm.2901 [Epub ahead of print].

112. Saeed M, Siddique N, Hung WY, et al. Paraoxonase cluster polymorphisms are associated with sporadic ALS. *Neurology* 2006; 67:771–776.

113. Ticozzi N, LeClerc AL,Keagle PJ, et al. Paraoxonase gene mutations in amyotrophic lateral sclerosis. *Ann Neurol* 2010; 68:102–107.

114. Van Blitterswijk M, Blokhuis A, van Es MA, et al. Rare and common paraoxonase gene variants in amyotrophic lateral sclerosis patients. *Neurobiol Aging* 2012; 33:1845.e1-3.

115. Van Es MA, van Vught PWJ, Blauw HM, et al. Genetic variation in DPP6 is associated with susceptibility to amyotrophic lateral sclerosis. *Nat Genet* 2008; 40(1):29–31.

116. Fogh I, D'Alfonso S, Gellera C, et al. No association of DPP6 with amyotrophic lateral sclerosis in an Italian population. *Neurobiol Aging* 2011; 32:966–967.

117. Daoud H, Valdmanis PN, Dion PA, et al. Analysis of DPP6 and FGGY as candidate genes for amyotrophic lateral sclerosis. *Amyotroph Lateral Scler* 2010; 11:389–391.

118. Rainier S, Bui M, Mark E, et al. Neuropathy target esterase gene mutations cause motor neuron disease. *Am J Hum Genet* 2008; 82:780–785.

119. Simpson CL, Lemmens R, Miskiewicz K, et al. Variants of the elongator protein 3 (ELP3) gene are associated with motor neuron degeneration. *Hum Mol Genet* 2009; 18:472–481.

120. Chow CY, Landers JE, Bergren SK, et al. Deleterious variants

of FIG4, a phosphoinositide phosphatase, in patients with ALS. *Am J Hum Genet* 2009; 84:85–88.

121. Gros-Louis F, Andersen PM, Dupre N, et al. Chromogranin B P413L variant as risk factor and modifier of disease onset for amyotrophic lateral sclerosis. *Proc Natl Acad Sci USA* 2009 Dec 22; 106:21777–21782.

122. Van Vught PWJ, Veldink JH, van den Berg LH. P413L CHGB is not associated with ALS susceptibility or age at onset in a Ducht population. *Proc Natl Acad Sci USA* 2010; 107:E77.

123. Blasco H, Corcia P, Veyrat-Durebex C, et al. The P413L chromogranin B variation in French patients with sporadic amyotrophic lateral sclerosis. *Amyotroph Lateral Scler* 2011; 12:210–214.

124. Van ES MA, Veldink JH, Saris CGJ, et al. Genome-wide association study identifies 19p13.3 (UNC13A) and 9p21.1 as susceptibility loci for sporadic amyotrophic lateral sclerosis. *Nat Genet* 2009; 41:1083–1087.

125. Diekstra FP, van Vught PW, van Rheenen W, et al. UNC13A is a modifier of survival in amyotrophic lateral sclerosis. *Neurobiol Aging* 2012; 33:e3-38.

126. Mitchell J, Paul P, Chen HJ, et al. Familial amyotrophic lateral sclerosis is associated with a mutation in D-amino acid oxidase. *Proc Natl Acad Sci USA* 2010; 107:7556–7561.

127. Seibenhener ML, Babu JR, Geetha T, et al. Sequestosome 1/p62 is a polyubiquitin chain binding protein involved in ubiquitin proteasome degradation. *Mol Cell Biol* 2004; 24:8055–8068.

128. Michou L, Collet C, Laplanche JL et al. Genetics of Paget's disease of bone. *Joint Bone Spine* 2006; 73:243–248.

129. Fecto F, Yan J, Vemula SP, et al. SQSTM1 mutations in familial and sporadic amyotrophic lateral sclerosis. *Arch Neurol* 2011; 68:1440–1446.

130. Blauw HM, Barnes CP, van Vught PW, et al. SMN1 gene duplications are associated with sporadic ALS. *Neurology* 2012; 78:776–780.

131. Landers JE, Melki J, Meininger V, et al. Reduced expression of the kinesin-associated protein 3 (KIFAP3) gene increases survival in sporadic amyotrophic lateral sclerosis. *Proc Natl Acad Sci USA* 2009; 106:9004–9009.

132. Traynor BJ, Nalls M, Lai SL et al. Kinesin-associated protein 3 (KIFAP3) has no effect on survival in a population-based cohort of ALS patients. *Proc Natl Acad Sci USA* 2010; 107:12335–12338.

133. Orsetti V, Pegoraro E, Cima V, et al. Genetic variation in KIFAP3 is associated with an upper motor neuron-predominant phenotype in amyotrophic lateral sclerosis. *Neurodegener Dis* 2011; 8:491–495.

134. Couthouis J., Hart M.P., Shorter J, et al. A yeast functional screen predicts new candidate ALS disease genes. *Proc Natl Acad.Sci USA* 2011; 108:20881–20890.

135. Al-Saif A, Al-Mohanna F, Bohlega S. A mutation in sigma-1 receptor causes juvenile amyotrophic lateral sclerosis. *Ann Neurol* 2011; 70:913–999.

CHAPTER **49**

Amyotrophic Lateral Sclerosis

Tamara S. Greene, Ericka P. Simpson, Stanley H. Appel

Motor neuron disease (MND) was separately described in the span of 25 years more than a century ago by the founders of modern neurology, appreciating the clinicopathologic significance of the anterior horn cells (AHC) of the anterior grey substance and anterolateral corticospinal tracts (CST). In classic accounts, progressive muscular atrophy (PMA) was described by Aran in 1850 (1), progressive bulbar palsy (PBP) by Duchenne in 1860 (2), and amyotrophic lateral sclerosis (ALS) by Charcot and Joffroy in 1869 (3), followed by primary lateral sclerosis (PLS) in 1875 by Erb (4). To this day, it is not clear whether use of the inclusive term MND is always appropriate to describe each of the separate entities. However, in the absence of a single applicable clinical marker for MND, most experts would agree that upper motor neuron (UMN) signs of hyperreflexia, Hoffman, Babinski signs, and clonus indicative of selective degeneration of the anterolateral corticospinal tracts (CST) combined with lower motor neuron (LMN) features of weakness, wasting, and fasciculation reflecting spinal motor neuron cell loss, assures the presumptive diagnosis of typical ALS in life with 98% accuracy in the hands of experienced clinicians, leaving the remainder to be deciphered at postmortem examination. Non-lethal disorders that may masquerade as ALS include multifocal motor neuropathy (MMN), inclusion body myositis (IBM), chronic inflammatory demyelinating polyneuropathy (CIDP), and atypical forms of MND due to widespread LMN involvement, alone or in association with compressive cervical spondylotic myelopathy (CSM). The spectrum of MND is shown in Table 1.

EPIDEMIOLOGY

The estimated incidence of sporadic ALS is four to six per 100,000, with a male-to-female ratio of 1.5:1, and a combined average age at onset of 56 years, with fewer patients presenting before age 40 years. Although the duration of disease may vary between three to five years, rarely, patients may survive decades while others expire shortly after diagnosis (5, 6). In 5 to 10% of patients, there is a discernible genetic basis termed familial *ALS* (FALS).

CLASSIFICATION

The revised diagnostic criteria of The World Federation of Neurology El Escorial Conference shown in Table 2 (7) provide a useful clinical benchmark for the diagnosis and classification of ALS. For classification purposes LMN signs include weakness, wasting or atrophy, and fasciculation. Overactive deep tendon reflexes (DTR), spasticity, and clonus, along with Hoffmann, Babinski, and pseudobulbar signs are indicative of UMN involvement. The regions of the body are classified into bulbar, cervical, thoracic, and lumbosacral. Patients with definite ALS manifest definite UMN and LMN signs in at least three spinal regions, or bulbar and two spinal regions, while those with probable ALS demonstrate UMN and LMN signs in at least two regions. Possible ALS is defined by UMN and LMN signs together in one region or UMN signs alone in two or more regions, whereas suspected ALS manifests LMN signs alone in two or more regions.

TABLE 1. Forms of motoneuron disease

Typical	LMN signs only	progressive spinal muscular atrophy (PSMA)
	UMN signs only	primary lateral sclerosis (PLS)
	UMN + LMN signs	ALS, progressive bulbar palsy (PBP)
	Familial ALS	
	Juvenile ALS	
Atypical	Mills hemiplegic variant	
	Flail-arm syndrome	
	Unilateral upper limb involvement: benign asymmetrical focal amyotrophy of young males; monomelic amyotrophy	
	MADRAS	
	Wasted leg syndrome	
	Unilateral leg hypertrophy	

TABLE 2. El Escorial Criteria for the Diagnosis of ALS

Definite ALS	UMN as well as LMN signs in the bulbar region and at least two other spinal regions, or
	UMN and LMN signs in three spinal regions
Probable ALS	UMN and LMN signs in at least two regions.
Possible ALS	UMN and LMN signs in one region, or
	UMN signs alone in 2 or more regions, or
	LMN signs rostral to UMN signs
Suspected ALS	LMN signs in two or more regions (UMN-pathology may be demonstrated at autopsy but there are no clinical signs)

Abbreviations: UMN, upper motor neuron; LMN, lower motor neuron

PATHOPHYSIOLOGY AND RISK FACTORS

The often heterogeneous clinical expression of ALS suggests the likelihood of combined multiple pathways and mechanisms in pathogenesis resulting in protein misfolding with abnormal accumulation of intracellular motor neuron aggregates, mitochondrial dysfunction, oxidative stress linked to free radical formation, impaired axonal transport, disorganized neurofilaments, and excitotoxicity. Although several risk factors have been implicated in sporadic ALS, none have been definitively proven except certain gene polymorphisms and mutations that have been identified. Certain environmental factors have been proposed as having an increased risk for developing ALS. It was suggested that military personnel might be at higher risk of developing ALS as were those exposed to potentially toxic chemicals and metals, however neither association was revealing. A possible consequence of cigarette smoking on the risk of developing ALS risk was equivocal, as were several studies examining the trigger head trauma. Notwithstanding, head trauma might conceivably aggravate the early course of ALS. Certain plants, seeds, and fruits have been associated with MND in different parts of the world; as, for example, ingestion of the Cycas micronesica in Guamanian ALS-parkinsonism dementia complex (ALS-PDC) (8). Konzo, a disorder almost exclusive to Africa, is characterized by the abrupt onset of non-progressive symmetrical spastic paraparesis due to high dietary consumption of cyanide from unprocessed roots of the cassava plant. Ingestion of seeds belonging to plants of the genus Lathyrus, endemic to India, Ethiopia, and Bangladesh, which contain high concentrations of the glutamate analogue β-oxalyl-L-α,β-diaminoproprionic acid (ODAP) toxic to CNS motor neurons likewise leads to irreversible, non-progressive spastic paraparesis with the unique feature of gluteal muscle atrophy. While most authorities agree that such factors may contribute to the development of ALS, other questions regarding selective vulnerability and relentless progression require further investigation.

MUTATIONS ASSOCIATED WITH FAMILIAL AND SPORADIC ALS

Several mutated genes have been associated with FALS and sporadic ALS (Table 3). Mutation in the copper/zinc superoxide dismutase *(Cu/ZnSOD)* gene located on chromosome 21 displays autosomal dominant (AD) inheritance and similar age at onset and clinical course in successive generations (9). Autosomal dominant ALS and frontotemporal dementia (FTD/ALS) is linked to a heterozygous expanded hexanucleotide repeat (GGGGCC) located at the 9p21.2 locus, between the noncoding exons 1a and 1b of the *C9orf72* gene (10, 11). Three pathogenic mutations notably lead to AD FALS. One missense mutation occurs at the 1p36.22 locus of the *TARDBP* gene encoding the 43kd TAR DNA binding protein, originally identified as a transcriptional repressor binding to TAR DNA of human immunodeficiency virus type 1 (HIV-1) 12). A second missense mutation occurs at the 16p11.2 locus of the *FUS* gene in FALS with or without FTD, encoding the FUS protein involved in the regulation of transcription and RNA splicing and transport with functional homology to *TARDBP* (13). A third mutation is found in dominantly inherited X-linked ALS and ALS/dementia maps to the Xp11.21 locus of the *UBQLN2* gene encoding the ubiquitin-like protein ubiquitin 2, associated with abnormal protein degradation, aggregation, and CNS neurodegeneration (14). Basophilic *FUS* inclusions are found in the cytoplasm of motor neurons with phenotypes of typical ALS alone or in association with cognitive impairment, FTD, and Parkinsonism. Ubiquinated inclusions containing pathologic forms of the protein are found in the cytoplasm of sporadic ALS and non-SOD1 FALS motor neurons. The gene most commonly associated with an increased susceptibility to sporadic ALS is *ATXN2* which mapped to the 12q24 locus in association with an expanded CAG trinucleotide repeat.

CLINICAL PRESENTATION AND NEUROLOGICAL EXAMINATION

The onset of symptoms in ALS patients is believed to occur when approximately 50 to 80% of motor neurons are lost, with most patients complaining of some functional impairment such as difficulty writing, buttoning, or holding onto objects, indicative of arm or hand weakness, or stumbling, tripping, and falls reflecting leg involvement. The onset of weakness is often asymmetric and distal in one extremity progressing to the other side, and over time, more rostral along the limb. When signs and symptoms are restricted to a single limb and adjacent root, a mistaken diagnosis of painless radiculopathy can occur. Occasionally, patients will have isolated weakness of neck extension muscles with forward drooping of the head,

termed floppy or dropped head syndrome. Bulbar symptoms are the presenting feature in 20% to 25% of patients, resulting in hoarseness, slurred speech, and difficulty swallowing leading to choking and drooling due to pooling of secretions. Bulbar involvement leads to complaints of sleep disruption and easy fatigability. In women older than 60 years, bulbar onset is the most common presenting feature, and confers an overall poorer prognosis because respiratory muscle involvement is more likely to follow soon thereafter, as is pseudobulbar affect, characterized by involuntary or uncontrollable episodes of crying and/or laughter, noted in up to one-half of patients. Fasciculation, which may be seen in other disorders, are seldom the presenting feature, but when widespread and combined with lingual wasting and tongue fibrillations, are highly suggestive of ALS. Patients with ALS may display a spectrum of frontotemporal cognitive and behavioral deficits that vary from word fluency, executive dysfunction, impulsivity, and compulsiveness, noted in up to one-half of patients, to cognitive impairment with features indicative of frank FTD.

DIAGNOSTIC STUDIES

The recommended evaluation of patients suspected of ALS is summarized in Table 4. The role of testing in ALS is two-fold: to confirm the diagnosis and identify other concomitant disorders toward which effective therapy might be directed. Three limb nerve conduction studies (NCS) and needle electromyography (EMG) are performed in all suspected patients to confirm the diagnosis and exclude disorders that may mimic ALS. Although sensory NCS are typically normal throughout the course of ALS, some patients will have abnormal sural sensory indices. The LMN involvement in ALS is electrodiagnostically evident in reduction of compound muscle action potentials (CMAP) amplitudes and the loss of fastest conducting fibers resulting in mild slowing of motor nerve conduction velocities (NCV). There may be impairment of neuromuscular transmission, usually evident as abnormal decrement of less than 10% of successive CMAP to 3/second repetitive motor nerve stimulation, in contrast to patients with myasthenia gravis (MG) in which the decrement typically exceeds 12%. However, some patients with ALS may have a decremental response >10%. Electromyography is performed in at least three body regions although most experts will investigate portions of all four regions, among them bulbar, cervical, thoracic, and lumbar myotomes. Acute denervation in lingual, masseter, facial, and sternocleidomastoid muscles within the bulbar region, and T1 to T10 paraspinous muscles of thoracic myotomes provide evidence of motor neuron involvement. The classical electromyographic correlates of MND include widespread acute denervation in the form of

TABLE 3. Genetic Basis of ALS

Locus	Gene	Product	Inheritance	Protein function	Other associated phenotypes
ALS1; 21q22	SOD1	Copper/zinc superoxide dismutase (Cu/ZnSOD)	Dominant	Dismutation of superoxide into oxygen and hydrogen peroxide	Variable
ALS2; 2q33	ALS2	Alsin	Recessive	Guanine nucleotide exchange factor	Juvenile onset; HSP and PLS
ALS3; 18q21	Not yet identified	Unknown	Dominant	Unknown	
ALS4; 9q34	SETX	Senataxin	recessive	DNA and RNA metabolism	Juvenile onset; LMN predominant
ALS5; 15q21	SPG11	Spatacsin	recessive	Unknown	Juvenile onset; HSP and Parkinsonism
ALS6; 16q12	FUS	Fused in sarcoma	Dominant / recessive	DNA repair and RNA processing	Juvenile and adult-onset; FTD, parkinsonism
ALS7; 20p13	ALS7	Unknown	Dominant	Unknown	
ALS8; 20q13	VABP	Vesicle-associated membrane protein B	Dominant	Vesicle trafficking	Late-onset SMA
ALS9; 14q11	ANG	Angiogenin	Dominant	Angiogenesis	Typical
ALS10; 1p36	TARDBP	TDP-43	Dominant	RNA binding and exon skipping	FTD, PSP
ALS11; 6q24	FIG4	Fig4	Dominant	Possibly vesicular trafficking	CMT 4J, PLS
ALS12; 10p13	OPTN	Optineurin	Dominant / recessive	Signal transduction and inhibition of apoptosis	POAG
ALS13; 12q24	ATX2	Ataxin 2	Dominant	Possibly RNA processing and translation	ALS-FTD, SCA
ALS/FTD; 17q21	MAPT	Microtubule-associated protein tau	Dominant	Stabilizes microtubules and promotes microtubular assembly	FTD, Parkinson's disease, Pick's disease
ALS/FTD; 9p21	C9orf72	Unknown	Dominant	Unknown	FTD, ALS-FTD
ALS/FTD; 9p13	VCP	Valosin-containing protein	Dominant	Part of the ubiquitin-proteasome system	Cognitive impairment
Xp11.23 - Xq13.1	UBQLN2	Ubiquilin 2	X-linked dominant	Destruction of damaged or abnormal cellular proteins	Juvenile and adult onset; dementia

Abbreviations: CMT, Charcot-Marie-Tooth; FTD, frontotemporal dementia; HSP, hereditary spastic paraplegia; LMN, lower motor neuron; PLS, primary lateral sclerosis; POAG, primary open-angle glaucoma; PSP, progressive supranuclear palsy; SCA, spinocerebellar ataxia; SMA, spinal muscular atrophy

TABLE 4. Diagnostic Evaluation in ALS

Nerve conduction studies	Normal NCS; CMAP normal or reduced Demyelination points to MMN or CIDP.
Needle EMG	Acute and chronic dennervation
Serology	CBC, ESR, chemistries, LFT, CK, vitamin B_{12}, folate, thyroid function studies, parathyroid hormone, quantitative immunoglobulins, SPEP, IFE, HIV, HTLV1 and 2, ANA, Borrelia burgdorferi titers, anti-GM1 and anti-MAG antibody titers.
MRI of the brain and cervical spine	Typically normal Rule out brainstem and cervical pathology
Lumbar puncture	Typically normal in ALS patients Rule out autoimmune inflammatory neuropathy
Muscle biopsy	Small angular fibers and fiber type grouping Rule out inflammatory myopathy

Abbreviations: CBC, complete blood count; CIDP, chronic immune demyelinating polyneuroradiculopathy; CMAPs, compund motor action potential; ESR, erythrocyte sedimentation rate; BUN, blood urea nitrogen; AST, ALT, aspartate and alanine aminotransferase; LDH, lactate dehydrogenase; CK, creatine kinase; ANA, antinuclear antibodies; EMG, electromyography; HIV, human immunodeficiency virus, HTLV, human T-lymphotrophic virus, LFTs, liver function tests; MMN, multifocal motor neuropathy with conduction block, MRI, magnetic resonance imaging; NCS, nerve conduction studies; SPEP, serum protein electrophoresis; IFE, immunofixation electrophoresis.

fibrillation potentials and positive sharp waves, and chronic denervation in the form of fasciculation potentials in association with a neurogenic recruitment pattern comprised of voluntary motor unit potentials of increased duration, amplitude, and polyphasia, with complex morphology.

Selected autoimmune and infectious serology and screening metabolic indices should be considered in all patients, among them a GM1ganglioside panel, B_{12} and folate levels, human immunodeficiency virus (HIV) types 1 and 2, *Borrelia burgdorferi* and syphilis serologies, serum protein and immunofixation electrophoresis for monoclonal paraproteinemia, and thyroid and parathyroid hormonal studies. Neuromuscular serologies such as acetylcholine receptor (AChR) and muscle specific kinase (MuSK) antibodies should be evaluated to rule out myasthenia gravis. The serum creatine kinase (CK) is frequently elevated in proportion to LMN involvement, although by no means diagnostic of ALS. Examination of cerebrospinal fluid (CSF), while not ordinarily necessary, is warranted in patients with atypical findings such as diminished DTR, sensory involvement, or when other laboratory indices suggest a systemic inflammatory or paraneoplastic process. Skeletal muscle biopsy of an involved limb region confirms the presence of neurogenic denervation of that region, and establishes evidence of the expected widespread process in an otherwise asymptomatic limb. Those morphological findings include small angular and target fibers without evidence of reinnervation. Additionally, ALS patients can have some evidence of reinnervation, as demonstrated by the presence of fiber type grouping. Neuroimaging studies should be tailored to the clinical presentation available, especially magnetic resonance imaging of the brain and spinal cord, which are indispensable in excluding compressive and intramedullary lesions of the foramen magnum and spinal cord.

Patients with ALS should undergo baseline and follow-up pulmonary function testing of upright and supine forced vital capacity (FVC) and mean inspiratory pressures (MIP) in advance of frank respiratory distress, dietary and nutritionist consultations to assure adequate dietary support despite poor appetite and swallowing difficulty, speech therapy to forestall diminishing communication as a consequence of advancing bulbar involvement, and physical and occupational therapy evaluations to formulate an individualized exercise program, prevent inadvertent falls, and to inaugurate assistive devices to enhance mobility and assure safe transfers. Such services should ideally be concentrated within a multidisciplinary ALS clinic setting for the benefit of patients to maximize the impact of physicians and health providers (15).

DIFFERENTIAL DIAGNOSIS

Disorders to exclude before establishing the diagnosis of ALS are listed in Table 5. Concomitant lymphoma and lung malignancies are suggested by atypical clinical presentations (16, 17), including a significantly elevated CSF protein with plasma cell dyscrasia (18) and positive serum anti-Hu antibodies in association with a paraneoplastic peripheral nerve vasculitis (19). Multifocal motor neuropathy with motor conduction block (20) and subacute motor neuronopathy (SMN) (21) may be clinically indistinguishable from PSMA. Such patients may manifest circulating anti-GM1 antibodies (22) and dramatically respond to immunomodulating and immunosuppressant therapies. There are rare reports of HIV-1 seropositive patients with MND responsive to antiretroviral treatment (23–25). In myasthenia gravis, acetylcholine receptor (AChR) or muscle specific kinase (MuSK) antibodies are usually positive. Those with post-polio muscular atrophy (PPMA), compressive cervical myelopathy, myasthenia gravis, and IBM can present clinical and electrophysiologic challenges because of concomitant LMN signs and abnormal spontaneous activity.

Although most patients with PLS present with sustained UMN disease, some patients may present as a further diagnostic challenge because of limited spontaneous activity on needle EMG that rarely progresses to frank ALS (26). Magnetic resonance spectroscopy (MRS), which shows a decreased N-acetyl- aspartate (NAA) level (a marker of neuronal integrity) with reversal of the NAA/creatine ratio in frontal motor cortex where the CST originates; diffusion tensor imaging (DTI), and transcranial magnetic stimulation (TMS), respectively, can evaluate UMN anatomy and function in ALS, and provide valuable quantitative assessment (27, 28). Pure PMA patients tend to progress more slowly compared to ALS patients, however, MRS has revealed UMN involvement in a significant number of patients with PMA (29). Additionally, up to a quarter of patients initially diagnosed with PMA develop UMN signs within five years of disease onset. Thus, it is imperative that these patients be monitored regularly.

Genetic testing revealing more than 40 CAG repeats at the Xq12 locus of the androgen receptor (AR) gene in men identifies patients with X-linked spinal and bulbar muscular atrophy or Kennedy syndrome (30, 31) with the syndrome of perioral fasciculation, slowly progressive LMN bulbar, limb, and girdle weakness, muscle atrophy, absent DTR, gynecomastia, elevated serum CK and gonadotrophin levels, and normal serum testosterone levels.

PROGNOSIS

Long-term survival in ALS is most often associated with younger age at onset, male gender, and limb rather than bulbar-onset. Atypical forms of ALS also have a widely different prognosis, as do other MND syndromes, including monomelic amyotrophy, PMA, and PLS that does not convert to classic ALS, with slower rates of progression and survival measured in decades rather than years.

TABLE 5. Disorders That Mimic ALS

Idiopathic	Primary lateral sclerosis
	Progressive muscular atrophy
	Monomelic amyotrophy
Infectious	HIV-1, 2
	HTLV-1 and HTLV-2
	Lyme neuroborreliosis
	CMV
	Poliomyelitis
Inherited	
	Familial spastic paraparesis
	Hexosaminidase A deficiency
	Spinal muscular atrophy
	Kennedy disease
Acquired	
	Myelopathic disorders
	Postradiation injury
	CNS demyelinating disorders
	Syringomyelia
	Brainstem and cervical cord pathology (tumor, Chiari malformation, spinal cord compression)
	Endocrine disorders (thyrotoxicosis, hyperparathyroidism)
	Immune-mediated disorders (plasma cell dyscrasia, multifocal motor neuropathy, mononeuropathy multiplex, and vasculitic neuropathy)
	Paraneoplasic syndromes (Lymphoproliferative, small cell lung cancer anti-Hu associated paraneoplastic encephalomyelitis)
	Exogenous poisoning (lead, mercury, lathyrism, Konzo, Guamanian ALS)
	Post-polio syndrome
	Benign fasciculation syndrome
	Inflammatory myopathies (Inclusion body myositis)

SYMPTOMATIC THERAPY

While no cure is known for ALS, the associated quality of life can be significantly impacted using symptomatic therapies, shown in Table 6.

Sialorrhea

Patients with bulbar weakness have troublesome sialorrhea that can be managed most easily by a manual suction device and by medications beginning with an anticholinergic such as amitriptyline, glycopyrrolate, or hexyphenidyl; scopolamine patch, and the sympathomimetic pseudoephedrine. These can be followed by botulinum toxin type A injection of the salivary glands, and radiation of the parotid and salivary glands. Room air humidification, hydration, and the mucolytic guaifenesin can thin already thick secretions.

Cramps, Spasticity, and Fasciculation

Spasticity, spasms, cramps, and fasciculation can be annoying and even disabling but may respond to anti-spasticity agents such as baclofen and tizanidine, benzodiazepines, and gabapentin. However, severely spastic patients refractory to conventional measures should be considered for intrathecal baclofen via a computer-driven pump system.

Depression and Pseudobulbar Affect

Mild depression occurs in 29%, and is severe in 6% of ALS patients (32), warranting antidepressant medication with first-line therapy using a selective serotonin reuptake inhibitor (SSRI). The combination of dextromethorphan and quinidine is approved by the Food and Drug Administration for the treatment of pseudobulbar affect.

Dysphagia

Progressive dysphagia leads to weight loss and fatigue that can be forestalled with dietary supplementation and percutaneous endoscopic gastrostomy (PEG) to increase caloric intake, and for the safe ingestion of oral medication, food, and fluids. The latter, which ultimately improves survival, should be placed in consultation with a gastroenterologist or surgeon.

Respiratory Insufficiency

Respiratory function may be compromised in varying degrees throughout the course of the illness, leading to frequent awakenings, hypersomnolence, fatigue, and respiratory failure. Polysomnography can show a disrupted sleep pattern due to impaired diaphragmatic function, hypoventilation, and oxygen desaturation. The current standard of care for those with respiratory compromise, indicated by a measured MIP <-60, FVC <50%, and abnormal nocturnal oximetry is noninvasive positive pressure ventilation (NiPPV) (15). It improves overall survival but may be difficult to tolerate. Such patients may benefit from diphenhydramine, zolpidem, or zaleplon to induce sleep.

Classically, Bi-level Positive Airway Pressure (BiPAP) devices have been the primary mode of non-invasive ventilation utilized by ALS patients. However, due to various reasons such as a poorly fitting mask or volume of air, BiPAP may be difficult to tolerate. A newer type of BiPAP, known

TABLE 6. Symptomatic Therapeutic Interventions in ALS

Sialorrhea/thick secretions	Amytriptyline, trihexyphenidyl, glycopyrollate, scopolamine patch, botox, guaifenesin
Cramps/spasticity	Baclofen, tizanidine, gabapentin
Fasciculations	Benzodiazepines
Depression	SSRI, Amytriptyline
Pseudobulbar effect	Dextromethorphan hydrobromide and quinidine sulfate, amitriptylline
Insomnia	Zolpidem, zaleplon, diphenhydramine
Respiratory therapy	Suction machine, nebulizers, cough-assist device, NiPPV
Feeding	Caloric supplementation, PEG
Speech	Speech therapy, alphabet chart, computer-based communication devices
Skin care	Frequent turning/position changing, protective creams, hospital bed, air mattress

Abbreviations: ALS, amyotrophic lateral sclerosis; NiPPV, noninvasive positive pressure ventilation; PEG, percutaneous endoscopic gastrostomy; SSRI, selective serotonin reuptake inhibiter.

as average volume assured pressure support (AVAPS), attempts to combine the pressure and volume characteristics of ventilation. AVAPS use was shown to produce better subjective sleep efficiency in stable hypercapneic COPD patients (33), and a study is currently underway to compare adherence with AVAPS versus traditional non-invasive ventilation options in ALS patients.

End of life

The natural endpoint of ALS is respiratory failure. Intubation for sustained mechanical ventilation may be a meaningful option for some patients, including those with respiratory failure despite NiPPV, and others at risk for aspiration due to inadequate clearance of secretions. Some patients choose not to pursue intubation at the end of life because of physical, emotional, and financial considerations. All of these scenarios can be reasonably anticipated in multidisciplinary ALS clinics wherein patients and families collectively participate in end-of-life decisions.

MEDICAL THERAPY BASED ON DISEASE PATHOGENESIS

No known therapy halts the inexorable progression of disease. However, riluzole at the dose of 50 mg twice daily was granted FDA approval for the treatment of ALS after it demonstrated statistically significant prolonged survival in ALS patients. However, no significant change in strength, respiratory function, or bulbar function was demonstrated (34). The drug blocks the toxic effects of glutamate by inactivating voltage-dependent sodium channels on glutaminergic nerve terminals and non-competitively inhibits the postsynaptic effects at N-methyl-D-aspartic acid (NMDA) and α-amino-3-hydroxyl-5-methyl-4-isoxazole-propionate (AMPA) receptors.

Antioxidant Therapy

Oxidative stress may impact motor neuron survival through modification of DNA, lipids, proteins, signal transduction, receptor kinetics, and protein degradation and aggregation. However, it is unclear to what degree it impacts initiation, propagation, and amplification of the disease. A daily dietary regimen of 2,000 U of vitamin E, 2,000 mg of vitamin C, 25,000 U of beta-carotene, and 3,000 mg of coenzyme q10 (CoQ10) are safe and well tolerated. A phase 2 trial of 2,700 mg of CoQ10 for nine months did not demonstrate efficacy (35), despite a slightly beneficial effect in SOD1G93A transgenic mice (36). Despite the purported promise, the anti-oxidants selegiline (37), N-acetyl cysteine, and creatine did not demonstrate efficacy to justify routine administration in ALS. A phase 2 trial employing the neuroprotective bile acid tauroursodeoxycholic acid in conjunction with riluzole to slow the progression of a small cohort of ALS patients is underway, as is the phase 3 trial termed EMPOWER, employing the neuroprotective agent dexpramipexole.

Immune Mechanisms and Neuroinflammation

A role for immune-mediated mechanisms in human ALS and transgenic SOD1 mice is suggested by the observation of increased microglial activation, CD8 and CD4 lymphocytes, and wild-type microglia that potentiate inflammatory responses (38). Regulatory T-lymphocytes increase during the early phase of an ALS mouse model but decrease during rapid acceleration of the disease, likely through the loss of FoxP3 expression (38). The microglia in transgenic mice expressing mutant SOD1 appear to be neuroprotective to motor neurons, but injury and stress induced by the presence of misfolded mutant SOD1 instead cause them to release reactive oxygen species and proinflammtory cytokines. The consequences include further motor neuron stress, culminating in a self-propagating cycle of injury and cell death (39). Immune suppression with cyclophosphamide, predni-

sone, thalidomide, and total body radiation has not impacted upon disease progression in ALS patients. Glatiramer acetate also did not show any beneficial effect in ALS patients (40). The molecule NP001, designed to transform macrophages from activation and injury producing to neuroprotective cells, deemed safe and tolerable in four different doses in the treatment of ALS, is in an ongoing phase 2 study.

Excitotoxicity and Glutamate Receptor Blockade

The amino acid excitotoxin glutamate, which is present in increased CSF concentrations of patients with ALS, has been the target of a number of medications to block its receptors, thereby interfering with motor neuron toxicity. Such medications include talampanel, gabapentin, topiramate, arundic acid, and memantine, all without clinical efficacy in ALS. The noncompetitive modulator of the AMPA glutamate receptor, talampanel, prolonged median SOD1 G93A mouse survival and lessened the decline of revised ALS Functional Rating Scale (ALSFRS-r) scores of treated ALS subjects compared to placebo, without a difference in the rate of progression in either of two doses compared to placebo, thus proving unsuccessful (41). Phase 2 studies of daily gabapentin (42) and topiramate (43) were likewise negative, as was the European trial of the valproate enantiomer arundic acid (ONO-2506), which was prematurely discontinued.

Memantine prolonged the survival of transgenic ALS mice (44) and although well tolerated in phase 2 and 3 trials, had no efficacy in ALS patients (45). Cephalosporins, which increase promoter activity of the glutamate transporter excitatory amino acid transporter 2 and is neuroprotective against glutamate toxicity, prolonged the survival of transgenic ALS mice (46); a multicenter trial of the drug is nearing completion.

Neurotrophic Factor Deficiency

The hypothesis that ALS is associated with deficiency of one or more nerve growth factors (NGF) or neurotrophins critical for neuronal functioning is suggested by the many different types of neurotrophins that support motor neurons, sensory and sympathetic neurons, and muscle tissue, as well as the observation that NGF promotes survival of chick embryo motor neurons and impedes apoptosis (47). Both brain-derived (BDNF) and ciliary-derived neurotrophic factors (CNTF) were ineffective in ALS (48, 49); similarly, insulin-like growth factor type 1 (IGF-1) showed conflicting clinical trial results in improved quality of life yet without statistical significance in motor aspects (50); a two-year phase 3 trial of IGF-1 showed no difference in primary and secondary outcome measures among treated and control cohorts (51). Vascular endothelial growth factor (VEGF), which is essential for angiogenesis and neuroprotection, predisposes experimental mice and humans to ALS when present in reduced concentrations (52). VEGF was also shown to delay onset and prolong life expectancy by up to 30% in an ALS mouse model after delivery into muscles without toxic effects (53). Intramuscular injection of SB-509, which upregulates VEGF translation and delays loss of muscle strength, and the neuroprotective agents NN0029 and olesoxime, are all underway for possible benefit in ALS.

Heat Shock Proteins

Overexpression of heat shock proteins (HSP) reduces ischemic injury in the mammalian brain. Proteasome dysfunction and HSP expression have been implicated in the pathogenesis of ALS. Arimoclomol, an amplifier of HSP expression, has emerged as a potential therapeutic candidate in experimental SOD1 mouse MND (54). It was well tolerated in a phase 2 clinical trial (55); phase 2 and 3 randomized, placebo-controlled clinical trials are currently underway in SOD1 FALS.

Programmed Cell Death

Programmed cell death requires activation of specific intracellular signaling pathways, and inhibition at various levels can delay or prevent its occurrence.

Such observations have had potential importance in the final common pathway of motor neuron destruction in ALS. The B-cell lymphoma 2 (Bcl-2)-family of apoptosis regulator proteins encoded by the *BCL2* gene and cysteine-aspartic proteases (caspases) both contribute to motor neuron programmed cell death. Overexpression of Bcl-2 mitigates neurodegeneration and prolongs survival of SOD1 transgenic mice (56). Caspase inhibition attenuates mutant SOD1 mediated cell death and prolongs survival via cytokine interactions (57). Caspase activation, which is normally regulated by cytochrome c and Bcl-2, notably enhances the life span of transgenic SOD1 mice. Minocycline, which crosses the blood-brain-barrier, inhibits cytochrome c release, reduces caspase and inflammatory enzyme activation, and delays progression in ALS transgenic mice (58). Although minocycline was deemed safe in patients with ALS, a multicenter randomized placebo-controlled phase III trial showed faster deterioration of the ALSFRS-r score in the treated group than among placebo treated controls (59).

OTHER THERAPIES ON THE HORIZON

A stable non-hypermetabolic state correlates with improved survival in ALS. Moreover, animal models of reduced adiposity and increased rates of energy expenditure and increased dietary lipid content offers enhanced neuroprotection and extends survival in transgenic ALS mice (60). The frequency of hyperlipidemia was two-fold higher in those with ALS than in control patients, and an abnormally elevated LDL/HDL ratio significantly increased survival by more than 12 months (61). Respiratory impairment, but not worsened clinical status or a lower body mass index, was related to the decrease in blood lipids and LDL/HDL ratio (62). However, a recent study noted that body mass index (BMI), but not dyslipidemia, showed a positive correlation with survival in ALS patients (63). A phase 2 clinical study will be examining the safety, tolerability, and efficacy of a long-term high fat and caloric diet in patients with ALS.

Peripheral blood hematopoietic stem cell transplantation (HSCT) has been successfully performed in mouse models of ALS leading to prevention of motor neuron degeneration and improved motor function in ALS mouse models (64). However, such studies have not demonstrated improvement or prolonged survival in patients in ALS. Appel and colleagues (65) followed 6 patients with ALS who received HSCT from identically matched sibling donors in whom the donor stem cells entered the CNS, engrafting as immunomodulatory cells. However, there was no associated clinical benefit. A phase I study of the safety of surgical implantation of human-derived spinal cord stem cells in human ALS is currently underway.

The *Nogo A* gene encodes reticulon 4, which limits regenerative nerve fiber growth. It is hypothesized to be involved in the pathophysiology of ALS, appears to be increased in some patients. A phase I study of the humanized monoclonal antibody GSK1223249, which inhibits the release of Nogo-A, was recently completed.

The fast skeletal muscle troponin activator CK-2017357, which delays fatigue and increases muscle contractile force in animal and human subjects, completed phase 1 safety and tolerability studies and will be recruiting patients assessed by the ALSFRS-R rating scale, as well as measures of pulmonary function, muscle strength, and fatigue.

The antisense oligonucleotide, ISIS-SOD1-Rx directed against *SOD1* RNA blocks production of normal and abnormal SOD1 protein and has the conceivable expectation of benefitting ALS. A phase I safety trial of intrathecally-introduced SOD1-Rx is currently underway in SOD1 FALS.

CONCLUSION

The view of ALS has changed drastically over the past few years. Whereas it was previously considered a pure MND, ALS is now viewed as a heterogeneous disorder as to the nature of onset, rate of progression, etiology, and pathogenesis. Survival in ALS has significantly improved due to multidisciplinary care; in large part due to earlier recognition and treatment of respiratory dysfunction. Continuing advances will better care and a meaningful hope for rational therapy based on a greater causal understanding of the disease will eventually lead to improved survival and quality of life for ALS patients.

REFERENCES

1. Aran RA. Recherches sur une maladie non encore decrite du systeme musculaire (Atrophie musculaire progressive). *Arch Gen Med* 1850; 24:172–214.

2. Duchenne G. Paralysie musculaire progressive de la langue, du voile due palais et des levres. *Arch Gen Med* 1860; 16:283–296; 431–445.

3. Charcot JM, Joffroy A. Deux cas d'atophie musculaire progressive avec lesions de la substance grise et des faisceaux antero-lateraux de la moelle epiniere. *Arch Physiol* 1869; 2:354–367, 629–760.

4. Erb WH. Uber einen wenig bekannten spinalen Symptomen-Complex. *Berl Klin Wochenschr* 1875; 12:357–359.

5. Qureshi M, Schoenfeld DA, Paliwal Y, Shui A, Cudkowicz ME. The natural history of ALS is changing: improved survival. *Amytroph Lateral Scler* 2009; 10:324–331.

6. Haverkamp L, Appel V, Appel SH. Natural history of ALS in a database population: validation of a scoring system and a model for survival prediction. *Brain* 1995; 118:707–719.

7. Brooks BR et al. El Escorial revisited: Revised Criteria for the Diagnosis of Amyotrophic Lateral Sclerosis. *Amyotroph Lateral Scler Other Motor Neuron Disord* 2000; 1:293–299.

8. Marler T, Lee V, Shaw C. Cycad Toxins and Neurological Diseases in Guam: Defining Theoretical and Experimental Standards for Correlating Human Disease with Environmental Toxins. *HortScience* 2005 40(6):1598–1606.

9. Rosen DR, Siddique T, Patterson D, et al. Mutations in Cu/Zn superoxide dismutase gene are associated with familial amyotrophic lateral sclerosis. *Nature* 1993; 362:59–62.

10. DeJesus-Hernandez M, Mackenzie IR, Boeve BF, et al. Expanded GGGCC hexanucleotide repeat in noncoding region of C90RF72 causes chromosome 9p-linked FTD and ALS. *Neuron* 2011; 72:245–256.

11. Renton AE, Majounie E, Waite A, et al. A hexanucleotide repeat expansion in C90RF72 is the cause of chromosome 9p21-linked ALS-FTD. *Neuron* 2011; 72:257–268.

12. Gitcho MA, Baloh RH, Chakraverty S, et al. TDP-43 A315T mutation in familial motor neuron disease. *Ann Neurol* 2008; 63:535–538.

13. Millecamps, S. et al. SOD1, ANG, VAPB, TARDBP, and FUS mutations in familial amyotrophic lateral sclerosis: genotype–phenotype correlations. *J Med Genet* 2010; 47:554–560.

14. Deng HX, Chen W, Hong ST, et al. Mutations in UBZLN2 cause dominant X-linked juvenile and adult-onset ALS and ALS/dementia. *Nature* 2011; 477:211–215.

15. Miller RG, Jackson CE, Kasarskis EJ, et. al. Practive Parameter Update: The Care of the Patient with Amyotrophic Lateral Sclerosis: Drug, Nutritional, and Respiratory Therapies (An Evidence-Based Review): Report of the Quality Standards Subcommittee of the American Academy of Neurology. *Neurology* 2009; 73:1218–1226.

16. Younger DS, Rowland LP, Latov N, Hays AP, Lange DJ, Sherman W, Inghirami G, Pesce M, Knowles OM, Powers J, Miller JR, Fetell MR, Lovelace RE. Lymphoma, motor neuron disease, and amyotrophic lateral sclerosis. *Ann Neurol* 1991; 29:78–86.

17. Younger DS. Motor neuron disease and malignancy. *Muscle Nerve* 2000; 23:658–660.

18. Younger DS, Rowland LP, Latov N, Sherman W, Pesce M, Lange DJ, Trojaborg W, Miller JR, Lovelace RE, Hays AP, Kim TS. Motor neuron disease and ALS: relation of high CSF protein content to paraproteinemia and clinical syndromes. *Neurology* 1990; 40:595–599.

19. Younger DS, Dalmau J, Inghirami G, Hays AP. Anti-Hu-associated peripheral nerve and muscle microvasculitis. *Neurology* 1994; 44:181–183.

20. Parry GJ, Clarke S. Pure motor neuropathy with multifocal conduction block masquerading as motor neuron disease. *Muscle Nerve* 1988; 11:103–107.

21. Schold SC, Cho E-S, Somasundaram M, et al. Subacute motor neuronopathy: a remote effect of lymphoma. *Ann Neurol* 1979; 5:271–287.

22. Klnsella L, Lange OJ, Trojaborg W, Sadiq SA, Younger DS, Latov N. The clinical and electrophysiologic correlates of elevated anti-GM1 antibody titers. *Neurology* 1994; 44:1278–1282.

23. MacGowas DJ, Scelsa SN, Waldron M. An ALS-like syndrome with new HIV infection and complete response to antiviral therapy. *Neurology* 2001; 57:1094–1097.

24. Nishio M, Loizumi K, Moriwaka Koike T, et al. reversal of HIV associated motor neuron disease after highly active antiretroviral therapy. *J Neurol* 2001; 248:233–234.

25. Verma A, Berger JR. ALS syndrome in patients with HIV-1 infection. *J Neurol Sci* 2006; 240:59–64.

26. Younger DS, Chou S, Hays AP, et al. Primary lateral sclerosis: a clinical diagnosis reemerges. *Arch Neurol* 1988; 45:1304–1307.

27. Mitsumoto H, Ulug AM, Pullman SL, Gooch CL, Chan S, Tang MX, et al. Quantitative objective markers for upper and lower motor neuron dysfunction in ALS. *Neurology* 2007; 68:1402–1410.

28. Kaufmann P, Pullman SL, Shungu DC, et al. Objective tests for upper motor neuron involvement in amyotrophic lateral sclerosis (ALS). *Neurology* 2004; 62:1753–1757.

29. Kim WK, Liu X, Sandner J, et. al. Study of 962 patients indicates progressive muscular atrophy is a form of ALS. *Neurology* 2009; 73:1686–1692.

30. Kennedy WR, Alter M, Sung JH. Progressive proximal spinal and bulbar muscular atrophy of late onset. A sex linked recessive trait. *Neurology* 1968; 18:671–680.

31. Amato AA, Prior TW, Barohn RJ, et al. Kennedy's disease: a clinicopathologic correlation with mutations in the androgen receptor gene. *Neurology* 1993; 43:791–794.

32. Atassi N, Cook A, Pineda CM, Yerramilli-Rao P, Pulley D, Cudkowicz M. Depression in amyotrophic lateral sclerosis. *Amyotroph Lateral Scler* 2011; 12:109–112.

33. Crisafulli E, Manni G, Kidonias M, Trianni L, Clini EM. Subjective sleep quality during average volume assured pressure support (AVAPS) ventilation in patients with hypercapnic COPD: a physiological pilot study. *Lung* 2009 Nov–Dec; 187(6):427–428.

34. Lacomblez L, Bensimon G, Leigh PN, Guillet P, Meininger V. Dose-ranging study of riluzole in amyotrophic lateral sclerosis/Riluzole Study Group II. *Lancet* 1996; 347:1425–1431.

35. Kaufmann P, Thompson JL, Levy G, Buchsbaum R, et al. Phase II trial of CoQ10 for ALS finds insufficient evidence to justify phase III. *Ann Neurol* 2009; 66:235–244.

36. Matthews RT, Yang L, Browne S, Baik M, Beal MF. Coenzyme Q10 administration increases brain mitochondrial concentrations and exerts neuroprotective effects. *Proc Natl Acad Sci USA* 1998; 95:8892–8897.

37. Lange DJ, Murphy PS, Diamond B, et al. Selegiline is ineffective in a collaborative double-blind, placebo-controlled trial for treatment of amyotrophic latral sclerosis. *Arch Neurol* 1998; 55:93–96.

38. Beers DR, Henkel JS, Zhao W, et al. Endogenous regulatory T lymphocytes ameliorate amyotrophic lateral sclerosis in mice and correlate with disease progression in patients with amyotrophic lateral sclerosis. *Brain* 2011; 134:1293–1314.

39. Appel SH, Zhao W, Beers DR, and Henkel JS. The microglial-motoneuron dialogue in ALS. *Acta Myologica* 2011; 30:4–8.

40. Meininger V, Drory VE, Leigh PN, et al. Glatiramer acetate has no impact on disease progression in ALS at 40 mg/day:

a double-blind, randomized, multicentre, placebo-controlled trial. *Amyotroph Lateral Scler* 2009; 10:378–383.

41. Pascuzzi R et al. A phase II trial of talampanel in subjects with amyotrophic lateral sclerosis. *Amyotroph Lateral Scler* 2010; 11:266–271.

42. Miller RG, Moore DH 2nd, Gelinas DF, et al. Phase III randomized trial of gabapentin in patients with amyotrophic lateral sclerosis. *Neurology* 2001; 56:843–848.

43. Cudkowicz ME, Shefner JM, Schoenfeld DA, et al. A randomized, placebo-controlled trial of topiramate in amyotrophic lateral sclerosis. *Neurology* 2003; 61:456–464.

44. Joo IS, Hwang DH, Seok JI, Shin SK, et al. Oral administration of memantine prolongs survival in a transgenic mouse model of amyotrophic lateral sclerosis. *J Clin Neurol* 2007; 3:181–186.

45. de Carvalho M, Pinto S, Costa J, et al. A randomized, placebo-controlled trial of memantine for functional disability in amyotrophic lateral sclerosis. *Amyotroph Lateral Scler* 2010; 11:456–460.

46. Rothstein JD, Patel S, Regan MR, et al. Beta-lactam antibiotics offer neuroprotection by increasing glutamate transporter expression. *Nature* 2005; 433:73–77.

47. Oppenheim RW, Maderdrut JL, Wells DJ, et al. Cell death of motoneurons in the chick embryo spinal cord. VI. Reduction of naturally occurring cell death in the thoracolumbar column of Terni by nerve growth factor. *J Comp Neurol* 1982; 210:174–189.

48. Kalra S, Genge A, Arnold DL. A prospective, randomized, placebo-controlled evaluation of corticoneuronal response to intrathecal BDNF therapy in ALS using magnetic resonance spectroscopy: feasibility and results. *Amyotroph Lateral Scler* 2003; 4:22–26.

49. Miller RG, Armon C, Barohn RJ, et al. A placebo controlled trial of recombinant human ciliary neurotrophic factor (rhCNTF) in amyotrophic lateral sclerosis. *Ann Neurol* 1996; 39:256–260.

50. Lai EC, Felice KJ, Festoff BW, et al. Effect of recombinant human insulin-like growth factor-I on progression of ALS. A placebo-controlled study. The North America ALS/IGF-I Study Group. *Neurology* 1997; 49:1621–1630.

51. Sorenson, EJ, Windbank AJ, Mandrekar JN, et al. Subcutaneous IGF-1 is not beneficial in 2-year ALS trial. *Neurology* 2008; 71:1770–1775.

52. Lambrechts D, Storkebaum E, Morimoto M, et al. VEGF is a modifier of amyotrophic lateral sclerosis in mice and humans and protects motoneurons against ischemic death. *Nature Genet* 2003; 34:383–394.

53. Azzouz M, Ralph SG, Storkenbaum E, et al. VEGF delivery retrogradely transported lentivector prolongs survival in a mouse ALS model. *Nature* 2004; 429:413–417.

54. Kalmar B, Novoselov S, Gray A, Cheetham ME, Margulis B, Greensmith L. Late stage treatment with arimoclomol delays disease progression and prevents protein aggregation in the SOD1 mouse model of ALS. *J Neurochem* 2008; 107:339–350.

55. Cudkowicz ME, Shefner JM, Simpson E, Grasso D, Yu, Zhang H, Shui A, Schoenfeld D, Brown RH, Wieland S, Barber JR, Northeast ALS Consortium. Arimoclomol at dosages up to 300 mg/day is well tolerated and safe in amyotrophic lateral sclerosis. *Muscle Nerve* 2008; 38:837–844.

56. Kostic V, Jackson-Lewis V, DeBilbao F, et al. Prolonging life in a transgenic mouse model of amyotrophic lateral sclerosis. *Science* 1997; 277:559–562.

57. Friedlander RM, Brown RH, Gagliardini V et al. Inhibition of ICE slows ALS in mice. *Nature* 1997; 388:31.

58. Zhou S, Stavrovskaya I, Drozda M et al. Minocycline inhibit cytochrome c release and delays progression of amyotrophic lateral sclerosis in mice. *Nature* 2002; 417:74–78.

59. Gordon PH, Moore DH, Miller RG, et al. Western ALS Study Group. Efficacy of minocycline in patients with amyotrophic lateral sclerosis: a phase III randomised trial. *Lancet Neurology* 2007; 6:1045–1053.

60. Dupuis L, Oudart H, Rene F, Gonzalez de Aguilar JL, Loeffler JP. Evidence for defective energy homeostasis in amyotrophic lateral sclerosis: benefit of a high-energy diet in a transgenic mouse model. *Proc Natl Acad Sci USA* 2004; 101:11159–11164.

61. Dupuis L, Corcia P, Fergani A, et. al. Dyslipidemia is a protective factor in amyotrophic lateral sclerosis. *Neurology* 2008; 70:1004–1009.

62. Chio A, Calvo A, Ilardi A, et. al. Lower serum lipid levels are related to respiratory impairment in patients with ALS. *Neurology* 2009; 73:1681–1685.

63. Paganoni S, Deng J, Jaffa M, Cudkowicz ME, Wills AM. Body mass index, not dyslipidemia, is an independent predictor of survival in amyotrophic lateral sclerosis. *Muscle Nerve* 2011 Jul; 44(1):20–24.

64. Lepore AC, Rauck B, Dejea C, Pardo AC, Rao MS, Rothstein JD,et al. Focal transplantation-based astrocyte replacement is neuroprotective in a model of motor neuron disease. *Nat Neurosci* 2008; 11:1294–301.

65. Appel SH, Engelhardt JI, Henkel JS, et al. Hematopoietic stem cell transplantation in patients with sporadic amyotrophic lateral sclerosis. *Neurology* 2008; 71:1326–34.

CHAPTER 50

Parkinsonian Syndromes and Multisystem Atrophies

Samay Jain, Steven J. Frucht

Parkinsonism refers to the clinical presentation of tremor at rest, rigidity, bradykinesia, loss of postural reflexes, flexed posture, and freezing. It is "definite" when tremor or rigidity is present with one other feature, "probable" when rest tremor or rigidity are present alone, and "possible" when two features other than rest tremor or rigidity are present. Traditionally, Parkinsonian disorders have been classified Parkinson disease (PD), multisystem atrophy (MSA), progressive supranuclear palsy (PSP), and corticobasal degeneration (CBD), wherein MSA encompasses the formally separate disorders of striatonigral degeneration (SND), sporadic olivopontocerebellar atrophy (SOPCA), and Shy-Drager Syndrome (SDS). Clinical and pathologic studies suggest that these syndromes represent a spectrum of a single neurodegenerative disorder linked by common pathology. Hence MSA incorporates syndromes of MSA with predominant Parkinsonian features (MSA-P) and prominent cerebellar dysfunction (MSA-C). The pathological classification of Parkinsonian disorders differentiates synucleinopathies and tauopathies. Synucleinopathy refers to neurodegenerative proteinopathies unified by the common pathological lesion of fibrillary aggregates of conformational and post-translationally modified alpha-synuclein. Alpha-synuclein is a major component of Lewy bodies seen in PD, and Papp-Lantos filaments seen in MSA. Thus, MSA and PD are examples of synucleinopathies in which Lewy bodies may appear diffusely in the cortex associated with dementia, in the brainstem with Parkinsonism, or in the brainstem, spinal cord, sympathetic ganglia, peripheral autonomic nerves, enteric nervous system or end organs. Such lesions may be associated with Parkinsonism and other non-motor features, including autonomic dysfunction, sleep disorders, depression, anxiety, or olfactory disturbances.

Tauopathy is distinguished from synucleinopathy by the absence of Lewy bodies and prominent intracellular filamentous tau inclusions. Tau is a microtuble-associated protein and abnormalities in the tau gene are directly responsible for many tauopathies. Both PSP and CBD fall under the category of a tauopathy. Data from human PSP brains and experimental models suggest that tau is hyperphosphorylated by kinases leading to detachment from microtubules. The unbound phoshphorylated tau has an intrinsic propensity to form cytotoxic aggregates. Microtubules are unstable after detachment of tau and lose their function. Mitochondrial dysfunction accelerates pathological tau aggregation.

This chapter reviews advances in the clinical recognition, etiopathogenesis, and management of idiopathic PD, MSA, PSP, and CBD emphasizing the distinguishing features of each and disorders that may mimic them.

PARKINSON DISEASE

PD comprises approximately 80% of all cases of Parkinsonism, making it the most common Parkinsonian syndrome, and the second most common neurodegenerative disorder after Alzheimer disease. The clinical aspects, genetic and environmental causes, and neuropathology of PD have recently been reviewed (1–3). The prevalence of PD in industrialized countries is 0.3% of the general population and approximately 1% of people older than 60. Onset generally occurs is 60 in the seventh decade with a higher frequency in men, and a male-to-female ratio of 3:2. Juvenile-onset PD (JPD) presents in the second decade of life before age 20, while young-onset patients present in the third to sixth decades from 21 to 50 years of age with 5 to 10% of patients overall having young-onset disease.

The three main features of PD are rest tremor, rigidity, and bradykinesia. Postural instability is also considered a cardinal feature, but is often absent early in the course of the disease unless freezing of gait is present. Tremor at rest is the presenting symptom in the majority of patients, and is almost always asymmetric in onset. It typically worsens with anxiety, movement of the contralateral side, and in walking. The arms are more commonly involved than the legs, and although rest tremor is seldom disabling, it is often of major concern to patients because of its social appearance.

Rigidity refers to increased resistance to passive stretch independent of velocity, which in Parkinsonism is likened to cogwheeling. Bradykinesia is often the most disabling sign of early PD, affecting fine motor tasks such as buttoning and writing. Postural instability develops gradually, causing an increased risk of falling. Gait also becomes slower, and shuffling, with en-block turning. Freezing also occurs, referring to difficulty initiating a motor task or sudden spontaneous hesitation or stopping of a motor activity. Both gait and postural abnormalities are rarely prominent early in the course of the disease, and if seen initially should raise suspicion of another Parkinsonian syndrome such as PSP or MSA.

Non-motor abnormalities are commonly seen in PD including dysautonomia, dementia, depression, sensory symptoms, and sleep disorders. Dementia occurs in 40 to 80% of patients, although more often in advanced stages of the disease. Depression is common, occurring in up to one-half of patients. Sleep disorders are exceedingly common in PD, including insomnia, early-morning awakening, restless leg syndrome (RLS), and rapid eye movement (REM) sleep behavior disorder.

Both pathological and clinical studies demonstrate that non-motor symptoms are intrinsic to PD, occur earlier, and impact quality of life more than motor symptoms. Of these, dysautonomia, REM sleep-behavior disorder, and olfactory disturbance have been recognized to often predate the onset of motor signs in PD. Autonomic physiology in PD is of particular interest because it underlies several non-motor symptoms, including orthostatic dizziness, constipation, urinary problems, erectile dysfunction, drooling, sweating, and swallowing problems. Autonomic nervous system (ANS) pathways are also of interest because such studies suggest PD neuropathology occurs early in the course of disease in peripheral structures, and may spread along autonomic pathways to involve the central nervous system.

The etiopathogenesis of PD is unknown and is likely to be multifactorial. Several mechanisms have been implicated including oxidative injury, mitochondrial or proteasome dysfunction, inflammation, or abnormal kinase signaling.

There is degeneration of the dopaminergic pathways from the substantia nigra pars compacta to the striatum. Clinical signs of PD become apparent when 80% of striatal dopamine and 50% of nigral neurons are lost. The pathology of PD is characterized by eosinophilic intraneuronal inclusions that contain α-synuclein known as Lewy neuritis, Lewy bodies and Lewy-related pathology. The presynaptic protein α-synuclein maintains synaptic integrity and is involved with regulation of dopamine synthesis. Although often seen in the absence of neuronal loss, evidence suggests that α-synuclein aggregation is a precursor to neurodegeneration. The pathological features of PD are observed in a chain of neurons forming autonomic pathways, including: the hypothalamus, preganglionic parasympathetic projection neurons in the dorsal motor nucleus of the vagus, and pre-ganglionic and post-ganglionic sympathetic projection neurons including the intermediomedial and interomediolateral nuclei of the spinal cord. Notwithstanding, they are also found in several end-organs including the submandibular gland, lower esophagus, duodenum, pancreas, bronchus, larynx, pericardium, adrenal medulla, parathyroid, and ovary. Pathological evidence that the ANS is involved early in the course of PD derives from studies of incidental Lewy body disease (ILDB), a diagnosis applied to those without a clinical history of PD, instead demonstrating the presence of Lewy-related pathology in the substantia nigra and/or locus coeruleus on autopsy. ILDB may be a precursor of PD since 70% to 100% of patients with pathological findings in the sacral and thoracic segments of the spinal cord, as well as paravertebral sympathetic ganglia, are similar to PD; moreover patients with ILDB demonstrate involvement of autonomic innervation in the cardiovascular, urinary, and gastrointestinal systems.

REM sleep behavior disorder is characterized by lack of normal muscle tone that occurs during sleep, leading to a patient moving about, "acting out a dream" during REM sleep. It often occurs in PD and other neurodegenerative disorders prior to onset of apparent motor signs. There is an estimated 12 year risk of a neurodegenerative disease of at least 50% in patients manifesting idiopathic REM sleep behavior disorder that includes PD followed by Lewy body dementia, Alzheimer disease, and MSA. Based on animal models, corresponding neuropathology is thought to take place in the brainstem, specifically in the region of the pontine subcaeruleus nucleus. Olfactory disturbances are common in PD as the olfactory bulb is probably one of the earliest involved structures with Lewy-related pathology in PD. In fact, olfactory deficits often predate motor signs by 2 to 5 years, as may psychiatric manifestations, including depression and anxiety. The non-motor features of PD appear to relate more closely to widespread Lewy-related pathology than previously acknowledged, opening future possibilities to the recognition of PD by the non-or "premotor" manifestations, facilitating treatment before overt motor signs develop.

Genetic and environmental factors are thought to interact and affect the risk of developing PD. The factors that initiate PD may differ from those involved in disease progression. In the past decade, the role of genetic factors in the development of PD have been established with the identification of 16 "PARK" genetic loci to date, and at least six disease-causing genes, including α-synuclein (*SNCA*); leucine-rich repeat kinase 2 (*LRRK2*), Parkin (*PARK2*); PTEN-induced putative kinase-1 (*PINK1*); DJ-1 (*PARK7*); and ATPase type 13A2 (*ATP3A2*) genes. Monogenic PD is estimated to account for 5% or more of PD patients with autosomal dominant (AD) or autosomal recessive (AR) inheritance. A causative mutation in *PARK2*, which is responsible for most cases of AR PD, encodes parkin, a ubiquitin protein ligase that ubiquinates α-synuclein; both α-synuclein and ubiquitin are components of Lewy bodies. Mutations in *PARK2* are thought to account for up to one-half of all JPD, however it should be noted that while monogenic PD may present in younger patients, it may present as a late-onset Parkinsonism. Of note, the AD *PARK8* locus corresponds to the *LRRK2* gene with the phenotype of classical Parkinsonism.

Environmental causes have also been implicated in PD, including acute levodopa-responsive Parkinsonism following exposure to methylphenyltetrahydropyridine (MPTP), a contaminant of illicit street drugs. Other putative environmental exposures include carbon monoxide, manganese, carbon disulfide, and cyanide. Although patients exposed to these substances may clinically resemble PD, they differ pathologically in that the globus pallidus, rather than the substantia nigra, is primarily involved. Exposure to pesticides constitute a risk for development of PD, while smoking, uric acid, and coffee consumption are in large part associated with a decreased risk of developing PD. Other dietary and biochemical factors have been explored, although the results have been inconsistent due to lack, in part, to methodological limitations. The mechanisms postulated to explain how an environmental exposure leads to development of Parkinsonism include mitochondrial injury, complex I deficiency, oxidative stress, autophagy, inflammation, and excitotoxicity.

Although PD is a clinical diagnosis without absolute laboratory or neuroimaging confirmation, functional neuroimaging employing positron emission tomography (PET) with flurodopamine provides a baseline and supportive evidence of the diagnosis, after which a treatment, chosen from among a variety of agents, can be established. Early intervention is aimed at slowing progression of the disease with the use of neuroprotective therapeutic modalities without ignoring the importance of providing prompt symptomatic relief. Although research in neuroprotective strategies for PD is highly active, to date there is no proven treatment that alters the progression of PD. Rasagline is a monamine oxidase type B (MAO-B) inhibitor that prevents the metabolism of dopamine, which may be neuroprotective.

Symptomatic treatment is first considered when symptoms become bothersome or cause disability such that the time from disease onset to treatment is variable and individualized according to a given patient's needs, and based on targeting specific symptoms, minimizing and avoiding unwanted side effects. Available symptomatic medications include anticholinergic and dopaminergic agents, and amantadine. Anticholinergic medications are used to treat tremor, especially in younger patients who tolerate the medication better than the elderly. Amantadine has weak anti-Parkinsonian action and may be used early in the disease, along with other dopaminergic treatment, especially when dyskinesia needs to be minimized. More potent symptomatic treatment requires treatment with levodopa or dopamine agonist. The dopamine agonists bromocriptine, pramipexole, and ropinirole are used in early young PD patients because they seldom develop adverse dyskinesia.

Dopamine agonists have less anti-Parkinsonian effects than levodopa, however common side effects of nausea, somnolence, sudden sleep attacks, vivid dreams, hallucinations, hypotension, and leg edema may limit use in the elderly. They are generally well tolerated and effective in relieving symptoms, especially in early PD, allowing a delay in the introduction of levodopa therapy, which is the most potent anti-Parkinsonian medication employed through much of the disease. It is not an exaggeration to assert that virtually every PD patient will eventually take levodopa. Most starting with a dopamine agonist treatment will eventually require levodopa by five years. Levodopa is less expensive than a dopamine agonist, and has a similar adverse side-effect profile with the exception of somnolence, hallucinations, and leg edema that occur less commonly and less severely. Levodopa is always combined with carbidopa or benserazide to prevent peripheral conversion to dopamine by dopa-decarboxylase to reduce side effects. Commencement of levodopa is often delayed in early-onset disease because of the occurrence of motor fluctuation, which begins as the effects of levodopa wear off, causing bradykinesia and tremor, which over time can fluctuate between "on" periods of increased mobility, and "off" periods of relative immobility. This can initially be predicted with end-of-dose fluctuation, but over time becomes less reliable. Motor fluctuations occur in more than 90% of young-onset patients treated with levodopa within five years, and in 25% to 50% of patients overall. Levodopa-induced dyskinesia is a major motor complication of therapy that occurs at the time of peak dose effect or diphasically in the beginning or end of a dose cycle. The dyskinesias are most often choreic but may also be dystonic. Since the most common cause of motor fluctuations is linked to the short half-life of levodopa, one strategy is to include a catechol-O-methyltransferase (COMT) inhibitor to extend the half-life of levodopa. High-protein meals reduce levodopa absorption, allowing patients to separate protein meals temporally from levodopa ingestion. Dopamine agonists can be used with levodopa, to enhancing its effectiveness and to reduce off time; amantadine can be used to suppress dyskinesia.

Surgical treatment of PD employing deep brain stimulation is another option for patients with persistent disabling motor fluctuations and intact cognition. Deep brain stimulation alleviates motor complications, and tremor and reduces the need for medication so that side effects can be minimized. The most common surgical targets are the subthalamic nucleus and the globus pallidus. Targeting of the ventral intermediate nucleus is reserved patients with essential tremor.

Multiple System Atrophy

MSA, which refers to degeneration of extrapyramidal, cerebellar, and ANS pathways accounts for up to 22% of tissues of the Parkinson Brain Bank. The clinical classification, clinical aspects, natural history, and etiopathogenetic factors have recently been reviewed (4–9). The mean age of onset is in the middle of the sixth decade, with an average survival of six years. A consensus statement recognized four domains for the clinical criteria of MS, including autonomic failure and urinary dysfunction, Parkinsonism, cerebellar ataxia, and corticospinal tract (CST) dysfunction (4). However, definitive diagnosis required pathological confirmation with the finding of glial cytoplasmic inclusions and degenerative changes in various brain regions. The clinical presentation is variable with 80% of patients manifesting Parkinsonism as a predominant feature (MSA-P), and less than 20%, a predominant cerebellar syndrome (MSA-C).

Patients with pathologically proven MSA show symptom presentation in the sixth decade. Parkinsonism is respectively seen in up to 87%, autonomic failure in 74%, cerebellar ataxia in 54%; and CST signs in 49% of affected patients. Dementia is uncommon, and a feature useful in distinguishing MSA from synucleinopathy. Parkinsonism presents with akinesia, rigidity, and tremor in two-thirds of patients, with postural instability and hypokinetic speech. Cerebellar features include limb ataxia, and impoverishment of gait and speech. Intention tremor may be evident along with abnormal extraocular movements, including square-wave jerks, saccadic pursuit, nystagmus, dysmetria, and slow pursuit. It may be challenging to discern cerebellar features when Parkinsonian akinesia and rigidity predominate, resulting in a disproportionate number of patients labeled as PD or MSA-P. Dysfunction of the ANS presents in men with impotence, urinary and fecal incontinence or retention, and orthostatic intolerance, leading to recurrent syncope. Signs of ANS also include constipation, hypohidrosis, and atrophy of the iris. CST signs noted in up to half of pathologically proven patients with MSA present with unilateral or bilateral Babinski signs, hyperreflexia and spasticity. Such patients may develop speech disorders, including a mixed dysarthria with hypokinetic, ataxic, and spastic features in association with dysphagia. Ocular signs include anisocoria or frank Horner syndrome, diplopia, hypometric saccades, and horizontal and vertical gaze palsies. Dystonia may present with anterocollis. Sleep disorders include daytime hypersomnolence, insomnia, arrhythmic respiration, respiratory stridor, and obstructive and central sleep apnea; a REM-sleep-behavior disorder occurs in up to two-thirds of patients even before development of motor signs. One-third of patients also experience sleep-related inspiratory stridor due to vocal cord paresis that is exceedingly rare but requires prompt management when stridor supervenes, warranting consideration of tracheostomy.

The terms MSA-P and MSA-C were adopted to reflect the variable clinical syndromes of MSA, although some prefer the older nomenclature in selected instances, as for example, SND in those with predominant Parkinsonian of the arms and legs, and signs of cerebellar degeneration, dysautonomia, and hyperactive deep tendon reflexes (DTR). Such patients that manifest neuronal degeneration in the SN similar to those with PD, and in the striatum accounting for Parkinsonian features, have a poor response to levodopa due to loss of striatal efferent fibers. However, before striatal efferent fibers degenerate, patients with SND respond partially to levodopa, although often requiring high doses to obtain a salutary response. By contrast, those with OPCA present with a predominant cerebellar syndrome, with less apparent Parkinsonism and dysautonomia. Histopathologic degeneration is concentrated in the pons, olives, and cerebellum. Such patients may present with speech disturbances and motor dysfunction restricted to the legs. Patients with SDS manifest ANS involvement and autonomic failure with Parkinsonian and cerebellar features, and pathological involvement of the intermediolateral cell columns. Signs of Parkinsonism and ANS involvement are not sufficient to diagnose SDS as they can occur in PD as well. Nonetheless, it is important to document cerebellar and CST signs, and poor responsiveness to levodopa in support of the diagnosis of SDS. A study of 16 patients with MSA had ANS involvement in advance of motor symptoms in 63%, with a median time to wheelchair-dependence of three years for MSA-P, and five years for MSA-C. The median survival after diagnosis was four years for MSA-P and nine years for MSA-C. A review of 203 pathologically confirmed patients showed that 48% died of bronchopneumonia and 21% died suddenly, often as a result of aspiration, sleep apnea, or cardiac arrhythmia. Although MSA, like PD, is a clinical diagnosis, laboratory evidence of ANS, neuroendocrine involvement, neuroimaging, and electrodiagnostic evaluation can be diagnostically supportive. Afferent and central ANS and neuroendocrine reflex pathways are selectively affected while postganglionic autonomic fibers are relatively spared; specific evaluation of these pathways can provide evidence of selective dysfunction. The centrally acting adrenoreceptor agonist, clonidine, normally stimulates the release of growth hormone but fails to do so in MSA, distinguishing it from PD in pure autonomic failure. Positron-emission tomography with fluorodopamine shows normal cardiac sympathetic innervation in most MSA patients, unlike PD. Magnetic resonance imaging (MRI) of the brain reveals striatal, cerebellar, and brainstem abnormalities in MSA, including putaminal atrophy and T_2-signal hypointensities, slit-like signal changes along the posterolateral putaminal margins, and pontine atrophy with a "hot cross bun" sign. Urodynamic studies and sphincter EMG studies are often abnormal due to the involvement of Onuf nucleus, which is present in the S2 through S4 segments of the spinal cord, innervating striated muscle of the external anal and urethral sphincter. Such dysfunction is rarely noted in PD.

The pathological features of MSA are unique degeneration of both pigmented catecholamine-containing cells in the brainstem and cholinergic cells in the intermediolateral columns, with distal ganglionic and postganglionic degeneration. Glial cytoplasmic inclusions found in the striatum, SN, inferior olives, pons, cerebellar Purkinje cells, intermediolateral cell columns, and Onuf nucleus provide a marker for the disorder, showing positive staining for ubiquitin, tau, and α-synuclein, indicating that MSA is a form of synucleinopathy. Such aggregated α-synuclein proteins form brain lesions that are hallmarks of neurodegenerative synucleinopathies. Antibodies to specific nitrated tyrosine residues in α-synuclein demonstrate extensive and widespread accumulation of nitrated α-synuclein in MSA inclusions found in primary motor and other regions of the cerebral cortex in MSA. It is hypothesized that MSA is a primary oligodendrogliopathy with glial cytoplasmic inclusions and secondary neuronal multisystem degeneration. Although Mendelian inheritance patterns have been noted in MSA pedigrees, no pathogenic mutations have been discerned.

MSA-P typically has poor responsiveness to levodopa, although one-third of patients may experience temporary benefit, along with axial-induced dyskinesia, which has the appearance of dystonia of the face and jaw with anterocollis. One reason for the variable response to levodopa in MSA is the absence of striatal efferent fibers necessary for its motor effects, particularly in those of older age, whereas patients with onset before age 50 have a good levodopa response, with only about 13% maintaining sustained benefit. Although cerebellar dysfunction predominates in less than 20% of patients, it eventually develops in half of all patients. Although several agents are being investigated, there is currently no proven neuroprotective treatment. Neuroprotective trials of minocycline, recombinant growth hormone and riluzole have been negative for slowing disease progression. Orthostatic hypotension is treated supportively with fludrocortisone, alternatively with the oral adrenergic vasoconstrictor midodrine, as well as knee-high support hose, increased salt diet, sleeping upright in bed, and small frequent meals. Instructing the patient to sit up slowly from a lying position and then standing after a few minutes is also useful. As ANS involvement worsens, the need for an antihypertensive or anti-arrhythmic in a given patient may change. Urinary incontinence, urgency, and erectile dysfunction are amenable to treatment. however those who choose to use sildenafil should be cautioned regarding the risk of significant hypotension.

Progressive Supranuclear Palsy

PSP is the commonest Parkinsonian disorder after PD and MSA. There are several recent reviews of the clinical features, natural history, and clinical genetics of PSP (10–12). The incidence of PSP increases with age, with men affected more frequently than women. In addition to Parkinsonism, clinical symptoms include early postural instability, supranuclear gaze palsy, and cognitive decline. The disorder is characterized by abundant neurofibrillary tangles, which differ in both distribution and composition from those associated with Alzheimer disease. Affected patients present with dysarthria, bradykinesia, postural instability, supranuclear vertical gaze palsy, bradykinesia, axial rigidity, pseudobulbar palsy, subcortical dementia, and lack of responsiveness to levodopa treatment.

Clues to PSP in patients with otherwise typical PD include early instability and falls, particularly during the first year of symptom onset, visual complaints such as double vision or difficulty driving, and vertical supranuclear gaze palsy. Marked slowing of vertical saccades precedes the development of vertical supranuclear gaze palsy and may be demonstrated by selective loss of vertical opticokinetic nystagmus. Spontaneous eye blinking is profoundly reduced in PSP patients. There may be retraction of the eyelids with sustained frontalis contraction in the presence of facial hypomimia, causing staring or startled facial expressions. Visual hallucinations, drug-induced dyskinesia and autonomic dysfunction are relatively uncommon, and help to discriminate it from PD and MSA.

Severe speech and swallowing difficulties may lead patients to overstuff their mouths while eating, which can be assessed by having the patient move their tongue rapidly from side to side and articulating labial and dental consonants. Pooling of secretions, loss of the gag reflex and choking while drinking can all be seen in the setting

Table 1. Differentiating Characteristics of Parkinsonian Syndromes

Feature	Parkinson disease	MSA	PSP	CBD
Response to dopaminergic therapy	Yes	Limited to small minority	No	No
Asymmetric or symmetric onset	Asymmetric	Symmetric	Symmetric	Asymmetric
Cerebellar ataxia	No	Yes	No	No
Dysautonomia	Late in disease	Yes	No	No
Dementia	40 to 80% (late)	Rare	Frontal lobe type	Common
Cortical sensory findings	No	No	No	Yes
Apraxia	No	No	No	Yes
Falls and instability	Late	Early	Within 1 year of onset	Can occur, especially if leg has apraxia
Eye movements	Decreased blink rate and paucity of movement	Square-wave jerks	Supranuclear gaze palsy, vertical gaze >> horizontal	Increased horizontal saccade latency
Abductor vocal cord weakness causing stridor	No	Yes	No	No
Decade of onset	Seventh	Sixth	Seventh	Seventh
Average life expectancy	Same as general population with treatment	Death 6 years after diagnosis	Death 5 to 6 years after diagnosis	Death 5 to 10 years after diagnosis

of dysphagia. The speech may have soft, monotonous, slow, slurred, or scanning quality. Disturbances of posture lead to an erect stance accompanied by backward veering with hyperextension of the neck and trunk. There may be frontal lobe apathy, impaired abstract thought, decreased verbal fluency, and imitative behaviors. Cognitive impairment occurs in up to half of PSP patients during early disease stages. Patients with PSP have a median survival of eight years from the time of onset of disease with pneumonia being the most common immediate cause of death.

Although the precise cause of PSP is not known, the disorder is associated with specific haplotypes of the tau gene that encodes a phosphoprotein in the family of microtubule-associated proteins involved with the assembly and stabilization of tubulin, a protein important in maintaining cell infrastructure. Hyperphosphorylated tau protein forms neurofibrillary tangles in various regions of the brain. Abundant neurofibrillary tangles or neutrophil threads occur in the basal ganglia and brainstem, with variable neuronal loss and gliosis. Lipid peroxidation appears to play a role in PSP as specific aldehydes have been found in a regional distribution coinciding with degenerative patterns in PSP. It has been suggested that reactive oxygen species can result in the creation of a version of tau that is resistant to dephosphorylation, resulting in abnormal accumulation.

The clinical characteristics of PSP coincide with the observed pathological changes in decreasing order of severity in the internal and external segment of the globus pallidus, subthalamic nucleus, SN, red nucleus, substantia innominate, dentate nucleus, pontine nuclei, inferior olivary nucleus, neostriatum, and nucleus of the oculomotor nerve. Cerebellar degeneration is seen in PSP but not PD, accounting for wider-based gait. Whereas involvement of the locus coeruleus is generally not as severe in PSP compared to PD accounting for less autonomic instability.

Although there are no specific tests for PSP, thinning of the quadrigeminal plate, reduced diameter, and atrophy of the midbrain with sparing the pons supports the diagnosis of PSP, differentiating from MSA that shows a normal midbrain and reduced pontine diameters.

Treatment of PDP is relatively ineffective due to the widespread involvement of dopaminergic and non-dopaminergic neurotransmitter systems; however, improvement in the quality of life is achievable through palliative therapy, including weighted walkers and physiotherapy for gait instability, dietary modification, and percutaneous endoscopic gastrostomy (PEG) to address dysphagia, optometric prisms for visual disturbances, botulinum toxin for blepharospasm, artificial tears for dry eyes caused by decreased blinking, antidepressant medication, and family counseling for depression and emotional incontinence.

Corticobasal Degeneration

This sporadic disorder with a mean of onset in the seventh decade is estimated to account for 1% of patients with Parkinsonism although the true incidence and prevalence is not known. The clinical, genetic, radiographic, and pathological aspects of CBD have recently been reviewed (13–15). Clinical onset is usually with asymmetric Parkinsonism of the akinetic-rigid type and limb clumsiness that progresses to akinesia, rigidity, and apraxia in more than 90% of patients, although a majority will have initial cognitive impairment. Patients manifest irregular action and postural tremor that responds poorly to levodopa, however less common features include gait disorder with postural instability, dysarthria, dysphasia, orofacial dyspraxia, masked fasces, unilateral painful paresthesia, pyramidal tract signs, and behavioral problems. Criteria have been established to include the initial presentation of predominant basal ganglia and CST signs, however clinical diagnosis is usually based upon the presence of limb rigidity and at least one cortical sign such as apraxia, cortical sensory loss, or alien limb phenomenon.

The tremulous movements of CBD differ from those of PD as they are typically up to 8 Hz and occur with action, posture, or tapping of the involved limb, and are often irregular occurring with superimposed focal myoclonus. Asymmetric limb dystonia presents in the arm with the hand and forearm flexed and the arm adducted at the shoulder. The fingers are generally flexed at the metacarpophalangeal joints and extended or flexed at the proximal and distal interphalangeal joints. Painful dystonia, rigidity, cortical sensory loss, ideomotor apraxia, choreoathetoid movement, and the alien limb phenomenon of the affected limb can be encountered. The latter, which refers to failure to recognize ownership of a limb in the absence of visual cues is pathognomic for CBD and is associated with autonomous activity of the extremity, including unconscious postures, levitation, occasionally cortical sensory loss, dystonia, apraxia, and dementia. Ideomotor apraxia is recognized by impaired timing, sequencing, spatial organization, and mimicking, whereas limb kinetic apraxia presents with impaired dexterity and fine movements. Cognitive and neuropsychological profiles are often abnormal in CBD, leading to difficulty in praxis, naming, digit span, and motor series examinations. Frontal subcortical dementia associated with impaired gesture, and preservation of recognition memory, immediate recall, and attention, and concomitant depression, apathy, irritability, and agitation can occur in CBD.

Abnormal eye movements are common in CBD, including increased latency of the horizontal saccade when compared to patients with PSP. However, extraocular movements are slow, hypometric, and unlike PSP, vertical saccades are usually normal. Speech changes that can be seen include slow production, dysphonia, echolalia, and palilalia. Speech problems are present in a majority of patients and language can be affected with paraphasic errors and aphasia, whereas late stages can evolve toward anarthria, aphonia, and swallowing disorders. Early-onset bilateral Parkinsonism and a frontal lobe syndrome both predict a poor prognosis; the disorder is progressive in all patients with progressive deterioration due to aspiration pneumonia and sepsis and fatal outcome 10 years or less after disease onset.

Neuroimaging is normal in early stages of CBD, however with progression there is asymmetric frontoparietal cortical atrophy and dilatation of the lateral ventricles on MRI with fluid attenuated inversion recovery (FLAIR) sequences. Electroencephalography (EEG) is typically normal early in the disease, but later reveals asymmetric slowing in the hemisphere contralateral to the involved limb.

Histopathology shows asymmetric frontoparietal cortical atrophy with neuronal loss, gliosis and swelling, and cell bodies devoid of Nissl substance, making them "achromatic." Pyramidal neurons in the third and fifth cortical layers have a swollen eosinophilic and hyaline appearance, while those of the substantial nigra lack pigmentation and appear ballooned, eosinophilic, and vacuolated with lack of Nissl substance. Such findings are not specific for CBD and can occur in Pick, Alzheimer, and Creutzfeld-Jakob disease, PSP, and amyotrophic lateral sclerosis.

Corticobasal degeneration is a tauopathy generated by transcripts of exon 10 on chromosome 17, further characterized by extensive phosphorylation of the tau protein which, normally unfolded, soluble, and heat stable, is rendered insoluble, forming filamentous structures less efficient in promoting tubulin polymerization. It has been suggested that CBD and PSP may both be different clinical manifestations of a similar pathology with over-representation of a similar tau protein haplotype.

Treatment for the disorder is challenging with a universally poor response to levodopa. Clonazepam benefits action tremor and myoclonus, however clonazepam, diazepam, and alprazolam have also been used, and baclofen and tizanidine improve rigidity and tremor. Botulinum toxin may be useful in the treatment of painful upper limb dystonia and blepharospasm. Atypical neuroleptics such as quetiapinne, olanzapine, or clozapine may be helpful for psychotic symptoms. Typical antipsychotics such as haloperidol worsen CBD symptoms and should be avoided. Selective serotonin reuptake inhibitors can be used to treat depression or obsessive-compulsive symptoms.

Dysphagia, constipation, and urinary symptoms, commonly seen in PD, also need to be carefully monitored and the patient safe-guarded for aspiration by dietary adjustments and PEG tube placement. Physiotherapy helps maintain mobility, prevents limb contracture, and alleviates pain related to dystonic posturing; occupational and speech therapy may also be of assistance in symptomatic patients.

DETERMINING THE ETIOPATHOGENESIS OF PARKINSONISM

When evaluating a patient with Parkinsonism, it is important to be aware of any features that can help determine whether a patient has PD or not. The family and social history, medications, and past illnesses may reveal factors that contribute to the Parkinsonian syndrome. Since Parkinsonism is the most common motor abnormality in MSA, such patients are routinely misdiagnosed as having PD. Up to 10% of patients diagnosed with PD have MSA, and given the differences in prognosis and treatment of PD, accurate clinical diagnosis is critical. Table 1 summarizes the salient distinguishing clinical features of Parkinsonism. The secondary causes of Parkinsonism should be systemically excluded, as treatment for another underlying disease may go unnoticed or contribute to further clinical deterioration.

Whereas Parkinson disease almost always responds well to levodopa, an absent, poor, or waning response to levodopa is characteristic of atypical Parkinsonian disorders such as MSA. Given the relatively early age of onset of MSA, the proportion of patients with Parkinsonism due to MSA will be greater around age fifty, roughly a decade earlier than the peak onset of PSP. The clinical features that favor MSA over PD include severe dysarthria, stridor due to abductor cord weakness, anterocollis, and poor response to levodopa. Dementia, while unusual in MSA, occurs in

PSP, yet when present in Parkinsonism should also raise suspicion of LBD.

A number of disorders can mimic MSA, including multiple myeloma, spinocerebellar ataxia (SCA) types 1, 2, and 3; Machado-Joseph disease, and dentatorubropallidoluysian atrophy, all of which can be associated with Parkinsonism. SCA2 presents with young-onset levodopa-responsive Parkinsonism, followed by ataxia for up to 25 years. Finally, MSA should be differentiated from pure autonomic failure, which does not have Parkinsonism or cerebellar signs. The diagnosis of PSP may be problematic since several of the classic symptoms and signs may be seen in other conditions. For example, supranuclear gaze palsy, typical of PSP, also occurs in CBD, dementia with Lewy bodies, CJD and, less commonly, MSA. Features that differentiate PSP from PD include supranuclear vertical gaze palsy, rapid disease progression, early postural instability, falls, symmetric pyramidal involvement, and akinetic-rigid Parkinsonism unresponsive to levodopa. Tremor is relatively uncommon in PSP and is rarely the presenting symptom. Fatures that distinguish PSP for CBD include alien limb syndrome, severe asymmetric Parkinsonism, cortical sensory deficits, severe ideomotor apraxia, myoclonus, and late-onset postural instability in the latter. CBD may be mistaken for Alzheimer, Pick disease, Wernicke encephalopathy, PSP, sudanophilic leukodystrophy and frontotemporal dementia.

REFERENCES

1. Lees AJ, Hardy J, Revesz T. Parkinson's disease. *Lancet* 2009; 373:2055–2066.
2. Warner TT, Schapira AHV. Genetic and environmental factors in the cause of Parkinson's disease. *Ann Neurol* 2003; 53(Suppl3):S16–S25.
3. Feany MB. New genetic insights into Parkinson's disease. *N Eng J Med* 2004; 351:1937–1940.
4. Gilman L, Low P, Albanese A, et al. Consensus statement on the diagnosis of multiple system atrophy. *Clin Auton Res* 1998; 8:359–362.
5. Schulz JB, Peterson KT, Jauch M, et al. Multiple system atrophy: natural history, MRI morphology, and dopamine receptor imaging with 123I BZM SPECT. *J Neurol Neurosurg Psychiatry* 1994; 57:1047–1056.
6. Wenning GK, Shlomo TF, Daniel YB, et al. Multiple system atrophy: a review of 203 pathologically proven cases. *Mov Disord* 1997; 12:133–147.
7. Bannister R, Mowbray J, Sidgwick A. Genetic control of progressive autonomic failure: evidence for an association with an HLA antigen. *Lancet* 1983; 321:1017.
8. Giasson BI, Duda JE, Murray IVJ, et al. Oxidative damage linked to neurodegeneration by selective alpha-synuclein in synucleinopathy lesions. *Science* 2000; 290:985–989.
9. Morris HR, Vaughan JR, Datta SR, et al. Multiple system atrophy/progressive supranuclear palsy: alpha-synuclein, synphilin, tau, and APOE. *Neurology* 2000; 55:1918–1920.
10. Nath U, Ben-Shlomo Y, Thomson RG, et al. Clinical features and natural history of progressive supranuclear palsy: a clinical cohort study. *Neurology* 2003; 60:910–916.
11. Rojo A, Pernaute RS, Fontan A, et al. Clinical genetics of familial progressive supranuclear palsy. *Brain* 1999; 122:1233–1245.
12. Tuite PJ, Clark HB, Bergeron C, et al. Clinical and pathologic evidence of corticobasal degeneration and progressive supranuclear palsy in familial tauopathy. *Arch Neurol* 2005; 62:1453–1457.
13. Kouri N, Whitwell JL, Josephs KA, et al. Corticobasal degeneration: a pathologically distinct 4R tauopathy. *Nat Rev Neurol* 2011; 7:263–272.
14. Josephs KA, Whitwell JL, Dickson DW, et al. Voxel-based morphometry in autopsy proven PSP and CBD. *Neurobiology of Aging* 2008; 29:280–289.
15. Yamaguchi H, Fukuyama H, Nagahama Y. Atrophy of the corpus callosum, cortical hypometabolism, and cognitive impairment in corticobasal degeneration. *Arch Neurol* 1998; 55:609–614.

CHAPTER 51

Poliomyelitis and the Post-Polio Syndrome

Burk Jubelt, Laura Simionescu

In the first half of the 20th century, epidemics of poliomyelitis (polio) ravaged the world. In the epidemic of 1952, over 20,000 Americans developed paralytic polio. With the introduction of the Salk inactivated polio vaccine (IPV) in 1954 and the Sabin oral polio vaccine (OPV) in 1961, the number of paralytic cases decreased to a handful per year. Polio had vanished and no longer was on the consciousness of Americans. The elimination of polio was a tremendous achievement for science and American medicine. However, in the late 1970s, survivors of paralytic polio began to notice new health problems that included fatigue, pain, and new weakness not considered "real" by the medical establishment. The term "post-polio syndrome" (PPS) was later coined to emphasize the new health problems. This chapter reviews acute poliomyelitis and the related syndrome, PPS.

POLIOMYELITIS

History

The history of polio has been extensively reviewed (1). Epidemic polio is a modern disease related to improved sanitation and human hygiene in the Western world with occurrences in Europe during the mid-19th century, and somewhat later in North America, during which resulting flaccid paralysis was ascribed to anterior horn cell (AHC) damage and intracerebral inoculation of brain tissue homogenates transmitted the disease to primates. By the mid-20th century, the three poliovirus serotypes had been identified and the virus was cultured in non-neural tissues, eliminating the need for pathogenic animal studies.

Aggressive vaccination programs have eliminated paralytic polio due to indigenous wild type poliovirus in the United States (US). In 1988, the World Health Organization (WHO) announced the initiative for the global eradication of polio, and since then, three regions were certified as polio-free, including the Region of the Americas in 1994, the Western Pacific Region in 2000 and, most recently, the European Region in 2002 (2). Several further developments included the cloning and sequencing of several strains of the three serotypes, resolution of the viral structure to 29 nm by x-ray crystallography, delineation of the amino acid sequence of the viral coat and receptor attachment site important in the induction of the antibody response, and the molecular cloning of the nucleotide sequences of the CD155 immunoglobulin superfamily-derived cellular receptor. The enteroviruses and picornaviruses were genomically reclassified (3), leading to the designation of human enterovirus C species.

Clinical Manifestations

Definitions and Nomenclature

Poliovirus infections are divided into minor and major forms (Figure 1). The minor illnesses occur 1 to 3 days before the onset of paralysis, with gastrointestinal complaints of nausea and vomiting, abdominal cramps and pain, and diarrhea and the systemic manifestations of sore throat, fever, malaise, and headache.

The major illness includes all forms of central nervous system (CNS) disease caused by poliovirus, including aseptic meningitis or non-paralytic polio, polioencephalitis, bulbar polio, and paralytic poliomyelitis, alone or in

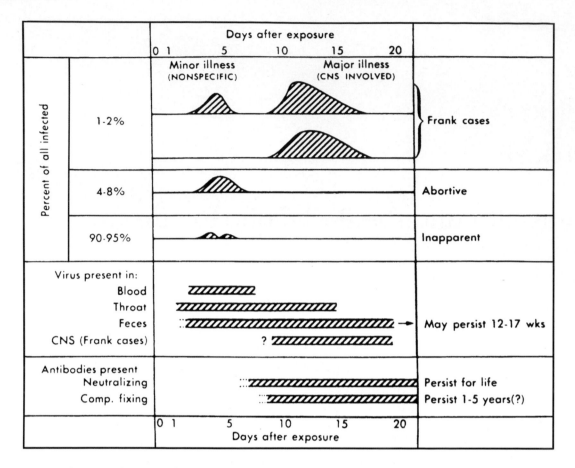

FIG. 1. Schematic diagram of the clinical forms of poliomyelitis correlated with the times at which virus is present in various sites and the development of serum antibodies. From, Horstmann DM. Epidemiology of poliomyelitis and allied diseases, 1963. *Yale J Biol Med* 1963; 36:5–26, with permission.

combination. It can follow the minor illness immediately or, more often, within 3 to 4 days or occur without the minor illness. It is common for patients to have aseptic meningitis recognized by a stiff neck, back pain, photophobia, and headache before the onset of paralytic polio. Polioencephalitis precedes paralysis and rarely occurs alone. It can manifest as tremulousness, obtundation, agitation, and autonomic dysfunction. The latter is recognized by labile hypertension, hypotension, tachycardia, arrhythmias, and excessive sweating. Upper motor neuron signs of spasticity, hyperreflexia and Babinski signs are usually lost as paralytic disease ensues (4). Muscle pains, muscle cramps, fasciculation, and radicular pain rarely occur without paralysis, but when they do occur, they usually precede paralysis by 24 to 48 hours. Paralytic disease is due to poliovirus infection of the motor neuron. Spinal cord anterior horn cells and other motor neurons are selectively vulnerable to poliovirus infection (5). Infection by poliovirus results in a variable distribution and variable extent of paralysis.

Clinical Symptoms and Signs

Paralytic polio, which accounts for 0.1 to 2.0% of all epidemic poliovirus infections, can be of bulbar, spinal, or bulbospinal types, leading to asymmetric, flaccid, patchy, and more proximal than distal progressive paralysis affecting the arms more than legs, typically spreading over 5 to 6 days with incipient wasting and areflexia. Rarely, transverse myelitis characterized by paraparesis, urinary retention, sensory, and autonomic involvement occurs.

Predominant bulbospinal polio in adults, and isolated bulbar involvement in children, which occurs in 10 to 15% of paralytic cases, most frequently involves cranial nerves VII, IX, and X, resulting in facial weakness, swallowing, and phonatory disturbances, and the medullary reticular formation leading to ataxic breathing, lethargy, obtundation, as well as hypotension, hypertension, and cardiac arrhythmias.

Chronic and persistent poliovirus infection occasionally occurs in children with agammaglobulinemia and cellular immunodeficiency several months after receipt of the live oral vaccine leading to lower motor neuron paralysis and fatal progressive CNS dysfunction.

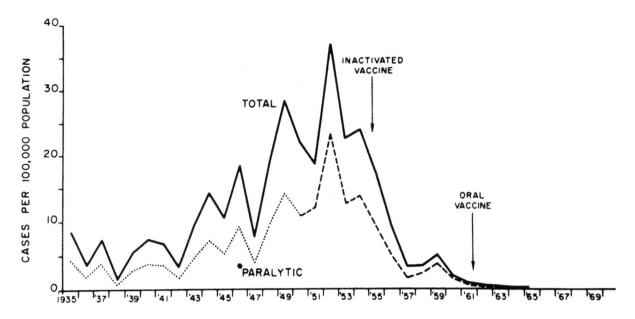

FIG. 2. Incidence of poliomyelitis in the United States, 1935–1964. From: Paul JR. *History of poliomyelitis*. New Haven: Yale University, 1971, with permission.

Epidemiology

Incidence

Although the incidence of paralytic polio peaked in the US in 1952 at about 20,000 cases (6), cycles of polio epidemics in the US and other developed countries stopped with introduction of the IPV and OPV (Figure 2). While there was little threat of polio epidemics in most countries, as of 2010, the WHO still listed 15 countries with endemic polio (7).

The overall reduction in global poliomyelitis, from over 300,000 cases in 1988 to fewer than 1,500 cases in 2010, was achieved through very aggressive vaccination campaigns utilizing OPV (8). While a given country can be declared poliovirus-free, any lapse in the vaccination protocol can precipitate epidemics (7, 9) and the ease with which poliovirus is reintroduced into a population underscores the need to continue vigilant vaccination programs.

Transmission

The poliovirus is primarily spread by fecal-hand-oral transmission from one host to another and shed in oral secretions for several weeks and in the feces for several months. It is often introduced into the household by small children who are not toilet trained and spreads rapidly in a family, infecting other household members in 4 to 5 days depending upon prior immunity, household size, sanitary hygiene conditions (10), and environmental factors such as sanitation, level of hygiene, crowded conditions, geography, season of the year, and host characteristics.

Endemic Versus Epidemic Activity

The geographic location and temperature changes are factors that result in endemic or epidemic poliovirus activity. In tropical and semitropical areas, poliovirus circulates endemically year-round, whereas in temperate zones, epidemics peak in the summer and early fall. From ancient times until the late 1800s, endemic poliovirus activity was due to crowding, poor personal hygiene, and poor public sanitation. By early childhood, most individuals were infected by all three serotypes and infrequent sporadic cases of paralytic polio or true infantile paralysis, a pattern that still occurs in semitropical and tropical underdeveloped areas of the world.

By the late 1800s, epidemic activity occurred in developed temperate areas of the world due to improved personal hygiene and public sanitation (11). Infants and small children, not previously exposed to poliovirus, created a large pool of susceptible older children, adolescents, and adults. The latter were more likely to develop severe disease when poliovirus infection swept through this virgin population, within which a high rate of paralysis occurred (1).

Predisposing Factors

There are other predisposing factors for paralytic polio, including age at onset, such that older children, adolescents, and adults have more severe and potentially fatal paralysis than infants and young children, and male sex appears to enhance susceptibility to paralytic polio. Preceding or contemporaneous tonsillectomy is associated with a higher incidence of bulbar polio, while traumatic and injected extremities are more likely to become paralyzed, a so-called provoking effect. While physical exertion predisposes to more severe paralysis, pregnancy increases the incidence of paralytic disease by three-fold.

Pathogenesis and Pathology

Following spread by fecal-hand-oral transmission and viral replication in the oropharynx, intestinal mucosae, and sub-mucosal lymphatic tissues, a primary viremia occurs followed by replication in non-neural target tissues and CNS invasion. Two factors mitigating CNS invasion include defects in the blood–brain barrier, particularly the area postrema, and possible viral entry at the neuromuscular junction during viremia, the latter along distal axons with retrograde axonal transport to the CNS. The poliovirus may reach the neuro-muscular junction during viremia, entering the distal axon and transported in a retrograde manner to the CNS.

After several days of poliovirus CNS infection, pathologic changes are seen in AHC, including shrinkage and dissolution leading to diffuse chromatolysis and loss of basophilic staining, that proceeds to further shrinkage, eosinophilic type B inclusions, and cell membrane disintegration if the infection does not resolve. The inflammatory response further engenders meningeal, perivascular, and parenchymal infiltrates initially composed of polymorphonuclear leukocytes over the first 24 to 48 hours, followed by mononuclear and microglial cell responses with neuronophagia.

Laboratory Studies

General laboratory tests are generally uninformative. The complete blood count may reveal a peripheral leukocytosis. Poliovirus can be isolated from the oropharynx for several weeks and from stool for several months. Since several enteroviruses may be isolated from the stool, serologic testing and polymerase chain reaction (PCR) DNA amplification is needed to confirm the responsible virus type. A four-fold or greater rise in the serum poliovirus antibody titer between acute and convalescent specimens is considered diagnostic of infection, however it is important to obtain the acute phase specimen as early as possible in the course of the illness, and the convalescent phase sample at four weeks to detect the diagnostic four-fold rise. Cerebrospinal fluid (CSF) examination shows findings similar to those of other CNS viral infections with certain caveats (1). The cell count is increased, often comprised initially of polymorphonuclear leukocytosis followed by a shift to mononuclear cells in 12 to 48 hours of hundred to several thousand cells per mm^3 prompting consideration of bacterial meningitis. The CSF protein is normal or mildly elevated in the range of 100 to 300 mg/dL for several weeks and remaining high for months; hypoglycorrhachia is rarely encountered. While an increased CSF/serum antibody ratio exceeding 1:150 with increased titers of IgM-specific antibody supports the diagnosis of CNS poliovirus infection, PCR remains the preferred method to confirm the diagnosis (12, 13). Magnetic resonance imaging (MRI) studies may localize inflammation to the spinal cord anterior horns (14).

Diagnosis

The combination of fever, headache, stiff neck, and asymmetric flaccid paralysis without sensory loss, in conjunction with a compatible CSF profile, makes the diagnosis of paralytic polio very likely. However, other viruses, including herpes and non-polio enterovirus(1, 15) can lead to asymmetric flaccid paralysis, although typically not as severe. Other disorders may be considered if the major manifestations of polio are lacking or if unusual features are present.

Management

Treatment

Patients with acute polio paralysis should be hospitalized to assure stability of cardiovascular, respiratory, and autonomic nervous system functions, food and nutritional status. Appropriate positioning and placement of splints prevent muscle contracture, while foot boards prevent foot drop, and turning prevents decubiti ulcer. Physical therapy commencing with passive movement, followed by active physical therapy with non-fatiguing muscle-strengthening exercises and hydrotherapy are necessary and recommended. Braces and other orthotics facilitate ambulation after paralysis peaks and strength begins to return, while orthopedic consultation for arthrodesis, tendon transference, and leg-shortening procedures are generally deferred for up to two years until maximum recovery occurs.

Prevention

Vaccination is the mainstay of prevention. The IPV and OPV have been very effective in decreasing the incidence of poliomyelitis, and the advantages and disadvantages of each vaccine have been reviewed (1). The IPV results in a shorter term immunity, which might necessitate revaccination if outbreaks occur, but it does not cause paralysis. A high level of vaccination of the population is required with the IPV to prevent the spread of wild-type virulent viruses in the community in contrast to the OPV, which produces long-term and possibly lifelong immunity by exposure to vaccine strains circulating in the population via secondary spread, thus eliminating wild-type virulent strains without the risk of vaccination related paralysis. Both meticulous personal, family, and public hygiene, including clean water and sewage treatment, hand washing, and availability of clean utensils decrease person-to-person and fecal-hand-oral transmission.

Prognosis and Complications

The expected low mortality rate of 7% to 8% results from prompt initiation of adequate respiratory and supportive care. Patients surviving an acute attack of paralytic polio have significant recovery of motor function, although permanent and severe residual paralysis of one or two extremities is not uncommon. Motor improvement starts within weeks after onset, although in rare cases extension of localized paralysis can be seen as late as the third or fourth week of illness. One-half of patients recover in three months, and 75% in six months, with minimal further improvement occurring slowly over the next two years.

Acute and subacute complications result from immobility and resulting decubiti, contractures, foot and wrist drop, and urinary tract infections. Pneumonia results from bulbar muscle dysfunction and respiratory insufficiency. Other complications include osteoporosis, skeletal deformities such as scoliosis, reduced extremity growth, and PPS for up to 40 years after acute polio.

POST-POLIO SYNDROME

Epidemiology

New muscle weakness as a late sequela of poliomyelitis was recognized in the late 19th century. Between 1875 and 1975, about 200 cases were reported in the world literature (4). Since then, an epidemic of several thousand cases of PPS occurred (4) related to the large epidemics of polio that occurred during the first half of this century. The estimated prevalence of PPS in those with prior polio varies from 22% to 64% depending upon the definition. A cross-sectional survey showed the prevalence of PPS to be 8.0 per 100,000 population (16). The risk factors predisposing to development of PPS are similar to those of paralytic polio, including severity of the prior polio, age at onset of polio, with adolescents and adults developing more severe PPS than infants and small children. The more complete the degree of recovery of paralytic polio, the more likely PPS is to occur.

Clinical Manifestations

Post-polio syndrome is a neurologic disorder that produces a cluster of symptoms in individuals with prior acute para-

lytic polio, often 30 to 50 years earlier. The time to development of PPS after initial polio ranges from 8 to 71 years, with an average interval of 35 years, and more severe acute polio prompting earlier onset of new weakness. Arthralgia and myalgia are due to the long-term effects of residual weakness and excessive stress on joints, ligaments, and tendons.

Fatigue, the most prominent manifestation, occurs in up to 80% of patients (4), most often described as disabling exhaustion, likened to a wall that precludes even minimal physical activity, as well as increasing physical weakness, tiredness, lack of energy, and loss of strength during exercise, affecting mental and physical functioning. The pathophysiology of fatigue is not well understood but several hypotheses include impairment of the brain activating system resulting from age-, and prior polio-related neuronal attrition, dysfunction of the neuromuscular junction as in myasthenia gravis, and intervening psychological and social factors (4).

New onset of weakness and wasting are the signature features of PPMA (4), the formal criteria of which are documented paralytic polio and partial recovery thereof followed by a period of stabilization, and progressive and persistent neurologic deterioration without alternative cause (Table 1) (17, 18). Such findings which appear to be due to disintegration of the motor unit (19), occur in muscles previously affected, that are partially or fully recovered, as well as clinically unaffected muscles, the latter of which may have been subclinically involved during the acute polio. Previously affected muscles are more likely than unaffected muscles to later become weak. The distribution of the new weakness, which is usually asymmetric, proximal, distal, or patchy, correlates with the severity of paralysis at the time of the acute polio and with the degree of recovery, thus with the number of surviving motor neurons. New onset of wasting, rare as an isolated manifestation of PPS, occurs in no more than one-

Table 1. Diagnostic Criteria for PPS*

1. A prior episode of paralytic poliomyelitis with residual motor neuron loss (which can be confirmed through a typical patient history, a neurologic examination and, if needed, an electrodiagnostic exam).

2. A period of neurologic recovery followed by an interval (usually 15 years or more) of neurologic and functional stability.

3. A gradual or abrupt onset of new weakness or abnormal muscle fatigue (decreased endurance), muscle atrophy, or generalized fatigue.

4. Exclusion of medical, orthopedic, and neurologic conditions that may be causing the symptoms mentioned in 3.

*Consensus statement of the 1997 Post-Polio Task Force Roundtable Meeting

half of patients with new-onset weakness. The latter may be accompanying fasciculation, cramps, and pseudohypertrophy. Weakness may involve specific muscle groups or function, such as respiratory muscles, especially in those that had prior ventilator support during acute polio. Such patients with PPS and chronic respiratory failure may lose an average of 1.9% of their vital capacity per year due to superimposed central hypoventilation due to residual bulbar motor neuron involvement, cardiac disease, and scoliosis, requiring nighttime or continuous ventilatory support.

Bulbar muscle weakness, a recognized component of PPS, is associated with dysphagia, which occurs in up to 20% of polio survivors due primarily to pharyngeal and laryngeal muscle weakness. Videofluoroscopic studies reveal impaired tongue movements, delayed pharyngeal constriction, pooling in the valleculae or pyriform sinuses, and mild aspiration. Other bulbar muscles, such as those of the face and vocal cords, may be affected, and dysarthria may occur. Upper motor neuron signs were noted in 8.3% of a PPS cohort, a frequency similar to that seen in acute poliomyelitis.

Sleep apnea in PPS may be due to central causes in those with a history of bulbar polio due to residual damage of the brainstem reticular formation, while an obstructive sleep pattern may instead be related to pharyngeal muscle weakness, obesity, and musculoskeletal deformities.

The continuous progression of weakness during the 12 years of follow-up of PPS patients was noted to proceed in a stepwise or continuous pattern at an average rate of 1% per year (20), although higher rates of progression of up to 11% per year for those in their 40s and 17% for others in their 60s or 70s (21).

Laboratory Studies

Like polio, routine blood tests are typically uninformative except for the serum creatine kinase (CK), which may be mildly elevated, so noted in one large cohort with progressive weakness. A mild CSF protein elevation may be encountered (4).

Electromyography

Concentric needle electromyography (EMG) of patients with prior polio (4) show chronic denervation and reinnervation with increased amplitude of voluntary motor unit potentials (MUP) and neurogenic patterns of reduced recruitment in previously involved, as well as uninvolved muscles. New weakness was associated with active and chronic denervation, however nerve conduction studies were typically normal.

Single fiber EMG of newly symptomatic muscle shows increased fiber density and neuromuscular transmission defects of increased jitter and blocking, the latter varying with the number of years since acute poliomyelitis. Macro-EMG shows large reinnervated motor units that develop by collateral sprouting and decrease over time from recovery of acute polio, most likely due to loss of terminal sprouts due to less efficient reinnervation.

Motor unit number estimation is abnormal in patients with a history of prior polio and in those with PPS, with no clear distinction between the patient's groups with respect to either the number of motor units measured or the rate of decline of motor units.

Muscle Biopsy

The biopsy findings of patients with old poliomyelitis (4) reveal evidence of chronic denervation and reinnervation, indicated by fiber type grouping, and active denervation evidenced by small angulated fibers often associated with neural-cell adhesion molecules on the surface of muscle fibers. Large group atrophy, noted in motor neuron disease, is a much less common finding in PPS. Notwithstanding, chronic denervation and reinnervation, and acute denervation do not discriminate between symptomatic and asymptomatic PPS. Superimposed myopathic features occur in patients with partial recovery of originally affected muscles so studied, less so in muscles originally spared but newly affected, compared with those originally affected yet fully recovered. The finding of frank myopathy and lymphocytic infiltrates in patients with PPS is not well understood.

Etiopathogenesis

The likeliest mechanisms for the development of PPS are shown in Table 2 (4). The loss of AHC and motor units with normal aging does not become prominent until after the age of 60 years. More important than chronologic age in PPS is failure of compensation of progressive motor neuron loss by reinnvervation and collateral sprouting with progressively larger motor unit territories, especially in patients with longer intervals of recovery from prior polio. Novel candidate protein biomarkers for PPS that are believed to be involved in different pathways of neurodegeneration and apoptosis, and found in CSF of affected patients, contributing to the etiopathogenesis of PPS include gelsolin, hemopexin, peptidylglycine α-amidating monooxygenase, glutathione synthetase, and kallikrein 6 (22).

The role of chronic persistent poliovirus infection (4) has been suggested by poliovirus infection in experimental mouse motor neuron studies (23) and persistence of poliovirus and other enteroviruses in immunodeficient children (4), human neuroblastoma cells (24), and fetal brain cells (25). However, isoelectric focusing and enzyme linked immunoassay (ELISA) techniques did not reveal poliovirus antibodies in serum or CSF in patients with antecedent poliomyelitis or evidence of persistent infection (26, 27).

Inflammatory immune-mediated mechanism for PPS

Table 2. Possible Etiologies of PPS*

Death of remaining motor neurons with normal aging, coupled with the previous loss from poliomyelitis

Premature aging of cells permanently damaged by poliovirus

Premature aging of remaining normal motor neurons due to an increased metabolic demand (increased motor unit size after poliomyelitis)

Premature exhaustion of new terminal sprouts with advancing age in the large reinnervated motor units that developed after polio (possibly also excessive metabolic demand)

Chronic poliovirus infection

Predisposition to motor neuron degeneration because of the glial, vascular, and lymphatic changes caused by poliovirus

Poliomyelitis-induced vulnerability of motor neurons to secondary insults

Genetic predisposition of motor neurons to both poliomyelitis and premature degeneration

Immune-mediated etiopathogenesis

*Modified from reference 4.

Table 3. Evidence-Based Treatment of PPS*

Generalized fatigue
  Institute lifestyle changes, including energy conservation measures and weight-loss programs
  Prescribe appropriate lower extremity orthoses or other assistive devices
Musculoskeletal pain and joint instability
  Decrease mechanical stress on joints and muscles
    Lifestyle changes, such as weight-loss programs and pacing activities
    Using assistive devices (including canes, crutches, orthoses, wheel chairs, and adaptive equipment)
  Prescribe anti-inflammatory medications, heat, and massage
Bulbar muscle weakness
  Dysphagia
    Instruction on compensatory swallowing techniques
  Dysphonia
    Instruction on voice therapy techniques
  Respiratory failure
    Noninvasive positive pressure ventilation at night and as needed
    Tracheotomy and permanent ventilation
    Administer influenza and pneumococcal vaccines
  Sleep disorders
    Use of continuous or bilevel positive airway pressure or nasal ventilation
Muscle weakness and fatigue
  Institute a nonfatiguing strengthening exercise program
  Institute physical activity pacing with rest periods
  Avoid overuse of weakened muscles
Cardiopulmonary conditioning
  Institute cycle or arm ergometer exercise programs
  Institute aquatic nonswimming exercise training

*Modified from reference 33.

have been suggested by the finding of inflammatory cell mediated immune inflammatory foci in the spinal cords of affected PPS patients (28–30), including several neuronal degeneration and active gliosis (28), more pronounced in the patients with new weakness. Further evidence of a dysimmune etiopathogenesis derives from the increased expression of CSF and serum tumor necrosis factor TNF-α and interferon-γ, and serum interleukin-6 and leptin (31, 32) in affected patients with PPS.

Management

The management of PPS is primarily symptomatic and supportive (33, 34) (Table 3). A 2006 report of the Task Force of the European Federation of Neurological Societies (EFNS) (35) concluded that a small number of controlled studies of potential specific treatments for PPS employing pyridostigmine (36), corticosteroids (37), and amantadine (38) showed no significant effect on muscular strength or fatigue, similar to the findings of two controlled trials of modafinil (39, 40).

The 2008 report of the 2008 Task Force of the EFNS (41) concluded that two randomized controlled trials (42, 43), one open, another uncontrolled study (44), and one case report (45) evidenced an 8.3% increase in mean muscle strength after two IVIg cycles during three months, along with improved physical activity and subjective vitality in the IVIg treated group (42). Whereas another study noted significant improvement of pain but not muscle strength and fatigue in the actively treated group (43). The open study reported a positive benefit on quality of life (44). An atypical patient with rapid progression of weakness showed marked improvement with IVIg (45). Moreover, IVIg treatment reduced pro-inflammatory cytokines in the CSF (43). The optimal dose and IVIg cycle frequency have not been systemically examined to allow specific recommendations.

Respiratory insufficiency is managed with non-invasive respiratory support with intermittent positive pressure ventilation using nasal masks and mouthpieces (46, 47), averting acute respiratory failure and tracheal intubation.

Pneumococcal and influenza flu vaccination is recommended for affected adults, especially those with chronic respiratory illness.

Excessive generalized fatigue, described as exhaustion with minimal exertion, has been treated with energy conservation measures and may be improved by decreasing physical activity, pacing daily activities, and taking frequent rest periods and naps. Fatigue in PPS responds better to sleep than that of the chronic fatigue syndrome, although frequent rest periods are also helpful. Pacing of physical activities with work–rest programs decreased local muscle fatigue, increased work capacity, and results in recovery of strength in symptomatic PPS, as do measures to prevent or treat obesity and use of assistive devices to conserve energy.

Dysphagia is improved by swallowing techniques (48), and dysphonia responds to voice therapy and amplification devices. Musculoskeletal pain, muscle pain, and joint instabilities also respond to pacing of activities, prevention or treatment of obesity, use of assisted devices, and the judicious use of anti-inflammatory medications (4).

Patients with PPS may have increased sensitivity to local anesthetics and parenteral administered non-depolarizing muscle blockers, leading to recommendations include the use of shorter-acting anesthetic agents, and avoidance of long-acting agents with the propensity to affect the neuromuscular junction, in patients undergoing surgery and other procedures (49). There are no reports of hyperkalemia associated with anesthesia in patients with PPS.

REFERENCES

1. Jubelt B, Lipton HL. Enterovirus infections. *Handb Clin Neurol* 1989; 56:307–347.
2. Smith J, Leke R, Adams A, Tangermann RH. Certification of polio eradication: process and lessons learned. *Bull World Health Organ* 2004; 82:24–30.
3. Stanway G, Brown F, Christian P, et al. Family Picornaviridae. In: Fauquet CM, Mayo MA, Maniloff J, Desselberger U, Ball LA, eds. *Virus taxonomy, Eighth Report of the International Committee on the Taxonomy of Viruses.* London: Elsevier Academic Press, 2005.
4. Jubelt B, Cashman NR. Neurological manifestations of the post-polio syndrome. *Crit Rev Neurobiol* 1987; 3:199–220.
5. Ford DJ, Ropka SL, Collins GH, et al. The neuropathology observed in wild-type mice inoculated with human poliovirus mirrors human paralytic poliomyelitis. *Microb Pathog* 2002; 33:97–107.
6. *Poliomyelitis surveillance summary 1980–1981,* Atlanta: Centers for Disease Control, 1982.
7. Centers for Disease Control and Prevention. Wild poliovirus type 1 and type 3 importations—15 countries, Africa, 2008–2009. *MMWR* 2009; 58:357–362.
8. Centers for Disease Control and Prevention. Progress toward interruption of wild poliovirus transmission-worldwide, January 2010–March 2011. *MMWR* 2011; 60:582–586.
9. Aylward B, Yamada T. The polio endgame. *N Engl J Med* 2011; 364:2273–2275.
10. Pallansch MA, Roos RP. *Enteroviruses: polioviruses, coxsackieviruses, echoviruses and newer enteroviruses.* In: Knipe DM, Howley DM, eds. Fields Virology, 5th ed. Philadelphia: Lippincott, 2007.
11. Nathanson N, Martin JR. The epidemiology of poliomyelitis: enigmas surrounding its appearance, epidemicity and disappearance. *Am J Epidemiol* 1979; 110:672–692.
12. Noordhoek, GT, Weel JF, Poelstra E, et al. Clinical validation of a new real-time PCR assay for detection of enteroviruses and parechoviruses, and implications for diagnostic procedures. *J Clin Virol* 2008; 41:75–80.
13. Archimbaud C, Chambon M, Bailly JL, et al. Impact of rapid enterovirus molecular diagnosis on the management of infants, children, and adults with aseptic meningitis. *J Med Virol* 2009; 81:42–48.
14. Kornreich L, Dagan O, Grunebaum M. MRI in acute poliomyelitis. *Neuroradiology* 1996; 38:371–372.
15. Li J, Loeb JA, Shy ME, et al. Asymmetric flaccid paralysis: a neuromuscular presentation of West Nile virus infection. *Ann Neurol* 2003; 53:703–710.
16. Takemura J, Saeki S, Hachisuka K, et al. Prevalence of post-polio syndrome based on a cross-sectional survey in Kitakyushu, Japan. *J Rehabil Med* 2004; 36:1–3.
17. Halstead LS. Diagnosing post-polio syndrome: inclusion and exclusion criteria. In, Silver JK, Gawne AC, eds. *Post-polio Syndrome.* Philadelphia: Hanley & Belfus, 2004.
18. Halstead LS. A brief history of post-polio syndrome in the United States. *Arch Phys Med Rehabil* 2011; 92:1344–1349.
19. Dalakas M, Illa I. Post-polio syndrome: concepts in clinical diagnosis, pathogenesis, and etiology. *Adv Neurol* 1991; 56:495–511.
20. Dalakas MC, Elder G, Hallett M, et al. A long-term follow-up study of patients with post-poliomyelitis neuromuscular symptoms. *N Engl J Med* 1986; 314:959–963.
21. Klein MG, Whyte J, Keenan MA, et al. Changes in strength over time among polio survivors. *Arch Phys Med Rehabil* 2000; 81:1059–1064.
22. Gonzalez H, Ottervald J, Nilsson KC, et al. Identification of novel candidate protein biomarkers for the post-polio syndrome—implications for diagnosis, neurodegeneration and neuroinflammation. *J Proteomics* 2009; 71:670–681.
23. Destombes J, Couderc T, Thiesson D, et al. Persistent poliovirus infection in mouse motor neurons. *J Virol* 1997; 71:1621–1628.
24. Colbere-Garapin F, Christodoulou C, Crainic R, et al. Persistent poliovirus infection of human neuroblastoma cells. *Proc Natl Acad Sci USA* 1989; 86:7590–7594.
25. Pavio N, Buc-Caron NH, Colbere-Garapin F. Persistent poliovirus infection of human fetal brain cells. *J Virol* 1996; 70:6395–6401.
26. Salazar-Grueso EF, Grimaldi LM, Roos RP, et al. Isoelectric focusing studies of serum and cerebrospinal fluid in patients with antecedent poliomyelitis. *Ann Neurol* 1989; 2 6:709–713.
27. Jubelt B, Salazar-Grueso EF, Roos RP, et al. Antibody titer to poliovirus in blood and cerebrospinal of patients with post-polio syndrome. *Ann NY Acad Sci* 1995; 753:201–207.
28. Pezeshkpour GH, Dalakas MC. Long-term changes in the spinal cords of patients with old poliomyelitis: signs of continuous disease activity. *Arch Neurol* 1988; 45:505–508.
29. Miller DC. Post-polio syndrome spinal cord pathology. *Ann NY Acad Sci* 1995; 753:185–193
30. Kaminski JH, Tresser N. Hogan RE, et al. Pathological analysis of spinal cords from survivors of poliomyelitis. *Ann NY Acad Sci* 1995; 753:390–393.

31. Gonzalez H, Khademi M, Andersson M, et al. Prior poliomyelitis-evidence of cytokine production in the central nervous system. *J Neurol Sci* 2002; 205:9–13.

32. Fordyce CB, Gagne D, Jalifi F, et al. Elevated serum inflammatory markers in post-poliomyelitis syndrome. *J Neurol Sci* 2008; 271:80–86.

33. Jubelt B. Post-polio syndrome. *Curr Treat Options Neurol* 2004; 6:87–93.

34. Gonzalez H. Olsson T, Borg K. Management of post-polio syndrome. *Lancet Neurol* 2010; 9:634–642.

35. Farbu E, Gilhus NE, Barnes MP, et al. EFNS guideline on diagnosis and management of post-polio syndrome. Report of an EFNS task force. *Eur J Neurol* 2006; 13:795–801.

36. Trojan DA, Collet J-P, Shapiro S, et al. A multicenter, randomized, double-blinded trial of pyridostigmine in post-polio syndrome. *Neurology* 1999; 53:1225–1233.

37. Dinsmore S, Dambrosia J, Dalakas MC. A double-blind, placebo-controlled trial of high dose prednisone for the treatment of post-poliomyelitis syndrome. *Ann NY Acad Sci* 1995; 753:303–313.

38. Stein DP, Dambrosia JM, Dalakas MC. A double-blind, placebo-controlled trial of amantadine for the treatment of fatigue in patients with the post-polio syndrome. *Ann NY Acad Sci* 1995; 753:296–302.

39. Vasconcelos OM, Prokhorenko OA, Salajegheh MK, et al. Modafinil for treatment of fatigue in post-polio syndrome: a randomized controlled trial. *Neurology* 2007; 68:1680–1686.

40. Chan KM, Strohschein FJ, Rydz D, et al. Randomized controlled trial of modafinil for the treatment of fatigue in post-polio patients. *Muscle Nerve* 2006; 33:138–141.

41. Elovaara I, Apoltolski S, van Doorn P, et al. EFNS guidelines for the use of intravenous immunoglobulin in treatment of neurological diseases. *Eur J Neurol* 2008; 15:893–908.

42. Gonzalez H. Sunnerhagen KS, Sjöberg I, et al. Intravenous immunoglobulin for post-polio syndrome: a randomized controlled trial. *Lancet Neurol* 2006; 5:493–500.

43. Farbu E, Reckland T, Vik-Mo E, et al. Post-polio syndrome patients treated with intravenous immunoglobulin: a double-blinded randomized controlled pilot study. *Eur J Neurol* 2007; 14:60–65

44. Kaponides G, Gonzalez H, Olsson T, et al. Effect of intravenous immunoglobulin in patients with post-polio syndrome-an uncontrolled pilot study. J *Rehabil Med* 2006; 38:138–140

45. Farbu E, Reckand T, Gilhus NE, et al. [Intravenous immunoglobulin in post-polio syndrome]. *Tidsskrift for den Norske Laegeforening* 2004; 124:2357–2358

46. Bach JR. Management of post-polio respiratory sequelae. *Ann NY Acad Sci* 1995; 753:96–102.

47. Gillis-Haegerstrand C, Markström A, Barle H. Bi-level positive airway pressure ventilation maintains adequate ventilation in post-polio patients with respiratory failure. *Acta Anaesthesiol Scand* 2006; 60:580–585

48. Silbergleit AK, Waring WP, Sullivan MJ, et al. Evaluation, treatment, and follow-up results of post-polio patients with dysphagia. Otolaryngol *Head Neck Surg* 1991; 104:333–338

49. Lambert DA, Giannouli E, Schmidt BJ. Post-polio syndrome and anesthesia. *Anesthesiology* 2005; 103:638–644.

CHAPTER 52

Paraneoplastic Disorders and Motor Dysfunction

Myrna R. Rosenfeld, Josep Dalmau

Paraneoplastic neurologic disorders (PND) are immune-mediated disorders associated with systemic cancers. The PND may affect any portion of the nervous system, resulting in relatively isolated disorders such as paraneoplastic cerebellar degeneration (PCD) or more complex symptomatology such as that seen in paraneoplastic encephalomyelitis (PEM). Motor dysfunction is often a component of a PND and rarely may be the only symptom. As motor dysfunction may have many etiologies and occurs frequently in the absence of cancer, it may be difficult to exclude that motor dysfunction in a patient with cancer is merely coincidental. The determination of a paraneoplastic pathogenesis is dependent on several factors, including rate of onset, type of syndrome, and detection of specific antineuronal antibodies. Most PND present acute or subacutely as opposed to the more insidious and chronic presentation of neurodegenerative disorders. There are some syndromes that associate with cancer much more frequently than others, or the clinical features, as for example, the acute onset of a cerebellar syndrome in an adult, are so characteristic that they readily suggest a paraneoplastic pathogenesis. Other syndromes may result from paraneoplastic mechanisms but occur more frequently in the absence of cancer and may require a more extensive differential diagnosis. For example, chorea, motor neuron disease (MND), and the Guillain-Barré syndrome (GBS) may be paraneoplastic manifestations of cancer or lymphoma but are usually non-cancer related. The presence of paraneoplastic antibodies that serves as a marker of the paraneoplastic origin of a neurologic syndrome confirms the diagnosis of PND. These antibodies, however, are not present in about 40% of patients and, therefore, their absence does not rule out that a syndrome could be paraneoplastic. Additionally, there are antibodies that associate with specific neurologic syndromes that occur with or without cancer. In these cases, the antibodies serve as markers for the neurologic syndrome but do not distinguish between a paraneoplastic or non-paraneoplastic etiology. This chapter reviews the antibody-associated paraneoplastic motor disorders, which are summarized in Table 1.

PARANEOPLASTIC CEREBELLAR DEGENERATION

This disorder is characterized by the subacute development of cerebellar dysfunction that initially manifests with dizziness, nausea, vomiting, dysarthria, oscillopsia, and diplopia. Within a few weeks or months the patient is incapacitated with a pancerebellar syndrome often accompanied by a superimposed tremor of the head and extremities. The diagnosis of PCD should be suspected in any patient older than 50 years with subacute development of cerebellar dysfunction. The antibodies most typically associated with predominant PCD are anti-Yo, anti-Tr and anti-voltage-gated calcium channels (VGCC), although any of the well-characterized antibodies may be found (1). Patients with Yo antibodies are typically postmenopausal women and about 75% have cancer of the ovary and 20% cancer of the breast (2). Patients with Tr antibodies are usually young men with Hodgkin's lymphoma (HL) or, rarely, non-Hodgkin's lymphoma (NHL), and symptoms may develop before the diagnosis of the lymphoma or when the tumor is in remission (3). Patients with VGCC antibodies usually have a small cell lung cancer (SCLC) and about half of these patients will also have Lambert Eaton myasthenic syn-

Table 1. Paraneoplastic Neurologic Disorders Causing Abnormal Movements

Dominant Paraneoplastic Syndrome	Abnormal Movement	Common Antibody Association	Common Tumor Association
PCD[1]	Ataxia, oscillopsia, tremor	Yo Tr , mGluR1 VGCC[2]	Breast, ovary and other gynecological tumors HL SCLC
PEM	PCD, MND, myelopathy Prominent chorea	Hu CRMP5, amphiphysin	SCLC SCLC, Thymoma SCLC
Brainstem encephalitis	Hypokinesis, rigidity, gaze paralysis, orofacial dyskinesias, trismus Trismus, laryngospasm	Ma2 Ri	Germ-cell tumor of testis in young men, non-SCLC in older men or women Breast, ovary, SCLC
NMDA receptor encephalitis	Orofacial dyskinesias, chorea, dystonia, choeoathetoid movements	Antibodies to the NR1 subunit of NMDAR	Teratoma of the ovary
Stiff-person syndrome and PERM	Axial rigidity and muscle spasms; progressive encephalomyelitis with myoclonus	Amphiphysin[3] GAD, GlyR	SCLC, thymoma, breast, HL Rarely paraneoplastic
MND	UMN LMN	None None	Breast HL and NHL, SCLC
Myelopathy	Isolated syndrome rare; more commonly associated with encephalomyelitis or PCD	Amphiphysin, CRMP5	Lung, breast
POM	Predominant opsoclonus myoclonus (children)	Not characterized	Neuroblastoma
	With additional brainstem and cerebellar dysfunction (adults)	Ri	Breast, ovary, SCLC
PSN	Sensory ataxia, pseudoathetoid movements	Hu	SCLC
Subacute and chronic sensorimotor neuropathy	Distal polyneuropathy	CRMP5, Hu None	Lung Plasma cell dyscrasias
Neuromyotonia Morvan sydnrome	Muscle cramps, stiffness, delayed muscle relaxation +/- CNS involvement	Caspr2	Thymoma
LEMS	Proximal weakness that improves with exercise; muscle aches and stiffness	VGCC, SOX1[4]	SCLC

PCD: Paraneoplastic cerebellar degeneration; PEM: Paraneoplastic encephalomyelitis; mGluR1: Metabotrophic glutamate receptor type 1: VGCC: Voltage-gated calcium channels; SCLC: Small-cell lung cancer; MND: Motor neuron disease; GAD: Glutamic-acid decarboxylase; CRMP5: Collapsin response-mediated protein 5; PSN: Paraneoplastic sensory neuronopathy; NMDAR: N-methyl-D-aspartate receptor; PERM: Progressive encephalomyelitis with myoclonus; GlyR: Glycine receptor; UMN: Upper motor neuron; LMN: Lower motor neuron; HL: Hodgkin lymphoma; NHL: Non-Hodgkin lymphoma; Caspr2: Contactin-associated protein-like 2; MND: Motor neuron disorders; POM: Paraneoplastic opsoclonus myoclonus; LEMS: Lambert-Eaton myasthenic syndrome.

[1]These antibodies are typically found when PCD is the predominant syndrome although almost all known antibodies can associate with PCD.
[2]About one-half of patients with PCD and VGCC antibodies will also have LEMS.
[3]Antibodies to glutamic acid decarboxylase are found in non-paraneoplastic stiff-person syndrome.
[4]SOX1 antibodies are highly associated with the presence of a SCLC and are markers for paraneoplastic LEMS.

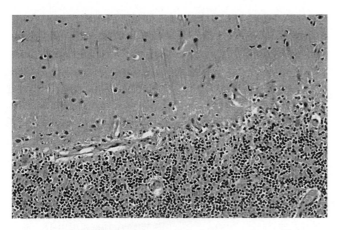

FIG. 1. Paraneoplastic cerebellar degeneration. Absence of Purkinje cells in a patient with small-cell lung cancer and cerebellar degeneration associated with paraneoplastic encephalomyelitis and anti-Hu antibodies.

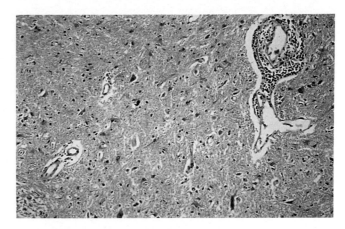

FIG. 2. Paraneoplastic motor neuron dysfunction. Anterior horn of the spinal cord of a patient with anti-Hu–associated encephalomyelitis and predominant lower motor neuron dysfunction. Note the absence of motor neurons and the presence of perivascular inflammatory infiltrates.

drome (LEMS) (4,5). Antibodies against the metabotropic glutamate receptor type 1 (mGluR1) have been identified in a few patients with idiopathic or paraneoplastic cerebellar ataxia associated with HL(1). Autopsy studies of patients with PCD show complete or near complete loss of Purkinje cells with relative preservation of other cerebellar neurons (Figure 1), explaining why response to therapy is most often minimal. However, some patients who receive anti-tumor treatment, with or without immunosuppressive therapy, may stabilize or improve, especially if treatment is started while symptoms are still progressing. Patients that undergo treatment for the underlying tumors live longer than those with untreated cancers. Some patients with Tr and mGluR1 antibodies will improve with immunotherapy.

Paraneoplastic Encephalomyelitis

Paraneoplastic encephalomyelitis describes patients with cancer who develop signs and symptoms of multifocal involvement of the nervous system that gives rise to several syndromes that can occur alone or in association (6). Paraneoplastic sensory neuronopathy (PSN) presents in 75% of patients with PEM. Other syndromes include limbic and/or brainstem encephalitis, cerebellar degeneration, myelopathy and autonomic dysfunction. PEM may be associated with virtually all types of tumors; however, in more than 75% of patients the underlying tumor is a SCLC. Such patients usually have high titers of anti-Hu antibodies in serum and cerebrospinal fluid (CSF) (7). Less frequently, anti-CRMP5 antibodies, with or without anti-Hu, are found in association with SCLC, thymoma, renal or lymphoma (6, 8). Anti-amphiphysin antibodies, which often associate with paraneoplastic stiff-person syndrome can also occur with PEM (9). Motor neuron dysfunction is a predominant symptom in 20% of patients with anti-Hu-associated PEM and

may be the presenting symptom (10). (Figure 2). Symptoms usually start with proximal loss of strength in the arms, sometimes in an asymmetric pattern. Weakness of neck extensor muscles has been reported in a few patients. Muscle wasting and fasciculation are common. Contemporaneous weakness and sensory neuronopathy may initially suggest GBS, and when spinal cord involvement predominates, a diagnosis of atypical motor neuron disease may be considered until other areas of the nervous system become involved (11). Patients with PEM and CRMP5 antibodies often present with prominent choreic movements that may initially be asymmetric or unilateral (12, 13) with later cerebellar ataxia, uveitis, optic neuritis, and peripheral symptoms due to sensorimotor axonal neuropathy (8). PEM is often refractory to treatment; however, there are patients who respond to treatment of the tumor, immunotherapy including corticosteroids, intravenous immunoglobulins (IVIg), or rituximab, and often both, especially if treatment is instituted while the patient's symptoms are still progressing. Treatment-responders should be considered for maintenance B-, and T-cell immunosuppressive therapy.

Paraneoplastic Limbic and Brainstem Encephalitis

Patients with limbic encephalitis develop short-term memory loss with relative preservation of other cognitive functions. Antibodies usually found in paraneoplastic limbic encephalitis include anti-Hu, anti-Ma2, and anti-CRMP5. In those with anti-Hu or CRMP5 autoantibodies, the limbic encephalitis is a fragment of PEM with a presentation characteristic of that disorder. Detection of anti-Ma2 antibodies in young men usually associates with testicular neoplasms while the commonest neoplasm of elderly men and women is non-SCLC (14). Patients with anti-Ma2 antibodies often manifest brainstem encephalitis (15) with several types of motor disturbances, including Parkinsonism, severe hypokinesis, and gaze paralysis (16). Upward and downward gaze can be affected early, along with forceful jaw opening and closing, and involuntary masticatory movements that result in lip and tongue injuries (17). Involuntary tremor is uncommon, but hypokinesis, hypophonesis, and rigidity commonly occur. Brainstem symptoms may progress in a rostral to caudal direction involving cranial nerve nuclei, cerebellar and horizontal gaze neural pathways (18). The disorder may be confused with Whipple disease and progressive supranuclear palsy (19). Prompt diagnosis of anti-Ma2 encephalitis is important because up to one-third of patients respond to immunotherapy and specific treatment of the tumor.

N-methyl-D-aspartate (NMDA) receptor encephalitis

Anti- N-Methyl-D-Aspartate (NMDA) receptor encephalitis most commonly occurs in young women and children (20, 21). Patients initially develop psychiatric symptoms and memory loss that progresses to seizures, decreased consciousness, autonomic instability and frequent hypoventilation necessitating intubation. Movement disorders occur in up to 80% of patients, including orofacial dyskinesia, choreoathetoid movements of the limbs, dystonia, rigidity, and opisthotonic postures (20, 22). Such movements are described as kissing, pouting, fish, and rabbit-like motions with tongue protrusion and rolling, which when synchronous with forceful jaw opening and closing, frequently results in tongue injury. The limb movements present with a dancing, milking, bicycling, floating, flailing, or pill-rolling appearance, often accompanied by pelvic thrusting (23). Some of the movements may suggest a relation to seizures but EEG monitoring fails to confirm an epileptogenic basis. The pathogenic antibody is directed against cell surface epitopes of the NR1 subunit of the NMDA receptor regardless of the presence of an associated tumor. Whether the disorder is paraneoplastic depends upon the age of the patient, with benign or malignant unilateral or bilateral ovarian teratomas found in over one-half of women older than 18 years, but in less than 15% of women younger than 14 years (20). About 5% of men will have a tumor, usually a testicular germ-cell tumor. Prompt treatment with corticosteroids, IVIg, or plasma exchange (PE) alone or in combination, with removal of the tumor often results in substantial neurologic recovery (24). Patients refractory to these treatments may respond to second-line therapy with cyclophosphamide or rituximab (25). Relapses occur in one quarter of patients, most often in patients without a tumor or whose tumor was not removed.

Paraneoplastic Stiff-Person Syndrome

Stiff-person syndrome is characterized by progressive rigidity involving axial and proximal limb muscles with muscle ache and muscle spasm triggered by sensory and emotional stimuli. The rigidity consists of a board-like contraction of the affected muscles, which improves during sleep and with benzodiazepines. Non-paraneoplastic stiff-person syndrome may be associated with antibodies against glutamic acid decarboxylase (GAD), while paraneoplastic stiff-person syndrome is often associated with antibodies to amphiphysin (26, 27). The most common cancers are breast, lung, colon, and HL. Some patients with cancer, mostly SCLC, develop progressive encephalomyelitis with rigidity and spinal myoclonus (PERM) that is likely a variant of stiff-person syndrome (28) with additional brainstem dysfunction. Some patients with PERM have antibodies to the α-1 subunit of the glycine receptor (GlyR), however none to date have had an associated cancer (29). Paraneoplastic stiff-person syndrome may respond to immune therapy and treatment of the tumor and symptomatically to benzodiazepine medication and baclofen. IVIg is useful in patients with non-paraneoplastic stiff-person syndrome, and is likely effective in the paraneoplastic form of the disorder.

Paraneoplastic Motor Neuron Syndromes

The concurrence of cancer with MND is usually coincidental, however rare patients whose symptoms of the MND improved with treatment of the tumor suggest the possibility of a paraneoplastic pathogenesis (11). Some patients with breast cancer have developed a predominant upper motor neuron disorder (UMN) mimicking primary lateral sclerosis (PLS) while pure lower motor neuron (LMN) disease has been observed in patients with HL, NHL, and SCLC. Reports of the latter have declined, suggesting non-paraneoplastic mechanisms, including viral infections that are now managed more effectively. In a series of patients with NHL and MND, no antibodies were identified and none of the patients improved with treatment of the underlying cancer (30).

Paraneoplastic Myelopathy

Paraneoplastic myelopathy usually occurs in association with neurologic dysfunction of other levels of the neuraxis. Isolated paraneoplastic myelopathy is rarely described in patients with lung or breast cancer. The more commonly associated antibodies are anti-amphiphysin, CRMP5 and Hu. Onset is insidious or subacute and usually precedes the detection of cancer. In one series, 23% of patients were initially diagnosed with primary progressive multiple sclerosis (MS), in part due to the presence of CSF oligoclonal bands

(31). This series found that the presence of symmetric longitudinally extensive tract or gray matter-specific changes on spinal MRI was characteristic of paraneoplastic myelopathy. Systemic immunotherapy and specific treatment of the underlying tumor may provide mild improvement or stabilization but the majority of patients fail to respond and become wheelchair dependent within one year of onset.

PARANEOPLASTIC OPSOCLONUS-MYOCLONUS

In children, opsoclonus-myoclonus (POM) usually occurs in association with neuroblastoma with the neurological symptoms preceding the tumor diagnosis in 50% of cases. In adults, several underlying tumors have been reported, with SCLC and cancers of the breast and ovary most common. Most of the well-characterized paraneoplastic antibodies have been reported in isolated cases but the majority of patients, both adults and children, are antibody negative (32). Some adult patients, in particular those with SCLC and 5% of children with neuroblastoma, have anti-Hu antibodies while a small subset of adults, predominantly those with breast and ovarian cancer, have anti-Ri antibodies (33). Such patients have additional symptoms of brainstem and cerebellar dysfunction including truncal and gait ataxia, vertigo, nausea, dysphagia, ocular paresis, axial rigidity, trismus, laryngeal spasms, and confusion (34).

Some children with neuroblastoma have uncharacterized antibodies against post-synaptic or cell surface antigens located on cerebellar granular cells (35). Children with neuroblastoma-associated POM respond to tumor treatment along with immunomodulatory therapies such as prednisone, adrenocorticotropic hormone, IVIg, or rituximab. In many cases, the responses are partial and the children are left with residual behavioral, psychomotor, and sleep disorders. Adult POM is less responsive to immunotherapy but nonetheless may be helpful, but improvement is mild or not sustained unless the tumor is treated (36). Those whose tumors are treated promptly have better neurological outcome than those whose tumors are not treated, in those cases the disorder often progressed to severe encephalopathy and death (37).

Paraneoplastic Sensory Neuronopathy

PSN most commonly occurs in association with PEM in patients with SCLC and anti-Hu antibodies but may be an isolated syndrome is some cases. Patients present with the subacute and often asymmetric onset of numbness or pain that initially may mimic a radiculopathy or multifocal neuropathy that progresses to involve all extremities and all modalities of sensation. As a result, patients develop a severe sensory ataxia and dystonic or pseudoathetoid postures of the extremities. The disorder is often refractory to treatment; however, patients whose tumors are treated with or without concomitant immunotherapy are more likely to have symptom stabilization or improvement than those whose tumors are not treated (6). In the absence of a tumor or if tumor therapy is not feasible immunotherapy is warranted as some patients may have transient responses.

GUILLAIN-BARRÉ SYNDROME

Some patients with NHL and solid tumors have been reported with concurrent GBS, but the small number of cases precludes distinguishing a paraneoplastic pathogenesis (38). Neurologic symptoms have been reported during active disease, in remission, and in some patients before cancer relapse. Such patients have the same response to plasma exchange and IVIg as those with idiopathic GBS. Patients with hematopoietic disorders treated with bone marrow transplant are at increased risk of GBS. Several pathogenic factors have been considered, including iatrogenically suppressed T-cell function, humoral factors, graft versus-host disease, and cytomegalovirus infection.

SUBACUTE AND CHRONIC SENSORIMOTOR NEUROPATHY

In patients with cancer, peripheral neuropathy is common but a paraneoplastic origin is rare. When it does occur, it is most commonly associated with lung cancer. The onset of the neuropathy usually follows the diagnosis of the cancer but may precede it by several years (39). Most patients present with a distal symmetric polyneuropathy characterized by weakness, wasting, sensory loss, and decreased deep tendon reflexes that slowly worsen over the course of the disease with rare cranial nerve involvement. Neurologic symptoms may rarely stabilize, but more often slowly worsen or progress in a remitting or relapsing course. Some patients harbor anti-CRMP5 antibodies alone or combined with anti-Hu antibodies. In patients with sensorimotor neuropathy, the presence of anti-Hu antibodies indicates that the sensory deficits derive from dorsal root ganglia involvement. Treatment with corticosteroids or IVIg may lead to neurological improvement, particularly when demyelinating features predominate. Up to 10% of patients with a peripheral sensorimotor neuropathy of unknown etiology have a monoclonal gammopathy. Plasma cell dyscrasias associated with peripheral neuropathy include monoclonal gammopathy of uncertain significance (MGUS), multiple myeloma, Waldenstrom macroglobulinemia, cryoglobulinemia, monoclonal gammopathy with solid tumors, monoclonal gammopathy with angiofollicular lymph node hyperplasia (Castleman disease) and the combination of peripheral neuropathy, organomegaly, endocrinopathy, M-protein, and skin changes of so-called, POEMS syndrome.

Neuromyotonia and Morvan syndrome

Peripheral nerve hyperexcitability (PNH) is characterized by muscle cramps, stiffness, myokymia, fasciculation, and delayed muscle relaxation or neuromyotonia. It is often found in association with a sensorimotor polyneuropathy and in patients with thymoma and SCLC. A subgroup of patients with neuromyotonia have antibodies to contactin-associated protein-like 2 (Caspr2) and, in some instances, additional involvement of the CNS with cognitive impairment, memory loss, hallucinations, seizures, and autonomic dysfunction (40, 41). The combination of neuromyotonia and CNS dysfunction is termed "Morvan syndrome." Anti-Caspr2-associated syndromes occur with or without an associated tumor, usually thymoma. Patients with Caspr2- associated symptoms may have other immune mediated disorders such as myasthenia gravis (MG) with acetylcholine receptor (AChR) or muscle specific tyrosine-kinase receptor (MuSK) antibodies. The combination of symptoms related to neuromyotonia and those due to other autoimmunities, such as fasciculation and muscle atrophy, has resulted in some patients with Caspr2 antibodies being diagnosed with atypical MND. The detection of Caspr2 antibodies is therefore important as the associated symptoms often respond to immunotherapy.

LAMBERT-EATON MYASTHENIC SYNDROME (LEMS)

About 60% of patients with Lambert-Eaton myasthenic syndrome (LEMS) have an associated SCLC that is usually detected within two years of onset of neurologic symptoms (42). Tumors other than SCLC are rare, but lymphomas have been reported in some patients. In the majority of patients, the first symptom is proximal lower extremity weakness. Less frequently, presenting symptoms include generalized weakness, autonomic dysfunction, aching, and stiffness of muscles. Autonomic dysfunction eventually affects 80% of the patients and includes dry mouth, erectile dysfunction,

Table 2. The Dutch-English LEMS Tumor Association Prediction (DELTA-P) Score[1]

Clinical and Demographic Information	Yes	No
Dysarthria, dysphagia, masticatory, bulbar or neck muscle weakness	1	0
Erectile dysfunction*	1	0
Loss of weight > 5%	1	0
Tobacco: Active Smoker	1	0
Age > 50	1	0
Performance Status (KPS < 60)	1	0

[1]Adapted from reference 45
* Women receive of a score of 0
KPS: Karnofsky Performance Status

constipation, and blurred vision. Cranial nerve involvement as manifested by diplopia, ptosis, slurred speech, and dysphagia is commonly mild or transient.

Antibodies to VGCC are found in almost all patients with paraneoplastic and non-paraneoplastic LEMS while 10% of non-paraneoplastic LEMS patients have no detectable antibodies. The presence of antibodies to SOX1 is strongly associated with SCLC and therefore these antibodies are markers for paraneoplastic LEMS (43, 44). A simple clinical scoring system based on age, weight loss, smoking, Karnofsky performance status, presence of bulbar symptoms, and erectile dysfunction calculated within three months of LEMS onset helps to distinguish cancer and non-cancer associated LEMS patients (Table 2) (45). Scores directly correlate with increasing risk of SCLC such that patients with the lowest scores have little to no risk of SCLC, while those with higher scores have close to 100% certainty of an SCLC. In patients with paraneoplastic LEMS, treatment of the tumor usually results in improvement of the neurologic disorder. Plasma exchange and IVIg can lead to short-term benefits in those with acute deterioration, whereas long-term improvement can occur with maintenance 3, 4-diaminopyridine (DAP), a drug that enhances release of ACh, or immune suppression with corticosteroids, azathioprine, and cyclosporine. Acute worsening of neurologic symptoms usually heralds tumor recurrence.

REFERENCES

1. Shams'ili S, Grefkens J, De Leeuw B, et al. Paraneoplastic cerebellar degeneration associated with antineuronal antibodies: analysis of 50 patients. *Brain* 2003; 126:1409–1418.
2. Peterson K, Rosenblum MK, Kotanides H, et al. Paraneoplastic cerebellar degeneration. I. A clinical analysis of 55 anti-Yo antibody-positive patients. *Neurology* 1992; 42:1931–1937.
3. Bernal F, Shams'ili S, Rojas I, et al. Anti-Tr antibodies as markers of paraneoplastic cerebellar degeneration and Hodgkin's disease. *Neurology* 2003; 60:230–234.
4. Graus F, Lang B, Pozo-Rosich P, et al. P/Q type calcium-channel antibodies in paraneoplastic cerebellar degeneration with lung cancer. *Neurology* 2002; 59:764–766.
5. Mason WP, Graus F, Lang B, et al. Small-cell lung cancer, paraneoplastic cerebellar degeneration and the Lambert-Eaton myasthenic syndrome. *Brain* 1997; 120:1279–1300.

6. Graus F, Keime-Guibert F, Rene R, et al. Anti-Hu-associated paraneoplastic encephalomyelitis: analysis of 200 patients. Brain 2001; 124:1138–1148.

7. Dalmau J, Furneaux HM, Rosenblum MK, et al. Detection of the anti-Hu antibody in specific regions of the nervous system and tumor from patients with paraneoplastic encephalomyelitis/sensory neuronopathy. Neurology 1991; 41:1757–1764.

8. Yu Z, Kryzer TJ, Griesmann GE, et al. CRMP-5 neuronal autoantibody: Marker of lung cancer and thymoma related autoimmunity. Ann Neurol 2001; 49:146–154.

9. Ishii A, Hayashi A, Ohkoshi N, et al. Progressive encephalomyelitis with rigidity associated with anti-amphiphysin antibodies. J Neurol Neurosurg Psychiatry 2004; 75:661–662.

10. Dalmau J, Graus F, Rosenblum MK, et al. Anti-Hu-associated paraneoplastic encephalomyelitis/sensory neuronopathy. A clinical study of 71 patients. Medicine (Baltimore) 1992; 71:59–72.

11. Forsyth PA, Dalmau J, Graus F, et al. Motor neuron syndromes in cancer patients. Ann Neurol 1997; 41:722–730.

12. Vernino S, Tuite P, Adler CH, et al. Paraneoplastic chorea associated with CRMP-5 neuronal antibody and lung carcinoma. Ann Neurol 2002; 51:625–630.

13. Samii A, Dahlen DD, Spence AM, et al. Paraneoplastic movement disorder in a patient with non-Hodgkin's lymphoma and CRMP-5 autoantibody. Mov Disord 2003; 18:1556–1558.

14. Mathew RM, Vandenberghe R, Garcia-Merino A, et al. Orchiectomy for suspected microscopic tumor in patients with anti-Ma2-associated encephalitis. Neurology 2007; 68:900–905.

15. Rosenfeld MR, Eichen J, Wade D, et al. Molecular and clinical diversity in paraneoplastic immunity to Ma proteins. Ann Neurol 2001; 50:339–348.

16. Matsumoto L, Yamamoto T, Higashihara M, et al. Severe hypokinesis caused by paraneoplastic anti-Ma2 encephalitis associated with bilateral intratubular germ-cell neoplasm of the testes. Mov Disord 2007; 22:728–731.

17. Dalmau J, Graus F, Villarejo A, et al. Clinical analysis of anti-Ma2-associated encephalitis. Brain 2004; 127:1831–1844.

18. Hoffmann LA, Jarius S, Pellkofer HL, et al. Anti-Ma and anti-Ta associated paraneoplastic neurological syndromes: 22 newly diagnosed patients and review of previous cases. J Neurol Neurosurg Psychiatry 2008; 79:767–773.

19. Castle J, Sakonju A, Dalmau J, et al. Anti-Ma2-associated encephalitis with normal FDG-PET: a case of pseudo-Whipple's disease. Nat Clin Pract Neurol 2006; 2:566–572.

20. Dalmau J, Lancaster E, Martinez-Hernandez E, et al. Clinical experience and laboratory investigations in patients with anti-NMDAR encephalitis. Lancet Neurol 2011; 10:63–74.

21. Florance NR, Davis RL, Lam C, et al. Anti-N-methyl-D-aspartate receptor (NMDAR) encephalitis in children and adolescents. Ann Neurol 2009; 66:11–18.

22. Kleinig TJ, Thompson PD, Matar W, et al. The distinctive movement disorder of ovarian teratoma-associated encephalitis. Mov Disord 2008; 23:1256–1261.

23. Iizuka T, Sakai F, Ide T, et al. Anti-NMDA receptor encephalitis in Japan: long-term outcome without tumor removal. Neurology 2008; 70:504–511.

24. Dalmau J, Gleichman AJ, Hughes EG, et al. Anti-NMDA-receptor encephalitis: case series and analysis of the effects of antibodies. Lancet Neurol 2008; 7:1091–1098.

25. Ishiura H, Matsuda S, Higashihara M, et al. Response of anti-NMDA receptor encephalitis without tumor to immunotherapy including rituximab. Neurology 2008; 71:1921–1923.

26. Raju R, Foote J, Banga JP, et al. Analysis of GAD65 autoantibodies in Stiff-Person syndrome patients. J Immunol 2005; 175:7755–7762.

27. De Camilli P, Thomas A, Cofiell R, et al. The synaptic vesicle-associated protein amphiphysin is the 128- kD autoantigen of Stiff-Man syndrome with breast cancer. J Exp Med 1993; 178:2219–2223.

28. Meinck HM, Thompson PD. Stiff man syndrome and related conditions. Mov Disord 2002; 17:853–866.

29. Mas N, Saiz A, Leite MI, et al. Antiglycine-receptor encephalomyelitis with rigidity. J Neurol Neurosurg Psychiatry 2011; 82:1399–1401.

30. Briani C, Vitaliani R, Grisold W, et al. Spectrum of paraneoplastic disease associated with lymphoma. Neurology 2011; 76:705–710.

31. Flanagan EP, McKeon A, Lennon VA, et al. Paraneoplastic isolated myelopathy: clinical course and neuroimaging clues. Neurology 2011; 76:2089–2095.

32. Sabater L, Xifro X, Saiz A, et al. Analysis of antibodies to neuronal surface antigens in adult opsoclonus-myoclonus. J Neuroimmunol 2008; 196:188–191.

33. Casado JL, Gil-Peralta A, Graus F, et al. Anti-Ri antibodies associated with opsoclonus and progressive encephalomyelitis with rigidity. Neurology 1994; 44:1521–1522.

34. Pittock SJ, Lucchinetti CF, Lennon VA. Anti-neuronal nuclear autoantibody type 2: paraneoplastic accompaniments. Ann Neurol 2003; 53:580–587.

35. Blaes F, Pike MG, Lang B. Autoantibodies in childhood opsoclonus-myoclonus syndrome. J Neuroimmunol 2008; 201–202:221–226.

36. Erlich R, Morrison C, Kim B, et al. ANNA-2: an antibody associated with paraneoplastic opsoclonus in a patient with large-cell carcinoma of the lung with neuroendocrine features—correlation of clinical improvement with tumor response. Cancer Invest 2004; 22:257–261.

37. Bataller L, Graus F, Saiz A, et al. Clinical outcome in adult onset idiopathic or paraneoplastic opsoclonus-myoclonus. Brain 2001; 124:437–443.

38. Vigliani MC, Magistrello M, Polo P, et al. Risk of cancer in patients with Guillain-Barre syndrome (GBS). A population-based study. J Neurol 2004; 251:321–326.

39. Antoine JC, Mosnier JF, Absi L, et al. Carcinoma associated paraneoplastic peripheral neuropathies in patients with and without anti-onconeural antibodies. J Neurol Neurosurg Psychiatry 1999; 67:7–14.

40. Lancaster E, Huijbers MGM, Bar V, et al. Investigations of Caspr2, an autoantigen of encephalitis and neuromyotonia. Ann Neurol 2011; 69:303–311.

41. Irani SR, Alexander S, Waters P, et al. Antibodies to Kv1 potassium channel-complex proteins leucine-rich, glioma inactivated 1 protein and contactin-associated protein-2 in limbic encephalitis, Morvan's syndrome and acquired neuromyotonia. Brain 2010; 133:2734–2748.

42. Titulaer MJ, Wirtz PW, Kuks JB, et al. The Lambert-Eaton myasthenic syndrome 1988–2008: a clinical picture in 97 patients. J Neuroimmunol 2008; 201–202:153–158.

43. Sabater L, Titulaer M, Saiz A, et al. SOX1 antibodies are markers of paraneoplastic Lambert Eaton myasthenic syndrome. Neurology 2007; 70:4260–4267.

44. Titulaer MJ, Klooster R, Potman M, et al. SOX antibodies in small-cell lung cancer and Lambert-Eaton myasthenic syndrome: frequency and relation with survival. J Clin Oncol 2009; 27:4260–4267.

45. Titulaer MJ, Maddison P, Sont JK, et al. Clinical Dutch-English Lambert-Eaton Myasthenic syndrome (LEMS) tumor association prediction score accurately predicts small-cell lung cancer in the LEMS. J Clin Oncol 2011; 29:902–908.

CHAPTER 53

Human Immunodeficiency Virus Infection

David S. Younger

INTRODUCTION

Disorders of the motor system due to central and peripheral nervous system (CNS and PNS) involvement can be a major or minor feature of the neurologic syndromes associated with human immunodeficiency virus (HIV) infection and the acquired immune deficiency syndrome (AIDS).

CLASSIFICATION AND STAGING OF HIV INFECTION

According to the Centers for Disease Control and Prevention (CDC) (1), the criteria for HIV infection include a repeatedly reactive screening enzyme-linked immunosorbent assay (ELISA), which is an extremely sensitive test for the antibody confirmed by the more specific Western blot analysis. Both are important to perform since false positive tests do occur, albeit in 1 of 135,187 (.0007%) persons in populations with low prevalence rates of HIV, such as military recruits (2). Other criteria include direct identification of virus in host tissue by virus isolation and HIV antigen detection, or a positive result on any other highly specific licensed HIV test. The revised classification system replaced the one proposed in 1986 (3) that was developed before widespread use of CD4+ T-cell testing (4). It categorizes patients of age >13 years on the basis of clinical conditions associated with HIV infection and CD4+ T-lymphocyte counts. Three ranges, expressed in T-lymphocyte counts of blood per microliter (uL) were CD4+ T-lymphocyte counts > or = to 500 cells (Category 1); 200–499 cells (Category 2); and < 200 cells (Category 3), with equivalent CD4+ percentages for the stratifying values of Category 1 (29%) and Category 3 (14%), which in contrast to CD4+ counts were subject to less variation on repeated measures (5, 6). This classification system was considered useful in guiding clinical and therapeutic action in the management of HIV-infected adolescents and adults (7). Antimicrobial prophylaxis and anti-retroviral therapies, shown to be most effective within certain levels of immune dysfunction (8–13), would be considered not only for individuals with CD4+ T-lymphocyte counts <500/uL, but as prophylaxis against common serious opportunistic infection such as *Pneumocystis carinii* pneumonia (PCP) in those with CD4+ T-lymphocyte counts <200/uL. The revised CDC guidelines recognized clinical categories of HIV infection, namely asymptomatic, persistent generalized lymphadenopathy and acute primary infection despite another accompanying illness (Category A); symptomatic conditions in an HIV-infected adolescent or adult attributed to HIV or a defect in cell-mediated immunity (Category B) and AIDS (Category C). The CDC surveillance case definition for AIDS was expanded to include all HIV-infected individuals with CD4+ T-lymphocyte counts <200 cells/uL or the equivalent percentage while retaining the 23 clinical conditions in the previous AIDS surveillance definition (3). The World Health Organization (WHO) proposed a classification and staging system for HIV based primarily on clinical criteria and included use of CD4+ T-lymphocyte determinations (14), incorporating a performance scale and total lymphocyte counts to be used instead of CD4+ T-lymphocyte determinations in countries where the latter testing is not available.

EPIDEMIOLOGY

According to a joint report of the WHO, United Nations Programme on HIV/AIDS (UNAIDS), and the United Nations Children's Fund (UNICEF) (15), in 2010 there were an estimated 34 million people living with HIV globally and 2.7 million new cases, with an estimated 1.8 million individuals dying from AIDS-related cause (Table 1) Since 2005, there has been a three-fold increase in the number of facilities providing anti-retroviral therapy in low and middle income countries. This has been combined with both a seven-fold increase in the percentage of women tested for HIV and the number of children taking anti-retroviral therapy, and a five-fold similar increase in all individuals so treated worldwide, these statistics demonstrate a significant trend toward control of the global epidemic. This trend was explained by the joint commitment of member states of the United Nations and its agencies as fostering access of HIV testing, counseling, highly active anti-retroviral therapy (HAART) and combination antiretroviral therapy (cART) to infected pregnant women and children, particularly in the poorest developing countries such as sub-Sahara Africa, which bears 90% of the global HIV burden. There are an estimated 1.2 million HIV infected individuals in the United States accounting for approximately 17,000 HIV-related deaths, a statistic that has remained relatively stable over the past decade because of continued access to HAART. The incidence of CNS-AIDS-related events detected pathologically in over 90% of patients so studied (16–21), is favorably correlated with the introduction and widespread use of HAART as was observed for the risk of a first event of CNS-AIDS, AIDS-dementia complex (ADC) between 1993 and 1994 (22), and CNS opportunistic infections, notably primary CNS lymphoma and progressive multifocal leukoencephalopathy (PML) from 1990 to 1998 (23).

CENTRAL NERVOUS SYSTEM DISORDERS

The CNS manifestations of HIV may be divided into generalized disorders, among them HIV encephalopathy (HIVE), HIV-associated cerebellar disease, HIV-myelopathy, and focal disorders including HIV-associated toxoplasmosis, primary CNS lymphoma, and PML.

HIV-Associated Dementia

The ADC (24), HIV-1–associated cognitive/motor complex (25), and HIVE are synonyms for HIV-associated dementia (HAD), one of many HIV-associated neurocognitive disorders (HAND) (26), with an estimated annual incidence of 7% among persons with AIDS, and affecting up to 16%

of all persons with AIDS (27), leading to cognitive, functional, and focal neurological and behavioral impairments. Of 271 HIV-positive men and women with CD4+ counts of <200 cells/υL or demonstrated cognitive impairment, 56 (21%) met criteria for a minor cognitive/motor disorder, including mental and memory slowing, motor dysfunction, incoordination, emotional lability, and a deficit in role function, while 65 (24%) were moderately demented with only three patients mildly affected; and the remaining 150 (55%) unimpaired (28).

Disease progression is associated with an increased number of extrapyramidal signs reflecting subcortical primarily, basal ganglia involvement, similar to that of gay men and intravenous drug users with a decline in the CD4+ T-lymphocyte cell count and concomitant frontal release signs including glabellar, snout, suck, and palmomental, reflexes and extrapyramidal signs including rigidity, bradykinesia, salivation, gait, hypomimia, speech tremor, and impaired alternating movements (29). The AIDS Task Force of the American Academy of Neurology (AAN) (30) suggested formal separation of HAD from minor cognitive motor disorder (MCMD), distinguishing three subtypes of HAD depending upon demonstration of motor, behavioral, or psychological symptoms or both, with MCMD defined by the essential features of a history of impaired cognitive/behavioral function in two areas, causing mild impairment in work or activity of daily living (ADL). Magnetic resonance imaging (MRI) of the brain demonstrates prominent symmetrical periventricular non-enhancing white matter hyperintensities that spare subcortical U-fibers, with secondary lateral ventriculomegaly *ex vacuo* (Figure 1) (31), mild to moderate neocortical and caudate atrophy (32), and reduced basal ganglia volume on quantitative neuroimaging (33), which correlate with cognitive impairment.

The pathologic hallmark of HAD is inflammation marked by microglial nodules and multinucleated giant cells (Figure 2) (34) with predominant affliction in periventricular white matter and basal ganglia, in particular the globus pallidus (35). Neocortical atrophy is less prominent (36), although there is an association between synaptic markers of neurologic damage and intra-CNS HIV burden, reflecting a reduction in cortical neuronal synaptic density and arborization (37). The neuropathology of the white matter lesions is heterogeneous, consisting of vacuolar leukoencephalopathy, angiocentric foci of hemosiderin laden macrophages, multinucleated giant cells, and microglial nodules (38).

Experimental infection of neurons using *in situ* polymerase chain reaction (PCR) hybridization techniques (39) is accompanied by inflammation and macrophage activation that contributes to, and worsens, HAD independent of viral replication wherein clinical disease severity correlates with the amount of monocytic infiltration and macrophage microglia activation than the quantity of infected neurons

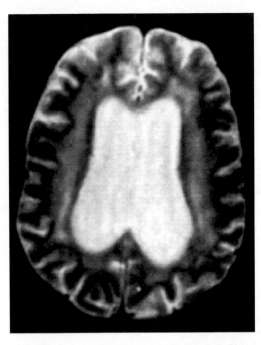

FIG. 1. HIV-associated dementia. T$_2$-weighted magnetic resonance image of the brain of a 34-year-old HIV-infected man with dementia. There is diffuse enlargement of the lateral ventricles and hyperintense signal throughout the periventricular white matter consistent with leukoencephalopathy. From: Simpson D, Tagliati M. Neurologic manifestations of HIV infection. *Ann Intern Med* 1994; 121:771, with permission.

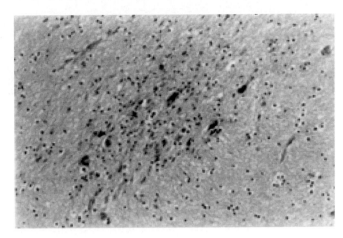

FIG. 2. HIV-associated dementia. Photomicrograph showing a microglial nodule with multinucleated giant cells within the centrum semiovale. Hematoxylin-eosin, original magnification x25. From: Simpson D, Tagliati M. Neurologic manifestations of HIV infection. *Ann Intern Med* 1994; 121:769–785, with permission.

or viral load, suggesting that indirect mechanisms rather than direct infection are important factors in etiopathogenesis (40). Postulated mechanisms of neuronal dysfunction related to the direct effects of HIV-infected macrophage infiltration and activation have included glutamate-mediated excitotoxicity by the gp120 HIV envelope glycoprotein, induction of neuronal apoptosis by cytokine release of tumor necrosis factor-alpha (TNF-α), and the excitatory metabolic effects of quinolinate and eicosanoids (41).

HAART employing a protease inhibitor (PI) (indinavir, ritonavir, or saquinavir) plus two reverse transciptase inhibitors (nRTI) (zidovudine, didanosine, zalcitabine, lamivudine, or stavudine) in naïve patients so treated, produced a positive and sustained effect on neurocognitive impairment in 116 patients with advanced HIV-infection, including reducing the prevalence from baseline of 80.8% to 50% at six months, and 21.7% at 15 months, notably in measures, concentration and speed of mental processing, mental flexibility, memory, fine motor functions, and visuospatial and constructional abilities (42). After six months of HAART, those with normal neuropsychological examination had lower mean plasma viremia and greater mean log plasma HIV RNA changes from baseline than matched neuropsychological impaired subjects. The severity of HIV-related

neurocognitive impairment (NCI) at initiation of HAART was the strongest predictor of persistent neuropsychological (NP) deficits among 94 patients with NCI so studied, in whom 62.8% experienced persistent NP deficits despite HAART controlling for HIV risk category, CD4+ T-lymphocyte count, plasma viral load, and use of CNS-penetrating drugs (43). The stable or increased prevalence of neurological disease suggests that treatment of CNS disease may be suboptimal due to poor antiretroviral penetration across the blood-CSF (BCB) and blood-brain barriers (BBB) (44), a factor that was subsequently analyzed in 467 HIV seropositive patients who reported antiretroviral drug use. Each drug was assigned a penetration rank based upon the reported chemical properties, concentration in CSF, and established clinical efficacy in clinical studies (45): low penetration as, for example, saquinavir, enfuvirtide, nelfinavir, didanosine; intermediate penetration, as in atazanavir, stavudine, efavirenz; or high penetration as for nevirapne, ritonavir-boosted lopinavir, zidovudine, and efavirenz.

In multivariate regression analysis, antiretroviral drug regimens with lower CPE rank were not surprisingly associated with detectable CSF viral loads even after adjusting for total number of antiretroviral drugs, with poorer penetration of the certain antiretroviral drugs into the CNS appearing to allow continued HIV replication in the CNS, as indicated by higher CSF HIV viral loads.

Current antiretroviral management in patients with HAN should consist of a combination of two or three medications monitored by clinical response and measurement of CSF viral RNA load. Apart from the positive role of HAART in reducing opportunistic infections (OI) in AIDS, some patients so treated may suffer a paradoxical deterioration as their immune function improves. The so-called immune restoration disease (IRD) (46) or immune reconstitution inflammatory syndrome (IRIS) (47), occurs in patients treated for a known OI, and while recovering from it deteriorates after starting HAART, alternatively, in those previously asymptomatic on starting HAART, develop an inflammatory response to an occult infection with subsequent development of symptoms such as PML, cryptococcal meningitis, cerebral toxoplasmosis, and cytomegalovirus (CMV) retinitis, or other seemingly unrelated disorders, including CNS lymphoma, ischemic and ischemic stroke. The IRIS characteristically occurs in patients with low pre-CART CD4+T-cell counts <100/μL and an increase of >four-fold or to >200 CD4⁺ T-cells/μL.

Alternative experimental therapeutic approaches to HAD have employed non-antiretroviral agents to prevent the neurotoxic effects of factors secreted by HIV-infected or HIV-activated-macrophages that could potentially contribute to neuronal dysfunction and cell death, however none have shown sustained convincing benefit. A randomized double-blind, placebo-controlled trial of the neuroprotective agent peptide T in HIV-positive patients with cognitive impairment did not show significant difference from placebo on study endpoints of a comprehensive neuropsychological battery score (48). A randomized, placebo-controlled trial of the voltage-dependent calcium channel antagonist nimodipine was well tolerated but only one patient reached the endpoint, and there was no statistical difference in a Neuropsychological Percent Change score among the cohorts receiving placebo, or high and low doses of the study drug (49). A randomized, double-blind, placebo-controlled tolerability trial of the monoamine oxidase B inhibitor and putative anti-apoptotic agent deprenyl, and the antioxidant thioacetic acid in patients with HIV-associated cognitive impairment, showed encouraging improvement in verbal memory with trends for improvement in other components of auditory verbal learning. However, the study was not designed to test efficacy. Thioacetic acid had no benefit in cognitive function (50). A randomized double-blind, placebo-controlled study of minocycline, with both anti-inflammatory and neuroprotective effects, was well-tolerated in a cohort of patients with HIV-associated cognitive impairment, but cognitive improvement was not observed (51). Developing neuroprotective strategies for the treatment of HIV-associated neurocognitive dysfunction is summarized by Rumbaugh and colleagues (52).

HIV-RELATED CEREBELLAR DISEASE

AIDS-related causes of cerebellar disease include PML and CMV infection, both of which can be associated with brainstem signs and oculomotor disturbances. Pancerebel-

lar degeneration caused by HIV was described in a patient without opportunistic infection or secondary cause (53) and in association with inhaled heroin termed "chasing the dragon" (54, 55).

HIV-ASSOCIATED MYELOPATHY

The most frequently encountered spinal cord pathology in AIDS is slowly progressive vacuolar degeneration of the lateral and posterior white matter tracts, with clinical and pathologic features similar to the subacute combined degeneration caused by B$_{12}$ deficiency (56). HIV vacuolar myelopathy is clinically apparent in 27% of patients with HIV infection and in up to 55% of patients at postmortem examination (57). The clinical features include progressive spastic paraparesis, sensory and spinocerebellar ataxia, erectile dysfunction, and detrusor sphincter dyssynergia. Vacuolar myelopathy may coexist with distal sensory polyneuropathy (DSP) with progressive stocking sensory loss and absent ankle reflexes. MRI of the spine typically shows normal or nonspecific T$_{2}$-posterolateral white matter hyperintensities and normal or nonspecific atrophy. Fibular and posterior tibial somatosensory evoked potentials show prolongation of central conduction times. Asymptomatic HIV-infected patients with CD4+T-cell counts <200/mm^3 can be shown to have subclinical myelopathy, which in the early stages is accompanied by normal or mild cerebrospinal fluid (CSF) abnormalities. The pathological findings of vacuolar myelopathy (Figure 3) include macrophage infiltration and demyelination and vacuolation of the posterolateral white matter tracts of the thoracic cord, with little

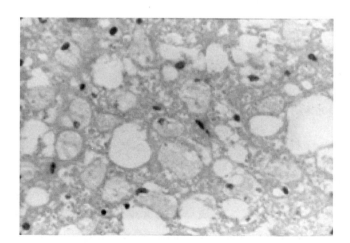

FIG. 3. Vacuolar myelopathy in AIDS. High-power photomicrograph from the white matter of the spinal cord, showing large vacuoles. Macrophages are evident within the vacuoles. Hematoxylin-eosin, original magnification x250. From: Simpson D, Tagliati M. Neurologic manifestations of HIV infection. *Ann Intern Med* 1994; 121:769–785, with permission.

or no axonal degeneration. The clinical severity of vacuolar myelopathy correlates closely with the degree of pathologic involvement. There is no evidence of direct HIV infection of the cord in vacuolar myelopathy, and HIV-infected macrophages, present in the gray matter of the cord in the typical form of multinucleated giant cells and microglial nodules, were not demonstrated in regions of vacuolar change. Tyor and colleagues (58) found increased numbers of major histocompatibility (MHC) class I and II macrophages expressing TNF-α and IL-1 in regions of vacuolation, with increased level of neopterin, B_2-microglobulin, and TNF-α in the CSF. A unifying hypothesis of HIV neuropathogenesis, which includes cytokine-induced injury to neurons, oligodendrocytes, and Schwann cells by infiltrating HIV-infected macrophages (59), plausibly explains vacuolar myelopathy, as does metabolic injury associated with B_{12} deficiency (60) and persistent immune activation, leading to significant local production of cytokines, toxins, and oxygen radicals that cause membrane and myelin damage in the setting of secondary methyl group deficiency. Remission of vacuolar myelopathy, which may occur after commencement of antiretroviral therapy (61), was associated with functional, clinical, and radiological improvement after HAART (62).

FOCAL BRAIN LESIONS

Focal brain lesions (FBL), which have been a leading diagnostic problem in HIV-infective patients, can present with motor manifestations of hemiparesis, hemiataxia, dysmetria, rigidity, cogwheeling, chorea, and hemiballismus. The commonest cause of FBL in this population is toxoplasmic encephalitis (TE) caused by the parasitic protozoan *Toxoplasma (T.) gondii*, a food and water-borne pathogen that infects humans and animal hosts. Common sources of *T. gondii* include ingestion of oocysts from cat feces from cat litter and gardening, or ingestion of tissue cysts in undercooked meat.

Toxoplasma cysts form in the host and remain latent; in the immunocompromised state in association with HIV/AIDS, they reactivate in the host, resulting in disseminated toxoplasmosis, including encephalitis, typically presenting as headache, confusion, fever, altered mental status, hemiparesis, psychomotor retardation, seizures, and cranial nerve palsies (63–65). Approximately 90% of TE cases are due to reactivation of a latent infection, most commonly in those with CD4+ T-cell counts<100/uL. Other causes of FBL include primary CNS lymphoma (PCNSL); the microbiologic agents *Mycobacterium tuberculosis, Cryptococcus (C.) neoformans*, and *Treponema (T.) pallidum*; the Jacob Creutzfeldt (JC) virus that causes PML and CMV (Figure 4).

The identification of disease patterns in AIDS-related FBL was facilitated by a prospective analysis employing the clinical variables of mass effect of FBL on CT and MRI, Toxoplasma serology, anti-Toxoplasma prophylaxis, and the results of PCR assays for the amplification of Epstein Barr virus (EBV)–DNA, JCV-DNA, and T. gondii-DNA. In a prospective analysis (66) of 136 consecutive HIV-infected patients with a diagnosis of a FBL causing enhancement and mass effect on neuroimaging, the probability of TE was 0.87 in Toxoplasma-seropositive patients not receiving empiric anti-Toxoplasma prophylaxis consisting of pyrimethamine-sulfadiazine or pyrimethamine-clindamycin in sulfonamide-intolerance patients, but only 0.59 if prophylaxis was performed. Treatment of TE, which can result in tissue destruction via massive inflammation and brain abscess formation, has repeatedly been shown to respond to 50mg mg of pyrimethamine, 4 g/day of sulfadiazine, 25 mg of folinic acid for up to 6 weeks (67, 68) without added benefit of 10 mg/kg/day of trimethoprim (TMP), and 50 mg/kg/day of sulfamethoxazole (SMX). Sulfonamide-intolerant patients can be treated with a combination of clindamycin, pyrimethamine, and folinic acid, with comparable efficacy (67) and, alternatively atovaquone, azithromycin, and clarithromycin.

If EBV-DNA or *T. gondii*-DNA tests were positive, the probability of PCNSL or TE increased to more than 0.96; however, the absence of *T. gondii*-DNA did not exclude the possibility of a TE diagnosis, inasmuch as the was 100% specific but only 50% sensitive. In those with FBL without mass effect and typically non-enhancing, the probability of PML was 0.81, increasing to 0.99 if JCV-DNA testing was positive. The latter had a respective sensitivity and specificity of 90% and 98%. Brain biopsy, with a sensitivity of 93% and perioperative morbidity and mortality respectively, of 12% and 2%, was a necessary procedure in EBV-DNA positive cases and in seronegative patients with FBL, displaying mass effect and enhancement. Positive JCV-DNA obviated the necessity of brain biopsy in patients with FBL without mass effect.

A later analysis of FBL correctly identified the etiology of FBL in 26 patients based upon the CD4+T-lymphocyte count, serum toxoplasma immunoglobulin G (IgG) serology, chest radiography, and routine lumbar puncture (LP) studies, including India ink smear, cryptococcal antigen assay, stain and culture for acid-fast bacilli and fungi, cytology, adenosine deaminase (ADA) and Mycobacterium tuberculosis PCR testing, serum and CSF syphilis serology, and single photon emission-computer tomography (SPECT) for enhancing lesions (69). The etiology of FBL included tuberculosis brain abscess in 14 patients, PCNSL in four, toxoplasmosis in four, neurosyphilis in one, PMP in one, cryptococcosis in one, and toxoplasmosis and tuberculosis in one case. The diagnosis of tuberculous brain abscess was ascertained by acute or chronic chest X-ray changes,

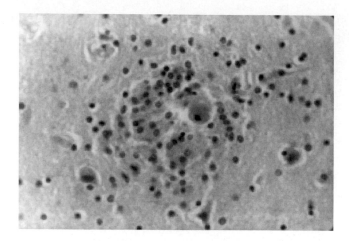

FIG. 4. Cytomegalovirus encephalitis. High-power photomicrograph showing a microglial nodule with associated CMV inclusion. Hematoxylin and eosin, original magnification x250. From: Simpson D, Tagliati M. Neurologic manifestations of HIV infection. *Ann Intern Med* 1994; 121:769–785, with permission.

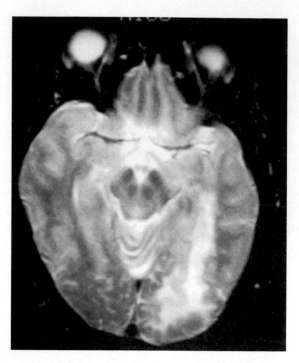

FIG. 5. Progressive multifocal leukoencephalopathy. T_2-weighted MRI shows a large confluent area of increased signal within the white matter of the right cerebral hemisphere. From: Simpson D, Tagliati M. Neurologic manifestations of HIV infection. *Ann Intern Med* 1994; 121:769–785, with permission.

diffuse reticulonodular, interstitial radiographic pattern, with fibrosis, scarring, calcified scarring, detectable CSF ADA levels, and when performed, growth of CSF culture for *M. tuberculosis*, and response to treatment. The diagnosis of PCNS in four patients was made on the basis of a characteristic SPECT scan that showed increased [201]Th uptake, which according to an algorithm, was performed in all patients with solitary mass lesions to differentiate it from TE (70, 71). Brain positron emission tomography (PET) (72, 73), abnormal CSF cytology, flow cytometry, and immunocytologic staining for B-cell markers to demonstrate monoclonality, so noted in 80% of patients with PCNSL (74) and CSF EBV-DNA (75), were all useful surrogate markers for PCNSL to obviate the need for brain tissue sampling.

In patients with FBL without mass effect upon CT and MRI, PML was the most likely focal CNS disorder, with a probability of .81. PML develops in up to 4% of patients with AIDS, and is the initial manifestation of AIDS in up to 29% of patients (76) who present with altered mental status, speech and visual disturbances, gait difficulty, hemiparesis, and limb incoordination. Neuroimaging with T_2-weighted spin-echo MRI scan shows extensive and numerous white matter lesions that appear hypointense on T_1-weighted images and hyperintense on T_2-weighted sequences, but typically do not enhance with administration of intravenous contrast (77) (Figure 5).

Neuropathological findings are characterized by multiple areas of pronounced white matter demyelination with frequent involvement of the gray-white matter junction and cortical gray matter in severe cases, in association with ballooned oligodendroglial cells, with nuclear inclu-

sions containing many virions (Figure 6) (78). Although a positive CSF JCV-DNA determined a probability of PML of >.098, its negativity did not exclude the possibility of PML. Accordingly among 27 patients with PML and FBL, four (15%) had mass effect, and seven (28%) had contrast enhancement of causative lesions which were multiple in 13 (48%) and found in the basal ganglia in five (19%), differentiating it from either TE with respective frequencies of 95%, 95%, 67%, and 69% for the occurence of mass effect, contrast enhancement, multiplicity, and localization in the basal ganglia; similarly in PCNSL in 97% 95%, 56%, and 41%. In patients with suspected PML and negative PCR for JCV-DNA in CSF, the diagnosis remained PML with a probability of .27. Such patients should be considered for repeated lumbar punctures to increase the yield of JCV-DNA sensitivity (79), and amplification of other potentially causative agents in the CSF, including CMV, Herpes simplex (HSV), Varicella zoster virus (VZV), and HIV-1, followed by brain biopsy only after a careful consideration.

Cytomegalovirus infection of the nervous system occurs in patients with AIDS presents with one of several characteristic CNS syndromes (80). CMV retinitis (CMV-R) begins in the peripheral retina but may be a harbinger of encephalitis (81). Diffuse micronodular encephalitis (CMV-E) (82), is

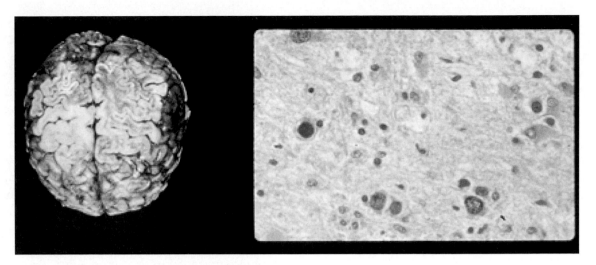

FIG. 6. Progressive multifocal leukoencephalopathy. Brain tissue shows confluent demyelinated foci in the left hemisphere on ultrastructural horizontal sections and a histopathologic photomicrograph of the same lesion containing atypical astrocytes and oligodendroglia with intranuclear inclusions characteristic of JC virus, the etiologic agent of PML. From: Hair LS, Symmans F, Powers JM, et al. Progressive multifocal leukoencephalopathy in patients with human immunodeficiency virus. *Hum Pathol* 1992; 23:663–667, with permission.

further separable into a more common multifocal, diffusely scattered micronodular type that histologically resembles HIV encephalitis (Figure 4), and another with small microglial nodules and inclusion-bearing cytomegalic cells, both of which have an anatomical distribution suggesting hematogenous invasion. Ventriculoencephalitis (83) occurs in advanced AIDS and severely depressed CD4+ T-cell counts. Two-thirds were already taking anti-CMV therapy with ganciclovir or foscarnet at the onset of ventriculoencephalitis. It is clinically distinguished from CMV-E by a more acute onset of lethargy, disorientation, cranial nerve palsy, nystagmus, and ventriculomegaly on brain imaging. Both lumbosacral polyradiculopathy and ventriculoencephalitis have an etiopathogenesis of spread via CSF.

HIV-associated cryptococcal infection, most often caused by *Cryptococcus (C.) neoformans*, commences as an initial pulmonary infection, which depending upon the host immune response, number, and virulence of the organism, is cleared, contained within granulomata as a latent infection, or disseminates. HIV-seropositive patients develop reactivation of latent infection, presenting as sub-acute meningoencephalitis (84). Dilated perivascular spaces, especially in the basal ganglia, can be filled with viable cryptococci, followed by a granulomatous reaction and gelatinous material that lead to the formation of cryptocommas. Abnormal enhancement on neuroimaging studies may be absent and there may be only mild mass effect (85). Small multiple enhancing cortical nodules can also occur (86). Cryptococcomas are generally unassociated with focal symptoms and signs (85, 86).

The hematogenous dissemination and local spread of TB from the subarachnoid space, with or without meningeal involvement and acute meningitis, leads to focal granulomatous abscesses and tuberculomas (87). They occur at the corticomedullary junction, are multiple in one-third of patients, more commonly in the supratentorial fossa (88). There is abnormal ring enhancement on neuroimaging studies with a central area of calcification giving a target appearance (89). Cerebral tuberculomas resolve after several months of antituberculous therapy, depending upon the size of the lesions (90). Expansion of the mass can occur despite initial therapy and may be accompanied by neurologic worsening, which when present, may require treatment with adjuvant corticosteroids (91). Tuberculous meningitis can also lead to cerebral infarction in up to 27% of HIV infected patients, compared to 6% of HIV negative patients (92). Positive CSF TB cultures are detected in 50 to 64% of symptomatic HIV patients compared to 10 to 30% of immunocompetent cases. The sensitivity of CSF cultures in symptomatic HIV cases of TB increases to nearly 100% with a specificity of 94% when PCR analysis of TB DNA is added (93).

Localized syphilitic granulomatous masses in the CNS are termed *gummas* (94). They demonstrate abnormal ring enhancement and can be associated with significant mass effect on neuroimaging studies (95). Meningovascular syphilis presents with multifocal cerebral infarction (96). A positive serum VDRL and fluorescent treponemal antibody absorption (FTAabs) test is suggestive of neurosyphilis, which can be confirmed by seropositivity of the VDRL result in the CSF. The sensitivity of the CSF VDRL is 30 to 70% (97) and its specificity can be altered by potential contamination of the CSF with the blood. Most authors, therefore, recommend treatment for neurosyphilis when the CSF shows elevation of the protein content and pleocytosis, in spite of a negative VDRL result (97). Absence of the CSF FTAabs can be used to exclude the diagnosis of neurosyphilis when the CSF analysis is normal (98). Treatment includes 12 million to 14 million units of intravenous aequous penicillin G daily for 10 days (98) with a goal of achieving a negative serum and CSF VDRL. However, some HIV-infected patients may have a persistent low positive titer.

NEUROMUSCULAR DISORDERS

Neuromuscular disorders associated with HIV-1 infection occur at all stages of the disease and affect all parts of the PNS and motor unit, from the anterior horn cell (AHC) to muscle leading to motor neuron disease (MND), progressive polyradiculopathy, cranial neuropathy (CN), distal symmetrical polyneuropathy (DSP), and acute and chronic inflammatory demyelinating polyneuropathy (AIDP and CIDP), mononeuritis multiplex (MNM), autonomic neuropathy (AN), neuromuscular junction (NMJ) disturbances, and myopathy. These disorders have diverse etiologies, including the retrovirus itself, immunodeficiency, autoimmunity, the effect of comorbid disorders and OI, and those of medications. A recent review has been published (99).

Motor Neuron Disease

Different forms of MND that occur in association with HIV infection have been described, including amyotrophic lateral sclerosis (ALS) (100, 101), primary lateral sclerosis (PLS) (102, 103), and bulbar palsy (104), however the causal relationship remains uncertain. In Patient 1 of Almeida and colleagues (104), PML may have been a cause for pseudobulbar syndrome, and in Patient 2, ALS may have occurred by chance.

Progressive Polyradiculopathy

The clinical and laboratory features of progressive lumbar polyradiculopathy due to cauda equina infection resulting in inflammation and necrosis of lumbosacral nerve roots, has a characteristic presentation, recognition of which, especially in advanced HIV, should prompt consideration of CMV infection (105, 106). Affected patients present with leg pain, paresthesia, flaccid leg weakness, areflexia, sphincter incontinence, and urinary retention. Electrodiagnostic

studies show evidence of acute and subacute axonopathy with absent sensory nerve action potential (SNAP). Contrast MRI of the lumbosacral spine may show enhanced clumped roots. The CSF in CMV-infected cases typically shows polymorphonuclear pleocytosis, reduced glucose, and raised protein content, although these typical features may also be absent and should not be used as strict criteria in a decision to employ ganciclovir or foscarnet therapy. Culture for CMV is positive in up to 50% of patients. Previous or current systemic CMV disease, especially retinitis, supports an association with active infection (80). The demonstration of CMV-DNA in CSF by PCR confirms the diagnosis, with a sensitivity and specificity of close to 100% (107). Ganciclovir, foscarnet, and cidofovir monotherapy were recommended treatment options while awaiting CSF PCR results for CMV-DNA, as a delay in treatment can result in irreversible axonal degeneration and a lack of subsequent response to treatment.

Cranial Neuropathy

Cranial neuropathies occur frequently in HIV infection alone and in AIDS. The facial nerve is the most commonly affected, followed by the abducens, oculomotor, hypoglossal, trigeminal, vestibulocochlear, optic, trochlear, glossopharyngeal, and vagal nerves (108). The etiopathogenesis of cranial neuropathy in AIDS may be related to concurrent cryptococcal disease, tuberculosis, neurosyphilis, and lymphomatous meningitis (108). HIV infected patients with facial nerve palsy are indistinguishable from immunocompetent patients with Bell's palsy except for the likelihood of detecting CSF pleocytosis (109, 110). The prognosis for facial motor recovery is excellent. Hoarseness due to recurrent laryngeal nerve involvement has been reported (111). Intra-axial causes of AIDS associated with cranial neuropathy occurs with PML, PCNSL, and CMV-E, further separable by contrast brain MRI and lumbar CSF analysis (112).

Distal Sensory Polyneuropathy

Distal symmetrical polyneuropathy, which usually occurs in late immune-suppressed stages of HIV infection, is the most common neurologic complication of AIDS, presenting in up to one-third of patients (113). The frequency of DSP increases with the fall in CD4+ T-cell count.

The clinical features of DSP include distal symmetrical numbness, paresthesia, and dysesthesia, beginning in the legs that spread to the arms in association with mild weakness, usually confined to ankle dorsiflexor and evertor and intrinsic foot muscles, and absent ankle reflexes. Electrodiagnostic studies reveal symmetric sensorimotor axonal polyneuropathy with small or absent sural SNAP, and mild to moderate chronic neurogenic changes in distal limb muscles on needle electromyography (EMG) (114).

Postmortem examination reveals pathologic evidence of DSP in nearly all patients with AIDS. Inflammatory, non-inflammatory, and the direct effects of HIV contribute to the pathogenesis of DSP (115). There are excitotoxicity effects of HIV protein gp120 on dorsal root ganglia (DRG) that in affected patients show macrophages and T cell infiltration on postmortem examination. Nerve biopsy tissue shows endoneurial infiltration by HIV-infected macrophages with increased TNF-α mRNA levels and, like vacuolar myelopathy and HIV encephalopathy, DSP appears to result from infiltrating activated HIV-infected macrophages (59). However, one reported patient with primarily sensory neuropathy (116) had evidence of necrotizing arteritis and expression of HIV viral antigens in infiltrating macrophages. Several additional factors may contribute to the development of DSP in AIDS including diabetes mellitus, alcoholism, thiamine, pyridoxine, and B$_{12}$ deficiency, and toxicity of isoniazid and nucleoside analogue therapy (117). The latter leads to axonal polyneuropathy in a dose-dependent fashion several months after treatment, and is generally reversible within two to three months of discontinuation of the drug. Discontinuation of the offending drug may be the only useful means of differentiating this toxic neuropathy from DSP. However, patients may experience an intensification of neuropathic symptoms termed the "coasting period," while others tolerate challenge with lower doses of the anti-retroviral agents. Sural nerve specimens from four patients with ddC-induced polyneuropathy showed mitochondrial DNA depletion with increased numbers of abnormal mitochondria in axons and Schwann cells (117). The primary treatment of DSP is supportive, with consideration of a trial of analgesics, tricyclic antidepressants, and anticonvulsant medication.

Inflammatory Demyelinating Polyneuropathy

Acute IDP, resembling Guillain-Barré syndrome (GBS) and CIDP, occur early in the course of HIV infection and resemble the clinical disorders of uninfected patients (118). However, the mean CSF white blood cell count of HIV-related CIDP was 14 cells/mm³ compared with 1 cell/mm³ in patients without HIV-1 infection (119). Sural nerve biopsy reveals macrophage-mediated demyelination and intense inflammatory cell infiltrates that do not stain for HIV RNA by in situ hybridization (118). Nerve conduction studies fulfill criteria for demyelination (120). The prognosis of GBS and CIDP in HIV infection is as favorable as patients without HIV infection employing plasma exchange, and intravenous immune globulin (IVIg), and immunosuppressant medications alone and in combination.

Mononeuritis Multiplex

Mononeuritis multiplex presents with acute, painful, asymmetric sensorimotor deficits in the distribution of individual peripheral and cranial nerves, often in association with fever, weight loss, and lymphadenopathy. Electrodiagnostic studies typically reveal asymmetric sensorimotor axonopathy neuropathy with frequent superimposed DSP (121, 122). Patients with CD4+T-cell counts less than 100 cells/mm³ can have an etiopathogenesis of MNM due to systemic infection by CMV with intraneural invasion (123). Primary vasculitic neuropathy, which occurs in the early stages of HIV infection when there is heightened immune activation, and presents with typical asymmetric features, becomes symmetrical in later stages owing to overlapping and confluence of lesions (124). Laboratory evaluation in affected patients should include investigation for hepatitis B antigenemia and circulating antibody, hepatitis C serology, circulating immune complexes, and cryoglobulins. Corticosteroid therapy may lead to clinical improvement of vasculitic neuropathy in early HIV infection (125).

Autonomic Neuropathy

Autonomic neuropathy was reported in HIV-positive patients in the pre-HAART era (126, 127). In 2000, the overall prevalence of cardiovascular AN (CVAN) and DSP were similarly assessed at 15%, with correlation to changes in CD4+ T-cell counts, more advanced stage of disease, and intake of neuropathogenic drugs dideoxycytidine, dideoxyinosine, and 2′, 3′ didehydro-2′, 3′ dideoxythymidine. The presence of CVAN was believed to place affected patients at risk for unexpected cardiorespiratory arrest with progression of CVAN. This was later questioned in HIV-positive African (128) and Indian patients (129).

Neuromuscular Junction Disorders

There are numerous reported patients with the concordance of HIV/AIDS and myasthenia gravis (MG) (130–134), including several with circulating acetylcholine receptor (AChR) (133) or anti-muscle specific tyrosine kinase (MuSK) (132) antibodies, most of whom followed a benign clinical course with a favorable response to anticholinesterase therapy. In several patients (130–132, 134), MG followed institution of HAART for HIV, with response to immunosuppressive therapy (132), suggesting an impact of IRIS. One HIV-positive African man with two years of fluctuating weakness developed further symptoms after initiation with HAART that was associated with clinical, electrophysiological, and serologic features of Lambert-Eaton Myasthenic syndrome (LEMS), including circulating antibodies to voltage-gated calcium channels (VGCC) without a detectable tumor (135), and a positive response to IVIg therapy.

Myopathy

HIV-associated myopathy resembles sporadic inflammatory myopathy in uninfected patients (136, 137) and shares similar clinical and laboratory criteria for diagnosis, including progressive proximal weakness, elevation of the serum creatine kinase (CK), myopathic EMG, and inflammation in muscle biopsy tissue. HIV-associated myopathy occurs at any stage of infection, but it is most often encountered in the early stages of HIV infection when autoimmunity is highest. Although the prevalence is unknown, postmortem data suggests involvement in up to one-quarter of HIV/AIDS patients. Serum CK levels are often several-fold normal, and electrodiagnostic studies show fibrillation and positive sharp wave activity in up to 79% of patients on needle EMG, with a typical myopathic recruitment pattern exhibiting early rapid recruitment of motor unit potentials (MUP) upon graded maximal effort. Muscle biopsy tissue typically shows scattered myofiber degeneration, necrosis, and phagocytosis, with inflammatory cell infiltration, although less than that in HIV-seronegative polymyositis (Figure 7). Immunohistochemical studies show endomysial T-cell infiltrates of the CD8 phenotype, with MHC class 1 expression consistent with a primary T-cell–mediated cytotoxic process. *In situ* investigation employing PCR of muscle tissue detected amplified HIV-1 nucleic acids (138). Consideration should be given to standard immunomodulating and immunosuppressant therapy in non-HIV patients to induce a remission and improve weakness, weighing the risks of systemic immunosuppression in the propensity to develop opportunistic infection.

Very high levels of CK, sometimes in the hundreds of thousands, have been reported during all stages of HIV infection (139) such that HIV should be considered in patients with myoglobinuria and known risk factors for AIDS. Affected patients present with fever, local muscle swelling, compartment syndromes, and renal failure. One reported patient demonstrated isolated necrotic fibers without inflammation (140), but studies for HIV antigens were not performed. Myoglobinuria may be precipitated by systemic infections, malignancy, limb compression, local pyomyosits, neuroleptics, sulfonamides, and didanosine. Management consists of hydration, alkalinization, and careful monitoring of renal function.

Pathological variants of HIV-associated myopathy include nemaline rod myopathy (141) and microvasculitis (142). Nemaline rods appears as electron-dense filamentous bodies on electron microscopy with crystalline period-

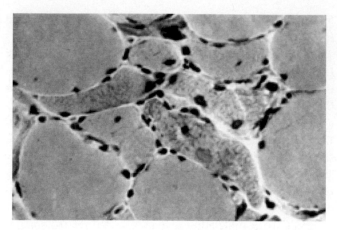

FIG. 7. HIV-associated myopathy. Photomicrograph of a quadriceps muscle biopsy reveals basophilic degenerating fibers without significant inflammatory cell infiltration. Hematoxylin-eosin, original magnification x100. From: Simpson D. Neuromuscular complications of human immunodeficiency virus infection. *Semin Neurol* 1992; 12:39, with permission.

icity characteristic of nemaline rods. Similar findings were reported in zidovudine (AZT)-related myopathy.

Co-infection with HTLV-I may be a proximate and contributory factor in HIV-related polymyositis (PM) (143), the pathology of which differs in the predominance of infiltrating CD4+ cells, some of which show productive infection with HTLV-I (144). *In situ* hybridization of affected cases revealed localization of HTLV-1 to myocytes (145). Three biopsy-proven patients with inclusion body myositis (IBM) were described (137). Two had HIV-1, and one HTLV-I seropositivity, the pathological presentations of which were identical to other sporadic cases, evidencing rimmed vacuoles, MHC type 1 sarcolemmal expression, infiltration of CD8+ cells, and retroviral-infected macrophages.

An HIV-wasting syndrome is characterized by unexplained weight loss of at least 10% of premorbid weight, and 30 days or more of diarrhea. Limb weakness is typically painless, progressive, proximal, and associated with marked muscular wasting (146). The pathologic changes in skeletal muscle are nonspecific, including scattered myofiber degeneration, neurogenic atrophy of myofibers, and mononuclear inflammatory cell infiltration (147). The cause of the wasting syndrome has been ascribed in part to anorexia, nutritional, endocrinologic, concurrent gastrointestinal disorders, and unexplained catabolism. Management includes correction of contributing systemic abnormalities.

Dalakas and colleagues (148) described myopathy associated with AZT therapy at doses of 1,000 mg to 1,200 mg, two-fold normally used in clinical practice. Progressive painful, proximal weakness and elevated serum are the usual presenting features. Muscle biopsy showed 5 to 50% of myofibers with small ragged red fiber morphology on the modified Gomori Trichrome stain, with variable mononuclear inflammatory cell infiltration and increased sarcolemmal MHC type 1 expression, cytoplasmic bodies, and nemaline rods. Electron microscopy in 13 cases showed abnormal swollen mitochondria with paracrystalline inclusions. AZT is believed to inhibit mitochondrial DNA polymerase, resulting in depletion of mitochondrial DNA, reduced respiratory cycle enzyme activity, and subsequent energy failure. Withdrawal of AZT results in improvement in clinical weakness preceded by a fall in the CK level. Further evidence for a primary mitochondrial disorder followed demonstration of skeletal muscular carnitine deficiency, increased glycogen and lipid deposition, cytochrome oxidase deficiency, mitochondrial DNA depletion, reduced phosphocreatine levels with delayed recovery post-exercise as measured by MR spectroscopy (MRS) of the gastrocnemius muscle (149). A primary role for HIV infection in AZT myopathy is based on the finding of inflammatory cell infiltrates, increased staining of myofibers for IL-1, IL1 mRNA (150). The conflicting data on AZT myopathy has led to confusion as to the practical management of patients taking AZT who complain of muscular symptoms and demonstrated elevation of serum CK. A survey of the frequency of documented weakness, myalgias, and elevated CK was taken as part of the ACTG 016 trial comparing 1,000 mg AZT versus placebo for 711 patients with CD4+T-cell counts between 200 and 800 mm^3 (151). Myalgia and elevation of CK were reported in 20 to 40% in both patient groups. Limb weakness occurred in fewer than 2% of patients, all taking AZT, and improved with commensurate fall of the CK with discontinuation of AZT. Discontinuation of AZT is recommended solely because of myalgia or elevation in the CK, even the absence of documented weakness and myopathy demonstrated on electrophysiological studies. The significance of mitochondrial-type pattern abnormalities on biopsy in the absence of weakness is similarly uncertain because continued AZT use may not be associated with the development of weakness (152). Stavudine (d4T) which is now uncommonly used in resource-rich nations, causes HIV-associated neuromuscular weakness syndrome (HANWS) (153) that results in rapidly progressive weakness resembling GBS, with lactic acidosis, nausea, vomiting, weight loss, abdominal distension, hepatomegaly, and lipoatrophy. Muscle biopsy in affected patients show evidence of mitochondrial dysfunction, including ragged red fibers (RRF) and mitochondrial DNA (mtDNA) depletion.

ACKNOWLEDGMENTS

The author wishes to express appreciation to Jennifer Werely, MD, for research assistance. David M. Simpson, MD, and Daniel J.L. MacGowan, MD, MRCPI, participated in prior versions of this chapter.

REFERENCES

1. CDC. 1993 Revised classification system for HIV infection and expanded surveillance case definition for AIDS among adolescents and adults. *MMWR Morb Mortal Wkly Rep* 1992; 41:961–962.
2. Update: serological testing for HIV-1 antibody-United States, 1988 and 1989. *MMWR Morb Mortal Wkly Rep* 1990; 39:380–383; Burke DS, Brundate JF, Redfield RR, et al. Measurement of the false positive rate in a screening program for human immunodeficiency virus infections. *N Engl J Med* 1988; 319:961–964.
3. CDC. Classification system for human T-lymphotrophic virus type III/lymphadenopathy-associated virus infection. *MMWR Morb Mortal Wkly Rep* 1986; 35:334–339.
4. CDC. Classification system for human T-lymphotrophic virus type III/lymphadenopathy-associated virus infections. *MMWR Morb Mortal Wkly Rep* 1987; 36:1–15S.
5. Lange MA, de Wolf F, Goudsmit J. Markers for progression of HIV infection. *AIDS* 1989; 3:S153–S160.
6. US Congress, Office of Technology Assessment. The CDC's case definition of AIDS: implications of the proposed revisions. Background paper, OTA-BP-H-89. Washington, DC: US Government Printing Office, August 1992.
7. Fernandez-Cruz E, Desco M, Garcia Montes M, et al. Immunological and serological markers predictive of progression to AIDS in a cohort of HIV-infected drug users. *AIDS* 1990; 4:987–994.
8. National Institutes of Health. State-of-the-art conference on azidothymidine therapy for early HIV infection. *Am J Med* 1990; 89:335–344.
9. CDC. Guidelines for prophylaxis against Pneumocystis carinii pneumonia for persons infected with human immunodeficiency virus. *MMWR Morb Mortal Wkly Rep* 1992; 41:1–11.
10. Fischl MA, Richman DD, Hansen N, et al. The safety and efficacy of zidovudine (AZT) in the treatment of subjects with mildly symptomatic human immunodeficiency virus type 1 (HIV) infection: a double-blind, placebo controlled trial. *Ann Intern Med* 1990; 112:727–737.
11. Volderding PA, Lagakos SW, Koch MA, et al. Zidovudine in asymptomatic human immunodeficiency virus infection: a controlled trial in persons with fewer than 500 CD4-positive cells per cubic millimeter. *N Engl J Med* 1990; 322:941.
12. Lagakos S, Fischl MA, Stein DS, et al. Effects of zidovudine therapy in minority and other subpopulations with early HIV infection. *JAMA* 1991; 266:2709–2712.
13. Easterbrook PJ, Keruly JC, Creagh-Kirk T, et al. Racial and ethnic differences in outcome in zidovudine-treated patients with advance HIV disease. *JAMA* 1991; 266:2713–2718.
14. CDC. Guidelines for preventing the transmission of tuberculosis in health-care settings, with special focus on HIV-related issues. *MMWR infection Morb Mortal Wkly Rep* 1990; 39:1–29.
15. WHO, UNAIDS, UNICEF. Global HIV/AIDS response. Epidemic update and health sector progress towards universal access. *Progress Report* 2011.

16. Levy RM, Bredesen DE, Rosenblum ML. Neurologic manifestations of the acquired immunodeficiency syndrome (AIDS): experience at UCSF and review of the literature. *J Neurosurg* 1985; 62:475–495.

17. Petito CK. Review of central nervous system pathology in human immunodeficiency virus infection. *Ann Neurol* 1988; 23:S54–S57.

18. Gray F, Gherardi R, Scaravilli F. The neuropathology of the acquired immunodeficiency syndrome (AIDS). *Brain* 1988; 111:245–266.

19. Kure K, Llena JF, Lyman WD, et al. Human immunodeficiency virus-1 infection of the nervous system: an autopsy study of 268 adult, pediatric and fetal brains. *Hum Pathol* 1991; 22:700–710.

20. de la Monte SM, Gabuzda DH, Ho DD, et al. Peripheral neuropathy in the acquired immunodeficiency syndrome. *Ann Neurol* 1988; 23:485–492.

21. Snider WD, Simpson DM, Nielsen S, et al. Neurological complications of acquired immune deficiency syndrome: analysis of 50 patients. *Ann Neurol* 1983; 14:403–418.6–11.

22. D'Armino Forte A, Duca PG, et al. Decreasing incidence of CNS AIDS-defining events associated with anti-retroviral therapy. *Neurology* 2000; 54:1856–1859.

23. Sacktor N. The epidemiology of human immunodeficiency virus-associated neurological disease in the era of highly active antiretroviral therapy. *J Neurovirol* 2002; 8:115–121.

24. Price RW, Brew BJ. The AIDS dementia complex. *J Infect Dis* 1988; 158:1079–1083.

25. McArthur JC, Hoover DR, Bacellar H, et al. Nomenclature and research case definitions for neurological manifestations of human immunodeficiency virus type-1 (HIV-1) infection: report of a Working Group of the American Academy of Neurology AIDS Task Force. *Neurology* 1991; 41:778–785.

26. Antimori A, Arendt G, Becker JT, et al. Updated research nosology for HIV-associated neurocognitive disorders. *Neurology* 2007; 69:1789–1799.

27. McArthur JC, Hoover DR, Bacellar H, et al. Dementia in AIDS patients: incidence and risk factors. *Neurology* 1993; 43:2245–2252.

28. The Dana Consortium on Therapy for HIV Dementia and Related Cognitive Disorders. Clinical confirmation of the American Academy of Neurology algorithm for HIV-1-associated cognitive/motor disorder. *Neurology* 1996; 47:1247–1253.

29. Marder K, Liu X, Stern Y, et al. Neurological signs and symptoms in a cohort of homosexual men followed for 4.5 years. *Neurology* 1995; 45:261–267.

30. Janssen RS, Cornblath DR, Epstein LG, et al. Nomenclature and research case definitions for neurological manifestations of human immunodeficiency virus type-1 (HIV-1) infection. Report of a Working Group of the American Academy of Neurology AIDS Task Force. *Neurology* 1991; 41:778–785.

31. Kieburtz K, Ketonen L, Cox C, et al. Cognitive performance and regional volume in human immunodeficiency virus type 1 infection. *Arch Neurol* 1996; 53:155–158.

32. Dal Pan GJ, McArthur JC, Aylward E, et al. Patterns of cerebral atrophy in HIV-1 infected individuals: results of a quantitative MRI analysis. *Neurology* 1992; 42:2125–2130.

33. Aylward EH, Henderer JD, McArthur JC, et al. Reduced basal ganglia volume in HIV-1-associated dementia: results from quantitative neuroimaging. *Neurology* 1993; 43:2099–2104.

34. Wiley CA, Achim C. Human immunodeficiency virus encephalitis is the pathological correlate of dementia in acquired immunodeficiency syndrome. *Ann Neurol* 1994; 36:673–676.

35. Brew BJ, Rosenblum M, Cronin K, et al. AIDS dementia complex and HIV-1 brain infection: clinical-virological correlations. *Ann Neurol* 1995; 38:563–570.

36. Seilhean D, Duyckaerts C, Vazeux R, et al. HIV-1 associated cognitive-motor complex: absence of neuronal loss in the cerebral neocortex. *Neurology* 1993; 43:1492–1499.

37. Wiley CA, Masliah E, Morey M, et al. Neocortical damage during HIV infection. *Ann Neurol* 1991; 29:651–657.

38. Schmidbauer M, Huemer M, Cristina S, et al. Morphological spectrum, distribution and clinical correlation of white matter lesions in AIDS brains. *Neuropathol Appl Neurobiol* 1992; 18:489–501.

39. Bagasra O, Lavi E, Boboroski L, et al. Cellular reservoirs of HIV-1 in the central nervous system of infected individuals: identification by the combination of in situ polymerase chain reaction and immunohistochemistry. *AIDS* 1996; 10:573–585.

40. Glass JD, Fedor H, Wesselingh SL, et al. Immunocytochemical quantitation of human immunodeficiency virus in the brain: correlations with dementia. *Ann Neurol* 1995; 38:755–762.

41. Lipton SA. Human immunodeficiency virus infected macrophages, gp120 and N-methyl-D-aspartate neurotoxicity. *Ann Neurol* 1993; 33:227–228.

42. Tozzi V, Balestra P, Galgani S, et al. Positive and sustained effects of highly active antiretroviral therapy on HIV-1 associated neurocognitive impairment. *AIDS* 1999; 13:1889–1897.

43. Tozzi V, Balestra P, Ballagamba R, et al. Persistence of neuropsychological deficits despite long-term highly active antiretroviral therapy in patients with HIV-related neurocognitive impairment: prevalence and risk factors. *J Acquir Immune Defic Syndr* 2007; 45:174–183.

44. Aweeka F, Jayewardene A, Saprans S, et al. Failure to detect nelfinavir in the cerebrospinal fluid of HIV-1-infected patients with and without AIDS dementia complex. *J Acquir Immune Defic Syndr Hum Retrovirol* 1999; 20:39–43.

45. Letendre S, Marquie-Beck J, Capparelli E, et al. for the CHARTER Group. Validation of the CNS penetration-effectiveness rank for quantifying antiretroviral penetration into the central nervous system. *Arch Neurol* 2008; 65:65–70.

46. Price P, Mathiot N, Krueger R, et al. Immune dysfunction and immune restoration disease in HIV patients given highly active antiretroviral therapy. *J Clin Virology* 2001; 22:279–287.

47. Subsai K, Kanoksri S, Siwaporn C, et al. Neurological complications in AIDS patients receiving HART: a 2-year retrospective study. *Eur J Neurol* 2006; 13:233–239.

48. Heseltine PNR, Goodkin K, Hampton Atkinson J, et al. Randomized double-blind placebo-controlled trial of peptide T for HIV-associated cognitive impairment. *Arch Neurol* 1998; 55:41–51.

49. Navia BA, Dafni U, Simpson D, et al.; and the AIDS Clinical Trial Group. A phase I/II trial of nimodipine for HIV-related neurological complications. *Neurology* 1998; 51:221–228.

50. The Dana Consortium on the Therapy of HIV Dementia and Related Cognitive Disorders. A randomized double-blind, placebo-controlled trial of deprenyl and thioacetic acid in human immunodeficiency virus-associated cognitive impairment. *Neurology* 1998; 50:645–651.

51. Sacktor N, Miyahara S, Deng I, et al., On behalf of the ACTG A5235 team. Minocycline treatment for HIV-associated cognitive impairment. Results from a randomized trial. *Neurology* 2011; 77:1135–1142.

52. Rumbaugh JA, Steiner J, Sacktor N, et al. developing neuroprotective strategies for treatment of HIV-associated neurocognitive dysfunction. *Futur HIV Ther* 2008; 2:271–280.

53. Tagliati M, Simpson D, Morgello S, et al. Cerebellar degeneration associated with human imunodeficiency virus infection. *Neurology* 1998; 50:244–251.

54. Wolters EC, Van Wijngaarden GK, Stam FC, et al. Leucoencephalopathy after inhaling heroin pyrosylate. *Lancet* 1982; 2:1233–1237.

55. Krigstein A, Armitage B, Kim PY. Heroin inhalation and progressive spongiform leukoencephalopathy. *N Engl J Med* 1997; 336:589–590.

56. Petito CK, Navia BA, Cho ES, et al. Vacuolar myelopathy pathologically resembling subacute combined degeneration in patients with the acquired immunodeficiency syndrome. *N Engl J Med* 1985; 312:874–879.

57. Dal Pan GJ, Glass JD, McArthur JC. Clincopathologic correlations of HIV-1 associated vacuolar myelopathy. An autopsy-based case-control study. *Neurology* 1994; 44:2159–2164.

58. Tyor WR, Glass JD, Baumrind N, et al. Cytokine expression of macrophages in HIV-1 associated vacuolar myelopathy. *Neurology* 1993; 43:1002–1009.

59. Tyor WR, Wesselingh SL, Griffin JW, et al. Unifying hypothesis for the pathogenesis of HIV-associated dementia complex, vacuolar myelopathy, and sensory neuropathy. *J Acq Immun Def Syndr Hum Retrovirol* 1995; 9:379–388.

60. Kieburtx KD, Giang DW, Schiffer RB, et al. Abnormal vitamin B12 metabolism in human immunodeficiency infection. Association with neurological dysfunction. *Arch Neurol* 1991; 48:312–314.

61. Eyer-Silva WA, Couto-Fernandez JC, et al. Remission of HIV-associated myelopathy after initiation of lopinavir in a patient with extensive previous exposure to highly active antiretroviral therapy. *AIDS* 2002; 16:2367–2369.

62. Bizaare M, Dawood H, Moodley A. Vacuolar myelopathy: a case report of functional, clinical, and radiological improvement after highly active antiretroviral therapy. *Int J Infect Dis* 2008; 12:442–444.

63. Luft BJ, Remington JS. Toxoplasmic encephalitis in AIDS. *Clin Infect Dis* 1992; 15:211–222.

64. New LC, Holliman RE. Toxoplasmosis and human immunodeficiency virus (HIV) disease. *J Antimicrob Chemother* 1994; 33:1079–1082.

65. Porter SB, Sande MA. Toxoplasmosis of the central nervous system in the acquiring immunodeficiency syndrome. *N Engl J Med* 1992; 327:1643–1648.

66. Antinori A, Ammassari A, De Luca A, et al. Diagnosis of AIDS-related focal brain lesions: A decision making analysis based on clinical and neuroradiologic characteristics combined with polymerase chain reactive assays in CSF. *Neurology* 1997; 48:687–694.

67. Luft BJ, Hafner R, Korzun AH, et al. Toxoplasmic encephalitis in patients with the acquired immunodeficiency syndrome. *N Engl J Med* 1993; 329:995–1000.

68. Kongsaengdao S, Samintarapanya K, Oranratnachai K, et al. Randomized controlled trial of pyrimethamine plus sulfadiazine versus trimethoprim plus sulfamethoxazaole for toxoplasma encephalitis in AIDS patients. *J Int Assoc Physician AIDS Care* 2008; 7:11–16.

69. Smego RA, Orlovic D, Wadula J. An algorithmic approach to intracranial mass lesions in HIV/AIDS. *Int J of STD & AIDS* 2006; 17:271–276.

70. Ruiz A, Ganz WI, Post MJD, et al. Use of thallium-201 brain SPECT to differentiate cerebral lymphoma from Toxoplasma encephalitis in AIDS patients. *Am J Neuroradiol* 1994; 15:1885–1894.

71. D'Amico A, Messa C, Castagna A, et al. Diagnostic accuracy and predictive value of 201Th SPECT for the differential diagnosis of cerebral lesions in AIDS patients. *Nucl Med Comm* 1997; 18:741–750.

72. Pierce MA, Mahlan D, Maciunas RJ, et al. Evaluating contrast-enhancing brain lesions in patients with AIDS by using positron emission tomography. *Ann Intern Med* 1995; 123:594–598.

73. Heald AE, Hoffman JM, Barlett JA, et al. Differentiation of central nervous system lesions in AIDS patients using positron emissions tomography (PET). *Int J STD AIDS* 1996; 7:337–346.

74. So YT, Beckstead JH, David RL. Primary central nervous system lymphoma in acquired immune deficiency syndrome. A clinical and pathological study. *Ann Neurol* 1986; 20:566–572.

75. Arribas JR, Clifford DB, Fichtenbaum CJ, et al. Detection of Epstein-Barr virus DNA in cerebrospinal fluid for diagnosis of AIDS-related central nervous system lymphoma. *J Clin Microbiol* 1995; 33:1580–1583.

76. Berger JR, Kaszovitz B, Post JD, et al. Progressive multifocal leukoencephalopathy associated with human immunodeficiency virus infection. A review of the literature with a report of sixteen cases. *Ann Intern Med* 1987; 107:78–87.

77. Simpson D, Tagliati M. Neurologic manifestations of HIV infection. *Ann Intern Med* 1994; 121:769–785.

78. Hair LS, Symmans F, Powers JM, et al. Progressive multifocal leukoencephalopathy in patients with human immunodeficiency virus. *Hum Pathol* 1992; 23:663–667.

79. De Luca A, Cingolani A, Linzalone A, et al. Improved detection of JC virus DNA in cerebrospinal fluid for diagnosis of AIDS-related progressive multifocal leukoencephalopathy. *J Clin Microbiol* 1996; 34:1343–1346.

80. McCutchan JA. Cytomegalovirus infections of the nervous system in patients with AIDS, *CID* 1995; 20:747–754.

81. Bylema S, Achim C, Wiley C, et al. The predictive value of cytomegalovirus retinitis for cytomegalovirus encephalitis in acquired immunodeficiency syndrome. *Ophthalmology* 1994; 112:1–8.

82. Morgello S, Cho E, Nielsen S, et al. Cytomegalovirus encephalitis in patients with acquired immunodeficiency syndrome: an autopsy study of 30 cases and a review of the literature. *Hum Pathol* 1987; 18:289–297.

83. Kalayjian RC, Cohen ML, Bonomo RA, et al. Cytomegalovirus ventriculoencephalitis in AIDS: a syndrome with distinct clinical and pathological features. *Medicine* 1993; 72:67–77.

84. Jarvis JN, Harrison TS. HIV-associated cryptococcal meningitis. *AIDS* 2007; 21:2119–2129.

85. Mathews VP, Alo PL, Glass JD, et al. AIDS-related CNS cryptococcosis: radiological-pathological correlation. *Am J Neuroradiol* 1992; 13:1477–1486.

86. Tien RD, Chu PK, Hesselink JR, et al. Intracranial cryptococcosis in immunocompromised patients: CT and MRI findings in 29 cases. *Am J Neuroradiol* 1991; 12:283–289.

87. Dube MP, Holtom PD, Larsen RA. Tuberculous meningitis in patients with and without human immunodeficiency virus infection. *Am J Med* 1992; 93:520–524.

88. Jinkins JR. Computed tomography of intracranial tuberculosis. *Neuroradiology* 1991; 33:126–135.

89. Van Dyk A. CT of intracranial tuberculosis with specific reference to the target sign. *Neuroradiology* 1988; 30:329–336.

90. Villoria MF, de la Torre J, Munoz L, et al. Intracranial tuberculosis in AIDS: CT and MRI findings. *Neuroradiology* 1992; 34:11–14.

91. Afghani B, Liberman JM. Paradoxical enlargement or development of intracranial tuberculomas during therapy: case report and review. *Clin Infect Dis* 1994; 19:1092–1099.

92. Berenguer J, Moreno S, Laguna F, Vicente T, et al. Tuberculous meningitis in patients infected with the human immunodeficiency virus. *N Engl J Med* 1992; 326:668–672.

93. Kox LKK, Sjoukje S, Kolk AHJ, et al. Early diagnosis of

tuberculous meningitis by polymerase chain reaction. *Neurology* 1995; 45:2228–2232.

94. Kaplan JG, Sterman AB, Horoupian D, et al. Luetic meningitis with gumma: clinical, radiographic, and neuropathologic features. *Neurology* 1981; 31:464–467.

95. Berger JR, Waskin H, Pall L, et al. Syphilitic cerebral gumma with HIV infection. *Neurology* 1992; 42:1282–1287.

96. Holland BA, Perrett LV, Mills CM. Meningovascular syphilis: CT and MR findings. *Radiology* 1986; 158:439–442.

97. Hart G. Syphilis tests in diagnostic and therapeutic decision making. *Ann Intern Med* 1986; 104:368–376.

98. Golden MR, Marra CM, Holmes KK. Update on syphilis: resurgence of an old problem. *JAMA* 2003; 290:1510–1514.

99. Robinson-Papp J, Simpson DM. Neuromuscular diseases associated with HIV-1 infection. *Muscle Nerve* 2009; 40:1043–1053.

100. Verma A, Berger J. ALS syndrome in patients with HIV-1 infection. *J Neurol Sci* 2006; 240:59–64.

101. Moulignier A, Roulonguet A, Pialoux G, et al. Reversible ALS-like disorder in HIV infection. *Neurology* 2001; 57:995–1001.

102. Verma A, Berger J. Primary lateral sclerosis with HIV-1 infection. *Neurology* 2008; 70:575–577.

103. Younger DS, Chou S, Hays AP, et al. Primary lateral sclerosis: a clinical diagnosis re-emerges. *Arch Neurol* 1988; 45:1304–1307.

104. Almeida V, Mestre T, De Carvalho M. Pseudobulbar syndrome in two patients with human immunodeficiency virus infection. *Amyotroph Lateral Scler* 2010; 11:220–222.

105. So YT, Olney RK. Acute lumbosacral polyradiculopathy in acquired immunodeficiency syndrome: experience in 23 patients. *Ann Neurol* 1994; 35:53–58.

106. Miller RF, Fox JD, Thomas P, et al. Acute lumbosacral polyradiculopathy due to cytomegalovirus in advanced HIV disease: CSF findings in 17 patients. *J Neurol Neurosurg Psychiatry* 1996; 61:456–460.

107. Cinque P, Vago L, Dahl H, et al. Polymerase chain reaction on cerebrospinal fluid for diagnosis of virus-associated opportunistic diseases of the central nervous system in HIV-infected patients. *AIDS* 1996; 10:951–958.

108. Serrano P, Hernandez N, Arroyo JA, et al. Bilateral Bell palsy and acute HN type 1 infection: report of 2 cases and review. *Clin Infect Dis* 2007; 44:e57–61.

109. Anonymous. Needlestick transmission of HTLV-III from a patient infected in Africa. *Lancet* 1984; 2:1376–1377.

110. Wiselka MJ, Nicholson KG, Ward SC, et al. Acute infection with human immunodeficiency virus associated with facial nerve palsy and neuralgia. *J Infect* 1987; 15:189–194.

111. Small PM, McPhaul LW, Sooy CD, et al. Cytomegalovirus infection of the laryngeal nerve presenting as hoarseness in patients with acquired immunodeficiency syndrome. *Am J Med* 1989; 86:108–110.

112. Berger JR, Flaster M, Schatz N, et al. Cranial neuropathy heralding otherwise occult AIDS-related large cell lymphoma. *J Clin Neurophthalmol* 1993; 13:113–118.

113. Barohn RJ, Gronseth GS, LeForce BR, et al. Peripheral nervous system involvement in a large cohort of human immunodeficiency virus-infected individuals. *Arch Neurol* 1993; 50:167–171.

114. Cornblath DR, McArthur JC. Predominantly sensory neuropathy in patients with AIDS and AIDS-related complex. *Neurology* 1988; 38:794–796.

115. Apostolski S, McAlarney T, Quattrini A, et al. The gp120 glycoprotein of human immunodeficiency virus type 1 binds to sensory ganglion neurons. *Ann Neurol* 1993; 34:855–863.

116. Younger DS, Rosoklija G, Hays AP. Sensory neuropathy in AIDS: Demonstration of vasculitis and HIV antigens in peripheral nerve. *J Neurol* 1994; 241 (Suppl):17.

117. Dalakas M, Semino-Mora C, Leon-Monzon M. Mitochondrial alterations with mitochondrial DNA depletion in the nerves of AIDS patients with peripheral neuropathy induced by 2'3'-dideoxycytidine (ddC). *Lab Invest* 2001; 81:1537–1544.

118. Cornblath DR, McArthur JC, Kennedy PGE, et al. Inflammatory demyelinating peripheral neuropathies associated with human T-cell lymphotropic virus type III infection. *Ann Neurol* 1987; 21:32–40.

119. Thornton CA, Latif AS, Emmanuel JC. Guillain-Barré syndrome associated with human immunodeficiency virus infection in Zimbabwe. *Neurology* 1991; 41:812–815.

120. Cornblath DR, Asbury AK, Albers JW, et al. Research criteria for diagnosis of chronic inflammatory demyelinating polyneuropathy (CIDP). *Neurology* 1991; 41:617–618.

121. Lange DJ, Britton CB, Younger DS, et al. The neuromuscular manifestations of human immunodeficiency virus infections. *Arch Neurol* 1988; 45:1084–1088.

122. Roullet E, Asseurus V, Gozlan J, et al. Cytomegalovirus multifocal neuropathy in AIDS: analysis of 15 cases. *Neurology* 1994; 44:2174–2182.

123. Said G, Lacroix C, Chemoulli P, et al. Cytomegalovirus neuropathy in acquired immunodeficiency syndrome: a clinical and pathological study. *Ann Neurol* 1991; 29:139–146.

124. Gherardi R, Lebargy F, Gaulard P, et al. Necrotizing vasculitis and HIV replication in peripheral nerves. *N Engl J Med* 1989; 321:685–686.

125. Bradley WG, Verma A. Painful vasculitic neuropathy in HIV-1 infection: relief of pain with prednisone therapy. *Neurology* 1996; 47:1446–1451.

126. Cohen JA, Laudenslager M. Autonomic nervous system involvement in patients with human immunodeficiency virus infection. *Neurology* 1989; 39:1111–1112.

127. Freeman R, Roberts MS, Friedman LS, et al. Autonomic function and human immunodeficiency virus infection. *Neurology* 1990; 40:575–580.

128. Compostella C, Compostella L, D'Elia R. The symptoms of autonomic dysfunction in HIV-positive Africans. *Clin Auton Res* 2008; 18:6–12.

129. Sakhuja A, Goyal A, Jaryal AK, et al. Heart rate variability and autonomic function tests in HIV positive individuals in India. *Clin Auton Res* 2007; 1:193–196.

130. Hung WL, Lin YH, Wang PY, et al. HIV-associated myasthenia gravis and impacts of HAART: one case report and brief review. *Clin Neurol Neurosurg* 2011; 113:672–674.

131. Knopf L, Menkes DL. Comorbid HIV and myasthenia gravis: case report and reviews of the literature. *J Clin Neuromuscul Dis* 2010; 12:80–84.

132. Kurokawa T, Nishiyama T, Yamamoto R, et al. Anti-MuSK antibody positive myasthenia gravis with HIV infection successfully treated with cyclosporine: a case report. *Rinsho Shinkeigaku* 2008; 48:666–669.

133. Gorthi SP, Shankar S, Johri S, et al. HIV infection with myasthenia gravis. *J Assoc Physicians India* 2005; 53:995–996.

134. Chiesa E, Bongiovanni M, Melzi S, et al. Efavirenz-containing highly active anti-retroviral therapy in an HIV-infected patient with myasthenia gravis. *AIDS* 2003; 17:2544–2545.

135. Truffert A, Allali G, Vokatch N, et al. Mild clinical expression of Lambert-Eaton Myasthenic syndrome in a patient with HIV infection. *BMJ Case Rep* 2009; pii:bcr08.2008.0649 Epub 2009 Jan 23.

136. Illa I, Nath A, Dalakas M. Immunocytochemical and virological characteristics of HIV-associated inflammatory myopathies: similarities with seronegative polymyositis. *Ann Neurol* 1991; 29:474–481.

137. Cupler EJ, Leon-Monzon M, Miller J, et al. Inclusion body

myositis in HIV-I and HTLV-I infected patients. *Brain* 1996; 6:1887–1893.

138. Seidman R, Peress N, Nuovo GJ. In situ detection of polymerase chain reaction-amplified HIV-1 nucleic acids in skeletal muscle in patients with myopathy. *Mod Pathol* 1994; 7:369–375.

139. Younger DS, Hays AP, Uncini A, et al. Recurrent myoglobinuria and HIV seropositivity: incidental or pathogenic association? *Muscle Nerve* 1989; 12:842–843.

140. Chariot P, Ruet E, Authier FJ, et al. Acute rhabdomyolysis in patients infected by human immunodeficiency virus. *Neurology* 1994; 44:1692–1696.

141. Dalakas MC, Pezeshkpour GH, Flaherty M. Progressive nemaline (rod) myopathy associated with HIV infection. *N Engl J Med* 1987; 317:1602–1603.

142. Said G, Lacroix-Ciaudo C, Fujimura H, et al. The peripheral neuropathy of necrotising arteritis: a clinicopathological study. *Ann Neurol* 1988; 23:461–465.

143. Wiley CA, Nerenberg M, Cros D, et al. HTLV-1 polymyositis in a patient also infected with the human immunodeficiency virus. *N Engl J Med* 1989; 320:992–995.

144. Dwyer BA, Mayer RF, Lee SC. Progressive nemaline rod myopathy as a presentation of human immunodeficiency virus infection. *Arch Neurol* 1992; 49:440.

145. Dickoff D, Simpson DM, Wiley CA, et al. HTLV-1 in acquired adult myopathy. *Muscle Nerve* 1993; 16:162–165.

146. Simpson DM, Bender AN, Farraye J, et al. Human immunodeficiency virus wasting syndrome may represent a treatable myopathy. *Neurology* 1990; 40:535–538.

147. Belec L, Mhiri C, Di Costanzo B, et al. The HIV wasting syndrome. *Muscle Nerve* 1992; 15:856–857.

148. Dalakas MC, Illa I, Pezeshkpour GH, et al. Mitochondrial myopathy caused by long-term zidovudine therapy. *N Engl J Med* 1990; 322:1098–1105.

149. Dalakas MC, Leon-Monzon ME, Bernardini I, et al. Zidovudine-induced mitochondrial myopathy is associated with muscle carnitine deficiency and lipid storage. *Ann Neurol* 1994; 35:482–487.

150. Gherardi RK, Florea-Strat A, Fromont G, et al. Cytokine expression in the muscle of HIV infected patients: evidence for interleukin-1a accumulation in mitochondria of AZT fibers. *Ann Neurol* 1994; 36:752–758.

151. Simpson DM, Slasor P, Dafni U, et al. Analysis of myopathy in a placebo-controlled zidovudine trial. *Muscle Nerve* 1997; 20:382–385.

152. Cupler EJ, Hench K, Jay CA, et al. The natural history of zidovudine (AZT)-induced mitochondrial myopathy. *Neurology* 1994; 44:A132.

153. HIV Neuromuscular Syndrome Study Group. HIV-associated neuromuscular weakness syndrome. *AIDS* 2004; 18:1403–1412.

CHAPTER 54

Growth Factors and Signals: Impact on Neurological Systems

Douglas W. Zochodne

Recognition of the central and peripheral nervous systems (CNS and PNS) as plastic and dynamic has led to hope that specific growth factors or their downstream signaling cascades might protect the nervous system from disease, resurrect impaired connections or support alternative pathways providing similar function. Advances in the understanding of growth factors and growth signals have identified several critical concepts. The first of these is the realization that, hitherto, systems, including motor systems, previously thought of as static in adults have surprising responsiveness following injury. The second concept is that a number of the growth factors are elaborated by targets or glial cells to signal the growth cone or cell body, either locally or at a distance. A third concept followed the important discovery that led to the recognition that growth factors can be synthesized by neurons and act on themselves by autocrine signaling. Fourth, is the recognition that growth factors have tremendous redundancy in their actions, frequently sharing common downstream signaling cascades. Exploiting these downstream pathways may allow direct manipulation of neuronal growth. While absence of a given factor or its receptor may render severe developmental deficits, in many instances loss can be compensated for by the actions of other factors.

This chapter summarizes the present understanding of nervous system growth factors, recognizing that any such review is selective and limited. The list of molecules with potential growth factor actions has expanded and the major families have undergone extensive investigation, including neurotrophin family of factors, the first identified of which was nerve growth factor (NGF) over 50 years ago, and non-neurotrophin growth factors, including ciliary neurotrophic factor (CNTF), insulin-like growth factors (IGF), and glial derived neurotrophic factor (GDNF). Newer ideas on how growth factor signaling may be utilized are reviewed as are selected animal disease models that utilize growth factors and their respective pathways. The findings of clinical trials utilizing these agents will be presented along with thoughts about the limitations these approaches have encountered.

NEUROTROPHINS

General Comments

The first member of the neurotrophin family, NGF was described in 1953 by Levi-Montalcini and Hamburger (1) as a soluble factor isolated from mouse sarcoma tumors capable of inducing hyperplasia in sympathetic ganglia by stimulating neurite outgrowth. The working definition of a neurotrophin was that of an endogenous soluble protein regulating survival, growth, morphological plasticity, or synthesis of proteins for differentiated function of neurons (2). An important property, though not an absolute requirement, was that the factor be transported retrograde by the axons of the neurons it supports. Five members of this family have been described, each acting on a related tyrosine kinase (Trk) receptor: NGF, brain derived neurotrophic factor (BDNF) (3, 4), neurotrophin-3 (NT-3) (5, 6), neurotrophin 4/5 (NT-4/5) (7), and neurotrophin 6 (NT-6) (8) (Table). NGF, NT-3, and BDNF are all transported retrograde into sensory neurons of the dorsal root ganglia (DRG) of adult rats (9-11). BDNF is also transported retrograde by motor neurons (11). The primary receptors for these proteins have been labeled Trk A for NGF, Trk B for BDNF, and NT 4/5 and Trk C for NT-3 with some promiscu-

TABLE. Neurotrophins and Other Growth Factors

	Receptor	Target tissue (PNS
Classical neurotrophins and their peripheral nerve targets		
Nerve growth factor (NGF)	TrkA, p75	small fiber sensory neurons sympathetic neurons
Brain-derived neurotrophic factor (BDNF)	TrkB, p75	motor neurons sensory neurons
Neurotrophin-3(NT-3)	TrkC, p75	large sensory neurons sympathetic neurons motor neurons
Neurotrophin-4/5 (NT-4/5)	TrkB, p75	motor neurons sensory neurons sympathetic neurons
Neurotrophin-6 (NT-6)	?	?

Other Growth Factors:

Factors that act on the gp 130 receptor complex
Ciliary neurotrophic factor (CNTF)
Leukemia inhibitory factor (LIF)
Cardiotrophin-1 (CT-1)
Growth factors discovered in other tissues with actions on the nervous system
Fibroblast growth factors (FGF)
Epidermal growth factor (EGF)
Platelet-derived growth factors (PDGF)
Erythropoietin
Transforming growth factor β (TGFβ)
Hepatocyte growth factor (HGF)
Macrophage stimulating protein (MSP)
Insulin related growth factors
Insulin
Insulin-like growth factor I and II (IGFI and IGFII)
Cytokines
Interleukin-1
Interleukin-6
Interleukin-11
Bone morphogenetic proteins (BMP)
Other
Glial-derived neurotrophic factor (GDNF)
Other GDNF family members (neurturin, artemin, persephin)
Semaphorins

ity in their specificity. Trk receptors mediate differentiation, survival, and loss of proliferative capacity of subpopulations of neuronal cells through a number of intracellular second messengers. The survival benefit is conferred by blocking apoptotic cell death. One of the primary experimental approaches toward understanding the role of neurotrophins and other growth factors utilizes axotomy, or a section of a neuron axon. In developing neurons, axotomy is associated with severe and widespread retrograde apoptosis that can be rescued with growth factors. In adults, this form of retrograde loss is far less prominent but there are changes in neuron morphology and gene expression.

An additional low affinity neurotrophin receptor, p75, originally described in relationship to NGF, is activated by all of the members of the neurotrophin family. The complexity of p75 actions has been more fully appreciated, including its role in guidance and apoptosis of neurons. At the membrane of a growth cone, p75 interacts with several proteins, including NOGO, the myelin protein that inhibits spinal cord regeneration. In the absence of Trk receptors, p75 signals neuron and Schwann cell (SC) apoptosis (12), but together with Trk receptors, enhance neurotrophin actions and transport (13).

At the level of the growth cone, p75 interacts with Rho GTPase, one of a family of interesting molecular switches that influence growth cone dynamics (14-16). When translocated to the growth cone membrane, RhoA acts through Rho kinase (ROCK) to enhance myosin II phosphorylation and actin mediated growth cone retraction (16). Other family members, such as Rac1 and CDC42, instead enhance growth cone extension. P75 has differing actions depending whether it is or not occupied by a ligand (17). When occupied, for example, by a pro-neurotrophin, a molecular precursor of a mature neurotrophin, it inhibits RhoA activation to thereby facilitate outgrowth (18, 19). P75 receptors bind with greater affinity to pro-neurotrophins, enabling them to support a wide range of axon types by signaling at growth cones independently of Trks (20, 21). Insulin also inhibits Rho signaling by a mechanism related to the facilitation of regeneration (22, 23). Finally, RhoGTPases likely play key roles in growth cone turning. The orientation of axons, for example after peripheral nerve transections, may play a crucial role in how well they regenerate (15, 24).

Neurotrophin molecular dimers bind to Trk receptors to cause Trk dimerization and tyrosine autophosphorylation (25). Autophosphorylation, in turn, activates intracellular pathways that influence not only survival of neurons, but outgrowth properties of their axons (26). While more than one pathway may promote survival in response to receptor tyrosine kinase (RTK) activation, two appear particularly important. PI3K activated by RTK is localized to plasma membranes, activates PDK1/2 then Akt (pAkt is the phosphorylated, active form). Akt, in turn, (also known as PKB) interrupts several components of the apoptosis cascade including BAD, caspase-9, p53, and the forkhead transcription factor FKHRL1. Moreover, the PI3K-PDK1/2-Akt pathway promotes axonal outgrowth (27, 28), the details of which are reviewed elsewhere (29, 30). Redundant support of neurons by RTKs, perhaps of lesser importance, occurs through the Ras-mitogen activated protein kinase (MAPK) pathway molecules, interacting with HSP27 and/or ATF-3 (31–33). All of these pathways may be amenable to newer downstream approaches toward enhancing growth factor actions.

Neuron populations and associated glial cells support themselves and their neighboring cells in several ways. These include autocrine, or self-supporting, and paracrine, or locally supporting fashions using neurotrophin-Trk interactions, retrograde support from targets, and support through the circulation (Figure 1). This has been described in DRG where both TrkC and NT-3 transcripts are produced, namely the factor and the receptor produced by the same population of cells (34) Indeed, evidence of the importance of this autocrine loop has been illustrated by Acheson and colleagues (35) demonstrating that adult sensory ganglia cells in culture had reduced survival when exposed to BDNF antisense oligonucleotides. Autocrine neurotrophin production may be used by adult neurons to resist retrograde apoptosis following axotomy because it compensates for variations in target tissue support of neurons (36).

There are complex interactions of the classical neurotrophins with other non-neurotrophin growth factors. For example, CNTF and LIF may antagonize the NGF action on DRG sensory neurons (37), and modulate chick embryonic sensory neuron NT-3 and NT-4-mediated survival by TGF-β and LIF (38).

Nerve Growth Factor

This growth factor and its high affinity receptor, Trk A, have trophic actions that appear to be largely, but not exclusively, confined to small sensory and sympathetic neurons. Trk A receptors are required for survival of developing sympathetic neurons (39). Since Trk A receptors are particularly expressed in sensory and sympathetic cell populations, the influence of NGF directly on motor systems may be limited. NGF-TrkA signals may act at several levels, including locally at growth cones, and retrograde by endosomal retrograde transport as a dimer to the cell body (40). There may be yet other mechanisms of very rapid retrograde signaling not involving actual transport of NGF or its receptor (41). Mice with TrkA knockout have severe neuronal loss in sensory and sympathetic ganglia as well as loss in the cholinergic forebrain, all incompatible with prolonged survival (42). There is evidence that NGF may stimulate BDNF transcription (43). The roles of NGF and TrkA in counteracting axotomy-induced changes in DRG neurons were reviewed

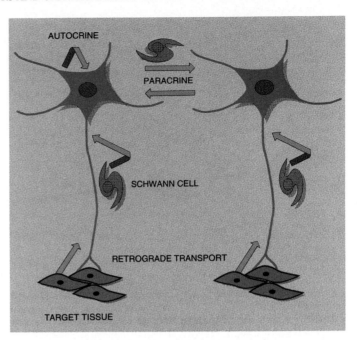

FIG. 1. An illustration of the potential routes of growth factor support of peripheral motor neurons. Growth factors may be elaborated by neurons themselves (autocrine support), between cell types in the spinal cord (paracrine), from glial cells such as Schwann cells or transported retrograde from the periphery (muscle). From, Zochodne DW, *Science and Medicine* 1999; 6:46–55, with permission.

in detail by Verge and coworkers (44). NGF is capable of reversing both declines in peptide and protein expression after axotomy (SP, α- and β CGRP, neurofilament M subunit, TrkA, p75, fluoride-resistant acid phosphatase) and neuronal atrophy. In addition, however, NGF prevents increases in other cellular constituents after axotomy such as galanin, NPY, VIP and CCK (44).

NGF administered in supraphysiological doses may have hyperplastic actions. Intraventricular administration of high doses of NGF induced sprouting of sensory fibers, sympathetic fibers, and SC hyperplasia in a curious subpial distribution in rats (45). Intraventricular administration of NGF into the rat CNS prompted sprouting of cerebrovascular perivascular catecholamine sympathetic fibers (46).

Brain Derived Neurotrophic Factor

First identified in conditioned media of glioma cell lines and subsequently isolated as a small basic protein from porcine central nervous system tissue (3, 47, 48), BDNF is transported retrograde to motor neurons from target muscle or from proliferating SC (11, 49–52). It is a potent motor neuron survival factor, rescuing neonatal spinal and cranial motor neurons from death after axotomy (53, 54). It also supports the survival of neurite outgrowth from neural placode-derived sensory ganglia, but unlike NGF, BDNF does not support sympathetic neurons (55). Some of the survival actions of BDNF involve facilitation of the anti-apoptotic factor Bcl-2 (56). Animals with a targeted disruption of the BDNF gene or BDNF knockout, survive postnatally for only a few weeks and have loss of vestibular neurons and DRG neurons, but not facial motor neurons (57). In contrast, knockout of the BDNF receptor gene, TrkB, is associated with yet earlier animal death after birth, and loss of both spinal and cranial facial motor neurons as well as DRG sensory neurons (58). This discrepancy indicates that BDNF alone is not required to support motor neuron survival, whereas other neurotrophins, such as NT 4/5, can compensate by activating the TrkB neurotrophin receptor.

The loss of cholinergic immunoreactivity in axotomized hypoglossal motor axons was prevented by central intraventricular infusions of BDNF or NT 4/5 but not NGF or NT-3 (59, 60). These findings correlated with the fact that the injured motoneurons expressed Trk B receptors and p75 but not Trk A or Trk C. Such central intraventricular delivery of BDNF is an approach that could allow direct access to neurons in central motor disorders. Ependymal cells however, express non-functional TrkB receptors capable of interrupting BDNF signaling. Such receptors, which are truncated and lack a tryrosine kinase component, form heterodimers with normal receptors and sequestrate BDNF (61–63).

Acting through TrkB, BDNF enhances synaptic efficacy in the hippocampus (64), and the maturation of NMDA receptors of cultured mouse cerebellar granule cells (65); and may play a role in the development of neuromuscular junctions (49, 66). BDNF, NT-3, and NT-4/5, but not NGF, increase the innervation of human muscle fibers co-cultured with rat spinal cord explants (67). BDNF mRNA is increased in rat brain after experimental cortical impact injury (68), and as discussed above, other trophic agents may influence BDNF, as for example, NGF acting through TrkA in the regulation of BDNF transcription in DRG cells (43, 69).

Neurotrophin-3

NT-3 is a 119 amino acid basic protein, that exerts its actions as a dimer (6, 70, 71). Although NT-3 primarily binds to Trk C and p75, there is also weak binding to TrkB (72). Like TrkB, Trk C also exists in truncated nonfunctional forms that may sequester the ligand and diminish its actions (73). NT-3 is essentially a sensory neurotrophin with supporting actions that differ from NGF because it supports large sensory neurons that relay such information as muscle spindle activity and proprioception. NT-3 thus promotes formation of proprioceptive, nodose sensory, auditory sensory, and possibly sympathetic neurons (74). NT-3, which reverses axotomy-related changes in neurofilament subunit expression (44), is transported retrograde by large sensory neurons that reside in DRG (11, 53). Motor neurons synthesize NT-3, (34) which is also expressed in muscle spindles (5, 75). In keeping with the complex actions of all of the neurotrophin family members, NT-3 supports the survival and differentiation of motor neurons and potentiates neuromuscular synapses in culture (76–78) but has no influence on adult sympathetic neurons (79). While the actions of NT-3 are mediated through Trk C, there is evidence that cooperative activation of Trk B and C, perhaps in part through NT-3, are important in promoting survival of other cell types such as hippocampal neurons and cerebellar granule neurons (80). During development, TrkB and TrkC transcripts appear in nigrostriatal neurons (81) and DRG sensory neurons. Mice lacking NT-3 or NT-3 knockouts have severe loss of spinal proprioceptive sensory neurons and peripheral sensory organs (82). TrkC deficient mice have loss of muscle sensory spindle sensory axons (83). During development, NT-3 also contributes to the development of neuromuscular junctions and enhances sprouting of corticospinal tracts (CST) (66). In adults, NT-3 promotes CST sprouting after injury and supports central noradrenergic cells (84, 85).

Other Neurotrophins

NT-4/5 supports the survival of developing sensory and sympathetic neurons (7). It has a more widespread distribution and its efficient signaling and retrograde transport depends on the presence of p75 receptors (86). NT4/5 derived from muscle acts as an activity-dependent trophic signal for adult rat motor neurons (87). Like BDNF, NT4/5 prevents retrograde facial motor neuron loss after axotomy in newborn rats and in adults, prevented alterations in adult motor neuron choline acetyltransferase after injury (88, 89).

NON-NEUROTROPHIN GROWTH FACTORS

Ciliary Neurotrophic Factor and Family

Ciliary neurotrophic factor is a 200 amino acid protein that was found to support the survival of sympathetic neurons in the embryonic chick ciliary ganglion. It is a member of the alpha helical cytokine superfamily that includes leukemia inhibitory factor (LIF), interleukin 6, granulocyte colony-stimulating factor and oncostatin M (90, 91). CNTF, LIF and a related growth factor, cardiotrophin-1 receptor, are linked to a signaling transducer known as gp130. In the case of CNTF, its receptor is made up of LIFRβ and CNTFRα, that complex with gp130. As is the case with many growth factors, SC are the primary source of CNTF in the PNS and their synthesis of the growth factor allows it to be taken up and transported retrograde by motor and sensory axons (92). The robust support that SC generally add to outgrowing axons, through a large menu of growth factors, is illustrated by the observation that adult sensory neurons in culture preferentially direct their outgrowing branches to a cluster of co-cultured SC and related satellite cells (Figure 2).

Retrograde transport of CNTF is accelerated after nerve injury. Levels of CNTF mRNA decline in SC if their contact with axons is lost; for example, distal to a nerve injury (93). It protects developing motor neurons from cell death (94, 95), and in the adult, CNTF offers a number of roles by preventing neuronal degeneration of axotomized medial septal neurons (96) and axotomized substantia nigra dopaminergic neurons (97); moreover, systemic injections induce sprouting by adult motor neurons (98, 99). Leukemia inhibitory factor (LIF) rescues neonatal motor and sensory neurons following axotomy (100, 101).

Insulin and Insulin-Like Growth Factors

Insulins and their cousins, the insulin-like growth factors (IGF), originally termed somatomedins, act as trophic molecules for neurons. Both IGF-1 and II are single-chain polypeptides with A and B domains resembling those of insulin, a connecting C domain resembling that of proinsulin, and D domain (102). Insulin and IGF-1 receptors share downstream transduction pathways and their ligands cross-occupy each other's receptors (103, 104). Insulin and IGF-1 receptors are autophosphorylated by ligand binding, develop tyrosine kinase activity, then activate downstream molecules through the IRS-1 and 2 docking protein pathways (105). Insulin receptor substrate (IRS)-1, frequently co-localizes with insulin and IGF-1 receptors, and contains multiple serine/threonine and tyrosine phosphorylation sites and activates the "survival" kinases PI-3K-Akt, as well as many other signals that include Shc, Grb-2,S6 kinase, PKCε kinase, MAP2 kinase, Raf1 kinase and cfos (106–108).

IGF circulates in the bloodstream, but is also synthesized by glial cells (109). Their actions are modulated by six IGF-binding proteins (IGFBP) in the circulation and in tissues (110). IGF-1 receptors (IGF-1R) are expressed on neurons and SC, allowing local support of regeneration in the microenvironment of injured peripheral nerves (111). They also promote myelination (112) whereas IGF-1 knockout mice have abnormalities of myelinated axons (113). IGF-1, which also supports neurons, blocked toxin-induced apoptosis in cerebellar neurons in culture (114), and hippocampal neuron survival through an interesting collaboration with BDNF (115).

Insulin supports the nervous system and may access neurons through the bloodstream or by local synthesis, as identified in neurons (116). In the PNS, insulin receptors (IR) are expressed on the perikarya of sensory neurons in DRG,

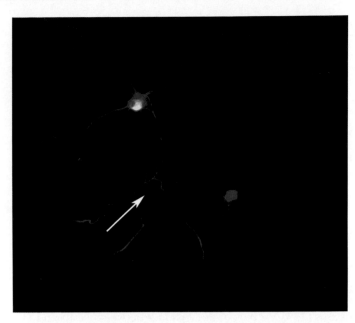

FIG. 2. Adult rat peripheral sensory neurons in vitro showing extensive neurite (axon precursor) formation. The arrow points to a collection of unstained glial cells in the culture that have attracted neurites to grow towards it. The image illustrates the robust impact that a menu of trophic factors, synthesized by glial cells, has on axon outgrowth. From Zochodne DW. *Neurobiology of Peripheral Nerve Regeneration,* Cambridge Press, 2008, with permission.

nodes of Ranvier and on regenerating axons (117, 118). Receptor expression rises after ipsilateral nerve injury and in diabetic neuropathy models (23, 119). Insulin promotes regeneration of peripheral axons and reverses features of experimental diabetic neuropathy independent of glucose levels following local near nerve or intrathecal administration (23, 119-122). Administration of insulin by the intranasal route accesses CSF and can also reverse features of experimental diabetic neuropathy (123). Intranasal insulin also reversed experimental diabetic leukoencephalopathy, a neurodegenerative disorder of white matter that develops in long-term models of diabetes (124, 125). Finally, IR is expressed in the terminals of sensory axons that innervate the skin (217).

GDNF

Glial cell line-derived neurotrophic factor (GDNF) belongs to the transforming growth factor β (TGFβ) family. Signaling occurs through receptors with two components: GPI-linked GFRα1-4, and the GDNF molecules neurturin, artemin and persephin, and receptor tyrosine kinase encoded by RET. GDNF interacts with the TGFβ family, tyrosine kinase and neural cell adhesion molecule (NCAM), reviewed elsewhere (126). In adults, GDNF is expressed in skeletal muscle and is retrograde transported by motor nerves (127, 128).

It supports several neuronal systems as, for example, dopaminergic neurons, indicating a potential role in Parkinson disease. It supports cerebellar Purkinje cells, spinal motor neurons, newborn rat facial motor neurons, axotomized adult facial nucleus motor neurons, and GABAergic embryonic neurons transplanted intraocular into adult rats (127–131). The actions of GDNF are more potent than those of BDNF, CNTF, or LIF, and together with its receptor, GFRα-I, rise to high levels of expression in SC during Wallerian-like degeneration distal to peripheral nerve injury (132). Failing reinnervation in distal nerve stumps over the long term, GDNF eventually declines to very low levels, indicating a limited ability to support regrowing axons (133). As part of its cross talk between axons and SC, GDNF may also influence the timing of axon myelination, as, for example, when exogenous GDNF administered to rats leads to proliferation of SC, as well as initiates inappropriate myelination of small caliber axons (134).

Growth Factors of Other Tissues

The fibroblast growth factor (FGF) family (135) now includes at least 23 members, but was originally divided into acidic FGF (aFGF) and basic FGF (bFGF) (136). FGF are bound in the extracellular matrix by heparan sulfate proteoglycans and, when released, act on receptor tyrosine kinases (137). They have been shown to have multiple roles during early brain development but also during adulthood and following injury. For example, FGF-1 is a known survival factor for injured rat spinal neurons (138). Alternatively, FGF-2 mRNA is increased in embryonic, but not adult, spinal cord injuries ·(139), possibly reflecting the better success of embryonic than adult spinal cord recovery post-injury. FGF influence cholinergic differentiation (135). Unilateral cortical infarction in rats treated with aFGF was associated with an increased concentration of NGF and NGF transcript ipsilateral to the lesion (140). They provide trophic support in survival and axon outgrowth for nerve regeneration. FGF receptors 2, 7, and 8, are expressed in sensory neurons (141–143). Additionally, the FGF receptor is upregulated in DRG neurons post-injury and these levels decrease following regeneration (144). bFGF potentiates motor neuron sprouting by CNTF (99) and rescues adult DRG cells in rats after a sciatic nerve section (145). One of the difficulties in studying FGF is the possibility that some of their apparent neuronal trophic actions may be indirect because they come from glial or supporting cells (135). Mice lacking the FGF receptors, Fgfr1 and Fgfr2, in SC developed abnormalities of nociceptive unmyelinated axons indicating a lack of trophic support by umyelinated SCs (146).

Additional growth factors not dealt with in further depth here but that have actions on the nervous system include epidermal growth factor (EGF) (147). EGF plays an important role in promoting stem cell development into neurons (148). Platelet-derived growth factors (PDGF) and their receptors are found on neurons and SC (149). Transforming growth factor β (TGFβ) is a large family of growth factors, of which types 1 and 2 are present in the peripheral nervous system (150–153). Erythropoietin (EPO) and its receptor are most often considered in the context of anemia associated with renal failure. However, both are expressed on neurons and SC (154). EPO may have potent actions on nerve regeneration. The expression of EPO and its receptor, EPO-R, rise in peripheral nerve axons and DRG neurons after injury (155). Local delivery of EPO by a conduit over two weeks to a rat sciatic nerve after crush injury increased the density and maturation of regenerating myelinated axons as well as the density and intensity of calcitonin gene-related peptide (CGRP) expression. Its action involves phosphorylation of Akt. One interesting facet of EPO is that its absence in patients with renal failure might account for uremic neuropathy, previously only reversible with transplantation (156). Interestingly, EPO is now routinely administered to renal patients whereas uremic neuropathy may be diminishing in prevalence.

The semaphorin family of molecules, widely express in the embryo, are secreted, membrane-associated, and influence the guidance, fasciculation, branching, and synapse formation of growing axons (157). Semaphorin 3A (Sema3A) acting on neuropilin receptors collapses growth cones. Sema3A and other family members however, may alternatively facilitate growth when acting in a different context. Overall, these actions may be influenced by the ambient intrinsic state of neuron or growth cone. Thus, it is possible that manipulation of semaphorin signaling in adults might have an impact both on regeneration or neuron degeneration. As inhibitory molecules, semaphorins may, for example, be critical in preventing inappropriate "wrong way" axon sprouting.

Pleiotrophin (PTN) belongs to the midkine (MK) family of heparin-binding growth factors (158) and is also known as heparin-binding growth associated molecule or heparin-binding neurotrophic factor. PTN and midkine are cysteine and basic amino-acid-rich proteins with 50% amino acid homology. They ligate low-density lipoprotein receptor-related protein (LRP-1), anaplastic lymphoma kinase (ALK), protein tyrosine phosphatase (PTP), and N-syndecan. PTN and MK promote neurite outgrowth (159, 160). In the peripheral nerve, PTN is acutely upregulated in nerve stumps distal to crush and is localized to SCs, macrophages, and endothelial cells (161, 162).

Hepatocyte growth factor (HGF), or "scatter factor" is a pleiotropic molecule that acts through the Met tyrosine kinase receptor (163). Macrophage stimulating protein (MSP) is a growth factor related to HGF (149). HGF supports spinal motor neurons through an autocrine loop (149, 163). HGF also acts as a mitogen in adult denervated SC cell populations, encouraging them to proliferate and support regenerative axon outgrowth (164, 165). Like other growth factors, HGF may have synergistic interactions with NGF through PI3K, PLC-γ, and Ras/MAPK pathways (163). c-Met, the HGF receptor, is expressed in small sensory neurons and in dermal cutaneous axons. In the skin, noninvasive stimuli are associated with local rises in HGF and in the downstream signaling molecule Rac 1 (166). This signaling pathway may contribute to the plasticity encountered in cutaneous axons. For example, after wounding or noninvasive stimulation, such as simple hair clipping, alterations in the density of cutaneous axons are associated with apparent activation of the HGF-c-Met-Rac1 pathway.

Vascular endothelial growth factor (VEGF) (167, 168) mediates vascular angiogenesis but it is also expressed in a subset of small ganglia neurons. Its receptor, fetal liver kinase receptor (flk-1), is also expressed in sensory ganglia neurons, their growth cones as well as SC. VEGF stimulates axon outgrowth from adult sensory ganglia and increases the survival of neurons and satellite cells (169). VEGF, like the neuregulins CGRP and HGF, also promotes SC proliferation, a critical event in facilitating axon regrowth. *In vivo*, local exogenous VEGF treatment increases outgrowth of axons, SC, or both (170, 171). Given the multiple roles of VEGF, it is possible that this signal promotes concurrent adjacent outgrowth of axons and blood vessels during nerve injuries.

Cytokines

Brain trauma activates expression of NGF through interleukin-1 β (IL-1β) (172). In peripheral nerves, IL-1 synthesized by macrophages stimulates NGF production in peripheral nerves by non-neuronal cells (173). In contrast, IL-6 has actions that differ from most cytokines in that it may act directly as a growth factor (174). Inflammation may generate several growth factors that have actions on neurons beyond those of the interleukins (175). Bone morphogenetic proteins (BMP) are cytokines that were initially discovered to support the formation of bone and cartilage but may have widespread actions, including an impact on nerve regrowth (176, 177) .

Novel Growth Factors

A number of other substances have been described as potential growth factors in the nervous system, including extracellular nucleotides and nucleosides (178), arachidonic acid

(179), and CGRP, which indirectly promote nerve regeneration by acting as a mitogen for SC cells (180, 181).

CGRP is upregulated in distal regenerating axon terminals from local axon synthesis despite decline in its cell body synthesis following axotomy injury. It offers several roles within injured nerves, including SC mitogen-related support for regenerative activity and potent vasoactive action on local nerve microvessels (182). Highlighting the importance of these roles, local knockdown of CGRP mRNA or its receptors dramatically attenuates axon outgrowth from the proximal stumps of transected peripheral nerves (181).

Cysteine-rich neurotrophic factor (CNRF) is a non-neurotrophin growth factor isolated from the mollusk *Lymnae stagnalis*, that promotes neurite outgrowth and influences motor neuron electrophysiological properties through its action on the p75 receptor (183).

Exploiting Growth Factor Signaling Cascades

Growth factor signals converge upon relatively few key pathways within neurons including MAPK-ERK, PLC-Υ1-IP3-DAG, JAK-STAT, and PI3K-Akt. Growth factor receptors interact with Ras that activates the protein kinase Raf, which in turn phophorylates MEK1 or MEK2 (MEK=MAPK and ERK kinases), and phosphorylates and activates ERK1 and ERK2. These second messenger pathways are of importance during peripheral nerve regeneration both within axons and in partnering SC (184).

The PI3K-Akt pathway has been of particular interest in regeneration. Its interruption impairs distal axon outgrowth in sensory neurons (185, 186). The p85 PI3K regulatory subunit interacts with phosphorylated epitopes of the cytoplasmic domain of activated receptor tyrosine kinases, utilized by many of growth factors, including insulin, IGF-1, and the neurotrophins. Subsequently, the p110 catalytic subunit (PIK3CA) of PI3K promotes the conversion of PI-4, 5-P2 (phosphoinosityl 4,5 diphosphate and PI(2)P) to PI-3,4,5-P3 [PI(3)P] that, in turn, phosphorylates to activate downstream Akt/PKB. pAkt has several targets, including glycogen synthase kinase 3β (GSK-3β), a multifunctional serine/threonine kinase, localized to leading edges of growth cones where it acts to suppress growth cone extension and axon formation (187). When phosphorylated through the PI3K-Akt/PKB signaling pathway, GSK-3β activity is shut down (188, 189). pAkt also inhibits FOXO3A nuclear signaling to suppress apoptosis. The overall PI3K-Akt pathway is illustrated in Figure 3.

Phosphatase and tensin homolog deleted on chromosome 10 (PTEN) is a phosphatase that inhibits the conversion of PI(2)P to PI(3)P. Pharmacological inhibition or siRNA knockdown of PTEN in the local microenvironment of regenerating peripheral nerves dramatically increases their outgrowth (190). Thus, by targeting an inhibitor of a central growth factor transduction pathway, growth signals within neurons are amplified as a potential new strategy to manipulate neuronal regrowth.

NEUROTROPHINS AND OTHER GROWTH FACTORS IN HUMAN DISEASE

Experimental Motor Disorders

The retrograde changes in motor neurons after axon section, or axotomy, have relevance in predicting the ability of human motor neurons to restore function after injury. For example, BDNF and NT-3 prevents axotomy-induced retrograde death of adult rat corticospinal neurons (191). Motor neuron degeneration in the wobbler mouse, a model of human motor neuron disease, is slowed by BDNF (192). In this autosomal recessive (AR) disease, there is muscle wasting and limb paralysis leading to difficulty with walking. Added CNTF had a synergistic benefit (193). Treatment of progressive motor neuronopathy (pmn) in mice, another AR

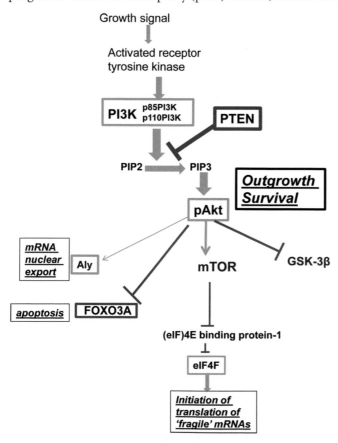

FIG. 3. A simplified version of the PI3K-Akt pathway that is important in the support and outgrowth of neurons. This pathway is activated by a number of growth factor ligands. Inhibition of the phosphatase PTEN offers a novel strategy to amplify growth factor signals.

model of human motor neuron disease, was more successful with CNTF than GDNF (194, 195). Gene therapy may provide another approach to drive local synthesis of specific growth factors in human motor neurons [see review (196)]. In transgenic ALS mice, retrograde delivery of IGF-1 in a recombinant adeno-associated virus (AAV) injected into muscle prolonged their lifespan by 30% (197).

Experimental Parkinsonism

The impact of growth factors on the substantia nigra of relevance to human Parkinson disease (PD) has been studied in a number of ways. Striatal neurons in culture have interesting but differential trophic support from several growth factors, including IGF-1, NT-3, and bFGF (198). Neurotrophins protect against experimental Parkinsonism induced by the toxin MPP+ in the striatum of neonatal rats. Kirschner and colleagues (199) reported that NGF, BDNF, bFGF, and NT-5, but not NT-3 were protective. NGF-producing neural stem cells transplanted into the striatum reduced damage from an excitotoxic lesion (200). The rat model of Parkinsonism induced by 6-hydroxydopamine (6-OHDA) has proven useful in identifying several potential roles for neurotrophic growth factors. In this model, infusion of NT-4/5, but not NT-3, enhanced the function of nigral grafts (201) whereas fibroblast grafts producing BDNF reduced loss of substantia nigra pars compacta domaninergic neurons (179). BDNF and NT4/5 also reversed alterations in neurotransmitter messages (202) while GDNF provided benefits both in this model and that of MPTP nigral injury in experimental Parkinsonism (202–205).

Nerve Regeneration

The impact of growth factors on regenerating nerves has been mixed (150). Since neurotrophins "turn off" features of the cell body regeneration program, their potential impact on fiber regeneration is uncertain. He and Chen (206) suggested that NGF improved motor nerve regeneration, and this finding was confirmed and extended to both motor and sensory recovery from sciatic lesions by Kemp and coworkers (207). High doses of NGF however inhibited regeneration. In another study, CNTF delivered locally by a mini-osmotic pump, improved regeneration of the rat sciatic nerve following transection whereas NGF was not effective (208). Insulin and IGF-II increases axon regeneration in rat sciatic nerves (23, 209)

To span sites of peripheral nerve transection, bioartificial grafts with embedded growth factors have been studied as an alternative to harvested sural nerve grafts. Lee and colleagues (210) used NGF in such a conduit or artificial graft and demonstrated improvements in rat axon regrowth. The benefits from NGF provided by this intervention were similar to that from the use of a nerve graft. As important as the delivery of the growth factor, there are two additional considerations. One is that a gradient is established to encourage new axons to grow in a directionally specific fashion to a distal stump (211). The second is the availability of growth factors delivered to injury sites.

Endogenous support by growth factors may vary depending on the axon type. For example, denervated and reinnervated cutaneous nerves, but not motor ventral roots, express mRNAs for NGF, BDNF, vascular endothelial growth factor, hepatocyte growth factor, and insulin-like growth factor-1. In contrast, motor ventral roots upregulated mRNAs for pleiotrophin (PTN) and glial cell-line-derived neurotrophic factor (164). PTEN inhibition enhances convergent downstream signaling, increasing the amount and extent of axon outgrowth from the proximal stumps of transected sciatic nerves (190).

Peripheral Neuropathy

Peripheral neuropathies with involvement of motor and sensory fibers may be treatable by neurotrophic factor and other agents. Axotomy or transection of peripheral nerves, has also provided an understanding of how retrograde changes influence the properties and gene expression of injured neurons. Such retrograde changes have important influences on how nerves may regenerate. NGF and NT-3 may benefit experimental diabetic neuropathy by reversing diabetes-related alterations in sensory neuron peptide expression and changes in axonal conduction velocity (212, 213). The expression of Trks may decline in long-term models of diabetic neuropathy, a change that may be important in promoting neurodegeneration (214). Both insulin and IGF may be important sources of trophic support to neurons and their availability is impaired in diabetes (215). Insulin itself, either by its actions on insulin receptors or by cross occupying IGF-1 receptors, is capable of reversing conduction abnormalities in experimental diabetes independently of blood levels of glucose, suggesting a direct trophic action (119, 120).

An important mechanism of recovery from neuropathies is collateral sprouting of axons from residual intact fibers into nearby denervated target organs. Collateral sprouting of motor and sensory fibers helps to reinnervate targets denervated from proximal lesions to nerves that are not likely to regenerate to their targets. Diamond and colleagues (216) have demonstrated that NGF supports collateral, but not regenerative, sensory axon sprouting in the skin. Local intraplantar doses of insulin, acting on insulin receptors expressed by cutaneous axons, reduced epidermal axon loss in experimental models of both type 1 and type 2 diabetes, without an impact on glucose levels (217).

NT-3 was found to be of benefit in the large fiber toxic sensory neuropathy caused by high doses of pyridoxine (218), and NGF repaired loss of peptides in DRG in experimental taxol neuropathy (219). NGF may benefit in cisplatin neuropathy (220).

Other

Interestingly, TrkB and TrkC mRNA transcripts decline in spinal motor neurons of rats with aging, suggesting that loss of trophic support could account for motor deficits observed in the elderly (221). In experimental cerebral infarcts of rats from middle cerebral artery occlusions, Kokaia and coworkers (222) noted transient rises in BDNF, NGF, and TrkB expression. The findings suggested that endogenous synthesis of BDNF and NGF play a role in recovery from human cerebral infarcts. FGFs have also been proposed for this indication (223). Primates with a quinolinic acid induced model of human Huntington's chorea given intrastriatal implants of polymer-encapsulated baby hamster kidney fibroblasts secreting human CNTF had evidence of neuroprotection (224). Growth factors may play a role in repair from spinal cord injury. Nakahara (225) implanted grafts of fibroblasts genetically modified to secrete NGF, NT-3, or bFGF into the central canal region of adult rat spinal cords. Sensory and noradrenergic dorsal root fibers were attracted into the graft. A separate report from the same group suggested NT-3 producing fibroblasts improved corticospinal tract regrowth and provided some functional recovery (226). Adding cAMP to NT-3 may confer additional benefits (227) whereas BDNF grafts had no influence. Liu and colleagues (228), in a separate work, noted regeneration of rubrospinal axons and recovery of forelimb function from implanted fibroblasts secreting BDNF in hemisected rat cervical spinal cords. Chronic infusion of NT-3 and BDNF promoted CNS axonal regeneration through semipermeable guidance channels bridging transected rat thoracic spinal cords (229). Finally, neurotrophins have been used to enhance the activity or survival of fetal neuronal grafts in adults. Sinson and coworkers (230) used this strategy in rats with fluid percussion brain injuries. NGF did not enhance transplant survival but improved memory.

CLINICAL TRIALS

An important criteria for the use of growth factors in human CNS and PNS is whether they can penetrate the blood-brain barrier and blood nerve barrier. Poduslo and Curran (231) provided information on the permeability-surface area of the trophins, noting the following order of permeability: BDNF approximately =NT-3>CNTF>>NGF for both the blood nerve and blood-brain barriers.

Motor Neuron Disease

Motor neuron disease (MND) has prompted particular interest in possible therapeutic benefits of neurotrophins and other growth factors. To date, human trials of specific growth factors have not been of clear benefit.

First, recombinant methionyl human BDNF in a Phase III trial had no overall benefit. Some post-hoc analyses of subgroups had improved survival i.e., those with gastrointestinal side effects that were classified as "responders" and those with respiratory vital capacities less than 91% (232).

Second, recombinant human insulin-like growth factor-1 (rhIGF-1) given subcutaneously for nine months had no benefit in one trial (233) and mild slowing of functional impairment and decline in health-related quality of life in another (234). A further two-year subcutaneous IGF-1 trial by Sorenson and coworkers (235) of 330 ALS patients from 20 medical centers was not beneficial. Some of the problems with subcutaneous IGF-1 in clinical trials have included tachycardia, dyspnea, hypoglycemia, hypotension, and microvascular proliferation (236).

Third, a Phase II-III trial of recombinant human CNTF (rHCNTF) given subcutaneously for nine months did not confer any benefit (237), similar to a second trial (238). CNTF was associated with injection site reactions, cough, asthenia, nausea, anorexia, weight loss, and unexpected increased salivation and there was an increased mortality rate with higher doses (238).

Fourth, Xaliproden, a non-petidic compound thought to have growth factor activity, given to 54 ALS patients for up to 32 weeks did not significantly slow their rate of deterioration in limb function but resulted in borderline slowing of deteriorating respiratory function in a subset of patients (239).

Lastly, a preliminary recent open labeled multicenter safety trial of granulocyte colony-stimulating factor in 24 patients with ALS reported a reduction in CSF levels of inflammatory markers. GCSF may recruit bone marrow cells to aid in CNS repair. There were few serious adverse events but no impact on the disease course was identified (240).

Polyneuropathy

A large multicenter trial of subcutaneous injections of recombinant human NGF (rhNGF) in diabetic neuropathy involving 1,019 patients did not identify benefits over a 48-month time period (241). This was a disappointing finding given that encouraging Phase II data had been reported earlier, possibly complicated by inadequate blinding from NGF-induced pain (242). In human immunodeficiency virus type 1- (HIV-1) related peripheral neuropathy rhNGF (200) improved measures of pain, but did not reduce analgesic use or increase epidermal skin axon innervation. Injection site discomfort was common (243).

A small trial of subcutaneous recombinant human BDNF (rhBDNF) involving 30 patients did not identify significant improvement in insulin–treated diabetic patients with neuropathy when administered over 85 days (244). A randomized pilot trial of subcutaneous BDNF in Guillain-Barre syndrome (GBS) patients was highly limited in scope but did not identify benefits of the neurotrophin over placebo (245).

Other

Benefits in manual muscle strength from recombinant human IGF-1 administration have been reported in a four-month Phase II trial of small numbers of patients with myotonic muscular dystrophy (246). NGF has been considered for Alzheimer disease, particularly its associated cholinergic neuron loss. Extensive primate studies have been completed, indicating that host fibroblasts engineered to produce NGF can remain viable and can rescue cholinergic cell loss or atrophy (247). Intranasal insulin accesses the CSF without the need for intrathecal administration and has been reported to improve cognition in patients with Alzheimer disease. Administration of 20 IU BID over 21 days improved attention, verbal memory, and functional status and increased the $A\beta40/42$ ratio in the serum of patients with early mild Alzheimer disease or mild cognitive impairment (248).

BDNF, NT-3, and GDNF have been considered for PD (249). A trial of GDNF given by intracerebroventricular catheters over eight months did not improve PD, but did induce nausea, vomiting, anorexia, weight loss, electrical sensations, and asymptomatic hyponatremia (250). It was uncertain whether this route of delivery accessed structures damaged in PD. An open labeled trial of intraputaminal injection of recombinant human GDNF in 34 patients with PD did not confer significant clinical benefit over six months despite an increase in ^{18}F Dopa uptake (251). Device and catheter related complications and the development of neutralizing antibodies were noted in three patients from each group. These findings contrasted with a smaller Phase I trial of ten patients with intraputaminal GDNF infusion that suggested a benefit of the approach (252). A more recent multicenter double-blinded randomized trial of AAV2- delivered intraputaminal neurturin, compared to sham surgery in 58 patients with advanced PD, did not demonstrate benefit over 12 months. Serious adverse effects were encountered in 13 of 38 AAV2-neuturin patients and four of 20 sham surgery patients that included myocardial infarction, pulmonary embolism, postoperative confusion, hemorrhage, seizures, mental changes, and urinary retention (253).

Summary and Overall Limitations in the Clinical Use of Growth Factors

Despite considerable enthusiasm for the direct use of growth factors, particularly neurotrophic factors, in the treatment of neurological disorders in mid to late 1990, enthusiasm for their use in trials has waned. Many investigators now realize that while such enthusiasm was appropriate, several critical aspects of the work contributed to disappointing results.

First, doses of trophic factors may have been several orders of magnitude too low to demonstrate efficacy. Delivery systems that can provide higher amounts of growth factors directly to the part of the nervous system where they may effect change may have better success. To this end, viral drug delivery systems, or the use of the intranasal delivery route, which directly accesses the CSF may be fruitful avenues for future work.

Second, target disease does not involve a growth factor-sensitive pathway: In many disorders, including ALS, it is uncertain whether the primary pathological derangement is reversible by any form of growth factor support. For example, in ALS, it is uncertain whether the central canonical survival pathway, PI3K-pAkt, is altered in targeted motor neurons, or whether the disorder compromises survival by as yet undefined, but separate, mechanisms (254, 255).

Third, when should growth factors be administered? For most neurological disorders and most growth factors, it is uncertain whether a preventive role or a regenerative role would best be served by their use. In the case of ALS, there may be substantial drop out of motor neurons before the disorder is recognized. Loss of the entire motor neuron tree only leaves the opportunity to prevent loss in remaining motor neuron populations.

Lastly, where are the receptors for the growth factor distributed? In the case of diabetic neuropathy, administration of rhNGF, for example, may only hope to influence the behavior of small nociceptive neurons expressing their high affinity receptor TrkA. Trial endpoints have not been designed to evaluate this specific population and there is no evidence that diabetic neuropathy is confined to this fiber population. Alternatively, it may be that NGF replenishment strategies signal, through low-affinity p75 receptors expressed in SCs that offer secondary support to a wider range of neurons. Despite these limitations, the widening range and repertoire of growth factors known to impact the nervous system offers hope for new therapeutic approaches. Exploiting their downstream signaling pathways selectively with targeted approaches may allow arrest or reversal of "permanent" neurological impairment.

ACKNOWLEDGMENTS

DZ has been supported by the Alberta Heritage Foundation for Medical Research (AHFMR) as an AHFMR Scientist and has received grant support from the Canadian Institutes of Health Research, the Canadian Diabetes Association, and the Juvenile Diabetes Research Foundation.

REFERENCES

1. Levi-Montalcini R, Hamburger V. A diffusible agent of mouse sarcoma, producing hyperplasia of sympathetic ganglia and hyperneurotization of viscera in the chick embryo. *J Exp Zool* 1953; 123:233–287.
2. Hefti F, Dento TL, Knusel B, et al. Neurotrophic factors: what are they and what are they doing? In: Loughlin SE, Fallon JH, eds. *Neurotropic factors*. Toronto: Academic Press, 1993; 25–49.
3. Barde YA, Edgar D, Thoenen H. Purification of a new neurotrophic factor from mammalian brain. *EMBO* 1982; 1:549–553.
4. Leibrock J, Lottspeich F, Hohn A, et al. Molecular cloning and expression of brain-derived neurotrophic factor. *Nature* 1989; 341:149–152.
5. Hory-Lee F, Russell M, Lindsay RM, et al. Neurotrophin 3 supports the survival of developing muscle sensory neurons in culture. *Proc Natl Acad Sci USA* 1993; 90:2613–2617.
6. Maisonpierre PC, Belluscio L, Squinto S, et al. Neurotrophin-3: a neurotrophic factor related to NGF and BDNF. *Science* 1990; 247:1446–1451.
7. Berkemeier LR, Winslow JW, Kaplan DR, et al. Neurotrophin-5: a novel neurotrophic factor that activates trk and trkB. *Neuron* 1991; 7:857–866.
8. Gotz R, Koster R, Winkler C, et al. Neurotrophin-6 is a new member of the nerve growth factor family. *Nature* 1994; 372:266–269.
9. Hendry IA, Stockel K, Thoenen H, et al. The retrograde axonal transport of nerve growth factor. *Brain Res* 1974; 68:103–121.
10. Schmidt RE, Yip HK. Retrograde axonal transport in rat ileal mesenteric nerves. Characterization using intravenously administered 125I-nerve growth factor and effect of chemical sympathectomy. *Diabetes* 1985; 34:1222–1229.
11. DiStefano PS, Friedman B, Radziejewski C, et al. The neurotrophins BDNF, NT-3, and NGF display distinct patterns of retrograde axonal transport in peripheral and central neurons. *Neuron* 1992; 8:983–993.
12. Rabizadeh S, Oh J, Zhong L-T, et al. Induction of apoptosis by the low-affinity NGF receptor. *Science* 1993; 261:345–348.
13. Chao MV, Hempstead BL. p75 and Trk: a two receptor system. *Trends Neurosci* 1995; 18:321–326.
14. Luo L, Jan LY, Jan YN. Rho family GTP-binding proteins in growth cone signaling. *Curr Opin Neurobiol* 1997; 7:81–86.
15. Yuan XB, Jin M, Xu X, et al. Signalling and crosstalk of Rho GTPases in mediating axon guidance. *Nat Cell Biol* 2003; 5:38–45.
16. Niederost B, Oertle T, Fritsche J, et al. Nogo-A and myelin-associated glycoprotein mediate neurite growth inhibition by antagonistic regulation of RhoA and Rac1. *J Neurosci* 2002; 22:10368–10376.
17. Kaplan DR, Miller FD. Axon growth inhibition: signals from the p75 neurotrophin receptor. *Nat Neurosci* 2003; 6:435–436.
18. Gehler S, Gallo G, Veien E, et al. p75 neurotrophin receptor

signaling regulates growth cone filopodial dynamics through modulating RhoA activity. *J Neurosci* 2004; 24:4363–4372.

19. Yamashita T, Tohyama M. The p75 receptor acts as a displacement factor that releases Rho from Rho-GDI. *Nat Neurosci* 2003; 6:461–467.

20. Lee R, Kermani P, Teng KK, et al. Regulation of cell survival by secreted proneurotrophins. *Science* 2001; 294:1945–1948.

21. Ibanez CF. Jekyll-Hyde neurotrophins: the story of proNGF. *Trends Neurosci* 2002; 2 5:284–286.

22. Begum N, Sandu OA, Duddy N. Negative regulation of rho signaling by insulin and its impact on actin cytoskeleton organization in vascular smooth muscle cells: role of nitric oxide and cyclic guanosine monophosphate signaling pathways. *Diabetes* 2002; 51:2256–2263.

23. Xu QG, Li X-Q, Kotecha SA, et al. Insulin as an in vivo growth factor. *Exp Neurol* 2004; 188:43–51.

24. Giniger E. How do Rho family GTPases direct axon growth and guidance? A proposal relating signaling pathways to growth cone mechanics. *Differentiation* 2002; 70:385–396.

25. Jing S, Tapley P, Barbacid M. Nerve growth factor mediates signal transduction through trk homodimer receptors. *Neuron* 1992; 9:1067–1079.

26. Glass DJ, Yancopoulos GD. The neurotrophins and their receptors. *Trends Cell Biol* 1993; 3:262–268.

27. Brunet A, Datta SR, Greenberg ME. Transcription-dependent and -independent control of neuronal survival by the PI3K-Akt signaling pathway. *Curr Opin Neurobiol* 2001; 11:297–305.

28. Namikawa K, Honma M, Abe K, et al. Akt/protein kinase B prevents injury-induced motoneuron death and accelerates axonal regeneration. *J Neurosci* 2000; 15; 20:2875–2886.

29. Franke TF, Hornik CP, Segev L, et al. PI3K/Akt and apoptosis: size matters. *Oncogene* 2003; 22:8983–8998.

30. Hanada M, Feng J, Hemmings BA. Structure, regulation and function of PKB/AKT—a major therapeutic target. *Biochim Biophys Acta* 2004; 1697:3–16.

31. Nakagomi S, Suzuki Y, Namikawa K, et al. Expression of the activating transcription factor 3 prevents c-Jun N-terminal kinase-induced neuronal death by promoting heat shock protein 27 expression and Akt activation. *J Neurosci* 2003; 23:5187–5196.

32. Campenot RB, Eng H. Protein synthesis in axons and its possible functions. J Neurocytol 2000; 29:793–798.

33. Kaplan DR, Miller FD. Neurotrophin signal transduction in the nervous system. *Curr Opin Neurobiol* 2000; 10:381–391.

34. Tojo H, Takami K, Kaisho Y, et al. Analysis of neurotrophin-3 expression using the lacZ reporter gene suggests its local mode of neurotrophic activity. *Neuroscience* 1996; 7 1:221–230.

35. Acheson A, Conover JC, Fandl JP, et al. A BDNF autocrine loop in adult sensory neurons prevents cell death. Nature 1995; 374:450–453.

36. Lindsay RM. Role of neurotrophins and trk receptors in the development and maintenance of sensory neurons: an overview. *Philos Trans R Soc Lond B Biol Sci* 1996; 351:365–373.

37. Mulderry PK. Neuropeptide expression by newborn and adult rat sensory neurons in culture: effects of nerve growth factor and other neurotorphic factors. *Neuroscience* 1994; 59:673–688.

38. Krieglstein K, Unsicker K. Distinct modulatory actions of TGF-beta and LIF on neurotrophin-mediated survival of developing sensory neurons. *Neurochem Res* 1996; 21:843–850.

39. Fagan AM, Zhang H, Landis S, et al. TrkA, but not TrkC, receptors are essential for survival of sympathetic neurons in vivo. *J Neurosci* 1996; 16:6208–6218.

40. Reichardt LF, Mobley WC. Going the distance, or not, with neurotrophin signals. Cell 2004; 118:141–143.

41. MacInnis BL, Campenot RB. Retrograde support of neuronal survival without retrograde transport of nerve growth factor. *Science* 2002; 295:1536–1539.

42. Smeyne RJ, Klein R, Schnapp A, et al. Severe sensory and sympathetic neuropathies in mice carrying a disrupted Trk/NGF gene. *Nature* 1994; 368:246–249.

43. Apfel SC, Wright DE, Wiideman AM, et al. Nerve growth factor regulates the expression of brain-derived neurotrophic factor mRNA in the peripheral nervous system. *Mol Cell Neurosci* 1996; 7:134–142.

44. Verge VMK, Gratto KA, Karchewski LA, et al. Neurotrophins and nerve injury in the adult. *Philos Trans R Soc Lond B Biol Sci* 1996; 351:423–430.

45. Winkler J, Ramirez GA, Kuhn G, et al. Reversible Schwann cell hyperplasia and sprouting of sensory and sympathetic neurities after intraventribular administration of nerve growth factor. *Ann Neurol* 1997; 41:82–93.

46. Isaacson LG, Billieu SG. Increased perivascular norepinephrine following intracerebroventricular infusion of NGF into adult rats. *Exp Neurol* 1996; 39:54–60.

47. Monard D, Stockel K, Goodman R, et al. Distinction between nerve growth factor anf glial factor. *Nature* 1975; 258:444–445.

48. Monard D, Solomon F, Rentsch M, et al. Glia-induced morphological differentiation in neuroblastoma cells. *Proc Natl Acad Sci USA* 1973; 70:1894–1897.

49. Kwon YW, Gurney ME. Brain-derived neurotrophic factor transiently stabilizes silent synapses on developing neuromuscular junctions. *J Neurobiol* 1996; 29:503–516.

50. Piehl F, Frisen J, Risling M, et al. Increased trkB mRNA expression by axotomized motoneurones. *NeuroReport* 1994; 5:697–700.

51. Meyer M, Matsuoka I, Wetmore C, et al. Enhanced synthesis of brain-derived neurotrophic factor in the lesioned peripheral nerve: different mechanisms are responsible for the regulation of BDNF and NGF mRNA. *J Cell Biol* 1992; 119:45–54.

52. Griesbeck O, Parsadanian AS, Sendtner M, et al. Expression of neurotrophins in skeletal muscle: quantitative comparison and significance for motoneuron survival and maintenance of function. *J Neurosci Res* 1995; 42:21–33.

53. Yan Q, Elliott JL, Matheson C, et al. Influences of neurotrophins on mammalian motoneurons in vivo. *J Neurobiol* 1993; 24:1555–1577.

54. Oppenheim RW, Yin QW, Prevette D, et al. Brain-derived neurotrophic factor rescues developing avian motoneurons from cell death. *Nature* 1992; 360:755–757.

55. Lindsay RM, Rohrer H. Placodal sensory neurons in culture: nodose ganglion neurons are unresponsive to NGF, lack NGF receptors but are supported by a liver-derived neurotrophic factor. *Dev Biol* 1985; 112:30–48.

56. Allsopp TE, Kiselev S, Wyatt S, et al. Role of Bcl-2 in the brain-derived neurotrophic factor survival response. *Eur J Neurosci* 1995; 7:1266–1272.

57. Jones KR, Farifias I, Backus C, et al. Targeted disruption of the BDNF gene perturbs brain and sensory neuron development but not motor neuron development. *Cell* 1994; 76:989–999.

58. Klein R, Smeyne RJ, Wurst W, et al. Targeted disruption of the trkB neurotrophin receptor gene results in nervous system lesions and neonatal death. *Cell* 1993; 75:113–122.

59. Tuszynski MH, Mafong E, Meyer S. Central infusions of brain-derived neurotrophic factor and neurotrophin-4/5, but not nerve growth factor and neurotrophin-3, prevent loss of the cholinergic phenotype in injured adult motor neurons. *Neuroscience* 1996; 71:761–771.

60. Yan Q, Matheson C, Lopez OT, et al. The biological responses of axotomized adult motoneurons to brain-derived neurotrophic factor. *J Neurosci* 1994; 14:5281–5291.

61. Yan Q, Matheson C, Sun J, et al. Distribution of intracerebral ventricularly administered neurotrophins in rat brain and its correlation with trk receptor expression. *Exp Neurol* 1994; 127:23–36.

62. Anderson KD, Alderson RF, Altar CA, et al. Differential distribution of exogenous BDNF, NGF, and NT-3 in the brain corresponds to the relative abundance and distribution of high-affinity and low-affinity neurotrophin receptors. *J Comp Neurol* 1995; 357:296–317.

63. Eide FF, Vining ER, Eide BL, et al. Naturally occurring truncated trkB receptors have dominant inhibitory effects on brain-derived neurotrophic factor signaling. *J Neurosci* 1996; 16:3123–3129.

64. Levine ES, Dreyfus CF, Black IB, et al. Selective role for trkB neurotrophin receptors in rapid modulation of hippocampal synaptic transmission. *Brain Res Mol Brain Res* 1996; 38:300–303.

65. Muzet M, Dupont JL. Enhancement of NMDA receptor maturation by BDNF in cultured mouse cerebellar granule cells. *NeuroReport* 1996; 7:548–552.

66. Wang T, Xie K, Lu B. Neurotrophins promote maturation of developing neuromuscular synapses. *J Neurosci* 1995; 15:4796–4805.

67. Braun S, Croizat B, Lagrange MC, et al. Neurotrophins increase motoneurons' ability to innervate skeletal muscle fibers in rat spinal cord--human muscle cocultures. *J Neurol Sci* 1996; 136:17–23.

68. Yang K, Perez-Polo JR, Mu XS, et al. Increased expression of brain-derived neurotrophic factor but not neurotrophin-3 mRNA in rat brain after cortical impact injury. *J Neurosci Res* 1996; 44:157–164.

69. Apfel SC, Wright DE, Dromia C, t al. Nerve growth factor stimulates BDNF mRNA expression the peripheral nervous system. *Soc Neurosci Abs* 1995; 21:196.Abstract

70. Hohn A, Leibrock J, Bailey K, et al. Identification and characterization of a novel member of the nerve growth factor/brain-derived neurotrophic factor family. *Nature* 1990; 344:339–341.

71. Radziejewski C, Robinson RC, DiStefano PS, et al. Dimeric structure and conformational stability of brain-derived neurotrophic factor and neurotrophin-3. *Biochemistry* 1992; 31:4431–4436.

72. Chao MV. Neurotrophin receptors: a window into neuronal differentiation. *Neuron* 1992; 9:583–593.

73. Valenzuela DM, Maisonpierre PC, Glass DJ, et al. Alternative forms of rat TrkC with different functional capabilities. *Neuron* 1993; 10:963–974.

74. Chalazonitis A. Neurotrophin-3 as an essential signal for the developing nervous system. *Mol Neurobiol* 1996; 12:39–53.

75. Copray JC, Brouwer N. Selective expression of neurotrophin-3 messenger RNA in muscle spindles of the rat. *Neuroscience* 1994; 63:1125–1135.

76. Wong V, Arriaga R, Ip NY, et al. The neurotrophins BDNF, NT-3 and NT-4/5, but not NGF, up- regulate the cholinergic phenotype of developing motor neurons. *Eur J Neurosci* 1993; 5:466–474.

77. Henderson CE, Camu W, Mettling C, et al. Neurotrophins promote motor neuron survival and are present in embryonic limb bud. *Nature* 1993; 363:266–270.

78. Lohof AM, Ip NY, Poo M-M. Potentiation of developing neuromuscular synapses by the neurotrophins NT-3 and BDNF. *Nature* 1993; 363:350–353.

79. Birren SJ, Lo L, Anderson DJ. Sympathetic neuroblasts undergo a developmental switch in trophic dependence. *Development* 1993; 119:597–610.

80. Minichiello L, Klein R. TrkB and TrkC neurotrophin receptors cooperate in promoting survival of hippocampal and cerebellar granule neurons. *Genes Dev* 1996; 10:2849–2858.

81. Jung AB, Bennett JR, Jr. Development of striatal dopaminergic function. III: pre- and postnatal development of striatal and cortical mRNAs for the neurotrophin receptors Trk BTK+ and Trk C and their regulation by synaptic dopamine. *Brain Res* 1996; 94:133–143.

82. Farinas I, Jones KR, Backus C, et al. Severe sensory and sympathetic deficits in mice lacking neurotrophin-3. *Nature* 1994; 369:658–661.

83. Klein R, Silos-Santiago I, Smeyne RJ, et al. Disruption of the neurotrophin-3 receptor gene trkC eliminates la muscle afferents and results in abnormal movements. *Nature* 1994; 368:249–251.

84. Schnell L, Schneider R, Kolbeck R, et al. Neurotrophin-3 enhances sprouting of corticospinal tract during development and after adult spinal cord lesion. *Nature* 1994; 3 67:170–173.

85. Arenas E, Persson H. Neurotrophin-3 prevents the death of adult central noradrenergic neurons in vivo. *Nature* 1994; 367:368–371.

86. Ibanez CF. Neurotrophin-4: the odd one out in the neurotrophin family. *Neurochem Res* 1996; 21:787–793.

87. Funakoshi H, Belluardo N, Arenas E, et al. Muscle-derived neurotrophin-4 as an activity-dependent trophic signal for adult motor neurons. *Science* 1995; 268:1495–1499.

88. Koliatsos VE, Cayouette MH, Berkemeier LR, et al. Neurotrophin 4/5 is a trophic factor for mammalian facial motor neurons. *Proc Natl Acad Sci USA* 1994; 91:3304–3308.

89. Friedman B, Kleinfeld D, Ip NY, et al. BDNF and NT-4/5 exert neurotrophic influences on injured adult spinal motor neurons. *J Neurosci* 1995; 15:1044–1056.

90. Bazan JF. Neuropoietic cytokines in the hematopoietic fold. *Neuron* 1991; 7:197–208.

91. Hall AK, Rao MS. Cytokines and neurokines: related ligands and related receptors. *Trends Neurosci* 1992; 15:35–37.

92. Curtis R, Adryan KM, Zhu Y, et al. Retrograde axonal transport of ciliary neurotrophic factor is increased by peripheral nerve injury. *Nature* 1993; 365:253–255.

93. Sendtner M, Stockli KA, Thoenen H. Synthesis and localization of ciliary neurotrophic factor in the sciatic nerve of the adult rat after lesion and during regeneration. *J Cell Biol* 1992; 118:139–148.

94. Arakawa Y, Sendtner M, Thoenen H. Survival effect of ciliary neurotrophic factor (CNTF) on chick embryonic motoneurons in culture: comparison with other neurotrophic factors and cytokines. *J Neurosci* 1990; 10:3507–3515.

95. Sendtner M, Kreutzberg GW, Thoenen H. Ciliary neurotrophic factor prevents the degeneration of motor neurons after axotomy. *Nature* 1990; 345:440–441.

96. Hagg T, Quon D, Higaki J, et al. Ciliary neurotrophic factor prevents neuronal degeneration and promotes low affinity NGF receptor expression in the adult rat CNS. *Neuron* 1992; 8:145–158.

97. Hagg T, Varon S. Ciliary neurotrophic factor prevents degeneration of adult rat substantia nigra dopaminergic neurons in vivo. *Proc Natl Acad Sci USA* 1993; 90:6315–6319.

98. Kwon YW, Gurney ME. Systemic injections of ciliary neurotrophic factor induce sprouting by adult motor neurons. *NeuroReport* 1994; 5:789–792.

99. Gurney ME, Yamamoto H, Kwon Y. Induction of motor neuron sprouting in vivo by ciliary neurotrophic factor and basic fibroblast growth factor. *J Neurosci* 1992; 12:3241–3247.

100. Cheema SS, Richards L, Murphy M, et al. Leukemia inhibitory factor prevents the death of axotomised sensory neurons in the dorsal root ganglia of the neonatal rat. *J Neurosci Res* 1994; 37:213–218.

101. Cheema SS, Richards LJ, Murphy M, et al. Leukaemia

inhibitory factor rescues motoneurones from axotomy-induced cell death. *NeuroReport* 1994; 5:989–992.

102. Le Roith D, Roberts CT, Jr. Insulin-like growth factors. *Ann NY Acad Sci* 1993; 692:1–9.

103. Ullrich A, Gray A, Tam AW, et al. Insulin-like growth factor I receptor primary structure: comparison with insulin receptor suggests structural determinants that define functional specificity. *EMBO* 1986; 5:2503–2512.

104. Steele-Perkins G, Turner J, Edman JC, et al. Expression and characterization of a functional human insulin- like growth factor I receptor. *J Biol Chem* 1988; 263:11486–11492.

105. White MF. The insulin signalling system and the IRS proteins. *Diabetologia* 1997; 40:S2–S17.

106. Heidenreich KA. Insulin and IGF-I receptor signaling in cultured neurons. *Ann NY Acad Sci* 1993; 692:72–88.

107. Fadool DA, Tucker K, Phillips, et al. Brain insulin receptor causes activity-dependent current suppression in the olfactory bulb through multiple phosphorylation of Kv1.3. *J Neurophysiol* 2000; 83:2332–2348.

108. Folli F, Bonfanti L, Renard E, et al. Insulin receptor substrate-1 (IRS-1) distribution in the rat central nervous system. *J Neurosci* 1994; 14:6412–6422.

109. Zochodne DW, Cheng C. Neurotrophins and other growth factors in the regenerative milieu of proximal nerve stump tips. *J Anat* 2000; 196:279–283.

110. Baxter RC, Martin JL. Binding proteins for the insulin-like growth factors: structure, regulation and function. *Prog Growth Factor Res* 1989; 1:49–68.

111. Cheng HL, Randolph A, Yee D, et al. Characterization of insulin-like growth factor-I and its receptor and binding proteins in transected nerves and cultured Schwann cells. *J Neurochem* 1996; 66:525–536.

112. Cheng HL, Russell JW, Feldman EL. IGF-I promotes peripheral nervous system myelination. *Ann NY Acad Sci* 1999; 883:124–130.

113. Gao WQ, Shinsky N, Ingle G, et al. IGF-1 deficient mice show reduced peripheral nerve conduction velocities and decreased axonal diameters and respond to exogenous IGF-1 treatment. *J Neurobiol* 1999; 39:142–152.

114. Fernandez-Sanchez MT, Garcia-Rodriguez A, Diaz-Trelles R, et al. A. Inhibition of protein phosphatases induces IGF-1-blocked neurotrophin-insensitive neuronal apoptosis. *FEBS Lett* 1996; 398:106–112.

115. Lindholm D, Carroll P, Tzimagiogis G, et al. Autocrine-paracrine regulation of hippocampal neuron survival by IGF-1 and the neurotrophins BDNF, NT-3 and NT-4. *Eur J Neurosci* 1996; 8:1452–1460.

116. Devaskar SU, Giddings SJ, Rajakumar PA, et al. Insulin gene expression and insulin synthesis in mammalian neuronal cells. *J Biol Chem* 1994; 269:8445–8454.

117. Sugimoto K, Murakawa Y, Sima AA. Expression and localization of insulin receptor in rat dorsal root ganglion and spinal cord. *J Peripher Nerv Syst* 2002; 7:44–53.

118. Sugimoto K, Murakawa Y, Zhang W, et al. Insulin receptor in rat peripheral nerve: its localization and alternatively spliced isoforms. *Diabetes Metab Res Rev* 2000; 16:354–363.

119. Brussee V, Cunningham FA, Zochodne DW. Direct insulin signaling of neurons reverses diabetic neuropathy. *Diabetes* 2004; 53:1824–1830.

120. Singhal A, Cheng C, Sun H, et al. Near nerve local insulin prevents conduction slowing in experimental diabetes. *Brain Res* 1997; 763:209–214.

121. Toth C, Brussee V, Martinez JA, et al. Rescue and regeneration of injured peripheral nerve axons by intrathecal insulin. *Neuroscience* 2006; 139:429–449.

122. Toth C, Brussee V, Zochodne DW. Remote neurotrophic support of epidermal nerve fibres in experimental diabetes. *Diabetologia* 2006; 49:1081–1088.

123. Francis G, Martinez J, Liu W, et al. Intranasal Insulin Ameliorates Experimental Diabetic Neuropathy. *Diabetes*; 58:934–945.

124. Toth C, Schmidt AM, Tuor UI, et al. Diabetes, leukoencephalopathy and rage. *Neurobiol Dis* 2006; 23:445–461.

125. Francis GJ, Martinez JA, Liu WQ, et al. Intranasal insulin prevents cognitive decline, cerebral atrophy and white matter changes in murine type I diabetic encephalopathy. *Brain* 2008; 131:3311–3334.

126. Sariola H, Saarma M. Novel functions and signalling pathways for GDNF. *J Cell Sci* 2003; 116:3855–3862.

127. Henderson CE, Phillips HS, Pollock RA, et al. GDNF: A potent survival factor for motoneurons present in peripheral nerve and muscle. *Science* 1994; 266:1062–1064.

128. Yan Q, Matheson C, Lopez OT. In vivo neurotrophic effects of GDNF on neonatal and adult facial motor neurons. *Nature* 1995; 373:341–344.

129. Lin LF, Doherty DH, Lile JD, et al. GDNF: a glial cell line-derived neurotrophic factor for midbrain dopaminergic neurons. *Science* 1993; 260:1130–1132.

130. Mount HT, Dean DO, Alberch J, et al. Glial cell line-derived neurotrophic factor promotes the survival and morphologic differentiation of Purkinje cells. *Proc Natl Acad Sci USA* 1995; 92:9092–9096.

131. Price ML, Hoffer BJ, Granholm AC. Effects of GDNF on fetal septal forebrain transplants in oculo. *Exp Neurol* 1996; 141:181–189.

132. Hoke A, Cheng C, Zochodne DW. Expression of glial cell line-derived neurotrophic factor family of growth factors in peripheral nerve injury in rats. *NeuroReport* 2000; 11:1651–1654.

133. Hoke A, Gordon T, Zochodne DW, et al. A decline in glial cell-line-derived neurotrophic factor expression is associated with impaired regeneration after long-term Schwann cell denervation. *Exp Neurol* 2002; 173:77–85.

134. Hoke A, Ho T, Crawford TO, et al. Glial cell line-derived neurotrophic factor alters axon Schwann cell units and promotes myelination in unmyelinated nerve fibers. *J Neurosci* 2003; 23:561–567.

135. Unsicker K, Grothe C, Ludecke G, et al. Fibroblast growth factors: their roles in the central and peripheral nervous system. In: Louglin SE, Fallon JH, eds. *Neurotrophic Factors*. Toronto: Academic Press, 1993:313–338.

136. Reuss B, von Bohlen, Halbach O. Fibroblast growth factors and their receptors in the central nervous system. *Cell Tissue Res* 2003; 313:139–157.

137. Lobb RR. Clinical applications of heparin-binding growth factors. *Eur J Clin Invest* 1988; 18:321–336.

138. Lee YS, Baratta J, Yu J, Lin VW, et al. AFGF promotes axonal growth in rat spinal cord organotypic slice co-cultures. *J Neurotrauma* 2002; 19:357–367.

139. Qi ML, Wakabayashi Y, Haro H, et al. Changes in FGF-2 expression in the distal spinal cord stump after complete cord transection: a comparison between infant and adult rats. *Spine* 2003; 28:1934–1940.

140. Figueiredo BC, Pluss K, Skup M, et al. Acidic FGF induces NGF and its mRNA in the injured neocortex of adult animals. *Brain Res Mol Brain Res* 1995; 33:1–6.

141. Li GD, Wo Y, Zhong MF, et al. Expression of fibroblast growth factors in rat dorsal root ganglion neurons and regulation after peripheral nerve injury. *NeuroReport* 2002; 13:1903–1907.

142. Tanaka A, Kamiakito T, Hakamata Y, et al. Extensive neuronal localization and neurotrophic function of fibroblast growth factor 8 in the nervous system. *Brain Res* 2001; 912:105–115.

143. Salvarezza SB, Lopez HS, Masco DH. The same cellular signaling pathways mediate survival in sensory neurons that switch their trophic requirements during development. *J Neurochem* 2003; 85:1347–1358.

144. Kato H, Wanaka A, Tohyama M. Co-localization of basic fibroblast growth factor-like immunoreactivity and its receptor mRNA in the rat spinal cord and the dorsal root ganglion. *Brain Res* 1992; 576:351–354.

145. Otto D, Unsicker K, Grothe C. Pharmacological effects of nerve growth factor and fibroblast growth factor applied to the transectioned sciatic nerve on neuron death in adult rat dorsal root ganglia. *Neurosci Lett* 1987; 83:156–160.

146. Furusho M, Dupree JL, Bryant M, et al. Disruption of fibroblast growth factor receptor signaling in nonmyelinating Schwann cells causes sensory axonal neuropathy and impairment of thermal pain sensitivity. *J Neurosci* 2009; 29:1608–1614.

147. Morrison R. Epidermal growth factor: structure, expression and functions in the central nervous system. In: Louglin SE, Fallon JH, eds. *Neurotrophic Factors*. Toronto: Academic Press, 1993; 339–357.

148. Reynolds BA, Weiss S. Generation of neurons and astrocytes from isolated cells of the adult mammalian central nervous system. *Science* 1992; 255:1707–1710.

149. Landreth GE. Growth Factors. In: Siegel GJ, Albers RW, Brady ST, Price DL, eds. *Basic Neurochemistry*, 7th ed. New York: Academic Press, 2006; 471–484.

150. Zochodne DW. *Neurobiology of peripheral nerve regeneration*. Cambridge: Cambridge, 2008.

151. Jiang Y, McLennan IS, Koishi K, et al. Transforming growth factor-beta 2 is anterogradely and retrogradely transported in motoneurons and up-regulated after nerve injury. *Neuroscience* 2000; 97:735–742.

152. Day WA, Koishi K, McLennan IS. Transforming growth factor beta 1 may regulate the stability of mature myelin sheaths. *Exp Neurol* 2003; 184:857–864.

153. Puolakkainen P, Twardzik DR. Transforming growth factors alpha and beta. In: Loughlin SE, Fallon JH, eds. *Neurotrophic factors*. Toronto: Academic Press, 1993; 359–389.

154. Campana WM, Myers RR. Erythropoietin and erythropoietin receptors in the peripheral nervous system: changes after nerve injury. *FASEB J* 2001; 15:1804–1806.

155. Toth C, Martinez JA, Liu WQ, et al. Local erythropoietin signaling enhances regeneration in peripheral axons. *Neuroscience* 2008; 154:767–783.

156. Bolton CF, Baltzan MA, Baltzan RB. Effects of renal transplantation on uremic neuropathy. A clinical and electrophysiologic study. *N Engl J Med* 1971; 284:1170–1175.

157. Gavazzi I. Semaphorin-neuropilin-1 interactions in plasticity and regeneration of adult neurons. *Cell Tissue Res* 2001; 305:275–284.

158. Kadomatsu K, Muramatsu T. Midkine and pleiotrophin in neural development and cancer. *Cancer Lett* 2004; 204:127–143.

159. Li YS, Milner PG, Chauhan AK, et al. Cloning and expression of a developmentally regulated protein that induces mitogenic and neurite outgrowth activity. *Science* 1990; 250:1690–1694.

160. Kaneda N, Talukder AH, Nishiyama H, et al. Midkine, a heparin-binding growth/differentiation factor, exhibits nerve cell adhesion and guidance activity for neurite outgrowth in vitro. *J Biochem* (Tokyo) 1996; 119:1150–1156.

161. Blondet B, Carpentier G, Lafdil F, et al. Pleiotrophin cellular localization in nerve regeneration after peripheral nerve injury. *J Histochem Cytochem* 2005; 53:971–977.

162. Mi R, Chen W, Hoke A. Pleiotrophin is a neurotrophic factor for spinal motor neurons. *Proc Natl Acad Sci USA* 2007; 104:4664–4669.

163. Maina F, Klein R. Hepatocyte growth factor, a versatile signal for developing neurons. *Nat Neurosci* 1999; 2:213–217.

164. Hoke A, Redett R, Hameed H, et al. Schwann cells express motor and sensory phenotypes that regulate axon regeneration. *J Neurosci* 2006; 26:9646–9655.

165. Krasnoselsky A, Massay MJ, DeFrances MC, et al. Hepatocyte growth factor is a mitogen for Schwann cells and is present in neurofibromas. *J Neurosci* 1994; 14:7284–7290.

166. Cheng C, Guo GF, Martinez JA, et al. Dynamic plasticity of axons within a cutaneous milieu. *J Neurosci* 2010; 30:14735–14744.

167. Carmeliet P, Storkebaum E. Vascular and neuronal effects of VEGF in the nervous system: implications for neurological disorders. *Semin Cell Dev Biol* 2002; 13:39–53.

168. Storkebaum E, Carmeliet P. VEGF: a critical player in neurodegeneration. *J Clin Invest* 2004; 113:14–18.

169. Sondell M, Lundborg G, Kanje M. Vascular endothelial growth factor has neurotrophic activity and stimulates axonal outgrowth, enhancing cell survival and Schwann cell proliferation in the peripheral nervous system. *J Neurosci* 1999; 19:5731–5740.

170. Sondell M, Lundborg G, Kanje M. Vascular endothelial growth factor stimulates Schwann cell invasion and neovascularization of acellular nerve grafts. *Brain Res* 1999; 846:219–228.

171. Hobson MI, Green CJ, Terenghi G. VEGF enhances intraneural angiogenesis and improves nerve regeneration after axotomy. *J Anat* 2000 Nov;197 Pt 4:591–605.

172. DeKosky ST, Styren SD, O'Malley ME, et al. Interleukin-1 receptor antagonist suppresses neurotrophin response in injured rat brain. *Ann Neurol* 1996; 39:123–127.

173. Lindholm D, Heumann R, Meyer M, et al. Interleukin-1 regulates synthesis of nerve growth factor in non- neuronal cells of rat sciatic nerve. *Nature* 1987; 330:658–659.

174. Gadient RA, Otten U. Postnatal expression of interleukin-6 (IL-6) and IL-6 receptor (IL-6R) mRNAs in rat sympathetic and sensory ganglia. *Brain Res* 1996; 724:41–46.

175. Richardson PM, Lu X. Inflammation and axonal regeneration. *J Neurol* 1994; 242:S57–S60.

176. Sampath TK, Muthukumaran N, Reddi AH. Isolation of osteogenin, an extracellular matrix-associated, bone-inductive protein, by heparin affinity chromatography. *Proc Natl Acad Sci USA* 1987; 84:7109–7113.

177. Wang YL, Wang DZ, Nie X, et al. The role of bone morphogenetic protein-2 in vivo in regeneration of peripheral nerves. *Br J Oral Maxillofac Surg* 2006; 45:197–202.

178. Neary JT, Rathbone MP, Cattabeni F, et al. Trophic actions of extracellular nucleotides and nucleosides on glial and neuronal cells. *Trends Neurosci* 1996; 19:13–18.

179. Katsuki H, Okuda S. Arachidonic acid as a neurotoxic and neurotrophic substance. *Prog Neurobiol* 1995; 46:607–636.

180. Cheng L, Khan M, Mudge AW. Calcitonin gene-related peptide promotes Schwann cell proliferation. *J Cell Biol* 1995; 129:789–796.

181. Toth CC, Willis D, Twiss JL, et al. Locally synthesized calcitonin gene-related Peptide has a critical role in peripheral nerve regeneration. *J Neuropathol Exp Neurol* 2009; 68:326–337.

182. Zochodne DW, Allison JA, Ho W, et al. Evidence for CGRP accumulation and activity in experimental neuromas. *Am J Physiol* 1995; 2 68:H584–H590.

183. Fainzilber M, Smit AB, Syed NI, et al. CRNF, a molluscan neurotrophic factor that interacts with the p75 neurotrophin receptor. *Science* 1996; 274:1540–1543.

184. Napoli I, Noon LA, Ribeiro S, et al. A central role for the ERK-signaling pathway in controlling Schwann cell plasticity and peripheral nerve regeneration in vivo. *Neuron* 2012; 73:729–742.

185. Mearow KM, Dodge ME, Rahimtula M, et al. Stress-mediated

signaling in PC12 cells - the role of the small heat shock protein, Hsp27, and Akt in protecting cells from heat stress and nerve growth factor withdrawal. *J Neurochem* 2002; 83:452–462.

186. Jones DM, Tucker BA, Rahimtula M, et al. The synergistic effects of NGF and IGF-1 on neurite growth in adult sensory neurons: convergence on the PI 3-kinase signaling pathway. *J Neurochem* 2003; 86:1116–1128.

187. Eickholt BJ, Walsh FS, Doherty P. An inactive pool of GSK-3 at the leading edge of growth cones is implicated in Semaphorin 3A signaling. *J Cell Biol* 2002; 157:211–217.

188. Chin PC, Majdzadeh N, D'Mello SR. Duplicate reference. Use 16803 Inhibition of GSK3beta is a common event in neuroprotection by different survival factors. *Brain Res Mol Brain Res* 2005; 137:193–201.

189. Dodge ME, Rahimtula M, Mearow KM. Factors contributing to neurotrophin-independent survival of adult sensory neurons. *Brain Res* 2002; 953:144–156.

190. Christie KJ, Webber CA, Martinez JA, et al. PTEN inhibition to facilitate intrinsic regenerative outgrowth of adult peripheral axons. *J Neurosci* 2010; 30:9306–9315.

191. Giehl KM, Tetzlaff W. BDNF and NT-3, but not NGF, prevent axotomy-induced death of rat corticospinal neurons in vivo. *Eur J Neurosci* 1996; 8:1167–1175.

192. Ikeda K, Klikosz B, Green T, et al. Effects of brain-derived neurotrophic factor (BDNF) on motor dysfunction in wobbler mouse motor neuron disease. *Ann Neurol* 1995; 37:505–511.

193. Mitsumoto H, Ikeda K, Klinkosz B, et al. Arrest of motor neuron disease in wobbler mice cotreated with CNTF and BDNF. *Science* 1994; 265:1107–1110.

194. Sagot Y, Tan SA, Baetge E, et al. Polymer encapsulated cell lines genetically engineered to release ciliary neurotrophic factor can slow down progressive motor neuronopathy in the mouse. *Eur J Neurosci* 1995; 7:1313–1322.

195. Sagot Y, Tan SA, Hammang JP, et al. GDNF slows loss of motoneurons but not axonal degeneration or premature death of pmn/pmn mice. *J Neurosci* 1996; 16:2335–2341.

196. Boillee S, Cleveland DW. Gene therapy for ALS delivers. *Trends Neurosci* 2004; 27:235–238.

197. Kaspar BK, Llado J, Sherkat N, et al. Retrograde viral delivery of IGF-1 prolongs survival in a mouse ALS model. *Science* 2003; 301:839–842.

198. Nakao N, Odin P, Lindvall O, et al. Differential trophic effects of basic fibroblast growth factor, insulin-like growth factor-1, and neurotrophin-3 on striatal neurons in culture. *Exp Neurol* 1996; 138:144–157.

199. Kirschner PB, Jenkins BG, Schulz JB, et al. NGF, BDNF and NT-5, but not NT-3 protect against MPP+ toxicity and oxidative stress in neonatal animals. *Brain Res* 1996; 713:178–185.

200. Martinez-Serrano A, Bjorklund A. Protection of the neostriatum against excitotoxic damage by neurotrophin-producing, genetically modified neural stem cells. *J Neurosci* 1996; 16:4604–4616.

201. Haque NS, Hlavin ML, Fawcett JW, et al. The neurotrophin NT4/5, but not NT3, enhances the efficacy of nigral grafts in a rat model of Parkinson's disease. *Brain Res* 1996; 712:45–52.

202. Sauer H, Wong V, Bjorklund A. Brain-derived neurotrophic factor and neurotrophin-4/5 modify neurotransmitter-related gene expression in the 6-hydroxydopamine- lesioned rat striatum. *Neuroscience* 1995; 65:927–933.

203. Sauer H, Rosenblad C, Bjorklund A. Glial cell line-derived neurotrophic factor but not transforming growth factor beta 3 prevents delayed degeneration of nigral dopaminergic neurons following striatal 6-hydroxydopamine lesion. *Proc Natl Acad Sci USA* 1995; 92:8935–8939.

204. Beck KD, Valverde J, Alexi T, et al. Mesencephalic dopaminergic neurons protected by GDNF from axotomy-induced degeneration in the adult brain. *Nature* 1995; 373:339–341.

205. Tomac A, Lindqvist E, Lin LF, et al. Protection and repair of the nigrostriatal dopaminergic system by GDNF in vivo. *Nature* 1995; 373:335–339.

206. He C, Chen Z. Enhancement of motor nerve regeneration by nerve growth factor. *Microsurgery* 1992; 13:151–154.

207. Kemp SW, Webb AA, Dhaliwal S, et al. Dose and duration of nerve growth factor (NGF) administration determine the extent of behavioral recovery following peripheral nerve injury in the rat. *Exp Neurol* 2011; 229:460–470.

208. Newman JP, Verity AN, Hawatmeh S, et al. Ciliary neurotrophic factors enhances peripheral nerve regeneration. *Arch Otolaryngol Head Neck Surg* 1996; 122:399–403.

209. Glazner GW, Lupien S, Miller JA, Ishii DN. Insulin-like growth factor II increases the rate of sciatic nerve regeneration in rats. *Neuroscience* 1993; 54:791–797.

210. Lee AC, Yu VM, Lowe JB, et al. Controlled release of nerve growth factor enhances sciatic nerve regeneration. *Exp Neurol* 2003; 184:295–303.

211. Kemp SW, Walsh SK, Zochodne DW, et al. A novel method for establishing daily in vivo concentration gradients of soluble nerve growth factor (NGF). *J Neurosci Methods* 2007; 165:83–88.

212. Tomlinson DR, Fernyhough P, Diemel LT. Neurotrophins and peripheral neuropathy. *Philos Trans R Soc Lond B Biol Sci* 1996; 351:455–462.

213. Zochodne DW. Neurotrophins and other growth factors in diabetic neuropathy. *Semin Neurol* 1996; 16:153–161.

214. Zochodne DW, Verge VMK, Cheng C, et al. Does diabetes target ganglion neurons? Progressive sensory neuron involvement in long term experimental diabetes. *Brain* 2001; 124:2319–2334.

215. Ishii DN. Implication of insulin-like growth factors in the pathogenesis of diabetic neuropathy. *Brain Res Rev* 1995; 20:47–67.

216. Diamond J, Holmes M, Coughlin M. Endogenous NGF and nerve impulses regulate the collateral sprouting of sensory axons in the skin of the adult rat. *J Neurosci* 1992; 12:1454–1466.

217. Guo G, Kan M, Martinez JA, Zochodne DW. Local insulin and the rapid regrowth of diabetic epidermal axons. *Neurobiol Dis* 2011; 43:414–421.

218. Helgren ME, Cliffer KD, Torrento K, et al. Neurotrophin-3 administration attenuates deficits of pyridoxine-induced large-fiber sensory neuropathy. *J Neurosci* 1997; 17:372–382.

219. Schmidt Y, Unger JW, Bartke I, et al. Effect of nerve growth factor on peptide neurons in dorsal root ganglia after taxol or cisplatin treatment and in diabetic (db/db) mice. *Exp Neurol* 1995; 132:16–23.

220. Apfel SC, Lipton RB, Arezzo JC, et al. Nerve growth factor prevents toxic neuropathy in mice. *Ann Neurol* 1991; 29:87–90.

221. Johnson H, Hokfelt T, Ulfhake B. Decreased expression of TrkB and TrkC mRNAs in spinal motoneurons of aged rats. *Eur J Neurosci* 1996; 8:494–499.

222. Kokaia Z, Zhao Q, Kokaia M, et al. Regulation of brain-derived neurotrophic factor gene expression after transient middle cerebral artery occlusion with and without brain damage. *Exp Neurol* 1995; 136:73–88.

223. Ay H, Ay I, Koroshetz WJ, Finklestein SP. Potential usefulness of basic fibroblast growth factor as a treatment for stroke. *Cerebrovasc Dis* 1999; 9:131–135.

224. Emerich DF, Winn SR, Hantraye PM, et al. Protective effect of encapsulated cells producing neurotrophic factor CNTF in a monkey model of Huntington's disease. *Nature* 1997; 386:395–399.

225. Nakahara Y, Gage FH, Tuszynski MH. Grafts of fibroblasts genetically modified to secrete NGF, BDNF, NT-3, or basic

FGF elicit differential responses in the adult spinal cord. *Cell Transplant* 1996; 5:191–204.

226. Grill R, Murai K, Blesch A, Gage FH, et al. Cellular delivery of neurotrophin-3 promotes corticospinal axonal growth and partial functional recovery after spinal cord injury. *J Neurosci* 1997; 17:5560–5572.

227. Lu P, Yang H, Jones LL, Filbin MT, et al. Combinatorial therapy with neurotrophins and cAMP promotes axonal regeneration beyond sites of spinal cord injury. *J Neurosci* 2004; 24:6402–6409.

228. Liu Y, Kim D, Himes BT, et al. Transplants of fibroblasts genetically modified to express BDNF promote regeneration of adult rat rubrospinal axons and recovery of forelimb function. *J Neurosci* 1999; 19:4370–4387.

229. Xu XM, Guenard V, Kleitman N, et al. A combination of BDNF and NT-3 promotes supraspinal axonal regeneration into Schwann cell grafts in adult rat thoracic spinal cord. *Exp Neurol* 1995; 134:261–272.

230. Sinson G, Voddi M, McIntosh TK. Combined fetal neural transplantation and nerve growth factor infusion: effects on neurological outcome following fluid-percussion brain injury in the rat. *J Neurosurg* 1996; 84:655–662.

231. Poduslo JF, Curran GL. Permeability at the blood-brain and blood-nerve barriers of the neurotrophic factors: NGF, CNTF, NT-3, BDNF. *Brain Res Mol Brain Res* 1996; 36:280–286.

232. Anonymous. A controlled trial of recombinant methionyl human BDNF in ALS: The BDNF Study Group (Phase III). *Neurology* 1999; 52:1427–1433.

233. Borasio GD, Robberecht W, Leigh PN, et al. A placebo-controlled trial of insulin-like growth factor-I in amyotrophic lateral sclerosis. European ALS/IGF-I Study Group. *Neurology* 1998; 51:583–586.

234. Lai EC, Felice KJ, Festoff BW, et al. Effect of recombinant human insulin-like growth factor-I on progression of ALS. A placebo-controlled study. The North America ALS/IGF-I Study Group. *Neurology* 1997; 49:1621–1630.

235. Sorenson EJ, Windbank AJ, Mandrekar JN, et al. Subcutaneous IGF-1 is not beneficial in 2-year ALS trial. *Neurology* 2008; 71:1770–1775.

236. Le Roith D. Seminars in medicine of the Beth Israel Deaconess Medical Center. Insulin-like growth factors. *N Engl J Med* 1997; 336:633–640.

237. Anonymous. A double-blind placebo-controlled clinical trial of subcutaneous recombinant human ciliary neurotrophic factor (rHCNTF) in amyotrophic lateral sclerosis. ALS CNTF Treatment Study Group. *Neurology* 1996; 46:1244–1249.

238. Miller RG, Petajan JH, Bryan WW, et al. A placebo-controlled trial of recombinant human ciliary neurotrophic (rhCNTF) factor in amyotrophic lateral sclerosis. *Ann Neurol* 1996; 39:256–260.

239. Lacomblez L, Bensimon G, Douillet P, et al. Xaliproden in amyotrophic lateral sclerosis: early clinical trials. *Amyotroph Lateral Scler Other Motor Neuron Disord* 2004; 5:99–106.

240. Chio A, Mora G, La B, V, et al. Repeated courses of granulocyte colony-stimulating factor in amyotrophic lateral sclerosis:

clinical and biological results from a prospective multicenter study. *Muscle Nerve* 2011; 43:189–195.

241. Apfel SC, Schwartz S, Adornato BT, et al. Efficacy and safety of recombinant human nerve growth factor in patients with diabetic polyneuropathy: A randomized controlled trial. rhNGF Clinical Investigator Group. *JAMA* 2000; 284:2215–2221.

242. Apfel SC, Kessler JA, Adornato BT, et al. Recombinant human nerve growth factor in the treatment of diabetic polyneuropathy. NGF Study Group. *Neurology* 1998; 51:695–702.

243. McArthur JC, Yiannoutsos C, Simpson DM, et al. A phase II trial of nerve growth factor for sensory neuropathy associated with HIV infection. AIDS Clinical Trials Group Team 291. *Neurology* 2000; 54:1080–1088.

244. Wellmer A, Misra VP, Sharief MK, et al. A double-blind placebo-controlled clinical trial of recombinant human brain-derived neurotrophic factor (rhBDNF) in diabetic polyneuropathy. *J Peripher Nerv Syst* 2001; 6:204–210.

245. Bensa S, Hadden RD, Hahn A, et al. Randomized controlled trial of brain-derived neurotrophic factor in Guillain-Barre syndrome: a pilot study. *Eur J Neurol* 2000; 7:423–426.

246. Vlachopapadopoulou E, Zachwieja JJ, Gertner JM, et al. Metabolic and clinical response to recombinant human insulin-like growth factor I in myotonic dystrophy—a clinical research center study. *J Clin Endocrinol Metab* 1995; 80:3715–3723.

247. Tuszynski MH. Growth-factor gene therapy for neurodegenerative disorders. *Lancet Neurol* 2002; 1:51–57.

248. Reger MA, Watson GS, Green P.S., et al. Intranasal insulin improves cognition and modulates B-amyloid in early AD. *Neurology* 2008; 70:440–448.

249. Ebendal T, Lonnerberg P, Pei G, et al. Engineering cells to secrete growth factors. *J Neurol* 1994; 242:S5–S7.

250. Nutt JG, Burchiel KJ, Comella CL, et al. Randomized, double-blind trial of glial cell line-derived neurotrophic factor (GDNF) in PD. *Neurology* 2003; 60:69–73.

251. Lang AE, Gill S, Patel NK, et al. Randomized controlled trial of intraputamenal glial cell line-derived neurotrophic factor infusion in Parkinson disease. *Ann Neurol* 2006; 59:459–466.

252. Slevin JT, Gash DM, Smith CD, et al. Unilateral intraputamenal glial cell line-derived neurotrophic factor in patients with Parkinson disease: response to 1 year of treatment and 1 year of withdrawal. *J Neurosurg* 2007; 106:614–620.

253. Marks WJ, Jr., Bartus RT, Siffert J, et al. Gene delivery of AAV2-neurturin for Parkinson's disease: a double-blind, randomized, controlled trial. *Lancet Neurol* 2010; 9:1164–1172.

254. Peviani M, Cheroni C, Troglio F, et al. Lack of changes in the PI3K/AKT survival pathway in the spinal cord motor neurons of a mouse model of familial amyotrophic lateral sclerosis. *Mol Cell Neurosci* 2007; 34:592–602.

255. Kirby J, Ning K, Ferraiuolo L, et al. Phosphatase and tensin homologue/protein kinase B pathway linked to motor neuron survival in human superoxide dismutase 1-related amyotrophic lateral sclerosis. *Brain* 2011; 134:506–517.

CHAPTER 55

Adult and Childhood Hydrocephalus

David S. Younger

Normal pressure hydrocephalus (NPH) is typified by the clinical triad of altered mentation, gait difficulty, and urinary sphincter disturbances in conjunction with ventricular dilatation of the brain and normal manometric pressure of the cerebrospinal fluid (CSF) at lumbar puncture. This chapter addresses the background, nosological concepts, etiopathogenesis, diagnostic laboratory studies, and management of adult and childhood NPH.

TERMINOLOGY

The term hydrocephalus refers to distention of the cerebral ventricles, usually as a result of obstruction of the CSF circulation. Communicating or non-obstructive hydrocephalus denotes patent CSF pathways from the ventricular system to lumbar subarachnoid space via the foramina of Luschka and Magendie, whereas non-communicating or obstructive hydrocephalus denotes blockage of the CSF circulation somewhere in the ventricular system. The onset of hydrocephalus may be at birth before union of the cranial sutures with enlargement of the head, or discovered later in adulthood wherein is it termed occult. Hydrocephalus is deemed to be idiopathic when there is no known cause for its occurrence, and secondary or symptomatic in the setting of another causative factor, including an encroaching ventricular tumor or infiltrating meningeal carcinomatosis, atresia, tumor, or ependymal gliosis of the Sylvian aqueduct, Arnold Chiari and other congenital malformations, meningeal fibrosis, bacterial meningitis, subarachnoid hemorrhage, head injury, and prior brain surgery. Whereas acute hydrocephalus is accompanied by symptoms of increased intracranial pressure (ICP), including headache, vomit-

ing, papilledema, and obtundation, with elevation of the CSF manometric pressure on lumbar puncture, an indolent onset of hydrocephalus can be symptomatic or not, with normal manometric pressures of 180 mm or less. The term hydrocephalus *ex vacuo* pertains to ventriculomegaly in association with prominent sulci, and marked cortical atrophy suggestive of an alternative etiopathogenesis, which in contrast to communicating and non-communicating hydrocephalus, is rarely if ever amenable to shunting.

BACKGROUND

Early pioneering papers (1–6) provided clinical and pathological descriptions of progressive symptomatic and idiopathic hydrocephalus without overt signs of ICP, some of which (7) described a beneficial response to shunting similar to that proposed later by Hakim and Adams (8), and Adams and colleagues (9). Although the historical choice of name NPH was based upon the finding of CSF pressures of 150 mm to 180 mm, the authors conceded that the ICP was probably higher in the early stages of the illness. However, once the increased pressure enlarged the ventricles, they maintained a distended state at a lower pressure in accordance with Pascal's Law for enclosed fluid in which the force (F) on the walls was equal to the product of the pressure (P) of the fluid and the area (A). Recognition and treatment of NPH by a surgical shunt procedure, according to Adams and coworkers (9), in their minds amounted to nothing less than a cure of a forme fruste of debilitating dementia among several patients, in association with akinetic mutism, another with breast-cancer-related meningeal carcinomatosis, and a third with no other cause thereof. Subsequent investigators did not observe similar encouraging results with CSF diversion based upon the proposed clinical triad, pneumoencephalographic, and intrathecal findings (10). However, two decades later, the disorder re-emerged as the cause of gait difficulty in those over age 60 years (11) as predicted by a ventricular span of greater than 12 mm on brain computed tomography (CT) and the clinical response to the withdrawal of CSF by lumbar puncture (LP).

EPIDEMIOLOGY

The incidence rate of shunted NPH was estimated to be 1.19 per 100,000 per year for the total population of Olmsted County in southeastern Minnesota, and 4.82 per 100,000 in those older than 50 years of age (12) based upon a cohort of 41 patients drawn from private and affiliated providers of the Mayo Health Systems between 1995 and 2003, in whom shunt placement was offered to patients with suspicion for NPH sufficient to justify an invasive diagnostic or therapeutic procedure, 32% of whom ultimately underwent ventriculoperitoneal (VP) shunting, all of whom had gait disturbance, 73% cognitive impairment, and 24% urinary incontinence.

CLINICAL PRESENTATION

Gait difficulty, mental impairment, and urinary incontinence classically appear in close or later succession, and are the most likely to improve after shunting. Gait difficulty may be the only apparent sign of NPH, manifested as difficulty in initiating walking as may be seen in the magnetic gait apraxia of frontal lobe disease, postural instability, and short-stepped and shuffling resembling parkinsonism. The mental impairment is of a subcortical type of dementia, which along with forgetfulness, inertia, inattention, decreased speed of complex information processing, and disturbed manipulation of acquired knowledge reflective of the loss of integrity of the frontal lobes, results instead in a discrepancy of delayed recall with normal or minimally affected recognition and encoding deficits, the inverse of which is seen in Alzheimer disease (AD). Urinary incontinence is of a spastic hyperreflexic urgency type associated with decreased inhibition of bladder contractions and detrusor instability, which in the most severe cases, is associated with a lack of concern for micturition due to severe frontal lobe involvement. Although a late sign, recognition of bladder incontinence completes the trial and prompts formal evaluation of NPH with the contemplation of inserting a shunt to avert further progression.

LABORATORY DIAGNOSIS

All patients should undergo a standard medical and neurological evaluation as may be deemed appropriate by the clinical presentation. Neuropsychological assessment should include a Mini-Mental State Examination (MMSE) (13) and more detailed cognitive evaluation, especially in those with an incomplete syndrome of NPH, such as gait or sphincter disturbance without overt dementia, recognizing that bedside cognitive screening may underestimate mental impairment of the subcortical type typical of NPH (14).

Magnetic resonance imaging (MRI) is the neuroimaging modality of choice in NPH. The MRI findings of NPH (Figure 1) classically include increased width of the frontal horns and third ventricle, corpus callosal thinning, enlargement of the temporal horns with a convexity sulcus pattern that is normal for age, increased lucency of the frontal and occipital periventricular horns on T_2-weighted images indicative of transependymal CSF movement, and a flow void sign indicative of high and pulsatile CSF flow through the aqueduct of Sylvius (15, 16). Those with AD differed on volumetric coronal MRI analysis of the hippo-

(A)

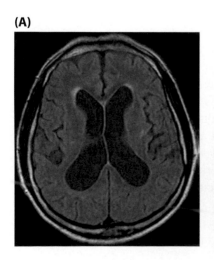

(B)

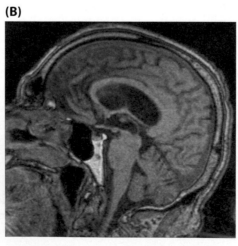

FIG. 1. Normal pressure hydrocephalus. Transaxial **(A)** and sagittal **(B)** T_1 Graded I-IV in increasing severity, -weighted MRI reveals moderate to severe enlargement of the ventricular system, patchy periventricular hyperintensities, flattening of cortical gyri, and thinning of the corpus callosum.

campus, especially in the CA1 region, due to presence of significant dilatation and atrophy of the perihippocampal fissure (17).

Although first eluded to by Adams and Hakim (9) as a therapeutic test in NPH and a predictor of response to shunting, and later emphasized by Wood and coworkers (18) and Fisher (19), the spinal tap or "tap-test" was standardized by Wikkelso and colleagues (20) and later studied in 27 patients with NPH undergoing VP shunt surgery, the removal of CSF from whom led to significant temporary improvement in psychometric and motor function in all 19 patients later benefited by shunt surgery (21). Although clinical improvement that follows LP confirms the suspicion of NPH in a given patient, lack thereof should not be considered exclusionary. Drainage of larger quantities of CSF via closed external lumbar drainage system for three to five days purportedly provides further accuracy in the prediction of potential responders to shunting. Among 32 patients with NPH (22), 10 demonstrated improvements after a single LP, however among the remaining 22 selected for study with external lumbar drainage, five patients experienced complications leading to exclusion, including displacement of the drain by the patient, root irritation, and meningitis. Of the remaining 17 patients, 12 showed a good response, and five did not. All 12 patients that benefited from external lumbar drainage also benefited from surgery, while none of the five lacking improvement from external lumbar drainage improved with shunting. Therefore, external lumbar drainage can select additional candidates for shunting beyond those identified by a CSF tap-test; however, there are potential complications, the magnitude of which may be reduced by removing the drainage system after improvement has occurred.

Three dynamic CSF measures, including conductance (23) and resistance to outflow of CSF (24), and quantification of abnormal ICP waves (25, 26), have been employed in the diagnosis of NPH but require more elaborate testing protocols available in only a few centers.

Isotope cisternography has been widely accessible in the evaluation of NPH (27, 28). An LP for the withdrawal of CSF and the subsequent injection of the radionuclear isotope is carried out under fluoroscopic guidance to minimize side effects. Its transit is followed for three days to determine whether there is a reversal of flow and a lack of migration of the isotope from the ventricles to the convexity as evidence of communicating hydrocephalus.

Single photon emission computed tomography (SPECT) by [133]xenon inhalation revealed patterns of aberrant cerebral blood flow that partly improved after shunting in accordance with changes in ventricular size on brain CT (27, 29).

NEUROPATHOLOGY AND ETIOPATHOGENESIS

The earliest two pathologically-proven patients with NPH presented with progressive dementia, weakness, and tremor likened to dementia paralytica, with subnormal CSF manometric pressure and ventriculographic evidence of a third ventricle tumor (1). At autopsy there was distention of the lateral and third ventricles, flattening of the cortical convulsions and quadrigeminal plates, with visible partially obstructing tumors. Four patients (30) presented, respectively, with occult hydrocephalus present only at postmortem examination associated with membranous obstruction of the foramina of Luschka, septated gliotic stenosis and forking of the acqueduct of Sylvius, membranous obstruction of the fourth ventricle, and near total gliotic occlusion of the acqueduct of Sylvius, consistent with symptomatic NPH.

From among a postmortem examination series of 1,000 patients with dementia (31) 1.3% had NPH of age ranging from 51 to 75 years, with associated ventriculomegaly, secondary thinning or rupture of the interventricular septum, subependymal gliosis, and rim-like periventricular demyelination. DiRocco and colleagues (32) reaffirmed the postmortem findings of NPH, including non-obstructive fibrosis, ventricular ependymal disruption, and subependymal glial reaction consistent with the pathogenic mechanism of defective CSF circulation and absorption. However, there was pronounced periventricular white matter edema and spongiosis presumed due to leakage of CSF across a disrupted ventricular ependymal wall into the cerebral parenchyma. Akai and colleagues (33) described seven additional patients with NPH at postmortem examination and noted similar prominent degeneration of periventricular and deep white matter parenchyma. As suggested, the development of NPH required not only a disturbance of CSF, but pre-, or coexisting vulnerability of the white matter caused by ischemia, hypoxia, and trauma. Newton and coworkers (34) provided evidence of the progression of cerebrovascular disease in a patient with shunted NPH in whom postmortem examination demonstrated multiple old and recent white matter infarcts, accompanied by widespread moderately severe arteriosclerosis in blood vessels, periventricular gliosis, macrophages with iron pigment in perivascular spaces, and état criblé, in addition to widely dilated ventricles. Leinonen and coworkers (35) did not identify unifying diagnostic neuropathological characteristics of NPH in frontal brain biopsy or postmortem brain tissue among 10 patients with clinical and neuroradiological features of NPH. Instead, three patients had AB aggregates of Thal phase 4 severity (36) in biopsied brain tissue, while seven others displayed AB only at postmortem examination of Thal phase 3 or less. One patient each had postmortem evidence of a primary tauopathy-type of corticobasal degeneration, one had AD with concomitant Lewy body changes not noted in biopsied brain tissue, and another had pathologically confirmed progressive supranuclear palsy (PSP) at postmortem examination. Subependymal gliosis was noted in all patients, as accompanied by multifocal vascular lesions considered sufficient to cause cognitive decline in three affected patients. With nearly one-half of patients given an alternative neurological diagnosis, and none of them realizing sustained improvement after shunting, it was questionable how many truly had NPH before developing the second disease. Moreover, a favorable early response to shunting did not exclude an underlying neurodegenerative condition, as evidenced by one patient with PSP who had early transient improvement after shunting followed by progressive worsening.

Toma and colleagues (37) analyzed the literature for study cohorts that examined the natural history of unshunted NPH, highlighting two series in particular (38, 39) that showed worsening of cognition, gait, and urinary incontinence, that commenced in up to two-thirds of patients as early as three to six months after initial assessment and steadily progressed for the study period of 24 months.

Whatever the contributing factors, brain dysfunction in NPH is a complex process that commences with hydrocephalic compression and stretching of arterioles and venules, that leads to variable disturbance of periventricular myelinated axons, white matter change, hypoperfusion, gliosis, limited neuronal death, and somewhat reversible brain dysfunction or subcortical disconnection. It is suggested that the ameliorative effects of shunting occur through restoration of cerebral blood flow and normalization of the extracellular periventricular environment.

TREATMENT

Neurologists referring patients with NPH for shunt placement should decide the appropriateness and timing of surgery, and review the types of pressure valves with the neurosurgeon. They should discuss the prospect of surgery with their patients, recognizing that shunt surgery may not be a panacea for the multifactorial nature of dementia and gait disturbances (40), and recognize the known inherent risks (41) that included new-onset seizures in four of 12 patients (33%), traumatic subdural hematoma shortly after shunt surgery in one patient, and death from pulmonary embolism in a fourth patient. It should not be difficult to advise shunt placement in a suitable surgical candidate with history of gait, cognitive, and urinary clinical disturbances, without another cause for hydrocephalus, and diagnostic features of NPH on CT, MRI, lumbar CSF tap-test or external lumbar drainage, and radioisotope cisternography.

Since the introduction of the one-way calibrated shunt system, a variety of valve systems have been used in the treatment of hydrocephalus with the common goal of draining off CSF that is not reabsorbed through natural CSF channels under physiological ICP. Currently available shunting systems can be categorized into those with low and high resistance, and mixed valves (42). The low-resistance valves include the Hakim spring ball variety and the Heyer-Schulte silicone rubber diaphragm systems that act as differential pressure valves. One high-resistance valve is the Holter silicone rubber slit valve. The mixed Orbis-Sigma valve is a 3-stage valve system that maintains flow rates at or close to CSF production under a range of pressures, first by acting as a conventional differential pressure valve, and later by variable resistance regulation, with a safety device at extreme differential pressures. In general, VP shunts are standard treatment while ventriculoatrial shunts are an option in those with a history of multiple laparotomy or defective peritoneal CSF resorption. Overdrainage of CSF is an expected complication of differential pressure valves in which flow is determined by the difference between the CSF input and output pressures. Certain positions, such as standing, leads to increased draining of the shunt that may exceed ventricular CSF secretion rate due to the height of the hydrostatic column between the inlet and the outlet of the shunt. Overdrainage can also occur in circumstances of temporary physiological ICP increases, such as in rapid eye movement sleep and exertion. Other potentially serious surgical complications, including hemorrhage, infection, seizures, and shunt obstruction can occur in up to a quarter of patients.

The followup in 12 of 41 patients with presumed NPH showed that at three to six months, 75% of patients demonstrated gait improvement, a rate that dropped to 50% improvement between six months and one year, and 33% maintained definite improvement. Compared to gait improvement, no patient had definite improvement in cognition without concomitant definitely improved gait and without known association of duration of symptom and shunt response.

Most authorities would agree that the anticipated surgical risk outweighs the anticipated benefit of shunting in the presence of a patient with prolonged severe dementia, especially bed-bound or near bed-bound patients. Each center that pursues a program in the management of hydrocephalus needs to monitor its own diagnostic approach with a multidisciplinary view to assure constancy in referral for surgery or other management strategies, with longitudinal blinded and quantitative outcomes of therapy.

HYDROCEPHALUS OF CHILDHOOD

Childhood hydrocephalus is a multifactorial disorder often with associated genetic predisposition. The syndrome of hydrocephalus due to congenital stenosis of the acqueduct of Sylvius (HSAS) is caused by mutation at the Xq28 locus of the *LICAM* gene encoding L1 cell adhesion molecule, and is estimated to occur in up to 25% of males with acqueductal obstruction corresponding to an incidence of 1 in 30,000 male births. Intraventricular (IVH), or germinal matrix hemorrhage (GMH), which occurs in up to 45% of premature infants of birth weight less than 1,500 gram, is associated with post-hemorrhagic ventricular dilatation in virtually all infants with severe IVH that resembles NPH (43, 44). Possible clues of an IVH include hypotonia, seizures, opthalmoplegia, irritability, and vomiting; however, small hemorrhages may go undetected and a high index of suspicion is needed, particularly in premature infants who may have coexisting health concerns. More significant IVH can have abnormal posturing, respiratory and cardiac sequel, asymmetrical pupillary size, and anemia.

Hydrocephalus results from obstructed CSF flow through the ventricular system due to arachnoiditis of the posterior fossa, which in a setting of increased compliance of immature periventricular tissue, leads to ventriculomegaly with initially normal ICP. Further worsening culminates with increased ICP, bulging of fontanelles, separation of sutures, upward gaze palsy, and rapid head growth. Ultrasound-based grading of GMH-IVH, wherein subependymal localization alone (Grade I GMH), is followed by increasing grades, depending upon the presence of intraventricular extension without (Grade II) or with associated ventricular dilatation (Grade III), and associated parenchymal hemorrhage (Grade IV). In those with IVH, abnormal MRI periventricular signals are indicative of active hydrocephalus, and distinguish both ventricular enlargement due to atrophy from dilatation resulting from CSF accumulation, and progressive from compensated hydrocephalus, which may impact upon a given treatment approach.

The concern for periventricular edema, astrocytosis, and alteration in periventricular white matter tissues with impairment of blood flow normally prompts consideration of CSF diversion via external ventricular drainage, subcutaneous reservoirs, medical, or pharmaceutical approaches to the removal or blood or blood products, serial LP and, finally, VP shunting, recognizing that the latter may incur undesirable side effects and long-term dependency.

Posterior fossa tumors and surgery can be complicated by NPH (45, 46). Hydrocephalus follows surgery or becomes insidiously evident over several days or up to a week after surgery. In some instances the ventricular dilatation may be evident preoperatively due to the presence of a brain stem or posterior fossa tumor. Two features appear to predict the need for permanent shunting, including those with resection of only a small volume of tumor and opening of the dura following tumor resection, with two-thirds to three-quarters of children otherwise managed perioperatively with external ventricular drainage (46).

Congenital hydrocephalus (47) can be associated with neural tube defects (NTD), the latter of which is divided into those that are open and, therefore, manifest visible neural tissue with leaking CSF, and the other closed, wherein there is no visible neural tissue or CSF leakage. Unlike closed NTD, open NTD are frequently associated with extensive CNS malformation and hydrocephalus. Examples of open NTD include myelomeningoceles, myeloschisis, and hemimyelomeningocele. Hydrocephalus, which may not be present at birth, becomes evident soon thereafter and, if significant, warrants shunting, which can be performed simultaneously with surgical close of the NTD, or delayed, depending upon the anticipated risk of shunt infection, a concept that is vigorously debated (48, 49). Chiari II malformation presents instead, in the weeks or months after birth, with signs due to lower cranial nerve palsy and brainstem compression and downward pressure from inadequately controlled hydrocephalus or syringomyelia. Placement of a shunt is of particular importance, followed by craniocervical decompression if needed. The diagnosis of an NTD is suggested by the clinical neurological signs, neuroimaging, including ultrasound and MRI, serum, and amniotic maternal alpha-fetoprotein levels.

Obstructive and communicating hydrocephalus accompanies acquired Sylvian aqueductal stenosis in association with vein of Galen malformation or venous hypertension, and in X-linked hydrocephalus due to congenital stenosis of the acqueduct of Sylvius (HSAS). Patients with vein of Galen malformation can present with neonatal high-output heart failure (50) requiring endovascular embolization before consideration of shunt placement (51) due to the inordinate frequency of potentially serious postoperative complications. The phenotype of HSAS consists of enlarged cerebral ventricles, mental retardation, spastic paraparesis, and adducted thumbs. The latter is not secondary to a neurological defect but instead appears to result from localized atrophy or agenesis of the abductor and extensor muscles of the thumbs.

Normocephalic children with ventriculomegaly can have stable arrested hydrocephalus discovered during the evaluation of other complaints without classical signs of elevated ICP, but with a historical insult that suggest prior injury and longstanding ventriculomegaly (52). Affected children show normal intelligence and abnormal neuropsychological findings characterized by difficulty in psychomotor function, with evidence of mild hyperreflexic diplegia when comparing reflexes of the arms with those of the legs. The onset of presence of intellectual retardation, focal neurological signs, especially spastic diplegia in such a child with arrested hydrocephalus, mitigates consideration of further evaluation and a possible trial of CSF removal or CSF diversion.

Factors relating to the quality of life in childhood hydrocephalus are being recognized as important factors in the outcome, of perhaps greater importance to the affected patient and parent, than the frequency of shunt infection or incompetence (53). They include cognitive disturbances that impact upon intelligence, school performance, lan-

guage and memory; physical dysfunction relating to disturbances in ambulation, pain, visual, speech and dexterity disturbances; chronic headache, and social, emotional, and psychological impairment and perception of self-competence. Quality of life measures and scores employing standardized questionnaires enable parents to participate in the social well being and decision-making process of their affected child.

REFERENCES

1. Riddoch G. Progressive dementia without headaches or changes in the optic disks due to tumors of the third ventricle. Brain 1936; 59:225–33.
2. Lhermitte J, Mouzon J. L'hydrocéphalie de l'adulte à forme paraplégique et à poussées successives. Rev Neurol 1942; 74:63–65.
3. Foltz EL, Ward AA. Communicating hydrocephalus from subarachnoid bleeding. J Neurosurg 1956; 13:546–66.
4. Kibler RF, Couch RSC, Crompton MR. Hydrocephalus in the adult following spontaneous subarachnoid hemorrhage. Brain 1961; 84:45–61.
5. Shulman K, Martin BF, Popoff N, et al. Recognition and treatment of hydrocephalus following spontaneous subarachnoid hemorrhage. J Neurosurg 1963; 20:1040–1049.
6. McHugh PR. Occult hydrocephalus. Q J Med 1964; 33:297–312.
7. Foltz EL, Ward AA. Communicating hydrocephalus from subarachnoid bleeding. J Neurosurg 1956; 13:546–66.
8. Hakim S, Adams RD. The special clinical problem of symptomatic hydrcephalus with normal cerebrospinal fluid pressure. Observations on cerebrospinal fluid hydrodynamics. J Neurol Sci 1965; 2:307–327.
9. Adams RD, Fisher CM, Hakin S, et al. Symptomatic occult hydrocephalus with "normal" cerebrospinal fluid pressure. A treatable syndrome. N Engl J Med 1965; 273:117–126.
10. Bannister CM. A report of 8 patients with low-pressure hydrocephalus treated by cerebrospinal fluid diversion with disappointing results. Acta Neurochir 1972; 27:11–15.
11. Fisher CM. Hydrocephalus as a cause of disturbances of gait in the elderly. Neurology 1982; 32:1358–1363.
12. Klassen BT, Ahlskog JE. Normal pressure hydrocephalus. How often does the diagnosis hold water? Neurology 2011; 77:1119–1125.
13. Folstein MF, Folstein SE, McHugh PR. "Mini-mental state": a practical method for grading the mental state of patients for the clinician. J Psychiatr Res 1975; 12:189–198.
14. Nelson A, Fogel BS, Faust D. Bedside cognitive screening instruments. A critical assessment. J Nerv Ment Dis 1986; 174:73–83.
15. Jack Jr CR, Mokri B, Laws ER, et al. MR findings in normal-pressure hydrocephalus: significance and comparison with other forms of dementia. J Comput Assist Tomogr 1987; 11:923–930.
16. Bradley WG, Scalzo D, Queralt J, et al. Normal-pressure hydrocephalus: evaluation with cerebrospinal fluid flow measurements at MR imaging. Radiology 1996; 198:523–529.
17. Kolodny AI, Waxman R, George AE, et al. MR differential diagnosis of normal-pressure hydrocephalus and Alzheimer disease: significance of perihippocampal fissures. AJNR 1998; 19:813–819.
18. Wood JH, Bartlet D, James AE, et al. Normal pressure hydrocephalus: diagnosis and patient selection for shunt surgery. Neurology 1974; 24:517–526.
19. Fisher CM. The clinical picture in occult hydrocephalus. Clin Neurosurg 1977; 24:270–284
20. Wikkelso C, Andersson H, Biomstrand C, et al. The clinical effect of lumbar puncture in normal pressure hydrocephalus. Description of a diagnostic CSF-TAP-TEST. J Neurol Neurosurg Psychiatry 1982; 45:64–69.
21. Wikkelso C, Andersson H, Biomstrand C, et al. Normal pressure hydrocephalus. Predictive value of the cerebrospinal fluid tap-test. Acta Neurol Scand 1986; 73:566–573.
22. Hann J, Thomeer TWM. Predictive value of temporary external lumbar drainage in normal pressure hydrocephalus. Neurosurgery 1988; 22:388–391.
23. Borgesen SE, Bjerris F. The predictive value of conductance to outflow of CSF in normal pressure hydrocephalus. Brain 1982; 105:65–86.
24. Boon AJW, Tans JTJ, Delwel EJ, et al. Dutch normal-pressure hydrocephalus study: prediction of outcome after shunting by resistance to outflow of cerebrospinal fluid. J Neurosurg 1997; 87:687–693.
25. Cardoso ER, Piatek D, Del Bigio MR, et al. Quantification of abnormal intracranial pressure waves and isotope cisternography for diagnosis of occult communicating hydrocephalus. Surg Neurol 1989; 31:20–27.
26. Symon L, Dorsch NWC. Use of long-term intracranial pressure measurement to assess hydrocephalic patients prior to shunt surgery. J Neurosurg 1975; 42:258–273.
27. Bannister R, Gilford E, Kocen R. Isotope encephalography in the diagnosis of dementia due to communicating hydrocephalus. Lancet 1967; 2:1014–1017.
28. James AE, Deland FH, Hodges FJ, et al. Normal pressure hydrocephalus. Role of cisternography in diagnosis. JAMA 1970; 213:1615–1622.
29. Vorstrup S, Christensen J, Gjerris F, et al. Cerebral blood flow in patients with normal pressure hydrocephalus before and after shunting. J Neurosurg 1987; 66:379–387.
30. McHugh PR. Occult hydrocephalus. Q J Med 1964; 33:297–312.
31. Jellinger K. Neuropathological aspects of dementias resulting from abnormal blood and CSF dynamics. Acta Neurol Belg 1976; 76:83–100.
32. Di Rocco C, Di Trapana G, Maira G, et al Anatomo-clinical correlations in normotensive hydrocephalus. J Neurol Sci 1977; 33:437-452.
33. Akai K, Uchigasaki S, Tanaka U, et al. Normal pressure hydrocephalus. Neuropathological study. Acta Pathol Jpn 1987; 37:97–110.
34. Newton H, Pickard JD, Weller RO. Normal pressure hydrocephalus and cerebrovascular disease: findings of post-mortem [Letter]. J Neurol Neurosurg Psychiatry 1989; 52:804.

35. Leinonen V, Koivisto AM, Savolainen S, et al. Post-mortem findings in 10 patients with presumed normal-pressure hydrocephalus and review of the literature. *Neuropathol Applied Neurobiol* 2012; 38:72–86.

36. Thal DR, Rub Urantes M, et al. Phases of AB-deposition in the human brain and its relevance for the development of AD. *Neurology* 2002; 58:1791–1800.

37. Toma AK, Stapleton S, Papadopoulos MC, et al. Natural history of idiopathic normal-pressure hydrocephalus. *Neurosurg Rev* 2011; 34:433–439.

38. Razay G, Vreugdenhil A, Liddell J. A prospective study of ventriculo-peritoneal shunting for idiopathic normal pressure hydrocephalus. *J Clin Neurosci* 2009; 16:1180–1183.

39. Scollato A, Tenebaum R, Bahol G, et al. Changes in aqueductal CSF stroke volume and progression of symptoms in patients with unshunted idiopathic normal pressure hydrocephalus. *AJNR* 2008; 29:192–197.

40. Bret P, Guyotat J, Chazal J. Is normal pressure hydrocephalus a valid concept in 2002? A reappraisal in five questions and proposal for a new designation of the syndrome as "chronic hydrocephalus." *J Neurol Neurosurg Psychiatry* 2002; 73:9–12.

41. Klassen BT, Ahlskog JE. Normal pressure hydrocephalus. How often does the diagnosis hold water? *Neurology* 2011; 77:1119–1125.

42. Vanneste JAL. Three decades of normal pressure hydrocephalus: are we wiser now? *J Neurol Neurosurg Psychiatry* 1994; 57:1021–1025.

43. Hill A, Volpe JJ. Normal pressure hydrocephalus in the newborn. *Pediatrics* 1981; 68:623–629.

44. Tsitouras V, Sgouros S. Infantile post-hemorrhagic hydrocephalus. *Childs Nerv Syst* 2011; 27:1595–1608.

45. Stein BM, Fraser RA, Tenner MS. Normal pressure hydrocephalus: complication of posterior fossa surgery in children. *Pediatrics* 1972; 49:50–58.

46. Dias MS, Albright AL. Management of hydrocephalus complicating childhood posterior fossa tumors. *Pediatr Neurosci* 1989; 15:283–289

47. Jeelani Y, McComb JG. Congenital hydrocephalus associated with myeloschisis. *Childs Nerv Syst* 2011; 27:1585–1588.

48. Miller PD, Pollack IF, Pang D, et al. Comparison of simultaneous versus delayed ventriculoperitoneal shunt insertion in children undergoing myelomeningocele repair. *J Child Neurol* 1996; 11:370–372.

49. Oktem IS, Menki A, Ozdemir A. When should ventriculoperitoneal shunt placement be performed in cases with myelomeningocele and hydrocephalus? *Turk Neurosurg* 2008; 18:387–391.

50. Jea A, Bradshaw TJ, Whitehead WE, et al. The high risks of ventriculoperitoneal shunt procedures for hydrocephalus associated with vein of Galen malformations in childhood: case report and literature review. *Pediatr Neurosurg* 2010; 46:141–145.

51. Schneider SJ, Wisoff JS, Epstein FJ. Complications of ventriculoperitoneal shunt procedures or hydrocephalus associated with vein of Galen malformations in childhood. *Neurosurgery* 1992; 30:706–708.

52. Torkelson RD, Leibrock LG, Gustavson JL, et al. Neurological and neuropsychological effects of cerebrospinal fluid shunting in children with assumed arrested ("normal pressure") hydrocephalus. *J Neurol Neurosurg Psychiatry* 1985; 48:799–806.

53. Dias MS, Albright AL. Management of hydrocephalus complicating childhood posterior fossa tumors. *Pediatr Neurosci* 1989; 15:283–289.

CHAPTER 56

Stroke and Motor Disorders

David S. Younger

Stroke is recognized by the sudden onset of neurological signs related directly to the sites of injury in the brain where the morbid process occurs (1). The associated motor dysfunction results from injury to areas of the brain subserving motor function. Although the clinical presentation of stroke is quite variable, about 80% of patients present with hemiparesis due to focal infarction along the pyramidal tract and its accompanying fibers (2) alone, or with cranial nerve, sensory, and extrapyramidal manifestations, owing to involvement of contiguous fiber tract and nuclear groups. Spasticity, stiffness, and hyperreflexia of the affected limbs, which supervene in up to one-half of patients in the paretic limbs, completes the upper motor neuron syndrome in a given patient, making the diagnosis apparent (3). Less commonly, hemiparesis can occur without upper motor neuron signs after a stroke, leading to initial diagnostic uncertainty (4).

This chapter considers the epidemiology, clinical presentation, laboratory evaluation, etiopathogenesis, and medical management of stroke, with an emphasis on pure motor syndromes. Acute stroke rehabilitation is considered in a later chapter.

EPIDEMIOLOGY

Stroke is the leading cause of morbidity and mortality in industrialized countries. The Northern Manhattan Stroke Study (NOMASS), which enrolled 924 stroke cases over a four year period from 1993 to 1997, provided insight into stroke in urban black, Hispanic, and white women and men (5, 6). The overall stroke incidence increased with age, primarily due to the increasing incidence of infarcts, less so intracranial hemorrhage (ICH), with only minimally increasing subarachnoid hemorrhage (SAH) frequency with age. However, compared to older individuals, the relative incidence risk ratio of hemorrhagic strokes to infarcts was greater among older adults, suggesting that increasing age or risk factors associated with increasing age, increased the likelihood of infarct more than ICH, and that of ICH more than SAH. In adults, age 20 to 44 years, 45% of strokes were caused by infarct, 31% ICH, and 24% SAH, compared with 80%, 14%, and 5%, respectively, in older individuals. A cryptogenic etiopathogenesis of stroke occurred more frequently in younger than older adults, 55% versus 42%; cardioembolic stroke occurred less frequency, 6% versus 22% in young versus older. However, extra-cranial, intracranial atherosclerosis and lacunar infarction occurred with about equal frequency. Men have a case fatality rate greater than women, 21% versus 11%. The relative risk of any stroke was greater in younger blacks and Hispanics than in whites, with an overall case fatality rate highest in ICH, followed by SAH and infarct.

From 1968 to 1996 there was a remarkable 60% decline in stroke mortality. Although it appears that stroke mortality is currently declining slowly for blacks more than whites, with persistence of geographic differences in stroke mortality around the nation, the rate of decline of stroke mortality has slowed to a plateau overall (7), making it imperative to stroke risk factors. Guidelines for the primary prevention of ischemic stroke have been provided (8). Important non-modifiable risk factors for ischemic stroke include age, gender, ethnicity, and heredity. Modifiable risk factors include hypertension, cardiovascular disease, diabetes mellitus (DM), hyperlipidemia, asymptomatic carotid stenosis, cigarette smoking, and alcohol abuse. Data from NOMASS provided new insights into these stroke risk factors (9). Physical activity had a protective effect against stroke, with relatively low levels of exercise, such as regular walking, producing this effect (10). Ingestion of five or more units of alcohol per day significantly increased risk for ischemic stroke, while consumption of one to two units per day conferred a lower ischemic stroke risk than those who did not drink at all (11). High density lipoproteins (HDL) were protective against stroke whereas lipoproteins increased stroke risk (12, 13). If stroke is subdivided into atherosclerotic, large artery carotid disease, and intracranial atherosclerotic disease, and non-atherosclerotic cryptogenic, lacunar, and cardio-embolic stroke categories, the protective effect of HDL was increased further in events of atherosclerotic origin. Drug treatment to lower low-density lipoprotein (LDL) and triglyceride levels, and increase HDL, reduce the risk for stroke as well as cardiovascular events.

There is evidence to suggest that blood vessel endothelial injury is involved in the atherosclerotic process and linked to increased incidence of stroke, the mechanisms of which could include elevated homocysteine levels and agents that infect the endothelium. Homocysteine, an important new risk factor for stroke is both genetically and environmentally controlled (14). Some individuals with hyperhomocysteinemia have a genetic defect in the enzyme cystathionine β synthetase. One-half of affected patients that are homozygous for the enzyme defect die at a young age from venous thrombosis and premature atherosclerosis, whereas heterozygous individuals are at risk for premature atherosclerosis. C. pneumoniae, a common cause of community-acquired pneumonia, pharyngitis, and sinusitis, and bacterial flora involved in periodontal disease, is theoretically capable of infecting the endothelium and inflicting injury, and may provide useful predictors of ischemic stroke. The sum total of these injurious events of the endothelium could stimulate platelet aggregation, adhesion, monocyte migration, and plaque formation to begin the atherosclerotic process, increasing the risk of stroke. Periodontal disease, which affects up to 20% of those age 60 years to 64 years, can be an important infectious agent and could, theoretically, elevate C-reactive protein (CRP) levels, increasing the risk of cardiovascular disease and stroke.

One epidemiological analysis (15) estimated that 37 to 42% of all ischemic strokes in blacks and whites could be attributable to the effects of DM alone or in combination with hypertension. However, those with ischemic strokes and DM tended to be younger and black, with hypertension, myocardial infarction, and higher cholesterol levels than non-DM. Early population-based epidemiological studies in elderly individuals revealed an association of carotid artery atherosclerosis with stroke risk, with the assumption that increasing age, hypertension, systolic blood pressure, DM, and smoking, but not lipids and lipoproteins, were

consistently related (16, 17). Data on elderly patients studied by NOMASS (18) demonstrated that apolipoprotein A-1 and B (apoA-1 and apoB) were significant determinants of moderate to severe carotid artery atherosclerosis; HDL was protective, while total cholesterol, triglycerides, and LDL cholesterol showed no association.

Hereditary factors in cerebral small vessel diseases are prominent in the cerebral microangiopathies (19). Cerebral autosomal-dominant arteriopathy with stroke and ischemic leukoencephalopathy (CADASIL) is caused by single base exchanges in the Notch3 gene on chromosome 19q, which plays a role in the embryonic development of vascular tissues, and endothelial and smooth muscle cell formation of arteries and veins. It affects younger and older adults between the ages of 40 and 60 years, sometimes in the third and fourth decade, and even in the seventh decade, irrespective of vascular risk factors. It leads to subcortical stroke and a slowly progressive, subcortical type of dementia, developing over a 5-year to 20-year period in 60% of affected patients. Later stages of the disease are characterized by pseudobulbar palsy, tetraparesis, urinary incontinence, and severe mental deterioration, although not reaching the severity of Alzheimer disease. Diagnosis can be made reliably by magnetic resonance imaging (MRI) of the brain, skin biopsy, and molecular genetic testing. Other cerebral microangiopathy syndromes include retinocerebral vasculopathy, which shares involvement of retinal, cerebral, and cochlear arterioles; cerebral amyloid angiopathy, and predisposes to lobar hemorrhage caused by rupture of affected small cortical vessels; and the mitochondrial cytopathies.

Although a single most likely cause of cerebral infarction is emphasized in leading stroke registries (20, 21), other investigators have emphasized the multiple potential causes of infarct (22–24). The Lausanne (22), Belsancon (23), and Ege Stroke Registries (24) noted rates of multiple potential causes of cerebral infarct of 7%, 4.7%, and 3.4%, respectively. This phenomenon has probably been underestimated in the literature, since several other stroke registries have sometimes included patients with two potential causes of infarct in "undetermined" subgroups (20, 21, 25). In ascertaining the frequency of multiple potential causes of cerebral infarct, The Lausanne Stroke Registry (22) distinguished subgroups of patients with large and small artery disease and cardiac embolism as follows: Large artery disease was diagnosed in those with one or more risk factors, including age >50 years, arterial hypertension, DM, cigarette smoking, hypercholesterolemia, stenosis of at least 50% of the lumen diameter in the appropriate large artery demonstrated by Doppler ultrasonography, three-dimensional magnetic resonance angiography (MRA), and conventional cerebral angiography. Small artery disease was presumed in those with longstanding arterial hypertension or DM and a cerebral infarct <15 mm in diameter limited to the territory of deep perforating vessels, in the absence of a cardiac or arterial source of embolism. Cardiac embolism was presumed in the presence of endocarditis, mitral stenosis, atrial fibrillation, sick sinus syndrome, intracardiac thrombus or tumor, prosthetic aortic or mitral values, left ventricular aneurysm or akinesia after myocardial infarct, and global cardiac hypokinesia or dyskinesia. Pure motor stroke, noted in 52% of patients, was the most common lacunar syndrome in the Lausanne stroke registry (22), followed by ataxic hemiparesis in 13% and dysarthria-clumsy hand syndrome in 3%. Pure motor stroke in 71% predominated in the patients with both large artery and cardiac embolic disease, as did ataxic hemiparesis and pure motor stroke, which occurred in one-third each of patients with combined large- and small-artery disease and cardiac embolism.

HISTORY

Patients that present with transient and fixed weakness due to presumed infarct should be evaluated expeditiously in the emergency room and later in a monitored stroke unit, recognizing that their condition may change abruptly. The goal is to identify the etiopathogenesis of the ischemia or infarction through a systematic history, examination, and laboratory evaluation, while contemplating empiric therapy to stabilize the condition and halt progression. The history obtained from the patient, family, or caregiver, should include all pertinent social and demographic information including age, gender, race-ethnicity, and possible contributory risk factors, including arterial hypertension, DM, hypercholesterolemia, cigarette smoking, alcohol use, known carotid bruits or carotid stenosis, hemachromatosis, cardiac ischemia and arrhythmia, previous transient ischemic attack (TIA) or stroke, oral contraceptive medication, and hereditary predisposition to stroke and ischemic heart disease. A prior chart, if available, may be useful to determine the patient's medical and neurological history findings of prior general and neurological examinations and laboratory studies. A preceding headache, loss of consciousness, seizure, weakness, vertigo, or syncope may be useful in dating the onset of ischemia.

PHYSICAL EXAMINATION

All patients should undergo detailed medical and neurological examination. The general medical examination should commence with an assessment of vital signs, recognizing that elevation of blood pressure may be secondarily elevated to support cerebral perfusion, followed by ascer-

tainment of neck bruits, cardiac murmurs, and the presence of peripheral pulses. The neurological examination should include ascertainment of the level of consciousness, verbal and written language, repetition, speech, prosody, possible word finding difficulty, aphasia, paraphasia, and neglect. Cranial somatic motor, sensory, and autonomic function, including visual field and oculomotor nerve function, should be assessed, recognizing that brainstem infarcts may present with supranuclear and lower motor neuron involvement mimicking peripheral nerve palsy. Examination of the limbs should include the strength testing graded 0 to 5 according to the Medical Research Council (MRC). Pronation and drift of the paretic arm should be so noted with the palm facing upward in active sustention, as well as cerebellar dysfunction, disturbances of which lead to nystagmus, axial and limb incoordination, tremor, and hypotonicity. Sensory loss, if present, will be demonstrable by assessment of vibration, proprioception, and light touch, pinprick, and temperature modalities. Cortical sensory loss may lead to asomatognosia with neglect and graphesthesia. Tendon reflexes can be examined in the seated or lying supine position, with elicitation of palmomental, finger flexor reflexes, and ascertainment of Hoffman, Babinski signs, and clonus.

STROKE EVALUATION AND CLASSIFICATION

Admission bloods should be sent for serum chemistries, including venous glucose, glycosylated hemoglobin, complete blood count (CBC), platelet and differential counts and serum osmolarity, lipids, lipoproteins and apolipoprotien constituents, ApoA and ApoB constituents of lipoproteins HDL and LDL, the former being cardioprotective and the latter atherogenic. The erythrocyte sedimentation rate (ESR), CRP, and venous homocysteine levels are potentially useful markers of injury and inflammation. Since stroke can be the result of connective tissue diseases involving the brain, it is not unreasonable to obtain appropriate serological studies to screen for antibodies to cardiolipin, antinuclear antibody (ANA), Sjogren Ro (SS-A) and La (SS-B), ribonucleoprotein (RNP) and Smith (Sm) antigens, antibodies to double-stranded (ds) deoxyribonucleic acid (DNA) and MPO and PR3 antigens found in nuclear cytoplasmic antibodies (c- and p-ANCA), as well as serological markers for spirochete infection due to *Tremponema pallidum* or syphilis, and *Borrelia burgdorferi*, the agent of Lyme neuroborreliosis. Venous levels of vitamin B_{12}, folic acid, and B_6 should be obtained because these vitamins have the capacity to alter homocysteine levels; as may physical inactivity and alcohol consumption. They can secondarily increase circulating plasma homocysteine levels; dietary supplementation may, in turn, return abnormal homocysteine levels to normal. The procoagulants Protein S, C, anti-thrombin III, and levels of other constituents of the classical and alternate complement cascade should be obtained in selected patients.

A 12-lead electrocardiogram (ECG) and continuous 3-lead electrocardiography monitoring, as well as chest radiographs, two-dimensional transthoracic and trans-esophageal echocardiography (TEE) should be performed in patients presenting with a stroke or TIA. Electroencephalography (EEG) is useful in selected patients, such as those who present with a focal seizure at onset of the ischemic event ascribed to embolism or hemorrhage of branch cortical vessels to assist in management.

Screening brain computed tomography (CT) and MRI employing T_1-, and T_2-weighted are equally sensitive to the detection of ischemic stroke and hematoma (26). However the additional of diffusion-weighted imaging (DWI) to the latter, detects ischemic regions within minutes of symptom onset, as well as relatively small cortical and sub-cortical lesions, including those in the brainstem and cerebellum, and other valuable information about the vascular territory with a sensitivity and specificity that approaches 100% (27). Additional available studies for stroke evaluation include three-dimensional MRA of arteries of the neck and cerebral circulation, extracranial and transcranial Doppler ultrasonography with frequency spectral analysis, and B-mode echo tomography of the carotid, vertebrobasilar, and selected intracranial arteries are all readily available at most centers and can provide useful information in stroke classification and management.

Acute stroke due to acute ischemic infarction (ACI) occurs when a cerebral vessel is occluded and a core of brain tissue dies, however the surrounding area, termed the ischemic penumbra, which is hypoperfused, remains at risk of further infarction. Deep brain ischemic leads to a cascade of Na^+/K^+ channels that results in cytotoxic edema, with the net uptake of water in affected brain tissue and narrowing of the extracellular matrix due to reduction in Brownian molecular motion (28). The categorization of subtypes of ischemic stroke is more than an academic exercise since it is inextricably linked to further management, the goal of which is to accurately ascertain the site, size, age, and vascular territory of an ischemic lesion within hours of symptom onset by early brain neuroimaging, and to consider one of the many treatment protocols, including intravenous recombinant tissue plasminogen activator (rt-PA) and other measures to restore or improve perfusion, without which the infarcted core may continue to enlarge and progressively replace ischemic tissue in the penumbra (28).

This categorization of subtypes of ischemic stroke, previously based upon risk factor profiles, clinical features of the stroke, and findings on brain imaging employing CT and MRI, has shifted in the direction of etiopathogenesis, recognizing the five essential types for purposes of acute management in clinical trials, including large-artery atherosclerotic, embolic and thrombotic, moderate and high-risk cardioembolic, small-vessel occlusive lacunar, and those due to other causes, undetermined, or with negative or incomplete evaluations (21).

Although non-contrast CT of the brain has been the standard for evaluation of patients with suspected stroke and to which all other brain imaging studies are compared, it is insensitive in detecting acute and small cortical or subcortical infarctions, especially in the posterior fossa. With advent of rt-PA treatment there has been interest in refining CT to identify subtle early signs of ischemic brain injury and arterial occlusion that might impact on the decision to treat with beyond the tissue clock criteria based upon a more favorable outcome of the ischemic penumbra, which dictates rt-PA be administered within three hours of symptom onset (29). Such refinements in CT imaging include perfusion-CT (PCT) employing whole-brain perfusion and dynamic perfusion that allow differentiation of reversible and irreversible ischemia and identification of the ischemic penumbra. Helical CT angiography (CTA) to rapidly and noninvasively evaluates vascular stenosis ad occlusions, all with the benefit of rapid data acquisition and performance with conventional CT equipment, however the disadvantage is the requirement for iodine contrast and additional radiation exposures (27).

The combination of perfusion-weighted imaging (PWI) to demonstrate areas of reduced cerebral perfusion, along with DWI to depict areas of irreversible injury, leads to mismatched areas, the PWI often being larger than DWI, representing the tissue at risk in the ischemic penumbra (26). In prospective studies of patients studied with sequential neuroimaging for ACI that included DWI, PWI, T_2-weighted MRI and MRA, 35 patients subjected to rt-PA with mismatch of PWI/DWI in the area of ischemic penumbra and cerebral arterial occlusion shown by MRA, showed significant reduction in infarct size and recanalization consistent with salvation of at-risk ischemic tissue (30).

The conventional brain imaging of lacunar infarction typically shows small, deep infarcts or a normal image, normal or minimal large artery stenosis, and no source of cardiac embolus. Infarcts related to extra-cranial stenosis demonstrate occlusion or moderate to severe stenosis of > 60% in the carotid, vertebral, or basilar artery correlates with expected territories of infarction. Infarcts related to intracranial atherosclerosis generally shows large artery stenosis or occlusion demonstrated by cerebral MRA, cerebral angiography, and transcranial Doppler studies. Cardioembolic infarction is suggested by concomitant atrial fibrillation or flutter, valvular heart disease, cardiac intraluminal thrombus, cardiomyopathy, recent myocardial infarction, bacterial or marantic endocarditis, atrial myxoma, or pulmonary vein thrombosis. Infarction associated with other causes requires consideration of dissection, fibromuscular dysplasia, vasculitis, sickle cell anemia, and migraine. Patients with primary ICH present with focal neurological symptoms and signs, and brain imaging evidence of intraparenchymal blood on brain imaging. The secondary causes of ICH include blood dyscrasia, anticoagulation, arteriovenous malformation, cavernous angiomata, trauma, and tumor. Those with SAH manifest the sudden onset of neurological deficits, headache, neck stiffness, and alteration of consciousness, with evidence of subarachnoid blood on brain imaging, as well as cerebrospinal fluid (CSF) xanthochromia and increased red blood cell counts.

PURE MOTOR STROKE

For more than 150 years since Dechambre (31) first employed the term *lacune*, derived from the Latin word *lacuna,* meaning cavity or hole, to describe a small area of cerebral infarction, and état criblé proposed by Durand-Fardel (32) for the multitude of small holes in the brain at postmortem examination, neurologists have struggled with the concept of predominant syndrome of motor weakness in stroke. The Harvard Cooperative Stroke Registry (33) ascertained that pure motor hemiparesis was the most frequent lacunar syndrome. Fisher and Curry (34) defined it as paresis involving the face, arm, and leg on one side, without sensory deficit, homonymous hemianopia, aphasia, agnosia, or apraxia. Fisher and Curry (34) described two patients with pure motor stroke and brainstem infarction associated with basilar artery atherosclerosis, however Fisher and Caplan (35) found occlusion by atheromatous plaque of a branch of the basilar artery in another patient with pure motor stroke. In a patient described by Ho (36) with pure motor hemiplegia due to infarction of the pontine cerebral peduncle, the basilar artery was patent but atherosclerotic without vascular occlusions, however the presence of hyalinized vessels close to the infarct suggested probable thrombosis of a small penetrating artery. One patient with medullary pyramidal infarction described by Chokroverty and colleagues (37) had diffuse large vessel atheromatous plaques as compared to the patient described by Ho and Meyer (38) who had patent vertebral and basilar arteries with narrowing of the lumen by patchy areas of calcified atheromatous plaque.

The concept of pure motor stroke was extended to include limited syndromes of faciobrachial and brachiocrural weakness (39–41). Whereas partial syndromes resulted from medullary, pontine, capsular, and cortical ischemic lesions, classical pure motor hemiplegia was usually due to small infarcts located in the internal capsule or brainstem (42). Pure motor strokes due to medullary and pontine infarction were not easily distinguished clinically and neuroradiologically from the capsular types (43). In addition to pure motor hemiparesis, Fisher (42) recognized 6 additional syndromes, including one of the medulla that spared the face; two of the pons associated with either horizontal gaze palsy or crossed sixth nerve palsy; one of the midbrain associated with crossed third nerve palsy; and two of the internal capsule, termed crossed hemiparesis with confusion, and another with motor aphasia.

Medullary Infarcts

Whereas lateral medullary infarction due to vertebral artery disease virtually never led to pure motor hemiparesis, lesions of the medial medulla may do so (Figure 1). Kumral and colleagues used MRI to investigate (44) unilateral medial medullary infarction in 10 patients, and bilateral lesions in one. Altogether, three clinical patterns were associated with unilateral lesions, including classical Dejerine syndrome of contralateral hemiparesis, lemniscal sensory loss, and ipsilateral lingual palsy altogether in seven; pure hemiparesis in two patients; and sensorimotor stroke in one with contralateral hemiparesis, hyperesthesia, and decreased pain sensation, without lingual palsy. A patient with bilateral medial medullary infarction presented with tetraparesis, bilateral deep sensation loss, dysphagia, dysphonia, and anarthria. Of 17 patients with unilateral medial medullary infarction, Kim and colleagues (45) noted two patients, or 12%, with pure motor stroke. Pure motor hemiparesis sparing the face was caused by an infarct of the medullary pyramid due to occlusion of either the vertebral artery itself or a penetrating branch (46), which at onset presented with slight vertigo and trace nystagmus.

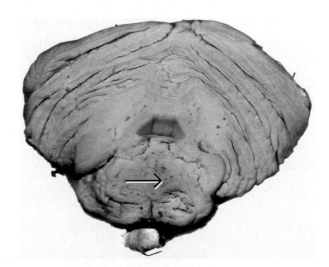

FIG. 1. Cross-section of the brainstem shows lacunar infarction of the medial medullary tegmentum in association with basilar thrombosis.

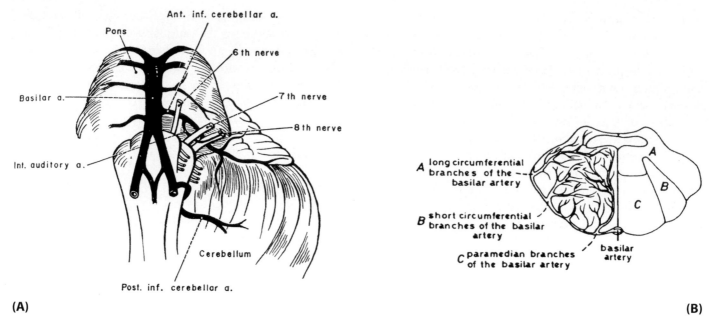

FIG. 2. (A) Vascular anatomy of the basilar artery. Reproduced from: Fisher CM. Vertigo in cerebrovascular disease. *Arch Otolaryngol* 1967; 85:531, with permission. **(B)** Basilar artery branch territories. From, Kappelle LJ, van Gijn J. Lacunar infarcts. *Clin Neurol Neurosurg* 1986; 88:4, with permission.

Pontine Infarcts

The vascular supply and territories of the basilar artery and its branch vessels in the brainstem are depicted in Figure 2A, 2B, underscoring the possible patterns of infarction. Huang and colleagues (47) studied nine patients with brainstem infarcts and two with hemorrhage diagnosed by CT, four of whom who presented with pure motor stroke due to ischemic infarction in the paramedian aspect of the pons in three, and hemorrhage in one. In the latter patient, as in the three original cases of pathologically-proven brainstem

infarct causing pure motor stroke, reported by Fisher and Curry (34), there was transient diplopia. Three of the four patients had progression of neurological deficits. Nighoghossian and colleagues (48) prospectively studied 21 patients with pure motor hemiparesis in whom CT demonstrated a causative capsular lesion in 15 patients or 71%, and was uninformative in six patients. Further evaluation by MRI revealed a paramedian pontine infarct as the notable cause of weakness. A combination of dysarthria and a history of previous transient gait abnormality or vertigo favored a pontine lesion. Outcome at three months was characterized by per-

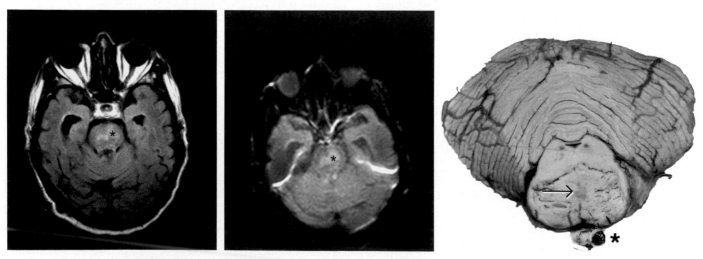

FIG. 3. Cross-section of the brainstem shows medial pontine lacunar infarction in association with basilar thrombosis. Note the thrombus in the basilar artery.

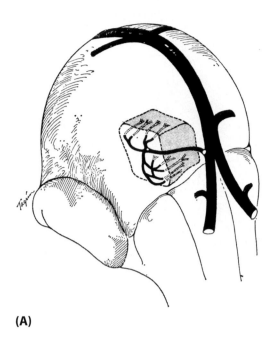

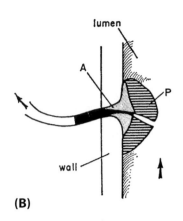

FIG. 4. (A) Schematic depiction of basilar artery branch occlusion. **(B)** Intravascular plaque narrows and occludes the ostium of the branch vessel. From, Fisher CM. Basilar artery branch occlusion: a cause of pontine infarction. *Neurology* 1971; 21:903, with permission.

sistent moderate to severe motor disability in 86% of patients with pontine infarcts. Kaps and colleagues (49) studied eight patients with isolated infarcts of the pons with pure motor hemiparesis that was severely progressive in the first three days, with overall relatively good outcome, but recurrence in two led to pseudobulbar palsy and tetraparesis. Brain MRI showed unilateral ventromedial pontine infarction in six patients, and bilateral lesions in two. Angiographic evaluation in four patients and color duplex examination in four showed atherosclerotic lesions without basilar occlusion. The progressive pattern of deterioration suggested propagating basilar thrombosis. An example of ventromedial pontine infarction due to basilar artery branch occlusion, in association with basilar thrombosis, is shown in Figure 3. The mechanism of branch vessel occlusion adjacent to the thrombosed basilar artery is depicted schematically in Figure 4A, 4B. Kunz and colleagues (50) studied 26 patients with progressive pure motor hemiparesis accompanied by dysarthria and homolateral ataxia due to paramedian pontine infarction. The weakness tended to be more marked distally in the arm following the somatotopic organization of the ventromedial pons and corticospinal tracts. Lesions located ventromedial in the pons affect corticospinal fibers associated with the arm and lead to predominant arm weakness.

Pontine lesions affecting corticopontine fibers that terminate upon facial motor nuclei and extrapyramidal and central tegmental tract fibers resulted in dysarthria, whereas those of the corticopontocerebellar fibers led to ataxia. Chan and Silver (51) reported a man with recurrent pure motor hemiparesis in whom MRI showed unilateral infarction of the ventral pons, and cerebral angiography confirmed a mid-basilar artery stenosis of >90% with ulcerated plaque, and diffuse irregularities along the entire length of the basilar artery representing atherosclerotic disease. The patient ultimately improved in spite of failed angioplasty and stenting due to plaque recoil.

Pure motor hemiparesis with horizontal gaze palsy was reviewed by Fisher (42). One pathologically proven case (35) had a causative paramedian infarct in the low pons with paresis of the face, arm, and leg combined with one-and-a-half syndrome of ipsilateral conjugate lateral gaze palsy and crossed internuclear ophthalmoplegia, leaving abduction of the opposite eye as the only horizontal eye movement, reflecting preservation of the opposite sixth nerve. The other syndrome described by Fisher (42) of pure motor hemiparesis with crossed sixth nerve palsy results from infarction of the paramedian inferior-most pons, catching the fibers of the ipsilateral sixth nerve as it exited from the brainstem.

Midbrain Infarcts

Bogousslavsky and colleagues (52) reported 22 patients with a first stroke and infarct limited to the midbrain on MRI. Two of the patients presented with pure motor hemiparesis, including one with hypertension and an infarct of the upper midbrain, and another with hypertension and diabetes with an infarct of the middle midbrain. In both patients, there was absence of localizing eye-movement abnormalities. Similar findings of a non-specific picture of pure motor hemiparesis from cerebral peduncle damage were described by Gaymard and colleagues (53). Fisher (42) described a syndrome of pure motor hemiparesis associated with crossed third-nerve palsy (Weber syndrome), a rare event in which an infarct involving the midportion of the cerebral peduncle caught the issuing fibers of the third nerve.

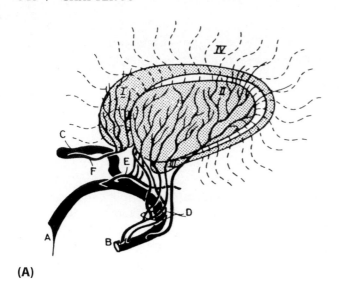

(A)

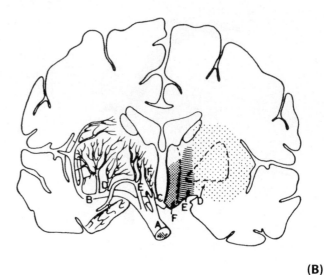

(B)

FIG. 5. Vascular supply of the internal capsule shown in lateral **(A)** and coronal **(B)** views. A, internal carotid artery; B, middle cerebral artery; C, anterior cerebral artery; D, lenticulostriate arteries; E, anterior choroidal artery; F, recurrent artery of Heubner. From, Kappelle LJ, van Gijn J. Lacunar infarcts. *Clin Neurol Neurosurg* 1986; 88:4, with permission.

Capsular Infarcts

The history of capsular lacunar infarction was reviewed by Mohr (54). Pierre Marie (55) used the term *lacune* in a description of 50 cases of capsular infarction, formulating a syndrome of sudden onset incomplete hemiplegia in which walking was disturbed in a permanent fashion, characterized as the small steps of "marche a petits pas de Dejerine." Considerable improvement in the paralysis occurred over hours to days, but complete recovery was unusual. A variety of modifiers were added to the original formulation. Ferrand in 1902 (56) noted that the same syndrome occurred whether the lesion was capsular or pontine in location. Foix and Levy (57) added the findings of equal affliction of the arm and leg. Foix and Hillemand (58) distinguished them from pontine lacunes in which arm weakness exceeded that of the leg. Fisher and colleagues revisited capsular infarcts between 1965 and 1979 (59), adding further syndromes of homolateral ataxia and crural paresis (60) and dysarthria-clumsy hand syndrome (61). To emphasize its frequency, 376 lacunes were found in 114 patients from among 1,042 consecutive patients examined postmortem, of whom 88, or 77%, had previous neurological symptoms (62). Another study noted that only 65% of lacunes diagnosed by CT were appropriate to the elicited neurological signs (63).

The blood supply of the internal capsule is derived from a number of small different arteries as depicted in Figure 5 A, B. Classical teaching suggested that capsular lesions leading to pure motor hemiplegia resulted from lacunes in the anterior part of the posterior limb of the internal capsule where pyramidal tract fibers were located (34). However that concept was revised with recognition that corticospinal tract fibers move to an increasing posterior position in the internal capsule as they descend from rostral to caudal levels to the posterior one-half of the posterior limb (64, 65, 66). Figure 6 demonstrates the neuroanatomical findings of a patient with capsular infarction.

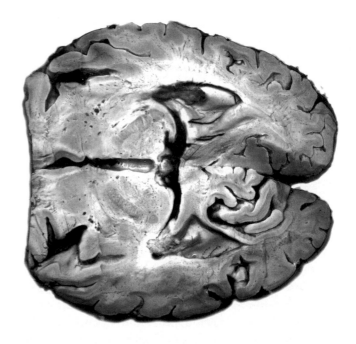

FIG. 6. Longitudinal section of the brain at the level of the internal capsule shows bilateral posterior capsular infarcts.

Kappelle and van Gijn (67) distinguished three types of capsular infarcts leading to pure motor hemiparesis based upon anatomical localization and presumed site of the arterial lesion: First, putaminal-capsulo-caudate infarct due to involvement of lateral lenticulostriate arteries. Second, capsule-pallidal infarct due to involvement of perforating branches of the anterior choroidal artery. And third, anterior capsule-caudate infarct resulting from a recurrent artery of Heubner lesion. However, it was not always possible to infer the origin of a given infarct or involved artery due to the branching pattern of the penetrating vessels and the presence of anastomosis channels that might exist between them (68).

Loeb (69) recorded 53 patients with pure motor hemiparesis and 34 patients with modified pure motor hemiparesis. In six patients, heralding symptoms surprisingly included paresthesias, headache, vertigo, and vomiting, with a faciobrachial-crural distribution of weakness in 42%. The lacunar cavity was located in the territories of lenticulostriate, thalamoperforating, anterior choroidal, paracentral lateral and medial branches of the posterior cerebral artery in decreasing order of frequency in 42 patients.

Russmann and colleagues (70) studied 13 patients with pure lenticular infarcts, all with faciobrachio-crural hemisyndromes, none of whom showed acute or delayed parkinsonism or abnormal movements. Nine of the patients had lesions restricted to the putamen. All infarcts were in the territory of the medial perforating branches of the middle cerebral artery (MCA). Presumed cause of infarct was small artery disease in five, artery-to-artery embolism in four and cardioembolism in three, and undetermined in one.

Kumral and coworkers (71) studied 11 patients with subinsular stroke located in a deep border zone between lenticulostriate arteries and small insular cortical penetrating branches of the MCA, and noted mainly motor deficits explicable by a lesion involving cortico-capsular motor pathways. In a study of 148 patients with acute isolated capsular stroke, reported by Arboix and colleagues (72), pure motor hemiparesis was found in 84 or 67.7% of patients, resulting from capsular infarction. Melo and colleagues (43) studied 255 patients with a first stroke and manifestation of isolated hemiparesis, and suggested a lacunar etiology of pure motor stroke in those with involvement of face, and upper and lower limb after logistic regression analysis of clinical variables. Less than one-half of patients had a deep infarct, and one-third had a potential source of embolism from the heart or large arteries. Fisher (42) delineated the syndrome of modified pure motor hemiparesis with motor aphasia in a pathologically studied patient that showed large softening of the genu and anterior limb of the internal capsule and the adjacent white matter of the inferior corona radiate. In addition, thrombotic occlusion of a lenticulostriate branch supplying the territory of the infarct

was identified. The patient manifested severe weakness of the right side of the face and moderate weakness of the right hand. The right leg was slightly weak and there was a Babinski sign elicited. Early in the illness there was dysarthria and the patient mispronounced words but corrected the errors. Later, he made single-syllable unintelligible sounds and finally was mute; however, comprehension remained normal. The only lesion in the brain was a 1.2 cm lacune in the anterior limb and anterior part of the posterior limb of the right internal capsule that ostensibly interrupted thalamofrontal connections.

Fisher (42) observed that the lacunar state, or l'etat lacunaire, first described by Marie (55), that included one or more lacunes associated with chronic progressive neurological decline marked by one or more episodes of slight hemiparesis and ending with dysarthria, small-step gait, imbalance, incontinence, pseudobulbar palsy, and some signs of dementia, were rarely, if ever, clinically encountered. Bilateral spastic hemiparesis was never part of the picture, adding doubt to the clinicopathologic correlation. Fisher (42) speculated that much of the clinical picture was probably due to unrecognized symptomatic normal pressure hydrocephalus (NPH). In Marie's patients (55) hydrocephalus was usually prominent pathologically, and illustrations showed enormous ventricular dilatation similar to that shown in the gross neuroanatomical specimen of Figure 7. Earnest (73) and Koto and coworkers (74) reported the association of lacunar infarcts and NPH. The general impression that multiple lacunes were distributed haphazardly, with some symptomatic and some not, was dubious to Fisher (42). The findings of nine patients with

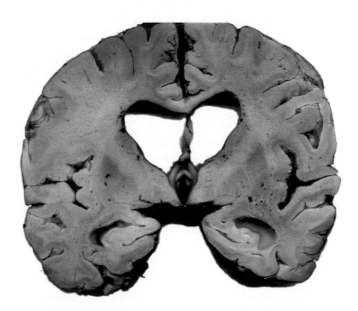

FIG. 7. Coronal section of the brain shows hydrocephalus and bilateral capsular infarcts.

lacunar infarction of the internal capsule associated with pure motor hemiparesis clearly indicated a tendency for the first lacunar infarct to be symptomatic (59). Of a total of 21 lacunes, 15 were capsular and were associated with pure motor hemiparesis. In these cases, survival for several years after the stroke was not unusual, providing ample time for other lacunar lesions to have occurred.

Several theories exist to explain the occurrence of capsular lacunes. The most prevalent cause appeared to be hypertension, which causes large vessels to elongate and dilate, resulting in displacement of the ostia of the smaller branches and subsequent branch occlusion (75). Hypertension alters the wall of small vessels less than 200 microns near sharp turns or at the origin of the penetrating branch (59) with initial focal deposits of fibrinoid material along the subintima, appearing as fine granular eosinophilic material (76), and later distributed through all layers of the vessel wall. This disorganization can eventually culminate in microaneurysms (77) as the cause of intracerebral hemorrhages arising in the internal capsule or basal ganglia, as well as lacunar infarcts, the latter by a thrombotic process extending from the aneurysm into the distal part of the artery (76, 78). Atherosclerotic plaque, sparing penetrating branches themselves, along the anterior, middle cerebral, and basilar artery could occlude penetrating vessels at their origin, resulting in infarction (35, 59). Emboli from extracranial sources such as the heart, or bifurcation of the internal carotid artery, may also be the source of lacunar infarction (59).

Hommel and colleagues (79) studied 100 patients with lacunar infarct, including 35 with pure motor stroke, and noted increased effectiveness overall in detection of a lacune appropriate to the symptoms in 89 patients when performed a few days after the stroke, suggesting that MRI was the imaging technique of choice in the study of lacunar syndromes. Toni and colleagues (80) found that clinical and CT indices of pure motor hemiparesis (81) yielded a positive predictive value of 56% among 123 patients with pure motor hemiparesis when applied in the first 12 hours of the stroke event. Other causes of pure motor hemiparesis that may mimic lacunar infarction clinically, warranting further specific laboratory investigation, included small hemorrhages in the internal capsule, pons, or putamen, demyelinating disease, subdural hematomas, solitary metastasis, and abscess. Cerebral angiography has a limited role in the evaluation of capsular lacunes because of its insensitivity in detecting occlusion of individual penetrating arteries in the internal capsule in all but giant lacunes (41), more often showing stenosis and occlusions of larger intracranial vessels, or the internal carotid artery. From a surgical standpoint, intervention for lacunar infarcts is indicated in only certain situations, such as when angiography demonstrates stenosis or mural irregularities of extracranial arteries as a possible source of tandem emboli that may be occluding penetrating vessels.

Cortical Infarcts

The literature is more limited concerning cortical motor infarcts. Ghika and colleagues (82) studied 32 patients with CT-, and MRI-proven pure parietal stroke and transient mild pseudoparesis of the hand associated with pyramidal signs, unilateral akinesia, non-awareness of muscle power, and motor hemineglect in non-dominant lesions, presumed to be due to loss of multiple sensory feedback to motor programs. De Freitas and colleagues (83) studied 895 patients with hemiparesis sparing the leg, comparing 1,644 stroke patients with paresis of the leg, and noted that in those with leg sparing weakness, a majority of lesions were caused by superficial infarcts, almost one-half of which were confined to superficial branches of the MCA territory, with twice the number in the anterior or superior division. More than half had a presumed embolic source from large artery disease or from the heart. Patients without leg involvement had a lower prevalence of small artery disease but a higher prevalence of migraine, TIA, atherosclerosis without stenosis, large artery disease, and left hemispheric stroke, with a lower frequency of hemorrhagic stroke.

STROKE OUTCOME

A recent study reported that 39% of patients with first-ever stroke were spastic after 12 months (84). Sommerfeld and colleagues (3) noted spasticity in 19% of patients investigated three months after stroke, however severe disabilities were seen in almost the same number of non-spastic as spastic patients, which included muscle stiffness and other measures of abnormal muscle tone and motor disability. It is well recognized that spasticity can interfere with motor and activity performance measures and lead to pain and secondary complications. However, there is no evidence that suppression of spasticity by either physiotherapy or medication results in parallel improvements in motor function (85).

Dethy and colleagues (86) studied a patient with right arm and leg tremor three months after a pure motor stroke. Brain MRI showed an ischemic lesion in the left centrum semiovale and a left caudate lacunar infarct. Brain positron emission tomography (PET) demonstrated glucose hypermetabolism in the left sensorimotor area. The authors concluded that unilateral tremor was related to the lacunar infarct in the caudate nucleus.

Staaf and colleagues (87) studied 180 patients with pure motor stroke and found that 60% of the patients died, most commonly as a result of coronary artery disease. After five years, the risk of death was increased among those with pure motor stroke compared to the general population, related independently to advanced age, male gender, and nonuse of aspirin. A risk of recurrent stroke was noted among those with risk factors of hypertension and diabetes. Steinke and Ley (88) studied 941 stroke patients with a severe motor deficit after lacunar infarct and noted progressive hemiparesis, presumably due to stepwise occlusion of branches of small penetrating arteries over a three-year period of observation.

Arauz and colleagues (89) investigated the collected risk factors and concomitant vascular disorders of 175 patients with a first symptomatic lacunar infarction defined by MRI over a 10-year period. Increased hemoglobin levels, DM, and leukoaraiosis (Figure 8), defined as the presence of bilateral symmetrical and diffuse abnormalities located in the white matter surrounding the frontal horn and parieto-occipital area encircling the ventricles, or hyperintense areas of the centrum semiovale, were important risk factors in patients with more than one lacunar infarct. The presence of multiple lacunar infarcts was considered an important indicator, not only for functional recovery but also for a higher rate of recurrence. Wenzelburger and colleagues (90) studied motor outcome following stroke of the internal capsule. There was a close correlation between posterior location of the posterior limb of the internal capsule and altered measures of timing and precision grip force of the hand. The more posterior the acute lesion was located with the posterior limb of the internal capsule, the more pronounced were chronic motor deficits.

STROKE MANAGEMENT

Treatment in stroke can be divided into acute stroke management and secondary prevention. Acute stroke carries a mortality of 20% due to the infarct or its complications,

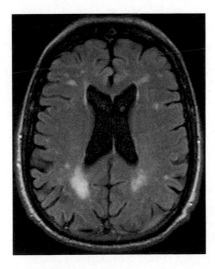

FIG. 8. Diffusion-weighted MRI in a patient with multiple lacunes that demonstrates leukoaraiosis. There are bilateral symmetrical and diffuse abnormalities located in the white matter surrounding the frontal horn and parieto-occipital area encircling the ventricles.

most commonly recurrent stroke, pneumonia, deep vein thrombosis, and pulmonary embolism. Care of the patient in a stroke unit appears to reduce overall mortality by 30% and improve outcome (91). Patients treated in a United Kingdom hospital with an acute stroke unit had an odds ratio of 0.89 for death after adjustment for age, sex, and length of stay (92). Although mortality did not differ in an analysis of 433 stroke patients admitted to a 10-bed university hospital Neurosciences Intensive Care Unit (NICU) before and after the appointment of a full-time neurointensivist (NI), 75% of patients were discharged home in the after period compared to 54% in the before period, indicating that direct patient care offered, and the organizational changes implemented by an NI, shortened the NICU and hospital length of stay (LOS) and improved disposition of patients. This may include aspects of supportive and physiological care as well as prevention of complications, that persists for many years after an acute stroke (93).

Early studies compared antithrombotic therapy employing antiplatelet or anticoagulant agents versus controls in ACI. The International Stroke Trial (IST) (94) was a large, randomized open trial of up to 14 days of antithrombotic therapy started as soon as possible after stroke onset. The aim was to provide reliable evidence of the safety and efficacy of aspirin and subcutaneous heparin. The primary outcomes were death within 14 days and death or dependency at 6 months. A total of 19,435 patients with suspected ACI entered 467 hospitals in 36 countries within 48 hours of symptom onset. Neither regimen of 5,000 International units (IU) nor 12,500 IU of twice-daily subcutaneous heparin offered any clinical advantages at six months. Moreover, there was a small but worthwhile benefit of 300mg of daily aspirin.

The Stroke Prevention in Reversible Ischemia Trial (SPIRIT) (95), which recruited patients with non-cardiac TIA and minor ischemic stroke, in a comparison of aspirin versus warfarin using a relatively high level of the international normalized ration (INR) of 3.0 to 4.5, was stopped early because of an excess of hemorrhagic events. A collaborative meta-analysis of 287 randomized trials involving 135,000 patients in comparisons of antiplatelet therapy versus control, and 77,000 patients in comparisons of different antiplatelet regimens though September 1997 (96), determined that low doses of daily aspirin in the range of 75 mg to 150 mg was an effective antiplatelet regimen for long-term use in high-risk patients in the prevention of non-fatal stroke, while in acute settings an initial loading dose of at least 150 mg was required. Adding a second antiplatelet drug to aspirin might produce additional benefits in some clinical circumstances, but more research into this strategy was needed.

The Warfarin-Aspirin Recurrent Stroke Study (WARSS) (97) compared warfarin with a target INR of 1.4 to 2.8 to 325 mg of daily aspirin in a multicenter, double-blind, randomized trial on the combined primary endpoint of recurrent ischemic stroke or death from any cause within two years, and found no difference between the two agents, regarding them as reasonable therapeutic alternatives. The European Stroke Prevention Study 2 (ESPS2) (98) undertook a randomized, placebo-controlled study to investigate the safety and efficacy of 25 mg of twice daily aspirin, 400 mg of modified-release daily dipyramidole, and the 2 agents in combination for secondary prevention of ischemic stroke, with the primary endpoints of stroke, death, and stroke or death together. Factorial pairwise comparisons showed that the risk of stroke or death was reduced by 13% with aspirin alone, 15% with dipyrimadol alone, and 37% with combination therapy. A meta-analysis of randomized trials testing antithrombotic agents to prevent stroke in patients with atrial fibrillation revealed that adjusted-dose warfarin reduced stroke by 62% compared to aspirin which reduced stroke by 22%, in which the benefit of either was not offset by the occurrence of major hemorrhage (99).

The Warfarin-Aspirin Symptomatic Intracranial Disease (WASID) Trial (100) randomly assigned 569 patients with TIA or stroke caused by 50 to 99% angiographically-proven stenosis of a major intracranial artery to receive a target INR of 2 to 3, or 1300 mg of daily aspirin, in a double-blind multicenter trial, the primary endpoint of which was ACI, ICH, or death from vascular causes other than stroke. Warfarin was associated with significantly higher rates of adverse events, including death in 9.7% compared to 4.3% for aspirin, with major hemorrhage, respectively, in 8.3% compared to 3.2%, and sudden death in 7.3% compared to 2.9%. Warfarin was not superior to aspirin in a population study, possibly due to inadequate time in a therapeutic INR target range. Moreover, stroke in this population, which probably occurred because of hypertensive vascular disease and a heightened risk of embolism from aortic, cardiac, and cerebrovascular sources associated with systemic atherosclerosis, further demonstrated that a delay in achieving a therapeutic level of anticoagulation in high-risk patients might have contributed to the failure of warfarin (101).

The practice of initially treating high-risk patients with a rapidly and consistently active anticoagulant, such as low molecular weight heparin, followed by a transition to antiplatelet therapy after an asymptomatic period, might prevent the accumulation of early adverse events. Warfarin reduces the rate of ischemic stroke in patients with atrial fibrillation but requires frequent monitoring and dose adjustment. Rivaroxaban, an oral factor Xa inhibitor, provided more consistent and predictable anticoagulation in the double-blind Rivaroxaban Once Daily Oral Direct Factor Xa Inhibition Compared with Vitamin K Antagonism for Prevention of Stroke and Embolism Trial in Atrial Fibrillation (ROCKET AF) trial of 14,264 patients randomly assigned to either rivaroxaban at a daily dose of 20 mg or dose-adjusted warfarin

(102). Rivaroxaban was also superior to dose-adjusted warfarin in preventing stroke or systemic embolism, with less bleeding and lower mortality with apixaban at a dose of 5 mg twice daily among 18,201 patients in the randomized double-blind trial of Apixaban for Reduction in Stroke and Other Thromboembolic Events in Atrial Fibrillation (ARISTOTLE) (103). In the double-blind Apixaban Versus Acetylsalicylic Acid to Prevent Stroke in Atrial Fibrillation Patients Who Have Failed or Are Unsuitable for Vitamin K Antagonist Treatment (AVEROES) study of 5 mg twice daily of apixaban versus 81 to 324 mg of daily aspirin in patients for whom vitamin K therapy was unsuitable, apixaban further reduced the risk of stroke or systemic embolism without significantly increasing the risk of major bleeding or intracranial hemorrhage. Whereas the oral direct thrombin inhibitor dabigatran administered at a dose of 110 mg in the Randomized Evaluation of Long-Term Anticoagulation Therapy (RE-LY) trial (104) was associated with a primary outcome rate of stroke of 1.53% as compared to 1.69% for warfarin, with a commensurately lower rate of bleeding for dabigatran of 2.71% per year as compared to 3.36% for warfarin, an adjustment in the daily dose of dabigatran to 150 mg was associated with a further reduction in the primary outcome of stroke to 1.11%.

The benefit of thrombolytic therapy with rt-PA in the treatment in ACI was first established by the NINDS rt-PA Stroke Study Group (29), in which randomized double-blinded administration of rt-PA was beneficial for ischemic stroke when treatment was begun within three hours of the onset of stroke as judged by four outcome measures, the National Institutes of Health stroke scale (NIHSS) (105), the modified Rankin Scale (mRS) (106), Barthel index (107), and the Glascow outcome scale (108), and resolution of the neurological deficit within 24 hours of the onset of stroke. However, symptomatic ICH occurred within 36 hours after the onset of stroke in 6.4% of patients given rt-PA, compared to 0.6% of placebo treated patients. Mortality at three months was 17% in the rt-PA group compared to 21% in the placebo group. The mechanism of benefit of rt-PA was ascribed to support of tissue in the ischemic penumbra that was hypoperfused, but not yet infarcted. Ultrasound has been used to accelerate thrombolysis with rt-PA (109). Although 75% of patients with mild or rapidly improving symptoms are expected to have a favorable outcome after three months, whether treated or not, thrombolysis with its potential risks does not seem to be justified in such patients. However, selected patients, especially those with proximal vessel occlusions and baseline NIHSS scores >or = to 10 points might be expected to derive a benefit from thrombolysis (110). Moreover, the poor outcome of patients who did not receive intravenous rt-PA because of relatively mild or improving ischemic stroke and were unable to be discharged home, suggested reevaluaton of the stroke severity criteria (111).

Treatment trials employing other thrombolytic agents beyond the three-hour window have had more disappointing results due to hemorrhagic sequel. Recognizing that detection of the neurological symptoms on awakening in so termed *wake-up stroke*, which occurred in 8 to 27% of patients with ischemic stroke (112–114), and the uncertainty about the time of onset of stroke in this situation, making them ineligible for thrombolytic treatment, the Abciximab in Emergency Stroke Treatment Trial (AbESTT) (115) randomized 400 patients within six hours of onset of ACI to either an abciximab bolus followed by a 12-hour infusion or placebo. Treatment with abciximab showed a non-significant shift in favorable outcome at three months, employing the mRS, and asymptomatic hemorrhagic transformation by brain imaging in 3.6% of patients so treated, compared to 33 placebo-treated patients. In a later study by the same investigators (116), study subjects who had a relatively higher rate of new stroke on CT, despite similar baseline characteristics of other stroke subjects, experienced a rate of bleeding in 13.6% of subjects, exceeding prespecified safety margins, and a 9.3% poorer outcome at three months as judged by the mRS, halting further recruitment.

Thrombolysis with alteplase administered at 3 to 4½ hours after ischemic stroke in 418 randomly assigned patients (117) had a more favorable outcome than 403 placebo-treated subjects (52.4% versus 45.2%) as judged by the mRS dichotomized as a favorable or unfavorable outcome, and a global outcome measure that combined the outcomes at day 90 on the mRS, Barthel index, NIHSS, and Glasgow Outcome scale (29). The incidence of any type of ICH was higher in the alteplase-treated subjects in 27% compared to 17.6% in placebo-treated subjects, with symptomatic ICH in 2.4% of alteplase-treated subjects compared to .2% of placebo-treated subjects, without mortality differences.

Among 180 patients with acute ischemic stroke of less than six hours duration caused by angiographically-proven occlusion of the MCA, and randomized to intra-arterial recombinant prourokinase (r-proUK) plus heparin, or heparin only in the Prolyse in Acute Cerebral Thromboembolism II (PROACT II) trial (118), 40% of r-proUK-treated subjects, and 25% of control subjects had an mRS of two or less. Respective mortality was 25% and 27%, with an MCA recanalization rate, respectively of 66% and 18%, and neurological deterioration that occurred within 24 hours, respectively in 10% and 2% of subjects. Despite an increase in early symptomatic ICH with IA r-proUK within six hours of the onset of ACI caused by MCA occlusion, there was a significantly improved clinical outcome at 90 days as judged by the modified Rankin scale (106). The Middle Cerebral Artery Embolism Local Fibrinolytic Intervention Trial (MELT) (119), which randomized intra-arterial infusion of UK to 114 study patients with angiographically-proven occlusions of the M1 or M2 portion of the MCA,

demonstrated a 90-day cumulative mortality of 5.3% in the UK-treated study group compared to 3.5% in the control group, with frequencies of ICH within 24 hours of 9% and 2%, respectively. The trial was aborted prematurely as the primary endpoint analysis of favorable outcome employing a modified NIHSS, mRS, and Barthel, did not reach statistical significance.

Two factors that appear to be important in the benefits of rt-PA are the lapse in time from onset of stroke symptoms to initiation of therapy, and the selection of patients for reperfusion therapy. Analyses of the major randomized placebo-controlled trials of rt-PA (alteplase) (120), including Parts 1 and 2 of the National Institute of Neurological Disorders and Stroke (NINDS-1, 2) trial in the USA, which tested treatment within three hours of stroke onset (29), 3 European Cooperative Acute Stroke Study (ECASS) trials (117, 121, 122), two Alteplase Thrombolysis for Acute Non-interventional Therapy in Ischaemic Stroke (ATLANTIS) trials (123, 124), and the Echoplanar Imaging Thrombolytic Evaluation Trial (EPITHET) (125) concluded that every effort should be taken to shorten the delay in initiation of treatment. Estimates of the number of patients needed to treat for each 90 minute epoch, that related the odds ratio (OR) of an excellent outcome with rt-PA compared with placebo, gradually decreased from 2.8 in those treated between zero and 90 minutes to 1.2 for 271 to 360 minutes (126), reflecting the biology of rt-PA such that beyond 4.5 to six hours, risk outweighed benefit. Recognizing that approximately five patients needed to be treated within 90 minutes, nine between 91 and 180 minutes, or 15 patients 181 to 270 minutes after symptom onset for one of them to have an excellent outcome attributable to rt-PA, every effort should be made to initiate treatment with rt-PA within 90 minutes of onset of symptoms of ACI (125, 127).

With the recognition that the typical patient loses 1.9 million neurons each minute in which strokes are untreated, the phrase "time is brain" emphasizes the need for emergent evaluation and therapy to prevent the loss in neural circuitry during ACI (128). Some authorities (129) advocate a "door-to-needle" time from onset of stroke symptoms to commencement of rt-PA of less than 60 minutes for current and future treatment studies, with others, including Members of the Brain Attack Coalition (BAC) (130), recommending a time from arrival in the emergency room to initiation of rt-PA of less than 60 minutes, and others, feasibly advocating a reduction of the time to 20 minutes by performing as much as possible during transport and only the basics after the patient has arrived, to curtail in-hospital delays (131).

The selection of subgroups of patients likely to benefit from reperfusion therapy would help the burden of stroke. The combination of PWI and DWI, yielding a mismatch between them, has served as an indicator of the ischemic penumbra. The Diffusion and Perfusion Imaging Evaluation for Understanding Stroke Evolution (DEFUSE) study (132) found that early reperfusion was associated with significantly increased odds of achieving a favorable clinical response in patients with a perfusion/diffusion mismatch on PW/DW-MRI, and an even more favorable response in those with a target mismatch profile. However, some contend that the penumbra and core of irreversible infarction, which has been based upon neurophysiological and functional studies in experimental models of focal ischemia, may be overestimated by MRI modalities (133). Pooled analysis of the EPITHET (125) and DEFUSE study (132) employing an automated MRI analysis software termed RAPID®, identified target mismatch patients in whom reperfusion was strongly associated with a favorable clinical outcome and attenuation of infarct growth, compared to those with a malignant profile in whom reperfusion was associated with an unfavorable clinical response and lack of infarct growth attenuation. With reprocessing and remeasuring the DWI and PWI lesion volumes using RAPID, the original DWI volumes in DEFUSE (132) were approximately 20% larger, and the original EPITHET (125) DWI volumes were almost 40% larger than those ascertained by RAPID, similar to PWI estimates wherein DEFUSE (132) and EPITHET (125) PWI volumes were, respectively, 25% and 55% larger than the RAPID volumes.

While reperfusion may reverse the ischemic cascade, the appropriately chosen population that will benefit from it represents, at most, a minority of all hospitalized acute ischemic strokes. Most are excluded from treatment because they present to the hospital after the three-hour time window. Pharmacologic reperfusion, which has the potential to induce further damage, makes the risk/benefit ratio of reperfusion dependent upon the amount of penumbral salvageable tissue. Accordingly, some authorities contend that it is time to explore neuroprotective agents in stroke prevention, recognizing that such agents may have the capacity to modulate the pathological ion transport over membranes, trap free-radical agents inside the penumbra, slow down the cascade for a limited period of time, enhancing the positive effects of reperfusion, and reduce reperfusion injury that might ensue (134). Such perspectives, which encouraged experimental designs that included rt-PA plus neuroprotective agent in combination have, however, been generally disappointing. Intravenous administration of the neuroprotectant NXY-059, a potent free-radical-trapping agent extensively tested in small- and large-animal models of focal ischemic stroke, was ineffective within six hours of onset of symptoms of ACI and in the prevention of alteplase-associated hemorrhage (135).

An open-label clinical study of 4 mg loading dose of intravenous magnesium sulfate neuroprotective therapy in the field by paramedics, followed by 16 grams over 24 hours in the hospital, was deemed to be feasible and safe, and showed good functional outcome at three months using the mRS in the Field Administration of Stroke Therapy-Magnesium (FAST-MAG) pilot trial (136).

An exploratory efficacy analysis of the intravenous administration of 2 grams per kilogram (g/kg) of 25% human albumin within five hours of onset of symptoms of ACI in the Albumin in Acute Stroke (ALIAS) trial (137) was halted for safety reasons, however it showed a trend toward a favorable primary outcome in the mRS and NIHSS scores up to 90 days after randomization in treated subjects suggesting the need for a Part 2 study.

The combination of thrombolysis plus the neuroprotectant hypothermia (HY) was given to 44 patients within six hours of onset of symptoms of ACI in the Intravenous Thrombolysis Plus Hypothermia for Acute Treatment of Ischemic Stroke (ICTuS-L) trial (138). The rationale of HY was its use in the reduction of brain edema and intracranial pressure after stroke (139). A comparison of outcome in the 28 patients randomized to HY and 39 to 30 to NT showed no significant differences in the two groups at 90 days using the mRS; however, pneumonia was more frequent after HY.

Neuroprotection with the statin agent lovastatin, which purportedly reduces neuronal injury in a dose-dependent fashion in experimental murine models, was administered at varied doses from 1 to 10 mg/k/day for three days to 33 patients in the Neuroprotection with Statin Therapy for Acute Recovery Trial (NeuSTART) study (140), with the result that 8 mg/kg for three days, which was associated with 13% toxicity, was deemed to be the final model for therapy. Further randomized studies are planned.

Another secondary prevention strategy has been the use of antihypertensive therapy. The Perindopril Protection Against Recurrent Stroke Study (PROGRESS) (141), designed to determine the effects of a blood-pressure- lowering regimen in hypertensive and non-hypertensive patients with a history of stroke or TIA, enrolled 6,105 individuals from 172 centers in Asia, Australia, and Europe. The subjects were randomly assigned to active treatment with 4 mg daily of the angiotensin-converting-enzyme (ACE) inhibitor perindopril in 3,051 patients, and placebo in the remainder, with the addition of the diuretic indapamide at the discretion of treating physicians. The primary outcome of trial was fatal or non-fatal stroke. The active treatment regimen reduced the risk of stroke, and combination therapy with perindopril and indapamide produced larger blood pressure reductions and larger risk reductions than did the single active drug therapy alone. The Losarten Intervention For Endpoint (LIFE) trial (142, 143) added further evidence to the concept that blockade of the renin-angiotensin system could provide cardiovascular protection beyond the blood-pressure-lowering effect. In 9,222 patients with primary hypertension and electrocardiographic evidence of left ventricular hypertrophy randomly assigned to losartan or atenolol at equal doses, both at

50 or 100 mg, to which diuretics and other antihypertensive agents could be added, blood pressure was reduced similarly in both groups and the primary composite endpoint of cardiovascular mortality, stroke, and myocardial infarction reached a rate of 23.8 per 1,000 patient-years of follow-up in the losartan group versus 27.9 in the atenolol group, yielding a decrease in the relative risk of 13%. The difference was due mainly to a significant reduction in frequency of stroke by 25% in the losartan group, without significantly different rates of myocardial infarction and cardiovascular mortality. Although at the end of follow-up, sitting systolic blood pressure was reduced with the angiotensin-1 receptor blocker losartan more effective than the beta-blocker atenolol despite similar pressure-lowering effects. In a combined analysis of the PReventiOn regimen For Effectively avoiding Second Strokes (PRoFESS) and Telmisartan Randomized AssessmeNt Study in aCE-iNtolerated subjects with cardiovascular Disease (TRANSCEND) trials (144) of renin-angiotensin II blockage-mediated reduction in stroke risk, independent of their blood-pressure-lowering effect, the incidence of the composite of stroke, myocardial infarction, or vascular death was 12.8% for telmisartan versus 13.8% for placebo.

The efficacy of carotid endarterectomy was investigated by the European Carotid Surgery Trial (ECST) (145) and the North American Symptomatic Carotid Endarterectomy Trial (NASCET) (146) that showed benefit of surgery with carotid stenosis of >70 %. Further analysis of the data suggested a lesser benefit in those with stenosis of 50% to 70% (147). The risk of recurrent stroke was increased in those with recent symptoms, ulcerated carotid plaque, hemispheric TIA, and stroke. Further analysis emphasized the benefit of operating within a few days of the event; in moderate stenosis of 50% to 69% there was benefit only if operations were carried out within two weeks of onset of symptoms (148).

Carotid angioplasty and stenting have been advocated as alternative therapies. Vascular disease medical interventions employing a combination of noninvasive strategies, including ongoing diagnosis, education, support of healthy lifestyle practices, and medications have been proposed for prevention of stroke associated with asymptomatic severe carotid stenosis (149).

In patients with a recent TIA or stroke attributed to 70% to 99% angiographically-proven stenosis in the diameter of a major intracranial artery, aggressive medical management was superior to percutaneous transluminal angioplasty and stenting (PTAS) with the use of the Wingspan stent system in the Stenting and Aggressive Medical Management for Preventing Recurrent Stroke in Intracranial Stenosis (SAMMPRIS) trial (150). The 30-day rate of stroke and death was 14.7% in the PTAS group and 5.8% in the group medically managed. By comparison, carotid stenting with use of an emboli-protection device was not inferior to carotid endarterectomy in high-risk patients with carotid artery stenosis of at least 50% of the luminal diameter, or an asymptomatic stenosis of at least 80% in the Stenting and Angioplasty with Protection in Patients at High Risk for Endarterectomy (SAPPHIRE) trial (151).

With primary endpoints of the cumulative risk of a major cardiovascular event at one year, and a composite of death, stroke, or myocardial infarction within 30 days after the intervention, or ipsilateral stroke between 31 days and one year, the primary endpoint occurred in 20 patients randomly assigned to carotid-artery stenting versus 32 patients assigned instead to endarterectomy. At one year, carotid revascularization was repeated in fewer patients who had received stents than in those who underwent endarterectomy. There were no significant differences between carotid artery stenting versus carotid endarterectomy by symptomatic status for the primary endpoint of stroke, myocardial infarction, or death within the periprocedural period or ipsilateral stroke for up to four years in the Carotid Revascularization Endarterectomy Versus Stenting Trial (CREST) (152), although periprocedural stroke and death rates were significantly lower for carotid endarterectomy in symptomatic patients.

The Endarterectomy Versus Angioplasty in Patients with Symptomatic Severe Carotid Stenosis (EVA-3S) trial (153) was prematurely stopped for reasons of safety and futility upon recognition that the 30-day incidence of any stroke or death was 3.9% after endarterectomy compared to 9.6% after stenting, and at six months, the respective incidence of any stroke or death was 6.1% and 11.7%. Among patients with recently symptomatic atherosclerotic internal carotid artery occlusion (AICAO) and hemodynamic cerebral ischemia, extracranial-intracranial (EC-IC) bypass surgery plus medical therapy did not reduce the risk of recurrent ipsilateral ischemic stroke at two years, compared to medical therapy alone in the Carotid Occlusion Surgery Study (COSS) (154).

Mechanical thrombectomy has been selectively used to treat large anterior circulation artery occlusions. Three reports (155–157) employing a new generation of mechanical devices demonstrated varied success in providing safe and effective revascularization for clot removal in intracranial large vessel occlusive disease in the anterior cerebral artery (ACA) and MCA and vertebrobasilar system (157). The Penumbra Pivotal Stroke Trial (155), which employed the Penumbra System® reperfusion catheter, enrolling 125 patients with neurological deficits and NIHSS > or = 8 within eight hours of symptom onset and angiographic occlusion of grade 0 or 1 (159) were followed clinically for 90 days. Revascularization was achieved in 81.6% of patients with a mortality of 32.8%, symptomatic ICH in 11.2% of patients, and procedural complications in 12.8%. Castano and colleagues (156) employed the Solitaire™ AB among 20 patients with stroke attributed to large artery occlusion of the anterior circulation vessels in the first eight hours of symptom onset.

The median NIHSS score was 19 and subjects demonstrated a cerebral infarction grade of 2b or 3 (159). Revascularization was achieved in 90% of patients with a mortality of 20% and symptomatic ICH in 10% with no procedural complications. The Multi MERCI Trial (157) employed both a first generation MERCI® device and the Merci®L5 Retriever to restore perfusion among 164 patients with large vessel territory stroke within eight hours of symptomatic onset, including those with persistent occlusion after intravenous rt-PA. With a median NIHSS of 19, recanalization was achieved in 57.3% of patients, with a mortality of 34%, symptomatic ICH in 9.8% of patients and procedural complications in 5.5%.

REFERENCES

1. Aho K, Harmsen P, Hatano S, et al. Cerebrovascular disease in the community: results of a WHO collaborative study. *Bull World Health Organ* 1980; 58:113–130.
2. Barker WH, Mullooly FP. Stroke in a defined elderly population, 1967–1985; a less lethal and disabling but no less common disease. *Stroke* 1997; 28:284–290.
3. Sommerfeld DK, Eek EU, Svensson AK, et al. Spasticity after stroke: +9 its occurrence and association with motor impairments and activity limitations. *Stroke* 2004; 35:134–139.
4. O'Dwyer NJ, Ada L, Neilson PD. Spasticity and muscle contracture following stroke. *Brain* 1966; 119:1737–1749.
5. Jacobs BS, Boden-Albala B, Lin IF, et al. Stroke in the young in the northern Manhattan stroke Study. *Stroke* 2002; 33:2789–2793.
6. Sacco RL, Boden-Albala G, Gan R, et al. Stroke incidence among white, black, and Hispanic residents of an urban community: the Northern Manhattan Stroke Study. *Am J Epidemiol* 1998; 147:259–268.
7. Howard G, Howard VJ, Katholi C, et al. Decline in US stroke mortality: an analysis of temporal patterns by sex, race, and geographic region. *Stroke* 2001; 32:2213–2220.
8. Goldstein LB, Adams R, Alberts MJ, et al. Primary prevention of ischemic stroke. A guidelines from the American Heart Association/American Stroke Association Stroke Council: Cosponsored by the Atherosclerotic Peripheral Vascular Disease Interdisciplinary Working Group; Cardiovascular Nursing Council; Clinical Cardiology Council; Nutrition, Physical Activity, and Metabolism Council; and the Quality of Care and Outcomes Research Interdisciplinary Working Group. *Circulation* 2006; 113:e873–923.
9. Sacco RL. Newer risk factors for stroke. *Neurology* 2001; 57(Suppl 2): S31–S34.
10. Sacco RL, Gan R, Boden-Albala B, et al. Leisure-time physical activity and ischemic stroke risk: the Northern Manhattan Stroke Study. *Stroke* 1998; 29:380–387.
11. Sacco RL, Elkind M, Boden-Albala B, et al. The protective effect of moderate alcohol consumption on ischemic stroke. *JAMA* 1999; 281:53–60.
12. Sacco RL, Benson RT, Kargman DE, et al. High-density lipoprotein cholesterol and ischemic stroke in the elderly: the Northern Manhattan Stroke Study. *JAMA* 2001; 285:2729–2735.
13. Kargman DE, Berglund LF, Boden-Albala B, et al. Increased stroke risk and lipoprotein (a) in a racially mixed area: the Northern Manhattan Stroke Study. *Stroke* 1999; 30:251.
14. Sacco RL, Roberts JK, Jacobs BS. Homocysteine as a risk factor for ischemic stroke: an epidemiological story in evolution. *Neuroepidemiology* 1998; 17:167–173.
15. Kissela BM, Khoury J, Kleindorfer D, et al. Epidemiology of ischemic stroke in patients with diabetes: the greater Cincinnati/Northern Kentucky Stroke Study. *Diabetes Care* 2005; 28:355–359.
16. Fine-Edelstein JS, Wolf PA, O'Leary DH, et al. Precursors of extracranial carotid atherosclerosis in the Framingham Study. *Neurology* 1994; 44:1046–1050.
17. Sutton-Tyrrell K, Alcorn HG, Wolfson SK Jr, et al. Predictors of carotid stenosis in older adults with and without systolic hypertension. *Stroke* 1993; 24:355–361.
18. Jeng JS, Sacco RL, Kargman DE, et al. Apolipoproteins and carotid artery atherosclerosis in an elderly multiethnic population: the Northern Manhattan stroke study. *Atherosclerosis* 2002; 165:317–325.
19. Ringelstein EB, Nabavi DG. Cerebral small vessel diseases: cerebral microangiopathies. *Curr Opin Neurol* 2005; 18:179–188.
20. Foulkes MA, Wolf PA, Price TR, et al. The Stroke Data Bank: design, methods, and baseline characteristics. *Stroke* 1988; 19:547–554.
21. Adams HP Jr., Bendixen BH, Kappelle LJ, et al. Classification of subtype of acute ischemic stroke. Definitions for use in multicenter clinical trial. TOAST. Trial of Org 10172 in Acute Stroke Treatment. *Stroke* 1993; 24:35–41.
22. Moncayo J, Devuyst G, Van Melle G, et al. Coexisting causes of ischemic stroke. *Arch Neurol* 2000; 57:1139–1144.
23. Moulin T, Tatu L, Crépin-Leblond T, et al. The Besançon Stroke Registry: an acute stroke registry of 2,500 consecutive patients. *Eur Neurol* 1997; 38:10–20.
24. Kumral E, Ozkaya B, Sagduyu A, et al. The Ege Stroke Registry: a hospital-based study in the Aegean region, Izmir, Turkey. Analysis of 2,000 stroke patients. *Cerebrovasc Dis* 1998; 8:278–288.
25. Yip PK, Jeng JS, Lee TK, et al. Subtypes of ischemic stroke. A hospital-based stroke registry in Taiwan (SCAN-IV). *Stroke* 1997; 28:2507–2512.
26. Mohr JP, Biller J, Hilal SK, et al. Magnetic resonance versus computed tomographic imaging in acute stroke. *Stroke* 1995; 26:807–812.
27. Adams HP Jr., del Zoppo G, Alberts MJ, et al. Guidelines for the early management of adults with ischemic stroke: a guideline from the American Heart Association/American Stroke Association Stroke Council, Clinical Cardiology Council, Cardiovascular Radiology and Intervention Council, and the Atherosclerotic Peripheral Vascular Disease and Quality of Care Outcomes in Research Interdisciplinary Working Groups: The American Academy of Neurology affirms the value of this guideline as an educational tool for neurologists. *Circulation* 2007; 115:e478–e534.
28. Wintermark M, Fiebach J. Imaging of brain parenchyma in stroke. *Handb Clin Neurol* 2009; 94:1011–1019.
29. The National Institute of Neurological Disorders and Stroke rtPA Stroke Study Group. Tissue plasminogen activator for acute ischemic stroke. *N Engl J Med* 1995; 333:1581–1587.
30. Jansen O, Schellinger P, Fiebach J, et al. Early recanalization in acute ischaemic stroke saves tissue at risk defined by MRI. *Lancet* 1999; 353:2036–2037.

31. Dechambre A. Memoire sur la curabilité du ramoulissment cerebral. *Gazette Medicale de Paris* 1838; 6:305–314.

32. Durand-Fardel M. Memoire sur une alteration particulaire de le substance cerebrale. *Gazette Medicale de Paris* 1842; 10:23–6, 33–8.

33. Mohr JP, Caplan LR, Melski JW, et al. The Harvard Cooperative Stroke Registry: a prospective registry. *Neurology* 1978; 28:754–762.

34. Fisher CM, Curry HB. Pure motor hemiplegia of vascular origin. *Arch Neurol* 1965; 13:30–44.

35. Fisher CM, Caplan LR. Basilar artery branch occlusion: A cause of pontine infarction. *Neurology* 1971; 21:900–905.

36. Ho KL. Pure motor hemiplegia due to infarction of the cerebral peduncle. *Arch Neurol* 1982; 39:524–526.

37. Chokroverty S, Rubino FA, Haller C. Pure motor Hemiplegia due to Pyramidal Infarction. *Arch Neurol* 1985; 32:647–648.

38. Ho KL, Meyer KR. The Medial Medullary Syndrome. *Arch Neurol* 1981; 38:385–387.

39. Bamford J, Sandercock P, Jones L, et al. The natural history of lacunar infarction. The Oxfordshire community stroke project. *Stroke* 1987; 18:545–551.

40. Arboix A, Martí-Vilalta JG, García JH. Clinical study of 227 patients with lacunar infarcts. *Stroke* 1990; 21:842–847.

41. Rascol A, Clanet M, Manelfe C, et al. Pure motor hemiplegia: CT study of 30 cases. *Stroke* 1982; 13:11–17.

42. Fisher CM. Lacunar stroke and infarcts: a review. *Neurology* 1982; 32:871–876.

43. Melo TP, Bogousslavsky J, van Melle G, et al. Pure motor stroke: a reappraisal. *Neurology* 1992; 42:789–798.

44. Kumral E, Afsar N, Kirbas D, et al. Spectrum of medial medullary infarction: clinical and magnetic resonance imaging findings. *J Neurol* 2002; 249:85–93.

45. Kim JS, Kim HG, Chung CS. Medial medullary syndrome. Report of 18 new patients and a review of the literature. *Stroke* 1995; 26:1548–1552.

46. Ropper AH, Fisher CM, Kleinman GM. Pyramidal infarction in the medulla: a cause of pure motor hemiplegia sparing the face. *Neurology* 1979; 29:91–95.

47. Huang C, Woo E, Yu YL, et al. Lacunar syndromes due to brainstem infarct and hemorrhage. *J Neurol Neurosurg Psychiatry* 1988; 51:509–515.

48. Nighoghossian N, Ryvlin P, Trouillas P, et al. Pontine versus capsular pure motor hemiparesis. *Neurology* 1993; 43:2197–2201.

49. Kaps M, Klostermann W, Wessel K, et al. Basilar branch disease presenting with progressive pure motor stroke. *Acta Neurol Scand* 1997; 96:324–327.

50. Kunz S, Griese H, Busse O. Etiology and long-term prognosis of unilateral paramedian pontine infarction with progressive symptoms. *Eur Neurol* 2003; 50:136–140.

51. Chan DK, Silver FL. Basilar artery stenosis mimicking the lacunar syndrome of pure motor hemiparesis. *Can J Neurol* 2003; 30:159–162.

52. Bogousslavsky J, Maeder P, Regli F, et al. Pure midbrain infarction: clinical syndromes, MRI and etiologic patterns. *Neurology* 1994; 44:2032–2040.

53. Gaymard B, Saudeau D, de Toffol B, et al. Two mesencephalic lacunar infarcts presenting as Claude's syndrome and pure motor hemiparesis. *Eur Neurol* 1991; 31:152–155.

54. Mohr JP. Lacunes. *Stroke* 1982; 13:3–11.

55. Marie P. Des foyers lacunaire de désintégration et de different-sautres états cavitaires du cerveau. *Rev Med* 1901; 21:281.

56. Ferrand J. Essai sur l'hémiplégie des veillards, les lacunes de désintégration cerebrale. Thesis, Rousset, Paris 1902.

57. Foix C, Levy M. Les ramollissements sylviens. *Rev Neurol* 1927; 11:1.

58. Foix C, Hillemand P. Contribution a l'etude des ramollissements proturberantiels. *Rev Med* 1926; 43:287.

59. Fisher CM. Capsular infarcts: the underlying vascular lesions. *Arch Neurol* 1979; 36:65–73.

60. Fisher CM, Cole M. Homolateral ataxia and crural paresis: A vascular syndrome. *J Neurol Neurosurg Psychiatry* 1965; 28:48–55.

61. Fisher CM. A Lacunar stroke. The dysarthria-clumsy hand syndrome. *Neurology* 1967; 17:614–617.

62. Fisher CM. Lacunes: Small, deep cerebral infarcts. *Neurology* 1965; 15:774–784.

63. Kinkel PR, Kinkel WR, Jacobs L. Clinical-computerized tomographic (CT) correlations of cerebral lacunes. *Neurology* 1980; 30:44–45.

64. Englander RN, Netsky MG, Adelman LS. Location of human pyramidal tract in the internal capsule: anatomic evidence. *Neurology* 1975; 25:823–826.

65. Hirayama K, Tsubaki T, Toyokura Y, et al. The representation of the pyramidal tract in the internal capsule and basis pedunculi. A study based on three cases of amyotrophic lateral sclerosis. *Neurology* 1962; 12:337–342.

66. Hanaway J, Young RR. Localization of the pyramidal tract in the internal capsule of man. *J Neurol Sci* 1977; 34:63–70.

67. Kappelle LJ, van Gijn J. Lacunar infarcts. Clin *Neurol Neurosurg* 1986; 88:3–17.

68. Umansky F, Gomes FB, Dujovny M et al. The perforating branches of the middle cerebral artery. A microanatomical study. *J Neurosurg* 1985; 62:261–268.

69. Loeb C. The lacunar syndromes. *Eur Neurol* 1989; 29(Suppl 2):2–7.

70. Russmann H, Vingerhoets F, Ghika J, et al. Acute infarction limited to the lenticular nucleus: clinical, etiologic, and topographic features. *Arch Neurol* 2003; 60:351–355.

71. Kumral E, Özdemirkiran T, Alper Y. Strokes in the subinsular territory. Clinical, topographical, and etiological patterns. *Neurology* 2004; 63:2429–2432.

72. Arboix A, Martinez-Rebollar M, Oliveres M, et al. Acute isolated capsular stroke. A clinical study of 148 cases. *Clin Neurol Neurosurg* 2005; 107:88–94.

73. Earnest MP, Fahn S, Karp JH, et al. Normal pressure hydrocephalus and hypertensive cerebrovascular disease. *Arch Neurol* 1974; 31:262–266.

74. Koto A, Rosenberg G, Zingesser LH, et al. Syndrome of normal pressure hydrocephalus: possible relation to hypertensive and arteriosclerotic vasculopathy. *J Neurol Neurosurg Psychiatry* 1977; 40:73–79.

75. Hughes W. Origin of lacunes. Lancet 1965; 2:19–21.

76. Fisher CM. The arterial lesions underlying lacunes. *Acta Neuropathol* 1969; 12:1–15.

77. Fisher CM. Cerebral miliary aneurysms in hypertension. *Am J Pathol* 1972; 66:313–330.

78. Ross Russel RW. Observations on intracérébrale aneurysms. *Brain* 1963; 86:425–441.

79. Hommel M, Besson G, Le Bas JF, et al. Prospective study of lacunar infarction using magnetic resonance imaging. *Stroke* 1990; 21:546–554.

80. Toni D, Del Duca R, Fiorelli M, et al. Pure motor hemiparesis and sensorimotor stroke. Accuracy of very early clinical diagnosis of lacunar strokes. *Stroke* 1994; 25:92–96.

81. Bamford J, Sandercock P, Jones L, et al. The natural history of lacunar infarction: the Oxfordshire Community Stroke Project. *Stroke* 1987; 18:545–551.

82. Ghika J, Ghika-Schmid F, Bogousslavsky J. Parietal motor syndrome: a clinical description in 32 patients in the acute phase of pure parietal strokes studied prospectively. *Clin Neurol Neurosurg* 1998; 100:271–282.

83. de Freitas GR, Devuyst G, van Melle G, et al. Motor strokes sparing the leg: different lesions and causes. *Arch Neurol* 2000; 57:513–518.

84. Watkins CL, Leathley MJ, Gregson JM, et al. Prevalence of spasticity post stroke. *Clin Rehabili* 2002; 16:515–522.

85. Aichner F, Adelwöhrer C, Haring HP. Rehabilitation approaches to stroke. *J Neurol Transm Suppl* 2002; 63:59–73.

86. Dethy S, Luxen A, Bidaut M, et al. Hemibody tremor related to stroke. *Stroke* 1993; 24:2094–2096.

87. Staaf G, Lindgren A, Norrving B. Pure motor stroke from presumed lacunar infarct: long-term prognosis for survival and risk of recurrent stroke. *Stroke* 2001; 32:2592–2596.

88. Steinke W, Ley SC. Lacunar stroke is the major cause of progressive motor deficits. *Stroke* 2002; 33:1510–1516.

89. Arauz A, Murillo L, Cantú C, et al. Prospective study of single and multiple lacunar infarcts using magnetic resonance imaging: risk factors, recurrence, and outcome in 175 consecutive cases. *Stroke* 2003; 34:2453–2458.

90. Wenzelburger R, Kopper F, Frenzel A, et al. Hand coordination following capsular stroke. *Brain* 2005; 128:64–74.

91. Govan L, Weird CJ, Langhorne P, et al. Organized inpatient (stroke unit) Care for Stroke. *Stroke* 2008 epub ahead of print.

92. Jarman B, Aylin P, Bottle A. Acute stroke units and early CT scans are linked to lower in-hospital mortality rates. *BMJ* 2004; 328:369.

93. Lincoln NB, Husbands S, Trescoli C, et al. Five-year follow-up of a randomised controlled trial of a stroke rehabilitation unit. *BMJ* 2000; 320:549.

94. International Stroke Trial Collaborative Group. The International Stroke Trial (IST): a randomized trial of aspirin, subcutaneous heparin, both, or neither among 19435 patients with acute ischaemic stroke. *Lancet* 1997; 349:1569–1581.

95. A randomized trial of anticoagulation versus aspirin after cerebral ischemia of presumed arterial origin. *Ann Neurol* 1997; 42:857–865.

96. Antithrombotic Trialists' Collaboration. Collaborative meta-analysis of randomized trials of antiplatelet therapy for prevention of death, myocardial infarction, and stroke in high risk patients. *BMJ* 2002; 324:71–86.

97. Mohr JP, Thompson JL, Lazar RM, et al. Warfarin-Aspirin Recurrent Stroke Study Group. A comparison of warfarin and aspirin for the prevention of recurrent ischemic stroke. *N Engl J Med* 2001; 345:1444–1451.

98. Diener HC, Cunha L, Forbes C, et al. European Stroke Prevention Study. 2. Dipyridamole and acetylsalicylic acid in the secondary prevention of stroke. *J Neurol Sci* 1996; 143:1–13.

99. Hart RG, Benavente O, McBride R, et al. Antithrombotic therapy to prevent stroke in patients with atrial fibrillation: a meta-analysis. *Ann Intern Med* 1999; 131:492–501.

100. Chimowitz MI, Lynn MJ, Howlett-Smith H, et al. Comparison of Warfarin and Aspirin for Symptomatic Intracranial Arterial Stenosis. *N Engl J Med* 2005; 352:1305–1316.

101. Koroshetz WJ. Warfarin, aspirin, and intracranial vascular disease. *N Engl J Med* 2005; 352:1368–1370.

102. Patel MR, Mahaffrey KW, Garg J, et al. Rivaroxaban versus warfarin in nonvalvular atrial fibrillation. *N Engl J Med* 2011; 365:883–891.

103. Granger CB, Alexander JH, McMurray JJV, et al. Apixaban versus Warfarin in patients with Atrial Fibrillation. *N Engl J Med* 2011; 365:981–992.

104. Connolly SJ, Ezekowitz MD, Yusuf S, et al. Dabigatran versus warfarin in patients with atrial fibrillation. *N Engl J Med* 2009; 361:1139–1151.

105. Lyden P, Brott T, Tilley B, et al. Improved reliability of the NIH Stroke Scale using video training. NINDS TPA Stroke Study Group. *Stroke* 1994; 25:2220–2226.

106. van Swieten JC, Koudstaal PJ, Visser MC, et al. Interobserver agreement for the assessment of handicap in stroke patients. *Stroke* 1988; 19:604–607.

107. Mahoney FI, Barthel DW. Functional evaluation: The Barthel Index. *Md State Med J* 1965; 14:61–65.

108. Teasdale G, Knill-Jones R, van der Sande J. Observer variability in assessing impaired consciousness and coma. *J Neurol Neurosurg Psychiatry* 1978; 41:603–610.

109. *Harvard Heart Letter.* A new wave in stroke treatment (using ultra-high sound waves). February 2005; 1.

110. Nedeltchev K, Schwegler B, Haefeli T, et al. Outcome of stroke with mild or rapidly improving symptoms. *Stroke* 2007; 38:2531–2535.

111. Smith EE, Abdullah AR, Petkovska I, et al. Poor outcomes in patients who do not receive intravenous tissue plasminogen activator because of mild or improving ischemic stroke. *Stroke* 2005; 36:2497–2499.

112. California Acute Stroke Pilot Registry (CASPR) Investigators. Prioritizing interventions to improve rates of thrombolysis for ischemic stroke. *Neurology* 2005; 64:654–659.

113. Fink JN, Kumar S, Horkan C, et al. The stroke patient who woke up: clinical and radiological features, including diffusion and perfusion MRI. *Stroke* 2002; 33:988–993.

114. Boode BS, Welzen V, Franke C, et al. Estimating the number of stroke patients eligible for thrombolytic treatment if delay could be avoided. *Cerebrovasc Dis* 2006; 23:294–298.

115. Abciximab Emergent Stroke Treatment Trial (AbESTT) Investigators. Emergency administration of abcizimab for treatment of patients with acute ischemic stroke. Results of a randomized phase 2 trial. *Stroke* 2005; 36:880–890.

116. Adams HP Jr, Leira EC, Torner JC, et al. Treatment patients with 'wake-up' stroke: the experience of the AbESTT-II Trial. *Stroke* 2008; 39:3277–3282.

117. Hacke W, Kaste M, Bluhmki E, et al. Thrombolysis with Alteplase 3 to 4.5 hours after Acute Ischemic Stroke. *N Engl J Med* 2008; 359:1317–1329.

118. Furlan A, Higashida R, Wechsler L, et al. Intra-arterial prourokinase for acute ischemic stroke. The PROACT II Study: a randomized controlled trial. Prolyse in Acute Cerebral Thromboelmbolism. *JAMA* 1999; 282:2003–2011.

119. Ogawa A, Mori E, Minematsu K, et al. Randomized trial of intraarterial infusion of urokinase within 6 hours of middle cerebral artery stroke: the middle cerebral artery embolism local fibinolytic intervention trial (MELT) Japan. *Stroke* 2007; 38:2633–2639.

120. Lees KR, Bluhmki E, von Kummer R, et al. Time to treatment with intravenous alteplase and outcome in stroke: an updated pooled analysis of ECASS, ATLANTIS, NINDS, and EPITHET trials. *Lancet* 2010; 375:1695–1703.

121. Hacke W, Kaste M, Fieschi C, et al. Intravenous thrombolysis with recombinant tissue plasminogen activator for acute hemispheric stroke: The European Cooperative Acute Stroke Study (ECASS). *JAMA* 1995; 274:1017–1025.

122. Hacke W, Kaste M, Fieschi C, et al. Randomised double-blind placebo-controlled trial of thrombolytic therapy with intravenous alteplase in acute ischaemic stroke (ECASS II). *Lancet* 1998; 352:1245–1251.

123. Clark WM, Albers GW, Madden KP, et al. The rt-PA (alteplase) 0- to 6-hour acute stroke trial, part A (A0267g): results of a double-blind, placebo-controlled, multicenter study. Thrombolytic therapy in acute ischemic stroke study investigation. *Stroke* 2000; 31:811–816.

124. Clark WM, Wissman S, Albers GW, et al. Recombinant tissue-type plasminogen activator (Alteplase) for ischemic stroke 3 to 5 hours after symptom onset: The ATLANTIS study: a randomized controlled trial. Alteplase Thrombolysis for Acute

Noninterventional Therapy in Ischemic Stroke. *JAMA* 1999; 282:2019–2026.

125. David SM, Donnan GA, Parsons MW, et al, for the EPITHET investigators. Effects of alteplase beyond 3 h after stroke in the Echoplanar Imaging Thrombolytic Evaluation Trial (EPI-THET): a placebo-controlled randomized trial. *Lancet Neurol* 2008; 7:299–309.

126. Lansberg MG, Schrooten M, Bluhmki E, et al. Treatment time-specific number needed to treat estimates for tissue plasminogen activator therapy in acute stroke based on shifts over the entire range of the modified Rankin scale. *Stroke* 2009; 40:2079–2084.

127. Hacke W, Donnan G, Fieschi C, et al. Association of outcome with early stroke treatment: pooled analysis of ATLANTIS, ECASS, and NINDS rt-PA stroke trials. *Lancet* 2004; 363:768–774.

128. Saver JL. Time is brain-quantified. *Stroke* 2006; 37:263–266.

129. Smith EE, von Kummer R. Door-to-needle times in acute ischemic stroke. How long can we go? *Neurology* 2012; 79:296–297.

130. Alberts MJ, Hademenos G, Latchaw RE, et al. Recommendations for the establishment of primary stroke centers. Brain Attack Coalition. *JAMA* 2000; 283:3102–3109.

131. Meretoja A, Strbian D, Mustanoja S, et al. Reducing in-hospital delay to 20 minutes in stroke thrombolysis. *Neurology* 2012; 79:306–313.

132. Abers GW, Thijs VN, Wechsler L, et al. Magnetic resonance imaging profiles predict clinical response to early reperfusion: The diffusion and perfusion imaging evaluation for understanding stroke evolution (DEFUSE) study. *Ann Neurol* 2006; 60:508–517.

133. Heiss WD. The ischemic penumbra: correlates in imaging and implications for treatment of ischemic stroke. The Johann Jacob Wepfer Award 2011. *Cerebrovasc Dis* 2011; 32:307–320.

134. Sacchetti ML. Is it time to definitely abandon neuroprotection in acute ischemic stroke? *Stroke* 2008; 39:1659–1660.

135. Diener HC, Lees KR, Lyden P, et al. NXY-059 for the treatment of acute stroke: pooled analysis of the SAINT I and II Trials. *Stroke* 2008; 39:1751–1758.

136. Saver JL, Kidwell C, Eckstein M, et al. Prehospital neuroprotection therapy for acute stroke: results of the Field Administration of Stroke Therapy-Magnesium (FAST-MAG) Pilot Trial. *Stroke* 2004; 35:e106–e108.

137. Hill MD, Martin RH, Palesch YY, et al. The Albumin in Acute Stroke Part 1 Trial: an exploratory efficacy analysis. *Stroke* 2011; 42:1621–1625.

138. Hemmen TM, Raman R, Guluma KZ, et al. Intravenous thrombolysis plus hypothermia for acute treatment of ischemic stroke (ICTuS-L): final results. *Stroke* 2010; 41:2265–2270.

139. Schwab S, Schwarz S, Spranger M, et al. Moderate hypothermia in the treatment of patients with severe middle cerebral artery infarction. *Stroke* 1998; 29:2461–2466.

140. Elkind MS, Sacco RL, MacArthur RB, et al. High-dose lovastatin for acute ischemic stroke: results of the phase I dose escalation neuroprotection with statin therapy for acute recovery trial (NeuSTART). *Cerebrovasc Dis* 2009; 28:266–275.

141. PROGRESS Collaborative Group. Randomized trial of a perindopril-based blood-pressure-lowering regimen among 6105 individuals with previous stroke or transient ischemic attack. *Lancet* 2001; 358:1033–1041.

142. Daholf B, Devereux RB, Kjeldsen SE, et al. Cardiovascular morbidity and mortality in the Losartan Intervention For Endpoint reduction in hypertension study (LIFE): a randomized trial against atenolol. *Lancet* 2002; 359:995–1003.

143. Brunner HR, Gavras H. Commentary. Angiotensin blockade for hypertension: a promise fulfilled. *Lancet* 2002; 359:990–992.

144. Diener HC. Preventing stroke: the PRoFESS, ONTARGET, and TRANSCEND trial programs. *J Hypertens Suppl* 2009; 27(Suppl 5):S31–S36.

145. European Carotid Surgery Trialists' Collaborative Group. Randomized trial of endarterectomy for recently symptomatic carotid stenosis: final results in the MRC European Carotid Surgery Trial (ESCT). *Lancet* 1998; 351:1379–1387.

146. North American Symptomatic Carotid Endarterectomy Trial Collaborators. Beneficial effect of carotid endarterectomy in symptomatic patients with high-grade stenosis. *N Engl J Med* 325:445–453.

147. Barnett HJM, Taylor DW, Eliaziw M, et al for the North American Symptomatic Carotid Endarterectomy Trial Collaborators. Benefit of carotid endarterectomy in patients with symptomatic moderate or severe stenosis. *N Engl J Med* 1998; 339:1415–1425.

148. Rothwell PM, Eliasziw M, Gutnikov SA, et al. Endarterectomy for symptomatic carotid stenosis in relation to clinical subgroups and timing of surgery. *Lancet* 2004; 363:915–924.

149. Abbott AL. Medical (nonsurgical) intervention Alone is now best for prevention of stroke associated with asymptomatic severe carotid stenosis: results of a systemic review and analysis. *Stroke* 2009; 40:e573–e583.

150. Chimowitz MI, Lynn MJ, Derdeyn CP, et al. Stenting versus aggressive medical therapy for intracranial arterial stenosis. *N Engl J Med* 2011; 365:993–1003.

151. Yadav JS, Wholey MH, Kuntz RE, et al. Protected carotid-artery stenting versus endarterectomy in high-risk patients. *N Engl J Med* 2004; 351:1493–1501.

152. Silver FL, Mackey A, Clark WM, et al. Safety of stenting and endarterectomy by symptomatic status in the Carotid Revascularization Endarterectomy Versus Stenting Trial (CREST). *Stroke* 2011; 42:675–680.

153. Mas J-L, Chatellier G, Beyssen B, et al. Endarterectomy versus stenting in patients with symptomatic severe carotid stenosis. *N Engl J Med* 2006; 355:1660–1671.

154. Powers WJ, Clarke WR, Grubb RL Jr, et al. Extracranial-Intracranial bypass surgery for stroke prevention in hemodynamic cerebral ischemia: the Carotid Occlusion Surgery Study randomized trial. *JAMA* 2011; 306:1983–1992.

155. The Penumbra Pivotal Stroke Trial Investigators. The penumbra pivotal stroke trial: safety and effectiveness of a new generation of mechanical devices for clot removal in intracranial large vessel occlusive disease. *Stroke* 2009; 40:2761–2768.

156. Castano C, Dorado L, Guerrero C, et al. Mechanical thrombectomy with the Solitare AB device in large artery occlusions of the anterior circulation: a pilot study. *Stroke* 2010; 41:1836–1840.

157. Smith WS, Sung G, Saver J, et al. Mechanical thrombectomy for acute ischemic stroke: final results of the Multi MERCI Trial. *Stroke* 2008; 39:1205–1212.

158. Chesebro JH, Knatterud G, Robert R, et al. Thrombolysis in Myocardial Infarction (TIMI) Trial, Phase 1: A comparison between intravenous tissue plasminogen activator and intravenous streptokinase. Clinical findings through hospital discharge. *Circulation* 1987; 76:142–154.

159. Higashida RT, Furlan AJ, Roberts, et al. Trial design and reporting standards for Intra-arterial Cerebral Thrombolysis for Acute Stroke. *J Vasc Interv Radiol* 2003; 14:S493–S494.

CHAPTER 57

Motor Sequela of Dementia

Gayatri Devi

Consideration of motor disorders in patients with dementia is of clinical importance in establishing the etiopathogenesis of dementia in affected patients and, in many instances, in determining disease progression and prognosis. The motor manifestations, which may vary from mild extrapyramidal rigidity to paralysis, depending on the type and the stage of the dementia, may offer clues to prognosis and differential diagnosis. For example, patients with Alzheimer disease (AD) who develop parkinsonian features and motor difficulties later in their illness may have a more aggressive type of illness associated with a worse prognosis, such symptoms at onset should prompt consideration of dementia due to Lewy bodies (DLB) (1, 2). This chapter addresses motor disorders in dementia of various causes.

ALZHEIMER DISEASE

AD can be divided into two clinically different phenotypes and genotypes, namely early-onset AD (EOAD) with age at onset prior to the age of 60, and late-onset AD (LOAD) with an onset after 60 to 65 years (3) and identical pathology of intracellular neurofibrillary tangles and extracellular plaques that accumulate in vulnerable brain regions. About 5% of cases of AD are of the EOAD type. Autosomal dominant mutations in the presenilin 1 (PSEN1) gene located on chromosome 14, in the PSEN2 gene on chromosome 1, or the APP gene located on chromosome 21, account for one-half of patients with EOAD. Patients with EOAD manifest early myoclonus, parkinsonian, and psychiatric features with rapid progression to infirmity and death (4). They may be misdiagnosed by virtue of relative youth.

In one kindred (5), the proband developed depression at 29 years, followed by dementia a year afterward, and dysarthria, aphasia, and myoclonus four years later. He developed seizures by age 36 years and died two years later. His brother developed cognitive impairment at age 27 years, and by 30 years had aphasia, myoclonus, and generalized seizures followed by limb rigidity at 32 years and death a year later. The father had mood swings from age 35 years followed by violent temper, dementia, generalized seizures and myoclonus from age 38 years. The clinical diagnosis of Creutzfeld-Jakob disease (CJD) was made although brain pathology subsequently revealed AD. This family, with an exceptionally early age of onset and a virulent course, characterized by early motor disturbances, was found to have a mutation in the PSEN1 gene on chromosome 14.

The molecular pathogenesis of EOAD reflects the acceleration of an abnormal accumulation of β-amyloid and tau protein. Genetic screens are commercially available to screen for the commonest mutations; however, since many families have a mutation unique to that family, a negative genetic screen for the commonest mutations for EOAD does not preclude the diagnosis. While the response to treatment in EOAD has been less well studied than late-onset AD, therapy with acetylcholinesterase inhibitors and N-methyl D-aspartate (NMDA) antagonists are warranted.

The course of LOAD is more indolent than that of EOAD, with a prevalence of 9% above the age of 65 years, rising to between 35% and 50% in persons above the age of 85 years (6, 7). Women are at a higher risk than men, even after controlling for greater longevity, although this issue is controversial. In contrast to EOAD, LOAD manifests a multi-factorial etiology with contributions from genetics and the environment (8, 9). The presence of the apoE4 isoform of the apolipoprotein-E (*APOE*) gene on chromosome 19, as well as α_{-2}-macroglobulin polymorphisms, significantly increases the risk for the disorder (10). Other associations with variants in the sortilin-related receptor 1 (*SORL1*) gene, complement components 3b and 4b, clusterin and phosphatidylinositol-binding clathrin assembly protein, have been reported (11, 12).

Environmental factors are of equal or greater importance in determining development of LOAD, including antecedent head trauma, early hysterectomies, lower educational levels, cardiovascular disease, and low levels of physical activity, whereas a higher premorbid intellect correlates with protection from dementia later in life.

Motor manifestations in LOAD are uncommon early in the course of the condition when the disease is confined to the temporal cortex. As the illness progresses, the earliest motor symptom is extrapyramidal rigidity, which if present early, implies another diagnosis or a poor prognosis. Five to 10 years into LOAD, patients may develop geggenhalten, apraxia, and other frontal release phenomena, as well as left hemibody neglect. Myoclonus, seizures, and spasticity occur in the later terminal stages.

Magnetic resonance imaging (MRI) of the brain reveals hippocampal and general cortical atrophy. Brain ^{18}F-fluorodeoxyglucose-positron emission tomographic (FDG-PET) imaging shows hypometabolism of the temporal and parietal lobes. There are new techniques available to image β–amyloid plaque burden and distribution, further assisting in confirming the antemortem diagnosis.

Treatment is directed at the cognitive symptoms and the psychiatric disturbances. Therapy of the cognitive disorder includes the use of cholinesterase inhibitors including donepezil, rivastigmine and galantamine in the early stages of the condition, which can be continued well into the disease as long as they are tolerated, although data regarding efficacy of these agents after the first 2 to 3 years is inconsistent (13). The NMDA receptor antagonist memantine reduces glutamate-mediated neurotoxicity of vulnerable neurons and has been approved for the treatment of moderate to severe AD (14). Patients treated with a combination of a cholinesterase inhibitor and memantine fared better than those given either drug alone (15). Atypical antipsychotic agents such as quetiapine are effective for associated psychotic symptoms and agitation and have fewer side effects, while serotonin reuptake agents are efficacious in treating depression in AD.

LEWY BODY DEMENTIA

DLB is the second most common dementia, accounting for 10 to 15% of cases at autopsy (16). Subcortical and cortical Lewy bodies are associated with a variable combination of cognitive, psychiatric, and extrapyramidal features. Men and women are affected at autopsy in a ratio of 1.5:1. The clinical definition of DLB includes fluctuation of cognition and early prominence of psychiatric symptoms, especially visual hallucination, in up to 75% of patients, and parkinsonian features that lead to frequent falls, rigidity, and gait impairment, whereas resting tremor infrequently occurs. Symptoms of restless leg syndrome can precede the diagnosis of DLB by several decades (17). While a quarter of patients demonstrate rigidity and bradykinesia, the frequency varies depending upon patient selection bias and the confounding effects of neuroleptics. Postural instability, falls, and syncope occur in up to one-third of patients and should prompt consideration of DLB. Autonomic phenomena are more common in patients with DLB than AD, particularly orthostatic hypotension, carotid-sinus hypersensitivity, and urinary incontinence, the latter of which is an early phenomenon in DLB.

In contrast to AD, cortical Lewy bodies are preferentially deposited in the cingulate gyrus, insular cortex, and temporal lobe, with sparing of the hippocampus in cases of DLB, and neocortical neurofibrillary tangles are sparse or absent, reflecting the difference in tau processing. β-amyloid protein levels are however, equally increased in both disorders. Patients with DLB and an excess of tangles demonstrate a clinical pattern more akin to AD, while those with fewer tangles present with the classical features of DLB (18).

Brain MRI of patients with DLB shows preservation of the volume of hippocampal and medial temporal lobes, and imaging with single photon computed tomography (SPECT) demonstrates occipital hypoperfusion (19). Electroencephalography (EEG) shows slowing of the background and posterior dominant rhythms. Dopamine transporter (DAT) imaging, which confers a diagnostic sensitivity of 83% and a specificity of 100% employing ^{123}I-radiolabeled fluoropropyl brain SPECT, demonstrates dopamine transporter loss similar to that seen in PD in the caudate and anterior and posterior putamen, but with a flatter rostrocaudal caudate-putamen gradient transporter loss in the caudate and putamen (20).

There are differences in the neuropsychological profile of DLB compared to AD. Patients with DLB perform quantitatively worse on learning and memory tasks when compared with AD patients of the same degree of dementia severity, and manifest differences in focal attentional ability on visual search tasks. Treatment of cognitive loss with cholinesterase inhibitors is associated with a consistently more robust response in DLB than AD. Extrapyramidal symptoms respond to anti-parkinsonian agents, although dopamine agonist, monoamine oxidase-B inhibitor, and anticholinergic medications have the potential to exacerbate psychiatric symptoms. Neuroleptics used to treat psychiatric symptoms can result in acute extrapyramidal reactions in up to one-half of patients due to loss of substantia nigra dopaminergic neurons and the failure of up-regulation of post-synaptic striatal D_2 receptors in response to the nigrostriatal deficit and the neuroleptic challenge (21). The atypical neuroleptic clozapine, which exerts its antipsychotic effects via the D_4 receptors, is generally better tolerated and low doses are sufficient for symptom control. The diagnosis of DLB should be considered in patients with suspected idiopathic Parkinson disease who develop psychotic symptoms in response to anti-parkinsonian agents.

PARKINSON DISEASE DEMENTIA

About 10 to 40% of patients with PD develop dementia (PDD) and a large number of such patients develop mild cognitive impairment. About 15% to 20% of patients in movement disorders clinics, and a quarter of those in one autopsy series diagnosed with idiopathic PD, had another neurodegenerative condition such as AD (22). Since the pathology of PDD and DLB is similar, the clinical designation should conform to the arbitrary one year rule that Parkinsonian features should antedate dementia by more than a year to evoke the diagnosis of PDD, whereas dementia 12 months after onset of parkinsonism, instead suggests DLB. Clues to accurate diagnosis include the presence of rest tremor seen in 90% of patients. The occurrence of PDD is associated with a worse prognosis and a less favorable response to anti-parkinsonian medication than PD without dementia.

Autosomal dominant progressive frontotemporal dementia (FTLD) and parkinsonism due to mutation at the 17q21.31 locus of the microtubule-associated protein tau (MAPT) gene leads to disinhibition, apathy, poor impulse control, psychosis, alcoholism, dystonia, eye movement abnormalities, eyelid opening and closing apraxia, and upper and lower motor neuron dysfunction (23). Neuropathological features include tau-positive cytoplasmic inclusions and ballooned neurons in some, but not all kindred. PDD may be treated with the available anti-cholinesterase medication (24).

FRONTOTEMPORAL LOBE DEMENTIA

Patients with frontotemporal lobe dementia (FTLD) have selective, although differential involvement of frontal and temporal lobe cortices, depending on the type of FTLD. Of the three types of FTLD, the most common is behavioral variant frontotemporal dementia (bvFTD), followed by semantic dementia (SD) and progressive non-fluent aphasia (PNFA). Onset is generally before age 65 with nearly one-half of patients having an affected first-degree relative. About 30 to 50% of FTD cases are familial with mutations at the 17q21.31 loci of the MAPT gene encoding tau, and the GRN gene encoding progranulin (25). Most patients have evidence of grasp, snout, and sucking reflex frontal release signs; however, motor neuron signs can accompany clinical syndromes of FTLD-TDP characterized by TDP43 ubiquitin-positive inclusions. The presence of TDP43-positive inclusions as the major disease protein in ubiquitin-positive, tau-, and α-synuclein-negative FTLD and ALS (26) suggests a common pathologic substrate linking these neurodegenerative disorders (27).

The bvFTD type of FTLD, known as Pick disease, is associated with a dramatic change in personality and social conduct, with apathy, loss of volition, social disinhibition and distractibility, and preservation of memory. Both PNFA and SD, previously known as primary progressive aphasia, are associated with significant language difficulties.

All three lack a significant spatial disorder as manifested by intact diagram copying and dot counting, and intact perception, as tested by naming challenges, functional object descriptions, and pantomime object use. Patients with FTD perform poorly on tests of frontal lobe function, including the Wisconsin card sort, Stroop and trail-making tests.

Brain neuroimaging employing MRI, FDG-PET, and SPECT demonstrate concordant atrophy and abnormal tracer uptake in frontal and anterior temporal cortices of either hemisphere, which may be bilaterally symmetric or asymmetric and affect the left or right hemisphere disproportionately. The slowing of the background often seen on EEG in AD is not generally seen in the FTLD syndromes. Asymmetric atrophy of the left frontal and temporal lobes is seen in forms of PNFA and SD associated with symmetrical atrophy of bilateral anterior temporal neocortex and inferior and middle temporal gyri. Microscopically, all forms of FTLD are associated with microvacuolar change without specific histological features and severe astrocytic gliosis with or without ballooned cells and Pick-type inclusions. There are currently no effective treatments for the FTLD syndromes.

VASCULAR DEMENTIA

The vascular dementias (VaD) are heterogeneous disorders encompassing lesions due to embolism, hemorrhage, and ischemia, affecting vessels of differing caliber, large and small, named and unnamed, with involvement of cortical and subcortical structures. Strategic large vessel strokes of the right posterior cerebral artery and anterior cerebral artery territories can result in a clinical dementia, as may single lacunes in the genu of the capsule, intralaminar thalamic nuclei, and head of the caudate. Subcortical ischemic VaD due to lacunar infarction and periventricular leukoariosis spares U fibers as in Binswanger disease. Autosomal dominant cerebral arteriopathy with subcortical infarcts and leukoencephalopathy (CADASIL) due to heterozygous mutation at the 19p13.12 locus of the *NOTCH3* gene is characterized clinically by relapsing strokes with neuropsychiatric symptoms in young adults of both sexes.

Three criteria for the clinical diagnosis of VaD include cognitive loss, cerebrovascular etiopathogenesis inferred by history, examination, and neuroimaging; and onset of dementia within three months of a symptomatic stroke, the latter criterion of which is not necessary for the diagnosis of subacute VaD. Clinical and motor manifestations vary depending on the site of the lesion.

A careful history may reveal memory loss antedating the stroke in up to 15% of patients, suggesting underlying AD inheritance worsened by stroke. Neuroimaging characterizes cerebral small vessel disease, such as lacunar infarcts and white matter changes (WMC), appearing as bilateral areas of confluent symmetric hyperintense hemispheric signal changes on T_2-weighted, fluid-attenuated inversion recovery sequences on brain MRI, and hypodense periventricular or subcortical areas on brain CT (28). The Leukoaraiosis and Disability (LADIS) study collaboration, which showed an association between the severity of baseline WMC and transition to disability in a cohort of elderly patients, showed progression to dementia in 15%, and cognitive impairment without dementia in 25% so studied, independent of age, education, and medial temporal atrophy (29). Binswanger-related subcortical pathology, found in up to one-third of normal subjects of age 65 years and older and in one-half of those with AD, has been characterized as a silent epidemic (30). The presence of one or more lacunes increases the risk for AD by 20-fold and reduces the plaque and tangle burden required for clinical signs to appear. The importance of the vascular component in dementia needs to be specifically recognized and treated. Patients with AD and seemingly trivial vascular lesions warrant treatment to control cerebrovascular risk factors and to promote stroke prevention. Antihypertensive therapy is associated with a 28% reduction in the risk of recurrent stroke and a 38 to 55% reduction in the risk of dementia (31), and may actually delay the development of clinical dementia in those with pathological signs of the disease.

Acetylcholinesterase inhibitor medication is useful in the management of VaD (32), and all the available cholinesterase agents approved for the treatment of AD have been efficacious in treating patients with VaD. Calcium channel blockers may benefit VaD and AD by improving calcium dysregulation and conferring neuroprotection.

CORTICOBASAL DEGENERATION

Corticobasal degeneration (CBD) is a rare progressive neurodegenerative 4-repeat (4R) tauopathy that presents in the fifth to seventh decades of life with basal ganglia and cortical involvement, including with parkinsonism, akinesia, and rigidity, accompanied by other basal ganglia and cortical dysfunction, including limb and oculomotor apraxia, cortical sensory loss, dystonic posturing, myoclonus, and alien limb phenomenon (33). Other motor signs include blepherospasm, hypomimia, dysarthria, orofacial dyspraxia, gait disorder, choreoathetosis, postural instability, percussion myoclonus, and action and postural tremor with a frequency of 6 to 8 Hz that is more irregular and jerkier than the rest tremor of PD. The arm is the most affected region in choreoathetosis and assumes an adducted shoulder and flexed elbow and wrist position. Eye movement abnormalities include bilateral horizontal saccades with slowed extraocular movements appearing to require multiple steps to reach a target, with normal vertical saccades that differentiate the condition from progressive supranuclear palsy (PSP). Depression occurs commonly in CBD followed by apathy, irritability, and agitation. Delusions and obsessive-compulsive behavior are less common.

Formal cognitive and neuropsychological testing shows particular affliction of executive function, with better performance on tests of immediate recall and attention in CBD as compared to tests of praxis, digit span, and unimanual and bimanual motor series, which are more pronounced in patients with AD and extrapyramidal disease. Recognition memory is generally spared, however there may be impairment of coding and recall strategies.

Distinctive patterns of atrophy on brain neuroimaging have been observed in patients with autopsy-confirmed CBD (34). T_1-weighted volumetric MRI showed predominant patterns of cortical atrophy involving the posterior inferior, middle, and superior frontal lobes, the superior premotor cortex, and the posterior temporal and parietal lobes compared to controls. Other areas of atrophy included insular cortex, the supplemental motor area, subcortical grey matter (GM) of the globus pallidus, putamen, head of the caudate, and a small region of the brainstem at the dorsal pontomedullary junction. White matter atrophy was additionally noted in the posterior frontal lobes at the corticomedullary junction and corpus callosum, involvement of the latter of which correlated well with impaired cognition (35).

Brain FDG-PET imaging shows global reduction of oxygen and glucose metabolism in the cerebral hemisphere contralateral to the most affected limb, and in the thalamus concordant with nigrostriatal dopaminergic dysfunction (36). A pattern of asymmetrically reduced frontoparietal cerebral cortical metabolism and cerebral blood flow, in conjunction with bilaterally reduced F-dopa uptake in the caudate and putamen, supports the diagnosis of early CBD (37).

The pathology of CBD is characterized by circumscribed cortical atrophy with spongiosis and ballooned neuron, the distribution of which correlates with the clinical presentation. Neuronal and glial tau pathology is extensive in gray and white matter of the cortex, basal ganglia, diencephalon, and rostral brainstem, with abnormal tau accumulation in astrocytes forming pathognomonic astrocytic plaques, the latter of which is associated with bvFTD, semantic dementia, and progressive nonfluent aphasia. The parkinsonian syndrome of CBD responds poorly to levodopa, which aids in differentiating it from idiopathic PD.

NEUROACANTHOCYTOSIS

Irregularly spaced erythrocytes with a thorny surface and terminal bulbs termed *acanthocytes* are a valuable clue to the presence of neuroacanthocytosis, a neurodegenerative disorder that includes choreoacanthocytosis (ChAc) and the phenotypically similar disorder, McLeod syndrome, both of which can be characterized by progressive neurocognitive deficits. Onset of ChAc occurs in the first to seventh decade with variable generalized weakness, involuntary movements including grimacing, dystonia, tic-like movements, chorea, and subtle parkinsonism; later neuropsychiatric features include subcortical dementia supervene with cognitive impairment, personality change, and depression.

Other major neurological signs include disturbed coordination, hyporeflexia, seizures, and peripheral neuropathy. Progressive chorea and dementia resembles Huntington disease (HD), which should be considered in the differential diagnosis of ChAc. Brain MRI demonstrates areas of abnormally increased signal in the caudate and putamen, and variably in periventricular and hemispheric white matter, including the corpus callosum (38). Brain FDG-PET imaging shows dysfunction of dopaminergic neurons in the ventrolateral substantia nigra, with reduced glucose metabolism in the basal ganglia (39). The disorder is caused by homozygous or compound heterozygous mutation at the 9q21.2 locus of the *VPS13A* gene encoding chorein.

Cognitive and psychiatric impairment occurs late in the course of McLeod syndrome that displays X-linked inheritance due to mutation at the Xp21.1 locus in the *XK* gene that encodes an antigen of the Kell blood group system. Involvement of the CNS was indicated by the occurrence of seizures, psychopathology, choreatic movements, and cognitive impairment, the latter of which was discerned on assessment of higher cortical function, including psychometric tests that showed abnormal memory and executive function in 15 of 22 men, age 27 to 72 years, with the diagnosis of McLeod neuroacanthocytosis (40).

Brain MRI in 13 patients showed a rim of increased T_2-intensity in the lateral putamen in four patients. Brain ^{123}I-idodobenzamide-SPECT and FDG-PET imaging performed in three patients showed reduced dopamine-D_2-receptor binding in the striatum of two patients, one of whom had reduction that was more widespread, without any clinical sign of cerebral involvement, and in the absence of a movement disorder and unimpaired dopamine-D_2-receptor binding, one other patient demonstrated subnormal glucose metabolism of the caudate nuclei.

WILSON DISEASE

Untreated, this autosomal recessive disorder of copper metabolism, which presents with hepatic, neurologic, and psychiatric disturbances, alone or in combination, also manifests subcortical dementia (41). Liver involvement, which consists of recurrent jaundice, hepatitis, and chronic liver disease, results from intracellular hepatic copper with subsequent hepatic and neurologic abnormalities due to homozygous or compound heterozygous mutation at the 13q14.3 locus of *ATP7B* gene encoding copper-transporting ATPase 2.

Neurological involvement includes a predominant movement disorder presenting with tremor, loss of fine motor control, chorea, choreoathetosis, or a rigid-dystonic condition with mask-like facies, rigidity, gait disturbance, and pseudobulbar involvement. Psychiatric disturbances include depression, neurotic behavior, disorganized personality and intellectual deterioration.

Kayser-Fleischer rings at the limbus of the cornea are found in all patients with CNS involvement. Early psychometric studies (42, 43) performed before treatment with a diet low in copper and pencillamine chelation in patients with severe motor involvement showed neuropsychological findings that were so pronounced and, combined with memory deficits, were consistent with dementia (43, 44). Although many such patients recovered neurological function and even showed reversible changes in CT imaging (45), one reported patient (46) with advanced WD, Mini-Mental Status score of 12/30, and T_2-hyperintense signal abnormalities in the basal ganglia and midbrain on MRI before commencement of chelation therapy with D-penicillamine, was noted to have progressive interim improvement but died. At postmortem examination there were WMC noted in the superior frontal gyri extending into the deep cortex associated with unbound copper, neuronal loss, capillary proliferation, Alzheimer type 1 and 2 astrocytes, and abundant Opalski cells. The cause of subcortical dementia in WD is not well understood. Reversible cerebral dysfunction, which could occur as a result of hepatic encephalopathy and neurotransmitter imbalance, would not explain white matter destruction; however, mitochondrial abnormalities, so noted in the liver of one patient with WD (46), suggested a contribution of mitochondrial injury to other organs, including the brain. Mutation of the WD protein, that results in accumulation of intracellular copper and lead to oxidative attacks and damage within target tissues, is suggested by the correlation between severity of the neuropathological findings and cerebral copper content (47).

ADULT NEURONAL CEROID LIPOFUSCINOSIS

This disorder belongs to the neuronal ceroid-lipofuscinoses (NCL) group of inherited neurodegenerative lysosomal-storage disorders categorized by patterns of intracellular accumulation of autofluorescent lipopigment storage material, age at onset, and order of appearance of common clinical features from infancy to adulthood, including progressive dementia, seizures, and visual failure (48), with each phenotype assigned a unique ceroid lipofuscinosis (CLN) gene symbol. Kufs disease or adult ceroid lipofussinase (ACLN) presents in patients ranging from teenagers to persons greater than age 50 years, has a typical age at onset of 30 years, and differs from other forms of NCL in preservation of vision due to lack of retinal involvement. Until recently, brain biopsy was required to confirm the diagnosis of ACLN because, unlike other forms of NCL in which electron microscopy (EM) can be performed on heparinized whole blood lymphocytes and tissue biopsy of skin, conjunctiva, or other tissue, the characteristic lipopigment in Kufs disease is largely confined to neurons. The two clinical subtypes of Kufs disease, classically designated type A and B for the differing clinical presentation, have since been categorized by their respective CLN designations, CLN4A and CLN4B, allowing further separation by mode of inheritance and causative genetic mutations, with minor phenotypic overlap. Kufs type A disease (CLN4A), which displays autosomal recessive inheritance, is caused by homozygous or compound heterozygous mutation at the 15q23 locus of the *CLN6* gene encoding ceroid-lipofuscinosis neuronal protein 6, presents generally with progressive myoclonic epilepsy, whereas CLN4B, manifesting autosomal dominant inheritance, is due to heterozygous mutation at the 20q13.33 locus of the *DNAJC5* gene encoding cysteine-string protein alpha, presenting instead with dementia and a variety of motor-system signs. Accordingly, among four families with Kufs disease for whom there was good evidence of an autosomal recessive inheritance, three were affected by Kufs type A disease, presenting with tonic-clonic seizures or action myoclonus, followed by ataxia, cognitive decline, or dementia (49). A four-generation Alabama family of CLN4B was characterized by seizures, dementia, and myoclonus, and several individuals had parkinsonism prior to known molecular genetic localization to *DNAJC5* (50). The same investigators (51) identified a heterozygous mutation in the *DNAJC5* gene in a Czech family with autosomal dominant ACLN manifesting progressive confusion and dementia as well as frequent medically refractory generalized seizures. Brain MRI in the proband, age 38 years, showed prominence of cortical sulci and cerebellar folds, and mild lateral ventricular enlargement consistent with diffuse cerebral and cerebellar atrophy. Concurrent neuropsychiatric testing showed a full-scale intelligence quotient (IQ) of 73 with ensuing ataxia and myoclonus. Frontal lobe brain biopsy showed numerous neurons containing homogenous eosinophilic material that stained intensely with the periodic acid-Schiff reaction and was found to be autofluorescent with multiple neurons distended by granular osmiophilic deposits by ultrastructural examination. While challenging and often requiring invasive brain biopsy, available mutation screening for CLN4A and B should now be considered as initial diagnostic steps in patients with suspected Kufs disease.

HUNTINGTON DISEASE

This phenotypically heterogeneous autosomal dominant disorder presents in previously healthy persons age five to eight years, but mainly in the fourth to fifth decades of life, with chorea, dystonia, incoordination, cognitive decline, and behavioral disturbances. The cause of the disorder is abnormally expanded trinucleotide CAG repeats in the *HTT* gene located on chromosome 4p16.3 encoding huntingtin. The detection of an expansion of 36 or more CAG repeats in HTT in the setting of a positive family pedigree, and characteristic clinical findings, makes the diagnosis essentially certain. The length of CAG repeats correlates with an earlier age of onset, a cognitive behavioral presentation, and an accelerated disease progression. Subcortical cognitive dysfunction in HD, which typically spares long-term memory but impairs executive functions such as organization, planning, checking, or adaptation of alternatives, and delays the acquisition of new motor skills (52), worsens over time with speech deteriorating faster than comprehension. Unlike cognitive disturbances, psychiatric and behavioral involvement seen in 98% of patients, including depression, apathy, aggression and disinhibition, do not proceed in a stepwise progression along with worsening disease severity.

Patients with juvenile HD (JHD), defined as onset before age 20 years (53), can have an insidious onset with nonspecific psychiatric and cognitive difficulties. Among a cohort of French JDH patients (54), the commonest signs at onset were cognitive and psychiatric in 65% of patients, including severe alcohol and drug addiction, psychotic behavior, and suicide attempts, with motor signs occurring an average of six years later, included among them atypical features such as myoclonic head tremor and progressive cerebellar dysfunction. Less than one-half of the patients had fewer than 60 CAG repeats or a known history of inheritance from an affected parent, leading to misdiagnosis or a delay in diagnosis of up to nine years. Preclinical HD patients have substantially decreased basal ganglia and cerebral white matter volumes on axial-3-dimensional volumetric spoiled gradient echo MRI representing early degenerative changes (55).

Brain FDG-PET demonstrates a decrease in glucose utilization in cortical and striatal regions of the brain in all patients with HD and in one of pre-HD patients, due to cortical abnormalities and functional deafferentation from subcortical regions (56). The use of D_1-, and D_2-receptor antagonist radiotracer elements to examine dopaminergic receptor binding and striatal neuronal loss show changes over time associated with clinical manifestations of the disease, including functional capacity and motor abnormalities. Functional brain MRI (fMRI) in HD, which is less expensive and less invasive than FDG-brain PET imaging, shows impaired task performance and lower task-related activation in several subcortical and cortical regions while functional connectively imaging addressing fMRI blood-oxygen level-dependent (BOLD) signal responses between brain regions, showed impairment between anterior cingulated and lateral prefrontal regions and poor task performance associated with reduced connectivity (57). The selective degeneration of neurons in the caudate and putamen provide the clinicopathological correlation for chorea, while intraneuronal inclusions containing huntingtin in other affected cortical regions of the brain, including hippocampus, appear begin to explain behavioral and cognitive disturbances. Treatment of HD is aimed primarily at treating depression and psychosis.

WHIPPLE DISEASE

Whipple disease, a rare systemic infectious disease, is caused by infection by *Tropheryma whippelii* (TW), a gram-positive Actinomicetes commensal gut organism. Systemic symptoms present in the majority of patients and include fever of unknown origin (FUO), gastrointestinal symptoms including steatorrhea, chronic diarrhea, abdominal distension or pain, chronic migratory arthralgia or polyarthralgias, and unexplained lymphadenopathy, night sweats, or malaise. Evidence of CNS involvement, present in about 5% of patients at presentation, eventually occurs in up to 43% of patients. Cognitive change or altered level of consciousness without other neurological signs occurred in 11% of

84 patients in a retrospective review (58), whereas 81% patients had either cognitive change or supranuclear palsy, and 42% had both. Altogether, 47% of those with cognitive change had psychiatric signs of depression, euphoria, anxiety, psychosis, or personality change. Other neurological signs, alone or in combination, in fewer than 50% of patients, included upper motor neuron signs, hypothalamic manifestations of polydipsia, hyperphagia, change in libido, amenorrhea, changes in the sleep-wake cycle, or insomnia; 3rd, 4th or 6th cranial nerve palsies, myoclonus, ataxia, oculomasticatory myorhythmia (OMM), oculo-facial-skeletal myorhythmia (OFSM), and either peripheral nervous system (PNS) or CNS sensory deficits.

Two reported patients with Whipple disease, confirmed by positive polymerase chain reaction (PCR) for the pathogen on serum and CSF, presented with progressive dementia confirmed by psychometric and MMSE scores in both, one of whom had cortical and subcortical atrophy and abnormal signal changes in periventricular white matter on T_1-, and T_2-weighted MRI (59) and another that met consensus criteria for FTD in association with brain SPECT imaging revealing regional frontal and temporal hypoperfusion (60). Both patients improved clinically and neuroradiologically following antibiotic therapy for up to two years.

The diagnosis of WD is facilitated by tissue biopsy of the small bowel, heart, brain, lymph nodes and vitreous fluid stained with periodic acid Schiff (PAS) followed by EM for isolation of the bacterium; such tissues in addition to peripheral blood and CSF are later processed by PCR for confirmation of Whipple disease.

Brain biopsy is a sensitive technique once clinical suspicion of Whipple disease has been established, however, recognizing the diagnostic accuracy of 89% for all tissue (58) renders it potentially unnecessary, especially when there is no obvious neurological involvement.

The neuropathological findings in Whipple disease classically include focally inflammatory lesions containing large numbers of macrophages that contain PAS-positive inclusions, EM of which reveal phagosomes with membranous, laminar, or rod-shaped bacterium structures (61). False negative results can be minimized by performing endoscopically guided intestinal biopsies of multiple jejunal sites with routine performance of EM to confirm the diagnosis.

If two small-bowel biopsies are not diagnostic, another tissue should be biopsied such as lymph node, brain, or vitreous fluid where appropriate. Brain MRI should be performed in all suspected patients because focal abnormalities ranging from focal lesions without mass effect to large numbers of enhancing lesions with mass effect, are noted in over one-half of patients, although they are not specific to Whipple disease.

Criteria for the diagnosis of definite WD include the presence of OMM or OFSM, positive tissue biopsy, and informative PCR analysis. Both OM and OFSM are pathognomonic for Whipple disease. However, while very specific, the sensitivity of OMM or OFSM are low. Patients with FUO, gastrointestinal symptoms, chronic arthralgia, unexplained constitutional symptoms, and lymphadenopathy, as well as supranuclear vertical gaze palsy, rhythmic myoclonus, dementia with psychiatric symptoms, or hypothalamic manifestations should undergo tissue biopsy for Whipple disease. Unrecognized and therefore untreated, the natural history of CNS Whipple disease is progressive deterioration culminating in death (62). Patients with definite Whipple disease should be treated with parenteral and oral antibiotics for up to a year or more to assure cure.

CREUTZFELDT-JAKOB DISEASE

Human prior diseases occur in inherited, acquired, and sporadic forms, with about 15% of the inherited cases due to coding mutations at the 20p13 locus of the prior protein (*PRNP*) gene. Acquired forms due to iatrogenic CJD and variant (vCJD) acquired from infected cattle. The remaining majority of human prior cases occur as sporadic (sCJD) (63). The classification of CJD is based on molecular and phenotypic presentations (63, 64). The pathological isoform of the prion protein (PrP), termed PrP^s, formed through a posttranslational event involving conformational changes of the normal cellular isoform (PrP^c), differs from the latter by the high content of β-sheet structure and partial resistance to protease digestion. PrP^{sc} is considered an essential or exclusive component of the transmissible agent or prion. Among 300 patients with immunoblot PrP^{sc} positive CJD who lacked pathogenic mutations in the coding region of *PRNP* and a negative history of familial diseases or exposure to known prion contaminants, 3 sCJD (abbreviated MM, MV, VV), and one vCJD were discerned, along with various subtypes reflecting clinical and neuropathologic differences and similarities, respectively, between and among patients (64). Cognitive impairment, including memory loss, confusion, disorientation, and intellectual decline, were the commonest clinical features at onset of the disease, noted in 70% of patients, followed by psychiatric, visual disturbances, aphasia, and myoclonus.

Brain neuroimaging, EEG, and CSF studies contribute accuracy to the diagnosis of early and established CJD. The accuracy of brain MRI in the diagnosis of rapidly progressive dementia due to sCJD is obtained when temporal, parietal, or occipital cortical regions, or both caudate and putaminal nuclei displayed high signal intensities in fluid attenuated inversion recovery FLAIR or DWI, so noted in 83% of confirmed sCJD patients (65). Typical EEG findings of periodic or pseudoperiodic sharp-wave complexes (PSWC), seen in up to 80% of affected patients, contributes to the triad of dementia, myoclonus, and PSWC, a common early feature of sCJD, which along with visual signs of field defects, distortions, abnormal color vision, and cortical blindness, precedes severe dementia in about one-third of patients. The presence of the 14-3-3 protein in the CSF, part of the family of regulatory molecules expressed in all eukaryotic cells and reflective of destruction of neurons, is a useful *in vivo* diagnostic test for CJD and, when used in the appropriate clinical context, shows a good correlation to CJD. Widespread spongiform degeneration, neuronal loss, gliosis, and PrP-positive plaques of the cerebral cortex, most severe in occipital regions, are the clinicopathologic correlates of dementia. There are no effective treatments available for this condition.

REFERENCES

1. McKeith IG, Dickson DW, Lowe J, et al. Diagnosis and management of dementia with Lewy bodies: third report of the DLB Consortium. *Neurology* 2005; 65:1863–1872.
2. Portet F, Scarmeas N, Cosentino S, et al. Extrapyramidal signs before and after diagnosis of incident Alzheimer disease in a prospective population study. *Arch Neurol* 2009; 66:1120–1126.
3. Mayeux R. Early Alzheimer's disease. *N Engl J Med* 2010; 362:21942201.
4. Devi G, Williamson J, Massoud F, et al. A comparison of family history of psychiatric disorders among patients with early- and late-onset Alzheimer's disease. *J Neuropsychiatry Clin Neurosci* 2004; 16:57–62.
5. Devi G, Fotiou A, Jyrinji D, et al. Novel presenelin 1 mutations associated with early-onset dementia in a family with both early-onset and late-onset Alzheimer disease. *Arch Neurol* 2000; 57:1454–1457.
6. Kukull WA, Higdon R, Bowen JD, et al. Dementia ad Alzheimer disease incidence. a prospective cohort study. *Arch Neurol* 2002; 59:1737–1746.
7. Fitzpatrick AL, Kuller LH, Ives DG, et al. Incidence and prevalence of dementia in the cardiovascular health study. *J Am Geriatr Soc* 2004; 52:195–204.
8. McDowell I. Alzheimer's disease: insights from epidemiology. *Aging* 2001; 13:143–162.
9. Bertram L, Tanzi RE. Dancing in the dark? The status of late-onset Alzheimer's disease genetics. *J Mol Neurosci* 2001; 17:127–136.
10. Zappia M, Manna I, Serra P, et al. Increased risk for Alzheimer's disease with the interaction of MPO and A2M polymorphisms *Arch Neurol* 2004; 61:341–344.
11. Rogaeva E, Meng Y, Lee JH, et al. The neuronal sortilin-related receptor SORL-1 is genetically associated with Alzheimer disease. *Nat Genet* 2007; 39:168–177.
12. Harold D, Abraham R, Hollingworth P, et al. Genome-wide association study identifies variants at CLU and PICALM associated with Alzheimer's disease. *Nat Genet* 2009; 41:1088–1093.
13. Cummings JL. Drug therapy: Alzheimer's disease. *N Engl J Med* 2004; 351:56–67.
14. Reisberg B, Doody R, Stoffler A, et al. Memantine in

moderate-to-severe Alzheimer's disease. *N Engl J Med* 2003; 348:1333–1341.

15. Tariot PH, Farlow MR, Grossberg GT, et al. Memantine treatment in patients with moderate to severe Alzheimer disease already receiving donepezil: a randomized controlled trial. *JAMA* 2004; 291:317–324.

16. McKeith IG, Galasko D, Kosaka K, et al. Consensus guidelines for the clinical and pathologic diagnosis of dementia with Lewy bodies (DLB): report of the consortium on DLB international workshop. *Neurology* 1996; 47:1113–1124.

17. Boeve B, Silber M, Ferman T, et al. Association of REM sleep behavior disorder and neurodegenerative may reflect an underlying synucleopathy. *Mov Disord* 2001; 16:622–630.

18. Lippa CF, McKeith I. Dementia with Lewy bodies: improving diagnostic criteria. *Neurology* 2003; 60:1571–1572.

19. Lobotesis K, Fenwick JD, Phipps A, et al. Occipital hypoperfusion on SPECT in dementia with Lewy bodies but not AD. *Neurology* 2001; 13:643–649.

20. O'Brien JT, Colloby S, Fenwick J, et al. Dopamine transport loss visualized on FP-CIT SPECT in the differential diagnosis of dementia with Lewy bodies. *Arch Neurol* 2004; 61:919–925.

21. Walker Z, Costa DC, Walker RW, et al. Striatal dopamine transporter in dementia with Lewy bodies and Parkinson disease: a comparison. *Neurology* 2004; 62:1568–1572.

22. Hughes AJ, Daniel SE, Kilford L, et al. Accuracy of clinical diagnosis of idiopathic Parkinson's disease: a clinicopathologic study of 100 cases. *J Neurol Neurosurg Psychiatry* 1992; 55:181–184.

23. Mackenzie IRA, Rademakers R. The molecular genetics and neuropathology of frontotemporal lobar degeneration: recent developments. *Neurogenetics* 2007; 8:237–248.

24. Burn DJ, McKeith IG Current treatment of dementia with Lewy bodies and dementia associated with Parkinson's disease. *Mov Disord* 2003; 6:S72–S79.

25. Seelaar H, Rohrer JD, Pijnenburg YAL, et al. Clinical, genetic and pahtologicla heterogeneity of frontotemporal dementia: a review. *J Neurol Neurosurg Psychiatry* 2011; 82:476–486.

26. Van Deerlin VM, Sleiman PMA, Martinez-Lage M, et al. Common variants at 7p21 are associated with fronto-temporal lobe degeneration with TDP-43 inclusions. *Nature Genet* 2010; 42:234–239.

27. Neumann M, Sampathu DM, Kwong LK et al. Ubiquinated TDP-43 I in frontotemporal lobe degeneration and amyotrophic lateral sclerosis. *Science* 2006; 314:130–133.

28. Pantoni L. Cerebral small vessel disease: from pathogenesis and clinical characteristics to therapeutic challenges. *Lancet Neurol* 2010; 9:689–701.

29. Inzitari D, Pracucci G, Poggesi A, et al., for the LADIS Study Group. Changes in white matter as determinant of global functional decline in older independent outpatients: three year followup of LADIS (leukoaraiosis and disability) study cohort. *BMJ* 2009; 339:b2477.

30. Roman GC. Binswanger disease: the history of a silent epidemic. *Ann NY Acad Sci* 2000; 904:19–23.

31. Kirshner HS. Vascular dementia: a review of recent evidence for prevention and treatment. *Curr Neurol Neurosci Rep* 2009; 9:437–442.

32. Erkinjutti T, Roman G, Gauthier S. Treatment of vascular dementia-evidence from clinical trials with cholinesterase inhibitors. *Neurol Res* 2004; 26:603–605.

33. Kouri N, Whitwell JL, Josephs KA, et al. Corticobasal degeneration: a pathologically distinct 4R tauopathy. *Nat Rev Neurol* 2011; 7:263–272.

34. Josephs KA, Whitwell JL, Dickson DW, et al. Voxel-based morphometry in autopsy proven PSP and CBD. *Neurobiology of Aging* 2008; 29:280–289.

35. Yamaguchi H, Fukuyama H, Nagahama Y. Atrophy of the corpus callosum, cortical hypometabolism and cognitive impairment in corticobasal degeneration. *Arch Neurol* 1998; 55:609–614.

36. Lutte I, Laterre C, Bodart JM et al. Contribution of PET studies in diagnosis of corticobasal degeneration. *Eur Neurol* 2000; 44:12–21.

37. Laureys S, Salmon E, Garraux G, et al. Fluorodopa uptake and glucose metabolism in early stages of corticobasal degeneration. *J Neurol* 1999; 246:1151–1158.

38. Nicholl DJ, Sutton I, Dotti MT, et al. White matter abnormalities on MRI in neuroacanthocytosis. *J Neurol Neurosurg Psychiatry* 2004; 75:1200–1201.

39. Selcuk NA, Fenercioglu A. Reduction of glucose metolism in basal ganglia diagnosed with FDG-PET scan. A neuroacanthocytosis case. *Clin Nucl Med* 2010; 35:557–558

40. Danek A, Rubio JP, Rampoldi L, et al. McLeod neuroacanthocytosis: genotype and phenotype. *Ann Neurol* 2001; 50:755–764.

41. Lang D, Muller D, Claus D, et al. Neuropsychological findings in treated Wilson's disease. *Acta Neurol Scand* 1990; 81:75–81.

42. Goldstein NR, Ewert JC, Randall RV, et al. Psychiatric aspects of Wilson's disease (hematolenticular degeneration): Results of psychometric tests during long-term therapy. *Am J Psychiatry* 1968; 124:1555–15561.

43. Rosselli M, Lorenzana P, Rosselli A, et al. Wilson's disease, a reversible dementia: case report. *J Clin Exp Neuropsychol* 1987; 9:399–406.

44. Medulla A, Isaacs-Glaberman K, Scheinberg IH. Neuropsychological impairment in Wilson's disease. *Arch Neurol* 1988; 45:502–504;

? Lang C. Is Wilson's disease a dementing condition? *J Clin Exp Neuropsychol* 1989; 14:569–570.

45. Williams FJB, Walshe JM. Wilson's disease: an analysis of the cranial computerized tomographic appearance in 60 patients and the changes in response to treatment with chelating agents. *Brain* 1981; 104:735–752.

46. Mikol J, Vital C, Wassef M, et al. Extensive cortico-subcortical lesions in Wilson's disease: clinic-pathological study of two cases. *Acta Neuropathol* 2005; 110:451–458.

47. Horoupian DS, Sternlieb I, Scheinberg IH. Neuropathological findings in penicillamine-treated patients with Wilson's disease. *Clin Neuropathol* 1988; 7:62–67.

48. Mole SE, Williams RE, Goebel HH. Correlations between genotype, ultrastructural morphology and clinical phenotype in the neuronal ceroid lipofuscinoses. *Neurogenetics* 2005; 6:107–126.

49. Arsov T, Smith KR, Damiano J, et al. Kufs disease, the major adult form of neuronal ceroid lipfuscinosis, caused by mutations in CLN6. *Am J Hum Genet* 2011; 88:566–573.

50. Burneo JG, Arnold T, Palmer CA, et al. Adult-onset neuronal ceroid lipofuscinosis (Kufs disease) with autosomal dominant inheritance in Alabama. *Epilepsia* 2003; 44:841–846.

51. Noskova L, Stranecky V, Hartmannova H, et al. Mutations in DNAJC5, encoding cysteine-string protein alpha, cause autosomal-dominant adult-onset neuronal ceroid lipofuscinosis. *Am J Hum Genet* 2011; 89:241–252.

52. Walker FO. Huntington's disease. *Lancet* 2007; 369:218–228.

53. Myers RH. Huntington's disease genetics. *NeuroRx* 2004; 1:255–262.

54. Ribai P, Nguyen K, Hahn-Barma V, et al. Psychiatric and cognitive difficulties as indicators of juvenile Huntington disease onset in 29 patients. *Arch Neurol* 2007; 64:813–819.

55. Paulsen JS, Hayden M, Stout JC, et al. Preparing form preventative clinical trials: the Predict-HD study. *Arch Neurol* 2006; 63:883–890.

56. Paulsen JS. Functional imaging in Huntington's disease. *Exp Neurol* 2009; 216:272–277.

57. Paulsen JS. Functional imaging in Huntington's disease. *Exp Neurol* 2009; 216:272–277.

58. Louis ED, Lynch T, Kaufmann P, et al. Diagnostic guidelines in central nervous system Whipple's disease. *Ann Neurol* 1996; 40:561–568.

59. Rossi T, Haghighipour R, Haghighi M, et al. Cerebral Whipple's disease as a cause of reversible dementia. *Clinical Neurology and Neurosurgery* 2005; 107:258–261.

60. Benito-Leon J, Sedano LF, Louis ED. Isolated central nervous system Whipple's disease causing reversible frontotemporal-like dementia. *Clinical Neurology and Neurosurgery* 2008; 110:747–749.

61. Kitamura T. Brain involvement in Whipple's disease. *Acta Neuropathol* 1975; 33:275–278.

62. Adams M, Rhyner PA, Day J, et al. Whipple's disease confined to the central nervous system. *Ann Neurol* 1987; 21:104–108.

63. Hill AF, Joiner S, Wadsworth JDF, et al. Molecular classification of sporadic Creutzfeld-Jakob disease. *Brain* 2003; 126:1333–1346.

64. Parchi P, Zou W, Wang W, et al. Classification of sporadic Creutzfeld-Jakob disease based on molecular and phenotypic analysis of 300 subjects. *Ann Neurol* 1999; 46:224–233.

65. Zerr I, Kallenberg K, Summers DM, et al. Updated clinical diagnostic criteria for sporadic Creutzfeldt-Jakob disease. *Brain* 2009; 132:2659–2668.

CHAPTER 58

Motor Disorders in Epilepsy

Anuradha Singh

Epilepsy affects about 1% of general the population and is most common at the extremes of age. It is defined as two or more transient paroxysmal, recurrent unprovoked seizures resulting from depolarization of hyper excitable neurons in a synchronous manner. Patients can present with a myriad of symptoms. The common ones include, but are not limited to motor, sensory, autonomic and psychic symptoms. The two main categories of seizures include generalized and partial seizures. The motor manifestations of seizures, the subject of this chapter, presents with variable clinical semiology depending on the areas of the cortex involved.

NEUROANATOMY OF THE MOTOR CORTEX

The motor areas of the cerebral cortex are located in the frontal lobes which occupy about 40% of the area of both cerebral hemispheres. There are four distinct motor areas of importance: the primary motor cortex (MI), the supplementary motor area (SMA), premotor cortex (PMC) and cingulate motor area (CMA). These areas are directly connected to the periphery through the corticospinal tracts (CST). The primary motor cortex has major efferent connections to the subcortical and spinal regions but not to the association motor areas. The association motor cortex initiates movement and provides motivational force for self-initiated planned and externally cued movements. The association motor cortices flow information to the primary motor cortex. Communication, coordination and synchronization of activity between multiple motor areas and related sensory, association, and subcortical areas is necessary for the flexibility of movement (1). Lesions of the primary motor cortex cause substantial weakness

distally but patients can still have some residual proximal functions of the extremities.

PRIMARY MOTOR CORTEX

This region of motor cortex (MI) or Brodmann area (BA 4) executes skilled voluntary movements and provides most of the fibers in the CST. The cytoarchitecture of the primary motor cortex is unique in being agranular in layer IV and densely populated by giant pyramidal or Betz cells in layer V. It is organized somatotopically by the body representation with the tongue and lips arranged near the sylvian fissure followed by the thumb, fingers, arm, and trunk, with the leg, foot and toes on the medial surface (2, 3). It has a large representation for laryngeal, tongue and speech function, and intrinsic hand muscles for dexterity. Motor cortex receives afferents from the premotor cortex (PMC) (MII), anterior BA 6 and posterior BA 8; CMA, MIII, BA 23c, BA 24c, BA 24d, BA 6c, primary and proprioceptive association somatosensory cortex, with ventral anterior (VA) afferents from basal ganglia and ventral lateral (VL) cerebellar afferent connections from thalamic nuclei (Figure 1).

ASSOCIATION MOTOR CORTEX

Association motor cortices consist of the lateral PMC (LPMC) including MII, anterior BA 6, posterior BA 8; medial PMC (SMA) including MII, anterior BA6, posterior BA 8; and portions of BA 44. The cingulate motor cortex including MIII, BA 23c, BA 24c, and BA 6c, has cytoarchitectural and functional similarities to association motor cortex in that the

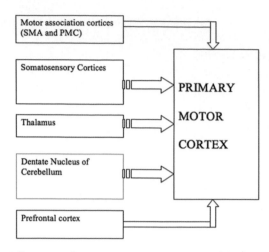

FIG. 1. Afferents of primary motor cortex. Abbreviations: PMC, premotor cortex; SMA, supplementary motor area.

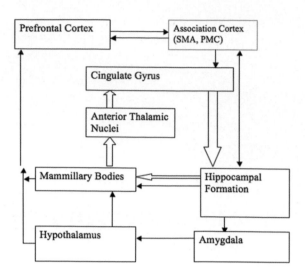

FIG. 2. Limbic pathways. Block arrows represent the Papez circuit. Abbreviations: PMC, premotor cortex; SMA, supplementary motor area.

latter exhibits gradual transition and imprecise demarcation from agranular MI to the granular prefrontal cortex, likewise, association motor and association sensory unimodal cortices have similar features. The former receives proprioceptive input from parietal association somatosensory cortex and thalamus, and projects to MI reciprocally and directly to subcortical and spinal areas in the CST.

SUPPLEMENTARY MOTOR AREA

Electrostimulation studies (4) contribute to the cytoarchitectural and physiological understanding of different cortices especially SMA which underlies spontaneous and self-initiated movements and plays important roles in motor repetitions and sequential processing of motor reversals and cues, and postural adjustments. Posterior SMA is demarcated as the mesial portion of premotor cortex and subdivided into two regions divided by the vertical anterior commissural line with the anterior portion termed pre-SMA or F6, and posteriorly SMA proper or F3 (5). The anterior pre-SMA anterior region joins prefrontal cortex with other premotor areas as does SMA proper with primary motor cortex and spinal cord (6), preparing and executing movements while pre-SMA is an internal selector of temporally oral movements and updated motor plans (7). Whereas pre-SMA monitors and switches between task performance possessing motor representation for the arms, neck, and face at high thresholds, SMA proper links component movements of a sequence possessing a complete somatotopic body representation at lower thresholds for stimulation-evoked movement (8, 9). The somatotopic representation of proximal and distal movements is better

segregated in MI than SMA (10) in spite of major cortical afferents from the ventral anterior (VA) nucleus of the thalamus carrying the majority of projections from the basal ganglia and prefrontal cortex. Each SMA projects to the PMC and to the contralateral SMA through the corpus callosum with bilateral efferents to striatum, CST and brainstem. The SMA plays an important part in bimanual coordination acting as a supplementary sensorimotor cortex extending across the medial precentral sulcus (11). The association motor cortex initiates movement and provides motivational force for self-initiated and externally cued movements related to acquisition rather than storage or execution of sequential motor tasks (12). Moreover, it facilitates the initiation of propositional speech and has a role in the suppression of non-propositional automatic speech, pacing both propositional and non-propositional speech, and contributing to articulation and phonation. Electrical stimulation elicits synergistic and complex movements of more than one joint (13–15).

LATERAL PREMOTOR CORTEX

The LPMC is located in area 6 where it receives major afferent connections from the cerebellum relayed from the ventral lateral (VL) nucleus of the thalamus while a portion of LPMC projects to the reticular formation. Owing to its rich connections with the parietal cortex important in all phases of motor action, LPMC is a virtual storage house for elementary motor acts, retrieving them for externally cued movements. Both PMC and prefrontal cortex prepare, initiate, select and learn movement patterns (16). Left hemispheric LPMC, Broca area and SMA store verbal information for working memory while spatial information is stored in the opposite side (17). The LPMC is bilaterally organized with strong relations to axial musculature with greater distal limb representation (18).

FRONTAL EYE FIELDS

The frontal eye fields (FEF) or BA 8, which are located in the caudal middle frontal gyrus, receive afferent input from peristriate, pulvinar, dorsomedial (DM) thalamic nuclei, and superior temporal and parietal cortex, triggering voluntary saccades, similar to those elicited after electrostimulation deviating the eyes to the contralateral side.

BROCA AREA

This area, which lies in the posterior portion of the inferior frontal gyrus and the frontal operculum, contains BA 44 and posterior BA 45 in the dominant hemisphere which it contributes to the motor programming of laryngeal, tongue and mouth movements during speech. It contains neural codes for the sequential relationships underlying grammar and electrostimulation of which causes speech arrest and impaired fluency, as well as more subtle receptive language deficits (19). The Wernicke area located in the superior temporal gyrus projects to the motor speech area via cortico-cortical association fibers termed the arcuate fasciculus.

LIMBIC MOTOR AREA

These C-shaped structures on the medial surface of the brain play important roles in memory, emotions, learning, and cognition (Figure 2). The limbic system comprises limbic association neocortex located on the medial surface of the frontal, parietal and temporal lobes; hippocampus formation or archicortex, a three-layered cortex located on the floor of the inferior horn of the lateral ventricle with efferent fornix tract fibers; and a portion of the amygdala or paleocortex and efferent fibers located in the stria terminalis; all three portions of which are interconnected with midbrain, diencephalon, septal nuclei and ventral striatum. Hippocampus circuits are important in the consolidating short-term into long-term memory and in visuospatial memory. It has three distinct subdivisions, the dentate gyrus, hippocampus, and the subiculum and receives major afferent input from entorhinal limbic association cortex. The output neurons of the hippocampal formation are located in the hippocampus and subiculum from which axons synapse in the mammillary bodies of the hypothalamus, and project to the anterior nuclei of the thalamus with branches to cingulate gyrus. Amygdala

circuits are involved more so with emotionality and overt behavioral expression. The limbic system contributes effector input to endocrine, autonomic and somatic motor systems. Although most of limbic association cortex is allocortex or neocortex, it consists of four gyri located on the medial and orbital surfaces of the cerebral hemisphere, including cingulate, medial orbital, parahippocampal, and those of the temporal pole. The limbic lobe and its connections contribute to emotion, memory, olfaction and visceral functions.

FRONTAL LOBE EPILEPSY

Frontal lobe epilepsy (FLE) is the second commonest epilepsy after temporal lobe epilepsy (TLE). Seizures emanating from SMA and perirolandic areas have been well studied, and present in any age group without gender differences. High resolution brain magnetic resonance imaging (MRI), positron emission tomography (PET), single photon emission computed tomography (SPECT), magnetic resonance spectroscopy (MRS), magnetoencephalography (MEG) and epilepsy monitoring units (EMU) have all contributed to improved diagnosis and understanding of FLE, as have subtraction SPECT co-registered to magnetic resonance imaging (SISCOM) (20) techniques in the evaluation of focal cortical dysplasia and other neuronal migrational disorders missed on the conventional MRI of the brain. Interictal discharges are less frequent in extra-temporal epilepsies including those with mesial frontal lobe seizure focus that are difficult to lateralize or localize on the scalp EEG. Intracranial EEG studies contribute more to the recognition of ictal frontal lobe seizure patterns, the salient features of which are summarized in Table 1. About 50% of the patients with frontal lobe seizures (FLS) have somatosensory auras, 20% have fear, distress or terror sensations, forced thinking and ideational manifestations termed psychical symptoms. About 50% of affected patients display autonomic symptoms including choking, throat and abdominal constriction, urge to urinate, chest pain and palpitation. Short-lasting repetitive gestural automatisms occur at the beginning of the seizure (21) with most sei-

Table 1: Characteristics of Frontal Lobe Epilepsy

Abrupt onset
Sudden cessation
Short duration of seconds to less than a minute
Frequent and tend to cluster
Nocturnal
Rapid secondary generalization
Focal clonic motor and tonic posturing
Minimal postictal confusion
Often confused with psychogenic seizures, movement or
  sleep disorders

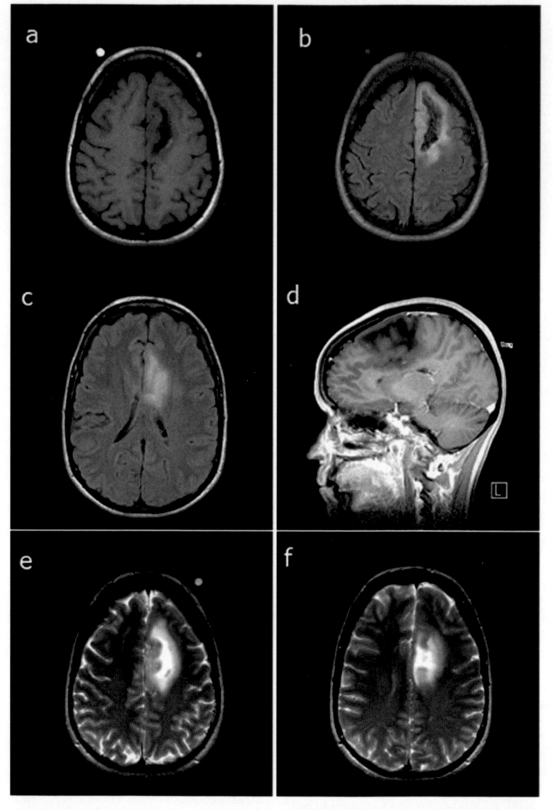

FIG. 3. Epileptogenic mass arising from the left medial frontal lobe as seen by brain MRI in different planes. a: Axial T$_1$-weighted pre-contrast images. b,c: Axial T$_2$-weighted FLAIR imaging showing peripheral hyperintensity with a low signal cystic core. d: Sagittal MPRAGE. e, f: Axial T$_2$-weighted pre-contrast images. g, h: Axial T$_1$-weighed post-contrast images show minimal enhancement.

zures originating from supplementary sensorimotor, peri-rolandic, dorsolateral, orbitofrontal, frontopolar, opercular and cingulate areas.

Supplementary Motor Area Seizures

These brief stereotyped, mainly nocturnal seizures last 10 seconds to 45 seconds with bizarre bilateral and often asymmetric tonic posturing, with arms more affected than legs, and associated vocalizations, speech arrest, proximal musculature involvement and fencing postures. Asymmetric tonic limb posturing presents which presents with tonic extension of one arm at the elbow with clenching of the fist and flexion at the wrist while the opposite extremity is flexed at the elbow, referred to as the figure 4 sign, is related to asymmetrical activation of the supplementary motor or prefrontal areas during the tonic phase of a generalized tonic-clonic seizure with ictal-onset contralateral to the extended arm in nearly all patients. By contrast, head turning can misleadingly be contralateral or ipsilateral to the ictal-onset. Patients respond immediately due to lack of a post-ictal period unless there is secondary generalization. Surgical resection of the seizure focus in the medial frontal lobe results in transient impairment of motor function. This condition, referred to as SMA syndrome, can be confused with pyramidal weakness wherein initiation of movement is particularly affected. The symptoms of SMA seizures, which include transient motor aphasia, hemi-neglect, apraxia, and speech, may be symptomatic of an epileptogenic structural lesion (Figure 3).

Opercular Seizures

These seizures include hyperkinetic and oral automatisms including lip-smacking, deglutition and laryngeal movements; and epigastric, visceral, gustatory and somatosensory aura. There may be asymmetric tonic-dystonic posturing, ballistic bimanual and bipedal movements, and associated speech arrest, hypersalivation and simple, focal facial clonic movements; speech difficulties can also occur in the post-ictal period. Complex motor seizures are a common feature of nocturnal frontal lobe epilepsy with origin in the insula and temporal pole.

Cingulate Seizures

These seizures have motor gestural automatisms at onset due to cingulate connections to the temporal lobe simulating TLE. Such patients who report changes in their mood and affect before the onset of seizures, later develop clonic mouth movement, tonic, atonic and tonic-clonic seizures., often associated with urinary incontinence.

Frontopolar Seizures

Such seizures are characterized by forced thinking behavior, adversive movements of the head and eyes followed by contraversive movements and loss of consciousness. Clinical manifestations may be minimal if seizures remain localized to this area. Axial clonic movements and falls can be seen in patients with secondary generalization.

Orbitofrontal Seizures

These seizures have complex motor gestural automatisms at onset due to connectivity with limbic and paralimbic areas, with a localization mistakenly attributed to the temporal lobe. Olfactory hallucinations, illusions, autonomic symptoms, bicyclical leg and axial automatisms are common, and clinical semiology may lag behind the electroencephalographic onset by several seconds.

Dorsolateral Seizures

These poorly-defined cephalic sensations present with non-specific vertiginous and epigastric auras, fear, anxiety, tonic-clonic movements, and versive movements of the eyes and head that differ from those with parasagittal seizures in whom head turning is easily recollected, and others with Broca area onset due to association with aphasia and speech arrest.

SEIZURES ORIGINATING IN MOTOR CORTEX

Simple focal motor seizures occur with a Jacksonian march due to spread across homunculus presenting with partial clonic or tonic-clonic movements that are asymmetric, unilateral or bilateral. Involvement of the motor strip representative of the arms leads to clonic activity of the distal muscles that moves up the arm, which with spread to primary motor

Table 2: Severe Epileptic Encephalopathy in Children

Lennox-Gastaut syndrome
West syndrome
Dose syndrome
Ohtahara syndrome
Severe myoclonic epilepsy of infancy
Progressive myoclonic epilepsies
Myoclonic epilepsy with ragged red fibers
Sialidosis
Inborn errors of metabolism
Neuronal carotid lipofuscinosis
Dentatorubral pallidoluysian atrophy
Rasmussen syndrome

Table 3: Etiopathogenesis of Symptomatic Myoclonus

Neuronal storage: Lafora body disease, lipid storage diseases, sialidosis, neuronal ceroid lipofuscinosis
Cancer: Neuroblastoma, small cell lung cancer
Dementia: Alzheimer disease, Lewy body dementia, Creutzfeldt-Jakob disease
Mitochondrial: Unverricht-Lundborg disease
Focal CNS insult: Stroke, abscess, tumor, vascular malformation, demyelinating plaque
Encephalopathy: Hypoxia, heat stroke, trauma
Metabolic disturbance: Hepatic and renal failure, hypoglycemia, hyponatremia, biotin deficiency
Malabsorption: Celiac disease, Whipple disease, Vitamin E deficiency
Drug: Psychotropic, anticonvulsant, anti-neoplastic, narcotic, cardiotonic, drug abuse
Toxin: Aluminium, bismuth, mercury, tetanus toxoid, strychnine
CNS System degeneration: Parkinson disease, Huntington disease, Wilson disease,
Multisystem atrophy, Progressive supranuclear palsy, Hallervorden-Spatz disease

cortex supero-mesially evoke similar movements of the contralateral leg. Ictal discharges spreading to contiguous SMA produce tonic movements of the ipsilateral leg. There may be simple or complex vocalizations, with the former varying from typical epileptic crying to bizarre screaming, howling, or moaning, and the latter depicted as palilalia, compulsive reiteration of words, phrases, commands, and gibberish sounds, words or phrases, all of which may be accompanied by swallowing movements, dysphasia, and contralateral tonic-clonic facial movements due to inferior peri-Rolandic cortical involvement. The most common areas of motor involvement are the distal arm, followed by the leg, and face. Todd paresis is common in seizures that originate in the precentral gyrus. Neuroimaging should be performed to exclude congenital vascular malformations and tumors of the peri-Rolandic region (22). Tonic postural motor seizures are associated with eye, head, and flexion movements of the trunk.

MYOCLONUS

These brief, abrupt, shock-like movements that occur in single or multiple muscles with a duration of less than 100 milliseconds, have a cortical, subcortical, thalamic, brainstem, spinal, peripheral nerve or root localization, and occur spontaneously, reflexively or prompted by action (23–26). There may be preferential involvement of the face or distal limbs, often in an asymmetrical, unilateral, focal-segmental, multifocal or generalized distribution, provoked by visual and auditory

stimuli, with irregular, rhythmic or repetitive characteristics. Physiologic myoclonus includes hiccups, and myoclonus associated with sleep, anxiety and strenuous exercise. Essential myoclonus is sporadic or genetic, and associated with ballistic movements or dystonia. Whereas epileptic myoclonus occurs in response to abnormal neuronal discharges of sensorimotor cortex (27) preceded by giant somatosensory evoked potentials and spikes discharges, those in relation to neonatal seizures can be benign or associated with severe refractory encephalopathy (28) (Table 2). Whereas myoclonus occurs in juvenile myoclonic epilepsy (JME) that typically presents with generalized bursts of irregular fast spikes, polyspikes, and after-going slow wave discharges measuring 4 to 6 Hz, it is also occurs in absence epilepsy of childhood presenting as eyelid myoclonus. The causes of symptomatic myoclonus are shown in Table 3.

EPILEPSIA PARTIALIS CONTINUA

This unique form of myclonus belongs to partial status epilepticus with clonic activity restricted to one body part involving the distal musculature, often refractory to medical treatment (29). The ictal activity can last hours, days, or even years without spread with associated rhythmic or arrhythmic movements that most often involve the hand, thumb, lips and face because of their large cortical representation. Frequently associated with focal weakness during an interictal or postictal phase, two types of EPC are recognized (30). The first is symptomatic and associated with a focal brain lesion and prognostically depends upon the underlying brain lesion; and the second is associated with Rasmussen encephalitis.

Rasmussen Syndrome

First encountered in three children with progressively refractory seizures and hemiplegia reminiscent of chronic viral encephalitis, this type of epilepsy presents in children age 14 months to 14 years with focal seizure onset (31–33). Although there is no propagation of the ictal process, noncontiguous foci and diffuse inter-ictal activity can spread bilaterally and asymmetrically with the seizure focus pointing toward the original involved hemisphere. Intractable seizures, progressive hemiparesis, and hemispheric atrophy can occur (Figure 4). Initially considered to be related to viral infection, polymerase chain reaction (PCR) and *in situ* hybridization studies have failed to isolate a causative viral agent. Brain histopatholgy which demonstrates perivascular cuffing with lymphocytic infiltration, microglial nodules and neuronophagia suggests a mechanism of dysimmunity as the cause of Rasmussen syndrome (RS). Treatment includes high dose corticosteroid medication, adrenocorti-

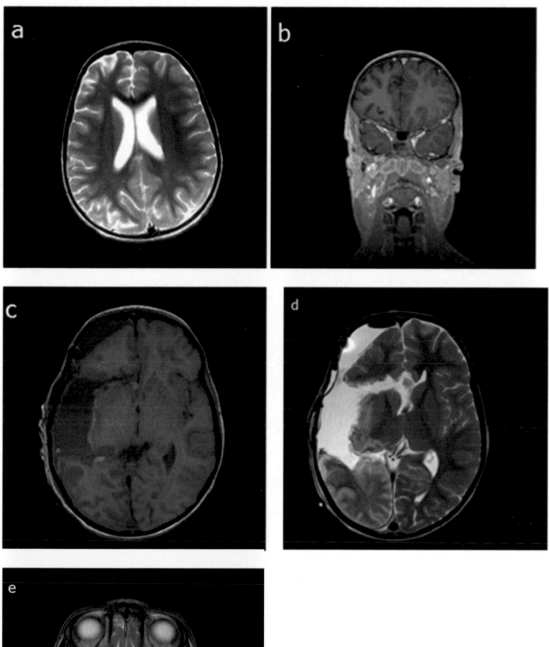

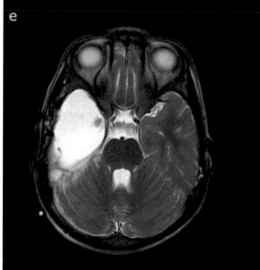

FIG. 4. A child with Rasmussen encephalitis and intractable partial seizures of the right hemisphere. MRI imaging of the brain shows progressive atrophy of the right hemisphere. **A:** Axial T_1-weighted images. **B:** Coronal T_1-weighted images. The patient underwent functional hemispherectomy. **C:** Postoperative axial T_1-weighted images. **D, E:** Axial T_2-weighted images.

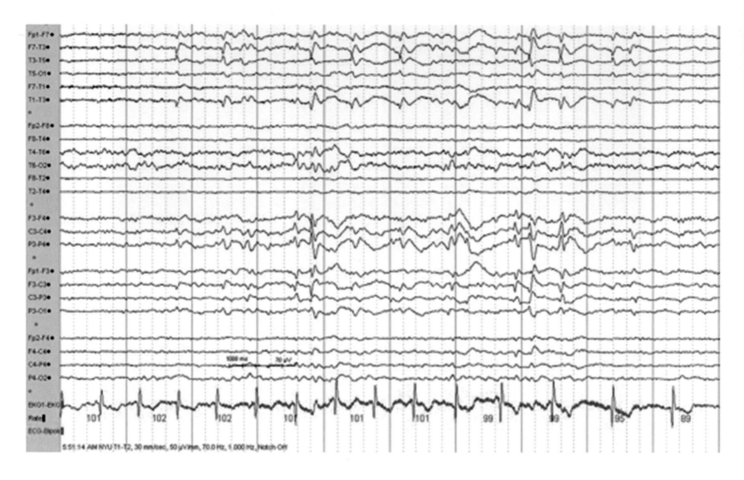

FIG. 5. Benign childhood epilepsy with centrotemporal spikes more prominent on the left side; Bipolar montage shows frequent high amplitude spikes with aftergoing slow waves in the left temporal and left central regions with phase reversal at T3 and C3; note few low amplitude right-sided central sharps maximal at C4.

cotrophin hormone (ACTH), intravenous immunoglobulin (IVIg) therapy, and plasmapheresis, alone or in combination. Seizures refractory to anti-epileptic medication can be treated by various approaches to surgical hemispherectomy.

BENIGN CHILDHOOD EPILEPSY WITH CENTROTEMPORAL SPIKES

This benign age-related and genetically determined syndrome leads infrequent focal sensorimotor and generalized tonic-clonic seizures in developmentally and neurologically normal children with an incidence of 10 to 20 per 100,000 people, with an age preference of 10 to 15 years. With up to 75% of seizures commencing between age 7 to 10 years and slight male gender preponderance (1.5:1), BCECTS is the commonest cause of generalized seizures in this age group. Focal seizures usually involve the inferior rolandic cortex leading to unilateral facial sensorimotor symptoms, speech arrest, and hypersalivation, oral dysesthesia, and lingual guttural and grunting. Up to three-quarters of seizures, most often generalized tonic-clonic with focal onset, occur at night; however diurnal episodes are shorter lasting. The interictal EEG shows frequent high amplitude multifocal, bilateral, independent synchronous sharp waves, spike and aftergoing slow-wave discharge complexes with a maximum along central and temporal regions during sleep (Figure 5), and a frequency, location and persistence that do not correlate with the frequency or severity of clinical seizures. The disorder has been mapped to the 11p13 locus of the *GRCh37* gene. Affected children can be managed with carbamazepine, limotrigene or gabapentin. The overall prognosis is usually excellent with most children reaching normal developmental milestones, remaining neurologically intact, and outgrowing their disease by age 12 to 15 years. The risk of developing epilepsy in adulthood is 2%.

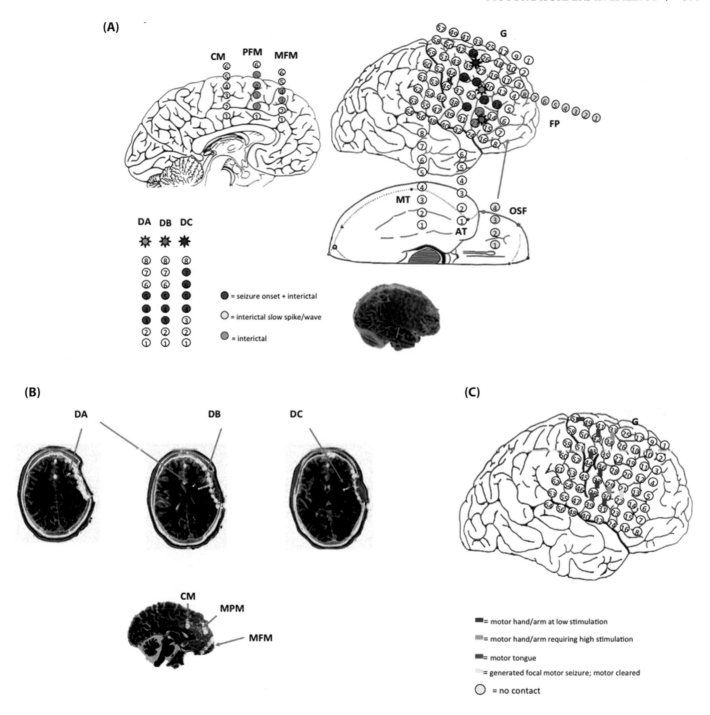

FIG. 6. Brain maps of a patient with frontal lobe epilepsy after right frontal grid and bilateral strips. **A:** Right frontal grid and seven right strips (indicated as modified 64 contact grid). Different seizure foci indicated by dark gray and black. **B:** Left frontal, central and parietal strips. **C:** Functional motor mapping in the same patient.
Abbreviations: FP: frontopolar; RAF: right anterior frontal; RMF: right midfrontal; RIF: right inferior frontal; RFP: right posterior frontal; RP: right parietal; RT: right temporal; LF: left frontal; LC: left center; LP: left parietal.

AUTOSOMAL DOMINANT NOCTURNAL FRONTAL LOBE EPILEPSY

Autosomal dominant nocturnal frontal lobe epilepsy (ADNFLE) (34–36) is a partial epilepsy characterized by onset of clusters of brief motor seizures asleep and upon awakening with peak onset from age 6 to 12 years and equal gender frequency. The seizures share some of the common characteristics of FLE with hyperkinetic, tonic, bipedal movements, dystonia, fencing and posturing that often lead to the misdiagnosis of a sleep disorder. Seizures tend to occur throughout life decreasing in frequency and intensity during the fifth to sixth decades whereupon they are termed fragmentary seizures. Brain MRI and interictal EEG are usually normal. The disorder is caused by a mutation at the 20q13.33 locus of the *CHRNA4* gene encoding the neuronal nicotinic receptor (nAChR) α-4 subunit.

INVASIVE MANAGEMENT OF EXTRA-TEMPORAL EPILEPSY

The surgical outcome and the inherent risk of surgery for epilepsy should always be weighed against the long-term consequences of intractable seizures, morbidity and mortality of recurrent untreatable seizures and the associated quality of life. Patients with operable lesions on brain MRI have the most favorable prognosis when undergoing complete lesionectomy. Intracranial monitoring with subdural grids, strips and depth electrodes assist in the determination of the epileptogenic focus in patients with a normal brain MRI (Figure 6). The extent of the epileptogenic zone determines the nature of resection. The various available surgical options include gyrectomy, topectomy or excision of a portion of cerebral cortex, partial and complete lobectomy. More aggressive intervention such as functional hemispherectomy is appropriate for selected patients with Rasmussen encephalitis, congenitally enlarged hemispheric porencephalic cysts, megalencephaly, and Sturge-Weber syndrome. Epilepsy surgery of the SMA region has been effective, with a success rate that varies from 25 to 75% in reducing the occurrence of seizures (37–40). Invasive EEG monitoring, extraoperative and intraoperative functional motor and language mapping procedures reduce the chance of postoperative deficits. Multiple subpial transaction (MST) should be performed when the epileptogenic focus overlaps eloquent motor cortex in the MI and motor speech areas. Transactions are made in such a way that the horizontal fiber system responsible for propagation of seizures is disrupted while preserving the columnar organization of the cortex thus minimizing the functional deficits as a result of transected cortex. At times, functional postoperative losses are accepted in order to reduce seizure burden. Corpus callosotomy is performed in FLE, those with drop attacks, and RS. Vagal nerve stimulator is also recommended for those with multifocal partial epilepsy.

REFERENCES

1. Rizzolatti G, Fadiga L; Grasping objects and grasping action meanings: the dual role of the monkey rostroventral premotor cortex (area F5). *Novartis Found Symp* 1998; 218:81–95.
2. Penfield W. Jasper H. *Epilepsy and the Functional Anatomy of the Human Brain*, Boston: Little Brown; 1954.
3. Penfield W, Rasmussen T. *The Cerebral Cortex of Man: A Clinical Study of Localization of Function*. New York: Macmillan; 1950.
4. Vogt C, Vogt O. Allgemeinere Ergebnisse Unserer Hirnforschung. *J Psychol Neurol* 1919; 25:279–439.
5. Picard N, Strick PL. Motor areas of the medial wall: A review of their location and functional activation. *Cereb Cortex* 1996; 6:342–353.
6. Vorobiev V, Govoni P, Rizzolatti G. Parcellation of human mesial area 6: cytoarchitectonic evidence for three separate areas. *Eur J Neurosci* 1998; 10:2199–203.
7. Shima K. and Tanji J. Both supplementary and presupplementary motor areas are crucial for the temporal organization of multiple movements. *J Neurophysiol* 1998; 80:3247–60.
8. Tanji J, New concepts of the supplementary motor area. *Curr Opin Neurobiol* 1996; 6:782–787.
9. Matsuzaka Y, Aizawa H. A motor area rostral to the supplementary motor area (presupplementary motor area) in the monkey: neuronal activity during a learned motor task. *J Neurophysiol* 1992; 68:653–62.
10. Luppino G, Matelli M, Rizzolatti G. Cortico-cortical connections of two electrophysiologically identified arm representations in the mesial granular frontal cortex. *Exp Brain Res* 1990; 82:214–218.
11. Lim SH, Dinner DS, Lüders HO. Cortical stimulation of the supplementary sensorimotor area. *Adv Neurol* 1996; 70:187–197.
12. Nakamura K, Sakai K, Hikosaka O. Effects of local inactivation of monkey medial frontal cortex in learning of sequential procedures. *J Neurophysiol* 1999; 82:1063–1068.
13. Fried I, Katz A, McCarthy G. Functional organization of human supplementary motor cortex studied by electrical stimulation. *J Neurosci* 1991; 11:3656–3666.
14. Penfield W, Welsch K. The supplementary motor area of the cerebral cortex; a clinical and experimental study. *Arch Neurol Psychiatry* 1951; 66:289–317.
15. Morris HH 3rd, Dinner DS, Lüders H. Supplementary motor seizures: clinical and electroencephalographic findings. *Neurology* 1988; 38:1075–1082.
16. Halsband U, Passingham RE. Premotor cortex and the conditions for movement in monkeys (Macaca fascicularis). *Behav Brain Res* 1985; 18:269–277.
17. Smith EE, Jonides J. Storage and executive processes in the frontal lobes. *Science* 1999; 283:1657–1661.
18. Strick PL, Dum RP, Picard N. Motor areas on the medial wall of the hemisphere. *Novartis Found Symp* 1998; 218:64–75.
19. Lim SH, Dinner DS, Pillay PK. Functional anatomy of the human supplementary sensorimotor area: results of extra

operative electrical stimulation. *Electroencephalogr Clin Neurophysiol* 1994; 91:179–193.

20. Cascino GD. Surgical Treatment for Extratemporal Epilepsy. *Curr Treat Options Neurol* 2004; 6:257–262.

21. Riggio S, Harner RN. Repetitive motor activity in frontal lobe epilepsy. *Adv Neurol* 1995; 66:153–164.

22. Beaumanoir A, Nahory A. Les epilepsies benignes partielles: 11 cas d'epilepsie partielle frontale a evolution favorable. *Rev Electroencephalogr Neurophysiol Clin* 1983; 13:207–211.

23. Fahn S, Marsden CD, Van Woert MH. Definition and classification of myoclonus. *Adv Neurol* 1986; 43:1–5.

24. Shibasaki H. Electrophyisological studies of myoclonus. *Muscle Nerve* 2000; 23:321–335.

25. Fahn S. Overview, history and classification of myoclonus. *Adv Neurol* 2002; 89:13–17.

26. Obeso JA. Classification, clinical features, and treatment of myoclonus. In: Watts RL, Koller WC, eds. *Movement disorders: neurologic principles and practice.* New York: McGraw-Hill Professional, 1997; 541–550.

27. Brown P. Myoclonus: A brief review of the phenomenology, pathophysiology, and underlying etiology of cortical, brainstem and spinal myoclonus. *Curr Opin Neurol* 1996; 9:314–316.

28. Volpe JJ. Neonatal seizures: current concepts and revised classification. *Pediatrics* 1989; 84:422–428.

29. Kojewnikoff AY: Eine besondere From von corticaler Epilepsie. *Neurologie Zentralblatt* 1895; 14:47–48.

30. Bancaud J, Bonis A, Trottier S. Continuous partial epilepsy: syndrome and disease, *Rev Neurol* (Paris). 1982; 138:803–814.

31. DeToledo JC, Smith DB. Partially successful treatment of Rasmussen's encephalitis with Zidovudine. *Epilepsia* 1994; 35:352 355.

32. Takahashi Y. Mori H. Mishina M. Autoantibodies to NMDA receptor in patients with chronic forms of epilepsia partialis continua. *Neurology* 2003; 61:891–896.

33. Maeda Y, Oguni H, Saitou Y. Rasmussen syndrome: multifocal spread of inflammation suggested from MRI and PET findings. *Epilepsia* 2003; 44:1118–1121.

34. Vining EP, Freeman JM, Pillas DJ. Why would you remove half a brain? *Pediatrics* 1997; 100:163–171.

35. Scheffer IE. Autosomal dominant nocturnal frontal lobe epilepsy. In: Berkovic SF, Genton P, Hirsch E, Picard F, eds. *Genetics of focal epilepsies*, 81-84. London: John Libbey, 1999.

36. Scheffer IE, Bhatia KP, Lopes-Cendes I. Autosomal dominant frontal epilepsy misdiagnosed as sleep disorder. *Lancet* 1994; 343:515–517.

37. Olivier A. Surgical strategies for patients with supplementary motor area epilepsy. The Montreal Experience. In: Lüders H, ed. *Supplementary Sensorimotor Area.* New York: Lippincott-Raven;1996; 429–443.

38. So N. Mesial frontal lobe epilepsy. *Epilepsia* 1998; 39(Suppl4):49–61.

39. Talairach J, Bancaud J, Bonis A, et al. Surgical therapy for frontal epilepsies. In: Chauvel P, Delgado-Escueta AV, Halgren E, et al, eds. *Frontal lobe seizures and epilepsy.* New York: Raven Press, 1992; 707–732.

40. Toczek M, Morrell M, Risinger M, et al. Intracranial ictal recordings in mesial frontal lobe epilepsy. *J Clin Neurophysiol* 1997; 14:499–506.

PART V

Neurorehabilitation

CHAPTER 59

Traumatic Brain Injury

Michal E. Eisenberg, Brian Im

EPIDEMIOLOGY

Traumatic brain injury (TBI) is defined as an impact to the head that results in disruption of brain functioning. While various forces cause TBI such as blunt trauma, acceleration and deceleration forces, and blast injures, the post-TBI motor, cognitive, emotional, and psychosocial sequelae can be just as devastating and long-lasting, leading to loss of independent function and safe performance of activities. Taken together, the long-term sequelae pose a significant challenge to recovery, requiring a multifaceted dynamic rehabilitative strategy.

EPIDEMIOLOGY

It is estimated that 10 million deaths and hospitalizations are related to TBI worldwide each year, with an estimated 57 million people who have been treated for one or more episodes of TBI. However, these figures likely underestimate the true burden of this condition as not all countries have TBI-specific treatment and reporting programs (1). Mortality due to TBI is greater in low to middle income countries, albeit lower related disability (2). By contrast, richer and more highly developed countries with advanced evaluation and treatment programs for TBI, have higher rates of chronic disability, probably reflecting improved survival with disability. Between 1995 and 2001, the Centers for Disease Control and Prevention (CDC) reported an average of 50,000 deaths, 235,000 hospitalizations, and 1,111,000 emergency department visits annually in the United States (U.S.) due to TBI. However, this data may also underestimate the full impact of TBI in the US as many mild injuries may go undiagnosed (3), and not all those experiencing TBI seek treatment (1).

Substance abuse plays an indirect role in TBI as greater than 50% of patients with TBI have elevated blood alcohol levels at the time of injury (4, 5). While uncertainty exists regarding the number of U.S. military personnel who sustain TBI and post-TBI stress disorders (6), one significant source of disability emerged from U.S. combatants of the Afghanistan and Iraq conflicts, and improved military equipment and acute trauma care in the field has increased the probability of survival from blast injuries leading to the expectation of increased non-fatal TBI (7).

Sports-related TBI is certainly underreported and underdiagnosed due to the lack of recognition of the significance of inadvertent concussion, especially when loss of consciousness is uncertain (8, 9), yet there may be significant impact on cognition (10, 11). The CDC estimates that 1.6 to 3.8 million sports-related concussions occur in the US annually, with many affected athletes failing to obtain expert subspecialty treatment (1). Sports-related concussions extend to both male and female contact sports, and across all age groups. Approximately 5 to 15% of individuals with documented mild TBI remain permanently symptomatic (12). A single concussion increases the risk of a second or subsequent event thereafter (13).

Approximately 2% of the U.S. population or 3 to 5 million persons, required assistance in the performance of activities of daily living (ADL) due to preceding TBI (14, 15). Taken together with the expected expense of 1 million dollars per individual in the cost of related care and medical expenditures associated with TBI, the staggering estimated financial burden of TBI was 60 billion dollars in the year 2000 (1, 16).

At Bellevue Hospital, a public facility in the City of New York, the societal impact is readily appreciated wherein victims of TBI are often uninsured and undocumented, and occasionally fall into the criminal system, with limited or no resources and meager caregiver support. Such patients may have inadequate follow-up care, limited resources, and a history of prior TBI that impacts on eventual outcome (17).

The leading causes of TBI include falls, motor vehicle accidents (MVA), intentional or unintentional injury, and assaults. When the causes of injury are examined in relation to different age groups, falls are a leading cause of TBI in young children and elderly adults, and MVA, sports concussion, bicycle accidents, and suicidal attempts are the most common in adolescents and young adults. While blast injury leads the causes of TBI in combat soldiers, the success of motor vehicle safely measures has led to an increase in the frequency of firearm-related TBI mortality (18).

HISTORY AND PHYSICAL EXAMINATION OF TBI

A thorough medical history and neurological examination are key to the evaluation and management of a patient with suspected TBI. The elicited history should include detailed premorbid health and functioning. For example, premorbid movement disorder and motor seizures may impact management (19). While many physical complaints will undoubtedly be the result of TBI, some may be unrelated to the trauma, such as incidental joint pain due to arthritis that exacerbates the impact of hemiparesis. The examination should focus on manual muscle testing to discern focal strength impairments, tone, incoordination, involuntary movements, and deficits of joint position sensation, and disturbances of stance and gait. Neuropsychological assessment should be performed in all patients with TBI to determine areas of cognitive weakness and guide therapy. Limited insight, impulsivity, memory impairments, or agitation due to brain injury can impair a patient's ability to follow the instructions of therapists, and carry over information from one session to another, without which the gains made on one day fail to continue to subsequent sessions.

Clues to TBI in a child with otherwise subtle or no involvement may be suggested by disturbances in grasping a pencil, clumsiness, poor performance on complex motor tasks for age, incomplete manual dominance, articulation, slowed reaction times, asymmetry of muscle tone, and disturbances of imitative finger drawing, hopping, and other sequential and alternating developmental screening tasks. Neuropsychological findings may instead suggest a developmental coordination disorder according to the Text Revised Diagnostic and Statistical Manual of Mental Disorders (DSM-IV-TR) (20), formally coded by the Ninth revision of the International Classification of Diseases (ICD-9) as 315.4.

The history and examination may provide important clues to anticipated therapies. Focal spasticity of a single limb or portion thereof, is often amenable to local maneuvers such as botulinum toxin (BoTN) or chemodenervation, whereas generalized spasticity requires management commencing with oral or intrathecal baclofen or other agents (21).

The physical deficits in mild TBI resolve more quickly than the associated cognitive and behavioral disturbances, including the often-overlooked disturbances of vestibular function, orthostasis, visuospatial and fine motor coordination, and postural control that significantly impact safety and functional independence more than overtly apparent cognitive and behavioral deficits. Gait disturbances resulting from injury to cortical and subcortical areas of central motor control and spatial organization are expected in TBI (22) and will often respond to short duration programs of gait and balance physiotherapy with the expectation of achieving independent ambulation by 5.5 weeks (23). Extrapyramidal disturbances that include tremor, focal dystonia, parkinsonism, ballismus, dyskinesia, dysphonia, myoclonus, opsoclonus, and tics due to injury of the basal ganglia are more responsive to pharmacological intervention (24, 25) than the motor sequel of cerebellar injury that instead results in ataxia, postural tremor, clumsiness, dysmetria, dysarthria, dysdiadochokinesia, hypotonia, and lateropulsion. Neurocognitive deficits that include disturbance of purposeful programmed movements due to ideomotor, ideational, constructive, conceptual, dissociative, and conduction apraxia, as well as deficits in body schema associated with asomatognosia, right-left confusion, finger agnosia, and neglect syndromes, improve with cognitive therapy.

MECHANISMS OF TBI

Primary TBI occurs at the moment of traumatic impact, leading to laceration, concussion, contusions, diffuse axonal injury (DAI), epidural, subdural, subarachnoid, intraparenchymal, and intraventricular hemorrhages, and cranial nerve injuries, the commonest of which is the olfactory nerve. Secondary injury may take the form of hypoxic or ischemic damage, hydrocephalus, cerebral edema, swelling, and metabolic cellular damage. Closed head injuries occur when the skull and lining of the brain remains intact, while open injury refers to those that occur when the intracranial vault is exposed to the outside environment; the latter is associated with an increased risk of central nervous system (CNS) infection. Depressed skull fractures are associated with more severe neurological deficits and outcomes compared to non-depressed fractures. In particular, temporal bone fractures pose a heightened risk for epidural hematoma due to the vascularity of the area, while basilar skull fractures are often associated with concomitant facial, acoustic, and vestibular cranial nerve injury. Projectile penetrating bullet-associated head injury leads to a fluid wave pattern of damage that exceeds that caused by the projectile itself when it enters the body with sufficient velocity. Blunt force trauma refers to impact caused by a relatively flat object or surface, but does not necessarily imply closed head injury. Such forces can cause skull fractures and soft tissue injury or sharp force trauma, due to objects with an edge or point, leading to penetrating injury. Those injuries with significant acceleration, deceleration, rotational effects, and high velocity can predispose to DAI due to shearing forces that disrupt the integrity of the brain. Patients with DAI present with variable severity of cognitive deficits depending on the severity of injury. Coup injuries refer to those caused by the initial impact of brain movement within the skull on the side of the external force, while contrecoup injury refers to those caused by the secondary impact on the brain against the skull bone, with the latter type often of greater severity depending upon the part of the skull involved and the inherent irregularity of the skull surface. A given mechanism of injury will not necessarily predict the anticipated severity of TBI as open skull sharp force injuries can be associated with proportionately less damage than closed skull, blunt force trauma in instances where the skull itself dissipates the forces interacting on the brain.

PROGNOSIS AND MANAGEMENT

TBI is categorized as mild, moderate, and severe, with only 15% of TBI moderate to severe and 85% mild, based upon the Glasgow Coma Scale (GCS) score, Galveston orientation and amnesia test (GOAT), and Orientation log (O-log). The GCS rapidly assesses the level of responsiveness of a patient by monitoring functioning as pertaining to eye opening, verbal response, and motor response. Aggregate scores of 3 to 8 are suggestive of a severe TBI, 9 to 12 of a moderate, and 13 to 15 of a mild degree of dysfunction. Motor response is the best predictor of long-term outcome, with the best GCS score in the first 24 hours of recovery classically considered the best predictor of recovery (26).

Post-traumatic amnesia (PTA), which is a state of acute confusion typified by perceptual, thinking, and concentrative disturbances, occurs during the early stages of TBI recovery, whether anterograde or retrograde, with a longer duration of PTA indicating a poorer prognosis. The GOAT is a standardized tool that evaluates the duration of PTA, with scores ranging from 0 to 100. A GOAT score of 75 or higher for two consecutive days is indicative of a longer state of PTA (27). The O-log assesses orientation and is considered by many to be easier to administer than the

GOAT, and is preferred for serial monitoring purposes. The JFK Coma Recovery Scale Revised-(R), which determines when a patient enters into and progresses beyond a minimally conscious state, consists of six subscales that investigate auditory, visual, motor, or motor, communicative, and arousal functions of a patient with an altered level of consciousness (LOC). Evidence of purposeful activity at any time indicates that the patient has entered the minimally conscious state (28, 29).

The Rancho Los Amigos Levels of Cognitive Function Scale is used both to categorize the level of post-TBI functioning and to characterize behavioral and cognitive patterns typically seen at different stages during TBI recovery (30). Brain neuroimaging employing computed tomography (CT) and magnetic resonance imaging (MRI) with diffusion tensor imaging is warranted in all patients with TBI (31). They reveal microhemorrhages in the corpus callosum, central subcortical white matter, and midbrain when associated with DAI. Somato-sensory evoked potentials (SSEP) have predictive value for TBI recovery (32), while cerebral perfusion with single photon emission computerized tomography (SPECT), positron emission tomography (PET) of the brain, and quantitative electroencephalography (QEEG) do not yet have a routine role in the care of affected patients. Moreover, there are no reliable biological markers for TBI.

Whereas non-pharmacological management should always be initially considered in patients with TBI due to anticipated heightened medication sensitivity, certain medications can have a favorable impact as, for example, in the prophylaxis of deep vein thrombosis and pulmonary embolism, treatment of sleep, autonomic, bowel and bladder dysfunctions, seizures, headache, and behavioral disturbances (33). The administration of amantadine to 184 vegetative or minimally conscious TBI patients a few weeks after sustaining a TBI accelerated the pace of functional recovery during the period more than placebo without engendering significant adverse side effects, however, the benefit declined after discontinuation (34).

Repetitive transcranial magnetic stimulation (rTMS) (35) and theta burst stimulation (TBS), employing very low-intensity combined-frequency rTMS (36), which has a possible role in stroke rehabilitation (36), can be associated with seizure induction (37) that makes it less practical in TBI.

The care of patients with TBI falls into a continuum, supervised by a physiatrist subspecialist, beginning with the acute management that progresses to inpatient rehabilitation, followed by community integration, and a lifetime of care-related issues afterward. While many patients with mild TBI can be managed as an outpatient without any inpatient care, specific programs in TBI rehabilitation attempt to address the comprehensive dysfunctional, physical, cognitive, and behavioral aspects. Those with altered LOC receive prophylactic measures to avert aspiration, pressure ulcers, and contracture, as well as cognitive stimulation, early postural retraining, and active and passive range-of-motion (ROM) exercises. Those who interact purposefully with their environment but are significantly impaired, focus on increasing self-awareness through retraining, while others less severely impaired work on transitioning into daily activities and, eventually, independence at home and in the community. Depression, anxiety, and labile emotion, all of which can follow TBI, are receptive to psychotherapy and psychiatric medical management.

As with most other medical conditions, the best treatment for TBI is to prevent its occurrence. Prevention of TBI is especially important given that many of these injuries are avoidable. Increasing the use of helmets and better safety equipment and rules in sports, developing better substance and alcohol abuse prevention programs, observing proper safety practices in motor vehicles, such as avoiding reckless driving and wearing seatbelts, removing tripping hazards and installing safety equipment in the homes of the elderly, implementing ideas to decrease TBI risk in children, including softer playground surfaces and education programs for both parents and children, and even simply paying closer attention to traffic laws when crossing the street are all simple, yet effective, ways to decrease the incidence of TBI.

REFERENCES

1. Langlois JA, Rutland-Brown W, Wald MM. The epidemiology and impact of traumatic brain injury: A brief overview. *J Head Trauma Rehabil* 2006; 21:375–378

2. De Silva MJ, Roberts I, Perel P, et al. Patient outcome after traumatic brain injury in high-, middle- and low-income countries: analysis of data on 8927 patients in 46 countries. *Int J Epidemiol* 2009; 38:452–458

3. Powell JM, Ferraro JV, Dikmen SS, et al. Accuracy of mild traumatic brain injury diagnosis. *Arch Phys Med Rehabil* 2008; 89:1550–1555

4. Kolakowsky-Hayner SA, Gourley EV 3rd, Kreutzer JS, et al. Pre-injury substance abuse among persons with brain injury and persons with spinal cord injury. *Brain Inj* 1999; 13:571–581

5. Levy DT, Mallonee S, Miller TR, et al. Alcohol involvement in burn, submersion, spinal cord, and brain injuries. *Med Sci Monit* 2004; 10:CR17–CR24

6. Hoge CW, Goldberg HM, Castro CA. Care of war veterans with mild traumatic brain injury—flawed perspectives. *N Engl J Med* 2009; 360:1588–1591

7. Okie S. Traumatic brain injury in the war zone. *N Engl J Med* 2005; 352:2043–2047

8. Guskiewicz KM, Weaver NL, Padua DA, et al. Epidemiology of concussion in collegiate and high school football players. *Am J Sports Med* 2000; 28:643–650

9. McCrea M, Hammake T, Olsen G, et al. Unreported concussion in high school football players: implications for prevention. *Clin J Sports Med* 2004; 14:13–17

10. Broglio SP, Macciocchi SN, Ferrara MS. Neurocognitive Performance of Concussed Athletes when Symptom Free. *J Athl Train* 2007; 42:504–508

11. Fazio VC, Lovell MR, Pardini JE, et al. The relation between post concussion symptoms and neurocognitive performance in concussed athletes. *NeuroRehabilitation* 2007; 22:207–216

12. Cassidy JD, Carroll LJ, Peloso PM, et al. Incidence, risk factors and prevention of mild traumatic brain injury: results of the WHO Collaborating Centre Task Force on Mild Traumatic Brain Injury. *J Rehabil Med* 2004; 43:28–60

13. Guskiewicz K, McCrea M, Marshall SW, et al. Cumulative effects associated with recurrent concussion in collegiate football players: the NCAA Concussion Study. *JAMA* 2003; 290:2549–2555

14. Thurman DJ, Alverson C, Dunn KA, et al. Traumatic brain injury in the United States: A public health perspective. *J Head Trauma Rehabil* 1999; 14:602–615

15. Zaloshnja E, Miller T, Langlois JA, et al. Prevalence of long-term disability from traumatic brain injury in the civilian population of the United States, 2005. *J Head Trauma Rehabil* 2008; 23:394–400

16. Finkelstein E, Corso P, Miller T, et al. *The incidence and economic burden of injuries in the United States.* New York (NY): Oxford University Press, 2006

17. Schofield PW, Butler TG, Hollis SJ, et al. Traumatic brain injury among Australian prisoners: rates, recurrence and sequelae. *Brain Inj* 2006; 20:499–506

18. Sosin DM, Sniezek JE, Waxweiler RJ. Trends in death associated with traumatic brain injury 1979 through 1992. Success and failure. *JAMA* 1995; 273:1778–1780

19. Ranjan N, Nair KP, Romaniski C, et al. Tics after traumatic brain injury. *Brain Inj* 2011; 25:629–633

20. Orlando, FL: Grune & Stratton; American Psychiatric Association. (2000). *Diagnostic and Statistical Manual of Mental Disorders*, 4th ed.-TR (Text revision). Washington, DC

21. Elovic EP, Simone LK, Zafonte R. Outcome assessment for spasticity management in the patient with traumatic brain injury: the state of the art. *J Head Trauma Rehabil* 2004; 19:157–177

22. Williams G, Galna B, Morris ME, et al. Spatiotemporal deficits and kinematic classification of gait following a traumatic brain injury: a systematic review. *J Head Trauma Rehabilitation* 2010; 25:366–374

23. Katz DI, White DK, Alexander MP, et al. Recovery of ambulation after traumatic brain injury. *Arch Phys Med Rehabil* 2004; 85:865–869

24. Weiner WJ. Can peripheral trauma induce dystonia? No! *Mov Disord* 2001; 16:13–22

25. O'Suilleabhain P, Dewey RB Jr. Movement disorders after head injury: diagnosis and management. *J Head Trauma Rehabil* 2004; 19:305–313

26. Jennett B. Defining brain damage after head injury. *J R Coll Physicians Lond* 1979; 4:197–200

27. Levin HS, O'Donnell VM, Grossman RG. The Galveston Orientation and Amnesia Test. A practical scale to assess cognition after head injury. *J Nerv Ment Dis* 1979; 167:675–684

28. Giacino JT, Ashwal S, Childs N, et al. The minimally conscious state: definition and diagnostic criteria. *Neurology* 2002; 58:349–353

29. Kalmar K, Giacino JT. The JFK Coma Recovery Scale, Revised. *Neuropsychol Rehabil* 2005; 15:454–460

30. Kay T, Lezak M. *Nature of head injury. Traumatic brain injury and vocational rehabilitation.* Menomonie, WI: University of Wisconsin-Stout Research and Training Center, 1990.

31. Manolakaki D, Velmahos GC, Spaniolas K, et al. Early magnetic resonance imaging is unnecessary in patients with traumatic brain injury. *J Trauma* 2009; 66:1008–1012

32. Houlden DA, Taylor AB, Feinstein A, et al. Early somatosensory evoked potential grades in comatose traumatic brain injury patients predict cognitive and functional outcome. *Crit Care Med* 2010; 38:167–174

33. Neurobehavioral Guidelines Working Group, Warden DL, Gordon B, et al. Guidelines for the pharmacologic treatment of neurobehavioral sequelae of traumatic brain injury. *J Neurotrauma* 2006; 23:1468–1501

34. Giacino JT, Whyte J, Bagiella E, et al. Placebo-controlled trial of amantadine for severe traumatic brain injury. *N Eng J Med* 2012; 366:819–826

35. Wassermann EM, Zimmermann T. Transcranial magnetic brain stimulation: therapeutic promises and scientific gaps. *Pharmacol Ther* 2012; 133:98–107

36. Corti M, Patten C, Triggs W. Repetitive transcranial magnetic stimulation of motor cortex after stroke: a focused review. *Am J Phys Med Rehabil* 2012; 91:254–270

37. Rossi S, Hallett M, Rossini PM, et al. Safety, ethical considerations, and application guidelines for the use of transcranial magnetic stimulation in clinical practice and research. *Clin Neurophysiol* 2009; 120:2008–2039

CHAPTER 60

Traumatic Spinal Cord Injury

Barry Rodstein, David S. Younger

The ancient Egyptians, followed by Hippocrates and the Romans recognized the combination of paralysis, sensory loss, incontinence, and priapism ascribed to spinal cord injury (SCI) invariably leading to death. The mortality for SCI, which was 80% during World War I (WWI), was impacted by the establishment of dedicated SCI centers, first at Boston City Hospital and later in a multidisciplinary unit in the British National Health Service at Stoke Mandevile Hospital to treat WWII veterans. The American Board of Physical Medicine and Rehabilitation (ABPMR), which grants specialty board certification in spinal cord medicine (SCM), defines this as the subspecialty that addresses the prevention, diagnosis, treatment, and management of traumatic spinal cord injury and non-traumatic etiologies of spinal cord dysfunction by working in an inter-specialty manner.

EPIDEMIOLOGY

The estimated annual incidence of survivors of SCI in the United States (U.S.) in 2009 was 40 per million population, or 12,000 cases, and the prevalence in 2008 was estimated at 259,000 persons alive with SCI. It disproportionately affects younger adults. The average age at injury in the U.S. in 2005 was 40.2 years, with 80.9% of those injured of the male sex. According to the National Spinal Cord Injury Database, which captures data from an estimated 13% of cases in the U.S., the commonest cause of traumatic SCI is motor vehicle crashes, noted in 42.9%, followed by falls in 20.9%, violence in 17.8%, sports and recreational injuries in 10.4%, and other or unknown causes in the remaining 8.0% of cases. About 30.6% have incomplete tetraplegia,

25.3% complete paraplegia, 20.0% complete tetraplegia and 18.6% incomplete paraplegia. From 1970 to 2010, the average length of stay in an acute hospital setting declined from 24 to 12 days, with a commensurate reduction in time in a rehabilitation unit from 98 to 37 days. About 51.9% of patients were unmarried at the time of injury, 32.1% had intact marriages, and 9.3% were divorced. The likelihood of getting married after SCI was 59% that of comparable persons in the general population. For the first three years after SCI the annual divorce rate was 2.3-fold higher, included among those who married after SCI, wherein the rate was also 1.7-fold higher.

ETIOLOGY

Although traumatic SCI can result from indirect insults such as hematoma or infarct, the cause is often direct trauma to the cord due to instability. Denis (1) proposed a "three-column" concept that evolved from a retrospective review of 412 thoracolumbar spine injuries and observations on spinal instability, the disruption of which led to an unstable spine. The posterior column consisted of the posterior ligamentous complex. The middle column consisted of the posterior longitudinal ligament, posterior annulus fibrosus, and posterior wall of the vertebral body. The anterior column consisted of the anterior vertebral body, anterior annulus fibrosus, and anterior longitudinal ligament. Non-traumatic causes of SCI include cervical spondylotic myelopathy (CSM), multiple sclerosis (MS), neoplasms, vascular abnormalities, syringomyelia, and transverse myelitis.

CLASSIFICATION

The anatomical or skeletal level of injury may be different from the neurological level of injury (NLI), which refers to the most cephalid intact level. Those with a C8 or higher NLI typically manifest tetraplegia, while others with T1 level or lower NLI show paraplegia.

International standards for the neurological classification of SCI (ISNCSCI) have been published (2, 3). The sensory NLI signifies the most caudal dermatome with normal sensation, while the motor level refers to the most caudal myotome with normal innervation. Practically, the myotomal innervation of an involved muscle with Medical Research Council (MRC) strength of 3/5 or more would be preceded cephalid by one that would instead be MRC strength 5/5.

The American Spinal Injury Association Impairment Scale (AIS) was developed to enhance the definition of neurological levels and the extent of incomplete injury in a given patient, as well as consistent and reliable data among centers participating in a National Database. Summed scores for motor, light touch, and pinprick assessment in complete SCI have high inter-rater reliability, making them useful in a given patient and in clinical trials involving serial neurological examinations (4). Complete spinal injury includes those without sacral sensory or motor sparing whereas those with incomplete injury have sensory sparing to light touch or pinprick in the S4 and S5 dermatome or intact deep anal pressure sensation, or preservation of voluntary anal sphincter reflexes contraction. Even in complete SCI, there may be a zone of partial preservation (ZPP).

EXAMINATION

In the acute phase of SCI, a detailed neurological and physiatric examination may be difficult due to a patients limited ability to cooperate, as well as the multiplicity of intravenous and electrical wires, tubes, and catheters typical of acute intensive care, and concomitant pain. In addition, patients may automatically substitute muscles and gravity to compensate for weakness. For example, a C6 tetraplegic patient with normal deltoids, biceps, and wrist extensor muscles may employ gravity for elbow extension, wrist flexion, and passive flexion of the long-finger flexors with active wrist extension when performing movement of gross hand grasp. This could be mistaken for paraplegia or incomplete tetraplegia. Other notable SCI syndromes include central cord syndrome, which occurs during hyperextension injury in those with pre-existing, asymptomatic, or subclinical cervical spondylosis and stenosis characterized by arm, greater than leg, weakness, variable sensory deficit, and bladder dysfunction. The prognosis of central cord syndrome is generally favorable with non-surgical treatment, especially in those with absent cord edema or other spinal cord abnormality on magnetic resonance imaging (MRI). Damage to a lateral half of the spinal cord, which results in the Brown–Sequard syndrome (BSS), leads to dissociation of weakness and impairment of proprioception that occurs ipsilateral to the side of the lesion, with contralateral interruption of pain and temperature sensation. There may be interruption of unilateral descending autonomic fiber tracts from the hypothalamus. The causes of BSS include knife and bullet injuries, MS, spinal cord tumors, disc herniation, vascular infarction, and central nervous system (CNS) or vertebral infections. The prognosis of BSS is extremely favorable, with most patients recovering to ambulatory, continent, and independent activities of daily living (ADL). Posterior cord syndrome is the least common and is notable for absence of proprioception with preservation of pain, temperature, and touch with variable motor function. Ambulation is usually impaired due to the proprioceptive deficit.

Injury to the conus medullaris located at the L1 vertebral level, which represents the terminal portion of the adult spinal cord containing sacral spinal segments, above which spinal segments for L4 through S1 emerge, produces characteristic clinical syndromes depending upon the location. Upper conus lesions produce an upper motor neuron (UMN) syndrome of symmetric weakness, dermatomal sensory impairment and sensory level, and normal anal and bulbocavernosus reflexes. A lesion at the conus leads to variable lower motor neuron (LMN) leg weakness, saddle anesthesia, dissociated pain and temperature sensory, absent anal and bulbocavernosus reflexes, and a neurogenic bladder. Lesions below the conus medullaris are polyradiculopathic and not true spinal cord injuries, presenting instead with asymmetric LMN weakness, flaccid bowel and bladder dysfunction, and sensory disturbances in multiradicular distribution, with pronounced radicular pain. The prognosis for improvement in lower conus lesions, which depends upon resolution of neuropraxic and axonotmesis, is more favorable than those due to underlying intramedually SCI.

PROGNOSIS

Among 3,585 individuals with traumatic SCI studied between 1988 and 1997, the neurological exam 72 hours after injury was more predictive of prognosis than that at presentation especially in those with complete paraplegia (5). Neurologic recovery after SCI was influenced by etiology and severity of injury, such that individuals who were motor-complete with extended zones of sensory preservation, but without sacral sparing, were less likely to convert to motor-incomplete status than those with sacral sparing. Those with complete paraplegia have the least improvement in motor scores; and recovery of leg paralysis is uncommon when the neurological level is complete at one month after injury.

Patients with tetraplegia show more improvement than paraplegics, with many gaining recovery of two to three segments within the initial NLI, and the majority gaining at least one myotomal level. A retrospective cohort of 70 patients with cross-sectional follow-up to determine the factors that predicted local recovery of complete SCI between 1994 and 2001 (6) showed that motor recovery did not occur below the zone of injury, although varying degrees of local recovery can be expected in tetraplegic individuals. For example, functional gains were achieved in two-thirds of patients who achieved useful strength at one level, 16% at two levels, and 3% at three levels below the NLI. In a study of 142 paraplegics (7) who remained complete injuries at follow-up, none with an initial NLI above T9 regained any leg motor function. However, 38% of those with an initial NLI at or below T9 had some return of leg motor function, primarily in hip flexors and knee extensors. About 20% of the patients with an initial NLI at or below T12 regained sufficient hip flexor and knee extensor strength to reciprocally ambulate using conventional orthoses and crutches. Unlike motor function, recovery of light touch and sharp-dull discrimination was independent of the initial NLI. Altogether, 4% of the patients demonstrated late conversion at more than four months after injury, from complete to incomplete SCI status; two of the six patients with an initial NLI at T12 and subsequent annual NLI at L1 and L2, reciprocally ambulated. Three of the six patients regained voluntary bladder and bowel control. Patients essentially unimpaired prior to the SCI and without other major injuries usually have predictable outcomes based on NLI and, in the case of paraplegia, should be able to achieve independent functioning.

PHASES OF CARE

Acute Phase

Specialized care of patients with SCI begins at the scene of the injury with early recognition of the process. Since up to 10% with loss of consciousness due to motor vehicle injuries can harbor a spine injury, all such patients should be considered a potential SCI victim, prompting boarding and collaring of the neck and observing for apparent neurological deficits. Initial goals are maintenance of airway, ventilation, and hemodynamic stability. Among 77 patients who presented with acute neurological deficits as a result of SCI occurring from C1 through T12, in an effort to maintain spinal cord blood flow and prevent secondary injury (8), early and aggressive medical management, including volume resuscitation and blood pressure augmentation optimized the potential for neurological recovery after sustaining trauma. Meticulous attention

must be paid to respiratory status, pulmonary hygiene, and risk for aspiration. A forced vital capacity (FVC) of 1.5 liters suggests adequate inspiratory strength whereas an FVC <1 liter often precedes ventilator failure. Spinal shock, which generally refers to the initial loss of spinal reflexes and recovery in a caudal to rostral sequence, is of limited clinical utility in the prognosis of SCI (9). In fact, among 50 subjects admitted consecutively over a nine-month period and observed for the presence of the bulbocavernosus reflex, delayed planter reflex, and cremasteric reflex, ankle and knee jerks for up to eight weeks, and assessed for ambulation of 200 feet at the time of discharge, fewer than 8% of subjects had no reflexes on the day of injury and reflexes did not follow a caudal to rostral pattern of recovery.

Patients should be assessed for traumatic brain injury (TBI) as it concomitantly occurs in up to three-quarters of patients with traumatic SCI. Also, the entire spinal column should be imaged as non-contiguous traumatic spinal fractures occur in up to 40% of patients with traumatic SCI. In children, however, spinal cord injury may occur without detectable radiological abnormalities.

Although the administration of a bolus 30 mg per kilogram (mg/kg) dose of methylprednisolone followed by methylprednisolone at a dose of 5.4 mg/kg for 24 to 48 hours was the standard of care for those with potential neurological SCI (10–12), some consider it inappropriate treatment (13), citing that in the strictest sense, administration of methylprednisolone within 24-hours should be considered experimental.

Post-Acute Rehabilitation and Transition Home

Once medically stable, the patient with SCI should be discharged to an acute inpatient rehabilitation facility with specialization in SCM. Exceptions include those with medical comorbid disorders who are frail, elderly, or too severely ill to participate in physical therapy. Patients with incomplete SCI and those functioning at a high level geographically amenable to outpatient services, may be discharged home. Patients in need of subacute nursing care may be discharged to a nursing facility. Ultimately, the transition home can be difficult when the patient goes from an environment with a very high level and intensity of specialized services to one in which the patient and family are largely on their own. Bowel and bladder management may need adjustment and emotional issues can be very significant when the focus changes from participating in physical and occupational therapy to the daily challenges of a more secluded and potentially more challenging experience at home. This transition can be facilitated by follow-up visits with a physiatrist, and the continuation of outpatient or home physical and occupational therapy.

SEQUELAE OF SPINAL CORD INJURY

Autonomic Disturbances

There are current guidelines describing international standards for the documentation of autonomic function after spinal cord injury (ISAFSCI) (14). Although typically considered cardioprotective, persons with SCI represent a model of autonomic nervous system (ANS) dysfunction that affects 24-hour hemodynamics and predisposes to increased cardiovascular disease by increasing 24-hour, daytime and nighttime, heart rates (HR) and altering heart rate variation (HRV) compared to normal controls (15). Hypothermia, more common in patients with tetraplegia, is another important problem, especially for those who reside in cold climates. Orthostasis may be problematic and require compression stockings, hydration, and the vasopressors midodrine and fludrocortisone. An important rehabilitation intervention in the acute phase of hospitalization is accommodation to the upright posture. Autonomic dysreflexia (AD) (16) typically occurs after spinal shock has resolved or at any time along the course of acute SCI, particularly in those with NLI at or above the T6. AD is manisfested by unopposed stimulation of sympathetic neurons in the intermediolateral gray matter of the spinal cord below the NLI, resulting in inappropriate release of norepinephrine (NE), dopamine-β-hydroxylase, and dopamine (DA), resulting in piloerection, pallor, vasoconstriction, hypertension, and pounding headache. Carotid and aortic baroreceptors respond to the elevation in BP by increasing vagal or parasympathetic ANS tone, resulting in bradycardia. Increased sympathetic inhibitory outflow above the lesion causes profuse sweating and vasodilation with flushing of the skin. The commonest triggers of AD are bladder distention, fecal impaction, and skin breakdown, however other noxious stimuli may precipitate an attack. The management of AD includes sitting the patient up, followed by loosening of tightly fitted clothing, assessment for bladder distension, kinking of a urinary catheter, need for intermittent catheterization, and fecal impaction. Short-acting antihypertensive medication such as topical nitrate, which can be removed once the trigger for the AD has been addressed, should be administered, or oral nifedepine (bite and swallow) can also be used.

Coagulation Disorders

Hypercoagulability, intimal vascular injury, and stasis are the main risk factors for venous thrombosis. Patients with SCI are hypercoagulable due to release of procoagulant factors. The trauma itself may lead to intimal vascular injury while paralysis and the initial bed-bound state cause stasis. Accordingly, patients with SCI are at increased risk for venous thromboembolism and deep venous thrombosis (DVT), the risk of which peaks at about seven to ten days after injury. Mechanical compression in SCI patients for the first two weeks, the initiation of anticoagulation within the first 72 hours, screening for procoagulopathy, and monitoring for DVT are all recommended in SCI. Low-molecular-weight heparin, such as enoxaparin, administered 30 mg every 12 hours or 40 mg daily by subcutaneous injection, or unfractionated heparin with the dose adjusted to achieve an activated partial thromboplastin time (APTT) of 1.5-times normal, should be used. Anticoagulation is generally continued for a total of at least eight weeks in patients with uncomplicated complete SCI and discontinued when the patient is ambulatory. An inferior vena cava filter is inserted when anticoagulation is contraindicated, and in patients with high cervical lesions and poor cardiopulmonary reserve.

Metabolic Disturbances

Osteoporosis is a predictable occurrence in the long bones below the level of injury in individuals with chronic SCI (17) due to increased bone absorption relative to deposition that results in hypercalcemia, fractures and renal calculi. Acute hypercalcemia is most common in children and adolescents, especially males. There may be deficiency of vitamin D and secondary hyperparathyroidism. (18). Contrary to the extremities and pelvis, several cross-sectional studies have found that the vertebral column does not appear to lose bone mass after paralysis, but rather tends to gain bone mass with age or longer duration of injury (19). A study employing lateral dual-energy radiographic absorptiometry (DXA) showed significantly reduced bone mineral density (BMD) compared to posterior-anterior (PA) DXA imaging that was normal, underestimating the potential risk for vertebral fracture (20).

Pulmonary Aspects

SCI can have a profound effect on respiration, especially when the diaphragm, which is responsible for two-thirds of resting VC, is impaired. The phrenic nerve and diaphragm, which derive innervation from the anterior primary rami (APR) of the C3 to C5 roots, may be disturbed in SCI at or above the C5 level, leading to the need for ventilator support. The internal intercostals, which aid in coughing, and external intercostal muscles, which assist in forced inhalation, derive their innervation from the APR of thoracic root, and may be disturbed in thoracic SCI. Similarly, the abdominal muscles, important in forced expiration and cough, may be denervated by thoracic SCI, leading to increased risk of aspiration. Further, flaccid paralysis of the external intercostal muscles results in paradoxical chest wall contraction during inspiration as the diaphragm descends, causing a decrease in FVC and maximal inspiratory force by about 70% and shallow breathing pattern.

As spinal shock resolves, these parameters often improve to about 60% of pre-injury expectations. Maximum expiratory force may peak at only 33% of predicted normal values (21). With rapid breathing and use of accessory muscles there can sometimes be an initially normal blood gas and oxygenation but fatigue or medical complications may lead to delayed respiratory failure. A VC of <1 liter is an indication for intubation and mechanical ventilator support. The factors of complete tetraplegia, age >45 years, high cervical NLI, premorbid lung disease, and pneumonia are associated with the propensity for tracheostomy.

Of 134 patients with tetraplegia due to SCI (22), 57% of those initially requiring respiratory support were weaned off of the ventilator by the time of discharge, with the most favorable prognosis of independent ventilation noted in 78% of those with NLI at the C4 level or lower. Up to 90% of patients requiring prolonged support survived one year, while 56% survived three years, and 33% for five years.

Of patients with NLI at C2 to C6 (23), 71% with NLI at C4 or below were weaned successfully compared to 20% of those with NLI of C3 or above. Spirometry evidencing an FVC ≥ 800 ml or NIF ≥40 mm H_2O, diaphragm fluoroscopy, normal phrenic nerve conduction studies, and diaphragm needle EMG are all measures of a favorable outcome.

Aspiration pneumonia is a leading cause of death for tetraplegic, making preventive care crucial for long-term survival. Influenza and pneumococcal vaccinations (24) can lead to protective levels and functional reactivated antibodies that persist for up to five years when received before age 65 years. Accordingly, vaccination of patients with SCI is recommended for those >65 years, especially if initially vaccinated at age <65 years, with a lapse of five years. Annual influenza vaccination is also recommended for patients with SCI.

An important concern is dysphagia, with estimates in tetraplegia that ranges from 7 to 80% of patients that endure SCI. Videofluoroscopy and fiberoptic endoscopic evaluation of swallowing (FEES) testing, and prior tracheostomy are useful predictors of dysphagia (25).

Sleep disordered breathing (SDB), which is associated with partial collapse of the pharyngeal airway during respiratory and leads to daytime sleepiness and cognitive dysfunction, is estimated to occur in 25 to 45% in tetraplegic SCI patients. Possible risk factors include obesity, neurological changes, abnormal craniofacial anatomy, alcohol use, obstructive sleep apnea, gastroesophogeal reflux disease (GERD), and baclofen use. Those with severe snoring or unexplained and significant daytime sleepiness should undergo a sleep study with polysomnography and electroencephalographic (EEG) monitoring, and endoscopic upper airway studies. The chronic use of a proton pump inhibitor increases the risk of Clostridium difficile infection and community acquired pneumonia.

Bladder Disturbances

Normal voiding is under the influence of the brainstem and spinal cord and is facilitated by synchronous contraction of the bladder and relaxation of the external urethral sphincter. A lesion situated between the brainstem and thoracic cord results in detrusor-sphincter dyssynergia leading to simultaneous contractions and the generation of elevated urinary tract pressures and incontinence, the treatment of which includes periodic catheterization to reduce post-void residual bladder accumulation, as well as anti-muscarinic medications and intravesical botulinum toxin injection to relax the bladder. Patients with paraplegia and individuals with C8 NLI and tetraplegia may self-catheterize, but for those unable to do so, they and their caretakers need to decide whether to implement intermittent catheterization, insert an indwelling catheter, or undergo ileal diversion or sphincterotomy with a condom catheter. During spinal shock and in sacral lesions, neurogenic bladder dysfunction leads to a flaccid and atonic bladder, which combined with reduced tone of the external sphincter, results in bladder distension and overflow incontinence. Treatment includes insertion of an indwelling Foley catheter or catheterization to maintain bladder volume at less than 500 milliliters.

Bowel Disturbances

Bowel sequela of SCI problems are also of the UMN and LMN type, typically with preservation of sphincter tone and continence in the former. Reflex voiding can occur with digital rectal stimulation and after meals to take advantage of the gastrocolic reflex such that evacuation can occur with reasonable predictability and continence can be achieved. Initially, a daily regimen is suggested but every other day is acceptable for the long term. An LMN bowel disturbance is more difficult to manage since reflex evacuation is not present, and the atonic external anal sphincter does not allow continence. The usual approach is to use medications to administer stool softeners, laxatives, and supplement with digital evacuation.

A minority of patients with neurogenic bowel may opt for a colostomy, allowing easy bowel maintenance without requiring a transfer to the toilet and virtually eliminating episodes of incontinence. This may be particularly appropriate in the case of chronic sacral ulceration.

Sexual Function and Fertility

SCI can have profound effects on sexual function and fertility. About 52% of women with SCI were able to achieve orgasm through stimulation as compared to 100% of normal control women (26); similar percentages exist for men. Whereas female fertility rates in SCI are believed to be close to normal, those for men decline markedly within the first two weeks of SCI, accompanied by erectile dysfunction (ED), ejaculatory dysfunction, and oligospermia, such that only 10% of men sustaining SCI are able to conceive a child through sexual intercourse. The relatively recent advent of phosphodiesterase-5 (PDE-5) inhibitors for ED, *in vitro* fertilization, and assisted reproductive technologies lead to improved rates of conception. It is estimated that about 80% of men with SCI can be treated with a PDE-5 inhibitor. Pregnancy in women sustaining SCI needs to be monitored closely as typical signs and symptoms of pregnancy-related complications may not appear. Those with T6 or higher NLI are at greatest danger due to the potential for AD and may be required delivery by Caesarian section.

Pressure Ulcers

Decreased and impaired mobility and reduced protective sensory barriers place patients with SCI at higher risk for developing pressure ulcers. Once present, they may be difficult to treat or reverse, and may even be life-threatening. Ulcer prevention begins in the acute phase of care with frequent repositioning and pressure relief surfaces, and continues with the proper selection of a wheelchair with an appropriate seat back, cushioning, and selection of sleeping surfaces. The most common affected areas of the skin lie beneath the bony ischii, sacrum, coccyx, trochanters and heels; those related to the occiput, ear, shoulders and malleoli also occur. Once home, the patient and care provider should be educated to regularly inspect all at-risk areas. Proper nutrition is important at all stages of care and cigarette smoking should be strongly discouraged. Pressure ulcers are staged as erythematous or non-blanching, partial-thickness skin loss or blister, full-thickness skin loss with visible fat, and full thickness skin loss with visible muscle or bone. An attempt should be made to find the cause of the pressure ulcer, and developing wounds should be treated promptly to avert progression including the development of osteomyelitis. Although suggested by the implication of peripheral vascular disease as a cause for pressure ulcers, and myocutaneous flaps and amputation after SCI, there was no significant difference in ankle brachial indices among individuals with SCI and controls (27).

Pain

Complaints of musculoskeletal, visceral, and neuropathic pain are common in SCI, the latter of which are typically described as burning, electrical, or dermatomal in distribution. Neuropathic SCI pain is treated with non-steroidal anti-inflammatory, anti-epileptic drugs such as pregablin or gabapentin, and a tricyclic antidepressant. Alterations in biomechanics and functional adaptations can place very high stresses on joints and muscles, with the shoulders particularly susceptible as those joints are highly mobile and relatively unstable and used for wheelchair and bed transfers, often leading to rotator cuff tear. While the principles of managing musculoskeletal injuries in SCI are similar to those for other patients, an aggressive approach is often warranted to restore arm function as quickly as possible. Caution should be exercised in the administration of opioid medication for pain as they are highly addictive and may pose a risk for young adults and children.

Spasticity and Contractures

Most patients have some degree of spasticity that commences at about one month after onset of SCI, that can be controlled with medications such as baclofen, tizanidine, benzodiazepine, and chemodenervation with botulinum toxin, alcohol or phenol. For those in whom spasticity cannot be controlled, or medication side effects are inordinate, intrathecal baclofen delivered by an implantable pump (28) may be an excellent option. Spasticity can be exaggerated by urinary tract infection, constipation, skin breakdown or other noxious stimulus, or syringomyelia. Contractures are easier to prevent by prophylactic stretch than to treat and can lead to discomfort, positioning problems, hygiene problems, and skin breakdown.

Bracing

Upper limb bracing is used to prevent contractures at the metacarpal phalangeal joints and long-finger flexor muscles, and at the wrists and elbows. Lower limb bracing for mobility is usually of limited use except in cauda equina lesions or very motivated low thoracic or conus paraplegics as the energy to ambulate is otherwise too high for functional ambulation.

Post-Traumatic Syringomyelia

The most common cause of neurological worsening after SCI is post-traumatic syringomyelia (29), with more than a quarter of patients with SCI developing syrinxes and some suffering progressive neurological deficits as a result of cyst enlargement. The mechanism of extension of a cavity has been attributed to pressure changes in the venous system, by the action of intraspinal veins on cerebral spinal fluid pressure, and fixation of the cord by adhesions and arachnoiditis at the site of SCI. The first symptoms in most patients is pain, which is increased with straining, coughing, or sneezing followed by sensory deficit, motor loss, and increase in spasticity, with autonomic symptoms such as abnormal sweating or hypertension occurring less frequently; an early clinical sign is probably loss of reflexes. Treatment can be conservative or surgical, the latter including techniques to reduce pressure inside the cyst, correction of bony deformities, decompression of the spinal cord, division of adhesions, and shunting (30).Long-term improvement occurs in fewer than one-half of patients so treated, and imaging evidence of a reduction in the size of the syrinx does not assure symptomatic resolution or even prevention of further neurological loss (30).

Psychiatric and Social Issues

SCI can lead to profound disruption of patients physical abilities, body image, sexuality, independence, and basic functioning. About one-third of affected patients are at risk for depression while in acute rehabilitation, while another one-third succumbs to depression after returning home to their communities. Patients with SCI have an increased risk of suffering debilitating levels of psychological morbidity, describing high levels of anxiety and feelings of helplessness and rating themselves lower on perceived quality of life (31). Not surprisingly, post-traumatic stress disorder (PTSD) occurs with an estimated incidence of 14 to 44%. Furthermore, SCI may be associated with an over-representation of those with substance abuse and other premorbid psychosocial disorders. It is incumbent upon health care providers treating those with SCI to be vigilant regarding mental health and psychosocial issues to offer supportive services as appropriate.

REFERENCES

1. Denis F. Spinal instability as defined by the three-column spine concept in acute spinal trauma. *Clin Orthop Relat Res* 1984; 189:65–76.
2. Kirshblum SC, Burns SP, Biering-Sorensen F, et al. International standards for neurological classification of spinal cord injury (revised 2011). *J Spinal Cord Med* 2011; 34:535–546.
3. Kirshblum SC, Waring W, Biering-Sorensen F, et al. Reference for the 2011 revision of the international standards for neurological classification of spinal cord injury. *J Spinal Cord Med* 2011; 34:547–554.
4. Marino RJ, Jones L, Kirshblum S, et al. Reliability and repeatability of the motor and sensory examination of the international standards for neurological classification of spinal cord injury. *J Spinal Cord Med* 2008; 31:166–170.
5. Marino RJ, Ditunno JF Jr, Donovan WH, et al. Neurologic recovery after traumatic spinal cord injury: data from the Model Spinal Cord Injury Systems. *Arch Phys Med Rehabil* 1999; 80:1391–1396.
6. Fisher CG, Noonan VK, Smith DE, et al. Motor recovery, functional status, and health-related quality of life in patients with complete spinal cord injuries. *Spine* 2005; 30:2200–2207.
7. Waters RL, Yakura JS, Adkins RH, et al. Recovery following complete paraplegia. *Arch Phys Med Rehabil* 1992; 73:784–789.
8. Vale FL, Burns J, Jackson AB, et al. Combined medical and surgical treatment after acute spinal cord injury: results of a prospective pilot study to assess the merits of aggressive medical resuscitation and blood pressure management. *J Neurosurg* 1997; 87: 239–46.
9. Ko HY, Ditunno JF Jr, Graziani V, et al. The pattern of reflex recovery during spinal shock. *Spinal Cord* 1999; 37:402–409.
10. Bracken MB, Collins WF, Freeman DF, et al. Efficacy of methylprednisolone in acute spinal cord injury. *JAMA* 1984; 251:45–52.
11. Bracken MB, Shepard MJ, Collins WF, et al. A randomized, controlled trial of methylprednisolone or naloxone in the treatment of acute spinal-cord injury: Results of the Second National Acute Spinal Cord Injury Study. *N Engl J Med* 1990; 322:1405–1411.
12. Bracken MB, Shepard MJ, Holford TR, et al. Methylprednisolone or tirilazad mesylate administration after acute spinal cord injury: 1-year follow up. Results of the third National Acute Spinal Cord Injury randomized controlled trial. *J Neurosurg* 1998; 89:699–706.

13. Hurlbert RJ. Methylprednisolone for acute spinal cord injury: an inappropriate standard of care. *J Neurosurg* 2000; 93:1–7.
14. Krassioukov A, Biering-Sorensen F, Donovan W, et al. International standards to document remaining autonomic function after spinal cord injury. *J Spinal Cord Med* 2012; 35:202–211.
15. Rosado-Rivers D, Radulovic M, Handrakis JP, et al. Comparison of 24-hour cardiovascular and autonomic function in paraplegia, tetraplegia, and control groups: implications for cardiovascular risk. *J Spinal Cord Med* 2011; 34:395–403.
16. Consortium for Spinal Cord Medicine. Acute management of autonomic dysreflexia: Individuals with spinal cord injury presenting to health-care facilities. 2nd ed. *J Spinal Cord Medicine*, 2002; 25(Suppl l):567–588.
17. Garland DE, Stewart CA, Adkins RH, et al. Osteoporosis after spinal cord injury. *J Orthop Res* 1992; 10:371–378.
18. Roberts D., Lee W., Cuneo R.C., et al: Longitudinal study of bone turnover after acute spinal cord injury. *J Clin Endocrinol Metab* 1998; 83:415–422.
19. Bauman WA, Spungen AM, Schwartz E, et al. Continuous loss of bone in chronic immobilization: a monozygotic twin study. *Osteoporosis Int* 1999; 10:123–127.
20. Bauman WA, Krishblum S, Cirnigliaro C, et al. Underestimation of bone loss of the spine with posterior-anterior dual-energy X-ray absorptiometry in patients with spinal cord injury. *J Spinal Cord Med* 2010; 33:214–220.
21. Ball PA. Critical care of spinal cord injury. *Spine* 2001; 26(Suppl):S27–S30.
22. Wicks AB, Menter RR. Long-term outlook in quadriplegic patients with initial ventilator dependency. *Chest* 1986; 90:406–410.
23. Chiodo AE, Scelza W, Forchheimer M. Predictors of ventilatory weaning in individuals with high cervical spinal cord injury. *J Spinal Cord Med* 2008; 31:72–77.
24. Waites KB, Canupp KC, Chen YY, et al. Revaccination of adults with spinal cord Injury using the 23-valent pneumococcal polysaccharide vaccine, *J Spinal Cord Med* 2008; 31:53–59.
25. Kirshblum S, Johnston MV, Brown J, et al. Predictors of dysphagia after spinal cord injury. *Arch Phys Med Rehabil* 1999; 80:1101–1105.
26. Sipski ML, Alexander CJ, Rosen RC. Orgasm in women with spinal cord injuries: a laboratory-based assessment. *Arch Phys Med Rehabil* 1995; 76:1097–1102.
27. Grew M, Kirshblum SC, Wood K, et al. The ankle brachial index in chronic spinal cord injury: a pilot study. *J Spinal Cord Med* 2000; 23:284–288.

28. Penn RD. Intrathecal baclofen for spasticity of spinal origin: seven years of experience. *J Neurosurg* 1992; 77:236–240.

29. Umbach I, Heilporn A. Review article: post-spinal cord injury syringomyelia. *Paraplegia* 1991; 29:219–221.

30. Brodbelt AR, Stoodley MA. Post-traumatic syringomyelia: a review. *J Clin Neurosci* 2003; 10:401–408.

31. Craig A, Tran Y, Middleton J. Psychological morbidity and spinal cord injury: a systematic review. *Spinal Cord* 2009; 47:108–114.

CHAPTER 61

Stroke Rehabilitation

Jung Ahn, John-Ross Rizzo, Ana-Marie Rojas

The neurological deficits caused by a stroke can impede the return to normal everyday life that existed before the illness, and even functionality in the activities of daily living (ADL). Spacicity is a notable aspect of the motor disturbances associated with stroke. Poststroke spasticity (PSS), is a recently recognized and quantifiable contributor to central paresis, ataxia, stance and gait disturbances, and other coordinated activities (1). This chapter considers the multifaceted and multidisciplinary aspects of stroke rehabilitation.

INPATIENT REHABILITATION

Stroke Rehabilitation Team

The first team encountered by the patient in stroke recovery is provided by the inpatient rehabilitation facility (IRF) consisting of physiatry, rehabilitation nursing, physical therapy (PT), occupational therapy (OT), speech-language pathology (SLP), swallowing therapy, orthotics, social work, psychology, recreational therapy, vocational counseling, and dietetics. The physiatric assessment begins with the identification of stroke deficits and residual neurologic function, in addition to concurrent medical issues that may include comorbid cardiovascular, pulmonary, renal disease, endocrinopathy, sphincter incontinence, autonomic disturbances, venous disease, skin breakdown, and speech and swallowing disturbances that pose a risk for aspiration. Although the role of the attending physiatrist is to communicate with the patient and family regarding functional progress, rehabilitation goals, future discharge planning, and day-to-day care, other specialists may be called upon to contribute expertise in managing complicated medical and surgical issues. Rehabilitation nurses provide continuous, around-the-clock nursing care and education. Physical therapists assess range of motion (ROM), muscle strength, mobility, balance, and ambulation, in addition to providing therapeutic exercises and functional training to improve skills and safety in transfer activities and ambulation. At discharge home, a variety of durable medical equipment (DME) may be available to assure safe mobility at home. Occupational therapists focus on hand motor skills, visual perception, cognitive function, self-care health maintenance activities, including brushing teeth, feeding, grooming and dressing activities, toileting, bathing and homemaking; the production of splints to assure proper functioning, and the assurance of a barrier-free home environment. A social worker evaluates the psychosocial history and the support system rendered by family members and caretakers toward safe discharge planning. A psychologist assures the evaluation and treatment of psychological issues and cognitive disturbances. A speech and language pathologist identifies and treats disturbances in verbal communication and language. A swallowing disorder specialist supervises the swallowing evaluation, utilizing video-fluoroscopic modified barium swallowing studies with various food textures to assess pharyngeal function. These later contribute to an appropriate diet that prevents or minimizes aspiration pneumonia. Recreational therapists facilitate the patient's reintegration into leisure and social activities while improving motor skills, coordination, and attention. A vocational counselor integrates the educational background with prior employment to explore later work opportunities. A nutritionist evaluates the nutritional status and diet, and offers recommendation appropriate to the neurological and medical condition.

TABLE 1. PULSES Profile

P	Physical Condition including diseases of viscera (cardiovascular, pulmonary, gastrointestinal, urologic, and endocrine) and cerebral disorders which are not enumerated in the lettered categories below.	
	No gross abnormalities considering the age of the individual	1 point
	Minor abnormalities not requiring frequent medical or nursing supervision	2 points
	Moderately severe abnormalities requiring frequent medical and nursing attention, yet still permitting ambulation	3 points
	Severe abnormalities requiring constant medical and nursing supervision confining individual to bed or wheelchair	4 points
U	Upper extremities including shoulder girdle, cervical and upper dorsal spine	
	No gross abnormalities considering the age of the individual	1 point
	Minor abnormalities with fairly good range of motion and function	2 points
	Moderately severe abnormalities but permitting the performance of daily needs to a limited extent	3 points
	Severe abnormalities requiring constant nursing care	4 points
L	Lower extremities including the pelvis, lower dorsal and lumbosacral spine	
	No gross abnormalities considering the age of the individual	1 point
	Minor abnormalities with fairly good range of motion and function	2 points
	Moderately severe abnormalities but permitting limited ambulation	3 points
	Severe abnormalities confining the individual to bed or wheelchair	4 points
S	Sensory components related to speech, vision, and hearing	
	No gross abnormalities considering the age of the individual	1 point
	Minor deviations insufficient to cause any appreciable functional impairment	2 points
	Moderate deviations sufficient to cause appreciable functional impairment	3 points
	Severe impairment causing complete loss of hearing, vision, or speech	4 points
E	Excretory function (sphincter function), either bowel or bladder	
	Complete control	1 point
	Occasional stress incontinence or nocturia	2 points
	Periodic bowel and bladder incontinence or retention alternating with control	3 points
	Total incontinence, either bowel or bladder	4 points
S	Sensorium (mental and emotional status)	
	No deviations considering the age of the individual	1 point
	Minor deviation in mood, temperament, and personality not impairing environment adjustment	2 points
	Moderately severe deviations requiring some supervision	3 points
	Severe variations requiring complete supervision	4 points
	Each of these areas can be scored by circling the appropriate number and summing the total.	Total

Stroke Rehabilitation in the Acute Neurological Setting

Stroke rehabilitation can be initiated and a program devised by the consulting physiatrist shortly after admission to the neurological ward or stroke unit, initially aimed at integration of acute therapeutic modalities while later focusing on the appropriate time to admit the patient to the acute IRF. The PULSES profile calculates a score that assists in determining the need for admission to an IRF (2) (Table 1), wherein a score of 6 indicates no functional impairment and probably no need for admission to an IRF, compared to a score of 24 that instead suggests too severe an impairment for admission.

Stroke Rehabilitation in the Inpatient Rehabilitation Facility

An IRF admission provides medical services and nursing care 24 hours per day, seven days per week; and rehabilitation therapy three hours per day, five days per week. Patients unable to tolerate that intensity of therapy can be managed in a skilled nursing facility (SNF), long-term nursing home care, or discharged home with referrals to a home care agency for skilled home services (3). An Individualized Overall Plan of Care (IOPOC) is compiled based upon the recommendations of the interdisciplinary team conference, and the initial functional assessment ensues. Multidisciplinary team evaluation conferences share the progress achieved in each of the stroke rehabilitation disciplines. It is useful to employ a functional independent measurement (FIM System®) score when assessing the patients status and in communicating with interdisciplinary team members.

NEUROLOGIC IMPAIRMENTS

Hemiplegia

A stroke involving the homunculus of the motor cortex results in upper motor neuron (UMN) paralysis of the contralateral side corresponding to the location of vascular insult. A stroke in the anterior cerebral artery (ACA) territory will likely spare motor function of the contralateral arm, whereas a lesion in the territory of the middle cerebral artery (MCA) will impair the contralateral arm more than the leg. A vascular event in the basal ganglia and internal capsule can result in contralateral weakness, while insult to the thalamus typically leads to contralateral hemi-body sensory deficits. Brainstem stroke lead to multimodality motor and sensory deficits, whereas cerebellar lesions impair coordination, equilibrium, and balance. A therapeutic exercise and functional training program focuses upon improving and compensating for these neurologic deficits.

Speech Disturbances

A stroke may impair speech production, and verbal or written language content. Insult to frontal operculum cortex leads to acute mutism, whereas localized lesions in the inferior frontal gyrus lead to disturbances in output of verbal and written language. A lesion in the superior and inferior branches encompassing the dominant MCA territory leads instead to global aphasia adding receptive disturbances of comprehension and repetition. Non-fluent or Broca type output aphasia is characterized by slow, hesitant, labored speech, decreased vocabulary in word finding, impaired grammar and writing deficits, reflecting difficulty in communication with normal or near normal auditory comprehension. A fluent or Wernicke type aphasia, results from a lesion in the dominant superior temporal gyrus leading to normal flow of verbal speech with a semblance of normal vocabulary and grammar, although verbal output is typically inappropriate and nonsensical.

Various instruments are available for measuring communication skills, such as the Functional Communication Profile (FCP), Communicative Abilities of Daily Living (CADL), Communicative Effectiveness Profile (CEP), or Functional Assessment of Communication Skills (FACS). Acquired aphasia lasting more than two months has little chance of recovery to premorbid levels, although post-stroke speech recovery may continue for six or more months. Fluent aphasia improves most in the first six months, whereas non-fluent aphasia may make gradual improvement over a year. Comprehension improves to a greater degree than verbal or written language expression in global aphasia following a stroke in the Broca area. Dysarthria is amenable to speech therapy employing an FCP.

Cognitive Deficits

Cognitive changes after a stroke, particularly in non-dominant hemispheric lesions, impact upon rehabilitation. Affected patients may not be aware of their deficits and are more liable to experience unsafe situations interfering with functional progress in performing self-care activities, prolonging the rehabilitation period. One complex pattern of altered cognition is apraxia, which impairs the ability to perform learned movements in the absence of weakness or sensory deficits. Two types, ideomotor and ideational, are commonly observed after a stroke due to damage along frontal and parietal cortex. Ideomotor apraxia is suggested by inability to imitate a series of movements, whereas ideational apraxia is suggested by disturbances in manipulating objects for a stated purpose. Restorative and compensatory methods can be utilized to improve cognitive impairments and apraxia involving the processes of revitalizing the lost ability while compensating with retained abilities. Noninvasive cortical stimulation and a variety of pharmacologic interventions can improve arousal and memory (4). Improvement in cognitive function occurs in up to 20% of those with mild cognitive impairment following a stroke, typically beginning at one month (5).

Visual Defects

It is estimated that 30 to 85% of stroke patients will experience some type of visual dysfunction following stroke (6–8). Vision problems hinder ADL, increase the risk of falling, and impede the overall outcome of rehabilitation (9), highlighting the importance of early intervention and evaluation for stroke-related visual disturbances (9, 10). The visual changes associated with stroke can be categorized into sensory, motor, and perceptual impairments. Sensory deficits include disturbances of visual acuity and the visual field, while motor impairments include ocular dysmotility. Perceptual disturbances include agnosia, alexia, figure-ground discrimination problems, defects in spatial relation, and unilateral neglect (Figure 1) (11). Recognition and treatment employing neurovisual rehabilitation employs compensation, substitution, and restitution-based approaches (7, 9). The first approach involves the utilization of unaffected aspects of the visual system to compensate for the deficit, while substitution employs environmental adaptations and low-vision devices to assist in visual disability. Restitution involves restoration of lost function. (7, 12). The risk of falling is closely related to visual impairment, in both normal aging and stroke (13).

THERAPEUTIC EXERCISES AND MODALITIES:

Range of motion (ROM) exercises and positioning are useful for early mobilization and to increase cognitive perceptual skills and sensory reintegration. Proprioceptive neuromuscular facilitation theory encourages diagonal and spiral components of repeated movements in a more natural pattern. There are techniques to inhibit primitive reflex activity by placing the affected joints in various positions naturally assumed after a stroke, while encouraging joint maintenance, inhibiting detrimental postures, and suppressing abnormal reflex patterns induced by spastic muscle tone.

Body-weight-supported-treadmill training is used in low functioning hemiplegic patients to improve gait function. The patient takes steps on the treadmill with a reciprocally-weighted harness for body-weight support. The treadmill initiates the involved leg in a gait generator reflex as it moves slowly over the conveyor belt. Extrinsic feedback mechanisms use mirrors, weight shifting and verbal cueing during therapy. This training improves the quality of therapy and allows for more steps to be taken by the patient during the session (14).

Mirror therapy integrates a mirror in fine motor planning and coordination. The patient, seated in front of the mirror oriented parallel to the midline blocking the view of the affected side, sees the reflection of the unaffected side in place of the affected side. This visual illusion enhances self-awareness, spatial attention, and insight on neglect (15).

Constraint-induced muscle training (CIMT) promotes use of the affected arm to acquire or reacquire a lost skill following the stroke. Relearning tasks promote cortical reorganization and recovery of motor function. To be qualified for this therapy the patient should have at least partial wrist and finger extension, adequate proximal limb control, and adequate balance with a constrained arm. Original CIMT programs consisted of two-week periods for 90% of waking hours, each six hours per day, designed to force the impaired limb in performing specific tasks. A modified CIMT program provides a less intense treatment over a longer period consisting of constraint to the intact limb five days per week, each day for five hours, with three hours of therapy three times per week for ten weeks.

Mental imagery was adapted to stroke rehabilitation to promote arm function and improve neglect. This modality, which employs picture cards and videotapes, has a positive effect on relearning of daily tasks following a stroke (16–18).

Neuromuscular electrical stimulation (NMES) refers to electrical lower motor neuron (LMN) stimulation to facilitate activation of muscle activity in plegic and paretic limbs. A therapeutic current is delivered via electrodes placed or implanted near peripheral nerves of interest to initiate functional movement.

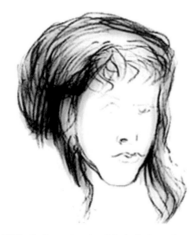

FIG. 1. A patient with left hemiparesis and unilateral neglect portrayed an image of his therapist demonstrating asymmetry of facial features less complex on the left side.

ORTHOSES, ASSISTIVE DEVICES, AND DURABLE MEDICAL EQUIPMENT

Therapeutic equipment is available to maximize independence in self-care activities and locomotion.

Orthoses

Orthoses are employed to prevent joint contracture of the wrist, fingers and ankle, and pressure ulcers on the heel and lateral malleolus of the involved limbs, including a resting hand splint, a cock-up wrist splint, and posterior ankle-foot splint with the rotatable bar. Spastic foot drop can be treated with different types of custom made ankle-foot orthosis (AFO). There are new types of AFO that utilize functional electrical stimulation including Bioness® and WalkAide®, recently introduced for improving quality in walking of hemiplegics.

Self-Care Assistive Devices and Durable Medical Equipment

Self-care assistive equipment can be ordered after discharge to aid adaptation of the patient with disability to environmental challenges. They include small utensils such as a swiveled spoon, a rocker knife and a cup adapter to assist in self-feeding. A universal cuff can be utilized for feeding, grooming, and brushing teeth. Velcro shoes, elastic shoelaces, button hook, reacher, a leg-lifter, sock donning aid, long shoehorn and others are useful in assistive dressing. Bathroom equipment crucial to enhance safety during toileting and bathing include grab bars for safe transfers, commode chair and seat elevator, anti-slip gripping bathtub mat, shower stall, dual hand-held showerhead, tub shower bench, and shower chair. During bathroom activities, a long handle sponge, a specialized soap dispenser or a soap-on-a-rope can be used to decrease dependency. The use of assistive bathroom equipment allows hemiplegics to be less dependent and safer during bathroom activities. A bedside commode chair should be prescribed for those with difficulty walking who may fall while traveling to the bathroom at night. A wheelchair should be obtained for ADL at home and in the community that includes a foam cushion, anti-tippers, swing-away detachable leg-foot rests and toggle brakes. A one-arm drive manual wheelchair is available for those who perform self-wheelchair locomotion on an even surface, and a simple transport chair for the caretaker. Power wheelchairs can be used by non-ambulatory patients with normal cognitive function, intact visual scanning skills, and reliable arm function.

Walking Aid

A cane and walker are used in the ambulation training for hemiplegic patients. The former include single-point, tripod, narrow-based, and wide-based quad canes. Available walkers include standard folding, hemi-, rolling, and 3-wheel and 4-wheel rolling walkers with seats. A hemi-walker is prescribed to patients with paralysis of the arm who require a wider base of support.

STROKE SEQUELAE

Subluxation of the Hemiplegic Shoulder

Shoulder subluxation may be noted in the seated or standing position, which although not typically painful, should be empirically supported with tape or a sling to reduce the gap between the glenoid and the head of the humerus.

Shoulder Pain

Pain may be due to pre-existing adhesive capsulitis, impingement, degenerative arthropathy, and tendinosis. However, in the absence thereof, it should nonetheless be treated with moist heat, gentle massage, ROM exercises, and transcutaneous electric nerve stimulation (TENS). Adhesive capsulitis in the hemiplegic shoulder can result from stroke-related spasticity, decreased ROM, muscle paralysis, and pain-limiting movement, as well as inappropriate use of a hemi-arm sling for shoulder subluxation. The latter should be exchanged for Swath-type slings, and underlying spasticity improved, with reduction of inflammation. Steroid injections can intermittently be used if no contraindications and warranted in the specific clinical situation.

Shoulder-Hand Syndrome

Also known as reflex sympathetic dystrophy (RSD) and complex regional pain syndrome (CRPS) type 1, and with an estimated prevalence of up to 70% in post-stroke hemiplegia, this syndrome leads to pain in the shoulder and hand, sparing the elbow, with associated signs of sympathetic overflow in the hand including swelling, puffiness, temperature change, erythema, and palmar perspiration. There may be osteoporotic findings on hand x-ray. Treatment includes symptomatic measures for control of pain and edema, including short-term oral corticosteroids, hand contrast baths, ROM, and massage.

Bowel and Bladder Dysfunction

Urinary sphincter dysfunction is common to all stroke patients, however, pre-existing conditions can lead to additional concerns including benign prosthetic hyperplasia, diabetic neuropathy, urinary tract infection, age-related stress incontinence, and concurrent in-dwelling catheterization. Treatment may be directed toward regulation of fluid intake, timed bladder emptying, clean intermittent catheterization (CIC), transfer training, and uropharmacological management. Men with urinary incontinence, condom external catheters should be treated individually. A urodynamic evaluation should be obtained to objectify the nature of the disturbance. Bowel incontinence is managed by a toileting schedule, stool softeners, laxatives, and enemas when needed.

Dysphagia

Dysphagia transiently occurs in up to 80% of acute stroke (19) and is monitored with swallowing studies so as to upgrade the diet as swallowing improves. Video fluoroscopic modified barium swallowing study reveals clinically significant tracheal aspiration. Unrecognized and unprotected, such patients are at risk for aspiration pneumonia, respiratory distress, dehydration, and malnutrition, the latter of which can impact upon outcome of rehabilitation (20). Mild dysphagia is treated with dietary modification, while more severe affliction is treated with a permanent feeding tube.

Spasticity

With a prevalence of PSS greater than 40%, and disabling PSS noted in up to 13% of patients (20), it is emerging as a significant health issue for stroke survivors in the United States and globally. The pathophysiology, epidemiology, motor interactions, assessment of functional impairment, and treatment of PSS is reviewed extensively elsewhere. (1). Spasticity due to unopposed UMN involvement is supportively managed with stretching, cold application, and splinting to decrease tone, improve ROM, and prevent joint contractures, in addition to pharmacological intervention with first, oral anti-spasticity medications such as baclofen, dantrolene sodium and tizanidine, and botulinum toxin administered via local injection into specific muscle groups under ultrasound and electromyographic guidance.

Venous Thromboembolism

Venous thromboembolism (VTE) increases after acute stroke due to lack of mobility and hemiplegia. Vigilance should begin at the time of admission and prevented by the application of intermittent pneumatic devices that provide sequential compression, and prophylactic subcutaneous anticoagulation or low molecular weight heparin. Inferior vena cava filter can be inserted if VTE prophylaxis is contraindicated or ineffective.

Infection

Infection is most often associated with inadvertent or clinically apparent aspiration pneumonia or urinary tract infection and should be treated with antibiotic therapy. Recurrent antibiotic therapy can lead to stool colonization with Clostridium difficile toxin.

Depression

Post-stroke depression (PSD), which is estimated to occur in up to 50% of patients in the year following a stroke, with an increase in mortality during the first decade, leads to depressed mood, anxiety, and adjustment disorder, with persistent feelings of sadness, feelings of hopelessness, guilt, lack of motivation, anhedonia, and even suicidal ideation (21–24). Other psychological manifestations of PSD include insomnia, impulsivity, confusion, agitation, emotional instability, and apathy. Prophylactic use of antidepressants is advised for patients with predisposing factors, including those with frontal lesions (21). The tricyclic medication nortriptyline is superior to the selective serotonin re-uptake inhibitor (SSRI) fluoxetine in the treatment of PSD to improve FIM scores (25), improve clinical outcome, and decrease mortality (23, 25).

FUNCTIONAL PROGNOSIS

Numerous factors contribute to the prognosis of stroke-related rehabilitation outcome including the lesion volume, location, and clinical neurological outcome (26, 27), with eventual return of strength and absence of apraxia significant predictors for return to work (28). Those unimproved after six months are unlikely to improve further.

REFERENCES

1. Brainin M. Poststroke spasticity. Treating to the disability. *Neurology* 2013; 80 (Suppl 2):S1–S4.

2. Moskowitz E, McCann CB. Classification of disability in the chronically ill and aging. *J Chronic Dis* 1957; 5:342–346.

3. Frank M, Conzelmann M, Engelter S. Prediction of discharge destination after neurological rehabilitation in stroke patients. *Eur Neurol* 2010; 63:227–233.

4. Zorowitz RD, Smout RJ, Gassaway JA, et al. Neurostimulant medication usage during stroke rehabilitation: the Post-Stroke Rehabilitation Outcomes Project (PSROP). *Top Stroke Rehabil* 2005; 12:28–36.

5. Rasquin SM, Lodder J, Verhey FR. Predictors of reversible mild cognitive impairment after stroke: a 2-year follow-up study. *J Neurol Sci* 2005; 229–230:21–25.

6. Kapoor N, Ciuffreda KJ. Vision disturbances following traumatic brain injury. *Curr Treat Options Neurol* 2002; 4:271–280.

7. Kerkhoff G. Neurovisual rehabilitation: recent developments and future directions. *J Neurol Neurosurg Psychiatry* 2000; 68:691–706.

8. Macintosh C. Stroke re-visited: visual problems following stroke and their effect on rehabilitation. *Br Orthopt J* 2003; 60:10–14.

9. Khan S, Leung E, Jay WM. Stroke and visual rehabilitation. *Top Stroke Rehabil* 2008; 15:27–36.

10. Jones SA, Shinton RA. Improving outcome in stroke patients with visual problems. *Age Aging* 2006; 35:560–565.

11. Jutai JW, Bhogal SK, Foley NC, et al. Treatment of visual perceptual disorders post stroke. *Top Stroke Rehabil* 2003; 10:77–106.

12. Riggs RV, Andrews K, Roberts P, et al. Visual deficit interventions in adult stroke and brain injury: a systematic review. *Am J Phys Med Rehabil* 2007; 86:853–860.

13. Harwood RH. Visual problems and falls. *Age Ageing* 2001; 30 (Suppl4):13–18.

14. Ada L, Dean CM, Vargas J, et al. Mechanically assisted walking with body weight support results in more independent walking than assisted overground walking in non ambulatory patients early after stroke: a systematic review. *J Physiother* 2010; 56:153–161.

15. Rothgangel AS, Braun SM, Beurskens AJ, et al. The clinical aspects of mirror therapy in rehabilitation: a systematic review of the literature. *Int J Rehabil Res* 2011; 34:1–13.

16. Page SJ, Levine P, Sisto S, et al. A randomized efficacy and feasibility study of imagery in acute stroke. *Clin Rehabil* 2001; 15:233–240.

17. Stevens JA, Stoykov ME. Using motor imagery in the rehabilitation of hemiparesis. *Arch Phys Med Rehabil* 2003; 84:1090–1092.

18. Liu KP, Chan CC, Lee TM, et al. Mental imagery for promoting relearning for people after stroke: a randomized controlled trial. *Arch Phys Med Rehabil* 2004; 85:1403–1408.

19. Flamand-Roze C, Cauquil-Michon C, Denier C. Tools and early management of language and swallowing disorders in acute stroke patients. *Curr Neurol Neurosci Rep* 2012; 12:34–41.

20. Wissel J, Manack A, Brainin M. Toward a epidemiology of poststroke spasticity. *Neurology* 2013; 80 (Suppl 2):S13–S19.

21. Dafer RM, Rao M, Shareef A, et al. Poststroke depression. *Top Stroke Rehabil* 2008; 15:13–21.

22. Williams LS, Ghose SS, Swindle RW. Depression and other mental health diagnoses increase mortality risk after ischemic stroke. *Am J Psychiatry* 2004; 161:1090–1095.

23. Jorge RE, Robinson RG, Arndt S, et al. Mortality and poststroke depression: a placebo-controlled trial of antidepressants. *Am J Psychiatry* 2003; 160:1823–1829.

24. Morris PL, Robinson RG, Samuels J. Depression, introversion and mortality following stroke. *Aust N Z J Psychiatry* 1993; 27:443–449.

25. Robinson RG, Schultz SK, Castillo C, et al. Nortriptyline versus fluoxetine in the treatment of depression and in short-term recovery after stroke: a placebo-controlled, double-blind study. *Am J Psychiatry* 2000; 157:351–359.

26. Ganesan V, Ng V, Chong WK, et al. Lesion volume, lesion location, and outcome after middle cerebral artery territory stroke. *Arch Dis Child* 1999; 81:295–300.

27. Wozniak MA, Kittner SJ, Price TR, et al. Stroke location is not associated with return to work after first ischemic stroke. *Stroke* 1999; 30:2568–2573.

28. Saeki S, Ogata H, Okubo T, et al. Return to work after stroke. A follow-up study. *Stroke* 1995; 26:399–401.

CHAPTER 62

Principles of Neuromuscular Rehabilitation

John R. Bach

Once the diagnosis of a progressive neuromuscular disease is made, there is a tendency to inform the patient or family that there is no effective intervention. This is done despite the availability of physical medicine interventions that can in many instances prolong life without hospitalization or tracheostomy and, in virtually all instances, enhance patient function. The worst case scenario is advanced amyotrophic lateral sclerosis (ALS), in which 88 to 97% (1–2) of lives can be prolonged and function maximized by physical medicine interventions. Eye blink alone can be used for communication and environmental control. Continuous ventilator users with advanced ALS or other severe neuromuscular conditions can continue sedentary gainful employment and have a positive attitude about their lives (2). Optimism can be encouraged by making aspects of neuromuscular rehabilitation available in a multidisciplinary care program to optimize patient options.

Those with neuromuscular impairments can have disability due to breathing dysfunction, skeletal muscle dysfunction, musculotendinous contractures, primary skeletal or cardiopulmonary pathology, poor endurance, other associated disorders or a combination thereof. The patient can be further handicapped by architectural barriers, public policies, inadequate finances, family support, or deficiencies in education.

Clinicians should identify and differentiate the disease process, impairments, disabilities, and handicaps faced by the patient so that physical medicine interventions and psychosocial support can be instituted and the person returned to the fullest possible physical, mental, social, and economic independence. Physical medicine interventions pertain to the use of equipment and activities that include non-invasive methods of ventilatory support and cough

facilitation, exercises, range-of-motion, and surgical interventions based on pathokinesiologic principles to maximize breathing, coughing, nutrition, and physical functioning. It is useful to consider the example of the three clinical stages of Duchenne muscular dystrophy (DMD) (Table 1). The clinician who understands the management principles for DMD can apply them to patients with other neuromuscular conditions.

AMBULATORY STAGE

In this stage, the diagnosis of DMD is established and the patient and family are told about family planning options, about possible treatment interventions, and the major options in each subsequent management stage are discussed. This is particularly important for optimizing compliance for later surgical therapies to maintain leg function, prevent scoliosis, avoid later hospitalizations for pulmonary morbidity and tracheostomy, and to prolong survival without invasive measures. Psychological support is important to prevent parental feelings of guilt, disrupted family psychodynamics, alienated family members, and to avert overprotection to the point of delaying the patient's emotional maturity and the assumption of self-directed activities and decision making.

Musculotendinous Contracture Management

The pathokinesiology of progressive gait difficulty has been described for DMD (3, 4), but it applies equally well to other myopathies, childhood polymyositis, and spinal muscular atrophy (SMA). Asymmetric hip extensor weakness leads to anterior and lateral pelvic tilt, asymmetric hip flexor con-

TABLE 1. Management Principles for Neuromuscular Disease

Ambulatory stage
1. Genetic counseling
2. Early counseling regarding future physical medicine options
3. Psychological support to prevent counterproductive family psychodynamics, to encourage goal-oriented activities, and to prepare the patient to be a self-directed individual
4. Early prevention or reduction of musculotendinous and chest wall and lung contractures
5. Supportive physical and occupational therapy and possibly splinting and therapeutic exercise
6. Pathokinesiologically justified surgical and bracing interventions
7. Prevention of cardiac complications

Wheelchair-dependent stage
8. Maintenance of proper nutrition
9. Facilitation of activities of daily living
10. Early surgical prevention or correction of back deformity
11. Prevention of cardiac complications
12. Maintenance of pulmonary compliance and normal alveolar ventilation

Stage of prolonged survival
13. Facilitation of independence with assistive devices and methods
14. Prevention of cardiac complications
15. Use of physical medicine respiratory muscle aids to assist alveolar ventilatory and clear airway secretions
16. Augmentative communication
17. Quality of life considerations

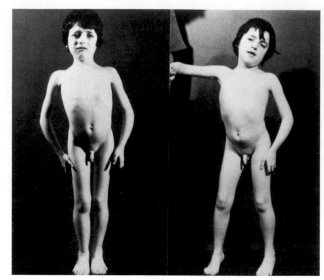

FIG. 1. Boy with Duchenne muscular dystrophy (DMD) unable to stand without assistance before (right) and able to walk without assistance or bracing after (left) extensive release of lower extremity contractures and transfer of tibialis posterior muscles. Photo courtesy of Dr. Yves Rideau.

tractures, and accentuated lumbar lordosis. Tensor fascia lata and iliotibial band contractures lead to a wide-based gait with internal rotation and flexion at the knees. With increasing quadriceps weakness, the patient stabilizes the knee by keeping the weight line anterior to the knee, but it must also be kept behind the hips because of weak hip extensors. Intact plantar flexors encourage toe walking and lead to equinus deformity that initially stabilizes the knees. Iliotibial tract tightness increases the torque on the femur and flexes the knee until the center of gravity shifts from behind the hip to the front of the knees. Strong foot evertor and tibialis posterior muscles destabilize the subtalar joint and lead to falls on uneven surfaces and later on level surfaces. Unless aggressively treated, the average age of wheelchair dependence in DMD is 8.6 to 9.5 years (range, 6 to 15 years) (5–8).

Although leg weakness plays a major role in the eventual loss of walking, musculotendinous contractures destabilize the gait prematurely, as seen by its prevention or early correction, resulting in prolongation of brace-free walking (9). An early prophylactic approach to preventing contractures depends on careful monitoring of the patient-strength, articular range-of-motion, speed of ambulation and rising from the floor (10). Surgically lengthening the Achilles tendon and hamstrings, resection of the iliotibial bands, lengthening of hip flexor muscles, and tibialis posterior tendon transfer to the dorsum of the foot generally performed between age four to seven years, increases and equalizes ankle dorsiflexor function (Figure 1) (10). These procedures are safer, better tolerated, and require less physical therapy (PT) afterward when performed at an earlier age. They interrupt the vicious cycle of weakness and contractures that lead to loss of standing balance. Earlier performed surgery and rehabilitation prolongs brace-free ambulation without long-term PT, burdensome splinting, and bracing (9, 10).

Similar management principles apply to patients with mild myopathy with better proximal strength because they require only certain elements of the surgical intervention such as possible tendo-achilles lengthening and tibialis posterior tendon transfer. Other approaches to the management of leg contractures include daily muscle stretching with bracing and PT (9, 10). Paul (11) noted that one-third of patients with DMD stopped walking before age six years when contractures were prevented by early surgery and a short course of postoperative PT, rendering continued therapy and splinting unnecessary. Nighttime leg splinting, combined with home PT, is an alternative approach. However, effective programs place considerable long-term burdens on patients and their families and night splints are often poorly tolerated. It has been suggested that this approach can maintain ambulation until age 10.3 years (12, 13).

The performance of late musculotendinous release when the patient is approaching wheelchair dependence often necessitates post-operative long-leg bracing but can prolong ambulation and the ability to stand (14, 15). However, late interventions are less well tolerated and require intensive postoperative PT with cumbersome, expensive, and often poorly tolerated long-leg braces.

Simple ankle-foot orthoses are not indicated for assisted ambulation in patients with neuromuscular disease unless the muscle weakness is limited to the ankles and knees. They can sometimes be used along with Lofstrand crutches after a late surgical contracture release, but they slow the speed of walking and make rising from a chair or going up steps more difficult because of reduced knee flexion and ankle extension. Patients with hereditary sensory-motor neuropathies (HSMN), and other similar conditions with distally predominant motor and sensory involvement, benefit from polypropylene ankle–foot orthoses to relieve toe dragging and to support pes cavus supinated feet; they also compensate for distal sensory deficits. A plastic or metal ankle–foot orthosis with an adjustable locked ankle enhances knee and ankle control by improving tibial stability.

Maintaining Pulmonary Compliance

Just as frequent passive range-of-motion is necessary to maintain the integrity and mobility of peripheral extremity articulations, deep insufflation is important for patients with diminished vital capacity (VC) to maintain pulmonary compliance and adequate volumes for an effective cough (16). Stacking of consecutively delivered volumes of air from a manual resuscitator or volume-cycled ventilator to the maximum lung insufflations that can be held with a closed glottis, termed "air stacking," increases cough flow and prevents pneumonia.

Exercise

Increased functional demands are potentially damaging to immature and dystrophic muscles susceptible to overuse (17). Greater weakness was found in the preferred dominant upper (18) and lower (19) limbs compared to the opposite non-preferred dystrophic side. Serum creatine kinase (CK) levels increase more after exercise of dystrophy muscles than in normal subjects. It is speculative whether patients with advanced weakness can engender overuse atrophy in the course of routine physical activity.

DeLateur and Giaconi (20) noted that strengthening and endurance training improved strength and slowed progression of weakness early in the course of DMD. Vignos and Watkins (21) further noted a 50% increase in strength over 4 months with gains that were maintained for one year after resistance exercise training of antigravity muscles, as did Milner-Brown and Miller (22) in 20-year-old to 53-year-old patients with facioscapulohumeral dystrophy (FSH), myotonic muscular dystrophy (DM), Becker muscular dystrophy (BMD), limb-girdle muscular dystrophy (LGMD), SMA, and diverse polyneuropathies. However, the initial strength had to be greater than 15 to 20% of normal. Fowler (23) suggested that dynamic high-resistance exercise training was potentially beneficial and resulted in gains in strength if the degree of weakness was not so severe and the rate of clinical progression was relatively slow. However, the period of daily exercise was limited and adapted to the individual's daily physical activity level.

Exercise programs may not benefit patients that need the most assistance. For example, there is little evidence that muscles with less than anti-gravity strength Medical Research Council (MRC) grade 3/5 will further strengthen with exercise that have lost most of the functionality. There is little evidence that temporarily strengthened muscles with MRC strength greater than 3/5 will have prolongation of function. Fowler and Goodgold (24) recommended commencing exercise early in the course of individuals with slowly progressive disorders, employing submaximal resistance and high-repetition aerobic exercise, as did Similarly and coworkers (21) who advocated two to three hours of daily standing, walking, and swimming per day as long as the patient felt rested after a night's sleep. All such patients should be encouraged to participate in individually enjoyable activities with avoidance of muscle strain.

Cardiac Considerations

Cardiac monitoring should be empirically delayed until the stage of wheelchair dependence and is considered there.

Nutritional Considerations

Undernourishment results from decreased appetite due to hypercapnia, impaired feeding ability, inpairment of taste, restrictions of food texture and flavor, dysphagia, choking sensation, tachypnea, aspiration, concomitant tracheostomy alone or combined with intermittent positive pressure ventilation (IPPV), and coexistent bowel disturbances (25). Specific nutritional interventions already exist for patients with SMA (26).

Patients should be weighed regularly and changes evaluated in the context of their disease as even a 10% reduction of ideal weight can be associated with loss of physiologic adaptability and increased morbidity (26), particularly in those with impaired pulmonary defense mechanisms. Food deprivation impairs respiratory muscle function by reducing available energy substrates. Diaphragmatic isometric strength endurance, maximum static inspiratory and expiratory pressures (MIPmax and MEPmax), maximum voluntary ventilation (MVV), oxygen tension, hypoxic and hypercapneic ventilator drive, all diminish with fasting (27–31). Ventilator failure likewise occurs with chronic starvation in normal subjects. Experimental rats restricted to one-third of the normal caloric intake for 6 weeks develop emphysema-like lung changes similar to starved individuals from Warsaw ghettos (32, 33). Malnutrition impairs cell-mediated and humoral immunity, alveolar macrophage phagocytic activity, while increasing bacterial adherence to the lower airways in patients with tracheostomy tubes (34–38).

Obesity complicates ventilator dynamics, however by the time a patient requires ventilator support, weight loss and undernutrition will supervene such that the weight of a patient with DMD and impending respiratory failure was an average of 70 pounds (39). Serum albumin and transferrin levels reflect the protein synthetic ability of the liver, both with half-lives under two weeks, and reflective of long-, but not short-term, protein status changes. Retinol-binding protein and prealbumin are more useful in the assessment of short-term nutritional competence because of the shorter half-life of 12 hours and two days, respectively (25). Other useful tests include total iron-binding capacity and serum vitamin A, C, and E levels.

Food intake can be assessed by use of a diary recording caloric and nutritional intake in comparison to ideal levels, however the latter may differ for inactive patients compared to the general population. The equation Kcal = 2,000 - age (years) – 50, yields the daily recommended caloric intake of children with DMD. (40). Those with advanced DMD or other neuromuscular disorders will have caloric requirements that may not exceed normal levels of resting energy expenditure, estimated to be 110% of the basal metabolic rate (BMR). The patients that transition from eating a diet of foods of diverse consistency to ones with soft and pureed texture, and later supplemented high-calorie liquid meals, should ultimately be referred for percutaneous endoscopy gastrostomy (PEG) tube placement, particularly when aspiration of upper airway secretions and food leads to oxygen desaturation, or caloric, fluids, and nutrient intake is inadequate to sustain normal metabolism (41).

STAGE OF WHEELCHAIR DEPENDENCE

Scoliosis Prevention

Severe scoliosis develops in all patients with SMA type I and II, and in up to 90% of those with DMD (42) and other childhood neuromuscular disorders. Scoliosis is less likely to develop in patients with a higher plateau VC, defined as the highest VC ever attained by the patient, and the least Cushingoid or obese the patient. Deflazatcort, an oxazoline derivative of prednisolone with fewer side effects than prednisone, given at a dose of 0.6 to 0.9 mg/kg daily for the first 20 days of the month, led to less scoliosis in DMD cohorts, improved cardiac and respiratory function and survival however the mechanism of improved bone health was not well understood (43).

Scoliosis-reduction surgery is generally indicated with curvatures of >40°, especially in a patient with failed thoracolumbar bracing and adequate cardiopulmonary function to safely tolerate surgical intervention. Surgical intervention may also be appropriate for patients with idiopathic and non-neuromuscular forms of scoliosis. One extubation protocol was associated with a favorably surgical outcome despite a marked reduction in lung volumes and respiratory muscle strength indices (44, 45).

Wheelchair seating modifications and thoracolumbar bracing preserves spine flexibility in small children but should be avoided in patients with DMD because such procedures have no ameliorative impact on the ultimate degree of curvature and can delay surgical intervention, leading to further weakness and longer postoperative recovery longer (46, 47). Up to one-third of patients with DMD and a relatively low plateau VC (Figure 2) may delay surgical intervention, awaiting deterioration of the scoliotic curve to more than 40° and diminishing the VC to values under 30% of predicted norms(47).

Scoliosis develops early in childhood in patients with SMA and the most common treatment approach is to limit progression of their irreversible curvature by total contact plastic thoracolumbar bracing, allowing normal early vertebral growth followed by spinal instrumentation and fusion (48–50). Failure to prevent scoliosis results in a variety of sequelae, including loss of the sitting ability concomitantly associated with protrusion of the ribs into the abdominal wall, loss of balance and comfort when seated, the need for custom seating, modifications, low back pain, compressive lumbar radiculopathy, ischial bone compression with acute discomfort, and skin breakdown (51–56). Spinal fusion should be reserved for children seeking a permanent solution to reduce a scoliotic curve.

Prevention of Cardiac Complications

Holter monitoring should be performed on a regular basis in conjunction with other standard studies of cardiac function such as chest radiographs, electrocardiography, and either echocardiography or radioscintigraphy scanning in patients with Emery-Dreifuss muscular dystrophy (EDMD), because they can have life-threatening cardiac arrhythmias, even in the presence of normal cardiac ejection. There is little, if any, evidence that cardiac arrhythmias pose a serious risk in patients with other dystrophies or myopathies, except when the ejection fraction (EF) is diminished, which is indicative of advanced cardiomyopathy.

Neuroendocrine activation triggered by subclinical heart failure (57, 58), norepinephrine (NE), and plasma atrial and brain natriuretic peptide concentrations, useful in the evaluation of heart failure and monitoring treatment, correlates with the severity of dilated cardiomyopathy and congestive heart failure (CHF) (58–64). Serum NE concentration is also an independent predictor of prognosis for patients with CHF (63, 64). Atrial natriuretic peptide levels, which are normally 10 pg./mL in young adults, increase as a function of cardiothoracic ratio and with the ratio of the pre-ejection period to left ventricular ejection time (LVEF). Atrial natriuretic peptide concentrations increase in DMD patients when LVEF decreases below 40% (65). Use of cardioprotective medications, including a beta-blocker, angiotensin-converting enzyme inhibitor, and possibly spironolactone for patients with decreased LV function, with or without CHF, significantly improves LVEF and normalizes neuroendocrine levels (66). These medications may need to be temporarily discontinued for patients in acute CHF, but once stabilized they should be carefully re-instituted (67).

Patients with severe LV dysfunction are at risk for developing mural thrombi and embolic complications. The correction of chronic hypercapnia with the use of inspiratory muscle aids is useful in reversing cor pulmonale and right ventricular failure (68). Patients with DMD rarely require anti-coagulation therapy because the absence of dystrophin in their platelet cell walls impairs blood clotting (69).

STAGE OF PROLONGED SURVIVAL

Facilitation of Activities of Daily Living

Arm Function

Arm weakness parallels leg and diaphragm weakness in patients with neuromuscular disease. By age 13 the strength of arm muscle groups in patients with DMD was only 4% of normal (70). Affected patients lose the ability to feed themselves by late adolescence when substituted movements, such as flexion of the trunk to meet the hand, balance of the forearm on the tip of the elbow, and use of the forearm to act as a lever using the fingers to crawl up the opposite arm, no longer work. A variety of mechanical systems are useful for

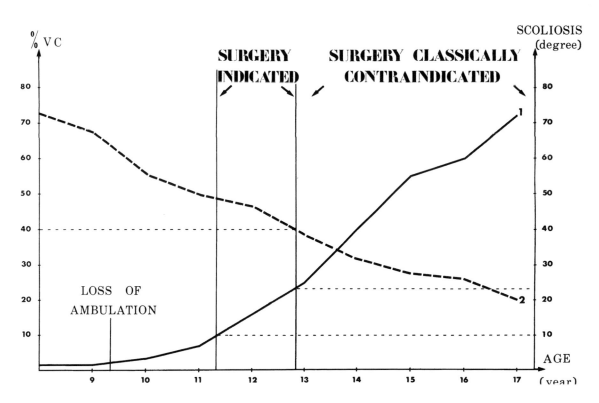

FIG. 2. This plot of vital capacity (VC) versus degree of scoliosis over time for boys with DMD and low plateau VCs. One in 3 DMD patients have VC plateau below 1,600 mL before 14 years of age demonstrating further that by the time scoliosis reaches 23°, the VC will have decreased to 40% of predicted normal. The ideal surgical window is presented (between the solid lines).

self-feeding, including a counterweighted overhead sling, motorized arm suspension system (70), ball-bearing forearm orthosis, and mobile arm support (71), the latter requiring adequate elbow flexor strength (69). When these are no longer adequate because of progressive weakness, finger-operated robotic arms mounted on a wheelchair (Figure 3) (72, 73), finger-controlled motorized wheelchairs, and environmental control systems allow patients to continue to feed themselves and perform many other arm activities.

Other useful adaptive aids include a long-handled comb, brushes and sponges, toilet paper holder, shoe horn, flexible shower hose, shower–tub transfer seat; grab bar, elevated toilet seat, and bedside commode chair, hos-

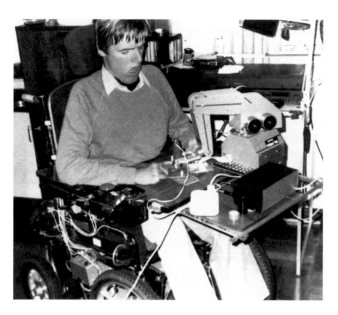

FIG. 3. DMD patient using a robot manipulator.

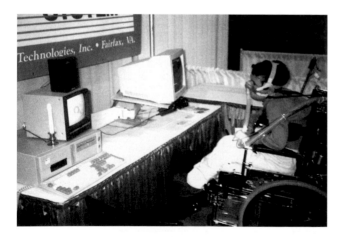

FIG. 4. The gaze of the user's eye on the computer screen (right monitor) is followed (left monitor) and triggers the computer.

pital bed, dressing and kitchen aids, and hydraulic lifts (74). The latter can be useful for transfers and to facilitate bowel evacuation. A patient placed onto a lift with a central cutout seat area, with the buttocks slowly lowered to the commode and the feet placed on the floor and thighs into an abdomen–bowel evacuation position, can greatly improve bowel evacuation function and time. Condom drainage systems can increase independence. Frequent turning of severely disabled patients in bed at night can be eliminated by use of a bed or mattress that slowly turns the patient from side to side. Occupational therapy home visits aid the physician in prescribing the most useful devices and home modifications. Other assistive devices promote, opportunities for professional education and employment (75). Patients with functional forearm musculature who have severe shoulder weakness, such as those with facioscapulohumeral (FSH) muscular dystrophy, may benefit from scapular stabilization to the ribcage and scapula-fixing orthoses to prevent winging, permitting arm abduction, and flexion to greater than 90°.

Communication

The selection of an appropriate communication system depends on the disease and stage of evolution. Non-electronic communication systems such as simple pencil and paper, letter and phrase boards, and direct selection techniques using eye movements are easily accessible to many patients and often adequate enough for most situations. Patients with SMA type I and ALS who become aphonic can learn to use a personal computer with keyboard emulator software to drive a voice synthesizer and printer (76). Simple blinking can operate an eye switch activated by infrared limbus pupil reflection, and electro-ocular switches may also be used (77). The Eye Gaze SystemTM (LC Technologies, Inc., Fairfax, VA) (Figure 4) is an integrated system that provides access to the electronic devices in the patient's environment but requires careful positioning for accurate use. Bach and coworkers (2) studied 22 patients with aphonia and ALS who were dependent on 24-hour ventilatory support for an average of 2.8 years while communicating with personal computer/voice synthesizer systems. Five patients used the system for over five years, among them one who used technologic aids for ten years earning a living by writing prose and poetry for a greeting card manufacturer. The ability to communicate no doubt enhances the psychological outlook and longevity of affected patients and may even have a salutary benefit on survival (78).

Mobility

Patients with good trunk stability and forearm function, particularly those with poor endurance, benefit from a motorized scooter with an elevated seat to facilitate transfers, attached baskets for carrying objects, and possibly ventilator trays. Scooters can be readily disassembled into three or four pieces of maximal weight 40 pounds and placed into the trunk or back seat of an automobile. Adapted strollers are available for children who are unable or too young to propel a wheelchair and require positioning support, however, their complexity varies. Like wheelchairs, the bases can have an option that allows the parent to recline a child as necessary, and with some, the base can be quickly reversed to permit parents to conveniently reposition children.

For maximal efficiency, wheelchairs should be of proper size and have accessories to increase the function and quality of life of the user. The value of the wheelchair to the physically challenged individual cannot be overstated. Wheelchair prescription is appropriate for long-distance travel, through shopping malls, along areas of uneven terrain, and at outdoor events for those with poor endurance, stance, and balance but who can otherwise walk with a cane, walker, or orthosis.

The ideal wheelchair is a light folding type for ease of transfer in an automobile. More substantial manual and powered wheelchairs are indicated for patients with greater walking difficulties. The patient must be measured for proper fit, and coat and orthotic use must be considered when applicable. Most wheelchairs have an overall width of 24 to 28 inches. Wider, more heavily constructed chairs can be made for obese individuals. A seat belt should be used for those with poor sitting balance or weak trunk musculature.

Two types of lightweight wheelchairs are available, one rigid and others with non-rigid frames. A rigid-framed chair has a solid immovable base and an axis that connects one wheel to the other. They are suited for the active individuals who expect to use it on a variety of uneven terrains. The solid axis provides more stability, a smoother ride, and is more durable. Such wheelchairs support more weight and accessories like ventilators and robot arms. A disadvantage of the rigid-frame wheelchair is that it cannot be folded and placed into a car. However, the pin-and-lock configuration of quick-release wheels permits rapid wheel removal to decrease the diameter of the chair in half for storage in the automobile trunk. Wheelchairs with a non-rigid frame have a cross-bar connecting one side of the wheelchair to the other. They fold to decrease their width in half. The cross-frame, however, wears out with use, compromising the integrity and stability of the wheelchair. Nevertheless, wheelchair users may prefer a cross-frame wheelchair because of its convenience. Both options should be tried to determine the one most appropriate for the user lifestyle and environmental restrictions.

Patients with neuromuscular conditions require adjustable removable leg rests with heel straps, offset foot plates and heel loops are used for those with severe ankle and foot deformities. The feet are maintained flat on the plates to discourage further deformity. Elevated foot rests increase the turning radius of the wheelchair and are generally used in conjunction with a reclining back in the presence of lower extremity edema, postural hypotension, and pressure sores that cannot be managed effectively in other ways. Individuals with poor endurance often benefit from a reclining seat because the ability to recline with extended knees reduces the tendency to develop flexion contractures of the knees and hips, and allows the user to rest more comfortably. Neck and head supports are necessary for individuals with advanced ALS, infantile SMA, and DMD. Neck rests with a forehead strap provide both lateral and anterior-posterior support. The user has the option of having full-length wheelchair arms or desk arms. Desk arms are preferable because they permit the user to approach and use tables. Full-length arms may be useful to support a lap board to facilitate the performance of schoolwork, gainful employment, and recreational activities. Elevated arm rests, rarely required by users with neuromuscular weakness, are fashioned to be removable to facilitate transfers. Special seating modifications are often required depending upon the type of weakness, instability, and deformity of the trunk, pelvis, and spine.

The individual must be positioned and aligned properly to discourage pelvic obliquity. A proper seating system can provide a stable surface while accommodating prominences or pelvic obliquity. The pelvis can be supported by a firm seat cushion supporting both ischia to keep the pelvis level and balanced. Several seating systems should be tried for comfort and function before one is prescribed. Commercially available seating systems include the RohoTM (Roho Inc., Belleville, IL), JayTM (Jay Medical Ltd., Boulder, CO), and Avant, MI (Invacare, Inc., Elyria, OH) systems. Wedges, padded inserts, and lateral trunk supports maximize comfort. The seats can be fully contoured for patients with severe deformity (79). Some seating systems permit the user to vary their sitting positions by adjusting the upright sitting posture to increase head and upper extremity control and to reduce skin pressure and pressure ulcers. The "Tilt-in-Space™" system (La Bac Systems, Inc., Denver, CO) shifts the user and the wheelchair seat and back simultaneously to change the seating orientation and shift skin pressures. Users can operate the tilt themselves via a switch.

Similar considerations for standard wheelchairs apply to motorized wheelchairs. Motorized wheelchairs have operation systems that must be chosen to satisfy the needs of the particular patient. For example, a front-wheel-drive wheelchair is more maneuverable in the confined spaces of the home, whereas a rear-wheel drive grips the ground better and is superior for outdoor use. When finger function is present, power wheelchairs can be operated by joystick controls. Tongue, chin, and sip-and-puff controls are usually used. When neck, finger, and lip musculature are inadequate, any volitional muscle activity can be adapted to

neck are too weak to grab a mouthpiece and IAPV is ineffective. A common mistake is not plugging the exhalation ports of a nasal interface designed for continuous and bi-level PAP delivery when using the same nasal interface on an active ventilator circuit. Although nasal interfaces are on the market without portals specifically used with active ventilator circuits and exhalation valves, there are many other styles of nasal interfaces with portals. During sleep, central nervous system-mediated reflex muscle activity cuts off excessive air leakage and reverses leakage-associated oxyhemoglobin desaturations, making open systems of mouthpiece and nasal IPPV more effective (55), while closed systems of noninvasive IPPV are possible by using lip seal retention with the nose plugged or an oral–nasal interface.

ORAL–NASAL IPPV

Covering both the nose and the mouth with an oral–nasal interface is usually unnecessary. With the ventilatory drive unblunted by oxygen therapy and sedating medications, a simple mouthpiece, lip seal, and nasal IPPV are generally effective for most patients, including those with little or no measurable VC. Nonetheless, comfortable strap-retained oral–nasal interfaces are commercially available (Respironics, Murrysville, PA) Oro-nasal "mask" interfaces can, in theory, provide a closed system of ventilatory support because they cover so much of the face. However, high strap pressures are required for retention and there is a strong tendency for air to leak into the eyes. These difficulties are solved by using a nasal prong interface with the lower edge descending to cover the lips to provide a closed NIV system that requires minimal strap pressures, thereby enhancing comfort. HybridTM (DeVilbiss Healthcare) and Mirage Liberty™ (ResMed, Inc.) interfaces are examples of such designs.

GLOSSOPHARYNGEAL BREATHING

Self-administered GPB indirectly assists expiratory muscles and supports ventilation by providing large volumes of air and increasing PCF (56). It also expands the lungs to maintain elasticity and raises the volume of one's voice. Patients who master GPB awaken from sleep only to discover that their ventilators are no longer functioning. The patient is instructed to take as deep a breath as possible and then augment it by GPB. The glottis captures boluses of air and projects them into the lungs. The vocal cords close with each gulp. One breath usually consists of six to eight gulps of 60 to 200 mL each. During the training period, the efficiency of GPB is monitored spirometrically by measuring the number of milliliters of air per gulp, the gulps per breath, and breaths per minute. An excellent training manual and video

is also available (57). A GPB rate of 12 to 14 per minute provides normal tidal volumes, minute ventilation, and hours of ventilator-free time (Figure 7) even in those with little or immeasurable VC (51). The maximum depth of a GPB should approach that of the maximum insufflation capacity. Most patients with polio and spinal cord injuries (44) and others with Duchenne muscular dystrophy (DMD), can use GPB for hours of ventilator-free breathing (58) The presence of a tracheostomy tube virtually precludes successful use of GPB because even with the tube plugged, gulped air leaks around the tube and out the tracheostomy site. The safety afforded by mastering GPB justifies removal of indwelling tracheostomy tubes, especially for those unweanable from ventilatory support (12).

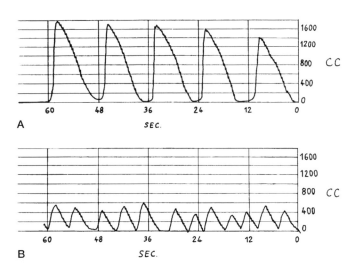

FIG. 7. Top: Glossopharyngeal breathing (GPB) minute ventilation of 8.39 L/min with GPB breaths averaging 1.67 L, 20 gulps, and 84 mL/gulp for each breath in a patient with a vital capacity of 0 mL. Bottom: Same patient using GPB at usual tidal volumes with minute ventilation of 4.76 L/min, 12.5 breaths, average eight gulps per breath, and 47.5 mL/gulp performed over a 1-minute period. From reference 51, with permission.

OXIMETRY MONITORING AND BIOFEEDBACK

Hypercapneic patients and those converted from tracheostomy to noninvasive IPPV can use oximetry as feedback to guide in the use of mouthpiece and nasal IPPV. The oxygen saturation pressure (SpO_2) alarm is set from 93 to 94%, and the patient is instructed to take a deeper breath to normalize the SpO_2 and then to take mouthpiece IPPV-assisted breaths when tired. Over time, patients with progressive muscular weakness spend longer periods of time on IPPV to maintain adequate ventilation and normal SpO_2, even up to 24 hours day, often without requiring hospitalization. In this manner, oximetry feedback can also be used to reset central ventilatory drive. Oximetry feedback can be particularly useful in the management of upper respiratory tract infections (6–8). In patients that use nasal IPPV during sleep, decreases in SpO_2 can be caused by obstruction to flow by nasal congestion and secretions. Oral nasal decongestants may be helpful. Patients can switch to lip seal IPPV or other noninvasive aids guided by nocturnal SpO_2 monitoring (12, 59).

Patients with a maximum assisted PCF of less than 5 L/sec should undergo continuous daytime SpO_2 monitoring during respiratory tract infections. When the SpO_2 decreases below 95%, either non-invasive IPPV or mechanically or manually assisted coughs are used as needed to eliminate airway secretions and return SpO_2 to normal. Thus, oximetry-guided use of respiratory aids prevents prolonged decrease in SpO_2 and respiratory failure. Oximetry screens for hypoventilation, mucous plugging, atelectasis, pneumonia, and other intrinsic lung conditions. Dehydration or decreases in SpO_2 baseline below 95% can indicate the need for more formal evaluation with chest x-ray and possible hospitalization.

EXTUBATION OF UNWEANABLE PATIENTS

Oximetry monitoring and biofeedback protocols prevents pneumonia and hospitalization for respiratory failure (6, 8). However, it is at times, insufficient (60). One extubation protocol (61) employing NIV support with mechanically assisted coughing was used to successfully extubate more than 150 unweanable patients, most of whom were transferred from another hospital that had failed multiple extubation attempts. Only two such patients with advanced bulbar-ALS failed extubation.

MAINTENANCE OF RESPIRATORY MUSCLE STRENGTH AND ENDURANCE

Inspiratory resistive exercise training improves respiratory muscle endurance but has not been shown to increase VC, maximum inspiratory, or expiratory pressures (62–64). The degree of improvement in endurance correlates with the level of VC and maximum inspiratory pressure (MIP) at the outset of training but no patient with less than 30% of predicted VC improved (62). This is the level of VC that correlates with risk of mucous plug-associated respiratory failure, often requiring nocturnal ventilatory assistance (36). Unfortunately, the improvement in endurance does not delay deterioration in respiratory muscle function or the need for ventilator use, especially patients in whom decreases in VC and inspiratory pressures may proceed rapidly despite training (65, 66).

COUNSELING

Counseling is needed to explain the options of early use and effective use of physical medicine respiratory muscle aids and other physical interventions to facilitate rehabilitation. Patients should be cautioned to avoid obesity, heavy meals, extremes of temperature and high humidity, excessive fatigue, home oxygen use, crowded areas, and exposure to respiratory tract pathogens and sedating medication. Early and appropriate attention during intercurrent respiratory tract infections with the oximetry-noninvasive IPPV-assisted coughing protocol should be reinforced. The need for influenza and bacterial vaccinations and even antiviral agents such as amantadine should be considered. Patients with progressive neuromuscular diseases can have now greatly increased survival and need to be counseled and encouraged to fulfill goal-oriented activities and future plans.

REFERENCES

1. Bach JR. Update and perspectives on noninvasive respiratory muscle aids. Part 1. The inspiratory muscle aids. *Chest* 1994; 105:1230–1240.
2. Bach JR. Ventilator use by muscular dystrophy association patients: an update. *Arch Phys Med Rehabil* 1992; 73:179–183.
3. Bach JR, Chaudhry SS. Management approaches in muscular dystrophy association clinics. *Am J Phys Med Rehabil* 2000; 79:193–196.
4. Bach JR. A comparison of long-term ventilatory support alternatives from the perspective of the patient and care giver. *Chest* 1993; 104:1702–1706.
5. Bach JR. Pulmonary rehabilitation. In: DeLisa JD, ed. *Rehabilitation Medicine: Principles and Practice.* Philadelphia: J.B. Lippincott, 1993; 952–972.
6. Bach JR, Baird JS, Plosky D, Nevado J, Weaver B. Spinal muscular atrophy type 1: management and outcomes. *Pediatr Pulmonol* 2002; 34:16–22.
7. Bach JR. Amyotrophic lateral sclerosis: prolongation of life by noninvasive respiratory aids. *Chest* 2002; 122:92–98.
8. Gomez-Merino E, Sancho J, Marin J, et al. Mechanical insufflation-exsufflation: pressure, volume, and flow relationships and the adequacy of manufacturer's guidelines. *Am J Phys Med Rehabil* 2002; 81:579–583.
9. Kang SW, Bach JR. Maximum insufflation capacity. *Chest* 2000; 118:61–65.
10. Miller WF: Rehabilitation of patients with chronic obstructive lung disease. *Med Clin North Am* 1967; 51:349–361.
11. Bach JR, Rajalaman R, Ballanger F, et al. Neuromuscular ventilatory insufficiency: the effect of home mechanical ventilator

use vs. oxygen therapy on pneumonia and hospitalization rates. *Am Phys Med Rehabil* 1998; 77:8–19.

12. Bach JR, Saporito LR. Criteria for extubation and tracheostomy tube removal for patients with ventilatory failure: a different approach to weaning. *Chest* 1996; 110:1566–1574.

13. Mohsenin V, Ferranti R, Loke JS. Nutrition for the respiratory insufficient patient. *Eur Respir J* 1989; 2:663s–665s.

14. Leonard C, Criner GJ. Swallowing function in patients with tracheostomy receiving prolonged mechanical ventilation. International Conference on Pulmonary Rehabilitation and Home Ventilation. Abstracts. 1991; 58.

15. Pineda HD. Rehabilitation management of pulmonary/respiratory diseases. In: Goodgold J, ed. *Rehabilitation Medicine*. St. Louis: C.V. Mosby, 1988; 374–383.

16. Graham WGB, Bradley DA. Efficacy of chest physiotherapy and intermittent positive-pressure breathing in the resolution of pneumonia. *N Engl J Med* 1978; 299:624–627.

17. Kirilloff LH, Owens GR, Rogers RM, Mazzocco MC. Does chest physical therapy work. *Chest* 1985; 88:436–444.

18. Make B. Pulmonary rehabilitation: myth or reality? *Clin Chest Med* 1986; 7:519–540.

19. van der Schans CP, Piers DA, Postma DS. Effect of manual percussion on tracheobronchial clearance in patients with chronic airflow obstruction and excessive tracheobronchial secretions. *Thorax* 1986; 41:448–452.

20. Connors AF, Hammon WE, Martin RJ, et al. Chest physical therapy: the immediate effect on oxygenation in acutely ill patients. *Chest* 1980; 78:559–564.

21. Eid N, Buchheit J, Neuling M, Phelps H. Chest physiotherapy in review. *Respir Care* 1991; 36:270–282.

22. De Boeck C, Zinman R. Cough versus chest physiotherapy: a comparison of the acute effects on pulmonary function in patients with cystic fibrosis. *Am Rev Respir Dis* 1984; 129:182–184.

23. Massery M. Manual breathing and coughing aids. *Phys Med Rehabil Clin North Am* 1996; 2:407–422.

24. Bach JR. Mechanical insufflation-exsufflation: comparison of peak expiratory flows with manually assisted and unassisted coughing techniques. *Chest* 1993; 104:1553–1562.

25. Bach JR, O'Brien J, Krotenberg R, et al. Management of end stage respiratory failure in Duchenne muscular dystrophy. *Muscle Nerve* 1987; 10:177–182.

26. Barach AL, Beck GJ, Bickerman HA, Seanor HE. Physical methods simulating cough mechanisms. *JAMA* 1952; 150:1380–1385.

27. Barach AL, Beck GJ, Smith RH. Mechanical production of expiratory flow rates surpassing the capacity of human coughing. *Am J Med Sci* 1953; 226:241–248.

28. Barach AL, Beck GJ. Exsufflation with negative pressure: physiological studies in poliomyelitis, bronchial asthma, pulmonary emphysema, and bronchiectasis. *Arch Intern Med* 1954; 93:825–841.

29. Suri P, Burns SP, Bach JR. Pneumothorax associated with mechanical insufflation-exsufflation and related factors. *Am J Phys Med Rehabil* 2008; 87:951–955.

30. Corrado A, Gorini M, De Paola E: Alternative techniques for managing acute neuromuscular respiratory failure. *Semin Neurol* 1995; 15:84–89.

31. Splaingard ML, Frates RC, Jefferson LS, et al. Home negative pressure ventilation: report of 20 years of experience in patients with neuromuscular disease. *Arch Phys Med Rehabil* 1985; 66:239–242.

32. Curran FJ, Colbert AP. Ventilator management in Duchenne muscular dystrophy and postpoliomyelitis syndrome: twelve years' experience. *Arch Phys Med Rehabil* 1989; 70:180–185.

33. Bach JR, Alba AS, Saporito LR. Intermittent positive pressure ventilation via the mouth as an alternative to tracheostomy for 257 ventilator users. *Chest* 1993; 103:174–182.

34. Goldstein RS, Molotiu N, Skrastins R, et al. Assisting ventilation in respiratory failure by negative pressure ventilation and by rocking bed. *Chest* 1987; 92:470–474.

35. Bach JR, Penek J. Obstructive sleep apnea complicating negative pressure ventilatory support in patients with chronic paralytic/restrictive ventilatory dysfunction. *Chest* 1991; 99:1386–1393.

36. Bach JR, Alba AS. Management of chronic alveolar hypoventilation by nasal ventilation. *Chest* 1990; 97:52–57.

37. Bach JR, Alba AS, Bohatiuk, et al. Mouth intermittent positive pressure ventilation in the management of post-polio respiratory insufficiency. *Chest* 1987; 91:859–864.

38. Baydur A, Gilgoff I, Prentice W, et al. Decline in respiratory function and experience with long-term assisted ventilation in advanced Duchenne's muscular dystrophy. *Chest* 1990; 97:884–889.

39. Bach JR. Prevention of morbidity and mortality with the use of physical medicine aids. In: Bach JR, ed. *Pulmonary Rehabilitation: the Obstructive and Paralytic Conditions*. Philadelphia: Hanley & Belfus, 1996; 303–329.

40. Bach JR, Alba AS. Total ventilatory support by the intermittent abdominal pressure ventilator. *Chest* 1991; 99:630–636.

41. Leger P, Jennequin J, Gerard M, et al. Home positive pressure ventilation via nasal mask for patients with neuromuscular weakness or restrictive lung or chest-wall disease. *Respir Care* 1989; 34:73–79.

42. Viroslav J, Rosenblatt R, Morris-Tomazevic S. Respiratory management, survival, and quality of life for high level traumatic tetraplegics. *Respir Care Clin North Am* 1996; 2:313–322.

43. McDermott I, Bach JR, Parker C, et al. Custom-fabricated interfaces for intermittent positive pressure ventilation. *Int J Prosthodont* 1989; 2:224–233.

44. Bach JR, Alba AS. Noninvasive options for ventilatory support of the traumatic high level quadriplegic. *Chest* 1990; 98:613–619.

45. Carroll N, Branthwaite MA. Control of nocturnal hypoventilation by nasal intermittent positive pressure ventilation. *Thorax* 1988; 43:349–353.

46. Ellis ER, Bye PTP, Bruderer JW, et al. Treatment of respiratory failure during sleep in patients with neuromuscular disease, positive-pressure ventilation through a nose mask. *Am Rev Respir Dis* 1987; 135:148–152.

47. Kerby GR, Mayer LS, Pingleton SK. Nocturnal positive pressure ventilation via nasal mask. *Am Rev Respir Dis* 1987; 135:738–740.

48. Bach JR, McDermott I. Strapless oral-nasal interfaces for positive pressure ventilation. *Arch Phys Med Rehabil* 1990; 71:908–911.

49. Ratzka A. Uberdruckbeatmung durch Mundstuck. In: Frehse U, ed. *Spatfolgen nach Poliomyelitis: Chronische Unterbeatmung und Moglichkeiten selbstbestimmter Lebensfuhrung Schwerbehinderter*. Munchen, West Germany: Pfennigparade eV, 1989; 149.

50. Goldstein RS, Avendano MA. Long-term mechanical ventilation as elective therapy: clinical status and future prospects. *Respir Care* 1991; 36:297–304.

51. Bach JR, Alba AS, Bodofsky E, et al. Glossopharyngeal breathing and non-invasive aids in the management of post-polio respiratory insufficiency. *Birth Defects* 1987; 23:99–113.

52. Bach JR. Alternative methods of ventilatory support for the patient with ventilatory failure due to spinal cord injury. *J Am Paraplegia Soc* 1991; 14 :158–174.

53. Delaubier A. Traitement de l'insuffisance respiratoire chronique

dans les dystrophies musculaires. In: Ridean Y, ed. *Memoires de Certificat D'etudes Superieures de Reeducation et Readaptation Fonctionnelles.* Paris: Universite R Descarte, 1984; 1–124.

54. Bach JR, Alba AS, Mosher R, et al. Intermittent positive pressure ventilation via nasal access in the management of respiratory insufficiency. *Chest* 1987; 92:168–170.

55. Bach JR. Noninvasive ventilation: mechanisms for inspiratory muscle substitution. In: Bach JR, ed. *Noninvasive Mechanical Ventilation.* Philadelphia, Hanley & Belfus. 2002; 83–102.

56. Sortor S, McKenzie M. *Toward independence: assisted cough* (video). Dallas, TX: BioScience Communications of Dallas. 1986.

57. Dail CW, Affeldt JE. *Glossopharyngeal Breathing* (video). Los Angeles, CA: Los Angeles Department of Visual Education, College of Medical Evangelists, 1954.

58. Bach JR, Bianchi C, Vidigal-Lopes M, et al. Lung inflation by glossopharyngeal breathing and "air stacking" in Duchenne muscular dystrophy. *Am J Phys Med Rehabil* 2007; 86:295–300.

59. Bach JR. Pulmonary rehabilitation considerations for Duchenne muscular dystrophy: the prolongation of life by respiratory muscle aids. *Crit Rev Phys Rehabil Med* 1992; 3:239–269.

60. Bach JR, Rajaraman R, Ballanger F, et al. Neuromuscular ventilatory insufficiency: the effect of home mechanical ventilator use vs. oxygen therapy on pneumonia and hospitalization rates. *Am J Phys Med Rehabil* 1998; 77:8–19.

61. Bach JR, Gonçalves MR, Hamdani I, et al. Extubation of unweanable patients with neuromuscular weakness: a new management paradigm. *Chest* 2010; 137:1033–1039.

62. DiMarco AF, Kelling JS, DiMarco MS, et al. The effects of inspiratory resistive training on respiratory muscle function in patients with muscular dystrophy. *Muscle Nerve* 1985; 8:284–290.

63. Martin AJ, Stern L, Yeates J, et al. Respiratory muscle training in Duchenne muscular dystrophy. *Dev Med Child Neurol* 1986; 28:314–318.

64. Rodillo E, Noble-Jamieson CM, Aber V, et al. Respiratory muscle training in Duchenne muscular dystrophy. *Arch Dis Child* 1989; 64:736–738.

65. Smith PEM, Coakley JH, Edwards RHT. Respiratory muscle training in Duchenne muscular dystrophy [Letter]. *Muscle Nerve* 1988; 11:784–785.

66. Schiffman PL, Belsh JM. Effect of inspiratory resistance and theophylline on respiratory muscle strength in patients with amyotrophic lateral sclerosis. *Am Rev Respir Dis* 1989; 139:1418–1423.

CHAPTER 65

Motor Aspects of Childhood Sleep Disorders

Thornton B.A. Mason II

Pediatric sleep medicine is a relatively new field that has advanced in the past decade with standardization of diagnostic studies and their evaluation, and the recognition that potentially treatable sleep disorders occur in all ages of childhood (1). This chapter is an overview of the motor sequelae of childhood sleep disorders.

EPIDEMIOLOGY

The overall frequency of an International Classification of Diseases, 9th Revision (ICD-9) diagnosis of sleep disorder (SD) was 3.7% in a large study cohort of mean age seven years, according to one epidemiological study (2). The prevalence of obstructive sleep apnea (OSA) syndrome (3) and restless legs syndrome (RLS) (4), each estimated to occur in about 2% of normal children, approaches 70% for sleep-related disorders in those with underlying neuromuscular disease such as spinal muscular atrophy (5) and Duchenne muscular dystrophy (DMD) (6). The prevalence of a specific pediatric sleep disturbance varies depending upon the stage of development of the child, which for research purposes may include five developmentally separate subgroups by age, including infancy (age 0 to 12 months), toddlers (12.1 to 47 months), preschool (4 to five years), school-aged children (6 to 12 years), and adolescence (13 to 18 years), each with associated characteristic sleep disorders. The commonest SD by ICD-9 code in a pediatric primary care study cohort of 154,957 children sub-grouped by age and developmental stage (2) was "sleep disorder not otherwise specified" (SD-NOS), perhaps reflecting a variety of sleep initiation and sleep maintenance issues. Other prominent diagnoses included nocturnal enuresis, sleep-disordered breathing, and infant apnea, which may be more common in those born prematurely.

Overall, sleep disorders increased respectively with age and developmental stages from 0.5% in infancy to 1.6% in preschool-aged children, emphasizing the challenge of parents and pediatricians alike to accurately report and document the occurrence of SD. In comparison, among one study cohort of 10,523 families, 1.9% of 8 to 11-year-olds met criteria for RLS as did 2% of 12 to 17-year-olds, the frequency of which decreased with moderately or severely distressing RLS symptoms, so noted, respectively in .5% and 1% of children in increasing age groups (4).

METHODS TO STUDY SLEEP

Sleep patterns can be evaluated subjectively employing questionnaires and objectively through polysomonography. Patterns of activity and inferred wakefulness can be demonstrated by actigraphy.

Questionnaires

Questionnaires have been developed specifically for pediatric sleep medicine to capture multiple aspects of sleep patterns, quality, and duration as well as specialized disturbances such as sleep disordered breathing (SDB) (7, 8). Depending upon the specific study design or clinical application as well as the patient's age and intellectual development, questionnaires can be administered to the patient directly or completed by a parent or guardian. Parental knowledge of the child's sleep patterns and features may be limited, in part due to infrequent observation of a segment of a given sleep cycle. While reported loud snoring, gasping, and pauses in breathing supports the diagnosis of OSA syndrome, hypoventilation indicative of central sleep apnea (CSA) syndrome may be much harder for parents to identify. Questionnaires also fail to reliably identify children with periodic limb movements in sleep. Observations of snoring and home-based pulse oximeter monitoring are also challenging since models of the latter typically do not store overnight data or provide graphic summaries. Small wristwatch-like accelerometers that record motion, termed actigraphs, infer periods of wakefulness and sleep over multiple days at home (9), and when paired with concurrent sleep diaries can help establish insufficient sleep duration due to inadequate sleep hygiene or circadian rhythm sleep disorders, such as delayed sleep phase syndrome. Those with SDB, however, can also have cycles of awakenings overnight with apparent sleep disruption. Moreover, some patients may have limited awakenings despite severe sleep apnea.

Polysomnography

The gold standard for evaluating sleep is overnight polysomnography ideally performed in an attended sleep laboratory (10). Standard pediatric polysomnography entails the noninvasive monitoring of multiple physiological signals, including electroencephalography (EEG), electo-oculograms (EOG), airflow by nasal pressure transducer and thermistor, electromyography (EMG) of the submentalis and tibialis anterior muscle groups, electrocardiography (EKG), chest and abdominal respiratory efforts, end-tidal and transcutaneous carbon dioxide (CO_2), and pulse oximetry, as well as therapeutic interventions such as the administration of supplemental oxygen or continuous positive airway pressure (CPAP). There are standardized protocols for analyzing polysomnograms, including the staging of sleep and scoring of discrete respiratory events (11). Although the simultaneous monitoring of so many parameters requires that a large number of sensors be attached to the head, face, chest, abdomen, and legs, and the child is then expected to sleep overnight in an unfamiliar environment, the vast majority of patients and families report the polysomnography experience to be satisfactory with no psychological sequel (12).

The total number of obstructive events, including obstructive apneas, hypopneas, and mixed apneas, divided by the total sleep time in hours, determines the obstructive sleep apnea index. An arousal index is calculated by counting the total number of arousals and awakenings in an hour of sleep, whereas sleep efficiency is calculated by dividing total sleep time by the duration of the study. Severe obstructive sleep apnea is defined by a high obstructive sleep apnea index; in many patients, there is also marked oxyhemoglobin desaturation, and elevated CO_2 values. Highly frag-

mented sleep, indicated by increased arousal and awakening indices, may also be seen, but sleep architecture is often less affected in children compared to adults. Although CO_2 values are not typically assessed in adult sleep labs, end-tidal and transcutaneous CO_2 measurements are important in the study of SDB. Polysomnographic examples of OSA, hypopnea, and CSA are shown in Figures 1 to 3.

Periodic Limb Movements in Sleep

Periodic limb movements in sleep (PLMS), once termed nocturnal myoclonus, occurs as rhythmic extensions of the great toe, with ankle dorsiflexion and knee and hip flexion. The movements occur in series, with clusters lasting minutes to hours. The diagnosis of PLMS is established through overnight polysomnography by scoring anterior tibialis EMG activity during sleep using standard criteria (11). Some movements are associated with definite EEG arousals while others may have related but subtle autonomic changes affecting heart rate and blood pressure. If frequent, the arousals may result in non-restorative sleep. The occurrence of PLMS may be related to other sleep and wake complaints such as insomnia and daytime sleepiness. PLMS is increasingly more common with advancing age, and is seen in 80 to 90% of adult patients with RLS (3).

Restless Legs Syndrome

Adults with RLS often report having had symptoms as children and case series have described children as young as 18 months of age with features of RLS (13). A consensus conference from the National Institutes of Health (NIH) summarized the diagnostic criteria for RLS in children (4), the essential features of which were all four criteria as follows: 1) Urge to move the legs accompanied by uncomfortable and unpleasant sensations in the legs; 2) Such symptoms are worse in the evening than during the day, or occur only as night begins; 3) Leg complaints worsen during periods of rest or inactivity; and 4) Symptoms are partially or total relieved by movement.

In addition to the afore mentioned essential criteria, the complaints of leg discomfort must be in the child's own words, or two of three supportive features must be met, among them: 1) A sleep disturbance for age; 2) A biological parent or sibling with RLS; or 3) The presence of periodic leg movements observed five or more times per hour on polysomnography. Children and adolescents with definite RLS were significantly more likely to have growing pains, emotional distress, falling or remaining asleep, and daytime sleepiness. RLS is uncommonly diagnosed in children, with only one in four confirmed patients who reported seeking medical care for symptoms ultimately receiving a diagnosis of RLS, and rarely if ever receiving a

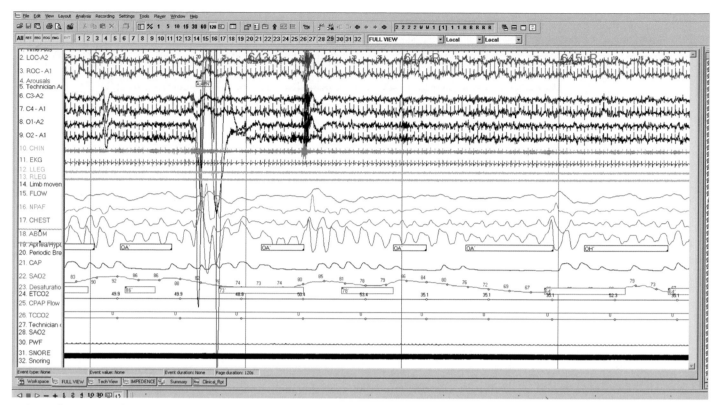

FIG. 1. Obstructive sleep apnea (OSA). Polysomnography shows severe OSA with repetitive obstructive apneic episodes (channel 19), oxygen desaturations (channels 22 and 23), and paradoxical breathing patterns (channels 17 and 18). There is further worsening of oxygen desaturations at the start of REM sleep in the second half of the figure (120 seconds view).

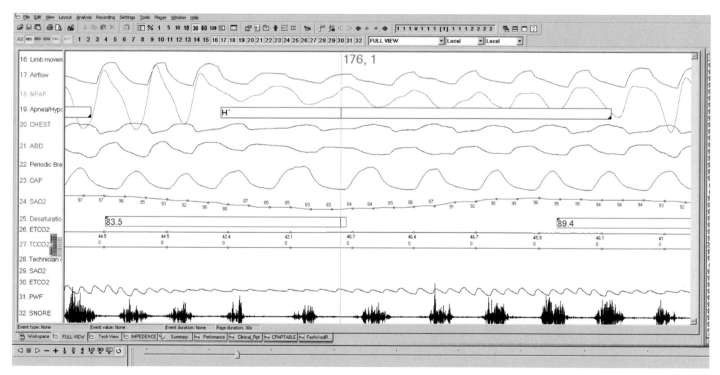

FIG. 2. Hypopnea. Polysomnography shows obstructive hypopnea (channel 19) with oxygen desaturation (channel 24) and reduced airflow amplitude of the nasal pressure transducer (channel 18). The snore signals (channel 32) are synchronous with chest and abdominal effort (channels 20 and 21).

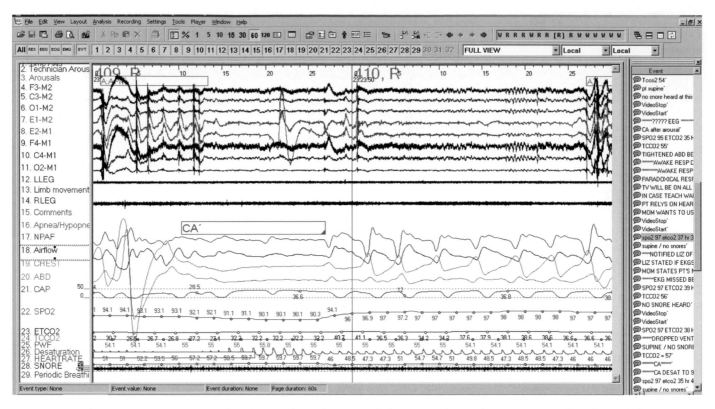

FIG. 3. Central apnea. Polysomnography shows physiologic central apnea (channel 16) associated with mild desaturation (channel 26) is evident during the first one-half part of the figure, followed by an arousal.

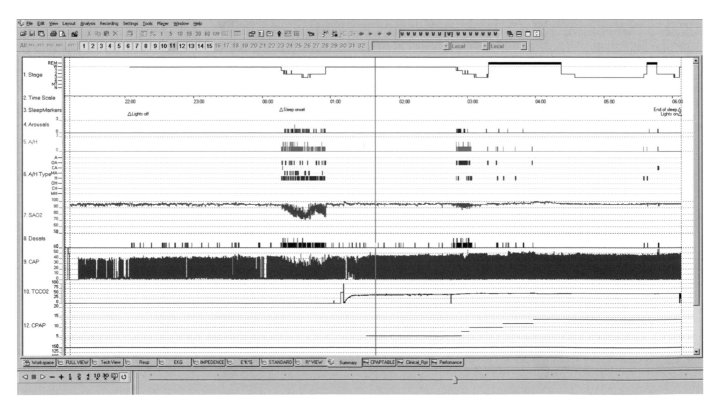

FIG 4. CPAP titration for severe obstructive sleep apnea. The hypogram tracing shows persistent desaturation (channel 7) due to OSA during the initial sleep episode, however with increasing CPAP pressures (channel 9), commencing at vertical marker, the episodes of OSA diminish concomitant with improved oxygen desaturation (channel 7).

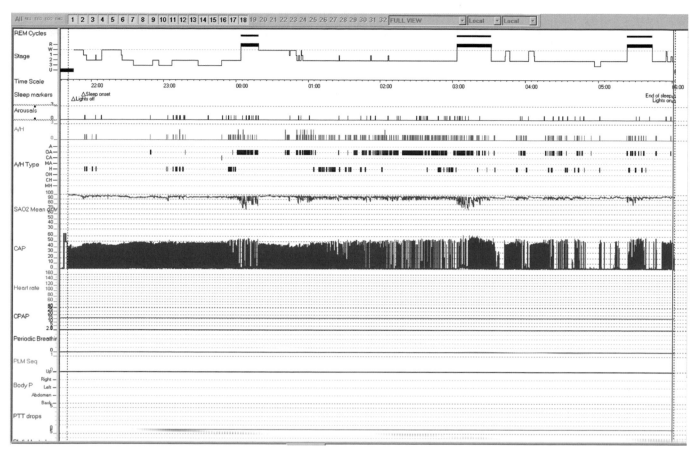

FIG. 5. Severe OSA in a teenager with Becker muscular dystrophy. The hypnogram tracing shows severe OSA with frequently scored events (OA channel) concomitant with oxygen desaturation (SAO2 channel) that cluster in REM sleep (REM cycle channel) when there is greatest physiologic vulnerability to airway obstruction. From a sleep architecture standpoint, sleep efficiency was normal as was the arousal/awakening index. There was no evidence of a surgically amenable upper airway lesion and he was rapidly initiated on CPAP therapy.

medication considered first-line treatment for RLS in the adult literature (14, 15). There have been no randomized, controlled medication trials in the pediatric population or Food and Drug Administration (FDA)-approved therapies for RLS for children. The non-pharmacologic management of children with RLS includes attention to good sleep hygiene, consideration of cognitive behavioral and relation therapies, exercise, restriction of caffeinated beverages, and screening for anemia and checking the serum ferritin level for responsiveness to elemental iron supplementation, followed by referral to a pediatric sleep center as needed to guide pharmacologic therapy. The latter in children includes the potential administration of dopaminergic agents in children with severe symptoms (16).

Sleep Apnea

Two essential types of sleep apnea are demonstrable by polysomnography, including central sleep apnea (CSA) and OSA; hypopnea is a related phenomenon. Sleep onset in normal individuals is typically accompanied by a shift in respiratory control from cortical to medullary respiratory centers with an associated 25% reduction in tidal volume (TV), a 2 to 4 Torr decrease in the partial pressure of oxygen (PaO2), and a commensurate rise in CO_2 (17). Central sleep apnea, which is defined as the absence or near absence of respiratory airflow in the setting of a decreased respiratory drive, is frequently accompanied by brief pauses in breathing that follow sighs, arousals, and movement with little or no oxygen desaturation, as well as frequent prolonged apneic episodes, increased periodic breathing, and high ventilator response to CO_2 (3).

The treatment of CSA is limited, with some patients responding to low-flow supplemental oxygen and bilevel positive airway pressure (BiPAP) and respiratory rate settings, and tracheostomy with ventilator support in the most severe patients. Central apnea of infancy usually resolves spontaneously in the first few months of life; some infants improve with methylxanthine or caffeine administration until interim brainstem maturation occurs.

The more common and treatable OSA syndrome is characterized by severely decreased or absent airflow despite progressive respiratory effort, often marked by paradoxical breathing and increasing negative intrathoracic pressures until airflow is restored, sometimes only after an arousal or awakening. Hypopneas are recognized as partially decreased airflow, particularly with snoring and labored breathing, followed by arousal and oxyhemoglobin desaturation.

Events that appear initially as a CSA due to absence of airflow and effort may be associated instead with subsequent restoration of effort with compromised flow, so-termed *mixed apneas* because of apparent central and obstructive components. Childhood OSA events are typically clustered during REM sleep, and accordingly, the partial pressure of carbon dioxide may peak during REM sleep intervals in the sleep cycle. Adenotonsillar hypertrophy, particularly in pre-school and school-aged children, macroglossia, retrognathia and micrognathia, low-lying soft palate, midface hypoplasia, nasal obstruction, deviated nasal septum, obesity, hypothyroidism, and occurrence of OSA in one or both parents, all appear to increase the risk of OSA (18). Adenotonsillectomy is the treatment of choice in otherwise healthy patients to eliminate or at least greatly improve OSA. However, since adenoidal tissue is not encapsulated and cannot be completed removed, regrowth can occur in the year after initial resection, leading to the need for reoperation, especially in children with initial symptomatic improvement. Uvulopalatopharyngioplasty and genioplasty may be performed in selected patients.

Secondary measures can include a 10 to 15% weight loss in obese patients, positional change when obstructive events occur nearly always in the supine position, maxillary expansion, and oral appliances. With progression, CPAP settings can be titrated to optimum levels using polysomnography (Figure 4), often employing respiratory flow data as well as pulse oximetry and transcutaneous CO_2 data, to accurately adjust flow rates. Continuous pressure through inspiration and expiration acts as a pneumatic splint to eliminate snoring and maintain airway patency. BiPAP therapy delivers pressures at two different settings, higher inspiratory and lower expiratory pressures, the difference between two pressures leading to improved respiratory gas exchange. It can be set to a timed mode such that a fixed number of breaths per minute are delivered during sleep for patients with significantly decreased or ineffective respiratory effort during sleep. A behavioral plan leading to gradual mask desensitization and acclimation is always necessary, commencing initially with lower pressures of 4 or 5 cm H_2O to promote acceptance, along with assurance of proper mask fit with a complete air seal. Incomplete fitting mask can lead to diminished efficacy and eye irritation. Nasal masks and nasal tubing designs are more appropriate for younger children because of concern for aspiration risk during emesis, in conjunction with a chin strap and appropriate head gear to assure optimal mask position, recognizing that overly tight ones can lead to skin breakdown and ulceration.

An ever-expanding variety of interface styles are available with a variety of styles specifically designed for younger children. Nightly CPAP units can be provided with heated humidification to reduce nasal stuffiness and irritation. Masks may need to be replaced semi-annually and tubing should regularly be inspected for damage and replaced to avoid air leaks. Secondary gastric distention can disturb sleep and may require special attention (19). A smart card technology permits download of home CPAP adherence data, such as the number of nights used and average duration of use, to help verify subjective reports of compliance, particularly when there is discordance between the parental assessment and suspected noncompliance (20).

Children with Neuromuscular Disease

Children with neuromuscular disease are at particular risk for SDB, evidenced by pulmonary function tests (PFT) that demonstrate a forced expiratory volume at one second (FEV_1) or forced vital capacity (FVC) <40% of predicted normal values, and inspiratory vital capacity (IVC) <60% predicted normal. Gradual worsening of OSA leads to digital clubbing, and right heart failure leads to cor pulmonale (17), while daytime hypercapnia with a PaCO2 level >45 Torr suggests concomitant nocturnal hypoventilation.

Children with neuromuscular diseases and weakness of pharyngeal dilator muscles of the upper airway develop increased upper airway resistance, while inspiratory muscle weakness and transient hypopnea and oxygen desaturations detected on overnight polysomnography evidences worsening OSA (Figure 5).

Patients with stable DMD can have OSA in the first decade of life followed by nocturnal hypoventilation in the second decade (17) while further disease progression is accompanied by deterioration of respiratory function with frank daytime respiratory failure and nocturnal hypoventilation (5). Accordingly, two-thirds of patients with DMD in one analysis SDB, and one-third of those with OSA improved with adenotonsillectomy, but statistical significance was only shown in improvement in the apnea-hypopnea index after commencement of CPAP (6). Children with clinically significant hypoventilation experience daytime lethargy, headaches, and anorexia (17). Their evaluation should include optimized end-tidal CO_2 recordings during polysomnography with comparison to initial waking blood gas. Polysomnography shows greater than 25% of sleep time with end-tidal CO_2 values >50 Torr range (11).

It may be difficult to separate children with coexistent non-obstructive hypoventilation and desaturation from OSA, however the former will have neither snoring nor paradoxical breathing (3). It is important to diagnose and treat

SDB since both OSA and nocturnal hypoventilation can be associated with significant morbidity and mortality. Pulmonary hypertension results from vasomotor recruitment in the pulmonary circulation in response to hypercapnia and hypoxemia, the latter of which can be managed with tracheostomy and ventilator support, whereas supplemental oxygen therapy alone should always be introduced with caution since the latter can lead to worsening of hypoventilation with CO_2 retention (19).

The cognitive and behavioral complications of OSA in children with neuromuscular disease include developmental delay, attentional difficulty, poor school performance, and aggressive behavior; less often seizures, asphyxial brain damage, and coma (3). Treatment with CPAP therapy in children with DMD leads to improved sleep quality, decreased daytime sleepiness, improved daytime gas exchange, increased independence, and a slower rate of decline in PFT indices than those untreated, along with longer survival in comparison with tracheostomy/mechanical ventilation management (21, 22). Overnight polysomnography is key in the effective titration of CPAP (10).

REFERENCES

1. Katz SL. Assessment of sleep-disordered breathing in pediatric neuromuscular diseases. *Pediatrics* 2009; 123(Suppl4):S222–S225.
2. Meltzer LJ, Johnson C, Crosette J, et al. Prevalence of diagnosed sleep disorders in pediatric primary care practices. *Pediatrics* 2010; 125:e1410–e1418.
3. AASM. International classification of sleep disorder. 2nd ed. Diagnostic and coding manual. Westchester, Illinois: *American Academy of Sleep Medicine*, 2005.
4. Picchietti D, Allen RP, Walters AS, et al. Restless legs syndrome: prevalence and impact in children and adolescents-The Peds REST Study. *Pediatrics* 2007; 120:253–266.
5. Mellies U, Dohna-Schwake C, Stehling F et al. Sleep disorderd breathing in spinal muscular atrophy. *Neuromuscul Disord* 2004; 14:797–803.
6. Suresh S, Wales P, Dakin C, et al. Sleep-related breathing disorder in Duchene muscular dystrophy: a disease spectrum in the paediatric population. *J Paediatr Child Health* 2005; 41:500–503.
7. Owens JA, Spirito A, McGuinn M. The Children's Sleep Habits Questionnaire (CSHQ): psychometric properties of a survey instrument for school-aged children. *Sleep* 2000; 23:1043–1051.
8. Chervin RD, Hedger K, Dillon JE, Pituch KJ. Pediatric sleep questionnaire (PSQ): validity and reliability of scales for sleep-disordered breathing, snoring, sleepiness, and behavioral problems. *Sleep Med* 2000; 1:21–32.
9. Souders MC, Mason TB, Valladares O, Bucan M, Levy SE, Mandell DS, et al. Sleep behaviors and sleep quality in children with autism spectrum disorders. *Sleep* 2009; 32:1566–1578.
10. Aurora RN, Zak RS, Karippot A, Lamm CI, Morgenthaler TI, Auerbach SH, et al. Practice parameters for the respiratory indications for polysomnography in children. *Sleep* 2011; 34:379–88.
11. Iber C, Ancoli-Israel S, Chesson A, Quan SF for the American Academy of Sleep Medicine. *AASM Manual fir the Scoring of Sleep and Associated Events: Rules, Terminology, and Technical Specifications.* 1st ed. Westchester, IL: American Academy of Sleep Medicine 2007.
12. Shubhadeep D, Mindell J, Millet GC, et al. Pediatric polysomnography: the patient and family perspective. *J Clin Sleep Med* 2011; 7:81–87.
13. Walters AS, Picchietti DL, Ehrenberg BL, et al. Restless legs syndrome in childhood and adolescence. *Pediatr Neurol* 1994; 11:241–245.
14. Early CJ. Clinical practice. Restless legs syndrome. *N Engl J Med* 2003; 348:2103–2109.
15. Silber MH, Ehrenberg BL, Allen RP, et al. An algorithm for the management of restless legs syndrome. *Mayo Clin Proc* 2004; 79:916–922.
16. Blum NJ, Mason TBA. Restless legs syndrome: What is a pediatrician to do? *Pediatrics* 2007; 120:438–439.
17. Katz SL. Assessment of sleep-disordered breathing in pediatric neuromuscular diseases. *Pediatrics* 2009; 123(Suppl4):S222–225.
18. Raizen DM, Mason TB, Pack AI. Genetic basis for sleep regulation and sleep disorders. *Semin Neurol* 2006; 26:467–83.
19. Wagner MH, Berry RB. Disturbed sleep in a patient with Duchenne muscular dystrophy. *J Clin Sleep Med* 2008; 4:173–175.
20. Marcus CL, Rosen G, Ward SL, Halbower AC, Sterni L, Lutz J, et al. Adherence to and effectiveness of positive airway pressure therapy in children with obstructive sleep apnea. *Pediatrics* 2006; 117:e442–451.
21. Finder JD, Birnkrant D, Carl J, Farber HJ, Gozal D, Iannaccone ST, et al. Respiratory care of the patient with Duchenne muscular dystrophy: ATS consensus statement. *Am J Respir Crit Care Med* 2004; 170:456–465.
22. Ishikawa Y, Miura T, Ishikawa Y, Aoyagi T, Ogata H, Hamada S, et al. Duchenne muscular dystrophy: survival by cardiorespiratory interventions. *Neuromuscul Disord* 21:47–51.

CHAPTER 66

Evaluation and Management of Swallowing and Voice Disorders

Celia F. Stewart, Andrew Blitzer

New and innovative perspectives and treatment have emerged in the areas of swallowing and voice treatments in motor disorders due to paralysis and paresis, Parkinson disease (PD), and hyperkinetic movement disorders (resulting in improve function and quality of life (1, 2). This chapter focuses on current methods, criteria, and outcome measures, and therapy for swallowing and voice disorders employing a team-oriented approach to management comprised of the diverse subspecialties of speech and language pathology, otolaryngology, neurology, nutrition, occupational therapy, physical therapy, and psychology.

The first section focuses on the methods for the assessment and management of dysphagia, and the second, specific issues related to flaccid, hypokinetic, and hyperkinetic voice disorders.

SWALLOWING DISORDERS

Normal Swallowing Physiology

Detailed aspects of swallowing physiology, evaluation and treatment are considered elsewhere (3). A normal swallow is a rapid, well-organized, precise, and well-synchronized process of muscle contraction and relaxations that moves the bolus of food from the lips over the tongue through the pharynx and into the esophagus. Disturbed efforts lead to coughing, choking, nasal reflux, aspiration, and regurgitation There are four swallowing phases; oral preparatory, oral proper, pharyngeal, and esophageal phases.

During the first phase, food enters the mouth and an oral seal is produced anteriorly by closing the lips and posteriorly by lowering the soft palate, preventing food or liquid from spilling out of the mouth while preparing it for later swallow. Mastication, shaping the bolus through pressing movements around the mouth, against the hard palate and teeth, and mixing it with saliva is facilitated by coordinated tongue movements. The duration of time the food remains in the mouth varies with individual preference.

During the oral or voluntary phase of swallowing the tongue holds the bolus against the palate and pushes the bolus posteriorly toward the oropharynx. Leakage into the nasopharynx is prevented by elevation of the soft palate and the opening of the entrance into the oropharynx. Sealing of the nasopharynx allows pressure to increase rapidly, moving the bolus toward the oropharynx such that when the bolus reaches the faucial pillars, the larynx is elevated, tilted anteriorly, and moved under the tongue, triggering a swallowing effort.

The pharyngeal phase classically begins when the bolus passes the point between the anterior faucial arches and where the tongue base crosses the lower rim of the mandible, interrupting respiration and inducing transient apnea until the bolus enters the esophagus, allowing the larynx to return to the resting position with abduction of the vocals. Several well-defined movements are triggered in the pharyngeal phase, including movement of the base of the tongue posteriorly as the epiglottis lowers to an inferior and posterior location and elevation of the larynx, causing the bolus to be delivered laterally away from the airway and posteriorly toward the upper esophageal sphincter (UES), while the epiglottis, aryepiglottic folds, false folds, and vocal folds protect the airway as the bolus descends into the hypopharynx.

A final involuntary phase begins as the bolus enters the esophagus, which closed at rest, pulls open, creating a negative pressure that sucks the bolus through the upper esophageal sphincter and into the esophagus. Food entering the esophagus triggers peristaltic motion, moving the bolus through the esophagus and into the stomach.

Assessment

Identification of the type of swallowing disorder and assessment of its severity requires the integration of information obtained from a detailed history of weight loss, changes in eating patterns, and food types that are difficult to swallow, as well as the findings of a targeted general and neurological examination, and instrumental assessment employing video fluoroscopic-modified barium swallow, and fiberoptic endoscopic evaluation of swallowing and sensation testing (FEESST).

Swallowing disorders associated with neurogenic disease, which impair motor control and sensory awareness, are difficult to identify due to decreased awareness of symptoms, reduced cough reflex, and impaired language skills without such detailed swallowing assessment. A cursory bedside assessment leads to incorrect estimates of aspiration (4), especially after stroke (5). A modified barium, or cookie swallow, during which the patient eats small amounts of food of different consistencies coated with barium, produces shadows of the food that are visualized. Radiographic assessment of the oral preparatory, oral, pharyngeal, and esophageal phases, that can be replayed frame-by-frame for more detailed assessment of dynamic areas of laryngeal elevation, tongue base motion, UES cricopharyngeal muscle opening or obstruction, and asynchronous muscular movements, as well as the observation and measurement of barium penetration below the glottis and into the larynx. Aspiration of more than 10% of the bolus after using compensatory strategies should prohibit consumption food with that texture type.

The efficacy of compensatory strategies such as changing position, posture, and the consistency of the bolus to facilitate swallowing can be examined. The technique of FEESST allows visualization of the pharynx, larynx, and trachea prior to, and following a swallow (6), including abnormal pooling of secretions, immobility of the vocal folds, and aspiration of secretions. It is a useful adjunctive technique to the barium swallow and in planning interventions and modification of diet (7, 8). Green dye food coloration improves visibility of the propulsion of food by the tongue base, the efficacy of the oropharyngeal contraction, clearance of the vallecula, hypopharyngeal contraction, and material from the pyriform sinuses into the larynx. FEESST performed after deliverance of a puff of air to the anterior wall of the pyriform sinus and aryepiglottic (9), predicts pharyngeal and supraglottic sensory deficits with aging (10), and silent (11) and symptomatic deficits (12) after a stroke.

Acute and Chronic Aspiration

The most dreaded outcome of a swallowing disorder is death due to aspiration pneumonia (13) triggered by aspiration of food, liquid, or secretions into the airway due to dysfunction of the normal phases of swallowing. Ill-fitting dentures, xerostomia, and disturbed motor coordination impact the oral preparatory phase. Frank aspiration during the oral phase of swallowing begins when an incohesive and improperly sized food bolus leaks posteriorly before the larynx is elevated, or if food particles remain in the mouth after the swallow. Pharyngeal dysphagia can be potentiated by cervical osteophytes, and lower (LMN) and upper motor neuron (UMN) weakness. Aspiration during the pharyngeal phase occurs when coordinated muscles fail to trigger, leading to opening of the airway, and spillage of the bolus into the valleculae, pyriform sinuses, and airway culminating in aspiration. Aspiration of the esophageal phase occurs if the upper esophageal sphincter fails to open and the food spills into the airway. Chronic aspiration into the tracheobronchial tree leads to life-threatening pulmonary disease manifested by cough, intermittent fever, recurrent tracheobronchitis, atelectasis, pneumonia, empyema, although milder symptoms of weight loss, cachexia, and dehydration may occur (14).

Treatment

In general, dysphagia therapy guides safe eating depending upon the results of the history, physical assessment, and instrumental exam. Such recommendations may change over time with objective improvement or progression of the underlying causes and compliance. Behavioral therapy includes motor exercises to strengthen the musculature; sensory stimulation, tactile and kinesthetic feedback to cue closure of the jaw and the amount and texture of the bolus. Postural changes direct the bolus toward stronger musculature while swallowing maneuvers benefit patients with mild to moderate dysphagia to maintain oral feeding. Medical and surgical treatment impacts upon the disturbed anatomy and physiology to safeguard airway function, such as surgical procedures to remove obstructing lesions, reconstruct the vocal folds, and tracheostomy. Other available options include chemodenervation and mechanical dilation of the esophagus. Carefully positioned prosthetic devices facilitate the oral preparatory and oral swallowing phases.

The type, location, and severity of the impairment will guide the different types of available therapy. Swallowing disorders restricted to the oral preparatory and oral phase can be treated initially with compensatory measures, including postural adjustments such as chin tucks to slow the movement of the food; head-up positions to speed up the flow of food, as well as improving sensory awareness, modification of food volume, texture, and degree of moisture; use of small spoons, cups, and straws; and isometric lingual exercises.

Although Individuals with unilateral hypoglossal nerve paralysis may be asymptomatic, bilateral lesions contribute to loss of bolus control and difficulty in swallowing initiation (15). Those with bilateral lingual paralysis or the secondary effects of cancer may elect placement of an intraoral prosthetic device to lower the palate and facilitate lingual contact during swallowing (16), or choose surgical correction (17). A jaw sling mechanically elevates the jaw, triggers closure of the lips and jaw, and places pressure placed on the base of the upper and lower teeth to stimulate the buccinator muscles and improve swallowing. A glide plane can attach to a lower denture further aligning the jaw. Such therapies can be supplemented with range-of- motion and strengthening exercises. Patients with PD demonstrate difficulty have with control of the food bolus due to repetitive upward and backward movements of the central portion of the tongue. This can be helped by behavioral swallowing therapy, such as laying on the stronger side, allowing gravity to pull the food toward the stronger side. Other helpful measures include reduction of the viscosity and resistance of the food bolus to move it along through the oral cavity, and gavage or nasogastric feeding.

The pharyngeal phase of swallowing may be impaired by acquired UMN, LMN, and peripheral nerve lesions. Vagal nerve deficits lead to delayed initiation of swallowing. Disturbances in the control of liquids as they pass through the pharynx, with spillage into the airway and penetration of the bolus into the nasal passages (15) are amenable to simple behavioral strategies such as turning the head toward the weakened side to direct the bolus toward the stronger side of the pharynx, and the consumption of soft and moist foods to promote adhesion of the food bolus and the facilitation of the pharyngeal phase. Mid-stage PD, is associated with delayed initiation of swallowing, incomplete closure of the laryngeal opening, food residual, and aspiration. This can be improved by the Shaker method that places patients on their backs with repetitive lifting of the head to strengthen pharyngeal muscle function and enhance opening of the upper esophageal sphincter (18). Velopharyngeal insufficiency, which results from an incomplete nasal seal, promoting decreased swallowing pressure with resultant backflow of food into the nasal passages. It is improved by the behavioral technique of thermal stimulation to increase movement of the soft palate and enhance the nasal seal, as well as, surgical pharyngeal flap, and placement of a palatal lift. The injection of space occupying material augments elevation of the soft palate and the posterior pharyngeal wall.

The pharyngeal muscles may be strengthened by thermal stimulation, supraglottic swallow procedures, and hyoid suspension with medialization, elevation, and anteriorization to improve the speed of swallowing. Incomplete closure of the laryngeal entrance is a separate risk for aspiration that can be ameliorated by vocal fold augmentation employing hyaluronic acid gel and hydroxyapatite paste, and other substances to improve vocal fold closure (19), however they are impermanent and reabsorb with time. Incomplete closure of the laryngeal entrance is treatable with thyroplasty performed under local anesthesia so the patient can phonate, swallow, and breathe while sizing and positioning for maximal efficacy. Concomitant fiberoptic instrumentation is used to observe the position of the vocal fold and the degree of closure of the glottal gap. (20). Some patients with a large posterior gap benefit from arytenoid adduction and arytenoidplasty (21). However there is divergent opinion regarding the efficacy of surgical to treat unilateral vocal cord immobility (22). Another approach to improve laryngeal closure is nerve graft employing the ansa cervicalis to improve muscle tone, glottic closure, and voice (23), which can be augmented by injection of collagen (24) and supplemented by hypopharyngeal pharyngoplasty to remove insensate and redundant pyriform sinus mucosa on the paralyzed side (25).

Patients with more severe pharyngeal phase disorders and intractable aspiration may be considered for placement of a glottic silicone prosthesis inserted via tracheostomy while sealing the glottis opening (26), or tracheo-esophageal diversion to separate the airway and food passages (27). Cuff or uncuffed tracheotomy does not improve swallowing but is the commonest way to separate and protect the airway from secretions and food substances, as well as providing direct access for good pulmonary toilet. The effectiveness of a tracheotomy tube decreases in cases of severe dysphagia when the tube restricts the elevation of the larynx (28). The airway may be surgically protected by reversible surgical separation of the larynx (29–31) but there is loss of phonation. With high tracheostomy, this separation can be done without diversion to the esophagus. When all else fails, a simple laryngectomy with externalization of the lower airway can be performed. Implantable laryngotracheal closure employing recurrent laryngeal nerve stimulation with maintenance of phonation has been described (32).

Disturbances of the esophageal phase of the swallow caused by UES dysfunction, can be treated with endoscopic botulinum toxin (BoNT) injection and endoscopic transection of the cricopharyngeal muscle at the midline via CO_2 laser at the midline. BoNT injection empirically leads to improved swallowing lasting up to 14 months. More than one-half of patients who undergo dilation experience some benefit. The effectiveness of cricopharyngeal myotomy depends upon accurate diagnosis of a hypertonic UES (33, 34).

VOICE DISORDERS

Neurologic voice disorders result from vocal fold weakness, lack of coordination, and involuntary movements and postures. They are further classifiable by age at onset, etiology, anatomic area of disturbance, and consequence on speech process. Current therapy focuses on rehabilitation of impacted respiration, phonation, resonation, and articulation. Neurological disorders may trigger disordered patterns of vocal fold vibration that result in changes in voice.

Voice Physiology

The myoelastic-aerodynamic theory provides a useful explanation for voice production (35). During quiet respiration, the vocal folds are abducted to the intermediate position by the posterior cricoarytenoid. Following inhalation and exhalation in preparation for phonation, the vocal folds simultaneously stiffen and adduct enough to vibrate without touching to prepare for phonation. As a puff of air passes between the vocal folds through a narrow opening, a slight negative pressure is generated and the vocal folds are sucked together. Medial movement of the membranous portion of the vocal folds close the glottis and block the flow of air. Building pressure under the vocal folds eventually blows them apart and elastically bringing them back together. Once oscillation begins, ongoing vibration results from the balance between transglottal pressure and stiffness of the vocal folds, with subtle changes of the vocal folds during voice production under control of the thyroarytenoid, lateral cricoarytenoid, and interarytenoid muscles for pitch, to adjust for loudness, and quality changes of voice.

Insights into the normal and abnormal muscular mechanisms underlying vocal fold mobility and phonation have been provided by needle electromyography (EMG), especially disorders due to flaccid muscle paralysis and mechanical vocal fold changes. Acute spontaneous activity at rest, including fibrillations and positive sharp waves, indicate acute or subacute LMN injury, although quiet baseline data of the laryngeal muscles may be technically difficult due to contemporaneous respiration, breath holding, and phonation. Laryngeal motor unit potentials (MUP) are optimally evaluated with a concentric needle, avoiding the necessity of a reference electrode, with electrode grounding over the sternum, employing a standard technique to study the thyroarytenoid-vocalis muscle complex, cricothyroid, lateral cricoarytenoid, posterior cricoarytenoid, and interarytenoid muscles at rest and with phonation.

Vagal and Recurrent Laryngeal Nerve Injury

Peripheral and LMN disorders exemplified by vagal and recurrent laryngeal nerve injury, are reviewed in detail elsewhere (36). They lead to reduced muscle tone associated sensory loss and pharyngeal paralysis with impaired vocal fold adduction and abduction, and a weak breathy voice that may be difficult to differentiate from mechanical changes that lead instead to joint fixation. Both may be associated with unilateral or bilateral absence of both adduction of the affected vocal fold during phonation and vocal fold abduction during respiration. There is rough, breathy diplophonia, poor glottal croup, and an out-of-breath sensation when talking because of the lack of glottal closure. Both laryngeal EMG and direct palpation assists in the diagnosis of vagal and recurrent laryngeal nerve injury. There may be acute and chronic denervation, and neurogenic MUP, associated with enhanced passive mobility, vocal fold bowing, abducted or paramedian positioned vocal folds, and anterior tipping of the arytenoid cartilage lowering the posterior vocal fold (37–40).

The therapy of flaccid vocal fold paralysis begins with behavioral and compensatory therapies focused on maximizing vocal fold vibration, reducing activity in extraneous muscles, optimizing breath flow and medical compression. This is balanced by decreasing the expiratory drive to match the strength of medial compression of the paralyzed vocal folds. Early injection augmentation can increase the bulk of the vocal fold and lead to optimal vocal fold repositioning. Other measures include arytenoid adduction and nerve graft. Fiberoptic-monitored surgical medialization is appropriate treatment after six months in the absence of significant reinnervation to augment closure of the glottis. The procedure is performed in the awake state to allow for optimal placement and size of the implant and to assure a louder voice, stronger cough, and improved swallow (41).

Parkinson Disease

Communicative defects and hypokinetic dysarthria occur in up to 90% of patients with PD (42). Mild dysphonia, which may a presenting feature of the disorder, occur intermittently, and are often ignored until awareness of voice symptoms develop and communication breaks. This leads to social isolation, need for repetition, and further disturbances in voice, articulation, and fluency over time (43, 44, 45).

The commonest voice symptoms associated with hypokinetic dysarthria include decreased voice loudness, monopitch and monoloud inflection, prosodic insufficiency, breathiness, hoarseness, roughness of the voice, shorter sustained phonation, and lower phonation quotients compared to normal (42, 46). Acoustic voice analysis shows increased shimmer, jitter, and harmonic-to-noise ratios. This is accompanied by excessive cycle-to-cycle variation in amplitudes of the vibrations, with excessive laryngeal noise (47) and a 4 to 7 Hz laryngeal rest tremor. Fiberoptic laryngeal examination reveals variable abnormalities, including bowing of the membranous portion of the vocal folds, incomplete adduction of the arytenoid cartilages, asymmetry of the position of the arytenoid from lack of coordinated posterior crico-arytenoid muscle activity, asymmetry of the cricothyroid muscle contraction, and tremor that coincide with a breathy voice, short phrasing, tremulous voice, weak cough, with reduced pitch and loudness (48). Individuals that attempt to compensate for these laryngeal variations and improve their voice suffer long-lasting fatigue (49). A disconnect between the timing and coordination of expiratory effort and phonation can lead to poor phonation. Intensive voice treatment leads to increased loudness and projection of their voices by improved vibratory patterns (1).

Disturbances in fluency and articulation are associated with imprecise consonants, inappropriate silences, short rushes of speech, variable speech rates, and repetition of words, phrases, and sentences. Imprecise articulation is related to improper tongue elevation to achieve complete closure on stops and inadequate constriction for fricatives. Some patients have progressive acceleration of words toward the end of a sentence similar to the festination of gait. With symptom progression, the patterns of inflection for expression of humor, sarcasm, concern, and emphasis may lessen, and talking can be laborious and frustrating. Disturbances in articulation may be accentuated by lingual weakness and fatigue (50) leading to altered range of motion, accuracy, steadiness, with increased tone of the facial, oral, and respiratory structures (51). There may be diadochokinesis of the lips, tongue, and jaw leading to imprecise and slowed articulation, even when the tempo of speech is increased. Respiration is impaired due to decreased vital capacity, irregular respiratory cycles, shallow breathing, poor synchronization, decreased voice loudness, and short phraseology.

Communication may also be impaired as a result of nonverbal spontaneous facial, hand, and body gestures, making it easier for the patient to sit passively and listen rather than participate by gesturing or speaking. Patients with PD can have word finding and fluency difficulty, resulting in excessive speech pauses, hesitations, and gaps. This decline in verbal fluency can also be related to aging (52). Despite the origin of the anomia, difficulty retrieving words can interfere with communication by causing vague speech, difficulty interjecting speech, and conversation gaps (53).

Behavioral treatment for parkinsonian hypokinetic dysarthria focuses on increasing loudness of the voice, decreasing the effort used during speech. Other means include improving respiratory support, enhancing precision of articulation, and hastening word retrieval. Reduced voice loudness, a common symptom in PD, responds well to speech therapy to increase loudness (50), and while not well understood, it is thought to be related to bowing and atrophy of the vocal folds, reduced expiratory drive, and diminished laryngeal control (50, 54). Tape recordings can be used to help the patient hear his voice and compare the loudness of his voice with that of the therapist. Breathing exercises can be employed to improve loudness by improving the speed and excursion of the muscles of respiration, as can modifications in posture to improve respiratory excursions. Strength and stamina can be enhanced by gradually lengthening utterances and increasing the complexity of the utterances, leading to a loud clearer voice. Electronic voice amplification is generally ineffective due to intelligible speech. Loudness may be affected by the Lombard effect of masking sounds in the ears. Articulation may be imprecise due to oral and facial muscle bradykinesia, decreased motor coordination, and increased pharyngeal secretions (51, 55).

Precise consonants and vowels are produced when the articulators make specific sequences of movements and make contact at specific locations. If the movements of the articulators are slow or imprecise, the lips, tongue, jaw, and soft palate will not reach their target positions and the resulting speech sounds will be imprecise. Exercises to increase the range, speed, and accuracy of the articulatory movements improves leads to improved speech intelligibility and decreases the stiffness of articulation. Articulation is adversely influenced by excessive saliva (1). Cognitive changes, which accompany PD in up to one-half of patients (56) and impact communication and word retrieval (57, 58) can be minimized by cognitive therapy.

Surgical interventions for vocal fold bowing and breathy dysphonia includes injection augmentation with hydroxyapatite paste, hyaluronic acid, and fat to improve speech loudness and maximum phonation time. However low pitch, dysarthria, and slowness of speech may persist. Type I thyroplasty or laryngeal framework surgery with medialization uses an implant to reversibly correct bowing of the vocal folds. Teflon augmentation may be employed along the middle third of the vocal fold. Respiratory involvement should prompt pulmonary function tests, room air arterial blood gas measurements, and sleep studies for potentially life-threatening apnea and respiratory dysrhythmia that may warrant tracheotomy.

HYPERKINETIC VOICE DISORDERS

Focal Laryngeal Dystonia

The dystonias are action-induced hyperkinetic motor disorders characterized by abnormal involuntary muscle contraction during skilled movement that disappears at rest. Cranial dystonias include blepharospasm, oromandibular dystonia, and spasmodic dysphonia, the latter of which is a focal laryngeal dystonia that leads to voice disturbances. It affects women more than men, typically in the fourth decade or afterward. There may be known trauma, exposure to phenothiazine drugs, head colds, flu, laryngitis, upper respiratory infections, or genetic predisposition, without known geographic, environmental, or occupational exposure. The onset may be gradual or abrupt, commencing with mild intermittent voice symptoms that gradually worsen, and persist one to three years later. Two categories of spastic dysphonia are recognized, adductor and abductor types, further discernible by direct observation of the vocal folds and the resulting voice quality. While smooth adduction and abduction movements of the vocal folds are present during quiet breathing, speech evokes involuntary adductor and abductor spasms.

The commonest symptoms of both categories of spasmodic dysphonia are a rough, breathy voice with frequent voice arrests and decreased loudness during connected speech. However, increased expiratory effort, strained-strangled voice quality, pressed voice, and increased symptoms on words initiating with vowels occur most often in adductor spasmodic dysphonia. There is often noted abductor spasmodic dysphonia including intermittent or continuous aphonic segments, and increased difficulty in words that start with voiceless sounds. Some patients with abductor spasmodic dysphonia use so much air during speech that they hyperventilate when they talk, and some speak on both inhalation and exhalation. Patients with true mixed adductor-abductor spasmodic dysphonia have both breathy and strained-strangled symptoms. They report increased effort in the throat, chest, and stomach that are, at times, more debilitating than the voice symptoms, all of which fluctuates over time and worsen in stressful speaking situations such as speaking on the telephone or in public speaking. Up to 90% of patients with spasmodic dysphonia have adductor spasmodic dysphonia leading to adductor spasms of the larynx, subclassifiable into four possible types (59). Type 1 is characterized by excessive adduction. Type II is hyperadducted vocal and ventricular folds. Type III, is forceful adduction and anterior movement of the arytenoid cartilages. Type IV is pulling forward of the arytenoid cartilages touching the pedicle of the epiglottis, causing sphincter closure of the glottis. Individuals with abductor spasmodic dysphonia have an appropriate position of the vocal folds at the start of phonation that pull open into an abducted posture during speech, and at times remain inappropriately abducted or involuntarily oscillates between abduction and adduction.

So-called mixed spasmodic dysphonia leads to a continuum of combined adductor and abductor laryngeal movements with strained, strangled, rough, and breathy voice quality with frequent breaks (60). Patients with compensatory abductor spasmodic dysphonia volitionally produce a breathy voice by whispering but do not fully contract their vocal folds to prevent the adductor spasms of strained-strangled voice production and voice breaks. The more common

compensatory adductor spasmodic dysphonia occurs in patients with abductor spasmodic dysphonia who attempt to prevent breathiness by hyper contracting the vocal folds. Adductor breathing dystonia is a rare variant of laryngeal dystonia that occurs during respiration and results in vocal stridor and air hunger. Such patients do not become hypoxic, and the stridor abates during sleep, however, two reported patients, in addition, had paradoxical diaphragmatic and chest wall movements (61). One type of laryngeal dystonia occurs during singing with spread to the speaking voice. Several such patients with singer dystonia developed dystonic symptoms in the midrange of their singing voice as it moved from the chest to the heard voice (62).

In 1992, Blitzer and Brin (63) described the treatment of adductor and abductor spasmodic dysphonia with BoNT. A subsequent report added 133 patients with spasmodic dysphonia treated with BoNT-A and BoNT-B (64). Standard practice commences with bilateral injections, each of 1.17 units of BoNT-A toxin diluted in 0.1mL for adductor spasmodic dysphonia, and 218.6 units each of BoNT-B, followed weeks later by additional bilateral doses, gauged to meet the individual needs for voice production while reducing side effects such as breathiness, shortness of breath, and mild choking with liquids associated with adductor injections. Most patients have a good response to the injections and suffer few side effects. The usual time to effect of the BoNT is two to three days, with a peak effect by nine days and average duration of benefit of ten to eleven weeks. Following the injection there is a period of decreased vocal function that lasts about 19 days, followed by improved voice. Local pain, sore throat, slight blood-tinged sputum, and dermal itchiness, with or without a rash, can occur after an injection.

The effect of injection of BoNT is not fully understood and the response to injections cannot be entirely explained by the injection alone. While the thyroarytenoid muscle is not a laryngeal adductor, injection therein diminishes adduction of the vocal folds. Diffusion of BoNT into the lateral cricoarytenoid likely explains weakening of adduction and associated dysphagia and breathiness. The occasional improvement of dystonia outside of the larynx that occurs after treatment is likely a result of interruption of the sensory component of gamma motor neurons. In addition to improved voice, there is concomitant change in several batteries of quality of life. Since the posterior cricoarytenoid muscle is the most mobile vocal fold in abductor spasmodic dysphonia, injection therein of an initial dose of 3.75 units leads to improved voice in up to 20% of patients without breathy breaks. Some patients with abductor spasmodic dysphonia require injections into other muscles or surgical procedures to improve their voices, the latter procedure of which was associated with overall improvement in 82% of patients (63).

Short periods of behavioral voice therapy combined with BoNT treatment can help maximize vocal quality and decrease breathiness after adductor injections by balancing expiratory drive and medial compression of the vocal folds. Such therapy focuses on decreasing expiratory drive, decreasing the effort at the level of the vocal folds, coordinating the expiratory drive and the effort levels, and decreasing extraneous muscle activity in the head and neck areas. Intense vocal exercise appears to enhance laryngeal BoNT injections in spasmodic dysphonia, resulting in improved phonation (65).

Gilles de la Tourette syndrome

This hyperkinetic disorder which has been reviewed elsewhere in detail (66), presents with sudden, rapid, recurrent, non-rhythmic motor sounds and tics, including facial grimacing, sudden movements of the trunk, head, neck, shoulders, arms, and legs. Phonic tics result from involuntary contractions in the respiratory, phonatory, and articulatory subsystems that trigger involuntary simple and complex utterances. Simple phonic tics, which involve a group of muscles, result in brief isolated involuntary utterances manifested as sniffing, throat-clearing, grunting, squeaking, screaming, coughing, blowing, sucking, and burping sounds. Complex involuntary motor tics are sequenced, repetitive movements, including linguistically meaningful utterances and verbalizations, such as the shouting of obscenities or profanities termed *coprolalia*, repetition of someone else's words or phrases termed *echolalia*, and repetition of one's own utterances, particularly the last syllable, word, or phrase of sentence, termed *palilalia*.

Loud phonic tics result in excessive forces at the level of the vocal folds, leading to focal irritation, swelling, hyperemia, and nodule and polyp formation that changes their structure and triggers dysphonia in speaking and singing, leading to overall roughness, breathiness, and voice stridor. Treatment of the thyroarytenoid muscle with BoTN interrupts the cycle by decreasing the strength with which the vocal folds contract (67).

VOCAL TREMOR

Vocal tremor has been reviewed in detail elsewhere (68). This action-induced tremor occurs during phonation and is obvious in both voice and laryngeal mechanism during sustained vowel production and connected speech. Tremor of the intrinsic and extrinsic laryngeal, pharyngeal, respiratory muscles, and articulator muscles leads to involuntary, rhythmic, oscillatory changes and rhythmical variations in frequency and amplitude of vocal fold vibrations. When the vocal structures are at rest, the tremor disappears. It

occurs alone or in association with essential tremor, orthostatic tremor, PD, cerebellar ataxia, dystonia, myoclonus, motor neuron disease, developmental speech, and language deficits. Tremor of the lateral cricoarytenoid, interarytenoid, and posterior cricoarytenoid muscles cause rhythmic abduction and adduction of the vocal folds, while those of the extrinsic laryngeal and pharyngeal muscles result in rhythmical vertical and horizontal laryngeal movements. Vocal tremor can also result from changes in subglottal air pressure induced by tremor in the external and internal intercostal muscles. Vibrations in the tongue, soft palate, and jaw contribute to vocal tremor, as may gross tremors elsewhere in the body.

An essential voice tremor occurs in up to 20% of patients with essential tremor, with rhythmical oscillatory movement of 4 to 12 Hz. Vocal tremor can be the first or only symptom of the disease or it can accompany tremors in other parts of the body. When vocal tremor occurs with tremors in other parts of the body, it may parallel the onset of the other symptoms or have a sudden independent onset. The voice symptoms associated with essential tremor include rhythmic quavering in pitch and loudness, especially during sustained vowel prolongation and continuant consonants, pitch, and phonating breaks, and degraded intelligibility. Pitch breaks occur when the pitch involuntarily and abruptly shifts to a lower or higher frequency. Phonation breaks occur when phonation involuntarily ceases and have been identified with visible vertical oscillations of the vocal folds, larynx, hypolaryngeal complex, or a combination of these structures. Vocal tremor worsens with emotional stress and fatigue, abates during movement, and disappears when at rest. Tremors are usually accentuated at the termination of a movement and maximal during maintenance of a posture. Essential voice tremor is treated with a combination of behavioral voice therapy and BoNT injected bilaterally into the thyroarytenoid and cricothyroid muscles to weaken the laryngeal (69, 70, 71, 72). Three behavioral strategies to lessen the tremor include increasing the speaking rate, higher pitch, and augmentation of breathiness.

Approximately 30% of the patients with spasmodic dysphonia have vocal tremor (73). The differentiation of a tremulous voice due to essential tremor and dystonia is particularly difficult. The vocal folds are never fully at rest, even during breathing, as one set of muscles or the other is always contracting and the laryngeal structures cannot twist or turn, only adduct or abduct, making it difficult to compare the structures at rest and with movement. A comparison of dystonic vocal tremor and essential vocal tremor reveals some differences (73, 74). Essential tremor has even rhythmical vocal arrests and vocal tremor, while those of spasmodic dysphonia have irregular vocal arrests and tremor. In essential tremor, frequency oscillations are more predominant that amplitude oscillations; moreover, those with spasmodic dysphonia can have significant improvement when whispering. Injection of BoNT into the cricothyroid muscle can be performed with the same technique used in spasmodic dysphonia.

Myoclonic movements, which occur as brief, sudden, involuntary jerks caused by muscular contractions, can be associated with abnormal involuntary movements of the soft palate and pharynx with a usual frequency of 1.5 to 3 Hz, while detailed assessment reveals synchronous jerks affecting the eyes, face, palate, larynx, diaphragm, neck, shoulders, and arm, giving rise to the syndrome of palato-pharyngo-laryngo-oculo-diaphragmatic myoclonus (75). The pharyngeal movements are classically unilateral and asymmetrical, with the palate and uvula drawn to one side, or bilateral and symmetric. The rhythmic myoclonic movements that nearly always persist in sleep, and while they can vary in rate with respiration and can often be suppressed, once begun, they rarely resolve. Patients complain

of clicking in their ears, broken speech patterns, and slow tremor. Myoclonic movements of the tensor veli palatini muscles of the soft palate result in opening of the Eustachian tube and the production of a faint clicking sound that can be heard by the patient and clinician. Treatment with tenotomy of the tensor veli palatini, stapedius, or tensor tympani muscles, and myringotomy and BoNT have had varying degrees of success (76). The broken speech pattern produced by laryngeal, palatal, pharyngeal, or diaphragmatic myoclonus simulates the dysphonia heard in laryngeal dystonia or tremor. Examination of the vocal folds frequently reveals slow rhythmic adduction and abduction of the vocal folds synchronized with other myoclonic movements in the palatal, pharyngeal, and possibly diaphragmatic muscles. While typically unresponsive to pharmacotherapy, some patients with palatal myoclonus respond to 5-hydroxytryptophan and decarboxylase-inhibition (77), carbamazepine (78), clonazepam, (79), tetrabenazine (79), and trihexyphenidyl (80).

REFERENCES

1. Sapir S, Ramig LO, Fox CM. Intensive voice treatment in Parkinson's disease: Lee Silverman Voice Treatment. *Expert Rev Neurother* 2011; 11:815–830.
2. Hartelius L, Jonsson M, Rickeberg A, et al. Communication and Huntington's disease: qualitative interviews and focus groups with persons with Huntington's disease, family members, and carergivers. *Int J Lang Commun Disord* 2010; 45:381–393.
3. Logemann, JE. *Evaluation and treatment of swallowing disorders.* San Diego: College Hill Press, 1983; 214–227.
4. Splaingard ML, Hutchins B, Sulton LD, et al. Aspiration in rehabilitation patients: videofluoroscopy versus bedside clinical assessment. *Arch Phys Med Rehabil* 1988; 69:637–640.
5. Baylow HE, Goldfarb R, Taveira CH, et al. Accuracy of clinical judgment of the chin-down posture for dysphagia during the clinical/bedside assessment as corroborated by videofluoroscopy in adults with acute stroke. *Dysphagia* 2009; 24:423–433.
6. Rees CJ. Flexible endoscopic evaluation of swallowing with sensory testing. *Curr Opin Otolaryngol Head Neck Surg* 2006; 14:425–430.
7. Langmore SE, Schatz K, Olsen N. Endoscopic and video fluoroscopic evaluations of swallowing and aspiration. *Ann Otol Rhinol Laryngol* 1991; 100:678–681.
8. Murray J, Langmore SE, Ginsberg S, et al. The significance of accumulated oropharyngeal secretions and swallowing frequency in predicting aspiration. *Dysphagia* 1996; 11:99–103.
9. Aviv JE, Martin JH, Keen MS, et al. Air pulse quantification of supraglottic and pharyngeal sensation: a new technique. *Ann Otol Rhinol Laryngol* 1993; 102:777–780.
10. Aviv JE, Martin JH, Jones ME, et al. Age-related changes in pharyngeal and supraglottic sensation. *Ann Otol Rhinol Laryngol* 1994; 103:749–752.
11. Aviv JE, Sacco RL, Thomson J, et al. Silent laryngopharyngeal sensory deficits after stroke. *Ann Otol Rhinol Laryngol* 1997; 106:87–93.
12. Aviv JE, Martin JH, Sacco RL, et al. Supraglottic and pharyngeal sensory abnormalities in stroke patients with dysphagia. *Ann Otol Rhinol Laryngol* 1996; 105:92–97.

13. Fernandez HH, Lapane KL. Predictors of mortality among nursing home residents with a diagnosis of Parkinson's disease. *Med Sci Monit* 2002; 8:CR241–246.
14. D'Amelio M, Ragonese P, Morgante L, et al. Long-term survival of Parkinson's disease: a population-based study. *J Neurol* 2006; 253:33–37.
15. Gillig PM, Sanders RD. Cranial Nerves IX, X, XI, and XII. *Psychiatry* 2010; 7:37–41.
16. Logemann J, Kahrilas P, Huyrst P, et al. Effects of intraoral prosthesis on swallowing in oral cancer patients. *Dysphagia* 1989: 4:118–120.
17. Davis JW, Lazarus C, Logemann J, et al. Effect of maxillary glossectomy prosthesis on articulation and swallowing. *J Prosthet Dent* 1987; 57:715–719.
18. Shaker R, Kern M, Bardan E, et al. Augmentation of deglutitive upper esophageal sphincter opening in elderly by exercise. *Am J Physiol* 1997; 272:G1518–1522.
19. Dursun G, Boynukalin S, Ozgursoy OB, et al. Long-term results of different treatment modalities for glottic insufficiency. *Am J Otolaryngol* 2008; 29:7–12.
20. Tateya I, Hirano S, Kishimoto Y, et al. Impacts and limitations of medialization thyroplasty on swallowing function of patients with unilateral vocal fold paralysis. *Acta Otolaryngol Suppl* 2010; 84–87.
21. Bielamowicz S, Gupta A, Sekhar LN. Early arytenoid adduction for vagal paralysis after skull base surgery. *Laryngoscope* 2000; 110:346–351.
22. Bhattacharyya N, Kotz T, Shapiro J. Dysphagia and aspiration with unilateral vocal cord immobility: incidence, characterization, and response to surgical treatment. *Ann Otol Rhinol Laryngol* 2002; 111:672–679.
23. Hassan MM, Yumoto E, Kumai Y, et al. Vocal outcome after arytenoid adduction and ansa cervicalis transfer. *Arch Otolaryngol Head Neck Surg* 2012; 138:60–65.
24. Hoffman H, McCabe D, McCulloch T, et al. Laryngeal collagen injection as an adjunct to medicalization laryngoplasty. *Laryngoscope* 2002; 112:1407–1413.
25. Mok P, Woo P, Schaefer-Mojica J. Hypopharyngeal pharyngoplasty

in the management of pharyngeal paralysis: new procedure. *Ann Otol Rhinol Laryngol* 2003; 112:844–852.

26. Eliachar I, Roberts JK, Hayes JD, et al. A vented laryngeal stent with phonatory and pressure relief capability. *Laryngoscope* 1987; 97:1264–1269.

27. Zietek E, Jach K, Matyja G. Treatment of chronic aspiration by Lindeman's tracheoesophageal diversion procedure. *Otolaryngol Pol* 2000; 54:373–378.

28. Ding R, Logemann JA. Swallow physiology in patients with trach cuff inflated or deflated: a retrospective study. *Head Neck* 2005; 27:809–813.

29. Biller HF, Lawson W, Baek SM. Total glossectomy: a technique of reconstruction eliminating laryngectomy. *Arch Otolaryngol* 1983; 109:69–73.

30. Montgomery WW. Surgery to prevent aspiration. *Arch Otolaryngol* 1975; 101:679–682.

31. Eisele DW. Surgical approaches to aspiration. *Dysphagia* 1991; 6:71–78.

32. Broniatowski M, Grundfest-Broniatowski S, Tyler DJ, et al. Dynamic laryngotracheal closure for aspiration: a preliminary report. *Laryngoscope* 2001; 111:2032–2040.

33. Robbins JA, Levine RL. Swallowing after lateral medullary syndrome plus. *Clin Comm Disord* 1993; 3:45–55.

34. Takes RP, van den Hoogen FJ, Marres HA. Endoscopic myotomy of the cricopharyngeal muscle with CO2 laser surgery. *Head Neck* 2005; 27:703–709.

35. Van den Berg J. Myoelastic-aerodynamic theory of voice production. *J Speech Hear Res* 1958; 1:227–244.

36. Younger DS. Neuromuscular disorders of the larynx. In, Blitzer A, Brin MF, eds. *Neurologic Disorders of the Larynx*, 2nd ed. New York:Thieme, 2009; 216–226.

37. Crumley RL. Unilateral recurrent laryngeal nerve paralysis. *J Voice* 1994; 8:79–83.

38. Chen D, Chen S, Wang W, et al. Spontaneous regeneration of recurrent laryngeal nerve following long-term vocal fold paralysis in humans: histologic evidence. *Laryngoscope* 2011; 121:1035–1039.

39. Roy N. Denervation of the external branch of the superior laryngeal nerve: laryngeal and phonatory features. *Curr Opin Otolaryngol Head Neck Surg* 2011; 19:182–187.

40. Pinto JA, de Mello Godoy LB, Pinto Marquis VW, et al. Bilateral vocal fold immobility: diagnosis and treatment. *Braz J Otorhinolaryngol* 2011; 77:594–599.

41. Vinson KN, Zraick RI, Ragland FJ. Injection versus medialization laryngoplasty for the treatment of unilateral vocal fold paralysis: follow-up at six months. *Laryngoscope* 2010; 120:1802–1807.

42. Logemann JA, Fisher H, Boshes B, et al. Frequency and concurrence of vocal tract dysfunctions in the speech of a large sample of Parkinson patients. *J Speech Hear Disord* 1978; 43:47–57.

43. Stewart C, Winfield L, Hunt A, et al. Speech dysfunction in early Parkinson's disease. *Mov Disord* 1995; 10:562–565.

44. Skodda S, Grönheit W, Schlegel U. Intonation and speech rate in Parkinson's disease: general and dynamic aspects and responsiveness to levodopa admission. *J Voice* 2011; 25:e199–205.

45. Plowman-Prine EK, Okun MS, Sapienza CM, et al. Perceptual characteristics of Parkinsonian speech: a comparison of the pharmacological effects of levodopa across speech and non-speech motor systems. *NeuroRehabilitation* 2009; 24:131–144.

46. Mueller PB. Parkinson's disease: motor speech behavior in a selected group of patients. *Folia Phoniatr* 1971; 23:333–346.

47. Tanaka Y, Nishio M, Niimi S. Vocal acoustic characteristics of patients with Parkinson's disease. *Folia Phoniatr Logop* 2011; 63:223–230.

48. Hanson DG, Gerbatt BR, Ward PH. Glottographic measurement of vocal dysfunction: a preliminary report. *Ann Otol Rhinol Laryngol* 1983; 92:413–420.

49. Solomon NP, Robin DA. Perceptions of effort during handgrip and tongue elevation in Parkinson's disease. *Parkinsonism Relat Disord* 2005; 11:353–361.

50. Sapienza C, Troche M, Pitts T, et al. Respiratory strength training: concept and intervention outcomes. *Semin Speech Lang* 2011; 32:21–30.

51. Silverman EP, Sapienza CM, Saleem A, et al. Tutorial on maximum inspiratory and expiratory mouth pressures in individuals with idiopathic Parkinson disease (IPD) and the preliminary results of an expiratory muscle strength training program. *NeuroRehabilitation* 2006; 21:71–79.

52. Sabbagh MN, Lahti T, Connor DJ, et al. Functional ability correlates with cognitive impairment in Parkinson's disease and Alzheimer's disease. *Dement Geriatr Cogn Disord* 2007; 24:327–334.

53. McDowd J, Hoffman L, Rozek E, et al. Understanding verbal fluency in healthy aging, Alzheimer's disease, and Parkinson's disease. *Neuropsychology* 2011; 25:210–225.

54. Gallena S, Smith PJ, Zeffiro T, et al. Effects of levodopa on laryngeal muscle activity for voice onset and offset in Parkinson disease. *J Speech Lang Hear Res* 2001; 44:1284–1299.

55. Haas BM, Trew M, Castle PC. Effects of respiratory muscle weakness on daily living function, quality of life, activity levels, and exercise capacity in mild to moderate Parkinson's disease. *Am J Phys Med Rehabil* 2004; 83:601–607.

56. Goldman JG, Litvan I. Mild cognitive impairment in Parkinson's disease. *Minerva Med* 2011; 102:441–459.

57. Cotelli M, Borroni B, Manenti R, et al. Action and object naming in Parkinson's disease without dementia. *Eur J Neurol* 2007; 14:632–637.

58. Cohn M, Moscovitch M, Davidson PS. Double dissociation between familiarity and recollection in Parkinson's disease as a function of encoding tasks. *Neuropsychologia* 2010; 48:4142–4147.

59. Blitzer A, Lovelace RE, Brin MF, et al. Electromyographic findings in focal laryngeal dystonia (spastic dysphonia). *Ann Otol Rhinol Laryngol* 1985; 94:591–594.

60. Cannito MP, Johnson JP. Spastic dysphonia: a continuum disorder. *J Commun Disord* 1981; 14:215–223.

61. Braun N, Abd A, Baer J, et al. Dyspnea in dystonia. A functional evaluation. *Chest* 1995; 107:1309–1316.

62. Chitkara A, Meyer T, Keidar A, et al. Singer's dystonia: first report of a variant of spasmodic dysphonia. *Ann Otol Rhinol Laryngol* 2006; 115:89–92.

63. Blitzer A, Brin MF, Stewart C, et al. Abductor laryngeal dystonia: a series treated with botulinum toxin. *Laryngoscope* 1992; 102:163–167.

64. Novakovic D, Waters HH, D'Elia JB, et al. Botulinum toxin treatment for adductor spasmodic dysphonia: longitudinal functional and quality of life outcomes. *Laryngoscope* 2011; 121:606–612.

65. Paniello RC, Edgar JD, Perlmutter JS. Vocal exercise versus voice rest following botulinum toxin injections: a randomized crossover trial. *Ann Otol Rhinol Laryngol* 2009; 118:759–763.

66. Jankovic J, Kurlan R. Tourette syndrome: evolving concepts. *Mov Disord* 2011; 26:1149––.

67. Salloway S, Stewart C, Israeli L, et al. Botulinum toxin for refractory vocal tics. *Mov Disord* 1996; 11:746–748.

68. Dromey C, Warrick P, Irish J. The influence of pitch and loudness changes on the acoustics of vocal tremor. *J Speech Lang Hear Res* 2002; 45:879–890.

69. Barkmeier-Kraemer J, Lato A, et al. Development of a speech

treatment program for a client with essential vocal tremor. Semin Speech Lang 2011; 32:43–57.

70. Warrick P, Dromey C, Irish J, et al. The treatment of essential voice tremor with botulinum toxin A: a longitudinal case report. *J Voice* 2000; 14:410–421.

71. Warrick P, Dromey C, Irish JC, et al. Botulinum toxin for essential tremor of the voice with multiple anatomical sites of tremor: a crossover design study of unilateral versus bilateral injection. *Laryngoscope* 2000; 110:1366–1374.

72. Finnegan EM, Luschei ES, Gordon JD, et al. Increased stability of airflow following botulinum toxin injection. *Laryngoscope* 1999; 109:1300–1306.

73. Wolraich D, Vasile Marchis-Crisan C, Redding N, et al. Laryngeal tremor: co-occurrence with other movement disorders. *ORL J Otorhinolaryngol Relat Spec* 2010; 72:291–294.

74. Kendall KA, Leonard RJ. Interarytenoid muscle botox injection for treatment of adductor spasmodic dysphonia with vocal tremor. *J Voice* 2011; 25:114–119.

75. Guillain G. The syndrome of synchronous and rhythmic palato-pharyngo-laryngo-oculo-diaphragmatic myoclonus. *Proc R Soc Med* 1938; 31:1031–1038.

76. Hanson B, Ficara A, McQuade M. Bilateral palatal myoclonus. Pathophysiology and report of a case. *Oral Surg Oral Med Oral Pathol* 1985; 59:479–481.

77. Magnussen I, Dupont E, Prange HA, et al. Palatal myoclonus treated with 5-hydroxytryptophan and decarboxylase-inhibitor. *Acta Neurol Scand* 1977; 55:251–253.

78. Sakai T, Murakami S. Palatal myoclonus responding to carbamazepine. *Ann Neurol* 1981; 9:199–200.

79. Jankovic J, Pardo R. Segmental myoclonus: clinical and pharmacologic study. *Ann Neurol* 1986; 43:1025–1031.

80. Jabbari B, Scherokman B, Gunderson CH, et al. Treatment of movement disorders with trihexyphenidyl. *Mov Disord* 1989; 4:202-212.

CHAPTER 67

Bladder, Bowel, and Sexual Disorders

David S. Younger

Disturbances of bladder and bowel continence and sexual function are common and can complicate the care of patients with central, peripheral and autonomic nervous system (CNS, PNS, and ANS) disorders (1). Urinary incontinence affects approximately 17 million Americans (2) and is a major cause of institutionalization in the elderly. The prevalence of fecal incontinence ranges from 10 to 17% of nursing home residents. Approximately 7% of men experience impotence, and as many as 37% complain of unsatisfactory erectile function. As many as one in three married women rarely or never achieve orgasm. These disorders have traditionally been considered together because the organs affected are physically proximate to each other and share a similar peripheral nerve innervation. Although disturbances of bladder, bowel, and sexual function may occur simultaneously as a result of a shared disease, they may occur separately with differing pathophysiology and thus need to be considered separately. They require examination techniques and expertise that are not part of the traditional neurologic examination and may not be familiar to many neurologists.

NEUROANATOMY AND NEUROPHYSIOLOGY

The relevant neuroanatomy and neurophysiology of the bladder, bowel, and sexual organs are reviewed elsewhere in detail (1–3) and portrayed in Figure 1. The storage and voiding of urine are performed by the coordinated function of the bladder, smooth muscle urethral sphincter, and striated muscle urethral sphincter. The bladder wall, formed by three layers of interdigitating detrusor smooth muscle, is comprised of an internal sphincter that is not anatomically isolated but functions as a physiological sphincter. Reflex bladder contractions are activated by sympathetic, parasympathetic, and somatic nerves from the spinal cord. Three sets of peripheral nerves, each with afferent and efferent components, innervate the bladder, urethra, and associated striated muscle of the urethra and pelvic floor. Sympathetic stimulation typically includes contraction of the sphincter muscle, relaxation of smooth muscle in the wall of hollow viscera, and constriction of blood vessels, while parasympathetic stimulation results instead in relaxation of sphincter muscles and contraction of smooth muscles of hollow viscera.

Parasympathetic innervation of blood vessels in erectile tissue of the genitals via pelvic splanchnic nerves, referred to as nervi erigentes, cause vasodilatation of vessels in erectile tissue upon stimulation. Visceral afferent fibers supplying the visceral peritoneum, pelvic organs, and vasculature transmit dull, aching, poorly localized pain via sympathetic afferent fibers, whereas bladder distention, rectal fullness, the urge to void or defecate, and sexual sensations are conveyed via parasympathetic afferent fibers. Parasympathetic efferent parasympathetic nerves originating in the intermediolateral cell column of the sacral spinal cord from the S2 to S4 segments, exit the spinal cord through the anterior roots, intermingle with somatic efferent fibers forming the spinal nerves, and continue in anterior primary rami reaching the pelvic splanchnic nerves to ganglion cells in the pelvic plexus, subsidiary vesical plexus, cavernous nerves, bladder wall, and urethra. While preganglionic synapses are generally nicotinic cholinergic, and further modifiable by muscarinic and adrenergic input, postganglionic parasympathetic fibers are generally microscopic, located intramurally in the detrusor, with muscarinic M3 receptor specificity.

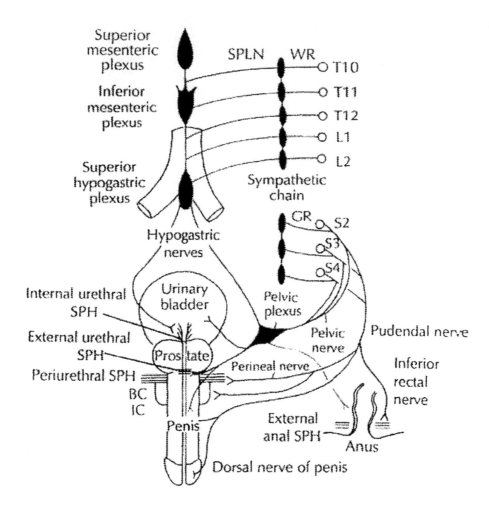

FIG. 1. Innervation of the pelvic bladder, rectum and genitalia. From, reference 2, with permission.

Sympathetic nerves supplying the bladder originate in the intermediolateral nuclei of the thoracic spinal cord from the T11 to L2 segments, and exit the spinal cord through the anterior roots, intermingled with somatic efferent fibers, forming spinal nerves and synapse in a nearby paravertebral ganglia in the sympathetic chain. Those destined for the bladder and urethra pass directly through paravertebral ganglia and exit as preganglionic visceral or splanchnic nerves synapsing on one of the prevertebral or collateral ganglia on the anterior aspect of the aorta or internal iliac vessels, such as the inferior mesenteric ganglia, before continuing inferiorly as the right and left hypogastric nerves, to the pelvic plexus. The latter give rise to subsidiary plexi and nerves including the vesical plexus to the bladder and urethra, and cavernous nerves to the urethral sphincter complex. Activation of postganglionic sympathetic fibers lead to excitation of the bladder base and urethra via α_1-adrenoceptors inhibit detrusor muscle located in the bladder dome via β-adrenoceptors and bladder parasympathetic ganglia via α_2-adrenoceptors, facilitate urethral smooth muscle contraction and bladder parasympathetic

ganglia via α_1-adrenoceptors. Somatic efferent fibers to the pelvis originate instead from motor neurons located in the anterior cell column of the lumbar spinal cord, exit the spinal cord as anterior roots forming spinal nerves with an adjacent posterior root and contribute fibers to the lumbar and sacral plexus.

Anococcygeal nerves are formed from lower sacral and coccygeal anterior rami and respective spinal nerves. Striated muscle of the external urethral and external anal sphincters are supplied by pudendal nerve branches that originate in α-motor neurons of Onuf nucleus in the anterior horn of sacral spinal cord segments from S1 to S3. The pudendal nerve exits the pelvic cavity below the piriformis via the greater sciatic foramen and re-enters the pelvic cavity, running along the lateral wall of the ischiorectal fossa in the pudendal canal supplying three major branches. One branch is distributed to the dorsal nerve of the penis or clitoris for cutaneous supply. A second branch, the inferior rectal nerve, supplies the lower anal canal, external anal sphincter and skin around the anus. A third branch, the perineal nerve, which divides into a cutaneous branch to the scrotum and ventral penis in men, or posterior labia and lower vagina in women, and distal urethra, innervates the superficial and deep perineal muscles, including the external urethral sphincter and levator ani.

Striated pelvic floor muscles, including the puborectalis and perivaginal are also supplied directly by pelvic nerve branches. The ascending and proximal colon derives parasympathetic innervation from the vagus nerve while the descending colon receives parasympathetic innervation via the pelvic nerves, and sympathetic innervation via the lumbar splanchnic and hypogastric plexuses. Internal anal smooth muscle sphincters possess both α-and β-adrenergic receptors. Penile erection is mediated via parasympathetic impulses that initiate the necessary penile vascular changes. In women, parasympathetic activity increases vaginal secretions in association with clitoral swelling. Sympathetic nerves supply the vas deferens, seminal vesicle, prostate, and bladder vesicle neck. The sympathetic efferent fibers in men close the proximal bladder neck to retrograde flow and induce the ejaculation of semen through rhythmic smooth muscle contraction and in women induce contraction of genital smooth muscle during orgasm. The complex CNS integration of somatic PNS and ANS function is accomplished in neuronal centers within the spinal cord, pons, midbrain, and other subcortical and cortical structures.

TERMINOLOGY AND CLASSIFICATION

There are three principal types of lower urinary tract (LUT) disturbances (4), those associated with storage, voiding, and post micturition. Those associated with the bladder storage phase relate to decreased contractility, decreased afferent function, or outlet obstruction (2) present with daytime frequency, urgency, nocturia, and incontinence, the latter of which may be stress, urgency-related, or mixed in nature. LUT disturbances associated with voiding and post micturition are most often associated with primary urological factors. The former includes slow stream, splitting, spraying, or intermittent stream, hesitancy, straining, and terminal dribbling, whereas the latter that relates to the sensation immediately after micturition and includes incomplete emptying and post micturition dribbling.

Neurogenic anorectal disorders fall into the broad categories of fecal incontinence due to primary neurological factors, and chronic constipation, often in association with colonic inertia or outlet obstruction. Disturbances of sexual function in men include disorders of libido, and erectile and ejaculatory function (5), while those in women relate to faulty vaginal lubrication and orgasm.

CLINICAL EVALUATION

The clinical evaluation of bladder, bowel, and sexual disturbances should commence with a directed history and physical examination. A history of chronic pain may be a useful clue to the presence of a genitourinary pain syndrome of LUT, bowel, sexual or gynecological nature. So-called painful bladder, urethral, vulval, vaginal, scrotal, perineal and pelvic pain syndromes (4) are relatively common, occur in the absence of proven infection or obvious pathology, and may be of neurological origin in some patients. Urgency with or without urge incontinence, often with frequency and nocturia, describe the overactive bladder and urge or urgency-frequency syndrome, for which there may be urodynamically demonstrable detrusor overactivity or other causes of urethra-vesical dysfunction in the absence of proven infection or other obvious pathology.

Objective signs of LUT disease may be provided by the patient when asked to record micturition and symptoms thereof for a period of days via a 24-hour micturition time chart, frequency volume chart, or bladder diary detailing the times of micturition, voided volumes, incontinence episodes, pad usage, fluid intake, and degree of urgency or incontinence.

Physical examination is essential in the assessment of all patients with LUT, bowel and sexual dysfunction, and should include abdominal, pelvic, perineal, and a focused neurological examination. The bladder can be felt by abdominal palpation or suprapubic percussion, and the perineal and genital organs can be manually inspected, including assessment of rectal sphincter, puborectalis muscle tone and contraction, perianal and perineal sensation, and elicitation of abdominal, cremasteric, bulbocavernosus, anal wink, and cutaneous reflexes. Visualization of the bladder, anorectum and internal pelvis of women are indispensable in the diagnosis of LUT disease. Urethral or extraurethral urine leakage may be seen during the examination, or with exertion, effort, sneezing, or coughing indicative of stress urinary incontinence. Vaginal examination, which assesses the pelvic floor musculature, may reveal prolapse or descent of one or more of the anterior vaginal wall, posterior vaginal wall, apex of the vagina, cervix, or uterus, or vault after hysterectomy. Pelvic floor muscle tone can be qualitatively defined by the tone at rest or during voluntary or reflex contraction by visual inspection, palpation, or perineometry. Rectal examination will exclude palpable anatomical abnormalities and is a means of assessing pelvic floor muscle function in children and men, and in excluding fecal impaction. The evaluation of bladder function includes conventional urodynamic techniques with artificial bladder filling via a catheter with a specific liquid at a specified rate, and measurements of intravesical pressure, abdominal pressure, and detrusor pressures employing filling cystometry and pressure flow studies of voiding. Filling cystometry gives information about pressure/volume relationships of the bladder during bladder filling, with determination of bladder sensation, detrusor function, bladder compliance, and bladder capacity, as well as urethral pressure measurements. Urine flow studies, defined as continuous or intermittent, can be illustrated on a flow curve detailing the flow rate, voided volume, maximum flow rate, voiding time, flow times, average flow rate, and maximum flow, as well as pressure measurements including premicturition pressure, opening pressure, maximal pressure, and closing pressure. Complete bladder emptying generally occurs in a normal time span and in the absence of obstruction, but may be abnormal due to underactivity, resulting in prolonged emptying or failure to achieve full emptying. So-called acontractile bladder is associated with a post-void residual demonstrated by ultrasound. Urethal function during voiding may reveal bladder outlet obstruction characterized by increasing detrusor pressure and reduced urine flow rate. Dysfunctional voiding may be due to involuntary intermittent contractions of periurethral striated muscle. Detrusor sphincter dyssynergia results from the concomitant contractions of urethral and periurethral striated muscle.

The neurological evaluation of male sexual dysfunction should include specific diagnostic testing for impotence, which can be divided into neuroendocrine and metabolic screening to exclude a contemporaneous systemic process, neurovascular insufficiency in those with systemic hypertension, advanced atherosclerotic disease, and possible underlying vasculitis, and electrodiagnostic studies in others with known or suspected PNS disturbances, and basic studies for erective capacity. The latter can be further divided into those that measure erectile function and others that measure neurological function directly (5).

Tests of noctural penile tumescence and rigidity (NPTR), which vary according to the methodology, include the postage stamp test, Poten test, and Snap-Gauge screening tests. These devices are wrapped around the flaccid penis and pasted or fastened at bedtime and give presumptive information about the evidence of nocturnal erections when properly examined the following morning if they are properly broken by the next morning. The measurement of penile expansion during a sleep study with direct visual monitoring and NPT testing and EEG confirmation of rapid eye movement (REM) sleep stages when tumescence and erection should occur, is considered the most accurate method of evaluating erectile dysfunction. Penile circumference and rigidity can be measured directly by a commercial rigidometer at home asleep, awake, or undergoing visual sexual stimulation. Erectile capacity can be investigated by intracorporeal injection of smooth muscle relaxants, which if followed by rigid erection, is considered strong evidence for neurogenic impotence. The most widely employed agents are papaverine, a papaverine-phentolamine combination, and prostaglandin E1. If papaverine leads to erection in an impotent patient, then additional testing for neurologic and psychogenic causes of impotence is required. Firm erection followed by various degrees of detumescence suggests venous leakage.

Anal manometry and cinedefecography can contribute information to the neurogenic basis of fecal incontinence and help direct therapy (6–9). Specialized tests for the neurologic evaluation of sexual dysfunction include studies of nocturnal penile tumescence and rigidity; vasoactive pharmacologic maneuvers to detect erectile capacity; and electrophysiologic studies of the pudendal nerve, bulbocavernosus reflex responses, pudendal somatosensory evoked potentials, and penile biothesiometry (5).

ELECTROPHYSIOLOGICAL TESTING

Neurological assessment of bladder, bowel, and sexual disorder requires the combined expertise of nerve conduction studies (NCS) and concentric needle electromyography (CNEMG) used in the physiological assessment of the spinal roots, lumbosacral plexus, and peripheral nerves of the PNS (2, 10); direct assessment of parasympathetic and sympathetic functions, including small nerve fiber electrophysiology and histopathological analysis of epidermal nerve fibers (ENF) in a punch skin biopsy; and selected aspects of central motor conduction employing transcranial magnetic stimulation (TMS) and somatosensory evoked responses (SSER).

There are protocols for the clinical neurophysiologic examination of the pelvic floor (11), which consists of several layers (2). The first layer is comprised of pelvic viscera and supporting endopelvic fascia. The second layer is formed by the muscular diaphragm and levator ani, innervated by small twigs arising directly from the S3 to S5 anterior primary rami (APR) and variably the pudendal nerve along its anterior portion, and the piriformis and obturator internus somatic musculature. Their fibers collectively run obliquely down and backward, inserting upon the anococcygeal ligament and coccyx posteriorly, and encircle the urethra, vagina, and anal canal inferiorly, forming a sling at the level of the anorectal angle, important in the maintenance of rectal continence. The third layer, comprised of the urogenital diaphragm along the anterior pelvic outlet, consists of deep transverse perineal muscles and the urethrovaginal sphincter in women. The most superficial layer of the pelvic floor is comprised anteriorly of the bulbocavernosus (BC), ischiocavernosus (IC), and superficial transverse perineal muscles, innervated along its inferior aspect by distal perineal branches of the pudendal nerve; and posteriorly by the external anal sphincter (EAS) that is comprised of subcutaneous, superficial, and deep layers, innervated variable or collectively by the inferior rectal or perineal branch of the pudendal or inferior rectal nerve.

In men, the external urethral sphincter (EUS) is composed of circular smooth muscle that is derived from the urethral wall at the base of the bladder, innervated by sympathetic fibers and striated type 1 muscle fibers, innervated by S2 to S4 efferent nerve fibers that course in the perineal branch of the pudendal nerve or others, somatic and parasympathetic motor fibers that transverse the pelvic plexus. Collectively, the muscle fibers encircle the urethra segment where peak urethral closure occurs and prevents retrograde ejaculation. It derives its innervation from the sympathetic nerves. The innervation proper of the urethra is via autonomic fibers derived from the pelvic plexus to the vesical plexus and cavernous nerves, with the periurethral sphincter, innervated by the perineal branch of the pudendal nerve.

Two reflexes, the bulbocavernosus reflex (BCR), manually elicited by compression of the glans penis or clitoris, and the anal reflex following pinprick of the mucocutaneous junction of the anus, can be recorded via surface electrodes placed along perineal muscles or sphincters following electrical stimulation to isolate and define the pathways more precisely (12). The evaluation of two sacral reflexes, the penilobulbocavernosus reflex in men and the homologous clitoroanal reflex (CAR) in women provide insight into the sacral segments and roots (13), whereas the urethroanal, vesicoanal, and anoanal reflexes have applicability to either sex (14). While peniloanal (PAR) and CAR traverse the pudendal nerve, afferent and efferent, sacral roots, and spinal cord pathways, they are subject to suprasacral modulation during voiding (15) and can be elicited following stimulation of the dorsal nerve of the penis with ring electrodes, with recording from the external anal sphincter with surface or needle electrodes on the glans and shaft or with a standard bipolar stimulator at the base of the penis (16). This reflex can also be recorded via surface electrode on an anal plug inserted into the anus to record from the anal sphincter (17), from the bulbocavernous muscle, or external urinary sphincter via surface or needle recordings (18).

A typical battery of perineal electrophysiological studies (5, 19–22) and recorded reflexes includes penile NCS, (23, 24), pudendal nerve responses (25–27), and the bulbocavernosus reflex (BCR) response (28). The bulbocavernosus reflex latency (BCRL) correlates with pudendal nerve-associated impotence. The pudendal nerve terminal motor latencies (PNTML) is recorded in the bulbocavernosus muscle and anal sphincter via special electrode (19). Pudendal nerve functioning is important in the evaluation of penile sensation and ejaculation, wherein the BCR is analogous to the ejaculation reflex. In the evaluation of impotence, an abnormal PNTML associated with normal BCRL indicates a distal lesion of the pudendal nerve.

CNEMG of the bulbocavernosus muscles and external anal sphincter (EAS) (10, 29) and other pelvic floor muscles is probably the most informative test in patients with suspected lower motor neuron (LMN) pelvic floor lesions affecting bladder and bowel function (11). Although amenable to a variety of electrodes including surface, fine wire, and needle types, CNEMG is amenable to computerized-assisted analysis of denervation and reinnervation signals, and the sampling of continuous motor unit potentials (MUP), firing during relaxation, MUP duration, area, and number of turns, with comparison to normative data (30). Absence of voluntary units and reflex recruited MUP are generally indicative of complete denervation or disruption.

One protocol for the evaluation of patients with pelvic floor dysfunction and suspected LMN disease commences with an evaluation of anal sphincter tone, anogenital sensation, BCR, and anal reflex. Positioned in the left lateral Sim's position, EMG of the subcutaneous EAS is performed with the needle directed perpendicular to the skin 1 cm inside the mucocutaneous junction, and directed medially toward the anal canal and advanced, if needed, until the superficial and deep muscle are entered (31). CNEMG is performed as part of the assessment of lumbosacral myotomes, including examination of the legs and paraspinal region, on the side with the more pronounced sensory deficit, if present, as in a cauda equina lesion. If no abnormality is found the need for further examination is questionable. In those with symmetrical involvement, as in conus or cauda equina lesions, and MSA, CNEMG assessment is carried out in the contralateral subcutaneous portion of the EAS to ascertain bilateral involvement. Patients of either sex with presumed distal lesions of the pudendal nerve, EAS muscle itself, and anal incontinence and suspected LMN disease, should undergo CNEMG of deep portions of the EAS muscle, in addition to the subcutaneous part, to ascertain the differences in the two sides. Patients with urinary incontinence of possibly neurogenic origin may optionally undergo examination of the EUS, even when the EAS has been found to be pathological, whereas in young women with unexplained urinary retention, CNEMG of the EUS with specific emphasis on the evaluation of muscle activity provoked by needle movements is mandatory, including a search for deceleration bursts. The EUS is approached transvaginally or periurethrally in women, 5 mm anterior or lateral, or through the urethral meatus and advanced while listening for CNEMG activity (32), and via transperineal approach in men, with the needle inserted anterior to the anus at the base of the penis and advanced toward the apex of the prostate (33).

Further examination of the pelvic floor may entail sampling of the BC and levator ani muscles to ascertain the integrity of the sacral roots, plexus, pudendal nerve and perineal nerve branch. The BC muscle, which is not tonically active at rest (11), lies superficially behind the scrotum on either side of the midline in the perineal region surrounding the bulb of the penis. It is approached via CNEMG 1 cm lateral to the bulb of the penis and advanced toward the midline until muscle activity is encountered. The levator ani, which has the advantage of sacral innervation and nonpudendal innervation, is approached by needle insertion at the mucocutaneous junction, and facilitated in localization by advising the patient to squeeze as if to delay urination.

Single fiber EMG (SFEMG), which provides information regarding fiber density, defined as the mean number of myofibers belonging to an individual motor unit per detection site, is a sensitive indicator of collateral reinnervation after partial denervation (10), but is less widely available.

Transcranial magnetic stimulation (TMS) of the motor cortex to record motor evoked potentials (MEP) to the EAS permits a determinant of central conduction time along the corticospinal tracts (CST), calculated by subtracting the response latency to sacral root stimulation from the total conduction time to motor cortex stimulation (34). The TMS technique can be employed to investigate the motor representation of the anal sphincter (35) to facilitate understanding of disorders in which the brain-gut axis is involved, such as anorectal outlet obstruction syndrome, irritable bowel syndrome, and anismus (10).

ANS testing (36, 37) and skin biopsy (38) should be considered in the evaluation of patients with bladder, bowel, and sexual dysfunction when there is evidence of PNS ANS disturbances. An evidenced-based review by the American Academy of Neurology (AAN) (39) suggested that composite autonomic scoring scale (CASS) integrating QSART, orthostatic blood pressure, heart rate response to tilt, heart rate response to deep breathing, the Valsalva ratio, and beat-to-beat blood pressure measurements during phases II and IV of the Valsalva maneuver, tilt, and deep breathing, provided a useful 10-point scale of autonomic function among those with graded autonomic failure and MSA, Parkinson disease, and autonomic neuropathy. Skin biopsy reliably detects both somatic and autonomic IENF density and morphology associated with small fiber sensory neuropathy (SFSN) and autoimmune autonomic ganglionopathy (40, 41).

TREATMENT

Urinary Incontinence

A variety of therapies are available for urinary incontinence, the choice of which depends upon the presence of concomitant detrusor instability, detrusor hyperreflexia, detrusor sphincter dyssynergia, and urethral instability (42–44).

Anticholinergic agents are effective in detrusor instability and hyperreflexia, and oxybutynin and tolterodine are the agents of choice due to their salutary anticholinergic effects on direct smooth muscle relaxation. Propantheline and dicyclomine are second-line agents. Side effects include urinary retention, xerostomia, blurred vision, constipation, nausea, and mental changes. The tricyclic antidepressant imipramine decreases bladder contractility and increases sphincter resistance and may be helpful but has side effects that limit its use in elderly patients. Bladder training, which incorporates patient education and scheduled voiding, in conjunction with pelvic floor exercises to strengthen periurethral and perivaginal striated muscles, reduces urgency and urge incontinence in men and women (45). Biofeedback using multi-measurement feedback such as simultaneous measurement of pelvic, abdominal, and detrusor activity can reduce incontinence and is useful in conjunction with pelvic muscle exercises and bladder training. Patients who participate in behavioral management programs derive maximal benefit when ongoing reinforcement and support are provided. Pelvic electrical stimulators that produce contraction of the sphincter and pelvic floor muscles employing vaginal-, anal-, and surface skin-stimulating electrodes, at varying frequency, intensity, and duration are clinically effective with minimal adverse side effects, and can be used in conjunction with other therapies. However, electrical stimulation for urge and stress incontinence may not improve outcome beyond that achieved with pelvic floor muscle training alone (45). Surgical treatment of detrusor instability that includes bladder denervation, augmentation intestinoplasty, and urinary diversion procedures are generally reserved for patients that are refractory to other treatments.

Stress incontinence may be associated with hypermobility of the bladder neck in women or with neurogenic sphincter deficiency. Pelvic floor exercises, biofeedback, and pelvic electrical stimulation improve stress urinary incontinence in older and younger patients (42). Pelvic exercises using vaginal weighted cones have been associated with reduction in incontinence episodes in premenopausal women. Patients with neurogenic sphincter deficiency respond with a decreased number of incontinent episodes to the α-receptor agonist phenylpropanolamine and pseudoephedrine (42). However, the latter is associated with a 16-fold increased risk of hemorrhagic stroke in women under age 50. Oral and vaginal estrogen therapy may benefit post-menopausal women with urgency and urge urinary incontinence but are ineffective in stress urinary incontinence (46, 47).

There are surgical therapies of bladder neck hypermobility that include retropubic suspension, needle bladder neck suspension, and anterior vaginal repair. Intrinsic sphincter deficiency may respond to sling procedures.

Both men and women may respond to periurethral injection of materials such as polytetrafluoroethylene, collagen, or autologous fat. Bladder hypocontractility in the absence of outlet obstruction due to overflow incontinence may respond to bethanechol. Alternative therapy includes intermittent straight catheterization.

Detrusor external sphincter dyssynergia, which represents the simultaneous contraction of the detrusor during simultaneous contraction of the external urethral sphincter, and interferes with bladder emptying seen in association with intrinsic spinal cord disease, responds to α-adrenergic blocking agents such as terazosin, as well as, baclofen and benzodiazepines, but none selectively relax sphincter striated muscle and adverse side effects limit their usefulness. Other therapeutic options include anticholinergic medication, intermittent catheterization, and intrathecal baclofen via an implantable pump, external sphincterotomy, sphincter stent prosthesis, and laser.

Sacral nerve stimulation by an implantable programmed neurostimulator device, approved for the treatment of urinary urgency, urgency-frequency, and non-obstructive urinary retention (48), can be used for treatment of patients who fail to achieve a satisfactory response to more conservative alternatives.

Fecal Incontinence

The treatment of fecal incontinence (6, 8) commences with institution of a high-fiber diet, stool-bulking agents, daily tap water enemas, and glycerin suppositories with a program of planned bowel evacuations (8). The anti-diarrheal synthetic opioid, loperamide, controls diarrhea by reducing urgency, stool frequency, and stool volume (49).

Biofeedback with intrarectal balloon distention and monitoring of anal external sphincter contraction reduces the frequency of incontinent episodes in patients who retain rectal sensation and voluntary sphincter contraction. Success correlates more with improvement in rectal sensation than with sphincter strengthening (6). Pelvic electrical stimulation with surface electrodes or an anal plug electrode and pelvic exercises, improves symptoms of mild incontinence (50, 51). Surgical approaches include direct repair of the external anal sphincter; posterior anal repair with plication of the levator ani, puborectalis, and levator ani muscles; anal encirclement to mechanically tighten the anus; implantation of an artificial sphincter; anal encirclement with portions of adjacent skeletal muscle; and colostomy, especially in refractory incontinence (52). Sacral nerve stimulation can be attempted by implantable programmed neurostimulattion (49).

Sexual Dysfunction

The therapy of sexual dysfunction in both sexes is equally challenging. Underlying and accompanying psychological disorders, including anxiety and depression, should be addressed and coexistent medical diseases identified and treated (53).

Specific therapies for male erectile dysfunction include the use of vasoactive medications, application of vacuum-constriction devices, and implantation of penile prostheses. Sildenafil is a phosphodiesterase type-5 inhibitor that increases cyclic guanosine monophosphate, relaxes penile smooth muscle, and improves erectile dysfunction in men with organic, psychogenic, and mixed causes (54). Adverse effects and complications include hypotension, headache, nasal congestion, flushing, dyspepsia, and transient visual disturbance (54). Alternatives with similar medications include vardenafil and tadalafil (54). The intracavernosal injection of alprostadil is an effective therapy in patients with neurogenic, vasculogenic, and psychogenic erectile dysfunction; however, side effects and complications include local pain, hematoma, or ecchymosis formation, priapism, and penile fibrosis (55). The efficacy of alprostadil was demonstrated with a transurethral preparation without the side effects of the injected form of the medication (56). A variety of other drugs have been used, including the α-adrenergic blockers phenoxybenzamine, phentolamine, and yohimbine and the smooth muscle dilator papaverine (53). Vacuum devices, which consist of a canister tube connected to a vacuum pump, draw blood into the penis, with tumescence maintained by a band placed at the base of the penis. However, adverse effects include decreased penile sensation, impaired ejaculation, ecchymosis, and rarely penile necrosis. Erectile function may also be restored by surgical placement of a semi-rigid or inflatable penile prosthesis; however, the possible complications include infection, erosion, penile gangrene, and malfunction of inflatable devices Ejaculatory dysfunction may respond to local mechanical vibration or to electrical stimulation of sympathetic outflow via intrarectal electrodes.

ASSOCIATED DISEASES

Stroke

The estimated incidence of urinary incontinence in stroke is 57 to 83% with gradual improvement over the ensuing six months (57), the causes of which include disruption of micturition pathways, stroke-related cognitive dysfunction, language deficits, concurrent neuropathy, and medication effects (58). Acute urinary retention may be the initial presenting feature but, over time, frequency, urgency, and urge incontinence become the primary complaints. Urinary incontinence was the single best predictor of moderate or severe disability at three and twelve months (59) and was associated with prolonged hospital stay (60). Overall, in a sample of 532 patients seen within seven days of an acute stroke (61), 53% of incontinent patients died within six months of their stroke. A prospective study cohort of 492 stroke patients (62) showed that urinary incontinence was an independent predictor of death at one year. Acute hemispheric lesions in the anteromedial frontal lobe, anterior paraventricular white matter, and internal capsule genu are predominant sites causing urinary dysfunction, but urinary dysfunction also accompanies leukoaraiosis in the elderly (63).

Variable patterns of urinary incontinence present on urodynamic testing probably reflect timing of the procedure after the stroke or the anatomic extent and location of the stroke (64). Cystometry performed in 39 patients (65) revealed uninhibited detrusor contractions in 18 of 21 patients with frontal, putaminal, or internal capsule lesions on brain computed tomography (CT) when examined at a mean of 19 months after stroke. Uninhibited sphincter relaxation is associated with internal capsule but not with putaminal lesions. Detrusor hyperreflexia and uninhibited sphincter relaxation occurs with cortical and internal capsule lesions (66, 67). Up to 21% of patients studied at a mean of 69 days after stroke (59) had bladder hyporeflexia, but the patients were either taking anticholinergic medications or had diabetes mellitus. Incomplete bladder emptying may also be present in continent post-stroke patients with a higher rate of urinary tract infections (68).

Patients under consideration for prostatectomy for symptoms of bladder outlet obstruction have a worse surgical outcome, with unsatisfactory results in up to 50% in those operated within a year of a stroke (69). Treatment of stroke-related urinary incontinence should be based on the underlying pattern of the incontinence, which is not always clinically apparent, and on the knowledge that this pattern may change with time. Fecal incontinence follows unilateral and bilateral frontal ischemic infarction (70, 71).

Fecal incontinence coexists with urinary incontinence in 80 to 98% of patients after stroke cases (72) with a frequency of 30% at 7 to 10 days that dropped to 11% at three months. Such patients are more likely to require long-term care.

Strokes resulting in hemiplegia are associated with a decline in coital frequency in men and women (73) due to erectile and ejaculatory dysfunction in men, and vaginal lubrication and orgasm in women. The prevalence of sexual dysfunction was greater in association with right hemisphere lesions than with left hemisphere lesions (74). An increased percentage of both men and women report diminished libido and moderate or complete dissatisfaction with sexual life after stroke.

Dementia

Disturbances of micturition and defecation are associated with lesions of the anteromedial frontal lobe, including the anterior cingulate gyrus and genu of the corpus callosum (75, 76). The presence of subcortical white matter lesions on magnetic resonance imaging (MRI) in those with Alzheimer disease (AD), selected for absence of vascular disease risk factors, symptomatic cerebrovascular disease, or cardiovascular disease, were associated with an increased frequency of urinary incontinence (77, 78). Bladder and bowel incontinence are frequent accompaniments of vascular dementia and Binswanger disease (79, 80). Urinary incontinence occurs earlier in vascular dementia than in AD (77). Whereas the temporal relationship of cognitive decline in AD is associated with urinary and fecal incontinence, similar to those with diffuse Lewy body disease (LBD), there is earlier decline in urinary and fecal incontinence when AD is associated with vascular lesions or Lewy bodies (81). The estimated prevalence of urinary incontinence in patients with AD varies from 16 to 40% and is related to the severity of dementia (82); its occurrence is predictive of later institutionalization (83). Urinary incontinence is also a symptom of normal pressure hydrocephalus (NPH), early symptoms of which consist of urgency and frequency, and late symptoms of urgency and fecal incontinence (84). Cystometrograms show uninhibited bladder contractions at small volumes (84, 85). Whereas side effects limit pharmacologic management in patients with NPH, other treatment options include prompt voiding with regularly scheduled toileting, simple alterations in environment, ambulation devices, strategies to improve ambulation; steps to eliminate bowel impaction; fluid restriction at night for nocturia, absorbent pads, external collection devices, and intermittent catheterization. Treatment of fecal incontinence in the elderly includes stool-bulking agents, anti-diarrhea agents, and scheduled toileting at a fixed time each day. Biofeedback and behavioral measures may be limited by patient comprehension of instructions (86). Sexual disinhibition occurs in 7% of affected patients with AD and incontinence (82).

Extrapyramidal Disorders

Parkinson disease (PD), multiple systems atrophy (MSA), Shy-Drager syndrome (SDS), and progressive supranuclear palsy (PSP) are all associated with urinary incontinence, the estimated incidence of which varies from 37 to 71% in PD alone (87). Symptoms include frequency, urgency, urge incontinence, hesitancy, and retention (87, 88). Detrusor hyperreflexia associated with sphincter relaxation is the most common urodynamic pattern in PD (87). Sphincter bradykinesia or failure of perineal floor muscle relaxation during detrusor contraction, and pseudo-dyssynergia or voluntary perineal floor muscle contraction in response to detrusor contraction, have also been described (87, 88). Urodynamic studies in patients receiving medication and repeated several hours after stopping medication are associated with both improvement and worsening of bladder hyperreflexia (89). A urodynamic study of 18 PD patients with wearing-off phenomena (90), performed before and one hour after treatment with L-dopa, showed increased detrusor hyperreflexia, worsened urgency, and increased static urethral closure pressure. The detrusor contractility increased more than urethral obstruction, producing improved voiding efficiency. Deep brain stimulation of PD patients increases the detrusor hyperreflexic contraction threshold and increased the initial desire to void bladder volume (91, 92). However, the urodynamic pattern of a studied cohort of L-dopa-treated and untreated men did not significantly differ (87).

Cystometry is indicated in those with obstruction considered for prostatectomy because normal preoperative voluntary sphincter control is associated with a lower risk of postoperative incontinence (93). Although stress incontinence is the most common cause of incontinence in non-parkinsonian women, a urodynamic study (94) revealed detrusor instability in 70.6% of women with PD so studied, who experience symptoms of urge and stress incontinence.

Age, severity of illness, and depression are important predictors of sexual function in men with PD, and the frequency of sexual dysfunction may be similar to that with other chronic illnesses (95). L-dopa may improve libido out of proportion to motoric improvement, and men are more likely to notice this than women (53). Male PD patients with low testosterone levels and decreased libido may improve with testosterone replacement therapy (96). Hypersexuality may uncommonly be associated with anti-parkinsonian medication therapy and has been described with high-frequency stimulation of the subthalamic nucleus (97, 98). A small improvement in satisfaction with their sexual life was shown in male PD patients after subthalamic nucleus deep brain stimulation (99). Slow colonic transit time, decreased phasic rectal contraction, weak abdominal strain, and paradoxical sphincter contraction are features of PD with frequent constipation (100).

Men with MSA experience urgency, frequency, and nocturia, and women experience stress incontinence. Patients with MSA have bladder hyperreflexia with later development of bladder atonia (101). Cystometry reveals detrusor hyperreflexia, but detrusor atonia and urinary retention can also occur (102). Women undergoing surgery for stress incontinence may fail to improve (103). Treatment with intermittent catheterization, anticholinergic medication, and desmopressin spray improve continence (103). Needle EMG of the ure-

thral and anal sphincter in MSA are abnormal, but not in idiopathic PD (104). An abnormal EMG study in combination with urodynamic findings of elevated post void residual urine, detrusor-external sphincter dyssynergia and open bladder neck at the start of bladder filling are all suggestive of MSA (105). Impotence is a common symptom of MSA and may be the presenting symptom (103, 106). An open bladder vesicle neck was present at rest in five patients undergoing cystometry, with evidence of external urethral sphincter denervation by CNEMG (107).

Urgency, urge incontinence, and obstruction are seen in patients with PSP, in whom urodynamic studies also reveal detrusor hyperreflexia, uninhibited striated sphincter relaxation, and detrusor sphincter dyssynergia (108). EAS CNEMG shows neurogenic abnormalities (108). Patients with MSA have abnormal colonic, transit time, sphincter EAS CNEMG, and videomanometry that correlates with fecal incontinence (109), while those with SDS show chronic reinnervation in EAS CNEMG studies (107, 110).

Multiple Sclerosis

Bladder dysfunction in multiple sclerosis (MS) arises as a result of interruption of pathways from the pontine micturition center to the sacral spinal cord (111). Common symptoms include urgency, frequency, and urge incontinence. Hesitancy, poor or interrupted urinary stream, dribbling, and incomplete emptying also occur. Urodynamic abnormalities include detrusor hyperreflexia, incomplete bladder emptying, and detrusor sphincter dyssynergia (112). Up to one-half of MS patients without urinary complaints have abnormal urodynamic studies. The presence of urinary symptoms correlates with longer duration of disease, the severity of pyramidal or sensory lesions, and the total disability score (113, 114). Bladder symptoms generally correlate poorly with any single urodynamic finding (115, 116). Irritative bladder symptoms may not be associated with uninhibited detrusor contractions, and some patients with obstructive symptoms may not have bladder areflexia (115). The pattern of urodynamic abnormality may change over time with development of new detrusor hyperreflexia or detrusor sphincter dyssynergia, the development of which is a urodynamic indicator of progressive MS (116). Sphincter dyssynergia in men may be associated with a higher risk of complications such as urosepsis and vesicoureteral reflux (117). Lack of response to treatment based on urodynamic assessment may be related to progression of MS (118). Patients with detrusor hyperreflexia respond well to treatment with oxybutynin or tolterodine (119). Refractory nocturia may respond to desmopressin. Bladder areflexia is treated with intermittent catheterization and is not usually responsive to bethanechol. Bladder hyperreflexia with dyssynergia is effectively managed with anticholinergic therapy in combination with intermittent catheterization. Detrusor sphincter dyssynergia has been reported to respond to intrathecal baclofen (120).

Constipation and fecal incontinence occur alone and in combination with urinary incontinence (121–123). In women, fecal incontinence may reflect a combination of factors, including CNS and pelvic PNS disease, and injury acquired with childbirth Evaluation of radiopaque marker transit and anorectal manometry has revealed increased colonic transit time and spontaneous rectal contractions and fecal incontinence in MS patients (124). Defacography shows evidence of rectal outlet obstruction with failure of the puborectalis and anal sphincter muscles to relax (125). Paradoxical contraction of the puborectalis muscle in constipated MS patients may be the anal equivalent of detrusor sphincter dyssynergia of the bladder (126). Patients with MS and fecal incontinence experience rectal sensation at a higher volume, increased thresholds of phasic external anal sphincter contraction, decreased maximal voluntary anal pressures, and require smaller volumes of rectal distention to inhibit internal sphincter tone than normal control subjects (127). Similar, less severe findings may be present in continent MS patients (128). Treatment is empiric and includes a high-fiber diet, bulking agents, adequate fluid intake, a regular defecation schedule with use of glycerin suppositories or digital stimulation, loperamide for loose stools, and regular exercise (129).

Sexual dysfunction in men includes erectile dysfunction, decreased penile sensation, inability to ejaculate, and premature ejaculation (128). Female patients report decreased vaginal lubrication and decreased vaginal sensation. Both men and women can have trouble achieving orgasm, and the presence of sexual dysfunction is associated with depression, bladder dysfunction, and bowel dysfunction. In a survey of 133 women with MS (130), over 70% reported that they enjoyed, felt aroused, and experienced orgasm with sexual activity. In this study, neurologic symptoms and lack of a sexual partner were the best predictors of sexual dysfunction (130). Some patients report improved sexual dysfunction after corticosteroid treatment (128). A double-blind placebo-controlled trial of sildenafil in men with MS and erectile dysfunction (129) showed significant improvement in erectile function and in quality of life.

Spinal Cord Disease

Spinal cord disease leads to upper motor neuron (UMN) dysfunction, however acute injury results in spinal shock and flaccid involvement associated with a non-contractile bladder that can last six to eight weeks. Abnormal external sphincter EMG activity returns before resumption of bladder activity, but as reflexive bladder activity returns, the urodynamic pattern of function demonstrates a hypercontractile bladder

alone or in association with external sphincter dyssynergia. Treatment includes intermittent catheterization to maintain low bladder pressures and to prevent upper urologic tract disease (131). Selected patients may benefit from pharmacologic therapy tailored to urodynamic findings, sphincterotomy, or augmentation cystoplasty. Autonomic dysreflexia, an exaggerated sympathetic outflow response to an afferent spinal stimulation, which usually manifests as a rise in blood pressure with slowing of heart rate, should be avoided through careful bladder management. Spinal cord transection results in bowel dysfunction that consists of intractable constipation, fecal impaction, overflow fecal incontinence, and distention-induced uncontrolled reflex defecation. Affected patients lack volitional control of defecation (132). Continence may be preserved without fecal impaction through avoidance of dehydration, a diet high in fiber, and a regular toileting regimen. Residual sexual function depends on the level of injury, with reflex sexual activity typically absent during spinal shock. Thoracic and cervical level lesions are generally associated with retention of reflex penile erections and occasional ejaculation in males, and with vaginal secretions as part of a genital reflex in females. Conus medullaris lesions are usually associated with absence of penile erections and vaginal secretions. A study of 68 premenopausal women with spinal cord injuries showed preservation of T11 to L2 dermatomal sensory function in association with pychogenically-mediated genital vasocongestion. Less than 50% of affected patients were able to achieve orgasm, with only 17% with complete S2 to S5 lesions and complete lower motor neuron dysfunction achieving orgasm, compared to 59% with other levels or degrees of injury (133).

Cauda Equina Injury

Cauda equina injury leads to LMN bladder and pelvic floor muscle dysfunction, resulting in voiding difficulties (134). Cauda equina compression resulting in acute disc rupture that leads to voiding and erectile dysfunction improves with surgical repair (135–137) and improves the likelihood of, or restores, erectile function. Cauda equina and conus lesions resulting in bladder areflexia show abnormal sphincter activity and denervation of pelvic floor muscles on needle CNEMG (138–140). Resulting bowel dysfunction consists of constipation and fecal incontinence, which improve over several months to years, even after effective decompression (141, 142). Acute cauda equina syndrome secondary to lumbar disc herniation may mimic pure conus medullaris syndrome with urinary retention, constipation, and impotence that too recovers with surgical decompression (143). Conservative treatment instead consists of intermittent catheterization guided by urodynamic abnormalities (144).

PERIPHERAL NEUROPATHY

Bladder, bowel, and sexual dysfunction result from PNS injury affecting somatic motor, sensory, and ANS function. Diabetes is perhaps the commonest etiologic factor in the peripheral neuropathic cause of bladder, bowel, and sexual dysfunction (1), with a prevalence rate of bladder dysfunction that increases with the duration of diabetes, which is estimated to be 25% after 10 years and >50% after 45 years of diabetes (145). Diabetic cystopathy is present in 26 to 87% of diabetic patients and correlates with the presence of a generalized polyneuropathy (146, 147). The onset is usually insidious, with impaired bladder sensation, delayed micturition reflexes, increased bladder capacity, and urinary retention, hesitancy, weak urinary stream, dribbling, and nocturia.

Common cystometric findings include detrusor areflexia with impaired sensation of bladder filling. However, patients with diabetes not uncommonly manifest detrusor hyperreflexia on urodynamic study, and men may exhibit features of bladder outlet obstruction (148). In elderly diabetic patients, the presence of bladder hyperreflexia and occasional detrusor sphincter dyssynergia may reflect coexistent associated neurologic diseases such as stroke or prior spinal trauma (149). Electromyography of perineal muscles can be used to show denervation and detrusor-sphincter dyssynergia (150), prolonged latency of evoked potentials in response to detrusor stimulation and prolonged latency of the BCR indicative of visceral neuropathy (151).

Treatment of resulting bladder areflexia includes scheduled voiding along with the Crede maneuver, cholinergic medications such as bethanechol, and intermittent catheterization. Intensive diabetic management (152) may favorably affect diabetic bladder dysfunction demonstrable on cystometry, and incontinence in those with urinary overflow.

Fecal incontinence occurs in up to 20% of diabetics, may be nocturnal, and can coincide with diarrhea (153). Sphincter tone may be diminished on examination, and incontinence may be related to abnormal internal or external anal sphincter function (154, 155). An increased perceptive threshold to rectal balloon distention suggests the presence of sensory dysfunction, and this may contribute to incontinence by impaired perception of rectal fullness (156). Biofeedback therapy can improve fecal incontinence in some patients (155).

Sexual dysfunction in male diabetic patients includes retrograde ejaculation, which is believed to be caused by contractile failure of the internal vesicle sphincter of the bladder during ejaculation. This may respond to sympathomimetic medications (157). Erectile dysfunction affects more than one-third of diabetic men and accounts for 9% of evaluations in a medical clinic for impotence (158, 159). Abnormalities of the BCRL and the dorsal nerve of the penis conduction velocity supports a PNS etiology for impotence

in diabetic men (159–161). Sexual dysfunction in diabetic women includes inadequate lubrication, anorgasmia, and dyspareunia (162). Both men and women can experience loss of libido, and psychological factors can play a role and need to be considered in the overall approach to treatment (163, 164). Therapeutic options include penile prosthetic insertion, vacuum constriction devices, and local pharmacologic injection therapy (165, 166).

Guillain-Barré syndrome (GBS) is a form of acute inflammatory demyelinating polyradiculoneuropathy (AIDP) characterized by symmetrical, ascending motor paralysis with or without sensory disturbances. ANS and bladder disturbances including urinary retention, voiding difficulty, and urinary urgency occur in up to one-quarter of patients (167, 168). The severity of GBS correlates with the occurrence of bladder dysfunction with three-quarters of intubated patients manifesting micturition problems (169), more common in those with severe weakness as compared to those with mild involvement (168). Underactivity or overactivity of the detrusor muscle, and hyperactive EUS activity were major urodynamic findings in 65 GBS patients (170). Management is usually supportive, with resolution of urinary symptoms in the natural course of the disease, however α-blocker medications may be necessary to ameliorate urinary dysfunction, and some patients need intermittent self-catheterization when recovery is slow or poor (170).

Hereditary sensory and autonomic neuropathies (HSAN) and transthyretin (TTR) familial amyloid neuropathy (171, 172) are associated with PNS and ANS bladder and bowel involvement (173). With differences in mode of inheritance, symptoms at onset, clinical course, and pathology of neurons or axons affected in individual subtypes, there has been increasing appreciation of the genetic, clinical neurophysiology, biochemical, and autonomic features of these disorders. Survivors with once fatal forms of HSAN, and TTR amyloid neuropathy experience varying autonomic disturbances that affect bladder, bowel, and sexual function, resulting from genetically mediated PNS and ganglionic neuronal degeneration in the former, and extracellular deposition of insoluble amyloid protein fibrils in the PNS of the latter. Lower urinary tract dysfunction in familial amyloidotic neuropathy of the Portuguese type (174) included dysuria, incontinence, sensitivity, and contractility disturbances of the detrusor muscle, non-relaxing urethral sphincter. Dyssynergia was found in one-quarter to one-half of patients so studied. Urinary retention was due to inadequate contraction of the detrusor, probably associated with non-relaxing of the internal and external sphincter, derived from deposition of an amyloid substance in the detrusor. Two other forms of systemic amyloidosis, immunoglobulin (AL) or primary amyloidosis associated with monoclonal paraproteinemic light chains as the amyloid fibrils; and reactive (AA) or secondary amyloidosis, occur in association with chronic inflammatory disorders wherein fibrils derived from amyloid A protein circulate as an acute phase reactant, both of which can be associated with ANS sequela.

Plexus Injury

Pelvic plexus injury may be a consequence of major pelvic surgery such as abdominoperineal resection or radical hysterectomy, as well as trauma and childbirth. Hysterectomy causes damage to the pelvic plexus and contributes to incontinence later in life (175). Features noticed in women undergoing radical hysterectomy and pelvic lymphadenectomy (176, 177) included decreased or altered awareness of bladder distention, stress incontinence, prolonged postoperative urinary retention, and hypertonicity on cystometric studies, reflecting excessive unopposed parasympathetic tone or an intrinsic increase in bladder myogenic tone secondary to surgical dissection adjacent to the bladder, with irritation from a indwelling bladder catheter. Tumor invasion of the pelvic plexus can lead to somatic, parasympathetic, and sympathetic nerve injury resulting in bladder areflexia with retention, constipation, and impotence (178, 179). Voiding dysfunction occurs after abdominoperineal resection of the rectum in more than two-thirds of patients (180, 181), symptoms of which usually subside over three to six months. Urodynamic findings are variable and include patients with areflexic and hyperreflexic bladder function, and decreased proximal urethral pressure. Bladder areflexia when present, is later replaced by hyperreflexia. Removal of the cardinal ligaments or a long cuff of the upper vagina during hysterectomy increases the likelihood of posterior pelvic plexus neuropathy with involvement of parasympathetic nerves during abdominoperineal resection with mobilization of the rectum (182). Women develop intractable constipation after hysterectomy associated with increased rectal compliance and volume reflective of incidental parasympathetic nerve injury (183). Functional obstruction of the colon may result from malignant tumor infiltration of the splanchnic nerves, celiac plexus, semilunar ganglia, and vagus nerves thought to reflect an imbalance of sympathetic and parasympathetic innervation, or Ogilvie syndrome (184). Surgery may be considered to prevent cecal rupture if conservative management failed to decompress the colon.

Sexual dysfunction may result from resection of the rectum with erectile and ejaculatory dysfunction in men and decreased vaginal secretions, dyspareunia, and diminished orgasm in women. The incidence is highest in abdominoperineal resection procedures and lower with anterior procedures, suggesting that the extent of local surgical trauma is an etiologic factor (185). The incidence of impotence is about 11% in men with lumbosacral plexus neuropathy secondary to tumor invasion (179).

Mononeuropathy

Stress urinary incontinence and genitourinary prolapse in women are associated with pudendal nerve injury, the diagnosis of which is ascertained with certainty when there is PNTML prolongation (186, 187). Single-fiber EMG of the pubococcygeus and anal sphincter muscles with genitourinary prolapse, with or without stress urinary incontinence, shows increased fiber density, consistent with reinnervation (187–189). These findings are more common in women who experience prolonged labor and vaginal delivery and may reflect direct pressure effect or stretching of the pudendal nerve (188). Vaginal dissection may be associated with perineal motor nerve injury and can worsen preexisting perineal neuropathy in patients with stress incontinence (190). CNEMG of pelvic floor muscles reveals asymmetric and uncoordinated levator muscle activation patterns in parous stress-incontinent women (191). Constipation, in addition to obstetric history, may be associated with the development of pudendal nerve damage and stress urinary incontinence (192). Fecal incontinence is commonly present in women with stress urinary incontinence and is associated with weakness of the internal and external anal sphincters, the puborectalis, and other striated muscles of the pelvic floor (193–195), and with prolongation of the PNTML measured to the rectal sphincter (196). This may result from injury to the pudendal nerves or direct injury to the pelvic nerves during vaginal delivery and is associated with multiparity, forceps delivery, and high birth weight (197).

Occult lacerations and direct muscle injury of the external anal sphincter may accompany neurogenic injury and contribute to incontinence (198, 199). PNTML measurement in patients with untreated fecal incontinence may progressively worsen but is not always associated with clinical worsening of incontinence (200). An association of PNTML with the extent of pelvic descent during straining has been suggested to represent the result of recurrent trauma to the pudendal nerves during perineal descent (201, 202); however, other studies have not suggested this relationship. Flaccid and non-contractile muscle movement abnormalities present on videoproctography in patients with neuropathic fecal incontinence were not present in those with chronic constipation without fecal incontinence and control patients (203). A prospective study of 213 patients with disturbances of defecation (204) did not demonstrate a correlation between perineal descent and PNTML. A sensory deficit of the rectum and anal canal may occur in isolation or accompany anorectal motor dysfunction and contribute to fecal incontinence (205, 206).

Conservative management includes pelvic electrical stimulation, pelvic floor exercises, and biofeedback therapy (207). Treatment of refractory patients includes surgical repair of the sphincter. The identification of extensive external striated sphincter injury by CNEMG may be valuable in predicting response to surgical sphincter repair (208). Unilateral or bilateral pudendal neuropathy is associated with a reduced likelihood of an excellent result from repair of anterior anal sphincter defects after obstetric delivery (209, 210). However, overlap does exist in preoperative PNTML values between patient groups achieving good versus poor long-term results (211).

Myopathy

Urinary and fecal incontinence are uncommon accompaniments of most myopathies. Fecal incontinence with myotonic muscular dystrophy may be increased with diarrhea. Needle CNEMG of the puborectalis and external anal sphincter muscle of patients with myotonic dystrophy reveals abnormalities consistent with both myopathy and reinnervation (212). Exercise-induced urinary incontinence and muscle weakness were the presenting features of a 68-year-old man with acid maltase deficiency (213). Stress incontinence with pelvic floor muscle involvement may be an early feature of limb girdle muscular dystrophy (214). Urinary incontinence is occasionally present in Duchenne muscular dystrophy but may instead be related to concomitant scoliosis or spinal fusion (215).

REFERENCES

1. Burakgazi AZ, Alsowaity B, Burakgazi ZA, et al. Bladder dysfunction in peripheral neuropathies. *Muscle Nerve* 2012; 45:2–8.
2. Roberts MM. Neurophysiology in neurourology. *Muscle Nerve* 2008; 38:815–836.
3. Blaivas JG. The neurophysiology of micturition: a clinical study of 550 patients. *J Urol* 1982; 127:958–963.
4. Abrams P, Cardozo L, Fall M, et al. The standardization of terminology of lower urinary tract Function: report of the Standardization Sub-committee of the International Continence Society. *Neurourol Urodyn* 2002; 21:167–178.
5. Assessment: neurological evaluation of male sexual dysfunction. Report of the Therapeutics and Technology Assessment Subcommittee of the American Academy of Neurology. *Neurology* 1995; 45:2287–2292.
6. Madoff RD, Williams JG, Caushaj PF. Fecal incontinence. *N Engl J Med* 1992; 326:1002–1007.
7. Henry MM. Pathogenesis and management of fecal incontinence in the adult. *Gastroenterol Clin North Am* 1987; 16:35–45.
8. Jorge JM, Wexner SD. Etiology and management of fecal incontinence. *Dis Colon Rectum* 1993; 36:77–97.
9. Wexner SD, Jorge JM. Colorectal physiologic tests: use or abuse of technology? *Eur J Surg* 1994; 160:167–174.
10. Lefaucheur JP. Neurophysiological testing in anorectal disorders. *Muscle Nerve* 2006; 33:324–333.
11. Podnar S, Vodusek DB. Protocol for clinical neurophysiologic examination of the pelvic floor. *Neurourol Urodyn* 2001; 20:669–682.
12. Podnar S. Nomenclature of the electrophysiologically tested sacral reflexes. *Neurourol Urodyn* 2006; 25:95–97.
13. Podnar S. Neurophysiologic studies of the penilo-cavernous reflex: normative data. *Neurourol Urodyn* 2007; 26:864–869.
14. Vodusek DB, Amarenco G, Batra A, et al. Clinical neurophysiology. In: Abrams P, Cardozo L, Khoury S, Wein A, eds. *Incontinence*, 3rd International Consultation on incontinence, June 26–29, 2004, Monaco, Plymouth, UK: Health Publications, 2005, 1:675–706.
15. Sethi RK, Bauer SB, Dyro FM, et al. Modulation of the bulbocavernous reflex during voiding: loss of inhibition in upper motor neuron disease. *Muscle Nerve* 1989; 12:892–897.
16. Vodusek DB, Janko M, Lokar J. Direct and reflex responses in perineal muscles on electrical stimulation. *J Neurol Neurosurg Psychiatry* 1983; 46:67–71.
17. Galloway NT, Chisholm GD, McInnes A. Patterns and significance of the sacral evoked response (the urologist's knee jerk). *Br J Urol* 1985; 57:145–147.
18. Galimberti V, Premoselli S, Passerini D, et al. Sacral reflexes normal values with monopolar short needle electrodes recording. *Electromyogr Clin Neurophysiol* 2001; 41:457–462.
19. Amarenco G, Ismael SS, Bayle B, et al. Electrophysiological analysis of pudendal neuropathy following traction. *Muscle Nerve* 2001; 24:116–119.
20. Fowler CJ. Pelvic floor neurophysiology. *Methods in Clinical Neurophysiology.* ed., Dantec; 1991; 2:1–24.
21. Swash M. Anorectal incontinence: electrophysiological tests. *Br J Surg* Suppl 1985; 72(Suppl):S14–S15.
22. Vodusek DB. Evoked potential testing. *Urol Clin North Am* 1996; 23:427–446.
23. Bradley W, Lin J, Johnson B. Measurement of the conduction velocity of the dorsal nerve of the penis. *J Urol* 1984; 131:1127–1129.
24. Clawson DR, Cardenas DD. Dorsal nerve of the penis nerve conduction velocity: a new technique. *Muscle Nerve* 1991; 14:845–849.
25. Haldeman S, Bradley WE, Bhatia NN. Evoked responses from the pudendal nerve. *J Urol* 1982; 128:974–980.
26. Haldeman S, Bradley WE, Bhattia NN. Pudendal evoked responses. *Arch Neurol* 1982; 39:280–283.
27. Dick HC, Bradley WE, Scott FB, et al. Pudendal sexual reflexes. Electrophysiologic investigations. *Urology* 1974; 3:376–379.
28. Siroky MB, Sax DS, Krane RJ. Sacral signal tracing: the electrophysiology of the bulbocavernosus reflex. *J Urol* 1979; 122:661–664.
29. Podnar S. Which patients need referral for anal sphincter electromyography? *Muscle Nerve* 2006; 33:278–282.
30. Podnar S, Vodusek DB, Stalberg E. Comparison of quantitative techniques in anal sphincter electromyography. *Muscle Nerve* 2002; 25:83–92.
31. Podnar S, Rodi Z, Lukanovic, et al. Standardization of anal sphincter EMG: technique of needle examination. *Muscle Nerve* 1999; 22:400–403.
32. Lowe EM, Lowe CJ, Osborne JL, et al. Improved method for needle electromyography of the urethral sphincter in women. *Neurourol Urodynam* 1994; 13:29–33.
33. DiBenedetto M, Yalla SV. Electrodiagnosis of striated urethral sphincter dysfunction. *J Urol* 1979; 122:361–365.
34. Welter ML, Dechoz S, Leroi AM et al. Reponses evoquees electriques et mecaniques du sphincter anal externe après stimulation magnetiques corticales et lombaires. *Neurophysiol Clin* 2000; 30:246–253.

35. Turnball GK, Hamdy S, Aziz Q, et al. The cortical topography of human anorectal musculature. *Gastroenterology* 1999; 117:32–39.

36. Ravits JM. AAEM minimonograph #48: autonomic nervous system testing. *Muscle Nerve* 1997; 20:919–937.

37. Petropouleas A, Younger DS. Autonomic reflex testing (ART). In, DJ Lynn, HB Newton, AD Rae-Grant, eds. *The 5-Minute Neurology Consult*. Lippincott Williams & Wilkins:New York, 2012; 39.

38. Lauria G, Cornblath DR, Johansson O, et al. EFNS Guidelines on the use of skin biopsy in the diagnosis of peripheral neuropathy. *Eur J Neurol* 2005; 12:1–12.

39. England JD, Gronseth GS, Franklin G, et al. Practice parameter: evaluation of distal symmetric polyneuropathy: role of autonomic testing, nerve biopsy, and skin biopsy (an evidence-based review): Report of the Amercan Academy of Neurology, American Association of Neuromuscular and Electrodiagnostic Medicine, and Amercan Academy of Physical Medicine and Rehabilitation. *Neurology* 2009; 72:177–184.

40. Lauria G, Lombardi R. Small fiber neuropathy: Is skin biopsy the holy grail? *Curr Diab Rep* 2012; 12:384–392.

41. Manganelli F, Dubbioso R, Nolano M, et al. Autoimmune autonomic ganglionopathy: a possible postganglionic neuropathy. *Arch Neurol* 2011; 68:504–507.

42. Huggins ME, Bhatia NN, Ostergard DR. Urinary incontinence: newer pharmacotherapeutic trends. *Curr Opin Obstet Gynecol* 2003; 15:419–427.

43. Fantl JA, Newman DK, Colling J, et al. Urinary incontinence in adults: acute and chronic management. Clinical Practice Guideline No. 2, 1996 update. Rockville, MD: *U.S. Department of Health and Human Services, Agency for Health Care and Policy Research*. AHPCR Publication No. 96-0682.

44. Chancellor MB, Blaivas JG, eds. *Practical neuro-urology-genitourinary complications in neurologic disease*. Boston, MA: Butterworth-Heinemann, 1995.

45. Burgio KL. Behavioral treatment options for urinary incontinence. *Gastroenterology* 2004; 126:S82–S89.

46. Diokno AC. Medical management of urinary incontinence. *Gastroenterology* 2004; 126:S77–S81.

47. Richardson DA. Conservative management of urinary incontinence—a symposium. *J Reprod Med* 1993; 38:659–661.

48. Pettit PDM, Thompson JR, Chen AH. Sacral neuromodulation; new applications in the treatment of female pelvic floor dysfunction. *Curr Opin Obstet Gynecol* 2002; 14:521–525.

49. Scarlett Y. Medical management of fecal incontinence. *Gastroenterology* 2004; 126:S55–S63.

50. Binnie NR, Kawimbe BM, Papachrysostomou M, et al. Use of the pudendo-anal reflex in the treatment of neurogenic faecal incontinence. *Gut* 1990; 31:1051–1055.

51. Keighley MRB, Fielding JWL. Management of faecal incontinence and results of surgical treatment. *Br J Surg* 1983; 70:463–468.

52. Madoff RD. Surgical treatment options for fecal incontinence. *Gastroenterology* 2004; 126:S48–S54.

53. Lechtenberg R, Ohl DA. *Sexual dysfunction. Neurologic, Urologic and Gynecologic Aspects*. Lea and Febiger: Philadelphia, 1994.

54. Rosen RC, McKenna KE. PDE-5 inhibition and sexual response: pharmacological mechanisms and clinical outcomes. *Annu Rev Sex Res* 2002; 13:36–88.

55. Linet OI, Ogring FG, for the Alprostadil Study Group. Efficacy and safety of intracavernosal alprostadil in men with erectile dysfunction. *N Engl J Med* 1996; 334:873–877.

56. Padma-Nathan H, Hellstrom WJ, et al, for the Medicated Urethral System for Erection (MUSE) Study Group. Treatment of men with erectile dysfunction with transurethral alprostadil. *N Engl J Med* 1997; 336:1–7.

57. Currie CT. Urinary incontinence after stroke. *Br Med J* 1986; 293:1322–1323.

58. Gelber DA, Good DC, Laven LJ, et al. Causes of urinary incontinence after acute right hemisphere stroke. *Stroke* 1993; 24:378–382.

59. Taub NA, Wolfe CDA, Richardson E, et al. Predicting the disability of first-time stroke sufferers at 1 year. *Stroke* 1994; 25:352–357.

60. Maguire PA, Taylor IC, Stout RW. Elderly patients in acute medical wards: factors predicting length of stay in hospital. *BMJ* 1986; 292:1251–1253.

61. Wade DT, Hewer RL. Outlook after an acute stroke: urinary incontinence and loss of consciousness compared in 532 patients. *Q J Med* 1985; 56:601–608.

62. Anderson CS, Jamrozik KD, Broadhurst RJ, et al. Predicting survival for 1 year among different subtypes of stroke. *Stroke* 1994; 25:1935–1944.

63. Sakakibara R, Takamichi H, Uchiyama T, et al. Urinary function in elderly people with and without leukoaraiosis: Relation to cognitive and gait function. *J Neurol Neurosurg Psychiatry* 1999; 67:658–660.

64. Brittain KR, Peet SM, Castleden CM. Stroke and incontinence. *Stroke* 1998; 29:524–528.

65. Tsuchida S, Noto H, Yamaguchi O, et al. Urodynamics studies on hemiplegic patients after cerebrovascular accidents. *Urology* 1983; 21:315–318.

66. Khan Z, Starer P, Yang WC, et al. Analysis of voiding disorders in patients with cerebrovascular accidents. *Urology* 1990; 34:265–270.

67. Khan Z, Hertanu J, Yang WC, et al. Predictive correlation of urodynamic dysfunction and brain injury after cerebrovascular accident. *J Urol* 1981; 126:86–88.

68. Garrett VE, Scott JA, Costich J, et al. Bladder emptying assessment in stroke patients. *Arch Phys Med Rehabil* 1989; 70:41–43.

69. Lum SK, Marshall VR. Results of prostatectomy in patients following a cerebrovascular accident. *Br J Urol* 1982; 54:186–189.

70. Ishii N, Nishihara Y, Imamura T. Why do frontal lobe symptoms predominate in vascular dementia with lacunes? *Neurology* 1986; 36:340–345.

71. Bogousslavsky J, Regli F. Anterior cerebral artery territory infarction in the Lausanne stroke registry. Clinical and etiologic patterns. *Arch Neurol* 1990; 47:144–150.

72. Harari D, Coshall C, Rudd AG, et al. New-onset fecal incontinence after stroke: Prevalence, natural history, risk factors and impact. *Stroke* 2003; 34:144–150.

73. Mankovic SP, Badlani G. Voiding and sexual dysfunction after cerebrovascular accidents. *J Urol* 2001; 165:359–370.

74. Coslett HB, Heilman KM. Male sexual function. Impairment after right hemisphere stroke. *Arch Neurol* 1986; 43:1036–1039.

75. Ishii N, Nishihara Y, Imamura T. Why do frontal lobe symptoms predominate in vascular dementia with lacunes? *Neurology* 1986; 36:340–345.

76. Andrew J, Nathan PW. Lesions on the anterior frontal lobes and disturbances of micturition and defecation. *Brain* 1964; 87:233–265.

77. Thal LJ, Grundman M, Klauber MR. Dementia: characteristics of a referral population and factors associated with progression. *Neurology* 1988; 38:1083–1090.

78. Bennett DA, Gilley DW, Wilson RS, et al. Clinical correlates of high signal lesions on magnetic resonance imaging in Alzheimer's disease. *J Neurol* 1992; 239:186–190.

79. Tarvonen-Schroder S, Roytta M, Raiha I, et al. Clinical features of leuko-araiosis. *J Neurol Neurosurg Psychiatry* 1996; 60:431–436.

80. Vascular dementia: diagnostic criteria for research studies:

report of the NINDS-AIREN International Workshop. *Neurology* 1993; 43:250–260.

81. Del-Ser T, Munoz DG, Hachinski V. Temporal pattern of cognitive decline and incontinence is different in Alzheimer's disease and diffuse Lewy body disease. *Neurology* 1996; 46:682–686.

82. Burns A, Jacoby R, Levy R. Psychiatric phenomena in Alzheimer's disease. IV. Disorders of behavior. *Br J Psychiatry* 1990; 157:86–94.

83. Newens AJ, Forster DP, Kay DW. Dependency and community care in presenile Alzheimer's disease. *Br J Psychiatry* 1995; 166:777–782.

84. Fisher CM. Hydrocephalus as a cause of disturbances of gait in the elderly. *Neurology* 1982; 32:1358–1363.

85. Jonas S, Brown J. Neurogenic bladder in normal pressure hydrocephalus. *Urology* 1975; 5:44–50.

86. Romero Y, Evans JM, Fleming KC, et al. Constipation and fecal incontinence in the elderly population. *Mayo Clin Proc* 1996; 71:81–92.

87. Pavlakis AJ, Siroky MB, Goldstein I, et al. Neurologic findings in Parkinson's disease. *J Urol* 1983; 129:80–83.

88. Berger Y, Blaivas JG, DeLarocha ER, et al. Urodynamic findings in Parkinson's disease. *J Urol* 1987; 138:836–838.

89. Fitzmaurice H, Fowler CJ, Rickards D, et al. Micturition disturbance in Parkinson's disease. *Br J Urol* 1985; 57:652–656.

90. Uchiyama T, Sakakibara R, Hattori T, et al. Short-term effect of a single levodopa dose on micturition disturbance in Parkinson's disease patients with the wearing off phenomenon. *Mov Disord* 2003; 18:573–578.

91. Finazzi-Agro E, Peppe A, D'Amico A, et al. Effects of subthalamic nucleus stimulation on urodynamic findings in patients with Parkinson's disease. *J Urol* 2003; 169:1388–1391.

92. Seif C, Herzog J, van der Horst C, et al. Effect of subthalamic deep brain stimulation on the function of the urinary bladder. *Ann Neurol* 2004; 55:118–120.

93. Staskin DS, Vardi Y, Siroky MB. Post-prostatectomy continence in the parkinsonian patient: the significance of poor voluntary sphincter contraction. *J Urol* 1988; 140:117–118.

94. Khan Z, Starer P, Bhola A. Urinary incontinence in female Parkinson disease patients. Pitfalls of diagnosis. *Urology* 1989; 33:486–489.

95. Lipe H, Longstreth WT Jr, Bird TD, et al. Sexual function in married men with Parkinson's disease compared to married men with arthritis. *Neurology* 1990; 40:1347–1349.

96. Okun MS, McDonald WM, DeLong MR. Refractory nonmotor symptoms in male patients with Parkinson disease due to testosterone deficiency: A common unrecognized comorbidity. *Arch Neurol* 2002; 59:807–811.

97. Uitti RJ, Tanner CM, Rajput AH, et al. Hypersexuality with antiparkinsonian therapy. *Clin Neuropharmacol* 1989; 12:375–383.

98. Romito LM, Raja M, Daniele A, et al. Transient mania with hypersexuality after surgery for high frequency stimulation of the subthalamic nucleus in Parkinson's disease. *Mov Disord* 2002; 17:1371–1374.

99. Castelli L, Perozzo P, Genesia ML, et al. Sexual well-being in parkinsonian patients after deep brain stimulation of the subthalamic nucleus. *J Neurol Neurosurg Psychiatry* 2004; 75:1260–1264.

100. Sakakibara R, Odaka T, Uchiyama T, et al. Colonic transit time and rectoanal videomanometry in Parkinson's disease. *J Neurol Neurosurg Psychiatry* 2003; 74:268–272.

101. Sakakibara R, Hattori T, Tojo M, et al. Micturitional disturbance in multiple system atrophy. *Jpn J Psychiatr Neurol* 1993; 47:591–598.

102. Wenning GK, Shlomo YB, Magalhaes M, et al. Clinical features and natural history of multiple system atrophy. An analysis of 100 cases. *Brain* 1994; 117:835–845.

103. Beck RO, Betts CD, Fowler CJ. Genitourinary dysfunction in multiple system atrophy: clinical features and treatment in 62 cases. *J Urol* 1994; 151:1336–1341.

104. Vodusek DB. Sphincter EMG and differential diagnosis of multiple system atrophy. *Mov Disord* 2001; 16:600–607.

105. Sakakibara R, Hattori T, Uchiyama T, Videourodynamic and sphincter motor unit potential analyses in Parkinson's disease and multiple system atrophy. *J Neurol Neurosurg Psychiatry* 2001; 71:600–606.

106. Gilman L, Low P, Albanese A, et al. Consensus statement on the diagnosis of multiple system atrophy. *Clin Auton Res* 1998; 8:359–362.

107. Salinas JM, Berger Y, De La Rocha RE, et al. Urological evaluation in the Shy Drager syndrome. *J Urol* 1986; 135:741–743.

108. Sakakibara R, Hattori T, Tojo M, et al. Micturitional disturbance in progressive supranuclear palsy. *J Auton Nerv Syst* 1993; 45:101–106.

109. Sakakibara R, Odaka T, Uchiyama T, et al. Colonic transit time, sphincter EMG, and rectoanal videomanometry in multiple system atrophy. *Mov Disord* 2004; 19:924–929.

110. Sakuta M, Nakanishi T, Toyokura Y. Anal muscle electromyograms differ in amyotrophic lateral sclerosis and Shy-Drager syndrome. *Neurology* 1978; 28:1289–1293.

111. Fowler CJ, van Kerrebroeck PEV, Nordenbo A, et al. Treatment of lower urinary tract dysfunction in patients with multiple sclerosis. Report from the Committee of the European Study Group of SUDIMS (Sexual and Urological Disorders in Multiple Sclerosis). *J Neurol Neurosurg Psychiatry* 1992; 55:986–989.

112. Hinson JL. Urodynamics and multiple sclerosis. *Urol Clin North Am* 1996; 23:475–481.

113. Bemelmans BLH, Hommes OR, Van Kerrebroeck PEV, et al. Evidence for early lower urinary tract dysfunction in clinically silent multiple sclerosis. *J Urol* 1991; 145:1219–1224.

114. Awad SA, Gajewski JB, Sogbein K, et al. Relationship between neurological and urological status in patients with multiple sclerosis. *J Urol* 1984; 132:499–502.

115. Blaivas JG, Bhimani G, Labib KB. Vesicourethral dysfunction in multiple sclerosis. *J Urol* 1979; 122:342–347.

116. Goldstein I, Siroky MB, Sax DS, et al. Neurologic abnormalities in multiple sclerosis. *J Urol* 1982; 128:541–545.

117. Blaivas JG, Barbalias GA. Detrusor-external sphincter dyssynergia in men with multiple sclerosis: an ominous urologic condition. *J Urol* 1984; 131:91–94.

118. McGuire EJ, Savastano JA. Urodynamic findings and long-term outcome management of patients with multiple sclerosis-induced lower urinary tract dysfunction. *J Urol* 1984; 132:713–715.

119. DasGupta R, Fowler CJ. Bladder, bowel, and sexual dysfunction in multiple sclerosis. *Drugs* 2003; 63:153–166.

120. Nanninga JB, Frost F, Penn R. Effect of intrathecal baclofen on bladder and sphincter function. *J Urol* 1989; 142:101–105.

121. Chia YW, Fowler CJ, Kamm MA, et al. Prevalence of bowel dysfunction in patients with multiple sclerosis and bladder function. *J Neurol* 1995; 242:105–108.

122. Swash M, Snooks SJ, Chalmers DHK. Parity as a factor in incontinence in multiple sclerosis. *Arch Neurol* 1987; 44:504–508.

123. Hinds JP, Eidelman BH, Wald A. Prevalence of bowel dysfunction in multiple sclerosis. A population survey. *Gastroenterology* 1990; 98:1538–1542.

124. Weber J, Grise P, Roquebert M, et al. Radiopaque markers transit and anorectal manometry in 16 patients with multiple sclerosis and urinary bladder dysfunction. *Dis Colon Rectum* 1987; 30:95–100.

125. Gill KP, Chia YW, Henry MM, et al. Defecography in multiple sclerosis patients with severe constipation. *Radiology* 1994; 191:553–556.

126. Chia YW, Gill KP, Jameson JS. Paradoxical puborectalis contraction is a feature of constipation in patients with multiple sclerosis. *J Neurol Neurosurg Psychiatry* 1996; 60:31–35.

127. Caruana BJ, Wald A, Hinds JP, et al. Anorectal sensory and motor function in neurogenic fecal incontinence—comparison between multiple sclerosis and diabetes mellitus. *Gastroenterology* 1991; 100:465–470.

128. Mattson D, Petrie M, Srivastava DK, et al. Multiple sclerosis. Sexual dysfunction and its response to medications. *Arch Neurol* 1995; 52:862–868.

129. DasGupta R, Fowler CJ. Bladder, bowel, and sexual dysfunction in multiple sclerosis. *Drugs* 2003; 63:153–166.

130. Borello-France D, Leng W, O'Leary M, et al. Bladder and sexual function among women with multiple sclerosis. *Mult Scler* 2004; 10:455–461.

131. Wheeler JS, Walter JW. Acute urologic management of the patient with spinal cord injury. Initial hospitalization. *Urol Clin North Am* 1993; 20:403–411.

132. Perkash I. Long-term urologic management of the patient with spinal cord injury. *Urol Clin North Am* 1993; 20:423–434.

133. Sipski ML, Alexander CJ, Rosen RC. Sexual arousal and orgasm in women: effects of spinal cord injury. *Ann Neurol* 2001; 49:35–44.

134. Goldman HB, Appell RA. Voiding dysfunction in women with lumbar disc prolapse. *Int Urogynecol J Pelvic Floor Dysfunct* 1999; 10:134–138.

135. Shapiro S. Caudae equina syndrome secondary to lumbar disc herniation. *Neurosurgery* 1993; 32:743–747.

136. O'Flynn KJ, Murphy R, Thomas DG. Neurogenic bladder dysfunction in lumbar intervertebral disc prolapse. *Br J Urol* 1992; 69:38–40.

137. O'Laoire SA, Crockard NA, Thomas DG. Prognosis for sphincter recovery after operation for caudae equina compression owing to lumbar disc prolapse. *Br Med J* 1981; 282:1852–1854.

138. Bradley WE, Andersen JT. Neuromuscular dysfunction of the lower urinary tract in patients with lesions of the caudae equina and conus medullaris. *J Urol* 1976; 116:620–621.

139. Sandri SD, Fanciullacci F, Politi P, et al. Urinary disorders in intervertebral disc prolapse. *Neurourol Urodyn* 1987; 6:11–19.

140. Pavlakis AJ, Siroky MB, Goldstein I, Krane RJ. Neurologic findings in conus medullaris and caudae equina injury. *Arch Neurol* 1983; 40:570–573.

141. Emmett JL, Love JG. Urinary retention in women caused by asymptomatic protruded lumbar disk: report of 5 cases. *J Urol* 1968; 99:597–606.

142. Hellstrom P, Kortelainen P, Kontturi M. Late urodynamic findings after surgery for cauda equina syndrome caused by a prolapsed lumbar intervetebral disk. *J Urol* 1986; 135:308–312.

143. Fujisawa H, Igarashi S, Koyama T. Acute cauda equina syndrome secondary to lumbar disc herniation mimicking pure conus medullaris syndrome-case report. *Neurol Med Chir* 1998; 38:429–431.

144. Appell RA. Voiding dysfunction and lumbar disc disorders. *Probl Urol* 1993; 7:35–40.

145. Sasaki K, Yoshimura N, Chancellor MB. Implications of diabetes mellitus in urology. *Urol Clin N Am* 2003; 30:1–12.

146. Frimodt-Moller C. Diabetic cystopathy: epidemiology and related disorders. *Ann Intern Med* 1980; 92:318–321.

147. Ellenberg M. Development of urinary bladder dysfunction in diabetes mellitus. *Ann Intern Med* 1980; 92:321–323.

148. Kaplan SA, Te AE, Blaivas JG. Urodynamic findings in patients with diabetic cystopathy. *J Urol* 1995; 153:342–344.

149. Starer P, Libow L. Cystometric evaluation of bladder dysfunction in elderly diabetic patients. *Arch Intern Med* 1990; 150:810–813.

150. Niakan E, Harati Y, Comstock JP. Diabetic autonomic neuropathy. *Metabolism* 1986; 35:224–234.

151. Bradley WE, Timm GW, Rockswold GL, et al. Detrusor and urethral electromyography. *J Urol* 1975; 114:891–894.

152. Diabetes Control and Complications Trial Research Group. The effect of intensive treatment of diabetes on the development and progression of long-term complications in insulin-dependent diabetes mellitus. *N Engl J Med* 1993; 329:977–986.

153. Valdovinos MA, Camilleri M, Zimmerman BR. Chronic diarrhea in diabetes mellitus: mechanisms and an approach to diagnosis and treatment. *Mayo Clin Proc* 1993; 68:691–702.

154. Schiller LR, Santa Ana CA, Schmulen AC, et al. Pathogenesis of fecal incontinence in diabetes mellitus. Evidence for internal-anal-sphincter dysfunction. *N Engl J Med* 1982; 307:1666–1671.

155. Wald A, Tunuguntla AK. Anorectal sensorimotor dysfunction in fecal incontinence and diabetes mellitus: modification with biofeedback therapy. *N Engl J Med* 1984; 310:1282–1287.

156. Caruana BJ, Wald A, Hinds JP, et al. Anorectal sensory and motor function in neurogenic fecal incontinence. Comparison between multiple sclerosis and diabetes mellitus. *Gastroenterology* 1991; 100:465–470.

157. Ellenberg M. Diabetes and sexual dysfunction. *NY State J Med* 1982; 82:927–930.

158. Price DE. Managing impotence in diabetes. *Br Med J* 1993; 307:275–276.

159. Slag MF, Morley JE, Elson MK, et al. Impotence in medical clinic outpatients. *JAMA* 1983; 249:1736–1740.

160. Kaneko S, Bradley WE. Penile electrodiagnosis. Value of bulbocavernosus reflex latency versus nerve conduction velocity of the dorsal nerve of the penis in diagnosis of diabetic impotence. *J Urol* 1987; 137:933–935.

161. Daniels JS. Abnormal nerve conduction in impotent patients with diabetes mellitus. *Diabetes Care* 1989; 12:449–454.

162. Campbell LV, Redelman MJ, Borkman M, et al. Factors in sexual dysfunction in diabetic female volunteer subjects. *Med J Aust* 1989; 151:550–552.

163. Schiavi RC. Psychological treatment of erectile disorders in diabetic patients. *Ann Intern Med* 1980; 92:337–339.

164. Lustman RJ, Clouse RE. Relationship of psychiatric illness to impotence in men with diabetes. *Diabetes Care* 1990; 13:893–895.

165. Williams G. Erectile dysfunction: diagnosis and treatment. *Br J Urol* 1987; 60:1–5.

166. Whitehead ED. Diabetes-related impotence and its treatment in the middle-aged and elderly. Part II. *Geriatrics* 1987; 42:77–80.

167. Sakakibara R, Hattori T, Kuwabara S, et al. Micturitional disturbance in patients with Guillain-Barré syndrome. *J Neurol Neurosurg Psychiatry* 1997; 63:649–653.

168. Lichtenfeld P. Autonomic dysfunction in the Guillain-Barré syndrome. *Am J Med* 1971; 50:772–780.

169. De Jager AE, Sluiter HJ. Clinical signs in severe Guillain-Barré syndrome: analysis of 63 patients. *J Neurol Sci* 1991; 104:143–150.

170. Sakakibara R, Uchiyama T, Kuwabara S, et al. Prevalance and mechanism of bladder dysfunction in Guillain-Barré syndrome. *Neurourol Urodynam* 2009; 28:432–437.

171. Hund, E., Linke RP, Willig F, et al. Transthyretin-associated neuropathic amyloidosis: pathogenesis and treatment. *Neurology* 2001; 56: 431–435.

172. Ando Y, Nakamura M, Araki S. Transthyretin-related familial amyloidotic polyneuropathy. *Arch Neurol* 2005; 62: 1057–1062.

173. Hilz MJ. Assessment and evaluation of hereditary sensory and autonomic neuropathies with autonomic and

neurophysiological examinations. *Clin Auton Res* 2002; 12(Suppl 1):I33–I43.

174. Andrade MJ. Lower urinary tract dysfunction in familial amyloidotic polyneuropathy, Portuguese type. *Neurourol Urodynam* 2009; 28:26–32.

175. Brown JS, Seeley DG, Fong J, et al. Urinary incontinence in older women: who is at risk? *Obstet Gynecol* 1996; 87:715–721.

176. Forney JP. The effect of radical hysterectomy on bladder physiology. *Am J Obstet Gynecol* 1980; 138:374–382.

177. Seski JC, Diokno AC. Bladder dysfunction after radical abdominal hysterectomy? *Am J Obstet Gynecol* 1977; 128:643–651.

178. Woodside JR, Crawford ED. Urodynamic features of pelvic plexus injury. *J Urol* 1980; 124:657–658.

179. Jaeckle KA, Young DF, Foley KM. The natural history of lumbosacral plexopathy in cancer. *Neurology* 1985; 35:8–15.

180. Blaivas JG, Barbalias GA. Characteristics of neural injury after abdomino-perineal resection. *J Urol* 1983; 129:84–87.

181. Yalla SV, Andriole GL. Vesicourethral dysfunction following pelvic visceral ablative surgery. *J Urol* 1984; 132:503–509.

182. Mundy AR. An anatomical explanation for bladder dysfunction following rectal and uterine surgery. *Br J Urol* 1982; 54:501–504.

183. Varma JS. Autonomic influences on colorectal motility and pelvic surgery. *World J Surg* 1992; 16:811–819.

184. Nanni G, Garbini A, Luchetti P, et al. Ogilvie's syndrome (acute colonic pseudo-obstruction): review of the literature (October 1948–March 1980) and report of four additional cases. *Dis Colon Rectum* 1982; 25:157–166.

185. Fegiz G, Trenti A, Bezzi M, et al. Sexual and bladder dysfunctions following surgery for rectal carcinoma. *Ital J Surg Sci* 1986; 16:103–109.

186. Snooks SJ, Badenoch DF, Tiptaft RC, et al. Perineal nerve damage in genuine stress urinary incontinence. An electrophysiological study. *Br J Urol* 1985; 57:422–426.

187. Smith ARB, Hosker GL, Warrell DW. The role of pudendal nerve damage in the aetiology of genuine stress incontinence in women. *Br J Obstet Gynaecol* 1989; 96:29–32.

188. Allen RE, Hosker GL, Smith ARB, et al. Pelvic floor damage and childbirth: a neurophysiologic study. *Br J Obstet Gynaecol* 1990; 97:770–779.

189. Anderson RS. A neurogenic element to urinary stress incontinence. *Br J Obstet Gynaecol* 1984; 91:41–45.

190. Zivkovic F, Tamussino K, Ralph G, et al. Long-term effects of vaginal dissection on the innervation of the striated urethral sphincter. *Obstet Gynecol* 1996; 87:257–260.

191. Deindl FM, Vodusek DB, Hesse U, et al. Pelvic floor activity patterns: comparison of nulliparous continent and parous urinary stress incontinent women. A kinesiological study. *Br J Urol* 1994; 73:413–417.

192. Spence-Jones C, Kamm MA, Henry MM, et al. Bowel dysfunction: a pathogenic factor in uterovaginal prolapse and urinary stress incontinence. *Br J Obstet Gynaecol* 1994; 101:147–152.

193. Swash M. Anorectal incontinence: electrophysiological tests. *Br J Surg* 1985; 72[Suppl]:S14–S15.

194. Lubowski DZ, Nicholls RJ, Burleigh DE, et al. Internal anal sphincter in neurogenic fecal incontinence. *Gastroenterology* 1988; 95:997–1002.

195. Snooks SJ, Henry MM, Swash M. Anorectal incontinence and rectal prolapse: differential assessment of the innervation to puborectalis and external anal sphincter muscles. *Gut* 1985; 26:470–476.

196. Kiff ES, Swash M. Slowed conduction in the pudendal nerves in idiopathic (neurogenic) faecal incontinence. *Br J Surg* 1984; 71:614–616.

197. Snooks SJ, Swash M, Henry MM, et al. Risk factors in childbirth causing damage to the pelvic floor innervation. *Int J Colorectal Dis* 1986; 1:20–24.

198. Sultan AH, Kamm MA, Hudson CN, et al. Anal-sphincter disruption during vaginal delivery. *N Engl J Med* 1993; 329:1905–1911.

199. Snooks SJ, Henry MM, Swash M. Faecal incontinence due to external anal sphincter division in childbirth is associated with damage to the innervation of the pelvic floor musculature: a double pathology. *Br J Obstet Gynaecol* 1985; 92:824–828.

200. Hill J, Mumtaz A, Kiff ES. Pudendal neuropathy in patients with idiopathic faecal incontinence progresses with time. *Br J Surg* 1994; 81:1494–1495.

201. Kiff ES, Barnes PRH, Swash M. Evidence of pudendal neuropathy in patients with perineal descent and chronic straining at stool. *Gut* 1984; 25:1279–1282.

202. Jones PN, Lubowski DZ, Swash M, et al. Relation between perineal descent and pudendal nerve damage in idiopathic faecal incontinence. *Int J Colorectal Dis* 1987; 2:93–95.

203. Pinho M, Yoshioka K, Keighley M. Are pelvic floor movements abnormal in disordered defecation? *Dis Colon Rectum* 1991; 34:1117–1119.

204. Jorge JMN, Wexner SD, Ehrenpries ED, et al. Does perineal descent correlate with pudendal neuropathy? *Dis Colon Rectum* 1993; 36:475–483.

205. Bielefeldt K, Enck P, Erckenbrecht JF. Sensory and motor function in the maintenance of anal continence. *Dis Colon Rectum* 1990; 33:674–678.

206. Rogers J, Henry MM, Misiewicz JJ. Combined sensory and motor deficit in primary neuropathic faecal incontinence. *Gut* 1988; 29:5–9.

207. Richardson DA. Conservative management of urinary incontinence. A symposium. *J Reprod Med* 1993; 38:659–661.

208. Cheong DMO, Vaccaro CA, Salanga VD, et al. Electrodiagnostic evaluation of fecal incontinence. *Muscle Nerve* 1995; 18:612–619.

209. Sangwan YP, Coller JA, Barrett RC. Unilateral pudendal neuropathy. Impact on outcome of anal sphincter repair. *Dis Colon Rectum* 1996; 39:686–689.

210. Laurberg S. Swash M, Henry MM. Delayed external sphincter repair for obstetric tear. *Br J Surg* 1988; 75:786–788.

211. Setti-Carrero PS, Kamm MA, Nicholls RJ. Long term results of postanal repair for neurogenic faecal incontinence. *Br J Surg* 1994; 81:140–144.

212. Herbaut AG, Nogueira MC, Panzer JM, et al. Anorectal incontinence in myotonic dystrophy: a myopathic involvement of pelvic floor muscles [Letter]. *Muscle Nerve* 1992; 15:1210–1211.

213. Chancellor AM, Warlow CP, Webb JN, et al. Acid Maltase deficiency presenting with a myopathy and exercise induced urinary incontinence in a 68-year-old male [Letter]. *J Neurol Neurosurg Psychiatry* 1991; 54:659–660.

214. Dixon PJ, Christmas TJ, Chapple CR. Stress Incontinence due to pelvic floor muscle involvement in limb-girdle muscular dystrophy. *Br J Urol* 1990; 65:653–654.

215. Carress JB, Kothari MJ, Bauer SB, et al. Urinary incontinence in Duchenne muscular dystrophy. *Muscle Nerve* 1996; 19:819–822.

CHAPTER 68

Motor Disorders Associated with Cerebral Palsy

Jilda N. Vargus-Adams, Jacob A. Neufeld, Pasquale Accardo

Cerebral palsy (CP) is defined as a group of developmental disorders attributed to non-progressive disturbances in the developing fetal or infant brain. There is often associated disturbances of sensation, cognition, communication, perception, behavior, and seizures (1). This definition acknowledges the non-progressive aspects of the motor disorder when identified during infancy that typically results from inherited and acquired lesions of the brain during early development, as well as the contribution of birth trauma, asphyxia, and prematurity. Improvements in obstetrical and neonatal care have not eradicated CP, which continues to be an important cause of infant and childhood disability. This chapter reviews the epidemiology, risk factors, classification and clinical subtypes, diagnosis and treatment options for childhood CP.

EPIDEMIOLOGY AND RISK FACTORS

Cerebral palsy is the commonest motor disorder of children with a prevalence of 3.9 per 1,000 in 3 to 17-year-olds in the United States (U.S.) with increasing prevalence (2, 3). Although black infants are more likely to develop CP, it is largely a result of lower birth weight rather than race, as low birth weight and prematurity are highly associated features (4). The disorder is slightly more common in boys than girls. Prenatal risk factors include lack of prenatal care, limited maternal education, infection or bleeding during pregnancy, maternal cigarette and illicit drug use, and history of multiple miscarriages. Perinatal risk factors include brain malformations, infection, perinatal adverse events and multiple gestation, and breech presentation for babies born at term (5, 6). Increased prematurity, cystic periventricular leukomalacia on brain imaging, and severe intraventricular

hemorrhage increases the risk of CP (7, 8). A birth weight less than 1500 grams results in a 25-fold increased risk of CP compared to infants with a normal birth weight (9). Prematurity is a major risk factor for CP, with an odds ratio greater than 50 for gestational age less than 32 weeks (10).

CLASSIFICATION

Cerebral palsy is classified by the associated movement disorder, topographical distribution, and functional ability. The physiological classification traditionally separated CP types by tone and movement patterns into spastic, dystonic, dyskinetic, hypotonic and mixed types. Spastic CP is the most common presentation, representing up to 90% of patients (11, 12), and reflective of corticospinal tract (CST) involvement. Dyskinetic CP presents with abnormal movements and disturbance of tone reflective of subcortical center involvement resulting from basal ganglia damage due to kernicterus in the extrapyramidal type. Pure hypotonia beyond infancy is atypical of CP. The topographical classification characterizes the distribution of motor dysfunction by the involved limbs, with monoparesis affecting one arm or leg, hemiparesis affecting one side of the body, diparesis affecting both legs, triparesis sparing one limb, and quadriparesis or total body involvement. The topographical classification is further simplified into bilateral and unilateral groups.

The functional classification has been the most popular and meaningful during the last decade. Movement disorders may be mixed and affected limbs may not be equally impaired, making classification challenging. Employing a scheme based on what a child can do is often easier and more reliable than physiological and topographical categories. Several functional classification schemes have been developed for CP children. One is the Gross Motor Functional Classification System (13), a second is the Manual Abilities Classification System (14), and the third is the Communication Function Classification System (15).

SPASTIC CEREBRAL PALSY

The most prevalent movement disorder in CP is a spastic or mixed, bilateral or unilateral type, presenting with predominant upper motor neuron signs manifested by hyperreflexia, Hoffman, Babinski signs, and ankle clonus, with velocity-dependent increases in resistance to movement and resistance that increases rapidly above a threshold speed and angle (16). Abnormal spastic tone may be consistent throughout the entire day, leading to a propensity for contractures and fixed limb deformity. Dystonia may be present, particularly when spasticity is inconstant, leading to abnormal posture or repetitive movement with involuntary contractions. Spastic-dystonic CP is common with wide-ranging degrees of dystonia and the onset is typically in infancy with persistence thereafter.

Older infants with spastic diparesis will bunny-hop, crawl non-reciprocally, and drag their legs in early walking, and develop a scissored or crouched gait pattern. Hip adduction, hip and knee flexion, and ankle plantar flexion may be accentuated by spasticity and dystonia. Those with spastic diparetic forms who sit by age two years will eventually walk (17). Absent sitting by four years of age is an unfavorable predictor of later ambulation. Spasticity accompanies weakness and reduced selective motor control in all affected limbs, and for children with upper extremity deficits it may be a primary contributor to limitations in self-care, writing, and recreational activities.

Spastic hemiparesis primarily affects full-term infants, and much like adults with middle cerebral artery strokes, those with hemiparesis often have greater impairment of the arm than the leg. Typical motor rehabilitative concerns focus on delayed walking; foot and ankle issues, including equinovarus deformity, and fine motor deficits in the affected arm leading to challenges in age-appropriate bimanual activities. At rest, the shoulder of an affected child will be adducted and internally rotated with the elbow flexed, the forearm pronated, and fingers clenched in a fist. This position may be exaggerated with running or other motor activity. Ambulation is delayed due to decreased spontaneous movement of the affected leg, usually until about 18 to 24 months, although most children with spastic hemiparesis walk by age three years.

Spastic quadriparesis is the most severe form of spastic CP, with an increased risk of epilepsy and intellectual disability likely due to more substantial brain damage and mal-

formation. Early evidence of spastic CP may be misleading. The National Collaborative Perinatal Project, which followed approximately 58,000 children with CP from 1959 to 1966, found that two-thirds were diagnosed with spastic diplegia in infancy and outgrew their motor signs by age 7 (18), whereas of those with early infantile hypertonicity, 16% ultimately developed CP, while the others had alternative diagnoses after intensive evaluation. Early developmental delay and hypertonicity are harbingers of the lifelong impairments due to CP, despite the provisional nature of the diagnosis before age four years (19).

DYSKINETIC CEREBRAL PALSY

The dyskinetic or extrapyramidal form accounts for approximately 10 to 20% of children with CP overall, and includes those with athetosis, pure dystonia, chorea, and ballismus. Infants and children with dyskinetic CP appear normal or mildly hypotonic in the first year of life or may be severely involved shortly after birth. Abnormal movements are often combined with hypotonia, poor head control, and speech difficulty, and associated athetosis is recognized as slow, writhing movements of the face and distal arms and legs. Dystonic postures can be intermixed with rhythmic twisting and slow involuntary movements. Chorea presents with rapid, regular jerking movements of the face and limbs. Those with ballismus have wide amplitude flailing of the limbs. Historically, dyskinetic CP and athetosis have been highly correlated with kernicterus and basal ganglia insult (20), however with more definitive management of neonatal hyperbilirubinemia, dyskinetic CP is becoming less prevalent. The needs of children with dyskinetic CP can be extensive, and their symptoms may prove exceptionally challenging to manage.

SCREENING AND DIAGNOSIS

Motor delay most often brings infants to the attention of a general pediatrician, and later to a pediatric neurologist, developmentalist or physiatrist. However, the traditional neurological examination of tone and reflexes, which may vary in the first year of life, may not be categorical proof of early CP. Recognizing that the age range for achieving individual motor milestones can vary, sequential motor milestones should be compared to standardized data to identify potentially significant impairments in most affected children, demonstrating significant delays from normative values. Traditional screening strategies include evaluation of abnormal movement patterns such as early handedness, bunny-hop crawling, and toe-walking; and primitive reflexes including obligatory atonic neck reflex or Moro that persist after six months. One sensitive measure of early CP is the general movement assessment (21, 22). Videotaped samples of spontaneous movements may predict development of CP in the majority of young infants.

Although hypotonia is common in presenting premature infants who ultimately manifest CP, all such infants admitted to a neonatal intensive care unit for prolonged care should be following carefully and screened for later CP because a previously floppy infant, especially one that is already rigid or spastic at discharge from the neonatal intensive care unit at age six months, is likely to have significant motor disability related to CP. Hypotonia and generalized motor delays are not specific to CP and may spontaneously resolve or may indicate other conditions such as motor neuron disease, genetic syndromes, or intellectual disability (23). Brain neuroimaging employing magnetic resonance imaging (MRI) is the preferred method of neuroimaging, although computerized tomography (CT) and ultrasound may be employed in the evaluation of children with suspected CP. Spastic bilateral CP associated with periventricular white matter lesions is common among premature infants with intraventricular hemorrhage. Neuroimaging in children with spastic hemiparesis may also reveal cortical dysplasia, porencephalic lesions, cortical or deep grey matter lesions contralateral to the side of hemiplegia in keeping with the *in utero* stroke etiology. Those with spastic diplegia will have extensive bilateral multicystic encephalomalacia on brain neuroimaging, while the brain findings of quadriparetic CP will likely be more severe and extensive; similarly, those with dyskinetic CP may manifest cortical and deep grey matter lesions (24).

TREATMENT AND OUTCOME

Children with CP should be managed in a multidisciplinary setting to the extent possible since it is a neurodevelopmental disorder with wide-ranging manifestations and co-morbidities, making it essential to incorporate the expertise of a pediatric physiatrist, neurologist, orthopedist, developmental pediatrician, and pediatric neurosurgeon, as well as other allied health professionals from the specialty fields of physical, occupational, speech, and recreational therapy and neuropsychology, dietary science, social work, and orthotics. Therapy and screening for co-morbid illnesses is paramount in infants and toddlers with CP, with most states having open access of early intervention CP programs. At three years of age, children can access therapy services through developmental preschool programs and, upon reaching school age, they may qualify for therapy services through public school. All such therapy addresses the motor disability of CP, including weakness, impaired control, movement disorders, spasticity, and dystonia, and the sequela thereof including contractures, dysarthria, dysphagia, and other impairments and limitations. Given the same degree of motor impairment, the child with less cognitive impairment is more likely to be able to cooperate with therapeutic programs including adaptation to assistive devices, powered mobility, and augmentative communication devices.

Spasticity is a primary target of interventions for CP. If conservative treatment with range of motion programs is ineffective, medical treatment may be pursued. Several medications can be useful in controlling tone, including baclofen, diazepam, dantrolene, and tizanidine, but the efficacy of these drugs is not well described (25). Botulinum toxin injections are useful in controlling focal hypertonicity and may benefit walking and functional skills before nerve blocks with phenol are pursued (26) via surgically implanted pump systems, while younger, ambulatory children with diparetic CP may be candidates for selective dorsal rhizotomy followed by intensive therapy (27).

Orthopedic procedures may be necessary for some children when bracing and casting are insufficient, including tendon lengthening and transfers and osteotomy to address motor imbalance, malalignment, contracture, hip subluxation, and other orthopedic complications of CP. Hip subluxation, dislocation, and scoliosis progresses silently such that regular radiographic surveillance is necessary, with their occurrence related to motor severity. Gait analysis can be used to guide surgical decision making, but does not always lead to consistent recommendations or predict outcome (28). Although a minority of children may be candidates for surgery of the arm, the benefits thereof are not as well established as those for the legs (29).

Bracing is important to sustain gross and fine motor skills, as well as maintain range of motion. Various forms of ankle foot orthoses (AFO) aid in standing and walking, and wrist-hand orthoses may facilitate grasping and hand use. Hip abduction bracing impacts progression of hip subluxation, especially when combined with spasticity management (30). Children with CP often utilize other durable medical equipment including a wheelchair, walker, cane, and crutches; lifts, specialized seating, bath equipment, and communication devices.

Medical issues should be addressed for all children with CP including bone demineralization associated with immobility and lack of weight bearing prompting calcium and vitamin D supplementation. Gastroesophageal reflux and constipation frequently require medical management, as do seizure disorders, for which appropriate specialist care should be obtained. Medical professionals caring for children with CP should be alert for signs of precocious puberty, learning difficulties, malnutrition, attention and behavior challenges, and visual impairment, and pursue appropriate evaluations for any such concerns. Fitness and wellness are important for children with CP similar to their normally developing peers, prompting the institution of appropriate, appealing activities to ensure their health and well-being.

REFERENCES

1. Bax M, Goldstein M, Rosenbaum P, et al. Proposed definition and classification of cerebral palsy, April 2005. *Dev Med Child Neurol* 2005; 47:571–576.

2. Boyle CA, Boulet S, Schieve LA, et al. Trends in the prevalence of developmental disabilities in US children, 1997–2008. *Pediatrics* 2011; 127:1034–42.

3. Winter S, Autry A, Boyle C, Yeargin-Allsopp M. Trends in the prevalence of cerebral palsy in a population-based study. *Pediatrics* 2002; 110:1220–1225.

4. Wu YW, Xing G, Fuentes-Afflick E, et al. Racial, ethnic, and socioeconomic disparities in the prevalence of cerebral palsy. *Pediatrics* 2011; 127:674–681.

5. O'Callaghan ME, MacLennan AH, Gibson CS, et al. Epidemiologic associations with cerebral palsy. *Obstet Gynecol* 2011; 118:576–582.

6. Himmelmann K, Ahlin K, Jacobsson B, et al. Risk factors for cerebral palsy in children born at term. *Acta Obstet Gynecol Scand* 2011; 90:1070–1081.

7. van Haastert IC, Groenendaal F, Uiterwaal CS, et al. Decreasing incidence and severity of cerebral palsy in prematurely born children. *J Pediatr* 2011; 159:86–91.

8. Ancel PY, Livinec F, Larroque B, et al. Cerebral palsy among very preterm children in relation to gestational age and neonatal ultrasound abnormalities: the EPIPAGE cohort study. *Pediatrics* 2006; 117:828–35.

9. Stanley FJ. Survival and cerebral palsy in low birthweight infants: implications for perinatal care. *Paediatr Perinat Epidemiol* 1992; 6:298–310.

10. Stanley F, Blair E, Alberman E. *Cerebral Palsies: Epidemiology and Causal Pathways*. London: Mac Keith Press, 2000.

11. Kirby RS, Wingate MS, Van Naarden Braun K, et al. Prevalence and functioning of children with cerebral palsy in four areas of the United States in 2006: a report from the Autism and Developmental Disabilities Monitoring Network. *Res Dev Disabil* 2011; 32:462–469.

12. Reid SM, Carlin JB, Reddihough DS. Distribution of motor types in cerebral palsy: how do registry data compare? *Dev Med Child Neurol* 2011; 53:233–238.

13. Palisano R, Rosenbaum P, Walter S, et al. Development and reliability of a system to classify gross motor function in children with cerebral palsy. *Dev Med Child Neurol* 1997; 39:214–223.

14. Eliasson AC, Krumlinde-Sundholm L, Rosblad B, et al. The Manual Ability Classification System (MACS) for children with cerebral palsy: scale development and evidence of validity and reliability. *Dev Med Child Neurol* 2006; 48:549–554.

15. Hidecker MJ, Paneth N, Rosenbaum PL, Developing and validating the Communication Function Classification System for individuals with cerebral palsy. *Dev Med Child Neurol* 2011; 53:704–710.

16. Sanger TD, Delgado MR, Gaebler-Spira D, et al. Classification and definition of disorders causing hypertonia in childhood. *Pediatrics* 2003; 111:89–97.

17. Molnar GE, Gordon SU. Cerebral palsy: predictive value of selected clinical signs for early prognostication of motor function. *Arch Phys Med Rehabil* 1976; 57:153–158.

18. Hardy JB. The Collaborative Perinatal Project: lessons and legacy. Ann Epidemiol 2003; 13:303–311; Nelson KB, Ellenberg JH. Children who "outgrew" cerebral palsy. *Pediatrics* 1982; 69:529–536.

19. Krageloh-Mann I, Cans C. Cerebral palsy update. *Brain Dev* 2009; 31:537–544.

20. Przekop A, Sanger TD. Birth-related syndromes of athetosis and kernicterus. *Handb Clin Neurol* 2011; 100:387–395.

21. Hadders-Algra M. General movements: A window for early identification of children at high risk for developmental disorders. *J Pediatr* 2004; 145(Suppl):S12–S18.

22. Hamer EG, Bos AF, Hadders-Algra M. Assessment of specific characteristics of abnormal general movements: does it enhance the prediction of cerebral palsy? *Dev Med Child Neurol* 2011; 53:751–756.

23. Paneth N. Establishing the diagnosis of cerebral palsy. *Clin Obstet Gyneco* 2008; 51:742–748.

24. Accardo J, Kammann H, Hoon AH, Jr. Neuroimaging in cerebral palsy. *J Pediatr* 2004; 145(Suppl):S19–S27.

25. Delgado MR, Hirtz D, Aisen M, et al. Practice parameter: pharmacologic treatment of spasticity in children and adolescents with cerebral palsy (an evidence-based review): report of the Quality Standards Subcommittee of the American Academy of Neurology and the Practice Committee of the Child Neurology Society. *Neurology* 2010; 74:336–343.

26. Fehlings D, Novak I, Berweck S, et al. Botulinum toxin assessment, intervention and follow-up for paediatric upper limb hypertonicity: international consensus statement. *Eur J Neurol* 2010; 17(Suppl 2):38–56.

27. McLaughlin J, Bjornson K, Temkin N, et al. Selective dorsal rhizotomy: meta-analysis of three randomized controlled trials. *Dev Med Child Neurol* 2002; 4417–4425.

28. Noonan KJ, Halliday S, Browne R, et al. Interobserver variability of gait analysis in patients with cerebral palsy. *J Pediatr Orthop* 2003; 23:279–287; Discussion 88–91.

29. Koman LA, Sarlikiotis T, Smith BP. Surgery of the upper extremity in cerebral palsy. *Orthop Clin North Am* 2010; 41:519–529.

30. Graham HK, Boyd R, Carlin JB, et al. Does botulinum toxin a combined with bracing prevent hip displacement in children with cerebral palsy and "hips at risk"? A randomized, controlled trial. *J Bone Joint Surg Am* 2008; 90:23–33.

CHAPTER 69

Management of Spasticity

James W. Stark, Saud A. Sadiq

Spasticity is a common clinical feature of a variety of central nervous system (CNS) disorders. Untreated, it can compound disability and negatively impact on functional activities of daily living (ADL). Current management is based upon an understanding of the pathophysiologic mechanisms underlying spasticity. The treating physician must choose among the various available therapeutic modalities alone and in combination. Oral medications are effective although associated adverse effects may restrict usage at therapeutic doses. Physical therapy (PT) programs remain important in integrated management of an individual patient. Botulinum neurotoxin (BoNT) is a well-established modality for the treatment of focal spasticity with intrathecal administration. Other less common agents are reserved for patients with more severe affliction.

DEFINITIONS AND KEY CLINICAL FEATURES

Spasticity results from upper motor neuron (UMN) lesions and the disinhibition of velocity-dependent increase in muscle tone during stretch. With rapid stretching of an affected muscle, there is a brief tone-free period, followed by an abrupt catch with increasing muscular tone to a peak, after which resistance dissipates like the opening of a clasped-knife. The associated positive clinical signs of resultant disinhibition include hyperreflexia, Babinski signs, and extensor and painful flexor spasms. The negative signs of spasticity are UMN weakness, fatigability, and incoordination (1–6).

Rigidity, which is usually associated with extrapyramidal disorders, may be mistaken for spasticity; however, it leads to increased constant muscle tone throughout the range of the muscle stretch response like bending a lead pipe. With few exceptions, such as secondary dystonia, in which signs of both rigidity and spasticity coexist, rigidity is generally not associated with hyperreflexia or the elicitation of Babinski signs (5, 6).

The most common causes of spasticity are traumatic brain injury (TBI) and spinal cord injury (SCI), multiple sclerosis (MS), cerebral palsy (CP), stroke, compressive myelopathy, transverse myelitis and autoimmune myelopathy due to human T-cell lymphotropic virus (HTLV) type I, human immunodeficiency virus (HIV), Lyme neuroborreliosis (LNB), spinal cord tumors, and dystonia. Less common causes are hereditary spastic paraplegia (HSP), stiff-person syndrome, primary lateral sclerosis (PLS), postencephalitic conditions, and spastic paraplegia in association with genetically distinct enzymatic and neurometabolic disorders. It is important to accurately determine the underlying condition resulting in spasticity when deciding upon optimal treatment.

PATHOPHYSIOLOGY

There is a recent review of spasticity (7). Normal muscle tone reflects the balance between inhibitory and excitatory inputs to the spinal alpha motor neuron (αMN). The rationale behind drug therapy is to correct this imbalance. Knowledge of the neuroanatomical pathways is essential to restoring normal resting muscle tone.

Basic Circuitry: The Stretch Reflex

A reflex consists of an input to the αMN and the resultant output. The input pathway is relatively complex and is modulated by several excitatory and inhibitory signals. Stretch reflex output is simple and occurs with the generation of an action potential and release of acetylcholine (ACh) at the neuromuscular junction (NMJ) that induces a muscle end-plate potential (EPP) with release of calcium ions from the muscle sarcoplasmic reticulum. An energy-requiring release of calcium enables myosin and actin filaments to slide over one another, the final outcome of which is myofiber contraction.

There are several inputs to the αMN including those from Ia spindle afferents from muscle spindle stretch receptors, which enter the dorsal horn of the spinal cord and synapse with the αMN in the ventral horn, and excitatory amino acids with glutamate and aspartate as neurotransmitters. These afferents synapse on the αMN of synergistic muscles to enhance contraction and on inhibitory interneurons in inhibiting contraction of antagonist muscles. The sensitivity of muscle spindle afferents is maintained by gamma motor neurons (γMN) that regulate fusimotor muscle spindle tone. Fusimotor discharges increase when a muscle is stretched, thereby regulating γMN activity and reflex muscle tone (8).

INCREASED EXCITATORY INPUT

On the basis of this simple circuitry, one could postulate several potential mechanisms for spasticity. For example, spasticity could result from hyperexcitability of the agonist αMN from a change in membrane properties (2, 9). However, disruptions of synaptic input to the αMN are more likely than intrinsic alterations (10). Excessive activity of the fusimotor system can lead to spindle that are overly sensitive to stretch although evidence for this is lacking (4, 6, 11–14). At the level of the αMN, potential therapeutic strategies could include interruption of afferent (anterior rhizotomy) or afferent (posterior rhizotomy) αMN pathways. A decrease in calcium ion release can be achieved with the medication dantrolene. A reduction in ACh release at the NMJ can be obtained with local injection of BoNT as well as a variety of physical therapy modalities.

Pathways Mediating Both Excitatory and Inhibitory Input

Several descending pathways contribute to spasticity, some of which influence fusimotor tone by increasing excitatory synapses on αMNs and transmitting their signals by the excitatory amino acid glutamate. However, the circuitry is complex and is not completely delineated. Two major descending pathways, an inhibitory norepinephrine (NE)-mediated dorsal reticulospinal tract and an excitatory serotonin (SE)-mediated medial reticulospinal tract, exert balancing influences on muscle tone. Other descending pathways, including the corticospinal tract (CST), rubrospinal, and vestibulospinal pathways exert important modulating influences on muscle tone. Spasticity results from a lack of UMN control on the inhibitory dorsal reticulospinal tract that shifts the balance toward the excitation of the medial reticulospinal tract and vestibulospinal tracts (2, 3). Potential therapies at this level include enhancement of adrenergic inhibitory activity with the use of clonidine and tizanidine, and reduction of SE excitatory activity with cyproheptadine.

Decreased Inhibitory Input

Many interneurons participate in the stretch reflex pathway, including Ia and Ib inhibitory interneurons and Renshaw neurons (15). The Ia inhibitory interneurons receive excitatory afferent input from Ia afferents and, in turn, inhibit αMN control of antagonistic muscles, known as reciprocal inhibition. The Ib inhibitory interneurons play an important integrative role in resting muscle tone, integrating the influence of Golgi tendon organs via Ib afferents with those of Ia afferents. Hence the phenomenon of interneurons mediating group I nonreciprocal inhibition is probably more accurate (9). Renshaw cells are another important interneuron that receives input from αMN branches as well as afferent input from descending spinal pathways and other interneurons and, in turn, synergistically inhibit αMN, γMN, Ia inhibitory interneurons, and other Renshaw cells. The latter have complex connections with many other cells via feedback loops that modulate αMN firing through the integration of signals from both descending pathways and afferent inputs (9).

Presynaptic inhibition of Ia afferents reduces the excitatory impact of Ia afferents on αMN, and both afferent inputs and descending pathways induce presynaptic inhibition (9), which when inadequate, contributes to spasticity. The transmitter γ-aminobutyric acid (GABA) is an important mediator of presynaptic inhibition. Enhancement of GABA or GABA-like transmission is one method of treatment (4). Medications such as baclofen, diazepam, clonazepam, and ivermectin exert much of their anti-spasticity effect by enhancement of GABA transmission.

THERAPEUTIC MODALITIES

The goal of treatment is to improve overall function and not just reduce spasticity while preventing or at the least, reducing its undesired consequences including decreased mobility, disabling pain, contractures, dependent ADL, inadequate hygiene, sexual dysfunction, sleep disturbances, and indirectly, low self-esteem and mood disorders. In some disorders, a certain degree of spasticity has functional value such as barely ambulatory patients with spastic paraparesis in whom overtreatment would render the patient non-ambulatory. The management of spasticity should ideally be based on ongoing clinical assessment leading to an appropriate therapeutic plan that includes 1 or more of the following options listed in order of least to most aggressive, namely PT, oral medications, BoNT injection, intrathecal therapies, and surgical ablative procedures. Table 1 summarizes the neuroanatomical and neurochemical elements of spasticity and the available therapeutic modalities that can selectively be employed.

Table 1. Pathophysiologic Basis of the Treatment of Spasticity

Site of Action	Neurotransmitter	Treatment
Muscle	Calcium	Dantrolene
NMJ	ACh	BoNT
(-) αMN	GABA	Baclofen, diazepam, clonazepam ivermectin
(-) Reticulospinal	NE	Tizanidine, clonidine
(+)Reticulospinal	SE	Cyproheptadine
(+) αMN		SDR

Abbreviations: NMJ, neuromuscular junction, ACh, acetylcholine; BoNT, botulinum neurotoxin; (-) and (+) αMN, inhibitory and excitatory αMN inputs; GABA, gamma-aminobutyric acid; NE, norepinephrine; SE, serotonin; SDR, selective dorsal rhizotomy

CLINICAL ASSESSMENT

A thorough clinical assessment is crucial in formulating a logical management plan. It requires a team approach with the input of a team of physician and non-physician health providers. A complete history and examination is performed to determine the severity of spasticity and its impact on function. The patient should be examined supine and erect and on more than one visit. Posture may have an effect on spasticity, the severity of which can vary in the course of hours or a day. The modified Ashworth Scale (22, 23), shown in Table 2, is a useful objective bedside measure of spasticity that can be easily employed in the initial assessment and determination of treatment benefit. However, functional assessments of other types such as ambulation, dressing, transferring, and turning in bed are also useful. The underlying neurologic condition causing spasticity and the associated complications, such as urinary tract infections and decubitus ulcers, which exacerbate the spastic condition, should be stabilized and optimally treated (2, 16–21). Acute worsening is almost always a manifestation of an associated medical change, such as a relapse in a patient with MS or unsuspected infection. The stepladder management approach to spasticity in these instances will lead to clearly defined and appropriately instituted goals. Treating physicians, therapists and, above all, the patient should agree on stated goals, and the patient should understand the limitations of treatment. For example, a therapy or manipulation that allows for easier transfer or relief of pain but does not strengthen a weak limb or restore lost function may not be the mutually desired goal (2).

Role of Physical Therapy

Physical therapy is effective without the side effects of medication and may be all that is needed at the outset of treatment. Spasticity leads to muscle immobilization and changes in muscle fiber length and number. Physical therapy interrupts this cycle, improves active function, patient comfort, and can enhance the effects of anticipated oral medications such as baclofen (24), although it is best initiated before the development of muscle shortening to maintain muscle length and elasticity. Accordingly, PT should be initiated as soon as possible, including passive

Table 2. Modified Ashworth Scale for Assessing Muscle Tone

Muscle Tone:	Spasm Score	Reflex Score
Scale-Definition	Scale-Definition	Scale-Definition
1-No increase in tone	0-No spasms	0-Absent reflexes
2-Minimal increased tone	1-Spasms upon stimulation	1-Hyporeflexia
3-Moderate increased tone	2-Occasional spasms: < 1/hr.	2-Normal reflexes
4-Severe increased tone	3-Frequent spasms: 1-10/hr.	3-Brisk reflexes; no clonus
5-Fixed-rigid muscle	4-Very freqent spasms: > 10/hr.	4- <4 beats of clonus
		5- >4 beats of clonus
		6- Sustained clonus

range-of-motion exercises, joint mobilization, positioning and stretching, bracing, strengthening, and serial casting (20, 25). Repetitive transcranial magnetic stimulation (rTMS) has been investigated as a treatment for spasticity from a variety of causes (26). It exerts its salutary effects by enhancing CST excitability, evident by the reduction of H reflex amplitudes on electrodiagnostic studies. The frequency of stimulation as well as duration and frequency of treatments may vary between studies. However, rTMS is more effective with frequent and brief treatments. Functional electrical stimulation (FES) (27, 28) induces active muscle contraction, leading to functional movements that enhance motor learning by reinforcing existing network connectivity. It delivers afferent as well as efferent stimulation, thereby improving regional blood flow and effectively reducing spasticity more than passive movement alone (28).

STANDARD ANTISPASTICITY AGENTS

Baclofen

When PT is not satisfactory, monotherapy for spasticity, oral baclofen is the drug of choice, especially when intrinsic spinal cord disease (20) and MS (18, 29) are the precipitating and sustaining cause, although one might consider others for those with hallucinations or seizures (21). Baclofen is a GABA analogue and although its precise mechanism of action is not known, it acts as a GABA-β agonist to inhibit spinal reflexes by hyperpolarizing afferent inputs.

The exact dose should be agreed upon by both the patient and physician as most patients will work out an individual schedule tailored to their needs. Physicians often give too low a dose to patients who can probably tolerate higher ones without incapacitating side effects (30). Higher doses tend not to be associated with treatment discontinuation, an observation that was noted in 20% of patients with MS that were taking more than 80 mg per day (31). Initiation of therapy should commence with a 10 mg nighttime dose to determine maximum efficacy while balancing side effects, to a total of 200 mg per day.

A double-blind study of baclofen treatment in MS showed a significant reduction in spasticity with concomitant relief of painful spasms, clonus, and improved range of joint motion that maintained functional status (32). Another study noted improved spasticity and reduction of painful spasms (33). A trial of 30 patients with MS treated with baclofen and stretching demonstrated the superiority of baclofen (24). Baclofen has been successfully used in the treatment of refractory stiff-person syndrome (34), and in a double-blind placebo-controlled trial of spasticity due to CP (35). It can provide benefit to patients with anxiety (36); however, not all spasticity-associated conditions respond to baclofen. A

double-blind placebo-controlled study of patients with SCI showed no significant reduction of spasticity with baclofen (37). Oral baclofen has poor penetration across the blood–brain barrier; therefore, patients may require high doses before unacceptable weakness, lethargy, somnolence, and other intolerable side effects occur (30). Weakness is usually an unmasking effect resulting from decreased resistance to muscular contraction (38) while frank toxicity signals subclinical renal insufficiency (39), the associated effects of which can lead to overdoses that can be life-threatening (40). When baclofen is discontinued after long-term use, it should be tapered gradually because rapid withdrawal has been associated with hallucinations, seizures, manic psychosis, dyskinesia, and hyperthermia (6, 41-48). Baclofen is distributed commercially in a racemic form and absorbed only in the upper small intestine (49). Arbaclofen placarbil is a prodrug of the active (R-isomer form which can be absorbed throughout the gastrointestinal tract with a longer half-life than racemic baclofen, which results in improved clinical efficacy and fewer side effects (49). A small study in patients with SCI demonstrated improved Ashworth scale scores with 20 or 30 mg tablets every 12 hours compared to placebo (50); side effects were minimal.

Diazepam and Clonazepam

The benzodiazepines diazepam and clonazepam are employed in the management of spasticity either as single agents or in combination due to synergistic actions (51). They facilitate presynaptic inhibitory action on GABA-β receptors, although there may be other independent anti-spasticity actions (4,6). Diazepam is effective in the treatment of spasticity associated with the stiff-person syndrome (6, 52). A study of 13 affected patients followed at the Mayo Clinic for 30 years demonstrated reduction in spasms, especially when combined with PT (53). The efficacy of clonazepam in treating spasticity from CP was demonstrated by a double-blind, placebo-controlled, crossover study of 12 children (54). One double-blind study of 22 children demonstrated that diazepam and dantrolene together were more effective than placebo, and the combination was more effective than either alone (55). However, benzodiazepines have undesirable sedative effects during waking hours and the potential for addiction and dangerous withdrawal symptoms when abruptly discontinued (6, 18, 56, and 57), as well as a deleterious effect on body weight gain (58). It is considered less preferable when compared with other medications (6, 51). In a double-blind study of 105 patients comparing diazepam and tizanidine, fewer adverse effects related to treatment discontinuation occurred with tizanidine (59). Similarly, when the adverse effect profile of diazepam was compared with dantrolene (60) and baclofen (61), diazepam was tolerated less well than either of the others. One study comparing clonazepam with baclofen found that both were equally effective, with clonazepam perhaps more beneficial in those with mild cerebral causes of spasticity, whereas baclofen was more effective in severe spinal spasticity (62).

In general, these agents are best used in small doses in combination therapy. The greatest efficacy is in patients with nocturnal spasms, and occasionally in treatment-resistant spastic dystonia wherein doses of 50 to 100 grams per day of diazepam are generally the last resort before commencement of intrathecal therapy.

Tizanidine and Clonidine

Tizanidine and clonidine are α_2-adrenergic agonists that inhibit the release of excitatory amino acids from spinal interneurons and the dorsal reticulospinal tract (63, 64). The effects of clonidine have been studied in chronic spinalized rats (65). It leads to reduced αMN excitability, decreased spontaneous electromyogram activity, diminished tonic activity, reduced amplitude of hind limb muscles and their respective reflexes, and an increase in the threshold for electronically induced reflexes (65).

Clonidine, alone and in combination with other agents, improves spasticity associated with SCI, brainstem infarction, MS, and TBI (66–71). However, its use is often limited because of adverse sympatholytic side effects including bradycardia, hypotension, sedation, dry mouth, and sexual dysfunction, which are generally reduced with transdermal delivery (70–75). Intrathecal clonidine (ITC) has been used with baclofen in the management of spasticity and neuropathic pain following spinal cord injury (76), and in patients with MS and spastic paraparesis (77).

Tizanidine is another α_2-adrenergic agonist with the advantage of less hypotension. Initial studies showed that patients who did not adequately improve on baclofen, dantrolene, or diazepam noted objective improvement with tizanidine (78, 79). Several studies have compared the two agents, including one double-blind trial of 12 patients with spasticity treated with baclofen or tizanidine with resultant decreased passive stretch responses compared with placebo, however tizanidine was more effective than baclofen (80). Another double-blind comparative study of 21 patients with MS showed similar efficacy of baclofen and tizanidine in reduction of spasms and clonus. However tizanidine was more effective in improving strength, bladder function, and ADL (81). Other studies have been less conclusive. Tizanidine and baclofen were minimally effective in improving spastic gait compared with placebo in one analysis (82) as were the results of four other trials that compared baclofen with tizanidine among 206 patients with spasticity in association with MS, cerebrovascular lesions, and other proximate causes wherein the reported improvement of two agents was not statistically significant (47, 83–85).

Nonetheless, some patients favor tizanidine over baclofen (83, 85). Nighttime dosing of sublingual tizanidine has been studied as more effective treatment for early morning spasticity with fewer side effects (86).

The subject of tizanidine efficacy was reviewed by Young (87). A randomized, placebo-controlled, double-blind clinical trial of spasticity due to MS showed that tizanidine was subjectively more effective than placebo in treating spasms and clonus. However, a reduction in muscle tone as measured objectively by the Ashworth Scale was not seen (88). Other studies of patients with MS (89) and SCI (90) showed an objective benefit in muscle tone by the Ashworth Scale but without functional improvement in activities of daily living. Despite a number of studies showing significant subjective or objective benefit with tizanidine, its efficacy in spasticity is still challenged (91). One important side effect of tizanidine is sedation (92), while others include hypotension, dizziness, asthenia, dry mouth and, less frequently, hepatic damage and hallucinations (79, 88–90, 92, 93). The conflicting data of efficacy and side effects renders it a second-line medication. The starting dose is 2 mg at bedtime, gradually increasing to a maximum of 36 mg per day in three to four daily divided doses. In all patients so treated, liver function tests should be carefully monitored (90).

Dantrolene

Dantrolene inhibits calcium release from muscle sarcoplasmic reticulum, disrupting contraction and reducing tone in spastic muscles (4, 30). The drug exerts its actions independent of neuronal circuitry. Early studies demonstrated improvement in some aspects of spasticity although not without caveats. Among 11 hemiplegic patients, dantrolene improved fine muscle control but did not significantly improve ADL (94). Among 23 treated patients with hemiplegia, clonus decreased and gait improved with treatment although patients > age 50 responded less well (95). In another study of 77 patients treated for up to two years with dantrolene, signs of muscle spasm, clonus, tone, and hyperreflexia improved, but functional improvement was less noticeable and side effects were common (96). One double-blind placebo-controlled study of dantrolene showed efficacy in about one-third of patients suffering from spasticity of various causes, but all reported adverse effects, some of which led to discontinuation of treatment (97). Patients with spasticity after stroke showed improvement in ADL with long-term administration (98). Dantrolene is the drug of choice for spasticity of cerebral origin (20, 71), notably in childhood CP (99); however, one double-blind study of 20 children with CP showed that dantrolene led to reduced muscle contraction force with little if any objective functional improvement (100). Others found similar results and questioned the preference of dantrolene as the drug of choice in CP (101). It is not recommended in spasticity of spinal origin due to MS (101, 102). The adverse effects of dantrolene include potentially severe liver toxicity, effusive pleural and pericardial disease, sedation, weakness, diarrhea, acne, and lymphoma. As with tizanidine, liver function studies should be performed before and during treatment, and discontinued if abnormalities arise (6, 18, 30, 60, 102–109). In doses of 25 to 400 mg per day, dantrolene should probably be reserved for patients who are unresponsive to other oral medications.

Cyproheptadine

Cyproheptadine is a seratonin or 5-hydroxytryptamine antagonist that exerts its antispasticity actions via the medial reticulospinal tract (110), evidence of which comes from experimental animal studies (111). In one small study of patients with SCI and MS, oral cyproheptadine significantly decreased clonus and spasms (112), whereas another study of 25 patients with SCI showed no difference between cyproheptadine, clonidine, and baclofen-associated improvement of leg tone by the Ashworth Scale or other objective measures of spasticity (113). Studies have also demonstrated the ability of cyproheptadine to improve gait and function in addition to reducing spasms (114,115). Cyproheptadine combined with clonidine and a locomotion training program in two patients, both wheelchair-bound by severe spasticity from SCI, became ambulatory with crutch assistance (116).

The adverse effects of cyproheptadine include sedation, dizziness, ataxia, tinnitus, blurred vision, hypotension, dry mouth, gastrointestinal upset, and fever. Anticholinergic side effects occasionally lead to urinary retention (117,118). Cyproheptadine is recommended in patients with MS and SCI, in conjunction with other antispasticity medications at the dose of 4 to 20 mg per day.

Botulinum Neurotoxin

The effects of overly active αMN, whatever the cause are treated with injections of BoNT directly into the endplate zone of affected muscles, impairing the NMJ release of ACh (119). Both open-label and double-blind placebo-controlled studies have demonstrated its clinical utility in restoring muscle tone and function in spasticity of diverse causes (120–131). However bruising at the injection site, weakness, flu-like symptoms, and antibody development limit its long-term use. Various formulations of BoNT are available including Botox® and Dysport® (both BoNT type A) and Myoblock® (BoNT type B). At bioequivalent doses, there seems to be few significant differences between the formulations. One newer formulation of BoNT type A (NT201 or Xeomin®) is highly purified and free of complex proteins (132) that reduce immunogenicity and antibody formation; NT201 has been used in blepharospasm, cervical dystonia, and stroke-associated spasticity (132,133).

Ivermectin

Ivermectin is an anti-parasitic agent with a mechanism of action in spasticity is due to the enhancement of GABA release, postsynaptic binding of GABA at parasite receptors (134,135), and possible GABA agonist activity (136). In an open-label pilot study of 10 patients with SCI spasticity, subcutaneous injection of an initial dose of 0.2 mg per kilogram followed two weeks later by an injection of 0.4 mg per kilogram, and maintenance doses of 0.4 to 1.6 mg per kilogram for several weeks, resulted in improved objective measures of spasticity in all 10 patients so treated, as well as decreased Ashworth Scores (in seven). There were no side effects, and some described improved mood, sphincter function, and sleep (136).

Cannabinoids

The efficacy of cannabis was demonstrated in an experimental murine model of MS (137) and has been employed clinically in the treatment of MS-associated spasticity (138, 139). Anecdotal reports of improved spasticity have resulted in several placebo-controlled double-blind trials (129,130,140–142), which in spite of lack of significant efficacy demonstrate, nonetheless, improvement on a variety of subjective assessments. Only one large study showed measurable reduction in the Ashworth scale of muscle tone (143). However, improvement in quality-of-life measures, such as reduction in nocturnal spasms and increased mobility, suggests a role in the treatment of patients with spasticity refractory to other medications. Various cannabis preparations demonstrated significant improvement in spasticity-associated pain assessments in MS, including urge incontinence and bladder overactivity (140–144).

Although illegal inhalation of marijuana is the most common route of administration of cannabis for the treatment of spasticity, several synthetic and cannabis-derived preparations exist. Marinol® is available in the United States for the treatment of chemotherapy-induced nausea and vomiting, as well as anorexia associated with aids but it has not been well studied in the treatment of spasticity. Nabilone, marketed as Cesamet® in the United States and Canada, is a synthetic cannabinoid indicated for chemotherapy-induced nausea and vomiting. It has been studied for the treatment of spasticity in small trials of patients with SCI with objective improvement in Ashworth scale scores (142). In one study, Nabilone was associated with improved spasticity-associated pain in a small group of MS patients (144). Sativex®, a newer cannabis-based or mucosal spray available in Canada and Europe, was approved for spasticity associated with MS, however in Canada the approval also extends to adjunctive relief of neuropathic pain associated with MS, as well as cancer-associated pain. These medications are generally well tolerated but dizziness; fatigue, mood change, and cognitive dysfunction are commonly reported side effects (140–143).

PRINCIPLES OF INTRATHECAL THERAPY

Administration of medication into the intrathecal space allows for careful titration of a very low dose of medicine directly to the site of action while eliminating systemic side effects. Intrathecal therapy, which requires surgical implantation of a programmable pump, is generally reserved for patients with severe spasticity that is intolerant of conventional medications at maximal therapeutic doses or show inadequate responsiveness to alternative treatments.

Intrathecal Baclofen

Intrathecal baclofen (ITB) therapy has been one of the most significant advances in the treatment of spasticity. It was approved by the U.S. Food and Drug Administration for use in spasticity of spinal cord origin in 1992 and of cerebral origin in 1996 and is employed most commonly in those with MS, SCI, CP, and TBI. The disorders responsive to ITB are summarized in Table 3.

McLean (145) reported 168 patients in nine independent studies demonstrating the effectiveness of ITB in spasticity that was ameliorated in 164 (98%), abolished in 130 (98%),

Table 3. Disorders Responsive to Intrathecal Baclofen

Spasticity of Spinal Origin	Spasticity of Cerebral Origin
MS	TBI
SCI	CP
Spinal cord infarction	Stroke
Transverse myelitis	Dytonia, especially secondary forms
Spinal cord tumor	MS
Compressive myelopathy	Axonic brain injury
PLS	Post-encephalitis
Stiff-Person Syndrome	Inheritied neurometabolic disorders
HSP	Miscellaneous: Arachnoid cyst, Laurence-Moon-Biedl syndrome

Abbreviations: MS, multiple sclerosis; TBI, traumtic brain injury; SCI, spinal cord injury; CP, cerebral palsy; PLS, primary lateral sclerosis; HSP, hereditary spastic paraplegia

as well as improved bladder function in 18 (78%) and overall functionality in 55 (71%). A consensus statement of MS experts concluded that ITB was effective and underutilized in the treatment of MS-associated spasticity (146) and advocated ITB early in the disease course in patients with severe spasticity, or those intolerant or unresponsive to oral therapies (146). Other studies have yielded similar results in spasticity from spinal trauma, MS, and other associated diseases (147–151). It has many advantages in the treatment of severe spasticity when compared with oral baclofen, as the latter penetrates the blood–brain barrier poorly, and lumbar cerebrospinal fluid (CSF) concentrations are low. For example, a 60 mg oral dose of baclofen yielded a CSF concentration of 24 mg per milliliter (mL), while direct delivery of 60 mg baclofen resulted in a spinal CSF baclofen concentration of 1,240 mg per mL (30). Thus, to obtain an adequate therapeutic response, patients require much higher and more frequent oral doses, leading to inconvenient and sometimes intolerable side effects. Since the current delivery device for delivery of ITB is a programmable pump, fine tuning of the clinical response is possible as is flexible-rate or pulsatile dosing. However, there are disadvantages to ITB, including the need for surgical implementation, frequent refilling follow-up visit, and obvious cosmetic issues. There is a general lack of awareness in the medical community about ITB, thus patients may be inappropriately referred or not at all, even when they might benefit from its use. Properly used, it is safe, with most difficulties related to pump implantation, catheter blocking, accidental overdose, and problems generally associated with inexperience. The commonest adverse effects include drowsiness, weakness, dizziness, and seizures; less frequently, there may be blurred vision, headaches, hypotension, numbness, constipation, slurred speech, lethargy, reversible coma, and respiratory depression with overdoses (30). One potential life-threatening complication is a withdrawal syndrome after sudden catheter or pump malfunction, which if untreated, may result in a syndrome resembling malignant hyperthermia (152).

The following criteria should be fulfilled before proceeding to catheter placement (145):

1. Disabling spasticity of a moderate to severe degree or intolerable pain.

2. Spasticity that is not due to reversible neurologic disease or trauma and has been present and stable for more than six months.

3. Failure of oral therapy despite maximal doses or unacceptable adverse effects. Treatment with three to four oral agents is advised before consideration of ITB. In cerebral origin spasticity, particularly in CP, oral treatment response is so poor that ITB may be indicated without a prolonged oral trial.

4. Patients or their caregivers that understand the risks and benefits involved with the intrathecal pump who can

participate in the necessary follow-up care of refilling the medication reservoir.

At the Multiple Sclerosis Research Center of New York, all patients that meet the above selection criteria for ITB therapy undergo a complete assessment and screening test, including a detailed neurologic history and physical examination with specific attention to grading of the spasticity and its associated features using the Ashworth and Spasm Scales (153). Eligible patients have a fall in their score by at least one point after the ITB screening test dose, given after lumbar puncture is performed. Two to 3 mL of CSF is withdrawn in a sterile manner for later reintroduction followed by instillation of 1 milliliter of baclofen at a concentration of 50 mg/ml mixed in a syringe with 1.5 mL of CSF via lumbar catheter, followed by 2 to 3 mL of CSF. In non-ambulatory patients with severe spasticity such as those with SCI, it is generally necessary to administer a higher screening dose of baclofen ranging from 75 mg to 100 mg. The patient is monitored hourly for adverse effects with particular attention to drowsiness and respiratory difficulties, while spasticity is reassessed at 2, 4, and 6 hours post procedure for improvement of signs and symptoms. The object of the screening process is to assess spasticity relief, not the achievement of functionality goals. Some patients may encounter profound weakness with the test dose, but this will not likely occur once the pump is implanted and the dose is given instead by continuous infusion. With careful titration of dose, muscle weakness can be avoided so as not to interfere with the current level of functioning.

A 2011 MS consensus panel (146) advocated consideration of ITB earlier than is common practice in symptomatic patients. A retrospective review of 36 mostly ambulatory MS patients with severe spasticity at a single institution found that all patients so studied had clinical improved spasticity and retained ambulatory function (154). Over several years, three such patients became paraplegic due to progression of their neurologic disease.

Patients who respond to ITB without serious side effects may be referred to neurosurgical care for pump implantation. Positive responders usually have dramatic subjective improvement in spasticity as judged by Ashworth scores after initial evaluation, and by the patient (155). Most authorities agree that ITB therapy should ideally be performed at centers specializing in spasticity treatment to minimize the risk of surgical implantation and post-implantation complications.

Intrathecal Clonidine

Although not FDA-approve for spasticity, ITC may be used alone or in combination with IT baclofen or IT morphine. The combination of ITC and ITB effectively reduced complications from spasticity in one reported patient with SCI,

after ITB alone was ineffective (76). A review of 21 patients treated with ITC at a single institution showed that ITC, alone or in combination with ITB or intrathecal morphine (ITM), was effective in treating severe spasticity due to a variety of conditions without additional safety concerns (77). The authors suggest the following five clinical criteria for the consideration of ITC:

1. As a single agent for relief of spasticity in patients who had an unacceptable degree of weakness with the use of ITB.

2. As a single agent for relief of spasticity in patients who developed tolerance to ITB after long-term use.

3. In patients with spasticity and significant weakness, addition of ITC to ITB enabled a reduction in the dose of ITB necessary for spasticity relief, thereby decreasing the degree of weakness and optimizing functionality.

4. In combination with ITB in patients with spasticity who also had a significant neuropathic pain syndrome and were intolerant to narcotics.

5. For relief of pain in patients with intractable pain and suboptimal response to ITM or ITN/ITB therapy.

In this study (77) the starting dose of ITC was 30 mg per day with most patients requiring a dose greater than 100 mg per day, and a maximum dose of 750 mg per day. Patients were managed for a long period of time (18 patients treated >5 years, and 6 patients >10 years) with minimal side effects. Uncommon side effects included hypotension, bradycardia, sedation, and sexual dysfunction (77).

Selective Dorsal Rhizotomy

Patients who do not benefit satisfactorily from PT or pharmacologic interventions should be referred for therapeutic neurosurgical procedures, including selective dorsal rhizotomy (SDR) (156, 157). This procedure reduces spasticity by removing the stimulating afferent input of muscle stretch receptors on motor neurons. The term "selective" refers to attempted sectioning of only those inputs that contribute to spasticity. However, SDR invariably leaves the patient with some undesirable sensory deficits. The history and details of the procedure are reviewed by Albright (158) and McLaughlin (159) and others. It is used in the pediatric population to improve muscle tone, range of motion, and gait (160). In a study of 178 children with CP, early SDR (at age 2 and 4 years) decreased the need for some, although not all, orthopedic procedures designed to correct leg deformities compared with SDR at ages 5 and 19 (161). Another study of 16 children with spastic diplegia due to CP experienced significantly improved cognitive function six months after SDR compared with those who failed to achieve the same improvement without SDR (162). However, a 10-year follow-up study after SDR in 19 children with CP revealed the benefits of the procedure were not as permanent as previously thought (163). Although SDR certainly provides relief to many patients, it is generally recommended only after other management modalities, including ITB. However, the case for childhood CP is more controversial with some

investigators preferring SDR (158) over ITB because of its definitive nature. However, neither therapy has emerged as clinically superior to the other (164–166).

REFERENCES

1. Landau WM. Spasticity: what is it? What is it not? In: Feldman RG, Young RR, Koella WP, eds. *Spasticity: Disordered Motor control.* Chicago: Mosby-Year Book, 1980; 17–24.

2. Young RR. Spasticity: a review. *Neurology* 1994;44(Suppl 9):S12–S20.

3. Brown P. Pathophysiology of spasticity. *J Neurol Neurosurg Psychiatry* 1994; 57:773–777.

4. Davidoff RA. Antispasticity drugs: mechanisms of action. *Ann Neurol* 1985; 17:107–116.

5. Adams RD, Victor M, Ropper AH. *Principles of Neurology.* New York: McGraw-Hill, 1997.

6. Young RR, Delwaide PJ. Drug therapy: spasticity. *N Engl J Med* 1981; 304:28–33, 96–99.

7. Burke D, Wissel J, Donnan GA. Pathophysiology of spasticity in stroke. *Neurology* 2013; 80:S20–S26.

8. Gordon J, Ghez C. Muscle receptors and spinal reflexes: the stretch reflex. In: Kandel ER, Schwartz JH, Jessell TM, eds. *Principles of Neural Science.* New York: Elsevier, 1991; 564–580.

9. Davidoff RA. Skeletal muscle tone and the misunderstood stretch reflex. *Neurology* 1992; 42:951–963.

10. Heckman CJ. Alterations in synaptic input to motor neurons during partial spinal cord injury. *Med Sci Sports Exerc* 1994; 26:1480–1490.

11. Hagbarth K-E, Wallin G, Löfstedt L. Muscle spindle responses to stretch in normal and spastic subjects. *Scand J Rehab Med* 1973; 5:156–159.

12. Hagbarth K-E, Wallin G, Löfstedt L, et al. Muscle spindle activity in alternating tremor of parkinsonism and in clonus. *J Neurol Neurosurg Psychiatry* 1975; 38:636–641.

13. Burke D. A reassessment of the muscle spindle contribution to muscle tone in normal and spastic man. In: Feldman RG, Young RR, Koella WP, eds. *Spasticity: Disordered Motor Control.* Chicago: Mosby-Year Book, 1980; 261–278.

14. Burke D. Critical examination of the case for or against fusimotor involvement in disorders of muscle tone. *Adv Neurol* 1983; 39:133–150.

15. Gordon J. Spinal mechanisms of motor coordination. In: Kandel ER, Schwartz JH, Jessell TM, eds. *Principles of Neural Science.* New York: Elsevier, 1991; 581–595.

16. Young RR. Role of tizanidine in the treatment of spasticity. *Neurology* 1994; 44[Suppl 9]:S4–S5.

17. Lindau WM. Spasticity: the fable of a neurological demon and the emperor's new therapy. *Arch Neurol* 1974; 31:217–219.

18. DeLisa JA, Little J. Managing spasticity. *Am Fam Physician* 1982; 26:117–122.

19. Ditunno JF, Formal CS. Chronic spinal cord injury. *N Engl J Med* 1994; 330:550–556.

20. Katz RT. Management of spasticity. *Am J Phys Med Rehabil* 1988; 67:108–116.

21. Merritt JL. Management of spasticity in spinal cord injury. *Mayo Clin Proc* 1981; 56:614–622.

22. Ashworth B. Preliminary trial of carisoprodol in multiple sclerosis. *Practitioner* 1964; 192:540–542.

23. Bohannon RW, Smith MB. Interrater reliability of a modified Ashworth scale of muscle spasticity. *Phys Ther* 1987; 67:206–207.

24. Brar SP, Smith MB, Nelson LM, et al. Evaluation of treatment protocols on minimal to moderate spasticity in multiple sclerosis. *Arch Phys Med Rehabil* 1991; 72:186–189.

25. Perry J. Rehabilitation of spasticity. In: Feldman RG, Young RR, Koella WP, eds. *Spasticity: Disordered Motor Control.* Chicago: Mosby-Year Book, 1980; 87–100.

26. Mori F, Kock G, Foti C, et al. The use of repetitive transcranial magnetic stimulation (rTMS) for the treatment of spasticity. *Progress Brain Research* 2009; 175:429–439.

27. Yan T, Hui-Chan C, Li L. Functional electical stimulation improves motor recovery of the lower extremity and walking ability of subjects with first acute stroke. *Stroke* 2005; 36:80–85.

28. Krause P, Szecsi J, Straube A. Changes in spastic muscle tone increase in patients with spinal cord injury using functional electical stimulation and passive leg movements. *Clinical Rehabilitation* 2008; 22:627–634.

29. Giesser B. Multiple sclerosis. Current concepts in management. *Drugs* 1985; 29:88–95.

30. Blanck TJ, Sadiq SA. General anesthetics and anesthesia-associated drugs. In: Rowland LP, Klein DF, eds. *Current Neurologic Drugs.* Philadelphia: Current Medicine, 1996; 239–308.

31. Smith CR, LaRocca NG, Giesser BS, et al. High-dose oral baclofen: experience in patients with multiple sclerosis. *Neurology* 1991; 41:1829–1831.

32. Feldman RG, Kelly-Hayes M, Conomy JP, et al. Baclofen for spasticity in multiple sclerosis. Double-blind crossover and three-year study. *Neurology* 1978; 28:1094–1098.

33. Sawa GM, Paty DW. The use of baclofen in treatment of spasticity in multiple sclerosis. *Can J Neurol Sci* 1979; 6:351–354.

34. Miller F, Korsvik H. Baclofen in the treatment of stiff-man syndrome. *Ann Neurol* 1981; 9:511–512.

35. Milla PJ, Jackson AD. A controlled trial of baclofen in children with cerebral palsy. *J Int Med Res* 1977; 5:398–404.

36. Hinderer SR. The supraspinal anxiolytic effect of baclofen for spasticity reduction. *Am J Phys Med Rehabil* 1990; 69:254–258.

37. Hinderer SR, Lehmann JF, Price R, White O, deLateur BJ, Deitz J. Spasticity in spinal cord injured persons: quantitative effects of baclofen and placebo treatments. *Am J Phys Med Rehabil* 1990; 69:311–317.

38. Smith MB, Brar SP, Nelson LM, et al. Baclofen effect on quadriceps strength in multiple sclerosis. *Arch Phys Med Rehabil* 1992; 73:237–240.

39. Asien ML, Dietz M, McDowell F, Kutt H. Baclofen toxicity in a patient with subclinical renal insufficiency. *Arch Phys Med Rehabil* 1994; 75:109–111.

40. Ghose K, Holmes KM, Matthewson K. Complications of baclofen overdose. *Postgrad Med J* 1980; 56:865–867.

41. Lees AJ, Clarke CR, Harrison MJ. Hallucinations after withdrawal of baclofen. *Lancet* 1977; 1:858.

42. Stien R. Hallucinations after sudden withdrawal of baclofen. *Lancet* 1977; 2:44–45.

43. Arnold ES, Rudd SM, Kirshner H. Manic psychosis following rapid withdrawal from baclofen. *Am J Psychiatry* 1980; 137:1466–1467.

44. Terrence CF, Fromm GH. Complications of baclofen withdrawal. *Arch Neurol* 1981; 38:588–589.

45. Kirubakaran V, Mayfield D, Regachary S. Dyskinesia and psychosis in a patient following baclofen withdrawal. *Am J Psychiatry* 1984; 141:692–693.

46. Garabedian-Ruffalo SM, Ruffalo RL. Adverse effects

secondary to baclofen withdrawal. *Drug Intell Clin Pharm* 1985; 19:304–306.

47. Stien R, Nordal HJ, Oftedal SI, et al. The treatment of spasticity in multiple sclerosis: a double-blind clinical trial of a new antispastic drug tizanidine compared with baclofen. *Acta Neurol Scand* 1987; 75:190–194.

48. Mandac BR, Hurvitz EA, Nelson VS. Hyperthermia associated with baclofen withdrawal and increased spasticity. *Arch Phys Med Rehabil* 1993; 74:96–97.

49. Lal R, Sukbuntherng J, Tai E, et al. Arbaclofen placarbil, a novel R-baclofen prodrug: Impoved absorption, distribution, metabolism, and elimination properties compared with R-baclofen. *J Pharmacology Experimental Therapeutics* 2009; 330:911–921.

50. Nance P, Huff F, Martinez-Arizala A, et al. Efficacy and safety study of arbaclofen placarbil in patients with spasticity due to spinal cord injury. *Spinal Cord* 2011; 49:974–980.

51. Lataste X, Emre M, Davis C, Groves L. Comparative profile of tizanidine in the management of spasticity. *Neurology* 1994; 44[Suppl 9]:S53–S59.

52. Kuhn WF, Light PJ, Kuhn SC. Stiff-man syndrome: case report. *Acad Emerg Med* 1995; 2:735–738.

53. Lorish TR, Thorsteinsson G, Howard FM Jr. Stiff-man syndrome updated. *Mayo Clin Proc* 1989; 64:629–636.

54. Dahlin M, Knutsson E, Nergardh A. Treatment of spasticity in children with low dose benzodiazepine. *J Neurol Sci* 1993; 117:54–60.

55. Nogen AG. Medical treatment of spasticity in children with cerebral palsy. *Childs Brain* 1976; 2:304–308.

56. Rall TW. Hypnotics and sedatives; ethanol. In: Gilman AG, Rall TW, Nies AS, Taylor P, eds. *Goodman and Gilman's The Pharmacological Basis of Therapeutics.* New York: McGraw-Hill, 1993; 345–382.

57. Waldman HJ. Centrally acting skeletal muscle relaxants and associated drugs. *J Pain Symptom Manage* 1994; 9:434–441.

58. Frisbie JH, Aguilera EJ. Diazepam and body weight in myelopathy patients. *J Spinal Cord Med* 1995; 18:200–202.

59. Bes A, Eyssette M, Pierrot-Deseilligny E, et al. A multi-centre, double-blind trial of tizanidine, a new antispastic agent, in spasticity associated with hemiplegia. *Curr Med Res Opin* 1988; 10:709–718.

60. Pinder RM, Brogden RN, Speight TM, et al. Dantrolene sodium: a review of its pharmacological properties and therapeutic efficacy in spasticity. *Drugs* 1977; 13:3–23.

61. Roussan M, Terrence C, Fromm G. Baclofen versus diazepam for the treatment of spasticity and long-term follow-up of baclofen therapy. *Pharmatherapeutica* 1985; 4:278–284.

62. Cendrowski W, Sobczyk W. Clonazepam, baclofen and placebo in the treatment of spasticity. *Eur Neurol* 1977; 16:257–262.

63. Coward DM. Tizanidine: neuropharmacology and mechanism of action. *Neurology* 1994; 44[Suppl 9]:S6–S11.

64. Delwaide PJ, Pennisi G. Tizanidine and electrophysiologic analysis of spinal control mechanisms in humans with spasticity. *Neurology* 1994; 44[Suppl 9]:S21–S28.

65. Tremblay LE, Bedard PJ. Effect of clonidine on motor neuron excitability in spinalized rats. *Neuropharmacology* 1986; 25:41–46.

66. Nance PW, Shears AH, Nance DM. Reflex changes induced by clonidine in spinal cord injury patients. *Paraplegia* 1989; 27:296–301.

67. Stewart JE, Barbeau H, Gauthier S. Modulation of locomotor patterns and spasticity with clonidine in spinal cord injured patients. *Can J Neurol Sci* 1991; 18:321–332.

68. Maynard FM. Early experience with clonidine in spinal spasticity. *Paraplegia* 1986; 24:175–182.

69. Sandford PR, Spengler SE, Sawasky KB. Clonidine in the treatment of brainstem spasticity. Case report. *Am J Phys Med Rehabil* 1992; 71:301–303.

70. Khan OA, Olek MJ. Clonidine in the treatment of spasticity in patients with multiple sclerosis. *J Neurol* 1995; 242:712–715.

71. Dall JT, Harmon RL, Quinn CM. Use of clonidine for treatment of spasticity arising from various forms of brain injury: a case series. *Brain Inj* 1996; 10:453–458.

72. Hoffman BB, Lefkowitz RJ. Catecholamines and sympathomimetic drugs. In: Gilman AG, Rall TW, Nies AS, Taylor P, eds. *Goodman and Gilman's The Pharmacological Basis of Therapeutics.* New York: McGraw-Hill, 1993; 187–220.

73. Gerber JG, Nies AS. Antihypertensive agents and the drug therapy of hypotension. In: Gilman AG, Rall TW, Nies AS, Taylor P, eds. *Goodman and Gilman's The Pharmacological Basis of Therapeutics.* New York: McGraw-Hill, 1993; 784–813.

74. Yablon SA. Sipski ML. Effect of transdermal clonidine on spinal spasticity. A case series. *Am J Phys Med Rehabil* 1993; 72:154–157.

75. Weingarden SI, Belen JG. Clonidine transdermal system for treatment of spasticity in spinal cord injury. *Arch Phys Med Rehabil* 1992; 73:876–877.

76. Middleton JW, Siddall PJ, Walker S, et al. Intrathecal clonidine and baclofen in the management of spasticity and neuropathic pain following spinal cord injury: a case study. *Arch Phys Med Rehabil* 1996; 77:824–826.

77. Ho J, Sadiq S. Use of intrathecal clonidine in patients with multiple sclerosis or spastic paraparesis. *J Neurology* 2012; 259:982–984.

78. Sie OG, Lakke JP. The spasmolytic properties of 5-chloro-4-(2-imidazolin-2-yl-amino)-2, 1,3-benzothiadiazole hydrochloride (DS 103-282): a pilot study. *Clin Neurol Neurosurg* 1980; 82:273–279.

79. Lapierre Y, Bouchard S, Tansey C, et al. Treatment of spasticity with tizanidine in multiple sclerosis. *Can J Neurol Sci* 1987; 14:513–517.

80. Hassan N, McLellan DL. Double-blind comparison of single doses of DS103-282, baclofen and placebo for suppression of spasticity. *J Neurol Neurosurg Psychiatry* 1980; 43:1132–1136.

81. Smolenski C, Muff S, Smolenski-Kautz S. A double-blind comparative trial of new muscle relaxant, tizanidine (DS 103-282), and baclofen in the treatment of chronic spasticity in multiple sclerosis. *Curr Med Res Opin* 1981; 7:374–383.

82. Corston RN, Johnson F, Godwin-Austen RB. The assessment of drug treatment of spastic gait. *J Neurol Neurosurg Psychiatry* 1981; 44:1035–1039.

83. Newman PM, Nogues M, Newman PK, et al. Tizanidine in the treatment of spasticity. *Eur J Clin Pharmacol* 1982; 23:31–35.

84. Eyssette M, Rohmer F, Serratrice G, et al. Multi-centre, double-blind trial of a novel antispastic agent, tizanidine, in spasticity associated with multiple sclerosis. *Curr Med Res Opin* 1988; 10:699–708.

85. Medici M, Pebet M, Ciblis D. A double-blind, long-term study of tizanidine ("Sirdalud") in spasticity due to cerebrovascular lesions. *Curr Med Res Opin* 1989; 11:398–407.

86. Vakhapova V, Auriel E, Karni A. Nightyl sublingual tizanidine HCl in multiple sclerosis: Clinical efficacy and safety. *Clinical Neuropharmacology* 2010; 33:151–154.

87. Young RR (supplement editor). Role of tizanidine in the treatment of spasticity. *Neurology* 1994; 44[Suppl 9]:S1–S80.

88. Smith C, Birnbaum G, Carter JL, et al. and The US Tizanidine Study Group. Tizanidine treatment of spasticity caused by multiple sclerosis: results of a double-blind, placebo-controlled trial. *Neurology* 1994; 44[Suppl 9]:S34–S43.

89. The United Kingdom Tizanidine Trial Group. A double-blind, placebo-controlled trial of tizanidine in the treatment

of spasticity caused by multiple sclerosis. *Neurology* 1994; 44[Suppl 9]:S70–S78.

90. Nance PW, Bugaresti J, Schellenberger K, et al. The North American Tizanidine Study Group. Efficacy and safety of tizanidine in the treatment of spasticity in patients with spinal cord injury. *Neurology* 1994; 44[Suppl 9]:S44–S52.

91. Lindau WM, Young RR. Tizanidine and spasticity. *Neurology* 1995; 45:2295–2296.

92. Miettinen TJ, Kanto JH, Salonen MA, et al. The sedative and sympatholytic effects of oral tizanidine in helathy volunteers. *Anesth Analg* 1996; 82:817–820.

93. Wallace JD. Summary of combined clinical analysis of controlled clinical trials with tizanidine. *Neurology* 1994; 44[Suppl 9]:S60–S69.

94. Jonsson B, Ladd H, Afzelius-Frisk I, et al. The effect of dantrium on spasticity of hemiplegic patients. *Acta Neurol Scand* 1975; 51:385–392.

95. Steinberg FU, Ferguson KL. Effect of dantrolene sodium on spasticity associated with hemiplegia. *J Am Geriatr Soc* 1975; 23:70–73.

96. Joynt RL. Dantrolene sodium: long-term effects in patients with muscle spasticity. *Arch Phys Med Rehabil* 1976; 57:212–217.

97. Luisto M, Moller K, Nuutila A, Palo J. Dantrolene sodium in chronic spasticity of varying etiology. A double-blind study. Acta Neurol Scand 1982; 65:355–362.

98. Ketel WB, Kolb ME. Long-term treatment with dantrolene sodium of stroke patients with spasticity limiting the return of function. *Curr Med Res Opin* 1984; 9:161–169.

99. Molnar GE. Long-term treatment of spasticity in children with cerebral palsy. *Int Disabil Stud* 1987; 9:170–172.

100. Joynt RL, Leonard JA Jr. Dantrolene sodium suspension in treatment of spastic cerebral palsy. *Dev Med Child Neurol* 1980; 22:755–767.

101. Whyte J, Robinson KM. Pharmacologic management. In: Glenn MB, Whyte J, eds. *The Practical Management of Spasticity in Children and Adults*. Philadelphia: Lea & Febiger, 1990; 201–226.

102. Ward A, Chaffman MO, Sorkin EM. Dantrolene, a review of its pharmacodynamic and pharmacokinetic properties and therapeutic use in malignant hyperthermia, the neuroleptic malignant syndrome and an update of its use in muscle spasticity. *Drugs* 1986; 32:130–168.

103. Mahoney JM, Bachtel MD. Pleural effusion associated with chronic dantrolene administration. *Ann Pharmacother* 1994; 28:587–589.

104. Miller DH, Haas LF. Pneumonitis, pleural effusion and pericarditis following treatment with dantrolene. *J Neurol Neurosurg Psychiatry* 1984; 47:553–554.

105. Petusevsky ML, Faling LJ, Rocklin RE, et al. Pleuropericardial reaction to treatment with dantrolene. *JAMA* 1979; 242:2772–2774.

106. Knutsson E, Martensson A. Action of dantrolene sodium in spasticity with low dependence on fusimotor drive. *J Neurol Sci* 1976; 29:195–212.

107. Meyler WJ, Bakker H, Kok JJ, et al. The effect of dantrolene sodium in relation to blood levels in spastic patients after prolonged administration. *J Neurol Neurosurg Psychiatry* 1981; 44:334–339.

108. Pembroke AC, Saxena SR, Kataria M, et al. Acne induced by dantrolene. *Br J Dermatol* 1981; 104:465–468.

109. Wan HH, Tucker JS. Dantrolene and lymphocytic lymphoma. *Postgrad Med J* 1980; 56:261–262.

110. Garrison JC. Histamine, bradykinin, 5-hydroxytryptamine, and their antagonists. In: Gilman AG, Rall TW, Nies AS, Taylor P, eds. *Goodman and Gilman's The Pharmacological Basis of Therapeutics*. New York: McGraw-Hill, 1993; 575–599.

111. Tremblay LE, Bedard PJ. Action of 5-hydroxytryptamine, substance P, thyrotropin releasing hormone and clonidine on spinal neuron excitability. *J Spinal Cord Med* 1995; 18:42–46.

112. Barbeau H, Richards CL, Bedard PJ. Action of cyproheptadine in spastic parapertic patients. *J Neurol Neurosurg Psychiatry* 1982; 45:923–926.

113. Nance PW. A comparison of clonidine, cyproheptadine and baclofen in spastic spinal cord injured patients. *J Am Paraplegia Soc* 1994; 17:150–156.

114. Wainberg M, Barbeau H, Gauthier S. Quantitative assessment of the effect of cyproheptadine on spastic paretic gait: a preliminary study. *J Neurol* 1986; 233:311–314.

115. Wainberg M, Barbeau H, Gauthier S. The effects of cyproheptadine on locomotion and on spasticity in patients with spinal cord injuries. *J Neurol Neurosurg Psychiatry* 1990; 53:754–763.

116. Fung J, Stewart JE, Barbeau H. The combined effects of clonidine and cyproheptadine with interactive training on the modulation of locomotion in spinal cord injured patients. *J Neurol Sci* 1990; 100:85–93.

117. Houang M, Leroy B, Forin V, et al. Acute urine retention: a rare mode of revelation of cervico-dorsal syringomyelia caused by cyproheptadine. *Arch Pediatr* 1994; 1:260–263.

118. Silberstein SD. Agents for migraine and other headaches. In: Rowland LP, Klein DF, Eds. *Current Neurologic Drugs*. Philadelphia: Current Medicine, 1996; 20–73.

119. Ford B, Fahn S. Agents for treating Parkinson disease and other movement disorders. In: Rowland LP, Klein DF, eds. *Current Neurologic Drugs*. Philadelphia: Current Medicine, 1996, 309–327.

120. Borg-Stein J, Pine ZM, Miller JR, et al. Botulinum toxin for the treatment of spasticity in multiple sclerosis. New observations. *Am J Phys Med Rehabil* 1993; 72:364–368.

121. Yablon SA Agana BT, Ivanhoe CB, et al. Botulinum toxin in severe upper extremity spasticity among patients with traumatic brain injury: an open-labeled trial. *Neurology* 1996; 47:939–944.

122. Bhakta BB, Cozens JA, Bamford JM, et al. Use of botulinum toxin in stroke patients with severe upper limb spasticity. *J Neurol Neurosurg Psychiatry* 1996; 61:30–35.

123. Simpson DM, Alexander DN, O'Brien CF, et al. Botulinum toxin type A in the treatment of upper extremity spasticity: a randomized, double blind, placebo-controlled trial. *Neurology* 1996; 46:1306–1310.

124. Hesse S, Lucke D, Malezic M, et al. Botulinum toxin for lower limb extensor spasticity in chronic hemiparetic patients. *J Neurol Neurosurg Psychiatry* 1994; 57:1321–1324.

125. Grazko MA, Polo KB, Jabbari B. Botulinum toxin A for spasticity, muscle spasms, and rigidity. *Neurology* 1995; 45:712–717.

126. Pierson SH, Katz DI, Tarsy D. Botulinum toxin A in the treatment of spasticity: functional implications and patient selection. *Arch Phys Med Rehabil* 1996; 77:717–721.

127. Burbaud P, Wiart L, Dubos JL, et al. A randomised, double blind, placebo controlled trial of botulinum toxin in the treatment of spastic foot in hemiparetic patients. *J Neurol Neurosurg Psychiatry* 1996; 61:265–269.

128. Koman LA, Mooney JF, Smith BP, et al. Management of spasticity in cerebral palsy with botulinum-A toxin: report of a preliminary, randomized, double-blind trial. *J Pediatr Orthop* 1994; 14:299–303.

129. Gooch JL, Sandell TV. Botulinum toxin for spasticity and athetosis in children with cerebral palsy. *Arch Phys Med Rehabil* 1996; 77:508–511.

130. Pullman SL, Greene P, Fahn S, et al. Approach to the treatment of limb disorders with botulinum toxin A. Experience with 187 patients. *Arch Neurol* 1996; 53:617–624.

131. Hesse S, Jahnke MT, Luecke D, et al. Short-term electrical stimulation enhances the effectiveness of Botulinum toxin in the treatment of lower limb spasticity in hemiparetic patients. *Neurosci Lett* 1995; 201:37–40.

132. Kanovsky P, Slawek J, Denes Z, et al. Efficacy and safety of treatment with incobotulinum toxin A (botulinum neurotoxin type A free from complexing proteins; NT 201) in post-stroke upper limb spasticity. *J Rehabil Med* 2011; 43:486–492.

133. Lippert-Gruner M, Svestkova O. Early use of Xeomin neurotoxin for local anti-spasticity therapy for pes equines after acquired brain injury (ABI). *Brain Inj* 2011; 25(12):1266–1269.

134. Webster LT Jr. Drugs used in the chemotherapy of helminthiasis. In: Gilman AG, Rall TW, Nies AS, Taylor P, eds. *Goodman and Gilman's The Pharmacological Basis of Therapeutics*. New York: McGraw-Hill, 1993; 959–977.

135. Kanwar RS, Varshneya C. Neuropharmacological effects of ivermectin in mice. *Ind J Physiol Pharmacol* 1995; 39:421–422.

136. Costa JL, Diazgranados JA. Ivermectin for spasticity in spinal-cord injury. *Lancet* 1994; 343:739.

137. Baker D, Pryce G, Croxford JL, et al. Cannabinoids control spasticity and tremor in a multiple sclerosis model. *Nature* 2000; 404:84–87

138. Zajicek J, Fox P, Sanders H, Wright D, et al. Cannabinoids for treatment of spasticity and other symptoms related to multiple sclerosis (CAMS study). *Lancet* 2003; 362:1517–1526.

139. Vaney C, Heinz M, Tschopp F, et al. Efficacy, safety and tolerability of an orally administered cannabis extract in the treatment of spasticity in patients with multiple sclerosis: a randomized, double-blind, placebo-controlled, cross-over study. *Mult Scler* 2004; 10:417–424

140. Novotna A, Mares J, Ratcliffe S, et al. and the Sativex Study Group. A randomized, double-blind, placebo-controlled, parallel-group, enriched-design study of babiximols (Sativex), as add-on therapy, in subjects with refractory spasticity cased by multiple sclerosis. *Eur J Neurol* 2011; 18:1122–1131.

141. Collin C, Ehler E, Waberzinek G, et al. A double-blind, randomized, placebo-controlled, parallel-group study of Sativex, in subjects with symptoms of spasticity due to multiple sclerosis. *Neurological Research* 2010; 32:451–459.

142. Pooyania S, Ethans K, Szturm T, et al. A randomized, double-blinded, crossover pilot study assessing the effect of nabilone on spasticity in persons with spinal cord injury. *Arch Phys Med Rehabil* 2010; 91:703–707.

143. Zajicek J, Sanders H, Wright D, et al. Cannabinoids in multiple sclerosis (CAMS) study: safety and efficacy data for 12 month follow up. *J Neurol Neurosurg Psychiatry* 2005; 76:1664–1669.

144. Wissel J, Haydn T, Muller J, et al. Low dose treatment with the synthetic cannabinoid Nabilone significantly reduces spasticity-related pain: a double-blind placebo-controlled cross-over trial. *J Neurology* 2006; 253(10):1337–41.

145. McLean BN. Intrathecal baclofen in severe spasticity. *Br J Hosp Med* 1993; 49:262–267.

146. Erwin A, Gudesblatt M, Bethoux F, et al. Intrathecal baclofen in multiple sclerosis: too little, too late? *Multiple Sclerosis* 2011; 17:623–629.

147. Penn RD. Intrathecal baclofen for spasticity of spinal origin: seven years of experience. *J Neurosurg* 1992; 77:236–240.

148. Coffey RJ, Cahill D, Steers W, et al. Intrathecal baclofen for intractable spasticity of spinal origin: results of a long-term multicenter study. *J Neurosurg* 1993; 78:226–232.

149. Abel NA, Smith RA. Intrathecal baclofen for treatment of intractable spinal spasticity. *Arch Phys Med Rehabil* 1994; 75:54–58.

150. Albright AL, Barron WB, Fasick MP, et al. Continuous intrathecal baclofen infusion for spasticity of cerebral origin. *JAMA* 1993; 270:2475–2477.

151. Akman MN, Loubser PG, Donovan WH, et al. Intrathecal baclofen: does tolerance occur? *Paraplegia* 1993; 31:516–520.

152. Coffey RJ, Edgar TS, Francisco GE, et al. Recognition and Management of a potentially life-threatening syndrome. *Arch Phys Med Rehabil* 2002; 83:735–41.

153. Gianino J. Intrathecal baclofen for spinal spasticity: implications for nursing practice. *J Neurosci Nurs* 1993; 25:254–264.

154. Sadiq S, Wang G. Long-term intrathecal baclofen therapy in ambulatory patients with spasticity. *J Neurology* 2006; 253:563–569.

155. Albright AL, Cervi A, Singletary J. Intrathecal baclofen for spasticity in cerebral palsy. *JAMA* 1991; 265:1418–1422.

156. Barolat G. Surgical management of spasticity and spasms in spinal cord injury: an overview. *J Am Paraplegia Soc* 1988; 11:9–13.

157. Kasdon DL, Abramovitz JN. Neurosurgical approaches. In: Glenn MB, Whyte J, eds. *The Practical Management of Spasticity in Children and Adults*. Philadelphia: Lea & Febiger, 1990; 259–267.

158. Albright AL. Neurosurgical treatment of spasticity: selective posterior rhizotomy and intrathecal baclofen. *Stereotact Funct Neurosurg* 1992; 58:3–13.

159. McLaughlin JF, Bjornson KF, Astley SJ, et al. The role of selective dorsal rhizotomy in cerebral palsy: critical evaluation of a prospective clinical series. *Dev Med Child Neurol* 1994; 36:755–769.

160. Thomas SS, Aiona MD, Pierce R, et al. Gait changes in children with spastic diplegia after selective dorsal rhizotomy. *J Pediatr Orthop* 1996; 16:747–752.

161. Chicoine MR, Park TS, Kaufman BA. Selective dorsal rhizotomy and rates of orthopedic surgery in children with spastic cerebral palsy. *J Neurosurg* 1997; 86:34–39.

162. Craft S, Park TS, White DA, Schatz J, et al. Changes in cognitive performance in children with spastic diplegic cerebral palsy following selective dorsal rhizotomy. *Pediatr Neurosurg* 1995; 23:68–75.

163. Tedroff K, Lowing K, Jacobson D, et al. Does loss of spasticity matter? A 10-year follow-up after selective dorsal rhizotomy in cerebral palsy. *Developmental Medicine and Child Neurology* 2011; 53:724-729.

164. Albright AL, Barry MJ, Fasick MP, et al. Effects of continuous intrathecal baclofen infusion and selective posterior rhizotomy on upper extremity spasticity. *Pediatr Neurosurg* 1995; 23:82–85.

165. Steinbok P, Daneshvar H, Evans D, et al. Cost analysis of continuous intrathecal baclofen versus selective functional posterior rhizotomy in the treatment of spastic quadriplegia associated with cerebral palsy. *Pediatr Neurosurg* 1995; 22:255–264.

166. Nance P, Schryvers O, Schmidt B, et al. Intrathecal baclofen therapy for adults with spinal spasticity: therapeutic efficacy and effect on hospital admissions. *Can J Neurol Sci* 1995; 22:22–29.

CHAPTER 70

Botulinum Toxin for Motor Disorders

David M. Swope, Ehsan Hadi, Mitchell F. Brin

Botulinum toxin (BoTN) is effective and often the primary and adjunctive therapy for a variety of diverse motor disorders manifested by dystonic and non-dystonic excessive muscle contraction and spasticity (Table 1), with the list continuing to grow. This chapter addresses the neuropharmacological and clinical aspects of BoTN.

BACKGROUND

The origin, structure, pharmacologic activity, and uses of BoTN have been extensively reviewed (1, 2). In essence, when botulinum neurotoxin is isolated from bacterial cultures, it is normally associated with non-toxic macromolecules such as proteins and nucleic acids. Administered parenterally for therapeutic use, the non-toxic proteins do not enhance the activity of the neurotoxin and may even interfere slightly. However, orally administered, they enhance its activity by protecting the neurotoxin from proteolytic enzymes in the gut.

The three steps involved in toxin-mediated paralysis include binding, internalization, and inhibition of acetylcholine (ACh) neurotransmitter release at the neuromuscular junction (NMJ). Internalization occurs via a receptor-mediated endocytotic and lysosomal vesicle pathway in which binding of toxin to nerves is selective and saturable, independent of Ca2+ concentration, and partially dependent on nerve stimulation. The toxin exerts its effect at the NMJ by inhibiting the release of ACh, and binding with increased affinity to cell ecto-acceptors, which allows it to enter target nerve cells. Although BoTN does not affect the synthesis or storage of ACh, non-physiological techniques can still induce release of ACh quanta, even at

nerve endings poisoned by BoTN. It has become increasingly clear that the primary action of BTX is the disruption of fusion proteins responsible for neurotransmitter vesicle release from the nerve terminal.

The preparations of BoTN used in clinical practice are distinct. Treating physicians should know which product they are using, especially in settings where multiple products and/or serotypes are available.

CLINICAL USES

Dystonia

This neurologic syndrome is dominated by involuntary muscle contractions that cause abnormal postures, including twisting, such as torticollis, flexion, or extension, as for example, anterocollis, retrocollis, writer's cramp, and adducting or abducting, such as blepharospasm and spasmodic dysphonia. It can be idiopathic or symptomatic of another disorder and can involve any voluntary muscle. The estimated prevalence of dystonia is 1 in 3,000 individuals, with cervical dystonia and writer's cramps the most common forms. Local injection of BoTN is primary therapy for many patients with dystonia, and is the secondary therapy for those that have failed other modalities.

Spasmodic dysphonia (SD) is characterized by action-induced spasm of the vocal cords causing excessive closing or opening of the vocal folds, leading to disturbances of voice and communication. Adductor SD, which accounts for 80% or more of affected patients, is far more common than abductor SD, and impacts upon quality of life. Injection of BoTN is used to treat SD, leading to improved

Table 1. Disorders Due to Excessive Muscle Contraction or Spasticity and Treated with BoTN

Dystonic spasms
    Blepharospasm
    Cervical dystonia
    Laryngeal dystonia
    Oromandibular dystonia
    Occupational cramps
    Limb dystonia
    Dystonic tremor
Non-dystonic excessive muscle contraction
    Back spasm
    Bladder: detrusor-sphincter dyssynergia
    Bruxism
    Cosmetic: Hyperfunctional facial lines
    Gastrointestinal: achalasia, anismus; cricopharyngeal, lower esophageal sphincter, rectal spasms and fissures
    Hemifacial spasm and synkinesis
    Cranial and myofascial pain
    Hyperhidrosis
    Presurgical spinal stabilization
    Tics
    Tremor: Parkinson disease, essential tremor, chin tremor
    Vaginismus
    Spasticity: Cerebral palsy, multiple sclerosis, spinal cord injury, stroke, traumatic brain injury

Modified from: Brin MF. Treatment of dystonia. In: Jankovic J, Tolosa E, eds. *Parkinson's Disease and Movement Disorders.* New York: Williams & Wilkins, 1998.

voice in up to 97% of patients (3). Patients so treated with BoTN and behavioral speech therapy experience a more favorable outcome than those who do not receive the latter. Other applications of BoTN-A include laryrngeal injection in those with chronic aspiration due to failure of reflexes that close the larynx (4) and injection of the posterior cricoarytenoid muscles and aryepiglottic folds to bring the vocal folds into apposition and protect the airway in preparation for surgical closure of the larynx, a procedure that is otherwise complicated by persistent abduction of the vocal folds. Injection of the cricopharyngeal component of the inferior constrictor of the pharynx is used to improve dysphagia, spasm, and herniation of posterior wall of the pharynx (5, 6).

Blepharospasm is a type of idiopathic focal dystonia that presents with involuntary eye blinking associated with contraction of bilateral orbicularis oculi, and eyelid closure. It varies from spasmodic intermittent to persistent and sustained eyelid closure, and is treated effectively with BoTN in up to 90% of patients. Although often misdiagnosed as blepharospasm, the peripheral myoclonic disorder of hemi-

facial spasm (HFS) presents with unilateral facial muscle contractions and is also improved by injection of BoTN into the affected muscles (7, 8). However, definitive treatment is provided by the search for compressive lesions of the 7th cranial nerve as it exits the brainstem. The anticipated cranial side effects of BoTN in blepharospasm and HFS include ptosis and blurred vision. Oromandibular dystonia is a rare focal dystonia that leads to involuntary jaw opening or jaw closing and involvement of the lower face, labial, and lingual muscles. It too shows significant improvement with BoTN (9, 10). Common side effects include mild breathiness and choking sensation (11). The management of upper limb dystonia can be challenging because of the variety of postures and the potential consequences of hand weakness, although many patients obtain relief from BoTN therapy. It has an expected onset at 72 hours, and peak effect by 1 week. Relief of symptoms lasts three to four months although some patients derive a longer periods of benefit. Toxin-related side effects include reversible weakness in the injected and adjacent muscles, as well as self-limited rash and flu-like syndrome.

Spasticity

Spasticity is recognized by increased muscle tone due to hyperexcitability of tendon stretch reflexes. Up to 70% of patients have symptomatic spasticity leading to pain, deformity, and reduced function. It is the most discernible component of the resultant upper motor neuron (UMN) syndrome in those with lesions of the corticospinal tract (CST) (12). Patients with spasticity and rigidity can have task and position-specific hypertonicity resembling dystonia. Adults with acquired spasticity that display a good range of motion early in the course of their disease do better than those with fixed or nearly-fixed contractures suggesting the importance of early BoTN intervention. A similar approach is suggested in pediatric patients to promote more normal limb growth and functionality. The outcome of BoTN combined with physiotherapy was three-fold more effective than baclofen and physical therapy, and ten-fold more effective than PT alone in stroke-related spasticity and prevention of contractures after stroke (13).

Gastrointestinal Disorders

Endoscopically guided BoTN is used to treat achalasia due to failure of relaxation of the lower esophageal sphincter during swallowing that leads to dysphagia, retrosternal pain, nocturnal regurgitation, non-cardiac chest pain, and secondary weight loss, the efficacy of which is evident after two treatments in up to 68% of patients (14). BoTN has also been used to treat diffuse esophageal spasm in non-achalasic esophageal dysmotility (15). Spasm of the sphincter of

Oddi leading to biliary obstruction was treated with BoTN via a long sclerotherapy needle (16) in two patients with usefulness limited by inaccessibility of the injected muscle. It has also been used in anismus due to chronic constipation (17) and outlet-type constipation attributed to focal dystonia of the pelvic floor and failure of relaxation of the puborectalis muscle (18), and in non-healing anal fissures caused by rectal spasm with efficacy of 92% compared to nitroglycerin in 70% (17, 19); and gastroparesis with superior result compared to placebo (17, 20).

Genitourinary Disorders

BoTN has not been used in the treatment of a variety of genitourinary disorders (21, 22), in particular neurogenic bladder and voiding disorders (23), prostatic pain, prostatism, benign prostatic hypertrophy (23–26), and refractory vaginismus (27). It has been shown to reduce post-void residual urine and urethra pressure in patients with detrusor sphincter dysnergia due to spinal cord injury, and may be considered in those with transient urinary retention following acute incomplete spinal cord injury that are expected to regain function and defer surgical sphincterotomy (28).

Visual Disorders

Pharmacotherapy-resistant acquired nystagmus is treated with retrobulbar injection of BoTN into the extraocular muscles of one eye every four to five months, while patching the other. It enables fixation of the injected retrobulbar injection of BoNT and improves visual fixation, as does BoTN in the treatment of strabismus, and childhood and infantile esotropia (29–31).

Cervical and Lumbar Spine Disease

Cervical disease may be associated with pain, dystonia, and motor tics for which the value of BoTN has been ascertained in random controlled trials (32–36). Preoperative treatment with BoTN-A facilitated management of movement disorder-induced cervical radiculopathy and myelopathy (37). Treatment of low back pain with BoTN therapy

leads to significant improvement in the intensity of pain and improvement of activities of daily living (33, 38).

Chronic Cranial and Myofascial Pain

BoTN has been used in treatment of myofascial pain, characterized by focal region of muscle tenderness and trigger points that provoke radiating pain upon pressure. This is based upon its presumed neuromodulatory effects, inhibiting neuropeptides and inflammatory mediators (33, 39, 40). Similar mechanisms have been postulated in the success of BoTN in the treatment of post-herpetic neuralgia (41). The benefit of BoTN in migraine headache (42), chronic tension and daily headache, the latter defined as >15 headache days per month and estimated to affect up to 5% of the population, has been attributed to mediation of nociceptive activity by the inhibition of release of neuropeptides glutamate and substance P, with reduced central sensitization (43). One large clinical trial demonstrated significant reduction in headache days in patients treated with BoTN compared to placebo (44).

Motor and Vocal Tics and Tremors

Use of BoTN has been reported in the treatment of refractory vocal tics, including those associated with Tourette syndrome (45), dystonic and simple motor tics (46), non-dystonic tremor (47), parkinsonian (48), and essential hand tremor (49), palatal tremor and ear clicks (50), and hereditary chin tremor (51).

Dermatologic Disorders

BoTN therapy is successful therapy in focal palm (52, 53) and axillary hyperhidrosis (54), and in the reduction of hyperfunctional facial (54) and cosmetic management of facial asymmetry following facial nerve palsy (56).

ACKNOWLEDGMENT

Supported in part by The Bachmann-Strauss Foundation.

REFERENCES

1. Dong M, Yeh F, Tepp WH, et al. SV2 Is the Protein Receptor for Botulinum Neurotoxin A. *Science* 2006; 312:592–596.
2. Aoki KR, Ranoux D, Wissel J. Using translational medicine to understand clinical differences between botulinum toxin formulations. *Eur J Neurol* 2006; 13:10–19.
3. Bhattacharyya N, Tarsy D. Impact on Quality of Life of Botulinum Toxin Treatments for Spasmodic Dysphonia and Oromandibular Dystonia. *Arch Otolaryngol Head Neck Surg* 2001; 127:389–392.
4. Pototschnig CA, Schneider I, Eckel HE, et al. Repeatedly successful closure of the larynx for the treatment of chronic aspiration with the use of botulinum toxin A. *Ann Otol Rhinol Laryngol* 1996; 105:521–524.
5. Schneider I, Pototschnig C, Thumfart WF, et al. Treatment of dysfunction of the cricopharyngeal muscle with botulinum A toxin: introduction of a new, noninvasive method. *Ann Otol Rhinol Laryngol* 1994; 103:31–35.
6. Blitzer A, Brin MF. Use of botulinum toxin for diagnosis and management of cricopharyngeal achalasia. *Otolaryngol Head Neck Surg* 1997; 116:328–330.

7. Evidente VG, Adler CH. An update on the neurologic applications of botulinum toxins. *Curr Neurol Neurosci Rep* 2010; 10:338–344.

8. Costa J, Espírito-Santo CC, Borges AA, et al. C. Botulinum toxin type A therapy for hemifacial spasm. *Cochrance Database Syst Rev* 2005; 25:CD004899.

9. Bhidayasiri R, Cardoso F, Truong DD. Botulinum toxin in blepharospasm and oromandibular dystonia: comparing different botulinum toxin preparations. *Eur J Neurol* 2006; 13:21–29.

10. Laskawi R, Rohrbach S. Oromandibular dystonia. Clinical forms, diagnosis and examples of therapy with botulinum toxin. *Laryngorhinootologie* 2001; 80:708–713.

11. Truong DD, Jost WH. Botulinum toxin: Clinical use. *Parkinsonism and related disorder* 2006; 12:331–355.

12. Shaw LC, Price Cl, can Wijck, et al. Botulinum Toxin for the Upper Limb After Stroke (BoTULS) Trial: effect on Impairment, Activity Limitation, and Pain. *Stroke* 2011; 42:1371–1379.

13. Bhakta BB. Management of spasticity in stroke. Rheumatology and Rehabilitation Research Unit, University of Leeds, Leeds, *UK British Medical Bulletin* 2000; 56:476–485.

14. De Looze DA. Botulinum toxin in the treatment of achalasia. *Eur J Neurol* 1997; 4:S85–S89.

15. Miller LS, Parkman HP, Schiano TD, et al. Treatment of symptomatic nonachalasia esophageal motor disorders with botulinum toxin injection at the lower esophageal sphincter. *Dig Dis Sci* 1996; 41:2025–2031.

16. Lacy BE, Weiser K, Kennedy A. Botulinum toxin and gastrointestinal tract disorder: panacea, placebo, or pathway to the future? *Gastroenterol Hepatol* 2008; 4:283–295.

17. Joo JS, Agachan F, Wolff B, et al. Initial North American experience with botulinum toxin type A for treatment of anismus. *Dis Colon Rectum* 1996; 39:1107–1111.

18. Sampaio C, Costa J, Joaquim JJ. Clinical comparability of marketed formulations of botulinum toxin. *Mov Disord* 2004; 19:S129–S136.

19. Kelly T, Ballal M, Khara G. Randomized clinical trial comparing botulinum toxin injections with 0.2 percent nitoglycerine ointment for chronic anal fissure. *Br J Surg* 2007; 94:162–167.

20. Arts J, Holvoet L, Caenepeel P, et al. Clinical trial: a randomized-controlled crossover study of intrapyloric injection of botulinum toxin in gastroparesis. *Aliment Pharmacol Ther* 2007; 26:1251–1258.

21. Frevert J, Dressler D. Complexing proteins in botulinum toxin type A drugs: a help or a hinderance? *Biologics: Targets and Therapy* 2010; 4:325–332.

22. Jankovic J. Botulinum toxin in clinical practice. *J Neurol Neurosurg Psychiatry* 2004; 75:951–957

23. Leippold T, Reitz A, Schurch B. Botulinum toxin as a new therapy options for voiding disorders: current state of the art. *Eur Urol* 2003; 44:165–174.

24. Rusnack SR, Kaplan SA. The use of Botulinum toxin in men with benign prostatic hyperplasia. *Rev Urol* 2005; 7:234–236.

25. Maria G, Brisinda G, Civello IM, et al. Relief by Botulinum toxin of voiding dysfunction due to benign prostatic hyperplasia: results of a randomized, placebo-controlled study. *Urology* 2003; 62:259–264.

26. Wein AJ. Prostate Botulinum A toxin injection—an alternative treatment for benign prostatic obstruction in poor surgical candidates. *J Urol* 2005; 174:1903.

27. Ghazizadeh S, Nikzad M. Botulinum toxin in the treatment of refractory vaginismus. *Obstet Gynecol* 2004; 104:922–925.

28. Schurch B, Stöhrer M, Kramer G, et al. Botulinum—A toxin for treating detrusor hyperreflexia in spinal cord injured patients: a new alternative to anticholinergic drugs? Preliminary results. *J Urol* 2000; 164:692–697.

29. Dutton JJ, Fowler AM. Botulinum toxin in ophthalmology. *Surv Ophthalmol* 2007; 52:13–31.

30. Tengtrisorn S, Treyapun N, Tantisarasart T. Botulinum A toxin therapy on esotropia in children. *J Med Assoc Thai* 2002; 85:1189–1197.

31. Spielmann AC. Botulinum toxin in infantile estropia: long-term results. *J Fr Ophtalmol* 2004; 27:358–365.

32. Comella CL. The treatment of cervical dystonia with botulinum toxins. *J Neural Transm* 2008; 115:579–583.

33. Jabbari B, Machado D. Treatment of refractory pain with botulinum toxins—An evidence-based review. *Pain Med* 2011; 12:1594–1606.

34. Truong D, Duane DD, Jankovic J, et al. Efficacy and safety of botulinum A toxin (dysport) in cervical dystonia: results of the first US randomized, double-blind, placebo-controlled study. *Mov Disord* 2005; 20:783–791.

35. Lew MF, Chinnapongse R, Zhang Y, et al. RimabotulinumtoxinB effects on pain associated with cervical dystonia: results of placebo and comparator controlled studies. *Int J Neurosci* 2010; 120:298–300.

36. Pappert EJ, Germanson T, Myobloc/Neurobloc European Cervical Dystonia Study Group. Botulinum toxin type B vs. type A in toxin-naïve patients with cervical dystonia: randomized, double-blind, noninferiority trial. *Mov Disord* 2008, 23:510–517.

37. Adler CH. Perioperative use of botulinum toxins. *Toxicon* 2009; 54:654–657.

38. Foster L, Clapp L, Erickson M, et al. Botulinum toxin A and chronic low back pain: a randomized double-blind study. *Neurology* 2001; 56:1290–1293.

39. Ferrante FM, Bearn L, Rothrock R, et al. Evidence against trigger point injection technique for the treatment of cervicothoracic myofascial pain with botulinum toxin type A. *Anesthesiology* 2005; 103:377–383.

40. Aoki KR. Review of a proposed mechanism for the antinociceptive action of botulinum toxin type A. *Neurotoxicology* 2005; 26:785–793.

41. Xiao L, Mackey S, Hui H, et al. Subcutaneous injection of botulinum toxin A is beneficial in postherpectic neuralgia. *Pain Med* 2010; 11:1827–1833.

42. Durham PL, Cady R, Cady R. Regulation of calcitonin gene related peptide secretion form trigeminal nerve cells by botulinum toxin type A: implications for migraine therapy. *Headache* 2004; 44:35–42.

43. Silberstein S. Botulinum neurotoxin: Origin and basic mechanism of action. *Pain Practice* 2004; 4:S19–S26

44. Dodick DW, Turkel CC, DeGryse RE, et al. OnabotulinumtoxinA for treatment of chronic migraine: pooled results from the double-blind, randomized, placebo-controlled phase of the PREEMPT clinical program. *Headache* 2010; 50:921–936.

45. Scott BL, Jankovic J, Donovan DT. Botulinum toxin injection into vocal cord in the treatment of malignant coprolalia associated with Tourette's syndrome. *Mov Disord* 1996; 11:431–433

46. Kwak CH, Hanna PA, Jankovic J. Botulinum toxin in the treatment of tics. *Arch Neurol* 2000; 57:1190–1193.

47. Henderson JM, Ghika JA, Van Melle G, et al. Botulinum toxin A in non-dystonic tremors. *Eur Neurol* 1996; 36:29–35.

48. Trosch RM, Pullman SL. Botulinum toxin A injections for the treatment of hand tremors. *Mov Disord* 1994; 9:601–609.

49. Brin MR, Lyons KE, Doucette J, et al. A randomized, double masked, controlled trial of botulinum toxin type A in essential hand tremor. *Neurology* 2001; 56:1523–1528.

50. Penney SE, Bruce IA, Saeed SR. Botulinum toxin is effective and safe for palatal tremor: A report of five cases and review of the literature. *J Neurol* 2006; 253:857–860.

51. Gordon K, Cadera W, Hinton G. Successful treatment of

hereditary trembling chin with botulinum toxin. *J Child Neurol* 1993; 8:154–156.

52. Schnider P, Moraru E, Kittler H. *Botulinum toxin in the treatment of focal hyperhidrosis.* Wienklin Wochenschr 2001; 113:S36–S41.

53. Saadia D, Voustianiouk A, Wang AK, et al. Botulinum toxin type A in primary palmar hyperhidrosis: randomized, single blind, two dose study. *Neurology* 2011; 57:2095–2099.

54. Heckmann M, Ceballos-Baumann AO, Plewig G, et al. Botulinum toxin A for axillary hyperhidrosis (excessive sweating). *N Engl J Med* 2001; 344:488–493.

55. Blitzer A, Binder WJ, Aviv JE, et al. The management of hyperfunctional facial lines with botulinum toxin. A collaborative study of 210 injection sites in 162 patients. *Arch Otolaryngol Head Neck Surg* 1997; 123:389–392.

56. Armstrong MW, Mountain RE, Murray JA. Treatment of facial synkinesis and facial asymmetry with botulinum toxin type A following facial nerve palsy. *Clin Otolaryngol Allied Sci* 1996; 21:15–20.

CHAPTER 71

Multidisciplinary Integrated Psychosocial and Palliative Care

Steven M. Albert

Despite commonalities in end-of-life trajectories and the institutional contexts in which we deliver end-of-life care, dying has an intensely personal quality. The optimal care of patients with progressive motor disorders includes attention to both personal psychosocial qualities and medical needs. Regardless of the diagnosis, the goals of psychosocial and palliative care are to enhance and maintain quality of life by keeping the disruptive features of the disease to a minimum, and allowing the dying patient to maintain individuality and aspects of personhood late into the disease. Such care reinforces independence and self-esteem and enhances useful coping strategies while actively identifying and modifying maladaptive behaviors. The progressive and ultimately fatal disorders without known cure or effective therapy, such as amyotrophic lateral sclerosis (ALS), are suited to integrated palliative and psychosocial models of care, which is the topic of this chapter.

GENERAL CONSIDERATIONS

The psychological and social needs of a patient with a progressive motor disorder should be ascertained as soon as possible after diagnosis and discussed with the patient and family, because the emotional reaction to the perceived loss of bodily integrity commences right away. Denial, fear, and anxiety are early reactions, which may be followed later by depression and anger. The intensity and duration of depressed mood is linked to the severity and rate of progression of the illness, but also to personality, family systems, and expectations about time remaining for closure and accomplishments.

There is a dynamic interchange between the patient and physician in the deliverance and receipt of a diagnosis of ALS. How a patient receives the diagnosis can vary with the differing styles of the communicating neurologist, from tolerating it surprisingly well to contemplations of helplessness and the inevitability of death.

Experienced ALS clinicians recommend as many visits as may be necessary to address personal concerns, treatment expectations, and other questions. Nonetheless, up to one-third of patients and their families complain that the diagnosis was withheld too long or crudely relayed, and despite the acknowledged accuracy that approaches 98% at experienced centers, most patients and families often express doubt and disbelief of the diagnosis of ALS. The leading concern in up to one-half of patients is the prospect of becoming disabled and dependent upon others, followed by the uncertainly in the length, mode of progression, and nature of the terminal phases of the illness. Recognizing that the course of ALS is inevitably progressive, and that the majority of patients succumb in 3 to 5 years of diagnosis, the American Academy of Neurology (AAN) (2) formulated practice parameter guidelines for the timing of psychological, sociological, and rehabilitative interventions in that disease. One treatment orientation tracks palliative care to families (3) in which care discussions are warranted when the patient shows clear psychological, social, or spiritual distress or suffering; analgesic medications. There is disease progression to the point of dysphagia requiring feeding tube intubation, dyspnea or symptoms of hypoventilation with a forced vital capacity of 50% or less. Virtually all patients lose function in two body regions from among bulbar, arm, or leg regions.

An integrated multidisciplinary approach (4) identifies early potential medical problems and provides an effective utilization of resources particularly in the managed care environment, without altering patient survival or disability outcome. The ideal team includes a neurologist, advanced care, clinical, or advanced practice nurse; physiatrist; physical, occupational, speech, swallowing, respiratory and vocational therapists; otolaryngologist, psychologist or psychiatrist; clergy, social worker, and nutritionist. Advanced-practice nurses can provide valuable leadership by virtue of their pivotal position as contact person for patients, their families, and other team specialists.

CHALLENGES OF PSYCHOSOCIAL CARE

The relationships between patient, family, and healthcare team can be optimized with recognition of several basic principles:

1. *Ensure that the relationship established with the patient and their family is professional, with clearly established boundaries and expectations.* Healthcare professionals should strive to create a warm, welcoming, hospitable environment. To offer hospitality in the true sense of the word is to offer an environment that restores the patient's spirit and physical nature (5). Hospitality and hospital are of the same Latin root, *hospitis*, meaning host, guest, or friend (6). Optimal relationships based on mutual respect should follow the adage of treating the patient as one would want to be treated if the situation were reversed. That includes inadvertent use of first names when referring to a patient, engendering a paternalistic relationship (7). While such an atmosphere of informality may well create a sense of ease, most patients find it difficult and of questionable utility unless everybody on the team, including the physician, adopts the convention (8). With increasing awareness of the need to empower patients, effort has been made toward fostering balanced gender-sensitive egalitarian models of team care (9) that conveys mutual dignity and respect.

2. *Identify coping strategies that take into account interpersonal communication styles of patients.* Patients draw on personal resources, trial and error, and professional guidance in developing coping and problem-solving strategies that do not rely upon escape or denial and with no single one effective for all patients (9). It is always useful to identify underlying emotional, spiritual, intellectual, and cultural factors that interfere with adequate communication, as well as ways in which a given patient has faced past challenges to assist in formulating successful treatment and coping strategies.

While many patients react somewhat traumatically to the diagnosis of ALS with denial, there may be an underlying sense of competence in the face of actual incompetence (10). The approach to the patient in denial is complex, with recognition of the positive and negative effects, including the psychological status, spiritual and cultural orienta-

tion, and eventual alignment with the medical team. Such an approach assists in reorienting patients and families to view the diagnosis of ALS as an ongoing challenge rather than a crisis (11). Support groups may be helpful in promoting reframing, and group facilitators are ever mindful that the emphasis is not what is happening to the family but how the family is relating to what is happening (12). Relationships with family and caregivers should be actively pursued, leading to insight into the system of family interdependence and identification of the members that will be the most influential in care decisions and use of certain assistive devices. Cultural factors may be important determinants of a successful relationship, and language barriers may hamper interpersonal communication.

3. *Ensure that an analysis of interdisciplinary treatment goals has been conducted to ascertain how psychosocial support might complement the medical plan of care.* The provision of psychosocial support can be facilitated or diminished by the behaviors and treatment goals of the interdisciplinary team. It is important that team members share common goals, establish close communicative ties, and that any tendency to do otherwise be discouraged.

4. *Ensure that the coping strategy and interpersonal communication of health professionals are continually self-assessed and open to outside counsel.* Healthcare professionals should be aware of their own behaviors, including dysfunctional or maladaptive patterns, as well as the promotion of collegial and collaborative relations among team members. Just as the patient and family are asked to meet the diagnosis of ALS as a continual challenge, so should the healthcare team. Self-assessment involves continued scrutiny of team behavior. It is useful to inquire whether the goals of the health professional team are realistic, if problem-solving and positive adaptation is promoted, and whether the psychological needs of the patient are being met. The supportive guidance from a psychiatric nurse clinician, psychologist, or psychiatrist can be indispensable in responding to the patient and family, particularly when psychological dysfunction is evident. The impact of an ALS case on the healthcare team should not be underestimated, as burn-out behaviors are common, and witnessing the decline and death of a patient with ALS can be dispiriting and difficult with affect upon the home life of clinicians.

INTEGRATED PALLIATIVE CARE

The focus of integrated palliative care, the timing of which varies among patients, should be offered at all stages of ALS to promote confidence, encourage independence, reduce the burden of physical handicaps, and sustain relationships with family, friends, and colleagues (13, 14).

Ambulation

The gradual loss of ambulation, that is a nearly universal feature of progressive ALS leads to consultation with physical medicine and physical and occupational therapy. These professionals, as well as other members of the interdisciplinary team, guide the patient in their increasing reliance on assistive devices to maintain independence as a result of weakness, spasticity, and imbalance. Mild to moderately affected patients benefit from a cane or walker. An ankle–foot orthosis and other bracing maneuvers improve balance, preserve energy, promote safety, and avert fatigue that might otherwise preclude the participation of patients in social activities. When frequent falls occur, a wheelchair may be necessary. Contemporary lightweight chairs are easy to operate and are portable. Self-propelled larger units offer the potential for continued independence, even in advanced disease, but they are more expensive and heavier than manually propelled ones.

Communication

Communication impairments resulting from dysarthria, anarthria, and dysphonia are challenges for patients with ALS and their healthcare providers. Speech difficulty leads to a sense of isolation, enhances preexisting dysfunctional communication styles, and can limit the ability to communicate basic needs, such as suctioning or repositioning. Consultation with an experienced speech pathologist is essential early in the diagnosis before problems in communication become overtly apparent. While speech remains possible through preserved action of the lips, tongue, palate, and larynx, ensuing bulbar weakness and spasticity lead to mixed patterns of dysarthria. The voice may have a raspy quality as a result of hyperadduction of the vocal cords and elevated laryngeal resistance in exhalation, whereas flaccid weakness of one or both vocal cords causes a breathy hypernasal voice due to escape of air into the nasal pharynx; slow, strained vocalizations result in poor pronunciation of consonants.

Bulbar Involvement

Management of bulbar symptoms in patients diagnosed with ALS begins with speech, language, and otolaryngologic assessments. It may be helpful to educate patients in oromotor exercises for mild impairments and to encourage early intervention for evaluation of augmentative aids. Verbal communication can be prolonged in tracheostomized patients as long as speech is intelligible and in spite of respiratory dependency through the use of cuffless tubes and intermittent positive pressure ventilation (IPPV). Computer-assisted aids and electronic communication systems are useful for maintaining communication to family, friends, and in allowing the patient to actively participate in the decision-making process even late in the illness.

Dysphagia and Nutrition

Optimal management of dysphagia and nutritional requirements is important in the psychosocial and physical well-being of patients with ALS and other progressive neuromuscular disorders. Dysphagia precedes ventilatory difficulty in three-fourths of patients with ALS and is present in virtually all others late in the illness (15). Normal swallowing requires the coordinated function of structures of the oral cavity, pharynx, larynx, and esophagus. Chewed food moves posteriorly in the oral cavity through constrictor muscles and other pharyngeal spaces to the esophagus where peristaltic movement carries it past the gastric sphincter and into the stomach. Alterations in smell, taste, and fear of aspiration and respiratory weakness can contribute to weight loss even before overt dysphagia is present. Whereas weakness of lip, cheek, lingual and neck muscles, hyperactive pharyngeal gag and cough reflexes, dyspnea, spinal hyperlordosis, and balance difficulty due to axial weakness all impair the early phase of swallowing, esophageal weakness and dysmotility compromise lower esophageal function. Clinical evaluation includes a review of clinical symptoms and signs of dysphagia and inspection of the nasopharynx, larynx, and esophageal paths by fiberoptic and video fluoroscopic studies. Liquids are generally more difficult to swallow than solids and pooling of liquids and secretions may be found along the vallecula and pyriform sinuses or in the laryngeal vestibule, increasing the likelihood for aspiration. The treatment of mild dysphagia includes dietary counseling, oromotor exercises, and positioning devices for the head and trunk. With bulbar involvement, aspiration can be improved by the management of secretions and abnormal breathing patterns, assisted coughing or chest physical therapy, oropharyngeal suctioning, and percutaneous endoscopic gastrostomy (PEG) placement. Nasogastric tubes are typically not used due to local irritation and an offensive appearance. The PEG is the most often used procedure for management of dysphagia due to its ease of implementation and low risk among individuals with a forced vital capacity of 50% of predicted and minimal anesthesia in placement (16). While it improves survival, running counter to the view that death due to starvation or malnutrition in ALS is a painless inevitable and merciful act (17, 18, 19), its effect on quality of life has not been well studied.

Pulmonary Function

Respiratory symptoms occur in all patients with ALS, often in association with ineffective cough, difficulty in clearing secretions, and in the aspiration of fluids and food. An astute clinician will recognize the signs of impending respiratory insufficiency, including agitation, lethargy, orthopnea, poor cough, increased use of accessory muscles, diminution of the volume of speech, and disturbed sleep. Pulmonary consultation can provide helpful information regarding respiratory muscle function. Pulmonary muscle function tests are the most reliable and sensitive measures of respiratory strength capacity and life expectancy and are optimally performed every 3 to 6 months. As vital capacity approaches 50% of predicted capacity, noninvasive intermittent positive-pressure aids (Bi-PAP, AVAPS) should be introduced. Some patients decide early in the course of their illness to pursue tracheostomy and are comfortable considering life assisted with ventilation, knowing that they may be unable to move and, at some point, unable to communicate (20, 21). The decision to proceed with endotracheal intubation or indwelling tracheostomy should be discussed as openly and supportively as possible with the patient and family members in advance of impending emergencies to remain in compliance with patient preferences for medical decision making. Similarly, documentation with respect to advance directives, healthcare proxy or, in the case of some states, durable power of attorney, should be completed and placed in the patient's chart and copies distributed to appropriate team members. The optimal situation for home ventilatory support includes adequate financial resources and psychosocial and medical support systems, including proximity to a clinic or hospital for the treatment of complications or emergencies (22).

Secretions

Drooling is a vexing problem in ALS and it is associated with oropharyngeal and lower lip muscle weakness and faulty containment and overflow of secretions, but not primary hypersalivation. Early in the disease, patients report a small pool of saliva on the pillowcase upon awakening or excessive secretions from the mouth requiring frequent dabbing of facial tissue. Beyond the embarrassment and social isolation it causes, drooling is associated with a heightened risk of aspiration. Medications such as tricyclic antidepressants and atropine-like drugs, with potent anticholinergic effects, reduce salivation by blocking parasympathetic outflow. However, they also have the potential for urinary retention, confusion, and hallucinations.

Mental Health

Care for the mental health of patients with ALS is a central challenge and includes recognition and treatment of clinically significant depression, anxiety, lability of mood, and dementia. The seemingly healthy adjustment to serious illness, which includes the denial of depression and anxiety, may be helped through referrals to psychiatry, psychology, social work, or pastoral care, and with pharmacotherapy. Yet depression is not as prevalent as might be expected. Our series suggested that up to 20% of patients with ALS met criteria for depression at the end of life (23), and it seems reasonable to treat depression in conjunction with facilitation of adaptive coping mechanisms. Anxiety and obsessive thought disorders associated with ALS have been less well studied, but experience suggests that they might also be amenable to counseling and pharmacologic intervention. Lability of mood, leading to extreme laughter or tearfulness, especially common in ALS, is related to pseudobulbar palsy and frontal lobe release mechanisms. Experience suggests a role for counseling to improve insight and pharmacotherapy for depression, anxiety, and lability.

Cognition

There is increasing awareness of clinical and pathologic syndromes of dementia in association with ALS. Mental disturbances in ALS-associated frontotemporal dementia are often minor compared with those with frank Alzheimer disease and can be easily overlooked by the busy clinician. Cognitive change is subtle and can include variable impairment in reasoning, abstraction, decision-making, goal-directed planning, and organizational ability (24). Subtle cognitive changes may be seen in the reluctance to introduce formal mechanisms of healthcare planning, such as institution of advance care directives or a healthcare proxy.

Social Contact

Contact with friends and family and satisfaction with that contact are important elements in the psychosocial well-being of patients with ALS. They are central after ambulation ceases and with loss of competency in the activities of daily living such as bathing, dressing, and grooming. Availability of the Internet and assistive devices that allow computer use after loss of hand function offers great benefit to patients who would otherwise face severe social isolation.

HOSPICE AND TERMINAL CARE

Attitudes about terminal or hospice care have varied over time, and such attitudes differ among physicians and patients. The term hospice has evolved from its medieval meaning as a place of rest for the sick and weary on a long journey. Today, hospice refers to supportive care in the period before death. It may be delivered at home, in skilled-care settings, or hospitals. Medicare hospice benefits require an election to forego certain kinds of curative medicine, but in practice, hospice is part of the continuum of palliative care, with palliative care ideally introduced long before the terminal period of the disease. Hospice care offers medical and social services for terminally ill patients and their families, which includes guidance in coping with physical, emotional, spiritual, and psychological distress. Patients can choose to forego tracheostomy in ALS and die with hospice support. The vast majority of patients with ALS in the United States elect this route, with only 5% to 20% choosing tracheostomy in clinical series (25). However, the situation is quite different in Japan, where between one-third and one-half receive tracheostomy (26, 27). At the other extreme are those who hasten to die, evident in perhaps 5 to 10% of (28) especially in the Netherlands and European regions wherein legal protection is in place for physicians who offer assisted dying (29). Such patients may receive help from families or clinicians, either taking medications themselves for assisted suicide and euthanasia. Patients who choose to hasten dying end life only a few weeks earlier than they would have died without such active measures (28). Spirituality and religiousness may also affect treatment decisions, with one study showing greater use of feeding tube placement among people reporting greater spiritual and religious orientation (30). The right to hasten death remains precarious as is the misfortunate use of tracheostomy is often introduced without patient consent (31). As a consequence, jurists and patient rights advocates have advocated legal and ethical standards to protect this right, as choice at the end of life is a central component of dignity when the patient is most vulnerable.

ACKNOWLEDGMENTS

Peregrine Murphy and Maura Del Bene prepared an earlier version of this chapter. We dedicate the chapter to the many families who have received psychosocial and palliative care at multidisciplinary ALS clinics, and to the staff who support such care.

REFERENCES

1. Mayer RF. Living with amyotrophic lateral sclerosis. In: Charash LI, Lovelace RE, Leach CF, et al, eds. *Muscular Dystrophy and other Neuromuscular Diseases: Psychosocial issues.* New York: Haworth Press, 1991; 23–30.
2. Miller RG, Jackson CE, Kasarskis EJ, et al. Practice parameter update: The care of the patient with amyotrophic lateral sclerosis: Multidisciplinary care, symptom management, and cognitive/behavioral impairment (an evidence-based review). Report of the Quality Standards Subcommittee of the American Academy of Neurology. *Neurology* 2009; 73:1227–1233.
3. Mitsumoto H. *Amyotrophic Lateral Sclerosis: A Guide for Patients and Families,* 3rd ed. New York: Demos Publishing, 2009.
4. Van den Berg JP, Kalmijn S, Lindeman E, et al. Multidisciplinary ALS care improves quality of life in patients with ALS. *Neurology* 2005; 65:1264–1267.
5. Koenig J. *New Testament Hospitality: Partnership with Strangers as Promise and Mission.* Philadelphia: Fortress Press, 1985.
6. Hendrick R. [Revised by Padol L.] *Latin Made Simple.* New York: Doubleday, 1992.
7. Campbell-Heider N, Hart C. Updating the nurse's bedside manner. *Image J Nurs Scholar* 1993; 25:133–139.
8. Henson RH. Analysis of the concept of mutuality. *Image J Nurs Scholar* 1997; 29:77–81.
9. Rabkin JG, Albert SM, Del Bene ML, et al. Prevalence of depressive disorders and change over time in late-stage ALS. *Neurology* 2005; 65:62–67.
10. Naugle RI. Denial in rehabilitation: its genesis, consequences, and clinical management. In: Marinelli RP, Dell Orto AE, eds. *The Psychological and Social Impact of Disability.* New York: Springer Publishing Company, 1991; 139–151.
11. Hulnick MR, Hulnick HR. Life's challenges: curse or opportunity? Counseling families of persons with disabilities. In: Marinelli RP, Dell Orto AE, eds. *The Psychological and Social Impact of disability.* New York: Springer Publishing Company, 1991; 258–268.
12. Noddings N. *Caring: A Feminine Approach to Ethics and Moral Education.* Berkeley: University of California Press, 1984.
13. Mitsumoto H, Rabkin JG. Palliative care for patients with amyotrophic lateral sclerosis: "prepare for the worst and hope for the best." *JAMA* 2007; 298:207–16.
14. Albert SM, Whitaker A, Rabkin JG, e al. Medical and supportive care among people with ALS in the months before death or tracheostomy. *J Pain Symptom Manage* 2009; 38:546–53.
15. Strand EA, Miller RM, Yorkston KM, et al. Management of oral-pharyngeal dysphasia symptoms in ALS. *Dysphasia* 1996; 11:129–139.
16. Mazzini L, Corra T, Zaccala M, et al. Percutaneous endoscopic gastrostomy and enteral nutrition in amyotrophic lateral sclerosis. *Neurology* 1995; 242:695–698.
17. Spataro R, Ficano L, Piccoli F, et al. Percutaneous endoscopic gastrostomy in amyotrophic lateral sclerosis. *J Neurol Sci* 2011; 304:44-48.
18. Sullivan RJ. Accepting death without artificial nutrition or hydration. *J Gen Intern Med* 1993; 8:220–224.
19. Bernat JL, Gert B, Mogielnicki RP. Patient refusal of hydration and nutrition: an alternative to physician-assisted suicide or voluntary active euthanasia. *Arch Intern Med* 1993; 153:2723–2728.
20. Albert SM, Murphy PL, Del Bene ML, et al. Prospective study

of palliative care in ALS: Choice, timing, outcomes. *J Neurol Sci* 1999; 169:108–113.

21. Albert SM, Murphy PL, Del Bene ML, et al. A prospective study of preferences and actual treatment choices in ALS. *Neurology* 1999; 53:278–283.

22. Moss AH, Casey P, Stocking CB, et al. Home ventilation for amyotrophic lateral sclerosis patients: outcomes, costs, and patient, family, and physician attitudes. *Neurology* 1993; 43:438–443.

23. Rabkin JG, Albert SM, Del Bene ML, et al. Prevalence of depressive disorders and change over time in late-stage ALS. *Neurology* 2005; 65:62–67.

24. Gordon PH, Goetz RR, Rabkin JG, et al. A prospective cohort study of neuropsychological test performance in ALS. *Amyotroph Lateral Scler* 2010; 11:312–20.

25. Rabkin JR, Albert SM, Tider T, et al. Predictors and course of elective long-term mechanical ventilation: A prospective study of ALS patients. *Amyotroph Lateral Scler* 2006; 7:86–95.

26. Hirano YM, Yamazaki Y, Shimizu J, et al. Ventilator dependence and expressions of need: A study of patients with amyotrophic lateral sclerosis in Japan. *Soc Sci Med* 2006; 62:1403–1413.

27. Ogino M. The survey report about the end-of-life care with ALS patients of ALS patients in Japan. *Rinsho Shinkeigaku* 2010; 50:1026–1028.

28. Albert SM, Rabkin JR, Del Bene ML, et al. Wish to die in end-stage ALS. *Neurology* 2005; 65:68–74.

29. Maessen M, Veldink JH, Onwuteaka-Philipsen BD, et al. Trends and determinants of end-of-life practices in ALS in the Netherlands. *Neurology* 2009; 73:954–961.

30. Murphy PL, Albert SM, Weber CM, et al. Impact of spirituality and religiousness on outcomes in patients with ALS. *Neurology* 2000; 55:1581–1584.

31. Kaub-Wittemer D, Steinbuchel N, Wasner M, et al. Quality of life and psychosocial issues in ventilated patients with amyotrophic lateral sclerosis and their caregivers. *J Pain Sympt Manage* 2003; 26:890–896.

INDEX

Note: Figures are indicated by the page number on which they occur, "f" interposed between the page number and the number of the figure itself: e.g., 58f2. Tables are indicated in a similar way using "t" between the page number and the table number: 98t2. Acronyms are included in parentheses following the full term, but are not listed separately in the index. Some very common medical acronyms (such as CNS for central nervous system, or CSF for cerebrospinal fluid) have been used without explanation in some index entries.